Anesthesia

Third Edition

Volume 1

Consulting Editors

Roy F. Cucchiara, M.D.
Professor, Department of Anesthesiology
Mayo Medical School
Chairman, Department of Anesthesiology
Mayo Clinic
Rochester, Minnesota

Edward D. Miller, Jr., M.D.
E. M. Papper Professor and Chairman
Department of Anesthesiology
Columbia University College of Physicians and Surgeons
New York, New York

J. G. Reves, M.D.
Professor, Department of Anesthesiology
Chief, Division of Cardiothoracic Anesthesia
Duke University School of Medicine
Director, Heart Center
Duke University Hospital
Durham, North Carolina

Michael F. Roizen, M.D.
Professor and Chairman, Department of Anesthesia
and Critical Care
Professor, Department of Medicine
University of Chicago Division of the Biological Sciences
Pritzker School of Medicine
Chicago, Illinois

John J. Savarese, M.D.
The Joseph F. Artusio, Jr., Professor and Chairman
Department of Anesthesiology
Cornell University Medical College
Anesthesiologist-in-Chief
The New York Hospital
New York, New York

LIBRARY

dose

WD 500

Subject

ANAESTHESIA

Anesthesia
Third Edition

Volume 1

Edited by

Ronald D. Miller, M.D.

Professor and Chairman, Department of Anesthesia
Professor, Department of Pharmacology
University of California, San Francisco, School of Medicine
San Francisco, California

Churchill Livingstone
New York, Edinburgh, London, Melbourne

Library of Congress Cataloging-in-Publication Data

Anesthesia / edited by Ronald D. Miller. — 3rd ed.
   p. cm.
  Includes bibliographical references.
  ISBN 0-443-08594-3 (set)
  1. Anesthesia. I. Miller, Ronald D., date
  [DNLM: 1. Anesthesia. WO 200 A573]
RD81.A54 1990
617.9′6 — dc20
DNLM/DLC
for Library of Congress   90-1543
                                                CIP

Distributed in the United Kingdom by Churchill Livingstone, Robert Stevenson House, 1–3 Baxter's Place, Leith Walk, Edinburgh EH1 3AF, and by associated companies, branches, and representatives throughout the world.

Accurate indications, adverse reactions, and dosage schedules for drugs are provided in this book, but it is possible that they may change. The reader is urged to review the package information data of the manufacturers of the medications mentioned.

The Publishers have made every effort to trace the copyright holders for borrowed material. If they have inadvertently overlooked any, they will be pleased to make the necessary arrangements at the first opportunity.

Acquisitions Editor: *Toni M. Tracy*
Assistant Editor: *Leslie Burgess*
Copy Editor: *David Terry*
Production Designer: *Marci Jordan*
Production Supervisor: *Sharon Tuder*
Indexer: *Irving Conde Tullar*

Printed in the United States of America

First published in 1990

Contributors

David D. Alfery, M.D.
Member, Anesthesiology Consultants of Nashville, P.C.; Staff Anesthesiologist, Centennial Medical Center and St. Thomas Hospital, Nashville, Tennessee

J. Jeffrey Andrews, M.D.
Assistant Professor, Department of Anesthesiology, University of Texas Medical School at Galveston, Galveston, Texas

William P. Arnold III, M.D.
Associate Professor, Department of Anesthesiology, University of Virginia School of Medicine, Charlottesville, Virginia

Michael J. Avram, Ph.D.
Associate Professor, Department of Anesthesia, Northwestern University Medical School; Affiliated Professional Staff Member, Department of Anesthesia, Northwestern Memorial Hospital; Research Consultant, Department of Anesthesia, Veterans Administration Lakeside Medical Center, Chicago, Illinois

Jeffrey M. Baden, M.B., B.S., F.F.A.R.C.S.
Associate Professor, Department of Anesthesia, Stanford University School of Medicine, Stanford, California; Chief, Anesthesiology Service, Veterans Administration Medical Center, Palo Alto, California

Peter L. Bailey, M.D.
Assistant Professor, Department of Anesthesiology, University of Utah School of Medicine, Salt Lake City, Utah

Steven J. Barker, Ph.D., M.D.
Associate Professor and Vice Chairman, Department of Anesthesiology, University of California, Irvine, College of Medicine, Irvine, California

Jonathan L. Benumof, M.D.
Professor, Department of Anesthesiology, University of California, San Diego, School of Medicine, La Jolla, California

Julien F. Biebuyck, M.B., D. Phil.
Eric A. Walker Professor and Chairman, Department of Anesthesia, Pennsylvania State University College of Medicine, Hershey, Pennsylvania

Susan Black, M.D.
Assistant Professor, Department of Anesthesiology, Loyola University of Chicago Stritch School of Medicine, Maywood, Illinois

David L. Brown, M.D.
Associate Clinical Professor, Department of Anesthesiology, University of Washington School of Medicine; Chief, Department of Anesthesiology, Virginia Mason Clinic, Seattle, Washington

Enrico M. Camporesi, M.D.
Professor and Chairman, Department of Anesthesiology, and Professor, Department of Physiology, State University of New York Health Science Center at Syracuse College of Medicine; Staff Anesthesiologist, University Hospital, Syracuse, New York

Roy D. Cane, M.B., B.Ch.(Rand), F.F.A.(S.A.)
Clinical Professor, Department of Anesthesia, and Associate Director, Division of Respiratory and Critical Care, Northwestern University Medical School, Chicago, Illinois

Norman J. Clark, M.D.
Senior Lecturer, Department of Anaesthetics, University of Zimbabwe School of Medicine, Harare, Zimbabwe

Charles J. Coté, M.D.
Associate Professor, Department of Anaesthesia, Harvard Medical School; Associate Anesthetist, Massachusetts General Hospital, Boston, Massachusetts

Benjamin G. Covino, Ph.D., M.D.
Professor, Department of Anaesthesia, Harvard Medical School; Chairman, Department of Anesthesia, Brigham and Women's Hospital, Boston, Massachusetts

Robert K. Crone, M.D.
Professor, Departments of Anesthesiology and Pediatrics, University of Washington School of Medicine; Director, Department of Anesthesiology, Children's Hospital and Medical Center, Seattle, Washington

Roy F. Cucchiara, M.D.
Professor, Department of Anesthesiology, Mayo Medical School; Chairman, Department of Anesthesiology, Mayo Clinic, Rochester, Minnesota

David J. Cullen, M.D.
Professor, Department of Anaesthesia, Harvard Medical School; Anesthetist, Massachusetts General Hospital, Boston, Massachusetts

John V. Donlon, Jr., M.D.
Associate Clinical Professor, Department of Anaesthesia, Harvard Medical School, Boston, Massachusetts

John C. Drummond, M.D., F.R.C.P.(C)
Associate Clinical Professor, Department of Anesthesiology, University of California, San Diego, School of Medicine; Staff Anesthesiologist, Veterans Administration Medical Center, La Jolla, California

Edmond I. Eger II, M.D.
Professor and Vice Chairman of Research, Department of Anesthesia, University of California, San Francisco, School of Medicine, San Francisco, California

Thomas W. Feeley, M.D.
Professor, Department of Anesthesia, Stanford University School of Medicine; Associate Medical Director, Intensive Care Unit, Stanford University Hospital, Stanford, California

Dennis M. Fisher, M.D.
Associate Professor, Departments of Anesthesia and Pediatrics, University of California, San Francisco, School of Medicine, San Francisco, California

Robert J. Fragen, M.D.
Professor of Clinical Anesthesia, Department of Anesthesia, Northwestern University Medical School; Attending Anesthesiologist, Northwestern Memorial Hospital, Chicago, Illinois

Thomas J. Gal, M.D.
Professor, Department of Anesthesiology, University of Virginia School of Medicine, Charlottesville, Virginia

Charles P. Gibbs, M.D.
Professor and Chairman, Department of Anesthesiology, University of Colorado School of Medicine, Denver, Colorado

Peter S. A. Glass, M.D.
Assistant Professor, Department of Anesthesiology, and Chief, Division of Orthopaedic Anesthesia, Duke University School of Medicine, Durham, North Carolina

William J. Greeley, M.D.
Assistant Professor, Departments of Anesthesiology and Pediatrics, Duke University School of Medicine; Medical Director, Pediatric Intensive Care Unit, Duke University Hospital, Durham, North Carolina

George A. Gregory, M.D.
Professor, Departments of Anesthesia and Pediatrics, University of California, San Francisco, School of Medicine, San Francisco, California

Eric J. Grigsby, M.D.
Anesthesiologist, Queen of the Valley Hospital; Private Practice, Napa Valley Pain Clinic, Napa, California

Gerald A. Gronert, M.D.
Professor, Vice Chairman, and Director of Research, Department of Anesthesiology, University of California, Davis, School of Medicine, Davis, California

Thomas F. Hornbein, M.D.
Professor and Chairman, Department of Anesthesiology, and Professor, Department of Physiology and Biophysics, University of Washington School of Medicine, Seattle, Washington

Carl C. Hug, Jr., M.D., Ph.D.
Professor, Departments of Anesthesiology and Pharmacology, Emory University School of Medicine; Director, Division of Cardiothoracic Anesthesia, The Emory Clinic, Atlanta, Georgia

James R. Jacobs, Ph.D.
Assistant Professor, Department of Anesthesiology, Duke University School of Medicine; Assistant Professor, Department of Biomedical Engineering, Duke University School of Engineering, Durham, North Carolina

Joel A. Kaplan, M.D.
Horace W. Goldsmith Professor and Chairman, Department of Anesthesiology, Mount Sinai School of Medicine of the City University of New York, New York, New York

Frank H. Kern, M.D.
Assistant Professor, Departments of Anesthesiology and Pediatrics, Duke University School of Medicine, Durham, North Carolina

Robert R. Kirby, M.D.
Professor, Department of Anesthesiology, University of Florida College of Medicine, Gainesville, Florida

Richard J. Kitz, M.D.
Henry Isaiah Dorr Professor, Department of Anaesthesia, Harvard Medical School; Anesthetist-in-Chief, Department of Anesthesia, Massachusetts General Hospital, Boston, Massachusetts; Co-Director, Division of Health Sciences and Technology, Harvard Medical School – Massachusetts Institute of Technology, Cambridge, Massachusetts

Donald D. Koblin, M.D., Ph.D.
Associate Professor, Department of Anesthesia, University of California, San Francisco, School of Medicine; Staff Anesthesiologist, Veterans Administration Medical Center, San Francisco, California

A. Joseph Layon, M.D.
Assistant Professor, Departments of Anesthesiology and Medicine, University of Florida College of Medicine, Gainesville, Florida

John B. Leslie, M.D.
Assistant Professor, Department of Anesthesiology, Duke University School of Medicine, Durham, North Carolina

Gershon Levinson, M.D.
Attending Anesthesiologist, Children's Hospital of San Francisco; Associate Clinical Professor, Department of Anesthesia, University of California, San Francisco, School of Medicine, San Francisco, California

J. Lance Lichtor, M.D.
Associate Professor, Department of Anesthesia and Critical Care, University of Chicago Division of the Biological Sciences Pritzker School of Medicine, Chicago, Illinois

Lawrence Litt, Ph.D., M.D.
Associate Professor, Department of Anesthesia, University of California, San Francisco, School of Medicine, San Francisco, California

Ronald A. MacKenzie, D.O.
Assistant Professor, Department of Anesthesiology, Mayo Medical School; Consultant, Department of Anesthesiology, Mayo Clinic, Rochester, Minnesota

Mervyn Maze, M.B., Ch.B., M.R.C.P.(U.K.)
Associate Professor, Department of Anesthesia, Stanford University School of Medicine, Stanford, California; Staff Physician, Anesthesiology Service, Veterans Administration Medical Center, Palo Alto, California

Richard I. Mazze, M.D.
Professor, Department of Anesthesia, Stanford University School of Medicine, Stanford, California; Staff Anesthesiologist, Anesthesiology Service, Veterans Administration Medical Center, Palo Alto, California

Robert G. Merin, M.D.
Professor, Department of Anesthesiology, University of Texas Medical School at Houston, Houston, Texas

Joseph M. Messick, Jr., M.D.
Professor, Department of Anesthesiology, Mayo Medical School; Consultant, Department of Anesthesiology, Mayo Clinic, Rochester, Minnesota

Edward D. Miller, Jr., M.D.
E. M. Papper Professor and Chairman, Department of Anesthesiology, Columbia University College of Physicians and Surgeons, New York, New York

Ronald D. Miller, M.D.
Professor and Chairman, Department of Anesthesia, and Professor, Department of Pharmacology, University of California, San Francisco, School of Medicine, San Francisco, California

Charles S. Modell, J.D.
Attorney, Larkin, Hoffman, Daly & Lindgren, Ltd., Minneapolis, Minnesota

Jerome H. Modell, M.D.
Professor and Chairman, Department of Anesthesiology, University of Florida College of Medicine, Gainesville, Florida

Richard E. Moon, M.D., F.R.C.P.(C), F.A.C.P., F.C.C.P.
Associate Professor, Department of Anesthesiology; Assistant Professor, Department of Pulmonary Medicine, Duke University School of Medicine; Staff Anesthesiologist and Pulmonologist, and Medical Director, Hyperbaric Center, Duke University Hospital, Durham, North Carolina

John Mott, M.D.
Assistant Professor of Clinical Anesthesia, Department of Anesthesiology, University of California, Davis, School of Medicine, Davis, California

Stanley Muravchick, M.D., Ph.D.
Associate Professor, Department of Anesthesia, University of Pennsylvania School of Medicine; Staff Anesthesiologist, Hospital of the University of Pennsylvania, Philadelphia, Pennsylvania

Terence M. Murphy, M.B., Ch.B., F.F.A.R.C.S.
Professor, Department of Anesthesia, University of Washington School of Medicine; Acting Director, Multidisciplinary Pain Center, University Hospital, Seattle, Washington

Michael Nugent, M.D.
Professor, Department of Anesthesiology, Medical College of Ohio, Toledo, Ohio

Fredrick K. Orkin, M.D., M.B.A.
Associate Professor, Department of Anesthesia, University of California, San Francisco, School of Medicine, San Francisco, California

P. Pearl O'Rourke, M.D.
Assistant Professor, Departments of Anesthesiology and Pediatrics, University of Washington School of Medicine; Director, Pediatric Intensive Care Unit, Children's Hospital and Medical Center, Seattle, Washington

Edward G. Pavlin, M.D.
Associate Professor, Department of Anesthesiology, University of Washington School of Medicine, Seattle, Washington

Marie Csete Prager, M.D.
Assistant Professor, Department of Anesthesia, and Director, Division of Liver Transplant Anesthesia, University of California, San Francisco, School of Medicine, San Francisco, California

L. Brian Ready, M.D., F.R.C.P.(C)
Assistant Professor, Department of Anesthesiology, University of Washington School of Medicine; Director, Acute Pain Service, University Hospital, Seattle, Washington

J. G. Reves, M.D.
Professor, Department of Anesthesiology, and Chief, Division of Cardiothoracic Anesthesia, Duke University School of Medicine; Director, Heart Center, Duke University Hospital, Durham, North Carolina

Susan A. Rice, Ph.D.
Associate Professor of Pharmacology and Toxicology in Anesthesia, Stanford University
School of Medicine; Associate Research Career Scientist, Veterans Administration Medical
Center, Palo Alto, California

Michael F. Roizen, M.D.
Professor and Chairman, Department of Anesthesia and Critical Care, and Professor, Department of Medicine, University of Chicago Division of the Biological Sciences Pritzker School
of Medicine, Chicago, Illinois

Alan F. Ross, M.D.
Assistant Professor, Department of Anesthesia, University of Iowa College of Medicine, Iowa
City, Iowa

John J. Savarese, M.D.
The Joseph F. Artusio, Jr., Professor and Chairman, Department of Anesthesiology, Cornell
University Medical College; Anesthesiologist-in-Chief, The New York Hospital, New York,
New York

Scott R. Schulman, M.D.
Assistant Professor of Cardiac Anesthesia, and Director, Division of Pediatric Anesthesia,
Department of Anesthesiology, University of California, Davis, School of Medicine, Davis,
California

Alan Jay Schwartz, M.D., M.S.Ed.
Associate Dean for Academic Affairs, and Professor, Departments of Anesthesiology and
Pharmacology, Hahnemann University School of Medicine, Philadelphia, Pennsylvania

Debra A. Schwinn, M.D.
Assistant Professor, Department of Anesthesiology, Duke University School of Medicine,
Durham, North Carolina

Daniel I. Sessler, M.D.
Assistant Professor, Department of Anesthesia, University of California, San Francisco,
School of Medicine, San Francisco, California

Barry A. Shapiro, M.D.
Professor of Clinical Anesthesia, and Director, Division of Respiratory and Critical Care,
Department of Anesthesia, Northwestern University Medical School, Chicago, Illinois

Harvey M. Shapiro, M.D.
Chairman, Department of Anesthesiology, and Professor, Departments of Anesthesiology
and Neurosciences, University of California, San Diego, School of Medicine, La Jolla, California

Nigel E. Sharrock, M.D.
Clinical Assistant Professor, Department of Anesthesiology, Cornell University Medical
College; Director, Department of Anesthesiology, Hospital for Special Surgery, New York,
New York

Sol M. Shnider, M.D.
Professor and Vice Chairman, Department of Anesthesia, and Professor, Department of
Obstetrics, Gynecology, and Reproductive Sciences, University of California, San Francisco,
School of Medicine, San Francisco, California

Frank G. Standaert, M.D.
Professor, Departments of Anesthesiology and Pharmacology, Medical College of Ohio,
Toledo, Ohio

Theodore H. Stanley, M.D.
Professor, Department of Anesthesiology, and Research Professor, Department of Surgery,
University of Utah School of Medicine, Salt Lake City, Utah

Thomas E. Stanley III, M.D., M.S.
Assistant Professor, Department of Anesthesiology, Division of Cardiac Anesthesia, Duke University School of Medicine, Durham, North Carolina

Donald R. Stanski, M.D.
Professor, Departments of Anesthesia and Medicine (Clinical Pharmacology), Stanford University School of Medicine, Stanford, California; Staff Anesthesiologist, Veterans Administration Medical Center, Palo Alto, California

Linda Stehling, M.D.
Professor and Deputy Chairman, Department of Anesthesiology, University of New Mexico School of Medicine, Albuquerque, New Mexico

John K. Stene, M.D., Ph.D.
Assistant Professor, Department of Anesthesia, Pennsylvania State University College of Medicine; Director, Perioperative Anesthesia Trauma Services, The Milton S. Hershey Medical Center, Hershey, Pennsylvania

David J. Stone, M.D.
Assistant Professor, Departments of Anesthesiology and Neurosurgery, University of Virginia School of Medicine, Charlottesville, Virginia

Gary R. Strichartz, Ph.D.
Professor of Anaesthesia (Pharmacology), Department of Anaesthesia, Harvard Medical School, Boston, Massachusetts; Professor of Pharmacology, Division of Health Sciences and Technology, Harvard Medical School–Massachusetts Institute of Technology, Cambridge, Massachusetts; Director, Neuroscience Research Laboratories, Department of Anesthesia, Brigham and Women's Hospital, Boston, Massachusetts

Judy Y. Su, Ph.D.
Research Professor, Department of Anesthesiology, University of Washington School of Medicine, Seattle, Washington

Daniel M. Thys, M.D.
Associate Professor, Department of Anesthesiology, and Director, Division of Cardiothoracic Anesthesia, Mount Sinai School of Medicine of the City University of New York, New York, New York

John H. Tinker, M.D.
Professor and Head, Department of Anesthesia, University of Iowa College of Medicine, Iowa City, Iowa

Alan S. Tonnesen, M.D.
Professor, Department of Anesthesiology, University of Texas Medical School at Houston; Medical Director, Surgical Intensive Care Unit, The Hermann Hospital, Houston, Texas

Kevin K. Tremper, Ph.D., M.D.
Associate Professor and Chairman, Department of Anesthesiology, University of California, Irvine, College of Medicine, Irvine, California

Leroy D. Vandam, M.D.
Professor Emeritus, Department of Anaesthesia, Harvard Medical School; Anesthesiologist, Department of Anesthesia, Brigham and Women's Hospital, Boston, Massachusetts

Jørgen Viby-Mogensen, M.D., Ph.D.
Professor and Chairman, Department of Anaesthesia, University of Copenhagen, Copenhagen, Denmark

W. David Watkins, M.D., Ph.D.
Professor and Chairman, Department of Anesthesiology, and Professor, Department of Pharmacology, Duke University School of Medicine, Durham, North Carolina

Denise J. Wedel, M.D.
Assistant Professor, Department of Anesthesiology, Mayo Medical School; Consultant, Department of Anesthesiology, Mayo Clinic, Rochester, Minnesota

Paul F. White, Ph.D., M.D.
Professor and Assistant to the Chairman, Department of Anesthesiology; Director, Division of Clinical Research, Washington University School of Medicine, St. Louis, Missouri

Roger D. White, M.D.
Professor, Department of Anesthesiology, Mayo Medical School; Consultant in Anesthesiology (Cardiovascular), Mayo Clinic, Rochester, Minnesota

Robert L. Willenkin, M.D.
Professor and Vice Chairman for Education, Department of Anesthesia and Critical Care Medicine, University of Pittsburgh School of Medicine, Pittsburgh, Pennsylvania

John Zelcer, B.Med.Sc.(Hon), F.F.A.R.A.C.S.
Clinical Instructor, Department of Anaesthesia, University of Melbourne School of Medicine, Melbourne, Australia

Preface to the Third Edition

Anesthesia has evolved into the standard text for training programs and practicing anesthesiologists since the publication of the first edition in 1980. Because of the prominent status *Anesthesia* has achieved in the eductional program of our specialty, the publishers and I felt a special responsibility to ensure that it continued to provide our specialty with the best possible reference.

When we began our discussions for this third edition, our first step was to critically evaluate the strengths and weaknesses of the previous edition. We invited eight leaders in anesthesia education, plus several members of the University of California, San Francisco, Department of Anesthesia to review the second edition in depth. They were asked to comment on specific chapters based on their area of expertise, and also to critique the book in general. Each was asked to consider several questions: Was each chapter a complete discussion of the topic? What were its strengths and weaknesses? Should the topic be repeated as a chapter in the third edition? What new material should be added to the third edition? Could the style and presentation be improved? Could the material be organized in a more efficient manner?

The answers to these questions provided us with a foundation upon which to develop the third edition of *Anesthesia*. Although the second edition was praised for excellence, significant changes in emphasis and authorship were necessary to reflect the increased knowledge and broader responsibility our specialty has achieved over the last several years. As a result, the third edition places greater emphasis on intravenously administered anesthetics, monitoring, subspecialty anesthesia, and the increasing importance of legal and socioeconomic issues.

New chapters include those on intravenous and inhaled anesthetic delivery systems; monitoring, including instrumentation, and cardiovascular, neurologic, respiratory, and temperature monitoring; and anesthesia for orthopaedics, hyperbaric medicine, pediatric cardiac surgery, and in remote locations. Monitored anesthesia care, autotransfusion, and hemodilution are discussed in separate chapters, and chapters on the management of general anesthesia and regional anesthesia techniques have been added. Clearly, with the development of patient-controlled anesthesia and epidural narcotics, postoperative pain management is a discipline in its own right; a chapter has been added to reflect this. Finally, the anesthesiologist's responsibilities in the legal, economic, and social issues of our time are discussed in the last section of the book. Chapters have been added on operating room management, the teaching of anesthesiology, and, importantly, environmental hazards including chemical dependency.

Our advisors were also requested to recommend the leading people in each area of anesthesia as contributors for the third edition. This led to contributor changes and additions designed to maintain the level of expertise expected in every chapter. As in the second edition, each chapter was written as a complete discussion of its topic, and is fully referenced. As a result, some overlap from chapter to chapter exists; this is intentional and allows the reader contrasting, but equally valid, views on many important topics in anesthesia.

In response to other readers' comments, we have changed the organization and format of *Anesthesia* in this edition. The most obvious of these changes are the larger pages and reduced number of volumes. These changes, combined with an exhaustive new index, make this new edition of *Anesthesia* simple and efficient to use without compromising its tradition of including all the information necessary for a thorough understanding of our specialty.

I am delighted to welcome to this edition Drs. Roy F. Cucchiara, Edward D. Miller, Jr., J. G. Reves, Michael F. Roizen, and John J. Savarese, who agreed to serve as consulting editors. To ensure intellectual and editorial integrity, each chapter was edited by one of them, by our editorial staff, and also myself. This intense review equals or exceeds that of most peer-reviewed journals, and it is my hope and intention that this vigorous editorial process will continue *Anesthesia's* role as the most complete reference text for the specialty.

With any large undertaking, many people, in addition to the authors, are required for success. At Churchill Livingstone I would like to acknowledge Toni M. Tracy, President; Leslie Burgess, Assistant Editor; and David Terry, Senior Copy Editor. I am also indebted to Pauline Snider for her editorial help, and Barbara Turner, my administrative assistant here at UCSF.

Ronald D. Miller, M.D.
San Francisco, California
February 1990

Preface to the First Edition

In recent years an ever-increasing number of monographs on specific aspects of anesthesia have appeared. However, there is still no comprehensive, up-to-date American reference work that covers the entire field of anesthesia. I felt that anesthesiologists would welcome a ready reference to which they could turn for a survey of the current state of the art. And so, when the publisher extended an invitation to organize and edit just such a book, the decision was made — after consultation with friends and colleagues — to accept this major challenge.

The reader will notice that this text, while comprehensive, is not encyclopedic. I assumed that the reader would be familiar with those aspects of elementary anesthesia practice not included in this book. The focus, therefore, is on major areas of new development in anesthesia that have ocurred in the last 20 years. While the emphasis of the book is clinical, the physiological and pharmacologic principles on which a sound anesthesia practice can be based are also presented.

The contributors were requested to provide a scholarly analysis of the topic on which they were writing. In some case, this analysis included challenging the efficacy of rarely challenged dictates in the practice of anesthesia, such as Dr. Roizen's analysis of the traditional preoperative evaluation (Ch. 1) and Dr. Kirby and Mr. Smith's analysis of intensive care units (Ch. 44). The contributors were given no restriction on the number of references that could be cited, and so the reader desiring a more detailed account of a particular subject will find a comprehensive list of references to the literature. Last and perhaps most important, I did not attempt to impose a uniform point of view. For example, the preoperative evaluation and treatment of the patient with hypertension is discussed in several chapters. This allows the reader to evaluate most of the points of view with special reference to the type of surgery being proposed (e.g., hypertension and vascular surgery).

The success of any multiauthored book is in large part dependent on the expertise of the contributors and the degree of their commitment. The contributors to this book were invited because they are acknowledged authorities in their fields. This has truly been a collaborative effort, and for that reason the names of the contributors join mine on the front cover. Without their support and participation, this book would not exist. They have my deepest thanks.

I appreciate the help and flexibility provided by the staff of Churchill Livingstone, especially Donna Balopole, during the entire project. And last — but certainly not least — I am especially grateful to my family and colleagues for their patience during the time *Anesthesia* was in preparation. Their encouragement and understanding were a continuing source of strength.

Ronald D. Miller, M.D.

Contents

SECTION III: ANESTHESIA MANAGEMENT

Volume 2

SECTION IV: SUBSPECIALTY MANAGEMENT

SECTION V: CRITICAL CARE MEDICINE

SECTION VI: ANCILLARY RESPONSIBILITIES AND PROBLEMS

Section I
INTRODUCTION

1
SCOPE OF MODERN ANESTHETIC PRACTICE

Richard J. Kitz
Leroy D. Vandam

HISTORY OF ANESTHETIC PRACTICE

Introduction

Anesthesia is considered an American invention, although innovations of such significance can hardly have arisen spontaneously. The individual's well-being was not genuinely considered until the need for surgical treatment of disease arose; attempts at relieving pain were hitherto sporadic. True, operations had been performed over the centuries but always for the superficial malady—a fracture, amputation, cataract extraction, trephination of the skull, or removal of bladder calculus. To these ends, the anesthetic properties of hypnosis and trance, pressure over peripheral nerves and blood vessels, application of cold, alcohol intoxication, or ingestion of herbal concoctions were used. A more influential approach to illness had been the Galenical concept of disease, in which an imbalance among four cardinal body humors, blood, phlegm, and yellow and black bile, was said to exist; this concept survived well into the present century.

3

Antecedents of Modern Anesthesia

The gastrointestinal tract long remained the only avenue for medicinal therapy. The inhalation of vapors became an alternative approach. With techniques of anesthetic administration more or less divided into schools, the choice now lies among inhalation, intravenous, or regional techniques, or combinations thereof. But the seeds of all three methodologies were implanted during the Middle Ages. Although this chapter mainly considers subsequent developments and the birth of a new medical specialty, anesthesiology, it is worthwhile to look to the antecedents.

Inhalational Anesthesia

Around 1540, Paracelsus, a Swiss physician and alchemist, sweetened the feed of fowl with sweet oil of vitriol, a substance earlier prepared by Valerius Cordus, then named Aether by Frobenius—the familiar diethyl ether that would later be inhaled by most surgical patients over a span of 100 years or more. Paracelsus was led to exclaim, "and besides, it has associated with it such sweetness that it is taken even by chickens and they fall asleep from it for a while but awaken later without harm."

Local Anesthesia

The coca leaf was believed to be a gift to the Incas from Manco Capac, son of the sun god, as a token of esteem and sympathy for their suffering. Initially used narrowly for religious and political purposes, the leaves achieved a more ominous significance with the destruction of the Incan civilization in the 16th century by Francisco Pizarro's conquistadores. The lower classes and slaves were paid off in coca leaves, an effective method of increasing and prolonging their productivity—low-cost, high-output labor. Customarily, coca leaves bound into a ball (cocada) with guano and cornstarch were chewed with lime or alkaline ash to release the active alkaloid. Anthropologic documentation of that era indicates that trephination was successful as the operator permitted cocaine-drenched saliva to drip from the mouth onto the wound, thereby providing creditable local anesthesia.

Intravenous Anesthesia

One can construe that Harvey's studies of the circulation enabled both Percival Christopher Wren and Daniel Johann Major (Fig. 1-1) to conceive the idea of injection of medicinals into the bloodstream. Consequently, in 1665, Wren wrote that he could

> easily contrive a way to convey any liquid thing immediately into the circulating mass of blood; thus, in pretty big and lean dogs, by making ligatures on the veins and then opening them on the side of the ligature towards the heart; and by putting into them slender syringes or quills, fastened to bladders containing the matter to be

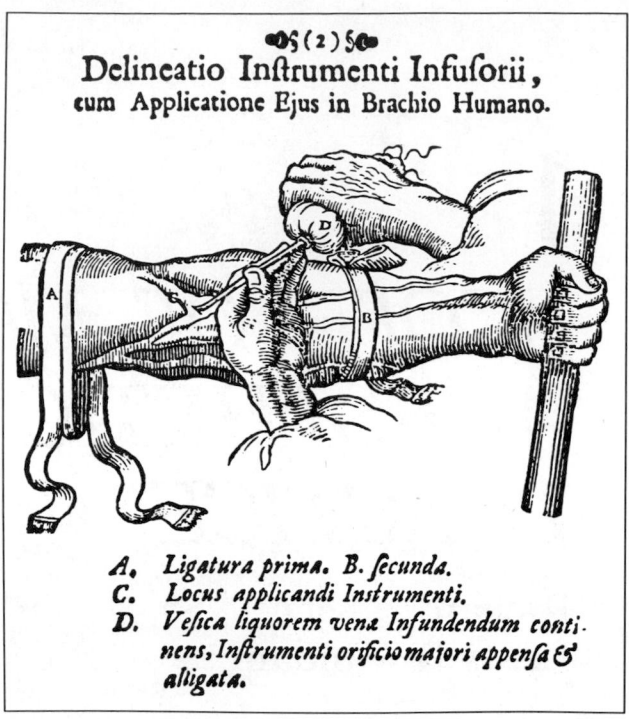

Fig. 1-1. A wood engraving illustrating the intravenous injection of medicinals, employing a quill and bladder and two tourniquets. (From Major DJ: Chirurgia Infusoria placidis CL: Virorium Dubiis impugnata, cum modesta, ad Eadem, Responsione. Kiloni, 1667.)

> injected . . . whereof the success was that opium, being soon circulated into the brain did within a short time stupefy, though not kill the dog: but a large dose of the crocus metallorum, made another dog vomit up life and all.

The dried crocus or saffron was at the time employed as a stimulant, antispasmodic, and emmenagogue.

The Rise of Inhalational Anesthesia

Primary observations on the physiology of the circulation and respiration eventually led to the discovery of gases and vapors and their experimental inhalation. In the mid-17th century, a Belgian, J. B. van Helmont, recognized a group of gases different from those of the atmosphere and attempted to classify them, while Harvey during his studies on the circulation noticed a difference in color, from dark to florid, when blood passed through the lungs. Robert Hooke opened the chest of a dog while sustaining lung inflation with a bellows, thereby proving that their rhythmic expansion is not immediately necessary for survival. A related conclusion was that some part of the atmosphere must enter the lungs, an essential ingredient named phlogiston by Stahl. Concurrently, Robert Boyle, in exhausting air from a bell jar containing a lighted taper and a living bird, extinguished the lives of both. In 1774, in the process of heating mercuric oxide, Joseph Priestley liberated oxygen, a gas with a "goodness" that sustained life, perhaps identical with the phlogiston of Becher and his pupil Stahl. Incidentally, Priestley also obtained nitrous oxide from nitric oxide. However, Antoine Lavoisier recognized phlogiston as the oxygen we breathe in the atmosphere and concluded that only a smaller share of it was concerned in respiration, the larger share being irrespirable (nitrogen). He also observed that exhaled air precipitated lime water, and concluded that it must also contain chalky air or carbon dioxide. Thus, the outlines of external respiration were delineated.

In the last decade of the 18th century a center for the pneumatic treatment of disease was established in Birmingham, England. Joseph Priestley, James Watt, Josiah Wedgewood, Dr. Richard S. Pearson, and Thomas Beddoes were among the founders. Ether could be inhaled by a sufferer via funnel to alleviate congestion and phlegm. Beddoes wrote that the medicinal use of these factitious airs was beneficial in the cure of bladder calculus, sea scurvy, and catarrhal fever. Realizing that more intensive experimentation was required, this group, with little knowledge of the causes of disease, established a Pneumatic Institute at Clifton, Bristol, and providentially appointed Humphry Davy, the youthful, brilliant chemist and physiologist, as superintendent. First, Davy disproved the theory proposed by the American, Samuel Latham Mitchell, that nitrous oxide was the contagium of disease. While himself breathing nitrous oxide for the relief of headache and the pain of an erupting third molar tooth, Davy experienced a "thrilling and an uneasiness swallowed up in pleasure." Thus originated his seminal pronouncement: "As nitrous oxide in its extensive operation appears capable of destroying pain, it may probably be used with advantage during surgical operations in which no great effusion of blood takes place." Not a surgeon, Davy failed to pursue the idea, but Henry Hill Hickman of Shifnal in Shropshire did so, a practitioner and surgeon who lamented that, "something had not been thought of whereby the fears [of a patient] may be tranquilized and suffering relieved." Having partially asphyxiated to a state of insensibility several animal species with carbon dioxide, Hickman in 1824 addressed his famous message to the Royal Society: "Letter on Suspended Animation — with the view of Ascertaining its Probable Utility in Surgical Operations on Human Subjects." Unfortunately and sadly, Hickman came the closest of all to the concept of surgical anesthesia, but utilizing an unlikely agent.

Davy's subjective experiences were duplicated among friends and visitors to the Institute and were soon taken up by the adventurous public in the form of frolics. In the United States, Crawford W. Long, while a student at the University of Pennsylvania in the late 1830s, could very well have observed and participated in such fantasies. Sometime after his return to Jefferson, Ga., as a general practitioner, Long probably not only introduced such frolics but surely persuaded a young man, James M. Venable, to inhale ether while a growth was excised from the nape of his neck. Even though this venture was repeated several times, the matter was kept secret until the first report appeared in 1848, in the *Southern Medical and Surgical Journal*, several years delayed by influential physicians who were utilizing mesmerism for surgical operations.

Within two years of this first clandestine surgical anesthetic,* on December 10, 1844, Gardner Quincy Colton took his itinerant medicine show to Hartford, Conn., where an audience could experience the exhilarating effects of nitrous oxide inhalation. So intoxicated, Samuel A. Cooley did not notice at first that he had injured a leg in the melee, but in the audience Horace Wells, a dentist, was quick to pick up the significance of this suggestion of analgesia. The next day, Wells had one of his own carious teeth painlessly extracted by a fellow dentist, while Colton administered the anesthetic. As the anguish of dental pain could now be assuaged, Wells set about to tell the world of his discovery. Circumstantially, a one-time student of Wells, William Thomas Green Morton, then in practice in Boston and enrolled in a course of lectures at Harvard Medical School, arranged for a demonstration by Wells in January 1845, before a group of medical students. However, the nitrous oxide demonstration proved a failure, as a student screamed out in pain as his tooth came out, even though later admitting to no recollection of pain. No doubt the time of induction was too brief and the gas reservoir too small to provide a surgical plane of anesthesia.

W. T. G. Morton, probably a witness to this abortive demonstration, also yearned to relieve pain, for a dental prosthesis of his invention could only be applied after the rotted roots of teeth were extirpated, an experience few patients would venture to endure. As a domiciliary student with Charles T. Jackson, eccentric geologist and chemist, Morton learned from him that pure ether applied to the gums would through evaporation yield a degree of cold anesthesia. Following experiments with inhalation of the vapor of ether in several animal species, Morton went a step further and on September 30, 1846, in his Boston office, painlessly removed a tooth from the mouth of Eben H. Frost, a merchant of that city. When notice of the operation appeared in a newspaper the next day, Henry Jacob Bigelow, a surgeon at the Massachusetts General Hospital, arranged to observe several additional anesthetics of the kind given by Morton. Suitably impressed and convinced of its surgical utility, Bigelow arranged for a trial of anesthesia at the hospital with John Collins Warren, a renowned surgeon, one-time dean of Harvard Medical School and founder of the hospital in 1821 with several others. Warren was also a progenitor of the *Bos-*

---

* Sometime before 1842, William E. Clarke of Rochester, N.Y., gave ether to a Miss Hobbie, as a carious tooth was removed by dentist Elijah Pope.

ton Medical and Surgical Journal, now the *New England Journal of Medicine*. On October 16, 1846, using a hastily devised glass reservoir incorporating the drawover principle of vaporization, Morton anesthetized Edward Gilbert Abbott, a young printer, while Warren deftly ligated a congenital venous malformation in the left cervical triangle. This feat culminated in J. C. Warren's memorable remark to the assembled gallery, "Gentlemen, this is no humbug" (Fig. 1-2).

The Massachusetts General Hospital has, to this day, designated the incident as the first public demonstration, rather than discovery, while Oliver Wendell Holmes, professor of anatomy and literateur extraordinary, chose the Greek-derived noun, anaesthesia, to characterize the process. He had also considered "neurolepsis," a term employed today to describe the drugs used in one variety of balanced anesthesia. With a medical discovery of universal significance, it was only natural that a prolonged period of controversy would ensue as to who might be given the credit. Fortunately, such an outcome did not impede further application of the method, enhanced by the prestige of the hospital and its Harvard-affiliated physicians, who knowledgeably reported on the pharmacology and physiology of the phenomenon.

In a situation of multiple discoveries as recounted here, sociologists of science would assert that the concept was "in the air," merely awaiting the appropriately receptive mind and social circumstance. Perhaps the Americans succeeded because of their pioneering spirit and lack of authoritative medical institutions. In England, on the brink of the industrial revolution, a medical hierarchy had already existed, made up of hospitals and societies, with public health a new concern and the general practitioner the dominant figure — here a revolutionary therapy might not be adopted so readily.

W. Stanley Sykes in an essay on "The Seven Foundation Stones, in Order of Merit" ranked the contenders for recognition in descending order of importance. First was Hickman who "above all others had the idea of anaesthesia most deeply and spontaneously engrained in him." Second was Horace Wells, who "given the stimulus and the sight of a man partly under the influence of gas failing to notice an injury . . . saw the possibility of it at once, as no one else had done." Third would be W. T. G. Morton "to whom belongs the undoubted credit of introducing successful anaesthesia with sufficient publicity to ensure that it immediately achieved world-wide acceptance." Fourth, "Humphry Davy discovered the analgesic properties of nitrous oxide by inhaling it and made his famous suggestion that it could be used for surgical operations." In fifth place is Crawford W. Long, "another pioneer who could easily have held a much higher place and had only himself to blame." "Long's place in the ranking order is low simply because of his extraordinary reticence." "There was no originality about James Young Simpson," and Charles T. Jackson, the last of the pioneers, "really does not deserve to be in the list at all. He did not have the idea of anaesthesia in the first place. All he did was to try and cash in upon it when it proved to be successful."

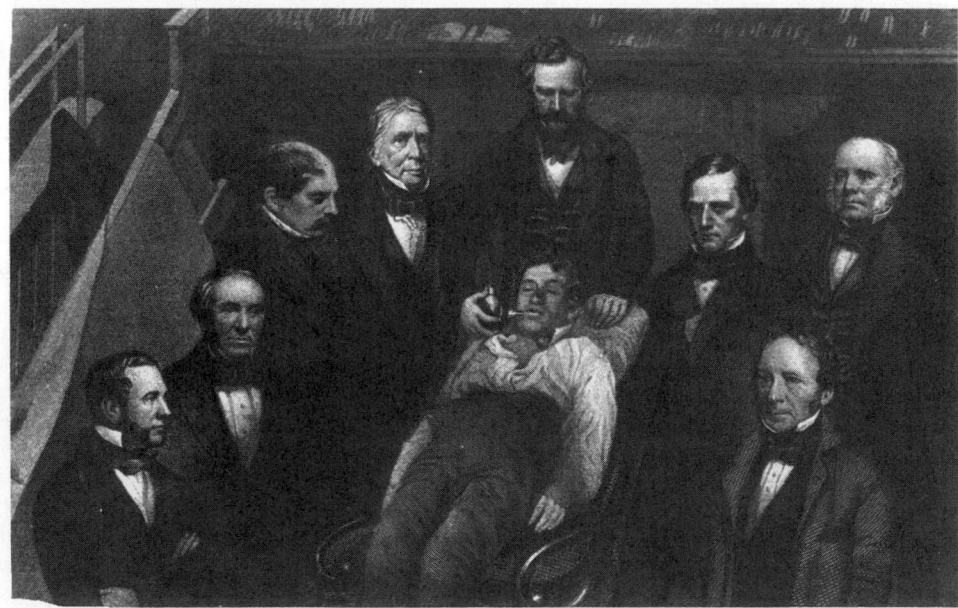

Fig. 1-2. William Thomas Green Morton giving the first public demonstration of etherization at the Massachusetts General Hospital, Boston, October 16, 1846. Physicians around Edward Gilbert Abbott, patient, are from left to right: H. J. Bigelow, A. A. Gould, J. Mason Warren, J. Collins Warren, Morton, Samuel Parkman, George Hayward, and S. D. Townsend. (From a steel engraving in Rice NP: Trials of a Public Benefactor, 1859.)

Professional Anesthesia in England: Application to Obstetrics

John Snow, general practitioner, clinical investigator, and epidemiologist (who halted a cholera epidemic in London), became the first of a long line of British physician anesthetists, in contrast to America, where that species was to blossom only around the turn of the century (Fig. 1-3). In 1847, Snow's text on *The Inhalation of the Vapour of Ether* appeared, containing case reports and an elaborate description of the traditional signs and stages of ether anesthesia. An earlier tract on ether written by Robinson, a dentist, had appeared, as well as an account by Plomley of the stages of anesthesia, but Snow's pronouncements were definitive. Likewise in Great Britain toward the end of 1847, James Young Simpson, obstetrician, who had first utilized ether to relieve the pain of labor, adopted chloroform for the purpose, as suggested to him by David Waldie. The compound had been independently synthesized by Samuel Guthrie of Sackett's Harbor, N.Y., Eugène Soubeiran of France, and Justus von Liebig of Germany. Although the clergy as well as other physicians opposed the concept of relieving pain during childbirth, the method took hold and achieved lasting status after Queen Victoria gave birth to Prince Leopold while given chloroform at the hands of John Snow, dubbed anesthesia à la reine. To further strengthen the princi-

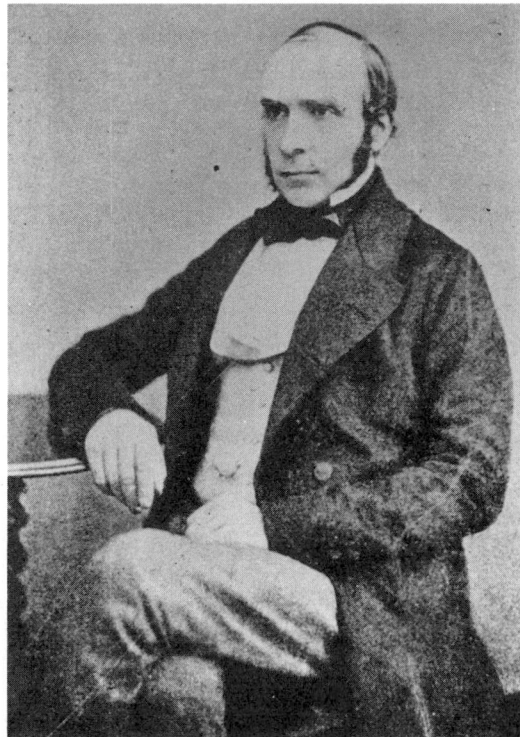

Fig. 1-3. John Snow (1813–1858). Physician, epidemiologist, and first specialist in anesthesia. (Reproduced from the Asclepiad, 1887, Vol. 4.)

ple of obstetric anesthesia, Walter Channing, professor of midwifery and medical jurisprudence at Harvard, in 1847, wrote a *Treatise on Etherization in Childbirth*, the results of a survey to settle the important issue of safety. Although the validity of the study is questioned, Channing cited the use of morphine during labor and also included cases in which chloroform had been employed. Because of its less objectionable properties, more pleasant odor, and rapid induction and emergence, chloroform superseded ether in Great Britain. And, in 1858, a second text by Snow was published, *On Chloroform and Other Anaesthetics*, completed posthumously, with a biography added by Benjamin Ward Richardson, Snow's successor.

Developments in Surgery

Surprisingly, the initial usage of both ether and chloroform led to little alteration in surgical practice, which remained largely of an external nature: trephining the skull, tapping the chest for fluid removal, relief of strangulated hernia, bladder calculus extraction, fracture reduction, and amputation of extremities. Surgical writings and lectures then pertained mostly to anatomy. Moreover, with an increase in the number of hospitals and their consequent use rather than the home to treat illness, a new problem arose, that of infection, which came to be known as hospitalism. The initial solution, listerism, or surgical antisepsis using carbolic acid, was not widely practiced until 1879, when it was acclaimed at an international conference. Then arose steam sterilization and true antisepsis.

Siegrist observed that the introduction of anesthesia was not the first attempt to render patients insensible to pain. Why then did surgery not have its great development before the mid-19th century, coincident with rather than resulting from anesthesia? The answer lies in studies of the development of concepts of disease, "for surgery is only one method of treatment and like any other method is largely determined by the concept of disease prevailing at the time." As noted in the introduction to this chapter,

> For over 2000 years disease was considered to be the result of a disturbed balance of the cardinal humors of the body which enjoyed health when in balance but showed symptoms of disease when upset.
>
> Then in the 18th and 19th centuries with Morgagni describing the results of large numbers of autopsies, it was learned that organic lesions were responsible for disease. It seemed, then, that if an organ were abnormal its function would also be abnormal. Consequently it became the purpose of diagnostics to perceive anatomic changes in the living patient, by the use of percussion and auscultation and the use of bulbs and mirrors to look into the body cavities. Roentgenology was the ultimate triumph in this direction. The surgeon by draining an abscess or excising an ulcer or tumor was removing the disease and correcting the organ. But without doubt surgery could not develop freely before the two bonds had been removed that enslaved it—pain and infection.

Local Anesthesia

Cocaine began to receive attention in Europe and America in mid-19th century. Around 1860, Albert Niemann, a pupil of Friedrich Wöhler, isolated the alkaloid in crystalline form. Twenty years later, von Anrep wrote an extensive review on the physiologic and pharmacologic properties of cocaine, clearly citing the locally numbing effect on the tongue and dilation of the pupil, the former leading him to suggest that some day cocaine might become of medical importance. Later, Sigmund Freud of Vienna began to study the properties of the drug when given samples for trial by the Merck Company. As a result of reviewing The Index Catalogue of the Library of the Surgeon General's Office of the United States Army, which referenced some 25 papers and 10 monographs under the heading Erythroxylin Coca, Freud, in 1884, wrote his classic paper, "Über Coca." Believing coca to be a worthy substitute for morphine, Freud first attempted to eliminate the morphine addiction of a close friend, Ernst von Fleischl–Marxow, who had long suffered from a painful posttraumatic thenar neuroma. von Marxow developed a new addiction as a consequence, as would many a cocaine user later on, but Freud himself never seemed to go down that path.

Freud and Koller

Freud and Karl Koller, an intern in the Department of Ophthalmology at the Allgemeinen Krankenhaus in Vienna, using a dynamometer to study the effect of coca on muscle strength, both noticed the numbing effect on the tongue as they swallowed the experimental drug. Koller had a burning desire to anesthetize the cornea and conjunctiva for ophthalmologic operations and had already tried morphine and chloral bromide. In Freud's absence, he and Joseph Gärtner dissolved a trace of the white powder in distilled water and instilled the solution into the conjunctival sac of a frog. After a minute or so, "the frog allowed his cornea to be touched and he also bore injury to the cornea without a trace of reflex action or defense." Koller wrote, "one more step had yet to be taken. We trickled the solution under each other's lifted eyelids. Then we placed a mirror before us, took pins, and with the head tried to touch the cornea. Almost simultaneously we were able to state jubilantly: 'I can't feel anything.'" A communication describing this finding, dated early September 1884, was read and a practical demonstration given by Joseph Brettauer at the Ophthalmological Congress at Heidelberg on September 15 of that year. Koller did not have the means to travel there. Koller gave full credit to Freud for the inspiration. Despite the latter's disappointment at not being first with the discovery, Freud is considered by many to be the founder of psychopharmacology because of his initial use of cocaine, the forerunner of mescaline, LSD, and the amphetamines, to modify behavior and subsequently to relieve mental illness.

James Leonard Corning

After Koller, James Leonard Corning deserves citation for his analytic approach to local anesthesia in humans based on laboratory experimentation. Having learned of Koller's report, Corning recalled the experiment in which, when strychnine is injected subcutaneously in the frog, the animal is thrown into violent spasms as a result of an effect on the spinal cord. Since, following laminectomy, a much smaller quantity of strychnine injected beneath the membranes is equally effective, he assumed that the poison must act via vascular absorption. Cognizant of the presence of the many small veins, venae spinosum, about the spinal column and cord, Corning reasoned that it might be possible to utilize cocaine therapeutically. Accordingly, in a young dog, about 20 minims of a 2 percent solution of cocaine were injected between the spinous processes of the dorsal vertebrae. After some minutes, incoordination of the posterior extremities developed, followed by insensibility. These results were almost immediately applied to a patient, a man suffering from spinal weakness and seminal incontinence. "To this end, I injected 30 minims of a 3 percent solution of the hydrochloride of cocaine into the space situated between the spinous processes of the 11th and 12th dorsal vertebrae." After a lapse of 6 to 8 minutes, when nothing happened, the injection was repeated. Finally, 10 minutes later, anesthesia began to appear in the lower extremities, and a sound could be passed through the urethra without pain. Corning concluded his report with the statement, "Whether the method will ever find application as a substitute for etherization in genito-urinary or other branches of surgery, further experience alone can show." This conclusion follows the pattern of statements made by Wren, Davy, and von Anrep in relation to intravenous, inhalational, and local anesthesia, respectively, thereby further confirming the evolutionary aspects of science. Corning's textbook on local anesthesia, published in 1886, was the first devoted to the subject.

Regional Anesthesia Techniques and Agents: Procaine and Epinephrine

In juxtaposition to inhalational anesthesia, and because of toxicologic problems with chloroform, a high anesthetic mortality, and lack of trained personnel to give general anesthesia, local anesthesia became highly popular with surgeons, especially in France and Germany, and to some extent in the United States. After a trial on himself that resulted in the first-known development of a lumbar puncture headache, August Bier of Germany began to give spinal anesthesia in 1898, followed by Matas in America and Tuffier in France. Then, because of the evident toxicity and tendency toward addiction of cocaine, a number of ester substitutes were synthesized, procaine (Novocain) by Einhorn becoming the more lasting of the group. As a result of pharmacologist John J. Abel's efforts at Johns Hopkins

Medical School, epinephrine was isolated from the capsule of the suprarenal gland in 1897 and was ultimately crystallized by Takamine. Heinrich Braun, a German surgeon, advocated the use of cocaine in conjunction with epinephrine, when, in 1903, he reported on its practical importance in inducing anemia of the mucosa in rhinolaryngologic and urologic surgery, thereby permitting the concentration of cocaine to be lowered and diminishing the dangers of intoxication.

Most currently used techniques of regional anesthesia were devised during that first decade: brachial plexus block, axillary and supraclavicular approaches; intravenous regional anesthesia (Bier); celiac plexus block; caudal anesthesia; hyperbaric and hypobaric techniques of spinal anesthesia; and all the presently employed nerve blocks about the head and neck as applied in dentistry and plastic surgery. Thereafter, aside from technical innovation and understanding of some of the physiologic and toxicologic responses to local anesthetics, the great impetus to regional anesthesia came from the synthesis of the amide local anesthetics and an understanding of their pharmacodynamic and especially pharmacokinetic properties.

Intravenous Anesthesia

We have cited the primitive experiments of Wren and Major in introducing medicinals into the circulation, quick upon Harvey's description of the circulation. Around the 1850s, the hypodermic hollow needle and glass and metal syringes were introduced via the inventions of Scotsmen Francis Rynd (1845) and Alexander Wood (1855), and Charles Gabriel Pravaz (1853). Although these improvements over the quill and bladder were to herald both intravenous and regional anesthesia, Rynd and Wood were making injections into the vicinity of nerves for the relief of neuralgia, while Pravaz injected ferric chloride via trocar into arterial aneurysms in an attempt to induce thrombosis.

Pierre-Cyprien Oré

W. Stanley Sykes, in a posthumously published essay, cited Pierre-Cyprien Oré as the true pioneer of intravenous anesthesia. Employing chloral hydrate for the purpose, his first report on the method was addressed, in 1872, to the Surgical Society of Paris. Utilizing a modification of the Pravaz syringe and needle, as he had found the latter likely to transfix the vein and cause the solution to be injected perivenously. Oré claimed that chloral hydrate was the most powerful of all anesthetics. As usual, opposition arose as critics raised the possibility of development of phlebitis and clotting. In a monograph published with a detailed account of 36 cases, some 18 for cataract surgery, others in treating tetanus, Oré claimed not to have encountered a single instance of clotting or phlebitis. Cardiac arrest occurred in one patient, an otherwise healthy, middle-aged man undergoing cataract extraction.

Anociassociation

Early in the 1900s, an essential concept was proposed toward the development of balanced anesthesia in which intravenous anesthesia is a major component. This was the anociassociation theory of George W. Crile, who in 1901 stated, "In conscious individuals, all noxious stimuli reach the brain. During general anesthesia only the traumatic stimuli are perceived centrally while with complete anociassociation all stimuli are blocked." Enlarged upon by Harvey Cushing in 1902, the idea of anociassociation became the basis for the use of opioids intravenously, so prominent in practice today. Incidentally, George Crile at the Cleveland Clinic and the Mayo brothers of Rochester were the first to employ nurse anesthetists in their surgical practices. Cushing had a number of "firsts" relative to the development of anesthesia: coinage of the term "regional anesthesia"; keeping of anesthesia records; the first in the United States to employ the Riva-Rocci technique for measurement of blood pressure intraoperatively; first user of a precordial stethoscope during operation; and a surgeon who first appointed a physician in charge of anesthesia at his clinic in Boston, Walter M. Boothby.

The Barbiturates

The major impetus for the subsequent development of intravenous anesthesia lay in the synthesis of the short-acting, water-soluble barbiturates. In 1903, long after von Baeyer had synthesized barbituric acid or malonylurea (1864), Fischer and von Mering prepared the first sedative barbiturate, diethyl barbiturate, or barbital, a long-lasting hypnotic soon to be succeeded by the sodium salt of phenobarbital. Then, as other soluble compounds were devised, a number of barbiturates of short, medium, and long duration became available. Pernoston, a shorter-acting agent, was first given intravenously in 1927, in 10 percent aqueous solution, while in 1928 John S. Lundy began to supplement inhalational anesthesia with amytal, then pentobarbital intravenously, a procedure he designated balanced anesthesia. As by current standards both drugs provide only a relatively slow onset of action, the advent of hexobarbital, or Evipal, in 1932 (Weese) resulted in the first rapidly acting intravenous anesthetic to receive wide usage. Ultimately, a sulfur derivative of barbituric acid yielded the necessary qualities with the result that thiopental, a derivative of pentobarbital, was adopted both by Lundy at the Mayo Clinic and by Waters at Wisconsin. Dundee noted how remarkable it is that this drug has survived and withstood the challenge of so many others. As in every intravenously given compound, no matter the therapeutic ends, the lasting effects of such drugs depends on specific pharmacodynamic and pharmacokinetic properties, as first shown by Brodie and colleagues around 1950.

The Evolution of Professionalism in America

The British were indeed fortunate in having physicians, beginning with John Snow, who specialized in anesthesia, a circumstance that eventually led in the 1890s to the formation of societies and publication of articles in such journals as the *Lancet, British Medical Journal,* then the *Proceedings of the Royal Society of Medicine,* in which the subject of anesthesia had its own section. By definition, professionalism is a calling in which one professes to have acquired some special knowledge used by way of instructing, guiding, or advising others, or in serving them in some art.

The Milieu

In America at the time of the first public demonstration, medicine was in a period of frontier expansion, in contrast to Great Britain. The general practitioner did all the work, and although the Easterners began to loom as specialists and leaders, a good deal of emphasis was placed on practice as a business, with medical education at a low level. The only medium for scientific publication in the first part of the 19th century was the Transactions of the Royal Society. At the turn of the century, a class of physicians emerged clearly identified with anesthesia. Interestingly, the primordial group was made up mostly of Middle Westerners and Canadians, who may have had as peculiar characteristics, "their pioneering traditions, their common purpose, devotion to equality and their struggle for success." Of the pioneers, Ralph Waters was to remark in a reflective mood that, "the development of a specialty could be traced in terms of men, publications and organizations." Three figures stand out in this regard, Waters among them.

Francis Hoeffer McMechan

F. H. McMechan, born in Cincinnati, son of a physician, excelled in college in oratory and dramatics and became a newspaper reporter upon graduation, before matriculation at the Cincinnati Medical School. There, as would be the custom for many a decade, he was required to administer anesthetics, for his father as well, so that he became a devotee of the method. Over the years 1903 to 1910, he combined anesthesia with general practice, but progressively crippling arthritis forced abandonment of practice and his subsequent preoccupation with the organization of anesthesia and medical editing.

In 1912, in conjunction with Bainbridge, a surgeon, Yandell Henderson, a physiologist, and James T. Gwathmey, an anesthetist, McMechan founded the American Association of Anesthetists. As a result of his persuasion, the *American Journal of Surgery* began in 1914 to publish a *Quarterly Supplement on Anesthesia* (Fig. 1-4), which survived until 1926, with McMechan as editor; he also served as editor of a *Year Book on Anesthesia and Analgesia.* His formation of one group after

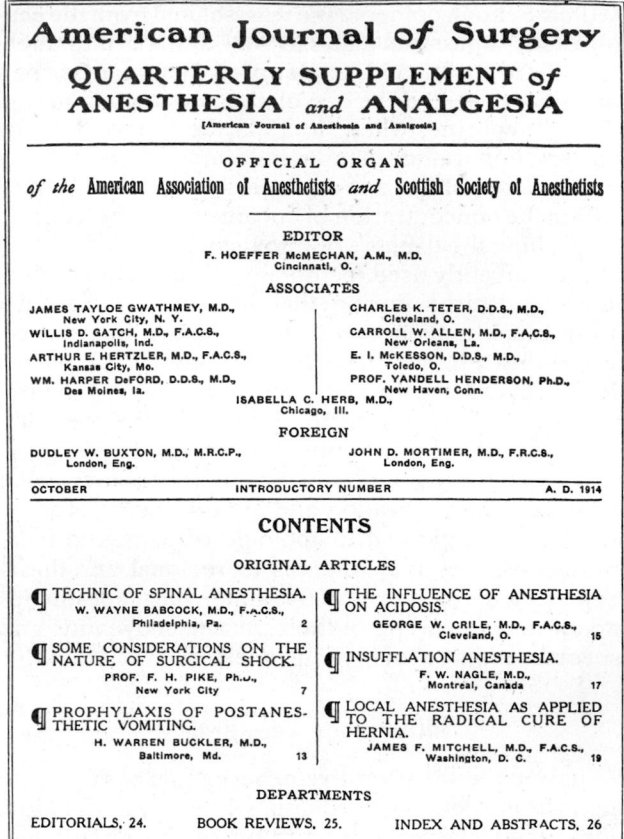

Fig. 1-4. Quarterly Supplement of Anesthesia and Analgesia, Introductory Number, October 1914, edited by F. Hoeffer McMechan, as it appeared in the American Journal of Surgery.

another in the United States and Canada led ultimately to the National Anesthesia Research Society, then to an International Society whose medium of reporting in 1922 became *Current Researches in Anesthesia and Analgesia,* the first publication devoted solely to those subjects. Assisted in these endeavors by his wife, McMechan, who died in 1939, would have been gratified to know that the International Society and its publication, *Anesthesia and Analgesia,* survive today.

Elmer I. McKesson

The second of the trio was an innovator, teacher, and inventor, E. I. McKesson, born in 1881 in Walkerton, Ind. A teacher at first, McKesson was graduated from Rush Medical School and while an intern in Toledo became attracted to anesthesia. Later, he would found the University of Toledo, where he served as associate professor of physiology and physiologic chemistry. McKesson invented and developed many pieces of apparatus: gas-oxygen machines, suction apparatus, metabolism-measuring devices, intermittent and demand gas flow valves, oxygen tents, and other instruments, all manufactured by the Toledo Technical Appliance Company. The Nargraf apparatus and the McKesson gas machine remained standard equipment until well into the 1950s.

Ralph M. Waters

Third, we return to R. M. Waters, who left his mark on several generations of anesthetists by way of far-reaching vision, combining in no small measure all the stellar attributes of the other early American anesthetists. Born in 1883 in Bloomfield, Ohio, he was graduated from Western Reserve University Medical School, served as an intern in Cleveland, and then practiced privately in Sioux City, Iowa, with obstetrics as a chief interest. He began to give anesthesia for operations performed by the other practitioners, although some of them employed nurses for that purpose. Self-trained and with only a few specialized writings at his disposal — *Proceedings of the Royal Society*, McMcchan's *Quarterly*, and Gwathmey's and Baskerville's *American Text Book of Anesthesia* — Waters in 1919 wrote an article, "Why The Professional Anesthetist." Such was his growing reputation that by 1927 he was invited to a post on the faculty of the University of Wisconsin as assistant professor of surgery in charge of anesthesia, one of a group of luminaries in surgery, physiology, and pharmacology. For the first time ever he established a resident training program in anesthesia coupled with an investigative effort that entailed among other things the examination of hydrocarbon-epinephrine cardiac arrhythmias, the pharmacology of cyclopropane, and a reexamination of the toxicology of chloroform. Many a piece of apparatus arose from this clinical-investigative milieu, some rediscovered, others new: cuffed endotracheal tubes, laryngoscopic blades and pharyngeal airways, carbon dioxide absorption canisters, and precision-controlled liquid anesthetic vaporizers.

True, there were other outstanding innovators in American anesthesia, among them Arthur A. Guedel, John Silas Lundy, and a later generation of university chairmen-professors, including E. A. Rovenstine (New York University), R. M. Tovell (Hartford Hospital), H. K. Beecher (Harvard), S. C. Cullen (Iowa and San Francisco), John Adriani (Tulane), R. D. Dripps (Pennsylvania), E. M. Papper (Columbia-Presbyterian Hospital), P. P. Volpitto (Georgia), and L. D. Vandam (Harvard).

THE DEVELOPMENT OF MODERN ANESTHESIA

The American Society of Anesthesiologists

In 1905, a group of physicians, with Adolf F. Erdman as the catalyst, formed the Long Island Society of Anesthetists, "to promote the art and science of anesthesia." As the membership grew in numbers the name of the organization was, in 1911, changed to the New York Society of Anesthetists, then augmented by out-of-state anesthe-

tists so that by 1916, 60 members were enrolled. On the 25th anniversary (1930) of the founding of the Society, a two-day scientific program was convened in New York City. In 1936 the name was once again changed to describe its breadth and character, The American Society of Anesthetists (ASA), Incorporated, with 484 adherents.

Over succeeding years all the attributes of a specialty society were fulfilled, and the designation anesthesiologist replaced the nondescript term, to indicate that anesthesiologists are physicians who have received formal training in anesthesia. A certification committee was appointed that led in 1940 to the acceptance of a section on anesthesiology into the hierarchy of the American Medical Association. That year marked the initial publication of its official journal, *Anesthesiology*. The stature of the Society was enhanced by incorporation of the Wood Library – Museum of Anesthesiology in 1950; to accommodate its multiple activities, a society headquarters was erected in Park Ridge, Ill., in 1962, with an addition two years later to house the Library – Museum. The ASA has dedicated itself to the following goals and endeavors: standards for equipment and patient care; education; repeated self-analysis via survey to crystallize the state and objectives of the Society; issues of manpower; affiliation with the World Federation of Societies of Anesthesiologists; and consideration of problems common to all kinds of medical practice. All these endeavors continue to progress with an eye toward discerning trends and future developments.

Progress since 1940

After a gestational period of approximately 100 years, modern anesthesia began around the 1940s. At that time, as Lewis Thomas asserted, medicine was about to undergo a second revolution, from a mere art into a powerfully effective science. First, in the later 19th century, rebellion against the Galenical tradition had resulted in a practice in which the history, physical examination, and establishment of a diagnosis provided a basis for prognosis, not cure. This transition was succeeded in the late 1930s by the discovery of effective new drugs, initially the sulfonamides and then the antibiotics, for treatment of infection. Inevitably, anesthesia would be caught up in the succeeding therapeutic and scientific ferment, as were all the specialties of medicine.

The first change in direction was the initial use during anesthesia of a curare product by Griffith and Johnson of Montreal in 1942. The muscle-paralyzing properties of the alkaloid derived from several preparations of South American plants had been known for centuries, and the site of action at the neuromuscular junction was graphically demonstrated by Claude Bernard. In the United States, crude extracts had been employed clinically to treat spasticity and to modify the convulsions induced during psychotherapy of depression and other psychoses. Initially, when given the extract for experimental trial, S. C. Cullen of Iowa City and E. M. Papper of New York, independently, had deemed the paralytic effects to be too much a physiologic trespass to be introduced to the anesthetic regimen. No one knows what subtle influence led Griffith to inject Intocostrin during the course of a cyclopropane anesthetic without prior experimentation. T. C. Gray of Liverpool was reminded of John Hunter's advice to Edward Jenner in regard to vaccination: "Do not think — try." Perhaps Griffith was affected by the therapeutic revolution under way, even as Horace Wells in another era had perceived the concept of anesthesia while witnessing a demonstration of the mental effects of nitrous oxide.

The subsequent general use of curare had widespread repercussions. As a result of the muscle paralysis induced, tracheal intubation became necessary for manual control of pulmonary ventilation during anesthesia, followed rationally by the development of mechanical ventilators, obligatory studies on the physiology of central and peripheral respiration, and the invention of postanesthetic recovery rooms where anesthesiologists would play a dominant role. In connection with this broadened participation in patient care, many physicians returning from World War II, where they had had introductory experience with anesthesia, sought further training in this developing branch of medicine.

Anesthesiologists, as they now designated themselves, were soon impelled to scrutinize the safety of their performance, and the use of curare no doubt sharpened the focus. Thus, following the findings of several American anesthesia study commissions and reminiscent of the Hyderabad Chloroform Commissions of late 19th century, H. K. Beecher of Boston initiated a prospective study of operating room deaths. This project incorporated the practice of some 10 university-associated hospitals during the years 1948 to 1952. From a total of approximately 600,000 anesthetic administrations, the overall anesthetic-associated death rate was adjudged to be about 1 : 1,560. In addition, many important epidemiologic data emerged. The most startling and controversial finding was a significantly higher mortality rate in patients given muscle relaxants, mainly curare, during anesthesia. While Beecher ascribed this occurrence to an inherent drug toxicity, more likely the explanation was to be found in residual postanesthetic muscle paralysis and the associated respiratory insufficiency, inadequately treated or unrecognized in those days. One of the conclusions derived from this study suggests the state of anesthesia of that era: "Great changes in the use of anesthesia agents and techniques occurred within the five years of this study. This suggests that the practice of anesthesia is far as yet from achieving stability."

Also in the 1950s, following the admonition of W. T. Salter, a pharmacologist of Yale, that, "without vision and research the professions die" (see below), research in anesthesia began, initially in conjunction with basic science departments in medical schools. Thus, S. S. Kety of Philadelphia and B. B. Brodie of New York inaugurated the science of pharmacokinetics in their respective studies on the uptake and distribution of inhaled anesthetics and the metabolism of thiopental. With this impetus, anesthesiologists enlarged on these basic concepts that today compose routine knowledge of the drugs we use. Soon thereafter, because of their unfavorable properties, most of the traditional inhaled anesthetics were replaced by the new anesthetics. Diethyl ether and cyclopropane were also abandoned, not only because of their flammability but also because of their poor pharmacodynamic and pharmacokinetic attributes. Only nitrous oxide maintained its place, while procaine was succeeded by local anesthetic agents of greater latitude.

The major inhaled anesthetic substitutions included the nonflammable, highly lipid soluble, and therefore potent vapors, halogenated inhalants, more versatile neuromuscular blockers, and local anesthetics with the amide rather than ester structure. In some instances, there were unforeseen events, as when halothane was associated with development of postanesthetic fatal hepatic necrosis, a phenomenon previously well-documented for chloroform. A multi-institutional cooperative endeavor supported by the National Institutes of Health led to the National Halothane Study. Although the conclusions of the survey were hotly debated, the data derived from some 34 institutions based on approximately 850,000 anesthetic administrations suggested an incidence of halothane-associated fatal hepatic necrosis approaching 1 in 10,000 anesthetics. Repeated administration of halogens for several anesthetics was an important contributing factor. While an altered sensitivity to halothane was deemed responsible by some, a more convincing explanation implicated toxic metabolites induced by hypoxia as the cause. Only recently has evidence reappeared for an immunologic basis of the lesion (see Ch. 6 for details).

Following these events, research on anesthesia began to reach its stride. First, the unsuspected fact emerged that inhaled anesthetics formerly considered inert were indeed metabolized to various degrees; for example, halothane was 20 percent metabolized and methoxyflurane was 50 percent metabolized. Not long after its introduction, methoxyflurane was discovered to induce a rare kind of renal failure with tubular necrosis, characterized by high urinary output unresponsive to vasopressin. Because of the pharmacokinetics and production of a toxic metabolite, the free fluoride ion, a condition once described by the French as diabetes insipidus fluorique, was found to occur after methoxyflurane anesthesia. Fluoroxene, another halogenated compound, was abandoned because of probable metabolite-induced hepatic necrosis. Investigations engendered by these events showed that the metabolism of halogenated anesthetics could be enhanced by hepatic enzymatic induction coincident with the use of barbiturates or phenytoin, with an actual proliferation of the endoplasmic reticulum and increase in cytochrome P-450. This discovery further emphasized the existing tenet that anesthesiologists in their choice of anesthetics must remember the possibility of interactions with drugs of all kinds.

After the short-acting intravenous barbiturates were introduced, J. S. Lundy of Rochester coined the term "balanced anesthesia" to describe his use of these agents in conjunction with general or regional anesthesia. These practices were further advanced when Laborit and Huguenard of France, during the French–Indo-Chinese warfare of the late 1940s, utilized a "lytic cocktail" to prevent development of circulatory shock in the wounded. The resulting "artificial hibernation" induced by simultaneous injection of a barbiturate, an analgesic, meperidine, and the tranquilizer chloropromazine (L'Arqactil), was typified by a state of stress-free, suspended animation. The tranquilizer was then succeeded by a butyrophenone, haloperidol, and meperidine was replaced by phenoperidine, one of a new class of potent opioids. The concept was characterized as neurolept-analgesia, a term Oliver Wendell Holmes had considered in 1846, before suggesting "anaesthesia" to describe the newly demonstrated phenomenon. In sequence, fentanyl (in combination with droperidol, known as Innovar) was succeeded by the more potent opioids alfentanil and sufentanil. Purely intravenous anesthesia became possible, as practiced in clinics on the continent, while the potent analgesics were also given intraspinally (subarachnoid and epidural) to treat postoperative pain. This extra-anesthetic practice ushered in the era of anesthesiologists' concern with relief of acute postoperative pain, on the foundation of their existing clinics that had mainly focused on chronic pain syndromes.

The profusion of unique agents and novel techniques introduced over the last 20 years naturally disclosed other unrecognized pharmacologic phenomena, some deleterious indeed. One category that pertains to all of drug therapy concerns pharmacogenetics, in which pharmacokinetic activity may be influenced by genetic factors. In this area, pharmacologists and anesthesiologists discovered that the metabolism of succinylcholine in plasma could be delayed or indeed prevented by the presence or absence of a variety of inherited pseudocholinesterases (see Ch. 12). Similarly, although elevations of body temperature and development of convulsions during ether anesthesia had long been noticed, a more malignant kind of hyperpyrexia came to be recognized. The malignant hyperthermia syndrome (MHS), often fatal, seemed to be triggered by a genetically determined response to agents such as succinylcholine and halothane (also see Ch. 28).

Related to genetics is the fetal loss or development of fetal malformations that may occur when a pregnant woman is exposed to a variety of drugs, with some anesthetics suspect at least in animal experiments. One consequence of the putative adverse fetal effects was the initiation of epidemiologic studies, which purported to show that the pregnant woman in the course of her operating room activities (nurses, anesthesiologists, and wives of anesthesiologists) could be exposed to trace anesthetic gases. A higher incidence of fetal loss was claimed, which led to the expensive installation of scavenging systems and the revival of closed system anesthesia techniques with all of their complexities (see Chs. 6 and 79).

The development of contemporary anesthesia can be embellished by citing the improvement in anesthetic apparatus and monitoring systems toward greater safety or, on the pharmacologic side, the continued search for the basis of narcosis at the molecular level. In this connection, a useful clinical yardstick was the concept of minimum alveolar concentration (MAC), which correlates closely with lipid solubility of anesthetics. Also, measurements of MAC permitted comparison of studies on the physiologic effects of anesthetics in terms of their relative potencies. Parenthetically, there is the seemingly heretical suggestion that nitrous oxide should once and for all be abandoned because of the ever-present liability of hypoxemia, because of its effect on essential bone marrow metabolic enzymes, and last, because of its well-known nonpharmacologic properties in relation to air-containing body cavities.

The modern era of anesthesiology is reflected in the many respected scientific publications now devoted to that specialty the world over. Thus, the designation *anesthesiologist* may have been merited only after its adherents began to record their clinical experience and the results of laboratory investigations. We quote once more the lofty language of Salter's editorial, the leaven of the profession, "Namely, that professions do not live by service alone but rather by the words of wisdom which issue out of the mouths of those few demigods who in every generation lead and inspire the multitude of their professional associates."

We have suggested that modern anesthesia emerged about 100 years after the founding of clinical anesthesia. The events of the last decades have not been merely a parochial anesthetic excursion, but a manifestation of medicine's second revolution, which proceeds at an ever-quickening pace, anesthesiology included.

THE SCOPE OF ANESTHETIC PRACTICE

Definition of Modern Anesthesia

What is anesthesiology—what is its content, what are its boundaries, and are they expanding or remaining static? Where are its current opportunities and what lies in the future? Although the practice of anesthesiology is constantly changing and further defining its unique role and special mission, a working definition is essential. We first depict the domains of knowledge and practice that are unique to the specialty. The American Board of Anesthesiology (ABA), the ultimate arbiter of our profession, has recently (1989) revised its definition of anesthesiology as a practice of medicine dealing with, but not limited to, the following:

1. **The assessment of, consultation for, and preparation of patients for anesthesia**

2. **The provision of insensibility to pain during surgical, obstetric, therapeutic and diagnostic procedures, and the management of patients so affected**

3. **The monitoring and restoration of homeostasis during the perioperative period, as well as homeostasis in the critically ill, injured, or otherwise seriously ill patient**

4. **The diagnosis and treatment of painful syndromes**

5. **The clinical management and teaching of cardiac and pulmonary resuscitation**

6. **The evaluation of respiratory function and application of respiratory therapy in all of its forms**

7. **The supervision, teaching, and evaluation of performance of both medical and paramedical personnel involved in anesthesia, respiratory and critical care**

8. **The conduct of research at the clinical and basic science levels to explain and improve the care of patients insofar as physiologic function and response to drugs are concerned**

9. **The administrative involvement in hospitals, medical schools, and outpatient facilities necessary to implement these responsibilities**

As the Board notes, "these criteria evolved largely from a chimera of the certified specialists created by successive generations of Board Directors." In an important and thought-provoking special article published by the Board entitled "Quality Anesthesia Care: A Model of Future Practice of Anesthesiology," the direction and content of anesthesia practice was predicted for the remainder of the second millenium. This was done for the Board's own guidance in planning both educational requirements and the evaluating and certifying processes, recognizing that its decisions may profoundly influence both the conduct of training programs and ultimately the nature of their product, the practitioner. In this planning document of the 1970s is clearly described the likelihood of an increasing use of a team approach toward the delivery of anesthesia care. But in the 1980s this model seems threatened by the serious rift between nurse anesthetists and anesthesiologists. The description then proceeds to detail training requirements essential for the anesthesiologist's performance as a consultant on the medical commons. Further, the Board recognized that the model described will be "continuously modified in the light of general medical developments." Indeed, the ABA mandated a full 4-year clinical program for all trainees in May 1986.

A complementary document is the Content Outline of the ABA-ASA In-Training Council. This outlines the domain of knowledge on which our specialty rests and is periodically revised by the Council to include the newest information essential to our practices and, putatively, the Board's examination system.

From this description of the anesthesiologists as consultants and their information base, we describe, in some cases to justify, and in others to predict, those aspects of anesthetic practice and associated scientific endeavors where consultant anesthesiologists can or should make contributions because of their special qualifications. Anesthesiology is thus construed as an interface where an anesthesiologist's unique qualifications are met by those of other medical practitioners. If ours is a narrow technical practice restricted to operating rooms, then the scope of the specialty we practice is limited. If, on the other hand, we have prepared well and acquired habits of continuing scholarship, then we have evolved in our specialty to provide all anesthetic and anesthesia-related services to the ill people of our institutions. We function as consultants among our peers, providing expert advice on diagnostic and therapeutic measures in those areas in which we are uniquely qualified. Because we are committed to this broader definition of the implications of anesthetic practice, the remainder of this chapter describes only our impressions of anesthesiologists in their expanded role as consultants.

The Operating Room

That the scope of anesthesia involves ministering to the anesthetic needs of surgical patients in operating rooms is indubitable. Yet, the concept as to how an anesthesiologist functions in that arena has been obfuscated by an historic tenet and a more recent attempt to further define the anesthesiologist's role. That all surgeons function as "captain of the ship" in the operating room was a tradition that assigned to them authority and responsibility for all aspects of the surgical experience, including those of which they might have little knowledge and less training. Anesthesia is a prime example of this. Recognizing that the care of a patient in an operating room is best rendered by a highly skilled team rather than a nonomniscient surgeon, the courts have relieved the surgeon of responsibility for anesthesia when conducted or supervised by an anesthesiologist (also see Ch. 75).

That an anesthesiologist is the "internist of the operating room" was perhaps an unfortunate definition as it seemed to compare us with a group of physicians having a different gestalt and who seldom frequent the operating theater. In addition, this may have suggested to surgeons that we are incapable of handling some of the more fundamental medical aspects of surgical care. Perhaps as a reaction to this philosophy, many anesthesiologists now see themselves primarily responsible for the noncutting aspects of a patient's surgical experience. This aligns us more appropriately with our surgical colleagues.

Fortunately, what emerged from the debate that accompanied the definition is the concept that an anesthesiologist is just that, an anesthesiologist, possessing neither solely medical nor solely surgical skills. Anesthesiologists are unique in keeping the patient alive by manipulating vital functions to provide the conditions essential for our colleagues to treat surgical disease. It is the continual practice of vital organ management that equips us so well to care for critically ill surgical patients in an associated arena, the intensive care unit.

In addition to direct provision of anesthesia services to surgical patients, most anesthesiologists assume responsibility for the efficient management of the operating room complex. Because they must orchestrate services for all surgical subspecialties and because they spend more time in the operating room theater than any other physician, it is rational that they assume the responsibility of allocating operating room resources. This requires that anesthesiologists in charge possess diplomatic skills and see clearly the universality of their duties, which transcend specialty allegiances, while enjoying the support and respect of colleagues from all services. Possession of these management characteristics should equip the anesthesiologist to conceptualize, plan, build, and supervise hospital units and freestanding surgical clinics as well.

In the past 5 years, the management of operating rooms has undergone major alterations imposed by economic imperatives. Although many ASA class I patients were suitable for surgery as outpatients, class II and III patients are now seen as outpatients with increasing frequency. Many more patients are admitted to the hospital on the day of surgery (also see Ch. 65). This has necessitated the establishment of unreimbursed preoperative evaluation clinics.

The technology of medical imaging is also affecting anesthesia practice in that supervision of care is required for many procedures. Computed tomography is being supplemented with magnetic resonance imaging and positron emission tomography. Extracorporeal shock-wave lithotripsy for renal and gallbladder calculi is increasingly common. Interventionist radiology utilizing embolization techniques to treat bleeding points and malformations in the gut and brain is now available. Percutaneous angioplasty is becoming more common. All too frequently these technologies are in a remote location from the operating theaters, further extending and stressing anesthesia services (also see Ch. 66).

The scope of anesthesia practice is approaching the boundaries of our skills, but the operating theater shall always remain the core of our practice and the principal source of our talents, now proving useful in other areas.

Postanesthesia Care Units
(Also See Ch. 68)

Although it can be argued that little good ultimately results from war among nations, it is now quite clear that the shock and resuscitation units organized during World War II, as well as during the Korean and Vietnam conflicts, resulted in the most efficient care of the wounded. Many studies revealed a reduction in morbidity and mortality in the care of those patients. Postanesthetic care units (PACU) had their genesis in these early experiences. Surgeons and anesthesiologists returning from World War II insisted that civilians enjoy similar standards of care. By the 1960s, all hospitals in the United States had specialized areas adjacent to operating theaters for the immediate postoperative recovery phase of the patient's treatment. Initially, there was no medical director of the PACU, which was administered by a nursing service. The nurse would call the surgeon or anesthesiologist as deemed appropriate. But it was more efficient for the nurses to seek the help of anesthesiologists in urgent situations requiring therapy because they were readily available, while the surgeon might not be. But the superior skills of anesthesiologists in expeditiously diagnosing and treating such potentially lethal conditions as respiratory insufficiency, arterial hypotension, cardiac arrhythmias, and loss of consciousness played a pivotal role. Because some of these complications may evolve from the anesthetic given, it was also natural for the anesthesiologist to assume interest in this kind of postoperative care. Later, when the Joint Commission on Accreditation of Healthcare Organizations (JCAHO) required appointment of a medical director for the PACU, virtually all hospitals turned to anesthesiology. Although a team effort involving surgeons, anesthesiologists, and nurses in the care of patients will always be the preferred model, the anesthesiologist is specially qualified to be the medical administrator responsible for establishing criteria for admission and discharge, general care of patients, and prime responsibility for emergency care, acquisition and use of equipment, triage, teaching, and those studies required to ensure the highest quality of care.

Perhaps because of a shortage of nurses in the past decade, the role of the PACU is changing. In the absence of adequate numbers of nurses, those especially skilled are assigned to the PACU and intensive care unit (ICU). Patients requiring more than routine care are frequently retained in these units, filling them to capacity and limiting elective surgery.

Measurement of the quality of anesthetic care is now a requirement in all phases of hospital activity. The PACU, a natural "choke point" in the process of anesthetic care, may be the best place to make these measurements. Nearly 100 percent of all anesthetized patients spend some time in the PACU, which allows for a systematic search for patterns of care that might be improved.

Care of the Critically Ill Patient

The Respiratory Care Unit
(Also See Ch. 71)

In the mid-1950s, the poliomyelitis epidemic that had started in Europe reached America. Over several years, in many European countries, Denmark particularly, physicians and students were mobilized to help support patients' vital functions, mainly respiration in the bulbar form of the disease. Simultaneously with the outbreak of bulbar poliomyelitis in New England, the major hospitals adopted the Danish model to deploy their resources and organize treatment protocols for patients with respiratory insufficiency . It is not surprising that the first respiratory ICU in the United States was established under the aegis of an anesthesia department at the Massachusetts General Hospital. Soon, respiratory physiotherapists who trained abroad were recruited and supporting laboratories were established. This type of multifold unit became a mecca for training other physicians, so that anesthesia's dominant role in the care of critically ill patients emerged.

Perhaps there has been no more worthy development over the past 20 years than involvement of the anesthesiologist in the care of those dangerously ill. Among the most seriously ill patients in hospitals are those who are anesthetized. All are affected by the drugs given and are often unconscious, apneic, and with manipulated cardiovascular and respiratory systems—all well monitored and modulated from minute to minute. If the degree of a critical illness is measured by vital function impairment, then anesthetized patients are indeed critically ill. It seems logical that anesthesiologists, perhaps by virtue of their training and daily practice, are uniquely qualified to care for critically ill surgical patients. Likewise, it would seem that those patients with major physiologic impairment not in the realm of surgery are probably better cared for by cardiologists, pulmonary physicians, and others.

Although the anesthesiologist's principal role in a surgical ICU entails the support of vital function, a team approach is clearly required and surely must include surgeons, nurses, medical consultants, administrators, and the clergy. In their roles as consultants in the therapy of multiorgan failure, anesthesiologists properly find themselves central to therapeutic measures employed. In general, they are given and accept the role of consultant in an ICU by invitation from a patient's surgeon or primary physician. At the moment the patient meets discharge criteria, their responsibilities cease.

In recognition of the special skills required by an anesthesiologist to assume responsibility for patients in ICUs, in 1986 the ABA defined the ingredients of a 1-year fellowship training period and required a written examination different from that used for primary certification. After the physician has achieved diplomate status, completing the fellowship and passing the special examination, the ABA may award a Certificate of Special Qualifications in Critical Care Medicine (CCM). By January 1989, 290 trainees were certified, second only to the American Board of Internal Medicine.

But all is not settled in the ICU. Specialists in other disciplines, especially trauma surgeons and pulmonologists, are vying with anesthesiologists for ICU control.

The surfeit of physicians in these specialties and their ability to gain hospital admission for their own patients are the principal reasons for this competition. It has been estimated that fewer anesthesiologists have primary responsibility for ICUs today compared with 5 years ago. Shared responsibility is likely to emerge as the preferred model for ICU management.

If health care is rationed in the United States, it may begin by limiting access to ICUs. Although numbering less than 10 percent of beds, they are the most expensive component of hospital care. Measures to predict outcome and determine cost effectiveness will be crucial (also see Ch. 70).

Resuscitation
(Also See Ch. 74)

In many hospitals over the past 20 years, anesthesiologists have often become solely responsible for organizing resuscitation teams to respond to emergencies. The medical community recognizes the appropriateness of their involvement in this activity. The anesthesiologist is usually a member of teams organized by the American Heart Association that offer programs to teach cardiopulmonary resuscitation to other physicians, hospital personnel, and the members of the community as well. This is one of the few instances in which an anesthesiologist accepts a highly visible, community responsibility. Few are more qualified.

Increasingly, anesthesiologists are being asked to participate as members of teams designed to transport the very ill from the community or far-off locations to tertiary referral centers. Except under unusual circumstances, it is the emergency medical technician who will assume that responsibility while relinquishing the role to the emergency medicine physicians to orchestrate the care after the patient has arrived at the hospital.

Emergency Room

The portal of entry for the seriously ill who are transported to a tertiary referral hospital is the emergency room (ER). An argument might be made that the anesthesiologist should be in charge of this facility. This might be appropriate were the patients indeed seriously ill, but as they often are not, an anesthesiologist is perhaps not the best choice. Often the care of the very ill or traumatized patient can best be effected by a team of experts, usually under the direction of trauma surgeons or an emergency medicine physician. Once vital organ function is stabilized via proper monitoring and life-support systems, the patient is usually triaged to an operating room or ICU where "anesthetic" care may continue until the patient can be released. In this arena, too, the essential role of the anesthesiologist lies in the care of the very ill surgical patient.

Trauma Centers
(Also See Ch. 63)

Under both national and state legislation, specific hospital complexes are being designated as trauma centers because they offer all the necessary manpower, equipment, and program resources essential to the efficient management of the traumatized patient. The role of the consultant anesthesiologist as a member of the trauma team emerges with the principal responsibility for vital organ stabilization in those patients in whom subsequent surgical intervention is required. Although not widely replicated, freestanding trauma centers have been established by commercial interests in some communities. Some are directed by anesthesiologists, and all have anesthesia personnel as key members of the trauma team. The relationship of these centers with local hospitals has not yet been clearly defined but will evolve until their appropriate position in the panoply of health care facilities is secured. Whenever that association is finally established, anesthesiologists will always be involved in those aspects of patient management appropriate to the scope of anesthesia practice.

Pain and Its Treatment
(Also See Chs. 60 and 69)

Ever since the era of Long, Wells, and Morton, anesthesiologists have been involved in the control of pain. No one would argue that this is an inappropriate mission for our specialty. But until recently, few pain control programs were developed in the United States within hospitals or among many residency programs. The demonstration that patients can safely manage their own postoperative analgesia needs in many circumstances has catalyzed the establishment of patient-controlled analgesia (PCA) services in most academic medical centers and many other community hospitals. With increasing evidence that PCA is patient adaptable, cost-effective, and may reduce the length of hospitalization, there may be dereliction in not providing this service to our patients.

The success of postoperative epidural analgesia to control postoperative pain has been reaffirmed. However, because it is labor intensive, this is not as likely to be as cost-effective, as safe, or as generally applicable as PCA. The method will probably be a therapy of choice in a few institutions and an ad hoc method in most others.

When trained personnel are available, every hospital with an anesthesia department should offer an organized program of pain control that may range from a mere consultation in diagnostic and therapeutic nerve blocks to a formalized pain clinic with regular hours, geographic site, and supporting staff, under the aegis of a pain management team composed of neurosurgeons, neurologists, radiologists, psychologists, and psychiatrists. The team concept is a community resource that,

with a few exceptions, has not been replicated throughout the country. At the very least, a pain consultation service and a PCA program should be established in all our institutions as they are so clearly within the realm of anesthesiology. Failure to do so narrows the scope of our specialty.

Clinical Pharmacology

Of the three basic disciplines—bioengineering, pathophysiology, and pharmacology—on which our clinical abilities depend, pharmacology is logically the most cogent. Anesthesia had its beginnings in the use of drugs (opioids, alcohol, coca, ether, chloroform) to produce the desired effects. Although an increasing number of anesthesiologists hold joint appointments in departments of pharmacology, it is perhaps odd that the most appropriate branch of pharmacology, clinical pharmacology, is seldom identified with our discipline. While classic pharmacology has become molecular biology, clinical pharmacology is defined as the study of drugs in humans and incorporates a body of knowledge that includes molecular mechanisms; biochemical alterations; action of drugs at receptors; the nature of the dose-response relationship; quantitating pharmacodynamic effects of drugs; molecular mechanisms of drug absorption, distribution, metabolism, and excretion; pharmacokinetics; the design, implementation, and interpretation of clinical trials; analytic methods for quantitating drugs in body compartments; and the epidemiology of adverse drug reactions.

Why are we not aligned with this endeavor and what does this portend for the future of our specialty? Whereas anesthesia had its beginnings in the operating room, obstetric suites, and dental establishments, having as its principal mission the attenuation of pain, clinical pharmacology has evolved principally from the efforts of academic internists in the United States to study cardiovascular drugs. More than 90 percent of the faculty of clinical pharmacology departments are affiliated with departments of medicine and pharmacology. Nevertheless, every anesthetization comprises an exercise in pharmacokinetics and dynamics. Most of the reports published in anesthesia journals can be classified in the sphere of clinical pharmacology. Soon we must share the results of our research on patients given potent drugs and monitored as they are in operating room and critical care situations and begin a fecund relationship with our clinical pharmacology colleagues whose origins, studies, and concepts too often exclude our participation. We must begin to expand the image of anesthesiology by attending clinical pharmacology meetings, by giving papers at those forums, by publishing in appropriate journals, and by participating in the activities of the clinical pharmacology divisions. Furthermore, and most importantly, we must seek research training opportunities in clinical pharmacology for our young investigators. In that way, the scope of anesthesiology can justifiably embrace the discipline of clinical pharmacology.

Biomedical Engineering

Our specialty is now technology dependent; notice the equipment required in modern operating rooms, ICUs, and pain clinics. It is no longer possible to care appropriately for the very ill patient without instrumentation. Further, many of the anticipated advances in our specialty will come from our colleagues in biomedical engineering. But the traditional relative isolation between hospitals and engineering schools will prove to be insufficient to meet requirements. Rather, those specialties dependent on technology, for example, anesthesiology, cardiology, radiation therapy, and radiology, should integrate engineering skills into their organizational structure. Engineers must abide with us to sense the most appropriate strategies to help solve our problems. Several of this country's anesthesiology departments have clinical engineering services and research groups as integral parts of their organizations. Logically, biomedical engineering that deals principally with patient interface technology and life support systems is well within the scope of anesthesiology. Among its responsibilities are the development of equipment specifications, acquisition, and maintenance; the determination of the cost-effectiveness of sophisticated equipment such as mass spectrometers, evoked potential monitors, automated record keepers, spectral array electroencephalographs, two-dimensional echocardiographs; the education of faculty and residents concerning the technology of anesthesia; and the provision of special anesthesia equipment for such current items as lithotripsy, magnetic resonance imaging, cyclotron therapy, and positron emission tomography.

The rigor with which engineers have approached our designated problems has been of immense help in defining the issues and identifying remedial strategies. The next step lies in educating our residents to work closely with engineers in the provision of expert care. Predictably, the anesthesiologist-gadgeteer of the past will be replaced by the anesthesiologist-engineer. Our specialty depends on defining issues in quantitative terms and developing solution-oriented strategies. Indeed, the scope of anesthesiology putatively includes biomedical engineering.

Education

The old adage that "knowledge is power" remains incontrovertible—the power to do good, to reduce the morbidity and mortality that attend anesthetic processes, thereby to improve the quality of care. Fortunately, the intellectual context of our practice undergoes constant revision as revealed in the Content Outline prepared for residents by the ABA-ASA Joint Council on In-Training Examinations. This document is available to all and is certainly the principal focus in identifying a body of anesthetic information appropriate for the medical community at large, for students of anesthesia at all levels, and for the continuing education of graduates.

Three organizations are entrusted with the responsibility of providing the educational and training requirements for those entering our specialty plus continuing educational programs for practicing anesthesiologists. The ABA (1989) has listed as its purposes the following:

A. **To maintain the highest standards of the practice of anesthesiology by fostering educational facilities and training in anesthesiology.**

B. **To establish and maintain criteria for the designation of a consultant in anesthesiology.**

C. **To inform the Accreditation Council for Graduate Medical Education (ACGME) concerning the training required of individuals seeking certification as such requirements relate to residency training programs in anesthesiology.**

D. **To establish and conduct those processes by which the Board may judge whether physicians who voluntarily apply should be issued certificates indicating that they have met the required standards for certifications as a consultant in anesthesiology.**

A consultant anesthesiologist possesses adequate measures of knowledge, judgment, clinical and character skills and personality suitable for assuming independent responsibility for patient care, for serving as an expert with the ability to deliberate with others providing advice and opinions in areas related to the practice of anesthesia and all subspecialties, and for serving as the leader of the anesthesia care team.

E. **To establish and conduct those processes by which the Board may judge whether physicians who voluntarily apply should be issued certificates indicating they have met the required standards for certification of special qualification in critical care medicine.**

F. **To serve the public, medical profession, hospitals and medical schools, by preparing for publication lists of physicians certified by the Board.**

Operationally, the Board establishes criteria for gaining entrance to its examination system, conducts both written and oral examinations, and certifies those who satisfy those training and examination requirements. It is clear that the ABA has dictated the very core of the specialty's educational process.

The Board is allied in this mission with the Residency Review Committee (RRC) for Anesthesiology. This tripartite group with representatives from the ABA, ASA, and American Medical Association (AMA) prescribes the General Requirements for Residency Training and prepares the Special Requirements for anesthesiology promulgated by the ACGME listed above. These documents describe the organizational arrangements and resources necessary to mount a residency training program but do not describe program content, conduct examinations, or certify specialists, which are within the purview of the Board. The RRC does, however, conduct periodic site inspections of all training programs to ascertain the extent to which they meet the General and Special Requirements. The RRC has the power to recommend approval, disapproval, or probationary status for residency programs.

As depicted earlier, the ASA also plays a vital role in the educational process, that of providing an organizational framework for meeting the political and continuing educational needs of its members. The Society provides for the scientific program and refresher courses at its annual meeting, conducts regional refresher courses nationwide, and distributes an updated, self-assessment examination for all practitioners, especially those unable to attend other continuing educational functions.

We must all continue self-education if we are to fulfill the role so long sought and so recently acquired as consultant anesthesiologists. The scope of anesthesiology is only as narrow or as broad as the knowledge, judgment, and skills that anesthesiologists apply to the ill people under their care.

Research

An anesthesia department in an academic medical center differs from that of the community hospital: the latter must strive to provide the highest quality of care to patients, while the former assumes an additional burden of constantly monitoring, revising, and improving that care. This obligation is discharged through education in residency programs and the identification and implementation of better means to care for the anesthetized ill patient. The better academic anesthesia departments offer an ingrained cultural medium in which an enquiring mind does think, solutions to problems in anesthesia are anticipated, and the discovery of new concepts is the reward.

Twenty-five years ago, W. T. Salter, professor of pharmacology at Yale, editorially issued a challenge to our specialty in his argument on "The Leaven of the Profession." For its sagacity, we quote the editorial in its entirety.

It is true for Anesthesiology as for any other profession that *service* must be leavened with progressive thought. Every profession has its corps of hewers of wood and drawers of water. It must also have its sprinkling of investigators to guide and lead it on its path forward. Without vision, the profession dies. At the present moment the progress of Anesthesia is limited almost exclusively by a lack of knowledge of the basic action of drugs as applied to human organisms which are abnormal. Greater strides must be made in elucidating the pathological pharmacology of such drugs as curare. The relative importance of analgesia as contrasted with relaxation must be reviewed on the basis of careful physiological measurement made at the bedside with modern methods. Who is to do such essential studies of Applied Pharmacology?

Obviously, a considerable knowledge of pathological

human physiology is involved. In this day and age there is a tendency for the routine anesthetist to "pass the buck" to the professor of physiology or the professor of pharmacology, in the vain hope that the answers can be learned from mice or monkeys. The respective professors named are usually only too eager to cooperate and interested in fostering the development of applied studies on man. They realize all too well, however, that such studies must be made by an applied pharmacologist, appointed by the Department of Anesthesiology. Such a man should be familiar with the everyday problems of the practicing Anesthesiologist. He should have basic training in the fundamental departments mentioned. He would do well perhaps to commence his work with experiments on animals performed under the aegis of the preclinical departments. Ultimately, however, the problem must be taken into the clinic and the definitive answers resolved there.

To this end, there must be trained a group of so-called "academic Anesthesiologists." These individuals must have the special training and sufficient leisure to advance the basic concepts of applied science. In their earlier years they must be supported by adequate fellowships. In their mature years they must receive adequate recognition in the form of staff appointments and university affiliation. They must not be run ragged with routine assignments, but must be protected from the irate surgeon who demands *service now* in the name of all humanity and the Trustees. At the present time the fellowships and funds available for this purpose are pitifully meager.

Part of the fault for this lack of opportunity lies in the diffidence of the routine anesthesiologist. The conscientious and overworked anesthetist, while rendering invaluable service to the community, fails to appreciate that his ultimate professional status cannot be guaranteed by *service* alone. Without vision and research, the professions die. It behooves every practicing member of the profession to exert his influence both in his local medical group and in his society of specialists to see to it that opportunities exist for progress.

Have we met that challenge? Surely we have come a long way. Over the past 10 years, especially, many of the principal advances in anesthetic practice and knowledge have come from within the specialty. But we are not yet at the knee of the curve leading to self-sufficiency. In fiscal year 1987, $13,573,272 of the $5.2 billion (0.27 percent) available for the support of extramural research by the National Institutes of Health was committed to anesthesia departments. Of the 88 principal investigators, 50 had the Ph.D. degree, 28 had an M.D. degree, and 10 had both M.D. and Ph.D. degrees. In 1988, the ASA, its associated foundations, and industrial collaborators committed close to $500,000 in direct support of research and research training. No data are available on research funding from other sources such as drug and equipment manufacturers and the departments themselves.

The paucity of long-term research funding and requirements for increased efficiencies in hospitals have virtually combined to preclude the kind of scholarship envisioned by Salter. And until we reach the plateau of self-sufficiency in meeting the needs of our specialty, we can only begin to mount an assault on the more generic issues and problems, those that have broad scientific and social implications, those that transcend our specialty. Studies are needed on the nature of consciousness; of memory; of central nervous system communication; of neural networks and artificial intelligence; of molecular biology, genetics, and immunology; of methods of measuring the quality of medical practice; of identifying just means for allocating limited medical resources; of determining the molecular mechanism of drug dependence. Although research and education germane to our specialty are clearly within grasp, we will have fully matured only when our vision and accomplishments exceed that scope.

Manpower

Why a section on manpower in a chapter dealing with the history and scope of anesthesiology? The history of our specialty is one of accomplishment by people, while the scope of anesthesiology ultimately is defined by the practice patterns and contributions of its practitioners. One wonders where our specialty would be positioned today if its protagonists had been leading surgeons rather than imaginative dentists. In England, this was a physician's specialty from the beginning only because anesthetists arose from the ranks of clinicians already practicing in a growing number of hospitals, specialty facilities among them. The burgeoning population of the United States far exceeded the capabilities of medical schools to meet the demands for any physician services, much less anesthesiology. Hence, it is not surprising that in the early years the conduct of anesthesia was assigned to general practitioners, medical students, and surgical junior house officers. Somewhat later, they in turn were replaced by nurse anesthetists usually working under the aegis of the hospital or surgeons but later under the supervision of anesthesiologists. The number of physicians entering our specialty has remained relatively constant at approximately 3 to 4 percent overall of graduating medical students. Together, nurse anesthetists and anesthesiologists were not able to meet the demands for anesthesia service. Simultaneously, this failure impaired the specialty's ability to respond to needs in other appropriate arenas, such as pain clinics, intensive care units, recovery rooms, and others that fall within the scope of our specialty.

For a 30-year period representing the 1950s, 1960s, and 1970s, this vacuum was partially filled by an influx of graduates from foreign medical schools—a phenomenon true for most specialty practices but perhaps not to the extent found in anesthesiology. The number of foreign medical graduates in American anesthesia training programs has fallen dramatically from a high of 58 percent in 1972 to 9 percent in 1988.

But over the past decade, two major events have signalled an approaching end to manpower shortages in anesthesia. One has been a steadily decreasing birthrate plus zero population growth. The other was a doubling of the number of medical schools in the United States and therefore an increase in student enrollment. Because of these trends, manpower in some specialties now exceeds the need and in most others is close to equilibrium; for a few such as anesthesiology, one can predict with some confidence that it is still unlikely we can meet the requirements for anesthesia services for the American people in the 1990s. Although the number of residents in training has risen from 2,421 in 1978 to 4,563 in 1988, the number of registered nurses in nurse anesthetist schools has fallen from about 1,200 to 600 over the same period. The physician trend is driven principally by the doubling of medical school graduates in the past decade and the relative attractiveness of the specialty; the nurse trend is in parallel with the general decline in nursing graduates.

In a recent study by the Committee on Manpower of the ASA, it was clear that over 90 percent of all anesthetics in the United States are given by anesthesiologists directly or by nurses under their supervision. The remainder are given by obstetricians, independently practicing certified nurse anesthetists (CRNAs), surgeons, general practitioners, and dentists. In 1988 there were 24,749 members of the ASA, including 15,562 diplomates of the ABA. Also in 1988 there were 24,068 members of the American Association of Nurse Anesthetists, of whom all are CRNAs. The total anesthesia manpower of almost 50,000 is responsible for an estimated 20,000,000 anesthetics per year exclusive of dental procedures.

A related and just as important issue is the quality of anesthesia manpower. Our specialty is now attracting an increasingly large number of the very best medical students and physicians with training in other specialties, particularly internal medicine and pediatrics. Others intrigued by anesthesiology in increasing numbers are physicians with graduate science degrees who see in our specialty many challenging research opportunities. So it is with some confidence that we enter the 1990s with the realization that for the first time, we will begin to approach the manpower needs with the best of practitioners. In turn, this should create the opportunity to move with vigor into those other areas described here where anesthesiologists are especially equipped to preside.

Standards in Anesthesia

One of the phenomena of the mid-1980s was the promulgation of practice standards in medicine as initiated by anesthesiology. Although surprising to some, the emergence of standards was both inevitable and predictable. Standards are an intimate part of a sophisticated society. Because of the infinite variations of our society, it is essential to its very existence that laws and regulations be promulgated in its best interests. In so doing, individual components yield a degree of freedom for the common good. The first standards in anesthesia, which are those describing minimal monitoring, were promulgated by nine teaching hospitals in Boston in 1987 (see Eichhorn et al.). Over the next several years, standards for an anesthetizing location in a non-operating room area, preanesthetic apparatus check-out systems, and care for postoperative care unit patients were issued. The monitoring standards were quickly endorsed by the ASA, state societies, and many an insurance carrier. The principal reasons cited by the Boston group in support of practice standards include the following:

1. **To improve patient care by attenuating individual variations in practice, thereby reducing the number of adverse outcomes arising from anesthesia accidents. Human beings are imperfect. We have our bad days, get tired daily, are frequently distracted, have uneven skills, and our senses are limited. Although monitors have other imperfections, they are human sense extenders, less error-prone, and more reliable and predictable. The Cooper critical incident studies have indicated that these very human characteristics are responsible for 90% of anesthetic accidents (1984). It follows that human errors can most probably be reduced by limiting these individual variations in medical practice patterns through the imposition of minimum standards.**

2. **To enhance detection of relatively low-frequency events, using principles derived from a large collective experience. Because serious injuries or death of patients occur very rarely in an individual's anesthesia practice, it seems unwarranted for individuals to develop standards of care based solely on their own adverse experiences.**

3. **To provide a means of objective evaluation. The individual practitioner or the chief can observe (and quantify, if desired) whether actual patient monitoring meets the standards. It is clear that this could lead to the identification of those anesthesia practitioners with a high-quality practice as compared to those with a higher level of morbidity and mortality. Peers and patients do not see us practice and there are no quantitative data available. Hence, it is not possible for patients, surgeons, or anesthesiologists to select an anesthesiologist. The measurement of the effect of standards on the outcomes of individual physician's practices could generate data useful in identifying the best. As threatening as this may seem, I believe this type of accountability will soon be sought by society. It behooves us to begin the process now to assure control of the mechanisms.**

Negative aspects of standards cited by Stoelting (in Gravenstein and Holzer) include the following:

1. **Objective data from which to derive standards may be lacking.**
2. **There may be reduced incentive to remain vigilant.**
3. **A false sense of security may be introduced.**
4. **Monitors may provide incorrect or unnecessary information.**
5. **Mandated requirements may be unrealistic.**
6. **We may stop looking for other ways to improve patient safety.**

In many states where minimal monitoring standards have been accepted, malpractice insurance rates have fallen, presumably in response to a reduction in the number of claims. It follows that the quality of anesthetic care may have been enhanced. Other specialties, too, are adapting to the leadership of anesthesiology.

Economics

In the early 1970s, the first public mutterings were heard that health care costs were excessive. And as those costs approached and then exceeded 10 percent of the country's Gross National Product (GNP), a change in the manner in which health care was managed and financed was mandated. The 1980s was a shift from free market enterprise to a regulated system much like that of the public utilities. Because two-thirds of health care dollars fund hospital care, hospital financing was the first to change to a diagnosis regulated group (DRG) system under Medicare. Hospital expansion was curtailed and outpatient care emphasized over that provided to inpatients. Length of hospital stay fell, some small hospitals were eliminated, and new systems of managed care were developed. These took the form of health maintenance organizations (HMO), preferred provider organizations (PPO), and independent practice associations (IPA), which negotiated contracts with patients, hospitals, and physicians to provide care and compensation at set rates. These and other measures only slightly attenuated the rate of rise in health care costs, which continues to substantially exceed that of inflation.

The regulators next turned to the matter of physician reimbursement in their efforts to control the cost of health care. The expense of reimbursing physicians has also at least doubled the inflation rates. The federal government mandated a change from the usual and customary physician-determined reimbursement scheme under Medicare to another mechanism. Resource-based relative value scales, physician DRGs, capitation, and other strategies are currently under debate. The 1990s will witness the installation of a new system to govern physician reimbursements, first under Medicare, followed in turn by other plans. The medical establishment explained its needs for reimbursement rates greater than inflation, arguing that the aging American population, expensive technology, and uncontrolled litigation were the principal determinants. In addition, the specter of decreasing quality of care was raised, surely attendant on the reduction of health care costs below an ill-defined limit. The public's reaction was to mandate measurement of the quality of hospital and physician care and to require publication of the data. This public accountability should reduce the number of marginal health care providers while allowing the public to choose their hospitals and physicians based in part on measures of quality.

These economic coercive measures will result in a seismic shift in patterns of practice and resource allocation in the 1990s. Anesthesiology will be similarly affected as our leaders struggle to ensure that our specialty is not treated unfairly and that the resources to be made available are adequate to meet the expectations of the American people. They will be severely tested and their success or failure on the new medical commons will be the quintessential factor in the shaping the scope of our specialty in the remainder of this century.

Academic anesthesia programs will be particularly hard-pressed. The economic imperative to increase output in academic medical centers is likely to curtail the time available for educational and research programs if faculty salaries are to be sustained, thus endangering our competitiveness for the best students and research funds. Mediocrity or, worse, the antithesis of excellence may prevail. It is not at all comforting to realize that other specialties will be similarly affected.

Future

We have reviewed briefly the history of our specialty and defined the scope of anesthesiology; our specialty seems secure but not yet mature and fully differentiated. While there has been a trend toward broadening our scope (e.g., chronic pain management, critical care medicine), increased subspecialty practice (e.g., neuroanesthesia, cardiac anesthesia, pediatric anesthesia) will make our specialty more mature and responsive to the changing health care scene. Yet, subspecialty practice will make allocation of anesthesia personnel even more complex. If we can accommodate to emerging economic constrains and implement the complete scope of anesthesia services in all hospitals, while developing the role of the consultant anesthesiologist and facilitating research in those areas germane to anesthetic practices and society in general, then we will have earned a permanent place at the high table of academe. It is on research and education that so much depends—the improvement of the quality of anesthetic care, the advancement of our specialty.

SELECTED READINGS

The History

Bonner TN: The social and political attitudes of midwestern physicians, 1840–1940. J Hist Med 8:133, 1953

Byck R (ed): Cocaine Papers. Sigmund Freud. New American Library, New York, 1974

Cartwright FF: The English Pioneers of Anaesthesia. John Wright and Sons, Bristol, 1952

Caws P: The structure of discovery: Scientific discovery is no less logical than deduction. Science 166:1375, 1969

Channing W: A Treatise on Etherization in Childbirth. William D. Ticknor, Boston, 1848

Duncum B: The Development of Inhalation Anaesthesia. Oxford University Press, London, 1947

Faulconer A, Keys TE: Foundations of Anesthesiology. Charles C Thomas, Springfield, IL, 1965

Keys TE: The History of Surgical Anesthesia. Schumans, New York, 1945

Laborit H, Huguenard P: Practique de l'hibernotherapie, en Chirurgie et en Medicine. Mason, Paris, 1954

Merton RK: Singletons and multiples in scientific discovery. A chapter in the sociology of science. Proc Am Philos Soc 105:470, 1961

Mortimer WG: History of Coca, "The Divine Plant" of the Incas. And/Or Press, San Francisco, 1974

Oré PC: Etudes, cliniques sur l'anesthesie chirurgicale par la methode des injections de chloral dans les veines. JB Baillière et Fils, Paris, 1875

Siegrist HE: Surgery before anesthesia. Bull School Med U Maryland 31:116, 1947

Smith WDA: Under the Influence. A History of Nitrous Oxide and Oxygen Anaesthesia. Macmillan, London, 1982

Snow J: On the Inhalation of the Vapour of Ether. John Churchill, London, 1847

Snow J: On Chloroform and Other Anaesthetics. John Churchill, London, 1858

Sykes WS: Essays on the First Hundred Years of Anaesthesia. Churchill Livingstone, Edinburgh. Vol I, 1960, Vol II, 1960, Vol III, 1982

The Development of Modern Anesthesia

Beecher H, Todd DP: A study of the deaths associated with anesthesia and surgery. Ann Surg 140:2, 1954

Brodie BB, Mark L, Papper EM, et al: The fate of thiopental in man and a method for its estimation in biological material. J Pharmacol Exp Ther 98:85, 1950

Bunker JP, Forrest WH, Mosteller F, et al: The National Halothane Study. A study of the possible association between halothane anesthesia and postoperative hepatic necrosis. U.S. Government Printing Office, Bethesda, MD, 1969

Cohen EN, Bellville JW, Brown BW: Anesthesia, pregnancy and miscarriage. A study of operating room nurses and anesthetists. Anesthesiology 35:343, 1971

Crandall WB, Pappas SG, Macdonald A: Nephrotoxicity associated with methoxyflurane. Anesthesiology 27:591, 1966

Griffith HR, Johnson GE: The use of curare in general anesthesia. Anesthesiology 3:418, 1942

Kety SS: The theory and application of the exchange of inert gas at the lungs and tissues. Pharmacol Rev 3:1, 1953

Mazze RI, Hitt BA, Cousins MJ: Effect of enzyme induction with phenobarbital on the in vivo and in vitro defluorination of isoflurane and methoxyflurane. J Pharmacol Exp Ther 190:523, 1974

Nilsson E: Origin and rationale of neurolept analgesia. Anesthesiology 24:267, 1963

Van Dyke RA, Chenoweth MB: Metabolism of volatile anesthetics. Anesthesiology 26:348, 1965

Whittaker M: Plasma cholinesterase variants and the anaesthetist. Anaesthesia 35:174, 1980

The Scope of Anesthetic Practice

American Association for the Advancement of Science: Frontiers in neuroscience. Science 242:633, 1988

American Board of Anesthesiology: Booklet of Information. American Board of Anesthesiology, Hartford, CT, 1989

American Board of Anesthesiology: Quality anesthesia care: A model of future practice of anesthesiology. Anesthesiology 47:488, 1977

Chernow B (ed): The Pharmacologic Approach to the Critically Ill Patient. Williams & Wilkins, Baltimore, 1988

Cooper JB: Anesthesiology and the engineer. Eng Med Biol 1:17, 1982

Cromwell J, Rosenbach ML: Reforming anesthesia payment under Medicare. Health Affairs 7:4, 1988

Eichhorn JH, Cooper JB, Cullen DJ, et al: Anesthesia practice standards at Harvard: A review. J Clin Anesth 1:55, 1988

Gravenstein JS, Holzer JF (eds): Safety and Cost Containment in Anesthesia. Butterworth, Boston, 1988

Hornbein TF: The setting of standards of care. JAMA 256:1040, 1986

Knaus WA, Zimmerman JE, Wagner DP, et al: APACHE — Acute Physiology and Chronic Health Evaluation: A physiologically-based classification system. Crit Care Med 9:591, 1981

National Institutes of Health: NIH Data Book. NIH Publication Number 88-1261, 1987

Salter WJ: The leaven of the profession. Anesthesiology 11:374, 1950

Starr P: The Social Transformation of American Medicine. Basic Books, New York, 1982

Zapol WM, Falke KJ (eds): Acute Respiratory Failure. Marcel Dekker, New York, 1985

Section II

SCIENTIFIC PRINCIPLES

2
BASIC PRINCIPLES OF PHARMACOLOGY AND ANESTHESIA

Debra A. Schwinn
John B. Leslie
W. David Watkins

INTRODUCTION

Anesthesia necessitates the administration of doses of drugs in such a manner as to produce desired effects yet avoid undesirable side effects or toxicity. In addition to analgesia and amnesia, pharmacologic control of the physiologic and pathophysiologic functions of all major organ systems is often required. These broad therapeutic objectives necessitate integration of the principles of physiology and pathophysiology with basic and clinical pharmacology. The resulting knowledge should form a rational basis for the appropriate administration of drugs to humans. In every instance, the therapeutic objective should be to maintain adequate drug concentrations at the desired sites of action to produce a specific effect. The anesthesiologist should therefore strive to select and administer drugs by routes and dosage regimens that will ensure tissue and receptor concentration levels between those that produce unacceptable toxicity and those that fail to provide effective therapy (i.e., within a range between toxic and subtherapeutic doses).

The empirical approach to drug administration consists of adjusting an initial dose in an amount and rate in accordance with the clinical response of an individual patient. The ability of the anesthesiologist to make these adjustments before administering a chosen dose has often been termed the art of anesthesia and will continue to reflect, in part, the important skill of establishing individualized dose-response relationships. With continued experience and research in anesthesiology, a variety of guidelines have emerged by which the science of anesthesiology will enhance the art.

This chapter is divided into two basic sections: pharmacokinetic principles and pharmacodynamic principles. The pharmacokinetic section describes the determinants of drug availability. Drug availability is, of course, determined in part by the dosage and rate at which it is administered. Additional important features of drug availability include the various modes of transport of molecules across biologic membranes and the extent to which drugs are bound to proteins present in the circulation and tissues. Availability of drug at its site of action is further influenced by blood flow to that site. The availability of an administered drug is influenced by the extent and speed of metabolic processes that chemically alter the parent compound to products possessing more or less biologic activity. Finally, the rate of removal of the drug and/or its metabolic products from the body influences the extent and the duration of the pharmacologic effect. Each of these concepts is explored in detail in the sections defining drug absorption, distribution, metabolism, and elimination. The latter portion of the pharmacokinetic section addresses the time course of drug effects.

The second major section of this chapter relates to pharmacodynamic principles. As stated above, the therapeutic objective is to maintain adequate drug concentration at a given site of action. Pharmacodynamics describes the relationship between plasma drug concentration and the pharmacologic effect. The broad areas of cellular mechanisms of drug action, clinical evaluation of drug effects, and biologic variability are covered in this section.

An understanding of pharmacokinetic and pharmacodynamic principles provides the anesthesiologist with a scientific foundation for achieving the therapeutic objectives associated with any drug. Selection of drugs should be based on individual patient variation, length and nature of surgical procedures, routes of administration, concurrent drug therapies, and other contributing variables.

PHARMACOKINETICS

Overview

Pharmacokinetics is the quantitative study of the absorption, distribution, metabolism, and elimination of chemicals in the body and the time course of these effects (Fig. 2-1). Simply stated, pharmacokinetics attempts to describe what the body does to a drug. The term was first used by Dost in 1953 in an attempt to quantitate the rate of change in drug concentrations in proposed compartments within the body. The mathematic complexity that has developed in pharmacokinetics to project the phases of drug absorption, distribution, and elimination has prevented many clinicians from developing a basic understanding of this science. It will become apparent, however, that as anesthesiologists begin to understand some of the basic principles of pharmacokinetics, the dose-response relationships of anesthetic drugs often can be predicted in normal or pathophysiologic states. These basic principles can be

applied to the great majority of drugs administered by anesthesiologists; and the addition of new drugs is rapidly assimilated by comparison with established compounds. A minimum of mathematics is included in this presentation in an attempt to emphasize principles rather than specific drugs or pharmacokinetic models. Several excellent in-depth reviews are listed in the reference section.

Absorption and Disposition of Drugs

General

Most drugs are intended to produce their effect systemically. For this to occur, they must circulate through the bloodstream to be present in their pharmacologically active forms at their sites of action. The process by which drugs are delivered to the blood in their active form is called absorption. Even drugs that are intended to act locally (i.e., local anesthetics) must cross membranes to produce an effect on their target tissue. Hence, absorption of drugs involves several physical processes, including ionization, route of administration, transport across membranes, bioavailability, and protein binding. Each of these processes contributes to the amount of active drug ultimately reaching the plasma or local tissue at a certain rate. This process is discussed below. The rate of absorption influences the time course of drug effect and is an important consideration in determining drug dosage. Also, the choice of the route by which a drug is administered is frequently influenced by rate and extent of drug absorption.

Ionization of Drugs

The chemical form of a drug determines the ease with which it may be absorbed. Most drugs are either weak acids or weak bases present in solution in both ionized and unionized forms. The unionized form is usually lipid soluble and will readily cross lipid membranes. By contrast, the ionized fraction is generally hydrophilic and does not easily cross membranes. The unionized fraction of a drug is controlled by the pK_a (the pH at which the compound is ionized 50 percent) and the pH gradient across the membrane. This relationship is defined by the Henderson-Hasselbach equation:

$$pH - pK_a = \log [A^-]/[HA] \quad \text{for an acid}$$

$$pH - pK_a = \log [B]/[BH^+] \quad \text{for a base}$$

where $[A^-]$ is the concentration of an ionized acid, $[HA]$ is the concentration of an unionized acid, $[B]$ is the concentration of an unionized base, and $[BH^+]$ is the concentration of an ionized base. Since pK_a is a constant for each drug, the pH of the local environment around the drug is important in its absorption. This means for a weak acid (pK_a above approximately 3), an acid environment such as the stomach (where pH is less than pK_a) will favor the denominator (or unionized form) and hence increase absorption. For a basic drug,

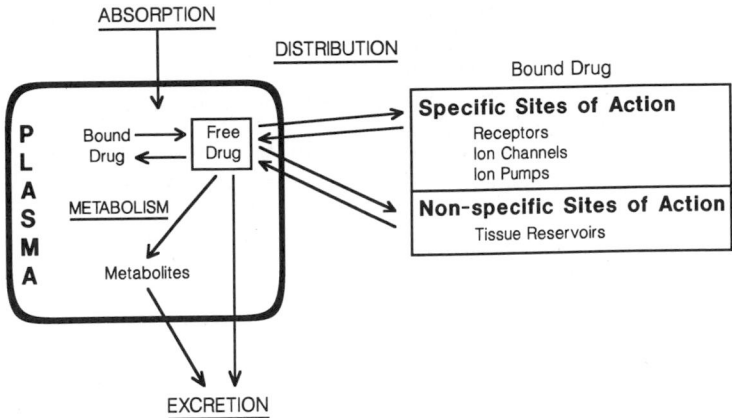

Fig. 2-1. Schematized depiction of various aspects of pharmacokinetics including absorption, distribution, metabolism, and excretion.

an acid environment such as the stomach (where pH is less than pK_a) will favor the denominator (or ionized form) and hence inhibit absorption. The relationship between pK_a, pH, and ionization percentages is shown in Fig. 2-2. This figure shows that significant changes in the ionized fraction of drugs will occur with drugs whose pK_a values are in the range of 3 to 8.

Clinical example of drug ionization. The gastric lumen has a pH of approximately 1, and the intestinal lumen a pH of 7 to 8. A weak acid such as acetylsalicylic acid, with a pK_a of 4.4, will be readily absorbed across the gastric membrane, whereas orally administered basic drugs will not be absorbed from the stomach but will be readily absorbed from the intestinal lumen. This phenomenon is the basis for the so-called ion trapping or concentration of weak acids in the stomach.

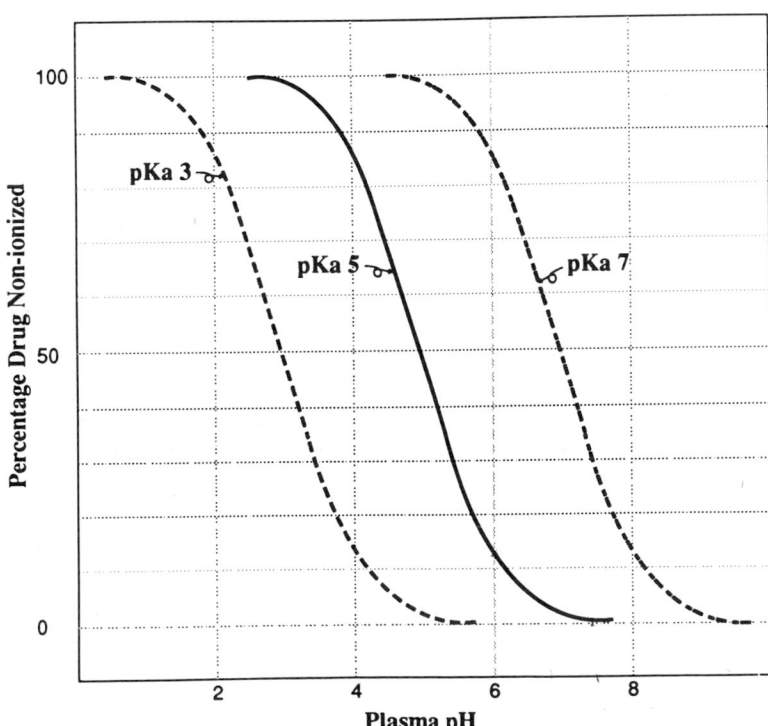

Fig. 2-2. Graphic display of the relationship between drug pK_a, the pH of solution, and the percentage of drug nonionized as determined by the Henderson-Hasselbach equation. Drugs with a pK_a nearest physiologic pH will show the greatest changes in percent ionization. At pH 7.4, drugs with a high pK_a will be essentially ionized and those with low pK_a nearly 100 percent nonionized (see text).

Local anesthetics are weak bases. When injected perineurally, the unionized form will cross the lipid neural membrane. To increase the fraction of local anesthetic present in the unionized form, sodium bicarbonate has been added to local anesthetic solutions prior to their injection. The addition of bicarbonate increases the pH above the pK_a of the local anesthetic, favoring the unionized form, which crosses the membrane more readily. This is the basis for the formulation of carbonated lidocaine. Once local anesthetic reaches the cytoplasm where a lower pH is present (below the pK_a of the local anesthetic), the ionized form of the drug is favored (also see Ch. 13).

Route of Administration

General

Drugs may be administered by many routes. The most common routes in anesthesia are enteral (oral), inhaled, intravenous, and intrathecal. However, clinical situations may exist in which other forms of administration of drugs must be considered. The rate of absorption of a drug is frequently related to its route of administration; hence, various routes of drug administration are discussed below.

Oral Administration

Oral administration of drugs is the most commonly used route in general therapeutics. The oral route is convenient, economic, and usually safe but requires a cooperative patient. Some of the orally administered drugs are absorbed from the stomach, but most are absorbed from the upper part of the small intestine. Drugs with pK_a values in the appropriate range for either the stomach or the small intestine will be readily absorbed. The simple premise that the stomach absorbs weakly acidic drugs is modified by the transit time through the stomach and the morphology of the organ (surface area). The absorbed drug is carried to the liver by the portal venous system, where a considerable fraction may be completely removed or altered by hepatic metabolism. Only a small fraction of the absorbed drug may escape the important influence of the liver to be distributed to the systemic circulation. This phenomenon has been termed the *first-pass effect of the liver*. Depending on the magnitude of this effect, oral dosage may have to be many times larger than the intravenous dosage to produce the same systemic concentrations of drugs and the same pharmacologic effects. In addition to the first-pass effect, orally administered drugs must first be dissolved before they can be absorbed. Drugs administered in aqueous solution are more rapidly absorbed than those administered in oily solution, suspension, or solid form. Many influences affect the rate of dissolution, including solubility, particle size, crystalline form and salt form of the drug, rate of disintegration of the solid dosage form into the gastrointestinal (GI) lumen, and the GI pH, mobility, and food content.

Sublingual Administration

A higher blood concentration of a drug may be achieved by permitting the drug to be absorbed in the mouth rather than swallowed and absorbed from a lower part of the GI tract. The first-pass effect of the liver can be minimized, and the drug is not subject to destruction by GI secretions.

Clinical example of sublingual administration. Nitroglycerin tablets are frequently given sublingually. Since they are readily absorbed via this route, nitroglycerin tablets do not need to be administered until chest pain is felt by the patient. The effect of pain relief may be achieved within minutes.

Rectal Administration

The rate of absorption from the rectum is rapid; this route may be useful in circumstances in which oral administration is precluded by vomiting. The first-pass effect of the liver is minimized by this route of administration.

Clinical example of rectal administration. In anesthesia, the most common rectally administered drug is methohexital (Brevital). In the absence of an intravenous catheter, this drug is frequently administered rectally to pediatric patients to achieve sedation prior to initiating general anesthesia (also see Ch. 59).

Subcutaneous Injection

The advantage of a subcutaneously administered drug is a relatively even and slow absorption, providing a relatively sustained effect. The rate of absorption may be further manipulated by altering the drug form, as is done with insulin. Also, the rate of absorption may be decreased by combining the drug with epinephrine, which reduces local blood flow, a procedure used commonly with infiltration of local anesthetics.

Intramuscular Injection

Slow absorption from an intramuscular injection site occurs when drugs are in solution in oil or in various suspensions. Aqueous solutions of drugs are rapidly and evenly absorbed.

Intrathecal Administration

When local and rapid effects on the central nervous system are desired, the limiting effects on rate and extent of drug absorption through the blood-brain barrier can be circumvented by intrathecal administration. However, access for this route requires considerably more skill and expertise than is needed for the oral, sublingual, rectal, subcutaneous, intramuscular, and intravenous routes.

Pulmonary Administration

Because of the large surface area of the alveoli, gases and volatile anesthetics that are inhaled are rapidly absorbed into the circulation (also see Ch. 4). Also, aerosols of sympathomimetic and other drugs are frequently used to relieve bronchospasm. In addition to pulmonary parenchyma, the pleura is capable of absorbing large quantities of pharmacologic agents.

Skin

Local effects can be achieved by application of ointments, creams, lotions, liniments, and pastes. Recently, controlled, sustained release of certain narcotic drugs from patches applied to the skin has been of interest to anesthesiologists involved in analgesia in ambulatory patients. Percutaneous absorption of ionized drugs can be enhanced by applying a drug solution to an electrode placed on the skin; a current is applied between the drug electrode and a neutral electrode. This is known as iontophoresis.

Perineural

Local anesthetics are injected in the space surrounding nerves. Regional anesthesia (also see Ch. 46), epidural anesthesia and spinal anesthesia (also see Ch. 45), all produce local effects on nerves. The rate of absorption of anesthetic locally determines the rate of onset of action. More details of the mechanism of action of local anesthetics may be found in Chapter 13.

Intravenous Injection

The main advantage of intravenous administration of drugs is the circumvention of the absorption process. Thus, the desired blood concentration is rapidly attained in a relatively accurate manner. This is also the ideal route for drugs that have to be given in large volumes or that are too irritant for intramuscular or subcutaneous injection. Nevertheless, there are dangers to intravenous administration of drugs. Once a drug is injected, it is irretrievable, and in the event of overdose or idiosyncratic reactions, the effects are immediate and often severe. Intravenous injection is the most common route of drug and fluid administration during anesthesia.

Drug Transport across Membranes

Once a route of administration for a drug has been chosen, all drugs must cross biologic membranes to reach their intended site of action. Biologic membranes consist of a central lipid bilayer core and a superficial covering consisting of proteins. Because of this combination of polar and nonpolar components in membrane structure, any drug must possess both lipid and water solubility to dissolve in, and thereby traverse, these cell boundaries. In addition to passive membrane transport, there are specialized mechanisms that enable a variety of substances to cross membranes and that are described below.

Aqueous Diffusion

The passive process of aqueous diffusion may also be described as filtration because it involves bulk flow of water that occurs as a result of hydrostatic or osmotic differences across the membrane. The rate of diffusion depends on such variables as drug concentration gradient, drug molecular weight, diffusion distance, diffusion surface area, and temperature. This process enables lipid-insoluble substances to pass through membrane pores. However, most drugs have a molecular size too large for passage through the pores. Pores in most cell membranes are not larger than 4 Å, permitting only small water-soluble molecules to pass. In general, molecules with molecular weights greater than 100 to 200 will not pass. A notable exception is the passage of large molecules such as albumin through the 40-A pores of capillary membranes.

Carrier-Mediated Active Transport

Carrier-mediated active transport is responsible for the rapid transfer of many organic substances such as amino acids and sugar across membranes. Characteristic features of this mode of transport are saturability, selectivity, and the requirement of energy. Substances may be mobilized by this means against an electrochemical or concentration gradient. Another form of carrier-mediated transport is facilitated diffusion, which does not require energy coupling but also does not transport compounds against a concentration gradient. This form of transport is, however, also saturable and selective.

Pinocytosis

Drugs of high molecular weight may be transported by pinocytosis, a process in which the molecule is enveloped in a small vesicle and as such crosses the membrane. This is characteristic of endothelial cells of the capillary wall. Proteins and glycoproteins may pass through cell membranes by this mechanism.

Bioavailability of Drugs

Bioavailability describes the rate and relative amount of an administered drug that reaches the systemic circulation. The formulation and route by which a drug is administered will affect its bioavailability. As previously mentioned, physical differences in crystal form, particle size, rates of disintegration of dosage form, and solubility of the drug will influence the rate and extent of absorption. Also, the influence of the liver on orally administered drugs affects systemic bioavailability. When a drug is administered intravenously, it is considered completely available systemically, so that bioavailability is one, or 100 percent. If it is injected in the form of an inactive pro-drug, for example, an ester that must be hydrolyzed to yield active product, then it may or may not be completely available systemically, depending on the completeness of the hydrolysis. The systemic availability and bioavailability are reflected by the area under the curves derived from plots of blood drug concentration versus time curves (Fig. 2-3). Bioequivalency is a comparative measure of bioavailability among different formulations of the same drug.

Protein Binding of Drugs

Since only the free, unbound portion of a chemical is usually pharmacologically active, binding of drugs to sites other than active sites, such as those found in plasma and tissue, may be of considerable importance. As far as absorption is concerned, binding of a drug may facilitate absorption by reducing the concentration in the aqueous phase of plasma. Binding is generally a reversible process, arriving at an equilibrium according to the law of mass action (total drug = bound drug + unbound drug). The unbound fraction is available for pharmacologic action and metabolism, while the bound fraction functions as a depot from which drug is made available as the equilibrium is reestablished after removal of free drug. The degree of drug binding is the ratio of bound drug to the total concentration of drug in the plasma. Drug binding depends on total drug concentration, plasma protein concentration, affinity of protein(s) for the drug, concomitant drug concentrations, plasma pH, and other pathophysiologic conditions that may alter these factors. (Protein binding is explained in greater detail below; see the section, *Drug Distribution*.)

Blood Flow — Relationship to Drug Disposition

The flow of blood to a tissue is important in the delivery of systemic drug to that site as well as the clearance of drugs from that tissue.

Drug Distribution

Once a drug has reached the systemic circulation (plasma), following absorption or directly by intravenous injection, it will be distributed throughout the body. Distribution refers to the reversible transfer of drug from one location to another and involves movement across lipid membranes and capillary walls as well as between active and inactive binding sites in different tissues of the body. The initial distribution is determined by the physicochemical characteristics of the drug, as well as cardiac output and regional blood flow to various organs. Lipid-soluble drugs are rapidly distributed to heart, brain, kidney, liver, and other extensively perfused organs. Less rapid distribution into muscle and still slower distribution into fat then occur

because these organs receive a smaller fraction of the cardiac output.

Drugs may achieve a higher concentration in peripheral tissues than in blood because of tissue binding and dissolution in fat. Protein binding profoundly affects drug distribution. Of the plasma proteins, albumin is quantitatively the most important; it has a high capacity for binding weakly acidic drugs. Another plasma protein, α-acidglycoprotein, binds weak bases. Both are of low specificity. The bound fraction of a drug, unavailable for specific pharmacologic action or metabolism, acts as a depot from which drug is regenerated as the equilibrium is reestablished after removal of free drug. The characteristics of this equilibrium and the rate at which the free fraction of drug is removed by metabolism and excretion determine the biologic half-life of a drug. Because albumin and the other plasma proteins possess a limited number of binding sites, drugs with similar affinities for albumin compete with one another for these sites, resulting in redistribution of a drug between plasma and tissue. A drug that displaces another albumin-bound drug from its binding sites forces the latter drug to diffuse into tissues, thereby causing the measured plasma concentration to decline. Although tissue binding of drugs is relatively difficult to measure, it is well known that some drugs have a greater affinity for certain tissues, and this can influence their onset and duration of action.

The uptake and distribution of inhaled anesthetics are discussed in detail in Chapter 4, and more detailed discussion of distribution as a determinant of pharmacologic activity is presented in succeeding specific chapters.

Clinical example of drug redistribution. Thiopental has a high lipid/water partition coefficient, hence it has a tendency to accumulate in fat, although this happens slowly because of generally limited blood flow to fat tissue. Thiopental, therefore, provides a good example of distribution and redistribution of a drug after intravenous administration. Initially, thiopental crosses lipid membranes rapidly and soon is almost undetectable in the plasma pool. High concentrations are reached in the organs of the vessel-rich group (brain, heart, liver, kidney). As the concentration gradient across the cell membranes reverses, thiopental leaves these organs just as quickly for redistribution to the intermediate vessel group (muscle) and finally into fat.

Drug Metabolism

Since many drugs are lipophilic substances that are not easily excreted in the aqueous urine, their removal from the body must be preceded by chemical changes to render them hydrophilic. This process usually leads to inactivation of the drug. Thus, lipophilic substances are modified by phase I *(functionalization)* processes (i.e., oxidation, reduction, or hydrolysis), rendering them more polar. Functional groups that decrease lipophilicity and allow hydrogen bonding to water include

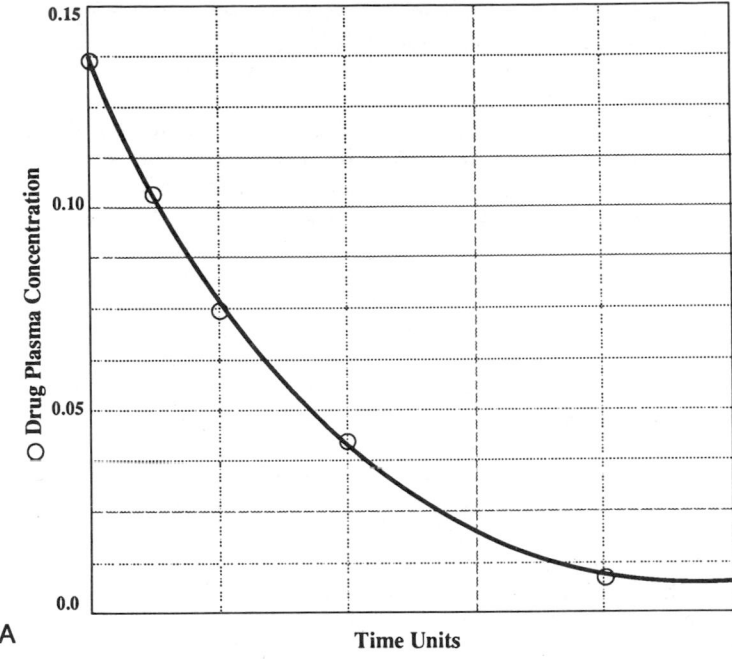

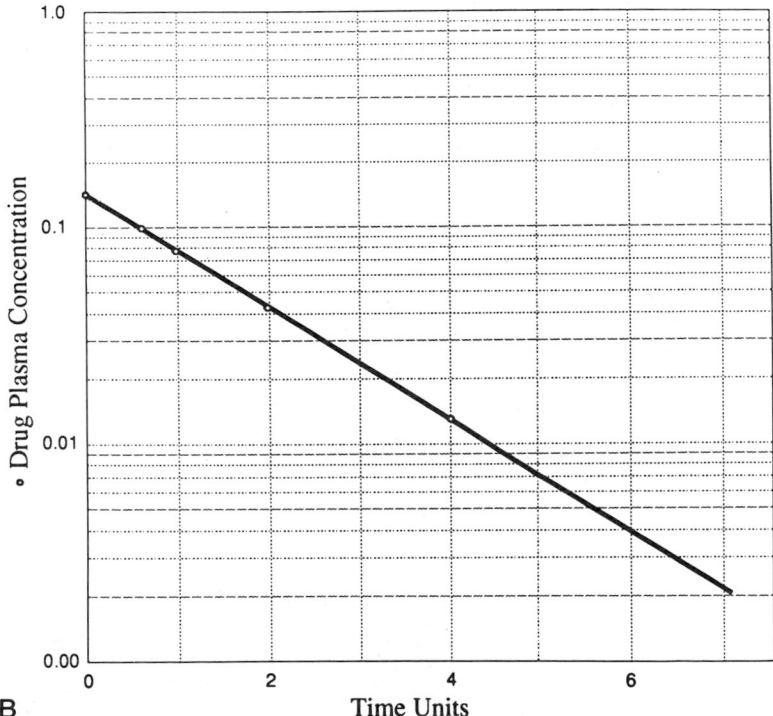

Fig. 2-3. (A) Computer simulation of a drug displaying one-compartment kinetics. The curve generated displays the expected plasma drug concentration on a linear concentration scale versus time. Ten units of drug were injected intravenously at time 0, and computer input variables were chosen to display an elimination half-life of 1 hour. **(B)** Computer simulation of the same one-compartment kinetics of the drug concentration versus time plot shown in Fig. A. In this graph, however, the plasma drug concentration is plotted on a logarithmic scale, thereby producing a straight line because of the single exponential decline of drug level over time.

—OH, —O—, —CHO, —COOH, —COOR, and others. These polar metabolites and other polar compounds are conjugated by phase II *(conjugation)* processes, rendering them hydrophilic. These hydrophilic substances may subsequently be excreted in the urine. Many of the more polar compounds, such as moderately strong bases or acids, may be excreted unchanged. We briefly review the most important metabolic processes.

Phase I (Functionalization) Reactions

Phase I metabolism consists of three types of chemical reactions: oxidation, reduction, and hydrolysis. This process is outlined with examples in Table 2-1.

Many of the oxidation-reduction reactions involving drugs administered to humans are catalyzed by the cytochrome P-450 systems located predominantly but certainly not exclusively in hepatic smooth endoplasmic reticulum. Enzymes located in this cell fraction are termed microsomal and are frequently subject to stimulation (induction) by exposure to a variety of drugs or environmental compounds. Microsomal drug-metabolizing activity may also be reduced in humans by other drugs that compete for microsomal enzyme activity or by direct inhibitors, such as the H_2-blocking drug cimetidine. Further numerous additional factors may modify the microsomal enzyme system such as age, hormones, nutrition, disease states, and multiple genetic factors.

Phase II (Conjugation) Reactions

Phase II metabolism consists of combining polar unchanged or metabolized compounds with a number of small endogenous substances. These reactions are called conjugations. Cofactors are usually involved, and energy is required. In humans, the most important conjugation is that with glucuronic acid, but conjugation also occurs with sulfate, acetate, amino acids, and many other endogenous groups. These transfers may be catalyzed by either microsomal or nonmicrosomal enzymes. Phase II metabolic reactions and therapeutics examples are presented in Table 2-2.

TABLE 2-1. Routes of Drug Biotransformation: Phase I (Functionalization) Reactions

Oxidations	Examples
Aliphatic hydroxylation	Thiopental, methohexital, pentobarbital, meperidine, ketamine
Aromatic hydroxylation	Lidocaine, bupivacaine, mepivacaine, phenobarbital, fentanyl, propranolol
Epoxidation (aromatic and alkane)	Phenytoin
O-Dealkylation	Pancuronium, codeine, phenacetin
N-Dealkylation	Ephedrine, isoproterenol Lidocaine, mepivacaine, bupivacaine, etidocaine, meperidine, ketamine, fentanyl, morphine, codeine, atropine, diazepam (ring amide)
S-Dealkylation	Methitural
N-Oxidation	Normeperidine Tetracycline, morphine, meperidine
S-Oxidation	Chlorpromazine
Oxidative deamination	Amphetamine, epinephrine
Desulfuration	Thiopental
Dehalogenation	Halothane, methoxyflurane, enflurane
Dehydrogenation	Ethanol
Reductions	**Examples**
Azoreduction	Fazadinium
Nitroreduction	Nitrazepam, dantrolene
Carbonyl reduction	Prednisone, warfarin
Alcohol dehydrogenase	Chloral hydrate
Hydrolysis	**Examples**
Ester hydrolysis (deesterification)	Procaine, chlorprocaine, tetracaine, cocaine, succinylcholine, propanidid, meperidine, pancuronium
Amide hydrolysis (deamidation)	Lidocaine, etidocaine, fentanyl, prilocaine

TABLE 2-2. Routes of Drug Biotransformation: Phase II (Conjugation, Synthetic) Reactions

Conjugation	Examples
O-Glucuronidation	Oxazepam, lorazepam, morphine, codeine, propranolol, nalorphine, naloxone, fentanyl
N-Glucuronidation	Sulfonamides
Sulfate conjugation	Morphine, fentanyl, lorazepam
Methylation	Morphine
Acetylation	Procainamide, sulfonamides, isoniazide
Conjugation with amino acids	Salicyclic acid
Mercapturic acid formation	Sulfobromophthalein (BSP)

Drug Elimination

General

Elimination is a general term signifying all processes that terminate the presence of a drug in the body. In addition to metabolism, major processes include renal excretion, hepatobiliary excretion, and, especially in anesthesia, pulmonary excretion. Minor routes of elimination are saliva, sweat, breast milk, and tears.

Renal Excretion

A major route of excretion of most chemicals, both metabolically changed or unchanged, occurs through the kidney. All substances of low molecular weight are filtered from the blood through the membrane of Bowman's capsule. The ultrafiltrate in the lumen of the proximal convoluted tubule contains both lipophilic and hydrophilic molecules. The hydrophilic molecules remain within the tubular lumen, while the lipophilic molecules are reabsorbed into the blood perfusing the tubule. Some substances are actively secreted from the blood into the proximal tubule by energy-consuming carrier-dependent processes.

As the renal tubular contents become more concentrated, unionized drug molecules are reabsorbed by diffusion across the tubular epithelium. Thus, in reabsorption, the passage of the lipophilic molecules back across the tubular membrane depends, as everywhere else, on lipid solubility, degree of ionization, and molecular shape and, in some cases, on special carrier mechanisms. Thus, weak acids are reabsorbed best from an acidic urine. As the urine pH varies, renal tubular reabsorption may be manipulated. In a patient who has had an overdose of acetylsalicylic acid, alkalinization of the urine will reduce renal tubular reabsorption and thus will enhance excretion of the drug, especially in combination with forced diuresis.

Hepatobiliary Excretion

Many metabolites of drugs formed in the liver are excreted into the intestinal tract with the bile. Some of these metabolites may be excreted in the feces, but most commonly they are reabsorbed into the blood and are ultimately excreted with the urine. This is called the enterohepatic cycle. A wide variety of organic cations and anions are actively transported into bile by carrier systems. At least three such systems for the transport of poorly lipid-soluble organic compounds have been identified. In these processes, the compounds are transported against a large concentration gradient from the plasma into the bile. Of note, some muscle relaxants are partially excreted via the hepatobiliary system (also see Ch. 12).

Pulmonary Excretion

Volatile anesthetics and anesthetic gases are in large part eliminated unchanged from the body through the lung. In this elimination process, the factors that determine uptake operate in a reverse manner. Alveolar partial pressure will depend on the amount of drug released into the alveoli by the blood, where insoluble agents will be readily released from blood and removed by alveolar ventilation.

Time Course of Drug Effects

General

Absorption, distribution, metabolism, and elimination all influence the onset and duration of action of drugs. These effects may be described by general mathematic principles. To derive mathematic models of pharmacokinetics, it is necessary to monitor drug concentrations over time (time zero being the point of drug administration). Although monitoring drug concentrations is helpful clinically in achieving therapeutic levels and preventing toxic levels (e.g., antiepileptic agents, antiarrhythmics, antibiotics, bronchodilators), it is also important in deriving pharmacokinetic parameters for a specific drug. In monitoring drug levels, the sensitivity and specificity of the drug assay and information about whether bound or free drug has been measured should be known. Serial measurements are always more useful than single measurements. For drugs that produce a clinical effect, plasma drug concentration measurements may be unnecessary because the drug dose can be titrated against the desired clinical response. However, if pharmacokinetic parameters are to be derived, the exact drug concentration over time is required. The most common mathematic models used to describe the relationship between plasma drug levels and clinical effect are described below.

Principles of Compartment Models

When a drug is administered to a patient, by whatever chosen route, the onset and duration of its pharmacologic effect depend on multiple factors, as outlined in the previous sections. Included are those factors affecting drug absorption, distribution, and the process of elimination. The various organ systems represent many combinations of perfusion, drug-binding affinity, drug solubility, drug ionization, and rates of metabolism. In physiologic pharmacokinetic modeling, organ systems having similar drug solubility and blood perfusion characteristics are grouped together, and an attempt is made to conceptualize the process of absorption, distribution, and elimination of the drug from these organ systems. These complex models have required extensive computer resources and are difficult to extrapolate to the individual patient. More applicable mathematic models have been derived from the assumption of pharmacokinetic compartments within the body. With each drug it is possible to utilize accessible drug concentration information from blood or urine and other tissues and to define relationships among drug dose, plasma concentration of the drug, and time. The actual pharmacokinetic compartment as defined may have no specific biologic correlation with a defined organ system or group of systems. The changes in drug concentration that take place over time within the conceptual compartments can be used to derive such parameters as half-life, volume of distribution, distribution characteristics, and other characteristics of drug elimination.

One-Compartment Model

Some drugs behave as though they are distributed into a single uniform compartment in the body from which a constant proportion of the drug in the body is eliminated within a chosen time period (e.g., 1 hour). Figure 2-3A represents a computer simulation of the administration of a drug distributing into one compartment and eliminated by first-order kinetics. At time 0, an intravenous bolus of 10 units of the drug was administered, and plasma concentrations were determined repeatedly over a 6-hour period. Figure 2-3A compares the decline in plasma concentration on a linear y-axis scale over time on the x axis. Examination of the drug concentration versus time plot demonstrates that drug concentrations decrease in constant proportion. At time 0, there was a plasma concentration of 0.14 units. The elimination half-life $t_{\frac{1}{2}}$ represents the time taken for the drug concentration to decline to one-half its original value. In this example, it can be seen that at the end

of 1 hour the concentration was 0.07 units; therefore, one-half of the drug was eliminated. Again, between the first and second hour, one-half of the remaining drug was eliminated. The half-life is independent of the amount of drug in the body. Table 2-3 illustrates that five half-lives are required to eliminate 96.9 percent of the administered drug. Elimination half-lives are also useful in selecting drug dosing intervals, in predicting the time required to reach a steady state of drug concentration, and in calculating drug accumulation. This is explained in more detail in the next section (see the section, *Two-Compartment Model*).

Mathematically, it has been shown that the elimination half-life is:

$$t_{\frac{1}{2}} = \ln 2/k = 0.693/k$$

where $\ln 2 = 0.693$ and k represents the first-order rate constant. This elimination rate constant, k, is a proportionality constant that describes the fraction of drug present at any given time that will be eliminated in that time unit. Simple mathematical rearrangement shows $k = 0.693/t_{\frac{1}{2}}$, thus k will have units of reciprocal time, that is, h^{-1}. In Figure 2-3A, therefore, $t_{\frac{1}{2}} = 1$ hour and $k = 0.693\ h^{-1}$.

If the same plasma drug concentration-time graph is replotted on a logarithmic concentration scale versus time, a straight line results (Fig. 2-3B). The graphing technique displays the exponential decline as a straight line because of the logarithmic scale. The slope of this line is equal to $-k/2.303$.

Two-Compartment Model

For most anesthetic drugs, the plot of the decline in the plasma concentration versus time is similar to the computer simulation of Figure 2-4. Figure 2-4 illustrates the decline in the plasma drug concentration on the logarithmic y-axis scale versus time on the x axis. There appear to be two distinct phases to the decline in plasma concentrations. The first phase in decline represents drug distribution that occurs immediately after injection when a very rapid rate of decline in plasma concentration is noted. This conceptually represents movement of the drug from the plasma to tissues. The second phase, which begins immediately after injection but becomes obvious only after completion of the relatively rapid distribution phase, is the slower decline of

TABLE 2-3. Elimination Half-Life

No. of Drug Half-Lives	Original Drug Remaining (%)	Original Drug Eliminated (%)
0	100	0
1	50	50
2	25	75
3	12.5	87.5
4	6.25	93.75
5	3.13	96.87
6	1.56	98.44

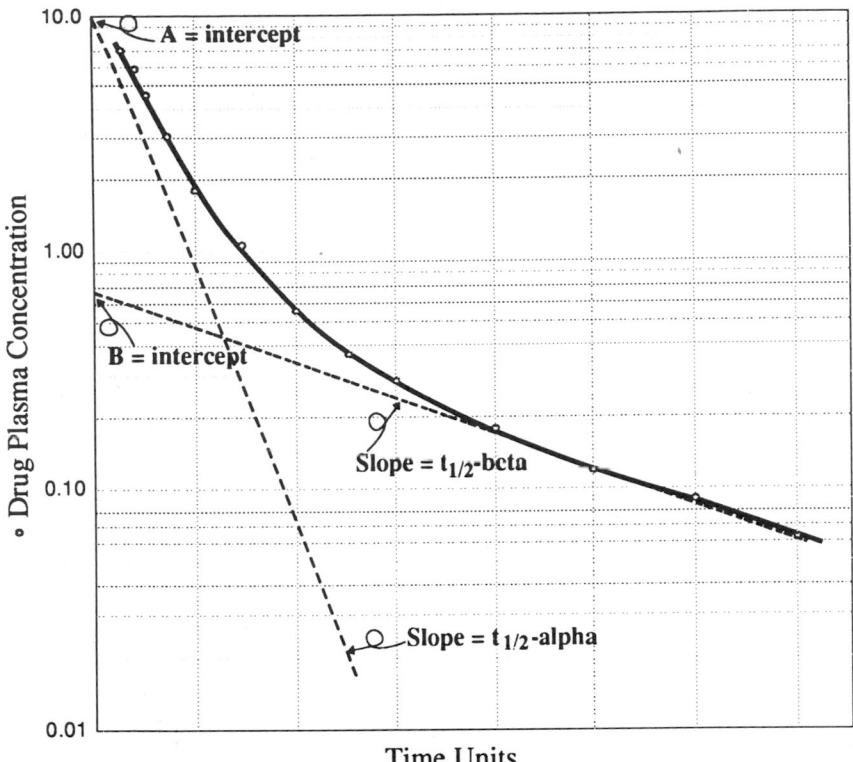

Fig. 2-4. Computer simulation of a drug with two-compartment kinetics. The curve displays the expected plasma drug concentrations on a logarithmic concentration scale versus time. Two distinct phases of drug plasma concentration changes are visually apparent: the initial rapid decline in drug level during the distribution phase and the slower decline in concentration during the elimination phase. The mathematic fit of the curve to the measured plasma drug levels is described in the text and is used to determine the various pharmacokinetic parameters for the drug.

plasma concentration resulting from drug elimination from plasma.

To explain this biphasic behavior, the body is divided conceptually into two compartments: a central compartment of small volume and a peripheral compartment of larger volume. As stated previously, these defined compartments represent pharmacokinetic compartments (black boxes), not specific organ systems or tissues. Conceptually, the central compartment generally represents the blood or plasma and the highly perfused tissues such as the heart, lungs, kidney, and liver. The peripheral compartment would represent drug present in other tissues.

For drugs with two-compartment pharmacokinetics, it is apparent from Figure 2-4 that the decline in drug level is a summation of two exponentially declining phases or parameters. These are again the generally shorter distribution phase and the longer elimination phase.

This two-compartment pharmacokinetic model can be defined mathematically by the formula:

$$Cp = Ae^{-\alpha t} + Be^{-\beta t}$$

where Cp = drug concentration in plasma at time t;

α = rate constant of the distribution phase; β = rate constant of the elimination phase; A = intercept at time 0 of the distribution phase line; B = intercept at time 0 of the elimination phase line; and t = time. Thus, the two-compartment model mathematically represents a biexponential equation in which the first exponential term ($Ae^{-\alpha t}$) summarizes the distribution phase and the second exponential term ($Be^{-\beta t}$) summarizes the elimination phase. The rate constants α and β can be determined from the slope of the graphs and are used to calculate the distribution and elimination half-lives.

Other Models

Some plasma drug concentration decay curves require three or more exponential terms to characterize the drugs decline from the plasma. A three-compartment model would therefore have three exponential terms and assume one central compartment and two conceptual peripheral compartments. Other techniques of pharmacokinetic analysis beyond the scope of this limited review include blood flow models, rate-limited models, membrane-limited models, nonlinear pharmacokinetic models, and noncompartmental analysis employing statistical moment theory. In practice, a basic understanding of first-order kinetics and one- and two-compartment models is often sufficient.

Derived Parameters

Further study of the one- and two-compartment pharmacokinetic models of drug concentration versus time plots demonstrates other valuable clinical pharmacology. These areas are covered briefly in the next four sections.

Absorption

Absorption has been previously described as the process by which a drug proceeds from the site of administration to a site of measurement, that is, the plasma or serum. For drugs administered by intravenous bolus, the concentration-time plots show an instantaneous peak. For drugs administered at a slower rate, the peak and time course of the distribution phase will be shifted to the right. Since various routes of drug administration have been described, we now explore the relationship between rate of administration and drug concentration-time plots.

Alteration of the rate of administration of a drug may produce dramatic changes in the drug concentration-time plots. Figure 2-5 represents a comparison of 10 mg of morphine administered intravenously in a two-compartment model either as a moderately rapid intravenous bolus (30 minutes) or by continuous infusion at rates requiring 4 hours. If it is accepted that the drug's primary or side effects depend on attaining a certain concentration at a site of action, then the differences in intensity of response produced by the different rates of administration are clear. It is especially important to note that the plasma concentrations are plotted on a logarithmic scale. If a specific plasma concentration is required for an effect, the more rapid intravenous injection would have yielded significantly higher plasma concentrations than the constant infusion method.

Figure 2-6 illustrates the differences in attained plasma drug levels of fentanyl when administered at the same total dose (10 μg/kg in a 70-kg patient) but by three different dosing methods. The single 700-μg bolus at time 0 produces significantly higher concentrations initially. The administration of smaller repetitive doses of fentanyl, although eventually supplying the same amount of drug, will produce markedly different drug levels over time. These simulations, based on actual

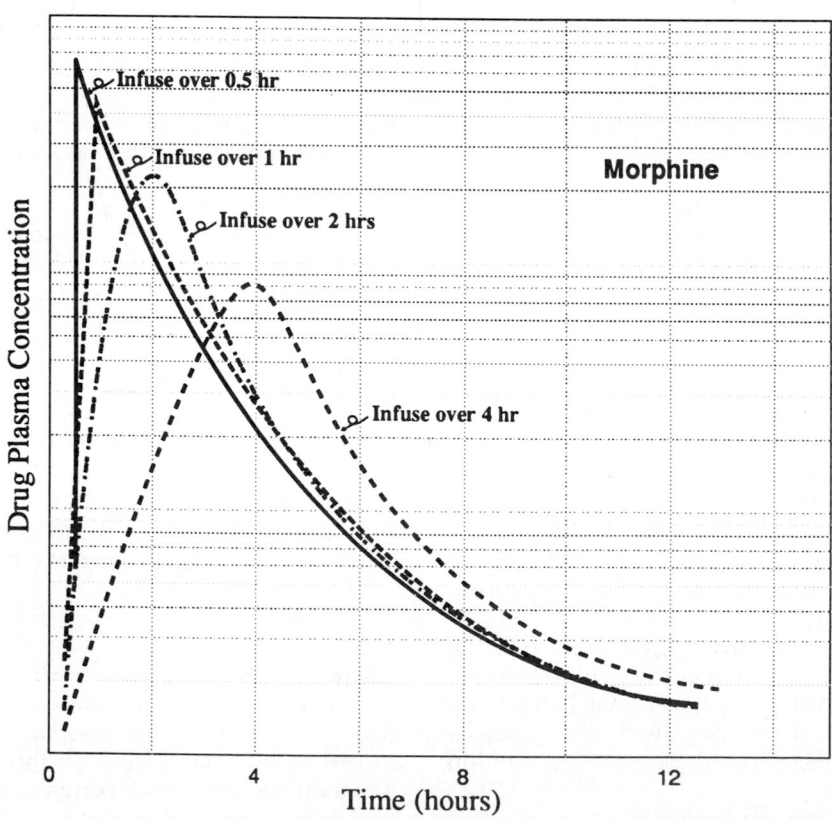

Fig. 2-5. Computer simulation of the differences between administration of 10 mg of morphine as a slow intravenous bolus (0.5-hour infusion) or as a slow intravenous infusion over variable time periods up to 4 hours. Modeling is performed with a predicted two-compartment fit displayed on a logarithmic scale against time (hours), and the total dose for all curves is 10 mg in a 70-kg patient.

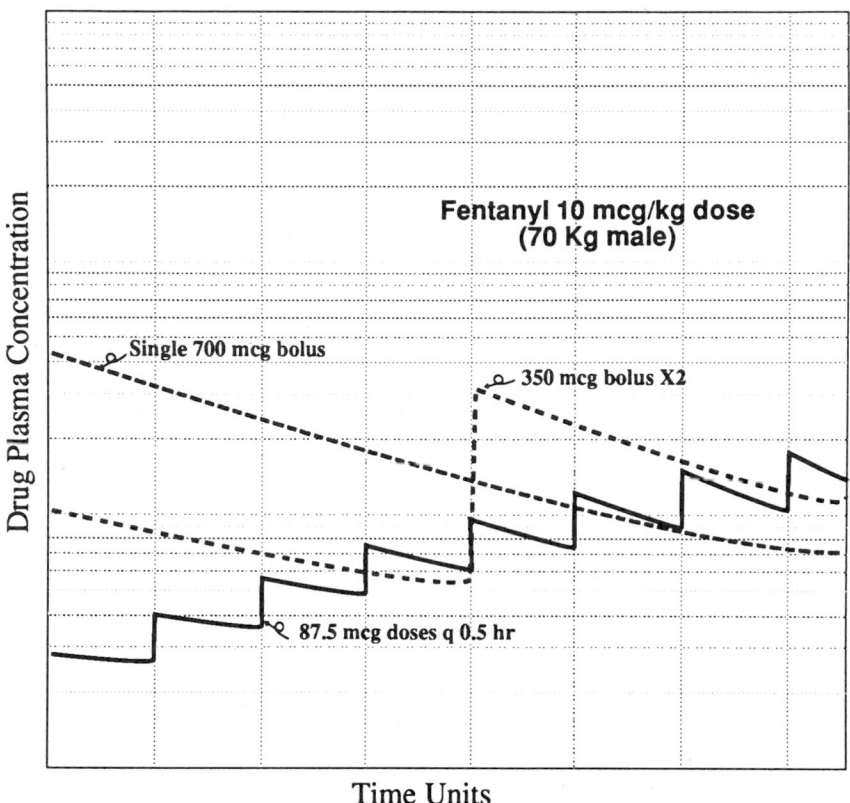

Fig. 2-6. Computer simulation of an anesthetic performed with the same total dose of fentanyl (10 μg/kg) administered by three different intravenous techniques. The y axis measures the predicted plasma drug level over time with the drug administered either as a single bolus at time 0 or in two or more doses. Note the significant differences in predicted plasma drug level by the three different administration techniques.

measured drug levels in blood, emphasize the principle of a combination of an initial bolus dose and continuous infusion or repetitive smaller boluses in maintaining therapeutic drug levels.

Figure 2-7 illustrates the combined bolus-constant infusion technique. In this simulation, the patient has received an initial bolus of alfentanil at 50 μg/kg. A continuous infusion is then begun at one of three infusion rates ranging from 1 to 3 μg/kg/min. If the drug is administered at a rate comparable to the rate of elimination, the amount of drug accumulation is minimal. However, if the drug is infused at a rate exceeding elimination, significant drug accumulation within the plasma will occur. As the science of anesthesiology progresses and the computer-assisted drug infusion systems develop, the clinician will be able to more closely titrate the rate of drug infusion to maintain the desired plasma level for an effect. A more in-depth discussion of continuous intravenous infusions is presented in Chapter 11.

The application of these principles, combined with the practical application of pharmacodynamics, is illustrated in Figure 2-8. The left axis (open circles) depicts the measured plasma drug level of vecuronium, and the right axis (hatched area) shows the twitch height of a train-of-four stimulus. The patient has been administered a bolus loading dose of 100 μg/kg followed by a continuous infusion of 100 μg/kg/h of vecuronium. The nondepolarizing effects of the relaxant administered by this technique continue until after termination of the infusion and elimination of the drug by metabolism and excretion.

As cautioned in the previous section, which outlined the factors affecting absorption, any disease process that alters protein binding, ionization, pH, tissue perfusion, blood volume, or other such factors will alter drug absorption, bioavailability, and pharmacokinetic profile. This requires the clinician continually to adjust the dose and rate of drug infusion based on individual patient responses and not on the group kinetics used for such simulations.

Distribution

Distribution is a dynamic process since it represents the process of reversible transfer of drug from one compartment to another compartment within the body. Important in this process is the concept of volume of distribution. The relationship between a measured plasma concentration and a known administered dosage de-

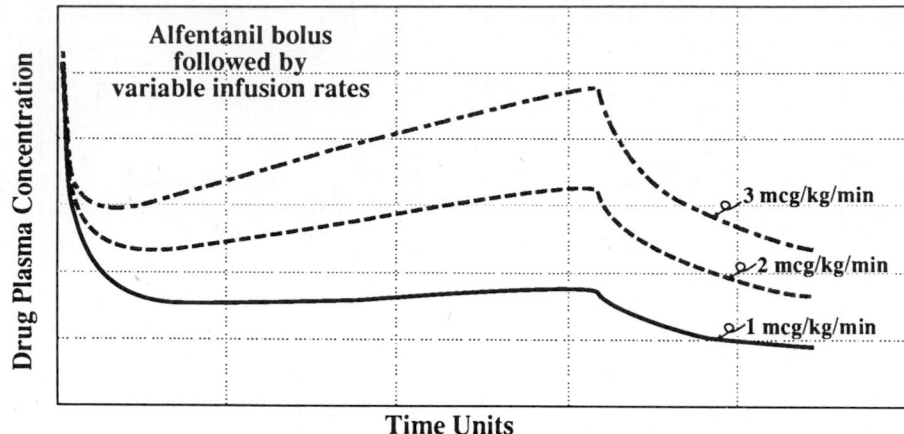

Fig. 2-7. Computer simulation of the differences between administration of alfentanil as an initial 50 μg/kg bolus loading dose followed by three different continuous intravenous infusion rates over time. The simulated higher infusion rate (3 μg/kg/min) results in potential drug accumulation.

fines an apparent volume of distribution, V_d. The apparent volume of distribution is the proportionality constant that relates the amount of drug in the body to the concentration in a reference compartment, usually the central compartment. Thus, V_d = total dose/plasma drug concentration. Again, no physiologic or anatomic significance may often be given to V_d. V_d may be as small as a plasma volume or as large as 10,000 times the plasma volume. A large volume of distribution suggests extensive tissue distribution and uptake. There are published tables of apparent volumes of distribution for most drugs. If the plasma concentration of a drug can be measured and the volume of distribution is established, it is simple to calculate the total amount of drug remaining in the body. If a given drug has a large volume of distribution, it may require a larger loading dose to achieve a given plasma level than if a similarly active drug has a smaller volume of distribution. Although the concept of an apparent volume of distribution has no

specific relationship to organ anatomy, many disease processes can significantly alter the volume of distribution. These alterations may occur in such states as renal failure, hepatic dysfunction, extremes of age, congestive heart failure, shock, and burns. Initiation or termination of cardiopulmonary bypass will also have significant effects on the volume of distribution and therefore on the circulating drug levels. Information about the volume of distribution may be useful in calculating a loading dose and in estimating changes in loading doses when predicted alterations in this volume are known to occur owing to disease processes.

Elimination

In pharmacokinetic terminology, elimination refers to the irreversible loss of drug from the site where the drug is measured. In mathematic terminology, elimination may represent the combination of the processes of

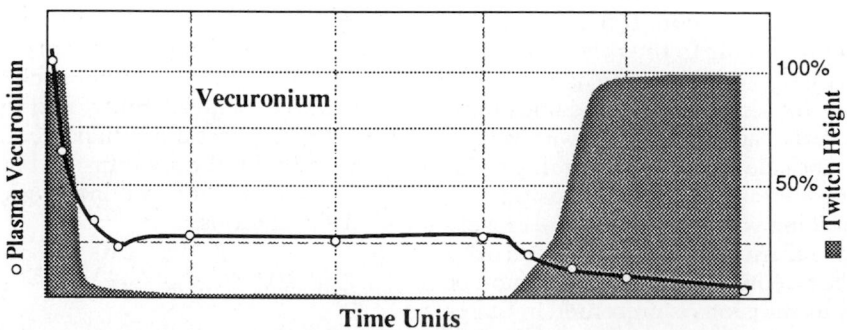

Fig. 2-8. Graphic representation of the relationship between the pharmacokinetic and pharmacodynamic effects of vecuronium in a patient. The vecuronium is administered as a 100 μg/kg bolus followed later by a continuous intravenous infusion at 100 μg/kg/h. The plasma drug levels are shown by the open circles. The train-of-four muscle twitch heights are shown by the hatched areas and demonstrate the measured clinical effects of this intravenous administration technique.

metabolism and excretion. The major sites of elimination, as previously described, are the kidney, liver, and lung. Important concepts in understanding the time course of elimination include elimination rate constants, elimination time constants, and clearance. These are described below.

Elimination Rate Constants. The derivation of the elimination rate constant k, as in the example of the one-compartment model, represents the fraction of drug that will be eliminated in that time unit. For example, if k = 0.05 minute, the plasma concentration will decrease by 5 percent each minute.

Elimination Time Constants. The pharmacokinetic parameters of some drugs, especially inhalational agents, are often expressed in time constants: $T_{1/e}$. The time constant estimates the time necessary for the concentration of the agent to change by a factor of $1/e$ and represents a 63 percent change per unit time. The relationship between the time constant and the elimination rate constant is $T_{1/e} = 1/k$. The time constant can be related to the drug's half-life by the equation: $t_{\frac{1}{2}} = 0.693\ T_{1/e}$.

Clearance. Total clearance represents that part of the volume of distribution that is cleared of the drug per unit of time. Total clearance is a summation of clearance by the various routes of elimination. Clearance is thus related to the volume of distribution and the rate of elimination from the total volume. Therefore, the units of clearance are volume per time, that is, milliliters per minute or, if corrected for weight, milliliters per minute per kilogram. This is expressed mathematically as follows:

$$\text{Clearance (Cl)} = V_d \times k$$

Conceptually, one may imagine a small box within a large box, where the small box is totally cleared of the drug in the unit time and instantaneously the remainder of the drug will redistribute into the volume of the large box. The small box will then be cleared again in unit time.

Renal. The practical significance of determining renal clearance (Cl_R) is to determine that fraction of the dose of the drug that is eliminated through renal mechanisms. This parameter is extremely useful in dosage adjustments in renal failure.

Hepatic. Hepatic clearance (Cl_H) represents the fraction of administered drug that is eliminated by the liver. Clearance by any organ depends on blood flow through the organ and the amount of drug that is removed with passage through the organ. Specific organ clearance values can therefore not exceed blood flow. Certain drugs such as propranolol and lidocaine have very high hepatic clearance rates. This results in high presystemic first-pass effect (elimination) if the drug is administered orally. As previously discussed, this occurs because the drug absorbed from the GI tract must first pass through the liver via the portal vein.

Total Body. Total body clearance (Cl) is the sum of the clearance rates by renal, hepatic, and other routes of elimination. The numeric value of total clearance and the two major components, Cl_H and Cl_R, may provide important insight into the elimination processes. As stated, this may be important in anticipating necessary adjustments in dosage regimens with different disease states. A drug with a large Cl_R value relative to the total clearance in the presence of renal failure will require a greater decrease in dose in the presence of renal failure than is necessary for the dose of a drug that has a larger Cl_H value. Large values of Cl and Cl_H often suggest significant elimination by the liver; such a drug may therefore have a greater systemic effect in patients with liver disease than in normal patients.

PHARMACODYNAMICS

Introduction

Pharmacodynamics describes the relationship between plasma drug concentration and pharmacologic effect. Simply stated, pharmacodynamics attempts to explain what effect a drug has in the body. Although the study of clinically important drug effects is multifaceted, pharmacodynamics may be divided into three general areas. These areas include transduction of biologic signals, clinical evaluation of drug effects, and biologic variability. Each of these aspects of pharmacodynamics is explored in greater detail in the sections which follow.

Transduction of Biologic Signals

General

Many clinically important drugs act on excitable cell membrane proteins such as receptors, ion channels, and ion pumps to initiate their clinical effect. Stimulation of excitable cell membranes results in activation or inhibition of chemical cascades that leads swiftly to clinical effects. This section explores the mechanisms by which excitable cell membranes couple to clinical effects. Receptors, ion channels, and ion pumps are defined and concepts such as receptor structure, classic receptor theory, second messengers, and new developments in molecular pharmacology are examined.

Characteristics of Excitable Cell Membranes

Receptors

Definition. In the broadest sense, a receptor is a component of a cell that interacts selectively with an extracellular compound to initiate a biochemical change or a cascade of biochemical alterations that represent the observed effects of the compound. Receptors function to determine (1) the quantitative relationship between a given dose of a drug and the produced effect, (2) the selectivity of a given drug's activity and effect, and (3) an explanation for the pharmacologic activity of receptor agonists and receptor antagonists. The receptor therefore serves to mediate or amplify the effect of the drug on the biologic system.

Historical Perspective. Although the concept of receptors is generally attributed to Paul Erhlich (1854–1915), earlier work done by Claude Bernard (1813–1878) paved the way for receptor theory. This earlier work is of particular interest to anesthesiologists because it centered on elucidation of the mechanism of action of curare, an arrow poison. In his experiments, Bernard ligated vessels leading to one hindlimb of a frog while leaving nerve input intact; then he administered curare. Pinching the paralyzed hindlimb produced reflex movements in the opposite, unparalyzed, vessel-ligated hindlimb. In this manner, Bernard showed that curare selectively paralyzed the muscles of a frog without affecting sensory nerve function. These experiments and others revealed the functional existence of the neuromuscular junction prior to its isolation anatomically. They also revealed that circulating substances produce selective effects on organ systems, a concept important in the development of receptor theory.

This concept of selectivity of effect eventually led Paul Erhlich to his conclusion that "agents cannot act unless they are bound," a cornerstone of receptor theory. Although Erhlich is attributed with discovering the concept of receptors, his contemporary J. N. Langley (1852–1926) coined the phrase receptive substance (or receptor). Langley extended Claude Bernard's work by showing that nicotine and curare had mutually antagonistic effects on the same receptive substance, that was neither nerve nor muscle. Today we recognize this receptive substance as being the nicotinic acetylcholine receptor in the neuromuscular junction. Several decades of research have refined receptor theory to the point where receptors are now recognized as discrete excitable proteins.

Receptor Structure. Overall physical structure of a receptor determines the three-dimensional configuration of the specific area of receptor protein that will bind a drug. The pharmacologic structure of a drug must match the three-dimensional configuration of the binding area of a receptor. Hence, subtle changes in drug structure may dramatically alter its ability to bind to a specific receptor population. In addition, two drugs with seemingly unrelated two-dimensional chemical structures may bind to the same receptor if their three-dimensional structures and charged areas are similar.

Recent advances in molecular biology have enabled researchers to deduce, from amino acid sequences, the primary structure of many receptors. Many receptors appear to belong to families of receptors in which several functionally similar receptors are related in physi-

cal structure. Common features of all membrane receptors appear to be hydrophobic transmembrane regions as well as intracellular and extracellular regions. The exact arrangement of these regions varies according to receptor type. It is beyond the scope of this review to detail even a list of currently proven receptor proteins. However, examples of the putative physical structure of three receptors important to the anesthesiologist, the β_2-adrenergic receptor, the γ-aminobutyric acid A (GABA$_A$) receptor, and the nicotinic acetylcholine receptor, are shown in Figures 2-9 and 2-10. It is important to note that both the GABA$_A$ and the nicotinic acetylcholine receptor are coupled to ion channels.

Receptor Agonists and Antagonists. Agonist drugs induce an effect that mimics endogenous hormones or neurotransmitters when bound to a receptor. This effect may be stimulatory or inhibitory. The term affinity as related to a given agonist is a measure of the attraction between the given drug and the receptor. A drug with low affinity for a given receptor will tend not to bind to the receptor and hence will produce no effect. A drug that binds avidly to a given receptor will produce the receptor-determined effect at a lower given dose of the receptor agonist.

Antagonist drugs inhibit or prevent receptor-mediated agonist effects by competing for receptor occupancy. A competitive antagonist can generally be displaced from the receptor complex by the administration of a receptor agonist if given in a large enough concentration, thus permitting the agonist to produce the expected effect. A noncompetitive antagonist, when bound to the receptor complex, will produce a loss of the expected effect that cannot be reproduced by the concurrent administration of a receptor agonist.

Clinical example of competitive antagonists. Acetylcholine mediates muscle contraction via the postsynaptic nicotinic acetylcholine receptor at the neuromuscular junction (also see Ch. 12). Vecuronium, a nondepolarizing muscle relaxant of moderate duration, is a competitive antagonist at this receptor. When vecuronium binds to the postsynaptic acetylcholine receptor, acetylcholine agonism is blocked and neuromuscular transmission is inhibited. The result is a flaccid paralysis. Neuromuscular transmission may be reinstated by administering an acetylcholinesterase inhibitor. Acetylcholinesterase inhibitors prevent the breakdown of acetylcholine, effectively raising the concentration of the agonist acetylcholine at the receptor, which displaces vecuronium from the receptor complex. When enough vecuronium is displaced, muscle contraction is reinstated. This principle is commonly used in anesthesia to antagonize drug-induced muscle relaxation at the end of a surgical procedure.

Ion Channels

In addition to receptors, pharmacologic agents act on other excitable cell membrane proteins such as ion channels. These channels mediate neural signalling by

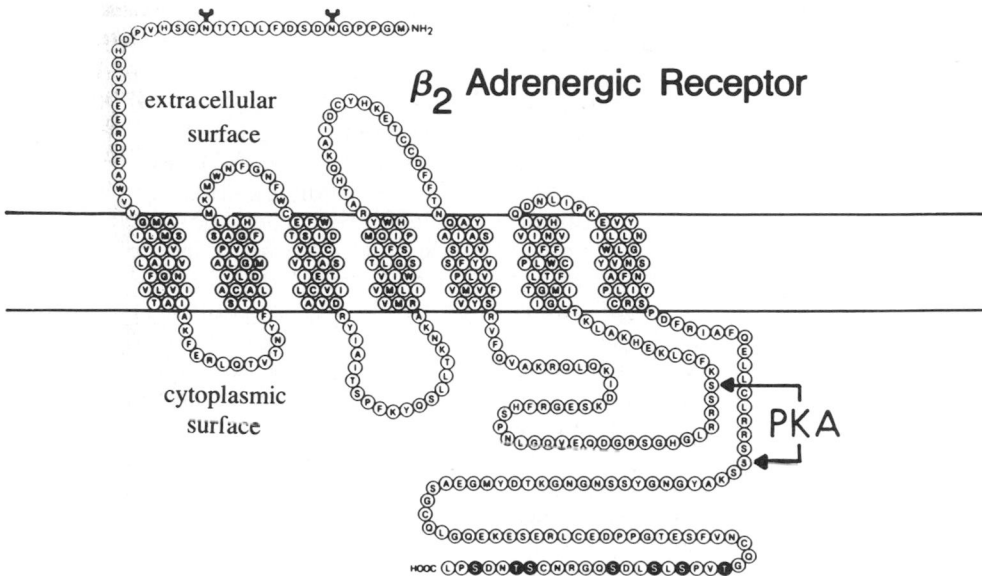

Fig. 2-9. Putative two-dimensional physical structure of the β_2-adrenergic receptor. There are seven hydrophobic transmembrane regions that span the cell membrane as well as extracellular and intracellular loops. The letters inside the circles are the standard representation for individual amino acids.

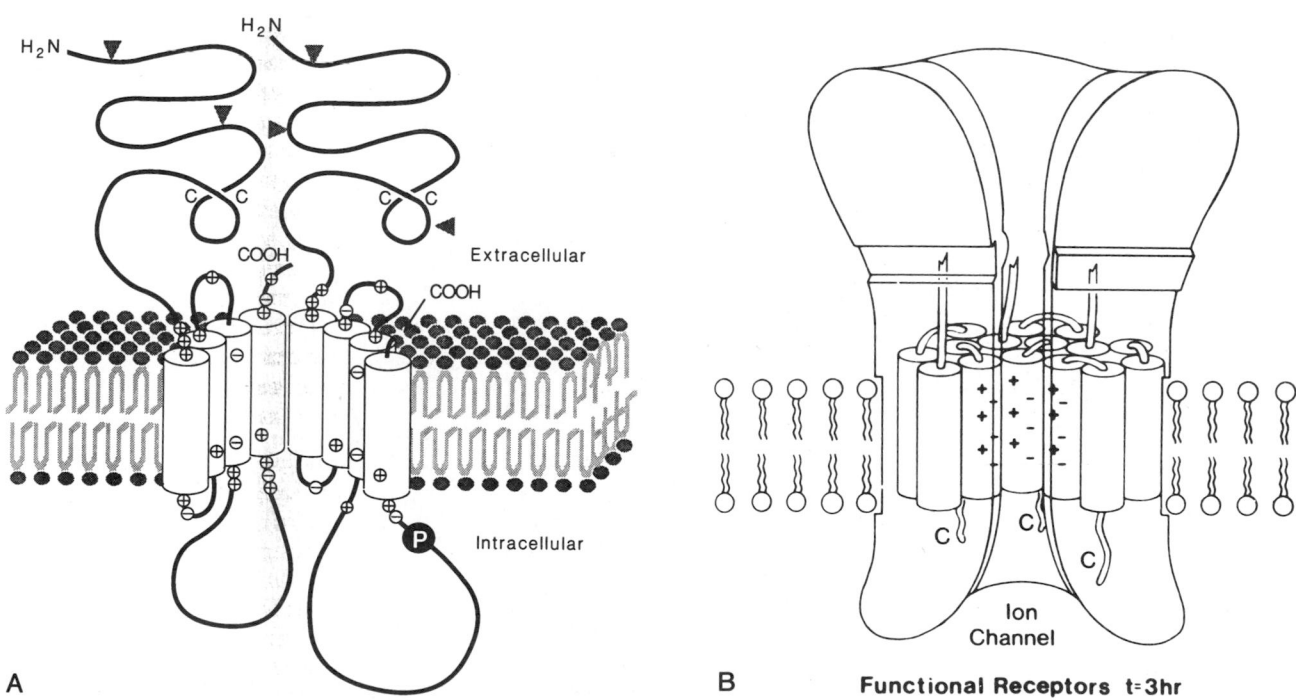

Fig. 2-10. Three-dimensional models of the structures of the GABA$_A$ receptor (**A**) and the nicotinic acetylcholine receptor (**B**) are shown in this figure. Only a portion of the receptor is illustrated to give a three-dimensional view. The GABA$_A$ receptor contains four large globular subunits ($\alpha_2\beta_2$), each of which contains four membrane-spanning helices. The structure of the nicotinic acetylcholine receptor is similar, with five large globular subunits ($\alpha_2\beta\gamma\delta$), each of which contains several membrane-spanning regions. Of note, the figures illustrate the presence of a central charged channel in both of these receptors that represents the ion channel to which the receptor is coupled.

modulating ion permeability of electrically excitable membranes. Since many drugs act directly or indirectly through ion channels, it is important to the anesthesiologist to review their function. Classic ion channels such as the sodium channel have charged areas that span the cell membrane. The formation of ion pairs between many positive and negative charges helps stabilize the channel in the membrane. Voltage-dependent gating of the sodium channel is made possible by the presence of a voltage sensor—a collection of charges that move under the influence of the cell membrane electrical field. During depolarization, these charges presumably move outward, causing conformational changes and rearrangement of ion pairs that results in sodium permeability. The putative physical structure of the sodium channel is shown in Figure 2-11.

Both the nicotinic acetylcholine receptor and the GABA$_A$ receptor are receptor-ion channel complexes. The combination of a classic receptor protein plus an ion channel gives ligand-gated ion channels the unique ability to have drugs directly alter membrane permeability to cations. This coupling is revealed in the physical structure of the receptor itself. While membrane receptors have hydrophobic transmembrane regions (Fig. 2-9) and ion channels have charged transmembrane regions (Fig. 2-11), ligand-gated ion channels have both hydrophobic and charged transmembrane regions (Fig. 2-10).

Ion Pumps

The third type of excitable membrane protein is the ion pump. The sodium-potassium-ATPase pump is perhaps the most familiar ion pump to the anesthesiologist since it is inhibited by the drug digitalis. To understand the function of the sodium-potassium-ATPase pump, it is important to review the cation composition of cells and extracellular fluid. Extracellular fluid is high in sodium and low in potassium, while intracellular fluid is high in potassium and low in sodium. Action potentials activate sodium channels, allowing sodium to rush intracellularly. The sodium-potassium-ATPase pump then rapidly pumps sodium out of the cell in exchange for potassium, returning the cell to its original cation composition. Drugs that act on ion pumps therefore alter intracellular/extracellular cation ratios, resulting in altered membrane electrical potential. This accounts for some drug effects.

Clinical example of a drug affecting ion pump function. The drug digitalis is sometimes used to treat myocardial failure. The mechanism of action of digitalis is inhibition of sodium-potassium-ATPase pump function. This is of special importance in the myocardial cell in which sodium-potassium-ATPase exchange is replaced by slower sodium-calcium exchange, thereby increasing intracellular calcium concentrations. Since calcium increases myocardial contractility, improved myocardial pump function results.

Classic Receptor Theory

To mediate effects, drugs must bind to receptors. Such drug-receptor interactions provide the basis for classic receptor theory. Classic receptor theory assumes that the compound or drug binds reversibly with the specific receptor site to produce a drug-receptor complex. The generation of this drug-receptor complex represents an intermediate step in producing a specific ef-

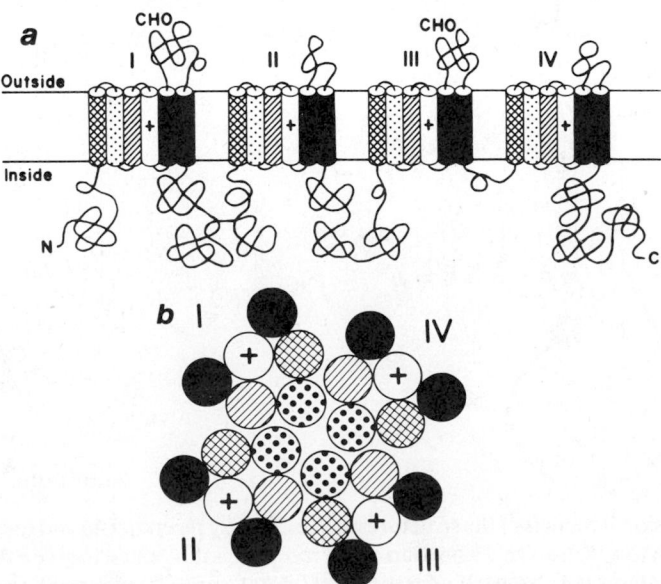

Fig. 2-11. (A & B) Physical structure of the sodium channel. There are four large globular units, each of which contains six membrane-spanning helices. The channel is charged and is present in the very center of the structure with the globular units surrounding it.

fect. The effect may cease when there is dissociation of the drug-receptor complex. This process is therefore analogous to the classic model of Michaelis-Menten enzyme kinetics. Mathematically, this may be expressed as

$$[D] + [R] \rightleftharpoons [DR]$$

where [D] = the concentration of drug, [R] = the concentration of receptor, and [DR] represents the concentration of drug-receptor complex. At equilibrium, one can define a K_d as the dissociation constant for that given drug. Thus, mathematically

$$K_d = \frac{[D][R]}{[DR]}$$

When an appropriate concentration of a drug is administered to occupy exactly 50 percent of the receptors, the measured K_d will be equal to the administered dose. Under these conditions, the K_d will have the dimensions of a concentration. A low dissociation constant indicates that less drug is required to occupy 50 percent of the receptors; therefore, the drug has high affinity for the receptor. The K_d has been determined for many of the drugs currently administered during anesthesia. The reciprocal of K_d, the association constant, is a measure of the affinity of the drug for the receptor.

In practice, it is difficult to measure precise drug-receptor occupancy. As stated, it is assumed that the drug-receptor complex represents an intermediate step in the production of a specific effect. It is, therefore, the practice to apply pharmacodynamic theory to compare a given dose of a drug with a resulting effect. An effect can be any biochemical or physiologic parameter that is measurable. A measured effect can be an alteration in a biochemical compound, an enzyme level, a physiologic parameter such as heart rate or blood pressure, or a response to any graded input into the biologic system. For example, in evaluating the pharmacodynamics of muscle relaxants, the measured effect is not a direct measurement of drug-receptor complexes but rather a response to a neuromuscular stimulus as delivered by a nerve stimulator. It is important that when a given effect is chosen relative to the drug of interest, there should be no measurable effect at zero concentration of the drug and a graded increase in effect to increasing doses of the drug.

From the discussion of pharmacokinetics, it is clear that the delivery of a drug to a given receptor will be time and dose dependent. If the receptor is located within the central compartment, where there may be instantaneous equilibration after an intravenous injection, the peak effect may occur immediately. Even in this example, if the effect depends on a drug-receptor complex-induced time-dependent change, the rate of production of an effect will be modified by this variable. If the drug-receptor complex occurs in a peripheral compartment, pharmacokinetic alterations in drug absorption and distribution may further alter the time course of a given drug effect.

Second Messengers

The binding of a hormone or drug to its receptor does not instantly produce clinical effects. Instead, a series of rapid biochemical events couple receptor binding to the ultimate clinical effect. These biochemical events are called second messengers. Since alterations in second messenger coupling can alter the effectiveness of a drug, it is important that the anesthesiologist understand general concepts about second messengers.

Many membrane receptors are coupled to their primary second messenger via membrane proteins called guanine nucleotide regulatory proteins (or G proteins; also sometimes called N proteins). The coupling of G proteins to receptor-hormone complexes requires energy in the form of guanosine triphosphate (GTP). Once this coupling occurs, then the stimulation (via stimulatory G proteins, Gs) or inhibition (via inhibitory G proteins, Gi) of the initial biochemical reaction in the effector cascade can occur. G proteins are composed of three subunits. One of these subunits, the α subunit, confers specificity for a specific receptor and effector. While the other two subunits, β and δ, are thought to anchor the G protein in the cell membrane, they may also have a role in modulating ion channels. Figure 2-12 shows a schematized interaction of receptors and G proteins.

Several receptor second messenger systems produce biologic effects in humans. The best understood second messenger system is the adenylate cyclase system. In this system, stimulatory G protein-receptor-hormone complexes increase the activity of the enzyme adenylate cyclase, resulting in increased levels of cyclic adenosine 3',5'-monophosphate (cyclic AMP) in the cell. Inhibitory G protein-receptor-hormone complexes decrease the activity of adenylate cyclase, resulting in decreased levels of cellular cyclic AMP. In general, increased levels of intracellular cyclic AMP activate enzymes called protein kinases that in turn phosphorylate proteins. Phosphorylated proteins are activated proteins that can ultimately manifest biologic effects. Examples of drugs or hormones that activate adenylate cyclase include glucagon, β-adrenergic agonists, and histamine. Muscarinic agonists, α_2-adrenergic agonists, and adenosine inhibit adenylate cyclase.

Another example of a second messenger system is the phosphatidylinositol system. Here, hydrolysis of phosphatidylinositol-4,5-bisphosphate in the cell membrane, catalyzed by phospholipase C, generates two second messenger molecules, inositol-1,4,5-triphosphate (IP_3) and 1,2-diacylglycerol (1,2-DG). The exact mechanism by which phosphatidylinositol breakdown leads to increased intracellular calcium levels is not known, but IP_3 appears to mobilize intracellular calcium directly, while 1,2-DG activates protein kinases. In any event, the resulting increased calcium levels intracellularly produce biologic effects. Examples of drugs that cause phosphatidylinositol breakdown are α_1-adrenergic agonists and muscarinic agonists.

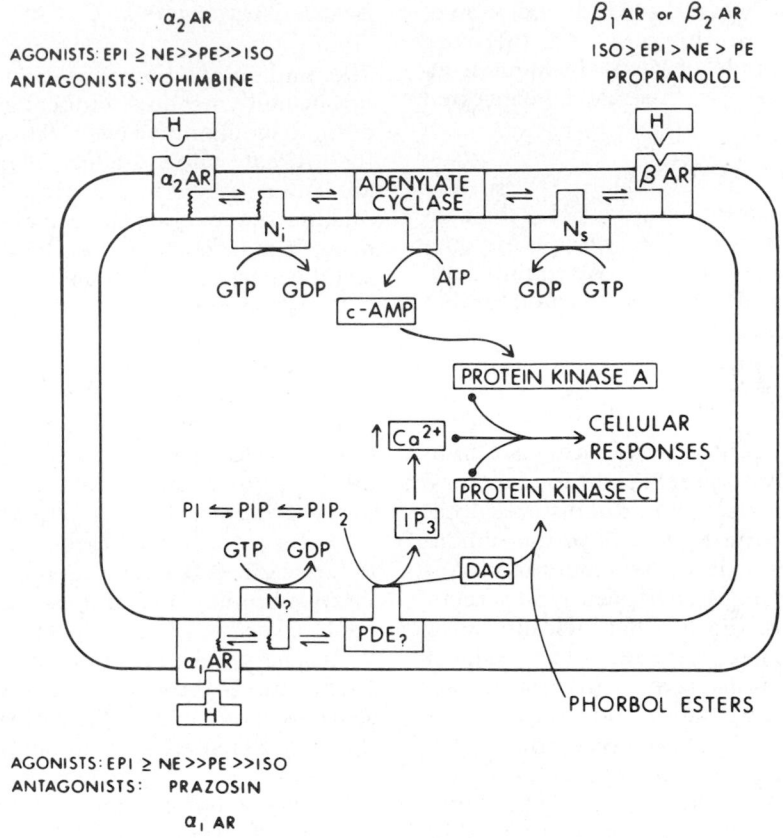

Fig. 2-12. Adrenergic receptors and their second messenger systems are shown in this figure. A hormone (*H*) or drug interacts with the receptor (*AR*, adrenergic receptor), which then binds to a stimulatory or inhibitory guanine nucleotide regulatory protein (*N*; *i*, inhibitory; *s*, stimulatory). This complex then binds to the first enzyme in the cascade of second messengers that leads to a biologic effect. β-Adrenergic and α_2-adrenergic receptors are coupled to the adenylate cyclase system, while the α_1-adrenergic receptor is coupled to the phosphatidylinositol system (see text). *ISO*, isoproterenol; *EPI*, epinephrine; *NE*, norepinephrine; *PE*, phenylephrine; *DAG*, diacylglycerol; IP_3, inositol -1,4,5-triphosphate; *PDE*, phosphodiesterase; *PI*, phosphatidylinositol; *PIP*, phosphatidylinositol 4-phosphate; PIP_2, phosphatidylinositol-4,5-bisphosphate.

Figure 2-12 depicts receptor-mediated adenylate cyclase stimulation and inhibition as well as phosphatidylinositol breakdown mediated by various adrenergic receptors.

New Developments in Molecular Pharmacology

The field of molecular pharmacology is rapidly advancing our understanding of excitable membrane proteins and their mechanism of action. Prior to the advent of molecular biology, most pharmacology research utilized tools such as binding experiments and protein purification techniques to elucidate the structure and mechanism of action of various drugs and receptors. Although important, these studies were tedious since many tissues contained more than one receptor subtype (some of which had not yet been discovered) and protein purification of receptors was a lengthy and complicated process. Molecular biology techniques

provide a unique opportunity to study receptors and their structure at the DNA level. This has rapidly advanced the field of molecular pharmacology in the last 10 years and will continue to do so for many years to come. Many new receptors and receptor subtypes have been discovered, paving the way for new pharmacologic agents that will eventually be used by the anesthesiologist. For this reason, molecular pharmacology is briefly described below.

Molecular pharmacology takes advantage of the fact that all proteins, including excitable membrane proteins, are encoded in the human genome as nucleic acids. Every amino acid present in a protein is coded for by a specific combination of three nucleotides in DNA. Therefore, if the DNA sequence that codes for a receptor protein can be found, the putative primary structure of the receptor is revealed. In addition, these fragments of DNA can then be inserted into special cells that will express (manufacture, assemble, and insert into the cell membrane) the receptor protein in high quantity.

This has several advantages. First, studies on the receptor itself can be done. By changing (mutating) the nucleotide sequence, an abnormal receptor can be formed. This abnormal receptor can be compared with the original receptor to see whether the changes made affect binding of drug to the receptor, or its coupling to second messengers. In this manner, the exact portions of the receptor that bind and couple the drug to its effect can be elucidated. G proteins have also been investigated in this manner. Second, new receptors and receptor subtypes can be discovered by searching for DNA sequences that are similar to those of known receptors. Several muscarinic acetylcholine receptor subtypes have been discovered by this technique. Once these new receptors are discovered, they can be characterized easily since their expression in high quantity in cells allows them to be screened by various pharmacologic agents. Last, and perhaps the most immediately clinically relevant, new investigational drugs can be rapidly screened for effects on various receptors. Cells that contain only a single highly expressed receptor can be tested with the new drug. In this way, pharmacologic effects of individual receptors can be studied in a controlled manner, isolated from other receptors and receptor subtypes. The discovery of new receptors, and the discovery of the structure of well-known receptors, will have implications on the pharmacologic agents used by anesthesiologists in the future.

Clinical Evaluation of Drug Effects

General

Once pharmacologic agents have stimulated excitable cell membrane proteins and produced an effect, it is important to evaluate this effect clinically. This section focuses on methods of evaluating drug effects such as dose-response curves, efficacy, potency, 50 percent effective dose (ED_{50}), 50 percent lethal dose (LD_{50}), and therapeutic index.

Dose-Response Curves

To simplify the correlation between drug dose and measured effect, this correlation is often expressed as a comparison of drug dose with the peak effect or equilibrium effect. This will yield a time-independent dose-response relationship. This simplification of expression of the dose-response relationship is the common presentation format for dose-response studies. The actual shape of the dose-response curves is determined by the choice of scales chosen for the two axes. For example, the effect scale can be either in absolute units (i.e., twitch height) or normalized to convert these units to a percentage of the maximum effect (i.e., percent twitch height depression). If the determined pairs (dose and resultant effect) are plotted on scales that are linear both on the x- and y-axes, the resultant curve will be hyperbolic. If the abscissa is changed to a log scale, the resultant curve, utilizing the same data, will be the classic sigmoid curve. This is shown in Figure 2-13. Many dose-response curves generated from clinical studies in humans will be linear when plotted with a logarithmic scale because, for ethical reasons, maximal doses (required to see the sigmoid shape of the curve) may not be administered.

Effect of Receptor Agonists on Log Dose-Response Curves

It can be demonstrated that two drugs that presumably act on the same receptor will display parallelism of their log dose-response curves in the presence or absence of antagonists. The log dose-response curve would be superimposed if the two drugs had the same molar affinity constant. The addition of two drugs with varying affinity constants might be predicted to have an effect dependent only on the total amount of drug-receptor complex generated. This suggests a direct linear relationship between receptor-drug complex and a measured effect. It is clear that this is not always the case in biologic systems. For example, in neuromuscular transmission, the measured change in effect on twitch height is not linear when receptor occupancy declines from 100 percent to 90 percent, as compared with the change from 80 percent to 70 percent occupancy.

A further distinction between agonists is based on achievement of the maximum measured pharmacologic response or effect. A full agonist will produce the maximal response at full receptor occupancy. A partial agonist will produce a lower maximal response or effect even at full receptor occupancy. The precise molecular mechanism explaining this blunting of the maximal response of partial agonists is under investigation. It is possible to imagine that the partial agonist produces a drug-receptor complex configuration that is slightly different from the full agonist drug-receptor complex.

Effect of Receptor Antagonists on Log Dose-Response Curves

The dose-response curve generated from the addition of an agonist in the presence of a competitive antagonist will demonstrate a different effect at every concentration of agonist used until the concentration of agonist is large enough to displace the antagonist from the receptors. At that concentration, the maximum effect produced by the dose is the same with or without the presence of the competitive antagonist. The dose-response curve generated by the addition of an agonist in the presence of a noncompetitive antagonist will show failure to attain the same effect with a given dose of agonist; at no concentration of agonist will the maximal effect be attained since the blockade of effect cannot be reversed.

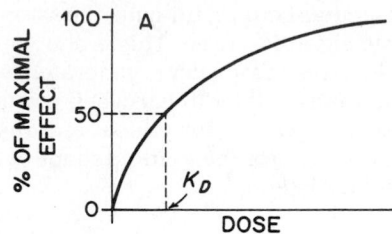
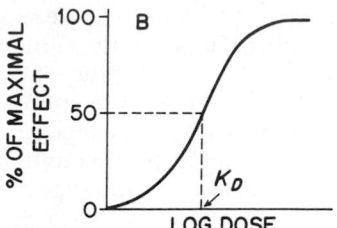

Fig. 2-13. Two representations of dose-response curves. **(A)** Dose is plotted on the x axis and effect is plotted on the y axis (as percent of maximal effect). When plotted on a linear scale, a typical hyperbolic curve results. **(B)** When the same data are plotted with a logarithmic scale on the x axis, the resulting curve is sigmoidal.

Efficacy

Efficacy refers to a measure of the intrinsic ability of a drug to produce a given effect. It is related to the maximum effect that can be produced by a given drug. Efficacy for a full agonist would be considered to be 1.0, while the efficacy of a pure antagonist is 0. Partial agonists will have efficacies of 0 to 1.0.

Potency

The term potency refers to the quantity of drug that must be administered to produce a maximum effect. Two drugs may have the same efficacy, but if one drug produces the maximum effect at 1 mg while the second drug produces the maximum effect only at 100 mg, the second drug is less potent. Figure 2-14 shows the relationship between efficacy, potency, and the dose-response curve.

Effective Dose and Lethal Dose

The ED_{50} is the dose of a drug required to produce a specific effect in 50 percent of individuals to whom it is administered. The LD_{50} is the dose of a drug required to produce death in 50 percent of individuals to whom it is administered. The therapeutic index of a drug is the ratio between the LD_{50} and the ED_{50} (LD_{50}/ED_{50}).

Hence, the higher the therapeutic index of a drug, the safer it is for clinical administration. The relationship between ED_{50}, and LD_{50}, and therapeutic index is shown in Figure 2-15.

Biologic Variability

Individual variation in response to an identical dose of administered drug occurs and is a phenomenon that is seen daily by the anesthesiologist. Individual variation

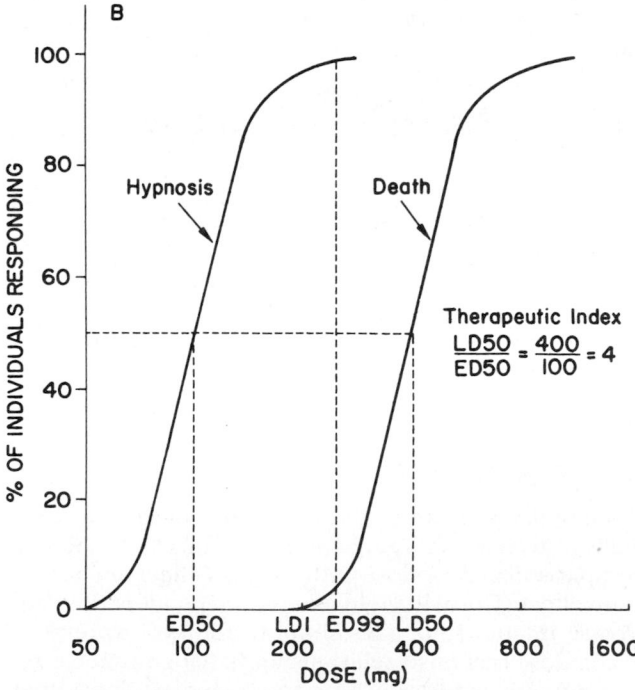

Fig. 2-15. Relationship among ED_{50}, LD_{50}, and therapeutic index. This curve was generated from data from experiments in which animals were injected with various doses of a sedative-hypnotic and the responses determined. ED_{50} is the dose of a drug required to produce a specific effect in 50 percent of individuals to whom it is administered. LD_{50} is the dose of a drug required to produce death in 50 percent of individuals to whom it is administered. The therapeutic index of a drug is the ratio between the LD_{50} and the ED_{50} (LD_{50}/ED_{50}).

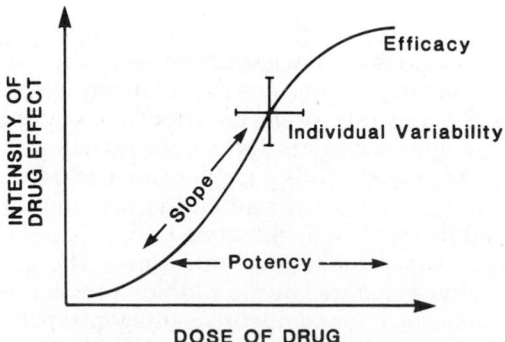

Fig. 2-14. Relationship between efficacy, potency, and individual variability shown on a typical sigmoidal dose-response curve. Note: the sigmoid shape is achieved by plotting log dose.

in response to a drug can occur as a result of differences in pharmacokinetic parameters such as absorption, distribution, metabolism, and excretion of a drug. Such pharmacokinetic differences were discussed earlier in this chapter. Individual variation in response to a drug can also be due to differences in pharmacodynamic responses. Hence, the exact same dose of anesthetic agent present at an effector site may produce different responses in different patients. The relationship between patient variability and the typical dose-response curve is shown in Figure 2-14. The clinician who wishes to produce a given therapeutic effect must therefore consider not only the choice of drug but also the parameters of time, pharmacokinetics, pharmacodynamics, and receptor dynamics. This section explores reasons for pharmacodynamic biologic variability including age, genetic variability, disease states, and receptor desensitization. Only an overview of these concepts will be presented since more detailed explanations will occur in ensuing chapters.

Age
(Also See Chs. 59 and 62)

Anesthesiologists treat patients of all ages. Clearly, the newborn, adult, and geriatric patient are different. While important age-related pharmacokinetic differences have been investigated, there is a paucity of data about pharmacodynamic differences among these age groups. Two drugs that have been examined for pharmacodynamic effects in adults and children are antiepileptic drugs and digoxin. The effective plasma concentration appears to be the same for children and adults, implying that no pharmacodynamic differences occur related to age with these particular drugs. Drugs with central nervous system effects such as benzodiazepines, however, do seem to have a stronger effect in the elderly; this effect cannot be explained by pharmacokinetic differences. Further research is needed in this important area in anesthesiology.

Genetic Variability

Examples of pharmacokinetic variability caused by genetic factors are common in anesthesia. They are usually related to absence or abnormal function of enzymes that metabolize drugs, as seen in atypical pseudocholinesterase. The most striking example of genetic variability causing pharmacodynamic differences in drug effect in anesthesia is the disease malignant hyperthermia.

Clinical example of pharmacodynamic variability caused by genetic variability. Malignant hyperthermia is manifested in approximately 1 in 20,000 anesthetics (also see Ch. 28). Various anesthetics, especially halothane, seem to trigger an abnormal hypermetabolic response that results in an uncontrolled increase in body temperature, muscle rigidity, metabolic acidosis, hyperkalemia, and hypercapnia. Although the exact cause

of malignant hyperthermia is unknown, it appears to be related to abnormal calcium release and uptake by the sarcoplasmic reticulum within cells. Since the disease does not influence the uptake and distribution of drug but is manifest once the drug interacts at the cellular level, it represents a classic genetic pharmacodynamic abnormality.

Disease States

Disease states may contribute to variation in drug response. Although disease states frequently result in pharmacokinetic variations (such as decreased perfusion in heart failure or decreased elimination in renal failure), pharmacodynamic variations are also seen. Diseases such as diabetes, thyroid disease, adrenal disease, myasthenia gravis, and hypertension alter receptor function.

Clinical examples of pharmacodynamic variability caused by disease states. In myasthenia gravis, antibodies to the postsynaptic nicotinic acetylcholine receptor effectively decrease the number of receptors present. Muscle weakness characterizes the disease. As a result, these patients are exquisitely sensitive to muscle relaxants that compete at this receptor. Clinically, the dose of muscle relaxants must be decreased or eliminated in this patient population (also see Ch. 12).

Heart failure alters myocardial pump function and also results in chronically elevated norepinephrine levels. Chronically elevated catecholamine levels in patients with heart failure decrease the responsiveness of myocardial β_1-adrenergic receptors without affecting β_2-adrenergic receptors. Hence, inotropic agents that have β_1-adrenergic agonism may not be as effective in this patient population.

Receptor Desensitization

Chronic stimulation of a receptor causes a decrease in responsiveness of the receptor to the agonist. This is called desensitization (also known as tachyphylaxis or tolerance). Desensitization occurs either by the uncoupling of the receptor-effector complex or by the physical removal (internalization) of receptors from the surface of a cell. There are two forms of desensitization—homologous and heterologous desensitization. In homologous desensitization, continuous stimulation of a receptor with an agonist drug causes the cell to decrease its responsiveness to the administered drug only. Heterologous desensitization occurs, however, when continuous stimulation of a receptor with an agonist drug or hormone causes the cell to decrease its responsiveness to other drugs in addition to the administered drug.

Clinical examples of desensitization. β-Adrenergic agonist drugs are occasionally administered chronically to patients with heart disease in the intensive care unit. Chronic administration of β-adrenergic agonists results in a decrease in β-receptor number in myocardial tissue. Thus, increasing concentrations of β-adrenergic agonists may be required over time to achieve the same effect. This is an example of homologous desensitization (also see Ch. 14).

Heterologous desensitization can be seen clinically in thyroid disease in which chronically elevated thyroid hormone levels occur. Although thyroid hormone binds to its own thyroid hormone receptor, chronic elevations in thyroid hormone levels also cause desensitization of the β-adrenergic receptor. Hence, higher doses of β-adrenergic agonist drugs may be necessary to achieve a desired effect in patients with hyperthyroidism.

Increased Receptor Sensitivity

The opposite of desensitization is increased sensitivity. When a receptor antagonist is chronically administered, receptor number may actually increase. If the receptor antagonist is suddenly discontinued, exaggerated responsiveness to the receptor agonist may occur.

Clinical example of increased receptor sensitivity. β-Adrenergic blocking drugs are often chronically administered to patients with hypertension and heart disease. Chronic administration of β-adrenergic blocking drugs results in an increase in β-receptor number in myocardial tissue. If β-adrenergic blocking drugs are abruptly discontinued (instead of being weaned), endogenous hormones such as epinephrine that act on β-adrenergic receptors may stimulate tachycardia and hypertension.

SUMMARY

In this chapter, the general area of pharmacology was reviewed by presenting the basic principles of pharmacokinetics and pharmacodynamics. Careful review of these principles will permit the anesthesiologist to conceptualize the movement of a drug from the site of administration through various body compartments to the site of action for a desired effect. Taking into account the pharmacologic effects of various disease states, the clinician should be able to individualize the choice of drugs for a particular patient. Hence, the current practice or art of administering certain anesthetic agents in given pathophysiologic states can be seen to have an important biologic basis. Further investigation of these practices will demonstrate not only a justification of methods but, more importantly, may suggest more appropriate therapeutic regiments.

Assimilation of drug-specific pharmacokinetic and pharmacodynamic parameters will maximize effective drug therapy. As a result, the empiric approach to the administration of many drugs can be replaced by a more rational scientific process. This enhancement of the anesthesiologist's understanding of the science of anesthesiology will find the greatest benefit in the ultimate outcome of optimal patient care.

SELECTED READINGS

Alberts B, Brey D, Lewis J, et al: Molecular Biology of the Cell. 2nd Ed. Garland, New York, 1989

Antonaccio MG (ed): Cardiovascular Pharmacology. 2nd Ed. Raven, New York, 1984

Bochner F, Carruthers G, Kampmann J, et al: Handbook of Clinical Pharmacology. 2nd Ed. Little Brown, Boston, 1983

Corssen G, Reves JG, Stanley TH: Intravenous Anesthesia and Analgesia. Lea & Febiger, Philadelphia, 1988

Galeassi RL, Benet LZ, Sheiner LB: Relationship between the pharmacokinetics and pharmacodynamics of procainamide. Clin Pharmacol Ther 25:358, 1979

Gibaldi M, Levy G: Dose-dependent decline of pharmacologic effects of drugs with linear pharmacokinetic characteristics. J Pharmaceut Sci 61:567, 1972

Gibaldi M, Levy G: Pharmacokinetics in clinical practice. 1. Concepts. JAMA 235:1864, 1976

Gibaldi M, Levy G: Pharmacokinetics in clinical practice. 2. Application. JAMA 235:1987, 1976

Gibaldi M, Perrier D: Pharmacokinetics. 2nd Ed. Marcel Dekker, New York, 1982

Goodman LS, Gilman A: The Pharmacological Basis of Therapeutics. 7th Ed. Macmillan, New York, 1985

Hull CJ: Pharmacokinetics and pharmacodynamics. Br J Anaesth 51:579, 1979

La Du BN, Mandel HG, Way EL (eds): Fundamentals of Drug Metabolism and Drug Disposition. Williams & Wilkins, Baltimore, 1977

Levy G: Correlation between drug concentration and drug response in man—pharmacokinetic considerations, pharmacology and the future of man. Proc 5th Int Congr Pharmacol 3:34, 1972

Rowland MR, Tozer TN: Clinical Pharmacokinetics: Concepts and Applications. Lea & Febiger, Philadelphia, 1980

Stanski DR, Watkins WD: Drug Disposition in Anesthesia. Grune & Stratton, Orlando, FL, 1982

Stoelting RK: Pharmacology and Physiology in Anesthetic Practice. JB Lippincott, Philadelphia, 1987

Tiengo M, Cousins MJ (eds): Pharmacological Basis of Anesthesiology: Clinical Pharmacology of New Analgesics and Anesthetics. Raven Press, New York, 1983

Wartak J: Clinical Pharmacokinetics: A Modern Approach to Individual Drug Therapy. Praeger Publishers, New York, 1983

Watson JD, Hopkins NH, Roberts JW, et al: Molecular Biology of the Gene. 4th Ed. Benjamin/Cummings Publishing, Menlo Park, CA 1987

Wood M: Plasma drug binding: Implications for anesthesiologists. Anesth Analg 65:786, 1986

3
MECHANISMS OF ACTION

Donald D. Koblin

INTRODUCTION

Although currently popular inhaled anesthetics include nitrous oxide, halothane, isoflurane, and enflurane, a far greater variety of inhaled agents can produce anesthesia (Fig. 3-1). The properties of these anesthetics vary considerably. For example, cyclopropane and diethyl ether are no longer used because of their explosiveness and flammability. Halothane is nonflammable but possesses a permanent dipole moment, can form hydrogen bonds, and is metabolized by the liver.

A. <u>AGENTS IN CLINICAL USE TODAY</u>

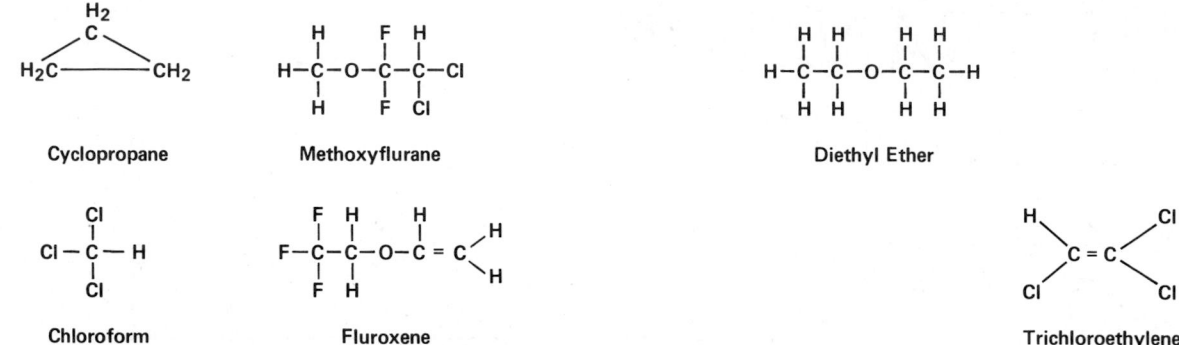

B. <u>AGENTS WHICH WERE ONCE IN COMMON CLINICAL USE:</u>

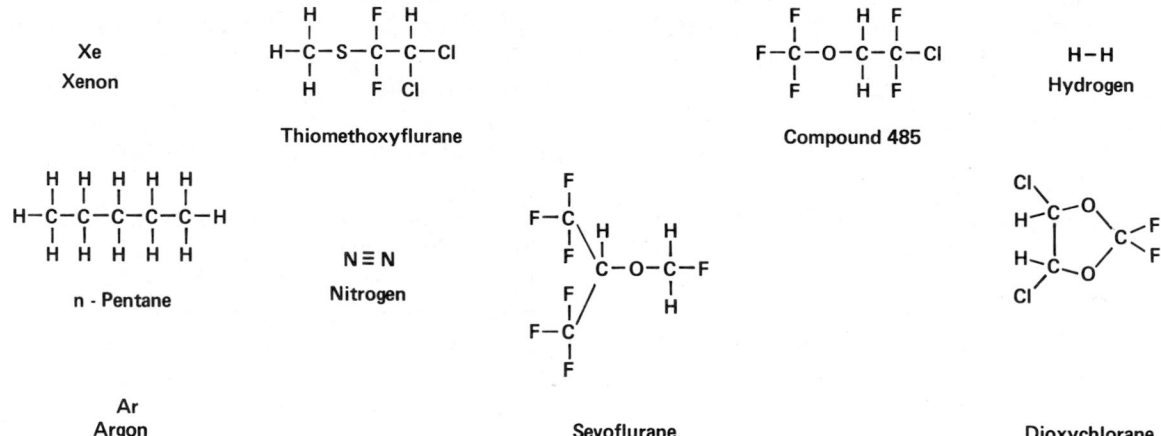

C. <u>SOME EXPERIMENTAL INHALED ANESTHETICS</u>

Fig. 3-1. Chemical structures of various inhaled anesthetics.

Xenon, an anesthetic more potent than nitrous oxide in humans,[1] is essentially inert and undergoes no known transformation in the body. The molecular size of inhaled anesthetics may differ by a factor of about 10.

The structural diversity of the inhaled anesthetics suggests that they do not interact directly with a single specific receptor site. However, some correlations of the potencies of anesthetics with their physicochemical properties do suggest a common (unitary) mechanism of general anesthetic action. An example is the striking relationship between anesthetic potency and lipid solubility (see the section, *Physicochemical Nature of the Site of Anesthetic Action*). Although such correlations do not provide a detailed mechanism of anesthesia, they have been helpful in defining the environment in which anesthetics act.

Any molecular hypothesis of anesthesia must explain the effects of anesthetics on the whole organism. For instance, since anesthetic administration can rapidly induce unconsciousness, and awakening can quickly occur following the discontinuation of anesthesia, physical or biochemical changes important to the mechanism of anesthesia must occur within seconds. Similarly, physical or biochemical alterations caused by anesthetics are meaningful only at clinical doses and physiologic temperatures and not at high anesthetic levels.[2] High levels may produce toxic effects unrelated to the mechanism by which inhaled anesthetics act. Furthermore, anesthetic requirement does not change with increasing duration of anesthesia.[3,4] Thus, any physical or biochemical change causally related to anesthesia should be stable for a period of hours or days.

Finally, the mechanism(s) by which inhaled anesthetics act may overlap the mechanism(s) of action of local anesthetics (Ch. 13), of intravenous narcotics (Ch. 10) and nonnarcotics (Chs. 8 and 9), and even of alcohols. This chapter considers only the inhaled anesthetics.

MEASUREMENT OF ANESTHETIC POTENCIES

An exploration of the mechanism by which anesthetics act requires a knowledge of relative anesthetic potencies for each of the agents. The best estimate of anesthetic potency is MAC—the minimum alveolar concentration (at 1 atmosphere [1 atm]) of an agent that produces immobility in 50 percent of those subjects exposed to a noxious stimulus.[5] For determination of MAC in humans, the stimulus is a surgical skin incision. In animals, the noxious stimulus is usually produced by clamping the tail or by passing electrical current through subcutaneous electrodes. The advantage of measuring the alveolar concentration is that after a short period of equilibration, this concentration directly represents the partial pressure of anesthetic in the central nervous system (CNS) and is independent of the uptake and distribution of the agent to other tissues. Another advantage of MAC is its consistency for a given animal or species or between different species or classes of animals.[5] This consistency makes it possible to discern small changes in anesthetic requirement that may give a clue as to how anesthetics act.

The anesthetic concentration that abolishes the righting reflex in 50 percent of the animals is often used to measure anesthetic potencies in smaller animals, that is, it is an anesthetic 50 percent effective dose (ED_{50}).[6] Since the inspired rather than the alveolar concentrations are measured, the method applies best to rapidly equilibrating (poorly blood-soluble) agents. Only with equilibration can it be assumed that the partial pressure of the inspired gas equals that at the site of action. The use of small animals and inspired concentrations facilitates work with agents at very high pressures (i.e., tens or hundreds of atmospheres). The anesthetic ED_{50} in the mouse, as determined by the rolling response (i.e., the righting reflex), correlates closely with MAC in humans over a 500-fold range in anesthetic requirements (Fig. 3-2).

However, the tail-clamp ED_{50} (MAC) and the righting-reflex ED_{50} are not identical. The tail-clamp ED_{50} is higher than the righting-reflex ED_{50}, and the ratio of these measurements averages approximately 1.8 (Table 3-1).[7-9] This ratio varies slightly with the anesthetic examined, implying that the righting reflex is depressed, at least in part, by a different mechanism from that which depresses the response to application of a tail clamp.[7,9] Thus, the relative potencies of inhaled anesthetics may depend on the end point measured.

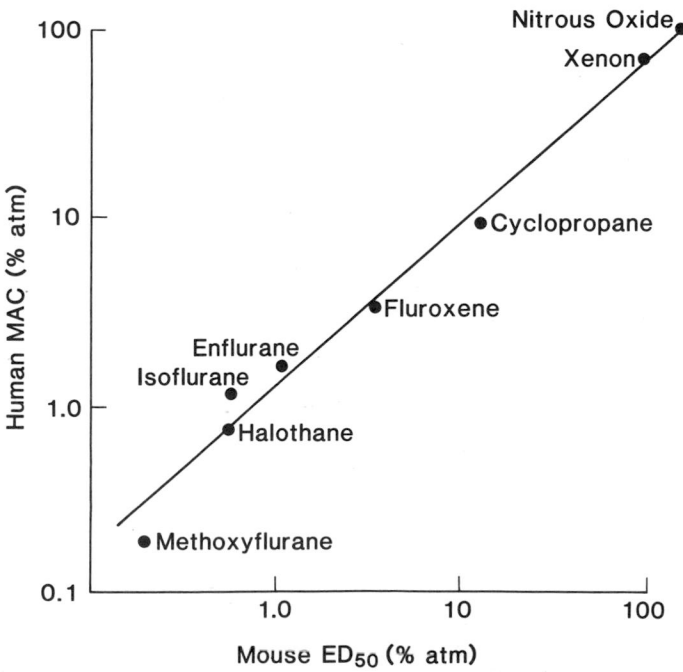

Fig. 3-2. A close correlation exists between the MAC of various anesthetics preventing a response to surgical incision in humans and the inspired dose of an anesthetic (ED_{50}) required to abolish the righting reflex in the mouse. (Data from Quasha et al.,[5] Koblin et al.,[8] and Smith et al.[286])

TABLE 3-1. Ratios of Anesthetic Potencies

	Tail-Clamp ED$_{50}$/Righting-Reflex ED$_{50}$	
Anesthetic	Mouse	Rat
Halothane	1.67	1.74
Enflurane	1.91	—
Isoflurane	2.10	2.41
Chloroform	1.61	—
Cyclopropane	1.97	—
Nitrous oxide	>1.82	—
Methoxyflurane	1.63–2.08	—
Diethyl ether	—	1.25

(Data from Deady et al.,[7] Koblin et al.,[8] and Kissin et al.[9])

ALTERATIONS IN ANESTHETIC REQUIREMENT PERTINENT TO THEORIES OF NARCOSIS

Effects of Temperature

In mammals, MAC decreases with decreasing body temperatures (from 41°C to 26°C) for all anesthetics, but the reduction per degree decrease in body temperature varies slightly from agent to agent.[4,10-12] The decrease in MAC varies from 2 percent per degree for cyclopropane to 5 percent per degree for halothane.

Effects of Pressure

In many species, the application of increasing hydrostatic pressures progressively increases the anesthetic dose required to bring about unresponsiveness, a phenomenon termed the *pressure reversal of anesthesia*.[13-16] In experiments with mammals, pressure is increased by the addition of helium, since helium does not produce anesthesia and possesses only a small inherent anesthetic effect at high pressures.[17] At a total pressure of 100 atm, a 30 to 60 percent increase in the partial pressure of inhaled anesthetics is required to abolish the righting reflex in the mouse.[15] However, not all species exhibit a pressure reversal of anesthesia. The reduction in swimming activity of freshwater shrimp induced by halothane, chloroform, and diethyl ether is not reversed by the application of high pressure.[18]

Effects of Age

In humans, halothane and isoflurane MACs are maximal in infants 1 to 6 months of age.[19,20] Halothane MAC is 1.20 percent atm in infants 1 to 6 months of age and decreases to 0.64 percent atm in patients with a mean age of 81 years.[21] Similar reductions in isoflurane and cyclopropane MACs occur in the elderly,[22] demonstrating that the greater susceptibility of older patients to

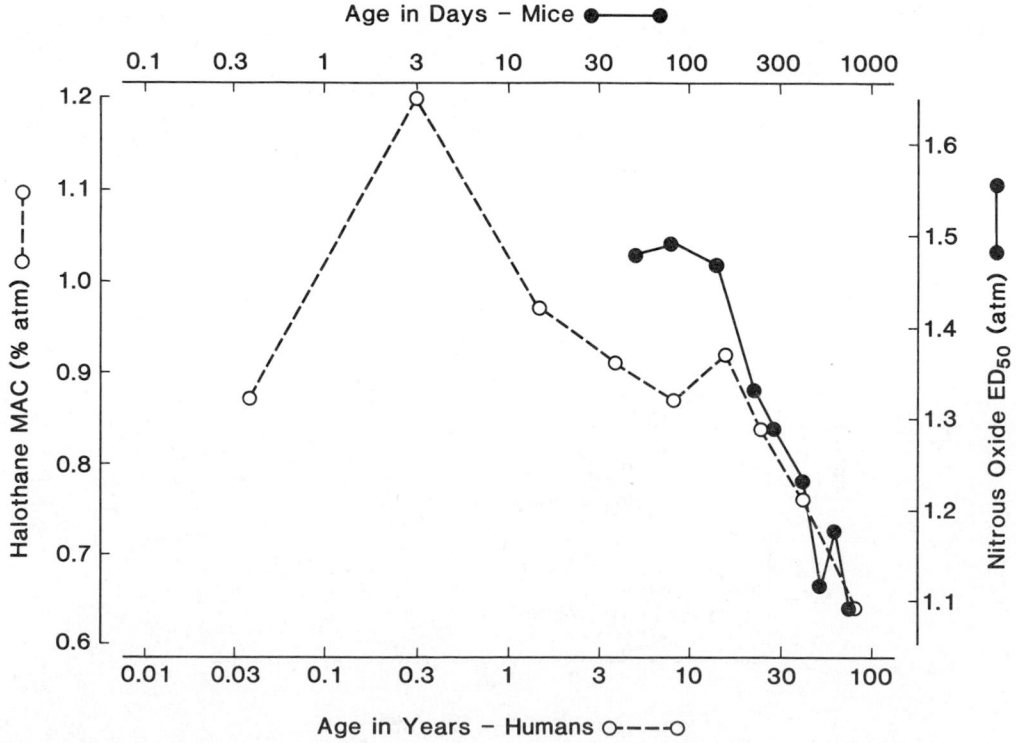

Fig. 3-3. Age-dependent alterations in anesthetic requirement in humans and mice over similar life spans. (Data for halothane in humans are from Lerman et al.[19] and Gregory et al.[21] Data for nitrous oxide in mice are from Koblin et al.[24])

CNS depression by inhaled anesthetics is not related to the absolute potency of the agent.

Rodent models may be useful for studying the mechanisms of change in anesthetic potency with age. The tail-clamp ED_{50} for halothane in the 28-month-old rat is 51 percent lower than in the 4-month-old animal.[23] In mice, the righting-reflex ED_{50} for nitrous oxide progressively decreases with age from 1.48 to 1.09 atm.[24] Comparison of mice and humans over similar life spans shows the decrease in anesthetic requirement of mice to parallel that clinically seen in humans (Fig. 3-3).

Effects of Ion Concentrations

Sodium

Hypernatremia increases sodium proportionately in cerebrospinal fluid (CSF) and increases halothane MAC in dogs by as much as 43 percent.[25] Conversely, hyponatremia dilutes CSF sodium and reduces halothane MAC.[25]

Calcium

Calcium infusions in dogs increase serum and CSF calcium by 2.6 and 1.3 times, respectively, without influencing halothane MAC.[26] However, calcium entry blockers (at relatively high concentrations) augment the potency of inhaled anesthetics. Verapamil (0.5 mg/kg) reduces halothane MAC by 25 percent in dogs,[27] and nitrendipine (50 mg/kg) decreases the righting-reflex ED_{50} of argon by 26 percent in mice.[28]

Magnesium

In dogs, a five-fold increase in serum magnesium is associated with a 12-percent increase in CSF magnesium and does not alter halothane MAC.[26] In rats, a 10-fold increase in plasma magnesium concentration above control levels decreases halothane MAC by approximately 60 percent.[29]

These effects of temperature, pressure, aging, and ion concentrations may be used to test the various models of anesthetic action. Any valid theory of anesthetic action must account for the influence of these physical and physiologic parameters on anesthetic requirement.

ACTIONS OF INHALED ANESTHETICS IN THE CENTRAL NERVOUS SYSTEM

Brain

General anesthetics may act by altering neuronal activity in selected regions of the CNS. Since the brain stem reticular formation plays a role in altering the state of consciousness and alertness and in regulating motor activity, it is often suggested that this structure is an important site of anesthetic action. Although the idea that anesthesia results from a decrease in "tone" in the ascending reticular system may be correct, it is most likely an oversimplification.[30] The effect of anesthesia on neuronal activity in the reticular formation is variable and can be increased, unchanged, or decreased, depending on the agent and the neuronal unit examined.[31] Thus, the anesthetic-induced disruption of nervous activity in the reticular formation probably depends on the specific interaction of a general anesthetic with specific structures within each neuronal unit. Moreover, consciousness cannot simply be equated with activity in the reticular formation, since gross lesions in the reticular formation can completely abolish the arousal reaction of the electroencephalogram while animals remain behaviorally awake.[32]

General anesthetics interrupt transmission in the CNS at sites other than the reticular formation. Clinical concentrations of inhaled agents may alter spontaneous and evoked activity in the mammalian cerebral cortex,[33,34] olfactory cortex,[35] and hippocampus.[36-38] Although inhaled anesthetics usually depress excitability of brain neurons, situations can be found in which anesthetics enhance excitability[38] (Fig. 3-4). In addition, inhibitory transmission may be influenced by volatile agents. Halothane prolongs γ-aminobutyric acid (GABA)-induced inhibition in the rabbit olfactory cortex.[39] In rat hippocampal slices, there are contrasting reports of a halothane-induced increase in the duration of inhibitory postsynaptic currents[40] and selective depression of inhibitory postsynaptic potentials by halothane, isoflurane, and enflurane.[41]

Spinal Cord

Excitatory postsynaptic potentials recorded in the ventral root are markedly depressed by volatile and gaseous agents.[42] Anesthetics may act on specific laminae of the spinal cord.[43] Wide dynamic range neurons in the dorsal horn are mainly associated with lamina V and exhibit, with halothane, a dose-dependent decrease in spontaneous and evoked discharge frequencies in the spinal cord-transected cat.[44] Both excitatory and inhibitory postsynaptic potentials are suppressed to approximately the same extent by 2 percent halothane in motoneurons of the newborn rat spinal cord.[45] In addition to a direct action on spinal neurons, inhaled agents may depress activity by activating the descending inhibition system from the brain.[46]

In summary, inhaled anesthetics interrupt transmission in many areas of the CNS, and anesthesia may not selectively influence one specific region. Although the most common action of anesthetics is to depress excitatory transmission, instances are known in which clinical concentrations of anesthetics have essentially no effect, prolong inhibitory transmission, or even potentiate excitatory or depress inhibitory transmission. Considering that the human brain consists of billions of neurons, each having thousands of synapses, the vari-

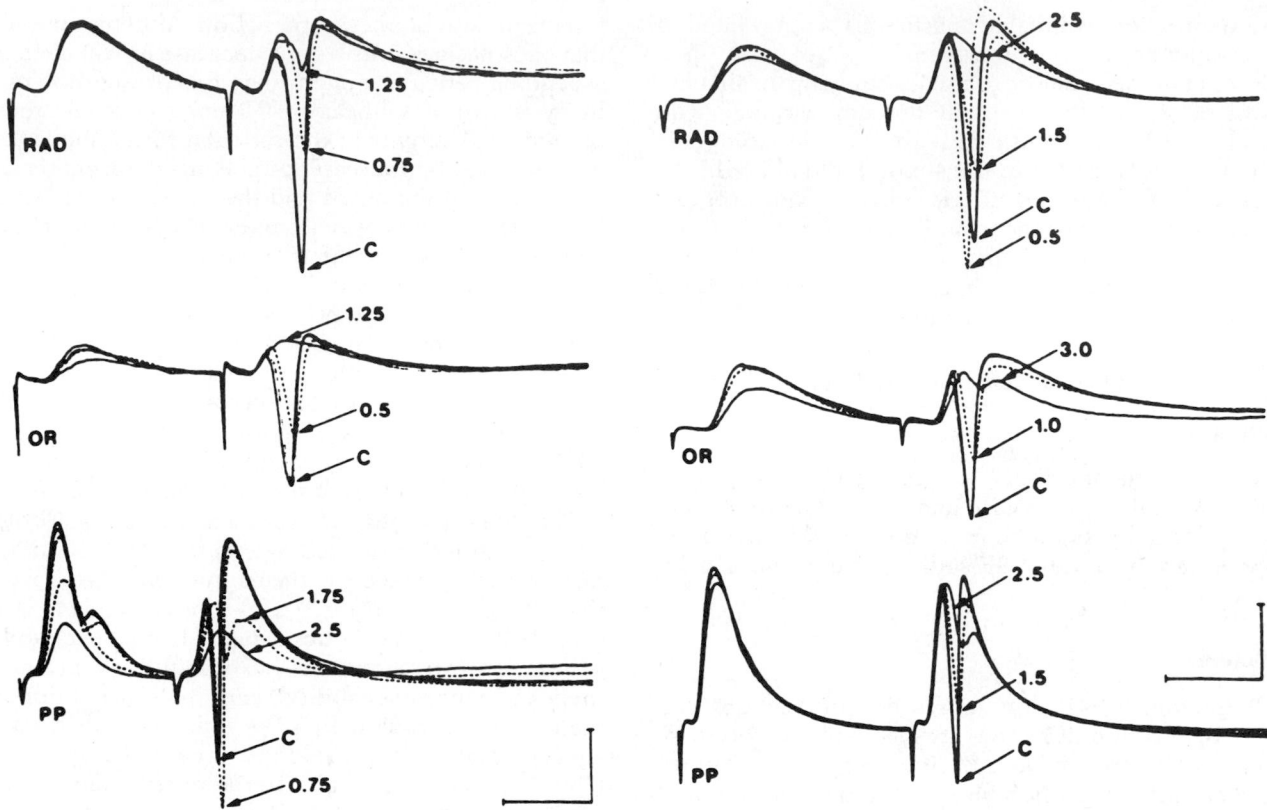

Fig. 3-4. The effects of halothane (**A**) and isoflurane (**B**) on three excitatory synaptic pathways in a rat hippocampal slice. The potential recordings were produced from stimulation of three discrete regions of the hippocampal slice: the stratum radiatum (RAD), the stratum oriens (OR), and perforant path (PP) fibers. Each superimposed series of records shows control (C) responses before (solid line) and after (light dotted line) washout together with two or three concentrations of anesthetic (numbers refer to volume percent). The horizontal calibration bar represents 20 milliseconds, and the vertical calibration bar represents 2.0 mV. These studies demonstrate that the ability of inhaled agents to depress or enhance neuronal excitability depends on the anesthetic, the anesthetic concentration, and the particular brain region examined. (From MacIver and Roth,[38] with permission.)

able nature of the effects of general anesthetics is not surprising. Attempts to reduce this complexity and to increase our understanding of general anesthetic action have led to experiments on isolated neuronal preparations.

INTERRUPTION OF NEURONAL TRANSMISSION BY INHALED ANESTHETICS

Peripheral Receptors

The action of inhaled anesthetics cannot be explained by an effect on peripheral receptors. In cats, anesthetizing concentrations of ether, halothane, or methoxyflurane do not alter cutaneous receptor responses to touch or movement of hair.[47] In monkeys, halothane can even sensitize cutaneous nociceptors by decreas-

ing the threshold to heat stimuli needed to stimulate A fibers and C fibers.[48]

Highly Sensitive Neurons

From the above discussion, it is apparent that inhaled agents can alter excitability in many different anatomic regions of the CNS. However, within each discrete area of the brain there may exist a relatively small number of neurons that are exquisitely sensitive to anesthetics. The existence of such highly sensitive cells is demonstrated in a molluscan ganglion consisting of 30 to 50 neurons having endogenous firing activity.[49] The firing activity is inhibited in only one of these neurons at a concentration of 0.80 percent atm halothane (Fig. 3-5). The other neurons in this cluster show little alteration in their steady-state firing activity when exposed to this concentration of halothane.[49] A possible mechanism for this increased sensitivity will be addressed later (see the section, *The Membrane as the Site of Anesthetic Action*).

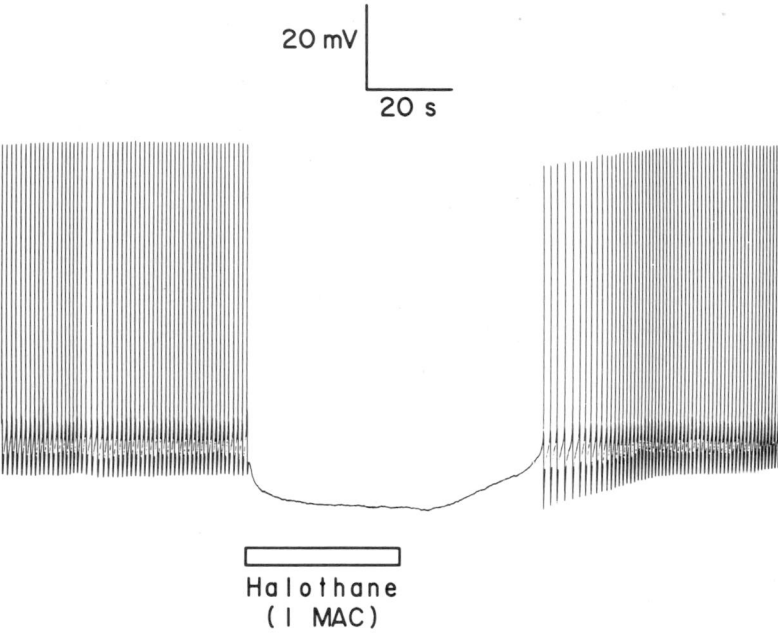

Fig. 3-5. Certain molluscan neurons having endogenous firing activity are extremely sensitive to volatile agents. The figure shows a continuous intracellular recording of membrane potential before, during (bar), and after exposure of a sensitive cell to normal saline solution containing halothane at a partial pressure of 0.0080 atmosphere. (From Franks and Lieb,[49] with permission.)

Axonal Versus Synaptic Transmission

Concentrations of inhaled anesthetics that alter synaptic transmission typically have a smaller effect on axonal transmission. The concentration of ether or chloroform that reduces the amplitude of the action potential in sympathetic nerve axons by one-half is three to five times the concentration that reduces synaptic transmission by one-half.[50] At halothane concentrations of 0.75 to 1.5 percent atm, there is a marked depression in synaptic transmission through the stellate ganglion, whereas axonal transmission is essentially unaltered.[51] Anesthetic concentrations close to 1.0 MAC do not alter the compound action potential of lateral olfactory tract fibers[52] or the electrical excitability of afferent fibers to the hippocampus.[53] Such concentrations do produce a 50 to 100 percent blockade of postsynaptic potentials. In these areas of the brain, compound action potentials in presynaptic fibers are little affected until concentrations of 2.0 MAC are obtained. The above findings are consistent with the idea that general anesthetics selectively block synaptic transmission in the CNS.

Nevertheless, at near-clinical concentrations, inhaled anesthetics may alter transmission through axons. For example, in the isolated rat superior cervical ganglion, 0.5 mM (approximately 1.5 percent atm) halothane decreases the amplitude of the compound action potential in preganglionic nerves by 12 percent (Fig. 3-6A).[54] Even partial blockade of axonal conduction could decrease the amount of neurotransmitter secreted and thereby influence synaptic transmission. That is, an apparent effect at the synapse may simply reflect depression of axonal transmission. Moreover, certain axons exhibit a biphasic effect following exposure to inhaled agents. In the squid giant axon, the minimum stimulus needed for excitation decreases over the first 2 to 3 minutes following exposure to halothane, chloroform, diethyl ether, or cyclopropane and then increases over the next 5 to 10 minutes.[55] An enhanced excitability of axons upon initial exposure to inhaled agents may explain the excitation sometimes observed upon induction of anesthesia.

The diameter of an axon may also influence its susceptibility to inhaled anesthetics. In the squid axon, the effect of *n*-hexane, *n*-heptane, and *n*-octane on the rate of action potential decline is inversely proportional to the square of axon diameter.[56] In the rat hippocampus, isoflurane (1.4 percent atm) depresses the activity of thin (0.16 μm) unmyelinated fibers but has little influence on the larger diameter (1 μm) myelinated fibers.[57] This greater susceptibility of smaller diameter axons to inhaled agents contrasts with the influence of local anesthetics, which appear to be as effective or more effective in blocking large compared with small diameter axons.[58,59]

The frequency at which axons transmit impulses may alter anesthetic potency. At relatively low impulse frequencies, an equilibrium concentration of volatile anesthetic produces a constant level of action potential

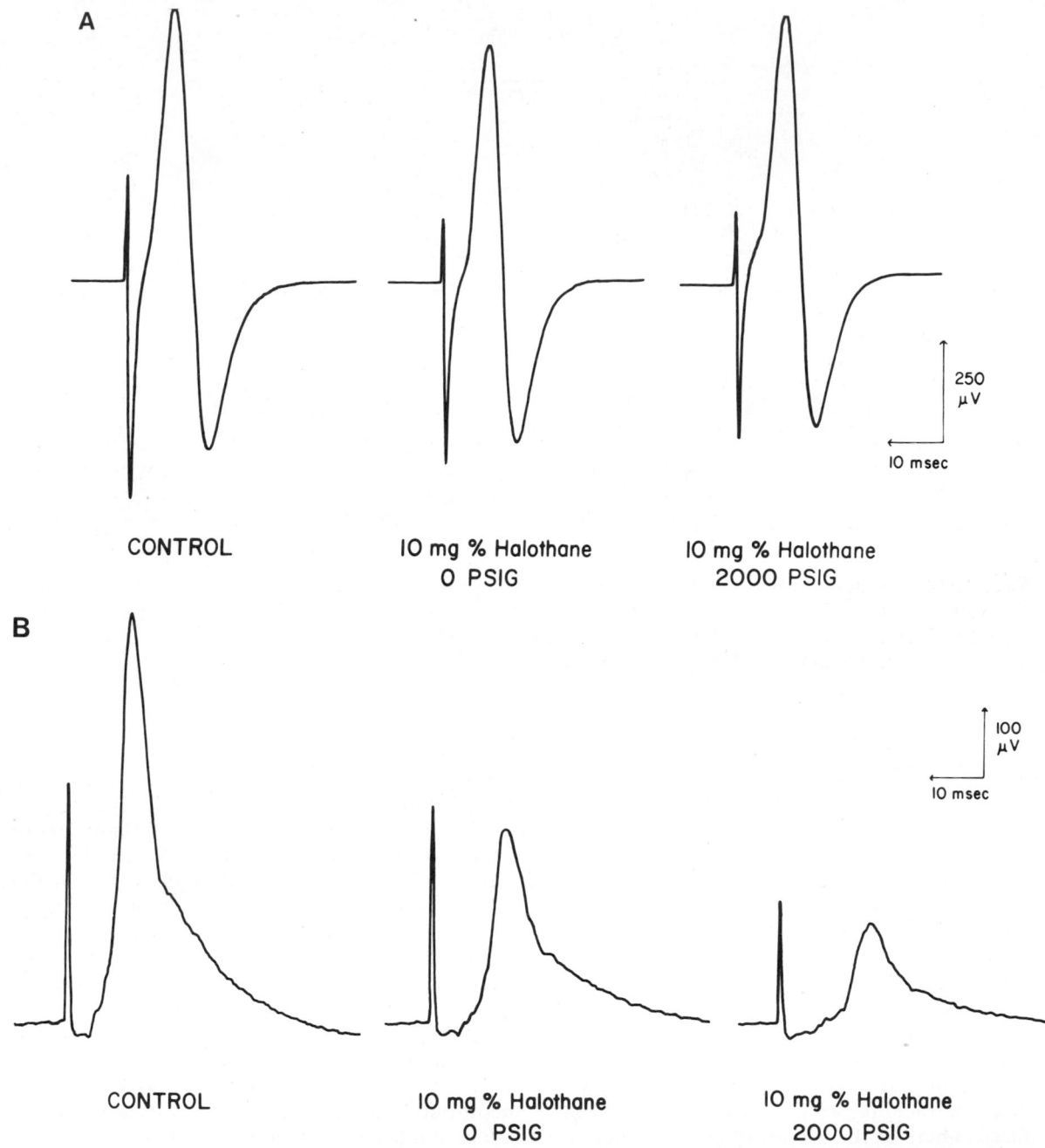

Fig. 3-6. **(A)** Halothane reduces the amplitude of the action potential measured in the preganglionic nerve from the superior cervical ganglion of the rat. The effect is reversed by the application of 2,000 psig (136 atm). **(B)** Recordings of the postganglionic action potential show that halothane depresses synaptic transmission and that high pressures add to this effect. (From Kendig et al.,[54] with permission.)

block.[60,61] However, at frequencies above 10 Hz, conduction block by halothane, methoxyflurane, and diethyl ether progressively increases, that is, it is use dependent.[61] Moreover, the branch points of axons exhibit a further increase in sensitivity to high-frequency conduction block.[62] This increased sensitivity may play a role in the mechanism of anesthesia, since even in the

absence of frank conduction block, partial or complete block can exist at axonal branches.[62]

Conversely, anesthetics may change the frequency pattern of firing activity. In isolated crayfish neurons, 3.5 percent atm enflurane induces irregular bursts of firing activity, halothane produces a transient increase in firing rate on initial exposure followed by a decrease in firing rate, and isoflurane only depresses the discharge rate without producing initial excitation.[63] Many of the findings in this model system mimic the clinical actions of these anesthetics.

Since high pressures antagonize anesthesia in the intact animal, the effects of pressure on axonal conduction and synaptic transmission in the presence of anesthetics may provide a clue to the cellular site of action. Compression of the isolated superior cervical ganglion of the rat by pressures of approximately 100 atm reverses the small depression of the compound action potential amplitudes in preganglionic sympathetic nerves treated with halothane or methoxyflurane at concentrations greater than 1.0 MAC[54] (Fig. 3-6A). By contrast, pressure alone depresses synaptic transmission and adds to the depressant effect of anesthetics (Fig. 3-6B). Thus, the results in this isolated model system imply conduction block as a possible mechanism of anesthesia, rather than blockade of excitatory transmission. This inference assumes that pressure produces its antagonism by acting at the same site at which the anesthetics produce their effect. However, this may not be the case. Evidence is available to explain the pressure reversal of anesthesia on an indirect basis, with pressure enhancing tetanic potentiation during repetitive stimulation of neurons.[64]

Synapses

Anesthetics may disrupt normal synaptic transmission by interfering with the release of neurotransmitter from the presynaptic nerve terminals into the synaptic cleft, by altering the reuptake of neurotransmitter following its release, by changing the binding of neurotransmitter to receptor sites on the postsynaptic membrane, or by influencing the ionic conductance change that follows activation of the postsynaptic receptor by neurotransmitter.[65]

Presynaptic Action

Intracellular recordings from lumbosacral motor neurons suggest a presynaptic site of diethyl ether action.[66] Ether decreases monosynaptic excitatory postsynaptic potentials evoked by impulses in single Ia afferent fibers but does not affect the postsynaptic potential change produced by one transmitter quantum.[66] These findings imply that ether presynaptically depresses excitatory transmitter release without altering the chemosensitivity of the postsynaptic membrane. However, in an in vitro preparation of the stellate ganglion of the cat, 1 to 2 percent atm halothane decreased acetylcholine release during low levels of synaptic transmission, but also seemed to produce a postsynaptic decrease in sensitivity to acetylcholine.[67]

Halothane decreases the release of norepinephrine from the guinea pig vas deferens secondary to hypogastric nerve stimulation.[68] Similarly, halothane (0.75 percent atm) inhibits release of norepinephrine from postganglionic sympathetic nerve endings located in the wall of the saphenous vein of dogs.[69] Halothane inhibits norepinephrine output evoked by activation of sympathetic nerve terminals in the heart[70] and in the adrenal medulla.[71,72] Cyclopropane inhibits agonist-induced release of catecholamines from the adrenal medulla but has no effect on spontaneous release.[73] In rat brain striatal slices, halothane decreases the release of dopamine following the application of a nicotinic agonist.[74]

In contrast to the above inhibitory effects on neurotransmitter release, inhaled agents may also promote the release of neurotransmitters. Nitrous oxide increases norepinephrine release from the pulmonary artery of the dog.[75] Halothane increases the release of GABA in the dorsal raphe nucleus of the cat.[76] Gaseous anesthetics increase both spontaneous and electrically evoked release of acetylcholine in the isolated guinea pig ileum preparation.[77] These increases in acetylcholine output are not reversed by adding helium to a total pressure of 136 atm, a pressure that reverses their anesthetic effect in vivo.[77]

In addition to an effect on the presynaptic release of neurotransmitters, it is conceivable that inhaled anesthetics may alter the duration of neurotransmitter action by influencing the reuptake of neurotransmitter into the nerve terminal. Halothane, isoflurane, and enflurane inhibit the uptake of 5-hydroxytryptamine by rat brain synaptosomes in a concentration-dependent manner.[78]

Postsynaptic Action

Evidence is also available for postsynaptic effects of inhaled anesthetics. Postsynaptic sites of anesthetic action may be studied by iontophoretic application of putative neurotransmitters thought to act directly on postsynaptic membrane receptors. Depending on the particular neuronal preparation and neurotransmitter examined, anesthetics may depress or enhance the postsynaptic response. For example, concentrations of ether that depress synaptic transmission depress the sensitivity of guinea pig olfactory cortical neurons[79] but increase the response of cortical neurons in cats[80] to the iontophoretic application of L-glutamate. In contrast, ether (and other volatile agents) augment the cortical neuron firing induced by iontophoretic application of acetylcholine to cortical neurons in the olfactory cortex of the guinea pig,[81] whereas ether reduces the response to acetylcholine in cortical neurons of cats.[80]

Inhaled anesthetics can alter the postsynaptic response at the neuromuscular junction. The ability of volatile anesthetics to depress the carbachol-induced depolarization at the end plate region of guinea pig lumbrical muscles closely correlates with their anesthetic potencies in humans.[82] Volatile agents increase the decay rate of endplate currents and decrease the amplitude of endplate potentials generated by glutamate at the crayfish neuromuscular junction[83] or by acetylcholine at the mouse diaphragm[84] (Fig. 3-7).

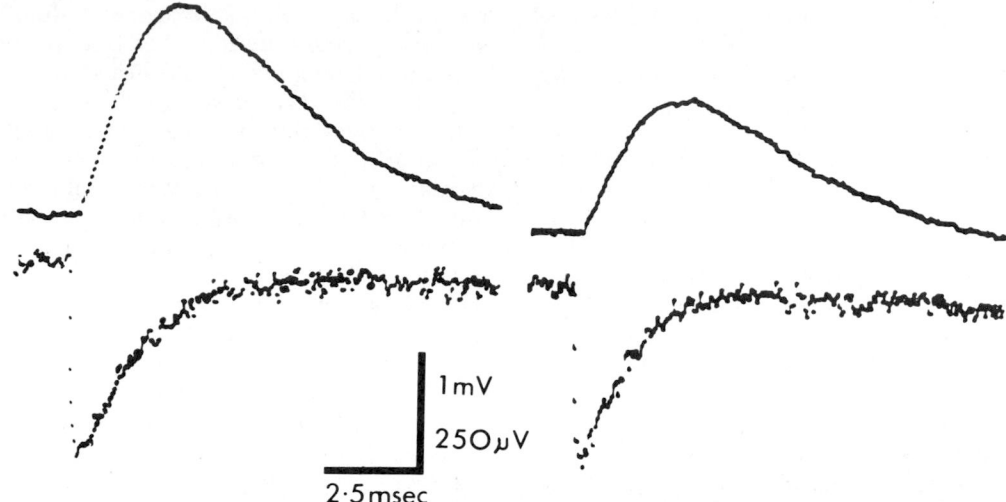

Fig. 3-7. Halothane (1 mM) reduces the amplitude of miniature endplate potentials (upper traces) by reducing the time constant of decay of miniature endplate currents (lower traces). Records are shown in control solution **(A)** and in 1 mM halothane **(B)**. (From Gage and Hamill,[291] with permission.)

Monosynaptic versus Polysynaptic Pathways

If anesthetics act by blocking synaptic transmission, it might be assumed that polysynaptic pathways would be more susceptible to anesthetic blockade than monosynaptic pathways, as the probability of blockade could increase with the number of connections. However, inhaled agents depress equally monosynaptic and polysynaptic responses recorded from the ventral root of the spinal cord[42,66] and may even depress the monosynaptic response to a greater extent.[85] Thus, the safety factor for transmission during anesthesia along a chain of neurons does not seem to be a function of synaptic chain length.

In summary, inhaled anesthetics act on synaptic regions, including afferent axons at the nerve terminal. Inhaled agents alter axonal and synaptic transmission in isolated neuronal systems and may have both presynaptic and postsynaptic effects. Clinical concentrations of inhaled agents can depress, leave unchanged, or enhance presynaptic neurotransmitter release and the postsynaptic response. The effect depends on the preparation, the frequency of neuronal transmission, the particular neurotransmitter, and the anesthetic examined.

ALTERATIONS IN NEUROREGULATORS ASSOCIATED WITH ANESTHESIA

The list of CNS transmitters and their subtypes is rapidly expanding. In addition to the "classical" transmitters (e.g., acetylcholine), endogenous amino acids and peptides may act as neurotransmitters or modulate the action of other neurotransmitters. Furthermore, the postsynaptic action of neurotransmitters may result in the formation of second messengers that mediate changes in neuronal transmission. Limited information is available concerning the relationship between the levels of neuroregulators in CNS and inhaled anesthetic requirement.

Acetylcholine

Neither halothane nor enflurane alters acetylcholine concentrations in rat brain.[86] However, these agents do decrease acetylcholine turnover rate, and the magnitude of this decrease varies with the region of the brain examined.[86] Synthesis of acetylcholine in rat brain is impaired by 70 percent nitrous oxide[87] or 3 percent atm halothane.[88]

Catecholamines

Rats anesthetized with halothane or cyclopropane have unaltered norepinephrine concentrations in most brain regions but may have an elevated norepinephrine content in the nucleus accumbens, locus ceruleus, and central gray catecholamine areas.[89] Although anesthesia does not deplete brain norepinephrine, a change in norepinephrine availability significantly influences anesthetic requirement. Drugs that decrease central levels of norepinephrine result in a dose-related decrease in halothane MAC, whereas agents that elevate central norepinephrine levels increase anesthetic requirement.[90] The ablation of certain norepinephrine-rich brain stem areas in rats lowers MAC by 16 to 35 percent compared with that in sham-operated littermate controls.[91]

In contrast to norepinephrine, central levels of dopamine appear to be inversely related to anesthetic requirement. Administration of levodopa to mice increases striatal dopamine content and produces a dose-dependent decrease in halothane MAC.[92] Conversely, chemical destruction of dopaminergic neurons lowers dopamine content and increases halothane MAC.[92]

The administration of α-adrenergic agonists markedly lowers anesthetic requirements. Clonidine (5 μg/kg) decreases halothane MAC by 42 percent in dogs.[93] D-Medetomidine, an agonist that is more selective for the α_2-adrenoreceptor than clonidine, produces a remarkable decrease in halothane MAC in dogs to less than 10 percent of the control value[94] (Fig. 3-8). This effect appears to be highly specific for the α_2-adrenoreceptor since the optical isomer L-medetomidine did not alter halothane MAC (Fig. 3-8). The lowering of anesthetic requirement by α_2-agonists may be mediated presynaptically by decreasing norepinephrine release and postsynaptically by depressing neuronal excitation.[94]

Serotonin

Serotonin levels are unaltered in most brain regions of rats anesthetized with halothane or cyclopropane but may increase in specific brain structures (e.g., substantia nigra, nucleus raphe dorsalis).[95] Destruction of the serotonin-rich nucleus raphe dorsalis in rats decreases anesthetic requirement by as much as 25 percent.[91]

γ-Aminobutyric Acid

Treatment of rat cerebral cortex slices with 3 percent atm halothane inhibits the metabolism of and increases the content of the inhibitory transmitter GABA but does not affect the uptake or release of GABA.[96] If the accumulation of GABA in inhibitory neurons is associated with an increase in inhibitory activity, the resulting decrease in synaptic transmission might contribute to the anesthetic state.[96] The finding that a GABA analog, THIP, crosses the blood-brain barrier and produces anesthesia in rodents is consistent with this hypothesis.[97]

Cyclic Nucleotides

The production of cyclic nucleotides may be influenced by neurotransmitters and anesthetics, and cyclic nucleotides may serve as second messengers in altering neurotransmission. Most studies demonstrate an increase in brain cyclic adenosine monophosphate

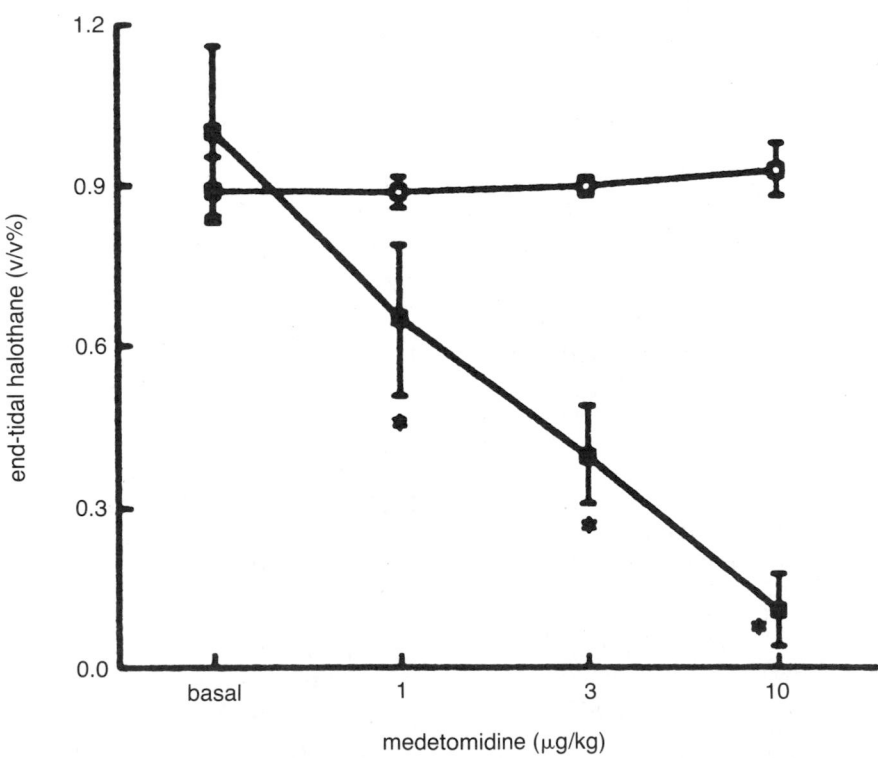

Fig. 3-8. The D stereoisomer (closed squares) of the α_2-adrenergic agonist medetomidine causes a dose-dependent decrease in halothane MAC in dogs, whereas the L stereoisomer (open squares) has little or no influence on halothane MAC. Asterisks indicate values that are significantly different from the controls. (From Vickery et al.,[94] with permission.)

(cAMP) content of rodents during the administration of volatile anesthetics, with the magnitude of the increase varying among different brain regions.[98-101] This increase in cAMP with anesthesia results, at least in part, from an anesthetic-induced activation of adenylate cyclase and inhibition of phosphodiesterase.[99,102] In contrast, levels of cyclic guanosine monophosphate (cGMP) in brain are decreased by volatile agents.[100,103] Such alterations in brain cyclic nucleotide content may chemically alter (e.g., via phosphorylation) neuronal macromolecules that are important in neurotransmission.

Endogenous Opiates

In the late 1970s, it was hypothesized that inhaled anesthetics may work through an action on the opiate receptor.[104,105] Consistent with this hypothesis, synthetic narcotics partially decrease the requirement for inhaled anesthetics in dogs[106] and rats.[107] Furthermore, the administration of naloxone (a narcotic antagonist) partially reverses the action of inhaled anesthetics when given either intravenously[104] or through the fourth cerebral ventricle.[105] However, this antagonistic effect of naloxone can be explained by a minor shift in the anesthetic dose-response curve. Anesthetic requirement, as measured by lack of response to a noxious stimulus[108-110] or by the ability to abolish the righting reflex,[111,112] is altered no more than a few percent by narcotic antagonists, even at doses of naloxone as high as 250 mg/kg.[108] The mild antagonism of inhalational anesthesia by high doses of naloxone probably results from a general increase in CNS excitation and not by pharmacologic competition for opiate receptors.[112]

Another prediction of the opiate theory of anesthesia is that inhaled agents may release an endogenous opiatelike substance in the CNS. Data are available to both support and refute this prediction. In rats, β-endorphin-like immunoreactivity increases in plasma following halothane anesthesia[113] and in the medial basal hypothalamus after brief exposure to 80 percent nitrous oxide.[114] Levels of methionine-enkephalin-like immunoreactivity may slightly increase in discrete brain regions with exposure to nitrous oxide,[115] although this is not always found.[116] In humans, plasma concentrations of β-endorphin-like or methionine-enkephalin-like immunoreactivity are reported to increase[117-119] or remain unchanged[119-121] during anesthesia with inhaled agents. There is no elevation in opioid peptides in CSF in patients anesthetized with a combination of halothane and nitrous oxide[122] or with isoflurane.[123] Thus, any contribution of the endogenous opiate system to the production of general anesthesia does not appear to require the release of opioid peptides.

Nevertheless, other experiments indicate a possible role for opiate receptors in anesthesia or analgesia. β-Endorphin administered into the cerebral ventricles of rats causes a sequence of behavioral and electroencephalographic responses similar to those produced with general anesthesia, and naloxone reverses these effects.[124] In addition, naloxone may partially antagonize the analgesic effect of nitrous oxide in rodents[125,126] and humans.[127,128] However, the antagonism of nitrous oxide-induced analgesia is not found in all studies, and there are even reports of naloxone enhancing the analgesic action of nitrous oxide.[129]

Thus, the available data concerning the role of endogenous opiates in the production of inhalational anesthesia is inconclusive. Although certain inhaled anesthetics may contribute to analgesia by releasing endogenous opiatelike compounds (or increasing the sensitivity to their effects), they do not appear to produce anesthesia by a simple action on or through an opiate receptor.

In summary, the predominant effects of inhaled anesthetics cannot at present be explained by the depletion, production, or release of a single neuromodulator in the CNS. In all likelihood, the anesthetic state involves a balance between many different neuromodulator systems.

PHYSICOCHEMICAL NATURE OF THE SITE OF ANESTHETIC ACTION

The preceding sections suggest that anesthetics may act at several gross (e.g., spinal cord versus reticular activating system) or microscopic (e.g., presynaptic versus postsynaptic) sites. The varied nature of these sites, however, does not preclude a unique action at a molecular level. For instance, depression of presynaptic neurotransmitter release and blockade of current flow through the postsynaptic membrane may arise from an anesthetic perturbation at an identical molecular site, even though the geographic locations of these sites differ. The thought that all inhaled anesthetics have a common mode of action on a specific molecular structure is called the *unitary theory of narcosis.* The nature of this presumed common site has been explored by correlating the physical properties of anesthetics with their potencies. The rationale behind this approach is that the best correlation between anesthetic potency and a physical property will suggest the nature of the anesthetic site of action. For example, the correlation of MAC and lipid solubility implies that the site of action is hydrophobic. Note that the correlations that depend on forces exerted between anesthetic molecules (e.g., the boiling point of an anesthetic) are not important to the study of anesthetic mechanisms, as such intermolecular forces cannot be representative of a single site of action. That is, such correlations are defined by the interaction of each anesthetic with itself rather than with a common site.

Hydrophobic Site: The Meyer-Overton Rule

The physical property that correlates best with anesthetic potency is lipid solubility[130-133] (Table 3-2 and Fig. 3-9). This correlation is termed the *Meyer-Overton rule,* after its two discoverers. The product of the an-

TABLE 3-2. Oil/Gas Partition Coefficients and Potencies of Inhaled Anesthetics in Dogs, Humans, and Mice

Anesthetic	Oil/Gas Partition Coefficient (37°C)	Dogs		Humans		Mice	
		MAC (atm)	MAC × Oil/Gas (atm)	MAC (atm)	MAC × Oil/Gas (atm)	Righting-Reflex ED$_{50}$ (atm)	Righting-Reflex ED$_{50}$ × Oil/Gas (atm)
Thiomethoxyflurane	7,230[a]	0.00035[a]	2.53				
Methoxyflurane	970[b]	0.0023[c]	2.23	0.0016[c]	1.55	0.0023[d]	2.23
Dioxychlorane	1,286[e]	0.0011[e]	1.41			0.0033[f]	4.24
Chloroform	265[b]	0.0077[c]	2.08			0.00357[g]	0.95
Halothane	224[b]	0.0087[c]	1.95	0.0074[c]	1.66	0.00645[g]	1.45
Enflurane	96.5[h]	0.0267[h]	2.58	0.0168[c]	1.62	0.0123[g]	1.19
Isoflurane	90.8[h]	0.0141[h]	1.28	0.0115[c]	1.04	0.00663[g]	0.60
Compound 485[h]	25.8[h]	0.125[h]	3.23				
I-653	18.7[i]	0.072[j]	1.35	0.0458[k]	0.86		
HFClCOCHFCF$_3$[h]	96.6[h]	0.0224[h]	2.16				
Iso-Indoklon	27.0[l]	0.460[l]	1.24			0.0255[l]	0.72
Aliflurane	124[m]	0.0184[m]	2.28				
Synthane	95[n]	0.012[n]	1.14				
Diethyl ether	65[b]	0.0304[c]	1.98	0.0192[c]	1.25	0.032[c]	2.08
Fluroxene	47.7[b]	0.0599[c]	2.86	0.034[c]	1.62	0.0345[o]	1.65
Sevoflurane	47.2[p]	0.0236[q]	1.11	0.0205[r]	0.97		
Cyclopropane	11.8[b]	0.175[c]	2.06	0.092[c]	1.09	0.142[g]	1.68
Xenon	1.9[b]	1.19[c]	2.26	0.71[c]	1.35	0.95[s]	1.80
Ethylene	1.26[b]			0.67[c]	0.84	1.30[o]	1.64
Nitrous oxide	1.4[b]	1.88[c]	2.63	1.04[t]	1.46	1.54[g]	2.16
Krypton	0.5[b]					4.5[s]	2.25
Sulfur hexafluoride	0.293[b]	4.9[c]	1.44			5.4[s]	1.58
Argon	0.15[b]					15.2[s]	2.28
Hexafluoroethane	0.126[b]					17.7[s]	2.23
Carbon tetrafluoride	0.073[b]	26[c]	1.90			18.7[u]	1.36
Nitrogen	0.072[b]	≥43.5[v]	≥3.13			34.3[u]	2.47
Mean ± standard error			2.04 ± 0.14		1.28 ± 0.09		1.82 ± 0.18

[a]Ref. 277; [b]ref. 278; [c]ref. 5; [d]ref. 8; [e]ref. 279; [f]ref. 280; [g]ref. 7; [h]ref. 144; [i]ref. 28 i;[j]ref. 282; [k]ref. 283; [l]ref. 147; [m]ref. 284; [n]ref. 285; [o]ref. 286; [p]ref. 287; [q]ref. 288; [r]ref. 289; [s]ref. 130; [t]ref. 290; [u]ref. 6; [v]ref. 163.

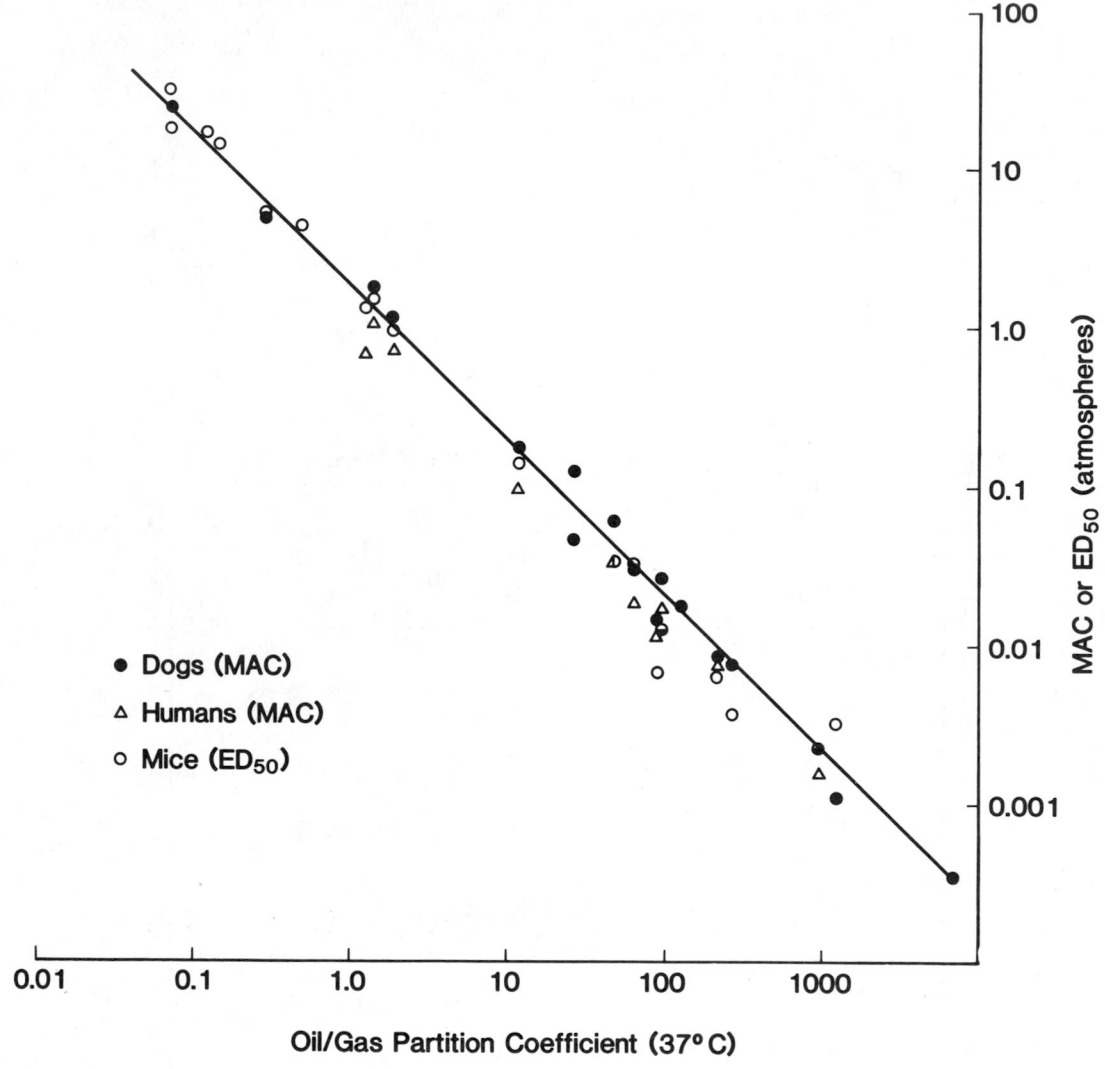

Fig. 3-9. Correlation of MAC in humans and dogs and the righting-reflex ED_{50} in mice with lipid solubility (i.e., the olive oil/gas partition coefficient.) Values are taken from Table 3-2.

esthetizing partial pressure of an inhaled agent and its olive oil/gas partition coefficient varies little over approximately a 100,000-fold range of anesthetizing partial pressures (Table 3-2, Fig. 3-9). For the correlation to be perfect, this product would have to be the same for all anesthetics for a given animal. Within a given species, the product of anesthetizing partial pressure and oil/gas partition coefficient varies only slightly. The product tends to be somewhat lower in humans (1.28 ± 0.09 atm) than in dogs (2.04 ± 0.14 atm) or mice (1.82 ± 0.18 atm for righting-reflex ED_{50}) (Table 3-2). The amazing closeness of this correlation implies a unitary molecular site of action and suggests that anesthesia results when a specific number of anesthetic molecules occupy a crucial hydrophobic region in the CNS. No other correlation employing the complete spectrum of inhaled agents approaches the excellent fit of that observed between anesthetic potency and lipid solubility. This finding has led many investigators to look for the molecular basis of anesthetic action in cellular hydrophobic regions.

Further Characterization of the Hydrophobic Site of Anesthetic Action

The correlation of potency to solubility in olive oil (Fig. 3-9 and Table 3-2) suggests that olive oil closely mimics the anesthetic site of action and that anesthesia occurs when a critical anesthetic concentration is attained at that site. However, since olive oil is a mixture of oils and is not very well characterized from a physicochemical point of view, attempts have been made to examine anesthetic solubility in simpler solvents to better define the nature of the site of anesthetic action. A pure solvent may be characterized by a solubility parameter, which is a measure of the intermolecular forces in that solvent.[130] Anesthetic potency correlates best with solubility in solvents having solubility parameters of about 8 to 11 (calories/cm^3)$^{1/2}$.[130,134] These values are representative of a solvent such as benzene and again imply a hydrophobic site of anesthetic action.

Franks and Lieb[135,136] have stated that an even better correlation between anesthetic potency and solubility is obtained when octanol, having a solubility parameter of approximately 10 (calories/cm^3)$^{1/2}$, is used as the model solvent. However, the improved correlation with octanol as the model solvent resulted from the inclusion of alcohols in the analyses.[135] For the inhaled anesthetics, the correlations between anesthetic potency in olive oil and octanol are essentially equivalent, suggesting either a hydrophobic or a combined polar and hydrophobic (i.e., amphipathic) site of anesthetic action.

Additive Effects of Inhaled Anesthetics

The Meyer-Overton rule postulates that it is the number of molecules dissolved at the site of anesthetic action, and not the types of molecules present, that causes anesthesia. Thus, 0.5 MAC of one agent and 0.5 MAC of another agent should have the same effect as 1.0 MAC of either agent. In general, this prediction has been confirmed in animals and humans.[1,137-141] In addition, binary combinations of methoxyflurane, halothane, enflurane, and trichloroethylene have an additive effect on evoked cortical responses in rats.[142] Nevertheless, slight antagonistic effects have been noted with nitrous oxide-containing mixtures in rats.[138,143] Furthermore, the administration of compound 485 (Fig. 3-1) produced a nonlinear decrease in the fraction of isoflurane MAC required to produce anesthesia in dogs,[144] indicating that the effect of isoflurane and compound 485 may be antagonistic. Such an antagonism might result from the convulsive activity of compound 485.[144] Overall, however, the evidence to date is consistent with an additive effect of anesthetics in whole organisms.

Apparent Exceptions to the Meyer-Overton Rule

Minor Deviations

Despite the close correlation between lipid solubility and anesthetic potency, deviations from this correlation do exist. For example, enflurane and isoflurane are structural isomers having approximately the same oil/gas partition coefficient, yet the anesthetic requirement for enflurane is 45 to 90 percent greater than that for isoflurane (Table 3-2). These differences in anesthetic requirements for agents having similar oil/gas partition coefficients suggest that the potency of an agent may depend on factors other than lipid solubility. One of these factors may be the convulsive properties of an agent. The possession of convulsive properties (e.g., as seen with enflurane) may oppose the anesthetic properties and increase the anesthetic requirement.

Convulsant Gases

Another apparent exception to the Meyer-Overton rule is the ability of certain lipid-soluble compounds to produce convulsions. Indeed, complete halogenation (or full halogenation of the end methyl groups) of alkanes and ethers tends to decrease the anesthetic potencies of these agents and to enhance convulsant activity.[145,146] For flurothyl ($CF_3CH_2OCH_2CF_3$), convulsions are produced in 50 percent of mice at a concentration of 0.122 percent atm.[147] However, higher concentrations of flurothyl have an anesthetic effect, and an ED_{50} for loss of the righting reflex is obtained at a flurothyl concentration of 1.22 percent atm.[147] The product of the oil/gas partition coefficient of flurothyl (46.9) and the righting-reflex ED_{50} in mice is 0.57 atm, a value that is close to but somewhat lower than the value for the conventional anesthetics (Table 3-2). Similarly, there is a biphasic pattern to the convulsive properties of enflurane in cats, with maximal seizure activity occurring between 3 and 4 percent atm enflurane and less seizure activity occurring both above and below this range of concentrations.[148]

Compound 485 (Fig. 3-1) possesses completely halogenated methyl groups and is a structural isomer of enflurane and isoflurane. It occasionally produced convulsions in dogs at concentrations near 6 percent atm.[144] As an isomer of enflurane and isoflurane, it was predicted to have a similar potency and solubility characteristics; however, its MAC was found to be 12.5 percent atm. This high value was balanced by a low oil/gas partition coefficient of 25.8 (approximately four times lower than the value for isoflurane or enflurane), again yielding a product (3.23 atm) similar to but slightly greater than that for other inhaled agents[144] (Table 3-2).

Oxygen is a convulsant gas at pressures of approximately 3 atm, with higher pressures producing a state very similar to anesthesia.[149] The product of its ED_{50} in mice (5.3 atm) and the oil/gas partition coefficient for oxygen (0.132) is 0.70 atm, a value that is also comparable to that for other anesthetics (Table 3-2).

Thus, the convulsant gases provide minor deviations from, but not marked exceptions to, the correlation between anesthetic potency and lipid solubility. Convulsant halogenated ethers may have different physical properties from the anesthetic halogenated ethers, since the convulsants are characterized by a low solubility parameter.[150] For example, flurothyl has a solubility parameter of 6.9, whereas the anesthetic halogenated ethers have values of approximately 8.0.[150] Furthermore, halogenated compounds that are anesthetics and convulsants may have different effects on synaptic transmission. Anesthetic agents block the excitatory glutamate response but not inhibitory transmission mediated by GABA at the crab neuromuscular junction, whereas convulsant agents block inhibitory but not excitatory transmission.[151] (However, both anesthetics and convulsants have a depressant effect on the postsynaptic action of acetylcholine.[152,153]) It has been speculated that the molecular microenvironment of the subregion that controls excitation has a different solubility parameter than the subregion involved with inhibitory transmission and that the different physiologic effects of the inhaled anesthetics and convulsants may be related to a differential distribution of these drugs in these subregions.[154]

Cutoff Effect

The highly lipid-soluble *n*-decane is nonanesthetic in animals, even though lower paraffin homologs such as *n*-pentane cause anesthesia.[155] Similarly, *n*-pentane is more potent in suppressing conduction in an isolated nerve than is its more lipid-soluble homolog *n*-octane.[56,156] This decrease in anesthetic potency in the higher members of a homologous series is known as the *cutoff effect* and is a characteristic that is not compatible with the Meyer-Overton rule. One postulate is that this phenomenon occurs because *n*-decane is too large to fit into the anesthetic site.[155] Another possibility is that the cutoff in potency with higher alkane homologs is due to limited solubilities of these anesthetics at the anesthetic site of action.[157] However, experimental evidence is available that disfavors the latter alternative.[158] Any unitary theory of narcosis involving a single hydrophobic site of action must eventually explain why such lipid-soluble compounds are not anesthetics.

Specific Receptors

As mentioned in the above section on neuroregulators, the administration of certain receptor-specific agonists can alter anesthetic requirement. Studies with a leucine enkephalin analogue indicate a possible dual mechanism of anesthetic action: one having an opiate receptor-specific mechanism that is reversible by an opiate antagonist, and the other having a nonspecific mechanism related to lipid solubility that is reversible with the application of high pressure.[159] This suggestion is consistent with the calculated levels in brain lipid of four synthetic narcotics (fentanyl, alfentanil, sufentanil, morphine) required to produce a 50 percent reduction in MAC in animals or a 50 percent reduction in maximal spectral edge frequency derived from the electroencephalogram in humans.[160] Although serum levels of these four narcotics associated with either endpoint of the anesthetic effect may vary by more than 5,000-fold, levels of these narcotics in brain lipid fall within a 10-fold range.[160] Thus, the sparing of inhaled anesthetic requirement by opiates may involve a hydrophobic site of action in addition to an action on specific receptors.

A greater challenge to the Meyer-Overton rule is presented by the marked decrease in anesthetic requirement caused by the α_2-agonist D-medetomidine[94] (Fig. 3-8). Its optical isomer, L-medetomidine, has an identical lipid solubility but has no effect on the potency of inhaled anesthetics (Fig. 3-8). Therefore, the sparing of anesthetic requirement by the D isomer is probably not mediated through an action at a nonspecific hydrophobic site.

Hydrophilic Site

Some investigators believe that the anesthetic site of action is not necessarily hydrophobic. For example, both Pauling[161] and Miller[162] suggested that anesthesia might be caused by the ability of anesthetics to precipitate the formation of hydrates. These hydrates are cage-like structures of water molecules surrounding a central anesthetic molecule, and it was speculated that hydrate microcrystals could alter the transmission of electrical charge through a neuron.[161,162] However, a unitary hydrate theory of anesthesia seems unlikely since there is a poor correlation between the ability of anesthetics to form hydrates and their anesthetic potency.[130,163]

Another hypothesis is that certain inhaled anesthetics act by disrupting hydrogen bonds.[164] (This cannot be a unitary hypothesis since compounds such as xenon and argon are anesthetics but do not form hydrogen bonds.) One suggestion is that inhaled agents disrupt the hydrogen bonding of water molecules neighboring the anesthetic site of action and thereby contribute to neuronal dysfunction[165] (e.g., by altering the transfer of current-carrying hydrated ions). If hydrogen bonds are important in anesthesia, then substitution of hydrogen for deuterium atoms in anesthetic molecules might alter the hydrogen-bonding capabilities of a compound and change its anesthetic potency. However, the findings of identical anesthetic potencies of chloroform and deuterated chloroform[166] and of halothane and deuterated halothane[167] do not support this prediction.

Volume Expansion by Inhaled Anesthetics

Although the Meyer-Overton rule postulates that anesthesia occurs when a sufficient number of anesthetic molecules dissolve at a certain site, it does not explain why anesthesia results. Mullins[134] took the lipid solubility correlation one step further and hypothesized that anesthesia occurs when the absorption of anesthetic molecules expands the volume of a hydrophobic region beyond a critical amount (critical volume hypothesis). Such an expansion might produce anesthesia by obstructing ion channels or by altering the electrical properties of neurons.

The volume expansion hypothesis of anesthetic action suggested several experiments. One prediction of the hypothesis was that anesthetizing partial pressures of inhaled agents should produce a consistent volume expansion in a model hydrophobic system. Indeed, anesthetizing doses of inhaled agents cause hydrophobic solvents to undergo a significant increase in volume.[168] The hypothesis also predicts that anesthesia should be reversed by compressing the volume of the expanded hydrophobic region, and high pressures do reverse many effects of anesthetics in vivo.[13-16,169] In addition, the critical volume theory is consistent with the observations that helium and neon, gases having low lipid solubilities, are not anesthetics. It also explains why hydrogen is not as potent as its lipid solubility-anesthetic potency correlation would predict; that is, the expansion caused by these agents is counterbalanced by the compression resulting from their high pressures.[13,15,17,169]

The critical volume hypothesis also suggests that a decrease in body temperature should antagonize the effect of anesthesia by contracting the volume of the expanded hydrophobic region. However, MAC does not increase but rather decreases as temperature decreases.[4,10-12] Although this fact seemingly contradicts the critical volume hypothesis, this prediction is complicated by the increased partitioning of anesthetics into nonpolar substances at decreased temperatures and the uncertainty of the effects of temperature per se on the organism.

Other arguments against the critical volume hypothesis include the finding of a nonlinear pressure antagonism for certain anesthetics and the fact that not all lipid-soluble compounds are anesthetics. These results have led to a *multisite expansion hypothesis*, which holds that general anesthesia results from expansion of several hydrophobic molecular sites, each having a finite size and somewhat different physical properties.[170] In sum, the critical volume hypothesis is a useful model for estimating the interactions between pressure and inhaled anesthetics, but it is probably an oversimplified view of the way in which anesthetics act.

THE MEMBRANE AS THE SITE OF ANESTHETIC ACTION

The electrical activity (i.e., transfer of ions) immediately underlying the transmission of nervous impulses occurs principally at the plasma membranes of nerves. Since inhaled agents disrupt this transmission, synaptic and/or axonal membranes are usually assumed to be the primary sites of anesthetic action. A membrane site of action is also consistent with the hydrophobic theories of anesthesia, since plasma membranes consist largely of hydrophobic components.

Electrophysiologic studies reveal the effects of anesthetics on the flow of ions through excitable membranes. In isolated axons, the conduction of the nervous impulse requires the sequential flow of sodium and potassium ions through selective transmembrane channels. Excitation produces a rapid increase in sodium conductance to a peak (the activation process) followed by a slower decline in sodium conductance to zero (the inactivation process). Inhaled anesthetics (al-

beit at relatively high concentrations) may decrease the magnitude of both sodium and potassium currents in isolated axons.[171] With recent advances in technology, electrophysiologic recordings of single membrane channels can now be obtained by forming a seal between the tip of a glass micropipette and a membrane patch of a few square micrometers. Using this "patch clamp" technique, unitary acetylcholine receptor channel currents have been measured in cultured cells in the absence and presence of isoflurane (Fig. 3-10).[172] Isoflurane decreases the average open duration of this membrane channel, and such an accelerated decay of the membrane current may decrease the net charge transferred across the membrane and impair transmission (Fig. 3-10).[172]

In contrast to the inhibitory effects of anesthetics on ion flow through membranes described above, other experiments suggest that anesthetics act by enhancing the conductance of certain ions through membranes. Inhaled agents hyperpolarize rat hippocampal[173] and human cortical[34] neurons, and this hyperpolarization may be related to an increase in potassium conductance.[34,173] Indeed, molluscan neurons that are highly sensitive to volatile agents (Fig. 3-5) exhibit a halothane-induced activation of potassium current that is associated with a marked hyperpolarization of the cell membrane and an inability to initiate firing of action potentials.[49] Moreover, it has been speculated that the sparing of inhaled anesthetic requirement by α_2-agonists (Fig. 3-8) may be related to their ability to bind to postsynaptic sites, increase potassium conductance, and induce hyperpolarization with consequent depression of neuronal excitability.[94]

The requirement of an intact plasma membrane for the transmission of nervous impulses and the abilities of anesthetics to disrupt the flow of ions through plasma membranes point to a membrane site of anesthetic action. Nevertheless, anesthetics could act indirectly at a cytoplasmic site. For example, anesthetics might alter the calcium-accumulating activity of cellular organelles (e.g., mitochondria[174]) and thereby alter the levels of intracellular free calcium. Such alterations in intracellular free calcium could in turn influence the conductance properties of excitable membranes and alter the presynaptic release of neurotransmitters.[80,175] Other cytoplasmic structures (e.g., microtubules) might have a linkage to the plasma membrane, and the reversible depolymerization of microtubules and microfilaments has been suggested as a mechanism of anesthetic action. However, not all inhaled anesthetics depolymerize microtubules.[176]

The above discussion suggests, but does not prove, that anesthesia results from an association of inhaled agents with plasma membranes of nerves. If so, which components of the plasma membrane are altered by the anesthetics? Biologic membranes consist of a cholesterol–phospholipid bilayer matrix having a thickness of approximately 4 nm. Peripheral proteins

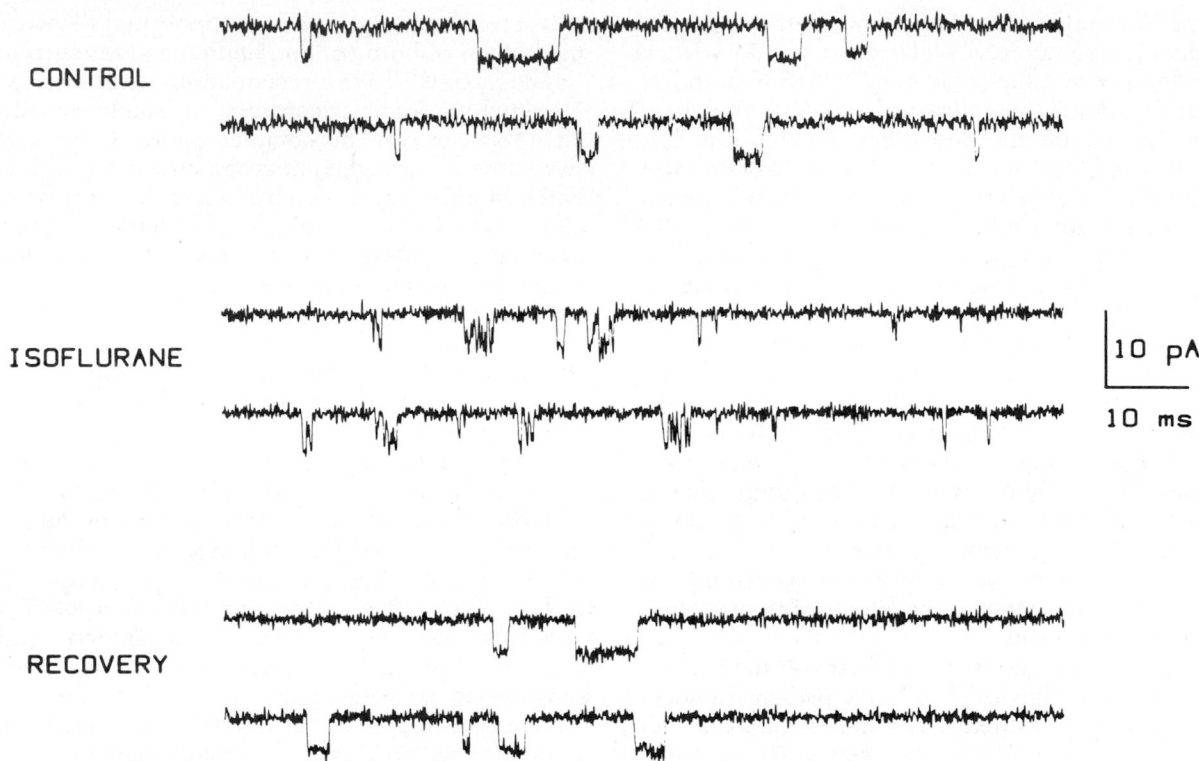

CONTROL

ISOFLURANE

RECOVERY

10 pA

10 ms

Fig. 3-10. Examples of unitary acetylcholine receptor channel currents before, during, and after local microperfusion with 5 mM isoflurane. Channel openings are represented by downward directions of the current trace. When isoflurane is removed (bottom panel), the channels are indistinguishable from those observed under control conditions. (From Brett et al.,[172] with permission.)

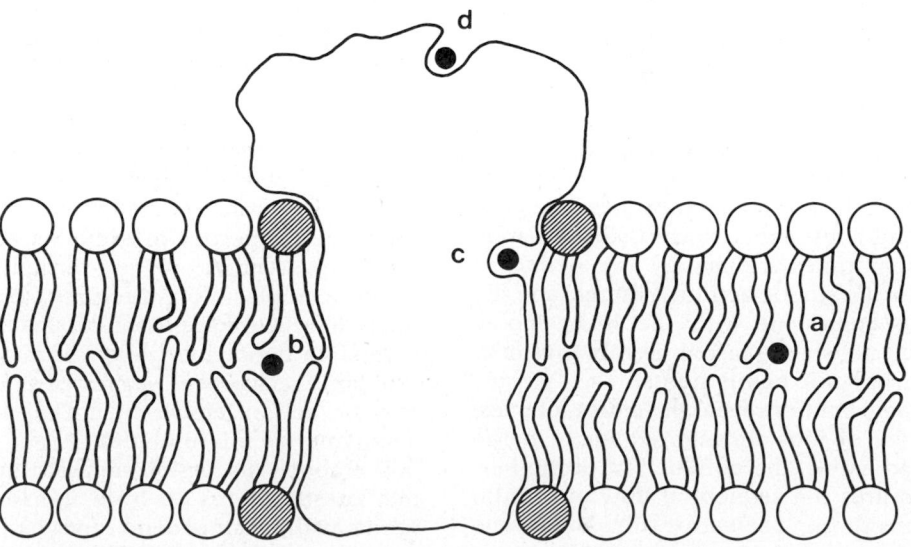

Fig. 3-11. Four possible target sites for inhaled anesthetic molecules (●) in a neuronal membrane include *(a)* the lipid bilayer as a whole, *(b)* lipids at a protein/lipid interface, *(c)* a protein site bounded by lipid, and *(d)* a protein site exposed to an aqueous environment. (From Franks and Lieb,[133] with permission.)

are weakly bound to the exterior hydrophilic membrane and integral proteins are deeply embedded in, or pass through, the lipid bilayer (Fig. 3-11). Synaptic plasma membranes are approximately 50 percent protein and 50 percent lipid by weight. If (as implied by the Meyer-Overton rule) inhaled agents bind to hydrophobic sites, anesthetics could act on the nonpolar interior of the lipid bilayer, at hydrophobic pockets in proteins extending outside or embedded into the lipid bilayer, or at the hydrophobic interface between intrinsic membrane proteins and the lipid matrix (Fig. 3-11).

Attempts to better understand the penetration of inhaled agents into, and their interaction with, membrane sites have led to an examination of isolated membrane components. These experiments were greatly aided by the discovery that phospholipids dispersed in an aqueous medium spontaneously form bilayers composing the surface of spherical structures (liposomes). These phospholipid bilayers act as a permeability barrier to ions and are similar to those found in biomembranes.[177] Liposomes have been extensively employed as model systems for the study of interactions between anesthetics and membrane lipids. In contrast, membrane proteins are often difficult to isolate and purify, and certain membrane proteins may exhibit an impaired function unless surrounded by a boundary layer of lipid. Nevertheless, recent advances have resulted in the biochemical characterization of several protein ionophores thought to permit the passage (tunneling) of ions through membranes during excitation.[178] However, only limited information is available concerning the interaction of inhaled agents with these membrane protein ionophores, and many experiments that examine anesthetic–protein interactions employ soluble proteins as model systems. Such proteins are easy to prepare in reasonable quantities but may not mimic precisely the natural proteins responsible for ion translocation.

INTERACTION OF INHALED ANESTHETICS WITH MEMBRANE LIPIDS

Binding of Anesthetics to Membrane Lipids

The solubility of gaseous and volatile agents in phospholipid bilayers correlates with their anesthetic potency. This correlation is at least as good as that obtained when olive oil is the model solvent.[157,179] The incorporation of cholesterol into phospholipid model membranes decreases the partitioning of inhaled agents but does not alter the good correlation between anesthetic potency and lipid membrane solubility.[157,179] The degree of saturation of lipid acyl chains[180] or the length of the acyl chains[181] has little effect on the partition coefficient. On the other hand, a decrease in temperature increases the partition coefficients of all agents, with the exception of carbon tetrafluoride.[157,179] Partitioning of inhaled anesthetics in lipid bilayers may increase as anesthetic concentrations increase.[182] At anesthetic concentrations close to 1.0 MAC, lipid membranes may contain as many as 80 phospholipid molecules for every anesthetic molecule.[133]

The interaction of inhaled agents with membrane lipids is a dynamic process, and anesthetic molecules may rapidly exchange between the membrane and aqueous phases.[183,184] Anesthetics may penetrate all depths of the lipid bilayer.[183] They may accumulate in the center of the bilayer[185] or may preferentially lodge at the polar head group region of a phospholipid membrane.[186] Thus, the precise location at which anesthetics bind in the lipid membrane is not known with certainty and may depend in part on the individual characteristics of the anesthetic or lipid composition of the bilayer examined.[187]

Effects on Membrane Permeability

Liposomes prepared in a salt solution entrap ions. The untrapped ions exterior to the liposomes can be removed, and the subsequent flux of ions from the interior to the exterior can be measured. Inhaled agents increase the cation permeability of liposomes in a dose-related manner.[188-190] These anesthetic-induced increases in cation permeability occur both in the presence of ionophores that facilitate the transport of ions through membranes and in the absence of ionophores.[188-190] Although all agents increase cation permeability, the magnitude of the increase depends on the lipid composition of the liposome and on the anesthetic examined.[188] The anesthetic-induced increases in cation permeability are reversed by the application of high pressures (approximately 100 atm).[188] This reversibility parallels the antagonism observed between anesthesia and pressure in vivo.

Inhaled anesthetics also increase the flow of protons across lipid vesicles.[190] The rate of proton transfer across the membrane may depend on lipid composition. The transfer of protons across liposomes with a cholesterol/phospholipid ratio of 1:2 is greater than that for liposomes prepared from phospholipids alone, whereas proton transfer across liposomes with a 1:1 cholesterol/phospholipid ratio is less than that for liposomes prepared from phospholipids alone.[191] It has been suggested that anesthetics act by increasing proton permeability across synaptic vesicles, collapsing the pH gradient required for retainment of catecholamines in their charged form and thereby depressing neurotransmission by releasing catecholamines from synaptic storage vesicles.[192] However, since marked depletion of brain catecholamines lowers MAC by a maximum of 40 percent (see section on neurotransmitters), this hypothesis could only partly explain the production of anesthesia.

Alterations in Membrane Dimension

Lipid monolayers adsorb inhaled agents, resulting in an increase in the lateral pressure of the monolayer that parallels the potency of the anesthetic.[193,194] This finding is consistent with the notion that anesthetics might expand membranes and exert pressure on the ionic channels needed for impulse transmission—a variation of the volume expansion theory of anesthesia—and thereby inhibit the opening or accelerate the closure of ionic channels. However, precise volume measurements show only a small (0.1 percent) expansion when suspensions of membranes in aqueous media are combined with inhaled agents at concentrations near 1.0 MAC.[195] Moreover, it has been suggested that this small volume expansion by anesthetics *(mean excess volume)* is not simply due to the volume occupied by anesthetics in the membrane but rather is caused by a combination of interactions: anesthetic molecules interacting with bulk water and water in the lipid phase, structural changes and volume changes in the lipid phase promoted by anesthetics, and anesthetic-induced changes in the interactions between lipid and water molecules.[196] Direct microscopic visualization of the erythrocyte surface shows an area of expansion ranging from 0.13 to 0.62 percent for halothane, methoxyflurane, ether, fluroxene, and isoflurane at concentrations of one to four times the MAC,[197] but long-chain alcohols that are not anesthetics also expand red cell surface area. This finding casts doubt on the role of membrane area expansion in anesthesia.[197]

It has been argued that part of the volume expansion produced by anesthetics is due to a thickening of the membrane lipid bilayer and that an anesthetic-induced increase in bilayer thickness could alter the electric field across the membrane and influence the flow of ions through membrane channels.[198] However, spectroscopic studies do not demonstrate an increase in lipid bilayer thickness by inhaled agents.[185,199] The estimated increase in membrane thickness at 0.1 atm cyclopropane (approximately 1.0 MAC in humans) is only 0.007 nm,[198] and it seems unlikely that such small changes in membrane thickness could play a role in anesthesia.

According to the critical volume hypothesis, an increase in pressure or a decrease in temperature should reverse anesthesia, because these physical changes compress membranes. However, a decrease in body temperature consistently increases anesthetic potency. This apparent contradiction is partly resolved by the increased partitioning of anesthetics into membranes at lower temperatures. Moreover, the expansion of membranes by anesthetics and an increase in temperature may not be equivalent. For example, anesthetics might expand membranes without changing thickness, and a decrease in temperature may cause a net contraction with an increase in membrane thickness.[157]

Alterations in Membrane Physical State

Further studies of the molecular changes occurring on the insertion of anesthetic molecules into lipid membranes led to the suggestion that anesthetics increase the mobility of membrane components (the fluidization theory of anesthesia).[200] Inhaled agents cause a dose-related increase in the mobility of fatty acid chains in a phospholipid bilayer.[201] High pressure reverses this "fluidization" of the bilayer,[202] a finding consistent with the previously described pressure reversal of anesthesia.

The ability of an anesthetic to *fluidize* a lipid bilayer depends on the structure of the agent examined and the composition of the lipid bilayer.[157] The incorporation of cholesterol[157] or gangliosides[203] into neutral phospholipid membranes enhances the membrane-disordering effects by a given partial pressure of inhaled anesthetic. At clinical concentrations, the increase in lipid fluidity by inhaled agents can be as small as 0.5 percent[204] or as large as 31 percent,[205] depending on the lipid system examined and the method of fluidity measurement. Moreover, the findings in model lipid membranes may not be applicable to biologic membranes. In synaptic membranes, the disordering effects of methoxyflurane and of diethyl ether (at concentrations of 2 to 5 MAC) are greater in the deeper regions of the bilayer than near the surface of the membrane.[206] Clinical concentrations of inhaled agents may actually *decrease* the fluidity of synaptic membranes.[207]

It has been suggested that even small changes in lipid fluidity may profoundly change membrane function. A 1 to 2 percent change in the fluidity structural parameter is associated with an increased efflux of cations from liposomes[189] and with an inhibition of sodium influx into mouse brain synaptosomes[208,209] and may be linked to the enhanced fusion of phospholipid vesicles promoted by inhaled agents.[210] Some investigators have speculated that the increased decay rate of postsynaptic currents (Fig. 3-7) and accelerated decay rate of open membrane channels (Fig. 3-10) caused by inhaled agents may result from an increased fluidity of the postsynaptic membrane, allowing a more rapid relaxation (i.e., return to the closed configuration) of the proteins involved in the conductance change after activation. However, incompatible with this hypothesis is the fact that hypothermia (which lessens the mobility of membrane lipids) potentiates nerve blockade by halothane[211] and that the raising of temperature does not mimic the pattern of accelerated channel-closing rates produced by an inhaled agent.[172]

Liposomes composed of a single type of phospholipid undergo a *phase transition*, that is, a sudden conversion of the lipids from a solid or gel phase to a liquid or fluid phase, as temperature increases past a critical point. Dipalmitoylphosphatidylcholine, a lecithin molecule possessing two saturated fatty acid chains 16 carbon atoms in length, undergoes a major transition at 41°C.

Clinical concentrations of halothane decrease the phase transition temperature of dipalmitoylphosphatidylcholine by about 0.5°C.[186] The composition and charge of the lipid bilayer determine the magnitude of the decrease in phase transition temperature by anesthetics, and the depression in transition temperature induced by inhaled agents can be reversed by the application of high pressure (100 atm).[212] According to one hypothesis, lipids surrounding an excitable membrane channel are normally exclusively in the more rigid gel phase, thereby helping maintain patency of the channel. It has been speculated that adding anesthetic may fluidize these lipids, impair the surrounding structural support, and allow the channel to close.[213] If a major phase transition is important in the production of anesthesia, one would predict a discontinuity in the relationship between temperature and MAC. However, there is no such discontinuity.[10]

An alternative proposal (the *lateral phase separation hypothesis*) is that the many different types of neuronal membrane lipids coexist in both fluid and gel forms and that anesthetics prevent the fluid to gel conversion that is needed for membrane excitation (Fig. 3-12).[214] The conversion of the fluid phase to the gel phase suppos-

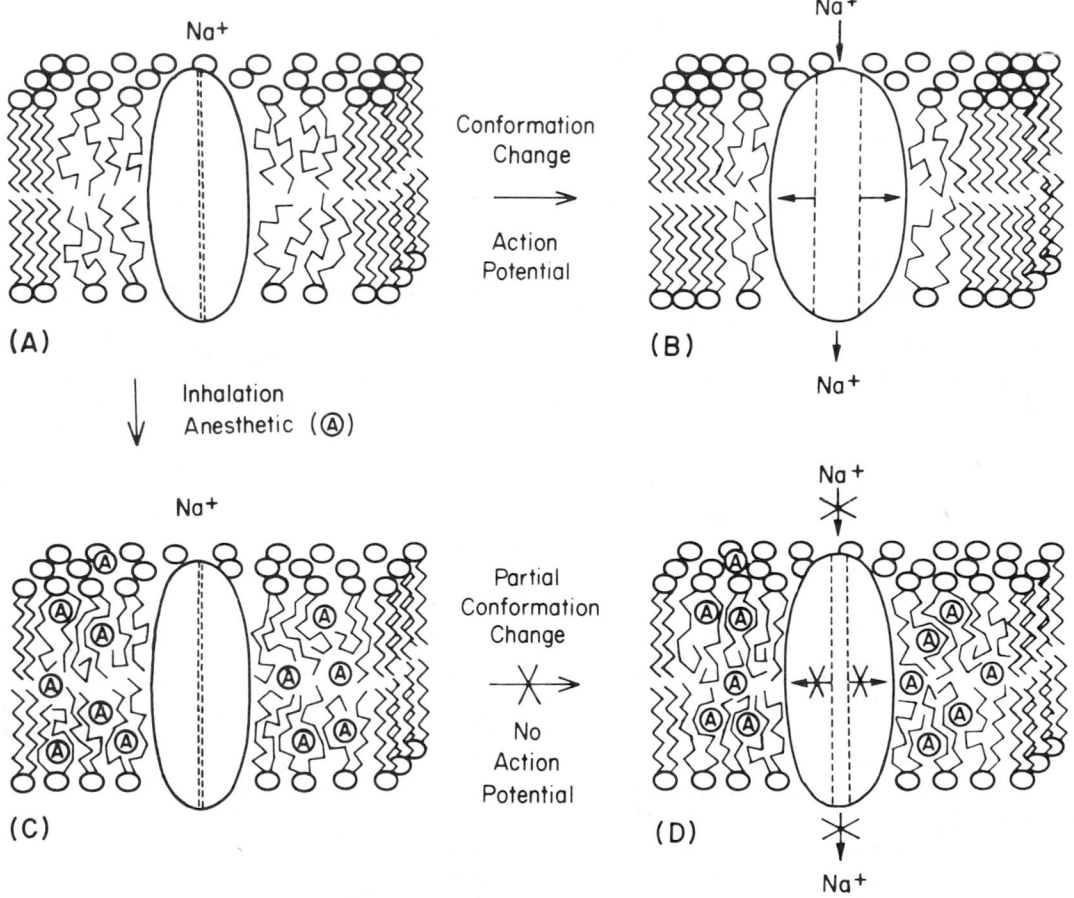

Fig. 3-12. (A) This representation of a neuronal membrane contains an integral membrane protein (the oval structure) that spans the phospholipid bilayer. The membrane protein has an ionic channel in the closed configuration. The small circles depict the phosphate head groups, and the zigzag lines depict fatty acid chains. On the left and right edges of the bilayer segment are regions in which the fatty acid chains are highly ordered. The phospholipids surrounding the intrinsic protein are disordered. **(B)** After a stimulus is received, the membrane protein expands (i.e., it undergoes a conformational change) and permits passage of ions through the channel. This expansion might be accomplished by converting some high-volume fluid-phase lipids into the low-volume solid phase. **(C)** Anesthetic molecules are pictured to invade both solid and fluid phases and convert much of the solid to a fluid phase. **(D)** After a stimulus is received, the membrane protein is unable to expand and open its channel, because the high-volume fluid-phase lipids cannot be converted into the low-volume solid-phase lipids in the presence of the anesthetic. The compression of the fluid phase without conversion is thought to require more lateral pressure than is immediately available. (From Trudell,[214] with permission.)

edly permits the expansion of a membrane protein to allow passage of ions through the protein channel (Fig. 3-12A & B). Anesthetic molecules are thought to sustain lipids in their fluid phase, block the formation of the low-volume gel phase, and thereby prevent the protein from changing its conformation to the open channel state (Fig. 3-12C & D). Support for this hypothesis comes from the finding that general anesthetics disrupt lateral phase separations in model membranes composed of two types of phospholipids and that these effects are partially reversed by the application of high pressure.[215]

Both the *fluidization* and *lateral phase separation* theories suggest that anesthetics act by making membranes more disordered or fluid and that the expansion in the membrane that accompanies this anesthetic perturbation can be counterbalanced by applying high pressures. These theories are compromised by the fact that small increases (1°C) in temperature increase membrane fluidity to approximately the same extent as clinical concentrations of inhaled anesthetics and therefore should augment anesthesia. However, an increase in body temperature decreases anesthetic potency. Furthermore, these theories imply that an age-dependent increase in membrane disorder should accompany the decrease in anesthetic requirement with age. In contrast, neuronal membranes tend to accumulate rigidifying lipids and the fluidity of neuronal membranes tends to decrease with age.[216]

THE INTERACTION OF INHALED AGENTS WITH PROTEINS

Most investigators agree that the ultimate action of inhaled anesthetics is on specific neuronal membrane proteins that permit the translocation of ions during membrane excitation. It remains a matter of debate, however, whether inhaled agents disrupt ion flow through membrane channels by an indirect action on the surrounding lipids or via a second messenger, or by a direct and specific binding to channel proteins. Specific binding sites for inhaled anesthetics are inferred from nuclear magnetic resonance measurements that suggest the existence of a saturable binding site for halothane in rat brain hemispheres at an inspired concentration of 2.5 percent atm.[217] In contrast, solubility measurements of halothane and isoflurane in rabbit brain and human brain homogenates provide no evidence for saturable anesthetic-binding sites at concentrations between 0.01 and 1.0 MAC.[218] Because of the complexity involved in searching for specific anesthetic-binding sites in whole brain or brain homogenate, attempts have been made to simplify this search by examining the interaction of anesthetics with isolated proteins.

Soluble Proteins

Distinct anesthetic-binding sites have been identified in several soluble proteins,[132] including hemoglobin,[219] myoglobin,[184,220] and serum albumin.[221] Anesthetics can move rapidly between their binding sites in soluble proteins and the surrounding aqueous solvent.[184] For myoglobin, the packing of protein side chains in the protein interior organizes a series of cavities, and these cavities may accommodate four xenon atoms per myoglobin molecule.[220] Cooperative protein motions may be required for an anesthetic to pass to its binding site, and anesthetics may be envisioned to pass through channels that connect the interior cavities to each other and to the surface of the protein molecule.[220] Conversely, the binding of inhaled agents to proteins may give rise to conformational changes, and these perturbations may be transmitted to a part of the protein molecule relatively distant from the anesthetic-binding site. The perturbation of hemoglobin[219] caused by an inhaled anesthetic is related to the lipid solubility and potency of that anesthetic. There is also speculation that an anesthetic-induced conformational change in the protein molecule could alter the ionic charge at the surface of the protein and disrupt clusters of structured water molecules at the protein surface.[221]

The interaction of inhaled anesthetics with soluble enzymes may be reflected indirectly by changes in enzyme activity. Many enzymes are resistant to even high concentrations of anesthetics. There is little or no inhibition of several glycolytic enzymes by saturated solutions of inhaled agents.[222,223] Concentrations much higher than the MAC are needed to inhibit acetylcholinesterase activity, and this inhibition does not bear a constant relationship to anesthetic potency.[224] The activity of purified choline acetyltransferase is unaltered by 4 percent atm halothane.[88] Serum cholinesterase activity is unchanged even by saturated solutions of volatile agents.[224]

Other soluble enzymes may be highly sensitive to clinical concentrations of inhaled agents. Halothane (0.8 percent atmosphere) and isoflurane (2.1 percent atmosphere) inhibit the enzyme-induced luminescence output of light-emitting bacteria, and application of high pressure may reverse this inhibition.[225] The purified firefly luciferase enzyme combines with its substrate (luciferin) to produce a photon of light, and a variety of inhaled anesthetics inhibit the activity (light intensity) of this enzyme by approximately 50 percent at concentrations near 1.0 MAC.[226] Halothane inhibits luciferase activity by competing with its substrate luciferin. The binding of one halothane molecule to the enzyme is sufficient to inhibit the enzyme, although the binding site appears large enough to accommodate two molecules of halothane.[226] The *cutoff effect* of anesthesia can also be mimicked by using the purified firefly luciferase enzyme as a model system. The concentrations of a homologous series of *n*-alkanes required to inhibit 50 percent of the luciferase activity decrease with an increasing number of carbon atoms until a chain length of six carbons is reached.[227] Beyond this chain length a cutoff in potency occurs, with the homologues hexane, heptane, and octane inhibiting luciferase activity to approximately the same extent as pentane. This cutoff seems to occur because the maximum aqueous solubilities of the poorly active agents are below the concentrations needed to inhibit one-half of the enzyme activity, but for certain homologues the cutoff effect may be related to the anesthetic binding to a protein pocket of circumscribed dimensions.[227] The above experiments with luciferase are consistent with a possible protein site of anesthetic action. One speculation is that inhaled anesthetics act by competing for protein binding with endogenous ligands that control neuronal excitability.[226]

Membrane Proteins

Two major obstacles are encountered when one attempts to study the influence of inhaled anesthetics on the purified protein ionophores involved in the membrane translocation of ions. First, the biochemical purification of such protein ionophores in adequate quantities is a difficult and time-consuming process. Second, even when these membrane proteins can be isolated, they need to be reincorporated into lipids for measurement of their functional ability to translocate ions. This reincorporation of the purified ionophore into a lipid membrane makes it difficult to distinguish whether an anesthetic affects ion flow through a direct action on the membrane protein or via an indirect action on surrounding lipids.

The acetylcholine receptor-ionophore complex is the best-characterized of the membrane proteins with regard to interaction with inhaled anesthetics. This protein complex is composed of five polypeptide chains that span the membrane and form the wall of the membrane channel. Volatile agents stabilize the acetylcholine receptor in a conformational form that binds agonists with high affinity and may be associated with a desensitized and thus inactive (closed channel) state.[228] Moreover, there is a fair correlation between anesthetic potency and the ability of volatile agents to increase the high-affinity binding of acetylcholine to its receptor[206,229] (Fig. 3-13), and the anesthetic-induced increase in acetylcholine binding is reversible by the application of high pressure.[230] Although an increase in agonist affinity and stabilization of the desensitized receptor state might be considered a possible mechanism of general anesthesia, there is relatively little enhancement of desensitization or increase in acetylcholine binding[206,229] (Fig. 3-13) at surgical concentrations of anesthetics. Furthermore, the finding that very high concentrations of inhaled anesthetics markedly *decrease* the binding of acetylcholine to its receptor (Fig. 3-13) demonstrates that there is no simple relationship between agonist binding and the anesthetic state.

The interaction of inhaled anesthetics with rhodopsin, another membrane protein that can be obtained in a fairly purified form, has also been examined. Clinical concentrations of inhaled agents produce a 10 percent inhibition of the light-induced proton uptake of retinal rod outer segment membranes, perhaps by altering the conformational changes of the rhodopsin molecule that normally occur during excitation.[231] Spectroscopic studies in a bacterial form of rhodopsin do indicate an anesthetic-induced conformational change in

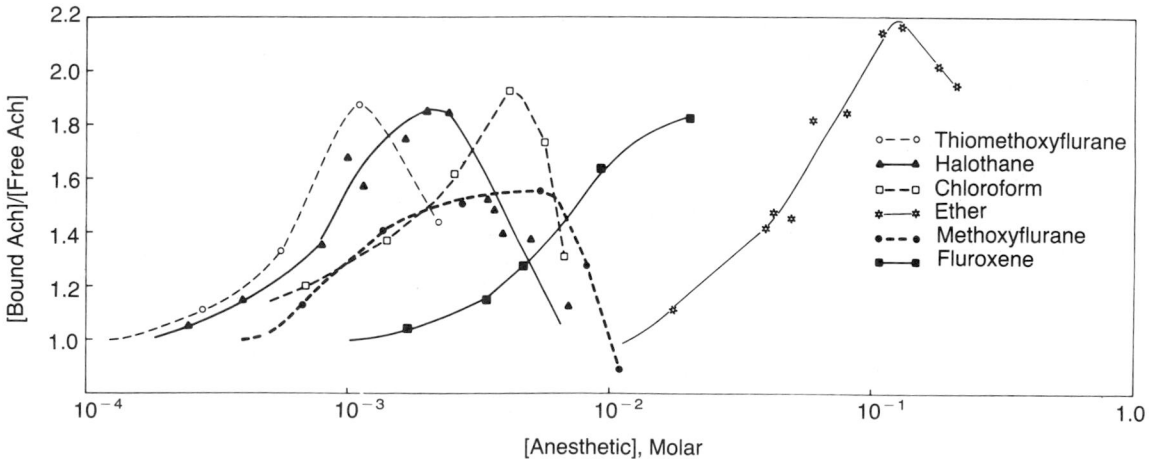

Fig. 3-13. The effect of six volatile anesthetics on the binding of [³H]acetylcholine to acetylcholine receptor-rich membranes prepared from the electric tissue of *Torpedo californica*. The abscissa represents the anesthetic concentration on a logarithmic scale, and the ordinate represents the ratio of acetylcholine bound to its receptor to the amount of free acetylcholine in solution at equilibrium. The volatile agents act in a biphasic manner, enhancing the binding at relatively low anesthetic concentrations and decreasing binding at higher concentrations. (From Firestone et al.,[229] with permission.)

the protein, but only at very high (approximately 10 times MAC) anesthetic concentrations.[232,233]

Using intact cellular preparations, a direct anesthetic-protein interaction may be inferred by the ability of inhaled agents to compete with ligands known to have specific binding sites on proteins. The Na^+-K^+-Cl^- cotransporter of rat glioma cells (a plasma membrane protein that simultaneously transports sodium, potassium, and chloride ions into the cell) is inhibited by halothane in a dose-dependent and competitive manner.[234] A 33 percent inhibition of activity occurs at 1.0 percent atm halothane.[234] In contrast, other inhaled agents (diethyl ether, enflurane, isoflurane, chloroform, methoxyflurane, trichloroethylene) do not inhibit the activity of this cotransporter at clinical concentrations. It was proposed from these experiments that the cotransporter membrane protein contained a hydrophobic pocket of circumscribed dimensions that allowed the binding of halothane, but not that of other inhaled agents.[234]

Recent studies have suggested that G proteins are potential membrane sites where anesthetics exert their functional effects. G proteins are guanine nucleotide-binding neuronal membrane proteins that couple many neurotransmitter receptors to ion channels in the brain.[235] That is, the binding of a neurotransmitter to its receptor can influence the activation state of a G protein, which in turn can control the opening or closing of an ion channel. G proteins are inactivated by pertussis toxin, and intracerebroventricular injection of pertussis toxin increases halothane MAC in rats by as much as 70 percent.[236] Furthermore, the reduction in halothane MAC promoted by an α_2-agonist is attenuated by treatment with pertussis toxin.[236] This implies that the halothane sparing effect of α_2-agonists is dependent on a G protein that is sensitive to pertussis toxin. Other experiments show that clinical concentrations of halothane and diethyl ether alter the interactions between the muscarinic acetylcholine receptor and G proteins in the rat brain stem.[237] Inhaled agents decrease the ability of a guanine nucleotide to depress the high-affinity binding of agonists to the muscarinic acetylcholine receptor.[237] Whether this alteration in agonist binding is due to a direct or indirect anesthetic action on membrane proteins remains to be determined.

USE OF ANIMAL MODELS: ATTEMPTS TO RELATE SUSTAINED ALTERATIONS IN ANESTHETIC POTENCY WITH NEUROCHEMICAL COMPOSITION

One approach to the mechanism of anesthetic action is to relate alterations in anesthetic requirement with biochemical and biophysical changes occurring in the CNS. A correlation between changes in anesthetic requirement and a structural change in the nervous system might indicate the critical properties of the anesthetic site of action and how anesthetics affect that site.

Tolerance Studies

Chronic Tolerance

Inhaled anesthetic requirement can be increased by the chronic exposure of mice to subanesthetic levels of nitrous oxide.[238-241] The maximal increase in the nitrous oxide righting-reflex ED_{50} for mice placed under 40 to 70 percent nitrous oxide is approximately 0.25 atm and occurs after 2 weeks of continuous exposure. Tolerance disappears within 6 days of removing the mice from the subanesthetic nitrous oxide environment.[238,239] Mice tolerant to nitrous oxide are also more tolerant to cyclopropane,[240] isoflurane,[240] and nitrogen.[241]

Chronic exposure to other anesthetics besides nitrous oxide can also produce tolerance. Mice continuously exposed to 18 atm of nitrogen for 2 weeks exhibit a 38 percent increase in the righting-reflex ED_{50} for nitrogen.[241] Intermittent and multiple exposures of mice to halothane, isoflurane, or enflurane result in an autotolerance for each of these anesthetics.[242] Rats intermittently exposed to halothane over a 56-day period develop a tolerance to acoustic evoked responses during the acute administration of halothane, as measured by permanent electrodes implanted in thalamic and hypothalamic regions.[243] In contrast, rats repeatedly exposed to anesthetic concentrations of cyclopropane and halothane for 1 hour every day for 20 and 30 days, respectively, did not develop a tolerance to cyclopropane.[244]

One possible mechanism for the tolerance that develops is that the continuous exposure to anesthetic alters the physical state of neuronal membranes and that the animals might adapt to this perturbation by adjusting the neuronal membrane lipid composition so that the physical state of the membrane is returned to that prior to anesthetic exposure. However, no significant differences in membrane order or in the composition of purified synaptic membrane fatty acid, phospholipid, or cholesterol occur in mice tolerant to nitrous oxide.[238,239] Other possible mechanisms behind tolerance development include alterations in neurotransmitter levels or their receptors. Prolonged exposure of rats to nitrous oxide decreases brain stem opiate receptor density by approximately 20 percent and may in part account for the analgesic action of nitrous oxide.[245]

Acute Tolerance

In humans, a tolerance to the analgesic effect of nitrous oxide is seen in some patients within 10 to 60 minutes of administration.[246,247] However, rat models have been inconsistent in demonstrating an acute tolerance to the analgesic action of nitrous oxide. No acute tolerance could be detected when rats were exposed to 75 percent nitrous oxide for 2 hours and analgesic potency was assessed by the time needed to induce a tail-flick to radiant heat.[248] In contrast, when rats were exposed to 70 percent nitrous oxide and analgesia was tested by pressure stimulation to the paw, tolerance to the effect of nitrous oxide developed within 45 minutes.[249] Tolerance was inhibited by the administration of an enkephalinase inhibitor, and it was suggested from these studies that endogenous opiates were involved in the development of tolerance.[249]

A tolerance to the anesthetic effects of nitrous oxide and ethylene (as measured by the righting reflex) is seen in mice within approximately 10 minutes after exposure.[250] Rapid tolerance to the effects of nitrous oxide is also manifested on the electroencephalogram,[251,252] on cerebral cortical responses to electrical stimuli applied to the forepaw of the rat,[33] and on blockade of sympathetic ganglia.[253] However, no clue has been found concerning the molecular mechanism behind this phenomenon.

Associated with the rapidly developing tolerance is a withdrawal syndrome that occurs in mice after exposure to nitrous oxide, ethylene, cyclopropane, and diethyl ether.[254] Exposures to nitrous oxide at partial pressures greater than 0.9 atm for 15 to 30 minutes produces the withdrawal syndrome.[255] This syndrome may be related to the emergence delirium occasionally seen in patients after general anesthesia. Although arguments have been made for cholinergic involvement[256] and for[257] and against[258] involvement of endogenous opiates, the mechanistic basis of this withdrawal syndrome remains to be explored.

Genetic Studies

One method of producing two groups of animals having different anesthetic potencies makes use of the fact that anesthetic requirement varies slightly among animals of a given species and that members resistant and vulnerable to anesthesia may be found in a normal population. Mice can be selected from a normal population with consistently high and consistently low nitrous oxide righting-reflex ED_{50}s.[259] Offspring from parents having consistently high nitrous oxide requirements also have high requirements (HI mice), whereas offspring from parents having low requirements similarly have low requirements (LO mice).[259] Repeating the process of selection, breeding, and testing for nitrous oxide requirement through 15 generations produced two lines of mice with nitrous oxide requirements separated by approximately 0.7 atm (Fig. 3-14).[8,259] The nitrous oxide righting-reflex ED_{50} for the population extremes of these HI and LO mice (i.e., those selected as breeders to produce the following generations) is approximately 1 atm apart.[8] The HI mice also have a higher anesthetic requirement for other inhaled anesthetics, but the separation in righting-reflex ED_{50} values between the two lines is inversely related to the lipid solubility of the anesthetic.[8] HI mice are more suscepti-

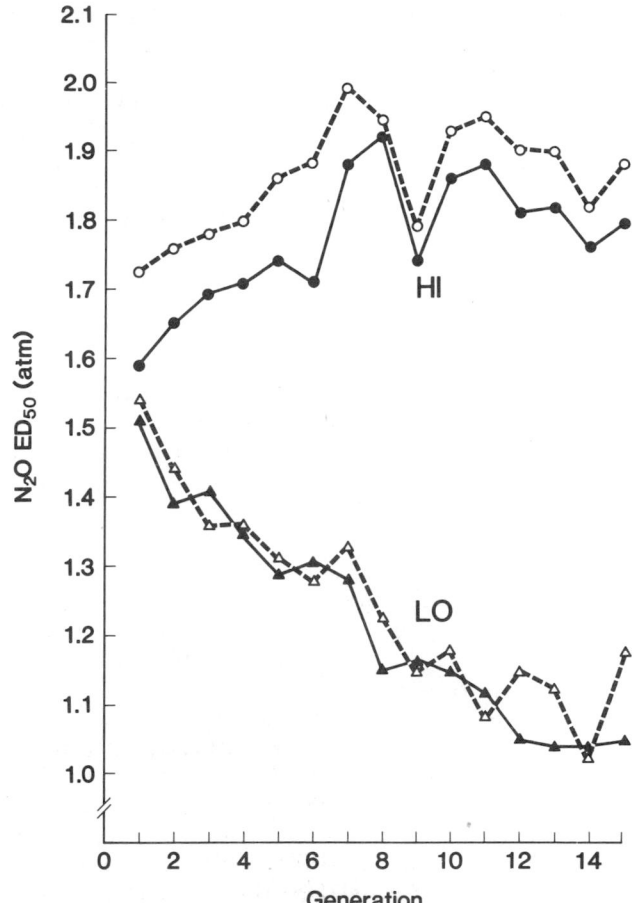

Fig. 3-14. Nitrous oxide righting-reflex ED_{50} values for male (closed symbols) and female (open symbols) offspring of mice selectively bred for resistance (HI group, circles) or susceptibility (LO group, triangles) to nitrous oxide anesthesia. The nitrous oxide requirements for HI and LO mice became progressively more separated over 15 generations of selective breeding. Standard errors about most points are less than 0.03 atmosphere. (Values for generations 1 through 10 are from Koblin et al.[8,259])

ble to the convulsant effects of high-pressure helium, flurothyl, pentylenetetrazole, strychnine, bicuculline, and picrotoxin than are LO mice.[260] Thus, the separation in anesthetic requirements between the two lines might be explained, at least in part, by a generalized increase in CNS excitability. Nitrous oxide ED_{50} values of offspring produced by cross-mating animals of the HI and LO lines approximate the average value of the parents, implying that the genetic control of resistance or susceptibility probably involves many genes.[261] For both lines of mice, the nitrous oxide requirement declines with age, with the HI mice having a greater age-related decrease in requirement.[24,262]

The discovery of the changes in the CNS that produce these differences in nitrous oxide requirement could provide an important insight into the mechanisms of anesthetic action. When the possibility that HI and LO mice differed in synaptic membrane lipid composition was examined, no differences could be found in synaptic membrane fatty acid, phospholipid, or cholesterol composition.[259] HI mice do have a 26 percent higher concentration of norepinephrine in whole brain than do LO mice.[262] Furthermore, in the medulla (but not in other brain regions), a significant correlation was found between norepinephrine content and nitrous oxide requirement of the selectively bred animals.[262] The age-related decrease in nitrous oxide requirements in the HI and LO mice paralleled the decline in norepinephrine levels in the medulla that occurred with aging.[262] Thus, the differences in anesthetic requirement between the HI and LO mice may arise, at least in part, from alterations in norepinephrine content in specific regions of the brain.

Mice selectively bred for their differential sensitivity to ethanol may also exhibit a differential sensitivity to inhaled anesthetics. Mice selectively bred for susceptibility to seizures upon withdrawal from ethanol are similarly prone to seizures following a 1-hour exposure to 75 percent nitrous oxide.[263] In addition, mice selectively bred for sensitivity (long-sleep mice) or resistance (short-sleep mice) to the hypnotic effect of ethanol have a differential sensitivity to certain but not all inhaled anesthetics.[264,265] However, the differential effect between short-sleep and long-sleep mice is greater for ethanol than for inhaled agents. Although the mechanisms for the differential sensitivities to ethanol and inhaled anesthetics may overlap, they are unlikely to be identical. For example, intracerebroventrical injection of the peptide neurotensin increases sensitivity to ethanol but not to halothane in short-sleep mice, whereas neurotensin enhances the sensitivity to halothane but not to ethanol in long-sleep mice.[266] The greater anesthetic requirement of the short-sleep mice is not associated with a different synaptic membrane fatty acid, phospholipid, or cholesterol composition.[264,267]

The above studies represent attempts to characterize the anesthetic site of action by using genetic techniques to produce animals that have sustained alterations in anesthetic requirement. An alternative approach is to examine for differences in anesthetic sensitivity in animals that are known to have alterations in brain structure. Quaking mice are autosomal recessive mutants with a deficiency in CNS myelin and a markedly altered myelin fatty acid and cholesterol composition compared with littermate controls.[268] The finding of similar ED$_{50}$s for inhaled anesthetics in quaking and control mice implies that the lipids in CNS myelin do not play a role in the production of anesthesia.[268]

Strains of *Drosophila melanogaster* that are resistant or sensitive to diethyl ether have also been obtained. Such strains are also resistant or sensitive to halothane and chloroform.[269] Resistance to halothane appears to be a sex-linked recessive trait, and resistance to chloroform is an incompletely dominant autosomal trait.

These two strains have different fatty acid and diglyceride contents in the phosphatidylethanolamine fraction but not in the phosphatidylcholine fraction.[270] However, these analyses were performed on lipids extracted from the whole organism, and it is uncertain how such lipid alterations might relate to the mechanisms of anesthesia.

Caenorhabditis elegans is a worm that has a completely defined nervous system and can be genetically manipulated with relative ease. Using immobility of the worm as the anesthetic endpoint, the potencies of inhaled agents in this organism parallel those found in higher animals.[271] Mutants of *C. elegans* have been developed that are hypersensitive to halothane, and additional mutations were discovered that could suppress this hypersensitivity to halothane.[272] The strains that are hypersensitive to halothane also exhibit an enhanced sensitivity to inhaled anesthetics that have an oil/gas partition coefficient greater than that of halothane, but not to anesthetics with lower oil/gas partition coefficients.[273] It was suggested from these studies that the mutant strains have an altered site of inhaled anesthetic action, the molecular basis of which remains to be determined.[273]

Dietary Studies

Mice fed diets of different fatty acid composition (saturated versus unsaturated) from birth have large alterations in certain synaptic membrane fatty acid components.[274] The most notable changes occur in the synaptic membrane phosphatidylethanolamine and phosphatidylserine fractions in mice fed the saturated fat diet, which exhibit a relative decrease in docosahexaenoic (22:6ω3) and increase in eicosatrienoic (20:3ω9) fatty acids. However, these alterations in synaptic membrane fatty acid composition have little or no influence on the righting-reflex ED$_{50}$s for nitrous oxide and isoflurane.[274] In contrast, diet-induced alterations in rat brain fatty acid composition can be correlated with alterations in anesthetic potency.[275] Compared with rats on a control diet, rats maintained on a fat-free diet exhibit lower levels of whole brain arachidonic acid (20:4ω6) and docosahexaenoic acid and an increase in eicosatrienoic acid. The fat-deprived animals exhibited a 10 to 33 percent decrease in MAC for methoxyflurane, halothane, isoflurane, and cyclopropane compared with control rats.[275] Furthermore, the enhanced sensitivity of the fat-deprived rats to inhaled agents could be reversed by supplementing the fat-deprived animals with linoleic acid (18:2ω6).[275] The alterations in anesthetic potency are correlated with changes in brain arachidonyl-phosphatidylinositol content, and one speculation is that such changes in arachidonyl-phosphatidyinositol content might alter the ability of neurotransmitters to synthesize chemical second messengers, thus altering neuronal excitability and anesthetic requirement.[276]

SUMMARY

Inhaled anesthetics disrupt neuronal transmission in many areas of the central nervous system. They may either enhance or depress excitatory or inhibitory transmission through axons or synaptic regions. Both pre- and postsynaptic effects have been found. Regardless of the macroscopic site of action, the ultimate action of inhaled agents is on neuronal membranes. Although a direct neuronal plasma membrane interaction seems likely, the possibility remains that inhaled anesthetics act indirectly via production of a second messenger. The excellent correlation between lipid solubility and anesthetic potency suggests that anesthetics have a hydrophobic or amphipathic site of action. Anesthetics bind to and perturb both membrane lipids and proteins, but it is presently uncertain which of these components is most important and how such perturbations might lead to the anesthetic state. Future advances in anesthetic mechanisms will go hand in hand with the development of molecular biology techniques used to clone and characterize excitable membrane channels and biophysical and biochemical advances used to study neuronal interactions. The development of animal models with sustained alterations in anesthetic potency will allow for the testing of hypotheses that specific molecular changes are important in the production of anesthesia.

REFERENCES

1. Cullen SC, Eger EI II, Cullen BF, Gregory P: Observations on the anesthetic effect of the combination of xenon and halothane. Anesthesiology 31:305, 1969
2. Trudell JR: Is there light at the end of the tunnel? Anesth Analg 64:385, 1985
3. Eger EI II, Saidman LJ, Brandstater B: Minimum alveolar anesthetic concentration: a standard of anesthetic potency. Anesthesiology 26:756, 1965
4. Eger EI II, Johnson BH: MAC of I-653 in rats, including a test of the effect of body temperature and anesthetic duration. Anesth Analg 66:974, 1987
5. Quasha AL, Eger EI II, Tinker JH: Determination and applications of MAC. Anesthesiology 53:315, 1980
6. Miller KW, Paton WDM, Smith EB: The anaesthetic pressures of certain fluorine-containing gases. Br J Anaesth 39:910, 1967
7. Deady JE, Koblin DD, Eger EI II, et al: Anesthetic potencies and the unitary theory of narcosis. Anesth Analg 60:380, 1981
8. Koblin DD, Deady JE, Eger EI II: Potencies of inhaled anesthetics and alcohol in mice selectively bred for resistance and susceptibility to nitrous oxide anesthesia. Anesthesiology 56:18, 1982
9. Kissin I, Morgan PL, Smith LR: Anesthetic potencies of isoflurane, halothane, and diethyl ether for various end points of anesthesia. Anesthesiology 58:88, 1983
10. Regan MJ, Eger EI II: Effect of hypothermia in dogs on anesthetizing and apneic doses of inhalation agents. Anesthesiology 28:689, 1967
11. Steffey EP, Eger EI II: Hypothermia and halothane MAC in the dog. Anesthesiology 41:392, 1974
12. Vitez TS, White PF, Eger EI II: Effects of hypothermia on halothane MAC and isoflurane MAC in the rat. Anesthesiology 41:80, 1974
13. Brauer RW, Hogan PM, et al: Patterns of interaction of effects of light metabolically inert gases with those of hydrostatic pressure as such—a review. Undersea Biomed Res 9:353, 1982
14. Halsey MJ: Effects of high pressure on the central nervous system. Physiol Rev 62:1341, 1982
15. Smith RA, Dodson BA, Miller KW: The interactions between pressure and anaesthetics. Philos Trans R Soc Lond [Biol] 304:69, 1984
16. Wann KT, MacDonald AG: Actions and interactions of high pressure and general anaesthetics. Prog Neurobiol 30:271, 1987
17. Dodson BA, Furmaniuk ZW, Miller KW: The physiological effects of hydrostatic pressure are not equivalent to those of helium pressure on *Rana pipiens*. J Physiol 362:233, 1985
18. Smith EB, Bowser-Riley F, Daniels S, et al: Species variation and the mechanism of pressure-anaesthetic interactions. Nature 311:56, 1984
19. Lerman J, Robinson S, Willis MM, Gregory GA: Anesthetic requirements for halothane in young children 0–1 month and 1–6 months of age. Anesthesiology 59:421, 1983
20. Cameron CB, Robinson S, Gregory GA: The minimum anesthetic concentration of isoflurane in children. Anesth Analg 63:418, 1984
21. Gregory GA, Eger EI II, Munson ES: The relationship between age and halothane requirements in man. Anesthesiology 30:488, 1969
22. Munson ES, Hoffman JC, Eger EI II: Use of cyclopropane to test the generality of anesthetic requirement in the elderly. Anesth Analg 63:998, 1984
23. Hoffman WE, Seals C, Miletich DJ, Albrecht RF: Plasma and myocardial catecholamine levels in young and aged rats during halothane anesthesia. Neurobiol Aging 6:117, 1985
24. Koblin DD, Lurz FW, Eger EI II: Age-dependent alterations in nitrous oxide requirements in mice. Anesthesiology 58:428, 1983
25. Tanifuji Y, Eger EI II: Brain sodium, potassium, and osmolarity: Effects on anesthetic requirement. Anesth Analg 57:404, 1978
26. Tanifuji Y, Nezu T, Kobayashi K, Eger EI II: Effect of brain calcium and magnesium on anesthetic requirement (MAC) in dogs. Jpn J Anesthesiol 29:741, 1980
27. Maze M, Mason DM, Jr., Kates RE: Verapamil decreases MAC for halothane in dogs. Anesthesiology 59:327, 1983
28. Dolin SJ, Little HJ: Augmentation by calcium channel antagonists of general anaesthetic potency in mice. Br J Pharmacol 88:909, 1986
29. Thompson, SW, Moscicki JC, DiFazio CA: The anesthetic contribution of magnesium sulfate and ritodrine hydrochloride in rats. Anesth Analg 67:31, 1988
30. Angel A: Processing of sensory information. Prog Neurobiol 9:1, 1977
31. Shimoji K, Fujioka H, Fukazawa T, et al: Anesthetics and excitatory/inhibitory responses of midbrain reticular neurons. Anesthesiology 61:151, 1984
32. Richards CD: In search of the mechanisms of anaesthesia. Trends Neurosci 3:9, 1980
33. Angel A, Gratton DA: The effect of anaesthetic agents on cerebral cortical responses in the rat. Br J Pharmacol 76:541, 1982

34. Berg-Johnsen J, Langmoen IA: Isoflurane hyperpolarizes neurones in rat and human cerebral cortex. Acta Physiol Scand 130:679, 1987

35. Richards CD: On the mechanisms of halothane anaesthesia. J Physiol (Lond) 233:439, 1973

36. Berg-Johnsen J, Langmoen IA: Isoflurane effects in rat hippocampal cortex: a quantitative evaluation of different cellular sites of action. Acta Physiol Scand 128:613, 1986

37. Saint DA, Quastel DMJ, Chirwa S: Effect of a volatile anesthetic upon presynaptic excitability in mammalian hippocampus. Can J Physiol Pharm 64:221, 1986

38. MacIver MB, Roth SH: Inhalation anaesthetics exhibit pathway-specific and differential actions on hippocampal synaptic responses *in vitro*. Br J Anaesth 60:680, 1988

39. Nicoll RA: The effects of anaesthetics on synaptic excitation and inhibition in the olfactory bulb. J Physiol (Lond) 223:803, 1972

40. Gage PW, Robertson B: Prolongation of inhibitory postsynaptic currents by pentobarbitone, halothane and ketamine in CA1 pyramidal cell in rat hippocampus. Br J Pharmacol 85:675, 1985

41. Fujiwara N, Higashi H, Nishi S, et al: Changes in spontaneous firing patterns of rat hippocampal neurons by volatile anesthetics. J Physiol (Lond) 402:155, 1988

42. deJong RH, Robles R, Corbin RW, et al: Effect of inhalation anesthetics on monosynaptic and polysynaptic transmission in the spinal cord. J Pharmacol Exp Ther 162:326, 1968

43. Heavner J: Jamming spinal sensory input: Effects of anesthetic and analgesic drugs in the spinal cord dorsal horn. Pain 1:239, 1975

44. Namiki A, Collins JG, Kitahata LM, et al: Effects of halothane on spinal neuronal responses to graded noxious heat stimulation in the cat. Anesthesiology 53:475, 1980

45. Takenoshita M, Takahashi T: Mechanisms of halothane action on synaptic transmission in motoneurons of the newborn rat spinal cord in vitro. Brain Res 402:303, 1987

46. Komatsu T, Shingu K, Tomemori N, et al: Nitrous oxide activates the supraspinal pain inhibition system. Acta Anaesthesiol Scand 25:519, 1981

47. de Jong RH, Nace RA: Nerve impulse conduction and cutaneous receptor responses during general anesthesia. Anesthesiology 28:851, 1967

48. Campbell JN, Raja SN, Meyer RA: Halothane sensitizes cutaneous nociceptors in monkeys. J Neurophysiol 52:762, 1984

49. Franks NP, Lieb WR: Volatile general anaesthetics activate a novel neuronal K^+ current. Nature 333:662, 1988

50. Larrabee MG, Posternak JM: Selective action of anesthetics on synapses and axons in mammalian sympathetic ganglia. J Neurophysiol 15:91, 1952

51. Bosnjak ZJ, Seagard JL, Wu A, et al: The effects of halothane on sympathetic ganglionic transmission. Anesthesiology 57:473, 1982

52. Richards CD, Russel WJ, Smaje JC: The action of ether and methoxyflurane on synaptic transmission in isolated preparations of the mammalian cortex. J Physiol (Lond) 248:121, 1975

53. Richards CD, White AE: Actions of volatile anaesthetics on synaptic transmission in the dentate gyrus. J Physiol (Lond) 252:241, 1975

54. Kendig JJ, Trudell JR, Cohen EN: Effects of pressure and anesthetics on conduction and synaptic transmission. J Pharmacol Exp Ther 195:216, 1975

55. Haydon DA, Simon AJB: Excitation of the squid giant axon by general anaesthetics. J Physiol (Lond) 402:375, 1988

56. Haydon DA, Hendry BM: Nerve impulse blockage in squid axons by *n*-alkanes: the effect of axon diameter. J Physiol (Lond) 333:393, 1982

57. Berg-Johnsen J, Langmoen IA: The effect of isoflurane on unmyelinated and myelinated fibers in the rat brain. Acta Physiol Scand 127:87, 1986

58. Wildsmith JAW, Gissen AJ, Takman B, Covino BG: Differential nerve blockade: Esters v. amides and the influence of pK_a Br J Anaesth 59:379, 1987

59. Fink BR, Cairns AM: Lack of size-related differential sensitivity to equilibrium conduction block among mammalian myelinated axons exposed to lidocaine. Anesth Analg 66:948, 1987

60. Kendig JJ, Courtney KR, Cohen EN: Anesthetics: Molecular correlates of voltage- and frequency-dependent sodium channel block in nerve. J Pharmacol Exp Ther 210:446, 1979

61. Strichartz G: Use-dependent conduction block produced by volatile anesthetic agents. Acta Anaesthesiol Scand 24:402, 1980

62. Kendig JJ, Grossman Y: Homogeneous and branching axons. Differing responses to anesthetics and pressure. p. 333. In Roth SH, Miller KW (eds): Molecular and Cellular Mechanisms of Anesthetics. Plenum, New York, 1986

63. Weston GA, Roth SH: Differential actions of volatile anaesthetic agents on a single isolated neurone. Br J Anaesth 58:1390, 1986

64. Kendig JJ, Grossman Y, MacIver MB: Pressure reversal of anaesthesia: a synaptic mechanism. Br J Anaesth 60:806, 1988

65. Richards CD: Actions of general anaesthetics on synaptic transmission in the CNS. Br J Anaesth 55:201, 1983

66. Zorychta E, Capek R: Depression of spinal monosynaptic transmission by diethyl ether: Quantal analysis of unitary synaptic potentials. J Pharmacol Exp Ther 207:825, 1978

67. Bosnjak ZJ, Dujic Z, Roerig DL, Kampine JP: Effects of halothane on acetylcholine release and sympathetic ganglionic transmission. Anesthesiology 69:500, 1988

68. Roizen MF, Thoa NB, Moss J, et al: Inhibition by halothane of release of norepinephrine, but not of dopamine-beta hydroxylase, from guinea-pig vas deferens. Eur J Pharmacol 31:313, 1975

69. Lunn JJ, Rorie DK: Halothane-induced changes in the release and disposition of norepinephrine at adrenergic nerve endings in dog saphenous vein. Anesthesiology 61:377, 1984

70. Gothert M, Duhrsen U, Rieckesmann JM: Ethanol, anaesthetics and other lipophilic drugs preferentially inhibit 5-hydroxytryptamine- and acetylcholine-induced noradrenaline release from sympathetic nerves. Arch Int Pharmacodyn Ther 242:196, 1979

71. Yashima N, Wada A, Izumi F: Halothane inhibits the cholinergic-receptor-mediated influx of calcium in primary culture of bovine adrenal medulla cells. Anesthesiology 64:466, 1986

72. Pocock G, Richards CD: The action of volatile anaesthetics on stimulus-secretion coupling in bovine adrenal chromaffin cells. Br J Pharmacol 95:209, 1988

73. Sumikawa K, Amakata Y, Kashimoto T, et al: Effects of cyclopropane on catecholamine release from bovine adrenal medulla. Anesthesiology 53:385, 1980

74. Westfall TC, DiFazio CA, Saunders J: Local anesthetic- and halothane-induced alteration of the stimulation induced release of ^{3}H-dopamine from rat striatal slices. Anesthesiology 48:118–124, 1978

75. Rorie DK, Tyce GM, Sill JC: Increased norepinephrine release from dog pulmonary artery caused by nitrous oxide. Anesth Analg 65:560, 1986

76. Soubrie P, Blas C, Ferron A, et al: Chlordiazepoxide reduces *in vivo* serotonin release in the basal ganglia of *Encephale isole* but not anesthetized cats: Evidence for a dorsal raphe site of action. J Pharmacol Exp Ther 226:526, 1983

77. Halliday DJX, Little HJ, Paton WDM: The effects of inert gases and other general anaesthetics on the release of acetylcholine from the guinea-pig ileum. Br J Pharmacol 67:229, 1979

78. Martin DC, Watkins CA, Adams RJ, Nason LA: Anesthetic effects on 5-hydroxytryptamine uptake by rat brain synaptosomes. Brain Res 455:360, 1988

79. Richards CD, Smaje JC: Anaesthetics depress the sensitivity of cortical neurones to L-glutamate. Br J Pharmacol 58:347, 1976

80. Krnjevic K: Cellular and synaptic effects of general anesthetics. p. 3. In Roth SH, Miller KW (eds): Molecular and Cellular Mechanisms of Anesthetics. Plenum, New York, 1986

81. Smaje JC: General anaesthetics and the acetylcholine-sensitivity of cortical neurones. Br J Pharmacol 58:359, 1976

82. Waud BE, Waud DR: Comparison of the effects of general anesthetics on the end-plate of skeletal muscle. Anesthesiology 43:540, 1979

83. Wachtel RE: Effects of some depressant drugs on synaptic responses to glutamate at the crayfish neuromuscular junction. Br J Pharmacol 83:387, 1984

84. Gage PW, McKinnon D, Robertson B: The influence of anesthetics on postsynaptic ion channels. p. 139. In Roth SH, Miller KW (eds): Molecular and Cellular Mechanisms of Anesthetics. Plenum, New York, 1986

85. Sugai N, Maruyama H, Goto K: Effect of nitrous oxide alone or its combination with fentanyl on spinal reflexes in cats. Br J Anaesth 54:567, 1982

86. Ngai SH, Cheney DL, Finck AD: Acetylcholine concentrations and turnover in rat brain structures during anesthesia with halothane, enflurane, and ketamine. Anesthesiology 48:4, 1978

87. Gibson GE, Duffy TE: Impaired synthesis of acetylcholine by mild hypoxic hypoxia or nitrous oxide. J Neurochem 36:28, 1981

88. Johnson GVW, Hartzell CR: Choline uptake, acetylcholine synthesis and release, and halothane effects in synaptosomes. Anesth Analg 64:395, 1985

89. Roizen MF, Kopin KJ, Thoa NB, et al: The effect of two anesthetic agents on norepinephrine and dopamine in discrete brain nuclei, fiber tracts, and terminal regions of the rat. Brain Res 110:515, 1976

90. Johnston RR, Way WL, Miller RD: The effect of CNS catecholamine-depleting drugs on dextroamphetamine-induced elevation of halothane MAC. Anesthesiology 41:57, 1974

91. Roizen MF, White PF, Eger EI II, Brownstein M: Effects of ablation of serotonin or norepinephrine brainstem areas on halothane and cyclopropane MACs in rats. Anesthesiology 49:252, 1978

92. Segal IS, Irwin I, Maze M: Modulating role of dopamine on anesthetic requirements. Anesthesiology 69A:640, 1988

93. Bloor BC, Flacke WE: Reduction in halothane anesthetic requirement by clonidine, an alpha adrenergic agonist. Anesth Analg 61:741, 1982

94. Vickery RG, Sheridan BC, Segal IS, Maze M: Anesthetic and hemodynamic effects of the stereoisomers of medetomidine, an α_2-adrenergic agonist, in halothane-anesthetized dogs. Anesth Analg 67:611, 1988

95. Roizen MF, Kopin IJ, Palkovits M, et al: The effect of two diverse inhalation anesthetic agents on serotonin in discrete regions of the rat brain. Exp Brain Res 24:203, 1975

96. Cheng SC, Brunner EA: Inhibition of GABA metabolism in rat brain slices by halothane. Anesthesiology 55:26, 1981

97. Cheng SC, Brunner EA: Inducing anesthesia with a GABA analog, THIP. Anesthesiology 63:147, 1985

98. Dedrick DF, Scherer YD, Biebuyck JF: Use of a rapid brain-sampling technique in a physiologic preparation: Effects of morphine, ketamine, and halothane on tissue energy intermediates. Anesthesiology 42:651, 1975

99. Triner L, Vulliemoz Y, Verosky M, et al: Action of volatile anesthetics on cyclic nucleotides in the brain. p. 229. In Fink BR (ed): Progress in Anesthesiology. Vol 2. Molecular Mechanisms of Anesthesia. Raven Press, New York, 1980

100. Kant GJ, Muller TW, Lanox RH, et al: In vivo effects of pentobarbital and halothane anesthesia on levels of adenosine 3',5'-monophosphate and guanosine 3',5'-monophosphate in rat brain regions and pituitary. Biochem Pharmacol 29:1891, 1980

101. MacMurdo SD, Nemoto EM, Nikki P, et al: Brain cyclic-AMP and possible mechanisms of cerebrovascular dilatation by anesthetics in rats. Anesthesiology 55:435, 1981

102. Narayanan TK, Confer RA, Dennison RL, et al: Halothane attenuation of muscarinic inhibition of adenylate cyclase in rat heart. Biochem Pharmacol 37:1219, 1988

103. Vulliemoz Y, Verosky M, Alpert M, Triner L: Effect of enflurane on cerebellar cGMP and on motor activity in the mouse. Br J Anaesth 55:79, 1983

104. Finck AD, Ngai SH, Berkowitz BA: Antagonism of general anesthesia by naloxone in the rat. Anesthesiology 46:241, 1977

105. Arndt JO, Freye E: Perfusion of naloxone through the fourth cerebral ventricle reverses the circulatory and hypnotic effect of halothane in dogs. Anesthesiology 51:58, 1979

106. Hall RI, Murphy MR, Hug CC: The enflurane sparing effect of sufentanil in dogs. Anesthesiology 67:518, 1987

107. Althaus JS, Difazio CA, Moscicki JC, Von Voigtlander PF: Enhancement of anesthetic effect of halothane by spiradoline, a selective κ-agonist. Anesth Analg 67:823, 1988

108. Harper MH, Winter PM, Johnson BH, et al: Naloxone does not antagonize general anesthesia in the rat. Anesthesiology 49:3, 1978

109. Pace NL, Wong KC: Failure of naloxone and naltrexone to antagonize halothane anesthesia in the dog. Anesth Analg 58:36, 1979

110. Levin LL, Winter PM, Nemoto EM, et al: Naloxone does not antagonize the analgesic effects of inhalation anesthesia. Anesth Analg 65:330, 1986

111. Smith RA, Wilson M, Miller KW: Naloxone has no effect on nitrous oxide anesthesia. Anesthesiology 49:6, 1978

112. Kraynack BJ, Gintautas JG: Naloxone: Analeptic action unrelated to opiate receptor antagonism? Anesthesiology 56:251, 1982

113. Maiewski S, Muldoon S, Mueller GP: Anesthesia and stimulation of pituitary β-endorphin release in rats. Proc Soc Exp Biol Med 176:268, 1984

114. Zuniga JR, Joseph SA, Knigge KM: The effects of nitrous oxide on the central endogenous pro-opiomelanocortin system in the rat. Brain Res 420:57, 1987

115. Quock RM, Kouchich FJ, Tseng LF: Influence of nitrous oxide upon regional brain levels of methionine-enkephalin-like immunoreactivity in rats. Brain Res Bull 16:321, 1986

116. Morris B, Livingston A: Effects of nitrous oxide exposure on met-enkephalin levels in discrete areas of rat brain. Neurosci Lett 45:11, 1984

117. Thomas TA, Fletcher JE, Hill RG: Influence of medication, pain and progress in labour on plasma β-endorphin-like immunoreactivity. Br J Anaesth 54:401, 1984
118. Cork RC, Hameroff SR, Weiss JL: Effects of halothane and fentanyl anesthesia on plasma β-endorphin immunoreactivity during cardiac surgery. Anesth Analg 64:677, 1985
119. Smith R, Besser GM, Rees LH: The effect of surgery on plasma β-endorphin and methionine-enkephalin. Neurosci Lett 55:17, 1985
120. Subaiya L, Rege A, Weng JT, et al: The influence of isoflurane on plasma beta-endorphin immunoreactivity. Anesth Analg 63:278, 1984
121. Evan SF, Stringer M, Bukht MDG, et al: Nitrous oxide inhalation does not influence plasma concentrations of β-endorphin or met-enkephalin-like immunoreactivity. Br J Anaesth 57:624, 1985
122. Way WL, Hosobuchi Y, Johnson BH, et al: Anesthesia does not increase opioid peptides in cerebrospinal fluid of humans. Anesthesiology 60:43, 1984
123. Sjostrom S, Tamsen A, Hartvig P, et al: Cerebrospinal fluid concentrations of substance P and (met)enkephalin-ARG^6-PHE^7 during surgery and patient-controlled analgesia. Anesth Analg 67:976, 1988
124. Havlicek V, LaBella FS, Pinsky C, et al: Beta-endorphin induces general anesthesia by an interaction with opiate receptors. Can Anaesth Soc J 27:535, 1980
125. Berkowitz BA, Finck AD, Ngai SH: Nitrous oxide analgesia: Reversal by naloxone and development of tolerance. J Pharmacol Exp Ther 203:539, 1977
126. Quock RM, Graczak LM: Influence of narcotic antagonist drugs upon nitrous oxide analgesia in mice. Brain Res 440:35, 1988
127. Chapman CR, Bendetti C: Nitrous oxide effects on cerebral evoked potential to pain: Partial reversal with a narcotic antagonist. Anesthesiology 51:135, 1979
128. Yang JC, Clark WC, Ngai SH: Antagonism of nitrous oxide analgesia by naloxone in man. Anesthesiology 52:414, 1980
129. Gillman MA, Lichtigfeld FA: Nitrous oxide analgesia is potentiated by low doses of naloxone: more possible evidence for a hyperalgesic opioid system. S Afr J Sci 83:560, 1987
130. Miller KW, Paton WDM, Smith EB, et al: Physicochemical approaches to the mode of action of general anesthetics. Anesthesiology 36:339, 1972
131. Seeman P: The membrane actions of anesthetics and tranquilizers. Pharmacol Rev 24:583, 1972
132. Miller KW: The nature of the site of general anaesthesia. Int Rev Neurobiol 27:1, 1985
133. Franks NP, Lieb WR: What is the molecular nature of general anesthetic target sites? Trends Pharmacol Sci 8:169, 1987
134. Mullins LJ: Some physical mechanisms in narcosis. Chem Rev 54:289, 1954
135. Franks NP, Lieb WR: Where do general anaesthetics act? Nature 274:339, 1978
136. Franks NP, Lieb WR: Molecular mechanisms of general anaesthesia. Nature 300:487, 1982
137. Miller RD, Wahrenbrock EA, Schroeder CF, et al: Ethylene-halothane anesthesia. Anesthesiology 31:301, 1969
138. DiFazio CA, Brown RE, Ball CG, et al: Additive effects of anesthetics and theories of anesthesia. Anesthesiology 36:57, 1972
139. Clarke RF, Daniels S, Harrison B, et al: Potency of mixtures of general anaesthetic agents. Br J Anaesth 50:979, 1978
140. Eger EI II (ed): MAC, Nitrous Oxide/N$_2$O. p. 57. Elsevier Science Publishing, New York, 1985
141. Skeehan TM, Larach DR, Hensley FA, et al: Anesthetic potency of co-administered halothane and isoflurane in the rat. Anesthesiology 67A:379, 1987
142. Angel A, Gratton DA: A possible mechanism for anaesthetic action. p. 1. In Tiengo M, Cousins MJ (eds): Pharmacological Basis of Anesthesiology: Clinical Pharmacology of New Analgesics and Anesthetics. Raven Press, New York, 1983
143. Cole DJ, Kalichman MW, Shapiro HM: The nonlinear contribution of nitrous oxide at sub-MAC concentrations to enflurane MAC in rats. Anesth Analg 68:556, 1989
144. Koblin DD, Eger EI II, Johnson BH, et al: Minimum alveolar concentrations and oil/gas partition coefficients of four anesthetic isomers. Anesthesiology 54:314, 1981
145. Rudo FG, Krantz JC: Anaesthetic molecules. Br J Anaesth 46:181, 1974
146. Burns THS, Hall JM, Bracken A, et al: Fluorine compounds in anaesthesia (9). Examination of six aliphatic compounds and four ethers. Anaesthesia 37:278, 1982
147. Koblin DD, Eger EI II, Johnson BH, et al: Are convulsant gases also anesthetics? Anesth Analg 60:464, 1981
148. Stevens JE, Fujinaga M, Oshima E, et al: The biphasic pattern of the convulsive property of enflurane in cats. Br J Anaesth 56:395, 1984
149. Smith RA, Paton WDM: The anesthetic effect of oxygen. Anesth Analg 55:734, 1976
150. Cohen S, Goldschmid A, Shtacher G, et al: The inhalation convulsants: A pharmacodynamic approach. Mol Pharmacol 11:379, 1975
151. Richter J, Landau EM, Cohen S: Anaesthetic and convulsant ethers act on different sites at the crab neuromuscular junction in vitro. Nature 266:70, 1977
152. Landau EM, Richter J, Cohen S: The mean conductance and open-time of the acetylcholine receptor channels can be independently modified by some anesthetic and convulsant ethers. Mol Pharmacol 16:1075, 1979
153. Gage PW, Sah P: Postsynaptic effects of some central stimulants at the neuromuscular junction. Br J Pharmacol 75:493, 1982
154. Landau EM, Richter J, Cohen S: Differential solubilities in subregions of the membrane: A non-steric mechanism of drug specificity. J Med Chem 22:325, 1979
155. Mullins LJ: Anesthetics. p. 395. In Lajtha A (ed): Handbook of Neurochemistry. Vol 6. Plenum, New York, 1971
156. Haydon DA, Requena J, Urban BW: Some effects of aliphatic hydrocarbons on the electrical capacity and ionic currents of the squid axon membrane. J Physiol (Lond) 309:229, 1980
157. Janoff AS, Miller KW: A critical assessment of the lipid theories of general anesthetic action. p. 417. In Chapman D (ed): Biological Membranes. Academic Press, London, 1982
158. Franks NP, Lieb WR: Partitioning of long-chain alcohols into lipid bilayers: Implications for mechanisms of general anesthesia. Proc Natl Acad Sci USA 83:5116, 1986
159. Dodson BA, Miller KW: Evidence for a dual mechanism in the anesthetic action of an opioid peptide. Anesthesiology 62:615, 1985
160. Stone DJ, DiFazio CA: Anesthetic action of opiates: Correlations of lipid solubility and spectral edge. Anesth Analg 67:663, 1988
161. Pauling L: A molecular theory of general anesthesia. Science 134:15, 1961
162. Miller SL: A theory of gaseous anesthetics. Proc Natl Acad Sci USA 47:1515, 1961
163. Eger EI II, Lundgren C, Miller SL, et al: Anesthetic potencies of sulfur hexafluoride, chloroform, and Ethrane in dogs. Anesthesiology 30:129, 1969
164. Buchet R, Sandorfy C: The effect of anesthetics on hydrogen

bonds: An infrared study at low anesthetic concentrations. Biophys Chem 22:249, 1985

165. Tsai YS, Ma SM, Kamaya H, Ueda I: Fourier transform infrared studies on phospholipid hydration: Phosphate-oriented hydrogen bonding and its attenuation by volatile anesthetics. Mol Pharmacol 31:623, 1987

166. Wood S, Wardley-Smith B, Halsey MJ, et al: Hydrogen bonding in mechanisms of anaesthesia tested with chloroform and deuterated chloroform. Br J Anaesth 54:387, 1982

167. Vulliemoz Y, Triner L, Verosky M, et al: Deuterated halothane—anesthetic potency, anticonvulsant activity, and effect on cerebellar cyclic guanosine 3′,5′-monophosphate. Anesth Analg 63:495, 1984

168. Miller KW: Inert gas narcosis, the high pressure neurological syndrome, and the critical volume hypothesis. Science 185:867, 1974

169. Miller KW, Paton WDM, Smith RA, et al: The pressure reversal of anesthesia and the critical volume hypothesis. Mol Pharmacol 9:131, 1973

170. Wardley-Smith B, Halsey MJ: Mixtures of inhalation and i.v. anaesthetics at high pressure. A test of the multi-site hypothesis of general anaesthesia. Br J Anaesth 57:1248, 1985

171. Urban BW, Haydon DA: The actions of halogenated ethers on the ionic currents of the squid giant axon. Proc R Soc Lond [Biol] 231:13, 1987

172. Brett RS, Dilger JP, Yland KF: Isoflurane causes "flickering" of the acetylcholine receptor channel: Observations using the patch clamp. Anesthesiology 69:161, 1988

173. Nicoll RA, Madison DV: General anesthetics hyperpolarize neurons in the vertebrate central nervous system. Science 217:1055, 1982

174. Branca D, Varotto ML, Vincenti E, Scutari G: The inhibition of calcium efflux from rat liver mitochondria by halogenated anesthetics. Biochem Biophys Res Commun 155:978, 1988

175. Daniell LC, Harris RA: Neuronal intracellular calcium concentrations are altered by anesthetics: Relationship to membrane fluidization. J Pharmacol Exp Ther 245:1, 1988

176. Saubermann AJ, Gallagher ML: Mechanisms of general anesthesia: Failure of pentobarbital and halothane to depolymerize microtubules in mouse optic nerve. Anesthesiology 38:25, 1973

177. Bangham AD: Liposome Letters. Academic Press, London, 1983

178. Catterall WA: Structure and function of voltage-sensitive ion channels. Science 242:50, 1988

179. Smith RA, Porter EG, Miller KW: The solubility of anesthetic gases in lipid bilayers. Biochim Biophys Acta 645:327, 1981

180. Janoff AS, Pringle MJ, Miller KW: Correlation of general anesthetic potency with solubility in membranes. Biochim Biophys Acta 649:125, 1981

181. Kamaya H, Kaneshina S, Ueda I: Partition equilibrium of inhalation anesthetics and alcohols between water and membranes of phospholipids with varying acyl chain-lengths. Biochim Biophys Acta 646:135, 1981

182. Lieb WR, Kovalycrik M, Mendelsohn R: Do clinical levels of general anesthetics affect lipid bilayers? Biochim Biophys Acta 688:388, 1982

183. Trudell JR, Hubbell WL: Localization of molecular halothane in phospholipid bilayer model nerve membranes. Anesthesiology 44:202, 1976

184. Miller KW, Reo NV, Schoot Uiterkamp AJM, et al: Xenon NMR: Chemical shifts of a general anesthetic in common solvents, proteins, and membranes. Proc Natl Acad Sci USA 78:4946, 1981

185. King GI, Jacobs RE, White SH: Hexane dissolved in dioleoyl-lecithin bilayers has a partial volume of approximately zero. Biochemistry 24:4637, 1985

186. Craig NC, Bryant GJ, Levin IW: Effects of halothane on dipalmitoylphosphatidylcholine liposomes: A Raman spectroscopic study. Biochemistry 26:2449, 1987

187. Washington K, Sarasua MM, Koehler LS, et al: Utilization of heavy-atom effect quenching of pyrene fluorescence to determine the intramembrane distribution of halothane. Photochem Photobiol 40:693, 1984

188. Johnson SM, Miller KW, Bangham AD: The opposing effects of pressure and general anaesthetics on the cation permeability of liposomes of varying lipid composition. Biochim Biophys Acta 307:42, 1973

189. Pang KY, Chang TL, Miller KW: On the coupling between anesthetic-induced membrane lipid fluidization and cation permeability of liposomes of varying lipid composition. Mol Pharmacol 15:729, 1979

190. Barchfeld GL, Deamer DW: The effect of general anesthetics on the proton and potassium permeabilities of liposomes. Biochim Biophys Acta 819:161, 1985

191. Fassoulaki A, Kaniaris P, Varonos DD: Do general anaesthetics perturb lipid membranes? The role of cholesterol. Br J Anaesth 56:1045, 1984

192. Bangham AD, Hill MW: The proton pump/leak mechanism of unconsciousness. Chem Phys Lipids 40:189, 1986

193. Clements JA, Wilson KM: The affinity of narcotic agents for interfacial films. Proc Natl Acad Sci USA 48:1008, 1962

194. Suezaki Y, Shibata A, Kamaya H, Ueda I: Atypical Langmuir adsorption of inhalation anesthetics on phospholipid monolayer at various compressional states: Difference between alkane-type and ether-type anesthetics. Biochim Biophys Acta 817:139, 1985

195. Franks NP, Lieb WR: Is membrane expansion relevant to anaesthesia? Nature 292:248, 1981

196. Mori T, Matubayasi N, Ueda I: Membrane expansion and inhalation anesthetics. Mean excess volume hypothesis. Mol Pharmacol 25:123, 1984

197. Bull MH, Brailsford JD, Bull BS: Erythrocyte membrane expansion due to the volatile anesthetics, the 1-alkanols, and benzyl alcohol. Anesthesiology 57:399, 1982

198. Elliott JR, Haydon DA, Hendry BM, Needham D: Inactivation of the sodium current in squid giant axons by hydrocarbons. Biophys J 48:617, 1985

199. Franks NP, Lieb WR: The structure of lipid bilayers and the effects of general anaesthetics. An x-ray and neutron diffraction study. J Mol Biol 133:469, 1979

200. Firestone LL, Kitz RJ: Anesthetics and lipids: Some molecular perspectives. Semin Anesth 5:286, 1986

201. Trudell JR, Hubbell WL, Cohen EN: The effect of two inhalation anesthetics on the order of spin-labeled phospholipid vesicles. Biochim Biophys Acta 291:321, 1973

202. Mastrangelo CJ, Trudell JR, Cohen EN: Antagonism of membrane compression effects by high pressure gas mixtures in a phospholipid bilayer system. Life Sci 22:239, 1978

203. Harris RA, Groh GI: Membrane disordering effects of anesthetics are enhanced by gangliosides. Anesthesiology 62:115, 1985

204. Mastrangelo CJ, Trudell JR, Edmunds HN, et al: Effect of clinical concentrations of halothane on phospholipid-cholesterol membrane fluidity. Mol Pharmacol 14:463, 1978

205. Ueda I, Hirakawa M, Arakawa K, Kamaya H: Do anesthetics fluidize membranes? Anesthesiology 64:67, 1986

206. Miller KW, Braswell LM, Firestone LL, et al: General anesthetics act both specifically and nonspecifically on acetylcholine receptors. p. 125. In Roth SH, Miller KW (eds): Mo-

lecular and Cellular Mechanisms of Anesthetics. Plenum, New York, 1986

207. Rosenberg PH, Alila A: GABA inhibits inhalation anaesthetic-induced membrane fluidization: A spin label study in synaptic and phospholipid membranes. Acta Pharmacol Toxicol 57:154, 1985

208. Harris RA, Bruno P: Effects of ethanol and other intoxicant-anesthetics on voltage-dependent sodium channels of brain synaptosomes. J Pharmacol Exp Ther 232:401, 1985

209. Harris RA, Bruno P: Membrane disordering by anesthetic drugs: Relationship to synaptosomal sodium and calcium fluxes. J Neurochem 44:1274, 1985

210. Simmonds AC, Halsey MJ: General and local anesthetics perturb the fusion of phospholipid vesicles. Biochim Biophys Acta 813:331, 1985

211. Rosenberg PH, Heavner JE: Temperature dependent nerve-blocking concentration of lidocaine and halothane. Acta Anaesthesiol Scand 24:314, 1980

212. Galla HJ, Trudell JR: Asymmetric antagonistic effects of an inhalation anesthetic and high pressure on the phase transition temperature of dipalmitoyl phosphatidic acid bilayers. Biochim Biophys Acta 599:336, 1980

213. Lee AG: Model for action of local anesthetics. Nature 262:545, 1976

214. Trudell JR: A unitary theory of anesthesia based on lateral phase separations in nerve membranes. Anesthesiology 46:5, 1977

215. Trudell JR, Payan DG, Chin JH, et al: The antagonistic effect of an inhalation anesthetic and high pressure on the phase diagram of mixed dipalmitoyl-dimyristoylphosphatidylcholine bilayers. Proc Natl Acad Sci USA 72:210, 1975

216. Shinitzky M: Patterns of lipid changes in membranes of the aged brain. Gerontology 33:149, 1987

217. Evers AS, Berkowitz BA, d'Avignon A: Correlation between the anaesthetic effect of halothane and saturable binding in brain. Nature 328:157, 1987

218. Coburn CM, Eger EI II: The partial pressure of isoflurane or halothane does not affect their solubility in rabbit blood or brain or human brain: Inhaled anesthetics obey Henry's law. Anesth Analg 65:960, 1986

219. Brown FF, Halsey MJ: Interactions of anesthetics with proteins. p. 385. In Fink BR (ed): Progress in Anesthesiology. Vol 2. Molecular Mechanisms of Anesthesia. Raven Press, New York, 1980

220. Tilton RF, Singh UC, Weiner SJ, et al: Computational studies of the interaction of myoglobin and xenon. J Mol Biol 192:443, 1986

221. Mashimo T, Kamaya H, Ueda I: Anesthetic-protein interaction: Surface potential of bovine serum albumin estimated by a pH-sensitive dye. Mol Pharmacol 29:149, 1986

222. Brammal A, Beard DJ, Hulands GH: Inhalation anaesthetics and their interaction *in vitro* with glutamate dehydrogenase and other enzymes. Br J Anaesth 46:643, 1974

223. Laverty DM, Fennema O: Effects of anesthetics and dichlorodifluoromethane on the activities of glyceraldehyde-phosphate dehydrogenase and pectin methylesterase. Biochem Pharmacol 34:2839, 1985

224. Braswell LM, Kitz RJ: The effect *in vitro* of volatile anesthetics on the activity of cholinesterases. J Neurochem 29:665, 1977

225. Nosaka S, Kamaya H, Ueda I: High pressure and anesthesia: Pressure stimulates or inhibits bacterial bioluminescence depending upon temperature. Anesth Analg 67:988, 1988

226. Franks NP, Lieb WR: Do general anaesthetics act by competitive binding to specific receptors? Nature 310:599, 1984

227. Franks NP, Lieb WR: Mapping of general anaesthetic target sites provides a molecular basis for cutoff effects. Nature 316:349, 1985

228. Young AP, Sigman DS: Conformational effects of volatile anesthetics on the membrane-bound acetylcholine receptor protein: Facilitation of the agonist-induced affinity conversion. Biochemistry 22:2155, 1983

229. Firestone LL, Sauter JF, Braswell LM, Miller KW: Actions of general anesthetics on acetylcholine receptor-rich membranes from *Torpedo californica*. Anesthesiology 64:694, 1986

230. Sauter JF, Braswell LM, Miller KW: Action of anesthetics and high pressure on cholinergic membranes. p. 199. In Fink BR (ed): Progress in Anesthesiology. Vol 2. Molecular Mechanisms of Anesthesia. Raven Press, New York, 1980

231. Mashimo T, Tashiro C, Yoshiya I: Effects of volatile anesthetics on light-induced proton uptake of rhodopsin in bovine rod outer segment disk membrane. Anesthesiology 61:439, 1984

232. Nishimura N, Mashimo T, Hiraki K, et al: Volatile anesthetics cause conformational changes of bacteriorhodopsin in purple membrane. Biochim Biophys Acta 818:421, 1985

233. Henry N, Beaudoin N, Baribeau J, Boucher F: Further characterization of anesthetic-treated purple membranes. Photochem Photobiol 47:85, 1988

234. Tas PWL, Kress HG, Koschel K: General anesthetics can competitively interfere with sensitive membrane proteins. Proc Natl Acad Sci USA 84:5972, 1987

235. Nicoll RA: The coupling of neurotransmitter receptors to ion channels in the brain. Science 241:545, 1988

236. Segal IS, Maze M: The role of pertussis toxin-sensitive G proteins in the anesthetic action of halothane in rats. Anesthesiology 69A:318, 1988

237. Anthony BL, Dennison RL, Narayanan TK, Aronstam RS: Diethyl ether effects on muscarinic acetylcholine receptor complexes in rat brainstem. Biochem Pharmacol 37:4041, 1988

238. Koblin DD, Dong DE, Eger EI II: Tolerance of mice to nitrous oxide. J Pharmacol Exp Ther 211:317, 1979

239. Koblin DD, Eger EI II, Smith RA, et al: Chronic exposure of mice to subanesthetic doses of nitrous oxide. p. 157. In Fink BR (ed): Progress in Anesthesiology. Vol 2. Molecular Mechanisms of Anesthesia. Raven Press, New York, 1980

240. Smith RA, Winter PM, Smith M, et al: Tolerance to and dependence on inhalational anesthetics. Anesthesiology 50:505, 1979

241. Brauer RW, Dutcher JA, Hinson W, et al: Effect of habituation to subanesthetic N_2 or N_2O levels on pressure and anesthesia tolerance. J Appl Physiol 62:421, 1987

242. Chalon J, Tank CK, Roberts C, et al: Murine auto- and cross-tolerance to volatile anaesthetics. Can Anaesth Soc J 30:230, 1983

243. Fuller GN, Rigor BM, Wiggins RC, et al: Prolonged daily inhalation of halothane modifies the dose-response pattern to acute administration of halothane. An electrophysiological study. Neuropharmacol 24:1033, 1985

244. Munson ES: Lack of tolerance to cyclopropane and cross-tolerance to halothane in rats. Can Anaesth Soc J 31:642, 1984

245. Ngai SH, Finck AD: Prolonged exposure to nitrous oxide decreases opiate receptor density in rat brainstem. Anesthesiology 57:26, 1982

246. Whitwam JG, Morgan M, Hall GM, et al: Pain during continuous nitrous oxide administration. Br J Anaesth 48:425, 1976

247. Rupreht J, Dworacek B, Bonke B, et al: Tolerance to nitrous oxide in volunteers. Acta Anaesthesiol Scand 29:635, 1985

248. Shingu K, Osawa M, Fukuda K, et al: Acute tolerance to the

analgesic action of nitrous oxide does not develop in rats. Anesthesiology 62:502, 1985

249. Rupreht J, Ukponmwan OE, Dworacek B, et al: Enkephalinase inhibition prevented tolerance to nitrous oxide analgesia in rats. Acta Anaesthesiol Scand 28:617, 1984

250. Smith RA, Winter PM, Smith M, et al: Rapidly developing tolerance to acute exposures to anesthetic agents. Anesthesiology 50:496, 1979

251. Mori K, Winters WD: Neural background of sleep and anesthesia. Int Anesthesiol Clin 13:67, 1975

252. Stevens JE, Oshima E, Mori K: Effects of nitrous oxide on the epileptogenic property of enflurane in cats. Br J Anaesth 55:145, 1983

253. Sauter JF: Electrophysiological activity of a mammalian sympathetic ganglion under hyperbaric nitrous oxide. Neuropharmacology 18:71, 1979

254. Smith RA, Winter PM, Smith M, et al: Convulsions in mice after anesthesia. Anesthesiology 50:501, 1979

255. Harper MH, Winter PM, Johnson BH, et al: Withdrawal convulsions in mice following nitrous oxide. Anesth Analg 59:19, 1980

256. Rupreht J, Dworacek B, Ducardus R, et al: The involvement of the central cholinergic and endorphinergic systems in the nitrous oxide withdrawal syndrome in mice. Anesthesiology 58:524, 1983

257. Manson HJ, Dyke G, Melling J, et al: The effect of naloxone and morphine on convulsions in mice following withdrawal from nitrous oxide. Can Anaesth Soc J 30:28, 1983

258. Milne B, Cervenko FW, Jhamandas KH: Physical dependence of nitrous oxide in mice: Resemblance to alcohol but not to opiate withdrawal. Can Anaesth Soc J 28:46, 1983

259. Koblin DD, Dong DE, Deady JE, et al: Selective breeding alters murine resistance to nitrous oxide without alteration in synaptic membrane lipid composition. Anesthesiology 52:401, 1980

260. Koblin DD, O'Connor B, Deady JE, et al: Potencies of convulsant drugs in mice selectively bred for resistance and susceptibility to nitrous oxide anesthesia. Anesthesiology 56:25, 1982

261. Koblin DD, Eger EI II: Cross-mating of mice selectively bred for resistance and susceptibility to nitrous oxide anesthesia: Potencies of nitrous oxide in the offspring. Anesth Analg 60:646, 1981

262. Roizen MF, Koblin DD, Johnson BH, et al: Mechanism of age-related and nitrous oxide-associated anesthetic sensitivity: the role of brain catecholamines. Anesthesiology 69:716, 1988

263. Belknap JK, Laursen SE, Crabbe JC: Ethanol and nitrous oxide produce withdrawal-induced convulsions by similar mechanisms in mice. Life Sci 41:2033, 1987

264. Koblin DD, Deady JE: Anaesthetic requirement in mice selectively bred for differences in ethanol sensitivity. Br J Anaesth 53:5, 1981

265. McIntyre TD, Alpern HP: Reinterpretation of the literature indicates differential sensitivities of long-sleep and short-sleep mice are not specific to alcohol. Psychopharmacology 87:379, 1985

266. Erwin VG, Korte A, Marty M: Neurotensin selectively alters ethanol-induced anesthesia in LS/Ibg and SS/Ibg lines of mice. Brain Res 400:80, 1987

267. Baker RC: Disassociation of cerebellar phospholipid composition and acute ethanol effects in mice selectively bred for differential sensitivity to ethanol. Alcohol Drug Res 7:291, 1987

268. Koblin DD: Anesthetic requirement in the quaking mouse. Anesthesiology 54:17, 1981

269. Gamo S, Ogaki M, Nakashima-Tanaka E: Strain differences in minimum anesthetic concentrations in *Drosophila melanogaster*. Anesthesiology 54:289, 1981

270. Gamo S, Nakashima-Tanaka E, Ogaki M: Alteration in molecular-species of phosphatidylethanolamine between anesthetic resistant and sensitive strains of *Drosophila melanogaster*. Life Sci 30:401, 1982

271. Morgan PG, Cascorbi HF: Effect of anesthetics and a convulsant on normal and mutant *Caenorhabditis elegans*. Anesthesiology 62:738, 1985

272. Sedensky MM, Meneely PM: Genetic analysis of halothane sensitivity in *Caenorhabditis elegans*. Science 236:952, 1987

273. Morgan PG, Sedensky MM, Meneely PM, Cascorbi HF: The effect of two genes on anesthetic response in the nematode *Caenorhabditis elegans*. Anesthesiology 69:246, 1988

274. Koblin DD, Dong DE, Deady JE, et al: Alteration of synaptic membrane fatty acid composition and anesthetic requirement. J Pharmacol Exp Ther 212:546, 1980

275. Evers AS, Elliott WJ, Lefkowith JB, Needleman P: Manipulation of rat brain fatty acid composition alters volatile anesthetic potency. J Clin Invest 77:1028, 1986

276. Haycock JC, Evers AS: Altered phosphoinositide fatty acid composition, mass and metabolism in brain essential fatty acid deficiency. Biochim Biophys Acta 960:54, 1988

277. Tanifuji Y, Eger EI II, Terrell RC: Some characteristics of an exceptionally potent inhaled anesthetic: Thiomethoxyflurane. Anesth Analg 56:387, 1977

278. Kent DW, Halsey MJ, Eger EI II, et al: Isoflurane anesthesia and pressure antagonism in mice. Anesth Analg 56:97, 1977

279. Eger EI II, Koblin DD, Collins PA: Dioxychlorane: A challenge to the correlation of anesthetic potency and lipid solubility. Anesth Analg 60:201, 1981

280. Uyeno ET, Denson DD, Simon RL, Jr., et al: Bioassay of fluorinated volatile anesthetics. Proc West Pharmacol Soc 20:357, 1977

281. Eger EI II: Partition coefficients of I-653 in human blood, saline, and olive oil. Anesth Analg 66:971, 1987

282. Doorley BM, Waters SJ, Terrell RC, Robinson JL: MAC of I-653 in beagle dogs and New Zealand white rabbits. Anesthesiology 69:89, 1988

283. Eger EI II: Personal communication, December, 1988

284. Munson ES, Schick LM, Chapin JC, et al: Determination of the minimum alveolar concentration (MAC) of Aliflurane in dogs. Anesthesiology 51:545, 1979

285. Mazze RI, Beppu WJ, Hitt BA: Metabolism of synthane: Comparison with in vivo and *in vitro* defluorination of other halogenated hydrocarbon anesthetics. Br J Anaesth 51:839, 1979

286. Smith RA, Koblin DD, Smith M, et al: The anesthetic potency of volatile agents in mice. p. 617. Abstracts of Scientific Papers. ASA Meeting, 1978

287. Strum DP, Eger EI II: Partition coefficients for sevoflurane in human blood, saline, and olive oil. Anesth Analg 66:654, 1987

288. Kazama T, Ikeda K: Comparison of MAC and the rate of rise of alveolar concentration of sevoflurane with halothane and isoflurane in the dog. Anesthesiology 68:435, 1988

289. Scheller MS, Saidman LJ, Partridge BL: MAC of sevoflurane in humans and the New Zealand white rabbit. Can J Anaesth 35:153, 1988

290. Hornbein TF, Eger EI II, Winter PM, et al: The minimum alveolar concentration of nitrous oxide in man. Anesth Analg 61:553, 1982

291. Gage PW, Hamill OP: Effects of several inhalation anesthetics on the kinetics of postsynaptic conductance changes in mouse diaphragm. Br J Pharmacol 57:263, 1976

4

UPTAKE AND DISTRIBUTION

Edmond I. Eger II

INTRODUCTION

To produce a brain anesthetic concentration sufficient for surgery requires proper manipulation of anesthetic delivery to the patient. Proper manipulation also requires that the delivered concentration not produce excessive depression. Thus, knowledge of the factors that govern the relationship between the delivered and brain (or heart or muscle) concentrations is indispensable to the optimum conduct of anesthesia. It is these factors that are the substance of anesthetic uptake and distribution.

THE INSPIRED TO ALVEOLAR ANESTHETIC RELATIONSHIP

Of the steps between delivered and brain anesthetic partial pressures, none is more pivotal than that between the inspired and alveolar gases. By use of high inflow rates (and hence conversion to a nonrebreathing system), the anesthetist can precisely control the partial pressure of anesthetic that is inspired. The alveolar partial pressure governs the partial pressure of anesthetic in all body tissues: all must approach and ultimately equal the alveolar partial pressure.

The Effect of Ventilation

Two factors determine the rate at which the alveolar concentration of anesthetic (FA) rises toward the concentration being inspired (FI): the inspired concentration (discussed in the section on the concentration effect) and the alveolar ventilation. The effect of ventilation is a powerful one. If unopposed on induction, ventilation rapidly increases the alveolar concentration (i.e., FA/FI quickly approaches 1). This is seen with preoxygenation to achieve nitrogen washout: normally a 95 percent or greater washout of nitrogen occurs in 2 minutes or less when a nonrebreathing (or high inflow rate) system is used.

However, the rapid washout of nitrogen or washin of oxygen is not mimicked by the inhaled anesthetics. The solubility of anesthetics is far higher than that of nitrogen and causes the transfer of substantial quantities of anesthetic to the blood passing through the lung. This uptake opposes the effect of ventilation to increase the alveolar anesthetic concentration. At low inspired concentrations, the FA/FI ratio ultimately is determined by the balance between the delivery of anesthetic by ventilation and its removal by uptake. The relationship is a simple one. For example, if uptake removes 1/3 of the inspired anesthetic molecules, then the FA/FI ratio will equal 2/3; if uptake removes 3/4 of the inspired molecules then FA/FI ratio will equal 1/4.

Anesthetic Uptake Factors

Anesthetic uptake itself is the product of three factors: solubility (λ), cardiac output ($\dot{Q}$), and the alveolar to venous partial pressure difference (PA − PV).[1] That is

$$\text{Uptake} = \lambda \cdot \dot{Q} \cdot (\text{PA} - \text{PV})/\text{BP} \qquad (1)$$

where BP is the barometric pressure. Being a product rather than a sum means that if any component of uptake approaches zero, then uptake must approach zero and the effect of ventilation to drive the alveolar concentrations rapidly upward will be unopposed. Thus, if the solubility is small (as for nitrogen), the cardiac output approaches zero (profound myocardial depression or death), or the alveolar to venous difference becomes inconsequential (as might occur after an extraordinarily long anesthetic), then uptake would be minimal and FA/FI would equal 1.

Solubility

The blood/gas partition coefficient (λ or *blood solubility*) described the relative affinity of anesthetic for two phases and hence how the anesthetic will *partition* itself between the two phases when equilibrium has been achieved. For example, enflurane has a blood/gas partition coefficient of 1.9, indicating that at equilibrium the concentration in blood will be 1.9 times the concentration in the gas (alveolar) phase. Remember that *equilibrium* means that no difference in partial pressure exists —that is, the blood/gas partition coefficient of 1.9 does *not* indicate that the partial pressure in blood will be 1.9 times that in the gas phase. The partition coefficient may be thought of in one other way: it indicates the relative capacity of the two phases. Thus, a value of 1.9 means that each milliliter of blood can hold 1.9 times as much enflurane as 1 ml of alveolar gas.

A larger blood/gas partition coefficient will produce a greater uptake and hence a lower FA/FI ratio. Since the anesthetic partial pressure in all tissues approaches that in the alveoli, the development of an adequate brain anesthetic partial pressure may be delayed in the case of highly blood-soluble agents such as ether or methoxyflurane (Table 4-1).[1] Even the moderate solubility of isoflurane, enflurane, or halothane would slow induction of anesthesia with these agents were it not for our use of "anesthetic overpressure." That is, we compensate for the uptake of anesthetic by delivering a far higher concentration than we hope to achieve in the alveoli. For example, on induction of anesthesia, we may use 3 to 4 percent halothane to produce an alveolar concentration of 1 percent.

Cardiac Output

The effect of altering cardiac output is intuitively obvious. The passage of more blood through the lungs will remove more anesthetic and thereby lower the alveolar anesthetic concentration. To the beginning student of uptake and distribution, this may appear to produce a conflict. It would seem that if more agent were taken up and delivered more rapidly to the tissues, then the tissue anesthetic partial pressure should rise more rapidly. In one sense this *is* true: an increase in cardiac output does hasten the equilibration of tissue anesthetic partial pressure with the partial pressure in arterial blood.[2] What this reasoning ignores is the fact that the anesthetic partial pressure in arterial blood is lower than it would be if cardiac output were normal.

The effect of a change in cardiac output is analogous to the effect of a change in solubility. As already noted, doubling solubility doubled the capacity of the same volume of blood to hold anesthetic. Doubling cardiac output also would double capacity, but in this case by increasing the volume of blood exposed to anesthetic.

The Alveolar to Venous Anesthetic Gradient

The alveolar to venous anesthetic partial pressure difference results from tissue uptake of anesthetic. Were there no tissue uptake, then the venous blood returning to the lungs would contain as much anesthetic as it had when it left the lungs as arterial blood. That is, the alveolar (equals arterial) to venous partial pressure difference would be zero. The presumption that alveolar and arterial anesthetic partial pressures are equal is reasonable in normal patients who have no barrier to diffusion of anesthetic from alveoli to pulmonary capillary blood and who do not have ventilation/perfusion ratio abnormalities. Later I shall consider the effect of

TABLE 4-1. Partition Coefficients at 37°C

Anesthetic	Blood/Gas	Brain/Blood	Liver/Blood	Kidney/Blood	Muscle/Blood	Fat/Blood
Desflurane (I-653)	0.42	1.3	1.4	1.0	2.3	30
Nitrous oxide	0.47	1.1	0.8	—	1.2	2.3
Sevoflurane	0.69	1.7	1.8	1.2	3.6	55
Isoflurane	1.4	1.6	1.8	1.2	3.4	52
Enflurane	1.8	1.4	2.1	—	1.7	36
Halothane	2.4	2.0	2.1	1.2	4.0	62
Diethyl ether	12	2.0	1.9	0.9	1.3	49
Methoxyflurane	15	1.4	2.0	0.9	1.6	61

(Data from Eger,[1] Eger and Eger,[70] Yasuda et al.,[71] Lerman et al.,[72] and Eger.[73])

ventilation/perfusion ratio abnormalities on anesthetic uptake.

The factors that determine the fraction of anesthetic removed from blood traversing a given tissue parallel those factors that govern uptake at the lungs: tissue solubility, tissue blood flow, and arterial to tissue anesthetic partial pressure difference. Again, uptake is the product of these three factors. If any one factor approaches zero, then uptake by that tissue becomes inconsequential. The succeeding paragraphs discuss the characteristics of each of these factors and then how uptake by individual tissues can be summed to give the venous component of the alveolar to venous anesthetic partial pressure difference.

Blood/gas partition coefficients span a range of values extending from 0.42 for I-653 (a new, experimental anesthetic that likely will be widely used in the future) to 15 for methoxyflurane (Table 4-1). In contrast, tissue/blood partition coefficients (i.e., tissue solubility) for lean tissues are close to 1, ranging from slightly less than 1 to a maximum of 4 (Table 4-1). That is, different lean tissues do not have greatly different capacities per milliliter of tissue. Put another way, a given anesthetic has roughly the same affinity for lean tissues and blood. As with blood/gas partition coefficients, tissue/blood partition coefficients define the concentration ratio of anesthetic at equilibrium. For example, a halothane brain/blood partition coefficient of 2.0 means that 1 ml of brain can hold 2.0 times more halothane than 1 ml of blood having the same halothane partial pressure.

Lean tissues differ in terms of their perfusion per gram — that is, the volume of tissue relative to the blood passing that tissue. A larger volume of tissue relative to flow confers a greater capacity to hold anesthetic. This has two implications. First, the large tissue capacity increases the transfer of anesthetic from blood to tissue. Second, it takes longer to fill up a tissue with a large capacity; that is, it will take longer for the tissue to equilibrate with the anesthetic partial pressure being delivered in arterial blood. In other words, a large tissue volume relative to blood flow will sustain the arterial to tissue anesthetic partial pressure difference (and hence uptake) for a longer time. Brain with its high perfusion per gram will equilibrate rapidly. Muscle, with about one-twentieth the perfusion of brain, will

take about 20 times longer to equilibrate. Uptake of anesthetic by muscle will continue long after uptake by brain has ceased.

Fat has a tissue/blood coefficient that is significantly greater than 1 (Table 4-1). Fat/blood coefficients range from 2.3 (nitrous oxide) to 62 (halothane). That is, each milliliter of fat tissue will contain 2.3 times more nitrous oxide or 62 times more halothane than 1 ml of blood having the same nitrous oxide or halothane partial pressure. This enormous capacity of fat for anesthetic means that most of the anesthetic contained in the blood perfusing fat will be transferred to the fat. Although most of the anesthetic will move from the blood perfusing fat into the fat, the anesthetic partial pressure in that tissue will rise very slowly. Both the large capacity of fat and the low perfusion per ml of tissue prolong the time required to narrow the anesthetic partial pressure difference between arterial blood and fat.

Tissue Groups

The algebraic sum of uptake by individual tissues determines the alveolar to venous partial pressure difference and hence uptake at the lungs. It is not necessary to analyze the effect of individual tissues to arrive at the algebraic sum. Instead, we can group tissues in terms of their perfusion and solubility characteristics, that is, in terms of those features that define the duration of a substantial arterial to tissue anesthetic partial pressure difference. Four tissue groups are the result of such an analysis (Table 4-2).[1]

The vessel-rich group (VRG) is composed of the brain, heart, splanchnic bed (including liver), kidney, and endocrine glands. These organs make up less than

TABLE 4-2. Tissue Group Characteristics

	Group			
	Vessel Rich	Muscle	Fat	Vessel Poor
Percentage of body mass	10	50	20	20
Perfusion as percentage of cardiac output	75	19	6	0

(Adapted from Eger,[1] with permission.)

10 percent of the body weight but receive 75 percent of the cardiac output. This high perfusion confers several features. Access to a large flow of blood permits the VRG to take up a relatively large volume of anesthetic in the earliest moments of induction. However, the small volume of tissue relative to perfusion produces a rapid equilibration of this tissue group with the anesthetic delivered in arterial blood. The time to half equilibration (i.e., the time at which the VRG anesthetic partial pressure equals one-half that in arterial blood) varies from about 1 minute for nitrous oxide to 2 minutes for halothane or enflurane. The longer time to equilibration with halothane or enflurane results from their higher tissue/blood partition coefficients (Table 4-1). Equilibration of the VRG with the anesthetic partial pressure in arterial blood is over 90 percent complete in 4 to 8 minutes. Thus, after 8 minutes, uptake by the VRG is too small (i.e., the arterial to VRG anesthetic partial pressure difference is too small) to significantly influence the alveolar concentration. Uptake after 8 minutes is principally determined by the muscle group.

Muscle and skin, which make up the muscle group (MG), have similar blood flow and solubility (lean tissue) characteristics. The lower perfusion (about 3 ml of blood per 100 ml of tissue per minute) sets this group apart from the VRG (70 ml per 100 ml per minute). Although about one-half of the body bulk is muscle and skin, this volume receives only 1 L/min blood flow at rest. The large bulk relative to perfusion means that during induction, most of the anesthetic delivered to the MG is removed from the MG blood flow. The time to half equilibration ranges from 20 to 25 minutes (nitrous oxide) to 70 to 90 minutes (enflurane or halothane). Thus, long after equilibration of the VRG has taken place, muscle continues to take up substantial amounts of anesthetic. This tissue approaches equilibration in 1 to 4 hours.

Once equilibration of muscle is complete, only fat (i.e., the fat group or FG) continues to serve as an effective depot for uptake. In a normal lean patient, fat occupies one-fifth of the body bulk and receives a blood flow of about 300 ml/min. That is, the perfusion per 100 ml of fat nearly equals the perfusion per 100 ml of resting muscle. Fat differs from muscle in its higher affinity for anesthetic, a property that greatly lengthens the time over which it absorbs anesthetic. The half-time to equilibration of fat ranges from 70 to 80 minutes for nitrous oxide to 19 to 37 *hours* for enflurane and halothane, respectively. It is apparent that equilibration with fat will not occur in the course of an ordinary halothane or enflurane anesthetic.

One tissue group, the vessel-poor group (VPG), remains to be defined. This group is composed of ligaments, tendons, bone, and cartilage—those lean tissues that have little or no perfusion. The absence of a significant blood flow means that this group does not participate in the uptake process despite the fact that it makes up one-fifth of the body mass.

Synthesis of the Factors Governing the Rise of the FA/FI Ratio

We may now consider the combined impact of ventilation, solubility, and the distribution of blood flow on the development of the alveolar anesthetic partial pressure. The initial rate of rise of FA/FI is rapid for all agents regardless of their solubility (Fig. 4-1).[3-5] The rapidity of this upswing results from the absence of an alveolar to venous anesthetic partial pressure difference (there is no anesthetic present in the lung to create a gradient) and hence the absence of uptake in the first moment of induction. Thus, the effect of ventilation to generate a sudden rise in FA/FI is unopposed. Obviously, the delivery of more and more anesthetic to the alveoli by ventilation produces a progressively greater alveolar to venous partial pressure difference. The increasing uptake that ensues will increasingly oppose the effect of ventilation to drive the alveolar concentration upward. Ultimately a rough balance is struck between the input by ventilation and removal by uptake. The height of the FA/FI ratio at which the balance is struck depends on the solubility factor in the uptake equation [eq. (1)]. A higher solubility produces a greater uptake for a given alveolar to venous partial pressure difference. Hence, the initial rapid rise in FA/FI will be halted at a lower level with a more soluble agent. This results in the first "knee" in the curve— higher for nitrous oxide than isoflurane, higher for isoflurane than enflurane, higher for enflurane than halothane, and higher for halothane than ether.

The balance struck between ventilation and uptake

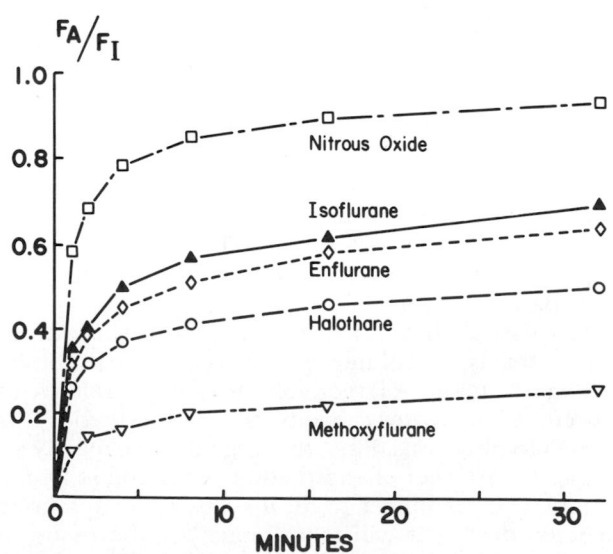

Fig. 4-1. The rise in alveolar (FA) anesthetic concentration toward the inspired (FI) concentration is most rapid with the least soluble anesthetic, nitrous oxide, and slowest with the most soluble anesthetic, diethyl ether. All data are from human studies.[1,3] (From Eger,[5] with permission.)

does not remain constant. FA/FI continues to rise, albeit at a slower rate than seen in the first minute. This rise results from the progressive decrease in uptake by the VRG, a decrease to an inconsequential amount after 8 minutes. Thus, by about 8 minutes, three-fourths of the cardiac output returning to the lungs (i.e., the blood from the VRG) contains nearly as much anesthetic as it had when it left the lungs. The consequent rise in venous anesthetic partial pressure decreases the alveolar to venous partial pressure difference and hence uptake, allowing ventilation to drive the alveolar concentration upward to the second knee at roughly 8 minutes.

With the termination of effective uptake by the VRG, muscle and fat become the principal determinants of tissue uptake. The slow rate of change of the anesthetic partial pressure difference between arterial blood and muscle or fat produces the relatively stable terminal portion of each curve in Figure 4-1. In fact, this terminal portion gradually ascends as muscle and, to a lesser extent, fat progressively equilibrate with the arterial anesthetic partial pressure. Were the graphs extended for several hours, a third knee would be found, indicating equilibration of the muscle group. Uptake after that time would principally depend on the partial pressure gradient between arterial blood and fat.

The Concentration Effect

The above analysis ignores the impact of the "concentration effect" on FA/FI. The inspired anesthetic concentration influences both the alveolar concentration that may be attained and the *rate* at which that concentration may be attained.[6,7] Increasing the inspired concentration accelerates the rate of rise. At an inspired concentration of 100 percent, the rate of rise is extremely rapid, since it is dictated solely by the rate at which ventilation washes gas into the lung. That is, at 100 percent inspired concentration, uptake no longer limits the level to which FA/FI may rise. The cause of this extreme effect is readily perceived. At 100 percent inspired concentration, the uptake of anesthetic creates a void that draws gas down the trachea. This additional "inspiration" replaces the gas taken up. Since the concentration of the replacement gas is 100 percent, uptake cannot modify the alveolar concentration.

The concentration effect results from two factors: a concentrating effect and an augmentation of inspired ventilation.[8] Both are illustrated in Figure 4-2. The first rectangle represents a lung containing 80 percent nitrous oxide. If one-half of this gas is taken up, the residual 40 volumes of nitrous oxide exists in a total of 60 volumes, yielding a concentration of 67 percent (Fig. 4-2A). That is, uptake of one-half of the nitrous oxide does not halve the concentration because the remaining gases are "concentrated" in a smaller volume. If the void created by uptake is filled by drawing more gas into the lungs (an augmentation of inspired ventilation), then the final concentration equals 72 percent (Fig. 4-2B).

The impact of the concentration effect on FA/FI may be thought of as identical to the impact of a change in solubility.[9] As the inspired concentration increases, the effective solubility decreases. That is, at 50 percent inspired nitrous oxide, FA/FI rises as rapidly as the FA/FI of an anesthetic that equals one-half the solubility of nitrous oxide and is given at 1 percent inspired concentration. Seventy-five percent inspired nitrous oxide acts like an anesthetic given at 1 percent that has one-fourth the solubility of nitrous oxide.

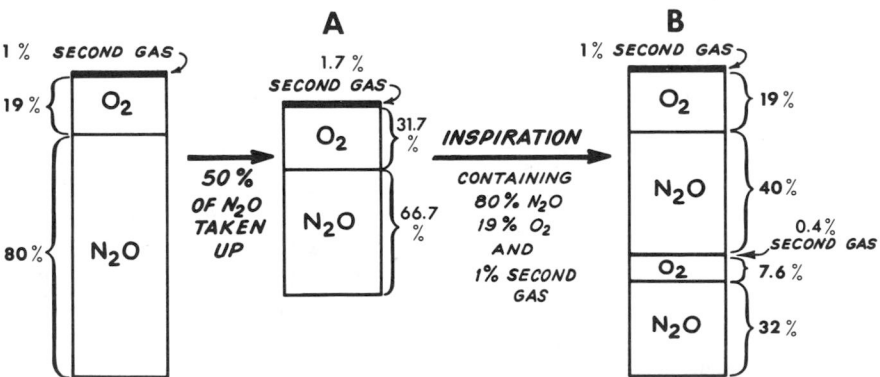

Fig. 4-2. The rectangle to the left represents a lung filled with 80 percent nitrous oxide plus 1 percent of a second gas. Uptake of one-half the nitrous oxide (**A**) does not halve the concentration of nitrous oxide and the reduction in volume concentrates and thereby increases the concentration of the second gas. Restoration of the lung volume (**B**) by addition of gas at the same concentration as that contained in the left-most rectangle will increase the nitrous oxide concentration and will add to the amount of the second gas present in the lung. (From Stoelting and Eger,[8] with permission.)

The Second Gas Effect

The factors that govern the concentration effect also influence the concentration of any gas given concomitantly.[8,10] This second gas effect applies to halothane or enflurane when administered with nitrous oxide. The loss of volume associated with the uptake of nitrous oxide concentrates the halothane or enflurane (Fig. 4-2A). Replacement of the gas taken up by an increase in inspired ventilation will augment the amount of halothane or enflurane present in the lung (Fig. 4-2B).

Both the concentration effect and second gas effect were demonstrated by the following experiments.[10] Dogs were given 0.5 percent halothane in either 10 percent nitrous oxide or 70 percent nitrous oxide. The F_A/F_I for nitrous oxide rose more rapidly when 70 percent nitrous oxide was inspired than when 10 percent was inspired (the concentration effect) (Fig. 4-3). Similarly, the F_A/F_I ratio for halothane rose more rapidly when 70 percent nitrous oxide was inspired than when 10 percent was inspired (second gas effect).

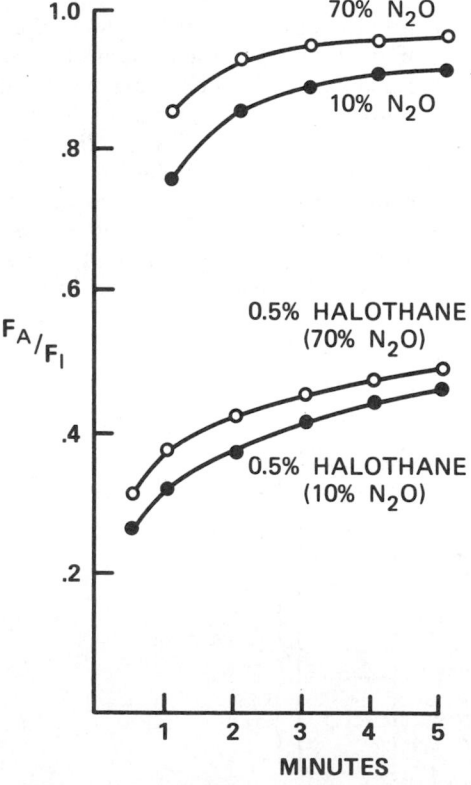

Fig. 4-3. In dogs, administration of 70 percent nitrous oxide produces a more rapid rise in F_A/F_I of nitrous oxide than administration of 10 percent (concentration effect, upper two curves). The F_A/F_I for 0.5 percent halothane rises more rapidly when given with 70 percent nitrous oxide than when given with 10 percent (second gas effect, lower two curves). (From Epstein et al.,[10] with permission.)

Percutaneous Anesthetic Loss

I have ignored two possible avenues by which anesthetics may be lost: transcutaneous movement and metabolism. Although transcutaneous movement occurs, the movement is small.[11,12] The greatest loss per alveolar anesthetic percent occurs with nitrous oxide. Loss of nitrous oxide might equal 5 to 10 ml/min with an alveolar concentration of 70 percent.

Metabolism of Anesthetic

Although percutaneous loss of anesthetic may not appreciably affect anesthetic uptake, loss of anesthetic by biodegradation can produce significant changes, particularly with agents that undergo extensive biodegradation. Berman et al.[13] found that phenobarbital pretreatment in rats decreased the arterial level of methoxyflurane. Carpenter et al.[14] found biodegradation of as much as one-half of the halothane and three-fourths of the methoxyflurane that was taken up. They speculated that this biodegradation could explain the finding that the alveolar concentration of halothane decayed more rapidly on recovery from anesthesia than did the alveolar concentration of enflurane and isoflurane, anesthetics that are significantly less soluble in blood.[15,16] Two reasons suggest that agents such as isoflurane or enflurane are less likely to be affected. First, they are not metabolized as readily as halothane or methoxyflurane.[17] Second, anesthetizing concentrations appear to saturate the enzymes responsible for anesthetic metabolism.[18] This particularly may limit the impact of metabolism during the washin as opposed to the washout of anesthetic. The combined effect of these factors remains to be determined, but it appears that metabolism is not a major determinant of F_A/F_I during anesthesia with more recently developed agents such as isoflurane and enflurane.

Intertissue Diffusion

Carpenter et al.[15,16] examined the washin and washout of isoflurane, enflurane, halothane, and methoxyflurane given simultaneously for fixed periods to young healthy patients. Washout was examined for several days after discontinuation of anesthetic administration. Analysis suggested that a model with five compartments best explained the resulting data for all the anesthetics (i.e., the model was independent of solubility and anesthetic metabolism). The time constants of four of these compartments were consistent with the model used earlier in this chapter. Thus, these compartments could be related to washin and washout of the lungs, vessel-rich group, muscle group, and fat group.

However, an additional important compartment was more difficult to explain. This compartment had a time constant of roughly 400 minutes, that is, between that for muscle and that for fat. This additional compartment was important because it accounted for almost one-third of the anesthetic taken up. In part, this compartment could be explained by uptake by highly perfused fat such as that found in bone marrow. However, the perfusion of such tissue is not sufficient to account for the major portion of uptake by this compartment. Carpenter et al.[15,16] speculated that this uptake resulted from diffusion of anesthetic from lean tissue to an adjacent thin layer of fat tissue. Such diffusion could be from the heart to pericardial fat, from the kidney to perirenal fat, from the intestine to mesenteric and omental fat, and from the dermis to subcutaneous fat.

FACTORS MODIFYING THE RATE OF RISE OF FA/FI

Alteration of those factors that govern the rate of delivery of anesthetic to the lungs or its removal from the lungs will alter the alveolar concentration of anesthetic. We have seen the importance of differences in solubility (Fig. 4-1). The succeeding sections examine the impact of differences in ventilation and circulation and the interaction of these differences with factors such as solubility.

The Effect of Ventilatory Changes

By augmenting the delivery of anesthetic to the lungs, an increase in ventilation accelerates the rate of rise of FA/FI (Fig. 4-4.)[1,19] A change in ventilation produces a greater relative change in FA/FI with a more soluble anesthetic. In Figure 4-4, an increase in ventilation from 2 to 8 L/min triples the ether concentration at 10 minutes, only doubles the halothane concentration, and scarcely affects the nitrous oxide concentration.

The impact of solubility may be explained as follows. With a poorly soluble agent such as nitrous oxide, the rate of rise of FA/FI is rapid even with hypoventilation. Since FA normally cannot exceed FI, there is little room for an augmentation of ventilation to increase FA/FI. With a highly soluble agent such as ether or methoxyflurane, most of the anesthetic delivered to the lungs is taken up. That is, if the uptake at 2 L/min ventilation equaled X, then the uptake at 4 L/min would approach 2X. Thus, if cardiac output is held constant, ventilation of 4 L/min produces an arterial ether concentration that is nearly twice the concentration produced by a ventilation of 2 L/min. Since arterial and alveolar concentrations are in equilibrium, our example suggests that doubling ventilation must nearly double the anesthetic concentration in lung or blood.

These observations imply that imposed alterations in ventilation (e.g., an increase produced by conversion from spontaneous to controlled ventilation) produce greater changes in anesthetic effect with more soluble agents. Since such effects include both anesthetic depth and depression of circulation, greater caution must be exercised when ventilation is augmented during anesthesia produced with a highly soluble agent.

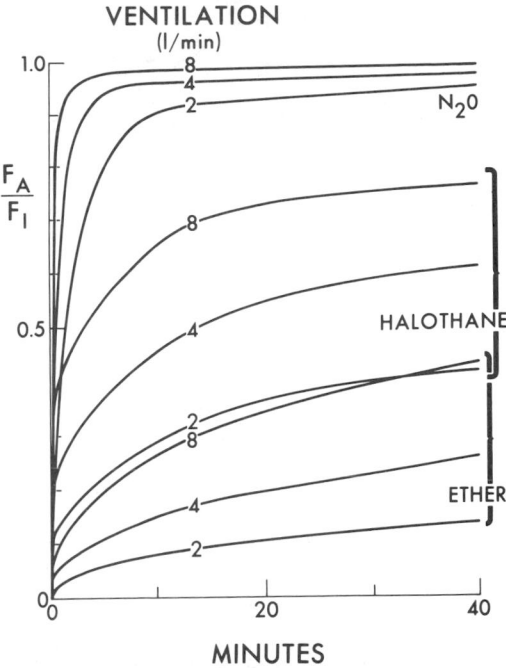

Fig. 4-4. The FA/FI ratio rises more rapidly if ventilation is increased. Solubility modifies this impact of ventilation: the effect on the anesthetizing partial pressure is greatest with the most soluble anesthetic (ether) and least with the least soluble anesthetic (nitrous oxide). (From Eger,[1] with permission.)

Anesthetics themselves may alter ventilation and thereby alter their own uptake.[2,20] Modern potent agents such as halothane, enflurane, or isoflurane all are profound respiratory depressants whose depression of ventilation is inversely related to anesthetic dose (Fig. 4-5).[21-23] At some dose, all the inhaled anesthetics probably produce apnea—a feature that must limit the maximum alveolar concentration that can be obtained if ventilation is spontaneous.

Thus, administration of an anesthetic concentration that produces significant respiratory depression progressively decreases delivery of anesthetic to the alveoli.[2,24] That is, doubling the inspired concentration does not double the alveolar concentration attained at a given point in time. At high inspired concentrations, further increases in inspired concentration produce little absolute change in the alveolar concentration (Fig. 4-6). Anesthetics thereby can exert a negative feedback effect on their own alveolar concentration, an effect that increases the safety of spontaneous ventilation by limiting the maximum concentration that is attained in the alveoli.

The Effect of Changes in Cardiac Output

The discussion in the previous section assumed a constant cardiac output and examined the effect of changes in ventilation. In this section the reverse process is dis-

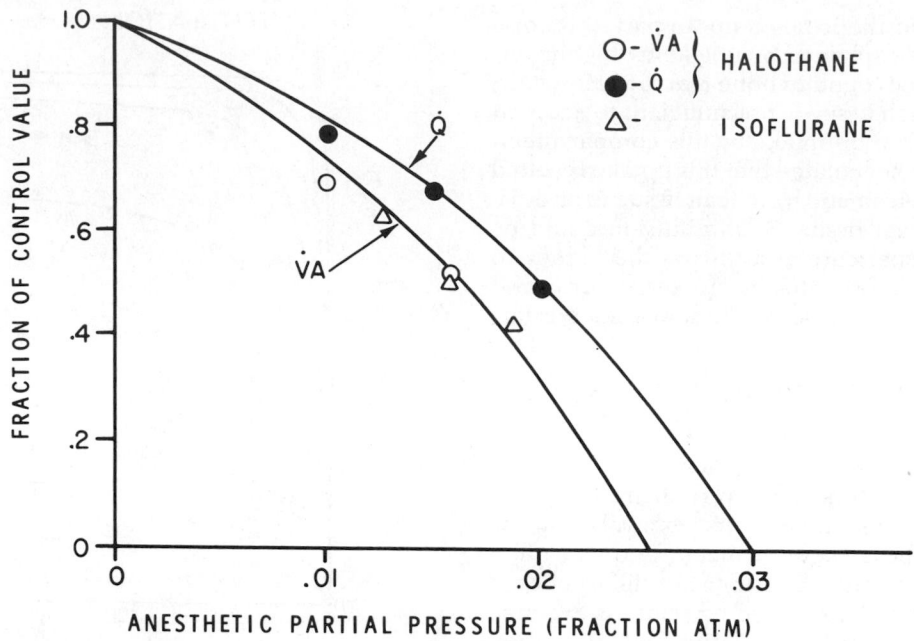

Fig. 4-5. Alveolar ventilation (VA) and cardiac output (Q̇) are expressed as a percentage of awake values. These data for halothane and isoflurane are taken from human studies.[20,21] (From Munson et al.,[2] with permission.)

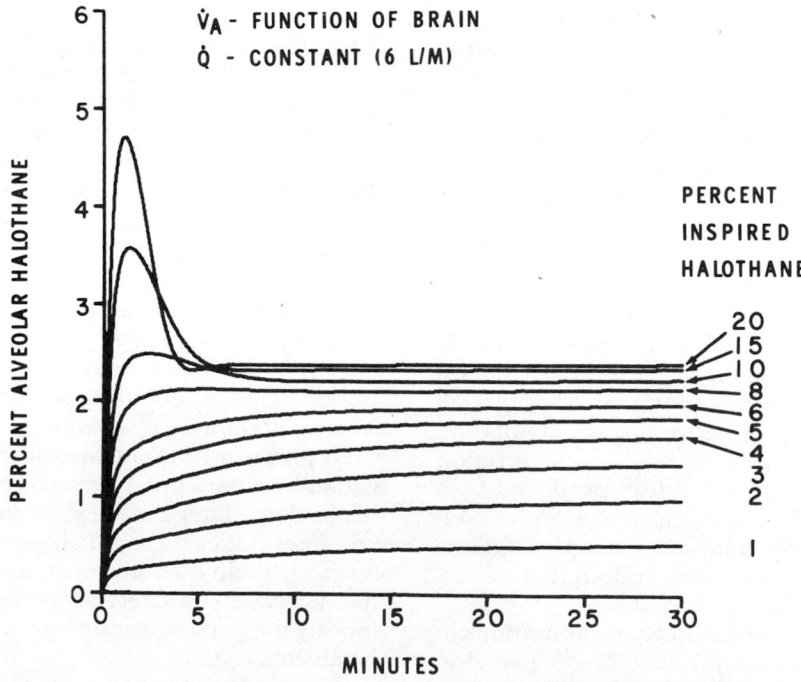

Fig. 4-6. An increase in inspired halothane concentration does not produce a proportional increase in the alveolar concentration because of the progressively greater depression of ventilation that occurs as alveolar halothane is increased. The initial "overshoot" seen with 10 to 20 percent inspired halothane results from the delay in the transfer of alveolar halothane partial pressure to the brain. (From Munson et al.,[2] with permission.)

cussed. An increase in cardiac output augments uptake and thereby hinders the rise in F_A/F_I.[1,25] As with a change in ventilation, a change in cardiac output scarcely affects the alveolar concentration of a poorly soluble agent; the alveolar concentration of a highly soluble agent will be much more influenced (Fig. 4-7). The reason for the impact of a change in solubility is similar to that which explains the effect of a change in ventilation. A decrease in cardiac output can do little to increase the F_A/F_I ratio of a poorly soluble agent, since the rate of rise is rapid at any cardiac output. In contrast, nearly all of a highly soluble agent will be taken up, and a halving of blood flow through the lungs must concentrate the arterial (equals alveolar) anesthetic (partial pressure), nearly doubling it is the case of an extremely soluble agent.

This effect of solubility suggests that conditions that lower cardiac output (e.g., shock) may produce unexpectedly high alveolar anesthetic concentrations if highly soluble agents are used. The higher F_A/F_I ratio should be anticipated and the inspired anesthetic concentration lowered accordingly to avoid further depression of circulation. Shock presents a two-pronged problem: an increase in ventilation usually accompanies the circulatory depression. Both an increase in ventilation and a decrease in cardiac output accelerate the rise in F_A/F_I. Perhaps this is why such heavy reliance is placed on the use of nitrous oxide in patients in shock.

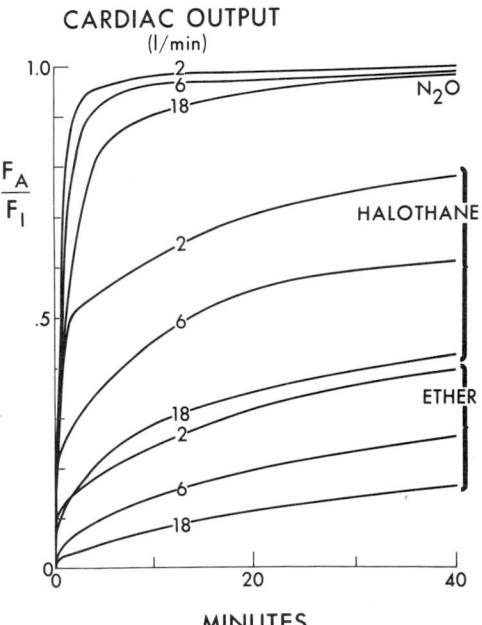

Fig. 4-7. If unopposed by a concomitant increase in ventilation, an increase in cardiac output will decrease alveolar anesthetic concentration by augmenting uptake. The resulting alveolar anesthetic change is greatest with the most soluble anesthetic. (From Eger,[1] with permission.)

In contrast to methoxyflurane or halothane, the alveolar concentration of nitrous oxide would be little influenced by the associated cardiorespiratory changes.

Anesthetics also affect circulation. Usually they depress cardiac output (Fig. 4-5),[26,27] although stimulation may occur with some agents (e.g., nitrous oxide, ether, or fluroxene). In contrast to the negative feedback that results from respiratory depression, circulatory depression produces a positive feedback: depression decreases uptake, and this increases the alveolar concentration, which in turn further decreases uptake. A potentially lethal acceleration of the rise in F_A/F_I results from the depression of cardiac output (Fig. 4-8).[2,20,24] The impact of this acceleration increases in importance with increasing anesthetic solubility. High inspired concentrations of agents such as enflurane or halothane should be administered with considerable caution, particularly if ventilation is controlled.

The Effect of Concomitant Changes in Ventilation and Perfusion

Consideration of the effects of ventilatory and circulatory alterations usually presumed that only one of these variables was changed while the other was held constant. In fact, both may change concomitantly. If both ventilation and cardiac output increase proportionately, an intuitive expection might be that F_A/F_I would be little altered. After all, uptake equals the product of solubility, cardiac output, and the alveolar to venous anesthetic partial pressure difference [eq. (1)]. In the absence of other changes, doubling cardiac output will double uptake, and this should exactly balance the influence of doubling of ventilation on F_A/F_I. That is, a doubling of both delivery of anesthetic to the lungs and removal of anesthetic from the lungs should produce no net change in the alveolar concentration.

The above reasoning ignores one other factor in the equation that defines uptake. By accelerating the rate at which tissue equilibration occurs, an increase in cardiac output accelerates the narrowing of the alveolar to venous partial pressure difference.[28] This accelerated narrowing of the alveolar to venous partial pressure difference reduces the impact of the increase in cardiac output on uptake. Thus, a proportional increase in ventilation and cardiac output will increase the rate of rise F_A/F_I.

The magnitude of the acceleration of rise in F_A/F_I will depend in part on distribution of the increase in cardiac output. If the increase is distributed proportionately to all tissues (e.g., if a doubling of output doubles flow to all tissues), then the increase is fairly small (Fig. 4-9).[28,29] Thus, conditions such as hyperthermia or thyrotoxicosis would only slightly influence the development of an anesthetizing anesthetic concentration through their influence on F_A/F_I. However, if the increase in cardiac output is diverted to the VRG, then a greater effect is seen.[28,30] Perfusion of the VRG nor-

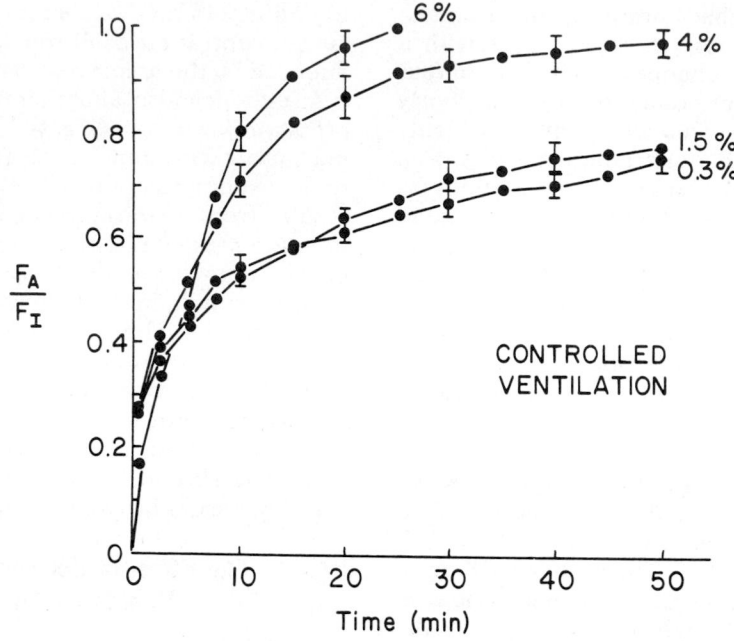

Fig. 4-8. Dogs given a constant ventilation demonstrate different rates of rise of F_A/F_I. The rates of rise depend on the inspired halothane concentration. The two higher concentrations accelerated the rate of rise by depressing cardiac output and thereby decreasing uptake. (From Gibbons et al.,[24] with permission.)

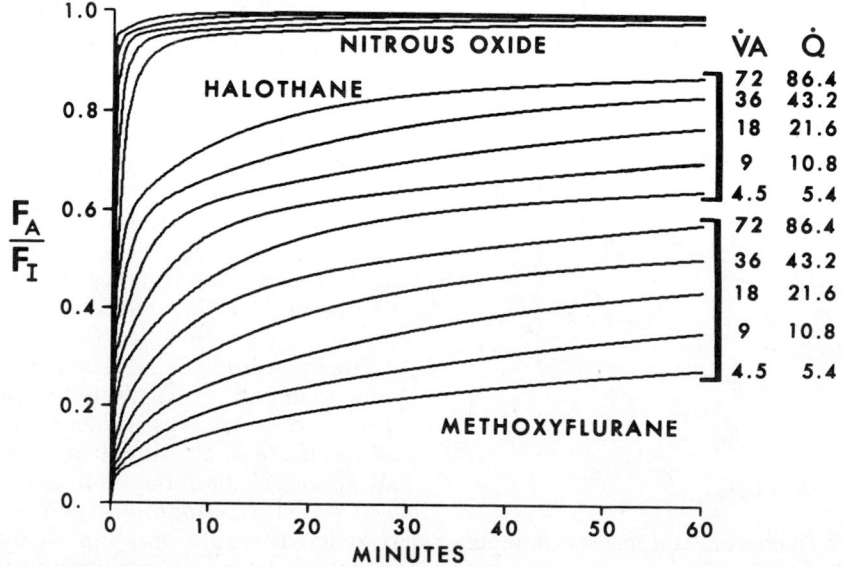

Fig. 4-9. Proportional increases in alveolar ventilation (V_A) and cardiac output ($\dot{Q}$) will increase the rate at which F_A/F_I rises. As indicated, the effect is relatively small if the increase in cardiac output is distributed proportionately to all tissues (i.e., if $\dot{Q}$ is doubled, then all tissue blood flows are doubled). The greatest effect occurs with the most soluble anesthetic. (From Eger et al.,[28] with permission.)

mally is high and results in rapid equilibration. Further increases in perfusion only hasten the rate of equilibration. Since blood returning from the VRG soon has the same partial pressure it had when it left the lungs, it cannot remove more anesthetic from the lungs. Thus, after a few seconds or minutes, the increase in ventilation will not be matched, even in part, by an increase in uptake. The result will be a considerable acceleration in the rise in Fa/Fi. This effect may be seen in a comparison of the Fa/Fi curves for children and adults (Fig. 4-10). Children (especially infants) have a relatively greater perfusion of the VRG and consequently show a significantly faster rise in Fa/Fi.[30] A clinical result of this accelerated rise is the more rapid development of anesthesia in young patients. The higher perfusion of the brain further accelerates the development of anesthesia.

Ventilation/Perfusion Ratio Abnormalities

To this point it has been assumed that alveolar and arterial anesthetic partial pressures are equal; that is, the alveolar gases completely equilibrate with the blood passing through the lungs. To some extent this assumption is incorrect, but the usual deviation from complete equilibration is small. Diseases such as emphysema, atelectasis, or congenital cardiac defects increase the deviation. The associated ventilation/perfusion ratio abnormality will do two things: increase the alveolar (end-tidal) anesthetic partial pressure, and decrease the arterial anesthetic partial pressure (i.e., a partial pressure difference will appear between alveolar gas and arterial blood). The relative change depends on the solubility of the anesthetic. With a poorly soluble agent, the end-tidal concentration is slightly increased, but the arterial partial pressure is significantly reduced. The opposite occurs with a highly soluble anesthetic.[31]

The considerable decrease in the arterial anesthetic partial pressure that occurs with poorly soluble agents may be explained as follows. Ventilation/perfusion ratio abnormalities increase ventilation relative to perfusion of some alveoli, while in other alveoli the reverse occurs. With a poorly soluble anesthetic, an increase in ventilation relative to perfusion does not appreciably increase alveolar or arterial anesthetic partial pressure issuing from those alveoli (see effect for nitrous oxide in Fig. 4-4). However, when ventilation decreases relative to perfusion, a significant effect can occur, particularly when ventilation is absent, as in a segment of atelectatic lung. Blood emerges from that segment with no additional anesthetic. Such anesthetic-deficient blood then mixes with the blood from the ventilated segments con-

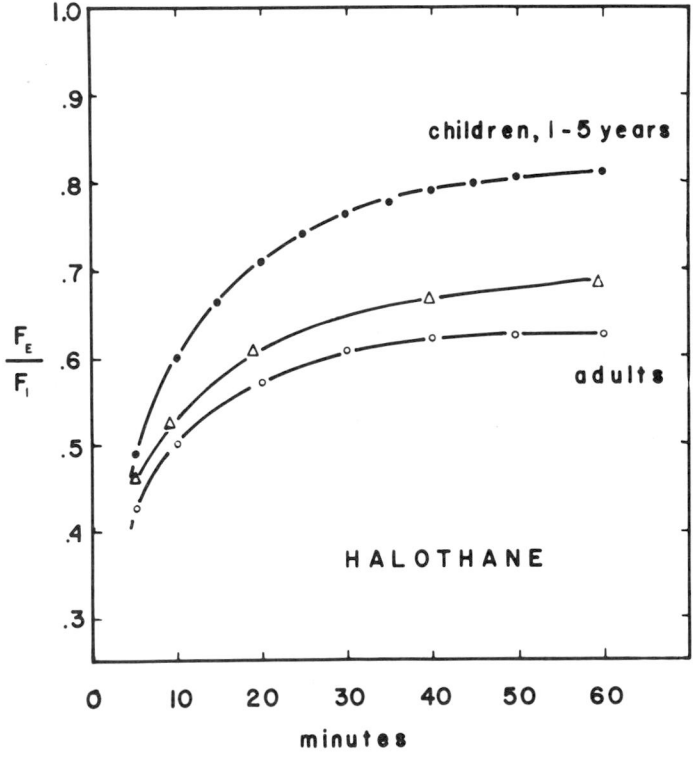

Fig. 4-10. The alveolar rate of rise of halothane is more rapid in children (uppermost curve) than adults (lower two curves, each from separate studies). The difference probably results from the greater ventilation and perfusion per kilogram of tissue in children and the fact that a disproportionate amount of the increased perfusion is devoted to the vessel-rich group. (From Salanitre and Rackow,[30] with permission.)

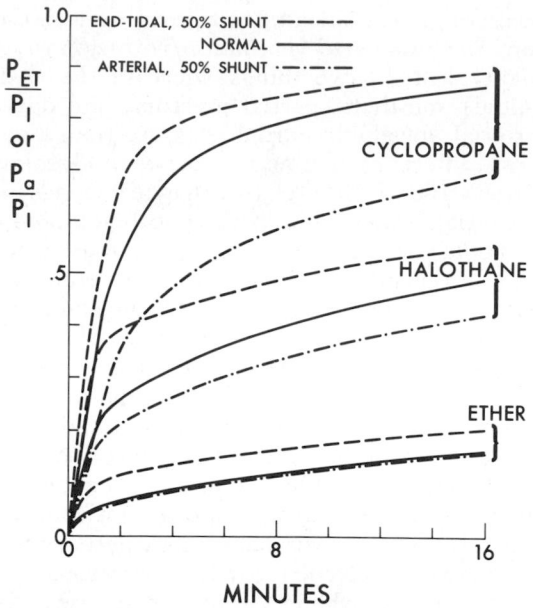

Fig. 4-11. When no ventilation/perfusion abnormalities exist then the alveolar (P_A or P_{ET}) and arterial (P_a) anesthetic partial pressures rise together (continuous lines) toward the inspired partial pressure (P_I). When 50 percent of the cardiac output is shunted through the lungs, then the rate of rise of the end-tidal partial pressure (dashed lines) is accelerated while the rate of rise of the arterial partial pressure (dot-dashed lines) is retarded. The greatest retardation is found with the least soluble anesthetic, cyclopropane. (From Eger,[1] with permission.)

taining a normal complement of anesthetic. The mixture produces an arterial anesthetic partial pressure considerably below normal.

With highly soluble agents, a different situation results from similar ventilation/perfusion ratio abnormalities. In alveoli receiving more ventilation relative to perfusion, the anesthetic partial pressure rises to a higher level than usual (see Fig. 4-4 for the effect on diethyl ether). That is, blood issuing from these alveoli has an increased anesthetic content, an increase that is nearly proportional to the increased ventilation. Assuming that overall (total) ventilation remains normal, this increase in the anesthetic contained by blood from the relatively hyperventilated alveoli will compensate for the lack of anesthetic uptake in unventilated alveoli.

These effects are illustrated in Figure 4-11 for a condition that may be iatrogenically produced: endobronchial intubation. Since all ventilation now is directed to the intubated lung, this lung will be hyperventilated relative to perfusion. F_A/F_I for this lung will be slightly increased (relative to the increase obtained in the absence of endobronchial intubation) with the poorly soluble cyclopropane and greatly increased with the highly soluble ether. As indicated earlier, the increase with ether will compensate for the absence of uptake from the unventilated lung—a compensatory mechanism not available with cyclopropane. The result is that the cyclopropane arterial partial pressure is well below normal, while the ether arterial partial pressure is scarcely changed.

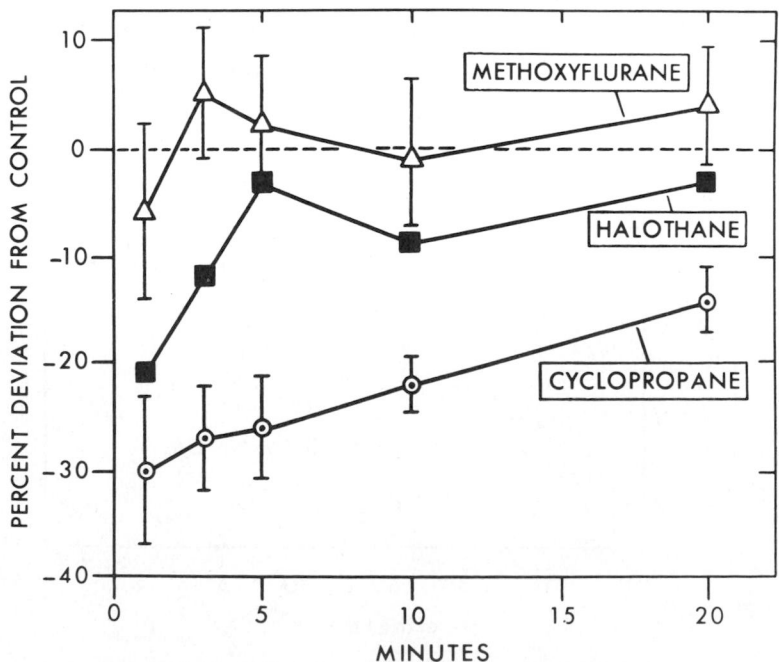

Fig. 4-12. In dogs when only the right lung was ventilated, the rise of the very soluble anesthetic, methoxyflurane, in arterial blood was normal (i.e., did not deviate from control), while the rise for the poorly soluble anesthetic, cyclopropane, was significantly slowed. (From Stoelting and Longnecker,[32] with permission.)

These concepts have been confirmed experimentally by comparing the rate of arterial anesthetic rise with and without endobronchial intubation in dogs.[32] Endobronchial intubation significantly slowed the arterial rate of rise of cyclopropane but did not influence the rise with methoxyflurane. An intermediate result was obtained with halothane (Fig. 4-12). These data suggest that in the presence of ventilation/perfusion ratio abnormalities, the anesthetic effect of agents such as cyclopropane or nitrous oxide may be delayed, whereas the effect of ether or methoxyflurane will be unaffected.

THE EFFECT OF NITROUS OXIDE ON CLOSED GAS SPACES

Volume Changes in Highly Compliant Spaces

During the course of anesthetic administration, appreciable volumes of nitrous oxide can move into closed gas spaces. Although this transfer does not influence F_A/F_I, it may have important functional consequences. There are two types of closed gas spaces in the body: compliant and noncompliant. Compliant spaces, such as bowel gas, pneumothorax, or pneumoperitoneum, are subject to changes in volume secondary to the transfer of nitrous oxide into these spaces.[33] These spaces normally contain nitrogen (from air), a gas whose low solubility (blood/gas partition coefficient = 0.015) limits its removal by blood. Thus, the entrance of

nitrous oxide (whose solubility permits it to be carried by blood in substantial quantities) is not countered by an equal loss. The result is an increase in volume. The theoretic limit to the increase in volume is a function of the alveolar nitrous oxide concentration, since it is this concentration that ultimately is achieved in the closed gas space. That is, at equilibrium the partial pressure of nitrous oxide in the closed gas space must equal its partial pressure in the alveoli. An alveolar concentration of 50 percent might double the gas space volume, while a 75 percent concentration might produce a fourfold increase.

These theoretical limits may be approached when equilibrium is rapidly achieved, as with a pneumothorax or gas emboli. The administration of 75 percent nitrous oxide in the presence of a pneumothorax may double the pneumothorax volume in 10 minutes and triple it by 30 minutes (Fig. 4-13).[33] This increase in volume may seriously impair cardiorespiratory function,[34] and the use of nitrous oxide is contraindicated in the presence of a significant pneumothorax.

A still more rapid expansion of volume occurs when air inadvertently enters the blood stream in a patient anesthetized with nitrous oxide. Expansion may be complete in seconds rather than minutes. Munson and Merrick[35] demonstrated that the lethal volume of an air embolus was decreased in animals breathing nitrous oxide as opposed to air (Fig. 4-14). The difference could be entirely explained by expansion of the embolus in the animals breathing nitrous oxide, that is, the pre-

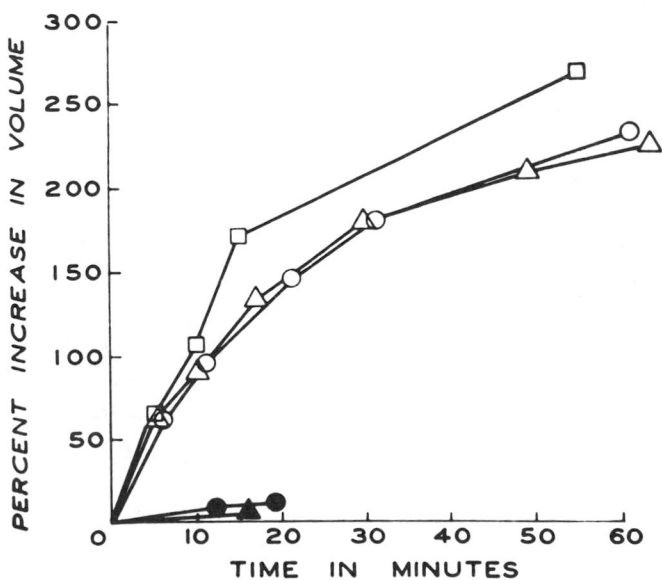

Fig. 4-13. The volume of a pneumothorax created by air injection is little affected when oxygen subsequently is breathed (filled triangle and circles). However, if 75 percent nitrous oxide is breathed, the volume doubles in 10 minutes and triples in a half-hour (open circles, squares, and triangles). (From Eger and Saidman,[33] with permission.)

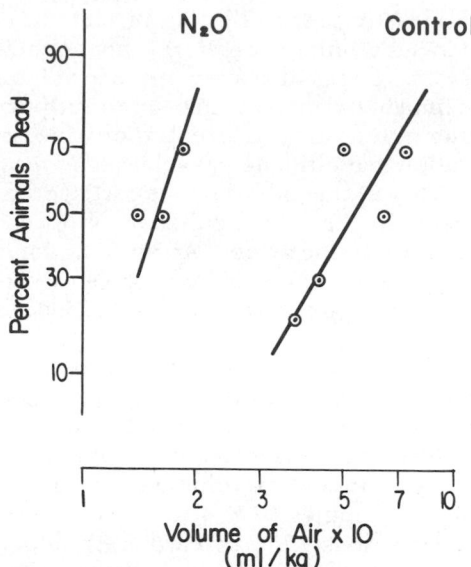

Fig. 4-14. Fifty percent of rabbits breathing oxygen were killed by an air embolus equaling 0.55 ml/kg. If the inspired gas mixture contained 75 percent nitrous oxide, then only 0.16 ml/kg was required to kill one-half of the animals. (From Munson and Merrick,[35] with permission.)

dicted total volume of air plus nitrous oxide in the embolus equaled the volume of air needed to produce death in animals breathing only air. These studies suggest caution in the use of nitrous oxide for procedures in which air embolization is a risk (e.g., posterior fossae craniotomies, laparoscopy). They also suggest that if air embolization is suspected, an immediate part of therapy should be the discontinuation of nitrous oxide. On the other hand, a nitrous oxide "challenge" may be used to test whether air embolization has occurred.[36]

The endotracheal tube cuff normally is filled with air. It, too, is susceptible to expansion by nitrous oxide.[37] The presence of 75 percent nitrous oxide surrounding such a cuff can double or triple the volume of the cuff. The result may be an unwanted increase in pressure exerted on the tracheal mucosa. Similarly, nitrous oxide may expand the cuffs of balloon-tipped (e.g., Swan-Ganz) catheters[38,39] when the balloons are inflated with air. The expansion is rapid, and a doubling of volume may occur within 10 minutes.

Pressure Changes in Poorly Compliant Spaces

Pressure can be produced by the entrance of nitrous oxide into gas cavities surrounded by poorly compliant walls. Unwanted increases in intraocular pressure may be imposed by nitrous oxide administration after intravitreal sulfur hexafluoride injection.[40] Other examples include the gas space created by pneumoencephalography and the natural gas space in the middle ear. Pressures in the head or middle ear may rise by 20 to 50 mmHg owing to the ingress of nitrous oxide at a faster rate than air can be removed.[41,42] Recognition of this problem decreased the use of nitrous oxide for pneumoencephalography, or for tympanoplasty, where the increased pressure may displace the graft. Increase in middle ear pressure may cause adverse postoperative effects on hearing.[43] The capacity of nitrous oxide to expand the gas in the middle ear also has been used to elevate an adherent atelectatic tympanic membrane off the promontory and ossicles.[44]

ANESTHETIC CIRCUITRY

The previous discussions generally have considered that the alveolar anesthetic concentration (F_A) was moving toward a constant inspired anesthetic concentration (F_I). In practice, the inspired concentration usually is not constant because a nonrebreathing system is not used. The rebreathing that results from the use of an anesthetic circuit causes the inspired concentration to be less than that in the gas delivered from the anesthetic machine. The inspired concentration thus is influenced by the delivered concentration, by the need to "washin" the circuit, and by the depletion of anesthetic in rebreathed gases produced by uptake of anesthetic.

Washin of the Circuit

To begin anesthesia, anesthetic must be "washed into" the volume of the circuit. At inflow rates of 1 to 5 L/min and a circuit volume of 7 L (3 L bag, 2 L carbon dioxide absorber, and 2 L in corrugated hoses and fittings), the washin of the circuit is 75 to 100 percent complete in 10 minutes (Fig. 4-15). Higher inflow rates produce a more rapid rise in the inspired concentration, suggest-

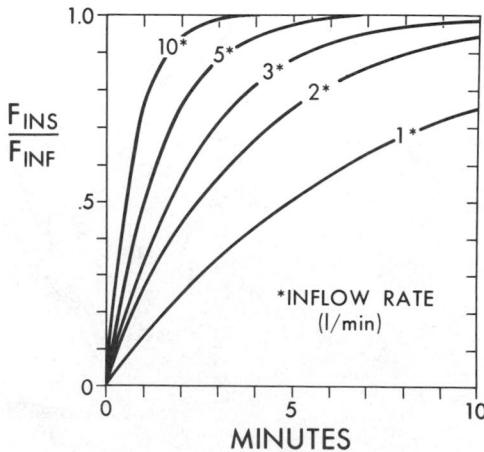

Fig. 4-15. The rate at which the inspired anesthetic concentration (F_{INS}) rises toward the inflowing concentration (F_{INF}) is determined by the inflow rate and circuit volume. In the case illustrated here, the circuit volume is 7 L. (From Eger,[1] with permission.)

ing that induction can be accelerated and made more predictable by use of high flow rates.

Anesthetic Loss to Plastic and Soda Lime

Uptake of anesthetic by several depots also hinders the development of an adequate inspired anesthetic concentration. The rubber or plastic components of the circuit may remove agent.[45] This is a significant problem in the case of methoxyflurane, which has a high solubility in rubber and plastic (Table 4-3). A lesser problem exists for halothane and isoflurane, and little or no problem results from the solution of nitrous oxide or the experimental anesthetics desflurane (I-653) and sevoflurane.

Similarly, uptake by soda lime is small unless the soda lime becomes dry, in which case substantial amounts may be absorbed.[47] Dry soda lime may slow induction by this mechanism and may also supply halothane subsequently.[48,49] Both dry and wet soda lime can destroy appreciable amounts of one anesthetic, the experimental agent sevoflurane.[50]

The Effect of Rebreathing

Inspired gas actually is two gases: that delivered from the anesthetic machine and that previously exhaled by the patient and subsequently rebreathed. Since the patient has removed (taken up) anesthetic from the rebreathed gas, the amount taken up *and* the amount rebreathed will influence the inspired anesthetic concentration. An increase in uptake or rebreathing will lower the inspired concentration of a highly soluble gas more than the inspired concentration of a poorly soluble gas. This effect of uptake can be diminished by decreasing rebreathing. Rebreathing is reduced by increasing the inflow rate. With a ventilation of 5 L/min, rebreathing can be essentially abolished by the use of a 5 L/min inflow rate.[51]

High inflow rates (i.e., 5 L/min or greater) have the advantage of increasing the predictability of the inspired anesthetic concentration. They have the disadvantage of being wasteful and of increasing the tendency toward atmospheric pollution. High inflow rates may be unacceptably costly in the case of the new (still

TABLE 4-3. Rubber/Gas and Plastic/Gas Partition Coefficients

Anesthetic	Polyethylene (Circuit Tube)	Rubber (Bag)	Polyvinyl chloride (Endotracheal Tube)
Nitrous oxide	—	1.2	—
Desflurane	16	19	35
Sevoflurane	31	29	68
Isoflurane	58	49	114
Enflurane	—	74	—
Halothane	128	190	233
Methoxyflurane	118	742	—

(Data from Eger et al.,[45] Titel and Lowe,[46] Targ et al.,[74] Munson and Eger,[75] and Eger and Brandstater.[76])

experimental) anesthetics desflurane and sevoflurane. High inflow rates also may result in drier inspired gas and greater difficulty in estimating ventilation from excursions of the rebreathing bag.

The Low Flow or Closed Circle Technique

These disadvantages of high inflow rates have led to a small but increasing application of closed circuit anesthesia.[52] Administration of closed circuit anesthesia has two requirements. First, if nitrous oxide is used, oxygen concentration must be measured and inflow adjusted to ensure adequacy of the inspired oxygen partial pressure. Second, there must be some gauge by which anesthetic is delivered from the machine. Ultimately this delivery is dictated by the response of the patient, but an initial estimate of the amount of anesthetic needed may be made from the "square root of time" formula (originally noted by Severinghaus[53]), which suggests that uptake decreases as a function of the square root of time. Application of this formula requires that anesthetic uptake for the first minute of anesthesia (U_1) be calculated. Uptake at subsequent times (U_t) is obtained as

$$U_t = U_1/(t)^{1/2} \qquad (2)$$

Uptake during the first minute may be estimated from the formula for uptake given earlier [eq. (1)]. Thus

$$U_1 = \lambda \cdot \dot{Q} \cdot (A)/BP \qquad (3)$$

The individual components are either known or can be easily estimated. For example, blood solubility (λ) for enflurane is 1.9. Cardiac output ($\dot{Q}$) in a normal adult is about 5,000 ml/min. During the first minute of anesthesia, the venous anesthetic partial pressure (v) is zero or low so that $(A) - v)/BP$ reduces to A/BP. We may assume that A/BP is the fractional alveolar concentration that we want to achieve. Since enflurane MAC with 60 percent nitrous oxide is about 0.8 percent enflurane (a fractional concentration of 0.008) and since we need something modestly in excess of MAC — say 1.2 times MAC — then A/BP equals 0.0096. Thus $U_1 = 1.9 \cdot 5,000 \cdot 0.0096$ or 91.2 ml/min. After 9 minutes of anesthesia, this reduces to 91.2/3 = 30.4 ml/min; after 25 minutes, it is 91.2/5 = 18.2 ml/min, and so on. Flow through the vaporizer then must be adjusted to give the above output; for example an 18.2 ml/min enflurane output at 20°C and 1 atmosphere pressure would require a flow through a Vernitrol or copper kettle of 62 ml/min (about 3.3 times as much as the amount of vapor desired; for halothane of isoflurane, the factor is about 2 times).

These calculations form a rough guide to the volume of anesthetic that must be delivered to sustain a given alveolar concentration. In practice, the volumes vary considerably,[54] in part as a function of variables such as body weight, fat-free body mass, and body surface area.[55] The estimate of the volume of anesthetic to be delivered should be modified by a knowledge of factors that might alter anesthetic requirement. Thus, the amount of anesthetic needed would be reduced by hypothermia, advanced age, or shock. The patient's response ultimately must govern the amount of anesthetic delivered: movement, hypertension, or tachycardia might indicate an increased need; hypotension might indicate a decreased need.

However, given the present trend toward monitoring anesthetic gas concentrations, all of the above calculations may be moot. If end-tidal concentration is known (e.g., by infrared or mass spectroscopic analysis), then a low flow or closed circuit administration can be controlled precisely. The delivered volume of anesthetic is adjusted to maintain the end-tidal concentration at whatever concentration is consistent with clinical needs, including those pertaining to surgery and the cardiovascular response of the patient.

RECOVERY FROM ANESTHESIA

General Principles

Nearly all the factors that governed the rate at which the alveolar anesthetic concentration rose on induction apply to recovery. Thus, the immediate decline is extremely rapid, since the washout of the functional residual capacity by ventilation is as rapid as the washin. It should be recalled that only 2 minutes are required to eliminate 95 to 98 percent of nitrogen from the lungs when pure oxygen is breathed.

Nitrogen, however, is a poorly soluble gas relative to the inhaled anesthetics. As ventilation sweeps anesthetic from the alveoli, an anesthetic partial pressure gradient develops from the returning venous blood to that in the alveoli. This gradient drives anesthetic into the alveoli, thereby opposing the tendency of ventilation to lower the alveolar concentration. The effectiveness of the venous to alveolar gradient in opposing the tendency of ventilation to decrease the alveolar anesthetic partial pressure is in part determined by the solubility of the anesthetic. A highly soluble agent such as methoxyflurane will be more effective than a poorly soluble agent such as nitrous oxide because a greater reserve exists in blood for the highly soluble agent. That is, far more methoxyflurane is available at a given partial pressure for transfer to the alveoli. Thus, the fall in the alveolar partial pressure of methoxyflurane is slower than the fall with halothane, and the latter in turn decreases less rapidly than nitrous oxide. The rate at which recovery occurs is similarly affected: it is rapid with nitrous oxide and may be slow with methoxyflurane. The rapidity of recovery thus in large part depends on the solubility of the anesthetic.[56]

Differences Between Induction and Recovery

Recovery differs from induction in two crucial ways. First, on induction, the effect of solubility to hinder the rise in alveolar anesthetic concentration could be overcome by increasing the inspired anesthetic concentration (i.e., by the application of "overpressure"). No such luxury is available during recovery: the inspired concentration cannot be reduced below zero. Second, on induction, all the tissues initially have the same anesthetic partial pressure—zero. On recovery, the tissue partial pressures are variable. The VGR has a pressure that usually equals that required for anesthesia. That is, the VRG has come to equilibrium with the alveolar anesthetic partial pressure. The muscle group may or may not have the same partial pressure as that found in the alveoli. A long anesthetic (2 to 4 hours) might permit equilibrium to be approached, but a shorter case would not. The high capacity of fat for all anesthetics except nitrous oxide precludes equilibration of the fat group with the alveolar anesthetic partial pressure with hours or even days of anesthesia.

The failure of muscle and fat to equilibrate with the alveolar anesthetic partial pressure means that these tissues initially cannot contribute to the transfer of anesthetic back to the lungs. In fact, as long as an anesthetic partial pressure gradient exists between arterial blood and that in a tissue, that tissue will continue to take up anesthetic. Thus, for the first several hours of recovery from halothane anesthesia, fat continues to take up halothane and by so doing accelerates the rate of recovery. Only after the alveolar (equals arterial) anesthetic partial pressure falls below that in a tissue can the tissue contribute anesthetic to the alveoli.

The failure of several tissues to reach equilibration with the alveolar anesthetic partial pressure means that the rate of decrease of alveolar anesthetic on recovery is more rapid than the rate of increase on induction and that recovery depends on part on the duration of anesthesia (Fig. 4-16).[57,58] A longer anesthetic puts more anesthetic into the slowly filling muscle and fat depots. Obviously, these reservoirs can supply more anesthetic to the blood returning to the lungs when they are filled than when they are empty and thereby can prolong the time to recovery.[56]

Solubility influences the effect of duration of anesthesia on the rate at which the alveolar anesthetic partial pressure declines.[58] The decline of the partial pressure of a poorly soluble agent such as nitrous oxide is rapid in any case, and thus the acceleration imparted by a less-than-complete tissue equilibration cannot significantly alter the rate of recovery. The approach to equilibration becomes important with halothane and even more important with methoxyflurane (Fig. 4-16). A rapid recovery may follow a short methoxyflurane anesthetic but may occur slowly after a prolonged anesthetic. This is one of the reasons why nitrous oxide is usually a component of an inhaled (or, for that matter, an injected) anesthetic regimen. The rapid elimination of this component permits at least a portion of recovery to be rapid. The recovery from anesthesia with the (still experimental) anesthetics desflurane and sevoflurane is more rapid than recovery from anesthesia with more soluble agents such as isoflurane or halothane.[56]

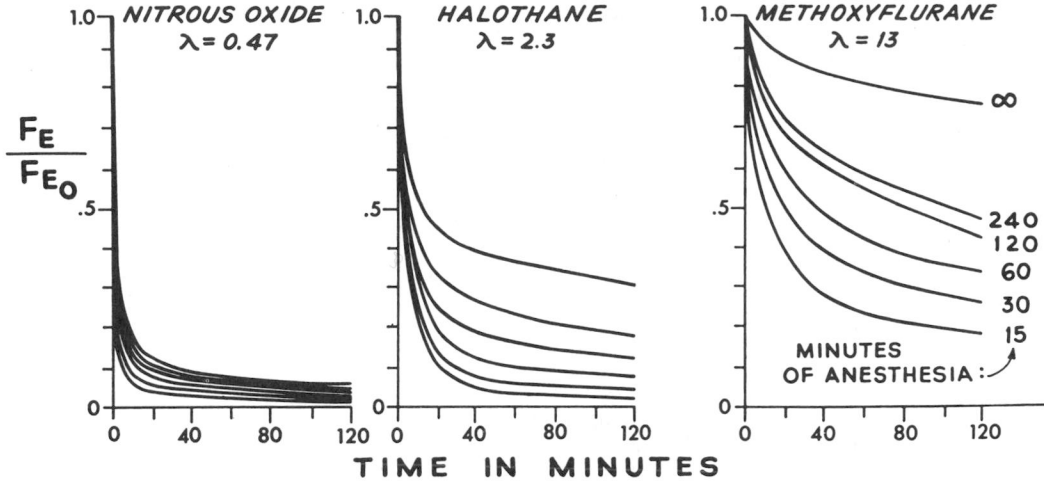

Fig. 4-16. Both solubility and duration of anesthesia affect the fall of the alveolar concentration (FE) from the alveolar concentration immediately preceding the cessation of anesthetic administration (FE$_o$). A longer anesthetic slows the fall, as does a greater solubility. (From Stoelting and Eger,[58] with permission.)

Recovery from anesthesia results from the elimination of anesthetic from the brain. This requires both that the arterial partial pressure of anesthetic decrease and that the decrease in arterial partial pressure is reflected in a decrease in the brain partial pressure of anesthetic. The high blood flow to brain combined with the limited brain/blood partition coefficient should ensure the second of these requirements.

Results from one study suggested that recovery from anesthesia might be prolonged because of binding of anesthetic (in this case, halothane) to the brain. Using nuclear magnetic resonance techniques, Wyrwicz et al.[59] believed that they found substantial amounts of halothane or a breakdown product of halothane remains in the brain of rabbits for as long as 98 hours after the administration of 1 percent halothane for 30 minutes.

The findings of Wyrwicz et al.[59] have been contradicted by several subsequent studies. Coburn and Eger[60] could not demonstrate binding of anesthetics to the brain in vitro. Using more conventional, invasive biochemical assays but the same experimental design, Strum et al. could not repeat the findings of Wyrwicz et al.[59] Similarly, autoradiographic studies indicate that 90 percent of the halothane introduced into the gray matter of the brain of monkeys by a brief anesthetizing exposure disappears from the brain within 20 minutes after exposure.[61] Finally, using nuclear magnetic resonance with better spatial localization than that used by Wyrwicz et al.,[59] Litt et al.[62] and Mills et al.[63] repeated the studies of Wyrwicz and colleagues. These subsequent studies demonstrated rapid washout of anesthetic from the brain, but a slow washout of anesthetic from fat adjacent to the brain. The slow washout was consistent with the washout attributed by Wyrwicz et al.[59] to washout from the brain.

Impact of Metabolism

The saturation of the enzymes responsible for the metabolism of anesthetics may limit metabolism from significantly altering the rate at which the alveolar anesthetic partial pressure rises. This limitation does not exist on recovery, and metabolism may be an important determinant of the rate at which the alveolar anesthetic partial pressure declines. The importance of metabolism to recovery is implied by results from Munson et al.,[4] who showed that contrary to what might be predicted from their respective solubilities, the alveolar washout of halothane is more rapid that than of enflurane. These results later were confirmed by the work of Carpenter et al.[15,16] This agrees with the relative ease with which these two agents are metabolized: 15 to 20 percent of the halothane taken up during the course of an ordinary anesthetic can be recovered as urinary metabolites.[64] Only 2 to 3 percent of enflurane can similarly be recovered.[65] Thus, there are two major routes by which halothane can be eliminated: the lung and the liver. With enflurane, elimination via the liver is relatively minor and explains why Munson et al.[4] found a more rapid fall in alveolar halothane.

Cahalan et al.[66] also have confirmed the results of Munson et al.[4] In addition, Cahalan et al. found that higher initial concentrations of enflurane and halothane did not alter the results. They also found that the metabolism of halothane may equal as much as 45 percent of the halothane taken up.

Diffusion Hypoxia

The uptake of large volumes of nitrous oxide on induction of anesthesia gives rise to the concentration and second gas effects. On recovery from anesthesia, the outpouring of large volumes of nitrous oxide can produce what Fink called *diffusion anoxia*.[67] These volumes may cause hypoxia (Fig. 4-17) in two ways. First, they may directly affect oxygenation by displacing oxygen.[67-69] Second, by diluting alveolar carbon dioxide, they may decrease respiratory drive and hence ventilation.[69] Both of these effects require that large volumes of nitrous oxide be released into the alveoli. Since large volumes of nitrous oxide are released only during the first 5 to 10 minutes of recovery, this is the period of greatest concern. This concern is enhanced by the fact that the first 5 to 10 minutes of recovery also may be the time of greatest respiratory depression. For these reasons, many anesthetists administer 100 percent oxygen for the first 5 to 10 minutes of recovery. This procedure may be particularly indicated in patients with pre-existing lung disease or when postoperative respiratory depression is anticipated (e.g., after a nitrous oxide-narcotic anesthetic).

Impact of the Anesthetic Circuit

The anesthetic circuit may limit the rate of recovery just as it limited induction. If the patient is not disconnected from the circuit on cessation of anesthetic delivery, the patient may continue to inspire anesthetic. To reduce the inspired level to zero or near zero, several factors must be taken into account. The anesthetic within the circuit must be washed out. In addition, the rubber or plastic components of the circuit and the soda lime within the circuit will have absorbed anesthetic (see Table 4-3) that can be released back into the gas phase,[64] and this too must be washed out. Finally, the patient's exhaled air contains anesthetic that cannot be re-

breathed if the inspired anesthetic concentration is to approach zero. The effect of each of these factors to raise the inspired anesthetic concentration can be overcome by the use of high inflow rates of oxygen, that is, 5 L/min or greater.

REFERENCES

1. Eger EI II (ed): MAC, Anesthetic Uptake and Action. Williams & Wilkins, Baltimore, 1974
2. Munson ES, Eger EI II, Bowers DL: Effects of anesthetic-depressed ventilation and cardiac output on anesthetic uptake. Anesthesiology 38:251, 1973
3. Cromwell TH, Eger EI II, Stevens WC, Dolan WM: Forane uptake excretion and blood solubility in man. Anesthesiology 35:401, 1971
4. Munson ES, Eger EI II, Tham MK, Embro WJ: Increase in anesthetic uptake, excretion and blood solubility in man after eating. Anesth Analg 57:224, 1978
5. Eger EI II: Isoflurane (Forane). A Compendium and Reference. 2nd Ed. Anaquest, Madison, WI, 1985
6. Eger EI II: Application of a mathematical model of gas uptake. p. 88. In Papper EM, Kitz RJ (eds): Uptake and Distribution of Anesthetic Agents. McGraw-Hill, New York, 1963
7. Eger EI II: The effect of inspired concentration of rise of alveolar concentration. Anesthesiology 24:153, 1963
8. Stoelting RK, Eger EI II: An additional explanation for the second gas effect: a concentrating effect. Anesthesiology 30:273, 1969
9. Eger EI II, Smith RA, Koblin DD: The concentration effect can be mimicked by a decrease in blood solubility. Anesthesiology 49:282, 1978
10. Epstein RM, Rackow H, Salanitre E, Wolf GL: Influence of the concentration effect on the uptake of anesthetic mixtures: the second gas effect. Anesthesiology 25:364, 1964
11. Stoelting RK, Eger EI II: Percutaneous loss of nitrous oxide, cyclopropane, ether and halothane in man. Anesthesiology 36:278, 1972
12. Cullen BF, Eger EI II: Diffusion of nitrous oxide, cyclopropane, and halothane through human skin and amniotic membrane. Anesthesiology 36:168, 1972
13. Berman ML, Lowe HJ, Hagler KT, Bochantin J: Uptake and elimination of methoxyflurane as influenced by enzyme induction in the rat. Anesthesiology 38:352, 1973
14. Carpenter RL, Eger EI II, Johnson BH, et al: The extent of metabolism of inhaled anesthetics in humans. Anesthesiology 65:201, 1986
15. Carpenter RL, Eger EI II, Johnson BH, et al: Pharmacokinetics of inhaled anesthetics in humans: Measurements during and after the simultaneous administration of enflurane, halothane, isoflurane, methoxyflurane, and nitrous oxide. Anesth Analg 65:575, 1986
16. Carpenter RL, Eger EI II, Johnson BH, et al: Does the duration of anesthetic administration affect the pharmacokinetics or metabolism of inhaled anesthetics in humans? Anesth Analg 66:1, 1987
17. Halsey MJ, Sawyer DC, Eger EI II, et al: Hepatic metabolism of halothane, methoxyflurane, cyclopropane, Ethrane and Forane in miniature swine. Anesthesiology 35:43, 1971
18. Sawyer DC, Eger EI II, Bahlman SH, et al: Concentration dependence of hepatic halothane metabolism. Anesthesiology 34:230, 1971
19. Yamamura H, Wakasugi B, Okuma Y, Maki K: The effects of

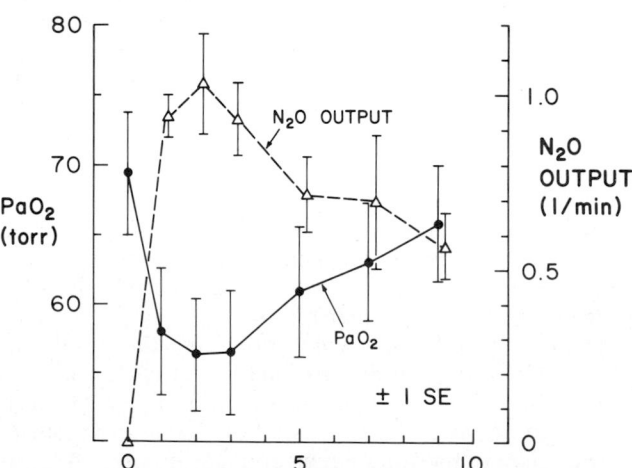

MINUTES AFTER END OF N₂O ANESTHESIA

Fig. 4-17. At time zero the inspired gas was changed from 21 percent oxygen/79 percent nitrous oxide to 21 percent/79 percent nitrogen. Arterial oxygen subsequently fell in association with the outpouring of nitrous oxide. (Adapted from Sheffer et al.,[68] with permission.)

ventilation on the absorption and elimination of inhalation anaesthetics. Anaesthesia 18:427, 1963

20. Fukui Y, Smith NT: Interactions among ventilation, the circulation, and the uptake and distribution of halothane — use of a hybrid computer multiple model. I. The basic model. Anesthesiology 54:107, 1981
21. Munson ES, Larson CP, Jr., Babad AA, et al: The effects of halothane, fluroxene and cyclopropane on ventilation: a comparative study in man. Anesthesiology 27:716, 1966
22. Fourcade HE, Stevens WC, Larson CP, Jr., et al: The ventilatory effects of Forane, a new inhaled anesthetic. Anesthesiology 35:26, 1971
23. Calverley RK, Smith NT, Jones CW, et al: Ventilatory and cardiovascular effects of enflurane anesthesia during spontaneous ventilation in man. Anesth Analg 57:610, 1978
24. Gibbons RT, Steffey EP, Eger EI II: The effect of spontaneous versus controlled ventilation on the rate of rise of alveolar halothane concentration in dogs. Anesth Analg 56:32, 1977
25. Yamamura H: The effect of ventilation and blood volume on the uptake and elimination of inhalation anesthetic agents. p. 394. In Progress in Anaesthesiology. Proceedings of the Fourth World Congress of Anesthesiologists. International Congress Series 200. Excerpta Medica, Amsterdam, 1968
26. Eger EI II, Smith NT, Stoelting RK, et al: Cardiovascular effects of halothane in man. Anesthesiology 32:396, 1970
27. Calverley RK, Smith NT, Eger EI II: Cardiovascular effects of enflurane anesthesia during controlled ventilation in man. Anesth Analg 57:619, 1978
28. Eger EI II, Bahlman SH, Munson ES: Effect of age on the rate of increase of alveolar anesthetic concentration. Anesthesiology 35:365, 1971
29. Wahrenbrock EA, Eger EI II, Laravuso RB, Maruschak G: Anesthetic uptake — of mice and men (and whales). Anesthesiology 40:19, 1974
30. Salanitre E, Rackow H: The pulmonary exchange of nitrous oxide and halothane in infants and children. Anesthesiology 30:388, 1969
31. Eger EI II, Severinghaus JW: Effect of uneven pulmonary distribution of blood and gas on induction with inhalation anesthetics. Anesthesiology 25:620, 1964
32. Stoelting RK, Longnecker DE: Effect of right-to-left shunt on rate of increase in arterial anesthetic concentration. Anesthesiology 36:352, 1972
33. Eger EI II, Saidman LJ: Hazards of nitrous oxide anesthesia in bowel obstruction and pneumothorax. Anesthesiology 26:61, 1965
34. Hunter AR: Problems of anaesthesia in artificial pneumothorax. Proc R Soc Med 48:765, 1955
35. Munson ES, Merrick HC: Effect of nitrous oxide on venous air embolism. Anesthesiology 27:783, 1966
36. Shapiro HM, Yoachim J, Marshall LF: Nitrous oxide challenge for detection of residual intravascular pulmonary gas following venous air embolism. Anesth Analg 61:304, 1982
37. Stanley TH, Kawamura R, Graves C: Effects of nitrous oxide on volume and pressure of endotracheal tube cuffs. Anesthesiology 41:256, 1974
38. Kaplan R, Abramowitz MD, Epstein BS: Nitrous oxide and air-filled balloon-tipped catheters. Anesthesiology 55:71, 1981
39. Eisenkraft JB, Eger EI II: Nitrous oxide anesthesia may double the balloon gas volume of Swan-Ganz catheters. Mt Sinai J Med 49:430, 1982
40. Wolf GL, Capuano C, Hartung J: Nitrous oxide increases intraocular pressure after intravitreal sulfur hexafluoride injection. Anesthesiology 59:547, 1983
41. Thomsen KA, Terkildsen K, Arnfred J: Middle ear pressure variations during anesthesia. Arch Otolaryngol 82:609, 1985
42. Saidman LJ, Eger EI II: Change in cerebrospinal fluid pressure during pneumoencephalography under nitrous oxide anesthesia. Anesthesiology 26:67, 1965
43. Waun JE, Sweitzer RS, Hamilton WK: Effect of nitrous oxide on middle ear mechanics and hearing acuity. Anesthesiology 28:846, 1987
44. Graham MD, Knight PR: Atelectative tympanic membrane reversal by nitrous oxide supplemented general anesthesia and polyethylene ventilation tube insertion. A preliminary report. Laryngoscope 41:1469, 1981
45. Eger EI II, Larson CP, Jr., Severinghaus JW: The solubility of halothane in rubber, soda lime and various plastics. Anesthesiology 23:356, 1962
46. Titel JH, Lowe HJ: Rubber-gas partition coefficients. Anesthesiology 29:1215, 1968
47. Titel JH, Lowe HJ, Elam JO, Grosholz JR: Quantitative closed-circuit halothane anesthesia. Anesth Analg 47:560, 1968
48. Grodin WK, Epstein MAF, Epstein RA: Mechanisms of halothane adsorption by dry soda-lime. Br J Anaesth 54:561, 1982
49. Grodin WK, Epstein RA: Halothane adsorption complicating the use of soda-lime to humidify anaesthetic gases. Br J Anaesth 54:555, 1982
50. Eger EI II: Stability of I-653 in soda lime. Anesth Analg 66:983, 1987
51. Harper M, Eger EI II: A comparison of the efficiency of three anesthesia circle systems. Anesth Analg 55:724, 1976
52. Altrete JA, Lowe HJ, Virtue RW: Low Flow and Closed System Anesthesia. Grune & Stratton, Orlando, FL, 1979
53. Severinghaus JW: The rate of uptake of nitrous oxide in man. J Clin Invest 33:1183, 1954
54. Ross JAS, Wloch RT, White DC, Hawes DW: Servo-controlled closed-circuit anaesthesia. Br J Anaesth 55:1053, 1983
55. O'Callaghan AS, Hawes DW, Ross JAS, et al: Uptake of isoflurane during clinical anaesthesia. Br J Anaesth 55:1061, 1983
56. Eger EI II, Johnson BH: Rates of awakening from anesthesia with I-653, halothane, isoflurane, and sevoflurane: a test of the effect of anesthetic concentration and duration in rats. Anesth Analg 66:977, 1987
57. Mapleson WW: Quantitative prediction of anesthetic concentrations. p. 104. In Papper EM, Kitz RJ (eds): Uptake and Distribution of Anesthetic Agents. McGraw-Hill, New York, 1963
58. Stoelting RK, Eger EI II: The effects of ventilation and anesthetic solubility on recovery from anesthesia: An in vivo and analog analysis before and after equilibration. Anesthesiology 30:290, 1969
59. Wyrwicz AM, Pszenny MH, Schofield C, et al: Noninvasive observations of fluorinated anesthetics in rabbit brain by fluorine-19 nuclear magnetic resonance. Science 222:428, 1983
60. Coburn CM, Eger EI II: The partial pressure of isoflurane or halothane does not affect their solubility in rabbit blood or brain or human brain. Anesth Analg 65:960, 1986
61. Cohen EN, Chow KL, Mathers L: Autoradiographic distribution of volatile anesthetics within the brain. Anesthesiology 37:324, 1972
62. Litt L, Ganzalez-Mendez R, James TL, et al: An in vivo study of halothane uptake and elimination in the rate brain with fluorine nuclear magnetic resonance spectroscopy. Anesthesiology 67:161, 1987
63. Mills P, Sessler DI, Moseley M, et al: An in vivo ^{19}F nuclear magnetic resonance study of isoflurane elimination from the rabbit brain. Anesthesiology 67:169, 1987
64. Rehder K, Forbes J, Alter H, et al: Halothane biotransformation in man: A quantitative study. Anesthesiology 28:711, 1967

65. Chase RE, Holaday DA, Fiserova-Bergerova V, et al: The biotransformation of Ethrane in man. Anesthesiology 35:262, 1971

66. Cahalan MK, Johnson BH, Eger EI II: Relationship of concentrations of halothane and enflurane to their metabolism and elimination in man. Anesthesiology 54:3, 1981

67. Fink BR: Diffusion anoxia. Anesthesiology 54:3, 1981

68. Sheffer L, Steffenson JL, Birch AA: Nitrous-oxide-induced diffusion hypoxia in patients breathing spontaneously. Anesthesiology 37:436, 1972

69. Rackow H, Salanitre E, Frumin MH: Dilution of alveolar gases during nitrous oxide excretion in man. J Appl Physiol 16:723, 1961

70. Eger RR, Eger EI II: Effect of temperature and age on the solubility of enflurane, halothane, isoflurane and methoxyflurane in human blood. Anesth Analg 64:640, 1985

71. Yasuda N, Targ AG, Eger EI II: Solubility of I-653, sevoflurane, isoflurane, and halothane in human tissues. Anesthesiology 69A:615, 1988

72. Lerman J, Schmitt-Bantel BI, Gregory GA, et al: Effect of age on the solubility of volatile anesthetics in human tissues. Anesthesiology 65:307, 1986

73. Eger EI II: Partition coefficients of I-653 in human blood, saline, and olive oil. Anesth Analg 66:971, 1987

74. Targ AG, Yasuda N, Eger EI II: Anesthetic plastic solubility. Anesthesiology 69A:297, 1988

75. Munson ES, Eger EI II: Methoxyflurane solubility in plastics. Anesthesiology 26:828, 1965

76. Eger EI II, Brandstater B: Solubility of methoxyflurane in rubber. Anesthesiology 24:679, 1963

5

CARDIOPULMONARY PHARMACOLOGY

Edward G. Pavlin
Judy Y. Su

Pulmonary Pharmacology of Inhaled Anesthetics
Effects of Inhaled Anesthetics on Bronchomotor Tone
Effects of Inhaled Anesthetics on Pulmonary Vascular Resistance
Effects of Inhaled Anesthetics on Mucociliary Function
Effects of Inhaled Anesthetics on Control of Ventilation

Cardiovascular Pharmacology of Inhaled Anesthetics
Effect of Inhaled Anesthetics on Circulation
Direct Effects of Inhaled Anesthetics on Contraction of Cardiac Muscle
Effect of Inhaled Anesthetics on Vascular Smooth Muscle
Effect of Inhaled Anesthetics on Baroreceptor Function

PULMONARY PHARMACOLOGY OF INHALED ANESTHETICS

Since inhaled anesthetics pervade the whole body, pulmonary function may be affected by both direct and indirect actions. The line between physiologic and pharmacologic effects may be very thin indeed. To avoid repetition of later chapters dealing with anesthesia and the lung, this chapter describes the more direct methods by which anesthetic gases and vapors alter the activities of various anatomic components of the lung. To this end, sections deal with airway resistance, pulmonary vascular caliber, mucociliary function, and ventilatory control. Although the latter involves discussion of receptors and the nervous system anatomically removed from the lung, dose-related depression of ventilation caused by anesthesia obviously is one of the most potent and important pulmonary side effects.

Effects of Inhaled Anesthetics on Bronchomotor Tone

The increase in airway resistance observed during an acute asthmatic attack may be both frightening and potentially lethal. Although a universally accepted definition of asthma is difficult to enunciate, in this discussion it is considered to be a transient state of increased airway resistance caused at least in part by an increase in bronchiolar smooth muscle tone. This increased muscle tone occurs in patients who exhibit clinical manifestations of extrinsic or intrinsic asthma as well as those with a pharmacologically reversible component of chronic obstructive lung disease. Indeed, with the proper stimulus, bronchospasm can occur in normal subjects who have no underlying history of lung disease of any kind. A mainstay of treatment is the administration of bronchodilating drugs. An excellent review of the mechanisms of action and clinical role of bronchodilating drugs has recently been published.[1] Because of legitimate concerns regarding anesthesia in these patients, the pharmacology of inhaled anesthetics with respect to their effects on bronchial smooth muscle is of great clinical importance. The effects of various anesthetics on airway resistance are summarized in Table 5-1.

Pharmacology of Bronchial Muscle

Some consideration must be given to the basic physiology and pharmacology of airways before the effects of inhaled anesthetics or other types of bronchodilating agents can be predicted or evaluated. The autonomic nervous system plays a key role in the control of bronchomotor tone both in normal airways and in those of patients with bronchospastic disease.

Airway smooth muscle, which extends as far distally as the terminal bronchioles, is under the influence of both parasympathetic and sympathetic nerves. Vagal innervation of the bronchial tree has been well documented, and sympathetic innervation, although less well defined, probably plays a role as well. The effects of the autonomic nervous system are thought to be mediated through their action on the stores of cyclic adenosine monophosphate (AMP) and cyclic guanosine monophosphate (GMP) in bronchial smooth muscle cells. Acetylcholine, or stimulation by the vagus nerve, is thought to provide an increase in the amounts of cyclic GMP relative to cyclic AMP, leading to smooth muscle contraction. Release of histamine in the airway or various forms of mechanical or chemical stimulation can result in an increase in afferent vagal activity with subsequent reflex bronchoconstriction. This increase in bronchomotor tone can be attenuated by atropine.

Adrenergic receptors in bronchial smooth muscle are classified into α and β types according to the classic description of Ahlquist.[2] While α-receptors are found in the bronchial tree in humans, their activity seems to be low and clinically unimportant. The β-receptors have been further refined into β_1 and β_2 types; the latter play the most significant role in bronchial muscle. Stimulation of β-receptors in bronchial smooth muscle causes relaxation of bronchial smooth muscle. This is probably mediated by an increase within muscle cells in levels of cyclic AMP relative to cyclic GMP. The result of these findings has been an increased interest in the formulation of β_2-specific drugs and potent bronchodilatory properties and a minimum of cardiac side effects (e.g., isoetharine, metaproterenol, terbutaline, salbutamol).

Specific Inhaled Anesthetics

Since its clinical introduction in 1956, halothane has been recommended as the anesthetic of choice in the presence of bronchospasm because of its bronchodilating characteristics. In a retrospective study, Shnider and Papper[3] found that in 49 patients with preanesthetic wheezing, halothane was clearly superior to ether, cyclopropane, ethylene, and regional anesthesia in decreasing this audible manifestation of bronchospasm. Despite its retrospective design and the use of a clinical sign, rather than objective measurements, this and other earlier clinical observations established halo-

TABLE 5-1. Effects of Inhaled Anesthetic on Airway Resistance

Anesthetic	Reference	Model	Measurement	Effect
Halothane	Shnider & Papper[3]	Human: (retrospective)	Wheezing	++
	Waltemath & Bergman[133]	Human: normal	Raw	0
	Brakensiek & Bergman[134]	Human: bronchospasm (aerosol)	Raw	++
	Hickey et al.[7]	Dog: bronchospasm (vagus, histamine)	Raw	++
	Coon & Kampine[8]	Dog: LL lobe bronchoconstriction ($\downarrow CO_2$)	Raw	++
	Klide & Aviado[5]	Dog: normal	Raw	++
	Fletcher et al.[6]	Guinea Pig: isolated tracheal muscle	Length	++
	Gold & Helrich[16]	Human: status asthmaticus	Raw	0
	Meloche et al.[15]	Human: cardiopulmonary bypass bronchoconstriction ($\downarrow CO_2$)	Raw	0
	Colgan[4]	Dog: normal	"Bronchial distensibility"	0
	Hirshman & Bergman[12]	Dog: bronchospasm (*Ascaris*)	Raw	++
Diethyl Ether	Shnider & Papper[3]	Human: (retrospective)	Wheezing	+
Cyclopropane	Hickey et al.[7]	Dog: bronchospasm (histamine, vagus)	Raw	+
	Colgan[4]	Dog: normal	"Bronchial distensibility"	0
Enflurane	Coon & Kampine[8]	Dog: LL Lobe bronchoconstriction ($\downarrow CO_2$)	Raw	+
	Hirshman & Bergman[12]	Dog: bronchospasm (*Ascaris*)	Raw	++
Methoxyflurane	Coon & Kampine[8]	Dog: LL Lobe bronchoconstriction ($\downarrow CO_2$)	Raw	+
Isoflurane	Hirshman et al.[13]	Dog: Bronchospasm (*Ascaris*)	Raw	++

Abbreviations and symbols: LL, left lower; Raw, airway resistance; ++, pronounced bronchodilation; +, bronchodilation; 0, no effect.

thane as the drug of choice for patients with either a history of asthma in the past or bronchospasm occurring during induction or maintenance of anesthesia.

The effects of inhaled anesthetics on airway caliber have been studied in vivo. Colgan[4] noted a decrease in "bronchial distensibility" in dogs anesthetized with halothane, ether, methoxyflurane, or trichloroethylene, with halothane having the most pronounced effect. Klide and Aviado[5] found a dose-dependent decrease in resting airway resistance with increasing concentrations of halothane in spontaneously ventilating dogs. However, the possibility of bronchodilation secondary to an increased resting $PaCO_2$ with deeper planes of anesthesia was not taken into account in either study.

In isolated guinea pig tracheal chains, halothane, diethyl ether, and thiopental caused relaxation of resting tone.[6] These drugs also attenuated tracheal muscle constriction induced by acetylcholine, but only halothane accomplished this in clinically relevant doses. In this instance, propranolol, a β-blocking drug, did not antagonize the relaxing properties of halothane on acetylcholine-induced bronchoconstriction, leading to a conclusion different from that of Klide and Aviado,[6] who had postulated a β-receptor stimulating action of halothane.

Hickey et al.[7] demonstrated the importance of controlled levels of $PaCO_2$ in evaluating the effects of agents on bronchial smooth muscle tone. In anesthetized, intubated dogs whose ventilation was controlled to achieve a $PaCO_2$ of approximately 40 mmHg, increasing concentrations of halothane and cyclopropane produced no change in resistance in the resting unstimulated airway. In the unstimulated airway, resting tone may be minimal and therefore the bronchodilating properties of any drug may be masked because no additional relaxation of bronchial musculature can be effected. By inducing a state of increased bronchial tone by use of either histamine administration or vagal stimulation, the superior bronchodilating qualities of halothane were well demonstrated when compared with cyclopropane at 1.5 minimal alveolar concentration (MAC) levels of anesthesia. Halothane, enflurane, and methoxyflurane were found to reverse the bronchoconstricting effects of hypocapnia in vivo in the isolated left lower lobe of the dog,[8] with halothane again proving the most efficacious at lower doses.

Patterson et al.[9] measured the resistive work of breathing during cardiopulmonary bypass and found that neither airway nor systemic administration of halothane caused significant changes in airway mechanics in the unstimulated state; however, the bronchoconstricting effects of low inhaled carbon dioxide mixtures were attenuated by inhaled halothane but not by halothane administered via the blood. A similar experiment by Meloche et al.[10] demonstrated that administration of halothane did indeed decrease the bronchoconstriction produced by hypocapnia, although not to the same extent as did the addition of 6.5 percent carbon dioxide to the inhaled mixture. That systemic administration of halothane via the bypass pump did not have similar effects suggests that halothane acts directly on the airway musculature and/or local reflex arcs rather than via centrally controlled reflex pathways.

Bronchoconstriction produced by the methods described may not be directly comparable to that which occurs in the asthmatic patient. A series of studies by Hirshman utilizing dogs sensitized to *Ascaris* antigen as an experimental testing model has contributed tremendously to our understanding of the effect of anesthetics on bronchospasm. Asthma was induced by intratracheal administration of an aerosol of *Ascaris* antigen. This model is perhaps more representative of the asthmatic patient with atopic bronchospasm.[11] Hirshman and Bergman[12] demonstrated attenuation of antigen-induced bronchospasm by concentrations of approximately 1 MAC of either halothane or enflurane with no significant difference between the two agents (Fig. 5-1). No attempt was made to describe a dose-response curve. The stimulus to bronchospasm was not continued throughout the administration of anesthetic gases, a condition that differs slightly from an "asthmatic" attack during anesthesia. Nonetheless, this is a very useful model for the investigation of the bronchodilating qualities of these and other anesthetic agents.

The same experimental preparation was utilized to examine the bronchodilating effects of isoflurane. Levels of 1.5 MAC of both isoflurane and halothane were found to produce a similar decrease in airway resistance in response to bronchospasm induced by *Ascaris* antigen (a mixed reflex and direct-acting stimulus).[13] Similar results were obtained with methacholine-induced (direct-acting stimulus) airway constriction. These data suggest that isoflurane and halothane act both by depressing airway reflexes *and* by direct bronchodilation. Halothane more effectively increased dynamic compliance (a measure of small airway resistance) than did isoflurane. Thus, isoflurane shares bronchodilating properties with halothane and enflurane.

The issue of histamine and inhaled anesthetics has also been addressed by Hirshman and colleagues in this same model. Antigen-induced asthma increased plasma histamine levels, which was not prevented if animals were previously anesthetized with halothane.[14] Thus, halothane does not inhibit histamine from mast cells. In another study of histamine-induced bronchospasm, halothane and topical atropine both decreased bronchoconstriction, but halothane did not add to the bronchodilating effects of atropine.[15]

Because of their bronchodilating effects, anesthetics such as halothane may be an effective method of treating status asthmaticus when other more conventional treatments have failed. However, documentation of this effectiveness is lacking. Gold and Helrich[16] evaluated the effect of halothane and tracheal intubation on six patients in status asthmaticus who had been treated for at least 72 hours with bronchodilators, steroids, and antibiotics. No significant change in airway resistance

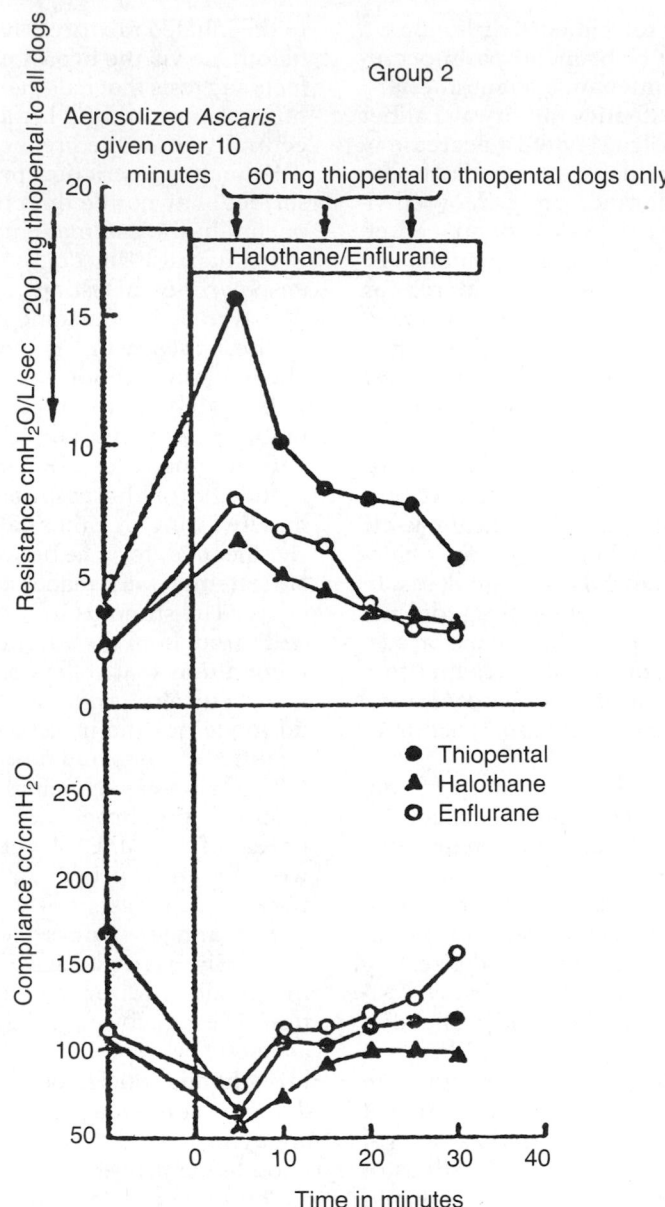

Fig. 5-1. The effect of halothane and enflurane on increased airway resistance in dogs: the airway resistance was triggered by prior administration of aerosolized *Ascaris*. This is a model of extrinsic asthma. Although the allergic stimulus was not maintained throughout the experiment, both halothane and enflurane appear to lower airway resistance compared with the control thiopental-anesthetized animals. (From Hirschman and Bergman,[12] with permission.)

was recorded in either the anesthetic or immediate postanesthetic period. Cardiac arrhythmias proved to be of some concern during the halothane therapy. Although all six patients improved within 3 days after treatment, the lack of a similar control group makes interpretation difficult. On the other hand, a recent publication[17] describes a patient who, although resist-

ant to other bronchodilators, promptly responded to the bronchodilating effects of halothane.

The use of more conventional bronchodilators in conjunction with anesthetics has not been extensively examined. Isoetharine was found to decrease severity of wheezing and peak airway pressure in 16 patients whose tracheas were intubated and who were anesthetized with different general anesthetics.[18] However, grading of the ausculatory changes was not done in a double-blind fashion. An excellent clinical study showed that a combination of subtoxic doses of aminophylline and isoetharine yielded greater relief of bronchospasm than either agent when used alone.[19]

Mechanisms of Action

General anesthetics may act at various sites to prevent or reverse bronchoconstriction resulting from a wide variety of stimulants. The possible mechanisms of action include direct dilatation of bronchial smooth muscle, blocking effects of various bronchoconstriction by central depression of the anesthetic state itself.

Klide and Aviado[5] showed that the reduction of airway resistance in dogs by halothane could be blocked by sotalol, a β-adrenergic antagonist. They concluded that halothane had β-agonist activity in bronchial smooth muscle. Later studies showed no effect of propranolol on halothane-induced relaxation of tracheal smooth muscle, in rabbit uterine smooth, or in rat aortic smooth muscle, all structures with β-receptor sites. Thus, Klide's earlier data were probably specific for sotalol, or it may have had smooth muscle-contracting properties of its own. It appears that halothane does *not* act as a β-agonist in this regard.

In both uterine and aortic smooth muscle strips, halothane is associated with an increase in cyclic AMP, suggesting stimulation of adenyl cyclase although not via β-receptor stimulation. In assessing the direct effects of halothane in vitro on dog tracheal smooth muscle, halothane suppressed the contraction of the muscle initiated by both direct and indirect electrical stimulation.[20] The investigators concluded that halothane inactivated or reduced free Ca^{++} in the cytoplasm and may suppress the influx of Ca^{++} across the cell membrane. This action of halothane is common to that of vascular smooth muscle and indeed cardiac muscle (see the section, *Cardiovascular Pharmacology of Inhaled Anesthetics*).

Isoflurane and halothane appear to act on airway reflexes and directly on smooth muscle[13] since airway constriction from both direct- and reflex-acting stimuli is relieved by these anesthetics. Histamine levels secondary to antigen challenge are not affected by halothane.[14] An in vitro study of dog tracheal muscle suggested that halothane acts directly on Ca^{++} stores in tracheal smooth muscle cells to interfere with the excitation-contraction coupling.[20]

In summary, inhaled anesthetics may act at several different sites in affecting bronchial smooth muscle relaxation. The direct action may involve the cyclic AMP mechanisms, although alternative actions on prostaglandins and Ca^{++} activity must be considered. While arguments for a specific β-agonist role of halothane exist, more recent data would suggest this is not the mechanism of halothane activity on smooth muscle mechanics.

Clinical Implications

The mechanisms by which increases in airway resistance may be stimulated have been summarized by Aviado.[21] Bronchospasm may occur in patients under conditions of disease other than asthma. Patients with chronic obstructive lung disease may present with elements of bronchospasm that contribute to their increased airway resistance, which may be discerned by demonstrating improvement in forced expiratory flow rates after administration of a bronchodilator. Normal healthy patients undergoing surgical stimulation of pulmonary arteries and parenchyma or trachea are known to be at risk of developing bronchospasm.[22] An isolated case report has described an episode of wheezing in a patient undergoing transurethral resection. Indeed, in a lightly anesthetized patient clinically discernible bronchospasm is not an unusual event following surgical stimulation or irritation of the trachea by endotracheal tubes. In anticipating such events in patients with known reactive airway disease or in the unexpected episode of bronchospasm, the choice of preoperative medication, induction agent, muscle relaxant, and the type and dosage of anesthetic drug are important in minimizing clinical symptoms. A review of anesthetic management of the asthmatic patient is suggested.[23]

The variety of studies previously described strongly suggest halothane as the anesthetic of choice. Although the preponderance of data suggest halothane as the most effective bronchodilator (Fig. 5-2), the work of Hirshman and colleagues would suggest that isoflurane and enflurane are as effective in decreasing airway resistance in their experimental preparation. Thus, isoflurane, and perhaps enflurane, are good alternatives to halothane when reactive airways are a concern. Thus,

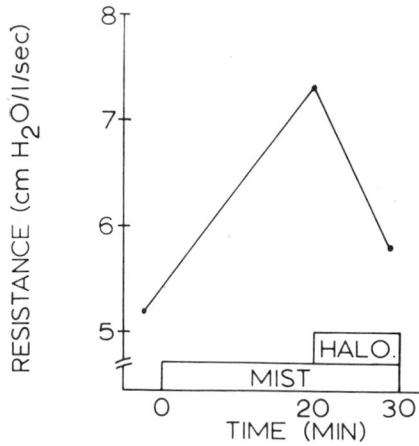

Fig. 5-2. The effect of halothane on increased respiratory resistance in humans provoked by inhalation of ultrasonic mist. Halothane effectively decreased airway resistance triggered by the irritation of ultrasonic droplets. (From Waltemath and Bergman,[133] with permission.)

the role of inhaled anesthetic is enhanced by sufficient depth of anesthesia to both depress airway reflexes and act as a direct bronchodilator. This is particularly true when instrumentation of the airway (e.g., endotracheal intubation) is to take place.

The high incidence of postanesthetic pulmonary complications in patients with chronic obstructive disease is well known. Studies of outcome with different anesthetics are not specific enough to evaluate the role of anesthetic drugs vis-à-vis effects on postoperative morbidity, airway resistance, or both. Thus, more objective studies are needed to evaluate effects of various inhaled anesthetics in patients who are at high risk of developing bronchospasm in the preoperative period.

Effects of Inhaled Anesthetics on Pulmonary Vascular Resistance

Interest in the pulmonary vasculature, sometimes referred to as the *lesser circulation*, has increased geometrically over the past 15 years. Techniques for easy measurement of pulmonary blood flow (cardiac output) and pulmonary vascular pressures have become commonplace. The role of the pulmonary vasculature in various disease states and its reaction to drugs including anesthetics has spurred much interest.

Determinants of Pulmonary Vascular Resistance

The role of pharmacologic agents in determining pulmonary vascular pressures and resistances is a complicated one, since many vasoactive agents have both direct effects on pulmonary blood vessels as well as indirect effects through alterations of cardiac output and pulmonary blood flow. Changes in pulmonary vascular resistance (PVR) and pressure may have significant effects on gas or fluid exchange in the lung. Increased PVR may give rise to an increase in pulmonary artery pressure if cardiac output is maintained constant and thereby promote increased transudation of fluid into the interstitium of the lung.

Regional changes in PVR are particularly important in that they may alter the relative distribution of blood flow within the lung, leading to altered ventilation-perfusion relationships and accompanying changes in gas exchange. Thus, a localized increase in PVR in an area of atelectasis may cause a shift of blood flow away from the atelectatic segment to better-ventilated regions of lung and thereby ultimately lead to improved gas exchange by decreasing blood flow to nonventilated lung. This increase in PVR in an area of atelectasis is believed to be partially due to localized tissue hypoxia. This phenomenon, termed *hypoxic vasoconstriction*, is of interest because of its importance in determining the magnitude of the effects of diseased and/or nonventilated areas of lung on gas exchange and $PaCO_2$. Hypoxic vasoconstriction appears to have protective value, and

drugs that interfere with this protective mechanism may adversely affect gas exchange. Many of the commonly used agents in anesthesia are included in the list of offenders.

PVR can be altered by several mechanisms. Passive changes in the diameter of the pulmonary blood vessels may be induced by increased cardiac output (increased pulmonary blood flow) or by elevations of left atrial pressure or both. The increased vascular distending pressure may cause an increase in cross-sectional diameter of the pulmonary vascular bed and hence a fall in PVR. Similarly, changes in lung volume may alter the dimensions of the vasculature and hence affect resistance. Increases of lung volume above functional residual capacity (FRC) caused by increased pressure in the airway are characteristically associated with passive increases in PVR; the latter are presumably caused by transmission of the higher alveolar pressures to blood vessels located in alveolar walls. On the other hand, reduction in lung volumes below normal FRC is also associated with passive increases in PVR. The latter are thought to be the result of a reduction in vascular dimensions as the lung shrinks. At low lung volumes, vessels are both shorter and narrower, apparently because of loss of a tethering effect of surrounding lung tissue. Additionally, vessels may become tortuous and crinkled at lower lung volumes. The net effect of these changes is a rise in PVR. It is of interest that resistance in the pulmonary circuit appears to be least at FRC.

Active changes in pulmonary vascular tone may also contribute to the level of resistance in the lesser circulation. These may be induced by changes in sympathetic tone, by local changes in PO_2 and/or PCO_2, or by changes in levels of catecholamines or other vasoactive substances released locally or in blood perfusing the lung. The pulmonary vasoconstrictor response to hypoxia, hypercarbia, or both is of interest in that it is opposite to that observed in most systemic vascular beds. Many anesthetic drugs tend to reduce lung volume and, therefore, may have additional effects on PVR through this mechanism as well.

A complete description of the ways in which anesthetics may affect pulmonary blood flow is well beyond the scope of this chapter. We confine ourselves to the much narrower question of how anesthetics may alter PVR with particular emphasis on the direct effects of anesthetics on hypoxic vasoconstriction. The effect of inhaled anesthetics on pulmonary blood flow and pulmonary artery pressure in humans in the absence of significant underlying pulmonary pathology is small. In general, the more potent agents such as halothane and enflurane simultaneously cause a decrease in PVR and an increase in left atrial pressure.[24,25] The net effect is usually little or no change in pulmonary artery pressure and a small decrease in pulmonary blood flow. Nitrous oxide and ether have less effect on cardiac output, and therefore, pulmonary blood flow is relatively unaffected. Overall, changes in PVR are small, tending to rise slightly during anesthetic administration.

Hypoxic Pulmonary Vasoconstrictor Response

The hypoxic pulmonary vasoconstrictor (HPV) response is believed to be mediated locally. The demonstration of this response in isolated perfused lungs reflects the local nature of this reflex. Furthermore, a similar response may be elicited in animals whose catecholamines have been depleted by reserpine or following α-adrenergic blockade. The sympathetic nervous system may, however, play a role in augmenting the response in certain circumstances, particularly in the presence of systemic hypoxemia.

Arteriolar constriction occurs in response to decreased oxygen tension in the alveolus. HPV responses in normal lung seem to appear when PaO_2 becomes less than 100 mmHg and maximal when PaO_2 is approximately 30 mmHg.[26,27] Mixed venous PO_2 ($P\bar{v}O_2$) may influence HPV in atelectatic lung since PaO_2 in the collapsed segment approaches $P\bar{v}O_2$.[28,29] Acidosis also appears to be a pulmonary vasoconstrictor both in intact animals and in isolated perfused lungs. With normal alveolar oxygen tensions, changes in PVR in response to acidosis are small, but in the presence of alveolar hypoxia they are greatly enhanced. Thus, vasoconstriction may be augmented by elevations in arterial hydrogen ion concentration, alveolar PCO_2, or both. The local mediator of the response to hypoxia and acidosis has not been identified.

The vasoconstrictor response of the pulmonary circulation to hypoxemia and acidosis is different from that of the systemic vasculature and appears to be suited to matching of lung perfusion to ventilation. Thus, hypoxic areas of the lung, because of local pulmonary vasoconstrictor reflexes, have reduced blood flow with a shift of blood flow to the better ventilated (less hypoxic and acidotic) areas of the lung. This selective redistribution of blood away from the poorly ventilated areas has been shown to decrease alveolar-arterial oxygen tension gradients [$P(A-a)O_2$].[30] The obliteration of this response by infusion of a pulmonary vasodilator, such as sodium nitroprusside, has been shown to decrease arterial PO_2 and increase pulmonary shunting in dogs with oleic acid-induced pulmonary edema.[31]

Inhaled Anesthetics and Hypoxic Pulmonary Vasoconstriction

A decrease in PaO_2 and an increase in $P(A-a)O_2$ has been frequently described during anesthesia. Many mechanisms exist by which this decrease in oxygenation may take place. Earlier explanations centered mostly on the effect of anesthesia on lung mechanics. Such effects as progressive pulmonary atelectasis and diminished FRC relative to closing capacity of the lung have been just two of the mechanisms suggested. In 1964, Buckley et al.[32] suggested that the local pulmonary vasoconstriction in response to hypoxia might be attenuated by halothane anesthesia. Since that time the effects of numerous inhaled anesthetics on HPV have been examined in a variety of animals and experimental models. Many of the studies have produced conflicting results regarding the effects of certain anesthetics, particularly halothane. A summary of experiments and results in this area is shown in Table 5-2. Sykes et al.[33] reported that halothane attenuated the rise in pulmonary artery pressure that recurred in isolated perfused denervated cat lungs in response to ventilation with an hypoxic gas mixture. However, these experiments were criticized because of instability of the vasoconstrictor response in the control preparation not exposed to anesthetics. When experiments were repeated in cat lungs in which sympathetic nervous innervation was preserved,[34] HPV was diminished by halothane only at inspired concentrations of 3 percent or greater. It is significant that in these latter experiments, there was no evidence that the hypoxic vasopressor response deteriorated with time as had been found by the previous investigations. Alveolar (end-expired) concentrations of anesthetic were not measured, and therefore, the true alveolar concentration of halothane was unknown. Thus, although the effect of halothane on hypoxic pulmonary constriction appeared to be attenuated in this model compared with the isolated denervated cat lung, it is difficult to compare equianesthetic doses of anesthetic because the alveolar concentrations were unknown.

Marshall et al.[35] utilized isolated perfused rat lungs to examine the effects of halothane, enflurane, and isoflurane on HPV. Dose-response curves were carefully established for each of these anesthetics. All three anesthetics depressed HPV in a dose-related manner and the 50 percent effective dose (ED_{50}) for HPV depression occurred at similar MAC values. This in vitro preparation allowed for control of lung perfusion and negated any effect of the sympathetic nervous system. Reversal of HPV by halothane has been substantiated by others in isolated perfused rat lungs.[36] Further conflicting experimental data exist in a series of studies performed on dogs.[37] Benumof and Wahrenbrock[38] tested the hypothesis that halogenated anesthetics and nitrous oxide cause local inhibition of HPV. Their experimental design consisted of isolating the left lower lobe of a dog and selectively ventilating this lobe with hypoxic gas mixtures containing MAC multiples of inhaled anesthetics while the remainder of the lung was ventilated with 100 percent oxygen. The effect on PVR was assessed by the measurement of blood flow to the isolated lobe, by use of an electromagnetic flowmeter, and by comparing it with total pulmonary blood flow. With constant pulmonary blood flow (cardiac output), pulmonary artery pressure, and left atrial pressure, a significant decrease in flow to the isolated left lower lobe was found in the presence of localized alveolar hypoxia. The administration of halothane or nitrous oxide did not diminish the magnitude of the hypoxic vasoconstrictive response (Fig. 5-3), although a profound dose-related effect could be demonstrated in the presence of fluroxene and isoflurane. The investigators then repeated these experiments[39] but administered the anesthetic to the whole animal as well as to the isolated lung

TABLE 5-2. Effects of Inhaled Anesthetics on Hypoxic Pulmonary Vasoconstriction

Anesthetic	Reference	Model	Effect
Halothane	Buckley et al.[32]	Dog: 5% O_2 whole lung	Inhibit
	Kaur et al.[135]	Dog: 10% O_2 whole lung	None
	Benumof & Wahrenbrock[38]	Dog: N_2 LL lobe	None
	Mathers et al.[39]	Dog: N_2 LL lobe	None
	Sykes et al.[33]	Cat: 3% O_2 isolated lung	Inhibit
	Bjertnaes et al.[36]	Rat: 2% O_2 isolated lung	Inhibit
	Loh et al.[34]	Cat: 3% O_2 innervated lung	Inhibit
	Sykes et al.[37]	Dog: whole lung	None
	Fargas-Babjak & Forrest[41]	Dog: 8% O_2 whole lung	None
	Bjertnaes[42]	Human: N_2 one lung	Inhibit
	Marshall et al.[35]	Rat: 3% O_2 isolated lung	Inhibit
Ether	Sykes et al.[33]	Cat: 3% O_2 isolated lung	Inhibit
	Sykes et al.[40]	Dog: N_2 left lung	Inhibit
	Loh et al.[34]	Cat: 3% O_2 innervated lung	Inhibit
	Bjertnaes[42]	Human: N_2 one lung	Inhibit
	Bjertnaes et al.[36]	Rat: 2% O_2 isolated lung	Inhibit
Trichlorethylene	Sykes et al.[33]	Cat: 3% O_2 isolated lung	Inhibit
	Sykes et al.[136]	Dog: N_2 one lung	Inhibit
Nitrous Oxide	Buckley et al.[32]	Dog: 5% O_2 whole lung	Enhanced
	Sykes et al.[40]	Dog: N_2 one lung	Inhibit
	Hurtig et al.[137]	Cat: 3% O_2 isolated lung	Inhibit
	Mathers et al.[39]	Dog: N_2 LL lobe	Inhibit (slight)
	Benumof & Wahrenbrock[38]	Dog: N_2 LL lobe	None
	Bjertnaes et al.[36]	Rat: 2% O_2 isolated lung	None
Fluroxene	Benumof & Wahrenbrock[38]	Dog: N_2 LL lobe	Inhibit
	Mathers et al.[39]	Dog: N_2 LL lobe	Inhibit
Methoxyflurane	Sykes et al.[33]	Cat: 3% O_2 isolated lung	Inhibit
	Bjertnaes et al.[36]	Rat: 2% O_2 isolated lung	Inhibit
Isoflurane	Benumof & Wahrenbrock[38]	Dog: N_2 LL lobe	Inhibit
	Mathers et al.[39]	Dog: N_2 LL lobe	Inhibit
	Marshall et al.[35]	Rat: 3% O_2 isolated lung	Inhibit
Enflurane	Mathers et al.[39]	Dog: N_2 LL lobe	None
	Marshall et al.[35]	Rat: 3% O_2 isolated lung	Inhibit
Cyclopropane	Tait et al.[138]	Cat: 3% O_2 isolated lung	None

Abbreviation: LL, left lower.

segment. In this preparation, cardiac output was diminished by halothane, isoflurane, and enflurane but the effects on blood flow to the isolated segment were almost identical to those obtained when administration of anesthetic was confined to the isolated lobe alone. Halothane at levels up to 2 MAC did not significantly interfere with hypoxic vasoconstriction of the test lobe, while isoflurane, enflurane, and fluroxene did lessen the vasoconstrictive effect of hypoxemia.

Sykes et al.[37] examined the effects of alveolar hypoxia in one lung on the relative distribution of pulmonary blood flow between both lungs in dogs. Blood flow distribution was measured by using xenon 133 in dogs whose tracheas were intubated with a double-lumen tube permitting independent ventilation of each lung. One lung was ventilated with nitrogen, while the other lung was ventilated with 100 percent oxygen. The PaO_2 was greater than 100 mmHg. A significant redistribution of flow to the well-oxygenated lung was found—

evidence of a brisk hypoxic vasoconstrictive response, which was preserved in the presence of halothane at inspired concentrations of up to 3 percent. Sykes et al.[40] in the same preparation demonstrated that ether profoundly affected the redistribution of pulmonary blood flow in response to hypoxia. Fargas-Babjak and Forrest[41] also found that increases in PVR in a nitrogen-ventilated lung were affected by inhalation of 1.5 percent halothane. Alveolar concentrations of halothane were not measured, however, and cardiac output was substantially reduced when compared with the unanesthetized state.

In a study of the effects of anesthetics on the phenomenon in humans, Bjertnaes[42] examined the effects of diethyl ether and halothane on the distribution of pulmonary blood flow during nitrogen ventilation of one lung while the opposite lung was ventilated with oxygen. Distribution of blood flow was assessed by lung perfusion scan. Hypoxic vasoconstriction was demon-

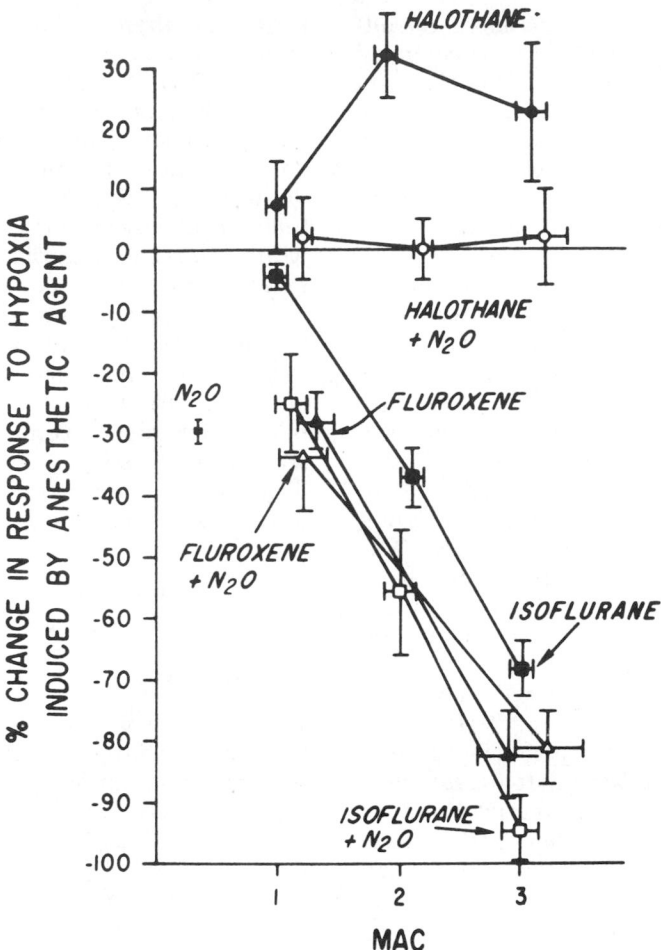

Fig. 5-3. The effect of anesthetics on the hypoxia-induced increase in PVR of an isolated left lower lobe of the dog. Zero on the vertical axis represents the normal distribution of pulmonary blood flow between the hypoxic left lower lobe and the remainder of the lung. A negative percentage change represents a decrease in the hypoxia-induced pulmonary vasoconstriction of the nitrogen-ventilated left lower lobe. In this preparation, halothane seems to have little effect on pulmonary vasoconstriction, but fluroxene, nitrous oxide, and isoflurane exhibit a dose-dependent decrease in hypoxic vasoconstriction. (From Benumof and Wahrenbrock,[38] with permission.)

strated in the nitrogen-ventilated lung during intravenous anesthesia with barbiturates but disappeared with the inhalation of either halothane or diethyl ether in the nitrogen-ventilated lungs. Abolishment of the HPV response was accompanied in most patients by a decrease in PaO_2. The method of measurement precluded the ability to demonstrate a return of hypoxic vasoconstriction to its former level after the withdrawal of the inhaled anesthetic. In addition, pulmonary artery and left atrial pressures were not measured, and it is known that changes in left atrial pressure may alter the pulmonary vascular response to hypoxia.

In contrast to this study, clinical observations in humans undergoing one-lung ventilation during thoracic surgery have failed to demonstrate changes consistent with attenuation of HPV by halothane. Comparing pulmonary gas exchange under intravenous anesthetics (ketamine) and isoflurane[43] or enflurane,[44]

no significant differences in $\dot{Q}s/\dot{Q}T$ or PaO_2 were found between the two anesthetics in two separate studies. Since ketamine is said to not affect HPV, this observation would suggest that halothane does not affect HPV when one lung is unventilated. However, several differences exist between these studies and others. Bjertnaes[42] ventilated one lung with oxygen and the other with nitrogen to demonstrate HPV, as opposed to the clinical situation of ventilating one lung with oxygen and allowing the unventilated nondependent lung to undergo various degrees of collapse. Thoracic surgery is done in patients with an open chest in the lateral position, altering distribution of perfusion pressures through the two lungs. The nondependent, or uppermost, lung may be diseased, altering pulmonary vascular responsiveness to hypoxia. It has been suggested that surgical manipulation of the lung and the pulmonary vessels may diminish HPV response, necessitating a prolonged exposure to hypoxia or possibly intermittent hypoxic exposure to reestablish HPV. The clinical observations of Rees and Gaines[44] and Anderson and Benumof[43] should not be interpreted as suggesting inhaled anesthetics do not alter HPV in humans. Rather, in this clinically important situation of thoracic surgery and one-lung anesthesia, HPV may be attenuated by other factors so the effect of inhaled anesthetics is not demonstrable.

The observed variations in response to administration of halothane may in part be due to species differences as well as to differences in experimental protocols. While diethyl ether has been found to have a profound effect on diminishing hypoxic pulmonary vasoconstriction in all models tested, the pulmonary vascular response to inhalation of nitrous oxide has been as varied as that measured during the administration of halothane. Sykes et al.[40] demonstrated in dog lung that nitrous oxide appeared to attenuate HPV. Other investigators have shown little or no effect from the addition of nitrous oxide to inhaled gas mixtures.[38] The effects of other less commonly used anesthetic agents are summarized in Table 5-2.

The mechanism by which some anesthetics appear to interfere with the pulmonary vasoconstrictor responses to hypoxia remains a mystery. If in fact pulmonary vascular smooth muscle responds to locally accumulated tissue metabolites, then anesthetics could act by interfering with the metabolic production of these vasoactive substances. It is also possible that anesthetics that have a direct relaxing effect on vascular smooth muscle may counteract locally or systemically mediated vasoconstrictive responses. Interference with calcium uptake by smooth muscle has also been suggested as one mechanism by which anesthetics may interfere with smooth muscle constriction. Similarly, increases in vascular tone in healthy lung caused by specific anesthetics or methods of ventilation might increase PVR in normal lung segments and thereby cause a redistribution of blood flow to the diseased lung.

One of the important factors involved in modulating the effects of hypoxic vasoconstriction may be the overall effect of pulmonary artery pressure. Thus, high pulmonary artery pressures, by increasing vascular distending pressure, may tend to cause passive distention of constricted vascular beds and thereby tend to reverse hypoxic vasoconstriction. Similarly, reflex pulmonary and systemic vasoconstriction in response to stimuli such as hypotension may increase PVR in healthy lung segments, again leading to a shift of blood flow to the diseased or "hypoxic" areas of lung. The net effect of anesthetics on HPV obviously depends on a number of other factors that commonly occur during surgery and anesthesia.

Clinically, despite some variation in experimental results, the effect of anesthetics on the pulmonary vasculature must be taken into account as one possible factor when considering the causes of hypoxemia under anesthesia. Although changes in distribution may account for some of these problems, attenuation of the hypoxic vasoconstrictor response may have a significant influence on PaO$_2$. In dogs with oleic acid-induced pulmonary edema, quite remarkable reversible increases in pulmonary shunting have been demonstrated by the administration of pulmonary vasodilators such as sodium nitroprusside[40] and nitroglycerine. Some anesthetics probably produce a similar response in patients with adult respiratory distress syndrome or with other types of pulmonary pathology associated with large right-to-left intrapulmonary shunts. The most likely effect of the various anesthetics in these patients remains to be defined. The selection of the appropriate type of anesthetic drugs may be of great importance in minimizing arterial hypoxemia in patients with wide alveolar to arterial oxygen tension differences. More work needs to be done, particularly in humans, before the effect of a particular anesthetic can be predicted.

Effects of Inhaled Anesthetics on Mucociliary Function

Normal Mucociliary Function

The clearance of mucus from the respiratory tract is an important defense mechanism of the lungs. Foreign particulate matter as well as the debris of pulmonary infection are removed by the upward and outward flow of mucus. Ciliated respiratory epithelium is located throughout the respiratory tract and extends distally as far as the terminal bronchioles, although the density of such cells decreases from trachea to alveoli.[45] Mucus-producing cells (goblet and submucous glands) are similarly distributed. The peculiar pattern of ciliary motion, consistent through various kinds of species, consists of a rapid stroke in a cephalad direction, followed by a slower recovery stroke in the opposite direction. Movements of distal cilia are followed closely by coordinated movements of those immediately proximal; the resulting wave of motion is referred to as metachronism.[46] The mechanism by which this coordination occurs has not been elucidated. In mammals, the sympathetic and parasympathetic nervous systems appear to play no role in the coordination of ciliary movement. The bending of individual cilia appears to be the result of an adenosine triphosphate (ATP)-dependent sliding of two parallel fibers within the ciliary filament.

Mucus represents a mixture of water, electrolytes, and macromolecules (lipids, mucins, enzymes) secreted by goblet cells and mucosal glands. Mucous secretions appear to provide a medium for entrapping and carrying foreign material and dead cells as well as for influencing the movement of the cilia. The blanket of mucus interacts with cilia and influences the rate and efficiency of ciliary movement. For instance, thicker layers of mucus appear to slow the removal of surface articles from the airway. The rheologic properties of mucus are very important and influence mucociliary function, with high elasticity and low viscosity appearing to be the characteristics required to promote the fastest transport by cilia.[47] The presence and characteristics of the mucous layer may also promote the coordination of ciliary beats.

Methods of Measurement of Mucociliary Function

Various methods have been used experimentally to assess mucociliary function in both normal animals and humans and to examine the effect of airway disease and drugs. The beat frequency of cilia is examined optically utilizing a microscope and high-speed photography in vitro, using either single cilia or tissue cultures of respiratory epithelium. In vivo techniques in animals have made use of a tracheal window, but in vivo measurements in humans would obviously pose some difficulty. The physical and chemical characteristics of mucus of expectorated specimens have also been studied extensively by Reid.[48] Characteristics may differ from those found in vivo because of contamination by salivary secretions and desiccation of expectorated secretions.

Techniques more applicable to humans include the measurement of movement of markers placed in the airway. Placement of radioactive markers in the airway is followed by measurement (utilizing external scintillation counters) of the velocity of movement of these particles in a cephalad direction in the trachea only. Sackner et al.[49] have developed a method of determining mucus velocity through a fiberoptic bronchoscope. Another technique involves the deposition of radiopaque or radioactive particles throughout the lung fields followed by sequential radiographic examinations of clearance of these inhaled particles. This allows an examination of mucociliary function in both peripheral as well as central airways.

Specific Effects of Inhaled Anesthetics

Postoperative hypoxemia and atelectasis are common findings in patients with many physiologic derangements contributing to pulmonary complications. The role of inhibited mucociliary function has sparked some recent interest and investigation. Gamsu et al.[50] compared the rate of tantalum clearance from the lungs of two groups of postoperative patients who had received general anesthesia with that of a control group consisting of awake patients undergoing tracheography. One group of patients, who underwent orthopaedic procedures, showed no significant differences from the control group. In contrast, in patients after intra-abdominal vascular surgery, retention of tantalum was demonstrated for as long as 6 days, with an average retention time threefold longer than in the control group. Retention of tantalum was correlated with the retention of mucus demonstrated in areas of atelectasis. Disappearance of tantalum from these areas of atelectasis occurred only after reexpansion of collapsed segments of lung.

Many factors other than anesthesia may affect and diminish mucociliary function, particularly in the mechanically ventilated patient. Dry inspired gases may both decrease ciliary beat frequency and cause a drying out of the mucous layer. In dogs, mucus flow rates measured by the rate of movement of a radioactive marker in the trachea were found to be maintained at normal rates for a 40-minute period if inspired air temperature was greater than 32°C with an inspired water vapor content of 33 mg/L.[51] A similar study demonstrated a complete cessation of flow of tracheal mucus after 3 hours of inhalation of dry air.[52] Mucus movement could be reinstituted by restoring inspired gases to 100 percent relative humidity at 38°C. Other factors diminishing the rate of mucus movement are high inspired oxygen concentration, inflation of the endotracheal tube cuff, and positive-pressure ventilation.[53]

In a study of tracheal mucus velocity in young anesthetized women undergoing gynecologic surgery, Lichtiger et al.[46] placed Teflon discs on the tracheal mucosa that were observed and filmed through a fiberoptic bronchoscope. Control values in awake volunteers had revealed a tracheal mucus velocity of 20 mm/min. Induction of anesthesia with halothane (1 to 2 percent) and nitrous oxide (60 percent) decreased the rate of mucus travel to 7.7 mm/min with little or no motion being seen by 90 minutes of anesthesia. Inspired gases were humidified, but the presence of higher than normal FiO_2, the use of a cuffed endotracheal tube, and the maintenance of ventilation by use of positive pressure could all have contributed to this dysfunction as well as the anesthetic.

In a study in which temperature and humidity of inspired gases and endotracheal tube cuff pressure were well controlled, Forbes[54] measured the effect of halothane anesthesia on mucociliary flow. Using external scintillation counters to measure the progression of radioactive droplets placed in the trachea, they found a dose-related depressant effect of halothane. Further studies showed a similar depressant effect in response to anesthesia with equipotent doses of enflurane and of nitrous oxide with halothane or nitrous oxide with narcotic anesthesia.[55] Conversely, ether anesthesia did not affect the velocity of mucus movement at concentrations of up to 2.4 MAC (Fig. 5-4).

Studying clearance of tantalum from the peripheral and central airways of anesthetized, intubated, mechanically ventilated dogs, Forbes and Gamsu[56] showed a delayed clearance of mucus both during and for at least 6 hours after anesthesia with halothane or ether at concentrations of 1.2 MAC. These same investigators[55] have recently found that controlled ventilation with oxygen in barbiturate-anesthetized dogs decreased tantalum clearance to approximately 50 percent of rates in awake spontaneously ventilating control animals. Since mechanical ventilation was utilized in the previously mentioned studies, its interaction with general anesthesia is unclear. Certainly the dose-related effects of halothane speak to a primary influence of halothane per se on mucus velocity.

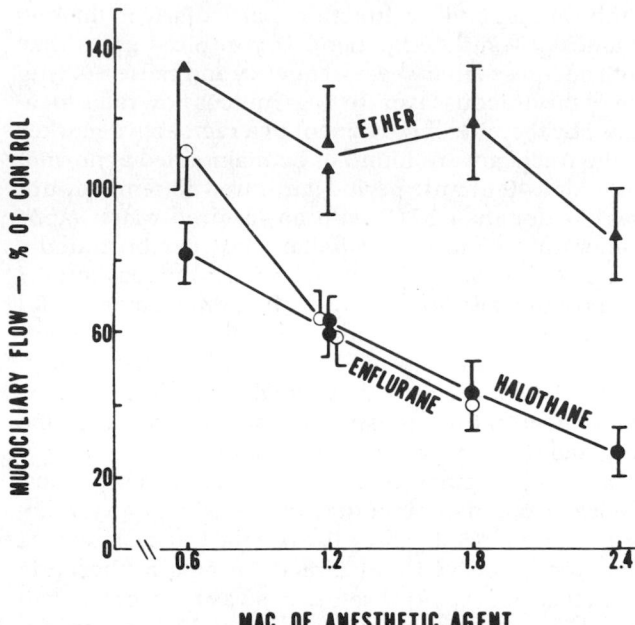

MAC OF ANESTHETIC AGENT

Fig. 5-4. Effects of various MAC levels of halothane, enflurane, and ether on mucociliary flow rates in dog tracheas. Each value is a mean ± standard error expressed as a percentage of the thiopental control. Note the dose-dependent depression of mucus velocity with enflurane and halothane anesthesia. (From Forbes and Horrigan,[55] with permission.)

Inhaled anesthetics could diminish rates of mucus clearance by diminishing ciliary beat frequency or by altering the characteristics or quantity of mucus produced during the anesthetized period. Nunn et al.[57] found dose-related decreases of ciliary activity and cellular mobility of the ciliated protozoan *Tetrahymena pyriformis* by exposure to six inhaled anesthetics including halothane. The ED_{50} for cessation of organism and ciliary movement corresponded closely to MACs of the various anesthetics. The mechanism by which cilia were affected was not clear, although the rapidity and reversibility of the depression suggested that metabolic depression of ATP stores was not involved. Extrapolation from the protozoan to the airway epithelia of mammals is hazardous but offers a very plausible explanation of observed slowing of mucus clearance.

In a recent study utilizing in vitro cultures of ciliated epithelium of dogs, Manawadu et al.[58] showed a depression of ciliary movement by halothane, but only at doses of 3 percent or more; these doses were well above usual clinical concentrations. These are substantially different sensitivities of cilia to halothane than that found by Nunn in *T. pyriformis*. The effects of anesthetics on ciliary beat frequency in humans have not been elucidated.

Clinical Significance

Because many factors contribute to postoperative pulmonary complications, the role of depressed mucociliary function is not known. It would seem clear that prolonged anesthesia could lead to pooling of mucus and thus result in atelectasis and respiratory infections. The patients at greatest risk would be those with excessive or abnormal mucus production: that is, those with chronic bronchitis, asthma, respiratory tract infection, or cystic fibrosis. Some evidence exists that patients with chronic obstructive lung disease anesthetized by regional block techniques show a lesser incidence of respiratory failure than those anesthetized with general anesthetics,[59] while other studies have failed to demonstrate this advantage. Controlled studies of the effects of inhaled anesthetics on mucociliary function in these already compromised groups of patients have not been done nor has the role of general anesthesia on their rate of pulmonary complications been clearly delineated. In animals, mucus pooling appears to occur in the intra-anesthetic and postanesthetic period; this suggests a need in the immediate postoperative period for vigorous pulmonary therapy directed toward enhancing clearance of secretions from the airways.

Effects of Inhaled Anesthetics on Control of Ventilation

Of the many derangements of lung function caused by anesthetics, alterations of minute ventilation are the most obvious. Many different stimuli interact in a complex manner to determine the level of ventilation in humans. The traditional approach to studying anesthetic effects on ventilation has been to measure ventilatory responsiveness before and after drug administration. The index of ventilatory response may be expired minute volume, frequency of respiration, or arterial carbon dioxide tension (a measure of alveolar ventilation). All of these offer some problem in interpretation of the effects on ventilatory control. Although it is an area of intense investigation, many aspects of ventilatory control are still unclear. Indeed, the precise origin of the normal respiratory pattern (the ventilatory pacemaker) remains a mystery. Investigations in humans are frequently hampered by being limited to measurements of expired gas volumes as an indicator of respiratory drive. Obviously, alterations in lung mechanics, such as those occurring during airway obstruction, may alter minute ventilation in the face of constant nerve traffic to the muscles of respiration. Similarly, a sufficient dose of muscle relaxant such as pancuronium will negate any ventilatory response to inhalation of carbon dioxide, but this would hardly constitute evidence of depression of ventilatory control.

A complete description of ventilatory control is beyond the scope of this chapter. Several excellent reviews of this subject already exist.[60] However, some understanding of normal ventilatory responses is necessary to appreciate the effects of drugs and the methods by which these effects are measured.

Control of Breathing

The volume of gas moving in and out of the lungs is matched to the oxygen consumed and carbon dioxide produced, which vary widely in disease, during exercise, and with alterations in environment (including differences in the chemical composition of inspired gases). A control system that modulates ventilation is necessary therefore to maintain stability in blood/gas tensions and acidity (Fig. 5-5) and to integrate frequency and tidal volume in such a manner as to minimize the work of breathing in response to variations in the total ventilatory requirements.

The system responsible for receiving and integrating the many input signals and ultimately producing movement of air in and out of the lungs is composed of *sensors*, which may be chemical (peripheral and central chemoreceptors) or mechanical (distortion receptors located in airways, alveoli, and respiratory muscles); a *respiratory control system*, which integrates the signal inputs from the receptor sites, centers of consciousness, and other influences (e.g., pain) and culminates in a level and pattern of nerve traffic to the muscles of respiration; and the *motor system*, composed of the chest wall and intercostal, diaphragmatic, and abdominal muscles, all of which respond to signals from the control center via the phrenic and spinal nerves.

Measurement of Respiratory Control Center Output

Detailed discussion of the respiratory control center may be found in the review of Berger et al.[60]

The *controller*, located in the medulla and pons, consists of two groups of neurons: the dorsal respiratory group (DRG), composed of cells active during inspiration; and the ventral respiratory groups (VRG), containing both inspiratory and expiratory neurons. The DRG may be the source of respiratory rhythm, and the apneustic center (VRG) may determine frequency and depth of ventilation and function as the off switch for inspiration. The exact site for integration of afferent

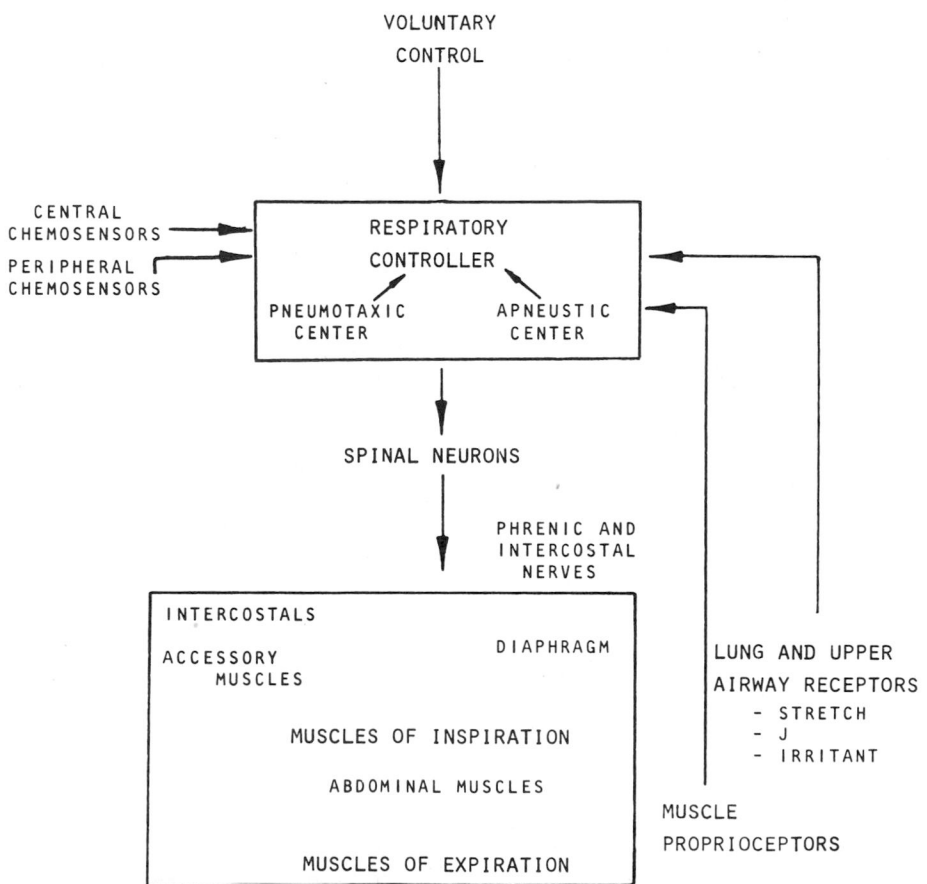

Fig. 5-5. Some aspects of the reflex control of ventilation. Inputs from many sources interact to alter ventilatory controller output and hence ventilation.

stimuli from pulmonary receptors is not clear, although the pneumotaxic center has been suggested.

The output of the respiratory control center may be assessed by measurement of cellular activity, phrenic nerve discharge, or various parameters of ventilation, of which minute ventilation (VE) is most commonly used clinically. VE is a useful measurement in normal humans but becomes a doubtful indicator of respiratory drive in patients with neuromuscular or mechanical impairment of breathing.

The search for a method of quantifying respiratory controller output led Whitelaw et al.[61] to develop a method measuring the pressure developed in the first 0.1 second of inspiration during the time that the airway is acutely obstructed immediately before inspiration. These investigators found that this parameter (P100) was independent of airway resistance and correlated well with phrenic nerve discharge. It was, however, sensitive to changes in lung FRC. A study involving the measurement of respiratory drive during methoxyflurane anesthesia showed an elevation of $PaCO_2$ but no change in P100.[62] One interpretation was that methoxyflurane did not decrease ventilatory drive but that the hypercapnia was caused by mechanical alterations in the lung or chest wall. A separation of controller output *(drive)* from VE is necessary to answer such questions as: Is ventilatory drive decreased in patients with chronic lung disease? Is the effect of anesthetics on such patients a decreased response to chemical stimuli or secondary to airway mechanical abnormalities?

Mechanoreceptors and Breathing

In the resting patient, the total amount of alveolar ventilation is believed to be determined by the partial pressures of oxygen and carbon dioxide as well as by acidity in arterial blood. The pattern of ventilation by which this minute volume is attained is determined by input signals emanating from the upper airways, lungs, and chest wall and mediated by the vagus nerve.

Lung and Airway Receptors

Pulmonary receptors that may have some relevance to the effect of anesthetics include irritant receptors and pulmonary stretch receptors. Irritant receptors are believed to be situated between airway epithelial cells. Such a location may explain the rapid response of the airways to various kinds of stimuli such as chemical irritants, smoke, and dust and to sudden mechanical deformation of the bronchial tree. These receptors are involved in coughing in response to many types of stimuli as well as in producing reflex tachypnea. They may also enhance the ventilatory response to inhaled carbon dioxide.

Pulmonary stretch receptors, located within the smooth muscle of small airways, respond to stretching or changes in lung volume. Increases in lung volume increase afferent nerve traffic via the vagus nerve to the respiratory control center, thereby inhibiting further inspiration (the Hering-Breuer reflex). This limitation of inspiration thereby determines the relationship between tidal volume and respiratory frequency. Thus, an attractive hypothesis is that although the level of alveolar ventilation is determined by chemical stimuli, the pattern of ventilation is determined by afferent mechanical signals from the lung and, to some extent, the chest wall. The pulmonary stretch receptors would therefore represent the off switch limiting tidal volume. This reflex has been demonstrated in animals at normal tidal volumes. In humans, however, tidal volumes in excess of 1 L are required to demonstrate an effect on ventilation. No change in normal breathing pattern has been observed in humans following bilateral vagal blockade. The data available would suggest that in awake, adult humans, many other factors in addition to pulmonary mechanoreceptors summate to determine the pattern of breathing.

The effects of common inhaled anesthetics on breathing patterns is depicted in Figures 5-6 and 5-7. With increasing depths of anesthesia, alveolar ventilation is progressively diminished; this is effected by a decrease in tidal volume with a simultaneous dose-related increase in breathing frequency. The rate of breathing is greatest with halothane anesthesia at higher MAC.[63]

The alteration in ventilatory pattern by anesthetics has been attributed to sensitization of pulmonary stretch receptors leading to lower tidal volumes and tachypnea. Vagal afferent activity was measured at various lung volumes in decerebrate cats with and without the intervention of various general anesthetics.[64] The presence of volatile anesthetics increased receptor discharge at any lung volume; that is, pulmonary stretch receptors did seem to be sensitized. Little evidence exists of such a mechanism in humans. Paskin et al.[65] examined the effect of elevation of FRC in anesthetized humans. The added volume and hence increased stimulus to pulmonary stretch receptors should have increased tachypnea. Instead, respiratory frequency decreased. Thus, the mechanism of production of tachypnea with decreased tidal volume in anesthetized humans remains unclear.

Mechanoreceptors in the Chest Wall

The force exerted by the muscles of inspiration is a function of afferent nerve traffic emanating from the control center. Although this may vary in response to chemical stimuli, mechanoreceptors in the chest wall also provide input to modify the pattern of breathing. Alteration in the position of the chest wall produces a change in efferent impulses from stretch receptors in tendons and intercostal muscle spindles. The effect of this input is to maintain tidal volume in the face of variations in inspiratory resistance. An increase in spindle discharge causes increased motor discharge to muscle fibers until muscle shortening relieves tension

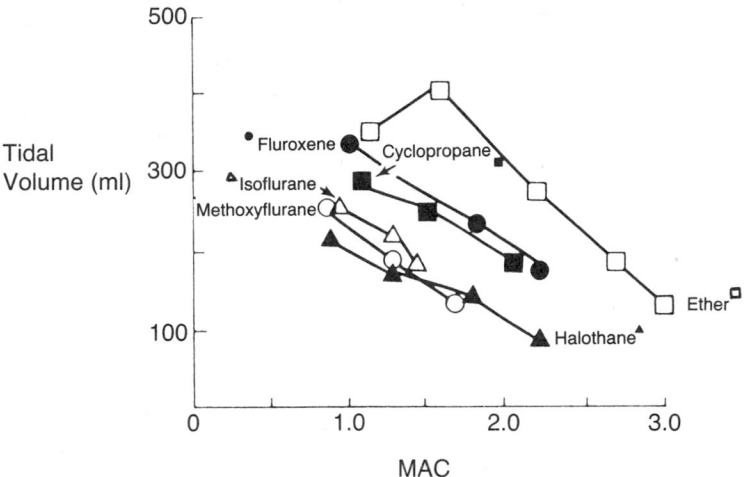

Fig. 5-6. Comparison of mean changes in tidal volume at multiples of MAC in patients anesthetized with one of five different anesthetics. Reduction of tidal volume was greatest for halothane and least for diethyl ether. (From Hickey and Severinghaus,[140] with permission.)

in the spindles. With increased inspiratory resistance, the muscle spindles detect a failure of shortening by the appropriate amount and therefore afferent signals are increased to the motor neuron pool. Accessory muscles of inspiration may be brought into use as well. This reflex increase in inspiratory effort results in sustained tidal volume and minute ventilation with increasing inspiratory resistive loading. These and other forces explain the ability of the body to maintain normal ventilation with different body positions, inspiratory resistance, and changes in compliance.

Anesthetics diminish but do not abolish ventilatory

responsiveness to inspiratory resistance.[66] During halothane anesthesia, ventilation is maintained in the face of increases in resistance or decrease in lung compliance until threshold is reached.[67] At that point, V_E is diminished with retention of carbon dioxide. At modest inspiratory resistances, ventilation is maintained even at 2 MAC halothane anesthesia.[68]

During normal quiet breathing, expiration is passively effected by the recoil characteristics of the lung. Expiratory pressures up to 10 cmH$_2$O do not bring abdominal muscles into play. Instead, lung volume is increased until increased lung recoil pressure offsets the

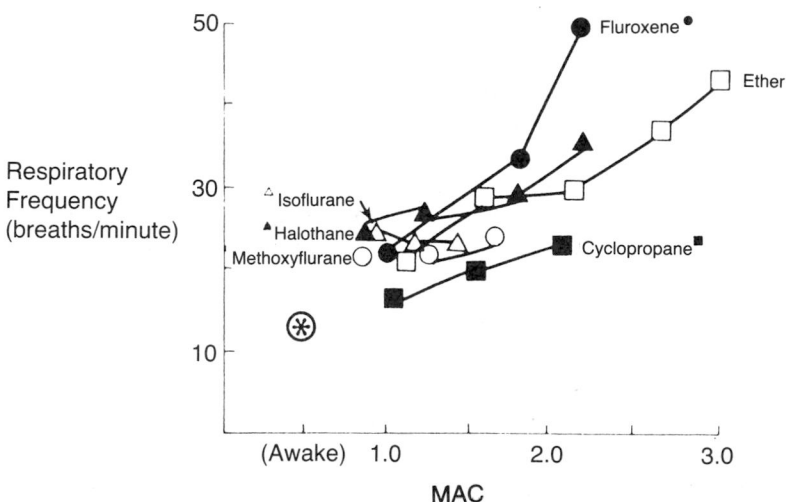

Fig. 5-7. Comparison of mean changes in respiratory frequency at multiples of MAC obtained in patients anesthetized with one of five different anesthetics. With all anesthetics, respiratory frequency increases as anesthesia is deepened. (From Hickey and Severinghaus,[140] with permission.)

elevation of expiratory resistance. In anesthetized patients[69] the ventilatory response to expiratory resistance is diminished more than that to inspiratory resistance. This is curious in light of the study by Freund et al.[70] demonstrating that the onset of anesthesia immediately produced activity of abdominal muscles during expiration (i.e., active muscular as well as passive lung recoil forces acted during the expiratory phase of ventilation).

Pietak et al.[71] found that patients with chronic obstructive lung disease who did *not* retain carbon dioxide while awake hypoventilated to a greater degree than normal patients under halothane anesthesia. The resting $PaCO_2$ was directly proportional to the severity of the obstruction (Fig. 5-8). Thus, patients with obstructive airway disease may have ventilatory responses obtunded to a greater degree by anesthesia than do patients with normal pulmonary function. These data clearly demonstrate the requirements for both close monitoring of alveolar ventilation and the use of mechanical ventilation in these patients.

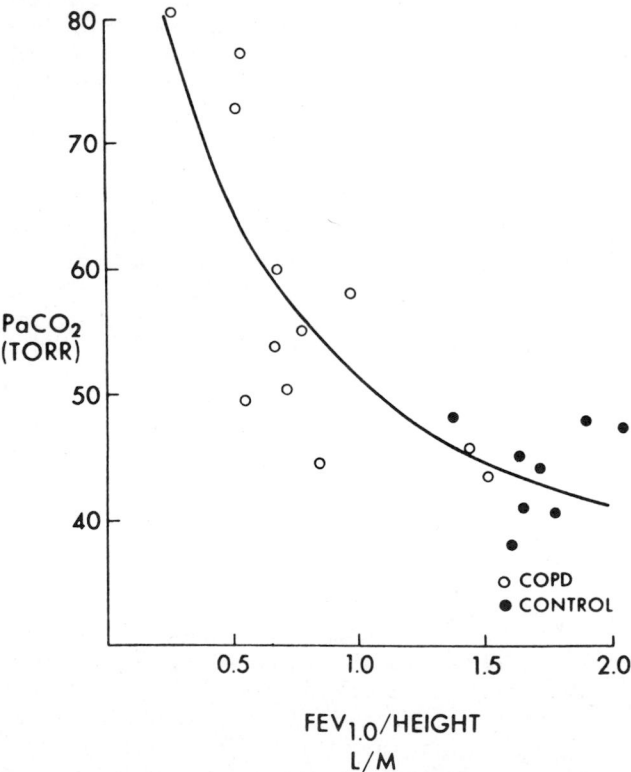

Fig. 5-8. Comparison of $PaCO_2$ during anesthesia during spontaneous ventilation relative to preoperative $FEV_{1.0}$. The chronic obstructive pulmonary disease (COPD) patients did not exhibit carbon dioxide retention before anesthesia, yet the degree of alveolar hypoventilation is much greater in the more severely obstructed patients. (From Pietak et al.,[71] with permission.)

Effects of Anesthetics on Ventilatory Response to Chemical Stimuli

Depression of ventilatory drive by anesthetics has been quantitated utilizing the physiologic principles of chemoreceptor function. These tests have usually involved varying of a chemical stimulus (arterial carbon dioxide or oxygen tension), measuring the ventilatory response to this variation, and then repeating this test after the administration of an anesthetic drug. The variation between the predrug and postdrug responses gives a measure of the depressant potential of the agent in question. Respiratory drive can thus be characterized by the ventilatory responsiveness to $PaCO_2$ (resting $PaCO_2$, apneic threshold, and ventilatory responses to an increase in CO_2 tension) or to a decrease in PaO_2. To obtain a more complete discussion of the basic elements of chemical ventilatory control, the reader is referred to other reviews.[72]

Responses to Carbon Dioxide

Changes in ventilation secondary to alterations in $PaCO_2$ are believed to be mediated chiefly via chemoreceptors located in the medulla. Patients whose peripheral chemoreceptor has been denervated by endarterectomy demonstrate approximately 85 percent of the increase in ventilation secondary to inhaled carbon dioxide observed prior to carotid body denervation.

Resting $PaCO_2$. The resting $PaCO_2$ is probably the most common index of ventilatory drive used clinically. Variation from the long-established normal value of 40 mmHg is interpreted as an indication of either interference with ventilatory drive or severe compromise of the mechanics of breathing. Indeed, elevation of the $PaCO_2$ is often used to define the presence of ventilatory failure. The effects of various concentrations of inhaled anesthetics on $PaCO_2$ are demonstrated in Figure 5-9.[73] Different anesthetics obviously depress resting ventilation to a different degree, with diethyl ether being the least depressant and halothane being the most depressant. Other investigators examining the effect of enflurane (Ethrane) on $PaCO_2$ demonstrated a $PaCO_2$ of over 60 mmHg at 1.0 MAC enflurane.[73] An explanation of the difference in elevation of $PaCO_2$ between diethyl ether and other inhaled anesthetics is lacking. The effect of surgical stimulation on ventilation in anesthetized patients has been noted by many clinical anesthesiologists and was documented for the anesthetic isoflurane by Eger et al.[74] (Fig. 5-10). At various multiples of MAC, these investigators demonstrated that the stimulation of surgical incision brought about a decrease in resting $PaCO_2$ of as much as 10 mmHg. The duration of anesthesia also plays a role in the level of ventilation. For both halothane and enflurane, the resting $PaCO_2$ after 6 hours of anesthesia was less than that measured after induction or after 3 hours of anesthesia.[75] $PaCO_2$ de-

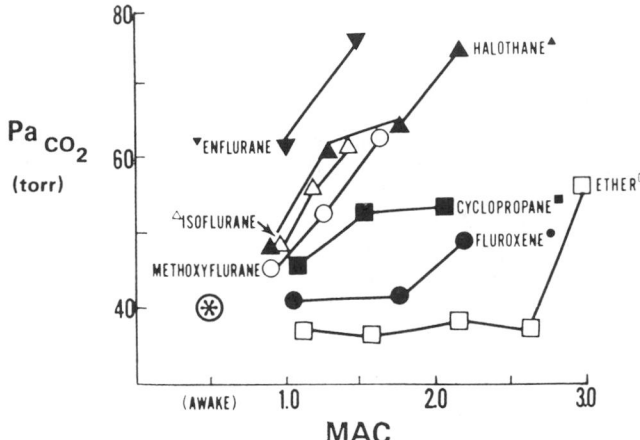

Fig. 5-9. Comparison of mean $PaCO_2$ values in patients anesthetized with one of seven different drugs. Patients were resting, spontaneously ventilating, and unstimulated. Enflurane elevated $PaCO_2$ to the greatest degree at equipotent doses of anesthetic, while ether produced the least change in alveolar ventilation. (From Hickey and Severinghaus,[140] with permission.)

creased from 63 mmHg to 53 mmHg over 6 hours of enflurane anesthesia. The reason for this apparent recovery of ventilatory drive is not clear.

Apneic Thresholds. Apneic threshold is defined as the highest arterial or alveolar PCO_2 at which a subject will remain apneic. It is not usually possible to demonstrate

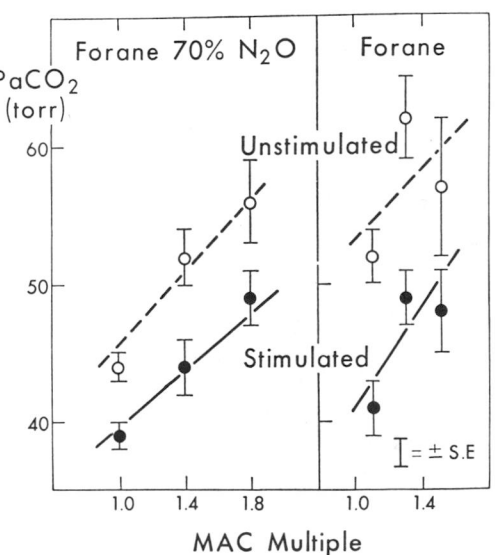

Fig. 5-10. The effect of surgical stimulation on the ventilatory depression of inhalational anesthesia with both nitrous oxide and Forane (isoflurane) or Forane alone. Surgical stimulation increased alveolar ventilation and decreased $PaCO_2$ at all depths of anesthesia examined. (From Eger et al.,[74] with permission.)

an apneic threshold in a conscious, unmedicated subject, who hyperventilates presumably because of stimuli from the cerebrum. However, one study reported apneic thresholds in awake humans approximately 5 mmHg below resting $PaCO_2$. A study by Hickey et al.[76] on the effects of ether, halothane, and isoflurane on apneic thresholds in humans demonstrated a similar relationship between apneic threshold and resting $PaCO_2$ for all three anesthetics and, remarkably enough, for various concentrations of the same anesthetics (Fig. 5-11). The difference between resting $PaCO_2$ and apneic threshold bore no relationship to the slope of carbon dioxide response curves or to the absolute level of resting $PaCO_2$. This phenomenon suggests that assisted ventilation under the influence of anesthetics is of little use in lowering $PaCO_2$. The effectiveness would be limited to a change of approximately 5 mmHg. Ventilation that lowered $PaCO_2$ below the apneic threshold would then in fact become controlled ventilation rather than assisted ventilation. Another clinically important aspect of this observation is in the reestablishment of spontaneous ventilation in the mechanically hyperventilated patient. On cessation of mechanical ventilation, carbon dioxide stores in the body must accumulate to raise the $PaCO_2$ level in the blood to the apneic threshold. The deeper the level of anesthesia, the longer the period of apnea necessary before the patient will commence spontaneous ventilation. An alternative method of management might be to decrease the anesthetic concentration by continuing mechanical ventilation with the anesthetic gases turned off. This maneuver will lower apneic threshold toward the patient's level of $PaCO_2$, thus diminishing the time of apnea required to initiate spontaneous ventilation.

Carbon Dioxide Response Curves. Measuring the minute ventilation in response to varying levels of $PaCO_2$ is a common method of quantitating the effects of drugs on ventilatory drive. In the presence of a high inspired concentration of oxygen, $PaCO_2$ is elevated by the investigator increasing concentrations of inspired carbon dioxide inhaled by the subject. This relationship of $\dot{V}E$ to $PaCO_2$ may be obtained either by the steady state technique, in which $PaCO_2$ is elevated and maintained at various constant levels for approximately 10 minutes, or by the rebreathing method of Read,[77] in which a subject rebreathes from a 5-L bag filled with 7 percent carbon dioxide in oxygen. In normal humans, inspiration of carbon dioxide increases minute ventilation approximately 3 L/min/mmHg $PaCO_2$, demonstrating a high gain from a central chemoreceptor in response to variations in $PaCO_2$. Thus, the slope of the plot is an index of ventilatory drive in response to carbon dioxide stimulus.

All inhaled anesthetics generally depress the carbon dioxide response curve at anesthetic levels (Fig. 5-12).[63] The degree of ventilatory depression varies both with the anesthetic and with the expired anesthetic concen-

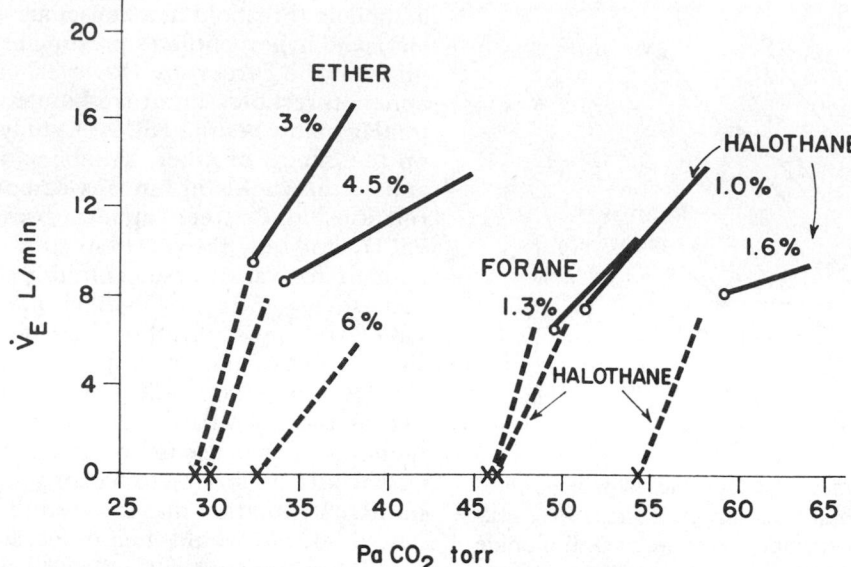

Fig. 5-11. Ventilatory responses to increased carbon dioxide and apneic thresholds during ether, Forane (isoflurane), and halothane anesthesia in patients. Apneic threshold in this study appeared to have a relative fixed relationship to resting $PaCO_2$. With an increase in ventilatory depression at increasing depths of anesthesia, resting $PaCO_2$ and apneic threshold increase approximately the same amount. (From Hickey et al.,[76] with permission.)

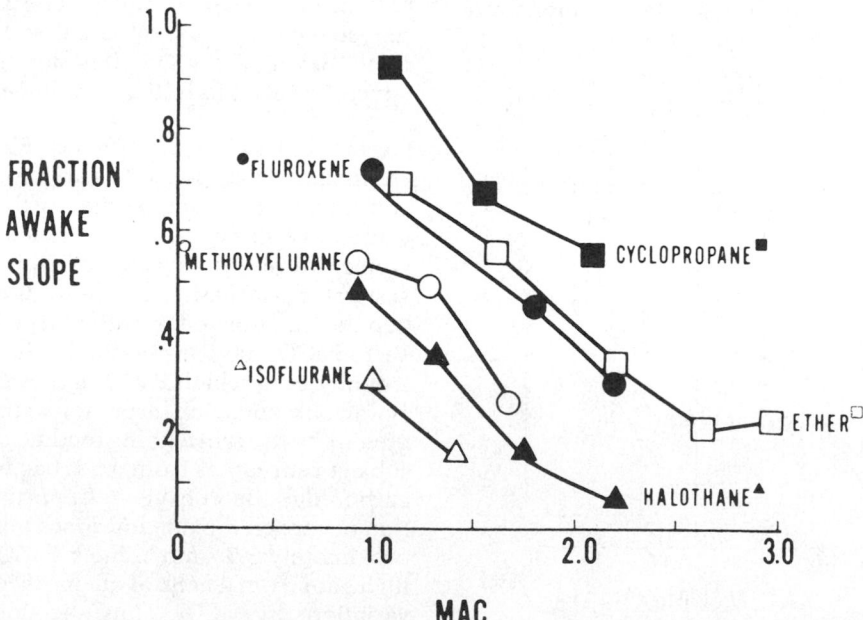

Fig. 5-12. Comparison of mean slopes of ventilatory response to inhaled carbon dioxide at multiples of MAC in an anesthetized patient. Values on the ordinate are expressed as a fraction of the awake slope. In this study, isoflurane depressed the ventilatory response to carbon dioxide to the greatest degree and cyclopropane was the least depressant. In all cases, increasing the depth of anesthesia diminished the ventilatory response to inhaled carbon dioxide. (From Hickey and Severinghaus,[140] with permission.)

tration. Ether diminished the ventilatory response to inhaled carbon dioxide at anesthetic depths at which $PaCO_2$ is maintained at normal levels. Although sedating concentrations of halothane and enflurane have little effect on carbon dioxide response slopes, 1 MAC halothane is a profound depressant of this measurement. Indeed, at levels of 2.5 MAC or more, no increase in ventilation to altered inspired carbon dioxide is observed. Isoflurane produces a similar degree of depression.[78] The slope of the ventilatory response curve during halothane anesthesia (like the resting $PaCO_2$) returns toward normal after 6 hours of anesthesia, although ventilatory responsiveness to carbon dioxide is still profoundly depressed.[75] In contrast to halothane, enflurane, and isoflurane, two other potent inhaled anesthetics, cyclopropane and methoxyflurane, produce much more modest depression. Nitrous oxide, a relatively weak inhaled anesthetic, did not depress the ventilatory response to carbon dioxide at concentrations of 50 percent. Studies by Hornbein et al.[79] showed that combined doses of nitrous oxide and halothane depressed ventilation less than an equipotent (same MAC) dose of halothane alone. It is somewhat surprising that in the only study performed at anesthetic concentrations of nitrous oxide (which took place under hyperbaric conditions), 1.5 MAC concentrations of nitrous oxide proved to be a potent respiratory depressant, which lowered the carbon dioxide response slope to 15 percent of that of the control.[80]

Depression of ventilatory responsiveness to inhaled carbon dioxide has great clinical relevance. Accumulation of carbon dioxide and the ensuing arterial and tissue acidosis may cause dysfunction in several organs, including the heart, where this condition may cause potentially dangerous cardiac arrhythmias. The attenuation of the normal ventilatory responses to elevated $PaCO_2$ (tachypnea, increased tidal volume) makes clinical diagnosis of hypercarbia difficult and necessitates the measurement of either arterial, alveolar, or end-tidal CO_2 tensions. During anesthesia, the ventilatory system will be less likely to compensate for carbon dioxide elevations secondary to rebreathing of carbon dioxide from malfunctioning anesthetic circuits or from increased metabolic production of carbon dioxide.

In their study on the effect of anesthesia on patients with chronic obstructive lung disease, Pietak et al.[71] clearly showed the decreased ability of these patients to respond to increased $PaCO_2$ (Fig. 5-13). This demonstrates the requirement for strict monitoring of arterial blood gases in these patients.

Ventilatory Responses to Hypoxemia

Increased ventilation in response to progressively lowered $PaCO_2$ is mediated entirely by the peripheral chemoreceptors. The hyperbolic response curve thus obtained rises most sharply at PaO_2 of approximately 40 mmHg. Various indices have been used to quantitate

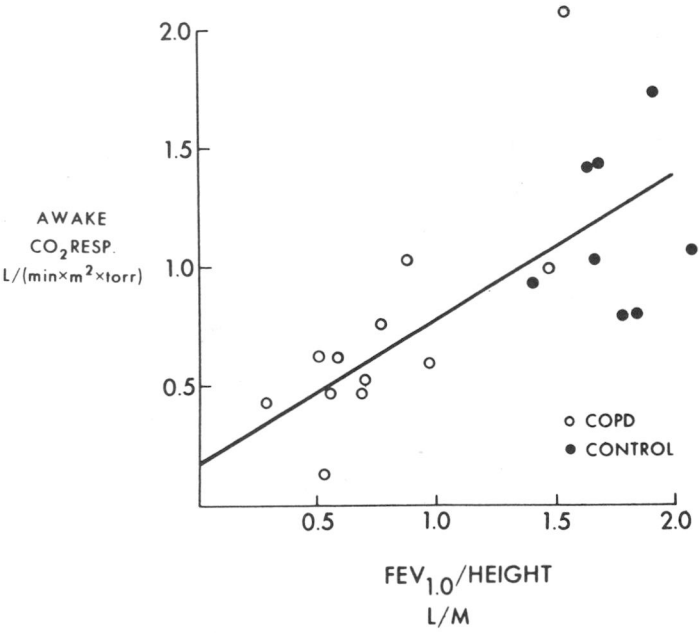

Fig. 5-13. Carbon dioxide response related to $FEV_{1.0}$ in awake patients breathing oxygen. Patients with chronic obstructive pulmonary disease (COPD) exhibit a diminished increase in ventilation to increases in inhaled carbon dioxide. The presence of airway obstruction makes the interpretation of "decreased ventilatory drive" difficult. (From Pietak et al.,[71] with permission.)

this response. A parameter "A" describes the curvature of the hyperbola; a low value of A is consistent with a flattened or lesser ventilatory response to progressive hypoxemia.

For some time the opinion was held that while the ventilatory responses to hypercarbia and acidosis were profoundly affected by anesthetics, the peripheral chemoreceptors were spared and the ventilatory response to hypoxemia was preserved. It is now evident from the results of studies performed during the 1970s that this belief is erroneous. Weiskopf and colleagues[81] studied the ventilatory response to hypoxia in three dogs during halothane anesthesia (1.1 percent end-tidal halothane concentration) and at different levels of $PaCO_2$. Significant depression of ventilatory responsiveness to hy-

poxia was observed at 1 MAC levels of halothane. In addition, the usual synergistic effect of hypoxia and hypercarbia on ventilation was profoundly attenuated. This work has subsequently been confirmed in dogs by Hirshman et al.,[82] who extended the study to demonstrate similar ventilatory depression by both enflurane and isoflurane. Furthermore, a dose-related attenuation of the hypoxic response was demonstrated. In an important study, Knill and Gelb[83] showed a similar response in humans to halothane anesthesia; however, the peripheral chemoreceptor function in humans was even more sensitive to the effects of anesthetics than in the dog. At 1.1 MAC halothane, the ventilatory response to hypoxemia was completely absent (Fig. 5-14). Furthermore, at very low anesthetic concentrations (0.1

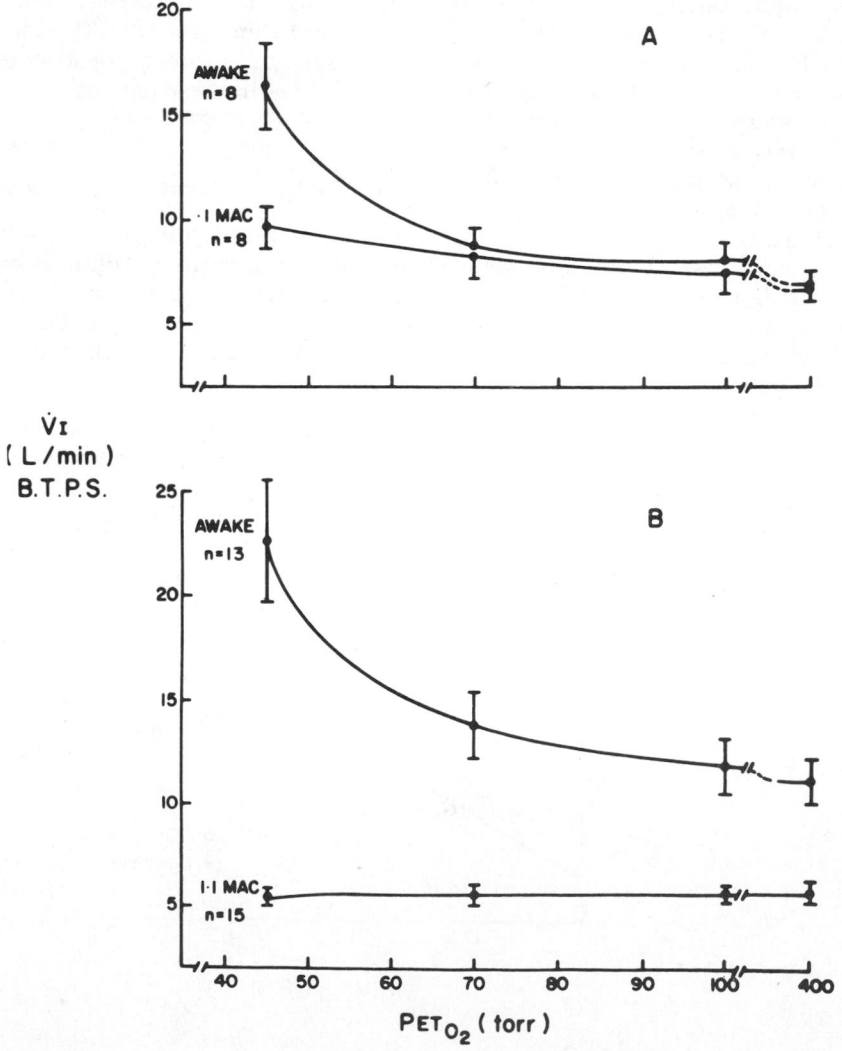

Fig. 5-14. Ventilatory response to hypoxia in human volunteers and patients anesthetized with halothane **(A)** The ventilatory increase to hypoxia is severely attenuated at levels of only 0.1 MAC halothane and **(B)** completely absent in this experiment at the 1.1 MAC halothane anesthesia. This represents a more significant depression of this measure of ventilatory drive during inhalation of anesthetics than that previously demonstrated in dogs. (From Knill and Gelb,[83] with permission.)

MAC halothane) ventilatory responsiveness was severely attenuated. At the same sedative levels of halothane, no change was seen in the carbon dioxide response curve. This profound depression of hypoxic responsiveness is clinically very important in that it suggests that patients will manifest a diminished ventilatory response to hypoxemia for some time after cessation of an anesthetic and at the arterial concentrations of halothane one would expect in a patient in the recovery room. The implications of this in patients who depend to some degree on a hypoxic drive to set their level of ventilation is obvious. The impaired function of the peripheral chemoreceptor in the presence of low levels of halothane was also demonstrated by a marked reduction in ventilatory responsiveness to doxapram or metabolic acidosis, both of which normally have a significant stimulatory effect on the peripheral chemoreceptor. Enflurane,[84] nitrous oxide,[85] and isoflurane have also been shown to depress hypoxic responsiveness in humans at subanesthetic concentrations.

These studies demonstrate that, in contrast to previous beliefs, the peripheral chemoreceptor is remarkably sensitive to the depressant effects of inhaled anesthetics as well as to many intravenous anesthetics, such as morphine and thiopental. Is hypoxic ventilatory response diminished by depression of chemoreceptor traffic or by the effect of anesthetics on the brain stem? An earlier study[86] suggested the former mechanism. This has been supported by two recent reports. Davies et al.[87] showed that 0.5 to 1.0 percent halothane administered to decerebrate cats reduced nerve discharge in the carotid sinus nerve when the peripheral chemoreceptor was stimulated by a variety of methods. Knill et al.[88] examined the ventilatory response to subanesthetic concentrations of halothane in normal volunteers breathing an isocapnic hypoxic gas mixture. Ventilatory response to hypoxia was depressed within 30 seconds of inhalation. They concluded that the peripheral chemoreceptors had to be the site of depression since pharmacokinetic calculations appeared to preclude a buildup of halothane in the brain within 30 seconds. These studies seem to indicate that anesthetics in subanesthetic doses depress the function of the carotid bodies by depressing their chemoreceptor response to stimuli such as hypoxia.

Greater concentrations of anesthetic depress brain stem function as well. It is clear that the tachypnea and increased ventilation seen with hypoxia under normal conditions would be absent or severely decreased during even light levels of anesthesia. Lack of these clinical signs mandates the frequent assessment of arterial oxygen tensions. Patients with chronic respiratory failure in whom the level of PaO_2 may represent an important determinant of minute ventilation may be drastically affected by even low doses of inhaled anesthetics. Thus, the ability of these patients to maintain adequate ventilation while breathing spontaneously may be severely impaired.

CARDIOVASCULAR PHARMACOLOGY OF INHALED ANESTHETICS

The output of the heart provides adequate perfussion of the body's organs through a wide range of perturbations and variations in requirements. For instance, a drop in arterial blood pressure through hemorrhage results in a reflex increase in cardiac output (through an increase in heart rate and contractile performance) such that perfusion in vital organs is maintained. This homeostasis in perfusion involves vascular reactivity, cardiac function (and the ability to vary it), and the reflexes that detect alterations and initiate adjustments in the cardiovascular system. Anesthetics may interfere in a dose-related way with the responsiveness of the cardiovascular system at nearly all sites in this interrelated system. In this portion of the chapter we discuss the mechanisms by which inhaled anesthetics act on myocardiac contractility, on vascular smooth muscle, and on the baroreceptor reflex that is so intimately involved in maintenance of arterial blood pressure. Other portions of this text describe the physiologic effects of these drugs on cardiovascular physiology in normal and diseased hearts.

Effect of Inhaled Anesthetics on Circulation

The overall impact of inhaled anesthetic is a decrease in mean arterial pressure (MAP). Halothane,[89] isoflurane,[90] and enflurane[91] depress MAP by 25% at 1 MAC in the isovolemic normal human. Halothane[89] and enflurane[90] reduce cardiac output, but isoflurane has little effect on output of the heart. Systemic vascular resistance is little changed by halothane, decreased by enflurane, and profoundly diminished by isoflurane. If the subject's arterial PCO_2 is allowed to rise under anesthesia, as in spontaneous ventilation, PVR is diminished even more, but cardiac output and MAP are enhanced. Thus, the overall effect of the potent inhaled anesthetics is a decrease in cardiac output (enflurane > halothane >> isoflurane) and a decrease in systemic vascular resistance (isoflurane > enflurane > halothane), leading to a drop in arterial pressure. Nitrous oxide at 1.5 MAC levels produces little change in any of the parameters.[92] Its direct effect is one of myocardial depression; however, indirectly it promotes an increase in sympathetic activity that diminished its depressant effect. Thus, nitrous oxide added to isoflurane increases PVR and MAP.[93]

Direct Effects of Inhaled Anesthetics on Contraction of Cardiac Muscle

The mechanics of cardiac muscle can be expressed as the amount of muscle shortening that occurs at various levels of preload (isotonic contraction) or as the isometric twitch force developed at a specified muscle length (isometric contraction). The parameters of an

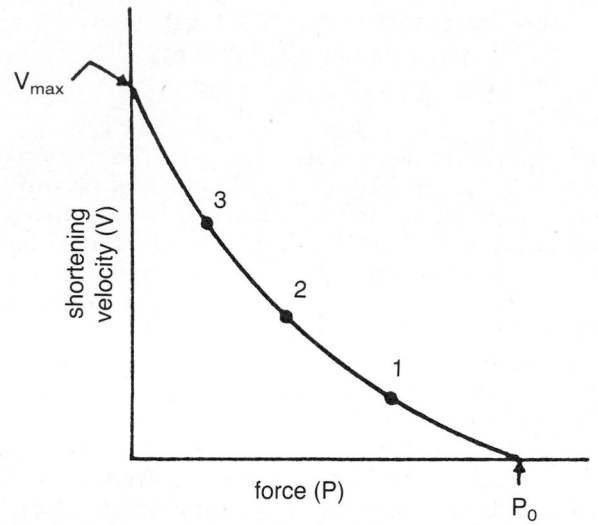

Fig. 5-15. Force-velocity relationship. *1, 2,* and *3* represent measured velocity at specific preload of muscle fiber. The curve is extrapolated to the force where zero shortening occurs (P_o = isometric twitch force). Vmax is the extrapolated theoretical maximum shortening velocity where preload is zero. (From Katz,[139] with permission.)

isometric twitch (Fig. 5-15) that can be analyzed are the peak developed force (F_o), maximum rate of rise ($+dF/dt$ max.) or fall ($-dF/dt$ max.) of the developed force, and time to the peak developed force (TPF). Inhaled anesthetics depress reversibly, and in a dose-dependent

manner, the F_o and $+dF/dt$ max. at steady state.[94] At 1 MAC, halothane decreases F_o and $+dF/dt$ max. to about 50 percent of control values. Measuring isotonic and isometric contraction in isolated papillary muscle of the ferret, the duration of the contraction has been shown to be decreased by inhaled anesthetics.[95] The order of potency for depression of the above parameters is enflurane > halothane > isoflurane >>> nitrous oxide.

Thus, inhaled anesthetics are direct and potent depressants of myocardial contraction. The steps by which a depolarization of excitable muscle membrane ultimately leads to a contraction of cardiac muscle must be understood before the interaction of the inhaled anesthetics can be appreciated.

Mechanism of Cardiac Contraction

A cardiac muscle cell is surrounded by a membrane called the *sarcolemma* or *plasma membrane*, and invaginations of the sarcolemma are called *transverse tubules* (T tubules) (Fig. 5-16). The intracellular membrane system is called the *sarcoplasmic reticulum* (SR) and can be isolated by differential centrifugation. The *isolated SR* consists of terminal cisternae (links between T tubule and sarcotubular network, mostly in the heavy fraction of isolated SR) and the sarcotubular network (longitudinal SR, mostly in the light fraction of isolated SR). The *contractile proteins* consist of myosin (in the thick filament) and actin (in thick and thin filaments) and the regulatory proteins (containing troponin and tropomyosin). *Troponin* is composed of three subunits: troponin C, troponin T, and troponin I.

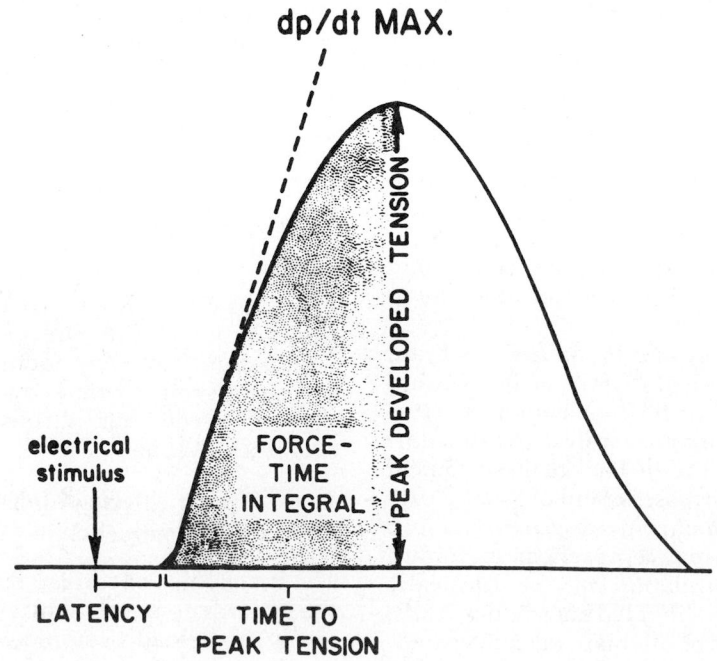

Fig. 5-16. Schematic illustration of typical muscle twitch recorded under isometric conditions. (From Brown and Crout,[94] with permission.)

When the muscle membrane is depolarized to threshold, an action potential is generated. The action potential travels through the sarcolemma and the T tubule, triggering release of calcium from the terminal cisternae of the SR and calcium influx through calcium channels in the sarcolemma, both resulting in increased free calcium in the cytoplasm (Table 5-3). The increased free calcium binds to troponin, resulting in conformational changes, and causes the interaction of myosin and actin. This interaction of the contractile proteins (cross-bridge interaction) can be demonstrated by measuring force development (isometric contraction) or muscle shortening (isotonic contraction). It is by measurement of this force that the depressant effects of inhaled anesthetics have been demonstrated.

Mechanisms of Cardiac Depression by Inhaled Anesthetics

Thus, inhaled anesthetics could depress contraction by (a) Decreasing free calcium concentration by (1) interfering with Ca^{++} movement through sarcolemma or by (2) decreasing availability or release of Ca^{++} from sarcoplasmic reticulum, and/or by (b) altering the sensitivity of regulatory and contractile proteins to available Ca^{++}. Relatively new experimental techniques have provided definitive information regarding the effects of the inhaled anesthetics on function.

Free Calcium Concentration

The intracellular free calcium concentration can be measured with Ca^{++} indicators such as bioluminescent proteins (e.g., aequorin)[96] or newly synthesized Ca^{++}-sensitive fluorescent dyes (e.g., fura-2).[97] Under physiologic conditions, aequorin generates light in the presence of calcium ions. The light intensity rises steeply as a function of calcium ion concentration between about 0.1 μM and 0.1 mM. The synthetic Ca^{++} indicators can be loaded into the muscle cells, and binding of the indicator by increased free calcium is indicated by an excitatory response to light with emission of fluorescent light of a longer wavelength. The time course of the light emission from aequorin or dyes can be translated into calcium concentration (calcium transient).

Using aequorin,[98] investigators have assessed simultaneously the effects of inhaled anesthetics on free calcium concentration and muscle contraction in isolated papillary muscle. They have found that the order of potency at equal MAC levels is halothane = enflurane > isoflurane in decreasing both isometric force and the associated calcium transient (Fig. 5-17). At high isoflurane concentration, no further decrease in calcium transient occurs[99] (Fig. 5-18). Thus, it is clear that a decrease in free calcium concentration by inhaled anesthetics is one cause of myocardial depression. The mechanism(s) of this decreased intracellular free calcium concentration could involve decreases in calcium influx through sarcolemma or calcium release from the SR during contraction.

Calcium Influx Through Sarcolemma. It is clear that calcium influx through the sarcolemma plays an important role in myocardial contraction because of the requirement for external calcium for myocardial contraction. One of the most important calcium influx pathways is through calcium channels in the sarcolemma. The direct measurement of calcium current through calcium channels (slow calcium inward current) by the patch clamp method has become feasible recently in isolated cardiac myocytes. Bosnjak and associates[100] have recently shown in canine myocytes that halothane, enflurane, and isoflurane all decrease the slow calcium inward current to a similar degree. Using an indirect method of measurement, a reduction of the maximal rate of rise of slow action potential in partially depolarized muscle by the inhaled anesthetics has also been observed. However, this effect on calcium channels differs in the order of potency in these three anesthetics.[100-102] Thus, there are some discrepancies that need to be resolved. It is clear, however, that decreased calcium inward current caused by the inhaled anesthetics would directly decrease the force of muscle contraction. No report is available as to the effects of the anesthetics on calcium influx through sarcolemma *other* than through calcium channels. The order of potency of the inhaled anesthetics in depressing myocardial contraction parallels that of changes in free calcium concentration but does not correspond to depression in slow calcium inward current, indicating that mechanisms other than calcium influx through muscle membrane play a role in anesthetic-induced myocardial depression.

TABLE 5-3. Structural and Functional Basis for Muscle Contractile Process

Structure	Function
Sarcolemma	Propagation of action potential; control of Ca^{++} fluxes across the sarcolemma
Transverse tubular system	Transmission of action potential to interior of cell; control Ca^{++} fluxes
Sarcoplasmic reticulum	Release of Ca^{++} to, and removal of Ca^{++} from, troponin C; storage of Ca^{++}
Terminal cisternae	Ca^{++} release from specific Ca^{++} release channels is initiated at the start of systole
Sarcotubular network	Relaxation site at which Ca^{++} is accumulated to terminate systole
Troponin C	Ca^{++} receptor of the contractile proteins
Actomyosin	Cross-bridge cycling for generation of force or shortening

(Modified from Katz,[139] with permission.)

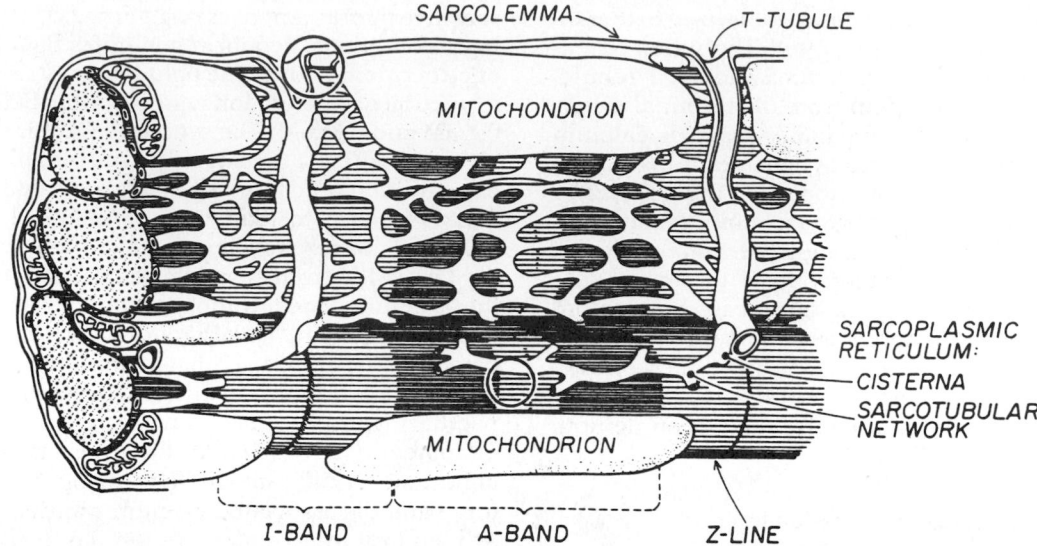

Fig. 5-17. Ultrastructure of the working myocardial cell. Contractile proteins are arranged in a regular array of thick and thin filaments (seen in cross-section at the left). The A band represents the region of the sarcomere occupied by the thick filaments into which thin filaments extend from either side. The I band is the region of the sarcomere occupied only by the thin filaments; these extend toward the center of the sarcomere from the Z lines, which bisect each I band. The sarcoplasmic reticulum, a membrane network that surrounds the contractile proteins, consists of the sarcotubular network at the center of the sarcomere and the cisternae, which abut on the T tubules and the sarcolemma. The transverse tubular system (T tubule) is lined by a membrane that extends from the sarcolemma and carries the extracellular space into the myocardial cell. Mitochondria are shown in the central sarcomere and in cross-section at the left side of the figure. (From Katz,[141] with permission.)

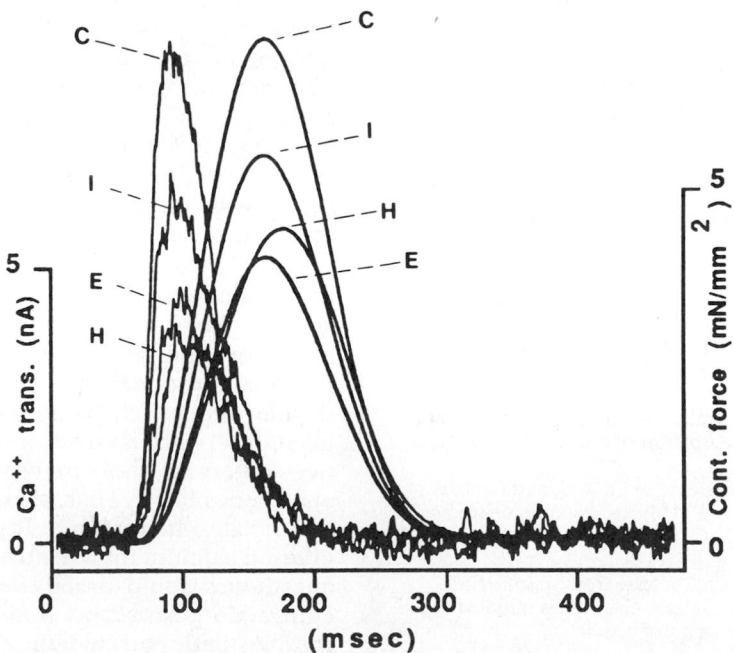

Fig. 5-18. Effects of halothane (H), enflurane (E), and isoflurane (I) on Ca^{++} transient and isometric force in isolated papillary muscle of the guinea pig. C, control in the absence of anesthetics. Ca^{++} transients (Ca^{++} trans.) (curves on the left side of the diagram) represent continuous measurement of free calcium concentration during the course of a twitch (Cont. force) shown on the right side of the diagram. The degree of twitch depression by the anesthetic correlates with the depression of free calcium in the cytoplasm. (From Bosnjak et al.,[99] with permission.)

Alterations of Cytoplasmic Ca^{++} by Interference of Ca^{++} Uptake Release from Sarcoplasmic Reticulum. Measurement of intracellular events has been made possible by development of a *skinned fibers* preparation. Skinned fibers refer to muscle fiber bundle with nonfunctioning sarcolemma created either by destroying the sarcolemma with detergents or by homogenization. This preparation, with intact myofibers, becomes permeable to ions and large molecules; thus, intracellular sites of muscle contraction can be studied. Depolarization of the sarcolemma is no longer required for muscle contraction. The advantages of the skinned fibers preparation are that the function of a specific organelle at intracellular sites can be studied and, at the same time, the physiologic measure force can be monitored. The intracellular mechanisms of action of the contractile process include Ca^{++} uptake and release from the SR and Ca^{++} activation of the contractile proteins.

In skinned fibers, different bathing solutions can be used to load Ca^{++} into the SR or to release Ca^{++} from the SR using a Ca^{++}-releasing agent (such as caffeine) to activate the myofibers and cause a tension transient.[103]

Using a caffeine-induced tension transient in skinned fibers from rabbit papillary muscle, Su and associates[103-105] have shown that the inhaled anesthetics decrease Ca^{++} accumulation and enhance Ca^{++} release from the SR in the following order of potency: halothane = enflurane $\gg$ isoflurane at equal MAC values. Decreased Ca^{++} accumulation in the SR in the skinned fibers is due to enhanced Ca^{++} release from the SR (increased SR membrane permeability to Ca^{++}) and/or due to decreased SR adenosine triphosphatase (ATPase) activity during loading, resulting in less SR Ca^{++} accumulation.

In isolated SR vesicles[106,107] and in isolated myocytes,[108] decreased calcium accumulation in the SR secondary to inhaled anesthetics has been demonstrated. Furthermore, at Ca^{++} concentrations comparable to those utilized in studies of skinned fibers, the isolated SR ATPase activity is also inhibited by halothane.[109] This decreased Ca^{++} accumulation in the SR could be the underlying mechanisms for myocardial depression, that is, it is due to less Ca^{++} available for subsequent contraction. The order of potency in causing Ca^{++} release from the SR and decreasing Ca^{++} accumulation in the SR is halothane = enflurane $>$ isoflurane. The degree of decreased Ca^{++} accumulation by halothane and enflurane is comparable to that depression observed in studies of isometric tension depression developed in isolated intact papillary muscle preparations.[94] Thus, anesthetic-induced Ca^{++} release from the SR may be the mechanism underlying the initial transient increase in twitch tension.[110] The subsequent decreased SR Ca^{++} accumulation may relate to the steady state twitch tension depression observed in isolated intact cardiac muscle.

Indirect approaches in isolated cardiac muscle also support the evidence accrued in the skinned fiber preparation. Measuring potentiated-state contraction as an index of the SR function in isolated cardiac muscle, Luk et al.[111] and DeTraglia[112] have shown that isoflurane is much less potent than halothane and enflurane in depressing the potentiated-state strength.

Influence of the Inhaled Anesthetics on Ca^{++} Activation of Contractile Proteins

To define the effect of contractile proteins, skinned fibers are studied in a bathing medium similar to intracellular fluid, but one in which the free Ca^{++} concentration is controlled and maintained constant by use of EGTA, a calcium buffer.

The Ca^{++}-activated force development of myofibers can be measured and is a direct function of free calcium concentration (Fig. 5-18). The Ca^{++}-force relationship can be expressed as submaximum and maximum force development. The submaximum force is sensitive to free Ca^{++} concentration, which can be interpreted as Ca^{++} binding to regulatory proteins, whereas the maximum force development relates to the strength or number of cross-bridge interactions. Studying rabbit papillary muscle, Su and associates[104,105,113] have shown that inhaled anesthetics cause a small amount of inhibition of the submaximum as well as the maximum Ca^{++}-activated tension development contractile proteins in a dose-dependent manner. There is also no difference in amounts of the depression of the maximum Ca^{++}-activated tension caused by halothane between newborn and adult rabbit myocardium.[114] The submaximum Ca^{++}-activated tension development is decreased by halothane to a greater degree in the adult myocardium than in newborn myocardium.

Biochemical methods, such as measuring myosin ATPase activity, can be used as an indication of muscle contraction since ATP provides energy for muscle contraction. These biochemical preparations include isolated actomyosin and myofibrils. Reports of small amount of inhibition of actomyosin ATPase activity of dog heart by halothane[115] are consistent with observed effects of halothane on maximum Ca^{++}-activated force development in skinned myocardial fibers of the rabbit. In isolated intact rabbit papillary muscle, the dynamic stiffness of Ca^{++} contractured muscle is decreased by all of the potent inhaled anesthetics,[116] suggesting a decreased number of cross-bridge interactions. This is again consistent with the finding of decreased maximum Ca^{++}-activated force development in the skinned fibers exposed to the same anesthetics. The myofibrillar ATPase activity of cat myocardium is inhibited by halothane at 1 MAC,[117] again agreeing with the effects of halothane on submaximum Ca^{++}-activated force development in skinned rabbit myocardium.[114]

In summary, from studies of the effects of inhaled anesthetics on the cellular mechanisms of contraction, it is clear that multiple steps are affected: decreases in calcium inward current, transient increases in calcium release from the SR, decreases in calcium accumulation thus affecting the availability of calcium released from Sr for subsequent contraction, decreases in calcium sensitivity of the contractile proteins and numbers of cross-bridge interactions. The order of potency in most of these steps is halothane > enflurane > isoflurane >> nitrous oxide.[118] Discrepancies exist mainly in the absolute rather than relative potency of the inhaled anesthetics.

Effect of Inhaled Anesthetics on Vascular Smooth Muscle

Hypotension induced by the inhaled anesthetics is in part due to decreases in peripheral vascular resistance. Direct effects of anesthetics on the vascular system can be studied in isolated vascular tissues analogous to those described for cardiac tissues. Study of the mechanisms of anesthetic action on the vasculature has become feasible because of the recent advance in understanding of mechanisms of smooth muscle contraction (for review[119,120]) and the role of endothelium (for review[121]).

In smooth muscle, as in skeletal and cardiac muscle, cytosolic Ca^{++} concentration is the principal regulator of contraction. The actin and myosin interaction develops the force generation in vascular smooth muscle contraction. However, there are at least two major aspects in the contractile process that are unique in smooth muscle: (1) the Ca^{++}-dependent process for initial force development by phosphorylation of myosin light chains resulting in cross-bridge interaction and force generation, and (2) the Ca^{++}-independent process for sustained force development (latch contraction). Briefly, upon depolarization, intracellular free Ca^{++} increases by either Ca^{++} influx through sarcolemma or by Ca^{++} release from the SR. This increase in free Ca^{++} activates protein kinase, which phosphorylates myosin light chains resulting in myosin-actin interaction and force generation. However, the mechanisms of sustained force generation are not clear (for review[119]).

Anesthetic influences on the microvasculature depend on anesthetic concentration and the particular vascular bed involved, especially at low anesthetic concentration. Deep halothane anesthesia, however, produces generalized arteriolar and venular dilatation in several vascular beds.[122]

In isolated rat aortic strips, halothane to a greater degree than isoflurane decreases phenylephrine-induced contraction in a dose-dependent manner.[123] In isolated dog coronary artery,[124] in which contraction was induced by prostaglandin $F_2\alpha$ and serotonin, isoflurane (2.3 percent) caused dose-dependent depression that was endothelium dependent. It was speculated that isoflurane either caused the release of endothelium-derived relaxation factor or facilitated its action on vascular smooth muscle. On the other hand, Muldoon et al.[125] have shown that 2 percent halothane, during contractions evoked by norepinephrine, causes decreases that

are mostly independent of endothelium in isolated canine carotid and rabbit aortic preparations, but increases tension in the canine femoral artery. They also have shown that halothane attenuates acetylcholine-induced relaxation. They speculated that halothane interferes with the synthesis, release, or transport of the endothelium-derived relaxing factor. However, an alternative hypothesis is that halothane causes production of endothelium-derived contracting factor, or has direct effects on the vascular smooth muscle, or both. Unfortunately, only one concentration of the anesthetic has been tested.

In the study of intracellular mechanisms of anesthetic action in detergent-treated (saponin) skinned (sarcolemma disrupted) aortic strips of the rabbit,[124] halothane increased Ca^{++} release from the SR and decreased calcium accumulation in the SR. The maximum Ca^{++}-activated tension development of the contractile proteins was only slightly diminished. Su and Zhang[126] have also shown that halothane causes force development in endothelium-dependent (norepinephrine-acetylcholine) or -independent (sodium nitroprusside) relaxed aortic rings of the rabbit. This evidence leads them to speculate that Ca^{++} release from the SR by halothane is the underlying mechanism for the initial contraction, whereas halothane decreases calcium accumulation in the SR, thus inhibiting KCl-induced tension development. A systematic investigation of the effects of the inhaled anesthetics on various vasculatures and their mechanisms of action is needed. Care should be taken as to the anesthetic concentration, types of vasculatures, endothelium dependence, animal species, and agonists used.

In summary, the effect of the inhaled anesthetics on the vascular system depends on the region of vasculature, experimental protocol (agonists, etc., used), endothelium, and animal species. From the intracellular sites of muscle contraction, halothane has similar mechanisms of action on vascular smooth muscle as well as cardiac muscle; that is, small depression on the contractile proteins, increases in Ca^{++} release from the SR, and decreases in Ca^{++} accumulation in the SR.

Effect of Inhaled Anesthetics on Baroreceptor Function

The baroreceptor reflex that is of interest to anesthesiologists consists of a sensor in the carotid bifurcation (which responds to pulse pressure and slope of systolic pressure rise), a central medullary integrating center that receives signals via the 9th cranial nerve, and output, which includes changes in heart rate, vascular and venous tone, and myocardial contraction. Thus, a drop in blood pressure invokes an increase in heart rate, peripheral vasoconstriction, and an increase in cardiac output, all of which attenuate the drop in blood pressure.

The particular reflex studied in the anesthetized state that involves changes is that of heart rate response. Injections of neosynephrine elevate blood pressure (plotted on the x axis), which quickly results in an increase in heart rate (1/h is plotted on the y axis). The slope of the resulting line is compared with one obtained during the awake state. A decrease in slope is an index of baroreceptor reflex depression.

Halothane,[127] enflurane,[128] and isoflurane[129] all depress the heart rate increase to hypotension. Isoflurane is the least depressive, which may explain the preservation of cardiac output during isoflurane anesthesia despite profound decreases in peripheral vascular resistance.

The mechanism of depression is not clear. The sites involved appear to be multiple. Output of carotid wall stretch receptor is altered by anesthetic-induced changes in wall tension.[130] Evidence exists for depression of central integration and efferent sympathetic and parasympathetic outflow.[131,132] Stimulation of sympathetic efferent nerves is much diminished under halothane anesthesia.[132]

Clinically, appreciation of attenuation of this reflex is most important. Hypovolemia is often countered by peripheral vasoconstriction and heart rate increase. Induction of anesthesia can cause profound decreases in blood pressure by diminishing baroreceptor responses. Furthermore, tachycardia utilized as a clue to the patient's intravascular volume is no longer a reliable clinical sign under inhalational anesthesia.

REFERENCES

1. Paterson JW, Woolcock AJ, Shenfield GM: Bronchodilator drugs. Am Rev Respir Dis 120:1149, 1979
2. Ahlquist RP: A study of the adrenotropic receptors. Am J Physiol 153:586, 1948
3. Shnider WM, Papper EM: Anesthesia for the asthmatic patient. Anesthesiology 22:886, 1961
4. Colgan FJ: Performance of lungs and bronchi during inhalation anesthesia. Anesthesiology 26:778, 1965
5. Klide AM, Aviado DM: Mechanism for the reduction in pulmonary resistance induced by halothane. J Pharmacol Exp Ther 158:28, 1967
6. Fletcher SW, Flacke W, Alper MH: The actions of general anesthetic agents on tracheal smooth muscle. Anesthesiology 29:517, 1969
7. Hickey RF, Graf PD, Nadel JA, et al: The effects of halothane and cyclopropane on total pulmonary resistance in the dog. Anesthesiology 31:334, 1969
8. Coon RL, Kampine JP: Hypocapnic bronchoconstriction and inhalation anesthetics. Anesthesiology 43:635, 1975
9. Patterson RW, Sullivan SF, Malm JR, et al: The effect of halothane on human airway mechanics. Anesthesiology 29:900, 1968
10. Meloche R, Norlander O, Norden I, Herzog P: Effects of carbon dioxide and halothane on compliance and pulmonary resistance during cardiopulmonary bypass. Scand J Thorac Cardiovasc Surg 3:69, 1969
11. Gold WM, Kessler GF, Yu DYC, et al: Pulmonary physiologic abnormalities in experimental asthma in dogs. J Appl Physiol 33:496, 1972
12. Hirshman CA, Bergman NA: Halothane and enflurane protect against bronchospasm in an asthma dog model. Anesth Analg 57:629, 1978
13. Hirshman CA, Edelstein G, Pectz S, et al: Mechanism of action of inhalational anesthesia on airways. Anesthesiology 56:107–111, 1982
14. Hermans JM, Edelstein G, Hanifen JM, et al: Inhalational anesthesia and histamine release during bronchospasm. Anesthesiology 61:69, 1984
15. Shah MV, Hirshman CA: Mode of action of halothane on histamine-induced airway constriction in dogs with reactive airways. Anesthesiology 65:170, 1986
16. Gold MI, Helfrich M: Pulmonary mechanics during general anesthesia. V. Status asthmaticus. Anesthesiology 32:422, 1970
17. Schwartz SH: Treatment of status asthmaticus with halothane. JAMA 251:2688, 1984
18. Sprague DH: Treatment of intraoperative bronchospasm with nebulized isoetharine. Anesthesiology 46:222, 1977
19. Wolfe JD, Tashkin DP, Calvares B, et al: Bronchodilator effects on turbutaline and aminophylline alone and in combination in asthmatic patients. N Engl J Med 298:363, 1978
20. Korenaga S, Tekeda K, Ho Y: Differential effects of halothane on airway nerves and muscle. Anesthesiology 60:309, 1984
21. Aviado DM: Regulation of bronchomotor tone during anesthesia. Anesthesiology 42:68, 1975
22. Bennett DJ, Torda TA, Horton DA, et al: Severe bronchospasm complicating thoracotomy. Arch Surg 101:555, 1970
23. Kingston HGG, Hirshman CA: Perioperative management of the patient with asthma. Anesth Analg 63:844, 1984
24. Price HL, Cooperman LH, Warden JC, et al: Pulmonary hemodynamics during general anesthesia in man. Anesthesiology 30:629, 1969
25. Marshall BE, Cohen PJ, Klingenmaier CH, et al: Some pulmonary and cardiovascular effects of enflurane (Ethrane) anesthesia with varying PaCO$_2$ in man. Br J Anaesth 43:996, 1971
26. Barer GR, Howard P, Shaw JW: Stimulus-response curves for the pulmonary vascular bed to hypoxia and hypercapnia. J Physiol 211:139, 1970
27. Marshall BE, Marshal C, Benumof J, Saidman LJ: Hypoxic pulmonary vasoconstriction in dogs: Effect of lung segment size and oxygen tension. J Appl Physiol 51:1543, 1981
28. Benumof JL, Pirho AF, Johansen I, Trousdale FR: Interaction of P$\bar{v}$O$_2$ with PaO$_2$ on hypoxic pulmonary vasoconstriction. J Appl Physiol 51:871, 1981
29. Domino KB, Wetstein L, Glasser SA, et al: Influence of mixed venous oxygen tension (P$\bar{v}$O$_2$) on blood flow to atelectatic lung. Anesthesiology 59:428, 1983
30. Haas F, Bergofsky EH: Effect of pulmonary vasoconstriction on balance between alveolar ventilation and perfusion. J Appl Physiol 24:491, 1968
31. Colley PS, Chency FW, Jr, Hlastala MP: Ventilation-perfusion and gas exchange effects of sodium nitroprusside in dogs with normal and edematous lungs. Anesthesiology 50:489, 1979
32. Buckley MJ, McLaughlin JS, Fort L III, et al: Effects of anesthetic agents on pulmonary vascular resistance during hypoxia. Surg Forum 15:183, 1964

33. Sykes MK, Davies DM, Chakrabarti MK, et al: The effects of halothane, trichlorethylene and ether on the hypoxic pressor response and pulmonary vascular resistance in the isolated, perfused cat lung. Br J Anaesth 45:655, 1973

34. Loh L, Sykes MK, Chakrabarti MK: The effects of halothane and ether on the pulmonary circulation in the innervated perfused cat lung. Br J Anaesth 49:309, 1977

35. Marshall C, Lindgren L, Marshall BE: Effects of halothane, enflurane and isoflurane on hypoxic pulmonary vasoconstriction in rat lungs in vitro. Anesthesiology 60:304, 1984

36. Bjertnaes J, Hauge A, Nakken KF, et al: Hypoxic pulmonary vasoconstriction: Inhibition due to anesthesia. Acta Physiol Scand 96:283, 1976

37. Sykes MK, Biggs JM, Loh L, et al: Preservation of the pulmonary vasoconstrictor response to alveolar hypoxia during the administration of halothane to dogs. Br J Anaesth 50:1185, 1978

38. Benumof JL, Wahrenbrock EA: Local effects of anesthetics on regional hypoxic pulmonary vasoconstriction. Anesthesiology 46:111, 1977

39. Mathers J, Benumof JL, Wahrenbrock EA: General anesthetics and regional hypoxic pulmonary vasoconstriction. Anesthesiology 46:111, 1977

40. Sykes MK, Hurtig JB, Tait AR, et al: Reduction of hypoxic pulmonary vasoconstriction during diethyl ether anesthesia in the dog. Br J Anaesth 49:293, 1977

41. Fargas-Babjak A, Forrest JB: Effect in halothane on the pulmonary vascular response to hypoxia in dogs. Can Anaesth Soc J 26:6, 1979

42. Bjertnaes LJ: Hypoxia-induced pulmonary vasoconstriction in man: Inhibition due to diethyl ether and halothane anesthesia. Acta Anaesthesiol Scand 22:570, 1978

43. Anderson MW, Benumof JL: Intrapulmonary shunting during one lung ventilation and surgical manipulation. Anesthesiology 45:A377, 1981

44. Rees ID, Gaines GY: One lung anesthesia—a comparison of pulmonary gas exchange during anesthesia with ketamine or enflurane. Anesth Analg 63:521, 1984

45. Leeson TS, Leeson CR: A light and electron microscope study of developing respiratory tissue in the rat. J Anat 98:183, 1964

46. Lichtiger M, Landa JF, Hirsch JA: Velocity of tracheal mucus in anesthetized women undergoing gynecologic surgery. Anesthesiology 42:753, 1975

47. Wanner A: Clinical aspects of mucociliary transport. Am Rev Respir Dis 116:73, 1977

48. Reid L: Natural history of mucous in the bronchial tree. Arch Environ Health 10:265, 1965

49. Sackner MA, Rosen MJ, Wanner A: Estimation of tracheal mucous velocity by bronchofiberoscopy. J Appl Physiol 34:495, 1973

50. Gamsu G, Singer MM, Vincent HH, et al: Postoperative impairment of mucous transport in the lung. Am Rev Respir Dis 114:673, 1976

51. Forbes AR: Temperature, humidity and mucous flow in the intubated trachea. Br J Anaesth 46:29, 1974

52. Hirsch JA, Tokayer JL, Robinson MJ, et al: Effects of dry air and subsequent humidification on tracheal mucous velocity in dogs. J Appl Physiol 39:242, 1975

53. Forbes AR, Gamsu G: Lung mucociliary clearance after anesthesia with spontaneous and controlled ventilation. Am Rev Respir Dis 120:857, 1979

54. Forbes AR: Halothane depresses mucociliary flow in the trachea. Anesthesiology 45:59, 1976

55. Forbes AR, Horrigan RW: Mucociliary flow in the trachea during anesthesia with enflurane, ether, nitrous oxide, and morphine. Anesthesiology 46:319, 1977

56. Forbes AR, Gamsu G: Mucociliary clearance in the canine lung during and after general anesthesia. Anesthesiology 50:26, 1979

57. Nunn JF, Sturrock JE, Wills EJ, et al: The effect of inhalational anaesthetics on the swimming velocity of *Tetrahymena pyriformis*. J Cell Sci 15:537, 1974

58. Manawadu BR, Mostow SR, LaForce FM: Impairment of tracheal ring ciliary activity by halothane. Anesth Analg 58:500, 1979

59. Tarhan S, Moffitt EA, Sessler AD, et al: Risk of anesthesia and surgery in patients with chronic bronchitis and chronic obstructive pulmonary disease. Surgery 74:720, 1973

60. Berger AJ, Mitchell RA, Severinghaus JW: Regulation of respiration. N Engl J Med 297:92, 138, 194, 1977

61. Whitelaw WA, Derenne JP, Milic-Emili J: Occlusion pressure as a measure of respiratory center output in conscious man. Respir Physiol 23:181, 1975

62. Dreen JP, Couture J, Iscoe S, et al: Occlusion pressures in man rebreathing CO_2 under methoxyflurane anesthesia. J Appl Physiol 40:805, 1976

63. Larson CP, Jr, Eger EI II, Muallem M, et al: The effects of diethyl ether and methoxyflurane on ventilation. Anesthesiology 30:174, 1969

64. Whittenridge D, Bulbring E: Changes in the activity of pulmonary receptors in anesthesia and their influence on respiratory behavior. J Pharmacol Exp Ther 81:340, 1944

65. Paskin S, Skovsted P, Smith TC: Failure of the Hering-Breuer reflex to account for tachypnea in anesthetized man: A survey of halothane, fluroxene, methoxyflurane and cyclopropane. Anesthesiology 29:550, 1968

66. Freedman S, Campbell EJM: The ability of normal subjects to tolerate added inspiratory loads. Respir Physiol 10:213, 1970

67. Moote CA, Knill RL, Clement J: Ventilatory compensation for continuous inspiratory resistive and elastic loads during halothane anesthesia in humans. Anesthesiology 64:582, 1986

68. Slee TA, Sharar SR, Pavlin EG, MacIntyre PE: The effects of airway impedance on work of breathing during halothane anesthesia. Anesth Analg (in press), 1989

69. Nunn JF, Ezi-Ashi TI: The respiratory effects of resistance to breathing in anesthetized man. Anesthesiology 22:174, 1961

70. Freund FG, Roos A, Dodd RB: Expiratory activity of the abdominal muscles in man during general anesthesia. J Appl Physiol 19:693, 1964

71. Pietak S, Weenig CS, Hickey RF, et al: Anesthetic effects on ventilation in patients with chronic obstructive pulmonary disease. Anesthesiology 42:160, 1975

72. Pavlin EG, Hornbein TF: Anesthesia and the control of ventilation. p. 793. In Handbook of Physiology, Respiratory System Section. American Physiologic Society, Bethesda, MD, 1987

73. Caverley RK, Smith NT, Jones CW, et al: Ventilatory and cardiovascular effects of enflurane anesthesia during spontaneous ventilation in man. Anesth Analg 57:610, 1979

74. Eger EI, Dolan WM, Stevens WC, et al: Surgical stimulation antagonizes the respiratory depression produced by Forane. Anesthesiology 36:544, 1972

75. Fourcade HE, Larson CP, Hickey RF, et al: Effects of time on ventilation during halothane and cyclopropane anesthesia. Anesthesiology 36:83, 1972

76. Hickey RF, Fourcade HE, Eger EI II, et al: The effects of ether, halothane and Forane on apneic threshold in man. Anesthesiology 35:32, 1971

77. Read DJC: A clinical method for assessing the ventilatory response to carbon dioxide. Aust Ann Med 16:20, 1967

78. Fourcade HE, Stevens WC, Larson CP, et al: The ventilatory effects of Forane, a new inhaled anesthetic. Anesthesiology 35:26, 1971

79. Hornbein TF, Martin WE, Bonica JJ, et al: Nitrous oxide effects on the circulatory and ventilatory responses to halothane. Anesthesiology 31:250, 1969

80. Winter PM, Hornbein TF, Smith G, et al: Hyperbaric nitrous oxide anesthesia in man. p. 103. Abstracts of Scientific Papers. 1972 ASA Meeting

81. Weiskopf RB, Raymond LW, Severinghaus JW: Effects of halothane on canine respiratory responses to hypoxia with and without hypercarbia. Anesthesiology 41:350, 1974

82. Hirshman CA, McCullough RE, Cohen PJ, et al: Hypoxic ventilatory drive in dogs during thiopental, ketamine, or pentobarbital anesthesia. Anesthesiology 43:628, 1975

83. Knill RL, Gelb AW: Ventilatory responses to hypoxia and hypercapnia during halothane sedation and anesthesia in man. Anesthesiology 49:244, 1978

84. Knill RL, Manninen PH, Clement JL: Ventilation and chemoreflexes during enflurane sedation and anaesthesia in man. Can Anaesth Soc J 26:5, 1979

85. Yacoub O, Doell D, Kryger MH, et al: Depression of hypoxic ventilatory response by nitrous oxide. Anesthesiology 45:385, 1976

86. Biscoe TJ, Millar RA: Effects of inhalation anesthetics on carotid body chemoreceptor activity. Br J Anaesth 40:2, 1968

87. Davies RO, Edwards MW, Jr, Lahiri S: Halothane depresses the response to carotid body chemoreceptors to hypoxia and hypercapnia in the cat. Anesthesiology 57:153, 1982

89. Knill RL, Clement JL: Site of selective action of halothane on the peripheral chemoreflex pathway in humans. Anesthesiology 61:121, 1984

89. Eger EI, Smith NT, Stoelting RK, et al: Cardiovascular effects in man. Anesthesiology 32:395, 1970

90. Calverley RK, Smith NT, Prys-Roberts C, et al: Cardiovascular effects of enflurane anesthesia during controlled ventilation in man. Anesth Analg 57:619, 1978

91. Stevens WC, Cromwell TH, Halsey MJ, et al: The cardiovascular effects of a new inhalation anesthetic, Forane, in human volunteers at constant arterial carbon dioxide tension. Anesthesiology 35:8, 1971

92. Winter PM, Hornbein TF, Smith G: Hyperbaric nitrous oxide anesthesia in man: Determination of anesthetic potency (MAC) and cardiorespiratory effects. p. 103. Abstracts of Scientific Papers. 1972 ASA Meeting

93. Dolan WM, Stevens WC, Eger EI, et al: The cardiovascular and respiratory effects of isoflurane-nitrous oxide anesthesia. Can Anaesth Soc J 21:557, 1974

94. Brown BR, Crout JR: A comparative study of the effects of five general anesthetics on myocardial contractility. I. Isometric conditions. Anesthesiology 34:236, 1971

95. Housmans PR, Murat I: Comparative effects of halothane, enflurane and isoflurane in equipotent anesthetic doses on isolated ventricular myocardium of the ferret. I. Contractility. Anesthesiology 69:451, 1988

96. Blinks JR, Mattingly PH, Jewell BR, et al: Practical aspects of the use of aequorin as a calcium indicator: Assay, preparations, microinjection, and interpretation of signals. Methods Enzymol 57:292, 1978

97. Grynkiewicz G, Poenie M, Tsien RY: A new generation of Ca^{2+} indicators with greatly improved fluorescence properties. J Biol Chem 260:3440, 1985

98. Bosnjak ZJ, Kampine JP: Effects of halothane on transmembrane potentials, Ca^{2+} transients, and papillary muscle tension in the cat. Am J Physiol 251:H374, 1986

99. Bosnjak ZJ, Aggarwal A, Turner LA, Kampine JP: Differential effects of halothane, enflurane and isoflurane on Ca^{2+} transients and papillar muscle tension in the guinea pig (abstract). Anesthesiology 69:A88, 1988

100. Bosnjak ZJ, Rusch NJ: Calcium currents are decreased by halothane, enflurane and isoflurane in isolated canine ventricular and purkinje cells (abstract). Anesthesiology 69:A452, 1988

101. Lynch C, Vogel S, Sperelakis N: Halothane depression of myocardial slow action potentials. Anesthesiology 55:360, 1981

102. Lynch C, Vogel S, Pratila MG, Sperelakis N: Enflurane depression of slow action potentials. J Pharmacol Exp Ther 222:405, 1982

103. Su JY, Kerrick WGL: Effects of halothane on caffeine-induced tension transients in functionally skinned myocardial fibers. Pflugers Arch 380:29, 1979

104. Su JY, Kerrick WGL: Effects of enflurane on functionally skinned myocardial fibers from rabbits. Anesthesiology 52:385, 1980

105. Su JY, Bell JG: Intracellular mechanism of action of isoflurane and halothane on striated muscle of the rabbit. Anesth Analg 65:457, 1986

106. Blanck TJJ, Thompson M: Calcium transport by cardiac sarcoplasmic reticulum: Modulation of halothane action by substrate concentration and pH. Anesth Analg 60:390, 1981

107. Blanck TJJ, Thompson M: Enflurane and isoflurane stimulate calcium transport by cardiac sarcoplasmic reticulum. Anesth Analg 61:142, 1982

108. Wheeler DM, Rice RT, Hansford RG, Lakatta EG: The effect of halothane on the free intracellular calcium concentration of isolated rat heart cells. Anesthesiology 69:578, 1988

109. Malinconico ST, McCarl RL: Effect of halothane on cardiac sarcoplasmic reticulum Ca^{2+}-ATPase at low calcium concentrations. Mol Pharmacol 22:8, 1982

110. Lynch C: Differential depression of myocardial contractility by halothane and isoflurane *in vitro*. Anesthesiology 64:620, 1986

111. Luk HN, Liu CI, Chang CL, Lee AR: Differential inotropic effects of halothane and isoflurane on dog ventricular tissues. Eur J Pharmacol 136:409, 1987

112. DeTraglia MC, Komai H, Rusy BF: Differential effects of inhalation anesthetics on myocardial potentiated-state contractions in vitro. Anesthesiology 68:534, 1988

113. Su JY, Kerrick WGL: Effects of halothane on Ca^{2+} activated tension development in mechanically disrupted rabbit myocardial fibers. Pflugers Arch 375:111, 1978

114. Krane EJ, Su JY: Comparison of the effects of halothane on skinned myocardial fibers from newborn and adult rabbit: Effects on contractile proteins. Anesthesiology 70:76, 1989

115. Merin RG, Kumazawa T, Honig C: Reversible interaction between halothane and Ca^{++} on cardiac actomyosin adenosine triphosphate: Mechanism and significance. J Pharmacol Exp Ther 190:1, 1974

116. Shibata T, Blanck TJJ, Sagawa K, Hunter W: The effect of halothane, enflurane, and isoflurane on the dynamic stiffness of rabbit papillar muscle. Anesthesiology 70:496, 1989

117. Ohnishi ST, Pressman GS, Price HL: A possible mechanism of anesthetic-induced myocardial depression. Biochem Biophys Res Commun 57:316, 1974

118. Su JY, Kerrick WGL, Hill SA: Effects of diethyl ether and nitrous oxide on functionally skinned myocardial cells of rabbits. Anesth Analg 68:451, 1984

119. Hai C-M, Murphy RA: Ca^{2+}, crossbridge phosphorylation, and contraction. Annu Rev Physiol 51:285, 1989
120. Van Breeman C: Cellular mechanisms regulating $[Ca^{2+}]$ smooth muscle. Annu Rev Physiol 51:315, 1989
121. Vanhoutte PM: Relaxing and contracting factors: Biological and clinical research. The Human Press, Clifton, NJ, 1988
122. Longnecker DE, Harris PD: Microcirculatory actions of general anesthetics. Fed Proc 39:1580, 1980
123. Sprague DH, Yang JC, Nagai SH: Effects of isoflurane and halothane on contractility and cyclic 3',5'-adenosine monophosphate system in the rat aorta. Anesthesiology 40:162, 1974
124. Blaise G, Sill JC, Nugent M, et al: Isoflurane causes endothelium-dependent inhibition of contractile responses of canine coronary arteries. Anesthesiology 67:513, 1987
125. Muldoon SM, Hart JL, Bowen KA, Freas W: Attenuation of endothelium-mediated vasodilation by halothane. Anesthesiology 68:31, 1988
126. Su JY, Zhang CC: Intracellular mechanisms of halothane's effect on isolated aortic strips of the rabbit. Anesthesiology (in press), 1989
127. Duke PC, Townes D, Wade JG: Halothane depresses baroreflex control of heart rate in man. Anesthesiology 46:A184, 1977
128. Morton M, Duke PC, Ong B: Baroreflex control of heart rate in man awake and during enflurane and enflurane-nitrous oxide anesthesia. Anesthesiology 52:B221, 1980
129. Kotrly KJ, Ebert TJ, Vucins E, et al: Baroreceptor reflex control of heart rate during isoflurane anesthesia in humans. Anesthesiology 60:C173, 1984
130. Seagard JL, Hopp FA, Bosnjak ZJ, et al: Extent and mechanism of halothane sensitization of the carotid sinus baroreceptors. Anesthesiology 58:D432, 1983
131. Behnia R, Koushanpour E: Local versus central effect of halothane on carotid sinus baroreceptor function. Anesthesiology 61:E161, 1984
132. Seagard JL, Hopp FA, Donegan JH, et al: Halothane and the carotid sinus reflex: Evidence for multiple sites of action. Anesthesiology 57:191, 1982
133. Waltemath CL, Bergman NA: Effects of ketamine and halothane on increased respiratory resistance provoked by ultrasonic aerosols. Anesthesiology 41:473, 1974
134. Brakensiek AL, Bergman JA: The effects of halothane and atropine on total respiratory resistance in anesthetized man. Anesthesiology 33:341, 1970
135. Kaur AE, Mazzic VV, Bergofski CH: Effect of anesthesia and neuromuscular blockers on pulmonary vascular responses to hypoxia and hypercapnia. Anesth Analg 51:402, 1972
136. Sykes MK, Arnot RN, Jastrzbski J, et al: Reduction of hypoxic pulmonary vasoconstriction during trichloroethylene anesthesia. J Appl Physiol 39:103, 1975
137. Hurtig JB, Tait AR, Sykes MK: Reduction of hypoxic pulmonary vasoconstriction by diethyl ether in the isolated perfused cat lung: The effect of acidosis and alkalosis. Can Anaesth Soc J 24:433, 1977
138. Tait AR, Chakrabarti MK, Sykes MK: Effect of cyclopropane on pulmonary vascular resistance and hypoxic pulmonary vasoconstriction in the isolated perfused cat lung. Br J Anaesth 50:209, 1978
139. Katz AM: Physiology of the Heart. Raven Press, New York, 1977
140. Hickey RF, Severinghaus JW: Chapter 21. In Hornbein TF (ed): Regulation of Breathing. Lung Biology in Health and Disease. Vol. 17. Part II. Marcel Dekker, New York, 1981
141. Katz AM: Congestive heart failure: Role of altered myocardial cellular control. N Engl J Med 293:1184, 1975

6
METABOLISM AND TOXICITY

Jeffrey M. Baden
Susan A. Rice

INTRODUCTION

The inhaled anesthetics initially were considered biochemically inert drugs. The occasional toxicity following their administration was attributed either to a direct effect on susceptible tissue or to a secondary effect resulting from unwanted physiologic changes. Now it is recognized that not only are the inhaled anesthetics metabolized in vivo, but also that their metabolites are responsible for both acute and chronic toxicities. In this chapter, we present the current status of information on the metabolism and toxicity of the inhaled anesthetics and discuss their known and presumed associations.

METABOLISM

Current concepts of drug biotransformation acknowledge that drug metabolism may produce varied results. The inherent pharmacologic and toxicologic actions of a drug may have potency equal to or greater or lesser than those of its metabolites. Alternatively, the type of pharmacologic and toxicologic actions exhibited by the parent drug may not be exhibited by the metabolites, but different actions may be apparent. Many factors, such as the extent of drug absorption, adsorption, excretion, secretion, and metabolism, affect drug efficacy and toxicity. These factors themselves are affected by chemical and physical properties of the drug. In the first few sections of this chapter, we discuss the properties of drugs and cellular membranes that influence drug availability at the cellular sites of metabolism.

PHYSICOCHEMICAL CONSIDERATIONS

Physicochemical Properties of Drug Molecules (Also See Ch. 2)

Three physicochemical properties primarily determine the distribution of a drug molecule and its availability for metabolism: ionization, lipid solubility, and molecular size and shape.[1] The degree to which a drug is ionized depends on the pK_a of the drug and the pH of the solution in which it is dissolved. Most drugs are weak bases or weak acids and have one or more functional groups that can be ionized. The pK_a for weak acids is high, while that for weak bases is low. The relationship between the degree of ionization, the pK_a, and the pH of a drug is described by the Henderson-Hasselbach equation:

$$pH = pK_a + \log \frac{[\text{dissociated drug}]}{[\text{undissociated drug}]} \quad (1)$$

The lipid solubility of a drug is determined by the presence or absence of lipophilic (hydrophobic) or nonpolar groups in the molecule. Alkyl groups (C_nH_{2n+1}-) such as the methyl group (CH_3—) are nonpolar. The lipophilic properties of a molecule increase as the length of the alkyl group increases. For example, the presence of an *n*-propyl group ($CH_3CH_2CH_2$—) makes the compound more lipophilic than the presence of a methyl group. Lipophilic properties increase when an alkyl group is inserted in the molecule, whether the substitution occurs on a carbon, nitrogen, oxygen, or sulfur atom. Substitution of oxygen by sulfur often markedly increases the lipophilic properties of a drug. The lipophilic properties are decreased and the hydrophilic or polar properties are increased when a molecule contains structural elements that allow hydrogen bonding to water (e.g., —OH, —O—, —CHO, —COOH, —Cl, and —Br). The presence of unsaturated bonds (e.g., —CH=CH—) further promotes the hydrophilic properties of a molecule.

Molecular size and shape also determine drug distribution. Various types of membranes have different pore sizes that allow the passage of different-sized molecules. For example, molecules up to about the size of albumin (molecular weight of 69,000; major axis, 150 Å; minor axis, 35 Å) can appear in the glomerular filtrate, but molecules larger than 4 Å in radius are excluded from the erythrocyte. All three physicochemical factors, ionization, lipid solubility, and molecular size and shape, influence the distribution of a drug and its ability to penetrate cellular membranes.

Properties of Cellular Membranes

Cellular and subcellular membranes are lipoid in nature and consist of a phospholipid bilayer and intercalated functional proteins.[2-4] They contain large quantities of phospholipids, cholesterol, and neutral lipids in association with proteins. Membrane phospholipids are amphoteric, that is, they have distinct polar and nonpolar regions. Nonpolar hydrocarbon chains are directed toward the center of the bilayer, while polar head groups remain in contact with the aqueous phase on the bilayer surface. The lipid structure is either completely or partially penetrated by membrane proteins that bind to interior and exterior surfaces of the bilayer. The proteins are necessary both for the maintenance of membrane integrity and for the specialized transport of endogenous (and structurally similar exogenous) molecules. In concert with drug properties, membrane properties determine the ability of a drug to enter cells.

Very small molecules and ions (e.g., Cl^-) apparently diffuse through aqueous membrane channels, while lipid-soluble molecules may diffuse freely through the membrane. Water-soluble molecules and ions of moderate size, including the ionic form of most drugs, can only enter the cell by specialized transport. The overall lipid solubility (i.e., the relative lipophilic and hydrophilic properties) of a drug molecule determines whether the drug will readily cross biologic membranes by a passive process. Membranes are generally permeable to the nonionized forms of lipid-soluble drugs. Ionized groups on a molecule (e.g., —COO⁻; —COOH is almost completely ionized at pH 7.4) interact strongly with water dipoles and as a result penetrate the lipoidal cell membrane poorly if at all. As a rule of thumb, the diffusion rate of a drug parallels the concentration gradient for the nonionized drug form. In general, the greater the lipid solubility, the greater the rate at which a drug will move through membranes.

Function of the Liver in Drug Metabolism

The inhaled anesthetics are primarily metabolized by the liver and, to a lesser extent, by other tissues (e.g., gastrointestinal tract, kidneys, lungs, skin). The following discussion of drug metabolism is limited to the liver because the vast majority of anesthetic biotransformation occurs in this organ and the principles of drug metabolism are similar from tissue to tissue.

Hepatic physiology is fully discussed in Chapter 17; however, a brief description is included in this discussion to aid in understanding the relationship between drug metabolism and toxicity. The liver is the largest organ in the body, weighing about 1,500 g in adult humans. It is a unique organ in that it has a double blood supply: 70 percent from the portal vein and 30 percent from the hepatic artery. Blood in the portal vein comes from the alimentary canal, pancreas, and spleen. Thus, any toxic material absorbed from the alimentary canal is processed by the liver before it enters the systemic circulation. The arrangement of portal veins and hepatic arteries defines the periphery of a roughly hexagonal zone of tissue, recognized histologically as the hepatic lobule. The lobule is composed of two cell types, the Kupffer cell and the liver cell (hepatocyte). The phagocytic Kupffer cell is part of the reticuloendothelial system, while the hepatocyte is primarily involved with homeostatic synthesis and metabolism. The cuboidal hepatic cells are arranged in one-cell-thick interconnecting sheets separated by sinusoidal capillaries (sinusoids). Blood flows through these sinusoids from the periphery of the lobule, fed by portal veins and hepatic arteries, to the centrally located hepatic venule (central vein).

The hepatocyte contains several structures that are involved in intermediary and drug metabolism, most notably the endoplasmic reticulum. This membranous matrix of lipoprotein is the major site of protein synthesis, electron transfer, lipid metabolism, and hormone and drug metabolism. It is also the main site for the synthesis of the lipoid and protein structural components for the cell and its organelles. Microscopically, the endoplastic reticulum appears as a series of vesicles and tubules suspended within the cytoplasm. Both the parallel arrays of rough endoplastic reticulum and the maze of smooth endoplasmic reticulum are part of one interconnected system that provides channels for the passive intracellular transport of proteins (including enzymes), lipids, and other compounds and provides intracellular storage for some of them. Under nonenzyme-induced conditions, the area of rough endoplasmic reticulum is about 25,000 μm^2, while the smooth endoplasmic reticulum is about 15,000 to 20,000 μm^2. The rough endoplasmic reticulum is identified by the presence of ribosomes (particles containing ribonucleic acid [RNA] and constituent proteins) adjacent to the tubular membrane and is the site of protein synthesis. It is extensively developed in protein-secreting cells. The smooth endoplasmic reticulum contains no granules and is the site of drug metabolism, bilirubin conjugation, steroid synthesis, and some enzyme synthesis. It is extensively developed in steroid-secreting cells.

In hepatocytes, both smooth and rough endoplasmic reticulum participate in drug metabolism. Many in vitro studies of the endoplasmic reticulum and its drug-metabolizing capabilities have been performed with microsomes. These are not naturally occurring organelles but are formed from the breakage and reformation of cisternal and tubular systems of the endoplasmic reticulum during cell fractionation.[5]

DRUG METABOLISM

Metabolism requires the interaction of drug (substrate) and enzyme. An enzyme-catalyzed chemical reaction proceeds at a rate approximately 10^9 times faster than a noncatalyzed reaction. Under appropriate conditions,

the enzyme molecule and the parent drug molecule form a complex resulting from intermolecular forces (e.g., van der Waals, ionic). The complex then decomposes, regenerating the enzyme and liberating a product (metabolite) different from the parent drug.

$$\text{enzyme} + \text{drug} \longrightarrow \text{enzyme–drug complex} \longrightarrow$$
$$\text{enzyme} + \text{metabolite} \quad (2)$$

Metabolism can be an important determinant of therapeutic activity and toxicity for a drug. It is affected by many factors including route of administration, species, strain, sex, age, diet, temperature, season, time of day, chronic administration, and the previous or concurrent administration of other drugs or chemicals. Unlike most drugs, the inhaled anesthetics are administered in great excess of the amount metabolized. Thus, biotransformation has little effect on pharmacologic activity but plays a significant role in determining anesthetic toxicity.

The major pathways of drug metabolism are oxidation, reduction, hydrolysis, and conjugation reactions. A drug may have a chemical structure suitable for simultaneous biotransformation in several metabolic pathways. The enzymes of these pathways compete for the drug (substrate). The ratio of metabolites depends on enzymatic reaction rates, drug concentration near the enzymes, and physicochemical reactions between metabolites and enzymes.

The overall pattern of drug metabolism is common to all animals species; it is biphasic in nature and consists of stepwise biotransformation and synthesis reactions. Figure 6-1 shows the general scheme of drug metabolism. Phase I (biotransformation reactions) consists of the oxidation (hydroxylation), hydrolysis, or reduction of a lipid-soluble or nonpolar drug. Phase II (synthesis reactions) consists of the conjugation of a drug or its metabolite with an endogenous compound (predominantly glycine, sulfate, or glucuronic acid). The net result of either phase of metabolism is the production of polar compounds that are more readily excreted in the bile or urine. Both phases are controlled by enzymes present in plasma, cytoplasm, mitochrondria, and endoplasmic reticulum. Quantitative and qualitative differences in metabolism seen among species lie mainly in the nature of these enzymes. Phase I metabolism occurs primarily in the environment of the endoplasmic reticulum, while phase II metabolism occurs primarily in the more aqueous environment of the cytoplasm. Substrates of phase I reactions are seldom substrates of phase II reactions, but products of phase I metabolism are often substrates for phase II reactions.

Phase I Reactions

Microsomal Drug-Metabolizing Enzymes

The cytochrome P-450-mediated monooxygenases are a collection of phase I enzymes. These hydroxylating enzymes are called mixed-function oxidases or mono-

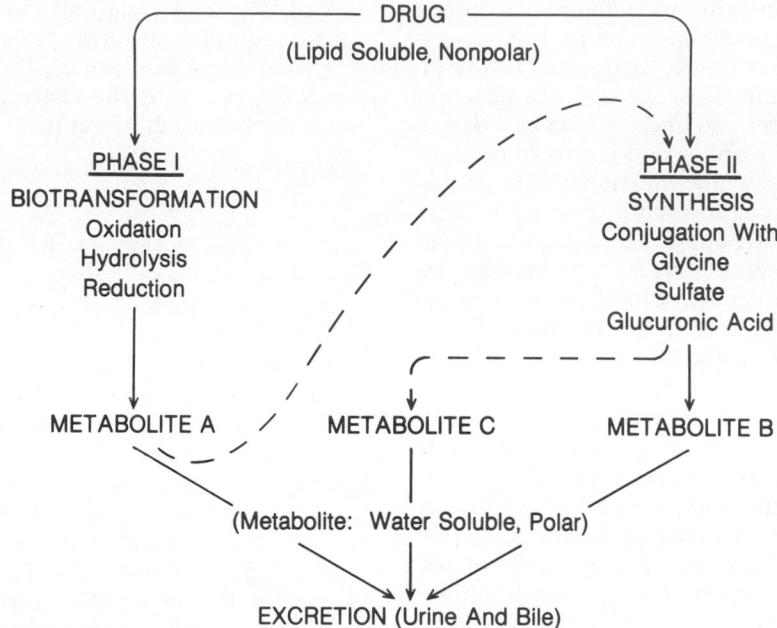

Fig. 6-1. Two phases of drug metabolism — biotransformation and synthesis — generally result in the formation of more water-soluble metabolites that are readily excreted in the urine and bile.

oxygenases because during metabolism one of the two atoms of molecular oxygen (O_2) is incorporated into cellular water (H_2O). The key enzyme components of this membrane-bound multicomponent system are the hemoproteins, cytochromes P-450, and the flavoprotein, NADPH-cytochrome P-450 reductase. Reactions of the monooxygenase system have been extensively studied in vitro by using microsomes and reconstituted systems. The monooxygenase system requires molecular oxygen (O_2) and NADPH. The overall reaction is a hydroxylation that can be represented as follows:

$$RH + NADPH + H^+ + O_2 \longrightarrow ROH + NADP^+ + H_2O \quad (3)$$

RH is the substrate, ROH is the hydroxylated product, and NADPH is the reduced form of nicotinamide adenine dinucleotide phosphate (NADP). The overall flow of electrons proceeds from NADPH to the flavoprotein (NADPH-cytochrome P-450 reductase) to molecular oxygen.[6] Under some circumstances, NADH can contribute an electron instead of NADPH. The intermediate electron carrier for NADH is the other microsomal hemoprotein, cytochrome b_5.

Figure 6-2 shows the steps in cytochrome P-450-mediated drug hydroxylation. Cytochrome P-450 is shown as Cyt P-450^{III} (the valence state of iron [Fe] in the hemoprotein is indicated), RH is the drug (substrate), and ROH is the hydroxylated drug metabolite. The flavoprotein NADPH-cytochrome P-450 reductase contains one flavin mononucleotide (FMN) and one flavin adenine dinucleotide (FAD). The first step of the hydroxylation reaction is assumed to be the formation of a ferric (Fe^{III}) cytochrome P-450-drug complex (Cyt P-450^{III}-R) by a rapid stoichiometric reaction of substrate with the oxi-

dized hemoprotein. This complex accepts one electron (e^-) from the FADH/FMNH$_2$ complex of NADPH-cytochrome P-450 reductase to form a ferrous (Fe^{II}) cytochrome P-450-substrate complex (Cyt P-450^{II}-R), which rapidly combines with oxygen to yield an oxygenated complex. Upon introduction of a second electron from the flavoprotein, or in some cases via NADH-cytochrome b_5 reductase, an activated iron-oxygen complex is formed (Fe$=$O^{III}). An internal electronic rearrangement occurs, oxygen is added to the drug (RO), the cytochrome P-450-drug complex decomposes, the hydroxylated product (ROH) is liberated, and the ferric cytochrome P-450 (Cyt P-450^{III}) is regenerated.

The cytochrome P-450-mediated monooxygenases, along with other metabolically linked enzymes, provide an important pathway by which the cell may metabolize and thus eliminate xenobiotics. They are responsible not only for deactivation of toxic compounds but also for the activation of drugs, chemicals, and environmental pollutants to toxic, mutagenic, and carcinogenic forms. These monooxygenases are arranged in a specific pattern in the endoplasmic reticulum to allow coordinated and side-directed reactions for the oxidation of a variety of substrates.

Numerous genetic and environmental factors (including chemicals and drugs) affect the endoplasmic reticulum and the performance of its drug-metabolizing complex. The phenomena of enzyme induction and inhibition are the most obvious examples; they depend on the rates of synthesis and degradation of the various membrane and enzyme system components. Hepatic microsomal membrane proteins have different turn-

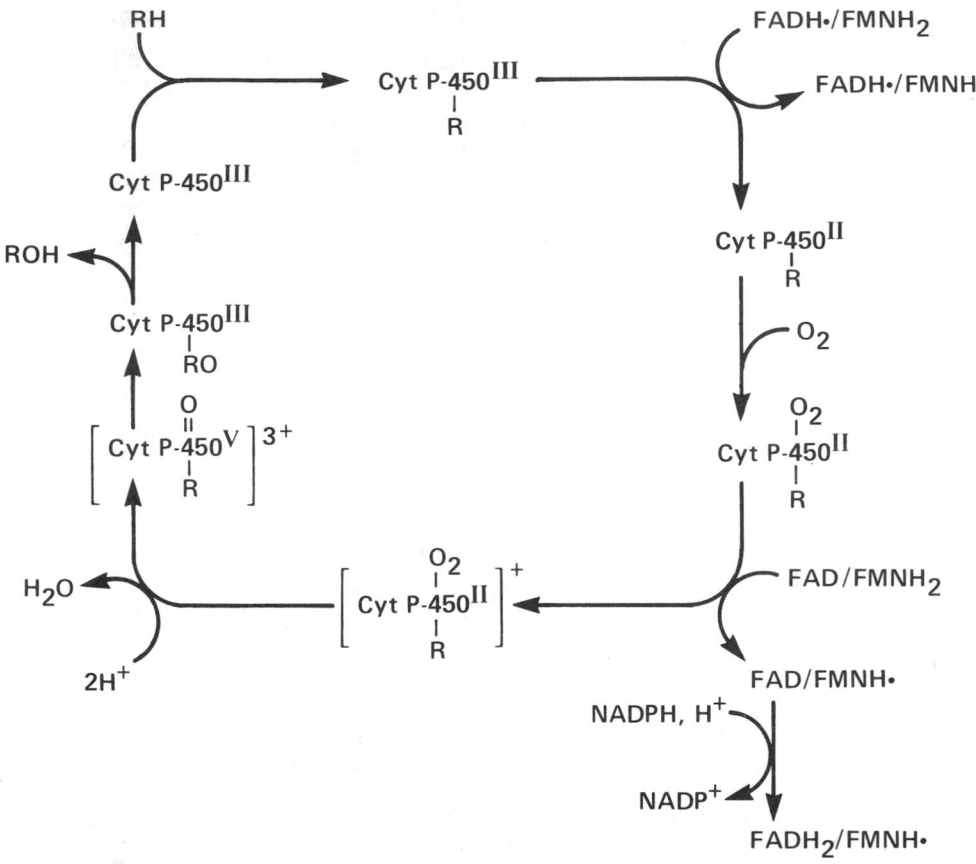

Fig. 6-2. A drug (RH), which is a substrate for the hepatic mixed-function oxidase system, interacts with cytochrome P-450 and is biotransformed to a hydroxylated product (ROH).

over rates. For example, the turnover rates of cytochromes P-450 and NADPH-cytochrome P-450 reductase are different, as are the turnover rates of cytochrome b_5 and NADH-cytochrome b_5 reductase. Thus, the microsomal membrane is not formed and degraded as a unit but rather by the random insertion of newly synthesized protein molecules into existing membranes.[7]

Human liver contains less cytochrome P-450 per gram of tissue (i.e., 10 to 20 nmol/g) than livers of other species. For example, rat liver contains approximately 30 to 50 nmol/g of liver. Furthermore, human liver is 2 percent of body weight, and rat liver is approximately 4 percent. These differences explain in part why humans metabolize drugs in vivo at rates that may be as much as 10 to 20 times slower than those of rats.[8,9]

Cytochrome P-450 is not a single entity but rather a mixture of isoenzymes having different substrate specificities. Along with differences in the hepatic content of cytochrome P-450 among mammalian species and individuals, these different cytochrome isoenzymes may be responsible for the variations in rates and pathways of anesthetic metabolism in vivo and in vitro that are observed among human subjects and laboratory animals.[9,10] For example, such variation has been demonstrated for cytochrome P-450-mediated dehalogenation

and dealkylation of the inhaled anesthetics.[11-21] The differences in metabolism between humans and animals must be carefully considered when evaluating potential toxicity.

Reactions Relevant to Inhaled Anesthetic Biotransformation

The most common types of drug biotransformation reactions are oxidations, reductions, and hydrolyses. The reactions that fall into these classifications are numerous and varied and are carried out by two classes of enzymes. The first primarily metabolizes naturally occurring (endogenous) substrates, although they can also metabolize foreign (exogenous) substrates. The second class consists of the so-called drug-metabolizing enzymes that reside mainly in the endoplasmic reticulum of the hepatocyte. It includes the cytochrome P-450-mediated monooxygenases, which are the primary means for biotransformation of foreign compounds. The inhaled anesthetics are metabolized by these enzymes primarily by oxidation reactions. Two types of oxidation reactions, dehalogenation and O-dealkylation, are responsible for the majority of anesthetic metabolism. One additional oxidation reaction, epoxidation, accounts for fewer anesthetic biotransformations but is important because of the toxic potential of epoxides. Reductive reactions result in substrate reduction by transferring electrons to the substrate rather than to molecular oxygen. The only inhaled anesthetic known to undergo a reductive reaction is halothane.[21-24] Hydrolysis reactions are not seen with the inhaled anesthetics because none possess the necessary ester linkage. Examples of the biotransformation reactions relevant to the inhaled anesthetics are shown below.

O-Dealkylation

O-Dealkylation results from hydroxylation of an alkyl group adjacent to the oxygen of an ether bond. The hemiacetal thus formed is a relatively unstable intermediate that rapidly decomposes to an alcohol and an aldehyde. The aldehyde may then either be reduced by alcohol dehydrogenase to an alcohol or be oxidized by aldehyde oxidase to form a carboxylic acid. The rate of the *O*-dealkylation reaction decreases as the length of the alkyl chain increases.

$$ROCH_2R' \xrightarrow{[O]} \left[\underset{\text{Hemiacetal}}{\overset{\displaystyle ROCHR'}{\underset{\displaystyle |}{\underset{\displaystyle OH}{}}}} \right] \longrightarrow ROH + R'CHO \tag{4}$$

Dehalogenation

Dehalogenation, contrary to what was previously believed, is not the result of a direct attack on the carbon-halogen bond. Rather, it results from hydroxylation of the halogen-containing carbon. A chemically unstable compound is formed that decomposes to a carboxylic acid, thus liberating halogen(s). Two halogens on the terminal carbon represent the optimal condition for dehalogenation, while a terminal carbon with three halogens is oxidized to a very limited extent.[25]

$$RCHX_2 \xrightarrow{[O]} \underset{|}{\overset{\displaystyle RCHX_2}{\underset{\displaystyle OH}{}}} \longrightarrow RCOOH + 2X^- \tag{5}$$

Epoxidation

An epoxide is formed when oxygen is attached to the adjacent unsaturated carbons of an olefin. Most epoxides are highly strained molecules and are extremely reactive because of the ease with which the ring can be opened. Some epoxides may be hydrated by the microsomal enzyme epoxide hydrase.[26]

$$R-CH=CH-R' \xrightarrow{[O]}$$

$$R-\underset{\overset{\displaystyle \diagdown}{}}{CH}-\underset{\overset{\displaystyle O}{\diagup}}{CH}-R' \xrightarrow{[H_2O]} R-\underset{\overset{\displaystyle |}{OH}}{CH}-\underset{\overset{\displaystyle |}{OH}}{CH}-R \tag{6}$$

Epoxide

Reduction

Reductive reactions catalyzed by the cytochrome P-450 enzyme system are very different from oxidative reactions. Because oxygen inhibits the reduction reaction, it is thought that one or more electrons are accepted directly by the substrate from cytochrome P-450. Reductive metabolism involving cytochrome P-450 has been confirmed for one anesthetic, halothane.[21-24]

$$CF_3CHBrCl \xrightarrow{e^-} CF_2=CHCl + F^- + Br^- \tag{7}$$

Phase II Reactions

Phase II reactions are conjugations. They occur when the drug contains a group suitable for combination with an endogenous compound (e.g., glycine, sulfate, glucuronic acid). The chemical groups on the drug molecule usually associated with these reactions are —OH, —COOH, —NH$_2$, and —SH. The product is generally a polar, water-soluble metabolite that is readily excreted. A typical conjugation reaction is illustrated below.

$$ROH + UDPGA \xrightarrow{\text{glucuronyl transferase}}$$
$$R\text{-}O\text{-glucuronide} + UDP \tag{8}$$

Conjugation of a drug (ROH) containing a hydroxyl (—OH) group to UDPGA (D-glucuronic acid in its "active" form; uridine diphosphate glucuronic acid) is catalyzed by glucuronyl transferase, which is located in the hepatic rough endoplasmic reticulum. The resulting glucuronide is more water soluble because of the presence of the polar sugar moiety. The free carboxyl (—COOH) group of the glucuronide, which is almost completely ionized at body pH, further enhances water solubility. Although a drug initially may not contain a chemical group suitable for conjugation reaction, one may be attained through a phase I reaction (i.e., by oxidation, reduction, or hydrolysis). Urochloralic acid is an example of an anesthetic metabolite that results from multiple consecutive biotransformations.[27-30] It is the glucuronic acid conjugate of trichloroethanol, a metabolite from the phase I metabolism of trichloroethylene.[30-32]

Enzyme Induction

Treatment of humans and animals with certain agents results in the enhanced metabolism of a variety of drugs and chemicals. This phenomenon, enzyme induction, is due to an increased de novo rate of enzyme synthesis and in some instances a decreased rate of enzyme degradation. The mixed-function oxidase drug-metabolizing enzymes can be induced by numerous agents in humans and by literally hundreds of agents in experimental animals.[33,34] Generally, enzyme inducers are highly lipophilic drugs and chemicals that are metabolized by the cytochromes P-450 that they induce. Induction is thought to be determined largely by the extent and duration of the interaction of the inducing agent with the enzyme concerned. The inducing properties of a drug are unrelated to the nature of its pharmacologic or toxicologic activity and may differ markedly from those of other drugs in the same class.

Induction of the mixed-function oxidase system by drugs such as phenobarbital results in proliferation of the smooth endoplasmic reticulum and an increase in liver weight.[35] With this type of inducer, NADPH-cytochrome P-450 reductase and specific cytochromes P-450 are preferentially increased. Other inducers, while increasing the synthesis of specific cytochromes P-450, do not affect cytochrome P-450 reductase or liver weight.

Many chemical and drug classes, including anticonvulsants, steroids, tranquilizers, sedatives, anesthetics, and insecticides, contain one or more compounds considered to be an enzyme inducer.[33-35] Even the inhaled anesthetics can induce drug-metabolizing enzymes in experimental animals with prolonged exposure.[36-38] In anesthetists exposed to approximately 19 ppm of halothane for 4 hours per week for 2 weeks, Duvaldestin et al.[39] demonstrated that salivary antipyrine clearance (a marker of drug metabolism) was increased by 29 percent.

In many case reports of drug toxicity, enzyme induction has been suggested to be a causative factor but often without good evidence. If a drug is toxic, its enhanced metabolism usually decreases but occasionally increases toxicity, if the metabolites are more toxic than the parent compound. Any enzyme-inducing agent has the potential to modify both the acute and the chronic toxicity of anesthetics. In view of the current practice of polypharmacy, enzyme induction may be common in patients undergoing surgery. But enzyme induction per se does not necessarily result in the increased metabolism of all drugs from the same class. For example, unlike methoxyflurane metabolism, enflurane metabolism is not significantly increased in vivo after phenobarbital or phenytoin treatment in humans[14] and animals[40-42] or in vitro in animals.[41,42] Furthermore, although anesthetics produce several toxic metabolites, when anesthetics are administered to surgical patients exposed to enzyme-inducing drugs, the production of toxic metabolites does not necessarily occur.[6,19,43]

Enzyme Inhibition

The consequences of enzyme inhibition for pharmacologic activity and toxicity can be just as great as those of enzyme induction. Many compounds can inhibit the activity of the drug-metabolizing enzymes and thereby alter the duration and intensity of pharmacologic and toxic effects. There are several mechanisms of inhibition.[44] Protein synthesis inhibitors such as cycloheximide decrease enzyme synthesis and thus reduce enzyme concentrations. Other agents are reversible inhibitors that compete for the active site of the same enzyme responsible for metabolism of the drug of inter-

est. Still others are irreversible inhibitors that degrade the heme in cytochromes P-450. Millimolar concentrations of methoxyflurane (5.8 mM), enflurane (13.3 mM), and halothane (18.8 mM) have been demonstrated to destroy cytochrome P-450 in microsomal preparations.[45]

Genetic-Species Variation

Genetic differences account for both the qualitative and quantitative differences in drug metabolism among species. Differences may be observed in the ratios or types of metabolites that are formed. Qualitative differences among species generally result from the presence or absence of specific enzymes in those species. Quantitative differences result from variations in the amount and localization of enzymes, the amount of natural inhibitors, and the competition of enzymes for specific substrates.

In humans, genetic factors that are otherwise undetected may be revealed in the expression of therapeutic activity and toxicity of a drug. For example, physiologic disposition of a drug may be unusual if there is structural variation in the serum protein that binds the drug. Even small changes in binding proteins can greatly affect a drug's disposition and ultimately its biologic activity. Genetic factors appear to be more important than environmental factors (such as diet and pollutant exposure) in determining the overall rate of drug metabolism and elimination in humans, although enzyme induction and inhibition may account for some unusual drug responses. Studies of halothane metabolism and elimination in twins have demonstrated far less variation in identical twins than in fraternal twins or in the normal population, even when environmental factors were quite dissimilar.[46]

METABOLISM OF SPECIFIC ANESTHETICS

The metabolism of virtually all inhaled anesthetics is described, although several of them are no longer in clinical use.

Nonhalogenated Inhaled Anesthetics

Diethyl Ether CH_3-CH_2-O-CH_2-CH_3 (See Eq. 9)

Van Dyke et al.[47] using ^{14}C-labeled diethyl ether in rats were the first to demonstrate metabolism of diethyl ether to carbon dioxide and nonvolatile urinary products. Presumably, enzymes of the hepatic mixed-function oxidase system cleave the ether linkage and produce two-carbon products such as ethanol, acetaldehyde, and acetic acid, which enter the general metabolic pool where they are further oxidized to carbon dioxide.[48,49] Diethyl ether metabolism has not been studied in vitro, but its in vivo metabolism is enhanced after phenobarbital treatment.[50] Chronic exposure of rats to subanesthetic concentrations of diethyl ether results in elevated concentrations of hepatic microsomal enzymes and increased metabolism of several drugs, including diethyl ether and other inhaled anesthetics.[36-38]

Ethylene $H_2C=CH_2$ (See Eq. 10)

Although initial experiments could not demonstrate ethylene metabolism, Van Dyke and Chenoweth[50] measured $^{14}CO_2$ and unidentified nonvolatile urinary products after the administration of ^{14}C-labeled ethylene to rats.

Cyclopropane

$$\begin{array}{c} CH_2 \\ \diagup \diagdown \\ H_2C-CH_2 \end{array}$$

Cyclopropane (C_3H_6) is the simplest cyclic compound that produces anesthesia. It is eliminated unchanged almost exclusively by the lungs. There are no data to suggest that it is metabolized.

Nitrous Oxide N_2O (See Eq. 11)

Nitrous oxide (N_2O) probably is not metabolized by human tissue. Hong et al.,[51] however, observed that N_2O was reductively metabolized in vitro to molecular nitrogen (N_2) by rat and human intestinal bacteria. They postulated that N_2O reduction in bacteria occurs via a single electron transfer process that results in the formation of free radicals and N_2. Evidence for N_2O induction of drug metabolism is contradictory. Enzyme induction in experimental animals has been reported after prolonged exposure to unspecified concentrations of N_2O.[52] Conversely, rats continuously exposed to 20 percent N_2O for 14 to 35 days exhibited inhibition of hepatic drug metabolism.[53] Pulmonary and testicular metabolism, however, were increased. Mice exposed to as much as 50 percent N_2O for 4 hours per day for 14 weeks showed no increase in hepatic microsomal cytochrome P-450 or defluorination of enflurane or methoxyflurane.[54] In another study, hexobarbital sleeping time was used as an indicator of drug metabolism in rats and was unchanged after exposure to 50 percent N_2O for 7 hours per day for 1 to 5 days.[37]

Halogenated Inhaled Anesthetics

Chloroform $CHCl_3$ (See Eq. 12)

Van Dyke et al.[47] demonstrated the metabolism of ^{36}Cl- and ^{14}C-labeled chloroform to $^{36}Cl^-$ and $^{14}CO_2$ in rats. Metabolism was later confirmed in two human volunteers in whom 50 percent of an administered dose of $^{13}CHCl_3$ was recovered as exhaled $^{13}CO_2$.[55] Elucidation of the mechanism has come largely from animal work by Pohl et al.[56-58] Cytochrome P-450-dependent oxida-

tion of the C-H bond of chloroform results in the formation trichloromethanol, which undergoes spontaneous dehydrochlorination to phosgene $(COCl_2)$.[56] Phosgene, in turn, reacts with water to form Cl^- and CO_2.[56,57] Phosgene can also react with two molecules of glutathione (GSH) to form diglutathionyl dithiocarbonate (GSCOSG).[58] GSCOSG can be rapidly metabolized via γ-glutamyl transpeptidase to N-(2-oxothiazolidine-4-carboxyl) glycine (OTZG), which is hydrolyzed to 2-oxothiazolidine-4-carboxylic acid (OTZ).[58] In the conversion of chloroform to CO_2, a reactive intermediate, presumably phosgene, can attack nucleophilic sites on tissue macromolecules and thus initiate toxic effects.[55,59-62] Metabolism and resultant increased metabolite binding to tissue is induced by phenobarbital[60] and 2-hexanone[62] and is inhibited by disulfiram.[60] Chronic exposure to chloroform increases in vivo metabolism of hexobarbital and presumably other anesthetics.[37]

Trichloroethylene $Cl_2C=CHCl$ (See Eq. 13)

As early as 1939, trichloroacetic acid had been isolated and identified as the primary urinary metabolite of trichloroethylene in dogs.[63] Six years later, Powell[31] quantitated the trichloroacetic acid in expired air, blood, and urine of species and suggested that trichloroethylene is metabolized at some site other than blood. It wasn't until 1965 that Byington and Leibman[29] and subsequently Leibman and McAllister[64] demonstrated that metabolism occurs primarily via the hepatic mixed-function oxidases. Trichloroethylene initially was believed to be transformed via an epoxide and a rearrangement of chlorine atoms to chloral hydrate.[27] More recent evidence from Miller and Guengerich[30,65] suggests that chlorine migration occurs within the oxygenated trichloroethylene-cytochrome P-450 complex to form chloral hydrate. This intermediate is further transformed by oxidation to trichloroacetic acid via a soluble enzyme (requiring nicotinamide adenine dinucleotide [NAD]) or by reduction to trichloroethanol via alcohol dehydrogenase (requiring the reduced form of NAD [NADH]).[28]

In vivo, the major metabolites of trichloroethylene are trichloroacetic acid, which is excreted unchanged in the urine; trichloroethanol, which is excreted in the urine either unchanged or as urochloralic acid, its glucuronic acid conjugate; and chloral hydrate.[65] The in vitro metabolism of trichloroethylene to chloral hydrate is increased after phenobarbital pretreatment.[64]

Fluroxene $CF_3-CH_2-O-CH=CH_2$ (See Eq. 14)

In humans, fluroxene is metabolized primarily in the liver to trifluoroacetic acid. Small quantities of trifluoroethanol and carbon dioxide also have been identified.[66] In mice, dogs, and rats, trifluoroethanol, a highly toxic metabolite, has been identified in sufficient concentrations to account for the chemical toxicity seen in

$$CH_3-CH_2-O-CH_2-CH_3 \xrightarrow{[O]} [?] \longrightarrow$$

$$CH_3-CHO + [?] + CH_3-CH_2OH \longrightarrow CH_3-COOH \longrightarrow CO_2 + ?- glucuronide$$

Eq. 9. Metabolism of diethyl ether.

$$H_2C=CH_2 \xrightarrow{[O]} [?] \longrightarrow CO_2 + [?]$$

Eq. 10. Metabolism of ethylene.

$$N_2O \longrightarrow [N_2O^-] \longrightarrow OH + OH^- + N_2$$

Eq. 11. Metabolism of nitrous oxide.

$$CHCl_3 \xrightarrow{[O]} CCl_3OH \longrightarrow Cl^- + COCl_2 \xrightarrow{HOH} CO_2 + 2Cl^-$$

$$\downarrow 2GSH$$

$$GSCOSG + 2Cl^-$$

$$\downarrow \gamma-glutamyl\ transpeptidase$$

$$OTZG$$

$$\downarrow HOH$$

$$OTZ$$

Eq. 12. Metabolism of chloroform.

$$Cl_2C=CHCl \xrightarrow{[O]} [?] \xrightarrow[migration]{Cl} CCl_3-CHO \xrightarrow{NAD} CCl_3-COOH$$

$$3Cl^- + CO \longleftarrow CCl_2-CHCl \qquad\qquad CCl_3-CH_2OH \Big\downarrow NADH$$

$$\overset{O}{\diagdown}$$

$$3Cl^- + CHO-COOH \quad [?] \qquad\qquad CCl_3-CH_2-O- glucuronide \Big\downarrow UDPG$$

Eq. 13. Metabolism of trichloroethylene.

these animals after fluroxene administration.[67,68] In humans, trifluoroethanol is produced in quantities too small to pose a clinical risk.[66] Fluroxene metabolism is increased in rats by pretreatment with the enzyme inducers phenobarbital, 3-methycholanthrene, 4-benzo[a]pyrene,[69,70] and pregnenolone-16α-carbonitrile.[68] Chronic exposure to fluroxene, like many other anesthetics, results in decreased hexobarbital sleeping time in rats.[37]

Halothane CF_3-$CHBrCl$ (See Eq. 15)

Halothane is extensively metabolized.[47,71,72] Its major metabolite in humans and animals is trifluoroacetic acid, which is formed during oxidative metabolism via cytochrome P-450. The urinary metabolites resulting from the oxidative pathway are the sodium salt of trifluoroacetic acid,[48,71] Cl^-, and Br^-.[72] Waskell and colleagues[20] demonstrated that two cytochromes P-450 are capable of oxidatively metabolizing halothane to trifluoroacetic acid. A presumed reactive intermediate of this oxidative pathway is trifluoroacetylchloride.[73] Other metabolites are speculative. Although significant amounts of trifluoroethanol have been identified in the urine of experimental animals, neither trifluoroethanol nor its glucuronide conjugates have been found in human urine. Likewise, another possible metabolite, trifluoroacetaldehyde, has not been isolated.

An alternative route of halothane metabolism is via a reductive pathway that requires the absence of oxygen and the presence of an electron donor. Both Br^- and F^- are metabolites of this pathway.[22,23,74,75] Two volatile metabolites (1,1-difluoro-2-chloroethylene [CDE] and 1,1,1-trifluoro-2-chloroethane [CTE]) and a volatile metabolite-decomposition product (1,1-difluoro-2-bromo-2-chloroethylene [DBE]) were first identified by gas chromatography-mass spectrometry in the exhaled gases of patients anesthetized with halothane.[76] The formation of CDE and the release of F^- in anaerobic hepatic microsomal incubations probably results from a cytochrome P-450-mediated two-electron reduction of halothane, while CTE formation and the production of free radicals results from a cytochrome P-450-mediated one-electron reduction.[24] The release of F^-, CDE, and DBE from halothane under anaerobic conditions can be catalyzed by reduced cytochrome P-450, hemoglobin, or hemin.[74] This finding suggests that the reaction is nonenzymatic and may only require reduced heme. In addition, suicidal inactivation of cytochrome P-450 has been demonstrated under hypoxic conditions (below 40 mmHg of O_2).[77] Presumably, inactivation is the result of cytochrome P-450 binding covalently to a reactive intermediate of CTE metabolism.

In experimental animals, increased halothane metabolism follows administration of inducing agents such as phenobarbital,[22,77,78] Aroclor 1254,[75,79] and isoniazid.[80] Prolonged exposure to subanesthetic concentrations of halothane results in increased drug metabolism in experimental animals[37,38] and humans.[39]

Methoxyflurane CH_3-O-CF_2-$CHCl_2$ (See Eq. 16)

Metabolism of methoxyflurane has been studied extensively, both in vivo and in vitro. The molecule can be oxygenated either at the methyl carbon or at the dichloroethyl carbon.[81,82] The major metabolites are F^-, dichloroacetic acid, and probably methoxydifluoroacetic acid, although the latter has not yet been isolated.[52,81,83] It is not known whether methoxydifluoroacetic acid is further metabolized in humans, although it would be expected to decompose in the acid environment of the kidneys and consequently release oxalic acid and additional F^-. Loew et al.[25] predicted from quantum mechanical calculations that the O-dealkylation of methoxyflurane occurs more rapidly than its dechlorination. The opposite was proposed by Holaday et al.[81] and was subsequently supported experimentally by Ivanetich et al.[84] Recently, Waskell et al.[11] identified two isozymes of cytochrome P-450 responsible for the O-demethylation of methoxyflurane. They also reported that cytochrome b_5 can act as the second electron donor and, at least in vitro, can stimulate significantly the metabolism of methoxyflurane by purified cytochromes P-450.[11,85]

In addition to cytochrome P-450-dependent metabolism, Warren et al. demonstrated that methoxyflurane can be defluorinated by both an enzymatic non-cytochrome P-450-dependent reaction[86] and a nonenzymatic[87] reaction. The enzymatic defluorination has been confirmed by Rice and colleagues[88,89] who suggested that the enzyme is glutathione-s-transferase. The nonenzymatic defluorination of methoxyflurane may not be significant in vivo; the reaction requires both glutathione and coenzyme B_{12} and shows an in vitro pH optimum of 10.[87]

Metabolism of methoxyflurane is increased in vivo and in vitro after treatment with enzyme-inducing drugs such as phenobarbital,[90,91] phenytoin,[42] ethanol,[15,16] diazepam,[92] and isoniazid.[17,18] Its metabolism is subject to inhibition in vivo and in vitro by SKF-525A[84,90,93] and in vitro by metyrapone.[84]

Enflurane CHF_2-O-CF_2-$CHClF$ (See Eq. 17)

Enflurane is slowly metabolized by the hepatic mixed-function oxidase system. The low reaction rate has complicated metabolism studies. Biotransformation releases F^- by oxidative dehalogenation. Initial oxidation may occur at the chlorofluoromethyl carbon or at the difluoromethyl carbon. Loew et al.[25] predicted that enflurane metabolism would occur primarily at the chlorofluoromethyl carbon. Studies of the metabolism of deuterated enflurane with rat hepatic microsomes[12] and the isolation of difluoromethoxy-difluoroacetic acid from rat liver[13] and human urine[13,94] support the prediction. Detection of insignificant amounts of chlorofluoroacetic acid suggest that there is very little metabolism at the difluoromethyl carbon.[13] The reactive intermediate formed from oxidation at the chlorofluor-

$$CF_3-CH_2-O-CH=CH_2 \xrightarrow{\text{[O]}} CF_3-CH_2OH + CH_2=CHO \longrightarrow \text{[?]} \longrightarrow CO_2$$

$$[CF_3-CH_2-O-CHOH-CH_2OH] \qquad [CF_3-CHO]$$

$$CO_2 + CF_3-CH_2OH \qquad CF_3-COOH$$

$$\downarrow \text{UDPG}$$

$$CF_3-CH_2-O-\text{glucuronide}$$

Eq. 14. Metabolism of fluroxene.

$$CF_3-CHBrCl \xrightarrow{\text{[O]}} [CF_3-COCl] + Br^- \xrightarrow{\text{HOH}} CF_3-COOH + Cl^-$$

$$\downarrow e^-$$

$$[CF_3-\overset{\cdot}{C}HBrCl] \longrightarrow CF_2=CBrCl + F^- \xrightarrow{\text{[GSH?]}} CH_2-S-CF_2CHBrCl$$

$$\underset{|}{CH-NHCOCH_3}$$

$$\xrightarrow{e^-} CF_2=CHCl + F^- + Br^- \qquad \underset{|}{COOH}$$

$$RH \diagdown \qquad [CF_3-\overset{\cdot}{C}HCl] + Br^- \qquad \downarrow \text{[O]}$$

$$R^\cdot \diagup \qquad CF_3-CH_2Cl \qquad \text{[?]} + F^-$$

Eq. 15. Metabolism of halothane.

$$CH_3-O-CF_2-CHCl_2 \xrightarrow{\text{[O]}} [CH_3-O-CF_2-CCl_2OH]$$

$$\downarrow \text{[O]} \qquad \qquad \downarrow$$

$$[CH_2OH-O-CF_2-CHCl_2] \qquad [CH_3-O-CF_2-CClO] + Cl^-$$

$$\downarrow \qquad \qquad \downarrow \text{HOH}$$

$$CH_2O + [CF_2OH-CHCl_2] \qquad CH_3-O-CF_2COOH + Cl^-$$

$$\downarrow$$

$$F^- + [CFO-CHCl_2]$$

$$\downarrow \text{HOH}$$

$$F^- + COOH-CHCl_2$$

$$\downarrow \text{[O]}$$

$$2Cl^- + COOH-COOH$$

Eq. 16. Metabolism of methoxyflurane.

omethyl carbon can either hydrolyze to produce difluoromethoxy-difluoroacetic acid or acetylate tissue protein to produce an adduct with immunogenic potential.[95]

Treatment with phenobarbital,[41,42,] phenytoin,[42] or ethanol[15,16] only slightly increases enflurane metabolism in rats. A study of surgical patients chronically consuming drugs such as phenobarbital, phenytoin, diazepam, and ethanol before anesthesia did not reveal enhanced F^- serum concentrations compared with untreated patients.[14] In contrast, about 50 percent of surgical patients on chronic isoniazid therapy demonstrated significantly elevated serum F^- concentrations.[19] Isoniazid also enhances enflurane metabolism in rats,[17,18] presumably by inducing a specific cytochrome P-450 isoenzyme. Deuteration studies have shown that isoniazid treatment in rats enhances metabolism only at the chlorofluoromethyl carbon.[12] From studies with phenobarbital and two enzyme inhibitors, SKF-525A and metyrapone, Ivanetich et al.[84] concluded that only one form of phenobarbital-induced cytochrome P-450 is involved in the metabolism of enflurane, while two forms are involved in the metabolism of methoxyflurane. This would explain in part the difference observed among anesthetics in the extent of in vitro defluorination after phenobarbital pretreatment. As with methoxyflurane, defluorination of enflurane is decreased after treatment with enzyme inhibitors SKF-525A and metyrapone.[84] Continuous exposure of rats to subanesthetic concentrations of enflurane significantly decreases hexobarbital sleeping time.[37] Exposure of mice to 0.5 percent enflurane for 5 days per week from 5 to 73 days did not alter hepatic microsomal cytochrome P-450 concentrations or defluorination rates of methoxyflurane, enflurane, or isoflurane; sevoflurane defluorination, however, was increased.[96]

Isoflurane CHF_2-O-$CHCl$-CF_3 (See Eq. 18)

Isoflurane was the most slowly metabolized of the fluorinated inhaled anesthetics[97-99] until the recent introduction of I-653 (CHF_2-O-CHF-CF_3).[100] What little metabolism there is results from oxidation of the α-carbon. As with enflurane, the difluoromethyl carbon of isoflurane is resistant to oxidation.[13] However, traces of trifluoroacetic acid may be excreted in the urine of rats and humans. Trifluoroacetaldehyde and trifluoroacetylchloride, expected intermediates between isoflurane and trifluoroacetic acid, may also be produced. Although phenobarbital,[91,99] phenytoin,[42] ethanol,[15] and isoniazid[17,18] pretreatments increase the defluorination of isoflurane, enzyme induction has not produced serum F^- concentrations of clinical significance.[97-99] Prolonged exposure to subanesthetic concentrations of isoflurane enhances the hexobarbital sleeping time of experimental rats.[37] Mice exposed to as much as 0.5 percent isoflurane for 4 hours per day, 5 days per week for 9 weeks had no significant changes in activity of hepatic microsomal cytochromes P-450 or b_5 or in de-

fluorination rates of methoxyflurane, enflurane, and isoflurane.[101]

Sevoflurane CH_2F-O-CH-$(CF_3)_2$ (See Eq. 19)

The in vitro rate of sevoflurane defluorination is approximately the same as that of methoxyflurane.[102,103] In vivo, however, there is far less serum F^- found with sevoflurane than with methoxyflurane.[102,104] The α-carbon is the most likely site of oxidation of sevoflurane rather than the trifluoromethyl carbons. In one study in human volunteers, nonvolatile organic fluoride (80 percent hexafluoroisopropanol) was detected in the blood and urine of volunteers anesthetized with sevoflurane.[104] Hexafluoroisopropanol is not subject to further degradation, although conjugation could be possible. Studies in patients and volunteers have shown that much of the metabolism to F^- occurs during exposure, presumably because of the low tissue solubility of sevoflurane and the stability of its metabolites.[104-107] Peak serum F^- concentrations are reached within a few hours of the end of anesthesia. In vivo studies have shown increased sevoflurane defluorination in rats after phenobarbital treatment.[103] In vitro, sevoflurane defluorination is increased in rat hepatic microsomes by pretreatment with phenytoin,[42] isoniazid,[17,18] ethanol,[16] and phenobarbital.[42,103]

Desflurane CHF_2-O-CHF-CF_3 (See Eq. 20)

Desflurane (I-653) is a new experimental volatile anesthetic with low lipid and blood solubility.[100] There is significantly less metabolism of I-653 to F^- and nonvolatile organic fluoride compounds in rats compared with isoflurane. Peak serum F^- concentrations in rats are seen about 4 hours after exposure. Routes of metabolism have not been published, but the molecule could be expected to be metabolized in a manner similar to isoflurane. Substitution of a fluorine in I-653 for the chlorine in isoflurane decreases the metabolism at the α-carbon. Pretreatment with phenobarbital or ethanol enhances serum F^- concentrations.[100]

TOXICITY

Mechanisms of Toxicity

The expression of drug toxicity is a function of various factors. In this section, we focus on mechanisms of tissue injury that are experimentally reproducible and consistent from one individual to another and not on those that are the result of a rare hereditary trait (i.e., inborn metabolic error). Three general mechanisms of drug toxicity apply to tissue injury associated with the inhaled anesthetics. They are the intracellular accumulation of metabolites in toxic amounts, the formation of haptens that can initiate systemic hypersensitivity or immune responses, and the production of reactive in-

$$CHF_2{-}O{-}CF_2{-}CHClF \xrightarrow{\quad [O] \quad} [CHF_2{-}O{-}CF_2{-}CClFOH]$$

$$\downarrow [O] \qquad\qquad\qquad\qquad\qquad \downarrow [O]$$

$$CF_2O + [CF_2OH{-}CHClF] \qquad\qquad CHF_2{-}O{-}CF_2{-}CFO + Cl^-$$

$$\downarrow HOH \qquad\qquad \downarrow \qquad\qquad\qquad\qquad \downarrow HOH$$

$$CO_2 + 2F^- \quad CFO{-}CHClF + F^- \qquad\qquad CHF_2{-}O{-}CF_2{-}COOH + F^-$$

$$\downarrow HOH$$

$$COOH{-}CHClF + F^-$$

Eq. 17. Metabolism of enflurane.

$$CHF_2{-}O{-}CHCl{-}CF_3 \xrightarrow{\quad [O] \quad} [CHF_2{-}O{-}CClOH{-}CF_3]$$

$$\downarrow [O] \qquad\qquad\qquad\qquad\qquad \downarrow$$

$$CF_2O + [CHClOH{-}CF_3] \qquad\qquad [CHF_2{-}O{-}CO{-}CF_3] + Cl^-$$

$$\downarrow HOH \qquad\qquad \downarrow$$

$$CO_2 + 2F^- \quad CHO{-}CF_3 + Cl^-$$

$$\downarrow$$

$$COOH{-}CF_3$$

Eq. 18. Metabolism of isoflurane.

$$CH_2F{-}O{-}CH{-}(CF_3)_2 \xrightarrow{\quad [O] \quad} CHOH{-}(CF_3)_2 + CH_2O + F^-$$

$$\downarrow$$

$$CO_2$$

Eq. 19. Metabolism of sevoflurane.

$$CHF_2{-}O{-}CHF{-}CF_3 \xrightarrow{\quad [O] \quad} [CHF_2{-}O{-}C\,FOH{-}CF_3]$$

$$\downarrow [O] \qquad\qquad\qquad\qquad\qquad \downarrow$$

$$CF_2O + [CHFOH{-}CF_3] \qquad\qquad [CHF_2{-}O{-}CO{-}CF_3] + F^-$$

$$\downarrow HOH \qquad\qquad \downarrow$$

$$CO_2 + 2F^- \quad [CHO{-}CF_3] + F^-$$

$$\downarrow$$

$$[COOH{-}CF_3]$$

Eq. 20. Metabolism of desflurane (I-653).

termediates that either adduct (form covalent bonds) to tissue macromolecules or initiate destructive free radical chain reactions. Additionally, there is a physicochemical reaction of N_2O with vitamin B_{12}.

Each of the above mechanisms, except for the vitamin B_{12} reaction, depends on metabolism of the parent anesthetic compound. Accumulation of metabolites in toxic quantities may occur because of increased production or decreased excretion. Other chemicals or pathologic states may modify drug metabolism and thereby initiate metabolite accumulation. When the concentration of a drug metabolite surpasses the intracellular threshold for toxicity, tissue injury results from the direct or indirect actions of the metabolite. Direct toxicity may result from the inhibition or modification of enzymatic and structural systems necessary for maintaining cellular integrity (e.g., membrane transport systems). Indirect toxicity may result from unwanted pharmacologic actions that are toxic to the target cell. An example is local tissue ischemia and cellular necrosis after accumulation of a metabolite possessing vasoconstrictive properties.

Probably the most important drug-mediated toxic mechanism is the production of reactive intermediates during drug metabolism. Reactive intermediates are thought to initiate toxicity in two ways: they can covalently bind with macromolecules to form adducts[108,109] or they can initiate aberrant free radical chain reactions.[110,111] Although few drugs are sufficiently reactive themselves to form covalent bonds with cell macromolecules (e.g., intracellular proteins, enzymes, nucleic acids), some drugs, including several inhaled anesthetics,[112] may produce reactive intermediates during phase I metabolism that are capable of doing so.

The binding of a reactive intermediate with tissue protein to produce a hapten-protein conjugate is one example of a potentially toxic covalent interaction. The conjugate may in turn induce the synthesis of drug or metabolite-specific antibodies and initiate hypersensitivity or immune responses.[113] Another way in which binding of reactive intermediates to tissue macromolecules might be harmful is by affecting cellular organelles such as the endoplasmic reticulum, mitochondria, lysosomes, and nucleus.[114] Yet other detrimental effects of covalent binding can result from depletion of endogenous cellular compounds necessary for normal cell function. Intracellular glutathione and other sulfhydryl-containing compounds function as natural cellular antioxidants and are necessary for cellular homeostasis.[115] When depleted of glutathione, the cell is susceptible to oxidant effects such as those produced by cytochrome P-450-mediated monooxygenases, which continue to function in the absence of intracellular substrate by transferring electrons to cell lipids.[116] Normally, glutathione can conjugate the free radical and thus interrupt destructive chain reactions. In the absence of glutathione, destructive reactions continue and cell death can ensue.

Highly reactive intermediates such as arene oxides (a type of epoxide) may covalently bind to proteins, nucleic acids, and other cellular components.[117] The chemically stable adducts formed with arene oxides and with many other classes of reactive intermediates may produce a variety of injuries such as hepatic necrosis,[115,118] mutagenesis, teratogenesis and carcinogenesis,[26,108,119,120] and drug allergies.[113]

In addition to producing nucleophilic intermediates, metabolism may produce intermediates with single unpaired electrons in their outer molecular orbital shells, known as free radicals. These are short-lived but highly reactive intermediates that can initiate chain reactions and produce pathologic damage.[110,121]

Free radical chain reactions consist of three phases. During the initiation phase, free radicals are generated by a single reaction or series of reactions. The propagation phase consists of a sequence of reactions that conserve or increase the numbers of free radicals. The termination phase is the destruction or inactivation of the generated free radicals. Once generated, radicals react with cellular components producing polymerization or cross-linking of enzymes and proteins, autoxidation of lipids within the organelle membranes, and damage to nucleic acids (e.g., main chain breaks in the nucleic acid strands or degradation of purine and pyrimidine rings).[114,122] Free radicals are generated during the normal course of cell metabolism,[116] but their concentration is stringently maintained at less than 10^{-9} M.[111,121] It is only when aberrant radical reactions occur and endogenous antioxidants (e.g., glutathione) are depleted that tissue injury results.[110]

Generally, reactions of free radical intermediates are assumed to be so rapid that no radicals escape the tissue in which they are formed.[114] Since the inhaled anesthetics are strongly lipophilic, damage from their reactive intermediates occurs mainly in lipid membranes, which are especially rich in unsaturated fatty acids. These unsaturated compounds are highly susceptible to damage because the presence of a double bond weakens the carbon-hydrogen bond of the α-methylene carbon atom (i.e., the carbon atom adjacent to the carbon with an unsaturated bond). Free radicals initiate peroxidation by abstracting hydrogen from the α-methylene carbon.[111,122] This results in rearrangement of double bonds and subsequent attack by oxygen and cleavage of the radical. Unless terminated, the oxidative damage will be transferred to adjacent fatty acids. Halothane and chloroform, at anesthetizing concentrations, stimulate lipoperoxidation in vivo in phenobarbital-pretreated rats and are thought by some to initiate tissue damage by this mechanism.[123]

The detrimental effects of reactive intermediates on cell integrity depend on the extent of free radical reactions and covalent binding and on the cellular functions that are impaired. The precise mechanism, however, by which specific reactive intermediates initiate cellular injury is seldom clear. One reason is that total binding of a reactive intermediate does not correlate well with the degree of toxicity. For example, although the metabolites of certain chemical carcinogens have been found to bind covalently to liver microsomes, there is no strict correlation between adduction and cell damage.[124] Furthermore, it is nearly impossible to determine experimentally which cellular function is impaired first because adduction to nontarget sites may be greater than to target sites.

Acute Toxicity

Effects on the Liver

Clinically, drug-mediated hepatotoxicity ranges in severity from slight dysfunction to massive hepatic necrosis. The cause may be hepatocellular damage, interference with bilirubin metabolism, or cholestasis. Direct hepatocellular damage is probably responsible for most cases of inhaled anesthetic-mediated hepatotoxicity. Direct hepatotoxins cause dose-related, consistent, and reproducible hepatic damage in humans and animals. Two examples are carbon tetrachloride and chloroform. Some hepatotoxins produce their toxic effects by hypersensitivity and humoral or cellular immune reactions. Examples are erythromycin, cloxacillin, and halothane.[113]

The extent of hepatotoxicity directly attributable to inhaled anesthetics is difficult to determine. Several factors may predispose the liver to postoperative dysfunction and necrosis, including chronic liver disease, viral infection (e.g., viral hepatitis and cytomegalovirus), septicemia, severe burns, pregnancy, nutritional deficiency, and previous or concomitant drug treatment. Additionally, hypoxia, hypercarbia, and hypotension may contribute to the liver damage. Strunin[125] suggests that anesthetics produce postoperative liver dysfunction indirectly by changing liver blood flow rather than directly by damaging liver cells. Certainly, many surgical procedures are followed by minor adverse changes in liver function that depend more on the site of surgery than on anesthetic technique.[126,127]

All anesthetic techniques reduce liver blood flow to some degree.[127] Although studies in healthy volunteers have demonstrated no evidence of hypoxia or anaerobic metabolism in the liver, this may not be the case for patients with pre-existing liver damage or other illnesses. In general, surgical manipulation appears to be a more important factor in decreasing liver blood flow than are the effects of the anesthetic agents.[127] Unfortunately, tests available to assess liver function are for the most part crude, not tissue specific, and only reflect abnormalities in the presence of severe disorders. Traditional measures of liver function are serum proteins, enzymes, and bilirubin. A change in serum enzymes may indicate leakage from damaged cells, failure of biliary secretion, or failure of synthesis. None of the enzymes routinely measured is entirely specific to the liver. Although isoenzymes are occasionally measured to improve tissue specificity, only the aminotransferases and alkaline phosphatase have stood the test of time for characterizing hepatic damage. Two aminotransferases routinely measured are aspartate aminotransferase (AsT), formerly called serum glutamate oxaloacetate transaminase (SGOT), and alanine aminotransferase (AlT), formally called serum glutamate pyruvate transaminase (SGPT). AsT is present in large amounts in the heart, liver, kidneys, and skeletal muscles. It is primarily a cytoplasmic enzyme and often is elevated after surgery, liver damage, and myocardial infarction. Although the concentration of AlT in the liver is less than of AsT, this enzyme is more specific to the liver, and significant elevations above normal concentrations are considered characteristic of hepatocellular damage. Hepatotoxicity associated with specific inhaled anesthetics is discussed in the following paragraphs.

Chloroform was discovered in 1831 and was first used in humans in 1847.[128] The first two cases of jaundice and death were observed in the same year.[129] In 1912, the Committee of Anesthesia of the American Medical Association recommended that chloroform no longer be used as an anesthetic because it produced an unacceptable incidence of liver and cardiovascular collapse.[130] Nevertheless, chloroform continued to be used until 1957.

Several investigators have observed covalent binding of chloroform or its metabolites to hepatic tissues. Cohen and Hood[59] performed low-temperature whole-body autoradiographic studies on mice administered $^{14}CHCl_3$ by inhalation. Nonvolatile radioactivity (i.e., metabolites) was confined to the liver. Illett et al.[60] measured increased covalent binding of ^{14}C after the administration of $^{14}CHCl_3$ to mice pretreated with phenobarbital. When animals were pretreated with piperonyl butoxide, another enzyme-inhibiting agent, decreased covalent binding was measured that closely paralleled decreased hepatocellular damage. Brown[123] demonstrated lipoperoxidation in rats pretreated with phenobarbital and subsequently treated with chloroform. When chloroform metabolism was inhibited by SKF-525A (2-diethylamine-2,2-diphenglyalerate HCl) or DPPD (N,N^1-diphenyl-p-phenylenediamine), lipoperoxidation was decreased. The enhanced covalent binding and lipoperoxidation in enzyme-induced animals provides strong circumstantial evidence for the formation of a reactive chloroform metabolite that initiates hepatotoxicity. More recent work has shown that chloroform is metabolized to phosgene ($COCl_2$) by hepatic microsomal cytochrome P-450.[56,57] $COCl_2$ probably attacks nucleophilic sites on hepatic macromolecules and initiates a cascade of unknown events that lead to hepatocellular damage.[57,58]

In 1905, Bevan and Favill[131] concluded that diethyl ether is hepatotoxic on the basis of four case reports. Later reviews of the cases, however, led to doubt about their conclusion. In experimental animals, diethyl ether has produced fatty changes and extensive degeneration in the liver but not to the extent observed with the classic hepatotoxin, chloroform.[132]

There are no case reports of hepatic necrosis after N_2O administration when hypoxia has been ruled out as a possible contributing factor. However, several cases of hepatic necrosis have been reported when N_2O was combined with intravenous barbiturate administration.[133-136] Continuous exposure of rats to 20 percent N_2O for as long as 35 days produced no significant changes in liver serum enzymes or in glutathione content.[53] The overwhelming evidence suggests that N_2O has little potential for producing hepatotoxicity.

Cyclopropane was first implicated as a possible hepatotoxin in a 1964 report of three patients who developed hepatic dysfunction after its use with other anesthetics.[137] Since then, there have been various case reports linking cyclopropane to hepatic damage.[134-136] The National Halothane Study reported that massive hepatic necrosis after cyclopropane administration occurred with an incidence of 1.70 in 10,000.[138] However, in 24 of the 25 cases cited, the patients were in shock and the outcome of hepatic necrosis might have been due to anesthetizing patients with already compromised blood flow rather than to the direct effect of cyclopropane.

Fluroxene was introduced in 1953 and was the first volatile fluorinated anesthetic used in humans.[139] In 1972, Reynolds et al.[140] reported that a patient treated with phenobarbital and phenytoin and then anesthetized with fluroxene died from massive hepatic necrosis. Further evidence implicating fluroxene in hepatic necrosis was provided by studies of experimental animals. Exposure to fluroxene produced no toxicity in enzyme-inhibited mice[141] but produced death from massive hepatic necrosis in enzyme-induced cats.[142] Necrosis after enzyme induction was presumed due to formation of free radicals or epoxidation of fluroxene's vinyl (—C=C—) moiety. Postanesthetic deaths in dogs, cats, and rabbits after exposure to trifluoroethanol, a known metabolite of fluroxene, suggested that this compound was responsible for the liver damage.[143] Recent work with various enzyme-inducing agents in rats has conclusively shown that the rate of metabolism of fluroxene to trifluoroethanol determines the severity of hepatic damage.[68] Fluroxene has now been withdrawn from clinical use.

Halothane was prepared by Suckling[144] in 1952 and was introduced into clinical practice in 1956.[145,146] Several clinical reports of postoperative jaundice and liver necrosis were published in 1963.[147-149] The clinical and pathologic findings resembled those of the classic hepatotoxin, chloroform. The reports prompted a number of retrospective studies, from which it was generally concluded that halothane was associated with the same incidence of postoperative hepatic damage as other anesthetics. Because some fault could be found in all the retrospective studies (e.g., lack of proper control groups or inadequate numbers), the U.S. National Halothane Study was undertaken.[138,150] A committee reviewed retrospectively the incidence of fatal massive hepatic necrosis occurring in approximately 850,000

surgical patients. The incidence of massive hepatic necrosis associated with halothane was 7 of 250,000 halothane anesthetics or about 1 in 35,000, and not 1 in 10,000 as is sometimes reported. The committee concluded that "unexplained fever and jaundice in a specific patient following halothane might reasonably be considered a contraindication to subsequent use." However, Dykes and Bunker[151] reported that there were no patients in the National Halothane Study who were jaundiced after halothane administration and who died following a second administration of halothane in whom necropsy documented a massive or intermediate hepatic necrosis.

In 1972, Strunin and Simpson[152] reviewed various reports and concluded that the data could be arranged to support or deny almost any hypothesis linking halothane anesthesia to liver damage. The situation is confused because much of the pre-1970s data supporting the hypothesis that halothane causes liver damage have not withstood critical examination. Nonetheless, it is now clear that halothane anesthesia is associated occasionally with liver damage in adults, especially after repeated administration.[153-156] Even children, once thought immune to "halothane hepatitis," are now known to be susceptible.[157,158] It now appears that there are two separate clinical entities, one a mild hepatoxicity occurring shortly after halothane exposure and the other a rare, severe, often fatal hepatoxicity with delayed onset.

Because halothane hepatitis is both rare and unpredictable, it has been speculated that some patients are predisposed to the condition either because they produce unusual levels of toxic metabolites or because they undergo an immunologic response that initiates hepatotoxicity. The latter mechanism has been proposed to explain the increased frequency and the overall reduced latency of hepatitis after repeated halothane exposure. The immunologic basis for halothane hepatitis has been discussed in several recent articles.[113,159,160] The first suggestive human data came in 1980 when it was demonstrated that sera from 7 of 11 patients with fulminant hepatic necrosis after halothane exposure contained an antibody that reacted with the surface of hepatocytes isolated from halothane-exposed rabbits.[161] The antibody, however, was not present in sera from patients with mild liver dysfunction after halothane exposure.[161,162] It was unclear whether this antibody initiated hepatocellular damage or was present as a result of the damage. More recent work has revealed that antibodies from patients with halothane hepatitis recognize antigens that contain the trifluoroacetyl group derived from oxidative halothane metabolism.[163]

The lack of a suitable animal model hampered early efforts to elucidate the mechanism of halothane-mediated hepatotoxicity. Unlike chloroform and fluroxene, which produce fatty infiltration, centrilobular necrosis, and elevated transaminase values in experimental animals, halothane did not produce hepatotoxicity in early animal studies. Even prolonged exposure to halothane did not consistently result in hepatic lesions.

Animal models of halothane-mediated hepatoxicity were eventually developed that proved useful in determining the role of biotransformation in hepatic injury. In several models, inducers of drug metabolism were used even though enhanced biotransformation has not been implicated in the pathogenesis of halothane hepatitis in humans. Centrilobular necrosis after halothane exposure occurs in rats pretreated with Aroclor 1254 (a mixture of polychlorinated biphenyls),[75,79] triiodothyronine,[167,168] and phenobarbital and isoniazid.[80,164-166]

The Aroclor 1254 model was abandoned because polychlorinated biphenyls themselves cause moderate alterations in liver ultrastructure and function. The halothane-hypoxic model is based on the observation that reductive metabolism of halothane occurs in vitro under hypoxic conditions[22-24,74] and is associated with increased covalent binding of reductive metabolites to liver protein and phospholipids.[22] Hepatic necrosis is produced in phenobarbital-pretreated rats exposed to halothane under hypoxic conditions ($FiO_2 = 7$ to 14 percent).[164-166] The hepatic lesion in this model is centrilobular in origin and similar to that seen in humans. The centrilobular area has the lowest oxygen concentration and the highest metabolic rate and thus is most susceptible to hypoxic injury. Lesion intensity depends on both the degree of enzyme induction and the degree of hypoxia for the production of reactive intermediates in the process of reductive metabolism. Although the model is reproducible and well defined, its clinical relevance is questionable because hypoxia is needed for lesion production. The mechanism by which reductive metabolism of halothane leads to hepatotoxicity remains obscure, although presumably it involves a one-electron reduction of halothane via cytochrome P-450, producing Br^- and a free radical that subsequently causes direct hepatocellular damage. However, some investigators have implicated hypoxia per se in the production of hepatic necrosis.[169-172] It is difficult to decide whether the reactive intermediates of reductive halothane metabolism[173] or hypoxia[171,172] and a halothane-induced decrease in liver perfusion[174] are responsible for the hepatic necrosis observed in the halothane-hypoxic rat model.

Several models have not utilized enzyme induction. The triiodothyronine (T_3) rat model does not rely on enhanced reductive halothane metabolism.[167,168] Thus, it appears that this model also may cause hepatotoxicity by producing relative cellular oxygen deprivation. Certainly, T_3-treated rats have a higher than normal oxygen consumption and develop hepatoxicity immediately after halothane exposure under normoxic conditions.[167] Another model not utilizing enzyme induction is the Institute of Medical and Veterinary Science (IMVS) guinea pig model.[175,176] A mild to severe hepatic injury was produced in 20 to 60 percent of male guinea pigs exposed for 4 hours to 1 percent halothane at an

FiO_2 of 0.21. The toxic mechanisms is unclear since 24-hour urinary excretions of both reductive (i.e., F^-) and oxidative (i.e., trifluoroacetic acid) metabolites were significantly elevated after halothane exposure.[175] Susceptibility to halothane-induced hepatotoxicity was not uniform among animals. Even repeated halothane exposure did not produce toxicity in guinea pigs not exhibiting elevated serum transaminases after initial halothane exposure.[176] A genetic predisposition to the development of hepatotoxicity in these animals was demonstrated; offspring of susceptible guinea pigs were susceptible themselves, while offspring of nonsusceptible animals were not.[176] The mechanism for hepatotoxicity in this model, however, remains obscure.

It now appears that neither hypoxia per se nor reductively generated reactive intermediates are the likely cause for the fulminant hepatic necrosis seen in humans. Recent evidence points to trifluoroacetylation of tissue protein, an oxidation-dependent reaction, as a causative factor. The isoniazid model has provided evidence that the oxidative pathway is involved in halothane hepatoxicity.[80] The model is characterized by significant elevations in serum transaminase levels and severe to moderate disruption in hepatic morphology in all rats treated with isoniazid after exposure to halothane under normoxic conditions. Oxidative but not reductive metabolism of halothane is stimulated in such rats, strongly suggesting that reactive intermediates of oxidative, not reductive, metabolism are responsible for the observed hepatoxicity.

Methoxyflurane was first synthesized in the United States in 1958 and introduced clinically in 1960.[177] Although none of the metabolites of methoxyflurane is known to be hepatotoxic, there have been a number of reports of hepatic dysfunction and death from hepatic coma after methoxyflurane exposure. In a review of 24 cases of methoxyflurane-associated hepatitis, Joshi and Conn[178] presented evidence for a syndrome similar to that described in 1976 by Walton et al.[156] for unexplained hepatitis following halothane administration. These workers concluded that a rare and indirect immunologic hepatic injury may occur that may have a direct effect on the liver by interfering with splanchnic circulation.[125,179,180] In humans, the adverse minor changes in liver function,[181] as well as the changes seen in isolated liver preparations,[125] appear to be reversible and may be dose related. It is still unclear whether hepatic dysfunction, as measured by Bromsulphalein (BSP) retention and serum hepatic enzyme elevation, was the result of the depth and duration of the anesthetic exposure, the type of operation, the extent of pre-existing hepatic disease, or methoxyflurane itself.

Enflurane was first used in North America in 1966.[182,183] Of the approximately 45 million enflurane anesthetics administered since that time, only a few isolated case reports of liver damage have been associated with its use.[184-187] In 1983, Lewis et al.[188] reported 24 cases of suspected enflurane-induced hepatoxicity. Seven of the cases had been previously published. The validity of their conclusions has been questioned because critical gaps in the individual case reports raise doubts of the accuracy of the information presented. Data on the duration of anesthetic exposure and the histologic confirmation of hepatic lesions were not presented for many subjects. Thus, the accuracy of other information (i.e., previous exposure to viral hepatitis or potential hepatotoxin) is in doubt. In addition, several patients were hypotensive and in shock and underwent operations with known potential for hepatic dysfunction. Eger et al.[189] concluded that the evidence did not support the existence of an enflurane-induced hepatic necrosis similar to that seen with halothane. Evidence from rat models of both enflurane and isoflurane hepatotoxicity suggests that liver dysfunction occurs only under conditions of severe hypoxia (FiO_2 = 7 to 10 percent).[170] These observations may be solely the result of hypoxic injury.[171]

Several case reports suggested that halothane exposure may have sensitized the patient and that subsequent anesthesia with enflurane resulted in hepatotoxicity.[190,191] Recently, Christ et al.[192] produced covalently bound acetylated protein adducts from halothane and enflurane in a rat model. The adducts were recognized by specific anti-trifluoroacetylated protein antibodies from the sera of six patients with halothane hepatitis. This cross-reactivity suggests that enflurane has the potential to produce an immune-mediated hepatotoxic response. Since the metabolism of enflurane is significantly less than that of halothane, presumably fewer antigenic tissue adducts are formed, with a correspondingly smaller likelihood of toxicity.

Sevoflurane is an experimental drug that was withdrawn from clinical testing in 1980. There have been several reports regarding its metabolism[102–107] and possible renal toxicity,[102–104,106] but only one reported an evaluation of hepatic function. In that study, five human volunteers showed no significant changes in transaminase and hepatic function measured up to 4 weeks after exposure.[104] The one animal study of untreated, phenobarbital-treated, and Aroclor 1254-treated rats exposed to sevoflurane likewise showed no significant changes in serum transaminases, liver triglycerides, or glutathione concentrations.[193]

Effects on the Kidney

Inhaled anesthetics depress renal function. They decrease urine flow, glomerular filtration rate, renal blood flow, and electrolyte excretion. These changes are usually secondary to effects on the cardiovascular, sympathetic, and endocrine systems and almost always return to normal shortly after anesthesia and surgery. If they persist for any length of time into the postanesthesia period, the cause is often a combination of factors such as prior existence of renal or cardiovascular disease, severe fluid and electrolyte imbalance, and the administration of mismatched blood; the choice of anesthetic is usually unimportant. Such causes should be recognized but are not true toxic reactions and as such

will not be considered further. Occasionally, however, the inorganic fluoride (F⁻) that is released during metabolism of fluorinated anesthetics may be directly nephrotoxic. Methoxyflurane is the classic example, and although this agent is seldom used in clinical practice, its nephrotoxicity is discussed as a basis for understanding the nephrotoxic potential of all current and future fluorinated anesthetics.

Methoxyflurane

Vasopressin-resistant polyuric renal insufficiency was first reported in 1966 in patients receiving prolonged methoxyflurane anesthesia for abdominal surgery.[194] Subsequently, evidence was gathered indicating that the causative agent was F⁻, an end product of the biotransformation of methoxyflurane. The evidence was based on three observations. First, serum F⁻ concentrations after methoxyflurane administration in humans show positive correlation with the degree of renal dysfunction.[195] Second, vasopressin-resistant polyuric renal insufficiency similar to that seen in humans after prolonged methoxyflurane anesthesia can be elicited easily in male Fischer 344 rats injected with sodium fluoride.[196] Finally, F⁻ is a potent inhibitor of many enzyme systems including those involving antidiuretic hormone.[197] Fischer 344 rats are excellent models for studying F⁻ nephropathy because they demonstrate renal changes after F⁻ administration similar to those seen in humans, including polyuria, hypernatremia, serum hyperosmolality, increased blood urea nitrogen (BUN) and creatinine (Cr) levels, and decreased BUN and Cr clearances. Furthermore, they have about the same serum F⁻ threshold for renal dysfunction as do humans.

The extent of nephrotoxicity in general surgical patients has been correlated with methoxyflurane dosage (in minimum alveolar concentration [MAC]-hours, that is, end-tidal concentration as a fraction of MAC times the duration of anesthesia, in hours) and peak serum F⁻ concentrations.[198] After 2.5 to 3.0 MAC-hours methoxyflurane, which corresponds to peak serum F⁻ concentrations of 50 to 80 μM, patients had subclinical toxicity characterized by a delayed return to maximum preoperative urinary osmolality, elevated serum urate concentration, and decreased urate clearance. Had a vasopressin resistance test been performed on these surgical patients, the threshold methoxyflurane dosage and serum F⁻ concentration to produce subclinical toxicity undoubtedly would have been lower. After 5 MAC-hours methoxyflurane, serum F⁻ concentrations were 90 to 120 μM, and patients had well-established but mild nephrotoxicity manifested by serum hyperosmolality, hypernatremia, polyuria, and urinary hypo-osmolality. Seven to 9 MAC-hours methoxyflurane led to serum F⁻ concentrations up to 175 μM and marked nephrotoxicity.

Despite the overall correlation between nephrotoxicity and peak serum F⁻ concentrations, individual patients given the same methoxyflurane dosage vary in their nephrotoxic susceptibility. Genetic heterogeneity, drug interaction, pre-existence of renal disease, and a host of other factors could account for the differences observed among patients. One example of a drug interaction is the additive nephrotoxic effect seen in patients receiving both methoxyflurane and the aminoglycoside antibiotic gentamicin.[199] The same effect is seen in Fischer 344 rats, in which concurrent administration of methoxyflurane and gentamicin produces greater nephrotoxicity than expected from either drug alone.[200]

Methoxyflurane is a potent anesthetic and an excellent analgesic and is still considered by some anesthetists to be a desirable drug. Its nephrotoxic potential, however, has all but eliminated it from clinical use. In an attempt to reduce the resultant production of F^-, several investigators have substituted deuterium (D) for hydrogen in the methoxyflurane molecule. The rationale is that the C-D bond is less chemically reactive than the C-H bond, and thus, metabolism is slowed if cleavage of the C-H bond is a rate-limiting reaction. Data from both in vitro and in vivo studies indicate that when all four hydrogens in methoxyflurane are replaced by deuterium, there is a significant but small decrease in F^- production.[201–203] Furthermore, unlike ordinary methoxyflurane, the metabolism of completely deuterated methoxyflurane is not enhanced after enzyme induction with phenobarbital.[203] Unfortunately, the overall reduction in F^- production and the possible benefit to enzyme-induced patients are not sufficient to offer a significant clinical advantage.

Other Fluorinated Anesthetics

Because modern volatile anesthetics are fluorinated to reduce their flammability, theoretically, they all possess nephrotoxic potential. Of those currently available, halothane, enflurane, and isoflurane are in widespread clinical use, whereas sevoflurane and I-653 are in the developmental stage. Halothane is not significantly defluorinated under normal clinical conditions and thus is not nephrotoxic. Defluorination is enhanced slightly under conditions of hypoxia and enzyme induction, but not to an extent associated with renal damage.[164,165] On the other hand, enflurane defluorination may occasionally result in serum F^- concentrations high enough to produce mild renal impairment. In a study with Fischer 344 rats, 6 to 10 hours of 2.5 percent enflurane anesthesia produced a mild vasopressin-resistant polyuric renal dysfunction.[40] Peak serum F^- concentrations were 40 to 57 μM, just reaching the threshold for renal toxicity.

Surgical patients almost never show renal dysfunction after enflurane anesthesia.[204] Although serum F^- concentrations postanesthesia are significantly higher than background concentrations, they seldom reach the threshold for nephrotoxicity. In comparison with methoxyflurane, serum F^- concentrations after enflurane anesthesia peak earlier and fall more rapidly, em-phasizing the important role that lipid solubility has in determining total F^- concentration production (Fig. 6-3). In one study, peak serum F^- concentrations from nine surgical patients averaged 22.2 μM following enflurane exposures averaging 2.7 MAC-hours.[205] The only controlled human study to show mild renal dysfunction after enflurane anesthesia involved 11 healthy volunteers.[206] After 9.6 MAC-hours of enflurane, maximum urinary osmolality following antidiuretic hormone administration was reduced from approximately 1,050 to 800 mOsm/kg; mean serum F^- concentration was 33.6 μM. The mild impairment of renal concentrating ability was not associated with hypernatremia, serum hyperosmolality, or increased serum creatinine or urea nitrogen and therefore was not regarded as clinically significant. Some clinicians have speculated that enflurane administered to patients with significant pre-existing renal disease could produce additional renal dysfunction. Such fears have not been borne out in studies of Fischer 344 rats with surgically induced chronic renal insufficiency.[207,208] Furthermore, results of a study of patients with mild to moderate renal insufficiency showed no clinically significant difference between preoperative and postoperative renal function after either enflurane or halothane administration.[209]

Isoflurane, an isomer of enflurane, is defluorinated much less than enflurane. In nine surgical patients, mean peak serum F^- concentration measured 6 hours after anesthesia was only 4.4 μM.[99] Thus, isoflurane is not associated with F^- nephrotoxicity.

Sevoflurane is a new fluorinated ether anesthetic with a low blood/gas partition coefficient of approximately 0.6. Results of in vitro studies indicate that it is defluorinated more than enflurane but less than methoxyflurane.[17,91] In a study of six healthy volunteers, serum F^- concentrations averaged 22 μM by the end of a 1-hour exposure to 3 percent sevoflurane and had fallen to low levels by 24 hours after anesthesia.[104] Peak serum F^- concentrations, however, were not measured, and anesthesia for longer than 1 hour was not performed. The clinical safety of this drug with respect to metabolism to fluoride ion has yet to be established in more extensive human studies.

I-653 is another new fluorinated volatile anesthetic that is being considered for clinical use. Preliminary animal studies indicate that its defluorination is even less than that of isoflurane, and it is therefore unlikely to have any nephrotoxic potential.[100]

Role of Enzyme Induction in Anesthetic Nephrotoxicity

Because the volatile inhaled anesthetics are defluorinated by the mixed-function oxidase system (cytochrome P-450), drugs that induce the enzymes of this system may lead to increased F^- production and nephrotoxicity. This effect has been clearly demonstrated with methoxyflurane; both Fischer 344 rats[210] and human volunteers[198] chronically pretreated with the classic enzyme inducers phenobarbital or pentobarbi-

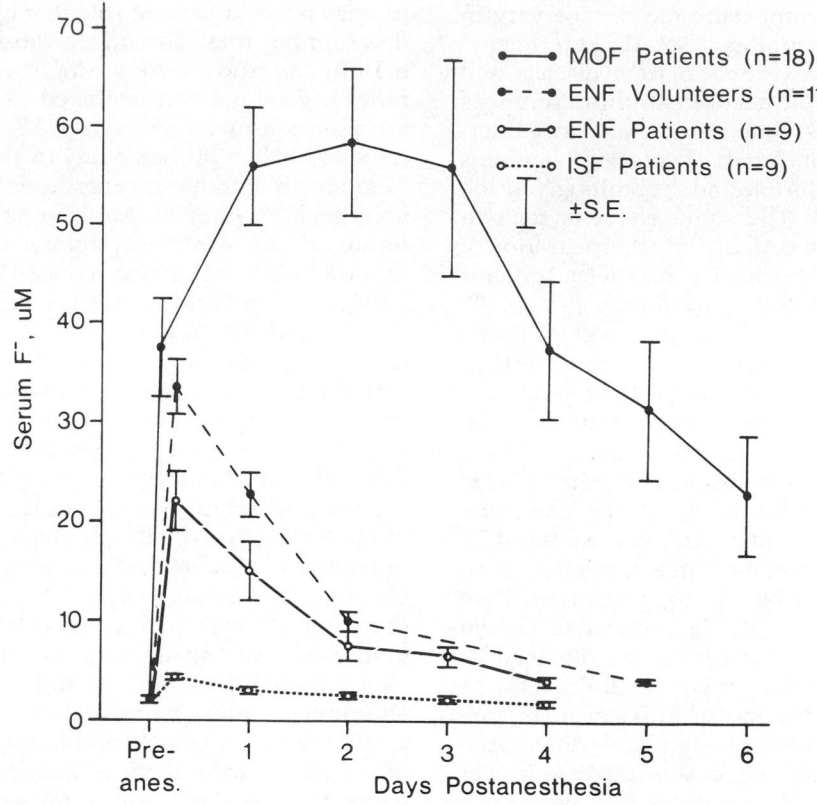

Fig. 6-3. Serum inorganic fluoride (F⁻) concentrations before and after administration of enflurane, isoflurane, and methoxyflurane anesthesia. A significant increase in F⁻ concentrations occurred immediately following enflurane anesthesia, reaching a mean peak value of 22.2 ± 2.8μM 4 hours after termination of anesthesia; mean duration of anesthesia was 2.7 ± 0.3 MAC-hours.[205] F⁻ levels in volunteers receiving enflurane anesthesia peaked at 33.6 ± 2.8μM; mean duration of exposure was 9.6 ± 0.1 MAC-hours.[206] Following 2 to 3 MAC-hours of methoxyflurane[198] mean peak serum F⁻ concentration was higher 61 ± 8μM, and declined more slowly than after enflurane. There was almost no increase in F⁻ following isoflurane administration.[47] (Modified from Cousins et al.,[205] with permission.)

tal show increased defluorination and nephrotoxicity. Other enzyme inducers such as phenytoin,[42] ethanol,[15,16] and diazepam[92] also increase methoxyflurane defluorination in rats.

The effects of phenobarbital and phenytoin on metabolism of other fluorinated anesthetics are less certain. Phenobarbital pretreatment of rats increases in vitro defluorination of sevoflurane[103] while only slightly increasing that of isoflurane.[41] Enflurane defluorination in vitro is not significantly increased.[41] The result with enflurane is surprising, but consistent with data obtained from a clinical study.[14] A series of 102 surgical patients were divided into four groups according to their drug intake histories: control (on no drug), 26 patients; chronic ethanol, 31 patients; chronic phenobarbital and/or phenytoin, 12 patients; and miscellaneous drugs, 33 patients. Regression lines of average peak serum F⁻ concentrations on enflurane dosage were not significantly different among the groups.

Thus, prior chronic treatment of surgical patients with these common enzyme-inducing drugs did not increase serum F⁻ concentrations after enflurane anesthesia. In contrast, prior chronic treatment with isoniazid may result in higher than expected serum concentrations of F⁻ and a transient urinary concentrating defect after enflurane anesthesia. Work with Fischer 344 rats has shown that unlike phenobarbital and phenytoin, isoniazid significantly increases enflurane defluorination.[17,18] In addition, a study of surgical patients has shown that approximately one-half of those chronically treated with isoniazid prior to enflurane anesthesia had significantly higher serum F⁻ concentrations than predicted,[19] but these elevated concentrations were not high enough or sustained long enough to produce clinically significant renal impairment. Patients with the higher concentrations of F⁻ are assumed to be slow acetylators of isoniazid, although this has not been substantiated.

Effects on the Gonads

Concern that inhaled anesthetics or their metabolites may damage germ cells has led to a number of studies. In one of the earliest, male LEW/Mai rats were exposed to 20 percent N_2O either continuously or for 8 hours per day for up to 35 days.[211] After only 2 days, minor damage to seminiferous tubules was noted, and after longer periods, atrophy of the seminiferous tubules, decreased sperm count, and decreased testicular weight were seen. Another study evaluated the effects of a low-dose N_2O/halothane mixture on spermatogonial cells.[212] Exposure was to air, to 50 ppm N_2O/1 ppm halothane, or to 500 ppm N_2O/10 ppm halothane for periods of 7 hours per day, 5 days per week over 52 weeks. The investigators reported that this chronic exposure to low-dose N_2O/halothane resulted in dose-dependent chromosomal damage in spermatogonial cells. In a study that examined mouse sperm morphology after exposure to anesthetics during early spermatogenesis, chloroform (0.08 percent and 0.04 percent), trichloroethylene (0.2 percent), and enflurane (1.2 percent) all slightly but significantly increased the number of sperm abnormalities above normal; other inhaled anesthetics studied gave negative results.[213]

In contrast to these positive studies, two studies have given negative results. In the first, Swiss/ICR mice were exposed to 0.3 percent enflurane, 4 hours per day, 5 days per week for 52 weeks; no increase in the rate of abnormal sperm or chromosomal aberration in spermatogonial cells was observed.[214] In the second study, male and female Swiss Webster mice were exposed to a maximum of 50 percent N_2O for 4 hours per day, 5 days per week for 14 weeks; no change in the percentage of abnormal sperm or number of oocytes was seen compared with control mice exposed only to air.[215]

In the only study in humans, semen was collected from 46 anesthesiologists who had worked for a minimum of 1 year in a scavenged operating suite.[216] Semen samples from 26 residents beginning an anesthesia training program were used as controls. The concentration of sperm and the percentage of abnormally shaped sperm in semen of working anesthesiologists were not different from those of beginning residents. Furthermore, sperm collected from 13 of the 26 residents after they had been working for 1 year was not different from the first sample.

Thus, despite some suggestive animal data, inhaled anesthetics have not been shown to have significant effects on germ cells in humans. However, studies have not been performed on patients exposed to high concentrations of anesthetics or on personnel working in unscavenged operating suites.

Hematopoietic and Neurologic Systems

Nitrous oxide interacts with vitamin B_{12} and disrupts several pathways involved in one-carbon chemistry. The biochemical basis of this effect is the oxidation of the cobalt in vitamin B_{12} by a physicochemical reaction with N_2O. The result in humans and animals is an irreversible inactivation of the enzyme methionine synthase, which requires vitamin B_{12} in the completely reduced form to act as its coenzyme. Methionine synthase catalyzes the conversion of methyltetrahydrofolate and homocysteine to tetrahydrofolate and methionine (Fig. 6-4). Failure to produce these products has a number of biochemical consequences including reduced synthesis of thymidine, which is an essential DNA base. The clinical syndrome associated with oxidation of vitamin B_{12} is essentially the same as that seen in pernicious anemia; there is megaloblastic hematopoiesis and subacute combined degeneration of the spinal cord.

The time for inactivation of methionine synthase is species dependent. In rats exposed to 50 percent N_2O, the half-time of inactivation is about 5 minutes.[217] Recovery of activity takes 3 to 4 days since oxidation of vitamin B_{12} is irreversible and vitamin B_{12} is covalently bound to the enzyme. Thus, new enzyme must be synthesized to restore activity. In humans, however, the half-time of inactivation is much longer, about 45 minutes.[217] Nevertheless, after several hours of routine anesthesia with N_2O, methionine synthase activity is very low. The decrease of thymidine synthesis takes somewhat longer to develop but also lasts several days. Experimental data suggest that there is a threshold concentration of about 1,000 ppm (0.1 percent) below which N_2O has no biochemical effect.[218]

The shortest exposure time required to produce megaloblastic hematopoiesis varies among patients and perhaps depends on their general state of health. In healthy patients undergoing routine surgery, mild megaloblastic bone marrow changes are not seen after 6 hours but are seen after about 12 hours of exposure to 50 percent N_2O; after 24 hours of exposure, changes are marked.[219] Limited evidence suggests that N_2O produces bone marrow changes earlier in seriously ill patients.[220] Evidence also suggests that the bone marrow changes are preventable by pretreating patients with large doses of folinic acid.[219] This drug is converted to the 5,10-methylene tetrahydrofolate needed for thymidine synthesis (Fig. 6-4).

The neurologic disease subacute combined degeneration of the spinal cord develops only after several months of daily exposure to N_2O. Thus, it occurs in those who chronically abuse N_2O and in those rare individuals who work for many months in an environment grossly contaminated with the gas. Dental personnel who are occasionally exposed to greater than 1,000 ppm waste N_2O in poorly ventilated dental operatories for long periods may be particularly at risk. In one study, 3 of 20 dentists exposed to mean concentrations up to 4,600 ppm had abnormal bone marrow.[221] Operating room personnel, however, are almost never exposed to such conditions in modern scavenged operating suites and would not be expected to have problems. Epidemiologic surveys confirm that dental but not operating room personnel have a higher incidence of

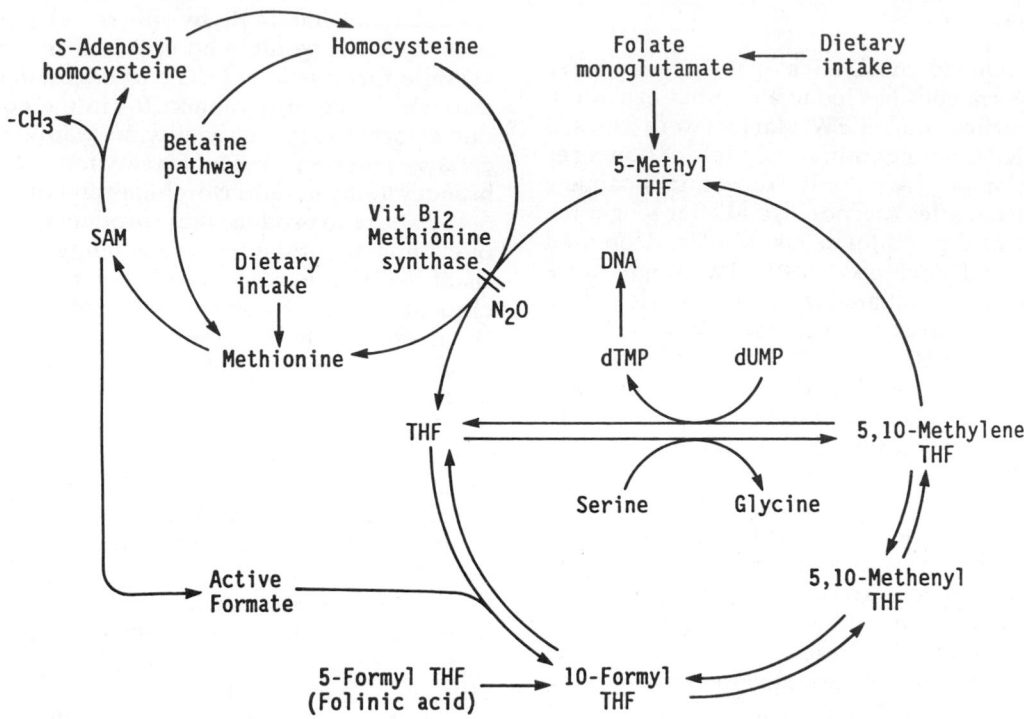

Fig. 6-4. Conversion of methyltetrahydrofolate and homocysteine to tetrahydrofolate and methionine.

neurologic disease, although exposure to waste N_2O has not definitely been shown to be the cause.[222]

Chronic Toxicity

From the time that chloroform hepatotoxicity was first recognized more than 100 years ago, great emphasis has been placed on anesthetic-induced acute organ toxicity. In recent years, proof that methoxyflurane causes nephrotoxicity and suspicion that halothane produces hepatotoxicity have enhanced interest in this topic. Historically, however, little thought has been given to possible long-term adverse effects on health from occupational exposure to trace concentrations of waste anesthetic gases.

Even if anesthetics have low potential for causing long-term toxicity, exposure of a large population may represent a considerable public health hazard. In the United States, about 50,000 hospital operating room personnel, including anesthesiologists, nurse anesthetists, and operating room technicians, are exposed daily to waste anesthetic gases.[223] In addition, surgeons, dental personnel, and veterinarians and their technical assistants have a variable but sometimes heavy exposure to anesthetics. For example, peak levels of at least 50 ppm halothane and 5,000 ppm N_2O have occasionally been recorded in operating room and dental operatory atmospheres.[224,225] The total number of exposed or potentially exposed personnel in the United States each year is about 225,000.[223] Of particular concern are reports that inhaled anesthetics possess mutagenic, carcinogenic, or teratogenic potential.

Mutagenicity

In recent years, investigators have become increasingly interested in the mutagenic potential of inhaled anesthetics for several reasons. First, chemical mutagenicity and carcinogenicity are closely correlated. Thus, finding that a particular anesthetic is a mutagen also implies that it is a potential carcinogen and should be studied in an animal test system. Because in vitro assays for mutagenicity require much less time and expense than in vivo assays for carcinogenicity, they have become popular screening methods for detecting carcinogens. A second reason for identifying mutagens present in the environment is that they may pose a threat to the integrity of the human genome (the totality of genes and chromosomes) and thus to future generations of humans.

Mutations are heritable changes in genetic information. Four types are generally recognized:

1. Base-pair mutation in which one of the four deoxyribonucleic acid (DNA) bases (adenine, guanine, thymine, or cytosine) is replaced by one of the others.
2. Frameshift mutation in which a base pair is added or deleted. In this case, all bases distal to the point of addition or deletion will be out of sequence, a potentially more serious mutation than the base-pair kind.
3. Large deletions or rearrangements of DNA segments.
4. Nondisjunction in which an unequal partition of chromosomes occurs between daughter cells.

A wide variety of test systems has been used to examine

the mutagenicity of inhaled anesthetics including assays with bacteria, yeast, mammalian cells in culture, and intact mammals. Most of these have been reviewed elsewhere and are only summarized here.[226,227]

Extensive work has been done with the Ames *Salmonella*/mammalian hepatic microsome system, which uses several strains of histidine-dependent *Salmonella typhimurium* as tester organisms. This system is a well-validated assay for mutagenicity and often is regarded as the standard against which other systems are compared. It has been used to test most current and former anesthetics. Only divinyl ether and fluroxene give unequivocally positive responses (Fig. 6-5), whereas trichlorethylene gives a weak mutagenic response. Other anesthetics including N_2O, halothane, and enflurane are not mutagenic when tested under a wide variety of experimental conditions and anesthetic concentrations. The general finding that anesthetics containing a double-bonded structure are mutagenic is consistent with knowledge about the high reactivity and mutagenicity of this class of chemicals.[228] Similarly, of all the metabolites of inhaled anesthetics that have been tested in the *Salmonella* assay, only 1,1-difluoro-2-bromo-2-chloroethylene (CF_2CBrCl) and 1,1-difluoro-2-chloro-ethylene (CF_2CHCl), both which contain a double-bonded structure, have been found to be even weakly mutagenic.

In general, results from numerous studies with other test systems have confirmed those from studies with *Salmonella* (Table 6-1). Some anomalous results exist, most notably the findings that N_2O and halothane are weakly mutagenic in *Drosophila*[229-231] and that N_2O is weakly mutagenic in *Tradescantia*.[232] Nonetheless, the overwhelming evidence from in vitro tests indicates that all currently used and most previously used anesthetics are not mutagens and therefore are probably not carcinogens. By contrast, anesthetics that contain a double-bonded structure are mutagens and potential carcinogens.

Mutagenicity studies in humans exposed to inhaled anesthetics have been uniformly negative. In an early study, no significant difference in the number of chromosomal aberrations could be detected between lymphocytes obtained from operating room nurses and those obtained from surgical outpatient nurses.[233] In another study, no mutagenic activity could be detected by *Salmonella* assay in urine of operating room personnel working in scavenged or unscavenged operating

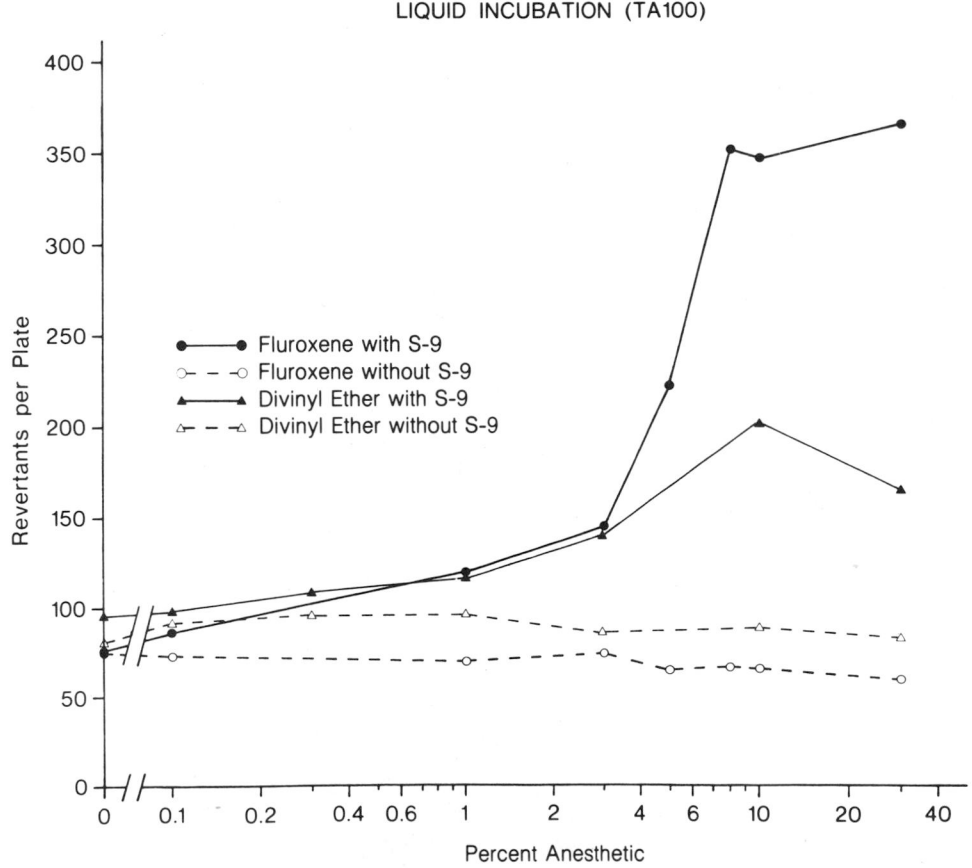

Fig. 6-5. Number of revertant colonies per plate of *Salmonella typhimurium*, TA100, after liquid suspension with fluroxene or divinyl ether, with or without S-9. Both fluroxene and divinyl ether showed a dose-dependent mutagenic response at concentrations greater than 1 percent in the presence of S-9.

TABLE 6-1. Tests of Mutagenicity

Anesthetic	Positive	Negative
Halothane	D	A,8-AzG,D,SCE,L,C
Nitrous oxide	D,T	A,8-AzG, SCE
Chloroform	—	A,8-AzG, SCE
Enflurane	—	A,8-AzG, D, SCE
Methoxyflurane	—	A, SCE
Isoflurane	—	A, D, SCE
Cyclopropane	—	A
Diethyl ether	—	D, SCE
Sevoflurane	—	A
Synthane	—	A
Dioxychlorane	—	A
Dioxyflurane	—	A
Trichloroethylene	A, M, S	A, SCE
Fluroxene	A, D, SCE	—
Divinyl ether	A, SCE	—

Abbreviations: A, Ames *Salmonella* or *Escherichia*/mammalian microsome; C, chromosomal mutations in mice; 8-AzG, 8-azaguanine in Chinese hamster lung fibroblasts; D, *Drosophila;* L, mouse dominant lethal test; M, mouse spot test; S, *Saccharomyces;* SCE, sister chromatid exchange in Chinese hamster ovary cells; T, *Tradescantia.*

rooms, or in urine of anesthesiology residents up to 15 months after the start of training.[234] Finally, lymphocytes from personnel exposed to waste anesthetic gases for durations up to 312 months had no higher incidence of chromosomal aberrations or sister chromatid exchange than those from unexposed individuals.[235] This later study was an extension of previous negative studies of sister chromatid exchanges in lymphocytes of operating room personnel exposed to waste anesthetic gases and patients anesthetized with halothane, enflurane, or fluroxene.[236-238] Thus, to date, no mutagenic effect of long-term or short-term exposure to inhaled anesthetics has been demonstrated in humans.

Carcinogenicity

The development of chemically induced tumors (chemical carcinogenesis) has three broad phases (Fig. 6-6). The first involves metabolic activation of the administered chemical to a positively charged reactive

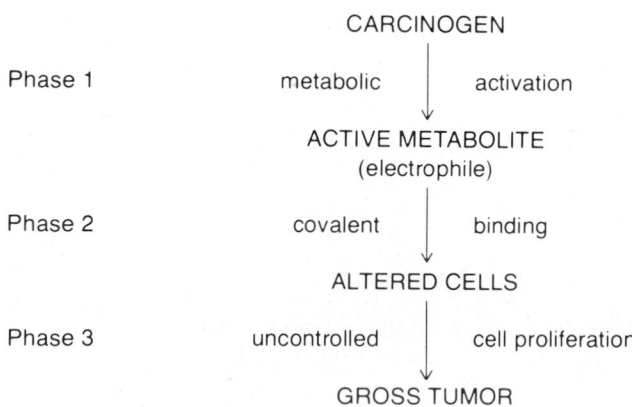

Fig. 6-6. Phases in chemical carcinogenesis.

intermediate or electrophile. The second is covalent binding of the electrophile to some critical tissue macromolecule. Although chemicals and metabolites bind to lipid, protein, RNA, and DNA, the latter is thought to be the target molecule for chemical carcinogenesis. After covalent binding has occurred, damaged macromolecules may be repaired or eliminated, remain dormant within the cell, or lead to the third phase, which involves cellular proliferation and development of clinically apparent tumors. This final phase, which occurs over a long time period and involves a multiplicity of mechanisms, is little understood.

Covalent binding of reactive intermediates to tissue macromolecules is presumed to be necessary but not to be the only requirement for chemical carcinogenesis. As indicated in the section on specific organ toxicity, covalent binding of anesthetic metabolites has been recognized for many years. Low-temperature whole-body autoradiography in mice has shown that both chloroform and halothane fragments bind covalently to liver and other body tissues.[59,239] Thus, some anesthetics satisfy at least one criterion for chemical carcinogenicity.

Structural similarity provides further circumstantial evidence of an association between anesthetics and chemical carcinogens (Fig. 6-7). Methoxyflurane, enflurane, and isoflurane are α-haloethers, as are the nonanesthetic but carcinogenic chemicals bis(chloromethyl)ether, chloromethyl methyl ether, and bis(α-chloroethyl)ether.[240,241] Halothane and chloroform are alkyl halides; methyl iodide, butyl bromide, and butyl chloride are from the same chemical group and are animal carcinogens.[242] Finally, the anesthetic and industrial solvent trichloroethylene is a halogenated alkene similar to the human[243] and animal[244,245] carcinogen vinyl chloride. Fluroxene and divinyl ether also contain the vinyl moiety. Although these observations on structure are interesting, they are by no means proof that anesthetics have carcinogenic potential. Minor structural differences often impart major changes in function, as has been clearly shown with aromatic hydrocarbons.[246] Epidemiologic surveys, animal studies, and in vitro carcinogenicity assays provide more definitive evidence of carcinogenic potential.

Despite the obvious advantage of surveying human populations to determine the carcinogenic risk of exposure to anesthetics, such surveys have provided little information on the carcinogenicity of specific anesthetics. The primary reason is that the dosages of anesthetics to which surveyed individuals have been exposed either have not been measured or at best have been estimated. Nonetheless, the studies so far performed should indicate whether working in a surgical or dental suite is associated with a higher incidence of cancer, regardless of the cause.

There have been a number of surveys of cancer incidence among exposed workers (Table 6-2).[247-255] In the largest, the American Society of Anesthesiologists (ASA) conducted a retrospective survey of 49,595 oper-

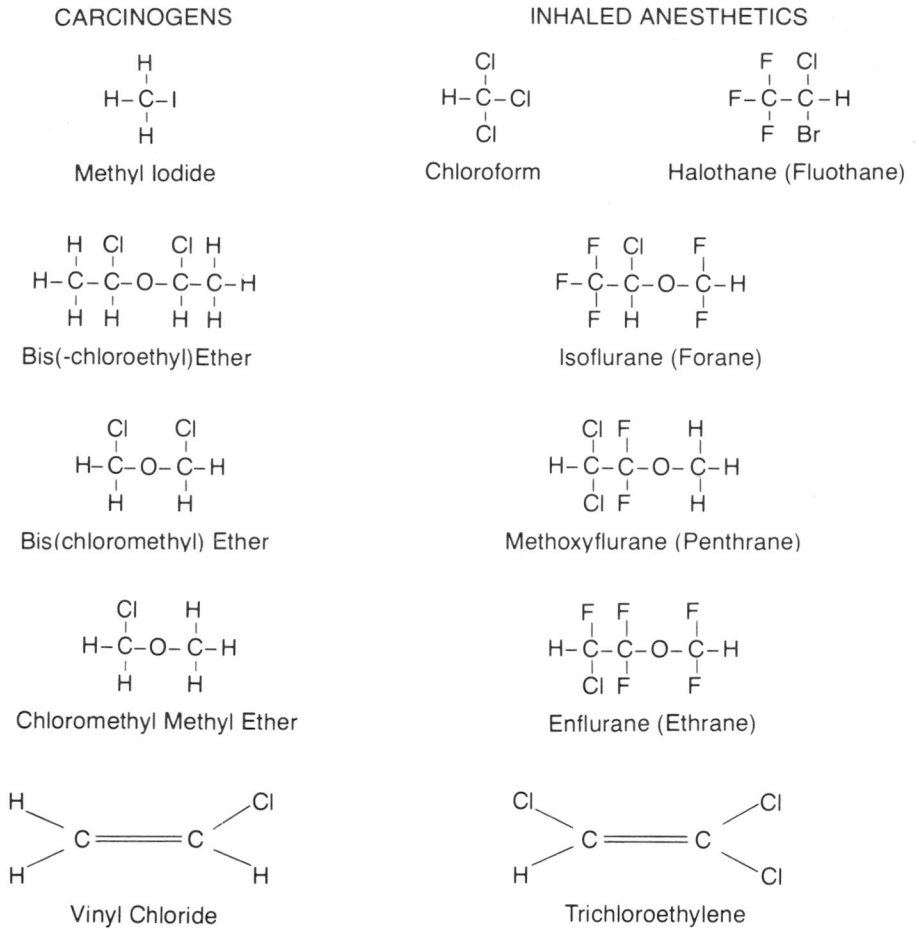

CARCINOGENS   INHALED ANESTHETICS

Methyl Iodide   Chloroform   Halothane (Fluothane)

Bis(-chloroethyl)Ether   Isoflurane (Forane)

Bis(chloromethyl) Ether   Methoxyflurane (Penthrane)

Chloromethyl Methyl Ether   Enflurane (Ethrane)

Vinyl Chloride   Trichloroethylene

Fig. 6-7. Structural formulas of several known human carcinogens and the inhaled anesthetics.

ating room personnel working throughout the United States.[249] A 1.3- to 2.0-fold increase in cancer incidence was noted among female members of the ASA and the American Association of Nurse Anesthetists compared with unexposed control female groups. No increase in cancer incidence was seen among surveyed males. In an earlier study, the incidence of cancer among 525 female nurse anesthetists in Michigan was compared with that of women participating in the Connecticut Tumor Registry.[248] The nurse anesthetists had a higher incidence of malignant cancers diagnosed during 1971 than did all the women of Connecticut during 1966 to 1969. In another large study, a national survey of health among dental personnel was reported.[254] The study

TABLE 6-2. Epidemiologic Surveys for Cancer Incidence or Deaths Among Personnel Exposed to Waste Anesthetic Gases

Studied	Population	Results	Investigators[a]
Deaths	ASA members	Negative	Bruce et al. (1968)[247]
Incidence	Nurse anesthetists	3.3-fold increase for 1971	Corbett et al. (1973)[248]
Incidence	ASA members	1.3- to 1.9-fold increase for women; negative for men	American Society of Anesthesiologists (1974)[249]
Deaths	ASA members	Negative	Bruce et al. (1974)[250]
Deaths	Anesthetists	Negative	Doll and Peto (1977)[251]
Deaths	ASA members	Negative	Lew (1979)[252]
Incidence	Anesthetists and offspring	Negative	Tomlin (1979)[253]
Incidence	Dental personnel	1.5-fold increase for women; negative for men	Cohen et al. (1980)[254]
Deaths	Anesthetists	Negative	Neil et al. (1987)[255]

[a] References are given as superscripts.
Abbreviation: ASA, American Society of Anesthesiologists.

population consisted of 30,650 dentists and 30,547 chairside assistants and was readily divided into those who used or did not use inhaled anesthetics to provide pain relief and sedation of patients. Otherwise, both groups did similar work under similar conditions. An estimate of anesthetic exposure was made by noting the number of hours per week spent by each respondent in the dental operatory. About 80 percent of inhaled anesthetic users were exposed to N_2O alone, while the remainder were exposed to potent volatile anesthetics in addition. The cancer incidence among female chairside assistants exposed to waste anesthetics for more than 8 hours per week was 50 percent greater than among those not exposed, although the increase was not statistically significant ($P = 0.056$). Analysis of various types of cancer showed that only cancer of the cervix occurred more frequently ($P = 0.06$) in exposed women than in unexposed women.

Collectively, the above studies of cancer incidence appear to show a small risk to females directly exposed to waste anesthetic gases. However, because of problems with study design and the low increase in cancer incidence observed, reviewers have generally been unconvinced of the existence of a hazard to humans.[256-259] Their lack of conviction is strengthened by the uniformly negative results from surveys of deaths from cancer (Table 6-2).

Because of the problems of interpreting epidemiologic surveys, many investigators have turned to animal studies to provide information on the carcinogenic potential of specific anesthetics. When administered in extremely large dosages by oral gavage, chloroform[260] produced liver cancer in B6C3F1 mice and renal tumors in male and female Osborne-Mendel rats, whereas trichloroethylene[261] caused liver tumors in mice but not in rats. Fifty animals were used in both studies for each treatment and control group. Although oral gavage may be appropriate for studying dietary and therapeutic intake of chloroform or trichloroethylene, this route of administration probably is not relevant to inhaled exposure of patients or operating room personnel. Indeed, administering a drug by an unusual route often leads to confounding carcinogenicity data.[262] Furthermore, when trichloroethylene was studied, the agent tested contained 0.19 percent 1,2-epoxybutane and 0.09 percent epichlorohydrin, both known mutagens.[263,264] Epichlorohydrin is also a rodent carcinogen.[265] The presence of these contaminants, although in small amounts, cast doubt on the significance of data gathered on trichlorethylene carcinogenicity.

In the only positive study of an anesthetic administered via inhalation, isoflurane led to an increased incidence of liver tumors in male, but not female, Swiss/ICR mice exposed in utero and for a short period postnatally.[266] Several factors, however, confound the interpretation of this finding, including the presence of high levels of polybrominated biphenyls in the livers of isoflurane-trated mice. In a more complete study in which a similar exposure regimen was used, no increased incidence of liver or other tumors could be demonstrated in mice exposed to isoflurane, halothane, enflurane, methoxyflurane, or N_2O.[267] In the most extensive study of isoflurane carcinogenicity, mice exposed to the maximum tolerated dose (0.4 percent ppm for 4 hours per day, 5 days per week) of isoflurane for 78 weeks showed no increase in cancer rate.[268] Halothane, enflurane, and nitrous oxide also have been tested at their maximum tolerated dose in three carcinogenicity studies in mice.[269-271] In the first, 161 mice were exposed to 500 ppm halothane for 2 hours per day both in utero and for 78 weeks after birth. In the second study, 250 weanling mice were exposed to 3,000 ppm enflurane for 4 hours per day for 78 weeks. In the final study, 303 weanling mice were exposed to concentrations of N_2O as high as 40 percent (vol/vol). Despite almost lifetime exposure to maximum tolerated doses, none of the anesthetics was carcinogenic. In a further study, groups of 50 rats exposed for 104 weeks to a N_2O/halothane mixture at concentrations of 50 ppm/1 ppm or 500 ppm/10 ppm showed no higher incidence of tumors than rats exposed to air alone.[272]

The overwhelming conclusion from both animal and human studies is that there is no carcinogenic risk either from working in the operating or dental suite or from exposure to anesthetics.

Teratogenicity

Teratology is the study of the production, anatomy and classification of congenital malformations. Although human development is remarkably consistent, it is not always perfect; congenital malformations, both severe and trivial, are found in 2 to 4 percent of all births in countries in which records are kept.[273] There are many mechanisms involved in abnormal development (Table 6-3). Some, such as mutations that result in specific biochemical abnormalities and chromosomal nondisjunction, are well established. Others, such as interference with abnormal cell membrane states, are less certain mechanisms of teratogenicity. Membrane changes have been observed with inhaled anesthetics at clinical concentrations.[274,275] Although the cause of most defects remains unknown, chemical teratogenesis in humans is well established (Table 6-4).

Most surveys that have examined the reproductive performance of operating room and dental personnel are listed in Table 6-5.[249,254,276-286] In a review of many of

TABLE 6-3. Teratogenic Mechanisms

Mutation[a]
Interference with cell division
Alteration of nucleic acid function
Removal of cell precursors and substrates
Lack of energy source
Enzyme inhibition
Change in cell membrane characteristics

[a] Four types—see text.
(Data from Wilson.[305])

TABLE 6-4. Known Human Chemical Teratogens[a]

Androgenic hormones (e.g., diethylstilbestrol)
Anticonvulsants (e.g., phenytoin)
Cancer chemotherapeutic agents (e.g., methotrexate)
Thalidomide
Organic mercury
Hypoglycemics (?) (e.g., tolbutamine)

[a] Account for only 2 to 3 percent of known causes of developmental defects in humans.
(Data from Schardein.[305])

these, an estimate was made of the relative risks for particular health hazards.[259] The magnitude of the relative risk for spontaneous abortion among exposed women was approximately 1.3, representing a 30 percent increase for this hazard. The increase was both consistent and statistically significant. For congenital abnormalities among offspring of exposed women, the relative risk was approximately 1.2. The overall data for wives of exposed males and for congenital abnormalities among their offspring were less consistent than for spontaneous abortion. For both spontaneous abortion and congenital abnormalities, the increases observed wcrc small and could not be attributed to a specific cause. Exposure to waste anesthetic gases, viruses, x-rays, a variety of chemicals other than anesthetics, or a combination of these factors could have accounted for the positive results. Furthermore, most surveys had serious methodologic faults, including failure to verify the medical data supplied by respondents. Interestingly, in the only three studies in which medical records were used to confirm medical data, negative results were obtained for a number of adverse reproductive hazards including spontaneous abortion.[284,286] The implication is that responder bias may be a factor in studies in which positive results have been reported.

Although some doubt remains concerning the ad-

verse reproductive effects of waste anesthetic gases, there is little doubt that surgery and anesthesia have detrimental effects on the pregnant patient. In the United States, at least 50,000 pregnant women (about 1.6 percent) undergo anesthesia and surgery during gestation for indications unrelated to pregnancy.[287] Operations for ovarian cysts, acute appendicitis, mammary tumors, and repair of incompetent cervix are most common. The risk of unexpected abortion or premature labor clearly is higher after an anesthetic. What is not immediately obvious is whether the patients' disease, surgery, anesthesia, or a combination of these is the precipitating cause. Another concern, although not yet substantiated, is that anesthesia during pregnancy leads to an increased incidence of congenital abnormalities. To assess the exact incidence of various anesthetic- and surgery-related hazards occurring during pregnancy, at least four major studied have been performed.[287-290]

In the earliest study, all obstetric records in the U.S. Naval Hospital in Portsmouth, Va., were examined for the period 1957 to 1961.[288] During this period, 18,248 live births and 255 stillbirths were recorded; 67 patients had surgery during pregnancy, 24 having general and 43 having regional anesthesia. Nine stillbirths or abortions occurred after anesthesia, but no congenital anomalies were noted. Of the nine fetal losses, four were associated with appendiceal abscesses and four with Shirodkar procedures for incompetent cervical os. All nine cases resulting in fetal loss received spinal anesthesia. This finding was attributed to sampling bias.

In a larger study, two sources of data were analyzed.[287] The first was records of 9,073 obstetric patients delivered at the University of California Medical Center, San Francisco, between July 1959 and August 1964. The second source was records of 60,912 obstetric patients from 17 hospitals taking part in an Obstetrical Statistical Cooperative Study. Of the first group, 147 women

TABLE 6-5. Results of Controlled Epidemiologic Surveys of Adverse Reproductive Effects Among Personnel Exposed to Waste Anesthetic Gases, and Their Spouses[a]

	Results			
	Exposed Women		Spouses of Exposed Men	
Investigators	Spontaneous Abortion	Major Anomaly in Offspring	Spontaneous Abortion	Major Anomaly in Offspring
Askrog and Harvald (1970)[276]	65%	Negative	170%	Negative
Cohen et al. (1971)[277]	270%	—	—	—
Knill-Jones et al. (1972)[278]	30%	160%	—	—
Rosenberg and Kirves (1973)[279]	70%	Negative	—	—
Corbett et al. (1974)[280]	—	190%	—	—
American Society of Anesthesiologists (1974[249]	30%	60%	Negative	30%
Knill-Jones et al. (1975)[281]	40%	Negative	Negative	Negative
Cohen et al. (1975)[282]	—	—	80%	Negative
Pharoah et al. (1977)[283]	Negative	Negative	—	—
Ericson and Kallen (1979)[284]	Negative	Negative	—	—
Cohen et al. (1980)[254]	160%	60%	50%	Negative
Axelsson and Rylander (1982)[285]	Negative	—	—	—
Hemminki et al. (1985)[286]	Negative	Negative	—	—

[a] Approximate percentage increase above control.

(1.6 percent) had operations during their pregnancies. In the second group, 50 appendectomies and 71 Shirodkar procedures were recorded. Premature delivery after operation occurred in 8.8 percent; perinatal mortality was 7.5 percent compared with 2 percent in the nonsurgical group. Detailed analysis of data obtained from these records indicated that premature labor after operation resulted mainly from the patient's surgical disease rather than from the surgical or anesthetic technique per se. In fact, no specific anesthetic technique, general or regional, had an advantage in lowering the incidence of premature labor, perinatal mortality, or congenital anomalies. As expected, there was a particularly high incidence of premature labor and perinatal mortality associated with operations for incompetent cervical os. Also noted was a normal incidence of congenital anomalies after operation, although the number of cases was too small to conclude with any degree of certainty that there was no hazard. Thus, it was recommended that anesthesia should not be administered during pregnancy or at least that it be delayed until after the period of maximum organogenesis (first trimester). Naturally, whether this advice can be heeded depends on the precise circumstances of each case.

In the third study, Brodsky et al.[289] used the results of the questionnaire survey of health among dental personnel[254] to determine fetal outcomes among 287 wives of dentists or female dental assistants who underwent surgery during the first or second trimester or pregnancy. Anesthesia for surgery during the first trimester in those not occupationally exposed to waste anesthetic gases was associated with a significantly increased rate of spontaneous abortion (from 5.1 to 8.0 percent) compared with the first control group. During the second trimester, the rate increased from 1.4 to 6.9 percent. There was no significant increase noted, however, in the number of congenital abnormalities in children born to these women.

In the final study, Duncan et al.[290] examined the health insurance data from the province of Manitoba for the years 1971 to 1978. They identified 2,565 women undergoing incidental surgery during pregnancy and paired them with pregnant women not undergoing surgery but with the same demographics. Both groups were assigned to a separately maintained congenital anomalies register. The incidence of spontaneous abortion was about twofold greater in those having general anesthesia for surgery during the first or second trimester compared with those not having surgery. In contrast, there was no significant difference in the incidence of congenital anomalies among offspring of the two groups. As with the other three studies of patients undergoing surgery and anesthesia, the causes of the adverse reproductive effects could not be identified.

Because of the difficulty in identifying causes and investigating mechanisms in humans, sophisticated animal studies have been developed over the last 30 years for examining the teratogenicity of chemicals. The complete assessment of a chemical now involves examining its effect on fertility, mating behavior, embryonic and fetal wastage, congenital anomalies, and postnatal survival and behavior. Despite their apparent thoroughness, animal studies are far from the perfect answer. Apart from the difficulty of extrapolating animal data to humans, the number of animals exposed in any experiment is small compared with the number of humans exposed; thus, there is usually insufficient statistical power to evaluate the presence of a weak teratogen. Nonetheless, because direct human experimentation is obviously not possible, animal studies are still necessary and continue to provide useful information.

Effects of inhaled anesthetics on reproductive processes of experimental animals have been the subject of many reports. Studies have been conducted at trace or subanesthetic concentrations of anesthetics to simulate occupational exposure and at anesthetic concentrations to simulate patient exposure. The large number of such studies precludes a complete discussion in the present chapter. The interested reader is referred to three more comprehensive reviews.[223,227,291]

In general, N_2O is the only inhaled anesthetic that has been convincingly shown to be directly teratogenic to experimental animals. High concentrations (50 to 75 percent) delivered to rats for 24-hour periods during organogenesis and low concentrations (0.1 percent) delivered to rats throughout pregnancy result in an increased incidence of fetal resorptions and visceral skeletal abnormalities.[292,293] Although effects in rodents are seen only after long periods of continuous exposure, it is not known whether humans are more sensitive than rodents and would show effects after shorter periods of exposure.

The mechanisms that produce these teratogenic effects with N_2O are unknown. The leading theory is that inhibition of methionine synthase causes critical shortages of intracellular methionine and DNA that are needed by the rapidly growing embryo. Certainly, both decreased DNA synthesis and decreased total DNA content have been observed in embryos immediately after N_2O exposure.[294,295] In recent years, however, some doubt has been cast on the methionine synthase theory of N_2O teratogenesis because maximum biochemical changes have been observed at concentrations that do not produce congenital malformations.[294] Furthermore, both halothane and isoflurane have been found to prevent most of the adverse reproductive effects of nitrous oxide without preventing the inhibition of methionine synthase. The whole subject of N_2O teratogenesis is being actively investigated, not only because of its relevance to patient and occupational safety but also because nitrous oxide can be used to determine the importance of vitamin B_{12}, folates, and one-carbon chemistry in developmental processes.

The other currently used inhaled anesthetics, halothane, enflurane, and isoflurane, are also teratogenic to rodents but only when administered at anesthetizing concentrations for many hours on several days during pregnancy. The consensus is that the teratogenic effects observed are caused by physiologic changes associated with the administration of these anesthetics rather than by the anesthetics themselves. Nonetheless, such findings emphasize the potential for anesthetics to cause teratogenic changes regardless of whether the mechanism is physiologic alteration or direct toxicity. Attention has recently focused on another aspect of teratogenesis, enduring behavioral deficits without any observable morphologic changes. While many organ systems are most sensitive to chemical teratogens during organogenesis, the central nervous system may be particularly vulnerable during myelination. In humans, this period is from the fourth intrauterine month through the second postnatal year. Thus, a chemical may produce behavioral teratogenesis if administered late in gestation or even after birth. Anesthetics have not escaped scrutiny as possible behavioral teratogens.

Rats exposed chronically to halothane (10 ppm) from conception to 60 days of age have been reported to have enduring learning deficits when tested on a shock-motivated light-dark discrimination task and a food-motivated symmetric maze.[296,297] Sampling of cerebral tissue showed electron microscopic evidence of neuronal degeneration and malformed synaptic membranes. In a more complete study, electron microscopic examination of cerebral cortical sections from rats exposed to halothane in utero showed central nervous system (CNS) damage such as synaptic malformation, disruption of the nuclear envelope, and cell death.[298] Exposure to various anesthetics during gestation or in the early postnatal period in rodents produced behavioral deficits. On days 3, 10, or 17 of pregnancy (roughly corresponding to the middle of first, second, or third trimester of pregnancy in humans), rats were anesthetized with 1.2 percent halothane for 120 minutes.[299] Activity of adult males and offspring as well as body weights and water intake were not different among groups. At 75 days of age, male offspring were tested on the shock-motivated Y-maze discrimination task. Rats exposed on the days 3 and 10 performed statistically less well than those exposed on day 17 or those not exposed (control animals). These same animals were also significantly more sensitive to footshock than were unexposed rats or those exposed on day 17.

Mice exposed to 0.5 percent halothane on gestational day 14 for 6 hours exhibited hypoactivity as young adults.[300,301] These results were similar to those observed for mice exposed to 75 percent N$_2$O for 4 hours on postnatal day 2. The interpretation of data are not obvious since different anesthetics, administered at different periods of development, produced essentially the same effects. Other studies in mice exposed to 5, 15, or 35 percent N$_2$O for 4 hours on days 6 to 15 of gestation produced significant hyporeactivity of the startle reflex to auditory and tactile stimuli on days 60 and 95 of age.[302] Rats exposed to 75 percent N$_2$O on gestational days 14 and 15 for 8 hours per day exhibited increased spontaneous motor activity at both 1 and 5 months of

age.[303] Offspring of Fischer 344 rats exposed to air or 1,500 ppm (0.15 percent) enflurane for 6 hours per day from conception to delivery have also been studied from 2 days to 90 weeks of age.[304] No significant treatment effects were observed.

Although a number of rodent studies have shown behavioral deficits after exposure to the inhaled anesthetics, the mechanism for these changes is not known and thus the applicability to humans is unclear.

Human studies have generally focused on long-term behavioral effects of maternal obstetric medication, including epidural anesthesia. Claims have been made that if the mother is given medication at delivery, the result will be depressed condition, motor skills, and language ability of offspring for at least the first 7 years of life. Such claims, however, are controversial. Behavioral abnormalities of offspring whose mothers received inhaled anesthetics at any time during delivery have not been well studied. Furthermore, studies have not been done to assess neurobehavior of children of operating room personnel who have been exposed to waste anesthetic gases. Firm conclusions about the risk of the occurrence of behavioral teratogenesis among the offspring of exposed personnel or in exposed patients therefore await further investigation.

REFERENCES

1. Daniels TC, Jorgensen EC: Physicochemical properties in relation to biologic action. p. 5. In Doerge RF (ed): Wilson and Gisvold's Textbook of Organic Medicinal and Pharmaceutical Chemistry. 8th Ed. JB Lippincott, Philadelphia, 1982
2. Singer SJ: The molecular organization of biological membranes. p. 146. In Rothfield L (ed): Structure and Function of Biological Membranes. Academic Press, Orlando, FL, 1971
3. DePierre JW, Ernster L: Enzyme topology of intracellular membranes. Annu Rev Biochem 46:201, 1977
4. Guidotti G: The structure of intrinsic membrane proteins. J Supramol Struct 7:489, 1977
5. DePierre JW, Dallner G: Structural aspects of the membrane of the endoplasmic reticulum. Biochim Biophys Acta 415:411, 1975
6. Guengerich FP, Macdonald TL: Chemical mechanisms of catalysis by cytochromes P-450: A unified view. Acc Chem Res 17:9, 1984
7. Omura T: Cytochrome P-450 linked mixed function oxidase: Turnover of microsomal components and effects of inducers on the turnover of phospholipids, protein and specific enzymes. p. 295. In Schenkman JB, Kupfer D (eds): Hepatic Cytochrome P-450 Monooxygenase System. Pergamon Press, New York, 1982
8. Quinn GP, Axelrod J, Brodie BB: Species, strain and sex differences in metabolism of hexobarbitone, amidopyrine, antipyrine and aniline. Biochem Pharmacol 1:152, 1958
9. Boobis AR, Davis DS: Human cytochromes P-450. Xenobiotica 14:151, 1984
10. Guengerich FP: Cytochrome P-450 enzymes and drug metabolism. p. 3. In Bridges JW, Chasseaud LF, Gibson GG (eds): Progress in Drug Metabolism. Vol. 10. Taylor and Francis, New York, 1987

11. Waskell L, Canova-Davis E, Philpot R, et al: Identification of the enzymes catalyzing metabolism of methoxyflurane. Drug Metab Dispos 14:643, 1986

12. Burke TR Jr, Martin JL, George JW, et al: Investigation of the mechanisms of defluorination of enflurane in rat liver microsomes with specifically deuterated derivatives. Biochem Pharmacol 29:1623, 1980

13. Burke TR, Branchflower RV, Lees DE, et al: Mechanism of defluorination of enflurane. Identification of an organic metabolite in rat and man. Drug Metab Dispos 9:19, 1981

14. Dooley JR, Mazze RI, Rice SA, et al: Is enflurane defluorination inducible in man? Anesthesiology 50:213, 1979

15. Van Dyke RA: Enflurane, isoflurane, and methoxyflurane metabolism in rat hepatic microsomes from ethanol-treated animals. Anesthesiology 58:22, 1983

16. Rice SA, Dooley JR, Mazze RI: Metabolism by rat hepatic microsomes of fluorinated ether anesthetics following ethanol consumption. Anesthesiology 58:237, 1983

17. Rice SA, Talcott RE: Effects of isoniazid treatment on selected hepatic mixed function oxidases. Drug Metab Dispos 7:260, 1979

18. Rice SA, Sbordone L, Mazze RI: Metabolism by rat hepatic microsomes of fluorinated ether anesthetics following isoniazid administration. Anesthesiology 53:489, 1980

19. Mazze RI, Woodruff RE, Heerdt ME: Isoniazid-induced enflurane defluorination in humans. Anesthesiology 57:5, 1982

20. Greunke LD, Konopka K, Koop DR, Waskell LA: Characterization of halothane oxidation by hepatic microsomes and purified cytochrome P-450 using a gas chromatographic mass spectrometric assay. J Pharmacol Exp Ther 246:454, 1988

21. Van Dyke RA, Baker MT, Jansson I, Schenkman J: Reductive metabolism of halothane by purified cytochrome P-450. Biochem Pharmacol 37:2357, 1988

22. Van Dyke RA, Gandolfi AJ: Anaerobic release of fluoride from halothane. Relationship to the binding of halothane metabolites to hepatic cellular constituents. Drug Metab Dispos 4:40, 1976

23. Maiorino RM, Sipes IG, Gandolfi AJ, et al: Factors affecting the formation of chlorotrifluoroethane and chlorodifluoroethylene from halothane. Anesthesiology 53:383, 1981

24. Ahr HJ, King LJ, Nastainczk W, et al: The mechanism of reductive dehalogenation of halothane by liver cytochrome P-450. Biochem Pharmacol 31:383, 1982

25. Loew G, Motulsky H, Trudell J, et al: Quantum chemical studies of the metabolism of the inhalation anesthetics methoxyflurane, enflurane, and isoflurane. Mol Pharmacol 10:406, 1974

26. Oesch F: Mammalian epoxide hydrases: Inducible enzymes catalyzing the inactivation of carcinogenic and cytotoxic metabolites derived from aromatic and olefinic compounds. Xenobiotica 3:305, 1973

27. Daniel JW: The metabolism of ^{36}Cl-labeled trichloroethylene and tetrachloroethylene in the rat. Biochem Pharmacol 12:795, 1963

28. Leibman KC, McAllister WJ: Metabolism of trichloroethylene in liver microsomes. I. Characteristics of the reaction. Mol Pharmacol 1:239, 1965

29. Byington KH, Leibman KC: Metabolism of trichloroethylene in liver microsomes. II. Identification of the reaction product as chloral hydrate. Mol Pharmacol 1:247, 1965

30. Miller RE, Guengerich FP: Metabolism of trichloroethylene in isolated hepatocytes, microsomes and reconstituted enzyme systems containing cytochrome P-450. Cancer Res 43:1145, 1983

31. Powell JF: Trichloroethylene: Absorption, elimination and metabolism. Br J Ind Med 2:142, 1945

32. Soucek B, Vlachova D: Excretion of trichloroethylene metabolites in human urine. Br J Med 17:60, 1960

33. Snyder R, Remmer H: Classes of hepatic microsomal mixed function oxidase inducers. p. 227. In Schenkman JB, Kupfer D (eds): Hepatic Cytochrome P-450 Monooxygenase System. Pergamon Press, New York, 1982

34. Conney AH: Pharmacological implications of microsomal enzyme induction. Pharm Rev 19:317, 1967

35. Remmer H, Merker HJ: Drug-induced changes in the liver endoplasmic reticulum. Association with drug-metabolizing enzymes. Science 142:1657, 1963

36. Brown BR, Jr., Sagalyn AM: Hepatic microsomal enzyme induction by inhalation anesthetics: Mechanism in the rat. Anesthesiology 40:152, 1974

37. Linde HW, Berman ML: Nonspecific stimulation of drug-metabolizing enzymes by inhalation anesthetic agents. Anesth Analg 50:656, 1971

38. Ross WT, Cardell RR: Proliferation of smooth endoplasmic reticulum and induction of microsomal drug-metabolizing enzymes after ether or halothane. Anesthesiology 8:325, 1978

39. Duvaldestin P, Mazze RI, Nivoche Y, et al: Occupational exposure to halothane results in enzyme induction in anesthetists. Anesthesiology 54:57, 1981

40. Barr GA, Cousins MJ, Mazze RI, et al: A comparison of the renal effects and metabolism of enflurane and methoxyflurane in Fischer 344 rats. J Pharmacol Ther 190:530, 1974

41. Hitt BA, Mazze RI: Effect of enzyme induction on nephrotoxicity of halothane related compounds. Environ Health Perspect 21:179, 1977

42. Caughey GH, Rice SA, Kosek JC, et al: Effect of phenytoin (DPH) treatment on methoxyflurane metabolism in rats. J Pharmacol Exp Ther 210:180, 1979

43. Greene NM: Halothane anesthesia and hepatitis in a high risk population. N Engl J Med 289:304, 1973

44. Ortiz de Montellano PR, Reich NO: Inhibition of cytochrome P-450 enzymes. p. 273. In Ortiz de Montellano PR (ed): Cytochrome P-450: Structure, Mechanism, and Biochemistry. Plenum, New York, 1986

45. Ivanetich KM, Lucas S, Marsh JA, et al: Organic compounds, their interaction with and degradation of hepatic microsomal drug-metabolizing enzymes in vitro. Drug Metab Dispos 6:218, 1978

46. Cascorbi HF, Vessel ES, Blake DA: Genetic and environmental influence on halothane metabolism in twins. Clin Pharmacol Ther 12:50, 1971

47. Van Dyke RA, Chenoweth MB, Van Poznak A: Metabolism of volatile anesthetics. I. Conversion in vivo of several anesthetics to $^{14}CO_2$ and chloride. Biochem Pharmacol 13:1239, 1964

48. Cohen EN: Metabolism of the volatile anesthetics. Anesthesiology 35:193, 1971

49. Green K, Cohen EN: On the metabolism of ^{14}C-diethyl ether in the mouse. Biochem Pharmacol 20:393, 1971

50. Van Dyke RA, Chenoweth MB: Metabolism of volatile anesthetics. Anesthesiology 26:348, 1965

51. Hong K, Trudell JR, O'Neill JR, Jr., et al: Metabolism of nitrous oxide by human and rat intestinal contents. Anesthesiology 52:16, 1980

52. Van Dyke RA: Biotransformation. p. 345. In Chenoweth MB (ed): Handbook of Experimental Pharmacology. Springer-Verlag, New York, 1972

53. Rao GS, Meridian DJ, Tong YS, et al: Biochemical toxicology

of chronic nitrous oxide exposures. Pharmacologist 21:216, 1979

54. Rice SA, Mazze RI, Baden JM: Effects of subchronic intermittent exposure to nitrous oxide in Swiss Webster mice. J Environ Pathol Toxicol Oncol 6:271, 1985

55. Charlesworth FA: Patterns of chloroform metabolism. Fed Cosmet Toxicol 14:59, 1976

56. Pohl LR, Bhooshan B, Whittaker NE, et al: Phosgene: A metabolite of chloroform. Biochem Biophys Res Commun 79:684, 1977

57. Pohl LR, Martin JL, George JW: Metabolic activation of chloroform by rat liver microsomes. Biochem Pharmacol 29:3271, 1980

58. Pohl LR, Branchflower RV, Highet RJ, et al: The formation of diglutathionyl dithiocarbonate as a metabolite of chloroform, bromotrichloromethane and carbon tetrachloride. Drug Metab Dipos 9:334, 1981

59. Cohen EN, Hood N: Application of low-temperature autoradiography to studies of the uptake and metabolism of volatile anesthetics in the mouse. I. Chloroform. Anesthesiology 30:306, 1969

60. Illett KF, Reid WD, Sipes GI, et al: Chloroform toxicity in mice: Correlation of renal and hepatic necrosis with covalent binding of metabolites to tissue macromolecules. Exp Mol Pathol 19:25, 1973

61. Scholler KL: Electron-microscopic and autoradiographic studies on the effect of halothane and chloroform on liver cells. Acta Anaesthesiol Scand (Suppl.) 32:5, 1968

62. Cowlen MS, Hewitt WR, Schroeder F: 2-Hexanone potentiation of [^{14}C]chloroform hepatotoxicity: Covalent interaction of a reactive intermediate with rat liver phospholipid. Toxicol Appl Pharmacol 73:478, 1984

63. Barrett HM, Johnson JH: The fate of trichloroethylene in the organism. J Biol Chem 127:765, 1939

64. Leibman KC, McAllister WJ: Metabolism of trichloroethylene in liver microsomes. III. Induction of the excretion of metabolites. J Pharmacol Exp Ther 157:574, 1967

65. Miller RE, Guengerich FP: Oxidation of trichloroethylene by liver microsomal cytochrome P-450: Evidence for chlorine migration in a transition state not involving trichloroethylene oxide. Biochemistry 21:1090, 1982

66. Gion H, Yoshimura N, Holaday DA, et al: Biotransformation of fluroxene in man. Anesthesiology 40:553, 1974

67. Blake DA, Rozman RS, Cascorbi HF, et al: Anesthesia. LXXIV. Biotransformation of fluroxene. I. Metabolism in mice and dogs in vivo. Biochem Pharmacol 16:1237, 1967

68. Murphy MJ, Dunbar DA, Kaminsky LS: Acute toxicity of fluorinated ether anesthetics: Role of 2,2,2-trifluoroethanol and other metabolites. Toxicol Appl Pharmacol 71:84, 1983

69. Ivanetich KM, Bradshaw JJ, Marsh JA, et al: The role of cytochrome P-450 in the toxicity of fluroxene. (2,2,2-trifluoroethyl vinyl ether) anesthesia in vivo. Biochem Pharm 25:773, 1976

70. Ivanetich KM, Bradshaw JJ, Marsh JA, et al: The interactions of hepatic microsomal cytochrome P-450 with fluroxene (2,2,2-trifluoroethyl vinyl ether) in vitro. Biochem Pharm 25:779, 1976

71. Stier A: Trifluoroacetic acid as a metabolite of halothane. Biochem Pharmacol 12:544, 1964

72. Stier A, Alter H, Hessler O, et al: Urinary excretion of bromide in halothane anesthesia. Anesth Analg 43:723, 1964

73. Satoh W, Fukuda Y, Anderson DK, et al: Immunological studies on the mechanism of halothane-induced hepatotoxicity. Immunohistochemical evidence of trifluoroacetylated hepatocytes. J Pharmacol Exp Ther 233:857, 1985

74. Baker MT, Nelson RM, Van Dyke RA: The release of inorganic fluoride from halothane and halothane metabolites by cytochrome P-450, hemin, and hemoglobin. Drug Metab Dispos 1:308, 1983

75. Sipes IG, Brown BR, Jr: An animal model of hepatotoxicity associated with halothane anesthesia. Anesthesiology 45:622, 1976

76. Sharp JH, Trudell JR, Cohen EN: Volatile metabolites and decomposition products of halothane in man. Anesthesiology 50:2, 1979

77. de Groot H, Harnisch U, Noll T: Suicidal activation of microsomal cytochrome P-450 by halothane under hypoxic conditions. Biochem Biophys Res Commun 107:885, 1982

78. Clauberg G: Untersuchugen uber den Einfluss von Inhalationsnarkose und Operation auf die Leberfunktion unter besonderer Berucksichtigung des Halothans. Anaesthesist 19:324, 1970

79. Reynolds ES, Molsen MT: Halothane hepatotoxicity: Enhancement by polychlorinated biphenyl pretreatment. Anesthesiology 47:19, 1977

80. Rice SA, Maze M, Smith CM, et al: Halothane hepatotoxicity in Fischer 344 rats pretreated with isoniazid. Toxicol Appl Pharmacol 87:411, 1987

81. Holaday DA, Rudofsky S, Treuhaft PS: Metabolic degradation of methoxyflurane in man. Anesthesiology 33:579, 1970

82. Van Dyke RA, Wood CL: Metabolism of methoxyflurane: Release of inorganic fluoride in human and rat hepatic microsomes. Anesthesiology 39:613, 1973

83. Yoshimura N, Holaday DA, Fiserova-Bergerova V: Metabolism of methoxyflurane in man. Anesthesiology 44:372, 1976

84. Ivanetich KM, Lucas SA, Marsh JA: Enflurane and methoxyflurane. Their interatction with hepatic cytochrome P-450 in vitro. Biochem Pharm 28:785, 1979

85. Canova-Davis E, Chiang JY, Waskell L: Obligatory role of cytochrome b_5 in the microsomal metabolism of methoxyflurane. Biochem Pharmacol 34:1907, 1985

86. Madelian V, Warren WA: Defluorination of methoxyflurane by a glutathione-dependent enzyme. Res Commun Chem Pathol Pharmacol 16:385, 1977

87. Warren W, Madelian V: Defluorination of methoxyflurane by glutathione and coenzyme B_{12}. Res Commun Chem Pathol Pharmacol 35:515, 1982

88. Wang S-L, Rice SA, Serra MT, Gross B: Purification and identification of rat cytosolic enzymes responsible for defluorination of methoxyflurane and fluoroacetate. Drug Metab Dispos 14:392, 1986

89. Rice SA, Wang S-L: Defluorination by hepatic gluthathione S-transferases? Toxicologist 7:217, 1987

90. Berman ML, Lowe HJ, Bochantin JS, et al: Uptake and elimination of methoxyflurane as influenced by enzyme induction in the rat. Anesthesiology 38:352, 1973

91. Mazze RI, Hitt BA, Cousins MJ: Effect of enzyme induction with phenobarbital on the in vivo and in vitro defluorination of isoflurane and methoxyflurane. J Pharmacol Exp Ther 190:523, 1974

92. Biermann JS, Rice SA, Gallagher EJ, West JA: Effect of diazepam treatment on hepatic microsomal anesthetic defluorinase activity. Arch Int Pharmacol Ther 283:181, 1986

93. Fiserova-Bergerova V: Changes of fluoride content in bone. An index of drug defluorination in vivo. Anesthesiology 38:345, 1973

94. Miller MS, Gandolfi AJ: Enflurane biotransformation in humans. Life Sci 27:1465, 1980

95. Christ DD, Satoh H, Kenna JG, Pohl LR: Potential metabolic

basis for enflurane hepatitis and the apparent cross-sensitization between enflurane and halothane. Drug Metab Dispos 16:135, 1988

96. Baden JM, Rice SA, Wharton RS, Laughlin NK: Metabolic and toxicologic studies with enflurane in Swiss/ICR mice. J Environ Pathol Toxicol 4:293, 1980

97. Mazze RI: Cousins MJ, Barr GA: Renal effects and metabolism of isoflurane in man. Anesthesiology 40:536, 1974

98. Holaday DA, Fiserova-Bergerova V, Latto IP, et al: Resistance of isoflurane to biotransformation in man. Anesthesiology 54:383, 1981

99. Hitt BA, Mazze RI, Cousins MJ: Metabolism of isoflurane in Fischer 344 rats and man. Anesthesiology 40:62, 1974

100. Koblin DD, Eger EI, Johnson BH, et al: I-653 resists degradation in rats. Anesth Analg 67:534, 1988

101. Rice SA, Baden JM, Kundomal YR: Effects of subchronic intermittent exposure to isoflurane in Swiss webster mice. J Environ Pathol Toxicol Oncol 6:285, 1986

102. Cook TL, Beppu WJ, Hitt BA, et al: Renal effects and metabolism of sevoflurane in Fischer 344 rats. An in vivo and in vitro comparison with methoxyflurane. Anesthesiology 43:70, 1975

103. Cook TL, Beppu WJ, Hitt BA, et al: A comparison of renal effects and metabolism of sevoflurane and methoxyflurane in enzyme induced rats. Anesth Analg 54:829, 1975

104. Holaday DA, Smith FR: Clinical characteristics and biotransformation of sevoflurane in healthy human volunteers. Anesthesiology 54:100, 1981

105. Fujii K, Morio M, Kikuchi H, et al: Pharmacokinetic study in excretion of inorganic fluoride ion, a metabolite of sevoflurane. Hiroshima J Med Sci 36:89, 1987

106. Kikuchi H, Morio M, Fujii K, et al: Clinical evaluation and metabolism of sevoflurane in patients. Hiroshima J Med Sci 36:93, 1987

107. Davidkova TI, Fujii K, Kikuchi H, et al: Urinary excretion of inorganic and organic fluoride after inhalation of sevoflurane. Hiroshima J Med Sci 36:99, 1987

108. Miller EC, Miller JA: Mechanisms of chemical carcinogenesis: Nature of proximate carcinogens and interactions with macromolecules. Pharmacol Rev 18:805, 1966

109. Anders MW (ed): Bioactivation of Foreign Compounds. p. 202. Academic Press, Orlando, FL, 1985

110. Demopoulos HB: The basis of free radical pathology. Fed Proc 32:1859, 1973

111. Demopoulos HB: Control of free radicals in biological systems. Fed Proc 32:1903, 1973

112. Brown BR, Jr., Sagalyn AM: Reactive intermediates of anesthetic biotransformation and hepatotoxicity. In Fink BR (ed): Molecular Mechanisms of Anesthesia. Progress in Anesthesiology. Vol. 1. Raven Press, New York, 1975

113. Pohl LR, Satoh H, Christ DD, Kenna JG: The immunologic and metabolic basis of drug hypersensitivities. Annu Rev Pharmacol 28:367, 1988

114. Myers LS, Jr: Free radical damage of nucleic acids and their components by ionizing radiation. Fed Proc 32:1882, 1973

115. DiLuzio NR: Antioxidants, lipid peroxidation and chemical induced liver injury. Fed Proc 32:1875, 1973

116. King MM, Lai EK, McCay PB: Singlet oxygen production associated with enzyme-catalyzed lipid peroxidation in liver microsomes. J Biol Chem 250:6496, 1975

117. Undenfriend S: Arene oxide intermediates in enzymatic hydroxylation and their significance with respect to drug toxicity. Ann NY Acad Sci 179:295, 1971

118. Recknagel RO: Alterations produced in the endoplasmic reticulum by carbon tetrachloride. Minerva Med 69:455, 1978

119. Undenfriend S, Bartl P: Symposium on the Biochemistry and Metabolism of Arene Oxides. Roche Institute of Molecular Biology, Nutley, NJ, 1972

120. Druckrey H: Specific carcinogenic and teratogenic effects of "indirect" alkylating methyl and ethyl compounds and their dependency on stages of ontogenic development. Xenobiotica 3:271, 1973

121. Pryor WA: Free radical reactions and their importance in biochemical systems. Fed Proc 32:1862, 1973

122. Bus JS, Gibson JE: Lipid peroxidation and its role in toxicology. p. 125. In Hodgson E, Bend JR, Philpot RM (eds): Review of Biochemical Toxicology. Elsevier/North-Holland, Amsterdam, 1979

123. Brown BR, Jr: Hepatic microsomal lipoperoxidation and inhalational anesthetics: A biochemical and morphologic study in the rat. Anesthesiology 36:458, 1972

124. Weinstein IB, Yamaguchi R, Gebert R, et al: Use of epithelial cell cultures for studies on the mechanisms of transformation by chemical carcinogens. In Vitro 11:130, 1975

125. Strunin L: The liver and anesthesia. p. 144. In Mushin WW (ed): Major Problems in Anaesthesia. Vol. 3. WB Saunders, London, 1977

126. Clarke RSJ, Doggart JR, Lavery T: Changes in liver function after different types of surgery. Br J Anaesth 48:119, 1976

127. Gelman SI: Disturbances in hepatic blood flow during anesthesia and surgery. Arch Surg 111:881, 1976

128. Simpson JY: On a new anaesthetic agent, more efficient than sulphuric ether. Lancet 2:549, 1847

129. Defalque RJ: The first delayed chloroform poisoning. Anesth Analg 47:374, 1968

130. Henderson Y, Cullen TS, Martin ED, et al: Report of the Committee on Anesthesia of the American Medical Association. JAMA 58:1908, 1912

131. Bevan AD, Favill HB: Acid intoxication, and late poisonous effects of anesthetics. Hepatic toxemia. Acute fatty degeneration of the liver following chloroform and ether anesthesia. JAMA 45:691, 754, 1905

132. Goldschmidt S, Ravdin IS, Lucke B: Anesthesia and liver damage. I. The protective action of oxygen against the necrotizing effect of certain anesthetics on the liver. J Pharmacol Exp Ther 59:1, 1937

133. Caravati CM, Wootton P: Acute massive hepatic necrosis with fatal liver failure. South Med J 55:1268, 1962

134. Gingrich TF, Virtue RW: Postoperative liver damage. Is anesthesia involved? Surgery 57:241, 1965

135. Herber R, Specht NW: Liver necrosis following anesthesia. Arch Intern Med 115:266, 1965

136. Slater EM, Gibson JM, Dykes MHM, et al: Postoperative hepatic necrosis. Its incidence and diagnostic value in association with the administration of halothane. N Engl J Med 240:983, 1964

137. Bennike KW, Hagelsten JO: Cyclopropane hepatitis. A Danish disease? Lancet 2:255, 1964

138. Bunker JP, Forrest WH, Mosteller F, et al: A Study of the Possible Association Between Halothane Anesthesia and Postoperative Hepatic Necrosis. National Halothane Study. US Government Printing Office, Washington, DC, 1969

139. Krantz JC, Carr CJ, Lu G, et al: Anesthesia. XL. The anesthetic action of trifluorethyl vinyl ether. J Pharmacol Exp Ther 108:488, 1953

140. Reynolds ES, Brown BR, Jr., Vandam LD: Massive hepatic necrosis after fluroxene anesthesia—a case of drug interaction. N Engl J Med 286:530, 1972

141. Cascorbi HF, Singh-Amaranath AV: Fluroxene toxicity in mice. Anesthesiology 37:480, 1972

142. Harrison GG, Smith JS: Massive lethal hepatic necrosis in cats anesthetized with fluroxene after microsomal enzyme induction. Anesthesiology 39:619, 1973

143. Johnston RR, Cromwell TH, Eger EI, et al: The toxicity of fluroxene in animals an man. Anesthesiology 38:313, 1973

144. Suckling CW: Some chemical and physical factors in the development of Fluothane. Br J Anaesth 29:466, 1957

145. Brennan RW, Hunter AR, Johnstone M: Halothane—a clinical assessment. Lancet 2:453, 1957

146. Johnstone M: The human cardiovascular response to Fluothane anaesthesia. Br J Anaesth 28:392, 1956

147. Brody GL, Sweet RB: Halothane anesthesia as a possible cause of massive hepatic necrosis. Anesthesiology 24:29, 1963

148. Bunker JP, Blumenfeld CM: Liver necrosis after halothane anesthesia. Cause or coincidence? N Engl J Med 268:531, 1963

149. Lindenbaum J, Leifer E: Hepatic necrosis associated with halothane anesthesia. N Engl J Med 268:525, 1963

150. Subcommittee on the National Halothane Study of the Committee on Anesthesia. National Academy of Sciences-National Research Council: Summary of the National Halothane Study: Possible association between halothane anesthesia and postoperative necrosis. JAMA 197:775, 1966

151. Dykes MHM, Bunker JP: Hepatotoxicity and anesthetics. Pharmacol Physicians 4:15, 1970

152. Strunin L, Simpson BR: Halothane in Britain today. Br J Anaesth 44:919, 1972

153. Bottinger LE, Dalen E, Hallen B: Halothane-inducd liver damage: An analysis of the material reported to the Swedish Adverse Drug Reaction Committee 1966–1973. Acta Anaesth Scand 20:40, 1976

154. Druckrey H: Specific carcinogenic and teratogenic effects of "indirect" akylating methyl and ethyl compounds and their dependency on stages of ontogenic development. Xenobiotica 3:271, 1973

155. Moult PJA, Sherlock S: Halothane related hepatitis. A clinical study of twenty-six cases. Q J Med (new series XLIV) 173:99, 1975

156. Walton B, Simpson BR, Strunin L, et al: Unexplained hepatitis following halothane. Br Med J 1:1171, 1976

157. Walton B: Halothane hepatitis in children. Anaesthesia 41:575, 1986

158. Kenna JG, Neuberger J, Mieli-Vergani G, et al: Halothane hepatitis in children. Br Med J 294:1209, 1987

159. Satoh H, Davies HW, Takemura T, et al: An immunochemical approach to investigating the mechanism of halothane-induced hepatotoxicity. p. 187. In Bridges JW, Chasseaud LF, Gibson GG (eds): Progress in Drug Metabolism. Vol. 10. Taylor and Francis, New York, 1987

160. Hubbard AK, Gandolfi AJ, Brown BR, Jr: Immunological basis of anesthetic-induced hepatotoxicity. Anesthesiology 69:814, 1988

161. Vergani D, Mieli-Vergani G, Albert A, et al: Antibodies to the surface of halothane-altered rabbit hepatocytes in patients with severe halothane-associated hepatitis. N Engl J Med 303:66, 1980

162. Davis M, Eddleston ALWF, Neuberger JM, et al: Halothane hepatitis. N Engl J Med 303:1123, 1980

163. Kenna JG, Satoh H, Christ DD, Pohl LR: Metabolic basis for a drug hypersensitivity: Antibodies in sera from patients with halothane hepatitis recognize liver neoantigens that contain the trifluoroacetyl group derived from halothane. J Pharmacol Exp Ther 245:1103, 1988

164. McLain GE, Sipes IG, Brown BR, Jr: An animal model of halothane hepatotoxicity. Anesthesiology 51:321, 1979

165. Jee R, Sipes IG, Gandolfi AJ, et al: Factors influencing an animal model of halothane hepatotoxicity. Toxicol Appl Pharmacol 52:267, 1980

166. Ross WT, Jr., Daggy BP Cardell RR: Hepatic necrosis caused by halothane and hypoxia in phenobarbital-treated rats. Anesthesiology 51:327, 1979

167. Wood M, Berman ML, Harbison RD, et al: Halothane-induced hepatic necrosis in triiodothyronine-pretreated rats. Anesthesiology 52:470, 1980

168. Uetrecht J, Wood AJJ, Phythyon JM, et al: Contrasting effects on halothane hepatotoxicity in the phenobarbital-hypoxia and triiodothyronine model: Mechanistic implications. Anesthesiology 59:196, 1983

169. Van Dyke RA: Hepatic centrilobular necrosis in rats after exposure to halothane, enflurane, or isoflurane. Anesth Analg 61:812, 1982

170. Harper MH, Collins P, Johnson B, et al: Hepatic injury following halothane, enflurane, and isoflurane in rats. Anesthesiology 56:14, 1982

171. Shingu K, Eger EI II, Johnson BH: Hypoxia *per se* can produce hepatic damage without death in rats. Anesth Analg 61:820, 1982

172. Shingu K, Eger EI II, Johnson BH: Hypoxia may be more important than reproductive metabolism in halothane-induced hepatic injury. Anesth Analg 61:824, 1982

173. Plummer JL, Beckwith ALJ, Bastin FN, et al: Free radical formation in vivo and hepatotoxicity due to anesthesia with halothane. Anesthesiology 57:160, 1982

174. Ross WT, Jr., Daggy BP: Hepatic blood flow in phenobarbital-pretreated rats during halothane anesthesia and hypoxia. Anesth Analg 60:306, 1981

175. Lunam CA, Cousins MJ, Hall PM: Guinea pig model of halothane-associated hepatotoxicity in the absence of enzyme induction and hypoxia. J Pharmacol Exp Ther 232:802, 1985

176. Lunam GA, Cousins MJ, de la Hall MP: Genetic predisposition to liver damage after halothane anesthesia in guinea pigs. Anesth Analg 65:1143, 1986

177. Artusio JF, Jr., Van Poznack A, Hunt RE, et al: A clinical evaluation of methoxyflurane in man. Anesthesiology 21:512, 1960

178. Joshi PH, Conn HO: The syndrome of methoxyflurane associated hepatitis. Ann Intern Med 80:395, 1974

179. Libonati M, Malsch E, Price HL, et al: Splanchnic circulation in man during methoxyflurane anesthesia. Anesthesiology 38:366, 1973

180. Cale JO, Parks CR, Jenkins MT: Hepatic and renal effects of methoxyflurane in dogs. Anesthesiology 23:248, 1962

181. Dahlgren BE, Goodrich BH: Changes in kidney and liver functions after methoxyflurane (Penthrane) anesthesia. Br J Anaesth 48:145, 1976

182. Botty C, Brown B, Stanley V, et al: Clinical experiences with compound 347—a halogenated anesthetic. Anesth Analg 47:499, 1968

183. Dobkin HB, Heinrich RG, Israel JS, et al: Clinical and laboratory evaluation of a new inhalation agent: Compound 347 (CHF$_2$-O-CF$_2$-CHFCl). Anesthesiology 29:275, 1968

184. Denlinger KJ, Lecky JH, Nahrwold ML: Hepatocellular dysfunction without jaundice after enflurane anesthesia. Anesthesiology 41:86, 1974

185. Van der Reis L, Askin SH, Freckner GN, et al: Hepatic necrosis after enflurane anesthesia. JAMA 227:76, 1974

186. Ona FV, Paranella H, Ayub A: Hepatitis associated with enflurane anesthesia. Anesth Analg 59:146, 1980

187. Paul JD, Fortune DW: Hepatotoxicity and death following two enflurane anaesthesias. Anaesthesia 42:1191, 1987

188. Lewis JH, Zimmerman HJ, Ishak KG, et al: Enflurane hepatoxicity. A clinicopathologic study of 24 cases. Ann Intern Med 98:984, 1983

189. Eger EI II, Smuckler EA, Ferrell LD, et al: Is enflurane hepatotoxic? Anesth Analg 65:21, 1986

190. Sadove MS, Reis L, Askin SH, et al: Hepatitis after use of two different fluorinated anesthetic agents. Anesth Analg 53:336, 1974

191. Sigurdsson J, Hriedarsson AB, Theodleifsson B: Enflurane hepatitis. A report of a case with a previous history of halothane hepatitis. Acta Anaesth Scand 29:495, 1985

192. Christ DD, Kenna JG, Kammerer W, et al: Enflurane metabolism produces convalently bound liver adducts recognized by antibodies from patients with halothane hepatitis. Anesthesiology 69:833, 1988

193. Lynch S, Martis L, Woods E: Evaluation of hepatotoxic potential of sevoflurane in rats. Pharmacologist 21:221, 1979

194. Crandell WB, Pappas SG, MacDonald A: Nephrotoxicity associated with methoxyflurane anesthesia. Anesthesiology 27:591, 1966

195. Mazze RI, Shue GL, Jackson SH: Renal dysfunction associated with methoxyflurane anesthesia. A randomized prospective clinical evaluation. JAMA 216:278, 1971

196. Mazze RI, Cousins MJ, Kosek JC: Dose-related methoxyflurane nephrotoxicity in rats: A biochemical and pathologic correlation. Anesthesiology 36:571, 1972

197. Smith FA (ed): Pharmacology of Fluorides. Handbook of Experimental Pharmacology. Springer-Verlag, New York, 1970

198. Cousins MJ, Mazze RI: Methoxyflurane nephrotoxicity: A study of dose response in man. JAMA 225:1611, 1973

199. Mazze RI, Cousins MJ: Combined nephrotoxicity of gentamicin and methoxyflurane anesthesia in man. A case report. Br J Anaesth 45:394, 1973

200. Barr GA, Mazze RI, Cousins MJ, et al: An animal model for combined methoxyflurane and gentamicin nephrotoxicity. Br J Anaesth 45:306, 1973

201. Hitt BA, Mazze RI, Denson DD: Isotopic probe of the mechanisms of methoxyflurane defluorination. Drug Metab Disp 7:446, 1979

202. McCarty LP, Malek RS, Larsen ER: The effects of deuteration on the metabolism of halogenated anesthetics in the rat. Anesthesiology 51:106, 1979

203. Baden JM, Rice SA, Mazze RI: Effects of deuterated methoxyflurane (d_4-MOF) on renal function in Fischer 344 rats. Anesthesiology 56:203, 1982

204. Mazze RI: The kidney: Anesthesia induced malfunction. p. 229. Twenty-Seventh Annual Refresher Course Lectures of the American Society of Anesthesiologists, San Francisco, 1976

205. Cousins MJ, Greenstein LR, Hitt BA, et al: Metabolism and renal effects of enflurane in man. Anesthesiology 44:44, 1976

206. Mazze RI, Calverley RK, Smith NT: Inorganic fluoride nephrotoxicity: Prolonged enflurane and halothane anesthesia in volunteers. Anesthesiology 46:265, 1977

207. Sievenpiper TS, Rice SA, McClendon F, et al: Renal effects of enflurane anesthetics in Fischer 344 rats with pre-existing renal insufficiency. J Pharmacol Exp Ther 211:36, 1979

208. Fish K, Sievenpiper TS, Rice SA, et al: Renal function in Fischer 344 rats with chronic renal impairment after the administration of enflurane and gentamicin. Anesthesiology 53:481, 1980

209. Mazze RI, Sievenpiper TS, Stevenson J: Renal effects of enflurane and halothane in patients with abnormal renal function. Anesthesiology 60:161, 1984

210. Cousins MJ, Mazze RI, Kosek JC, et al: The etiology of methoxyflurane nephrotoxicity. J Pharmacol Exp Ther 190:530, 1974

211. Kripke BJ, Kelman AD, Shah NK, et al: Testicular reaction to prolonged exposure to nitrous oxide. Anesthesiology 44:104, 1976

212. Coate WB, Kapp RW, Lewis TR: Chronic exposure to low concentrations of halothane-nitrous oxide: Reproductive and cytogenetic effects in the rat. Anesthesiology 50:310, 1979

213. Land PC, Owen EL, Linde HW: Mouse sperm morphology following exposure to anesthetics during early spermatogenis. Anesthesiology 51:S259, 1979

214. Baden JM, Land PC, Egbert B, et al: Lack of toxicity of enflurane on male reproductive organs in mice. Anesth Analg 61:19, 1980

215. Mazze RI, Rice SA, Wyrobeck AJ, et al: Germ cell studies in mice after prolonged exposure to nitrous oxide. Toxicol Appl Pharmacol 67:370, 1983

216. Wyrobeck AJ, Brodsky J, Gordon L, et al: Sperm studies in anesthesiologists. Anesthesiology 55:527, 1981

217. Royston BD, Nunn JF, Weinbren HK, et al: Rate of inactivation of human and rodent hepatic methionine synthase by nitrous oxide. Anesthesiology 68:213, 1988

218. Sharer NM, Nunn JF, Royston JP, Chanarin I: Effects of chronic exposure to nitrous oxide on methionine synthase activity. Br J Anaesth 5:693, 1983

219. O'Sullivan H, Jennings F, Ward K, et al: Human bone marrow biochemical function and megaloblastic hematopoiesis after nitrous oxide anesthesia. Anesthesiology 55:645, 1981

220. Amos RJ, Amess JAL, Hinds CJ, Mollin DL: Incidence and pathogenesis of of acute megaloblastic bone marrow change in patients receiving intensive care. Lancet 2:835, 1982

221. Sweeney B, Bingham RM, Amos RJ, et al: Toxicity of bone marrow in dentists exposed to nitrous oxide. Br Med J 291:567, 1985

222. Brodsky JB, Cohen EN, Brown BR, Jr., et al: Exposure to nitrous oxide and neurologic disease among dental professionals. Anesth Analg 60:297, 1981

223. NIOSH: Criteria for a recommended standard . . . occupational exposure to waste anesthetic gases and vapors. Department of Health, Education and Welfare (NIOSH) Publication No. 77-140, 1977

224. Millard RI, Corbett TH: Nitrous oxide concentration in the dental operatory. J Oral Surg 32:593, 1974

225. Pfaffli P, Nikki P, Ahlman K: Halothane and nitrous oxide in end-tidal air and venous blood of surgical personnel. Ann Clin Res 4:273, 1972

226. Baden JM, Simmon VF: Mutagenic effects of inhalation anesthetics. Mutat Res 75:169, 1980

227. Baden JM: Chronic toxicity of inhalation anaesthetics. Clin Anaesthesiol 1:441, 1983

228. Simmon VF, Baden JM: Mutagenic activity of vinyl compounds and derived epoxides. Mutat Res 78:227, 1980

229. Garrett S, Fuerst R: Sex-linked mutations in Drosophila after exposure to various mixtures of gas atmospheres. Environ Res 7:286, 1974

230. Kramers JC, Burm GL: Mutagenicity studies with halothane in Drosophila melanogaster. Anesthesiology 50:510, 1979

231. Kundomal Y, Baden JM: Mutagenicity of inhaled anesthetics in Drosophila melanogaster. Anesthesiology 62:305, 1985

232. Sparrow AH, Schairer LA: Mutagenic response of Tradescantia to treatment with x-rays, EMS, DBE, ozone, SO_2, N_2O and several insecticides. Mutat Res 26:445, 1974

233. Rosenberg PH, Kallio H: Operating-theatre gas pollution and chromosomes. Lancet 2:452, 1977

234. Baden JM, Kelly MJ, Cheung A, et al: Lack of mutagens in urine of operating personnel. Anesthesiology 53:195, 1980

235. Husum B, Niebuhr E, Wulf HC, et al: Sister chromatid exchanges and structural chromosome aberrations in lymphocytes in operating room personnel. Acta Anaesth Scand 27:262, 1983

236. Husum B, Wulf HC: Sister chromatid exchanges in lymphocytes in operating room personnel. Acta Anaesth Scand 24:22, 1980

237. Husum B, Wulf HC, Niebuhr E: Sister chromatid exchanges in lymphocytes after anesthesia with halothane or enflurane. Acta Anaesth Scand 25:97, 1981

238. Husum B, Wulf HC, Niebuhr E: Sister chromatid exchanges and structural chromosome aberrations in human lymphocytes after anaesthesia with fluroxene. Br J Anaesth 54:987, 1982

239. Cohen EN, Hood N: Application of low-temperature autoradiography to studies of the uptake and metabolism of volatile anesthetics in the mouse. III. Halothane. Anesthesiology 31:553, 1969

240. Leong BKJ, MacFarland HN, Reese WH: Induction of lung adenomas by chronic inhalation of bis(chloromethyl)ether. Arch Environ Health 22:663, 1976

241. Van Duuren BL, Goldschmidt BM, Katz C, et al: Alpha-haloethers: A new type of alkylating carcinogen. Arch Environ Health 16:472, 1968

242. Poirier LA, Stober GD, Shimkin MB: Bioassay of alkyl halides and nucleotide base analogs by pulmonary tumor response in strain A mice. Cancer Res 35:1411, 1975

243. Creech JL, Johnson MN: Angiosarcoma of the liver in the manufacture of polyvinylchloride. J Occup Med 16:150, 1974

244. Viola PL, Bigotti A, Caputo A: Oncogenic response of rat skin, lungs and and bone to vinyl chloride. Cancer Res 31:516, 1971

245. Maltoni C, Lefemine G: Carcinogenicity bioassays of vinyl chloride: Current results. Ann NY Acad Sci 246:195, 1975

246. Cavalieri E, Calvin M: Molecular characteristics of some carcinogenic hydrocarbons. Proc Natl Acad Sci USA 68:1251, 1971

247. Bruce DL, Eide KA, Linde HW, et al: Causes of death among anesthesiologists: A 20 year survey. Anesthesiology 29:565, 1968

248. Corbett TH, Cornell RG, Lieding K, et al: Incidence of cancer among Michigan nurse anesthetists. Anesthesiology 38:260, 1973

249. American Society of Anesthesiologists. Report of an ad hoc committee on the effect of trace anesthetics on the health of operating room personnel: Occupational Disease Among Operating Room Personnel: A National Study. Anesthesiology 41:321, 1974

250. Bruce DL, Eide KA, Smith NJ, et al: A prospective study of anesthesiologist mortality, 1967–1971. Anesthesiology 41:71, 1974

251. Doll R, Peto R: Mortality among doctors in different occupations. Br Med J 1:779, 1979

252. Lew EA: Mortality experience among anesthesiologists, 1954–1976. Anesthesiology 51:195, 1979

253. Tomlin PJ: Health problems of anesthetists and their families in the West Midlands. Br J Med 1:779, 1979

254. Cohen EN, Brown BW, Wu M: Occupational disease in dentistry and chronic exposure to trace anesthetic gases. J Am Dent Assoc 101:21, 1980

255. Neil HAW, Fairer JG, Coleman MP, et al: Mortality among male anesthetists in the United Kingdom, 1957–83. Br Med J 295:360, 1987

256. Walts LF, Forsythe AB, Moore JG: Critique: Occupational disease among operating room personnel. Anesthesiology 42:608, 1975

257. Fink BR, Cullen BF: Anesthetic pollution: What is happening to us? Anesthesiology 45:79, 1976

258. Vessey MP: Epidemiological studies of the occupational hazards of anesthesia—a review. Anaesthesia 33:430, 1978

259. Buring JE, Hennekens CH, Mayrent SL, et al: Health experiences of operating room personnel. Anesthesiology 62:325, 1985

260. Department of Health, Education and Welfare. Food and Drug Administration: Chloroform as an ingredient of human drug and cosmetic products. Fed Reg 14:15026, 1976

261. National Cancer Institute: Carcinogenesis technical report series. No. 2. Carcinogenesis bioassay of trichloroethylene. CAS No. 79-01-6, 1976

262. Oppenheimer BS, Oppenheimer ET, Danishefsky I, et al: Carcinogenic effect of metals in rodents. Cancer Res 16:439, 1956

263. Kucerova M, Zhurkov VS, Polivkova Z, et al: Mutagenic effect of epichlorohydrin. II. Analysis of chromosomal aberrations in lymphocytes of persons occupationally exposed to epichlorohydrin. Mutat Res 48:355, 1971

264. McCann J, Choi E, Yamasaki E, et al: The detection of carcinogens as mutagens in the Salmonella/microsome test: Assay of 300 chemicals. Part 1. Proc Natl Acad Sci USA 72:5135, 1975

265. Van Duuren BL, Goldschmidt BM, Katz C, et al: Carcinogenic activity of alkylating agents. J Natl Cancer Inst 53:695, 1974

266. Corbett TH: Cancer and congenital anomalies associated with anesthesia. Ann NY Acad Sci 271:58, 1976

267. Eger EI II, White AE, Brown CL, et al: A test of the carcinogenicity of enflurane, isoflurane, halothane, methoxyflurane and nitrous oxide in mice. Anesth Analg 57:678, 1978

268. Baden JM, Kundomal YR, Mazze RI, Kosek JC: Carcinogen bioassay of isoflurane in mice. Anesthesiology 69:750, 1988

269. Baden JM, Mazze RI, Wharton RS, et al: Carcinogenicity of halothane in Swiss/ICR mice. Anesthesiology 51:20, 1979

270. Baden JM, Egbert B, Mazze RI: Carcinogen bioassay of enflurane in mice. Anesthesiology 56:9, 1982

271. Baden JM, Kundomal YR, Luttropp ME, Jr., et al: Carcinogen bioassay of nitrous oxide in mice. Anesthesiology 64:747, 1986

272. Coate WB, Ulland BM, Lewis TR: Chronic exposure to low concentrations of halothane-nitrous oxide: Lack of carcinogenic effect in the rat. Anesthesiology 50:306, 1979

273. Klingberg MA, Weatherall JA (eds): Epidemiologic Methods for Detection of Teratogens. Karger AG, Basel S, 1979

274. Sturrock JE, Nunn JF: Mitosis in mammalian cells during exposure to anesthetics. Anesthesiology 43:21, 1975

275. Trudell JR: A unitary theory of anesthesia based on lateral phase separations in nerve membranes. Anesthesiology 46:5, 1977

276. Askrog V, Harvald B: Teratogen effect of inhalation anesthetics. Nord Med 83:498, 1970

277. Cohen EN, Bellville JW, Brown BW: Anesthesia, pregnancy and miscarriage: A study of operating room nurses and anesthetists. Anesthesiology 35:343, 1971

278. Knill-Jones RP, Moir DB, Rodrigues LV, et al: Anaesthetic practice and pregnancy: A controlled study of women anesthetists in the United Kingdom. Lancet 1:1326, 1972

279. Rosenberg P, Kirves A: Miscarriages among operating theatre staff. Acta Anaesthesiol Scand 53:37, 1973

280. Corbett TH, Cornell RG, Endres JL, et al: Birth defects among children of nurse anesthetists. Anesthesiology 41:341, 1974

281. Knill-Jones RP, Newman BJ, Spence AA: Anaesthetic practice and pregnancy: Controlled survey of male anaesthetists in the United Kingdom. Lancet 2:807, 1975

282. Cohen EN, Brown BW, Bruce DL, et al: A survey of anesthetic health hazards among dentists. J Am Dent Assoc 90:1291, 1975

283. Pharoah PO, Alberman E, Doyle P: Outcome of pregnancy among women in anaesthetic practice. Lancet 1:34, 1977

284. Ericson A, Kallen B: Survey of infants born in 1973 or 1975 to Swedish women working in operating rooms during their pregnancies. Anesth Analg 58:302, 1979

285. Axelsson G, Rylander R: Exposure to anesthetic gases and spontaneous abortion: Response in a postal questionnaire study. Int J Epidemiol 11:250, 1982

286. Hemminki K, Kyyronen P, Lindbohm M-L: Spontaneous abortions and malformations in the offspring of nurses exposed to anaesthetic gases, cytostatic drugs, and other potential hazards in hospitals, based on registered information of outcome. J Epidemiol Commun Health 39:141, 1985

287. Shnider SM, Webster GM: Maternal and fetal hazards of surgery during pregnancy. Am J Obstet Gynecol 92:891, 1965

288. Smith BE: Fetal prognosis after anesthesia during gestation. Anesth Analg 42:521, 1963

289. Brodsky JB, Cohen EN, Brown BW, et al: Surgery during pregnancy and fetal outcome. Am J Obstet Gynecol 8:1165, 1980

290. Duncan PG, Pope WDB, Cohen MM, Greer N: Fetal risk of anesthesia and surgery during pregnancy. Anesthesiology 64:790, 1986

291. Ferstandig LL: Trace concentrations of anesthetic gases: A critical review of their disease potential. Anesth Analg 57:328, 1978

292. Shepard TH, Fink BR: Teratogenic activity of nitrous oxide in rats. p. 308. In Fink BR (ed): Toxicity of Anesthetics. Williams & Wilkins, Baltimore, 1968

293. Vieira E, Cleaton-Jones P, Austin JC, et al: Effects of low concentration of nitrous oxide on rat fetuses. Anesth Analg 59:175, 1980

294. Mazze RI, Wilson AI, Rice SA, Baden JM: Reproduction and fetal development in rats exposed to nitrous oxide. Teratology 30:259, 1984

295. Fujinaga M, Mazze RI, Baden JM, et al: Rat whole embryo culture: An in vitro model for testing nitrous oxide teratogenicity. Anesthesiology 69:401, 1988

296. Quimby KL, Katz J, Bowman RE: Behavioral consequences in rats from chronic exposure to 10 ppm halothane during early development. Anesth Analg 54:628, 1975

297. Quimby KL, Aschkanase LJ, Bowman RE, et al: Enduring learning deficits and cerebral synaptic malformation from exposure to 10 parts of halothane per million. Science 185:625, 1974

298. Chang LW, Dudley AWJ, Katz J: Pathological changes in the nervous system following exposure to halothane. Environ Res 11:40, 1976

299. Smith RF, Bowman RE, Katz J: Behavioral effects of exposure to halothane during pregnancy. Anesthesiology 49:319, 1978

300. Koeter HBWM, Rodier PM: Behavioral effects in mice exposed to nitrous oxide or halothane: Prenatal vs. postnatal exposure. Neurobehav Toxicol Teratol 8:189, 1986

301. Rodier PM, Koeter HBWM: General activity from weaning to maturity in mice exposed to halothane or nitrous oxide. Neurobehav Toxicol Teratol 8:195, 1986

302. Rice SA: Prenatal N_2O exposure alters reflex to adult mice. Toxicologist 6:75, 1986

303. Mullenix PJ, Moore PA, Tassinari MS: Behavioral toxicity of nitrous oxide in rats following prenatal exposure. Toxicol Ind Health 2:273, 1986

304. Peters MA, Hudson AM: Postnatal development and behavior in offspring of enflurane exposed pregnant rats. Arch Int Pharmacol Ther 256:134, 1982

305. Wilson JE: Mechanisms of teratogenesis. p. 83. In: Environment and Birth Defects. Academic Press, Orlando, FL, 1973

306. Schardein JL: Principles of teratogenesis applicable to human exposure to drugs and chemicals. p.1 In: Chemically Induced Birth Defects. Marcel Dekker, New York, 1985

7

INHALED ANESTHETIC DELIVERY SYSTEMS

J. Jeffrey Andrews

Parts of this chapter have appeared in Barash PG, Cullen BF, Stoelting RK (eds): Clinical Anesthesia. JB Lippincott, Philadelphia, 1989. Reprinted with permission.

INTRODUCTION

Inhaled anesthetic delivery systems deliver a gas mixture of precisely known but variable composition to the patient. Delivery system components include the anesthesia machine, the vaporizers, the anesthetic circuit, and the ventilator. Removal of excess gas is accomplished by the scavenging system. A thorough understanding of these parts is essential to the safe practice of anesthesia. This chapter discusses the normal operation, function, and integration of major system components. More importantly, it illustrates some problems and hazards associated with each and describes appropriate preoperative checks.

ANESTHESIA MACHINES

Machine technology and emphasis on patient safety have increased over the years. The American National Standards Institute (ANSI) published the Z79.8-1979 machine standard in 1979.[1] The document was a landmark for the advancement of machine technology and patient safety because it provided guidelines to manufacturers regarding the minimum performance, design characteristics, and safety requirements for anesthesia machines. For almost 10 years, the ANSI Z79.8-1979 standard was the guideline, but it has recently been superseded by the American Society for Testing and Materials (ASTM) F1161-88 standard.[2]

The two documents share many similarities, but a few major differences exist. The ANSI Z79.8-1979 standard addressed both flowmeter-controlled vaporizers and electrically heated vaporizers. The new ASTM F1161-88 standard does not since these vaporizers are no longer manufactured in the United States. Several new requirements exist in the new document that were not present in the ANSI Z79.8-1979 standard. To meet the ASTM standard, newly manufactured anesthesia machines must have an oxygen analyzer, a breathing pressure monitor, and either an exhaled tidal volume monitor or a carbon dioxide monitor. These monitors must be in an enabled condition and functioning automatically when the machine is in use. The machine must have a prioritized alarm system that groups alarms into three categories: high priority, medium priority, and low priority.

Equipment does not automatically become obsolete when new standards are published and manufacturers are not forced to comply with them.[3] Nevertheless, the Ohmeda Modulus II Plus (Fig. 7-1) and the North American Drager Narkomed 3 (Fig. 7-2) meet and exceed the new ASTM F1161-88 standard.

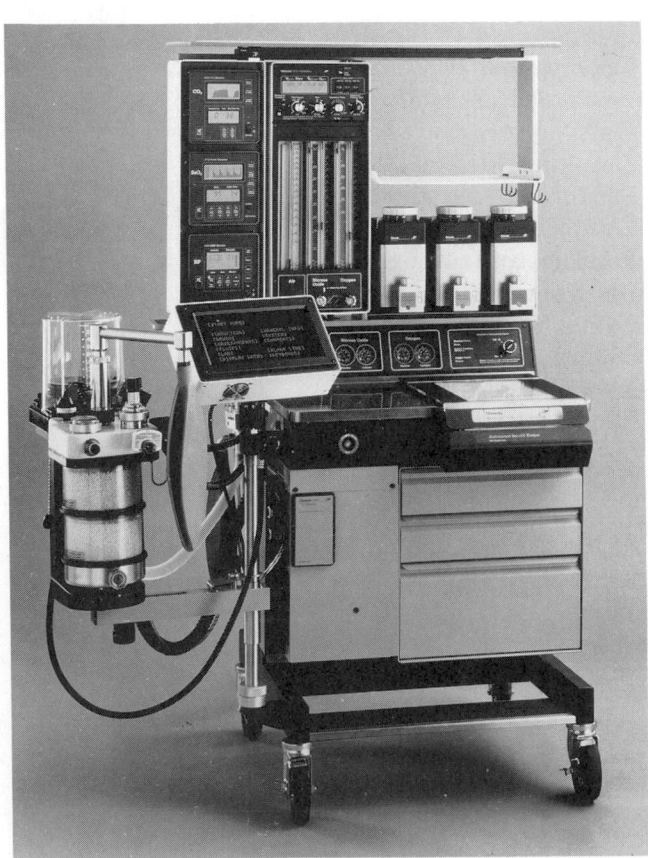

Fig. 7-1. Modulus II Plus anesthesia system. (Courtesy of Ohmeda, The BOC Group Inc., Madison, WI.)

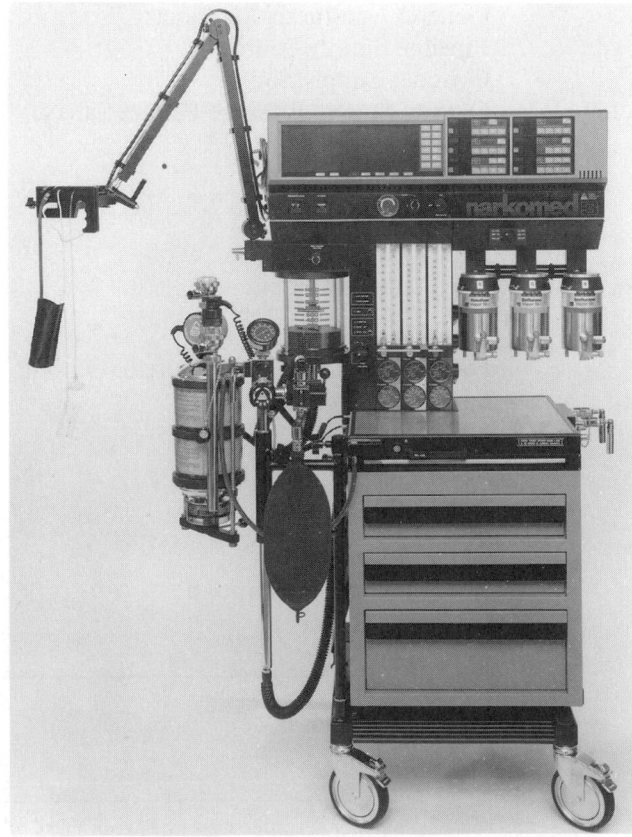

Fig. 7-2. Narkomed 3 anesthesia system. (Courtesy of North American Drager, Telford, PA.)

Generic Anesthesia Machines

A generic two-gas anesthesia machine is shown in Figure 7-3. Both oxygen and nitrous oxide have two supply sources. They consist of a pipeline supply source and a cylinder supply source. The pipeline supply source is the primary gas source for the anesthesia machine. The hospital piping system provides gases to the machine at approximately 50 pounds per square inch gauge (PSIG), which is the normal working pressure of most machines. The cylinder supply source serves as a backup if the pipeline fails. The oxygen cylinder source is regulated from 2,200 to approximately 45 PSIG, and the nitrous oxide cylinder source is regulated from 745 to approximately 45 PSIG.[4,5]

A safety device traditionally referred to as the fail-safe system is located downstream from the nitrous oxide supply source. It serves as an interface between the oxygen and nitrous oxide supply sources. This device shuts off or proportionally decreases the supply of nitrous oxide (and other gases) if the oxygen supply pressure decreases. Contemporary machines monitor the oxygen supply pressure using an alarm device that is actuated at a predetermined oxygen pressure such as 30 PSIG.[4–6]

Some machines have a second-stage oxygen regulator located downstream from the oxygen supply source. It is adjusted to a precise pressure level, such as 15 PSIG. This regulator supplies a constant pressure to the oxygen flow control valve regardless of fluctuating oxygen pipeline pressures. For example, the output from the oxygen flow control valve will be constant if the oxygen supply pressure is greater than 15 PSIG. The oxygen flow control valve allows the operator to con-

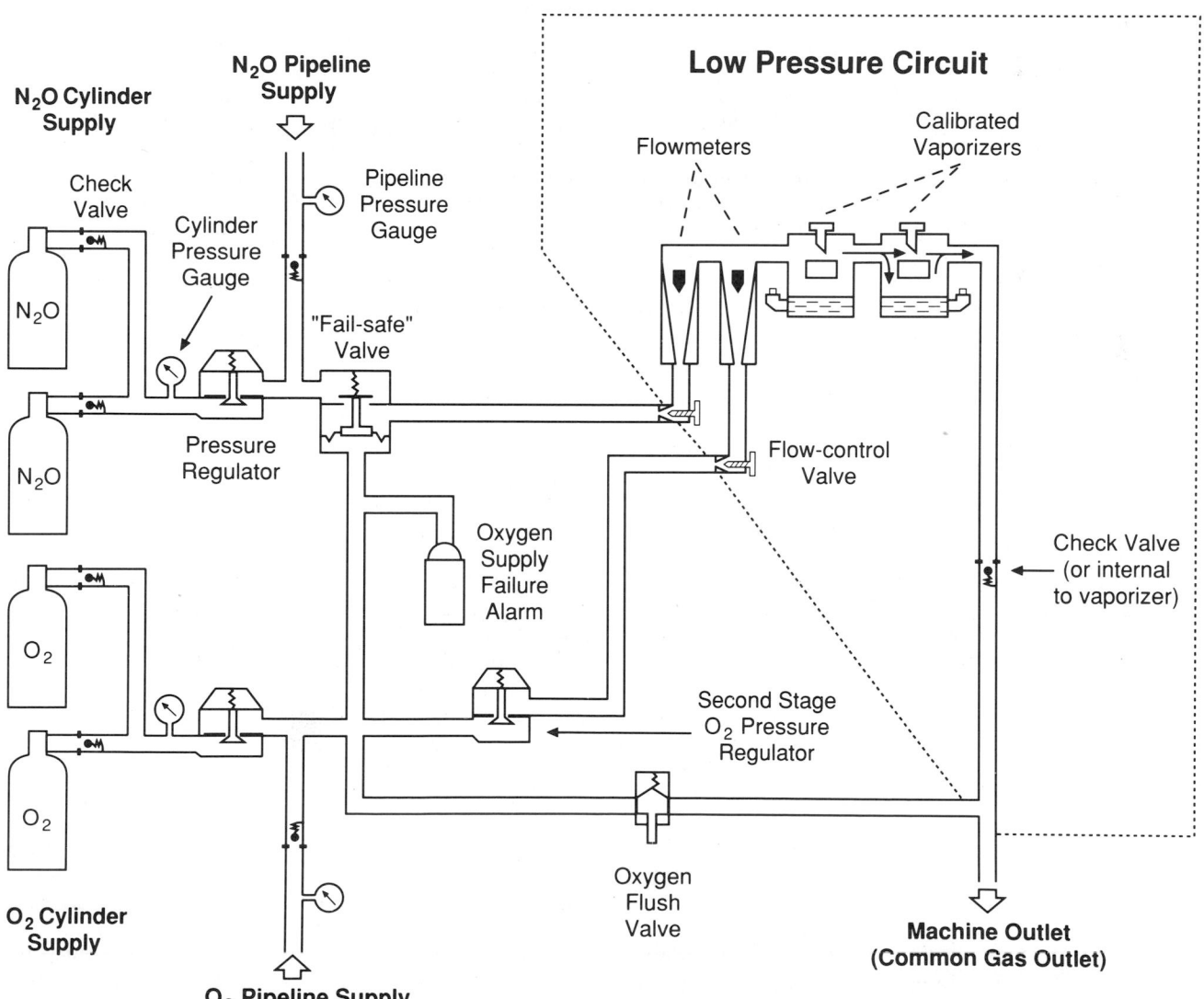

Fig. 7-3. Diagram of a generic two-gas anesthesia machine. (Modified from American Society of Anesthesiologists,[136] with permission.)

trol precisely the oxygen flow rate that is indicated on the oxygen flowmeter. The oxygen flow joins the flow from the nitrous oxide flowmeter in a common manifold and is directed to a calibrated variable-bypass vaporizer. Varying amounts of inhaled anesthetic can be added to the mixture, depending on the vaporizer setting. The mixture flows toward the common gas outlet.

Many machines have a machine outlet check valve between the vaporizers and the common gas outlet. Its purpose is to prevent backflow into the vaporizer, therefore minimizing the effects of downstream intermittent pressure fluctuations on agent concentration (see the section, *Vaporizers, Intermittent Back Pressure*). The presence or absence of a check valve *profoundly* influences the preoperative machine check (see the section, *Checking Anesthesia Machines*). The oxygen flush connection joins the mixed-gas pipeline between the one-way check valve and the machine outlet. Thus, the oxygen flush, when activated, has a "straight shot" to the common outlet.[4,5]

Pipeline Supply Source

The pipeline supply source is the primary gas source for the anesthesia machine. Most hospitals today have a central piping system to deliver medical gases such as oxygen, nitrous oxide, and air to the operating room. The central piping system must supply the anesthesia machine with the appropriate gas at the appropriate pressure for the machine to function properly. Unfortunately, this has not always occurred.

In a survey of approximately 200 hospitals in 1976, 31 percent reported difficulties with the pipeline systems.[7] The most common problem was inadequate oxygen pressure. This was followed by excessive pipeline pressures. The most devastating reported hazard, however, was accidental crossing of oxygen and nitrous oxide pipelines, which caused several deaths. The operator must take two actions if a pipeline crossover is suspected. First, the backup oxygen cylinder should be turned on. Then, the pipeline supply must be disconnected. This second step is mandatory because the machine will preferentially use the inappropriate 50 PSIG pipeline supply source instead of the lower pressure (45 PSIG) oxygen cylinder source.

Gas enters the anesthesia machine through the pipeline inlet connections (Fig. 7-3, see arrows). The pipeline inlet fittings are gas-specific Diameter Index Safety (D.I.S.S.) threaded body fittings. The D.I.S.S. provides threaded noninterchangeable connections for medical gas lines, and this minimizes the risk of misconnection. A check valve is located downstream from the inlet. It prevents reverse flow of gases from the machine to the pipeline or to the atmosphere.[2]

A pipeline pressure gauge is mandated by the ASTM F1161-88 standard. It must be located on the pipeline side rather than on the machine side of the check valve (Fig. 7-3).[2] Pressure measured in this location truly reflects pipeline pressure instead of pressure within the

machine. For example, the gauge will read zero if the pipeline supply source is not connected to the anesthesia machine, irrespective of the on/off status of the cylinders. A value of 50 PSIG, however, does not guarantee that the pipeline is supplying the machine. The gauge will read 50 PSIG even when the check valve is stuck in the closed position. The operator should open the backup cylinder if this problem is suspected.

Some older anesthesia machines had a "pipeline" pressure gauge located on the machine side of the check valve. The gauge read approximately 50 PSIG when the machine was connected to the pipeline source. However, if the cylinders were turned on, the gauge read 45 PSIG even when the pipeline source was disconnected. If the operator did not recognize this subtle difference (45 versus 50 PSIG), cylinder depletion potentially resulted in a zero gas source status.

Cylinder Supply Source

Anesthesia machines have reserve E cylinders if a pipeline supply source is not available or if the pipeline fails. Color-coded cylinders are attached to the anesthesia machine through the hanger yoke assembly. The hanger yoke assembly orients and supports the cylinder, provides a gas-tight seal, and ensures a unidirectional flow of gases into the machine.[4] Each hanger yoke is equipped with the Pin Index Safety System (P.I.S.S.). The P.I.S.S. is a safeguard introduced to eliminate cylinder interchanging and the possibility of accidentally placing the incorrect gas on a yoke designed to accommodate another gas. Two pins on the yoke are so arranged that they project into the cylinder valve. Each gas or combination of gases has a specific pin arrangement.[8]

Gas travels from the high-pressure cylinder source to the anesthesia machine when the cylinder is turned on (Fig. 7-3). A check valve is located downstream from each cylinder if a double-yoke assembly is used. The check valve has several functions. First, it minimizes gas transfer from a cylinder at high pressure to one with lower pressure. Second, it allows an empty cylinder to be exchanged for a full one while gas flow continues from the other cylinder into the machine with minimal loss of gas. Third, it minimizes leakage from an open cylinder to the atmosphere if one cylinder is absent.[4,5] A cylinder supply pressure gauge is located downstream from the check valves. The gauge will indicate the pressure in the cylinder having the higher pressure when two reserve cylinders of the same gas are opened at the same time.[9]

Each cylinder supply source has a pressure reducing valve known as the cylinder pressure regulator. It reduces the high and variable storage pressure present in a cylinder to a lower, more constant pressure suitable for use in the anesthesia machine. The oxygen cylinder pressure regulator reduces the oxygen cylinder pressure from a high 2,200 PSIG to approximately 45 PSIG. The nitrous oxide cylinder pressure regulator receives pressure of up to 745 PSIG and reduces it to approximately 45 PSIG.[4,5] Before the incorporation of cylinder pressure regulators into anesthesia machines, the operator had to progressively open the flow control valves to maintain a constant flow as the cylinder pressure declined.

The cylinders should be turned off except during the preoperative machine-checking period or when a pipeline source is unavailable. The reserve cylinder supply can be silently depleted if the cylinders are left on. This depletion occurs any time the pressure inside the machine decreases to a value lower than the regulated cylinder pressure. Oxygen pressure within the machine can decrease below 45 PSIG with oxygen flushing or with ventilator use, particularly at high peak flow rates. The pipeline supply pressures of all gases can be less than 45 PSIG if problems exist in the central piping system. If the cylinders are left on, they will eventually become depleted. Then, no reserve supply will be available if there is a pipeline failure.[5,10]

Oxygen Supply Pressure Failure Safety Devices

Oxygen and nitrous oxide supply sources existed as independent entities in older models of anesthesia machines, and they were not interfaced. Therefore, abrupt or insidious oxygen pressure failure had the potential to lead to the delivery of a hypoxic mixture. The ASTM F1161-88 standard states that "The anesthesia gas machine shall be designed so that whenever oxygen pressure is reduced from normal, and until flow ceases, the set oxygen concentration shall not decrease at the common outlet."[2] Contemporary anesthesia machines have a number of safety devices that act together in a cascade manner to minimize the risk of hypoxia as oxygen pressure decreases. Several of these devices are described below.

Pneumatic and Electronic Alarm Devices

Many older anesthesia machines have a pneumatic alarm device that sounds a warning when the oxygen supply pressure decreases to a predetermined threshold value such as 30 PSIG. The new ASTM F1161-88 standard mandates that both audible and visual indications occur when the oxygen pressure decreases below a manufacturer-specific pressure threshold.[2] Electronic alarm devices are now used to meet this guideline. The oxygen pressure threshold value for the Ohmeda Modulus II Plus is 27 PSIG, and it is 30 ± 3 PSIG for the Drager Narkomed 2B and the Narkomed 3.[9]

Fail-Safe Systems

A fail-safe valve is present in the gas line supplying each of the flowmeters except oxygen. The valve is controlled by oxygen pressure. It shuts off or proportionally decreases the supply of gases other than oxygen (nitrous oxide, air, carbon dioxide, helium, nitrogen) as the oxygen supply pressure decreases. Unfortunately, the misnomer of fail-safe has led to the misconception that the device prevents administration of a hypoxic mixture. This is not the case. Machines that are not equipped with a proportioning system (see the section, *Proportioning Systems*) can deliver a hypoxic mixture under normal working conditions. The oxygen flow control valve can be closed intentionally or accidentally. Normal oxygen pressure will maintain other gas lines open so that a hypoxic mixture can result.[4,5]

Ohmeda machines are equipped with a fail-safe valve known as the pressure-sensor shutoff valve. It is threshold in nature and is either open or closed. Figure 7-4 shows a nitrous oxide pressure-sensor shutoff valve with a threshold pressure of 20 PSIG. An oxygen pressure greater than the threshold value is exerted upon the mobile diaphragm in Figure 7-4A. This moves the

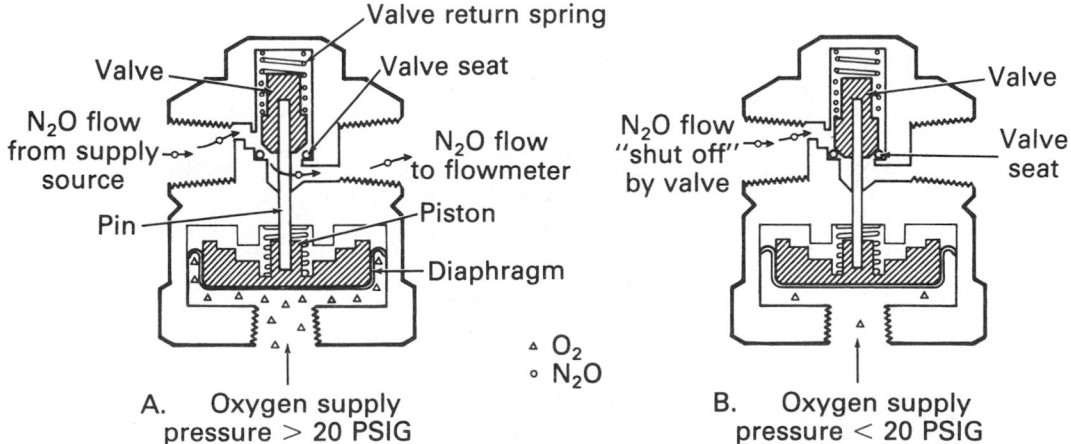

Fig. 7-4. Pressure-sensor shutoff valve. **(A)** The valve is open because the oxygen supply pressure is greater than the threshold value of 20 PSIG. **(B)** The valve is closed because of inadequate oxygen pressure. (Redrawn from Bowie and Huffman,[5] with permission.)

piston, pin, and valve off the valve seat. Nitrous oxide flow passes freely to the nitrous oxide flow control valve. The oxygen supply pressure in Figure 7-4B is less than 20 PSIG, and the force of the valve return spring completely closes the valve.[5]

Drager uses a fail-safe valve known as the Oxygen Failure Protection Device (OFPD) that interfaces the oxygen pressure with that of other gases, such as nitrous oxide, air, carbon dioxide, helium, and nitrogen. It differs from Ohmeda's oxygen pressure-sensor shut-off valve because the OFPD is based on a proportioning principle rather than a threshold principle. The pressure of all gases controlled by the OFPD will decrease proportionally with the oxygen pressure. The OFPD consists of a seat-nozzle assembly that is connected to a spring-loaded piston (Fig. 7-5). The oxygen supply pressure in the left panel is 50 PSIG. This pressure pushes the piston upward, forcing the nozzle away from the valve seat. Nitrous oxide (or other gases) advances toward the flow control valve at 50 PSIG. The oxygen pressure in the right panel is 0 PSIG. The spring is expanded and forces the nozzle against the seat, preventing flow through the device. Finally, the center panel shows an intermediate oxygen pressure of 25 PSIG. The force of the spring partially closes the valve. The nitrous oxide pressure delivered to the flow control valve is 25 PSIG. There is a vast continuum of intermediate configurations between the extremes (0 to 50 PSIG) of oxygen supply pressure. These intermediate configurations are responsible for the proportional nature of the OFPD.[6]

Second-Stage Oxygen Pressure Regulator

Most contemporary Ohmeda machines have a second-stage oxygen regulator set from 12 to 16 PSIG. Oxygen flowmeter output is constant when the oxygen supply pressure exceeds the set value. Ohmeda pressure-sensor shutoff valves are set at a higher threshold value (20 to 30 PSIG). This ensures that oxygen is the last gas flow to decrease if oxygen pressure fails.[11-15]

Oxygen Ratio Monitor Controller

The Oxygen Ratio Monitor Controller (ORMC) is a complex safety device used on contemporary Drager machines and is located downstream from the OFPD.[6,9,16,17] Both devices work together in a cascade manner when the oxygen supply pressure decreases. First, the OFPD proportionally decreases the pressure of the other gases such as nitrous oxide.[6] Then, the spring-loaded ORMC shuts off the nitrous oxide slave control valve when the oxygen pressure decreases below 10 PSIG. Thus, oxygen flow is the last to cease. This action represents only one function of the ORMC, which also serves as a proportioning device and an alarm system. The ORMC is discussed in detail in the section, *Proportioning Systems.*

Integration of Oxygen Pressure Failure Safety Devices

Different brands and models of anesthesia machines respond differently to an insidious decline in oxygen supply pressure.[18,19] Careful evaluation of a machine's response to a decline in oxygen supply pressure serves as a noninvasive fingerprint of the design of the internal anesthesia machine. Examples of such fingerprints are shown in Figure 7-6. They were generated in the following manner. All machine E cylinders were turned off, and a constant 50 PSIG nitrous oxide source was connected to the nitrous oxide pipeline inlet. With an initial oxygen pressure of 50 PSIG, the nitrous oxide and oxygen flow control valves were set to deliver 7 L/min nitrous oxide and 3 L/min oxygen. Total gas flow was calculated by adding the individual gas flows. An oxygen analyzer at the common outlet was used to determine the oxygen concentration of the fresh gas. The

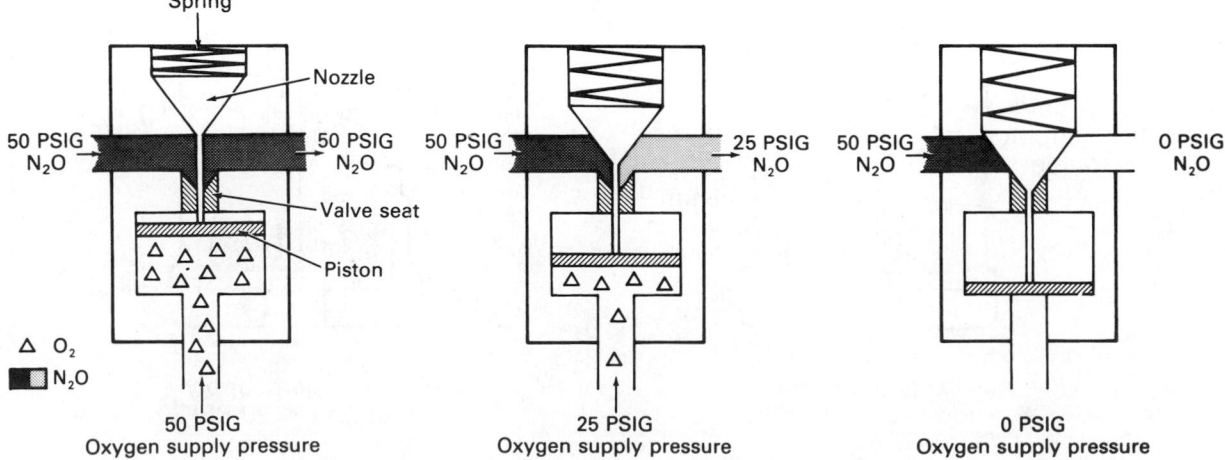

Fig. 7-5. Oxygen Failure Protection Device (OFPD). The OFPD responds proportionally to changes in oxygen supply pressure. (See text for details.) (Redrawn from Narkomed 2A Anesthesia System,[6] with permission.)

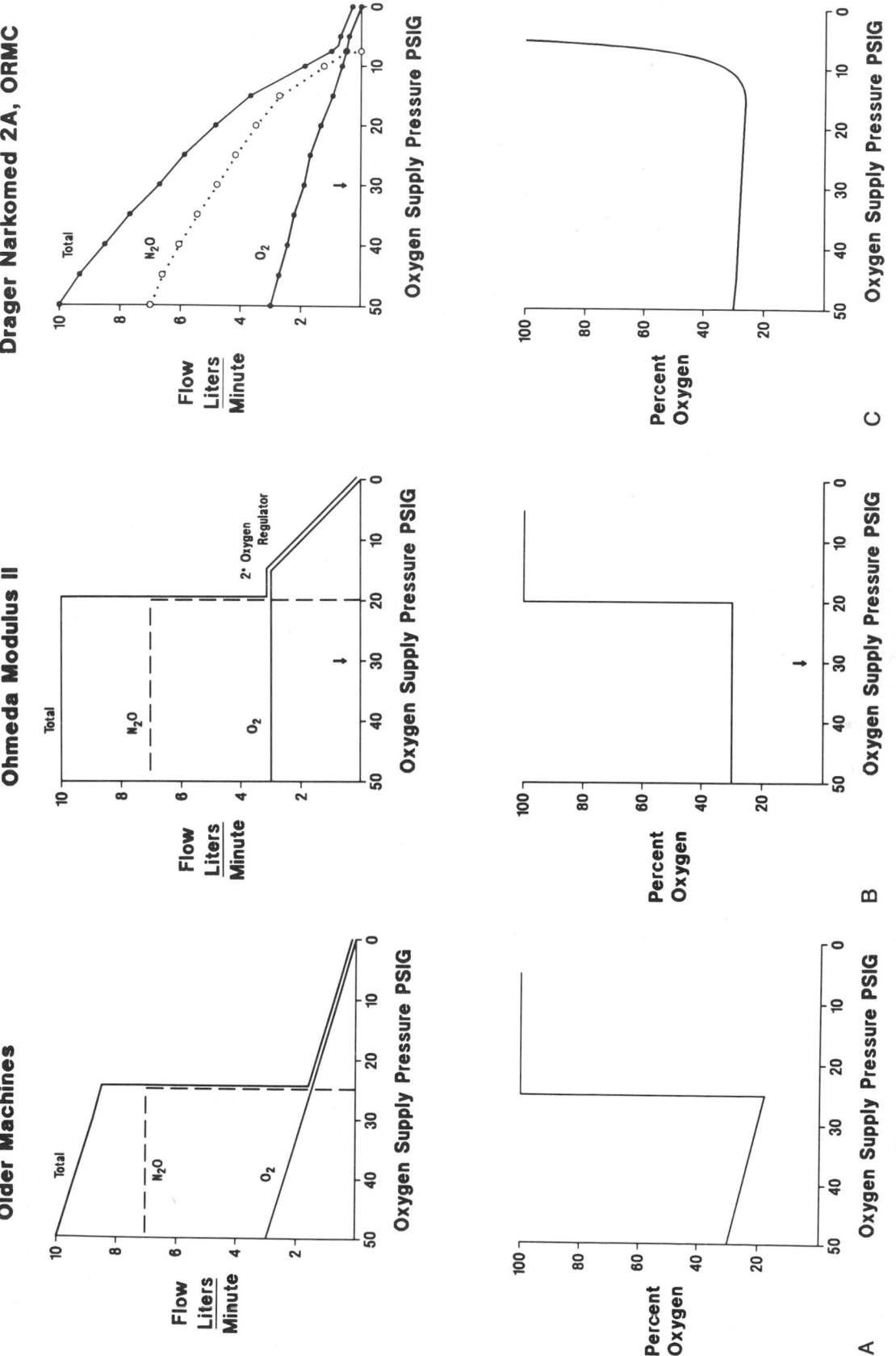

Fig. 7-6. Response of three anesthesia machines to a gradual decline in oxygen supply pressure. (A) The response of an older machine; (B) the response of an Ohmeda Modulus II; (C) the response of a Drager Narkomed 2A. Vertical arrows represent the oxygen supply pressure at which the low-oxygen pressure alarm sounds. (See text for details.) (From Andrews,[19] with permission.)

oxygen supply pressure was decreased in 5 PSIG decrements without changing the settings of the flow control valves. Gas flow and oxygen concentration were remeasured at each decrement, and the results were graphed.

Older Machines

Figure 7-6A represents the fingerprint of an older anesthesia machine that does not have a second-stage oxygen regulator. It does have, however, a threshold pressure-sensor shutoff valve set at 25 PSIG. A linear decline in oxygen flow occurs as the oxygen pressure decreases because of the absence of the second-stage regulator. Since the nitrous oxide supply pressure is adequate, the nitrous oxide flow remains constant at 7 L/min until the 25 PSIG oxygen pressure threshold is reached. A vulnerable oxygen pressure zone exists from 50 to 26 PSIG because the oxygen concentration of the fresh gas decreases and total flow decreases. The oxygen concentration increases to 100 percent below 25 PSIG oxygen pressure because the nitrous oxide is shut off by the oxygen pressure-sensor shutoff valve.

Ohmeda Modulus II

Figure 7-6B is the fingerprint of an Ohmeda Modulus II. It has a pneumatic low-oxygen-supply-pressure alarm set at 30 PSIG, a pressure-sensor shutoff valve set at 20 PSIG, and a second-stage oxygen regulator set at 14 PSIG.[12,13] The oxygen flow remains constant as long as the oxygen pressure is greater than 14 PSIG. This is unlike older machines without the second-stage oxygen regulator. As the oxygen supply pressure decreases from 50 to 21 PSIG, the flow of oxygen and nitrous oxide remains constant at 3 and 7 L/min, respectively. A pneumatic low-oxygen-pressure alarm sounds at 30 PSIG to alert the operator of a problem. It is important to note that when the alarm sounds, the oxygen concentration and the flows are identical to those at 50 PSIG. The nitrous oxide is shut off when the oxygen supply pressure decreases to 20 PSIG, which is the threshold pressure for the oxygen pressure-sensor shutoff valve. The oxygen concentration at that point increases to 100 percent. Oxygen flow remains constant at 3 L/min from 20 to 15 PSIG because the second-stage oxygen regulator is set at 14 PSIG. Finally, there is a linear decrease in oxygen flow with decreasing oxygen supply pressure below 14 PSIG.

The Ohmeda Modulus II response to loss of oxygen supply pressure has several advantages over older machines. The oxygen concentration remains constant or increases, and the operator is alerted to a problem before flows decrease. Oxygen flow remains constant because the value of the second-stage oxygen regulator is set at a low pressure until the oxygen supply pressure is almost depleted.

Drager Narkomed 2A ORMC

The Drager Narkomed 2A ORMC response to decreasing oxygen supply pressure is unique and is shown in Figure 7-6C. Several safety devices are recruited as the oxygen supply pressure decreases. These include the OFPD, the electronic low-oxygen-pressure alarm set at 30 PSIG, and the ORMC. First, the OFPD proportionally decreases nitrous oxide pressure in response to reduced oxygen pressure.[6] Flow reductions are proportional, and the oxygen concentration of the fresh gas mixture remains constant at 30 percent from 50 PSIG to approximately 10 PSIG. The spring-loaded ORMC shuts off nitrous oxide flow entirely when the oxygen pressure is below 10 PSIG. The oxygen concentration of the fresh gas then increases to 100 percent.

An attractive feature of the Narkomed 2A response to decreasing oxygen pressure is that the oxygen concentration is maintained or increased. A vulnerable oxygen supply pressure zone theoretically exists from 50 to 31 PSIG, because flows can decrease as much as 30 percent before the operator is alerted to an oxygen pressure problem. Clinically, however, this is probably insignificant because oxygen supply failure is usually complete and abrupt instead of gradual.

Flowmeter Assembly

The flowmeter assembly (Fig. 7-7) precisely controls and measures gas flow to the common gas outlet. The flow control valve regulates the amount of flow that enters a tapered, transparent flowtube known as a Thorpe tube. A mobile indicator float inside the flowtube indicates the amount of flow passing through the flow control valve. The quantity of flow is indicated on a scale associated with the flowtube.[4,5]

Physical Principles of Flowmeters

Opening the flow control valve allows gas to travel through the space between the float and the flowtube. This space is known as the annular space (Fig. 7-8). The indicator float hovers freely in an equilibrium position where the upward force resulting from gas flow equals the downward force on the float resulting from gravity at a given flow rate. The float moves to a new equilibrium position in the tube when flow is changed. These flowmeters are commonly referred to as *constant pressure flowmeters* because the pressure decrease across the float remains constant for all positions in the tube.[4,8,20]

Flowtubes are tapered, with the smallest diameter at the bottom of the tube and the largest diameter at the top. The term *variable orifice* designates this type of unit because the annular space between the float and the inner wall of the flowtube varies with the position of the float. The constriction created by the float can be tubular or orificial, depending on the flow rate (Fig. 7-9). The characteristics of a gas that influence its flow rate through a given constriction are (1) its density and (2) its viscosity. The annular space is tubular at low flow rates. Poiseuille's law applies in this situation, and *viscosity* becomes dominant in determining gas flow rate. The annular space simulates an orifice at high flow rates, and gas flow rate then depends predominantly on the *density* of the gas.[4,20]

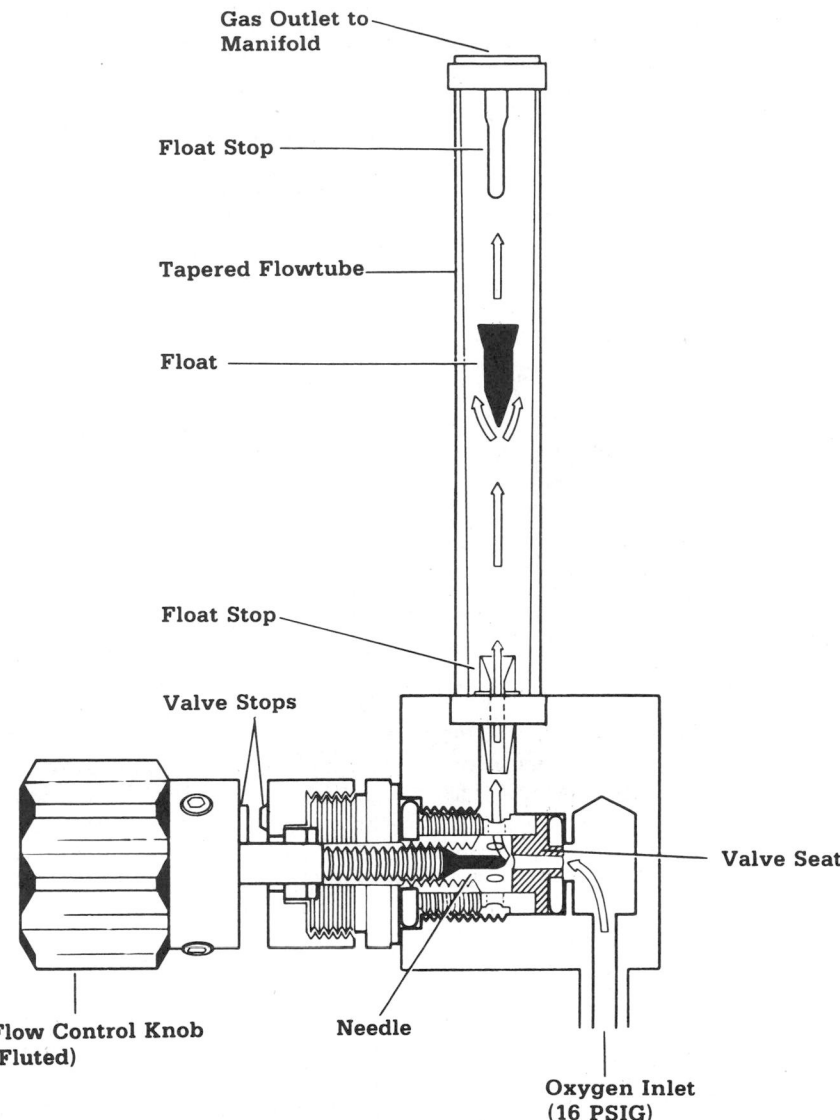

Gas Outlet to Manifold

Float Stop

Tapered Flowtube

Float

Float Stop

Valve Stops

Flow Control Knob (Fluted)

Needle

Valve Seat

Oxygen Inlet (16 PSIG)

Fig. 7-7. Oxygen flowmeter assembly. The oxygen flowmeter assembly is composed of the flow control valve assembly plus the flowmeter subassembly. (From Bowie and Huffman,[5] with permission.)

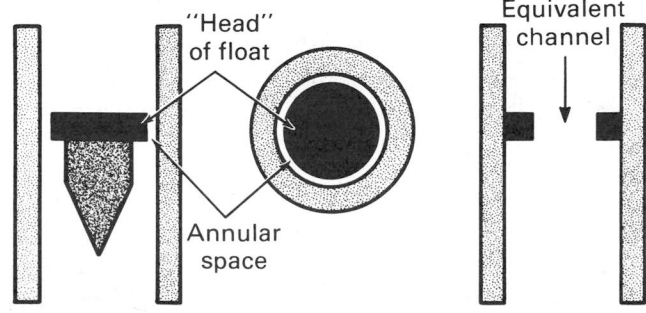

"Head" of float

Annular space

Equivalent channel

Fig. 7-8. The annular space. The clearance between the head of the float and the flowtube is known as the annular space. It can be considered an equivalent to a circular channel of the same cross-sectional area. (Redrawn from Macintosh et al.,[20] with permission.)

Components of Flowmeter Assembly

Flow Control Valve Assembly

The flow control valve assembly is composed of a flow control knob, a needle valve, a valve seat, and a pair of valve stops.[4] The assembly can receive its pneumatic input either directly from the pipeline source (50 PSIG) or from a second-stage pressure regulator.[5] The flow control valves are supplied by 50 PSIG on contemporary Drager machines such as the Narkomed 2A, Narkomed 2B, and Narkomed 3.[6,9,16,17] In contrast, the Ohmeda Modulus II oxygen and nitrous oxide flow control valves are supplied by 14 PSIG and approximately 26 PSIG, respectively.[13]

The location of the needle valve in the valve seat changes to establish different orifices when the flow control valve is adjusted. Gas flow increases when the

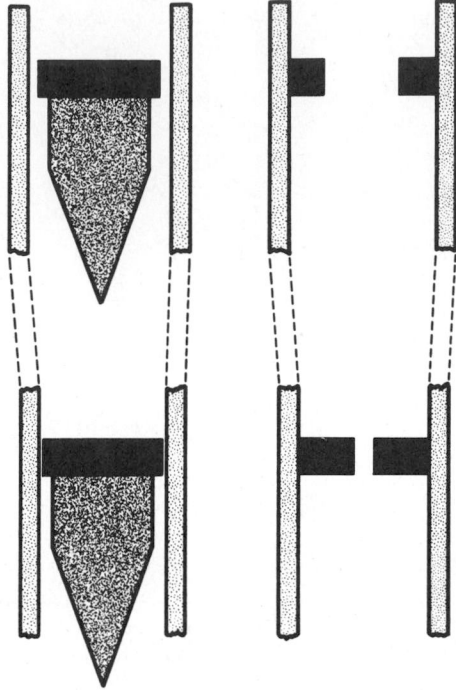

Fig. 7-9. Flowtube constriction. The lower pair of illustrations represents the lower portion of a flowtube. The clearance between the head of the float and the flowtube is narrow. The equivalent channel is tubular because its diameter is less than its length. Viscosity is dominant in determining gas flow rate through this tubular constriction. The upper pair of illustrations represents the upper portion of a flowtube. The equivalent channel is orificial because its length is less than its width. Density is dominant in determining gas flow rate through this orificial constriction. (Redrawn from Macintosh et al.,[20] with permission.)

flow control valve is turned counterclockwise, and it decreases when the valve is turned clockwise. Extreme clockwise rotation results in damage to the needle valve and valve seat. Therefore, flow control valves are equipped with valve stops to prevent this occurrence.[5] The stops come into contact with each other at zero flow on most flow control valves. However, the oxygen flow control valve stops of the Ohmeda Modulus I, Modulus II, Modulus II Plus, and Ohmeda 8000 are set at an oxygen flow rate of approximately 200 cc/min.[11-15] Thus, on contemporary Ohmeda machines, minimum oxygen flow results from incomplete closure of the oxygen flow control valve. On contemporary Drager machines, the oxygen flow control valve does close completely. Minimum oxygen flow enters the oxygen flow tube just downstream from the flow control valve.[6,9,16,17]

Safety Features. Contemporary flow control valve assemblies have numerous safety features. The oxygen flow control knob is physically distinguishable from other gas knobs. It is distinctively fluted, projects beyond the control knobs of the other gases, and is larger in diameter. All knobs are color coded for the appropriate gas, and the chemical formula or name of the gas is permanently marked on each. Flow control knobs are recessed or protected with a shield or barrier to minimize inadvertent change from a preset position. If a single gas has two flowtubes, the tubes are arranged in series and are controlled by a single flow control valve.[2]

Flowmeter Subassembly

The flowmeter subassembly consists of the flowtube, the indicator float with float stops, and the indicator scale.[4]

Flowtubes. Contemporary flowtubes are made of glass. Most have a single taper in which the inner diameter of the flowtube increases uniformly from bottom to top. Manufacturers provide double flowtubes for oxygen and nitrous oxide to provide better visual discrimination at low flow rates. A fine flowtube indicates flow from approximately 200 cc/min to 1 L/min, and a coarse flowtube indicates flow from approximately 1 L/min to 10 to 12 L/min. The two tubes are connected in series and supplied by a single flow control valve. The total gas flow is that shown on the higher flowmeter. Some older machines manufactured before the Z79.8-1979 standard have two flowtubes for a single gas arranged in parallel. Each of the tubes has a flow control valve. The total flow is the sum of the individual flows.[4]

Indicator Floats and Float Stops. Several different types of bobbins or floats are used to indicate flow on contemporary anesthesia machines. Ohmeda employs a plumb-bob type float on the Modulus I, Modulus II, and Modulus II Plus.[11-14] A rotating skirted float is used on the Excel series, and a ball float is used on the Ohmeda 8000.[15] Drager machines are equipped with sapphire ball floats.[6,9,16,17] Flow is read at the top of plumb-bob and skirted floats, but it is read at the center of the ball on the ball-type floats.[4]

Flowtubes are equipped with float stops at the top and bottom of the tube. The upper stop prevents the float from ascending to the top of the tube and plugging the outlet. It also ensures that the float will be visible at maximum flows instead of being hidden in the manifold. The bottom float stop provides a central foundation for the indicator when the flow control valve is turned off.[4,5]

Scale. The flowmeter scale can be marked directly on the flowtube or located to the right of the tube.[2] Gradations corresponding to equal increments in flow rate are closer together at the top of the scale because the annular space increases more rapidly than does the internal diameter from bottom to top of the tube. Rib guides are used in some flowtubes with ball-type indicators to minimize this compression effect. They are tapered glass ridges that run the length of the tube. There are usually three rib guides that are equally spaced around the inner circumference of the tube. In the presence of rib guides, the annular space from the bottom to the top of the tube increases almost proportionally with the internal diameter. This results in a nearly linear scale.[4] Rib guides are employed on Drager flowtubes.

Safety Features. The flowmeter subassembly for each gas on the Ohmeda Modulus I, Modulus II, and Modulus II Plus is housed in an independent, color-coded, pin-specific module. The flowtubes are adjacent to a gas-specific, color-coded backing. The flow scale and the chemical formula or name of the gas are permanently etched on the backing to the right of the flowtube.[11-14] Flowmeter scales are individually hand-calibrated by use of the specific float to provide a high degree of accuracy. The tube, float, and scale make an inseparable unit. The entire set must be replaced if any component is damaged.[5,11-13]

Drager does not use a modular system for the flowmeter subassembly. The flow scale, the chemical symbol, and the gas-specific color-coding are etched directly onto the flowtube.[6,9,16,17] The scale in use is obvious when two flowtubes for the same gas are used.

Problems with Flowmeters

Leaks

Flowmeter leaks are a substantial hazard because the flowmeters are located downstream from all machine safety devices except the oxygen analyzer.[21] Leaks can occur at the junction between the glass flowtube and the metal manifold because of problems associated with O-rings and gaskets. Glass flowtubes are the most fragile pneumatic component of the anesthesia machine. Gross damage is usually apparent, but subtle

cracks and chips may be overlooked resulting in errors of delivered flows.[22]

Eger et al.[23] in 1963 demonstrated that in the presence of a flowmeter leak, a hypoxic mixture is less likely to occur if the oxygen flowmeter is located downstream from all other flowmeters. Figure 7-10 is a contemporary version of the figure in Eger's original publication. The unused air flowtube has a large leak. Nitrous oxide and oxygen flow rates are set at a ratio of 3:1. A potentially dangerous arrangement is shown in Figure 7-10 A and B because the nitrous oxide flowmeter is located in the downstream position. A hypoxic mixture can result because a substantial portion of oxygen flow passes through the leak and all nitrous oxide is directed to the common gas outlet. A safer configuration that complies with the ASTM F1161-88 machine standard is shown in Figures 7-10 C and D. The oxygen flowmeter is located in the downstream position. A portion of the nitrous oxide flow escapes through the leak, and the remainder goes toward the common gas outlet. A hypoxic mixture is less likely because all the oxygen flow is advanced by the nitrous oxide.[23] Drager flowmeters are arranged as in Figure 7-10C, and Ohmeda flowmeters are as in Figure 7-10D.

A leak in the oxygen flowtube can produce a hypoxic mixture even when oxygen is located in the downstream position (Fig. 7-11).[21,22] Oxygen escapes through the leak and nitrous oxide flows toward the common outlet. This is particularly true at high nitrous oxide-to-oxygen flow ratios.

Inaccuracy

Flow error can occur even when flowmeters are assembled properly with appropriate components. Dirt or static electricity can cause a float to stick, and the actual flow may be higher or lower than that indicated. Stick-

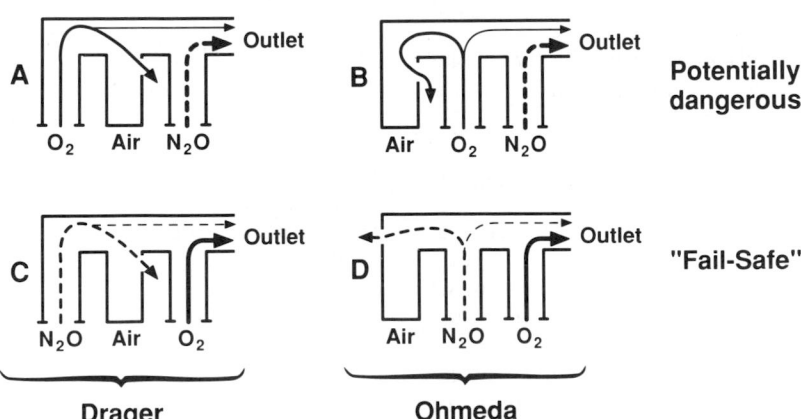

Fig. 7-10. Flowmeter sequence—a cause of hypoxia. In the event of a flowmeter leak, a potentially dangerous arrangement exists when nitrous oxide is located in the downstream position (**A & B**). The safest configuration exists when oxygen is located in the downstream position (**C & D**). (See text for details.) (Modified from Eger et al.,[23] with permission.)

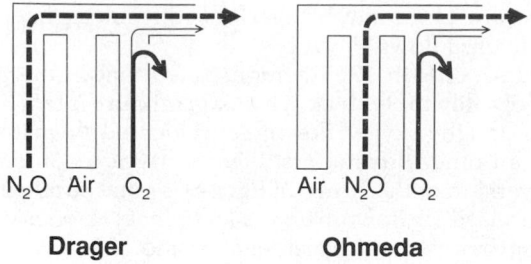

Drager **Ohmeda**

Fig. 7-11. Oxygen flowtube leak. An oxygen flowtube leak can produce a hypoxic mixture regardless of flowtube arrangement.

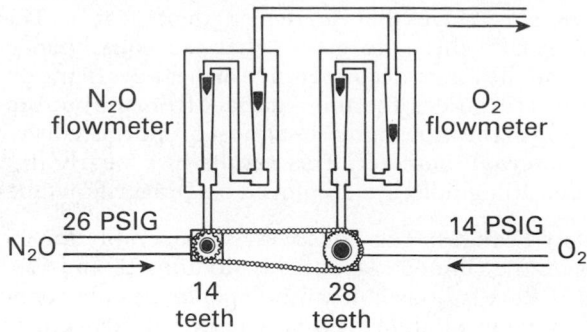

Fig. 7-12. Ohmeda Link-25 Proportion Limiting Control system. (See text for details.) (From Andrews,[19] with permission.)

ing is more common in the low-flow range because the annular space is smaller. A damaged float can cause inaccurate readings because the precise relationship between the float and the flowtube is altered. Back-pressure from the breathing circuit can cause a float to drop so that it reads less than the actual flow. Finally, if flowmeters are not aligned properly in the vertical position, readings can be inaccurate because tilting distorts the annular space.[4,22,24]

Ambiguous Scale

Before the standardization of flowmeter scales and the widespread use of oxygen analyzers, at least two deaths resulted from confusion created by ambiguous scales.[22,24,25] The operator read the float position beside an adjacent but erroneous scale in both cases. Today this is less likely to occur because contemporary flowmeter scales are marked either directly onto or to the right of the appropriate flowtube.[2] Confusion is minimized when the scale is etched directly onto the tube.

Proportioning Systems

Manufacturers have equipped newer machines with proportioning systems in an attempt to prevent delivery of a hypoxic mixture. Nitrous oxide and oxygen are interfaced either mechanically or pneumatically so that the minimum oxygen concentration at the common outlet is 25 percent.

Ohmeda Link-25 Proportion Limiting Control System

Contemporary Ohmeda machines use the Link-25 system. The heart of the system is the mechanical integration of the nitrous oxide and oxygen flow control valves. It allows independent adjustment of either valve, yet automatically intercedes to maintain a minimum 25 percent oxygen concentration with a maximum nitrous oxide/oxygen flow ratio of 3:1. An increased nitrous oxide flow beyond this maximum ratio results in a proportional 3:1 increase in oxygen flow.[11–15]

Figure 7-12 shows the Ohmeda Modulus II Link-25

system. The nitrous oxide and oxygen flow control valves are identical. A 14-tooth sprocket is attached to the nitrous oxide flow control valve, and a 28-tooth sprocket is attached to the oxygen flow control valve. A chain physically links the sprockets. When the nitrous oxide flow control valve is turned two revolutions, or 28 teeth, the oxygen flow control valve will revolve once because of the 2:1 gear ratio. The final 3:1 flow ratio results because the nitrous oxide flow control valve is supplied by approximately 26 PSIG, whereas the oxygen flow control valve is supplied by 14 PSIG. Thus, the combination of the mechanical and pneumatic aspects of the system yield the final oxygen concentration.[12,13]

Drager Oxygen Ratio Monitor Controller

Drager's proportioning system, the Oxygen Ratio Monitor Controller (ORMC), is used on the Drager Narkomed 2A, Narkomed 2B, and Narkomed 3. It is a pneumatic oxygen/nitrous oxide interlock system designed to maintain a fresh gas oxygen concentration of at least 25 ± 3 percent. The device controls the fresh gas oxygen concentration to levels substantially higher than 25 percent at oxygen flow rates less than 1 L/min (Fig. 7-13). The ORMC limits nitrous oxide flow to prevent delivery of a hypoxic mixture.[6,9,16,17] This is unlike the Ohmeda Link-25, which actively increases oxygen flow.

A schematic of the ORMC is shown in Figure 7-14. It is composed of an oxygen chamber, a nitrous oxide chamber, and a nitrous oxide slave control valve; all are interconnected by a mobile horizontal shaft. The pneumatic input into the device is from the oxygen and the nitrous oxide flowmeters. These flowmeters are unique because they have specific resistors located downstream from the flow control valves. These resistors create back-pressures that are directed to the oxygen and nitrous oxide chambers. The relative value of these resistors ultimately dictates the value of the controlled fresh gas oxygen concentration. The back-pressure in the oxygen and nitrous oxide chamber pushes against rubber diaphragms that are attached to the mobile horizontal shaft. Movement of the shaft regulates the ni-

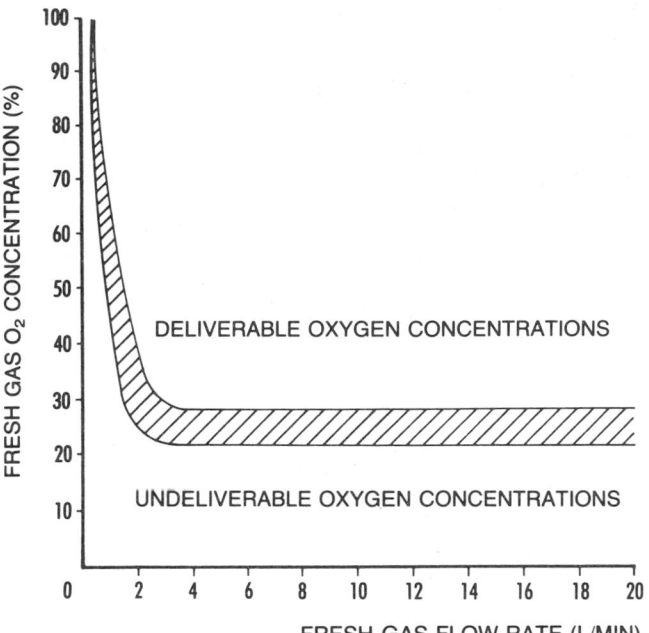

Fig. 7-13. Oxygen concentration control curve for the Drager Narkomed 2B and Narkomed 3. The Oxygen Ratio Monitor Controller (ORMC) maintains a minimal fresh gas oxygen concentration of at least 25 ± 3 percent at flow rates greater than 1 L/min. At flow rates less than 1 L/min, the device controls the fresh gas oxygen concentration to levels substantially higher than 25 percent. (Redrawn from Narkomed 3 Anesthesia System,[17] with permission.)

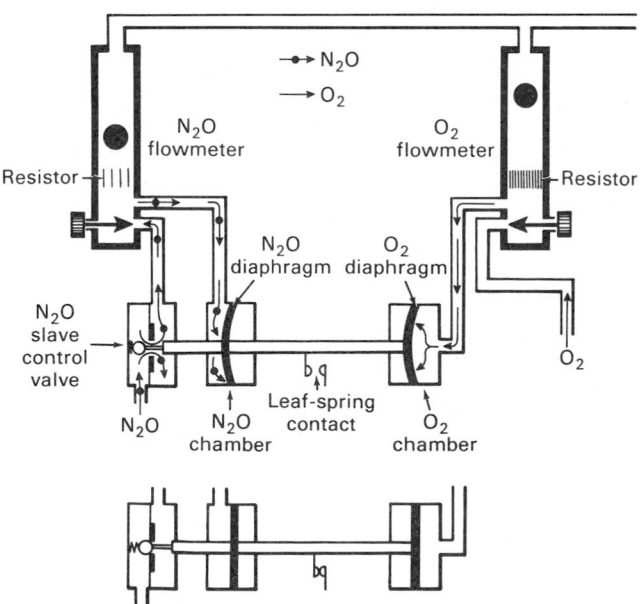

Fig. 7-14. Drager Oxygen Ratio Monitor Controller. (See text for details.) (Redrawn from Schreiber,[21] with permission.)

trous oxide slave control valve, which feeds the nitrous oxide flow control valve.[16,21]

If the oxygen pressure is proportionally higher than the nitrous oxide pressure, the nitrous oxide slave control valve opens to a larger degree, allowing more nitrous oxide to flow. As the nitrous oxide flow is increased manually, the nitrous oxide pressure forces the shaft toward the oxygen chamber. The valve opening becomes more restrictive and limits the nitrous oxide flow to the flowmeter. Figure 7-14 illustrates the action of a single ORMC under different sets of circumstances. The back-pressure exerted on the oxygen diaphragm, in the upper configuration, is greater than that exerted on the nitrous oxide diaphragm. This causes the horizontal shaft to move to the left, opening the nitrous oxide slave control valve. Nitrous oxide is then able to proceed to its flow control valve and out through the flowmeter. In the bottom configuration, the nitrous oxide slave control valve is closed because of inadequate oxygen back-pressure.[16,21]

The ORMC has a dual role. It serves as a proportioning device and a monitor. An electrical contact attached to the mobile horizontal shaft activates an alarm when the ORMC is limiting the nitrous oxide flow to prevent a hypoxic fresh gas mixture. The alarm is functional only in the "O_2/N_2O" mode and not in the "All Gases" mode. However, the ORMC continues to control the oxygen/nitrous oxide ratio regardless of the alarm status.[6,9,16,17]

Limitations

Proportioning systems are not foolproof. Machines equipped with proportioning systems still can deliver a hypoxic mixture under the following conditions.

Wrong Supply Gas

Both the Link-25 and the ORMC will be fooled if a gas other than oxygen is present in the oxygen pipeline. In the Link-25 system, the nitrous oxide and oxygen flow control valves will continue to be mechanically linked, and a hypoxic mixture will proceed to the common outlet. The oxygen rubber diaphragm of the ORMC will recognize adequate "oxygen" pressure, and flow of both the wrong gas plus nitrous oxide will result. The oxygen analyzer is the only machine monitor that will detect this condition in both systems.

Defective Pneumatics or Mechanics

Normal operation of the Ohmeda Link-25 and the Drager ORMC is contingent upon pneumatic and mechanical integrity. Pneumatic integrity in the Ohmeda system depends on properly functioning second-stage regulators. A nitrous oxide/oxygen ratio other than 3 : 1 will result if the regulators are not precise. The chain connecting the two sprockets must be intact. A 97 percent nitrous oxide concentration can result if the chain is cut or broken.[26] In the Drager system, a functional Oxygen Failure Protection Device (OFPD) is necessary to supply appropriate pressure to the ORMC. The mechanical aspects of the ORMC, such as the rubber diaphragms, the flowtube resistors, and the nitrous oxide slave control valve, must likewise be intact.

Leaks Downstream

The ORMC and the Link-25 function at the level of the flow control valves. A leak downstream from these devices such as a broken oxygen flow tube (Fig. 7-11) can result in the delivery of a hypoxic mixture. Oxygen escapes through the leak, and the predominant gas delivered at the common outlet is nitrous oxide. The oxygen analyzer is the only machine safety device that can detect the problem.[21] Drager recommends a preoperative positive-pressure leak test to detect such a leak.[6,9,16,17] Ohmeda recommends a preoperative negative-pressure leak test because of the check valve located at the common outlet[11,12,27,28] (see the section, *Checking Anesthesia Machines*).

Inert Gas Administration

Administration of a third inert gas, such as helium, nitrogen, or carbon dioxide, can result in a hypoxic mixture because contemporary proportioning systems link only nitrous oxide and oxygen.[6,9,11-17] Use of an oxygen analyzer is especially mandatory if the operator uses a third inert gas.

VAPORIZERS

Through the years, vaporizers have evolved from rudimentary ether inhalers to the present sophisticated variable-bypass, temperature-compensated vaporizers. Bubble-through copper kettle vaporizers are no longer manufactured in the United States, and they are not addressed by the ASTM F1161-88 standard. Therefore, this section is limited to newer variable-bypass vaporizers. Certain physical principles are reviewed briefly before the discussion so that the design, construction, and operation of these vaporizers can be understood.

Physics

Vapor Pressure

Inhaled volatile anesthetics exist in the liquid state at room temperature. When a volatile liquid is in a closed container, molecules escape from the liquid phase to the vapor phase until the number of molecules in the vapor phase is constant. These molecules bombard the wall of the container and create a pressure known as the saturated *vapor pressure*. As the temperature increases, more molecules enter the vapor phase and the vapor pressure increases (Fig. 7-15). Vapor pressure is

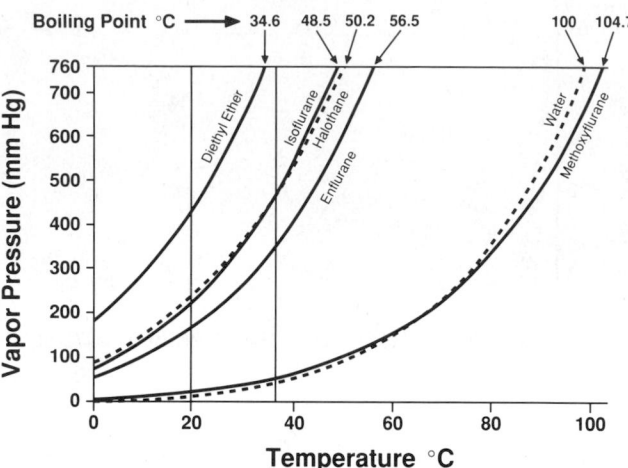

Fig. 7-15. Vapor pressure versus temperature curves. (Modified from Rodgers and Hill,[133] with permission.)

independent of atmospheric pressure and is contingent only on the physical characteristics of the liquid and the temperature. The *boiling point* of a liquid is that temperature at which the vapor pressure equals atmospheric pressure.[29-31]

Latent Heat of Vaporization

Energy must be expended to convert a molecule from the liquid to gaseous state because the molecules of a liquid tend to cohere. The *latent heat of vaporization* is defined as the number of calories required to change 1 g of liquid into vapor without a temperature change. The energy for vaporization must come from the liquid itself or from an outside source. The temperature of the liquid decreases during vaporization in the absence of an outside energy source. Energy loss can lead to significant decreases in temperature of the remaining liquid. This temperature drop will greatly decrease vaporization.[29,31,32]

Specific Heat

The *specific heat* of a substance is the number of calories required to increase the temperature of 1 g of a substance by 1°C.[29,31,33] The substance can be solid, liquid, or gas. The concept of specific heat is important to the design, operation, and construction of vaporizers because it is applicable in two ways. First, the specific heat value for an inhaled anesthetic is important because it indicates how much heat must be supplied to the liquid to maintain a constant temperature when heat is lost during vaporization. Second, manufacturers select vaporizer metals that have a high specific heat to minimize temperature changes associated with vaporization.

Thermal Conductivity

Thermal conductivity is a measure of the speed with which heat flows through a substance. The higher the thermal conductivity, the better the substance conducts heat.[29] Vaporizers are constructed of metals that have relatively high thermal conductivity, which helps maintain a uniform temperature.

Vaporizer Classification

The Ohmeda Tec 4 and the Drager Vapor 19.1 are classified as variable-bypass, flow-over, temperature-compensated, agent-specific, out-of-circuit vaporizers. *Variable bypass* refers to the method for regulating output concentration. After the total gas flow enters the vaporizer's inlet, the concentration control dial adjusts the amount of gas that goes to the bypass chamber and to the vaporizing chamber. The gas channeled to the vaporizing chamber flows over the liquid agent and becomes saturated. Thus, *flow-over* refers to the method of vaporization. The Tec 4 and the Vapor 19.1 are classified as *temperature-compensated* because they are equipped with an automatic temperature-compensating device that helps maintain a constant vaporizer output over a wide range of temperatures. These vaporizers are classified as *agent-specific* and *out-of-circuit* because they are designed to accommodate a single agent and to be located outside the breathing circuit. Conversely, copper kettle vaporizers are classified as measured-flow, bubble-through, non-temperature-compensated, multiple-agent, out-of-circuit vaporizers.[29]

Basic Design Principles

The total gas flow in a variable-bypass vaporizer enters the vaporizer's inlet and splits into two portions (Fig. 7-16). The first portion, which represents less than 20 percent of the total gas flow, passes through the vaporizing chamber where it is enriched or saturated with vapor of the liquid anesthetic. The second portion, which represents more than 80 percent of the total gas flow, goes directly through the bypass chamber. Finally, both partial gas flows rejoin at the vaporizer outlet. The ratio of the two partial gas flows depends on the ratio of resistances in the two paths; that is, the resistance in the bypass chamber compared with the resistance in the vaporizing chamber. The concentration control dial can be located in the bypass chamber or in the vaporizing chamber outlet. A change in the dial setting causes a change in resistance, which alters the gas flow ratio.[34]

Factors that Influence Vaporizer Output

The output of an ideal vaporizer would be constant at varying conditions such as flow rates, temperatures, back-pressures, and carrier gases. Designing such a va-

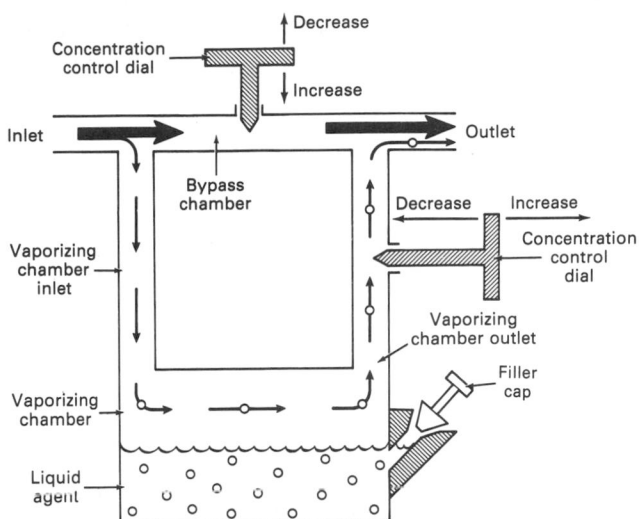

Fig. 7-16. Generic variable-bypass vaporizer. (See text for details.) (From Andrews,[19] with permission.)

porizer is difficult because as ambient conditions change, the physical properties of gases and of vaporizers themselves can change.[34] Contemporary vaporizers approach being ideal but still have some limitations. Several factors are listed below that can influence vaporizer output.

Flow Rate

Variable-bypass vaporizer output varies with the rate of gas flowing through them. This is particularly notable at extremes of flow rates. The output of all variable-bypass vaporizers is less than the dial setting at low flow rates (less than 250 cc/min). This results from the relatively high specific gravity of volatile anesthetic agents. Insufficient pressure is generated at low flow rates in the vaporizing chamber to upwardly advance the molecules. At extremely high flow rates such as 15 L/min, the output of most variable-bypass vaporizers is less than the dial setting. This is attributed to incomplete mixing and saturation in the vaporizing chamber. Also, the resistance characteristics of the bypass chamber and the vaporizing chamber can vary as flow increases. This can result in decreased output concentration.[34]

Figure 7-17 shows vaporizer output versus flow rate performance curves for three halothane vaporizers. These are the Fluotec Mark II, the Ohmeda Tec 4, and the Drager Vapor 19.1. In contrast to the older Fluotec Mark II, the output of contemporary vaporizers is nearly linear over a wide range of flow rates because of design improvements. An extensive wick and baffle system is used in the Tec 4 and Vapor 19.1 that increases the effective surface area of the vaporizing chamber.[5,35,36] Also, both vaporizers have constant resistance characteristics over clinically useful flow rates.

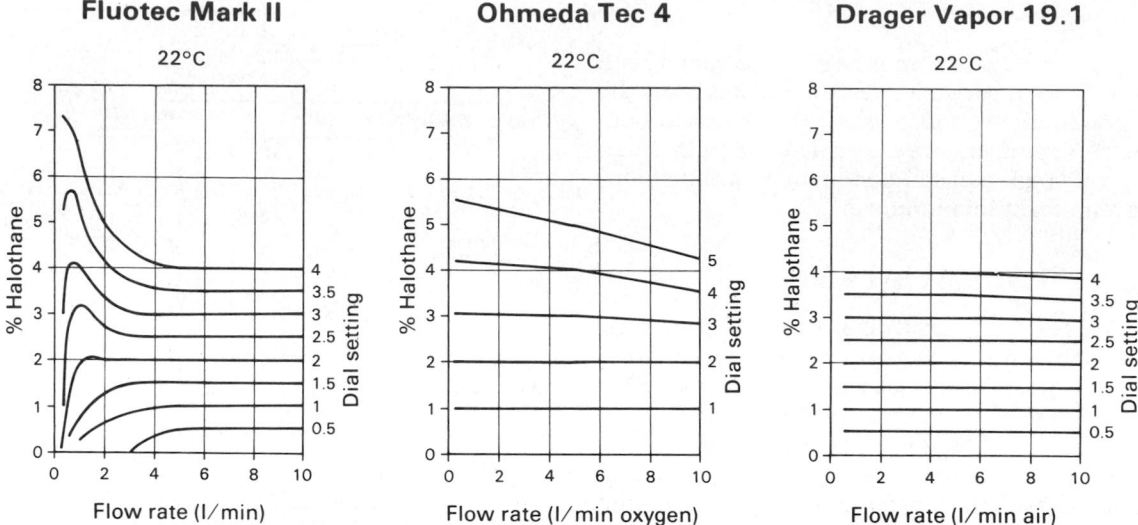

Fig. 7-17. Output versus flow rate performance curves of the Fluotec Mark II, the Ohmeda Tec 4, and the Drager Vapor 19.1. (Data from Ohmeda, The BOC Group Inc., Madison, WI, and North American Drager, Telford, PA.)

Temperature

The output of older non-temperature-compensated vaporizers varies considerably with changes in temperature. This occurs because vapor pressure is a function of temperature. The output of contemporary temperature-compensated vaporizers, however, is almost linear over a wide range of temperatures. Several improvements in design are responsible for this linearity. Manufacturers have incorporated an automatic temperature-compensating mechanism in the bypass chamber to help maintain a constant vaporizer output with varying temperatures.[5,35,36] The valve can be a bimetallic strip or an expansion element. In either case, gas flow is apportioned in favor of the bypass chamber as temperature increases.[34] Wicks are placed in direct contact with the metal wall of the vaporizer to help replace heat that

is used for vaporization. Vaporizers are constructed with metals having relatively high specific heat and high thermal conductivity to minimize heat loss.

Figure 7-18 shows vaporizer output versus temperature performance curves for the Ohmeda Tec 4. Within the temperature range of 20 to 35°C, there is only a slight increase in vaporizer output associated with an increase in temperature.[36] Accuracy cannot be ensured at temperatures outside this range because vapor pressure varies nonlinearly with temperature, whereas compensation varies linearly.

Intermittent Back-Pressure

Intermittent back-pressure associated with positive-pressure ventilation or with oxygen flushing can result in higher vaporizer output concentration than the

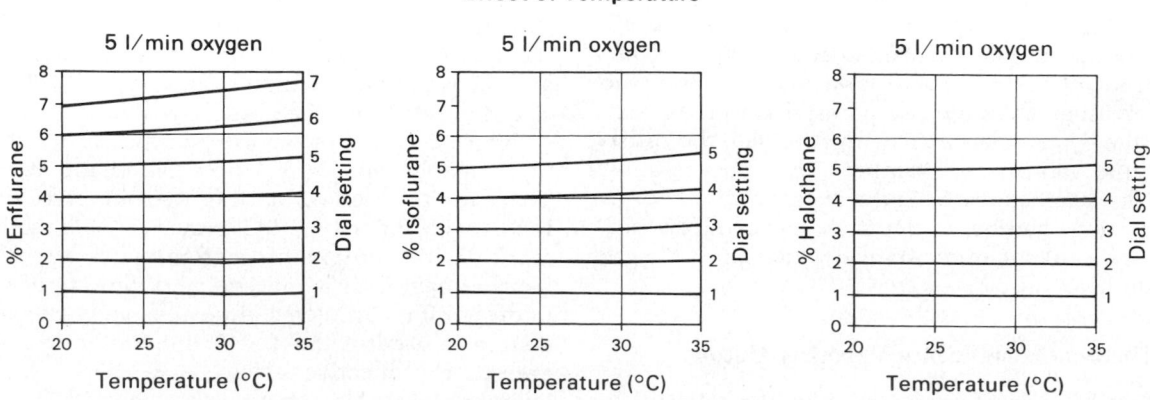

Fig. 7-18. Output versus temperature performance curves for Ohmeda Tec 4 vaporizers. (Redrawn from Tec 4 Continuous Flow Vaporizer Operator's Manual,[36] with permission.)

dialed setting. This phenomenon is known as the *pumping effect*.[29,34,37-39] It is more pronounced at low flow rates, low dial settings, and low levels of liquid anesthetic in the vaporizing chamber. Additionally, the ventilator settings themselves are important because the pumping effect is exacerbated at rapid respiratory rates, high peak pressures, and rapid drops in pressure during expiration.[35-39] The Ohmeda Tec 4 and Drager Vapor 19.1 are relatively immune from the pumping effect.[35,36] However, the pumping effect is clinically important to older variable-bypass vaporizers such as the Fluotec Mark II.[37]

One proposed mechanism for the pumping effect is described as follows. Pressure is transmitted in a retrograde manner from the patient circuit to the vaporizer during the inspiratory phase of positive-pressure ventilation. This produces a no-flow state within the vaporizer. Gas molecules are compressed in both the bypass chamber and the vaporizing chamber. Then, the backpressure is suddenly released during the expiratory phase of positive-pressure ventilation. Vapor exits the vaporizing chamber via two routes. One portion leaves in the conventional manner through the vaporizing chamber outlet. However, another portion exits in a retrograde manner through the vaporizing chamber *inlet* and joins the bypass flow. This occurs because the output resistance of the bypass chamber is lower than that of the vaporizing chamber, particularly at low dial settings. The enhanced output concentration results from the increment of vapor that travels in the retrograde direction.[34,37-39]

Ohmeda and Drager have addressed the pumping effect in the following manner. The vaporizing chambers of the Tec 4 and the Vapor 19.1 are smaller than those of older variable-bypass vaporizers such as the Fluotec Mark II (750 cc).[35,36,38] Therefore, no substantial volumes of vapor can be discharged from the vaporizing chamber into the bypass chamber during the expiratory phase. The Drager Vapor 19.1 has a patented long spiral tube that serves as the inlet to the vaporizing chamber.[35,38] When the pressure in the vaporizing chamber is released, some of the vapor enters this tube in a retrograde manner. The vapor does not enter the bypass chamber, however, because of tube length.[38] The Tec 4 has an extensive baffle system in the vaporizing chamber, and a one-way check valve has been inserted at the common outlet to minimize the pumping effect. This check valve may attenuate the pressure increase but does not prevent it, because gas still flows from the flowmeters during inspiration.[29,40]

Carrier Gas Composition

Vaporizer output is influenced by the composition of the carrier gas that flows through the vaporizer.[35,36,41-48] When the carrier gas is quickly switched from 100 percent oxygen to 100 percent nitrous oxide, there is a rapid transient decrease in vaporizer output followed by a slow increase to a new steady-state value (Fig. 7-19b).[46,47] The transient decrease in vaporizer output is attributed to nitrous oxide being more soluble than oxygen in halogenated liquid.[46] Therefore, the quantity of gas leaving the vaporizing chamber is transiently diminished until the inhaled anesthetic is totally saturated with nitrous oxide.

The explanation for the new steady-state output value is less understood.[48] With contemporary vaporizers such as the Drager Vapor 19.1 and the Ohmeda Tec 4, the steady-state output value is less when nitrous oxide is the carrier gas than when oxygen is (Fig. 7-19b).[35,36] Conversely, the output of some older vaporizers is enhanced when nitrous oxide is the carrier gas instead of oxygen.[41,43] The steady-state plateau is achieved more rapidly with increased flow rates, regardless of the ultimate output value.[47] Factors that contribute to the steady-state response include the viscosity and density of the carrier gas, the relative solubilities of carrier gases in the liquid anesthetic, the flow-splitting characteristics of the specific vaporizer, and the dial settings.[43,46-48]

Specific Vaporizers

Ohmeda Tec 4

The Ohmeda Tec 4 vaporizer system is used on all contemporary Ohmeda machines. As many as three Tec 4 vaporizers are attached to the vaporizer manifold that is located to the right of the flowmeters. Vaporizer and manifold mechanisms combine to form an interlock system. The function of the interlock system is to (1) ensure that only one vaporizer can be turned on at a

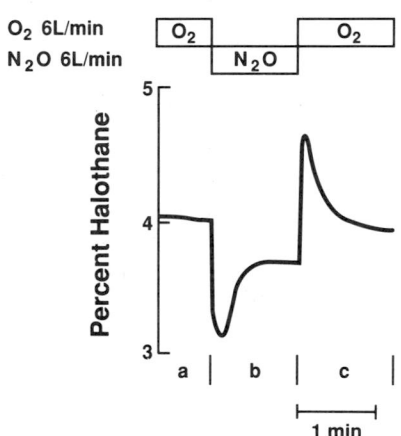

Fig. 7-19. Halothane output of a Drager 19.1 vaporizer with different carrier gases. The initial output concentration is approximately 4 percent halothane when oxygen is the carrier gas at flows of 6 L/min *(a)*. When the carrier gas is quickly switched to 100 percent nitrous oxide *(b)*, the halothane concentration decreases to 3 percent within 8 to 10 seconds. Then, a new steady-state concentration of approximately 3.5 percent is attained within 1 minute. (See text for details.) (Modified from Gould et al.,[46] with permission.)

time, (2) ensure that gas flow enters only the vaporizer that is turned on, (3) minimize unwanted trace vapor after a vaporizer is turned off, and (4) lock the vaporizers into the gas circuit, ensuring that the vaporizer inlet and outlet ports seal correctly. Flow from the flowmeters enters the vaporizer manifold and then moves only through the vaporizer, which is switched on, where it picks up a set concentration of anesthetic vapor. This gas mixture then flows out the vaporizer manifold to the common gas outlet.[14,36]

Each vaporizer has a single control dial with a concentration scale calibrated in percentage of anesthetic vapor per total volume. Turning on a vaporizer requires two simultaneous actions. The operator must depress the control dial release button, located to the left of the concentration control dial, and rotate the control dial counterclockwise. This prevents accidental displacement of the control dial from the off to the on position. A pair of mobile extension rods located behind the concentration control dial extend laterally when the vaporizer is turned on. If the lateral movement is transmitted either directly or indirectly to extension rods or another vaporizer on the manifold, that vaporizer cannot be turned on.[36]

Two different manifolds exist. An older version is present on the Ohmeda Modulus II and on the Ohmeda 8000. If the center vaporizer is removed from this manifold, the lateral two vaporizers can be turned on simultaneously because their extension rods do not communicate. Either the left or the right vaporizer should be moved to the center position to correct the problem as indicated by the manifold warning label. Then, the interlock mechanism will function because the extension rods of the two vaporizers are in contact with each other.[12,13,15] The Ohmeda Modulus II Plus has an improved manifold (Fig. 7-20). Only a single inhaled anesthetic can be delivered even when the center vaporizer is removed. The new manifold has a mobile bracket (Fig. 7-20, arrows) that is free to move left or right. When a side vaporizer is turned on, the lateral movement of its extension rod is transmitted through the bracket to the other vaporizer. This prevents the second vaporizer from being turned on.[14]

Two filling mechanisms are available including the screw-cap filler and the agent-specific keyed filler. The low location of the filler port minimizes overfilling in either case. The liquid capacity of the Tec 4 is 125 cc, and the amount retained by the wick system is 35 cc.[36]

A simplified diagram of the Ohmeda Tec 4 is shown in Figure 7-21. The total fresh gas flow enters the vaporizer's inlet and splits into two portions. The smaller first portion goes to the vaporizing chamber, which uses a wick and baffle system. The carrier gas becomes saturated with an agent and rejoins the larger bypass flow at the vaporizer outlet. The concentration control valve determines the relative flows through the vaporizing and bypass chambers. Temperature compensation is automatically accomplished by the bimetallic strip that influences flow through the bypass chamber. A one-way check valve is incorporated at the common outlet to minimize the pumping effect.[5]

Drager Vapor 19.1

The Drager Vapor Exclusion system is used on the Narkomed 2A, the Narkomed 2B, and Narkomed 3. As many as three vaporizers are attached semipermanently to the vaporizer mounting bracket, which is located to the right of the flowmeter bank (Fig. 7-22). A cam and lever interlock system is incorporated into the vaporizer bank, which prevents more than one vapor-

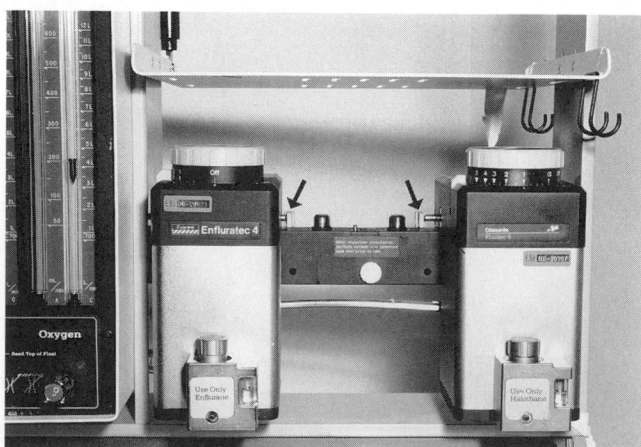

Fig. 7-20. Improved interlock system of the Ohmeda Modulus II Plus with center vaporizer removed. The new manifold has a mobile bracket (arrows) that allows communication between the extension rods of the two peripheral vaporizers. (See text for details.)

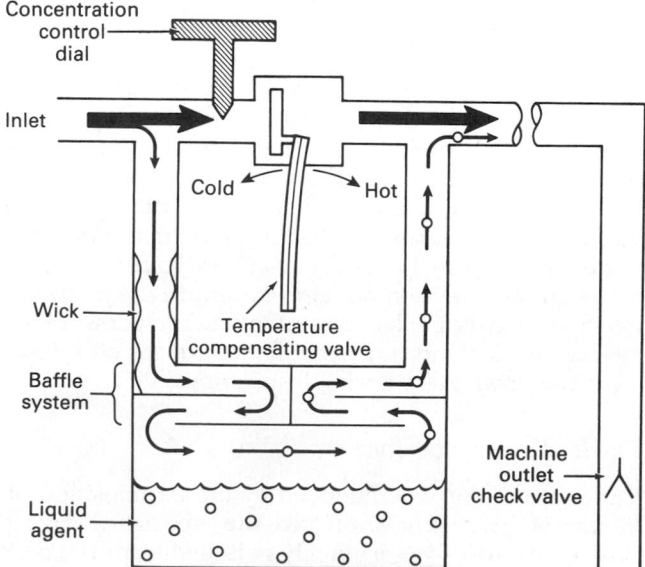

Fig. 7-21. Simplified schematic of the Ohmeda Tec 4 vaporizer. (See text for details.) (From Andrews,[19] with permission.)

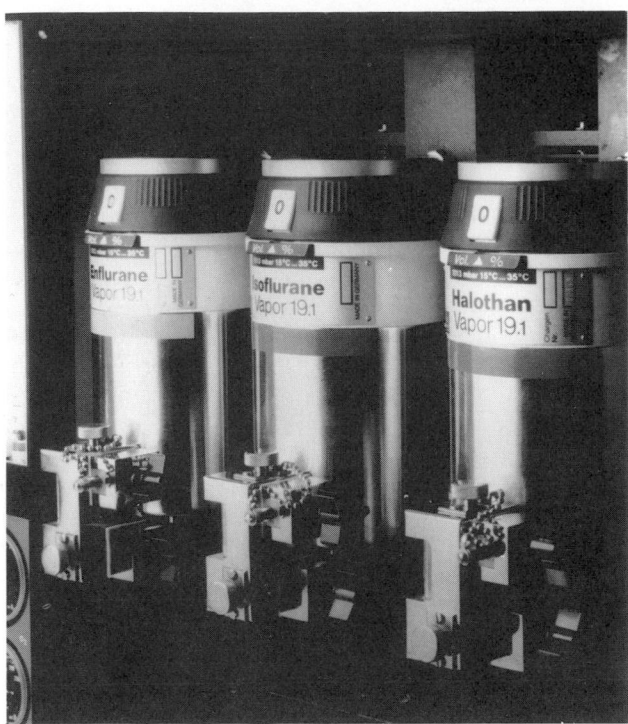

Fig. 7-22. Drager Vapor 19.1 vaporizers with keyed filling devices. (Courtesy of North American Drager, Telford, PA.)

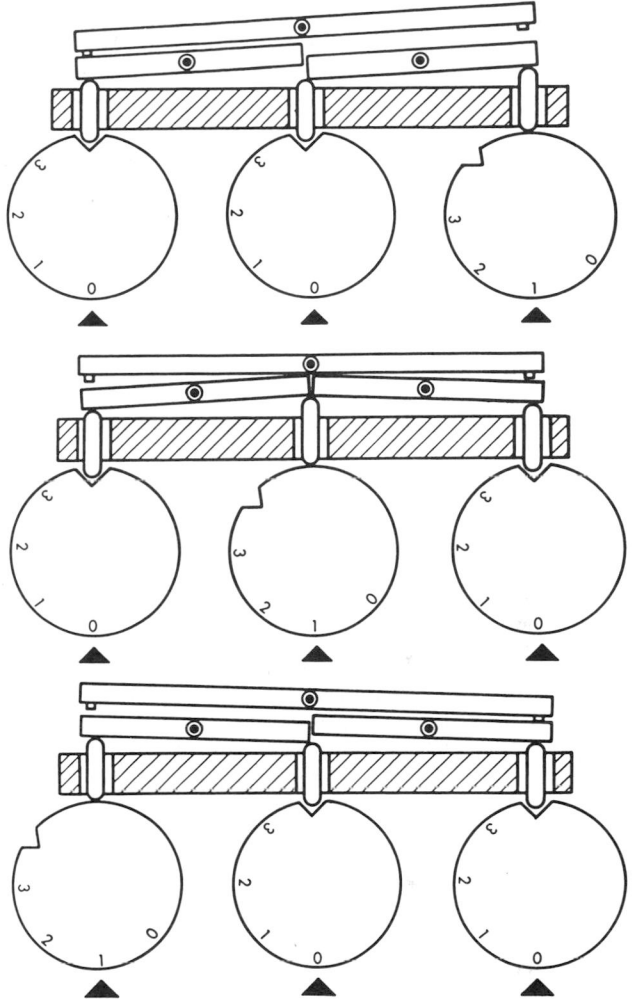

Fig. 7-23. Three top views of North American Drager's interlock system. A different vaporizer is turned on in each view. When one vaporizer is turned on, the other two are locked in the zero position. (Courtesy of North American Drager, Telford, PA.)

izer from being activated (Fig. 7-23). All unused vaporizers are locked in the zero position.[9,17] This external interlock system is different from the system used by Ohmeda in which the exclusion rods are an internal component of each vaporizer.[35] The Drager interlock system continues to function when any of the three vaporizers are removed. However, a short-circuit block must be installed in place of the vaporizer, or a leak will occur.

The output of the Drager Vapor 19.1 is regulated by a single concentration dial calibrated in percent and located on top of the vaporizer. When the control dial is set in the "0" position (off), fresh gas from the flowmeter passes with almost no resistance through a bypass inside the vaporizer directly to the common outlet. Thus, the actual vaporizing portion of the Vapor 19.1 is completely separated from the fresh gas flow. Also, in the "0" position, the inlet and the outlet of the vaporizing chamber are interconnected and vented through a hole. This ensures that no pressure builds in the vaporizing chamber. The anesthetic loss caused by venting in the off position is less than 0.5 cc/24 h at an ambient temperature of 22°C. Two types of filling mechanisms are available: the screw-cap filler or the safety, agent-specific, keyed filler. The liquid capacity of the Vapor 19.1 is 200 cc with a dry wick or 140 cc when the wick is wet.[35]

Figure 7-24 shows a simplified schematic of the Drager Vapor 19.1 in the on position. Flow through the

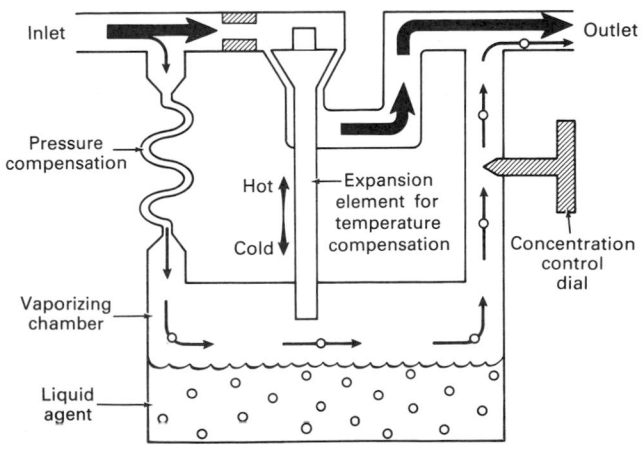

Fig. 7-24. Simplified schematic of the Drager 19.1 vaporizer. (See text for details.) (From Andrews,[19] with permission.)

Vapor 19.1 is similar to that through the Tec 4, but back-pressure and temperature compensation are different. The Vapor 19.1 uses a patented long spiral tube as the inlet to the vaporizing chamber, which acts as a buffer against the pumping effect. Some inhaled anesthetic gas molecules do travel in a retrograde manner up this tube during the expiratory phase of the pumping effect. However, they do not reach the bypass chamber because of the tube length. Drager does not employ a check valve at the common outlet because of this internal pressure compensation. Temperature compensation is achieved by an expansion element, which alters flow through the bypass chamber. The Vapor 19.1 has a wick and baffle system similar to that of the Tec 4.[35,36]

Safety Features

The Drager 19.1 and the Ohmeda Tec 4 have numerous safety features that have minimized or eliminated many hazards once associated with variable-bypass vaporizers. Agent-specific, keyed filling devices help prevent filling a vaporizer with the wrong agent. Overfilling of these vaporizers is minimized because the filler port is located at the maximum safe liquid level. Today's vaporizers are soundly secured to the vaporizer manifold, and there is little need to move them. Thus, problems associated with tipping are minimized. Contemporary interlock systems prevent administration of more than one agent.[35,36]

Hazards

Contemporary Variable-Bypass Vaporizers

Despite numerous safety features, some hazards are still associated with contemporary variable-bypass vaporizers.

Incorrect Agent

Many anesthesiologists prefer the screw-cap filler for convenience, although agent-specific, keyed fillers are available. A vaporizer can be filled with the wrong agent when the screw-cap filler is employed.

Tipping

Tipping can occur when vaporizers are incorrectly switched out or moved. However, tipping is unlikely when a vaporizer is attached to a manifold in the upright position. Excessive tipping can cause the liquid agent to enter the bypass chamber and can result in a high output concentration. The Tec 4 is slightly more immune to tipping than the Vapor 19.1 because of its extensive baffle system. However, if either vaporizer is tipped, it should not be used until it has been flushed for 20 to 30 minutes at high flow rates with the vaporizer set at a low concentration.[29]

Simultaneous Inhaled Anesthetic Administration

Two inhaled anesthetics can be administered simultaneously when the center Tec 4 vaporizer is removed from Ohmeda machines that have the older style vaporizer manifold. The left or right vaporizer should be moved to the central position if the central vaporizer is removed as indicated by the manifold label. The interlock system will then function properly because the two remaining vaporizers are adjacent.[12,13,15]

Leaks

Leaks often are associated with vaporizers.[29,49] A loose filler cap is the most common source of vaporizer leaks. They can occur at the O-ring junction between the vaporizer and its manifold. A vaporizer must be in the on position to detect a leak within it. Vaporizer leaks in the Drager system can be detected with a conventional positive-pressure leak test because of the absence of check valves. Ohmeda recommends a negative-pressure leak-testing device (suction bulb) to detect vaporizer leaks in the Modulus I and Modulus II because of the check valve at the machine outlet[11-13] (see the section, *Checking Anesthesia Machines*).

Freestanding (Add-On) Vaporizers

Freestanding, variable-bypass vaporizers have been added on to many anesthesia machines between the common outlet and the patient circuit. This practice is fraught with hazards. Tipping is a substantial possibility because the vaporizer is not permanently affixed to the machine. Furthermore, multiple agents can be administered because at least one agent from the machine plus the agent from the freestanding vaporizer can be delivered. Oxygen flushing (35 to 75 L/min) can deliver excess anesthetic from the freestanding vaporizer to the patient. Even though the inlet and outlet of freestanding vaporizers have different diameters, they can be connected in a reverse manner. Vaporizer output can be two times that indicated on the dial in this configuration.[50]

Many freestanding vaporizers have a check valve in the vaporizer outlet to minimize the pumping effect and to indicate reverse connection. This valve prevents detection of leaks in the low-pressure circuit when a traditional positive-pressure leak test is performed. Also, an intraoperative disconnection between the machine outlet and the vaporizer inlet can go unnoticed if positive-pressure ventilation is employed. The pressure from the breathing circuit closes the check valve during inspiration, and the disconnection is not detectable by conventional means.[51]

ANESTHETIC CIRCUITS

Gas exits the anesthesia machine at the common gas outlet, and it then enters an anesthetic circuit. The function of an anesthetic circuit is not only to deliver oxygen and anesthetic gases to the patient, but also to eliminate carbon dioxide. Carbon dioxide can be removed either by washout with adequate fresh gas inflow or by soda lime absorption. This discussion is limited to semiclosed rebreathing circuits and the circle system.

Mapleson Systems

Mapleson[52] described and analyzed five different arrangements of fresh gas flow, tubing, mask, reservoir bag, and the expiratory valve to administer anesthetic gases. They are now classically referred to as the Mapleson systems and designated from A to E. Willis et al.[53] added the F system to these original five. The Mapleson circuits are shown in Figure 7-25. The amount of rebreathing associated with each type is highly dependent on fresh gas flow rate. The performance of these circuits is best understood by studying the expiratory phase of the respiratory cycle.

Mapleson A

The Mapleson A is also known as Magill's circuit. It consists of a corrugated tube, a reservoir bag, a fresh gas inflow at the machine end, and a spring-loaded expi-

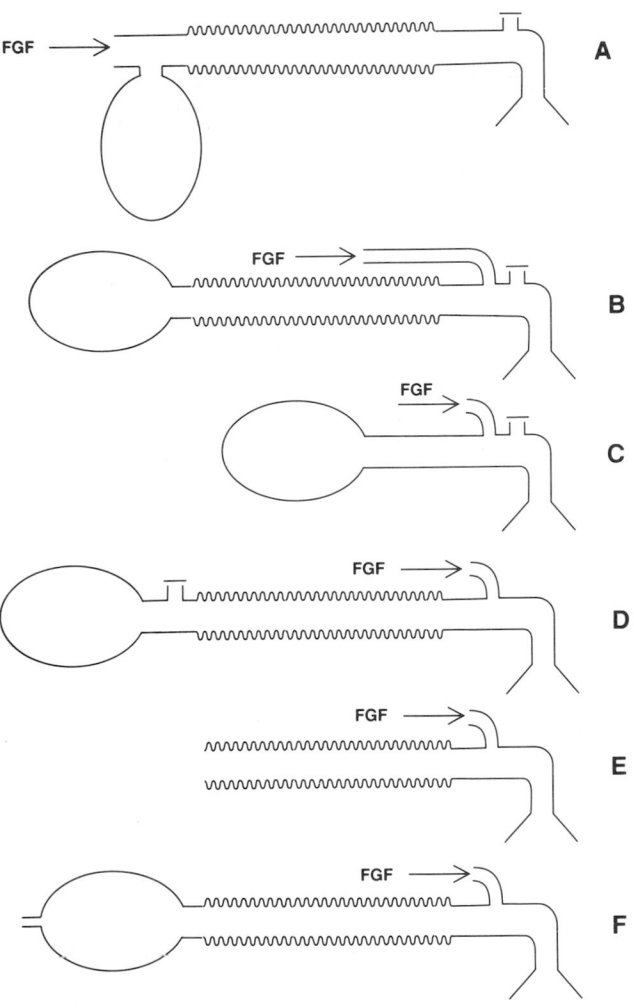

Fig. 7-25. (A–F) Mapleson breathing systems. FGF, fresh gas flow. (Redrawn from Willis et al.,[53] with permission.)

ratory valve near the patient end (Fig. 7-25). Rebreathing during spontaneous ventilation in this circuit can be prevented with relatively low fresh gas flows. Upon exhalation, the patient end of the tubing is filled with dead space gas followed by the alveolar gas. This stream travels up the tubing and meets the fresh gas flowing into the circuit (Fig. 7-26, left). The pressure in the circuit increases and forces the expiratory valve to open, allowing the alveolar gas to escape. Most of the dead space gas is washed out if the fresh gas flow is adequate. During the inspiratory phase, the fresh gas flushes the dead space gas through the tubing toward the patient. Rebreathing of dead space gas poses no problem because it does not contain carbon dioxide. Several studies have confirmed Mapleson's original finding that rebreathing of alveolar gas can be prevented if the fresh gas flow is equal to or exceeds the patient's minute ventilation.[54,55] Rebreathing does not occur until the fresh gas flow is below 70 percent of the patient's minute ventilation.

The Mapleson A circuit is inefficient during controlled ventilation.[56] Expiratory valve resistance must be increased to ventilate the patient. Venting the gas in the circuit occurs during the inspiratory phase, and the alveolar gases are retained in the tubing during the exhalation phase (Fig. 7-26, right). Thus, alveolar gas is rebreathed with the ensuing breath before the pressure in the system increases enough to force the expiratory valve open. This can cause an increase in arterial carbon dioxide tension. Adequate carbon dioxide elimination by using controlled ventilation with a Mapleson A system requires a fresh gas flow of greater than 20 L/min. In practice, controlled ventilation should be avoided with this system.

Mapleson B

The Mapleson B system features the fresh gas inlet near the patient end just distal to the expiratory valve (Fig. 7-25). This circuit functions similarly during both spontaneous and controlled ventilation, unlike the Mapleson A system. Location of the fresh gas inlet allows fresh gas to accumulate along with exhaled gases in the tubing (Fig. 7-26). The expiratory valve opens when pressure in the circuit increases, and a mixture of alveolar gas and fresh gas is discharged. During the next inspiration, the patient receives fresh gas flow from the machine and a mixture of retained fresh gas and alveolar gas from the tubing (Fig. 7-26). Composition of this inhaled mixture depends on fresh gas flow rate. Rebreathing can be prevented if the fresh gas flow rate is greater than twice the minute ventilation for both spontaneous and controlled ventilation.[56,57]

Mapleson C

The Mapleson C system is also known as the Water's circuit without an absorber. Arrangement of its components is similar to that of the Mapleson B, but the large-bore tubing is shorter (Fig. 7-25). This effectively re-

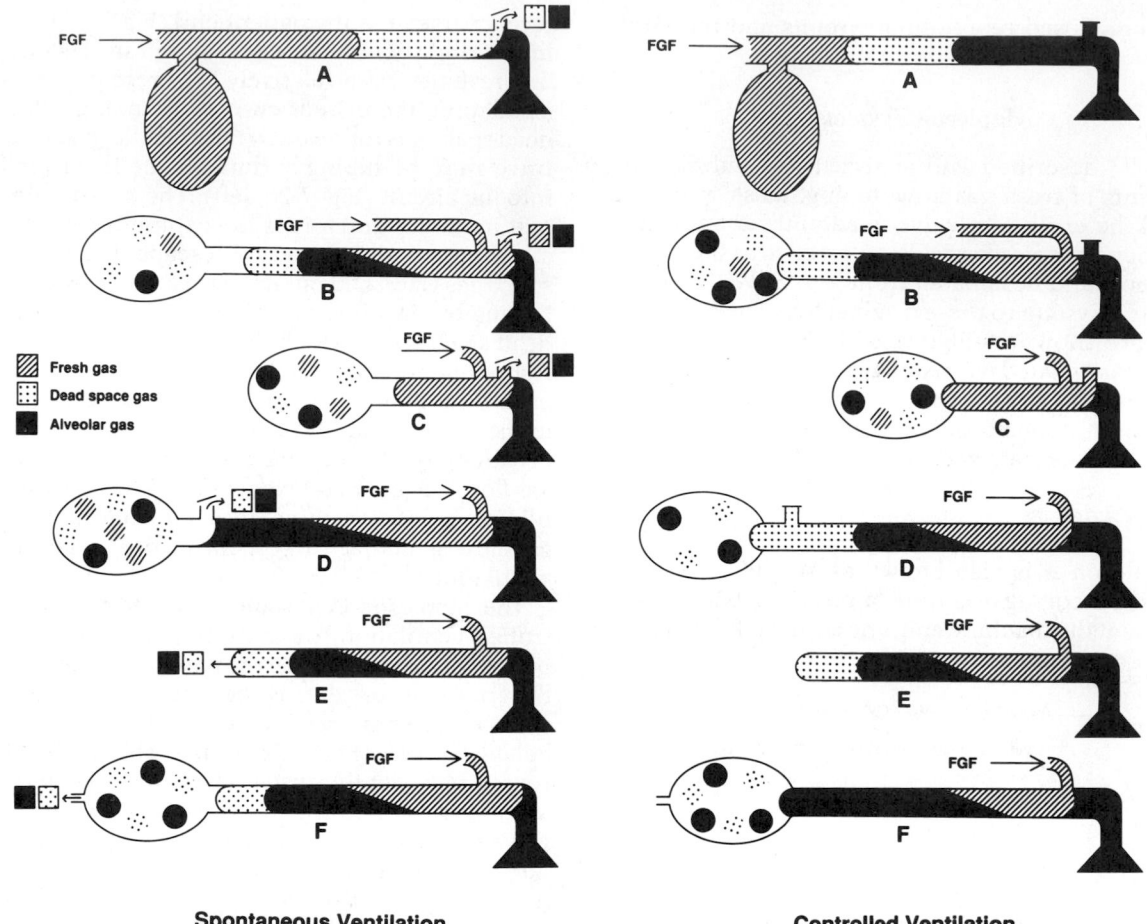

Spontaneous Ventilation   **Controlled Ventilation**

Fig. 7-26. Gas disposition at end-expiration during spontaneous (left) and controlled (right) ventilation in circuits A to F. FGF, fresh gas flow. (Modified from Sykes,[57] with permission.)

duces the reservoir volume and allows good mixing of fresh and exhaled gases. The inspired mixture contains more alveolar gas than the Mapleson B system. A fresh gas flow of twice the minute ventilation is required to prevent rebreathing.[57] Carbon dioxide will build up, although at a slower rate than with Mapleson B circuit, if rebreathing is allowed to occur.

Mapleson D

The Mapleson D circuit can be described as a T-piece with an expiratory limb. The fresh gas inlet is located near the patient end, but the expiratory valve is toward the machine end close to the reservoir bag (Fig. 7-25). During the expiratory phase of spontaneous ventilation, fresh gas and alveolar gas flow down the expiratory limb (Fig. 7-26). The expiratory valve opens as pressure increases in the circuit and a portion of this mixture is expelled. The patient receives a combination of fresh gas and mixed gas from the tubing during the next inspiration. The content of this inspired mixture is determined by the rate of fresh gas flow, the patient's

tidal volume, and the duration of the expiratory pause. A long expiratory pause (slow respiratory rate) allows the fresh gas to move down the tubing and flush the alveolar gas. A short expiratory pause (fast respiratory rate) provides inadequate time to flush the alveolar gas and allows rebreathing to occur. The amount of alveolar gas entering the tubing will increase if tidal volume is large. Rebreathing in this situation can be prevented by high fresh gas flows and a long expiratory pause. Mapleson determined that a fresh gas flow greater than two times the minute ventilation was enough to prevent rebreathing. Recently, it has been shown that normocapnia can be maintained during spontaneous ventilation if the fresh gas flow is 100 ml/kg/min despite rebreathing.[58] Soliman and Laberge[59] found that a flow rate of 206 ml/kg/min resulted in normocapnia in pediatric patients aged 1 to 5 years.

During the inspiratory phase of controlled ventilation, alveolar gas and dead space gas, instead of fresh gas, are forced out of the expiratory valve. Therefore, this system causes less rebreathing than the Mapleson B or C systems. Bain and Spoerel[58] have recommended the following fresh gas flow rates during controlled ventilation with the Mapleson D system:

2 L/min for infants weighing less than 10 kg
3.5 L/min for patients weighing from 10 to 50 kg
70 ml/kg/min for patients weighing more than 60 kg

In each of these cases, the recommended tidal volume is 10 ml/kg and the respiratory rate is 12 to 16 breaths/min.

Bain Circuit

The Bain circuit is a modification of the Mapleson D system. It is a coaxial circuit in which the fresh gas flows through a narrow inner tube within the outer corrugated tubing.[60] The central tube originates near the reservoir bag, but the fresh gas actually enters the circuit at the patient end (Fig. 7-27). Exhaled gases enter the corrugated tubing and are vented through the expiratory valve near the reservoir bag. The Bain circuit may be used for both spontaneous and controlled ventilation. The fresh gas flows necessary to prevent rebreathing are similar to those of the Mapleson D system. Normocarbia during spontaneous ventilation requires a fresh gas flow of 200 to 300 ml/kg, but a flow of only 70 ml/kg will produce normocarbia during controlled ventilation.[58,61,62]

There are many advantages to this circuit. It is lightweight, convenient, easily sterilized, and reusable. Scavenging of the gases from the expiratory valve is facilitated because it is located away from the patient. Exhaled gases in the outer reservoir tubing add warmth and humidity to inspired fresh gases. The hazards of the Bain circuit include unrecognized disconnection or kinking of the inner fresh gas hose. These problems can cause hypercarbia from inadequate gas flow or increased respiratory resistance.

The outer tube should be transparent to allow inspection of the inner tube. The integrity of the inner tube can be assessed as described by Pethick.[63] High-flow oxygen is fed into the circuit while the patient end is occluded until the reservoir bag is filled. The patient end is opened, and oxygen is flushed into the circuit. If the inner tube is intact, the Venturi effect occurs at the patient end. This causes a decrease in pressure within the circuit, and the reservoir bag deflates. Conversely, a leak in the inner tube allows the fresh gas to escape into the expiratory limb, and the reservoir bag will remain inflated. This test is recommended as a part of the preanesthesia check if a Bain circuit is used.

Mapleson E

The Mapleson E is a modification of Ayre's T-piece, which was developed in 1937 by Phillip Ayre[64] for use in pediatric patients undergoing cleft palate repair or intracranial surgery. It consists of a fresh gas inlet at the patient end and a long corrugated tubing (Fig. 7-25). It has minimal dead space, no valves, and very little resistance.[65]

The expiratory limb is the reservoir. Volume of the expiratory limb greater than the patient's tidal volume prevents entrainment of room air and thereby prevents dilution of anesthetic gases and oxygen. A fresh gas flow greater than three times the minute ventilation prevents rebreathing.

During spontaneous ventilation, the fresh gas and exhaled gas flow down the expiratory limb (Fig. 7-26, left). Peak expiratory flow occurs early in exhalation. Therefore, the proportion of fresh gas added to the exhaled gases increases. The fresh gas accumulates at the patient end. During the next breath, fresh gas is drawn both from the fresh gas inlet and the expiratory limb or the reservoir. Controlled ventilation can be accomplished by intermittently occluding the end of the expiratory limb.

Mapleson F

The most commonly used T-piece system is the Jackson-Rees[66] modification of Mapleson D. This is a T-piece arrangement with a reservoir bag and incorporates a relief mechanism for venting exhaled gases. The relief mechanism is either an adjustable valve at the distal end of the reservoir bag or simply a hole in the side of the bag. During spontaneous ventilation when the patient exhales, the gases pass down the expiratory limb and mix with the fresh gas (Fig. 7-26, left). The expiratory pause allows the fresh gas to push the exhaled gases down the expiratory limb. With the next inspiration, the inhaled gas mixture comes from the fresh gas flow and from the expiratory limb including the reservoir bag. Considerations for fresh gas flow rates are similar to those for the Bain circuit. Flow rates equivalent to three times the minute ventilation are recommended to prevent rebreathing.

The Jackson-Rees circuit is commonly used for controlled ventilation during an anesthetic procedure and for transportation of intubated patients. Fresh gas flow rates are similar to those in the Bain circuit. The degree of rebreathing is affected by the management of venting and ventilation.

The Jackson-Rees system is popular for pediatric an-

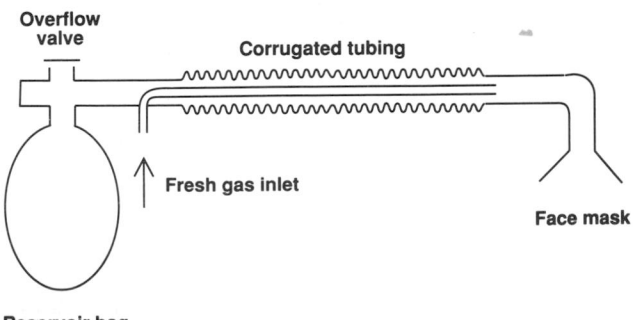

Fig. 7-27. The Bain circuit. (Redrawn from Bain and Spoerel,[60] with permission.)

esthesia, especially for head and neck surgery, because it is lightweight and can be positioned easily. It is simply constructed, inexpensive, and offers minimal resistance because there are no moving parts except the adjustable valve. Observation of the reservoir bag allows one to inspect respiratory excursions and judge the depth of anesthesia. Controlled ventilation can be instituted easily by squeezing the bag. Scavenging can be done either by enclosing the reservoir bag in a plastic chamber from which the waste gases are suctioned or by attaching various devices to the relief valves in the bag.

A disadvantage of this system is lack of humidification. However, this problem can be overcome by allowing the fresh gas to pass through an in-line heated humidifier. Incorporation of a water trap downstream from the humidifier accumulates condensed moisture from the fresh gas inlet tube. This prevents overhydration of the pediatric patient. Another disadvantage of the Jackson-Rees system is the need for high fresh gas flows. Finally, occlusion of the relief valve rapidly can increase the airway pressure, producing barotrauma.

Circle System

The circle system is the most popular breathing system in the United States. It is so named because its components are arranged in a circular manner. This system prevents rebreathing of carbon dioxide by soda lime absorption but allows partial rebreathing of other exhaled gases. The extent of rebreathing of the other exhaled gases depends on component arrangement and the inflow rate.

A circle system can be semiopen, semiclosed, or closed, depending on the amount of fresh gas inflow.[67] A semiopen system has no rebreathing and requires a very high flow of fresh gas. A semiclosed system is associated with rebreathing of gases and is the most commonly used system in the United States. A closed system is one in which the inflow gas exactly matches that being taken up, or consumed, by the patient. There is complete rebreathing of exhaled gases after absorption of carbon dioxide, and the overflow (pop-off) valve is closed.

The circle system (Fig. 7-28) consists of seven components including the following: (1) a fresh gas inflow source; (2) inspiratory and expiratory unidirectional valves; (3) inspiratory and expiratory corrugated tubes; (4) a Y-piece connector; (5) an overflow or pop-off valve; (6) a reservoir bag; and (7) a canister containing a carbon dioxide absorbent. The unidirectional valves are placed in the system to ensure unidirectional flow through the corrugated hoses. The fresh gas inflow enters the circle by a connection from the common gas outlet of the anesthesia machine.

Numerous variations of circle arrangement are possible depending on the relative positions of the unidirectional valves, the pop-off valve, the reservoir bag, the

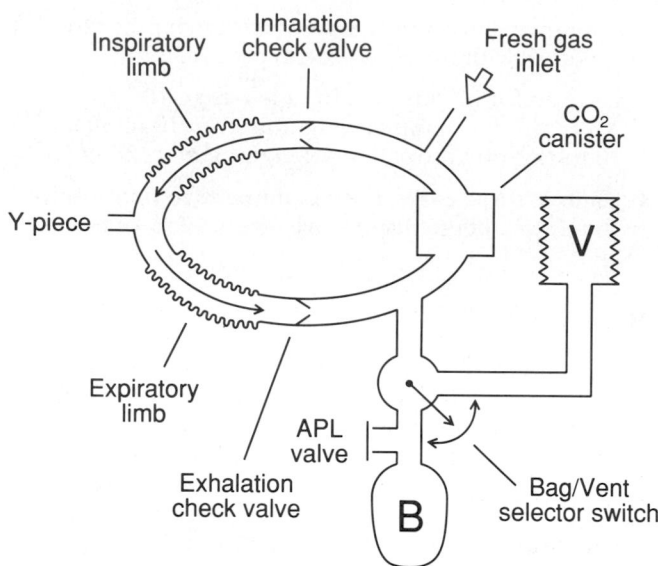

Fig. 7-28. Components of the circle system. *B*, bag; *V*, vent.

carbon dioxide absorber, and the site of fresh gas entry. However, to prevent rebreathing of carbon dioxide, three rules must be followed: (1) a unidirectional valve must be located between the patient and the reservoir bag on both the inspiratory and expiratory limbs of the circuit; (2) the fresh gas inflow cannot enter the circuit between the expiratory valve and the patient; and (3) the overflow (pop-off) valve cannot be located between the patient and the inspiratory valve. If these rules are followed, any arrangement of the other components will prevent rebreathing of carbon dioxide.[68]

The most efficient circle system arrangement that allows the highest conservation of fresh gases is one with the unidirectional valves near the patient and the pop-off valve just downstream from the expiratory valve. This arrangement conserves dead space gas and preferentially eliminates alveolar gas. A more practical but less efficient arrangement is the one used on all contemporary anesthesia machines (Fig. 7-28). It is less efficient because it allows alveolar and dead space gas to mix before venting.[68,69]

The advantages of the circle system include a relative constancy of inspired concentration, conservation of respiratory moisture and heat, and minimization of operating room pollution. Additionally, it can be used for closed-system anesthesia or with low oxygen flows. The major disadvantage of the circle system stems from its complex design. The circuit has approximately 10 connections, all of which can disconnect and leak. Malfunctioning valves can cause serious problems. Rebreathing can occur if the valves stick in the open position. Total occlusion of the circuit can occur if they are stuck closed. Finally, the bulk of the circle offers less convenience and portability than the Mapleson systems.

CARBON DIOXIDE ABSORPTION

Different anesthesia systems eliminate carbon dioxide with varying degrees of efficiency. This section is primarily concerned with the closed or semiclosed circle system, which requires carbon dioxide absorption to make rebreathing possible. Desirable features in the carbon dioxide absorption mechanism are lack of toxicity with common anesthetics, low resistance to air flow, low cost, ease of handling, and relative efficiency.

History

European scientists in the early 1900s were experimenting with the carbon dioxide absorptive properties of lime water and caustic sodas. However, the real impetus to develop efficient carbon dioxide absorptive techniques came from submarine and chemical warfare applications during World War I.[70] In 1915, Wilson[71] patented a new process to make soda lime that greatly increased its efficiency. Rebreathing techniques with carbon dioxide absorption were slow to gain in popularity until cyclopropane was introduced.[70] Cyclopropane was an expensive and explosive anesthetic agent. Many additions and refinements in soda lime have occurred since its invention, but the essential ingredients have remained unchanged.

Chemistry

Two formulations for carbon dioxide absorption are commonly used today. These are soda lime and baralyme. Soda lime consists of 94 percent calcium hydroxide, 5 percent sodium hydroxide, and 1 percent potassium hydroxide and an activator. Small amounts of silica are added to produce calcium and sodium silicate. This addition produces a hard compound and reduces dust formation. The efficiency of the soda lime absorption varies inversely with the hardness; therefore, little silicate is used in contemporary soda lime. Sodium hydroxide is the catalyst for the carbon dioxide absorptive properties of soda lime.[70,72]

Baralyme is composed of 80 percent calcium hydroxide and 20 percent barium hydroxide. Baralyme is more stable than soda lime and does not require a silica binder. Barium hydroxide is the catalyst. Baralyme is more dense than soda lime and is approximately 15 percent less efficient, based on weight, in absorbing carbon dioxide. Water is required for both formulations, but baralyme contains water as the barium hydroxide octahydrate salt. Therefore, it may perform better in a dry climate.[70,72]

The soda lime used in the early days of carbon dioxide absorption was noted to regenerate its efficiency to absorb carbon dioxide after being exhausted.[73] The explanation for this regeneration is complex, but it is of little concern today. Regeneration is rarely seen today because of improved soda lime with less silica and the addition of potassium hydroxide. Baralyme has no regeneration capability.[70,72]

The size of the absorptive granules has been determined by trial and error, which represents a compromise between resistance to air flow and absorptive efficiency.[74] The smaller the granules, the more surface area is available for absorption. However, air flow resistance increases. The granular size of soda lime and baralyme in anesthesia practice is between 4 and 8 mesh. Resistance to air flow at this size is negligible. Mesh refers to the number of openings per linear inch in a sieve through which the granular particles can pass. A 4-mesh screen means that there are four 1/4-inch openings per linear inch. An 8-mesh screen has eight 1/8-inch openings per linear inch.[70]

The absorption of carbon dioxide by soda lime is a chemical process, not a physical process.[73] Carbon dioxide combines with water to form carbonic acid. Carbonic acid reacts with the hydroxides to form sodium (or potassium) carbonate and water. Calcium hydroxide accepts the carbonate to form calcium carbonate and sodium (or potassium) hydroxide. The equations are as follows:

1. $CO_2 + H_2O \rightleftharpoons H_2CO_3$
2. $H_2CO_3 + 2NaOH$ (KOH) $\rightleftharpoons$ Na_2CO_3 $(K_2CO_3) + 2H_2O + Heat$
3. Na_2CO_3 $(K_2CO_3) + Ca(OH)_2$ $\rightleftharpoons$ $CaCO_3 + 2NaOH$ (KOH)

Some carbon dioxide may react directly with $Ca(OH)_2$, but this reaction is much slower.

The reaction with baralyme differs because more water is liberated by a direct reaction of barium hydroxide and carbon dioxide.

1. $Ba(OH)_2 + 8H_2O + CO_2 \rightleftharpoons BaCO_3 + 9H_2O + Heat$
2. $9H_2O + 9CO_2 \rightleftharpoons 9H_2CO_3$
   Then by direct reactions and by KOH and NaOH
3. $9H_2CO_3 + 9Ca(OH)_2 \rightleftharpoons CaCO_3 + 18H_2O + Heat$

Absorptive Capacity

The maximum amount of carbon dioxide that can be absorbed with the above equations is 26 liters of CO_2 per 100 g of absorbent. However, channeling of gas through granules may substantially decrease this efficiency and allow only 10 to 20 liters of carbon dioxide to actually be absorbed.[75]

Indicators

Ethyl violet is the pH indicator that is added to both soda lime and baralyme to help assess the functional integrity of the absorbent. It is a substituted triphenylmethane dye with a critical pH of 10.3.[72] Ethyl violet changes in color from colorless to violet when the pH of the absorbent decreases as a result of carbon dioxide absorption. The pH of fresh absorbent exceeds the critical pH, and the dye exists in its colorless form (Fig.

7-29A). As absorbent becomes exhausted, however, the pH decreases below 10.3, and ethyl violet changes to its violet (Fig. 7-29B) form through alcohol dehydration.

Historically, other pH indicators have been used to indicate absorbent exhaustion. All are acids or bases that change color when the hydrogen ion concentration changes. Other indicators and their respective colors are as follows: phenolphthalein (white → pink), clayton yellow (red → yellow), ethyl orange (orange → yellow), and mimosa Z (red → white).[76]

Incompatibilities

It is an important and desirable feature to have carbon dioxide absorbents that are not intrinsically toxic and that are not toxic when exposed to common anesthetics. Soda lime fits this description, but it is important to note that when using an uncommon anesthetic, trichloroethylene, toxicity may result. In the presence of alkali and heat, trichloroethylene degrades into the cranial neurotoxin dichloroacetylene. Phosgene, a potent pulmonary irritant, is also produced. The resulting toxicities are manifested by cranial nerve lesions, encephalitis, and adult respiratory distress syndrome (ARDS).[77] A newer anesthetic, sevoflurane, is somewhat unstable in soda lime, but this apparently does not produce any toxic effects.[78]

ANESTHESIA VENTILATORS

The anesthesia ventilator can substitute for the breathing bag of the circle system, the Bain circuit, and other breathing systems. Ten years ago anesthesia ventilators were mere adjuncts to the anesthesia machine. Today they have attained a prominent central role in newer anesthesia systems. This discussion focuses on the classification, operating principles, and hazards of anesthesia ventilators.

Classification

Ventilators can be classified according to the power source, the drive mechanism, the cycling mechanism,

and the bellows type. The following section briefly reviews ventilator classification and terminology prior to the discussion of individual anesthesia machine ventilators. For additional details, refer to texts such as *Mechanical Ventilation* by R. R. Kirby, R. A. Smith, and D. A. Desautels[79] and *Respiratory Therapy Equipment* by S. P. McPherson and C. B. Spearman.[80]

Power Source

The power source required to operate a mechanical ventilator is provided by either compressed gas, electricity, or both. Older pneumatic ventilators such as the Ohio Anesthesia Ventilator, the Ohio V5, and the Ohio V5A require only a pneumatic power source to function properly.[81-85] Contemporary electronic ventilators such as the Drager AV-E, the Ohmeda 7000, and the Ohmeda 7810 require both an electronic and a pneumatic power source.[6,9,14,16,17,86,87]

Drive Mechanism

Most anesthesia machine ventilators are classified as double-circuit, pneumatically driven ventilators. In a double-circuit system, a driving force compresses a bag or bellows that in turn delivers gas to the patient. Compressed gases provide the actual driving force. The ventilators are therefore pneumatically driven. The driving gas in the Ohmeda 7000 and the Ohmeda 7810 is composed of 100 percent oxygen.[14,86,87] In the Drager AV-E, it is a mixture of oxygen and air because a Venturi device is employed.[6,9,16,17]

Cycling Mechanism

Most anesthesia machine ventilators are time-cycled and provide ventilator support in the control mode. Inspiration is initiated by a timing device. Older pneumatic ventilators use a fluidic timing device. Contemporary electronic ventilators use a solid-state timing device and are thus classified as time-cycled and electronically controlled.

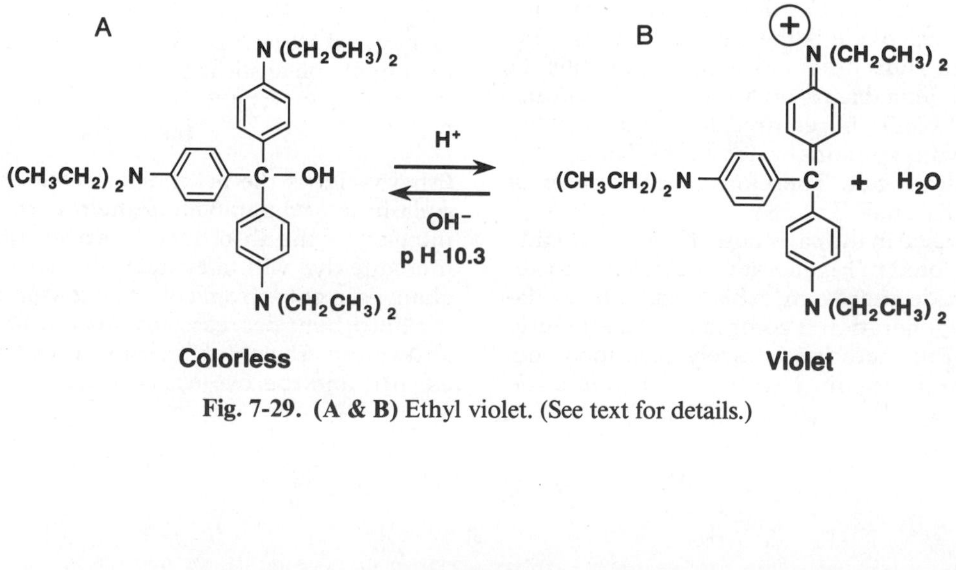

Fig. 7-29. (A & B) Ethyl violet. (See text for details.)

Bellows Classification

The direction of bellows movement during the expiratory phase determines the bellows classification. Ascending (standing) bellows ascend during the expiratory phase, whereas descending (hanging) bellows descend during the expiratory phase. Older pneumatic ventilators use weighted descending bellows, while most contemporary electronic ventilators have ascending bellows. Of the two configurations, the ascending bellows is safer. An ascending bellows will not fill if a disconnection occurs. The bellows of a descending bellows ventilator, however, will continue its upward and downward movement during a disconnection. The drive gas pushes the bellows upward during the inspiratory phase. During the expiratory phase, room air is entrained into the breathing system at the site of the disconnection because gravity acts on the weighted bellows. The disconnection pressure monitor and the volume monitor may be fooled even if a disconnection is complete[21] (see the section, *Breathing Circuit Problems*).

Operating Principles

A generic ascending bellows ventilator is shown in Figure 7-30. Simplified, it may be viewed as a breathing bag (bellows) located within a clear plastic box. The bellows physically separates the driving gas circuit from the patient gas circuit. The driving gas circuit is located outside the bellows, and the patient gas circuit is inside the bellows. During the inspiratory phase (Fig. 7-30A) the driving gas enters the bellows chamber, causing the pressure within it to increase. This increase in pressure is responsible for two events. First, the ventilator relief valve closes. This prevents anesthetic gas from escaping into the scavenging system. Second, the bellows is compressed, and the anesthetic gas within the bellows is delivered to the patient's lungs. This compression action is analogous to squeezing of the breathing bag by the anesthesiologist.[88]

During the expiratory phase (Fig. 7-30B), the driving gas exits the bellows chamber. The pressure within the bellows chamber and within the pilot line declines to zero, causing the mushroom portion of the ventilator relief valve to open. Exhaled patient gas fills the bellows before any scavenging. This occurs because a weighted ball similar to those used in ball-type positive end-expiratory pressure (PEEP) valves is incorporated into the base of the ventilator relief valve. The ball produces 2 to 3 cmH_2O of back pressure, so scavenging occurs only after the bellows fills completely and the pressure inside the bellows exceeds this pressure threshold. This design causes all ascending bellows ventilators to produce 2 to 3 cmH_2O pressure of PEEP within the breathing circuit. Scavenging occurs only during the expiratory phase since the ventilator relief valve is open only during expiration.[88]

Gas flow from the anesthesia machine into the breathing circuit is continuous, and it is independent of ventilator activity. During the inspiratory phase of mechanical ventilation, the ventilator relief valve is closed, and the breathing system adjustable pressure limiting valve (pop-off valve) is either closed or out of circuit. Therefore, the patient receives volume from the bellows and from the flowmeters during the inspiratory phase. Factors that influence the correlation between set tidal volume and exhaled tidal volume include the flowmeter settings, the inspiratory time, the compliance of the breathing circuit, external leakage, and the location of the tidal volume sensor.[14,86,87] Usually, the volume gained from the flowmeters during inspiration is counteracted by the volume lost to the breathing circuit compliance. The set tidal volume generally approximates the exhaled tidal volume. However, oxygen flushing during the inspiratory phase can result in barotrauma because excess volume cannot be vented.[88]

Pneumatic Ventilators

Pneumatic ventilators performed the majority of mechanical ventilation in the operating room until recent years. Although they have become less popular, many are still in use. Examples of pneumatic ventilators include the Ohio Anesthesia Ventilator, the Ohio V5, the Ohio V5A, and the Drager AV. They are classified as pneumatically powered, double-circuit, pneumatically driven, descending bellows, time-cycled, fluidically controlled, tidal-volume-preset ventilators that are generally used in the control mode. All use a Venturi drive-gas system. The entrained room air provides additional flow to the bellows chamber without substantially decreasing the oxygen supply pressure within the anesthesia machine.[81-85]

Pneumatic ventilators have several advantages. They require only a pneumatic power source. Therefore, they can be used effectively during an electrical power failure or in remote areas without electricity. The functional design of pneumatic ventilators is simple, and they are easy to operate. Most are mobile, freestanding units that can readily be moved from room to room. The fluidic control components have no moving parts and depend solely on gas flow and pressure to function. Maintenance is minimal, and a knowledge of electricity is not necessary to service the ventilators.

Disadvantages of pneumatic ventilators, however, outweigh the advantages. The major disadvantage is a possible unrecognized disconnection. This results from the descending bellows configuration coupled with a relatively low factory preset disconnection threshold pressure alarm limit such as 8 to 10 cmH_2O pressure. Most pneumatic ventilators have only one alarm: the low-pressure disconnection alarm. This is in marked contrast to newer electronic ventilators that may have multiple alarms. Finally, pneumatic ventilators have a limited number of controls and lack versatility.

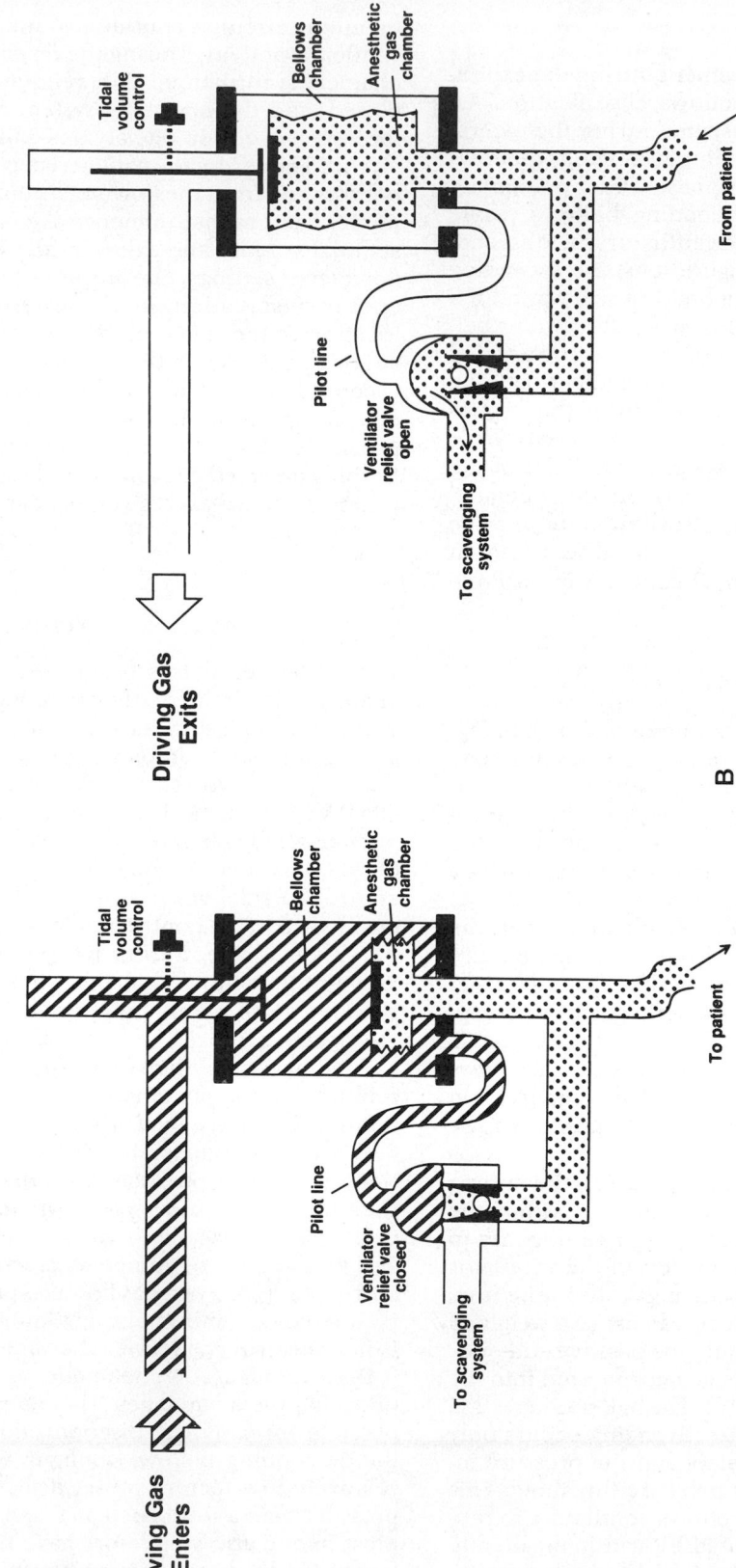

Fig. 7-30. (A) Inspiratory- and (B) expiratory-phase gas flows of a generic ascending bellows anesthesia ventilator. (See text for details.) APL, adjustable pressure-limiting. (From Andrews,[88] with permission.)

Electronic Ventilators

Contemporary electronic anesthesia machine ventilators such as the Drager AV-E, the Ohmeda 7000, and the Ohmeda 7810 are an integral portion of the global anesthesia system. Each is discussed below.

Drager AV-E Anesthesia Ventilator

The Drager AV-E is classified as a pneumatically and electronically powered, double-circuit, pneumatically driven, ascending bellows, time-cycled, electronically controlled, tidal-volume-preset controller. The AV-E is standard equipment on the Narkomed 2A, Narkomed 2B, and Narkomed 3, and it is not available as a free-standing ventilator. It consists of two major components: the control assembly and the bellows assembly. The control assembly contains the electronic and pneumatic components of the ventilator. It is located above the flowmeters and vaporizers, and it serves as a permanent shelf. The control assembly houses four controls. They include the ventilator power switch, the frequency control, the I:E ratio control, and the inspiratory flow control. The bellows assembly is located to the left of the flowmeters. The tidal volume scale on the plastic bellows housing ranges from 200 cc to 1,400 cc, and it increases from bottom to top. The tidal volume adjustment knob is above the bellows chamber. Adjustment of the knob determines the location of the bellows stop that limits the upward movement of the bellows within the bellows chamber to the desired tidal volume. The ventilator relief valve is behind the bellows chamber. The operator can observe the action of this valve because its dome is constructed of clear plastic.[6,9,16,17]

The operating principle of the AV-E is illustrated in Figures 7-31 and 7-32. Oxygen at 50 PSIG provides the pneumatic input to the driving gas circuit. Flow through this circuit is regulated by a solenoid valve that serves as an interface between the pneumatic and electric circuits of the ventilator. The electronic timing of the solenoid is determined by the settings of the frequency and I:E ratio controls. It is open during the inspiratory phase and closed during the expiratory phase.[6]

Inspiratory-phase gas flows are illustrated in Figure 7-31. Oxygen at 50 PSIG passes through the solenoid valve and opens the control valve. This allows the preset gas flow from the flow regulator to proceed through the control valve to the Venturi device. Back-pressure from the Venturi device is directed to the power relief valve and closes it. Then oxygen from the flow regulator passes through the Venturi device, and a substantial volume of room air is entrained through the muffler. The flow of the driving gas increases considerably without depleting the oxygen pressure within the anesthesia machine because a Venturi device is used.[6]

The driving gas is forced into the bellows chamber, causing the pressure within it to increase. The pressure increases causing two events. First, the ventilator relief valve closes. This prevents anesthetic gas from escaping into the scavenging system. Second, the bellows is compressed downward, and the anesthetic gas within the bellows is delivered to the patient's lungs. The ventilator relief valve remains closed as long as the bellows chamber contains pressure. The inspiratory pause time starts when the bellows is completely compressed, and it lasts until the bellows begins to ascend. The pressure in the bellows chamber, as preset by the flow regulator, cannot increase further. All excess pressure is released through the Venturi entrainment port, and the Venturi device simultaneously ceases to entrain room air.[6] The volume of driving gas that enters and exits the bellows chamber during the inspiratory phase may be substantially greater than the tidal volume delivered. This is particularly true with slow rates and with prolonged inspiratory pause times.

The expiratory phase gas flows of the Drager AV-E are shown in Figure 7-32. The expiratory phase begins when the electric signal to the solenoid terminates. As soon as the electric signal stops, the solenoid valve closes. This closure terminates the 50 PSIG gas supply to the control valve, which also closes. The preset gas flow from the flow regulator is interrupted by the control valve. This causes an immediate pressure decrease at the Venturi device, and no back-pressure is supplied to the power relief valve, which opens. Then the driving gas within the bellows chamber can exit through the power relief valve and through the entrainment port of the Venturi device.[6] Regardless of the route taken, all driving gas is discharged through the ventilator muffler.

The pressure within the bellows chamber and in the pilot line declines to zero, causing the mushroom portion of the ventilator relief valve to open. To prevent premature outflow of anesthetic gas into the scavenging system, a weighted ball similar to those used in ball-type PEEP valves is incorporated into the base of the ventilator relief valve. The ball produces 2 cmH$_2$O back-pressure. Thus, the bellows extends fully, and 2 cmH$_2$O pressure develops within the bellows chamber before anesthetic gas enters the scavenging system.[6]

Global examination of the inspiratory and expiratory gas flows of the Drager AV-E reveals the importance of a clean, functional muffler. Much of the driving gas is entrained through the muffler during the inspiratory phase. All the driving gas exits through the muffler during the expiratory phase. Pressure within the bellows chamber and within the pilot line increases if the muffler becomes occluded. The ventilator relief valve remains closed if there is pressure within the bellows chamber. As a result, excess anesthetic gas cannot vent into the scavenging system, and patient airway pressure increases.[89] Two alarms should quickly alert the anesthesiologist when this scenario occurs. These are the continuing system pressure alarm and the high-pressure alarm.

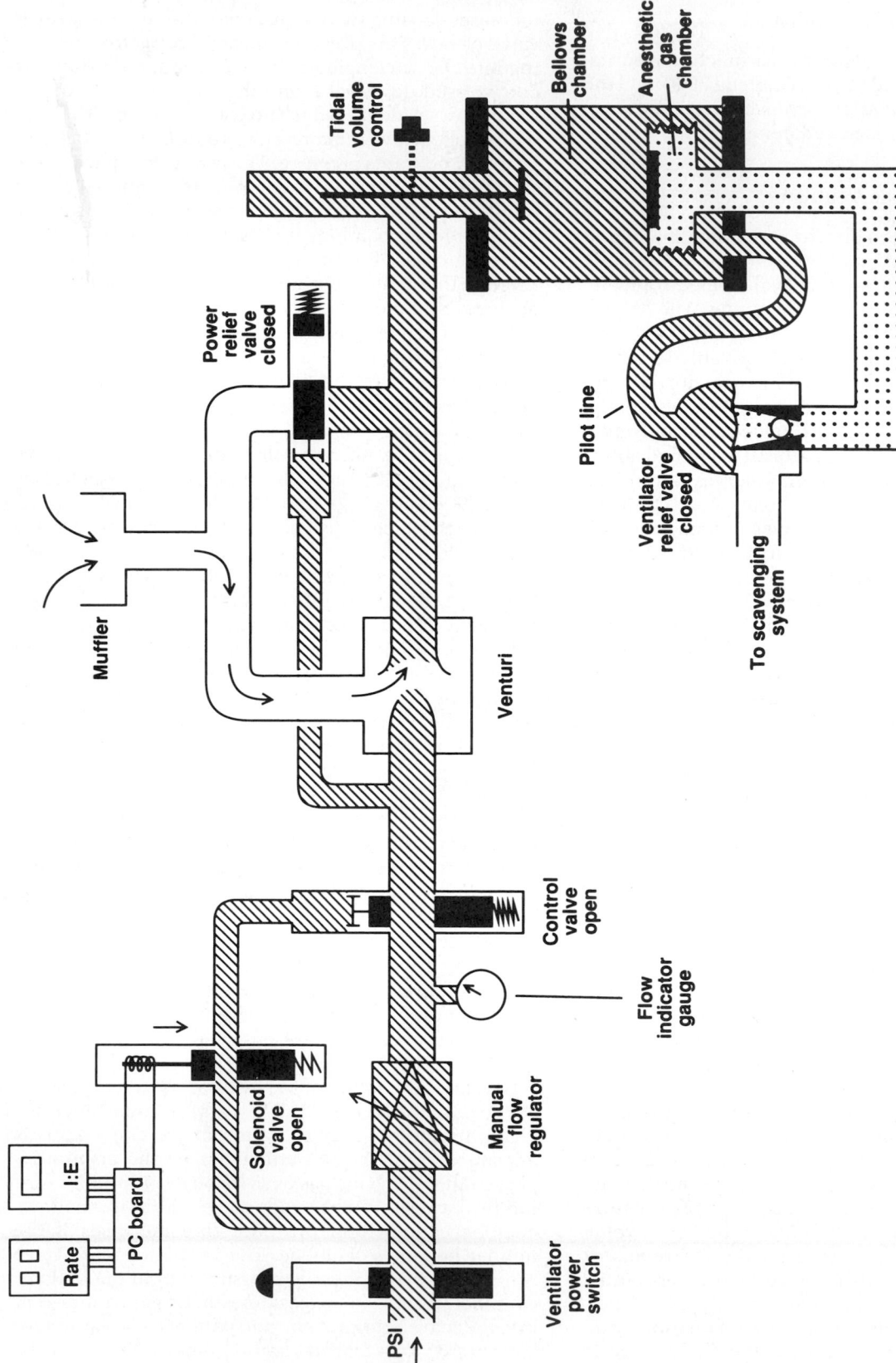

Fig. 7-31. Inspiratory-phase gas flows of the Dräger AV-E. (See text for details.) (From Andrews,[19] with permission.)

Tidal volume control

Bellows chamber

Anesthetic gas chamber

To patient

Power relief valve closed

Muffler

Pilot line

Venturi

Ventilator relief valve closed

To scavenging system

Flow indicator gauge

Control valve open

I:E

Rate

PC board

Solenoid valve open

Manual flow regulator

Ventilator power switch

50 PSI

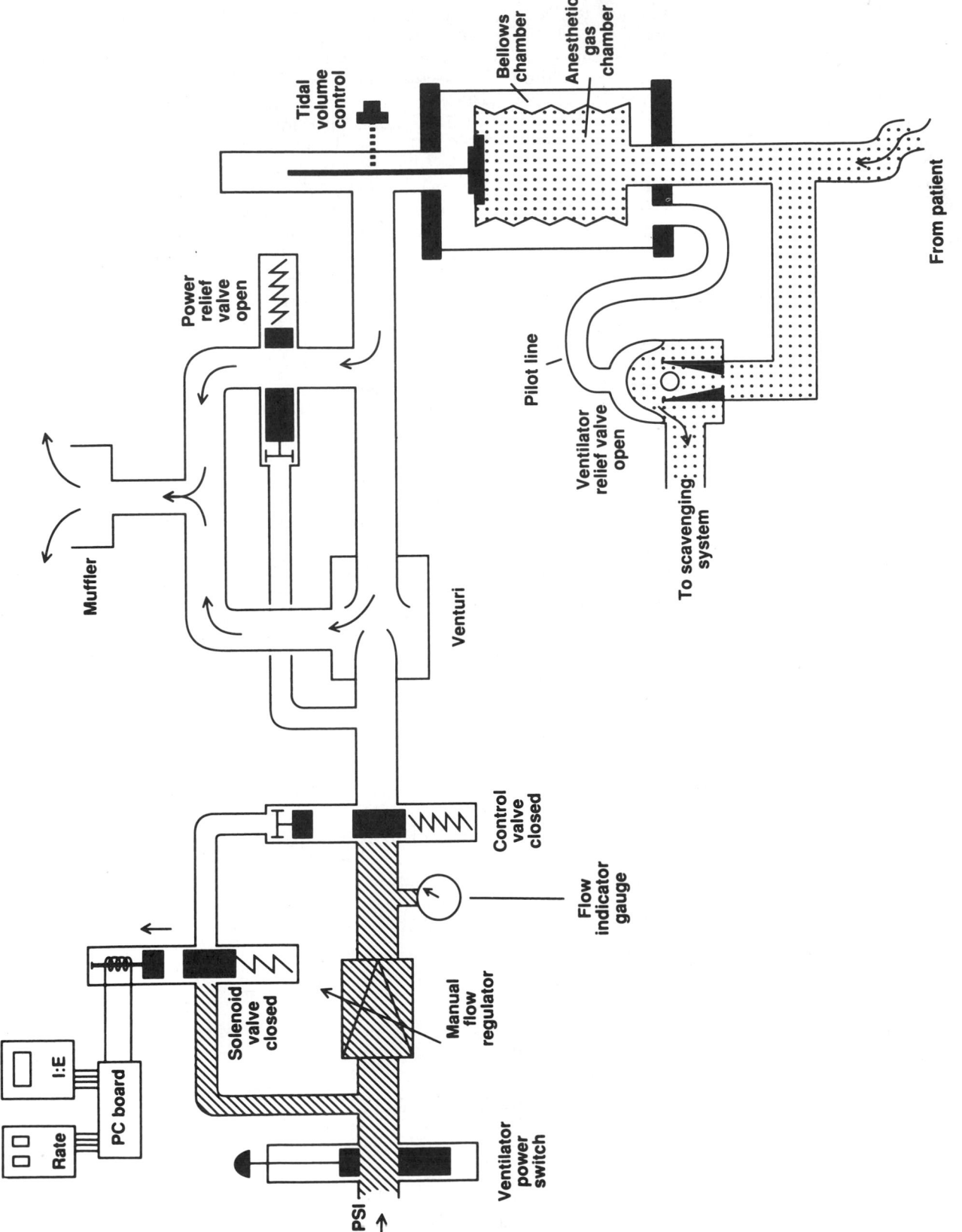

Fig. 7-32. Expiratory-phase gas flows of the Drager AV-E. (See text for details.) (From Andrews,[19] with permission.)

Two ventilator monitors are available on the Narkomed 2B and Narkomed 3. The breathing pressure monitor, or Baromed, is standard equipment. Pressure input from the patient circuit can be from either the carbon dioxide absorber or the Y-piece. Pressure versus time waveforms are displayed on a cathode ray tube. The operator sets a high-pressure alarm limit and a threshold pressure alarm limit if preset default values are not acceptable. Alarms are provided for high pressure, pressure below the threshold for 15 and 30 seconds (apnea), continuing pressure above the set threshold for 15 seconds, and subatmospheric (≤ -10 cmH$_2$O) pressure. The respiratory volume monitor, or Spiromed, is an optional monitor. The tidal volume sensor is located between the expiratory valve and the carbon dioxide absorber. Alarms are provided for low tidal volume (<70 cc), high respiratory rate (>99 breaths/min), and reverse flow through the sensor (>20 cc).[9,17]

Ohmeda 7000 Electronic Anesthesia Ventilator

The Ohmeda 7000 is classified as a pneumatically and electronically powered, double-circuit, pneumatically driven, ascending bellows, time-cycled, electronically controlled, minute-volume-preset controller. It consists of two units: the control module and the bellows assembly. The control module is mounted above the flowmeters on the Ohmeda Modulus II. It has six controls including the minute volume dial, the rate dial, the I : E ratio dial, the power switch, a sigh switch, and a manual cycle button. A tidal volume dial is not present on the Ohmeda 7000. The control module automatically calculates the tidal volume according to the setting of the minute volume and rate dials. The bellows assembly is mounted directly on the Ohmeda Gas Management system (GMS) absorber, using an interface manifold. The scale on the plastic bellows housing has a range of 100 to 1,600 cc, and it increases from top to bottom. The ventilator relief valve cannot be seen during ventilator operation because it is inside the bellows assembly base.[86,87]

The operating principle of the Ohmeda 7000 is similar to that of the Drager AV-E. Figure 7-33 is a schematic of the pneumatic circuitry of the Ohmeda 7000. The driving gas supply is 100 percent oxygen at 50 PSIG. A precision regulator reduces this pressure to 38 ± 0.5 PSIG. The regulated gas supply connects directly to a

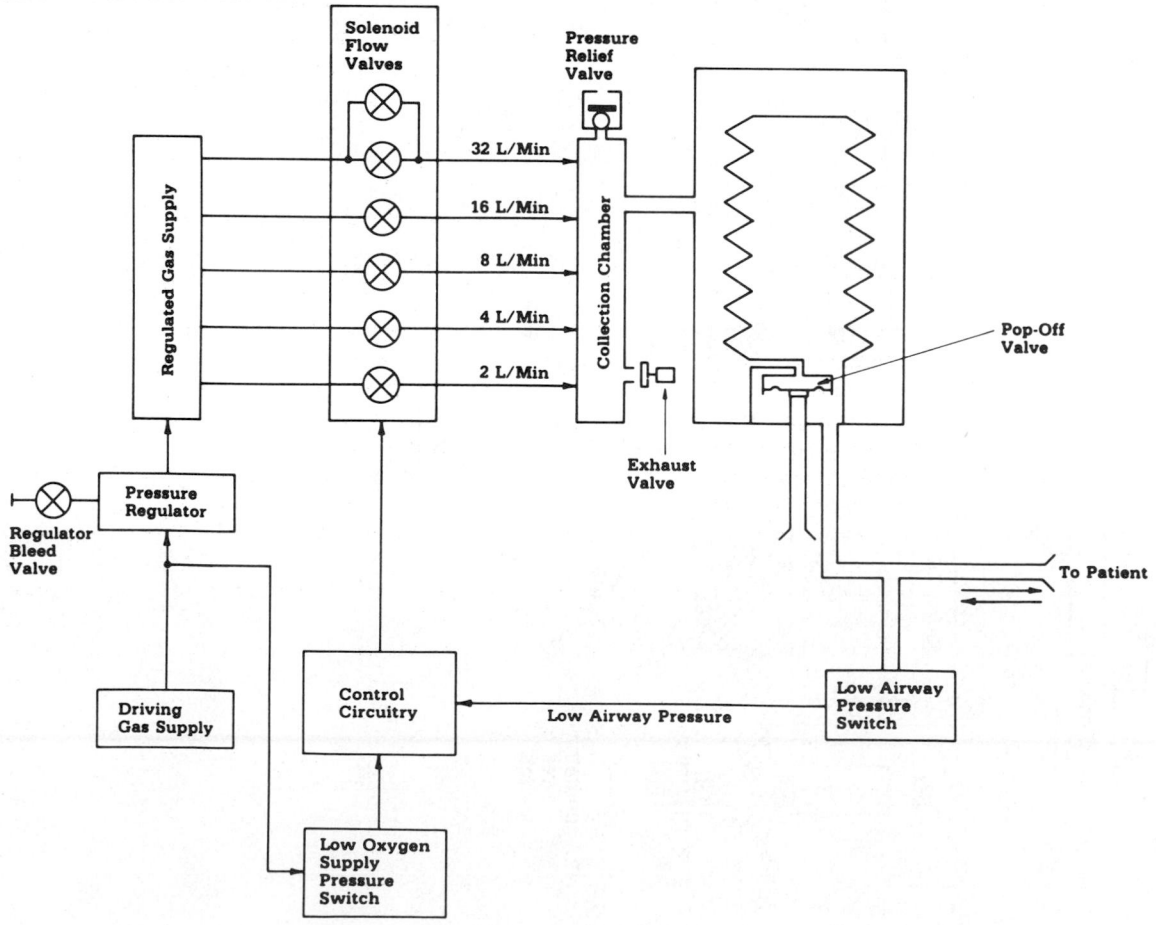

Fig. 7-33. Diagram of the Ohmeda 7000 Electronic Anesthesia Ventilator. (See text for details.) (Courtesy of Ohmeda, The BOC Group Inc., Madison, WI.)

manifold of five solenoid valves. The control box electronically regulates the solenoid valves during the inspiratory time. Gas flow is directed through tuned orifices that are calibrated for flows of 2, 4, 6, 8, 16, and 32 L/min. The range of flow selection is in 2 L/min increments from 4 to 60 L/min. A precise volume of driving gas equal to the tidal volume is delivered to the bellows chamber at a specific rate depending on the ventilator settings.[86,87]

During the inspiratory phase (Fig. 7-34A), the control module delivers its computed driving gas flow into the bellows chamber. The bellows is compressed as the driving gas volume and pressure increase within the housing. Anesthetic gas is forced out of the bellows, through the patient circuit, and into the patient's lungs. Flow stops when the full volume of driving gas has been delivered into the bellows chamber. A relief valve located within the control module opens and vents excess driving gas into the atmosphere if high pressure occurs during the inspiratory phase. The threshold for this relief valve is 65 cm H_2O pressure.[86,87]

Anesthetic gas enters the bellows chamber from the patient circuit during the expiratory phase (Fig. 7-34B and C). The ventilator relief valve, located inside the bellows chamber, has a threshold value of 2.5 cmH_2O pressure. Therefore, it opens only when the bellows is fully extended and the pressure within the bellows exceeds 2.5 cmH_2O pressure. Then, excess patient gas is popped off into the scavenging system.[86,87]

The operating principle of the Ohmeda 7000 is similar to that of the Drager AV-E, but some differences exist. The Ohmeda 7000 does not use a Venturi device, and the driving gas is composed of 100 percent oxygen. Driving gas inflow rate is regulated by five solenoids instead of one. The Ohmeda 7000 control module delivers a precise driving gas volume to the bellows assembly that displaces the bellows by the same amount. Therefore, the driving gas volume equals the tidal volume, and the bellows is only partially compressed during the inspiratory phase. The Drager's tidal volume, on the other hand, is derived from the position of a mechanical bellows stop. The driving gas volume may be substantially larger than the set tidal volume, and the bellows is fully compressed during inspiration. Because the two ventilators generate tidal volume by different means, the tidal volume scale on the plastic bellows housing differs. On the Ohmeda 7000, the scale increases from top to bottom, but on the Drager AV-E it increases from bottom to top.[6,9,16,17,86,87]

Ohmeda 7810 Electronic Anesthesia Ventilator

The Ohmeda 7810 is standard equipment on the Ohmeda Modulus II Plus anesthesia system. It is classified as a pneumatically and electronically powered, double-circuit, pneumatically driven, ascending bellows, time-cycled, electronically controlled, tidal-volume-preset, pressure-limited controller. The 7810 serves not only as a ventilator, but also as an oxygen analyzer, an airway pressure monitor, and a volume monitor. It combines

these monitors and provides an integrated ventilator alarm system.[14]

The Ohmeda 7810 consists of two basic units: the control module and the bellows assembly. The bellows assembly of the 7810 is almost identical to that of the 7000, but the control module is substantially different. The control module of the 7810 (Fig. 7-35) has four dials including the tidal volume dial, the rate dial, the inspiratory flow dial, and the inspiratory pressure limit dial. Other controls include the inspiratory pause button, the ventilator on/off switch, the alarm set pushwheels, the oxygen calibration thumbwheel, and the alarm silence button.[14]

The operating principle of the Ohmeda 7810 is very similar to that of the Ohmeda 7000, but the 7810 is more versatile. Many operators prefer the tidal volume preset feature of the 7810 compared with the minute volume preset of the 7000. The 7810 has more flexibility regarding I : E ratios. The 7000 is limited to I : E ratios of 1 : 1 through 1 : 3. The 7810, on the other hand, has a much broader continuum of I : E ratios that range from 1 : 0.33 (reverse I : E ratio) through 1 : 999. The 7810 has an inspiratory pause feature that increases the inspiration time by 25 percent. The 7000 does not have this feature. Probably the biggest advantage of the 7810 over the 7000 is the pressure-limiting feature. The 7810 uses an operator-adjustable, electronically controlled, automatic high-pressure relief system to manage excessive airway pressure. If the airway pressure exceeds the high-pressure threshold set by the operator, two events occur. The high-pressure alarm is activated, and the ventilator automatically releases the remaining driving gas into the atmosphere, terminating the inspiratory cycle. Active intervention is not required by the operator. If the high-pressure threshold is set appropriately, the possibility of barotrauma is minimized.[14,86,87]

Problems and Hazards

Numerous hazards are associated with anesthesia ventilators. They include problems with the breathing circuit, the bellows assembly, and the control assembly.

Breathing Circuit Problems

Breathing circuit disconnection is a leading cause of critical incidents in anesthesia.[90] The most common disconnection site is at the Y-piece. Disconnections can be complete or partial (leaks). A common source of leaks with older absorbers is failure to close the adjustable pressure-limiting valve (APL or pop-off valve) upon initiation of mechanical ventilation. The bag/ventilator switch on contemporary absorbers helps minimize this problem. As mentioned above, disconnections manifest more readily with the ascending bellows because the bellows will not fill.[21]

Several disconnection monitors exist. The most important monitor is a vigilant anesthesiologist using a precordial or esophageal stethoscope. Breath sounds should be auscultated continuously, and the chest wall

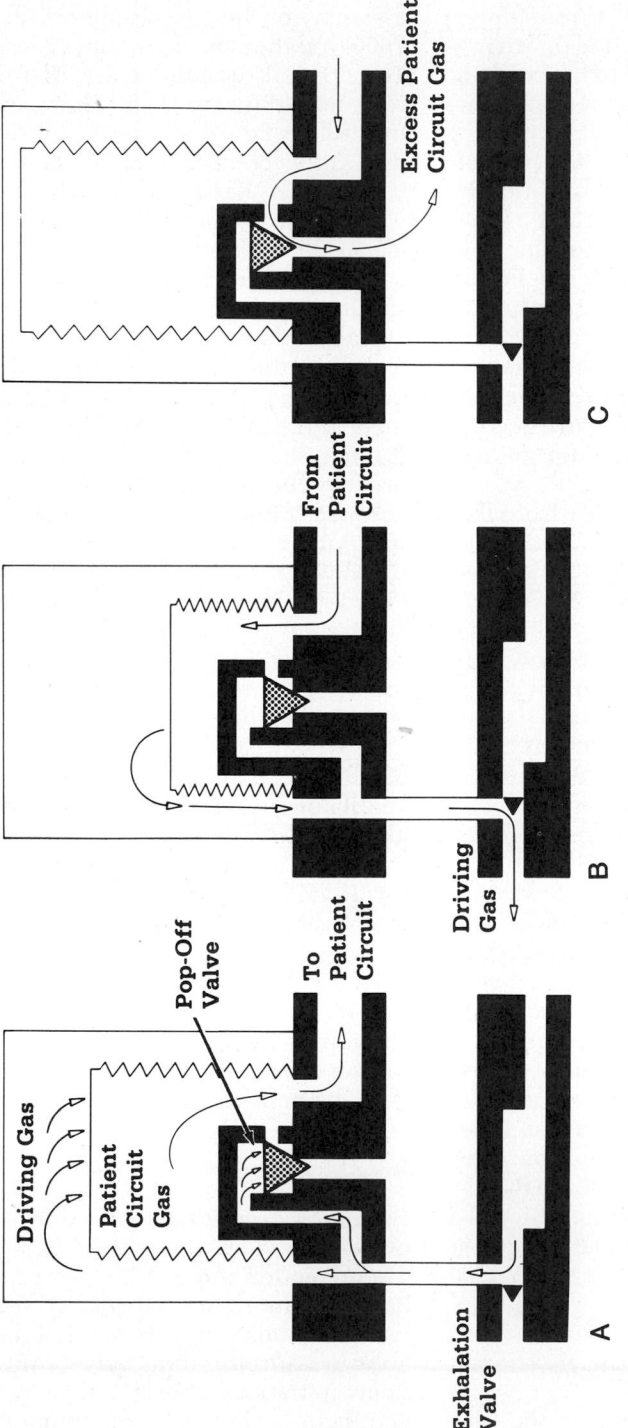

Fig. 7-34. Inspiratory- and expiratory-phase gas flows of the Ohmeda 7000 and 7810 Electronic Anesthesia Ventilator. **(A)** The start of inspiration. The control module closes the exhalation valve and delivers driving gas to the area around the bellows. **(B)** The beginning of expiration. The exhalation valve opens and gas flow in the breathing circuit and driving-gas circuit reverses. Driving gas is released into the atmosphere as the bellows extends. **(C)** If during the expiratory cycle (when the bellows has extended completely) the pressure inside the bellows exceeds about 2.5 cmH₂O, the pop-off valve opens, releasing any excess breathing system gas through the bellows assembly's exhaust port. (See text for additional details.) (Courtesy of Ohmeda, The BOC Group Inc., Madison, WI.)

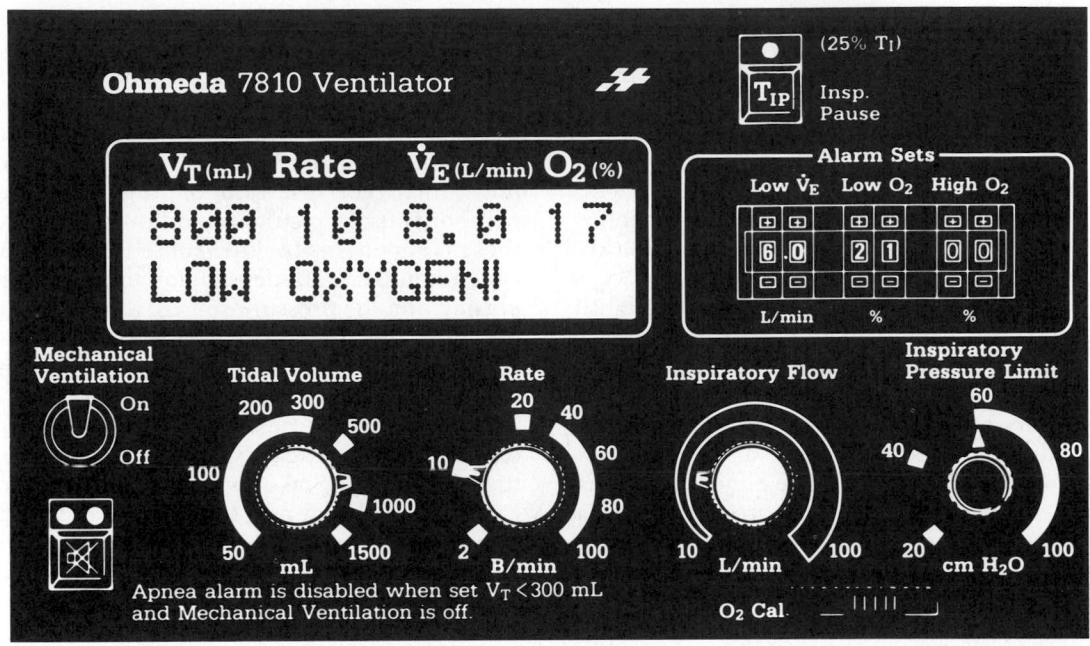

Fig. 7-35. Ohmeda 7810 control assembly. (Courtesy of Ohmeda, The BOC Group Inc., Madison, WI.)

excursion should be observed. Three other monitors include (1) pressure monitors, (2) respiratory volume monitors, and (3) carbon dioxide monitors.

Pneumatic and electronic pressure monitors are helpful in diagnosing disconnections. Factors that influence monitor effectiveness include the disconnection site, the pressure sensor location, the threshold pressure alarm limit, the inspiratory flow rate, and the resistance of the disconnected breathing circuit.[91,92]

Various anesthesia machines and ventilators have different locations for the pressure sensor and different values for the threshold pressure alarm limit (Table 7-1). The threshold pressure alarm limit may be factory preset or adjustable. An audible or visual alarm is actuated if the peak inspiratory pressure of the breathing circuit does not exceed the threshold pressure alarm limit. When an adjustable threshold pressure alarm limit is available, such as on the Drager Narkomed 2A,

TABLE 7-1. Disconnection Pressure Monitors[6,9,11–14,16,17,82–87]

Machine/Ventilator	Location of Pressure Sensor	Threshold Pressure Alarm Limit (cm H_2O)
Ohio Modulus I		
Model 21 Absorber	Patient side of	
Ohio Anesth Vent	expiratory	10
Ohio V5 or V5A	valve	8
Ohmeda Modulus II		
GMS Absorber	Patient side of	
Ohmeda 7000 Ventilator	expiratory valve	6
Ohmeda Modulus II Plus		
GMS Absorber	Patient side of	Δ4–9
Ohmeda 7810	inspiratory valve	PEEP compensated
Drager Narkomed 2A		
Drager AV-E	CO_2 absorber or Y-piece	8, 12, 26
Drager Narkomed 2B, 3		5 → 30
Drager AV-E	CO_2 absorber or Y-piece	(12 default)

Narkomed 2B, and Narkomed 3, the operator should set the pressure alarm limit to within 5 cmH₂O of the peak inspiratory pressure.[6,9,16,17] Figure 7-36 illustrates how a partial disconnection (leak) may be unrecognized by the low-pressure monitor if the threshold pressure alarm limit is set too low or if the factory preset value is relatively low.

Respiratory volume monitors are useful in detecting disconnections. Volume monitors sense exhaled tidal volume, minute volume, or both. The user should bracket the high- and low-threshold volumes slightly above and below the exhaled volumes. For example, if the exhaled minute volume of a patient is 10 L/min, reasonable alarm limits would be 8 to 12 L/min. Carbon dioxide monitors are probably the best devices to reveal patient disconnections. Carbon dioxide concentration is measured near the Y-piece either directly or by aspiration of a gas sample to the instrument. A drastic change in the difference between the inspiratory and end-tidal carbon dioxide concentration or the absence of carbon dioxide indicates a disconnection, a nonventilated patient, or other problems.[21]

Misconnections of the breathing system are not uncommon despite efforts by standards committees to eliminate this problem by assigning different diameters to various hoses and terminals. Anesthesia machines, breathing systems, ventilators, and scavenging systems incorporate a multitude of hose terminals. Hoses have been connected to inappropriate terminals and even to various solid cylindrically shaped protrusions of the anesthesia machine.[21]

Occlusion (obstruction) of the breathing circuit may occur. Tracheal tubes can become kinked. Hoses throughout the breathing circuit are subject to occlusion by external mechanical forces that can impinge on flow. Incorrect insertion of flow direction-sensitive components can result in a no-flow state.[21] Examples of these components include some PEEP valves and cascade humidifiers. Depending on the location of the occlusion and the pressure sensor, a high-pressure alarm may alert the anesthesiologist to the problem.

Excess inflow to the breathing circuit from the anesthesia machine during the inspiratory phase can result in barotrauma. The best example of this phenomenon is oxygen flushing. Excess volume cannot be vented from the system during inspiration because the ventilator relief valve is closed and the APL valve is either out of circuit or closed.[15] A high-pressure alarm, if present, may be activated when the pressure becomes excessive. In the Drager system, both audible and visual alarms are actuated when the high-pressure threshold is exceeded.[6,9,16,17] In the Modulus II Plus system, the Ohmeda 7810 ventilator automatically switches from the inspiratory to the expiratory phase when the adjustable peak pressure threshold is exceeded.[14] This minimizes the possibilities of barotrauma if the peak pressure threshold is set appropriately by the anesthesiologist.

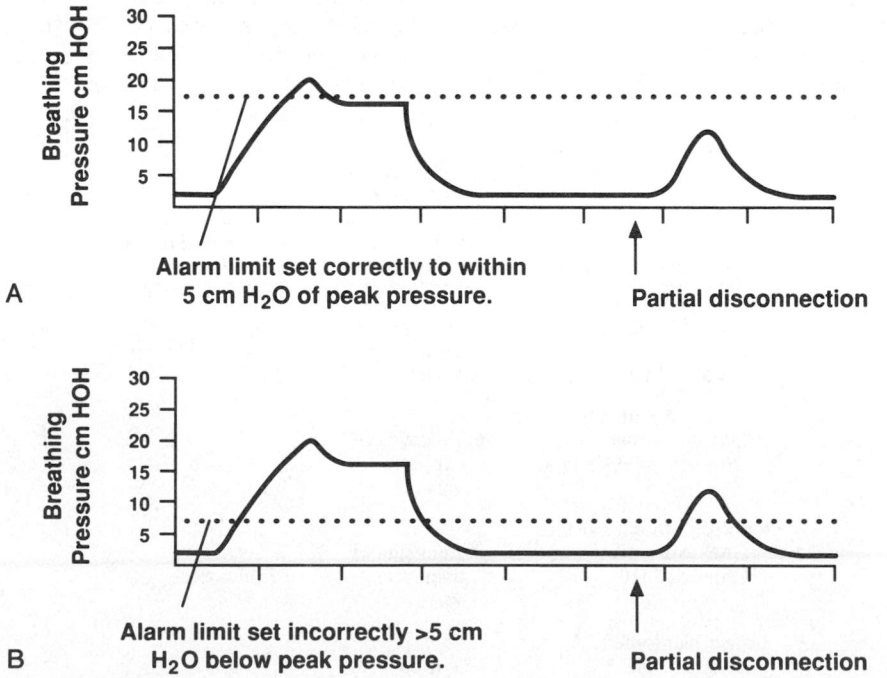

Fig. 7-36. Threshold pressure alarm limit. **(A)** The threshold pressure alarm limit (dotted line) has been set appropriately. An alarm is actuated when a partial disconnection occurs (arrow) because the threshold pressure alarm limit is not exceeded by the breathing circuit pressure. **(B)** A partial disconnection is unrecognized by the pressure monitor because the threshold pressure alarm limit has been set too low. (Redrawn from Baromed Breathing Pressure Monitor Operator's Instruction Manual,[134] with permission.)

Bellows Assembly Problems

Leaks can occur in the bellows assembly. Improper seating of the plastic bellows housing can result in inadequate ventilation because a portion of the driving gas is vented to the atmosphere. A hole in the bellows can lead to alveolar hyperinflation and possibly barotrauma in some ventilators because high-pressure driving gas can enter the patient circuit. The value on the oxygen analyzer may increase when the driving gas is 100 percent oxygen, or it may decrease if the driving gas is composed of an air-oxygen mixture.[93]

The ventilator relief valve can cause problems. Hypoventilation occurs if the valve is incompetent because anesthetic gas is delivered to the scavenging system during the inspiratory phase instead of to the patient. Gas molecules preferentially exit into the scavenging system because it represents the path of least resistance and the pressure within the scavenging system can be subatmospheric. Ventilator relief valve incompetency can result from a disconnected pilot line, a ruptured valve, or from a damaged flapper valve.[94,95] A ventilator relief valve stuck in the closed position can produce barotrauma. Excessive suction from the scavenging system can draw the ventilator relief valve to its seat and close the valve during both the inspiratory and expiratory phases.[21] Breathing circuit pressure escalates because excess anesthetic gas cannot be vented.

Control Assembly Problems

The control assembly can be the source of both electrical and mechanical problems. Electrical failure can be total or partial; the former is the more obvious. Some mechanical problems include leaks within the system, faulty regulators, and faulty valves. As mentioned previously, an occluded muffler can result in barotrauma (see the section, *Drager AV-E Anesthesia Ventilator*). Obstruction of driving gas outflow closes the ventilator relief valve, and excess patient gas cannot be vented.[89]

SCAVENGING SYSTEMS

The American National Standards Institute (ANSI) in 1982 released the Z79.11-1982 guideline entitled *Scavenging Systems for Excess Anesthetic Gases*. The document provided guidelines for manufacturers so that they could produce devices that safely and effectively scavenge excess anesthetic gas to reduce contamination in anesthetizing areas.[96] Scavenging is the collection and the subsequent removal of vented gases from the operating room.[97] Commonly, the amount of gas used to anesthetize a patient far exceeds the patient's needs. Therefore, scavenging minimizes operating room pollution.

Components

Scavenging systems have five components, which are (1) the gas-collecting assembly, (2) the transfer tubing, (3) the scavenging interface, (4) the gas disposal tubing, and (5) an active or passive gas disposal assembly.[96] An active system uses a central vacuum to eliminate waste gases. The pressure of the waste gas itself produces flow through a passive system.

Gas Collection Assembly

The gas collection assembly captures excess anesthetic gas and delivers it to the transfer tubing.[96] Excess gas is vented from anesthesia systems through the APL valve and through the ventilator relief valve. All excess gas passes through these valves, accumulates in the gas collection assembly, and is directed to the transfer tubing.

Transfer Tubing

The transfer tubing carries excess gas from the gas-collecting assembly to the scavenging interface. The tubing must be either 19 or 30 mm as specified by the ANSI Z79.11-1982 standard.[96] The tubing should be sufficiently rigid to prevent kinking, and it should be as short as possible to minimize the chance of occlusion. Some manufacturers color-code the transfer tubing with yellow bands to distinguish it from 22-mm breathing system tubing. Many machines have separate transfer tubes for the APL valve and for the ventilator relief valve. The two tubes frequently merge into a single hose before they enter the scavenging interface.

Scavenging Interface

The scavenging interface is the most important component of the system because it protects the breathing circuit or ventilator from excessive positive or negative pressure.[97] The interface should limit the pressures immediately downstream from the gas collection assembly to between -0.5 and $+10$ cmH$_2$O with normal working conditions.[96] Positive-pressure relief is mandatory, irrespective of the type of disposal system used, to vent excess gas in case of occlusion downstream from the interface. If the disposal system is active, negative-pressure relief is necessary to protect the breathing circuit or ventilator from excessive subatmospheric pressure. A reservoir is highly desirable with active systems since it stores excess waste gas until the evacuation system can eliminate it. Interfaces can be open or closed, depending on the method used to provide positive- and negative-pressure relief.[97]

Open Interfaces

An open interface contains no valves, and it is open to the atmosphere, allowing both positive- and negative-pressure relief. Open interfaces should be used only with active disposal systems that use a central vacuum system. Open interfaces require a reservoir because waste gases are intermittently discharged in surges, while flow to the active disposal system is continuous.[97]

Figure 7-37 shows four types of open interfaces used with active systems. The simplest is a T-tube shown in Figure 7-37A. Waste gas enters the top of the T-tube

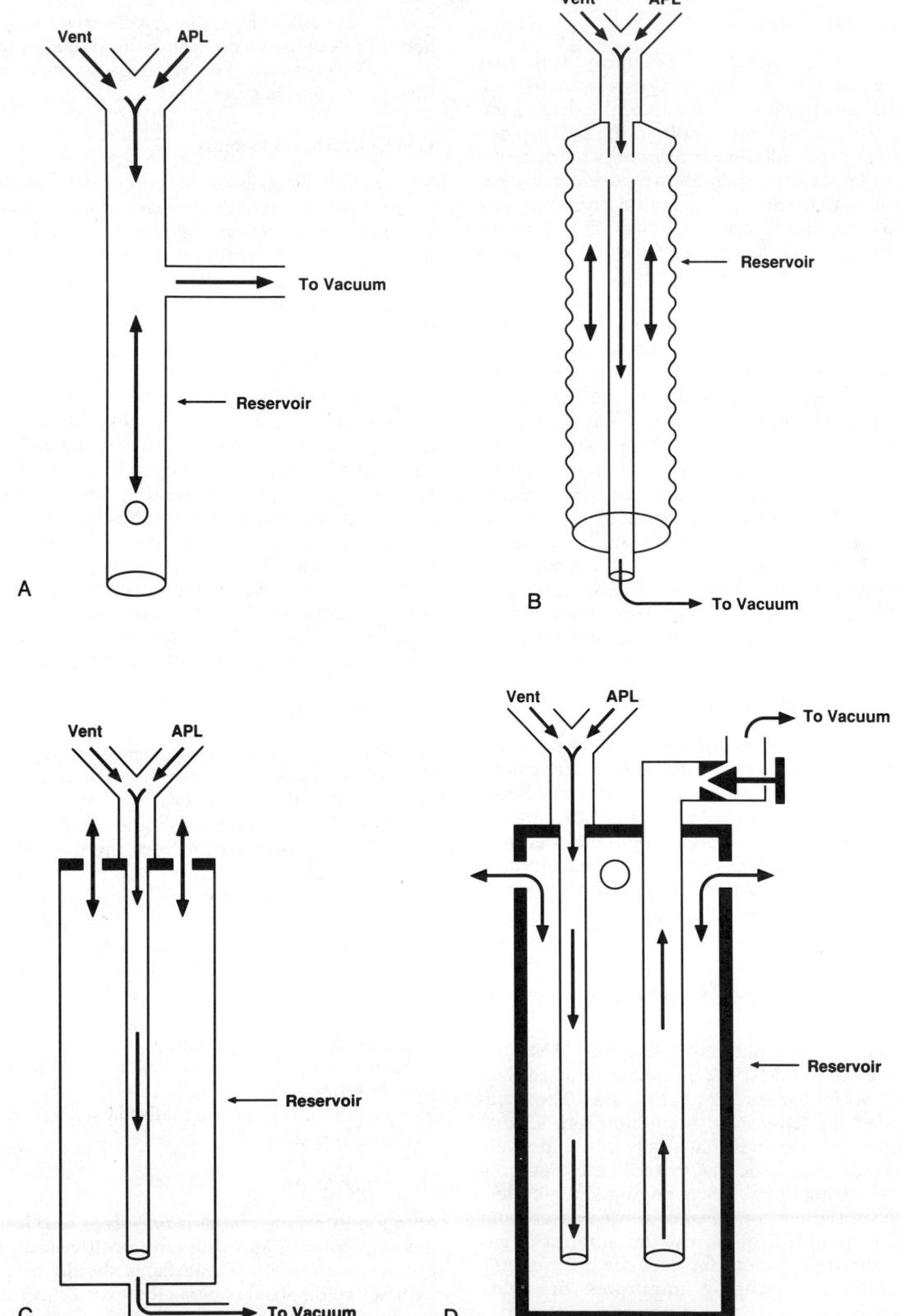

Fig. 7-37. (A–D) Open scavenging interfaces. Each requires an active disposal system. (See text for details.) (Modified from Dorsch and Dorsch,[97] with permission.)

through the transfer tubing. Some of the gas is scavenged immediately to the active disposal system, while another portion collects in the reservoir tubing. The gas in the reservoir is subsequently removed between breaths. Positive and negative relief occurs at the distal end of the reservoir tube. A safety hole in the reservoir provides positive- and negative-pressure relief if the distal end becomes occluded. Figure 7-37B is a coaxial system composed of a small inner tube and a large, corrugated outer tube. The proximal end of the small tube is open to the outer reservoir tube, and the distal end is connected to the active disposal system. Positive and negative relief occurs at the distal end of the corrugated hose, which is open to the atmosphere.[97]

Many contemporary anesthesia machines are equipped with open interfaces like those in Figures 7-37C and D.[98] An open canister provides reservoir capacity. The canister volume should be large enough to accommodate a variety of waste gas flow rates. Gas enters the system at the top of the canister and travels through a narrow inner tube to the canister base. Gases are stored in the reservoir between breaths. Positive- and negative-pressure relief is provided by holes in the top of the canister. The open interface shown in Fig. 7-37C differs somewhat from the one shown in Fig. 7-37D. The operator can regulate the vacuum by adjusting the vacuum control valve shown in Fig. 7-37D.[98]

The efficiency of an open interface depends on several factors. The vacuum flow rate per minute must equal or exceed the minute volume of excess gases to prevent spillage. The volume of the reservoir and the flow characteristics within the interface are important. Spillage will occur if the volume of a single exhaled breath exceeds the capacity of the reservoir. Leakage can occur long before the volume of waste gas delivered to the reservoir equals the reservoir volume if large-scale turbulence occurs within the interface.[99]

Closed Interfaces

A closed interface communicates to the atmosphere through valves. All closed interfaces must have a positive-pressure relief valve to vent excess system pressure if obstruction occurs downstream from the interface. A negative-pressure relief valve is mandatory to protect the breathing system from subatmospheric pressure if an active (disposal) system is used.[97] Two types of closed interfaces are commercially available. One has positive-pressure relief only; the other has both positive- and negative-pressure relief. Each type is discussed below.

Positive-Pressure Relief Only. This interface (Fig. 7-38A) has a single positive-pressure relief valve and is designed to be used only with passive disposal systems. Waste gas enters the interface at the waste gas inlets. Transfer of the waste gas from the interface to the disposal system relies on the pressure of the waste gas itself since a vacuum is not used. The positive-pressure

relief valve opens at a preset valve such as 5 cmH₂O if an obstruction between the interface and the disposal system occurs.[100] A reservoir bag is not necessary.

Positive- and Negative-Pressure Relief. This interface has a positive-pressure relief valve, at least one negative-pressure relief valve, and a reservoir bag. It is used with active disposal systems. Figure 7-38B is a schematic of North American Drager's closed interface for suction systems. A variable volume of waste gas intermittently enters the interface through the waste gas inlets. The reservoir stores transient excess gas until the vacuum system eliminates it. The operator should adjust the vacuum control valve so that the reservoir bag is properly inflated *(A)* and not overdistended *(B)* or completely deflated *(C)*. Gas is vented to the atmosphere through the positive-pressure relief valve if the system pressure exceeds +5 cmH₂O. Room air is entrained through the negative-pressure relief valve if the system pressure is more negative than −0.5 cmH₂O. A backup negative-pressure relief valve opens at −1.8 cmH₂O if the primary negative-pressure relief valve becomes occluded.[6]

Effectiveness of a closed system in preventing spillage depends on the inflow rate of excess gas, the vacuum flow rate, and the volume of the reservoir. Leakage of waste gases into the atmosphere occurs only when the reservoir bag becomes fully inflated and the pressure increases sufficiently to open the positive-pressure relief valve. In contrast, the effectiveness of an open system to prevent spillage depends not only on the volume of the reservoir, but also on the flow characteristics within the interface.[99]

Gas Disposal Tubing

The gas disposal tubing conducts waste gas from the scavenging interface to the gas disposal assembly. It should be collapse-proof and should run overhead if possible to minimize the chance of occlusion.[96]

Gas Disposal Assembly

The gas disposal assembly ultimately eliminates excess waste gas. There are two types of disposal systems: active and passive.

The most common method for gas disposal is the active assembly, which utilizes a central vacuum. The vacuum is a mechanical flow-inducing device that moves the waste gases. An interface with a negative-pressure relief valve is mandatory since the pressure within the system is negative. A reservoir is very desirable, and the larger the reservoir, the lower the suction flow rate needed.[97,99]

A passive disposal system does not use a mechanical flow-inducing device. Instead, the pressure of the waste gas itself produces flow through the system. Positive-pressure relief is mandatory, but negative-pressure relief and a reservoir are unnecessary. Excess waste gas

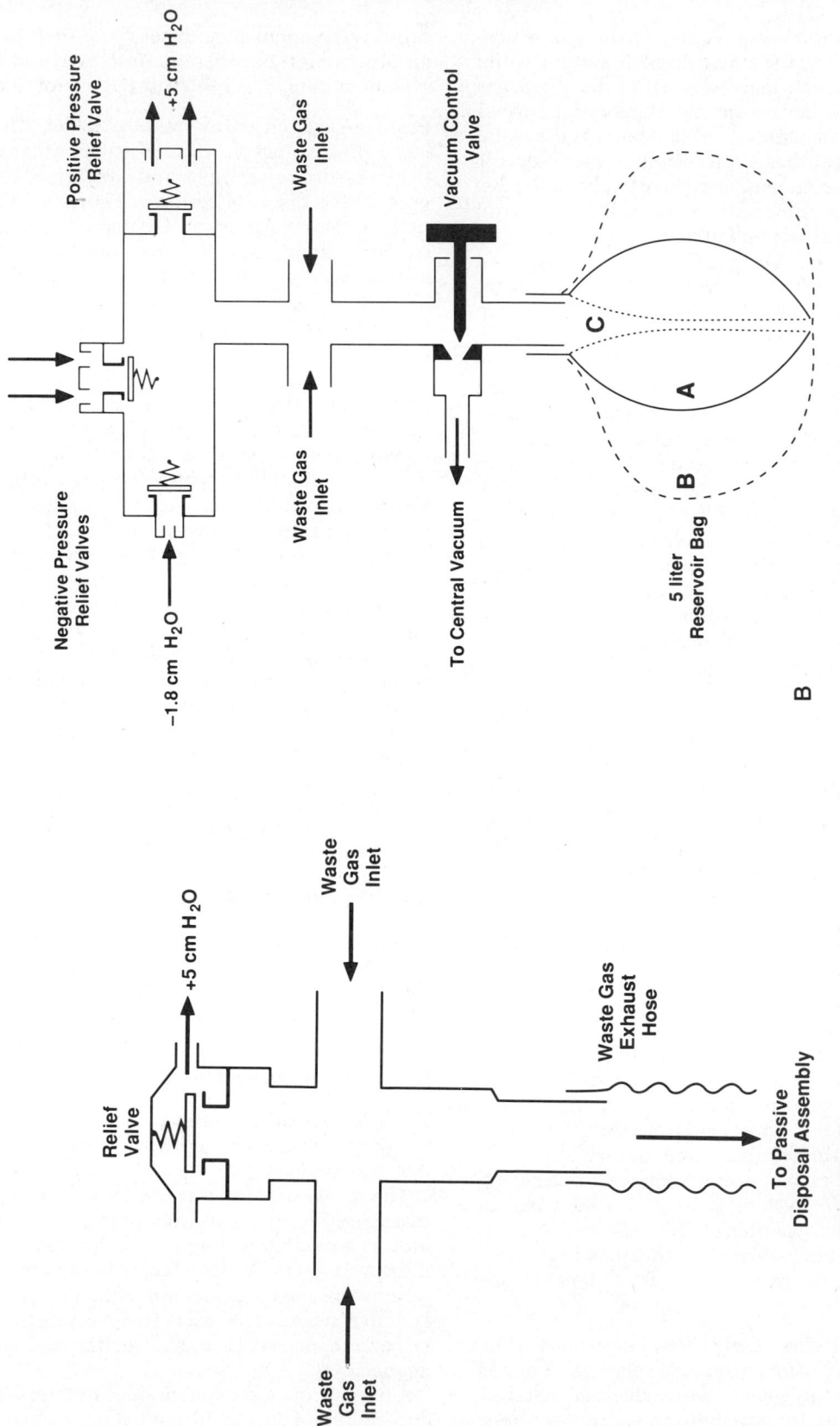

Fig. 7-38. Closed scavenging interfaces. (**A**) Interface used with an active system. (**B**) Interface used with a passive disposal system. (See text for details.) (Fig. A modified from: Scavenger interface for air conditioning. Instruction Manual[100]; Fig. B modified from Narkomed 2A Anesthesia System. Technical Service Manual,[6] with permission.)

Figure labels

B (upper portion):
- Positive Pressure Relief Valve
- +5 cm H₂O — rendered as $+5$ cm H_2O
- Waste Gas Inlet
- Vacuum Control Valve
- −0.5 cm H₂O — rendered as -0.5 cm H_2O
- Negative Pressure Relief Valves
- −1.8 cm H₂O — rendered as -1.8 cm H_2O
- Waste Gas Inlet
- To Central Vacuum
- 5 liter Reservoir Bag
- A, B, C

A (lower portion):
- +5 cm H₂O — rendered as $+5$ cm H_2O
- Waste Gas Inlet
- Relief Valve
- Waste Gas Exhaust Hose
- Waste Gas Inlet
- To Passive Disposal Assembly

can be eliminated in a number of ways. Some include venting through the wall, ceiling, floor, or to the room exhaust grill of a nonrecirculating air conditioning system.[97,99]

Hazards

Scavenging systems minimize operating room pollution, yet they add complexity to the anesthesia system. A scavenging system extends the anesthesia circuit all the way from the anesthesia machine to the ultimate disposal site. This extension increases the potential for problems. Pressure alterations produced by obstruction or unopposed vacuum can be transferred to the anesthesia circuit and potentially can harm the patient.[99] Hazards associated with scavenging are discussed below.

Transmission of Excessive Positive Pressure to the Breathing System

Obstruction of scavenging pathways can cause excessive positive pressure to be transmitted to the breathing system. Some causes for obstruction include (1) compression of flexible tubing by wheels of the anesthesia machine,[101–103] (2) kinking of flexible tubing,[104] (3) plugging of a gas disposal tube with ice,[105] and (4) misassembling of the exhaust connector of a passive disposal system.[106] Obstruction can occur anywhere in the scavenging system but is particularly hazardous if it occurs upstream from the scavenging interface because excess patient gas cannot be vented. Obstruction downstream from the interface is a lesser problem since excess gas will pop off through the positive-pressure relief valve of the interface and not jeopardize the patient.[104]

Prior to the implementation of the ANSI Z79.11-1982 standard, a specific type of circle system misconnection was another cause of dangerously high pressure. The 22-mm expiratory hose of the circle system was incorrectly connected to the exhaust port of the APL valve, rather than to the expiratory port of the carbon dioxide absorber.[102,107,108] This configuration prevented venting of excess gas, so the pressure rapidly increased. This hazard was minimized when the ANSI Z79.11-1982 standard mandated either a 19-mm or 30-mm male fitting for the outlet of the gas collection assembly.[96]

Application of Excessive Negative Pressure to the Breathing System

Excessive negative pressure can be applied to the breathing system if an active disposal system is used.[97] This condition can occur if the negative-pressure relief valve or port becomes obstructed or if the vacuum flow rate is excessive. Obstruction of the negative-pressure relief valve or port can be caused by dust accumulation,[109] tape,[110] plastic bags,[111] or other objects. Mechanical problems can cause the valve to stick in the closed position.[112] Excessive vacuum can result from improper adjustment of the vacuum control knob on a closed scavenging interface or from misassembly of scavenging components.[113,114]

The ultimate consequences of applying excessive negative pressure to the breathing system depend on the design of the APL valve or the ventilator relief valve.[97,115] When a strong vacuum is applied to the exhaust side of some APL valves, gas flows across from the patient circuit to the vacuum. This causes the breathing bag to collapse, and excessive negative pressure can develop within the patient circuit.[109,112,113,115] Application of unopposed vacuum to the exhaust side of some diaphragm-type APL valves, on the other hand, can produce excessive positive pressure within the patient circuit. The subatmospheric pressure sucks the diaphragm against its seat, and flow across the valve ceases. Waste gas from the patient circuit cannot escape, and barotrauma can result.[16,21] A similar scenario can occur with some diaphragm-type ventilator relief valves. Excessive suction draws the ventilator relief diaphragm to its seat, and the valve closes. Excess gas cannot be scavenged, and barotrauma can result.[21,114]

Loss of Means of Monitoring

Ironically, scavenging systems have been blamed for being too effective. Inhaled anesthetic overdose was undetected in two cases because of absence of smell of anesthetic.[104,116] The efficient scavenging system concealed the strong odor of the inhaled anesthetic.

CHECKING ANESTHESIA MACHINES

A complete anesthesia apparatus checkout procedure should be performed each day before the first case. An abbreviated version should be performed before each subsequent case. Several checkout procedures exist, but the most popular one is the August 1986 Food and Drug Administration (FDA) Anesthesia Apparatus Checkout Recommendations, reproduced in Appendix A.[117–120] The FDA checkout serves only as a generic guideline because the designs of different machines vary considerably. Also, many machines have been modified in the field. Therefore, specific checks must be performed on specific machines. The user must refer to the operator's manual for special procedures or precautions. The best example of the importance of performing the appropriate preoperative check is the low-pressure leak test (#16 FDA). Several mishaps have resulted from application of the wrong leak test to the wrong machine.[24,49,121]

The Low-Pressure Leak Test

The low-pressure leak test checks the integrity of the anesthesia machine from the flow control valves to the common outlet. It is the most important preoperative

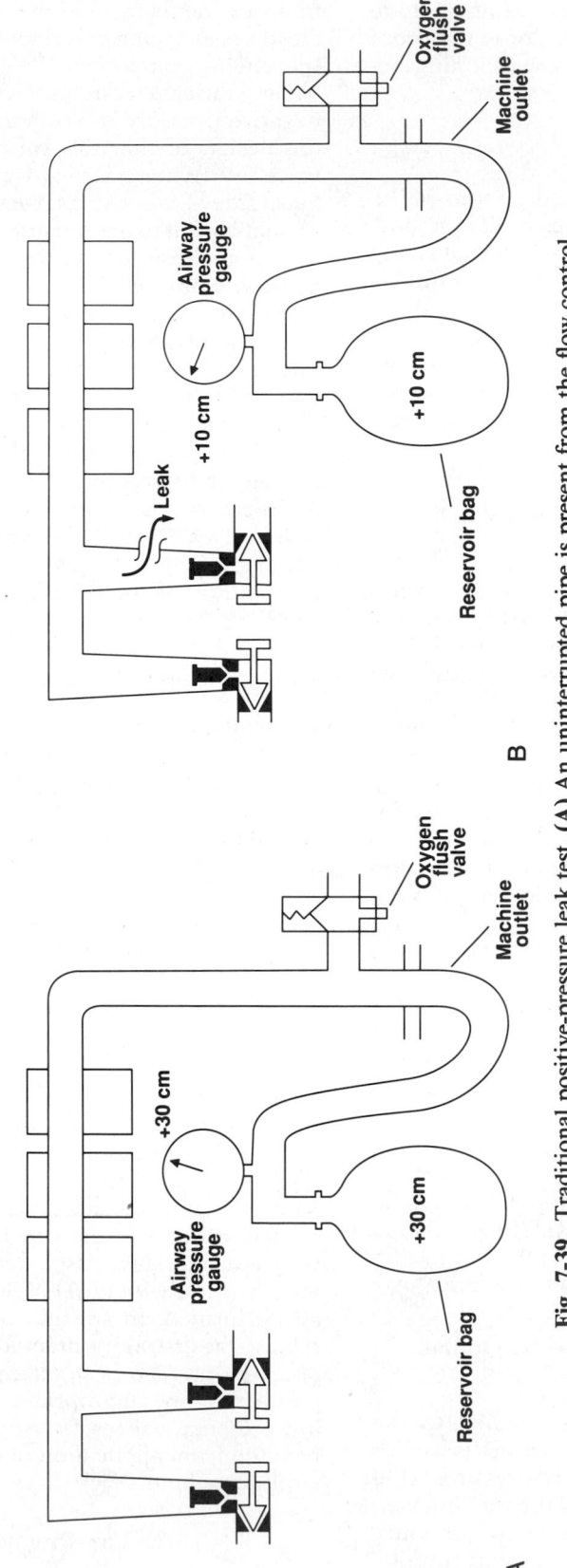

Fig. 7-39. Traditional positive-pressure leak test. (**A**) An uninterrupted pipe is present from the flow control valves to the circle system airway pressure gauge. The value on the airway pressure gauge does not decline when the low-pressure circuit is leak-free. (**B**) A leak in the low-pressure circuit is reflected by a decline in the value on the airway pressure gauge. (From Andrews,[135] with permission.)

check because it evaluates the portion of the machine that is downstream from all safety devices except the oxygen analyzer. The components located within this area are *precisely* the ones that are most subject to breakage and leaks. Flowtubes are the most delicate pneumatic component of the machine, and they can crack or break. Leaks can occur at the interface between the glass flowtube and the manifold because of problems associated with O-rings and gaskets. In fact, a typical three-gas anesthesia machine has 16 O-rings in the low-pressure circuit. Loose filler caps on vaporizers are a common source of leaks. Leaks can occur at the O-ring junction between the vaporizer and its manifold. Therefore, it is mandatory to perform the appropriate low-pressure leak test before every case. Most anesthesia machines have check valves located in the low-pressure circuit. The presence or absence of these check valves profoundly influences the type of leak test that should be used.[19] Each is discussed below.

Machines without Check Valves

A traditional positive-pressure leak test using the circle system can be performed on machines that do not have check valves in the low-pressure circuitry (Table 7-2). The pop-off valve is closed, and the system is pressurized by use of the oxygen flush and flow from the oxygen flow control valve. The exact details of the test are outlined in Appendix A, #16. An uninterrupted pipe is present from the flow control valves to the circle airway pressure gauge (Fig. 7-39). Therefore, a leak in the low-pressure circuit will be reflected by a decline in the value on the airway pressure gauge. This traditional test has two major advantages. First, it does not require accessory test devices. Second, it can be performed quickly. The main disadvantage of the traditional test is its lack of sensitivity when compared with leak tests using special devices (see below). This lack of sensitivity occurs because the traditional test is volume dependent. The pressurized volume in the breathing bag can mask leaks up to 250 cc/min.[19]

Drager recommends a more sensitive positive-pressure leak test for the Narkomed 2A, Narkomed 2B, and Narkomed 3 (Fig. 7-40). It is not volume dependent because a positive-pressure leak test device is substituted for the breathing bag. A no-flow state is created by turning the machine *off*. The pop-off valve is closed, and the inspiratory and expiratory valves are interconnected by a single breathing hose. The system is pressurized to 50 cmH_2O by use of a squeeze bulb. The pressure decrease from 50 to 30 cmH_2O should take 30 seconds or longer.[17]

Machines with Check Valves

Most Ohmeda machines have a machine outlet check valve (Table 7-2) to minimize the pumping effect. These include the Unitrol, the 30/70, the Modulus I, and the Modulus II.[11,12,27,28] The check valve is located downstream from the vaporizers and upstream from the oxygen flush. It is open (Fig. 7-41A) in the absence of back-pressure. Gas flow from the manifold moves the rubber flapper valve off its seat and allows gas to proceed freely to the common outlet. The valve closes (Fig. 7-41B) when back-pressure is exerted on it.[5] Intermittent positive pressure and oxygen flushing close the valve.

Ohmeda recommends the use of a negative-pressure leak test on the machines mentioned above (Fig. 7-42). It is performed with a negative-pressure leak-testing device. This is a suction bulb device, and it is included with all Ohmeda machines requiring it. A no-flow state is established. (The flow control valves are turned off when the Unitrol is tested. On the Modulus I and Modulus II the master switch is turned off, but the flow control valves are fully open.) The leak-testing device is attached to the common outlet. The bulb is compressed repeatedly until it remains collapsed. This action creates a vacuum in the low-pressure circuitry and opens the check valve. The machine is leak free if the hand bulb remains collapsed for 30 seconds, but a leak is present if the bulb reinflates during this time period.

TABLE 7-2. Check Valves and Recommended Leak Test

Anesthesia Machine	Machine Outlet Check Valve	Vaporizer Outlet Check Valve	Leak Test Recommended by Manufacturer	
			Positive Pressure	Negative Pressure (Suction Bulb)
Drager Narkomed 2A	No	No	X	
Drager Narkomed 2B	No	No	X	
Drager Narkomed 3	No	No	X	
Ohmeda Unitrol	Yes	Variable		X
Ohmeda 30/70	Yes	Variable		X
Ohmeda Modulus I	Yes	Variable		X
Ohmeda Modulus II	Yes	No		X
Ohmeda Excel series	Yes	No		X
Ohmeda Modulus II Plus	No	No		X

(Data from refs. 9, 11–14, 16, 17, 27, 28.)

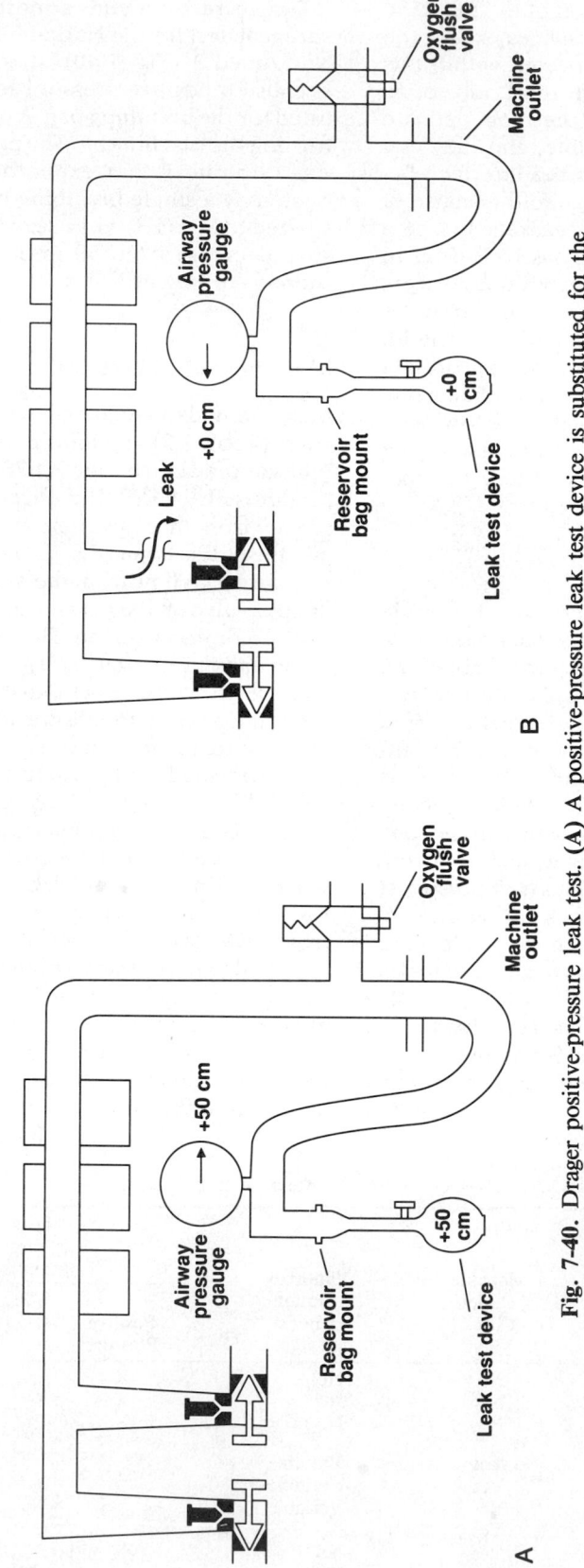

Fig. 7-40. Drager positive-pressure leak test. **(A)** A positive-pressure leak test device is substituted for the reservoir bag. The low-pressure circuit is pressurized to 50 cmH$_2$O by using the squeeze bulb. **(B)** A leak in the low-pressure circuit is reflected by a rapid decline in the value on the airway pressure gauge. (From Andrews,[135] with permission.)

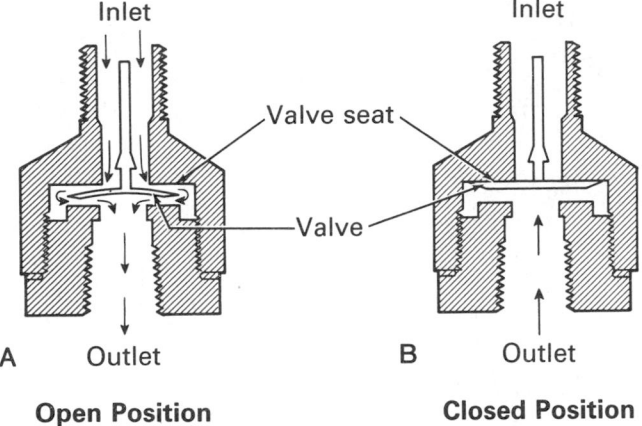

Fig. 7-41. (A & B) Machine outlet check valve. (See text for details.) (From Bowie and Huffman,[5] with permission.)

The leak test must be repeated with each vaporizer in the on position to detect vaporizer leaks.

Ohmeda's rationale for the negative-pressure leak test follows. First, the check valve separates the machine from the patient circuit. Pressurizing the circle system will only reveal leaks downstream from the check valve.[10] Second, the test is extremely sensitive because it is not volume dependent. It can detect leaks as small as 30 cc/min. Third, on the Modulus I and Modulus II, some components located *upstream* from the flow control valves are tested for leaks. These components include the oxygen flush, the pressure-sensing system, and the pneumatics of the master on/off switch.

Application of a traditional positive-pressure leak test to a machine equipped with a check valve can lead to a false sense of security despite the presence of a huge leak (Fig. 7-43).[24,49,121] Positive pressure from the patient circuit closes the check valve, and the value on the airway pressure gauge does not decline. The system appears to be tight, but in actuality, only the circuitry distal to the check valve is leak-free.[10] Thus, a vulnerable area exists from the check valve back to the flow control valves because this area is not tested by the traditional positive-pressure leak test. Addition of a freestanding vaporizer equipped with a check valve downstream from the common outlet creates an even larger vulnerable area.

Ohmeda Modulus II Plus

The new Ohmeda Modulus II Plus anesthesia system does not have a machine outlet check valve. Nevertheless, Ohmeda recommends the use of a negative-pressure leak test because the test is extremely sensitive.[14] Also, the recommendation of a negative leak test establishes a consistent method to check all currently manufactured Ohmeda machines.

HUMIDIFICATION

Precise administration of gases through modern anesthesia machines depends on clean and dry anesthetic gases. These are supplied as anhydrous gases free of particulate matter because the presence of moisture can cause the valves to malfunction, orifices to distort, and flowmeters to stray.[122] Inhalation of dry gases at room temperature or below imposes on the lower respiratory passages to humidify these gases.[123] In addition, endotracheal intubation bypasses nasopharyngeal air conditioning and compels the mucosa of the lower respiratory tract to perform the function of the nasopharynx.[124] Therefore, water and heat losses from the respiratory tract become clinically significant in patients receiving unhumidified gases during a general anesthetic for any but the shortest surgical procedure. Breathing dry air can lead to desiccation of mucus, impairment of ciliary function and mucus escalator activity, retention of secretions, atelectasis, bacterial colonization, and pneumonia. To minimize postoperative pulmonary complications, warmth and humidity must be added from external sources to these dry gases as they enter the patient's airway.

Humidity

Three terms are used to express water content of a gas.

Absolute humidity is the actual mass of water contained in a given volume of gas at a given temperature. Traditionally, this is measured as milligrams of water vapor per liter of gas (mg/L).

Maximum humidity is the maximum mass of water vapor that a given volume of gas can hold at a given temperature (saturated water content).

Relative humidity is a percent expression of the actual water vapor content of a gas compared with its capacity to carry water at a given temperature.

Humidity deficit is the lack of sufficient water vapor for saturation. Room air is rarely saturated, so additional moisture must be added when air enters the respiratory tree. A primary humidity deficit exists when inspired room air is less than saturated at a given temperature. A secondary humidity deficit occurs when inhaled air is warmed from room temperature to body temperature. This occurs because the capacity of air to carry moisture increases when the inspired air is warmed.[122,123,125] Under normal conditions, the nasal mucosa and the upper airways pay this deficit by giving up heat and water.

The water content to correct the humidity deficit at standard room air conditions can be calculated. Inspired air at 21°C and 50 percent humidity contains only 9 mg/L of water. Once inhaled, the water content must increase to 44 mg/L at 37°C, and the humidity deficit is 35 mg/L.

Humidity deficit (mg/L) = maximum humidity (37°C) − absolute humidity (21°C)

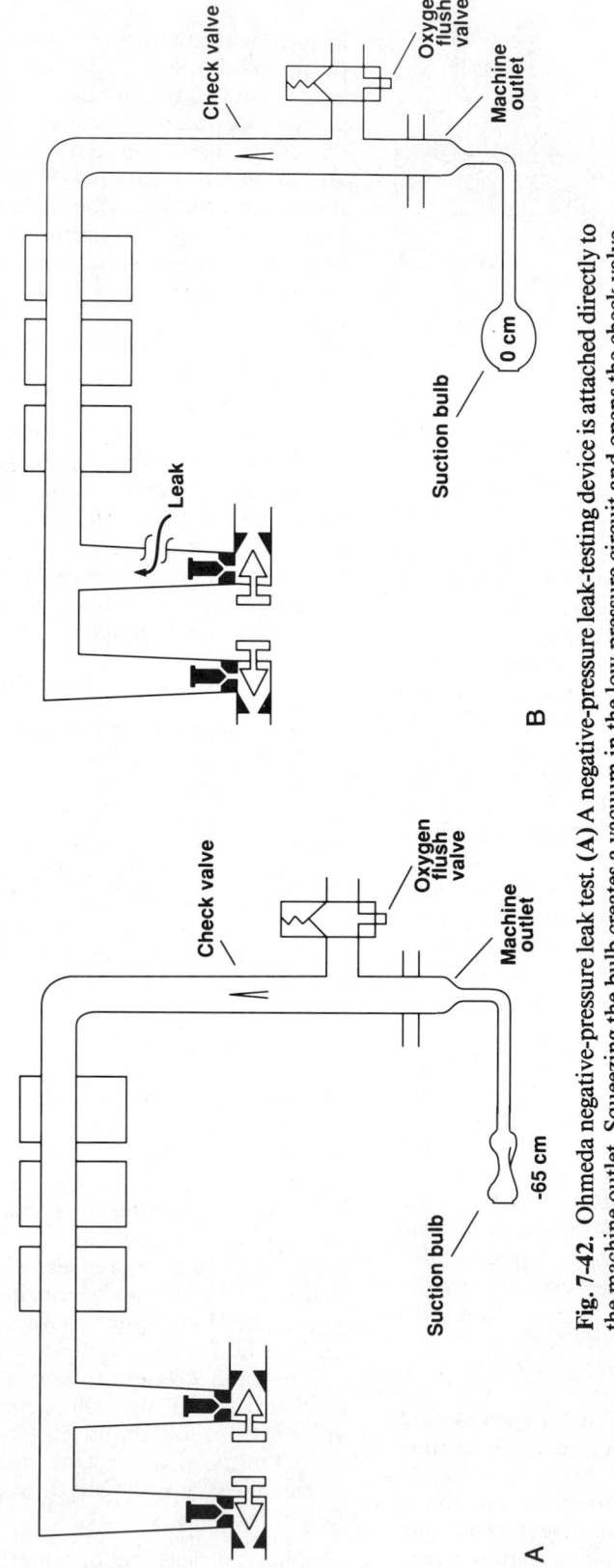

Fig. 7-42. Ohmeda negative-pressure leak test. (A) A negative-pressure leak-testing device is attached directly to the machine outlet. Squeezing the bulb creates a vacuum in the low-pressure circuit and opens the check valve. (B) When a leak is present in the low-pressure circuit, room air is entrained through the leak and the suction bulb inflates. (From Andrews,[135] with permission.)

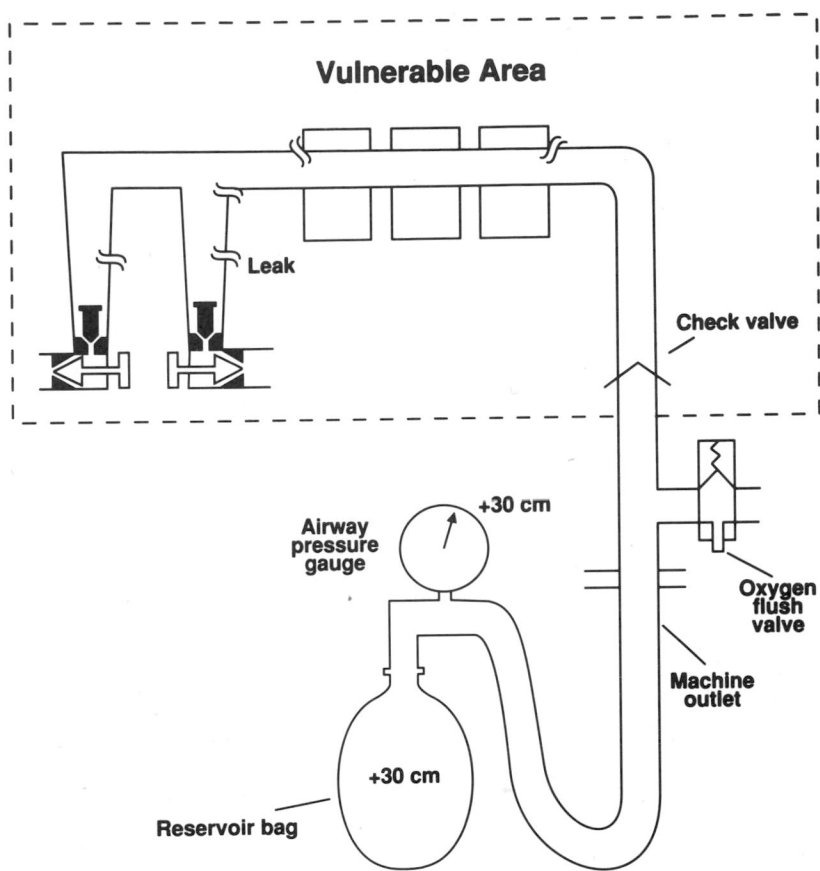

Fig. 7-43. Schematic of an anesthesia machine with a machine outlet check valve. The area within the rectangle is not checked by a traditional positive-pressure leak test. The components located within this area are precisely the ones that are most subject to breakage and leaks. Positive pressure within the patient circuit closes the check valve, and the value on the airway pressure gauge does not decline despite leaks in the low-pressure circuit. (From Andrews,[19] with permission.)

Compressed oxygen is 100 percent dry even at room temperature. Note that 44 mg of water vapor must be added to each liter of oxygen to achieve maximum humidity at 37°C. The relative humidity is zero in this instance. The humidity deficit is 44 mg/L because the difference between maximum water content (44 mg/L) and absolute water content (0 mg/L) is 44 mg/L.

The loss of respiratory water can be calculated by the following formula:

$$\text{Respiratory water loss (g/h)} = 60\dot{V}_E(44 - A_t)$$

Water loss is the product of the minute ventilation and the gradient of the inspired and exhaled water content. Minute ventilation, $\dot{V}_E$, can be measured or estimated from a nomogram. The water content of fully saturated exhaled air is 44 mg/L at 37°C. The absolute water content of the inspired air at a given temperature is expressed as A_t. The hourly water loss for a 70-kg adult breathing a standard room air mixture ($A_t = 9$ mg/L) approximates 13 g/h. This value is near the estimated insensible daily respiratory water loss of 250 cc/d. Total body water loss through this mechanism would in-

crease only to 16 g/h if 100 percent anhydrous oxygen were administered. Thus, respiratory water loss resulting from humidity deficits has a negligible effect on body water balance and is replaced easily even in children. The importance of humidification of inspired gases is best understood in terms of the local preservation of the protective mucus blanket and thermal regulation.[126-129] Gases delivered at 37°C and those that are 50 to 75 percent saturated will maintain the integrity of the mucus blanket.

Heat Loss

Humidity deficits require energy in two ways. The first way is the simple necessity of warming the inspired gases to body temperature. The heat loss for this activity depends on the minute ventilation, the temperature gradient between exhaled and inhaled gas, and the specific heat of the gas. It is expressed as follows:

$$\text{Humidity heat loss/min} = \dot{V}_E (37 - t) \text{ (specific heat)}$$

The caloric requirements for this activity are estimated

to be 40 cal/min for modern breathing systems in which the gases are delivered at room temperature.[125] The cooler the gases, the higher the delivered energy cost will be.

The most significant loss of heat and caloric debt results from the cost of vaporizing water to cover the humidity deficit. Heat is expended to vaporize enough water to saturate the inspired air at body temperature. The caloric expenditure for this activity has been estimated to be about 550 cal/g of water vaporized. Because anhydrous oxygen administration will require 16 g/h of water vapor, three times as many calories are expended per hour to humidify inhaled air. A depression of thermal regulation during general anesthesia compounds the heat loss and can produce a significant threat to anesthetized patients, particularly children. The administration of anesthetic gases at 37°C and 100 percent humidity can maintain body temperature in anesthetized patients and can even be used in some situations to rewarm patients who have been deliberately cooled. Warming by inhalation of heated and rehumidified air or oxygen by the mask or endotracheal tube is an effective method of increasing the patient's core temperature. The temperature of inspired gases at the mouth or endotracheal tube as well as the humidifier's inspiratory temperature reading should be monitored. Temperatures in excess of 40°C at the endotracheal tube can produce hemorrhagic, bronchospastic tracheobronchitis. Temperatures of 40°C or less at the endotracheal tube connection are safe for rewarming and allow a margin of safety in temperature regulation.

Anesthesia Circuits and Humidity

The minimum recommended humidity for anesthesia is 60 percent or 12 mg/L. Optimum values are between 14 and 30 mg/L of water vapor. Simple moistening of the insides of corrugated hoses and the reservoir bag has significantly increased the humidity in the circle system.[130] This achieves a water content of about 22 mg/L. The humidity declines with time as evaporation within the circuit produces cooling. The adult or pediatric closed-circle system can achieve a water content as high as 29 mg/L when the gases are passed through a soda lime canister.[126,131,132] The relative humidity approaches 100 percent because of water production by neutralization during the process of carbon dioxide absorption by soda lime. Some of the water vapor also comes from the exhaled air. However, the temperature is still less than 37°C, and the pressure gradient for water vapor is from the lungs to air. A closed circuit provides ideal inspired humidity. Humidification probably is not necessary in units designed for total rebreathing (closed system) because water loss is of small magnitude. Humidification is required for systems that are open or semiopen and in which high gas flows are used for protracted periods of time. Table 7-3 lists the humidity achieved with some anesthesia circuit systems.

TABLE 7-3. Relative Humidity of Gases in the Various Anesthetic Systems

Anesthetic System	Relative Humidity of Gases
Nonbreathing valve	0
T-piece	0
To and fro	40–100
Closed circle[a]	40–100
Bain modification	65–100
Human nose	65

[a] Higher relative humidity is achieved by low-flow, closed technique with a carbon dioxide absorber. Humidity is in the lower range with semiopen high-flow techniques.

Water Vaporizers

Three major types of heated water vaporizers are commonly used: the Hopkins, or pass-over, vaporizer; the bubbler; and the heated cascade humidifier.

1. The Hopkins, or pass-over, vaporizer is the simplest of the heated vaporizers. This type of humidifier is merely the heated version of the simple vaporizer. The large reservoir of the pass-over vaporizer is heated by an external hot plate element. It provides humidity by passing air over a relatively large surface area. This is the vaporizer used on the Emerson ventilator.[125]
2. Bubblers add vapor by evaporation by a stream of bubbles through a jar of water. A disadvantage of the bubbler is that the water in the jar is cooled as it evaporates. This lowers the temperature of the carrying gas and reduces its moisture-carrying capacity. The bubbler can only provide 20 percent relative humidity at body temperature unless it is heated. The deficit must be made up by the respiratory passages, and this may be poorly tolerated by a patient who already has lost mucociliary function. The addition of heat increases the performance of the bubbler, which is commonly used with nasal cannulas and oxygen masks.
3. Heated cascade humidifiers technically are bubblers. These devices deliver 100 percent humidity at body temperature. They break inspired gas into tiny bubbles and pass the bubbles through heated water. These are the mainstream humidifiers used with anesthesia systems and are the most effective of all the evaporative humidifiers. These vaporizers are typified by the Bennett cascade vaporizer. A potential hazard associated with the Bennett vaporizer is misconnection. It has a one-way check valve that retards the drift of humidity retrograde to the anesthesia machine.[125] Even though the inlet and outlet are labeled, they have the same diameter. Reverse hook-up results in a no-flow state.

The rationale for using heated humidity in anesthesia and respiratory therapy is to make the inspired gases comfortable for the patient, preserve the mucus blanket, heat inspired gases to provide 100 percent relative humidity, and counter the thermal loss resulting from water vaporization in the respiratory tree.

APPENDIX A

Anesthesia Apparatus
Checkout Recommendations†

This checkout, or a reasonable equivalent, should be conducted before administering anesthesia. This is a guideline that users are encouraged to modify to accommodate differences in equipment design and variations in local clinical practice. Such local modifications should have appropriate peer review. Users should refer to the operator's manual for special procedures or precautions.

*1. *Inspect anesthesia machine for:*
   Machine identification number
   Valid inspection sticker
   Undamaged flowmeters, vaporizers, gauges, supply hoses
   Complete, undamaged breathing system with adequate CO_2 absorbent
   Correct mounting of cylinders in yokes
   Presence of cylinder wrench

*2. *Inspect and turn on:*
   Electrical equipment requiring warm-up.
      (ECG/pressure monitor, oxygen monitor, etc.)

*3. *Connect waste gas scavenging system:*
   Adjust vacuum as required.

*4. *Check that:*
   Flow-control valves are off.
   Vaporizers are off.
   Vaporizers are filled (not overfilled).
   Filler caps are sealed tightly.
   CO_2 absorber bypass (if any) is off.

*5. *Check oxygen (O_2) cylinder supplies:*
   a. Disconnect pipeline supply (if connected) and return cylinder and pipeline pressure gauges to zero with O_2 flush valve.
   b. Open O_2 cylinder; check pressure; close cylinder and observe gauge for evidence of high-pressure leak.
   c. With the O_2 flush valve, flush to empty piping.
   d. Repeat as in b. and c. above for second O_2 cylinder, if present.
   e. Replace any cylinder less than about 600 PSIG. At least one should be nearly full.
   f. Open less full cylinder.

*6. *Turn on master switch (if present).*

*7. *Check nitrous oxide (N_2O) and other gas cylinder supplies:*
   Use same procedure as described in 5a. & b. above, but open and *CLOSE* flow-control valve to empty piping.

Note: N_2O pressure below 745 PSIG indicates that the cylinder is less than 1/4 full.

*8. *Test flowmeters:*
   a. Check that float is at bottom of tube with flow-control valves closed (or at min. O_2 flow if so equipped).
   b. Adjust flow of all gases through their full range and check for erratic movements of floats.

*9. *Test ratio protection/warning system (if present):*
   Attempt to create hypoxic O_2/N_2O mixture, and verify correct change in gas flows and/or alarm.

*10. *Test O_2 pressure failure system:*
   a. Set O_2 and other gas flows to mid-range.
   b. Close O_2 cylinder and flush to release O_2 pressure.
   c. Verify that all flows fall to zero. Open O_2 cylinder.
   d. Close all other cylinders and bleed piping pressures.
   e. Close O_2 cylinder and bleed piping pressure.
   f. **CLOSE FLOW CONTROL VALVES.**

*11. *Test central pipeline gas supplies:*
   a. Inspect supply hoses (should not be cracked or worn).
   b. Connect supply hoses, verifying correct color coding.
   c. Adjust all flows to at least mid-range.
   d. Verify that supply pressures hold (45 to 55 PSIG).
   e. Shut off flow-control valves.

*12. *Add any accessory equipment to the breathing system:*
   Add PEEP valve, humidifier, etc., if they might be used (if necessary remove after step 18 until needed).

13. *Calibrate O_2 monitor:*
   *a. Calibrate O_2 monitor to read 21% in room air.
   *b. Test low alarm.
   c. Occlude breathing system at patient end; fill and empty system several times with 100% O_2.
   d. Check that monitor reading is nearly 100%.

14. *Sniff inspiratory gas:*
   There should be no odor.

*15. *Check unidirectional valves:*
   a. Inhale and exhale through a surgical mask into the breathing system (each limb individually, if possible).
   b. Verify unidirectional flow in each limb.
   c. Reconnect tubing firmly.

---

* If an anesthetist uses the same machine in successive cases, the steps marked with an asterisk (*) need not be repeated or may be abbreviated after the initial checkout.

** A vaporizer leak can only be detected if the vaporizer is turned on during this test. Even then, a relatively small but clinically significant leak may still be obscured.

† From Food and Drug Administration.[120]

16. *Test for leaks in machine and breathing system:*
   a. Close APL (pop-off) valve and occlude system at patient end.
   b. Fill system via O_2 flush until bag just full, but negligible pressure in system. Set O_2 flow to 5 L/min.
   c. Slowly decrease O_2 flow until pressure *no longer rises* above about 20 cmH$_2$O. This approximates total leak rate, which should be no greater than a few hundred ml/min (less for closed-circuit techniques).
   CAUTION: Check valves in some machines make it imperative to measure flow in step c. above when pressure *just stops rising.*
   d. Squeeze bag to pressure of about 50 cmH$_2$O and verify that system is tight.

17. *Exhaust valve and scavenger system:*
   a. Open APL valve and observe release of pressure.
   b. Occlude breathing system at patient end and verify that negligible positive or negative pressure appears with either zero or 5 L/min flow and exhaust relief valve (if present) opens with flush flow.

18. *Test ventilator:*
   a. If switching valve is present, test function in both bag and ventilator mode.
   b. Close APL valve if necessary and occlude system at patient end.
   c. Test for leaks and pressure relief by appropriate cycling (exact procedure will vary with type of ventilator).
   d. Attach reservoir bag at mask fitting, fill system and cycle ventilator. Ensure filling/emptying of bag.

19. *Check for appropriate level of patient suction.*
20. *Check, connect, and calibrate other electronic monitors.*
21. *Check final position of all controls.*
22. *Turn on and set other appropriate alarms* for equipment to be used.
   (Perform next two steps as soon as is practical.)
23. *Set O_2 monitor alarm limits.*
24. *Set airway pressure and/or volume monitor alarm limits* (if adjustable).

REFERENCES

1. American National Standards Institute: Minimum Performance and Safety Requirements for Components and Systems of Continuous-Flow Anesthesia Machines for Human Use (ANSI Z79.8-1979). American National Standards Institute, New York, February, 1979
2. American Society for Testing and Materials: Minimum Performance and Safety Requirements for Components and Systems of Anesthesia Gas Machines (ASTM F1161-88). American Society for Testing and Materials, Philadelphia, 1988
3. Schreiber P, Schreiber J: Safety Guidelines for Anesthesia System Risk Analysis and Risk Reduction. North American Drager, Telford, PA, 1987
4. Dorsch JA, Dorsch SE: The anesthesia machine, p. 38. In Dorsch JA, Dorsch SE (eds): Understanding Anesthesia Equipment. 2nd Ed. Williams & Wilkins, Baltimore, 1984
5. Bowie E, Huffman LM: The Anesthesia Machine: Essentials for Understanding. Ohmeda, The BOC Group, Inc., Madison, WI, 1985
6. Narkomed 2A Anesthesia System. Technical Service Manual. North American Drager, Telford, PA, June, 1985
7. Feeley TW, Hedley-Whyte J: Bulk oxygen and nitrous oxide delivery systems: Design and dangers. Anesthesiology 44:301, 1976
8. Adriani J: Clinical application of physical principles concerning gases and vapors in anesthesiology. p. 58. In Adriani J (ed): The Chemistry and Physics of Anesthesia. 2nd Ed. Charles C. Thomas, Springfield, IL, 1967
9. Narkomed 2B Anesthesia System. Operator's Manual. North American Drager, Telford, PA, 1988
10. Dorsch JA, Dorsch SE: Equipment checking and maintenance. p. 401. In Dorsch JA, Dorsch SE (eds): Understanding Anesthesia Equipment. 2nd Ed. Williams & Wilkins, Baltimore, 1984
11. Modulus Anesthesia Gas Machine. Operation Maintenance. Ohio Medical Products, The BOC Group, Inc., Madison, WI, 1981
12. Modulus II Anesthesia System. Operation and Maintenance Manual. Ohmeda, The BOC Group, Inc., Madison, WI, 1985
13. Modulus II Anesthesia System. Service Manual. Ohmeda, The BOC Group, Inc., Madison, WI, 1985
14. Modulus II Plus Anesthesia System. Operation and Maintenance Manual. Ohmeda, The BOC Group, Inc., Madison, WI, 1988
15. Ohmeda 8000 Anesthesia Machine. Operation and Maintenance Manual. Ohmeda, The BOC Group, Inc., Madison, WI, 1985
16. Narkomed 2A Anesthesia System. Instruction Manual. North American Drager, Telford, PA, 1985
17. Narkomed 3 Anesthesia System. Operator's Instruction Manual. North American Drager, Telford, PA, 1986
18. Loeb RG, Ross WT, Lawson D: How modern anesthesia machines respond to a decrease in oxygen line pressure. Anesth Analg 66:S1, 1987
19. Andrews JJ: Anesthesia systems. p. 505. In Barash PG, Cullen BF, Stoelting RK (eds): Clinical Anesthesia. JB Lippincott, Philadelphia, 1989
20. Macintosh R, Mushin WW, Epstein HG: Flowmeters. p. 196. In Macintosh R, Mushin WW, Epstein HG (eds): Physics for the Anaesthetist. 3rd Ed. Blackwell Scientific Publications, Oxford, 1963
21. Schreiber P: Safety Guidelines for Anesthesia Systems. North American Drager, Telford, PA, 1985
22. Eger EI II, Epstein RM: Hazards of anesthetic equipment. Anesthesiology 24:490, 1964
23. Eger EI II, Hylton RR, Irwin RH, et al: Anesthetic flowmeter sequence—a cause for hypoxia. Anesthesiology 24:396, 1963
24. Rendell-Baker L: Problems with anesthetic and respiratory therapy equipment. Int Anesthesiol Clin 20:1, 1982
25. Mazze RI: Therapeutic misadventures with oxygen delivery systems: The need for continuous in-line oxygen monitors. Anesth Analg 51:787, 1972
26. Abraham ZA, Basagoitia B: A potentially lethal anesthesia machine failure. Anesthesiology 66:589, 1987

27. Ohmeda Unitrol Anesthesia System. Operation and Maintenance Manual. Ohmeda, The BOC Group, Inc., Madison, WI, 1985

28. 30/70 Proportionate Anesthesia Machine. Canadian Version. Ohio Medical Products, Madison, WI, 1982

29. Dorsch JA, Dorsch SE: Vaporizers. p. 77. In Dorsch JA, Dorsch SE (eds): Understanding Anesthesia Equipment. 2nd Ed. Williams & Wilkins, Baltimore, 1984

30. Macintosh R, Mushin WW, Epstein HG: Vapor pressure. p. 68. In Macintosh R, Mushin WW, Epstein HG (eds): Physics for the Anaesthetist. 3rd Ed. Blackwell Scientific Publications, Oxford, 1963

31. Adriani J: Principles of physics and chemistry of solids and fluids applicable to anesthesiology. p. 7. In Adriani J (ed): The Chemistry and Physics of Anesthesia. 2nd Ed. Charles C Thomas, Springfield, IL, 1962

32. Macintosh R, Mushin WW, Epstein HG: Vaporization. p. 26. In Macintosh R, Mushin WW, Epstein HG (eds): Physics for the Anaesthetist. 3rd Ed. Blackwell Scientific Publications, Oxford, 1963

33. Macintosh R, Mushin WW, Epstein HG: Specific heat. p. 17. In Macintosh R, Mushin WW, Epstein HG (eds): Physics for the Anaesthetist. 3rd Ed. Blackwell Scientific Publications, Oxford, 1963

34. Schreiber P: Anaesthetic Equipment: Performance, Classification, and Safety. Springer-Verlag, New York, 1972

35. Vapor 19.1 Operating Instructions. Dragerwerk, Lubeck, 1987

36. Tec 4 Continuous Flow Vaporizer. Operator's Manual. Ohmeda, The BOC Group, Inc., Steeton, England, 1987

37. Hill DW, Lowe HJ: Comparison of concentration of halothane in closed and semi-closed circuits during controlled ventilation. Anesthesiology 23:291, 1962

38. Hill DW: The design and calibration of vaporizers for volatile anaesthetic agents. p. 544. In Scurr C, Feldman S (eds): Scientific Foundations of Anaesthesia. 3rd Ed. William Heineman Medical Books, London, 1982

39. Hill DW: The design and calibration of vaporizers for volatile anaesthetic agents. Br J Anaesth 40:648, 1968

40. Morris LE: Problems in the performance of anesthesia vaporizers. Int Anesthesiol Clin 12:199, 1974

41. Stoelting RK: The effects of nitrous oxide on halothane output from Fluotec Mark 2 vaporizers. Anesthesiology 35:215, 1971

42. Diaz PD: The influence of carrier gas on the output of automatic vaporizers. Br J Anaesth 48:387, 1976

43. Nawaf K, Stoelting RK: Nitrous oxide increases enflurane concentrations delivered by Ethrane vaporizers. Anesth Analg 58:30, 1979

44. Prins L, Strupat J, Clement J, Knill RL: An evaluation of gas density dependence of anaesthetic vaporizers. Can Anaesth Soc J 27:106, 1980

45. Lin CY: Assessment of vaporizer performance in low-flow and closed-circuit anesthesia. Anesth Analg 59:359, 1980

46. Gould DB, Lampert BA, MacKrell TN: Effect of nitrous oxide solubility on vaporizer aberrance. Anesth Analg 61:938, 1982

47. Palayiwa E, Sanderson MH, Hahn CEW: Effects of carrier gas composition on the output of six anaesthetic vaporizers. Br J Anaesth 55:1025, 1983

48. Scheller MS, Drummond JC: Solubility of N_2O in volatile anesthetics contributes to vaporizer aberrancy when changing carrier gases. Anesth Analg 65:88, 1986

49. Peters KR, Wingard DW: Anesthesia machine leakage due to misaligned vaporizers. Anesth Rev 14:36, 1987

50. Marks WE, Jr., Bullard JR: Another hazard of free-standing vaporizers, increased anesthetic concentration with reversed flow of vaporizing gas. Anesthesiology 45:445, 1976

51. Capan L, Ramanathan S, Chalon J, et al: A possible hazard with use of the Ohio Ethrane Vaporizer. Anesth Analg 59:65, 1980

52. Mapleson WW: The elimination of rebreathing in various semiclosed anesthetic systems. Br J Anaesth 26:323, 1954

53. Willis BA, Pender JW, Mapleson WW: Rebreathing in a T-piece: Volunteer and theoretical studies of the Jackson-Rees modification of Ayre's T-piece during spontaneous respiration. Br J Anaesth 47:1239, 1975

54. Norman J, Adams AP, Sykes MK: Rebreathing with the Magill attachment. Anaesthesia 31:247, 1959

55. Kain ML, Nunn JF: Fresh gas economics of the Magill circuit. Anesthesiology 29:964, 1968

56. Sykes MK: Rebreathing during controlled respiration with the Magill attachment. Anaesthesia 31:247, 1959

57. Sykes MK: Rebreathing circuits: A review. Br J Anaesth 40:666, 1968

58. Bain JA, Spoerel WE: Flow requirements for a modified Mapleson D system during controlled ventilation. Can Anaesth Soc J 20:629, 1973

59. Soliman MG, Laberge R: The use of the Bain circuit in spontaneously breathing pediatric patients. Can Anaesth Soc J 25:276, 1978

60. Bain JA, Spoerel WE: A streamlined anaesthetic system. Can Anaesth Soc J 19:426, 1972

61. Ungerer MJ: A comparison between the Bain and Magill anesthetic systems during spontaneous breathing. Can Anaesth Soc J 25:122, 1978

62. Spoerel WE: Rebreathing and end tidal CO_2 during spontaneous breathing with the Bain circuit. Can Anaesth Soc J 30:148, 1983

63. Pethick SL: Letter to the editor. Can Anaesth Soc J 22:115, 1975

64. Ayre P: Endotracheal anesthesia for babies with special reference to hare-lip and cleft-palate operations. Anesth Analg 16:331, 1937

65. Ayre P: The T-piece technique. Br J Anaesth 28:520, 1956

66. Jackson-Rees G: Anaesthesia in the newborn. Br Med J 2:1419, 1950

67. Moyers J: A nomenclature for methods of inhalation anesthesia. Anesthesiology 14:609, 1953

68. Eger EI II: Anesthetic systems: Construction and function. p. 206. In Eger EI II (ed): Anesthetic Uptake and Action. Williams & Wilkins, Baltimore, 1974

69. Eger EI II, Ethans CT: The effects of inflow, overflow and valve placement on economy of the circle system. Anesthesiology 29:93, 1968

70. Adriani J: Carbon dioxide absorption. p. 151. In Adriani J (ed): The Chemistry and Physics of Anesthesia. Charles C Thomas, Springfield, IL, 1962

71. Wilson RE: Soda lime: An absorbent for industrial purposes. J Ind Eng Chem 12:1000, 1920

72. Dewey & Almy Chemical Division: The Sodasorb Manual of CO_2 Absorption. WR Grace, New York, 1962

73. Foregger R: The regeneration of soda lime following absorption of CO_2. Anesthesiology 9:15, 1948

74. Hunt HE: Resistance in respiratory valves and canisters. Anesthesiology 16:190, 1955

75. Brown ES: Performance of absorbents: Continuous flow. Anesthesiology 20:41, 1959

76. Adriani J: Soda lime indicators. Anesthesiology 5:45, 1944

77. Case History #39: Accidental use of trichloroethylene (Trilene, Trimar) in a closed system. Anesth Analg 43:740, 1964

78. Strum D, Eger EI II, Johnson BH, et al: Toxicity of sevoflurane in rats. Anesth Analg 66:769, 1987

79. Spearman CB, Sanders HG: Physical principles and functional designs of ventilators. p. 59. In Kirby RR, Smith RA, Desautels DA (eds): Mechanical Ventilation. Churchill Livingstone, New York, 1985

80. McPherson SP, Spearman CB: Introduction to ventilators. p. 230. In McPherson SP, Spearman CB (eds): Respiratory Therapy Equipment. CV Mosby, St. Louis, 1985

81. Ohio Anesthesia Ventilator. Operation Maintenance. Ohio Medical Products, The BOC Group, Inc., Madison, WI, 1982

82. Anesthesia Ventilator. Service Manual. Ohio Medical Products, The BOC Group, Inc., Madison, WI, 1983

83. Ohio V5 Anesthesia Ventilator. Operation and Maintenance Manual. Ohmeda, The BOC Group, Inc., Madison, WI, 1983

84. V5A Anesthesia Ventilator. Operation and Maintenance Manual. Ohmeda, The BOC Group, Inc., Madison, WI, 1986

85. V5/V5A Anesthesia Ventilator. Service Manual. Ohio Medical Products, The BOC Group, Inc., Madison, WI, 1983

86. 7000 Electronic Anesthesia Ventilator. Operation Maintenance. Ohmeda, The BOC Group, Inc., Madison, WI, 1985

87. 7000 Electronic Anesthesia Ventilator. Service Manual. Ohmeda, The BOC Group, Inc., Madison, WI, 1985

88. Andrews JJ: Understanding your anesthesia machine and ventilator. p. 59. In 1989 Review Course Lectures. International Anesthesia Research Society, 1989

89. Roth S, Tweedie E, Sommer RM: Excessive airway pressure due to a malfunctioning anesthesia ventilator. Anesthesiology 65:532, 1986

90. Cooper JB, Newbower RS, Kitz RJ: An analysis of major errors and equipment failures in anesthesia management. Considerations for prevention and detection. Anesthesiology 60:34, 1984

91. Raphael DT, Weller RS, Doran DJ: A response algorithm for the low-pressure alarm condition. Anesth Analg 67:876, 1988

92. Slee TA, Pavlin EG: Failure of low pressure alarm associated with use of a humidifier. Anesthesiology 69:791, 1988

93. Feeley TW, Bancroft ML: Problems with mechanical ventilators. Int Anesthesiol Clin 20:83, 1982

94. Khalil SN, Gholston TK, Binderman J, et al: Flapper valve malfunction in an Ohio Closed Scavenging System. Anesth Analg 66:1334, 1987

95. Sommer RM, Bhalla GS, Jackson JM, et al: Hypoventilation caused by ventilator valve rupture. Anesth Analg 67:999, 1988

96. American National Standard for Anesthetic Equipment: Scavenging Systems for Excess Anesthetic Gases (ANSI Z79.11-1982). American National Standards Institute, New York, 1982

97. Dorsch JA, Dorsch SE: Controlling trace gas levels. p. 247. In Dorsch JA, Dorsch SE (eds): Understanding Anesthesia Equipment. 2nd Ed. Williams & Wilkins, Baltimore, 1984

98. Open Reservoir Scavenger. Operator's Instruction Manual. North American Drager, Telford, PA, 1986

99. Gray WM: Scavenging equipment. Br J Anaesth 57:685, 1985

100. Scavenger interface for air conditioning. Instruction Manual. North American Drager, Telford, PA, 1984

101. Davies G, Tarnawsky M: Letter to the editor. Can Anaesth Soc J 23:228, 1976

102. Tavakoli M, Habeeb A: Two hazards of gas scavenging. Anesth Analg 57:286, 1978

103. Mantia AM: Gas scavenging systems. Anesth Analg 61:162, 1982

104. O'Connor DE, Daniels BW, Pfitzner J: Hazards of anaesthetic scavenging: Case reports and brief review. Anaesth Intensive Care 10:15, 1982

105. Hagerdal M, Lecky JH: Anesthetic death of an experimental animal related to a scavenging system malfunction. Anesthesiology 47:522, 1977

106. Hamilton RC, Byrne J: Another cause of gas-scavenging-line obstruction. Anesthesiology 51:365, 1979

107. Flowerdew RM: A hazard of scavenger port design. Can Anaesth Soc J 28:481, 1981

108. Mann ES, Sprague DH: An easily overlooked malassembly. Anesthesiology 56:413, 1982

109. Seymour A: Possible hazards with an anaesthetic gas scavenging system. Anaesthesia 37:1218, 1987

110. Rendell-Baker L: Hazard of blocked scavenge valve. Can Anaesth Soc J 29:182, 1982

111. Patel KD, Dalal FY: A potential hazard of the Drager scavenging interface system for wall suction. Anesth Analg 58:327, 1979

112. Mor ZF, Stein ED, Orkin LR: A possible hazard in the use of a scavenging system. Anesthesiology 47:302, 1977

113. Abramowitz M, McGill WA: Hazard of an anesthetic scavenging device. Anesthesiology 51:276, 1979

114. Malloy WF, Wightman AE, O'Sullivan D, Goldiner PL: Bilateral pneumothorax from suction applied to a ventilator exhaust valve. Anesth Analg 58:147, 1979

115. Sharrock NE, Leith DE: Potential pulmonary barotrauma when venting anesthetic gases to suction. Anesthesiology 46:152, 1977

116. Sharrock NE, Gabel RA: Inadvertent anesthetic overdose obscured by scavenging. Anesthesiology 49:137, 1978

117. Cooper JB: Toward prevention of anesthetic mishaps. Int Anesthesiol Clin 22:167, 1984

118. Spooner RB, Kirby RR: Equipment related anesthetic incidents. Int Anesthesiol Clin 22:133, 1984

119. Emergency Care Research Institute: Avoiding anesthetic mishaps through pre-use checks. Health Devices 11:201, 1982

120. Food and Drug Administration: Anesthesia apparatus checkout recommendations. Food and Drug Administration, Rockville, MD, 1986

121. Comm G, Rendell-Baker L: Back pressure check valves a hazard. Anesthesiology 56:327, 1982

122. Petty C: Anesthesia circuits. p. 81. In Petty C (ed): The Anesthesia Machine. Churchill Livingstone, New York, 1987

123. Forbes AR: Humidification and mucus flow in the intubated trachea. Br J Anaesth 45:874, 1973

124. Shapiro BA, Harrison RA, Kacmarek RM, Cane RD: Humidity and aerosol therapy. p. 90. In Shapiro BA, Harrison RA, Kacmarek RM, Cane RD (eds): Clinical Application of Respiratory Therapy. Year Book Medical Publishers, Chicago, 1985

125. McPherson SP, Spearman CB: Humidifiers and nebulizers. p. 119. In McPherson SP, Spearman CB (eds): Respiratory Therapy Equipment. CV Mosby, St. Louis, 1985

126. Chalon J, Ali M, Turndorf H, Fischgrund GK: Humidification of Anesthetic Gases. Charles C Thomas, Springfield, IL, 1981

127. Tausk HC, Miller R, Roberts RB: Maintenance of body temperature by heated humidification. Anesth Analg 55:719, 1976

128. Elder PT: Accidental hypothermia. p. 85. In Shoemaker WC, Thompson WL, Holbrook PR (eds): Textbook of Critical Care. WB Saunders, Philadelphia, 1984

129. Bernard JM, Pinaud M, Souron R: Perioperative hypothermia prevention. Acta Anaesthesiol Scand 31:521, 1987

130. Chase HF, Trotta R, Kilmore MA: Simple methods for humid-

ifying nonrebreathing anesthesia gas systems. Anesth Analg 41:249, 1962

131. Chalon J, Simon RS, Ramanathan S, et al: A high-humidity circle system for infants and children. Anesthesiology 49:205, 1978

132. Weeks DB: Humidification of anesthetic gases using heat-and-moisture exchangers. Anesth Rev 12:22, 1985

133. Rodgers RC, Hill GE: Equations for vapour pressure versus temperature: Derivation and use of the Antoine equation on a hand-held programmable calculator. Br J Anaesth 50:415, 1978

134. Baromed Breathing Pressure Monitor. Operator's Instruction Manual. North American Drager, Telford, PA, 1986

135. Andrews JJ: Understanding anesthesia machines. p. 78. In 1988 Review Course Lectures. International Anesthesia Research Society, 1988

136. American Society of Anesthesiologists: Check-out, a Guide for Preoperative Inspection of an Anesthesia Machine. ASA Patient Safety Videotape Program, Park Ridge, IL, 1986

8
BARBITURATES

Robert J. Fragen
Michael J. Avram

Introduction	Specific Organ Function Effects
Basic Pharmacology	Drug Interactions
Chemistry and Formulation	Recovery
Structure-Activity Relationships	Postoperative Sequelae
Mechanism of Action	**Administration of Barbiturates by Infusions**
Pharmacokinetics	**Other Uses of Barbiturates**
Clinical Pharmacology and Uses	Anticonvulsants
Pharmacokinetic Bases of Altered Dose	Brain Protection
Requirements	Wada Test
Nighttime Sedation and Premedication	Electroconvulsive Therapy
Induction of General Anesthesia	**Summary**

INTRODUCTION

For over 40 years barbiturates have been a standard element of anesthesia practice. Their use has profoundly affected the way anesthesiologists administer drugs, because barbiturates have a rapid but short action and are safe and effective when administered properly.

Although barbituric acid was first synthesized in 1864 by von Baeyer, it was not until 1903, when Fischer and von Mering synthesized diethylbarbituric acid, that a barbiturate with hypnotic activity became available. The many hypnotic barbiturates introduced between 1903 and 1932 had little impact on intravenous anesthesia because they had slow onsets and long durations of action.[1] In 1932, Weese and Scharpff introduced the methylated oxybarbiturate hexobarbital, bringing a new era to anesthesia, because hexobarbital had a rapid onset and short duration of hypnotic effect despite its excitatory side effects. Another barbiturate that is fast acting but devoid of excitatory side effects, thiopental,

was first administered in 1934 by Waters and Lundy.[1] Unfortunately, a lack of understanding of pharmacokinetics led to the use of hexobarbital and thiopental for the induction and maintenance of general anesthesia in the manner of diethyl ether and chloroform, sometimes with disastrous results including hypotension and prolonged sleeping times.[2] Administration of hexobarbital and thiopental in this manner to the casualties at Pearl Harbor resulted in so many deaths that intravenous anesthesia was described as "an ideal method of euthanasia."[3] The negative impact of this report was perhaps moderated by both an accompanying case report by Adams and Gray and an anonymous editorial suggesting that the method of drug administration rather than the drug's inherent toxicity caused the adverse outcomes.[4] Brodie and colleagues[5] provided further insight into the use of intravenous barbiturates by demonstrating that the effects of small doses of thiopental were terminated, not by metabolism, but by redistribution from their sites of action to other body tissues. Price[6] clarified this concept in 1960 and explained that during prolonged administration, distribution becomes less effective in terminating the drug's action because redistribution sites approach equilibrium.

An understanding of its pharmacokinetics[2,4-6] and its desirable pharmacologic properties[7] made thiopental the standard anesthetic drug to induce anesthesia.

BASIC PHARMACOLOGY

Chemistry and Formulation

The barbiturates are derivatives of barbituric acid (2,4,6-trioxohexahydropyrimidine) (Fig. 8-1), which is devoid of hypnotic activity, or of its 2-thio analogue. Although commonly called a cyclic ureide of malonic acid because of its synthesis from urea and malonic acid, barbituric acid is actually a pyrimidine nucleus.[8] Keto-enol tautomerization (Fig. 8-1) (or its sulfur equivalent) lends acidic character to the oxygen (or sulfur) at position 2 of the barbiturate nucleus; the predominance of the enol form, or its sulfur equivalent, in alkaline solution allows the formation of water-soluble barbiturate salts.[9]

The barbiturates commonly used for induction of anesthesia are the thiobarbiturates, thiopental [5-ethyl-5-(1-methylbutyl)-2-thiobarbituric acid] and thiamylal [5-allyl-5-(1-methylbutyl)-2-thiobarbituric acid], and the methylated oxybarbiturate, methohexital [α-dl-1-methyl-5-allyl-5-(1-methyl-2-pentynyl)barbituric acid] (Fig. 8-2). The sodium salts of these drugs, which are mixed with 6 percent by weight anhydrous sodium carbonate, are reconstituted with either water or 0.9 percent sodium chloride to produce 2.5 percent, 2.0 percent, or 1.0 percent solutions of thiopental, thiamylal, or methohexital, respectively. The buffering action of the sodium carbonate in the presence of atmospheric carbon dioxide maintains the moderate alkalinity (pH 10 to 11) of the barbiturate solutions. A decrease in the alkalinity of the barbiturate solutions can result in their precipitation as free acids; therefore, they should not be reconstituted with lactated Ringer's solution, nor should the reconstituted solutions be mixed with acidic solutions of other drugs. Properly reconstituted thiobarbiturate solutions are stable for 1 week if refrigerated. Sterile water solutions of methohexital can be used up to 6 weeks after reconstitution.

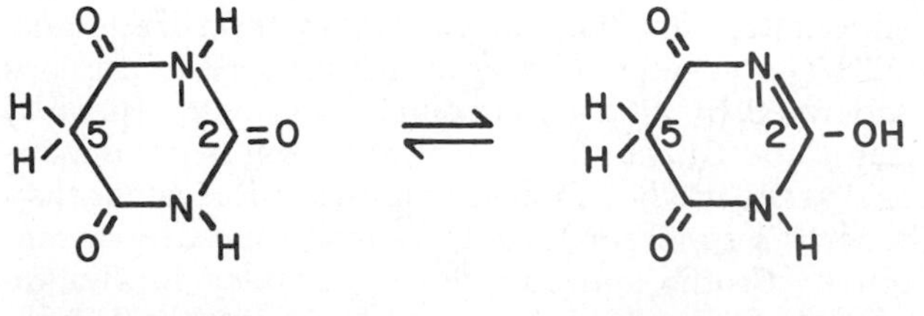

Structure-Activity Relationships

Modifying the structure of the hypnotically inactive barbituric acid (Fig. 8-1) can convert it into a hypnotic barbiturate with physicochemical properties that affect its ability to gain access to its sites of action and to interact with its receptor.

The structure-activity relationships of the barbiturates are well described.[8] Hypnotic activity is introduced to the barbituric acid molecule by the addition of side chains, especially if at least one of them is branched, in position 5 (Figs. 8-1 and 8-2). The length of the side chains in the 5 position influences both the potency and the duration of action of the barbituric acid derivatives; secobarbital and thiamylal are slightly more potent than pentobarbital and thiopental, respectively, because the former drugs have slightly longer (three versus two carbon) side chains in position 5 (Fig. 8-2). Replacing the oxygen atom with a sulfur atom at position 2 of an active barbiturate produces a barbiturate with a more rapid onset and a shorter duration of action; the thiobarbiturates, thiopental and thiamylal, have faster onsets and shorter durations of action than their oxybarbiturate analogues, pentobarbital and secobarbital (Fig. 8-2). Methylation of an active barbiturate in position 1 produces a drug like methohexital (Fig. 8-2) with not only a rapid onset and short duration of action but also an increased incidence of excitatory side effects. Therefore, any chemical modification that increases the lipophilicity of a hypnotic barbiturate will generally increase both its potency and its rate of onset while shortening its duration of action.

The effect of stereoisomerism on biologic activity is another important aspect of structure-activity relationships. Many barbiturates, including pentobarbital, secobarbital, thiopental, thiamylal, and methohexital, have asymmetric carbon atoms in one of the side chains attached to carbon 5 of the barbiturate ring (Fig. 8-2).[10] The *l* isomers of pentobarbital, secobarbital, thiopental, and thiamylal are nearly twice as potent as the *d* isomers, despite their similar access to the central nervous system (CNS). These barbiturates are marketed as racemic mixtures. Methohexital has four stereoisomers because it has an asymmetric center at carbon 5, as well as an asymmetric carbon atom on one of the side chains attached to carbon 5 (Fig. 8-2). The most potent hypnotic stereoisomer of methohexital is the *β-l*, which is four to five times as potent as the least active, *α-l*; however, the *β*-isomers produce excessive motor activity, so methohexital is marketed as a racemic mixture of *α*-isomers.[11] Differences in the potency of stereoisomers suggest interaction with the chiral active center of a receptor or enzyme rather than a nonspecific action; side effects are often due to nonspecific actions of drugs. Therefore, some consider the less active stereoisomer to be an impurity in the drug formulation.[12]

Fig. 8-1. The keto and enol tautomeric forms of barbituric acid with the sites of substitution in the hypnotically active barbiturates identified as 1, 2, and 5.

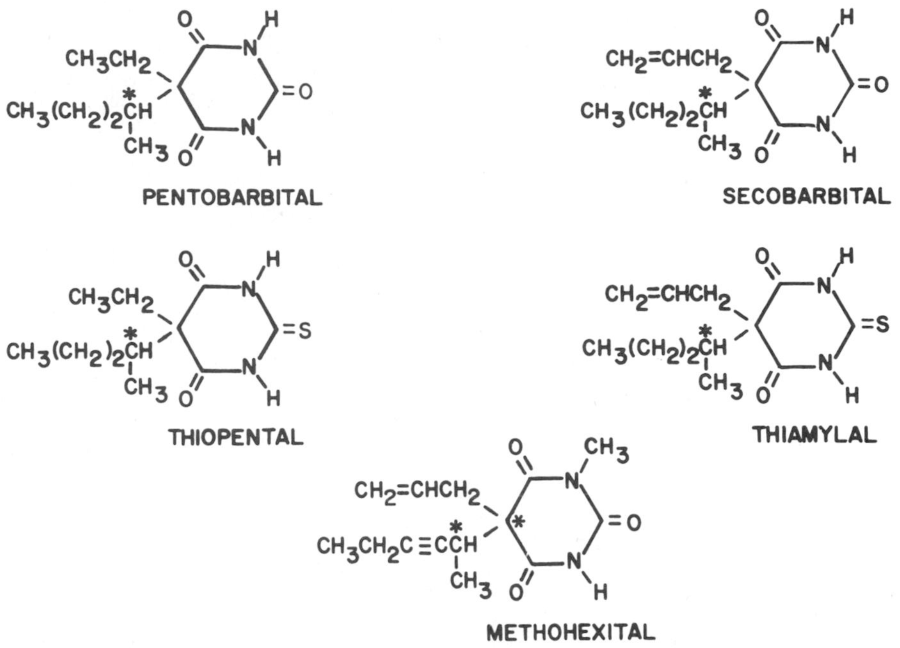

PENTOBARBITAL

SECOBARBITAL

THIOPENTAL

THIAMYLAL

METHOHEXITAL

Fig. 8-2. Hypnotically active barbiturates with asymmetric centers indicated by an asterisk.

Mechanism of Action

The γ-aminobutyric acid (GABA) receptor complex is the most likely site of barbiturate action.[13] Of the various effects of barbiturates at the cellular level, only their effects on the GABA receptor complex occur at clinical drug concentrations, correlate with anesthetic potency, and are stereospecific.

GABA is the principal inhibitory neurotransmitter in the mammalian CNS. The GABA receptor is an oligomeric complex consisting of a GABA receptor and its associated chloride ion channel, a benzodiazepine receptor, a barbiturate receptor, and a picrotoxin-binding site (Fig. 8-3).[14,15] Activation of the GABA receptor increases chloride conductance through the ion channel, hyperpolarizing and thereby inhibiting the postsynaptic neuron.

Barbiturates both enhance and mimic the action of GABA.[13] By binding to their receptor, barbiturates decrease the rate of dissociation of GABA from its receptor and increase the duration of GABA-activated chloride ion channel openings. At slightly higher but still clinically relevant concentrations, barbiturates directly activate chloride channels, even in the absence of GABA. Barbiturate enhancement of the action of GABA may be responsible for its sedative-hypnotic effects, while the GABA-mimetic effect at slightly higher concentrations may be responsible for "barbiturate anesthesia."[13]

Pharmacokinetics

The physiologic pharmacokinetic models of thiopental disposition developed by Price and colleagues[6,16] and by Bischoff and Dedrick[17] provide invaluable insight into the pharmacology of fast-acting drugs such as the barbiturates. Following intravenous administration, thiopental mixes rapidly within a central blood pool and is distributed by blood flow and molecular diffusion throughout the tissues of the body according to their rate of perfusion, their affinity for the drug, and the relative concentration of thiopental in the tissues and blood (Fig. 8-4). The highly perfused, relatively low volume tissues such as the brain equilibrate rapidly with the high, early concentrations of thiopental in the blood, resulting in the induction of anesthesia. Thiopental concentrations in the blood and highly perfused tissue then decrease rapidly as the drug redistributes to the large reservoir of less well perfused lean tissue such as muscle, terminating the effect of an induction dose.

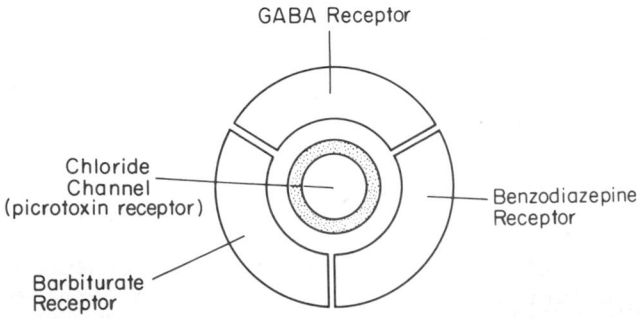

Fig. 8-3. The hypothetical GABA oligomeric complex. (From Olsen et al.,[14] with permission.)

% of dose

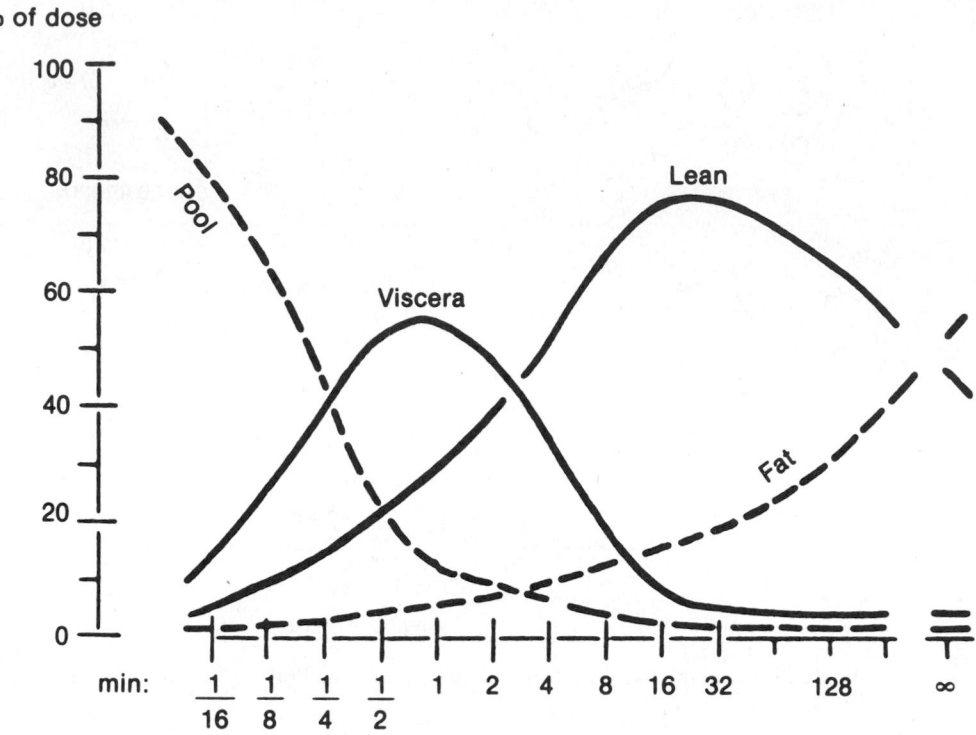

Fig. 8-4. Percentage of thiopental dose in the central blood pool, viscera, lean tissue, and fat after rapid intravenous administration. This model assumes there is no elimination clearance. (From Price et al.,[16] with permission.)

Despite its high affinity for thiopental, adipose tissue takes up drug slowly because of its poor perfusion; the amount of thiopental taken up by adipose tissue is not significant until long after its effects wane. The irreversible removal of thiopental from the body, the elimination clearance, like uptake into adipose tissue, is so slow relative to the uptake of drug by the lean tissue that it contributes minimally to the termination of the effect of an induction dose.

Compartmental pharmacokinetic models that mathematically characterize the blood drug concentration versus time relationships (Fig. 8-5) have largely replaced physiologic models[18] because physiologic models require extensive human data. Data from compartmental models of thiopental and methohexital disposition are presented in Table 8-1. The central volumes of distribution (V_C) of these drugs exceed intravascular space in these models; the rapid onsets of effect of the drugs suggest that the brain is part of their V_C. The action of an induction dose of thiopental or methohexital is terminated by redistribution from the relatively small V_C to the much larger total apparent volume of distribution, V_{dss}, suggesting extensive uptake by some body tissues. The low, restrictive elimination clearance (Cl_E) of thiopental is a reflection of its hepatic extraction ratio, which may be low because of its extensive protein binding. Methohexital has an intermediate hepatic extraction ratio and elimination

clearance despite extensive protein binding. Because the elimination half-life $(t\frac{1}{2}\beta)$ is a pharmacokinetic variable that depends directly on the volume of distribution and inversely on the Cl_E, the difference in $t\frac{1}{2}\beta$ between thiopental and methohexital is due to a difference in Cl_E.

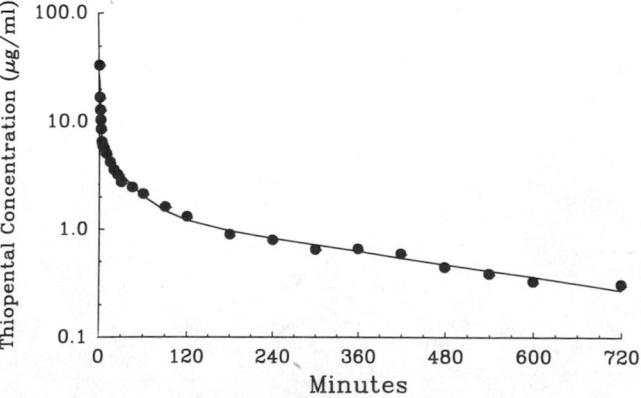

Fig. 8-5. Blood thiopental concentration versus time relationship after rapid intravenous drug administration. The circles represent measured thiopental concentrations, and the line represents a computer-generated fit to a quadriexponential equation. (Data from Henthorn et al.[18])

TABLE 8-1. Pharmacokinetics of Thiopental and Methohexital ($\bar{x} \pm$ SD)

Drug	V_C (L/kg)	V_{ss} (L/kg)	Cl_E (ml/min/kg)	$t\frac{1}{2}\beta$ (h)	Estimated Hepatic Extraction Ratio
Thiopental	0.38 ± 0.10	2.5 ± 1.0	3.4 ± 0.5	11.6 ± 6.0	0.15
Methohexital	0.35 ± 0.10	2.2 ± 0.7	10.9 ± 3.0	3.9 ± 2.1	0.50

Abbreviations: $\bar{x} \pm$ SD, mean $\pm$ standard deviation; V_C, central volume of distribution; V_{ss}, volume of distribution at steady state; Cl_E, elimination clearance; $t\frac{1}{2}\beta$ elimination half-life.
(Data from Hudson et al.[19])

Although Cl_E begins the moment a drug reaches its clearing organ(s), Cl_E becomes a dominant factor in the plasma drug concentration versus time relationship only after the end of the rapid decline in plasma drug concentrations during the redistribution phase (Fig. 8-5). Stanski and colleagues[19,20] determined the relative importance of Cl_E and redistribution to the termination of the effect of an induction dose of either thiopental or methohexital. They found that despite the threefold difference in the Cl_E of the drugs (Table 8-1), redistribution is the primary process terminating the effect of an induction dose of either drug; this is consistent with the results of physiologic models.[16,17] However, when methohexital or thiopental is administered in large doses, as multiple doses, or by continuous infusion, the capacity of the lean tissue to dilute the drugs decreases progressively as the tissue approaches equilibrium with the blood. Thus, termination of the drug action increasingly depends on the slower processes of uptake into adipose tissues and Cl_E, resulting in a prolonged drug effect.[6] As an extreme example, when thiopental was administered for 2 to 4 days of cerebral resuscitation, redistribution sites reached equilibrium with the blood, drug-metabolizing enzymes approached saturation, and recovery depended entirely on nonlinear (Michaelis-Menten) drug metabolism and took nearly 4 days[21] (Fig. 8-6).

The development of combined pharmacokinetic-

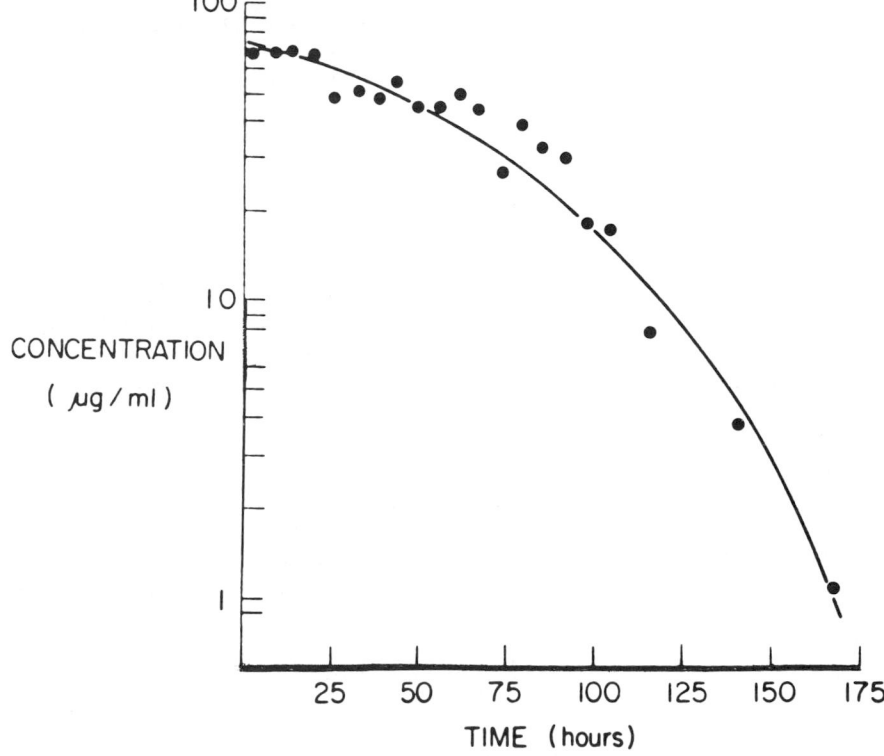

Fig. 8-6. Decline in plasma thiopental concentrations with time after a 42-hour infusion of 40.2 g of the drug for cerebral resuscitation, illustrating nonlinear (Michaelis-Menten) elimination clearance. Note the difference between this postdrug administration relationship and that for a standard dose of thiopental (Fig. 8-5), which has typical distributional phases followed by linear elimination clearance. (Modified from Stanski et al.,[21] with permission.)

pharmacodynamic models is a recent advance in the field of barbiturate pharmacokinetics. As measures of the CNS effect of thiopental in such models, Stanski and colleagues used the electroencephalogram (EEG) spectral edge, calculated by off-line power spectral analysis,[22] and the total number of waves per second, calculated from off-line aperiodic analysis of the EEG.[23] Combined pharmacokinetic-pharmacodynamic models can potentially establish the kinetic or dynamic basis of differences in the reactivity of individuals or groups of individuals (e.g., the elderly) to the barbiturates. With the availability of on-line effect analysis, combined pharmacokinetic-pharmacodynamic models can also provide the basis for adaptive feedback-controlled barbiturate infusions; Schwilden et al.[24] used the median frequency of the EEG power spectrum in this way to control a moderately successful methohexital infusion in volunteers. Pharmacodynamic modeling of anesthetic depth by using EEG variables, or other measures of effect, must be viewed with caution because there is no unequivocal measure of anesthetic depth.[25,26]

Henthorn et al.[18] recently developed a compartmental pharmacokinetic model of thiopental disposition that appears to reflect physiologic factors affecting early drug distribution. These investigators concomitantly administer thiopental and indocyanine green, a marker of intravascular space, and model their disposition on the basis of frequent early arterial blood samples. This technique characterizes the intravascular space by estimating total blood volume, resolving it into central and peripheral blood pools. Clearly, this model reflects cardiac output and its distribution during anesthesia and more accurately defines the initial pharmacokinetis of thiopental. This technique may be useful in establishing the pharmacokinetic basis of altered reactivity to initial doses of thiopental.

CLINICAL PHARMACOLOGY AND USES

Pharmacokinetic Bases of Altered Dose Requirements

Increased response to the barbiturates, exemplified by decreased dose requirements, is due to altered pharmacodynamics or early distribution pharmacokinetics because the barbiturates have rapid onsets of effect. Altered response to induction doses of the barbiturates is not due to changes in total volume of distribution, elimination clearance, or elimination half-life, since these minimally affect the plasma drug concentration versus time relationship when the barbiturates are exerting their effect and when their effect is being terminated. The classic example of increased response to thiopental is the decreased dose requirement in patients in hypovolemic shock, such as the Pearl Harbor casualties.[3] On the basis of his physiologic model, Price[6] reasoned that

the dose requirement is less in patients in hemorrhagic shock because in this condition the fraction of the dose received by the brain is very high and its rate of removal from the brain is very low owing to decreased blood flow to other tissues. Price's hypothesis was substantiated by a study showing changes in the physiologic kinetics of lidocaine in hypovolemic monkeys.[27]

The most extensively studied alteration in response to thiopental is the age-related decrease in dose requirement.[28,29] Using their effect model,[22] Homer and Stanski[30] found no change in the pharmacodynamics of thiopental with age. Investigators seeking a pharmacokinetic basis for the increased response of the elderly to thiopental found either no explanation[31] or an age-related decrease in the initial distribution volume[30] or rate of drug transfer from the central compartment to the rapidly equilibrating compartment.[32] While the latter observations could provide a pharmacokinetic rationale for the decreased dose requirements in the elderly, Krejcie and colleagues[33] could not find a kinetic explanation of the age-related increase in drug sensitivity when they closely examined early drug distribution using their new model.[18] Wulfsohn and Joshi[34] suggested that if the induction dose of thiopental is based on lean body mass rather than total body mass, there is no need to adjust the dose with age because the proportion of lean body mass decreases with increasing age. Termination of the effect of an induction dose of thiopental by redistribution to muscle[16] and the increase in the slowly equilibrating volume of distribution with age[31-33] is consistent with this suggestion. Furthermore, the apparently increased responses of the obese[29] and females[29] may be eliminated if the induction dose of thiopental is based on lean body mass, which represents a smaller proportion of total body mass in these patients.[34,35]

Acute tolerance to thiopental was first described by Brodie et al.[36] and, subsequently, by Dundee and associates[37] and by Toner et al.[38] According to these investigators, the plasma thiopental concentration at awakening is proportional to the dose used; that is, the depth of anesthesia is independent of the plasma thiopental concentration. This suggests that the higher the induction dose of thiopental, the less sensitive a patient will be to a subsequent dose. Hudson et al.[39] evaluated the relationship between venous plasma thiopental concentrations and the EEG spectral edge, going from light to moderately deep anesthesia and back during and after three infusions administered over approximately 1 hour; they found no acute tolerance. The consistency of plasma thiopental concentrations on awakening after exponential infusions delivering 0.8 to 2.6 g of thiopental led Crankshaw and colleagues[40] to conclude that there was no acute tolerance to thiopental. The discrepancies between these studies were at least partially explained by Barratt et al.,[41,42] who found that shortly after rapid intravenous drug administration, peripheral venous plasma thiopental concentrations poorly reflect brain (i.e., jugular venous) thiopental concentrations. This accounts for the apparent acute tolerance reported by Toner et al.[38]

Nighttime Sedation and Premedication (Also See Ch. 26)

Before benzodiazepines were available, pentobarbital and secobarbital were used orally for nighttime sedation prior to surgery and either orally, rectally, or intramuscularly for preoperative sedation. Barbiturates became popular because they provided drowsiness with minimal respiratory or cardiovascular depression and their use was rarely associated with nausea or vomiting. However, they occasionally caused disorientation, especially in the elderly, and they had no analgesic effect.

Barbiturates have now been displaced by benzodiazepines for these indications because barbiturates have lower therapeutic indices and patients develop tolerance to them more readily than to benzodiazepines. Although pentobarbital premedication also has a protective effect against local-anesthetic-induced seizures, benzodiazepines are preferable because they have less CNS-, cardiovascular-, and respiratory-depressant effects.[43] Pentobarbital and secobarbital produce dose-related drowsiness over a 50- to 150-mg dose range without relieving preoperative apprehension. Anesthetic induction is no easier in patients premedicated with barbiturates than in those given a placebo.[44]

Barbiturates have been administered to children by the oral, injectable, and rectal routes. When children receive pentobarbital for premedication, they are more uncooperative before surgery and more excitable in the recovery room than those who receive opioid premedication.[45] Rectally administered barbiturates have variable rates of absorption, onsets of effect, and durations of action.[46] Methohexital or the thiobarbiturates can be given intramuscularly to children for premedication but have no advantage over oral premedication or intramuscular midazolam, which causes less discomfort and requires a smaller volume.

Induction of General Anesthesia

Drugs and Dosage

Thiopental, thiamylal, and methohexital can be injected intravenously to induce general anesthesia and can also be used to maintain unconsciousness as the hypnotic component of a balanced anesthetic technique. These barbiturates continue to be the most popular anesthetic induction agents because they induce anesthesia rapidly and pleasantly. When injected intravenously, these lipid-soluble drugs act in one arm-brain circulation time and have their maximum effect in about 1 minute.[6] Because barbiturates redistribute rapidly from the brain to the lean body tissue, the duration of effect from a single induction dose is about 5 to 8 minutes. Induction doses produce the highest blood concentrations, and as a result, the most profound effects on body systems and the most side effects.

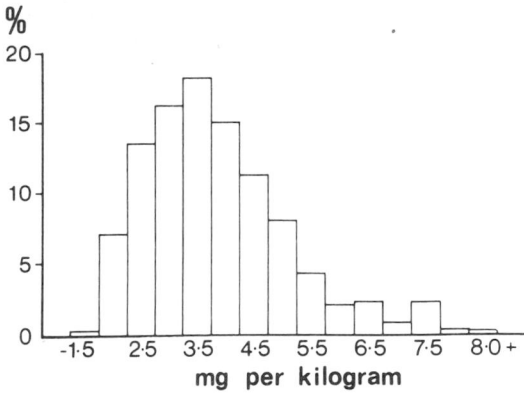

Fig. 8-7. This bar graph depicts the scatter of induction doses of thiopental (mg/kg) in 2,006 consecutive unselected anesthetic inductions. See the source reference for how the induction doses were determined. (From Dundee et al.,[48] with permission.)

The usual induction dose of thiopental for healthy adults is 2.5 to 4.5 mg/kg (Fig. 8-7) while a slightly higher dose, 5 to 6 mg/kg, is recommended for children, and 7 to 8 mg/kg is used for infants[47] (Fig. 8-8). To identify persons who might be particularly sensitive to the barbiturates, one can inject 25 percent of the calculated dose initially and then observe the patient's level of consciousness, respiration, and cardiovascular response. If this small dose has a great effect, the calculated dose should be reduced.

Both the patient's premedication and general health (ASA physical status) can influence the dose of thiopental necessary to induce anesthesia (Table 8-2).[48] Preme-

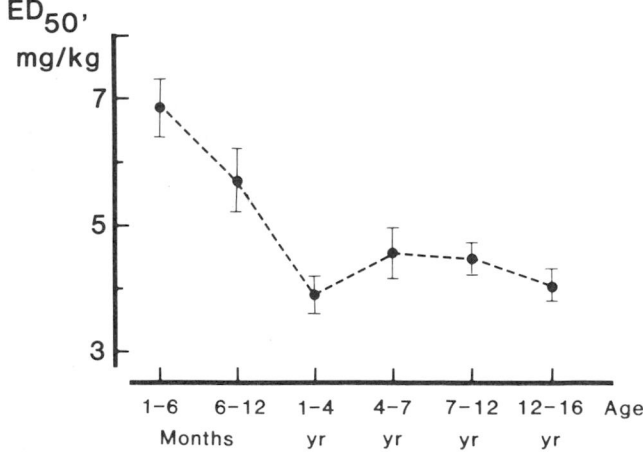

Fig. 8-8. Estimated $ED_{50} \pm SEM$ of thiopental in children of different ages from a dose-response study performed with the "up and down method." The ED_{50} is the dose at which anesthesia is induced in 50 percent of the children. The dashed lines do not represent data and are only added to facilitate visual observation of the actual data. (From Jonmarker et al.,[47] with permission.)

TABLE 8-2. Mean Thiopental Dose Following Various Premedicants

Premedication	Thiopental Dose (mg/kg)		
	ASA I	ASA II	ASA III & IV
None or atropine only	4.0	3.7	3.2
Benzodiazepine	3.4	3.3	3.1
Light opioid	3.4	3.1	3.0
Heavy opioid	3.1	2.8	2.7

(From Dundee et al.,[48] with permission.)

dicated geriatric patients require a 30 to 35 percent reduction in dose compared with younger patients.[28,29,48] Patients who have severe anemia or burns, malnutrition, advanced malignant disease, uremia, ulcerative colitis, or intestinal obstruction or are in shock require lower doses of any barbiturate to induce anesthesia. Hypothermia and circulatory failure slow the circulation time and prolong anesthetic induction; therefore, a much lower dose of barbiturate is necessary and its effect is greater. The acutely inebriated patient requires less barbiturate to induce anesthesia, while the chronic alcoholic requires a higher dose than normal.

An induction dose of 1.5 mg/kg of methohexital is equivalent to 4 mg/kg of thiopental; thus, methohexital appears to be about 2.7 times more potent. After reviewing a large number of cases with thiopental and thiamylal anesthetics, Tovall[49] concluded that there was no difference between the drugs in potency, incidence of laryngospasm and respiratory depression, cardiotoxicity, or recovery time. In the rest of this chapter, therefore, statements about thiopental also apply to thiamylal, unless stated otherwise.

Injection Complications

After injection of barbiturates, there may be an urticarial rash of the upper chest, neck, and face that fades after a few minutes. Anaphylactoid reactions such as hives, facial edema, bronchospasm, and shock occasionally occur after thiobarbiturate induction.[50] The absence of reactions to oral barbiturates does not ensure lack of sensitivity to intravenous barbiturates. Treatment of these reactions is symptomatic but should include 1-ml increments of 1 : 10,000 epinephrine and intravenous fluids. Aminophylline can be given to treat bronchospasm.

The incidence of pain on injection is 1 to 2 percent after thiopental and up to 5 percent after methohexital[51] when injected into small veins in the back of the hand or wrist and essentially none when injected into larger veins. If methohexital is injected into an artery or extravasated in the subcutaneous tissue, there is mild discomfort and no sequelae occur. However, if the thiobarbiturates[52] are extravasated, pain, edema, and erythema ensue; reactions ranging from slight soreness to extensive tissue necrosis can occur locally depending on the concentration and total amount injected.[4]

If the intravenous thiobarbiturates, especially in concentrations greater than 2.5 percent, are injected intraarterially, intense arterial spasm results and excrutiating pain can be felt from the injection site to the hand and fingers. The onset of pain and burning is immediate and can persist for hours. Within the first 2 hours, anesthesia or hyperesthesia of the hand, edema, or motor weakness can occur. Depending on the dose of drug injected, its concentration, volume, rate of injection, and the depth of the patient's sedation, a range of symptoms from mild discomfort to gangrene and loss of tissue in the hand can result.[4] The presence of a pulse does not rule out later development of thrombosis. The pathology is a chemical endarteritis that destroys the endothelium, subendothelial tissues, and possibly the muscle layer. To prevent permanent sequelae, treatment is necessary to dilute the barbiturate, relieve vascular spasm, and prevent thrombosis. Injection of papaverine (40 to 80 mg in 10 to 20 ml of normal saline) or 5 to 10 ml of 1 percent lidocaine or procaine into the artery may accomplish the first two objectives. Blocking the sympathetic nerves to the upper extremity with either a stellate ganglion block or a brachial plexus block can relieve spasm. Heparin can be given intravenously to prevent thrombosis.

Side Effects during Induction of Anesthesia

Besides producing unconsciousness, the barbiturates can cause mild muscular excitatory movements such as hypertonus, tremor, or twitching and respiratory excitatory effects including cough and hiccup. The dose-dependent incidence and severity of these effects are greater after methohexital than after thiopental, especially if the dose of methohexital is more than 1.5 mg/kg (Table 8-3).[53] Although these excitatory effects are not disturbing enough to limit the use of the barbiturates, atropine or opioids given just prior to anesthetic induction minimize the excitatory effects, while premedication with phenothiazines or scopolamine exaggerates them.[51] Inadequate induction doses can also evoke excitatory responses because inhibitory areas of the brain are the first to be depressed.

Specific Organ Function Effects

Central Nervous System Effects

The barbiturates may be hyperalgesic in subanesthetic concentrations, exaggerating the response to pain.[4] Clinical signs of their hyperalgesic effect include tachy-

TABLE 8-3. Incidence of Complications in Unpremedicated Patients

Anesthetic	Dose (mg/kg)	Excitatory (%)	Respiratory Upset (%)
Thiopental	4	9	6
Methohexital	1.6	33	26
Etomidate	0.3	80	19
Ketamine	3	24	4
Diazepam	0.8	0	10
Propofol	2	0	6

(Modified from Clark,[53] with permission.)

cardia, hypertension, diaphoresis, tearing, and tachypnea until pain becomes controlled.

Thiopental produces a dose-related depression of the EEG[54] (Fig. 8-9). The awake alpha pattern progresses to higher amplitude and slower frequency delta and theta waves until there is burst suppression and finally a flat EEG. A flat EEG can be maintained with a continuous infusion of thiopental (4 mg/kg/h)[55] or a pentobarbital infusion that maintains a plasma concentration of 3 to 6 mg/dl.[56] There is a dose-dependent depression of cerebral metabolism of oxygen ($CMRO_2$) that reaches a maximum of 55 percent when the EEG becomes flat. This reflects a decrease in neuronal, but not metabolic, need for oxygen; hypothermia is the only way to decrease the metabolic requirement. In addition, there is a parallel reduction in cerebral blood flow and intra-

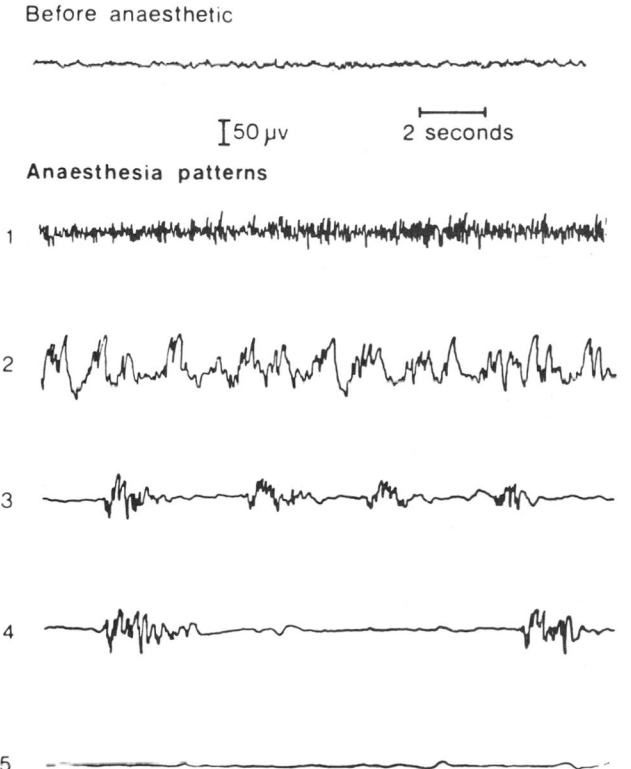

Before anaesthetic

I50 µv   2 seconds

Anaesthesia patterns

1

2

3

4

5

Fig. 8-9. Electroencephalographic changes with increasing doses of thiopental from an awake state to a flat EEG. (From Kiersey et al.,[54] with permission.)

cranial pressure (ICP)[57]; this is particularly beneficial for patients with increased ICP. Cerebral perfusion pressure is uncompromised because ICP decreases more than mean arterial pressure. The direction and magnitude of these changes are appropriate for patients with intracranial lesions, making thiopental an appropriate drug to induce anesthesia for neurosurgical operations (also see Ch. 54).

Thiopental is the preferred barbiturate for high dose or prolonged use for neuroanesthesia because patients had epileptiform seizures after very high doses of methohexital[58] and a 33 percent incidence of postoperative seizures when methohexital was given by continuous infusion.[59]

Thiopental is a satisfactory agent for use with somatosensory evoked potential (SSEP) monitoring. The evoked potential components remain even after administration of doses that cause a flat EEG. However, there is a dose-dependent change in median nerve SSEP response and brain stem auditory evoked response associated with the use of thiopental.[60,61]

Intravenous barbiturates are safe to use as anesthetic induction agents for ophthalmologic surgical procedures including those for open eye injuries. Intraocular pressure (IOP) decreases about 40 percent after an induction dose of thiopental or methohexital is injected. If succinylcholine is given immediately after thiopental, IOP returns to preinduction values, but if as much as 2 minutes elapse, IOP exceeds preinduction values.[62]

Respiratory Effects

The barbiturate induction agents cause central respiratory depression, the nature and duration of which depend on the dose, rate of injection, and type and dose of premedication; both the rate and depth of breathing can be depressed until apnea occurs. Although respiration returns toward normal in a few minutes, the responses to hypercarbia (Fig. 8-10) and hypoxemia (Fig. 8-11) are depressed for a longer time.[63] Even 2 mg/kg of pentobarbital, a dose used for premedication, depresses the ventilatory response to hypoxemia.[64]

There is a low incidence of hypersalivation and rarely bronchospasm or laryngospasm after barbiturate induction of anesthesia. Usually, these side effects are due to the insertion of artificial airways or tracheal tubes in lightly anesthetized patients; unless very large doses of barbiturates are used, laryngeal and tracheal reflexes

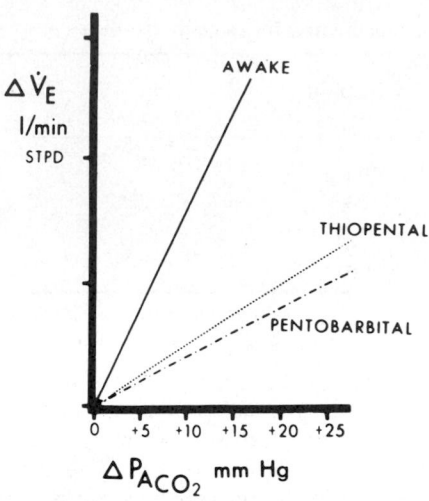

Fig. 8-10. Depression of the ventilatory response to carbon dioxide by pentobarbital and thiopental in the dog. The lines relate minute ventilation ($\dot{V}E$) to alveolar CO_2 tension (P_{ACO_2}). The slopes are normalized to the same starting point on the abcissa. STPD, standard temperature and pressure. (Modified from Hirshman et al.,[63] with permission.)

remain intact.[65] Thiopental and volatile anesthetic agents depress the mucociliary clearance of foreign material to the same degree.[66] Both methohexital[67] and thiopental are safe for asthmatic patients but do not cause bronchodilation, as ketamine does.

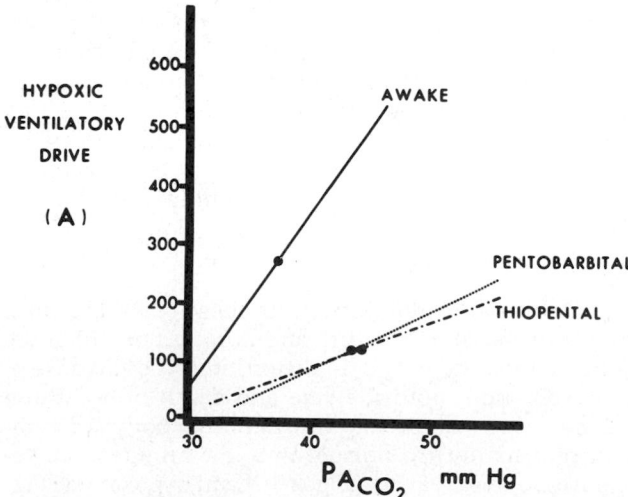

Fig. 8-11. Depression of O_2-CO_2 interaction by barbiturates. Hypoxic ventilatory drive (HVD[A]) is plotted as a function of the carbon dioxide tension (P_{ACO_2}) at which the studies were done. Each line represents the least-squares regression of about 40 studies. The circles represent the baseline P_{ACO_2} and HVD[A] obtained with each agent. (Modified from Hirshman et al.,[63] with permission.)

Cardiovascular Effects

The predominant cardiovascular effect of barbiturate induction is venodilation followed by pooling of blood in the periphery.[68] Myocardial contractility is depressed to a lesser degree than after volatile anesthetics,[69] but not by altering calcium uptake by cardiac sarcoplasmic reticulum.[70] Cardiac output decreases even though heart rate increases via the only slightly depressed baroreflex mechanism. Systemic vascular resistance usually remains unchanged. Heart rate increases more after methohexital than after equivalent doses of thiopental. No arrhythmias occur after induction of anesthesia by the barbiturates as long as hypoxemia and hypercarbia are avoided. The barbiturates also decrease sympathetic output from the CNS[71] and do not sensitize the heart to catecholamines.

Both thiopental and methohexital cause an increased heart rate, which results in an increased myocardial oxygen consumption. The arteriocoronary venous oxygen difference remains normal when aortic pressure is relatively unchanged because there is a proportional decrease in coronary vascular resistance and increase in myocardial blood flow.[72] However, if systemic pressure is low enough, coronary blood flow decreases. The barbiturates, therefore, must be used cautiously, if at all, in conditions in which an increased heart rate or a decrease in preload could be detrimental to the patient. Such conditions include pericardial tamponade, hypovolemia, congestive heart failure, ischemic heart disease, and heart block, as well as a high resting sympathetic tone or myocardial ischemia.

Hypotension from a given dose is greater in both treated and untreated hypertensive patients than in normotensive patients.[73] An exaggerated hypotensive effect probably occurs in the presence of a blunted baroreflex or β-adrenergic blockade.

Gastrointestinal, Renal, and Hepatic Effects

Normal patients and those with pre-existing liver disease have essentially no changes in gastrointestinal and liver function after barbiturate induction of anesthesia.[74] Hypoproteinemia in patients with hepatic or renal disease leads to a greater fraction of unbound thiopental than in normal patients.[75] Thus, for patients with chronic renal failure, induction doses of thiopental should be injected at a slower rate and maintenance doses should be decreased 50 to 75 percent but may have to be given more often than in healthy patients. A given dose can have a longer duration of effect in patients with hepatic failure and recovery can be more rapid in renal failure patients than in others.[76]

Thiopental can decrease urine output because it decreases blood flow to the kidney, causes renal artery constriction, and results in a small decrease in the glomerular filtration rate and urinary solute secretion.[7] Controversy exists about whether there is an increase in antidiuretic hormone secretion from the pituitary.[7,77]

Correcting hypotension and administering adequate intravenous fluids prevent the renal effects of barbiturate induction from becoming a clinical problem.

Metabolic Effects

Although there is a slight, clinically insignificant increase in blood glucose levels and impairment of the glucose tolerance test after thiopental injection, serum insulin levels do not change.[78] Heat loss results from barbiturate-induced vasodilation of cutaneous and skeletal muscle vessels, which may contribute to postoperative shivering.

Endocrine Effects

Thiopental decreases plasma cortisol concentrations but does not prevent adrenocortical stimulation from the stress of surgery[79] (Fig. 8-12). This contrasts with the effect of an induction dose of etomidate, which suppresses the adrenocortical response to stress.[79] Both thiobarbiturates cause a dose-related histamine release, in contrast to methohexital and pentobarbital[80] (Fig. 8-13), but histamine release is rarely of clinical consequence.

Obstetric Effects
(Also See Ch. 57)

Thiopental neither depresses nor increases the tone of the gravid uterus.[4] Thiopental is not harmful to the fetus when it is given for anesthetic induction for cesarean section in doses up to 6 mg/kg, but 8 mg/kg depresses the fetus.[81] Placental circulatory factors plus redistribution of thiopental in the mother and fetus protect the fetal brain and spinal cord from high concentrations of barbiturates and explain why the umbilical cord blood concentration of thiopental at delivery is one-half that in maternal blood. Safe delivery of the fetus by cesarean section is possible if accomplished within 10 minutes after anesthetic induction with either thiopental or ketamine.[82] The neonatal condition is better after thiopental induction than after midazolam induction.[83] Neurobehavioral tests showed that newborns were more depressed after mothers received thiopental than after they received ketamine or epidural anesthesia for vaginal deliveries.[84]

Drug Interactions

Barbiturates given to patients taking other CNS-depressant drugs such as ethanol, antihistamines, isoniazide, methylphenidate, and monoamine oxidase inhibitors

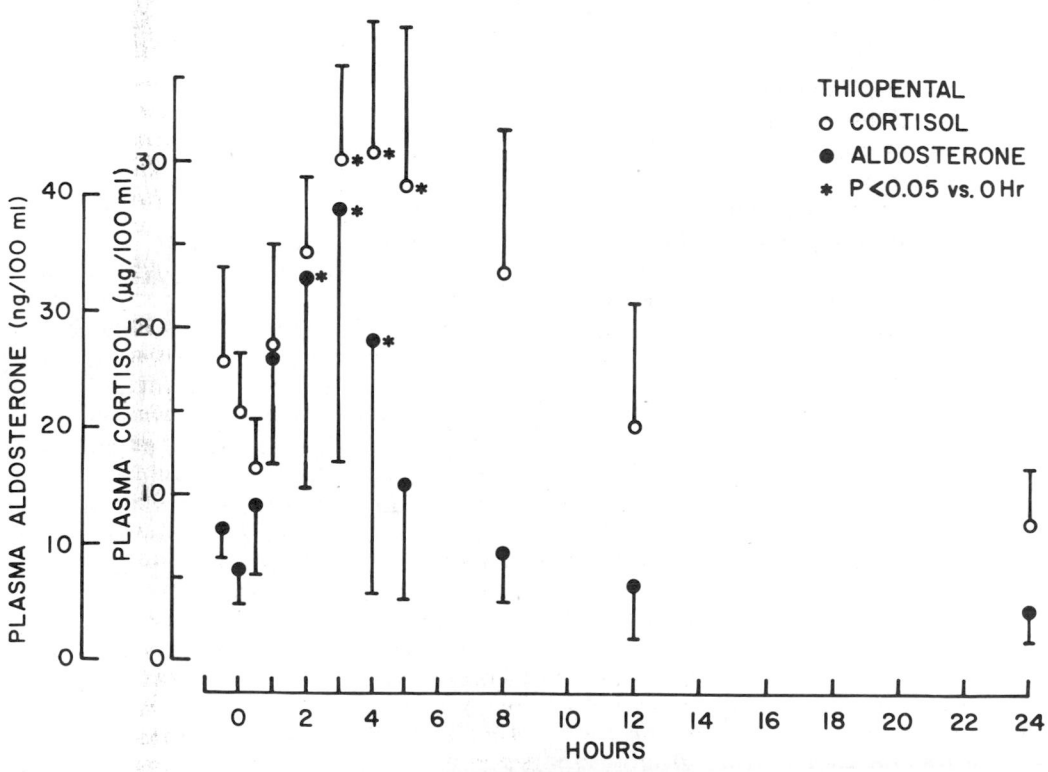

Fig. 8-12. Normal cortisol and aldosterone response after thiopental during and after general anesthesia. The adrenocortical response to stress is preserved after thiopental but is depressed after etomidate. (Data from Fragen et al.[79])

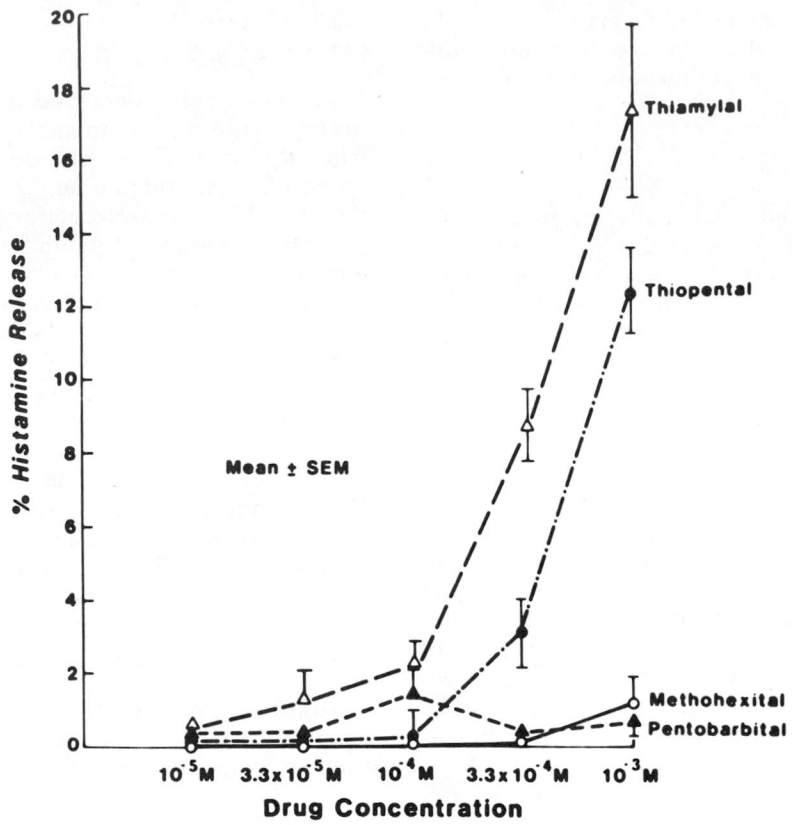

Fig. 8-13. Comparison of percent histamine release from human mast cells when in the presence of increasing concentrations of four barbiturates. Both thiobarbiturates produced significant dose-related histamine release. Histamine release by thiamylal was significantly greater than that by thiopental from 3.3×10^{-5} to 1×10^{-3} M ($P < 0.05$). (From Hirshman et al.,[80] with permission.)

cause greater CNS depression than when given alone. Concomitant administration of 5.6 mg/kg of aminophylline reduces both the depth and duration of sedation after thiopental administration.[85] Chronic barbiturate use induces hepatic microsomal enzymes, which accelerates the metabolism of other drugs metabolized by the P-450 system.[9]

Recovery

The time it takes for all CNS-depressant drug concentrations, not those of the intravenous hypnotic alone, to decrease below a particular threshold level determines the speed of recovery from general anesthesia. Recovery is rapid after many anesthetic regimens that include intravenous barbiturates. For example, if healthy patients have anesthesia induced with thiopental (4 mg/kg) and anesthesia maintained with 67 percent nitrous oxide, fentanyl (100 μg), and 50 to 100 mg increments of thiopental for operations lasting 30 minutes or less, they open their eyes in 3 to 4 minutes after the nitrous oxide is discontinued, and psychomotor tests

recover in 15 to 75 minutes.[86] This technique is satisfactory for outpatient or inpatient anesthesia.

Clinical recovery was faster in volunteers after single doses of methohexital (2 mg/kg) than after thiopental (6 mg/kg), but the ability to drive a motorized vehicle was impaired for 8 hours after methohexital compared with 6 hours after thiopental[87] (Fig. 8-14). Furthermore, psychophysiologic tests were impaired for 8 hours after thiopental, and abnormal sleep patterns on the EEG occurred for 12 hours after methohexital.[87] The recommendation that patients not drive for 24 hours after general anesthesia is based on these data.

Naloxone (0.05 mg/kg) fails to antagonize the effects of thiopental.[88] At this time, there are no specific pharmacological antagonists to treat barbiturate overdose; maintaining a patent airway, supporting ventilation, and supporting circulation are the appropriate symptomatic treatments.

Postoperative Sequelae

Venous sequelae include thrombosis and phlebitis and may not be seen until a few days postoperatively. Three

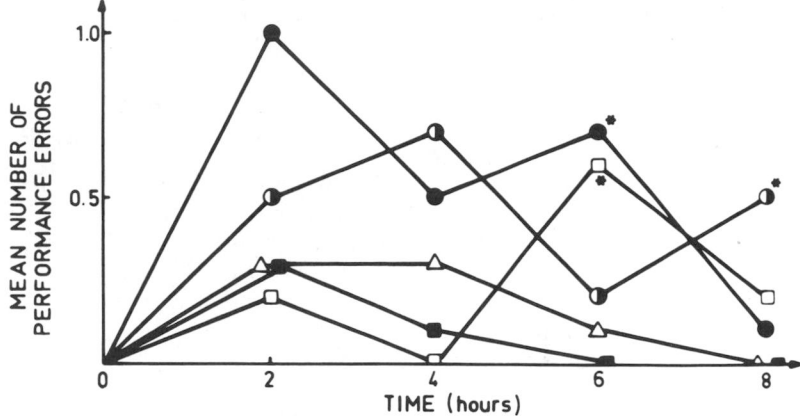

Fig. 8-14. Mean number of performance errors (neglected instructions, collisions, and driving off the road) during 30 minutes of simulated driving 2 to 8 hours after administration of 6 mg/kg of thiopental (●) 2 mg/kg of methohexital (◑), 6.6 mg/kg of propanidid (△), and 85 μl/kg of alphadione (□). Ten subjects in each group. *, $P < 0.05$ in comparison with control group (■). (From Korttila et al.,[87] with permission.)

to 4 percent of patients receiving thiopental and a slightly higher proportion after methohexital report venous thrombosis.[89] An idea of the overall incidence of venous sequelae after barbiturates compared with other induction agents is shown in Table 8-4. Venous sequelae are usually confined to an area of the vein in close proximity to the site of injection; they are treated symptomatically.

There are four reported cases of inadvertent epidural injections of up to 20 ml of 2 to 2.5 percent solutions of thiopental. The patients were successfully treated by injecting 0.5 percent bupivicaine into the epidural space to dilute thiopental and attempt to precipitate it.[90] Methohexital (1 percent) injected epidurally was treated with an epidural injection of saline plus methylprednisolone and hyaluronidase; no sequelae occurred.[91]

The low incidence of nausea and vomiting after barbiturate anesthesia is less than after inhaled anes-

thetics, ketamine, or etomidate, but the incidence is even lower after midazolam or propofol.[4]

Paralysis and death can occur if barbiturates are given to patients with acute intermittant porphyria or variegate porphyria. Barbiturates can precipitate acute and even fatal attacks of porphyria owing to the induction of δ-aminolevulinic acid synthetase, which catalyzes the rate-limiting step in the biosynthesis of porphyrins.[92]

ADMINISTRATION OF BARBITURATES BY INFUSIONS

Barbiturates administered by a continuous infusion for maintenance of hypnosis are seldom used for anesthesia because they may prolong recovery if improperly used. Crankshaw et al.[40] believe that thiopental can be used successfully as a major component of an anes-

TABLE 8-4. Incidence of Venous Sequelae after Intravenous Injection of Anesthetics

Drug	Solvent	Concentration (%)	No. of Patients Studied	Venous Sequelae	
				Day 3	Day 10
Thiopental	Water	5	307	6	0
Thiopental	Water	2.5	252	8	0
Methohexital	Water	2	251	6	NA
Methohexital	Water	1	203	3	NA
Etomidate	Propylene glycol	0.2	109	23	NA
Diazepam	Propylene glycol	0.5	44	23	39
Midazolam	Water	0.5	50	2	8
Lorazepam	Propylene glycol Polyethylene glycol	0.1	40	8	15

Abbreviation: NA, data unavailable.
(Modified from Clarke,[53] with permission.)

thetic technique when it is given as an exponential infusion based on lean body mass to prevent overdose in heavier patients. A successful infusion achieves a blood concentration of 15 to 20 μg/ml on induction and 10 to 20 μg/ml during maintenance. The mean plasma concentration at awakening is 5.9 ± 1.1 μg/ml. By determining "plasma drug efflux," which takes into consideration all drug movement from the plasma, Crankshaw et al.[93] could rapidly achieve and maintain a steady plasma concentration of thiopental and methohexital. Schwilden et al.[24] developed a combined pharmacokinetic-pharmacodynamic model to provide a closed-loop feedback control method of delivering methohexital to maintain a set EEG level and unconsciousness. Thiopental infusions of 2 to 3 mg/kg/h have been used to treat refractory aminophylline seizures and to control a hyperdynamic state after coronary bypass surgery.[94]

OTHER USES OF BARBITURATES

Anticonvulsants

Both thiopental and phenobarbital can stop seizures abruptly in patients refractory to other anticonvulsant drugs,[95] but benzodiazepines have largely replaced them for the acute treatment of seizures. GABA augmentors have anticonvulsant effects, and both barbiturates and benzodiazepines facilitate the action of GABA[96] to prolong hyperpolarization of the postsynaptic membrane. Other postsynaptic effects include altered membrane conductance of chloride ions and antagonism of glutaminergic and cholinergic excitation. Presynaptically, these drugs block calcium entry into nerve terminals and diminish transmitter release.[97] Barbiturates also increase the threshold of normal brain structures during electrically induced afterdischarges and inhibit the kindling process more effectively than do other antiepileptic drugs. Furthermore, small barbiturate doses can reduce seizure activity by increasing beta activity in the EEG.[97] Table 8-5 shows a dose schedule for phenobarbital treatment of seizures in different age groups with or without concomitant phenytoin therapy. The phenobarbital dose should be reduced in patients with hepatic or renal disease because a given dose can produce significantly higher blood concentrations in those patients.

Brain Protection
(Also See Chs. 19 and 54)

A number of actions of the barbiturates on the CNS can protect the brain in some clinical situations.[4] They decrease cerebral metabolism in areas of high brain activity until the EEG becomes flat, after which no further suppression occurs even with an increased dose. This decrease is nonlinear (Fig. 8-15) during a thiopental infusion.[98] Other barbiturate protective actions include an inverse steal in which vasoconstriction in healthy areas of the brain shunts blood to diseased areas; a reduction of intracranial pressure and an increase in cerebral perfusion pressure; stabilization of liposomal membranes; free radical scavenging; and an anticonvulsant effect. However, arterial hypotension must be avoided to maintain adequate cerebral perfusion pressure. The depression of cerebral metabolism neither alters the concentration of lactate, pyruvate, phosphocreatine, or adenosine triphosphate (ATP) nor does it have important effects on the pathways of cerebral glucose metabolism.[99]

In animals, doses of thiopental sufficient to suppress EEG activity are more likely to cause hypotension or ventricular fibrillation than are equivalent doses of pentobarbital.[100] High doses of methohexital cause depression of mean arterial pressure, cerebral blood flow, and cerebral metabolism; thiopental has similar effects at equivalent EEG suppression. Methohexital causes less cerebral vasoconstriction, has less effect on cerebral metabolism, and causes blood flow to return toward control values more rapidly than equivalent doses of thiopental.[101]

In primates, barbiturates decrease cerebral infarction size after focal cerebral artery occlusion but offer no benefit after stroke or cardiac arrest.[99] In humans, thiopental provides protection if a 40 mg/kg dose, sufficient to maintain a flat EEG, is given to patients having cardiac valvular surgery likely to have neuropsychiatric complications of emboli after normothermic cardiopulmonary bypass. However, these patients awaken more slowly and need more ionotropic support than untreated patients.[102] Thiopental may also protect

TABLE 8-5. Dose Structure of Antiseizure Phenobarbital Therapy

Age of Patient	t½β (h)	Loading Dose (IV) (mg/kg)[a]	Maintenance Dose (PO) (mg/kg/d)
Neonate (<1 mon)	63–98	15–20	3–4[b]
Infant (<1 yr)	47 ± 8	8–15	3–4
Child (<15 yrs)	37–73	8–20	1–4
Adult	64–141	8–20	1–3

[a] Can be administered at a rate of less than 100 mg/min not to exceed a total dose of 1,500 mg.
[b] Can also be given intramuscularly.
Abbreviations: IV, intravenous; PO, orally.
(From Vining,[97] with permission.)

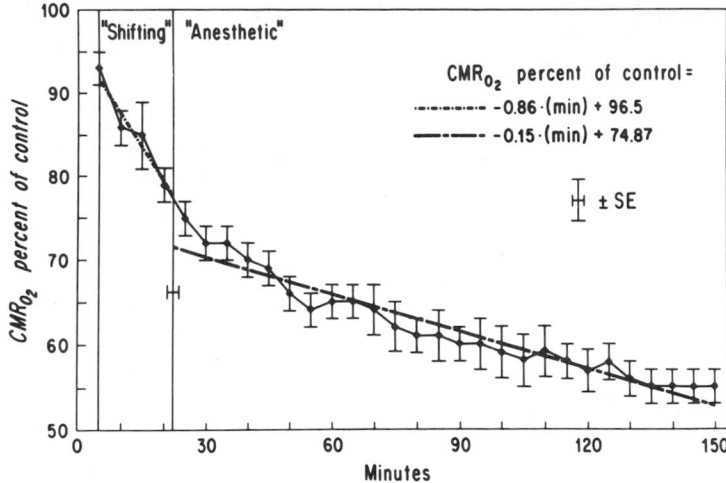

Fig. 8-15. Effect of thiopental on $CMRO_2$. $CMRO_2$ (percent of control) is plotted versus total dose of thiopental infused over time. Regression lines from changes in $CMRO_2$ are drawn for each EEG-determined area; for example, a decrease to 77 percent of control when the EEG is shifting and a slower decrease when an anesthetic pattern appears. (From Stulken et al.,[98] with permission.)

poorly perfused areas of the brain in patients with increased ICP secondary to carotid endarterectomy, thoracic aneurysm, and profound controlled hypotension.[103] Barbiturates may provide important brain protection for young patients by reducing hyperemic response to head injury,[104] but in adults they have failed to protect the brain after head trauma[105] and cardiac arrest.

Wada Test

A small dose of sodium amytal can be injected into the carotid artery to lateralize cerebral speech dominance in neurosurgical patients; this is known as the Wada test.[106] An alternative is injection of methohexital (3 to 5 mg) after a 1-mg test dose.[107]

Electroconvulsive Therapy

Methohexital is a better intravenous hypnotic for electroconvulsive therapy than propofol because propofol shortens the seizure duration.[108] It is better than thio-pental because transient premature atrial and ventricular contractions occur less frequently after methohexital whether or not atropine is used for pre-medication.[109]

SUMMARY

The actions of thiopental and other barbiturates have not changed since they were first used by anesthesiologists. However, our understanding of their pharmacokinetics and mechanisms of action have changed. We also have a better understanding of how the barbiturates affect the various body systems, enabling us to use these drugs most effectively, yet with minimum side effects. Comparing the anesthetic barbiturates to other sedative-hypnotics used to induce general anesthesia (Table 8-6) puts in perspective their important clinical properties.[110] Although thiopental is not the ideal intravenous drug to induce general anesthesia, its long-standing position as the standard anesthetic induction agent stems from its lack of major disadvantages.

TABLE 8-6. Summary of the Important Clinical Properties of the Intravenous Sedative-Hypnotics Used for Anesthetic Induction[a]

	Predictability of Induction	Induction Pain and Excitement	Cerebral Effects	Respiratory Effects	Cardiovascular Effects	Recovery Characteristics
Thiopental	+	0	+	−	−	+
Thiamylal	+	0	+	−	−	+
Methohexital	+	−	+	−	−	+
Etomidate	+	− −	+	0	+	−
Propofol	+	−	+	−	−	++
Ketamine	+	0	−	+	−	− −
Diazepam	−	− −	+	0	0	+
Midazolam	0	0	+	0	0	+

[a] ++ to − − is a five-point qualitative scale describing the relative positive (+, ++), neutral (0), or negative (−, − −) effect of each agent in each category. (From Fragen and Avram,[110] with permission.)

REFERENCES

1. Dundee JW: Historical vignettes and classification of intravenous anesthetics. p. 1. In Aldrete JA, Stanley TH (eds): Trends in Intravenous Anesthesia. Year Book Medical Publishers, Chicago, 1980

2. Dundee JW: Fifty years of thiopentone. Br J Anaesth 56:211, 1984

3. Halford FJ: A critique of intravenous anesthesia in war surgery. Anesthesiology 4:67, 1943

4. Dundee JW, Wyant GM: Intravenous Anaesthesia. 2nd Ed. Churchill Livingstone, New York, 1988

5. Brodie BB, Mark LC, Papper EM, et al: The fate of thiopental in man and a method for its estimation in biological material. J Pharmacol Exp Ther 98:85, 1950

6. Price HL: A dynamic concept of the distribution of thiopental in the human body. Anesthesiology 21:40, 1960

7. Guerra F: Thiopental forever after. p. 143. In Aldrete JA, Stanley TH (eds): Trends in Intravenous Anesthesia. Year Book Medical Publishers, Chicago, 1980

8. Dundee JW: Molecular structure-activity relationships of barbiturates. p. 16. In Halsey MJ, Millar RA, Sutton JA (eds): Molecular Mechanisms in General Anesthesia. Churchill Livingstone, New York, 1974

9. Harvey SC: Hypnotics and sedatives. p. 339. In Gilman AG, Goodman LS, Rall TW, Murad F (eds): Goodman and Gilman's The Pharmacological Basis of Therapeutics. MacMillan, New York, 1985

10. Andrews PR, Mark LC: Structural specificity of barbiturates and related drugs. Anesthesiology 57:314, 1982

11. Gibson WR, Doran WJ, Wood WC, Swanson EE: Pharmacology of steroisomers of 1-methyl-5-(1-methyl-2-pentynyl)-5-allyl barbituric acid. J Pharmacol Exp Ther 125:23, 1959

12. Ariëns EJ: Stereochemistry, a basis for sophisticated nonsense in pharmacokinetics and clinical pharmacology. Eur J Clin Pharmacol 26:663, 1984

13. Olson RW: Barbiturates. Int Anesthesiol Clin 26:254, 1988

14. Olson RW, Fischer JB, Dunwiddie TV: Barbiturate enhancement of γ-aminobutyric acid receptor binding and function as a mechanism of anesthesia. p. 165. In Roth SH, Miller KW (eds): Molecular and Cellular Mechanisms of Anesthetics. Plenum, New York, 1986

15. Olson RW: GABA-benzodiazepine-barbiturate receptor interactions. J Neurochem 37:1, 1981

16. Price HL, Kovnat PJ, Safer JN, et al: The uptake of thiopental by body tissues and its relation to the duration of narcosis. Clin Pharmacol Ther 1:16, 1960

17. Bischoff KB, Dedrick RL: Thiopental pharmacokinetics. J Pharm Sci 57:1346, 1968

18. Henthorn TK, Avram MJ, Krejcie TC: Intravascular mixing and drug distribution: The concurrent disposition of thiopental and indocyanine green. Clin Pharmacol Ther 45:56, 1989

19. Hudson RJ, Stanski DR, Burch PG: Pharmacokinetics of methohexital and thiopental in surgical patients. Anesthesiology 59:215, 1983

20. Burch PG, Stanski DR: The role of metabolism and protein binding in thiopental anesthesia. Anesthesiology 58:146, 1983

21. Stanski DR, Mihm FG, Rosenthal MH, Kalman SM: Pharmacokinetics of high dose thiopental used in cerebral resuscitation. Anesthesiology 53:169, 1980

22. Stanski DR, Hudson RJ, Homer TD, et al: Pharmacodynamic modeling of thiopental anesthesia. J Pharmacokinet Biopharm 12:223, 1984

23. Bührer M, Maitre PO, Ebling WF, Stanski DR: Defining thiopental's steady state plasma concentration-EEG effect relationships. Anesthesiology 67A:399, 1987

24. Schwilden H, Schüttler J, Stoeckel H: Closed-loop feedback control of methohexital anesthesia by quantitative EEG analysis in humans. Anesthesiology 67:341, 1987

25. Thomas DW, Runciman WB: Monitoring depth of anesthesia. Anaesth Intensive Care 16:69, 1988

26. Dingemanse J, Danhof M, Breimer DD: Pharmacokinetic-pharmacodynamic modeling of CNS drug effects: An overview. Pharmacol Ther 38:1, 1988

27. Benowitz N, Forsyth RP, Melmon KL, Rowland M: Lidocaine disposition kinetics in monkey and man. II. Effects of hemorrhage and sympathomimetic drug administration. Clin Pharmacol Ther 16:99, 1974

28. Dundee JW: The influence of body weight, sex and age on the dosage of thiopentone. Br J Anaesth 26:164, 1954

29. Christensen JH, Andreasen F: Individual variation in response to thiopental. Acta Anaesthesiol Scand 22:303, 1978

30. Homer TD, Stanski DR: The effect of increasing age on thiopental disposition and anesthetic requirement. Anesthesiology 62:714, 1985

31. Jung D, Mayersohn M, Perrier D, et al: Thiopental disposition as a function of age in female patients undergoing surgery. Anesthesiology 56:263, 1982

32. Christensen JH, Andreasen F, Jansen JA: Pharmacokinetics and pharmacodynamics of thiopentone a comparison between young and elderly patients. Anaesthesia 37:398, 1982

33. Krejcie TC, Henthorn TK, Avram MJ, Morton DL: Thiopental kinetics and age: A reassessment. Anesthesiology 57A:664, 1987

34. Wulfsohn NL, Joshi CW: Thiopentone dosage based on lean body mass. Br J Anaesth 41:516, 1969

35. Bruce Å, Andersson M, Arvidsson B, Isaksson B: Body composition. Prediction of normal body potassium, body water and body fat in adults on the basis of body height, body weight, and age. Scand J Clin Lab Invest 40:461, 1980

36. Brodie BB, Mark LC, Lief PA, et al: Acute tolerance to thiopental. J Pharmacol Exp Ther 102:215, 1951

37. Dundee JW, Price HL, Dripps RD: Acute tolerance to thiopentone in man. Br J Anaesth 28:344, 1956

38. Toner W, Howard PJ, McGowan WAW, Dundee JW: Another look at acute tolerance to thiopentone. Br J Anaesth 52:1005, 1980

39. Hudson RJ, Stanski DR, Saidman LJ, Meathe E: A model for studying depth of anesthesia and acute tolerance to thiopental. Anesthesiology 59:301, 1983

40. Crankshaw DP, Edwards NE, Blackman GL, et al: Evaluation of infusion regimens for thiopentone as a primary anaesthetic agent. Eur J Clin Pharmacol 28:543, 1985

41. Barrett R, Graham GG, Torda TA: The influence of sampling site upon the distribution phase kinetics of thiopentone. Anaesth Intensive Care 12:5, 1984

42. Barratt RL, Graham GG, Torda TA: Kinetics of thiopentone in relation to the site of sampling. Br J Anaesth 56:1385, 1984

43. deJong RH, Heavner JE: Local anesthetic seizure prevention: Diazepam versus pentobarbital. Anesthesiology 36:449, 1972

44. Forrest WH, Jr., Brown CR, Brown BW: Subjective responses to six common preoperative medications. Anesthesiology 47:241, 1977

45. Eger EI II, Kraft ID, Keasling HH: A comparison of atropine or scopolamine, plus pentobarbital, meperidine, or morphine as preanesthetic medication. Anesthesiology 22:962, 1961

46. Liu LMP, Gaudreault P, Friedman PA, et al: Methohexital plasma concentrations in children following rectal administration. Anesthesiology 62:567, 1985

47. Jonmarker C, Westrin P, Larsson S, Werner O: Thiopental requirements for induction of anesthesia in children. Anesthesiology 67:104, 1987

48. Dundee JW, Hassard TH, McGowen WAW, Henshaw J: The 'induction' dose of thiopentone. A method of study and preliminary illustrative results. Anaesthesia 37:1176, 1982

49. Tovall RM: A comparative clinical and statistical study of thiopental and thiamylal in human anesthesia. Anesthesiology 16:910, 1965

50. Thompson DS, Eason CN, Flacke JW: Thiamylal anaphylaxis. Anesthesiology 39:556, 1973

51. Whitwam JG: Methohexitone. Br J Anaesth 48:641, 1976

52. Stone HH, Donnelly CC. The accidental intra-arterial injection of thiopental. Anesthesiology 22:995, 1961

53. Clarke RSJ: Adverse effects of intravenously administered drugs used in anaesthetic practice. Drugs 22:26, 1981

54. Kiersey DK, Bickford RG, Faulkner A: Electroencephalographic patterns produced by thiopental sodium during surgical operations: Description and classification. Br J Anaesth 23:141, 1951

55. Turcant A, Delhumeau A, Premel-Cabic A, et al: Thiopental pharmacokinetics under conditions of long-term infusions. Anesthesiology 63:50, 1985

56. Rockhoff MA, Marshall LF, Shapiro HM: High dose barbiturate therapy in humans. Ann Neurol 6:194, 1979

57. Albrecht RF, Miletich DJ, Rosenberg R, et al: Cerebral blood flow and metabolic changes from induction to onset of anesthesia with halothane or pentobarbital. Anesthesiology 47:252, 1977

58. Gumpert J, Paul R: Activation of the electroencephalogram with intravenous brietal (methohexitone): The findings in 100 cases. J Neurol Neurosurg Psychiatry 34:646, 1971

59. Todd MM, Drummond JC, Sang H: The hemodynamic consequences of high-dose methohexital anesthesia in humans. Anesthesiology 61:495, 1984

60. Drummond JC, Todd MM, U HS: The effect of high-dose sodium thiopental in brain stem auditory and median nerve somatosensory evoked responses in humans. Anesthesiology 63:249, 1985

61. McPherson RW, Sell B, Traystman RJ: Effects of thiopental, fentanyl, and etomidate in upper extremity somatosensory evoked potentials in humans. Anesthesiology 65:584, 1986

62. Joshi C, Bruce DL: Thiopental and succinylcholine action on intraocular pressure. Anesth Analg 54:471, 1975

63. Hirshman CA, McCullough RE, Cohen PJ, et al: Hypoxic ventilatory drive in dogs during thiopental, ketamine, or pentobarbital anesthesia. Anesthesiology 43:628, 1975

64. McCullough RE, Cohen PJ, Weil JV: Effect of pentobarbitone on hypoxic ventilatory drive in man: Preliminary study. Br J Anaesth 47:963, 1975

65. Harrison GA: The influence of different anesthetic agents on the response to respiratory tract irritation. Br J Anaesth 34:804, 1962

66. Forbes AR, Gamsu G: Depression of lung mucociliary clearance by thiopental and halothane. Anesth Analg 58:387, 1979

67. Taylor C, Stoelting VK: Methohexital sodium—a new ultrashort acting barbiturate. Anesthesiology 21:29, 1960

68. Eckstein JW, Hamilton WK, McCammond JM: The effect of thiopental on peripheral venous tone. Anesthesiology 22:525, 1961

69. Frankle WS, Pool-Wilson PA: Effects of thiopental on tension development, action potential, and exchange of calcium and

70. potassium in rabbit ventricular myocardium. J Cardiovasc Pharmacol 3:554, 1981

70. Blank TJJ, Stevenson RL: Thiopental does not alter Ca^{2+} uptake by cardiac sarcoplasmic reticulum. Anesth Analg 67:346, 1988

71. Skovsted P, Price ML, Price HL: The effects of short-acting barbiturates on arterial pressure, preganglionic sympathetic activity and barostatic reflexes. Anesthesiology 33:10, 1970

72. Kettler D, Sonntag H, Wolfram-Donath U, et al: Haemodynamics, myocardial function, oxygen requirements, and supply of the human heart after administration of etomidate. p.81. In Doenicke A (ed): Anesthesiology and Resuscitation. Etomidate, an Intravenous Hypnotic Agent. Springer-Verlag, Berlin, 1977

73. Prys-Roberts C: Cardiovascular and ventilatory effects of intravenous anaesthetics. Clin Anaesth 2:203, 1984

74. Bittrick NM, Kane AVR, Mosher RE: Methohexital and its effect on liver function tests. Anesthesiology 24:81, 1963

75. Ghoneim MM, Pandya H: Plasma protein binding of thiopental in patients with impaired renal or hepatic function. Anesthesiology 42:545, 1975

76. Hudson RJ, Stanski DR: Barbiturates—pharmacokinetics and pharmacodynamics. Clin Anaesth 2:27, 1984

77. Marsland AR, Bradley JP: Anaesthesia for renal transplantation—5 years experience. Anaesth Intensive Care 11:337, 1983

78. Kaniaris P, Katsilambros N, Castanas E, et al: Relation between glucose tolerance and serum insulin levels in man before and after thiopental intravenous administration. Anesth Analg 54:718, 1975

79. Fragen RJ, Shanks CA, Molteni A, Avram MJ: Effects of etomidate on hormonal responses to surgical stress. Anesthesiology 61:652, 1984

80. Hirshman CA, Edelstein RA, Ebertz JM, Hanifin JM: Thiobarbiturate-induced histamine release in human mast cells. Anesthesiology 63:353, 1985

81. Kosaka Y, Takahashi T, Mark LC: Intravenous thiobarbiturate anesthesia for cesarean section. Anesthesiology 31:489, 1969

82. Bernstein K, Gisselsson SL, Jacobson L, Ohrlander S: Influence of two different anaesthetic agents on the newborn and the correlation between foetal oxygenation and induction-delivery time in elective caesarean section. Acta Anaesthesiol Scand 29:157, 1985

83. Bland BAR, Lawes EG, Duncan PW, et al: Comparison of midazolam and thiopental for rapid sequence anesthetic induction for elective cesarean section. Anesth Analg 66:1165, 1987

84. Hodgkinson R, Marx GF, Kim SS, et al: Neonatal neurobehavioral tests following vaginal delivery under ketamine, thiopental, and extradural anesthesia. Anesth Analg 56:548, 1977

85. Krintel JJ, Wegmann F: Aminophylline reduces the depth and duration of sedation with barbiturates. Acta Anaesthesiol Scand 31:352, 1987

86. Fragen RJ, Caldwell N: Comparison of a new formula of etomidate with thiopental—side effects and awakening times. Anesthesiology 50:242, 1979

87. Korttila K, Linnoila M, Ertama P, et al: Recovery and simulated driving after intravenous anesthesia with thiopental, methohexital, propanidid, or alphadione. Anesthesiology 43:291, 1975

88. Duncalf D, Nagashima H, Duncalf RM: Naloxone fails to antagonize thiopental anesthesia. Anesth Analg 57:558, 1978

89. O'Donnell JF, Hewitt JC, Dundee JW: Clinical studies of in-

duction agents. XXVIII. A further comparison of venous complications following thiopentone, methohexitone and propanidid. Br J Anaesth 41:681, 1969

90. Cay DL: Accidental epidural thiopentone. Anaesth Intensive Care 12:61, 1984

91. Wells D, Davies G, Wagner D: Accidental injection of epidural methohexital. Anesthesiology 67:846, 1987

92. Remmer H: The role of the liver in drug metabolism. Am J Med 49:617, 1970

93. Crankshaw DP, Boyd MD, Bjorksten AR: Plasma drug efflux —a new approach to optimization of drug infusion for constant blood concentration of thiopental and methohexital. Anesthesiology 67:32, 1987

94. Katz RI, Skeen JT, Quartararo C, Poppers PJ: Varied uses of a thiopental infusion. Anesth Analg 66:1328, 1987

95. Young GB, Blume WT, Bolton CF, Warren KG: Anesthetic barbiturates in refractory status epilepticus. J Sci Neurol 7:291, 1980

96. Olsen RW, Snowman AM, Lee R, et al: Role of the gamma-aminobutyric acid receptor-ionophore complex in seizure disorders. Ann Neurol 16:S90, 1984

97. Vining EPG: Uses of barbiturates and benzodiazepines in treatment of epilepsy. Neurol Clin 4:617, 1986

98. Stulken EH, Jr., Milde JH, Michenfelder JD, Tinker JH: The nonlinear response of cerebral metabolism to low concentrations of halothane, enflurane, isoflurane and thiopental. Anesthesiology 46:28, 1977

99. Smith AL: Barbiturate protection in cerebral hypoxia. Anesthesiology 47:285, 1977

100. Roesch C, Haselby KA, Paradise RP, et al: Comparison of cardiovascular effect of thiopental and pentobarbital at equivalent levels of CNS depression. Anesth Analg 62:749, 1983

101. Boarini DJ, Kassel NF, Coester HC: Comparison of sodium thiopental and methohexital for high-dose barbiturate anesthesia. J Neurosurg 60:602, 1984

102. Nussmeier NA, Arlund C, Slogoff S: Neuropsychiatric complications after cardiopulmonary bypass. Cerebral protection by a barbiturate. Anesthesiology 64:165, 1986

103. Bedford RF, Persing JA, Potereskin L, Butler A: Lidocaine or thiopental for rapid control of intracranial hypertension. Anesth Analg 59:435, 1986

104. Aitkenhead AR: Do barbiturates protect the brain? Br J Anaesth 53:1011, 1981

105. Ward JD, Becker DP, Miller DJ, et al: Failure of prophylactic barbiturate coma in the treatment of severe head trauma. J Neurosurg 62:383, 1985

106. Wada J, Rasmussen T: Intracarotid injection of sodium amytal for the lateralization of cerebral speech dominance. Experimental and clinical observations. J Neurosurg 17:266, 1960

107. Willmore LJ, Wilder BJ, Mayersdorf A, et al: Identification of speech lateralization by intracarotid injection of methohexital. Ann Neurol 4:86, 1978

108. Simpson KH, Halsall PJ, Carr CME, Stewart KG: Propofol reduces seizure duration in patients having anaesthesia for electroconvulsive therapy. Br J Anaesth 61:343, 1988

109. Mokriske BLK, Nagle SE, Cohen SM, et al: ECT induced cardiac arrhythmias during anesthesia with different barbiturates. Anesthesiology 69A:617, 1988

110. Fragen RJ, Avram MJ: Comparative pharmacology of drugs used for the induction of anesthesia. p. 303. In Stoelting RR, Barash PG, Gallagher TJ (eds): Advances in Anesthesia. Year Book Medical Publishers, Chicago, 1986

9
NONBARBITURATE INTRAVENOUS ANESTHETICS

J. G. Reves
Peter S. A. Glass

INTRODUCTION

The introduction of thiopental into clinical practice in 1934 was the advent of intravenous anesthesia. Thiopental and other barbiturates, however, are not ideal intravenous anesthetics primarily because they provide only hypnosis (see Ch. 8). The ideal intravenous anesthetic would provide hypnosis, amnesia, and analgesia. Thus, many other drugs have been used that offer some of or all these properties. These drugs have been introduced steadily into clinical practice with varying degrees of acceptance, but none has truly replaced thiopental as the most widely used intravenous anesthetic drug. With the increasing number of compounds, the use of intravenous anesthetics continues to grow.

The future of anesthetic management probably involves the use of several drugs used together, including inhaled anesthetics with intravenous drugs. A recent survey of mortality in 100,000 anesthetics reveals that practice of combined anesthetic drug use may be safer than the use of only one or two drugs,[1] the relative odds of dying within 7 days was 2.9 times greater when two or one anesthetic drugs were used compared to three or more. Although it is exceedingly difficult to interpret these data, the use of several drugs may be beneficial to anesthetic care. Thus the skillful use of multiple intravenous anesthetics is not only possible but perhaps preferable in the optimal care of patients. The purpose of this chapter is to provide information on the major nonbarbiturate and nonopioid intravenous anesthetic drugs available for use in practice today.

BENZODIAZEPINES

History

Benzodiazepines were discovered accidentally to be effective sedative-hypnotic drugs.[2] Sternbach synthesized chlordiazepoxide (Librium) in 1955, but it was discarded without testing because it was considered inert. However, in 1957 it was discovered to have entirely unexpected "hypnotic, sedative, and antistrichnine effects in mice."[3] This first benzodiazepine was released for oral use in 1960, and in that year it was clear that with sufficiently large doses, chlordiazepoxide possessed profound hypnotic and amnestic properties, al-

though it was not available in parenteral form for use in anesthesia. A patient who was taking chlordiazepoxide was reported to fall and fracture her sacrum accidentally,[4] thus anticipating the use of benzodiazepines for anesthesia before trauma surgery. Diazepam was synthesized by Sternbach in 1959 in search of a new and better compound. Oxazepam (Serax) is a metabolite of diazepam (Valium) that was synthesized in 1961 by Bell, and was marketed by a different pharmaceutical company. Lorazepam (Ativan) is a 2'-chloro substitution of oxazepam that was synthesized in 1971 in an attempt to produce a more potent benzodiazepine. The next major achievement was the synthesis of midazolam (Versed) in 1976 by Fryer and Walser as the first clinically used water-soluble benzodiazepine.[5] It is not certain when benzodiazepines were first used to induce anesthesia, but in 1966 several groups reported the use of diazepam for anesthesia.[6-8] Midazolam was the first benzodiazepine that was produced primarily for use in anesthesia.[9]

The benzodiazepines as a class of drugs produce many of the characteristics sought by anesthesiologists for anesthesia. They produce their actions by occupying the benzodiazepine receptor. The benzodiazepine receptor (BZR) was first discussed in December 1971 in Milan.[10] Barnett and Fiore explained experimental observations termed "diazepam acute tolerance," as mediated by a less-active metabolite occupying a benzodiazepine receptor so that subsequent administrations of diazepam were less effective.[11] In 1977, specific benzodiazepine receptors were described when ligands were found to interact with a central receptor.[12,13] The discovery and understanding of the mechanism of the benzodiazepine receptor has enabled chemists to develop many agonist compounds and even produce a specific antagonist for clinical use.

Physicochemical Characteristics

Three benzodiazepine receptor agonists are commonly used in the practice of anesthesia in the United States. These are midazolam, diazepam, and lorazepam (Fig. 9-1 and Table 9-1). All of these compounds are relatively small and are lipid soluble at physiologic pH. Each milliliter of diazepam solution (5 mg) contains propylene glycol 0.4 ml, alcohol 0.1 ml, benzyl alcohol 0.015 ml, and sodium benzoate/benzoic acid in water for injec-

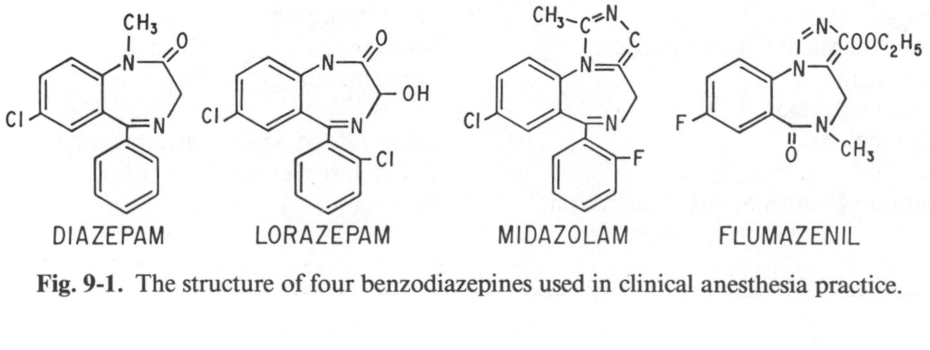

Fig. 9-1. The structure of four benzodiazepines used in clinical anesthesia practice.

TABLE 9-1. Physicochemical Characterization of Three Benzodiazepines

	Diazepam	Lorazepam	Midazolam
Mol. wt.	284.7[a]	321.2[a]	362[a]
pKa	3.3 (20°)	11.5 (20°)	6.2 (20°)[a]
Water soluble	No[a]	Almost insoluble	Yes[b]
Lipid soluble	Yes,[a] highly lipophilic	Yes (less no however), relatively less lipophilic	Yes,[b] highly lipophilic

[a] Data from Moffet.[370]

[b] pH dependent: pH > 4 = lipid soluble, pH < 4 = water soluble.

tion (pH 6.2–6.9). Lorazepam solution (2 or 4 mg/ml) contains 0.18 ml polyethylene glycol with 2 percent benzyl alcohol as a preservative. Midazolam solution contains 1 mg or 5 mg of midazolam per ml with 0.8 percent sodium chloride and 0.1 percent disodium edetate with 1 percent benzyl alcohol as a preservative. The pH is adjusted to 3 with hydrochloric acid and sodium hydroxide. Midazolam is the most lipid soluble of the three in vivo,[14] but because of its pH-dependent solubility, it is water soluble as formulated in a buffered acidic medium (pH 3.5). The imidazole ring of midazolam accounts for its stability in solution and rapid metabolism. The high lipophilicity of all three accounts for the rapid central nervous system (CNS) effect as well as their relatively large volumes of distribution.[15]

Metabolism

Biotransformation of the benzodiazepines occurs in the liver. The two principal pathways involve either hepatic microsomal oxidation (*N*-dealkylation or aliphatic hydroxylation) or glucuronide conjugation.[2,16] The difference in the two pathways is significant because oxidation is susceptible to outside influences and can be impaired by certain population characteristics (such as old age), disease states (such as hepatic cirrhosis), or the coadministration of other drugs that can impair oxidizing capacity (such as cimetidine). Conjugation is less susceptible to these factors.[2] Both midazolam and diazepam undergo oxidation-reduction or phase I reactions

in the liver.[17] Lorazepam is less affected by enzyme induction and some of the other factors known to alter the cytochrome P-450 and other phase I enzymes. For example, cimetidine inhibition of oxidative enzyme function impairs the clearance of diazepam,[18] but has no effect on lorazepam.[17] Age decreases and smoking increases the clearance of diazepam,[19] but neither have a significant effect on midazolam biotransformation.[19] Habitual alcohol consumption increases the clearance of midazolam,[20] meaning that patients with chronic ethanol use may require more midazolam for maintenance of anesthesia. The fused imidazole ring of midazolam is oxidized very rapidly by the liver, much more rapidly than the methylene group of the diazepine ring of other benzodiazepines. This accounts for the greater hepatic clearance of midazolam compared to diazepam.

The metabolites of the benzodiazepines can be important. Diazepam forms two active metabolites, oxazepam and desmethyldiazepam, both of which add to and prolong its effects. Midazolam is biotransformed to hydroxymidazolams, which have little activity.[21] Lorazepam has five metabolites, but the principal one is conjugated to glucuronide. This metabolite is inactive, water soluble, and rapidly excreted via the kidney.

Pharmacokinetics

The three benzodiazepines used in anesthesia are classified as short (midazolam), intermediate (lorazepam), and long lasting (diazepam) according to their metabolism and plasma clearance.[19,22] (Table 9-2) All the benzodiazepines plasma disappearance curves can be fitted to a two or three compartment model. Protein binding and volumes of distribution are not importantly different among these three benzodiazepines, but the clearance is significantly different. The clearance of midazolam ranges between 6 and 11 ml/kg/min whereas lorazepam is 0.8 to 1.8 ml/kg/min and diazepam is 0.2 to 0.5 ml/kg/min.[19] Because of these differences in clearances the drugs have predictably different plasma half-lives (Figs. 9-2 through 9-4). Although the termination of action of these drugs is primarily a result of redistribution of the drug from the central nervous sys-

TABLE 9-2. Pharmacokinetic Variables of Commonly Used Intravenous Anesthetics

	$t_{\frac{1}{2}}\beta$ (h)	Clearance (ml/kg/min)	V_{dss} (L/kg)	Reference
Diazepam	20–50	0.2–0.5	0.7–1.7	19
Droperidol	1.7–2.2	14	2.0	337,338
Etomidate	2.9–5.3	18–25	2.5–4.5	178–182
Fentanyl	2.5–5	5–15	3–5	
Flumazenil	0.7–1.3	5–20	0.6–1.6	71
Ketamine	2.5–2.8	12–17	3.1	99
Lorazepam	11–22	0.8–1.8	0.8–1.3	19
Midazolam	1.7–2.6	6.4–11	1.1–1.7	19
Propofol	4–7	20–30	2–10	234–240

Abbreviation: V_{dss}, volume of distribution at steady state.

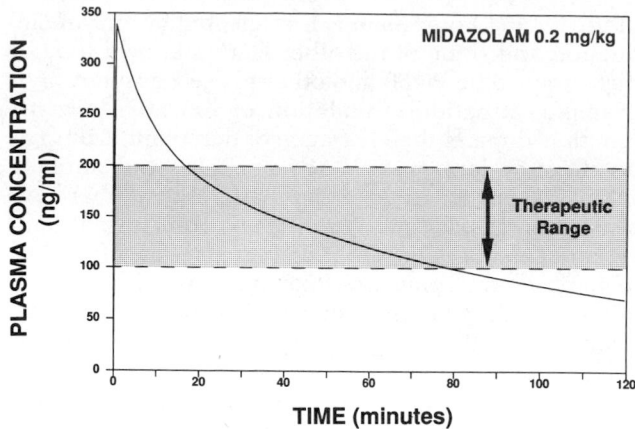

Fig. 9-2. Simulated time course of plasma levels of midazolam following an induction dose of 0.2 mg/kg. Plasma levels required for hypnosis and amnesia during surgery are 100 to 200 ng/ml, with awakening usually occurring below 50 ng/ml.

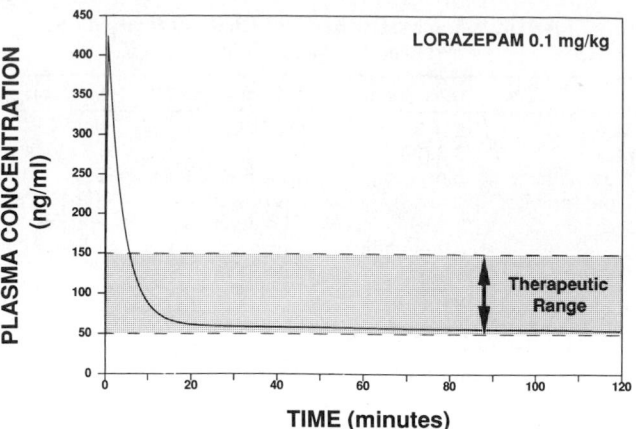

Fig. 9-4. Simulated time course of plasma levels of lorazepam following an induction dose of 0.1 mg/kg. Plasma levels required for hypnosis and amnesia during surgery are between 50 and 150 ng/ml, with awakening usually occurring below 50 ng/ml.

tem to other tissues, after repeated administration or after continuous infusion, midazolam blood levels will decrease more rapidly than the others because of its greater hepatic clearance. Thus patients given continuous infusions of midazolam should awaken faster than those given an infusion of diazepam.

Factors known to influence the pharmacokinetics of benzodiazepines are age, gender, race, enzyme induction, and hepatic and renal disease. Diazepam is very sensitive to some of these factors, particularly age. Age tends to reduce the clearance of diazepam significantly[23] and to a lesser degree the clearance of midazolam.[24] Lorazepam is resistant to the effects of age, gender, and renal disease on pharmacokinetics. These drugs are all affected by obesity. The volume of distribution is increased as the drug goes from the plasma into the adipose tissue. Although clearance is not al-

tered, elimination half-lives are prolonged owing to the delayed return of the drug to the plasma in the obese.[24] Based on pharmacokinetics, complex and seemingly contradictory dosing recommendations are required. For example, the induction dose of midazolam (and other benzodiazepines) should take into consideration a large weight (increased dose) because of the increased fat depot for the drug; however, dosing for continuous infusion in obese patients should be based on lean body weight because clearance is unaffected by weight.[19] In general, sensitivity to benzodiazepines in some groups, like the elderly, is greater despite relatively modest pharmacokinetic effects; thus, factors other than the pharmacokinetics of these drugs must be considered when they are used.

Pharmacology

All benzodiazepines have hypnotic, sedative, anxiolytic, amnestic, anticonvulsant, and centrally produced muscle relaxant properties. The drugs differ in their potency and efficacy with regard to each of the pharmacodynamic actions. The chemical structure of each drug dictates its particular physicochemical properties and pharmacokinetics as well as receptor-binding characteristics. The binding of benzodiazepines to their respective receptors is of very high affinity and is stereospecific and saturable. The rank order of receptor affinity (thus potency) of the three agonists is lorazepam > midazolam > diazepam. Although there are subtle differences between the benzodiazepines and their relative potencies with relation to each of the effects and side effects, an approximate relative potency is to diazepam (1 ×), midazolam (3 to 4 ×), and lorazepam (5 ×).

The mechanism of action of benzodiazepines is reasonably well understood.[25] The interaction of ligands

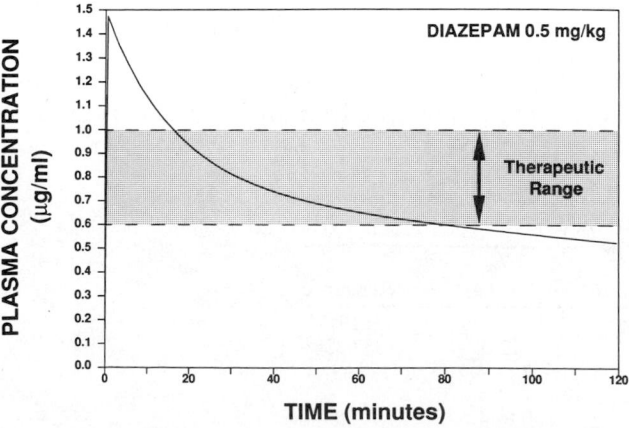

Fig. 9-3. Simulated time course of plasma levels of diazepam following an induction dose of 0.5 mg/kg. Plasma levels required for hypnosis and amnesia during surgery are 0.6 to 1.0 μg/ml, with awakening usually occurring below 0.5 μg/ml.

with the benzodiazepine receptor represents one of the few examples in which the complex systems of biochemistry, molecular pharmacology, and clinical behavioral patterns can be explained. More is understood about the mechanism of action of benzodiazepines than many other general anesthetics, although it is still not known how the different effects (amnesia, anticonvulsant, anxiolysis, and sleep) are mediated. It could be that these different effects are simply a result of absolute receptor occupancy. Using plasma concentration data and pharmacokinetic simulations, it has been estimated that a benzodiazepine receptor occupancy below 20 percent may be sufficient to produce the anxiolytic effect; sedation is observed with 30 to 50 percent receptor occupancy; and unconsciousness requires ≥ 60 percent benzodiazepine agonist receptor occupation.[26] It is generally agreed that benzodiazepines exert their effects by occupying the benzodiazepine receptor that modulates gamma-aminobutyric acid (GABA), the major inhibitory neurotransmitter in the brain. GABAergic neurotransmission counterbalances the influence of excitatory neurotransmitters. The benzodiazepine receptors are found in highest densities in the olfactory bulb, cerebral cortex, cerebellum, hippocampus, substantia nigra, and inferior colliculus, but lower densities are found in the striatum, lower brain stem, and spinal cord. Although there are two GABA receptors, it appears that the benzodiazepine receptor is part of the $GABA_a$ receptor complex on the subsynaptic membrane of the effector neuron. The $GABA_a$ receptor complex is made up of two protein subunits, α and β, arranged as hetero-oligomers, in a $\alpha_2\beta_2$ configuration

(Fig. 9-5). These proteins contain the various ligand-binding sites of the $GABA_a$ receptor, such as the benzodiazepine, GABA, and barbiturate binding sites. The benzodiazepine binding site is located on the α subunit, and the β subunit is thought to contain the binding site for GABA. With activation of the $GABA_a$ receptor, gating of the channel for chloride ions is triggered. The cell becomes hyperpolarized and therefore resistant to neuronal excitation. The degree of modulation of GABA-receptor function has a built-in limitation; this explains why there is a relatively high degree of safety with benzodiazepines.

A fascinating and therapeutically significant discovery regarding the benzodiazepine receptor is that among the pharmacologic spectrum of ligands are three different types or classes.[25] These classes of ligands have been called agonists, antagonists, and inverse agonists (Fig. 9-6). Their names connote their actions: the agonist (e.g., midazolam) alters the confirmation of the $GABA_a$ receptor complex so that binding affinity for GABA is increased with a resultant opening of the chloride channel. Agonist and antagonist bind to a common (at least overlapping) area of the receptor by forming differing reversible bonds with the receptor.[27] The well-known effects of an agonist then occur (anxiolysis, hypnosis, and anticonvulsant action). The antagonist (e.g., flumazenil) occupies the benzodiazepine receptor but produces no activity and therefore blocks the actions of both the agonists and inverse agonists. Inverse agonists reduce the efficiency of GABA-ergic synaptic transmission, and, because GABA is inhibitory, the result of decreased GABA is

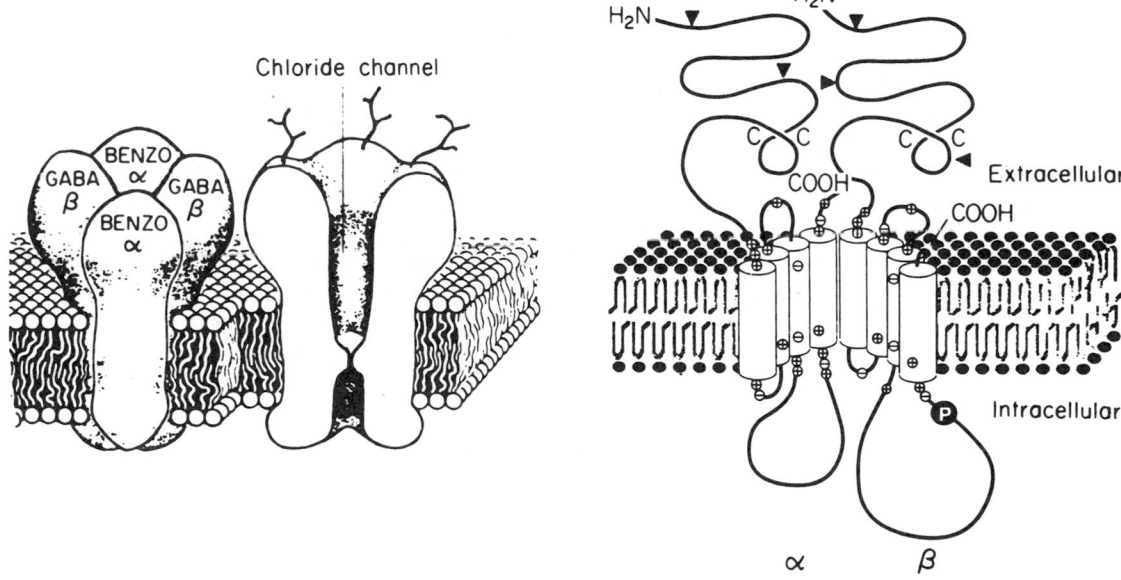

Fig. 9-5. Model of the $GABA_a$-receptor. (**A**) Comparison of the receptor of α- and β-subunits ($\alpha_2\beta_2$). By photoaffinity labeling benzodiazepine binding sites can be attributed to the α-subunit, high affinity GABA sites to the β-subunit. (**B**) Topology of the polypeptide chains according to the primary amino acid sequences deduced from cDNAs of the α- and β-subunit and their hydropathy profiles. (From Mohler and Richards,[25] with permission.)

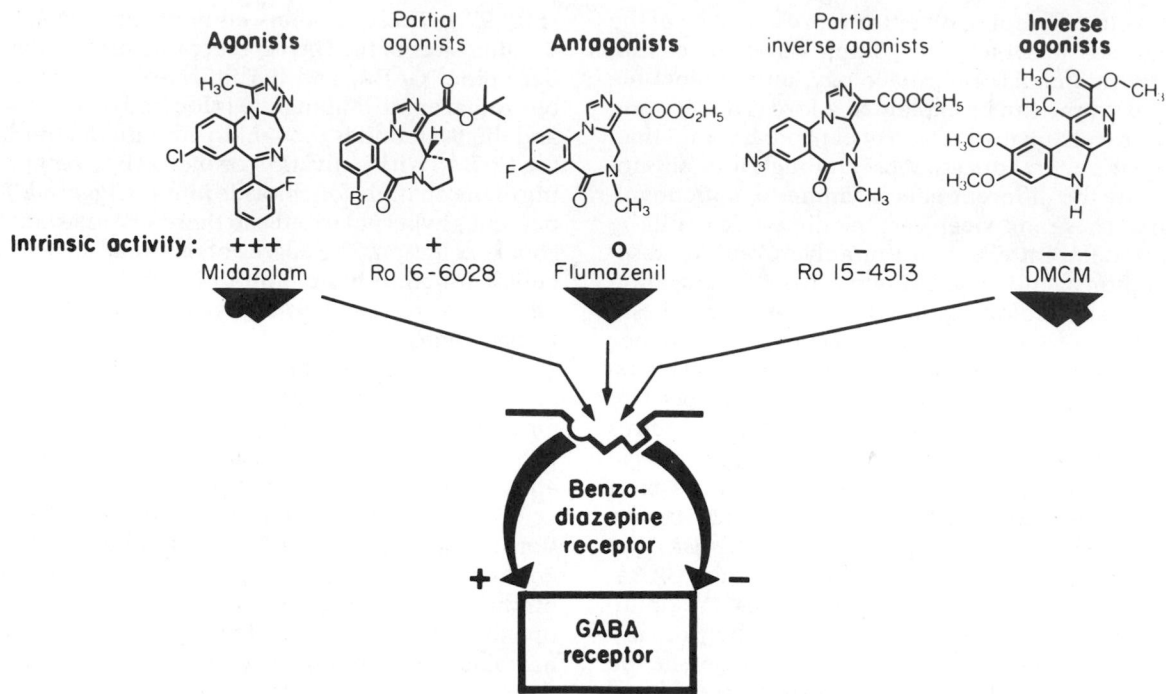

Fig. 9-6. Spectrum of intrinsic activities of benzodiazepine-receptor ligands. Benzodiazepine-receptor ligands range from agonists to inverse agonists. Structures of agonists, partial agonists, antagonists, partial inverse agonists, and inverse agonists compounds are shown. Intrinsic activity is greatest among the agonists and least among inverse agonists. Intrinsic activities are schematically indicated by + as positive, − as negative, o indicates a lack of intrinsic activity. (From Mohler and Richards,[25] with permission.)

CNS stimulation. The potency of the ligand is dictated by the affinity for the benzodiazepine receptor and the duration of effect by the rate of clearance of the drug from the receptor.

The onset and duration of action of a single bolus administration of a benzodiazepine depends on the lipid solubility, which probably explains the differences in onset and duration of action of the three benzodiazepines used in clinical practice in the United States. Midazolam and diazepam have a more rapid onset (usually within 30 to 60 seconds) of action than lorazepam (60 to 120 seconds). The duration of effect is also related to lipid solubility and blood level. The more rapid redistribution of midazolam and diazepam than lorazepam (presumably because of the lower lipid solubility of lorazepam)[14] accounts for the shorter duration of their actions.

Central Nervous System Effects

The benzodiazepines in a dose-related manner reduce cerebral metabolic rate for oxygen consumption ($CMRO_2$) and cerebral blood flow (CBF). Midazolam and diazepam maintain a relatively normal ratio of CBF to $CMRO_2$. In normal human volunteers midazolam, 0.15 mg/kg, induces sleep and reduces CBF 34 percent, despite a slight increase in $PaCO_2$ from 34 to 39

mmHg.[28] Brown et al.[29] studied electroencephalographic (EEG) tracings following 10 mg of midazolam intravenously and showed the appearance of rhythmic β activity at 22 Hz within 15 to 30 seconds of administration in healthy volunteers. Within 60 seconds there was a second β rhythm at 15 Hz. Alpha rhythm started to reappear at 30 minutes; however after 60 minutes there was resistant rhythmic β activity at 15 to 20 μV amplitude. The EEG changes are similar to diazepam EEG effects and not typical of light sleep, although the patients were clinically asleep.

Midazolam, diazepam, and lorazepam all increase the seizure threshold to local anesthetics and lower the mortality rate in mice exposed to lethal doses of local anesthetics.[30] Midazolam and diazepam cause a dose-related protective effect against cerebral hypoxia demonstrated by extending mouse survival time when mice were placed in 5 percent oxygen. The protection afforded by midazolam is superior to diazepam but less than pentobarbital.[30]

Respiratory System Effects

Benzodiazepines, like most intravenous anesthetics, produce dose-related central respiratory system depression. The respiratory depression of midazolam may be greater than that of diazepam and lorazepam, although comparative studies of the three do not exist. Lorazepam (2.5 mg IV) produces a similar but shorter-lasting decrease in tidal volume and minute ventilation compared to diazepam (10 mg IV) in patients with lung disease.[31] Peak decrease in minute ventilation after midazolam (0.15 mg/kg) is almost identical to that produced in normal patients given diazepam (0.3 mg/kg) as determined by CO_2 response data.[32] The slopes of the ventilatory response curves to CO_2 are flatter than normal (control), but not shifted to the right as seen with opioids. Judging from the plasma level and steepness of the dose-response effect on $PaCO_2$ curves (Fig. 9-7),[33] midazolam is about five- to ninefold more potent than diazepam, but it must be remembered that $PaCO_2$ is not a particularly sensitive measure of respiratory effect of a drug on the respiratory center. The peak onset of ventilatory depression with midazolam (0.2 mg/kg) is rapid (about 3 minutes), and significant depression remains for 15 minutes.[34] The respiratory depression of midazo-

lam is more pronounced and of longer duration in patients with chronic obstructive pulmonary disease, and the duration of ventilatory depression is longer with midazolam (0.19 mg/kg) than thiopental (3.3 mg/kg).[34] CO_2 response to lorazepam (0.05 mg/kg) is not depressed, but when combined with meperidine there is predictable respiratory depression.[35] The interactions of benzodiazepines with the many opioids on respiration has not been fully studied. It is probable that benzodiazepines and opioids produce additive or supra-additive respiratory depression even though they act at different receptors.

Apnea occurs with benzodiazepines. The incidence of apnea after thiopental or midazolam when given for induction of anesthesia is similar. Apnea occurred in 20 percent of 1130 patients given midazolam for induction and 27 percent of 580 patients given thiopental in the clinical trials with midazolam.[9] The incidence of apnea with diazepam and lorazepam is not known, but probably is lower than that for midazolam. Apnea is related to dose of benzodiazepine and is more likely to occur in the presence of opioids. Old age, debilitating disease, and other respiratory depressant drugs probably also increase the incidence and degree of respiratory depression and apnea with benzodiazepines.

Cardiovascular System Effects

The benzodiazepines used alone produce very modest hemodynamic effects. The hemodynamic changes reported with anesthetic induction doses of diazepam, midazolam, and lorazepam are listed in Table 9-3. These values represent the peak hemodynamic effect in the first 10 minutes after administration and come from studies of both healthy subjects and those with ischemic and valvular heart diseases.[36-43] The predominant hemodynamic change is a slight reduction in arterial blood pressure resulting from a decrease in systemic vascular resistance. The mechanism by which benzodiazepines maintain relatively stable hemodynamics involves the preservation of homeostatic reflex mechanisms,[44] but there is evidence that the baroreflex is somewhat impaired by both midazolam and diazepam.[45] Midazolam causes a slightly greater decrease in arterial blood pressure than do the other benzodiazepines, but the hypotensive effect is minimal and about the same as seen with thiopental.[46] Despite the hypotension, midazolam (0.2 mg/kg) is safe and effective for induction of anesthesia even in patients with severe aortic stenosis.[47] The hemodynamic effects of midazolam and diazepam are dose related: the higher the plasma level the greater the decrease in systemic blood pressure[33]; however, there is a plateau plasma drug effect above which little change in arterial blood pressure occurs. The plateau plasma level for midazolam is 100 ng/ml and for diazepam is about 900 ng/ml.[33] Heart rate, ventricular filling pressures, and cardiac output are maintained after induction of anesthesia with benzodiazepines. In patients with elevated left ventricular

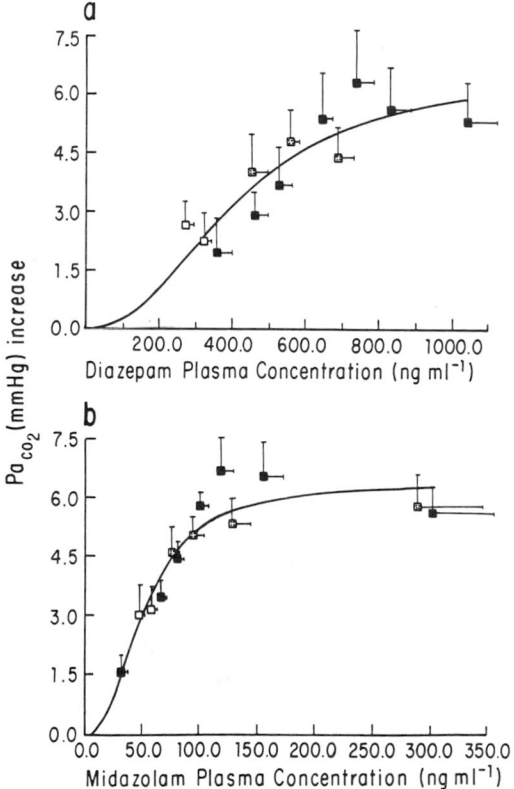

Fig. 9-7. (A) The increase of $PaCO_2$ form baseline versus the plasma concentration after 3 IV bolus doses of diazepam (0.15 mg/kg) given at 20-minute intervals. **(B)** The increase of $PaCO_2$ from baseline versus the midazolam plasma concentration after 3 IV bolus doses of midazolam (0.05 mg/kg) given at 20-minute intervals. The solid line represents a best fit model of the data from the three injections. Mean values are represented plus or minus SE mean; open boxes are data from injection 1; cross-hatched boxes from injection 2; and solid boxes from injection 3. (From Sunzel et al.,[33] with permission.)

TABLE 9-3. Hemodynamic Changes after Induction of Anesthesia with Nonbarbiturate Hypnotics

	Diazepam	Droperidol	Etomidate	Ketamine	Lorazepam	Midazolam	Propofol
HR	−9 to +13%	Unchanged	0 to +22%	0 to 59%	Unchanged	−14 to +12%	−10 to +10%
MBP	0 to −19%	0 to −10%	0 to −20%	0 to +40%	−7 to −20%	−12 to −26%	−10 to −40%
SVR	−22 to +13%	−5 to −15%	0 to −17%	0 to +33%	−10 to −35%	0 to −20%	−15 to −25%
PAP	0 to −10%	Unchanged	0 to −17%	+44 to +47%	—	Unchanged	0 to −10%
PVR	0 to −19%	Unchanged	0 to +27%	0 to +33%	Unchanged	Unchanged	0 to −10%
PAO	Unchanged	+25 to +50%	0 to −11%	Unchanged	—	0 to −25%	Unchanged
RAP	Unchanged	Unchanged	Unchanged	+15 to +33%	Unchanged	Unchanged	0 to −10%
CI	Unchanged	Unchanged	0 to +14%	0 to +42%	0 to +16%	0 to −25%	−10 to −30%
SV	0 to −8%	0 to −10%	0 to −15%	0 to −21%	Unchanged	0 to −18%	−10 to −25%
LVSWI	0 to −36%	Unchanged	0 to −27%	0 to +27%	—	−28 to −42%	−10 to −20%
dP/dt	Unchanged	—	0 to −18%	Unchanged	—	0 to −12%	—
References	36–38, 361–364	138, 153	205, 207, 209–212	127, 358–360	365, 366	36, 214, 367–369	213, 279–282, 284–289

Abbreviations: HR, heart rate; MBP, mean blood pressure; SVR, systemic vascular resistance; PAP, pulmonary artery pressure; PVR, pulmonary vascular resistance; PAO, pulmonary artery occluded pressure; RAP, right atrial pressure; CI, cardiac index; SV, stroke volume; LVSWI, left ventricular stroke work index; dP/dt, left ventricular stroke work.

filling pressures, diazepam and midazolam produce a "nitroglycerin" effect by lowering the filling pressure and increasing cardiac output.[39,41]

The stresses of endotracheal intubation (and surgery) are not blocked by midazolam.[36] Thus, adjuvant anesthetics, usually opioids, are often combined with benzodiazepines. The combination of benzodiazepines with opioids and N₂O has been investigated in patients with ischemic and valvular heart diseases.[38,43,47–51] Whereas the addition of N_2O to midazolam (0.2 mg/kg) and diazepam (0.5 mg/kg) has trivial hemodynamic consequences, the combination of benzodiazepines with opioids does produce a supra-additive effect.[52] The combinations of diazepam with fentanyl or sufentanil; midazolam with fentanyl[49] or sufentanil[51]; and lorazepam with fentanyl[43] or sufentanil[50] all produce greater decreases in systemic blood pressure than the drugs alone. The mechanism for this synergistic hemodynamic effect is not completely understood, but is probably related to a reduction in sympathetic tone when the drugs are given together.[48] There is evidence that diazepam and midazolam decrease catecholamines,[45] which is consistent with this hypothesis.

Uses

Intravenous Sedation

Benzodiazepines are used for sedation as preoperative premedication and intraoperatively during regional or local anesthesia. The anxiolysis, amnesia, and elevation of the local anesthetic seizure threshold are desirable benzodiazepine actions. The drugs should be given by titration for this use; endpoints of titration are adequate sedation or dysarthria (Table 9-4). The onset of action is more rapid with midazolam, usually with peak effect within 2 to 3 minutes of administration and slightly longer with diazepam and even more delayed with lorazepam. The duration of action of these drugs depends primarily on the dose used. Although the onset is more rapid with midazolam than diazepam after a single ad-

ministration, the recovery is similar,[53] probably because the drugs have similar early plasma decay (redistribution) patterns (Figs. 9-2 and 9-3). Lorazepam sedation, particularly amnesia, is slower in onset[54] and longer lasting than for the other two benzodiazepines.[55] There is often a disparity in the level of sedation compared to presence of amnesia (patients seem conscious and reasonably coherent, yet they are amnestic for events and instructions) with all three benzodiazepines. Lorazepam is particularly unpredictable with regard to duration of amnesia and this is undesirable in patients who wish or need to have recall in the immediate postoperative period.[54] The degree of sedation and the reliable amnesia as well as preservation of respiratory and hemodynamic function is overall better with benzodiazepines than with most other sedative hypnotic drugs used for conscious sedation. Despite the wide safety margin with benzodiazepines, respiratory function must be monitored when they are used for sedation to prevent undesirable degrees of respiratory depression.

Induction and Maintenance of Anesthesia

Midazolam is the benzodiazepine of choice for use in anesthetic induction. Although both diazepam and lorazepam have been used for induction of general anesthesia, the faster onset and lack of venous complications make midazolam better suited for this use. With midazolam, induction of anesthesia is accomplished when there is unresponsiveness to command and loss of the eyelash reflex. When used in appropriate doses (Table 9-4) induction occurs less rapidly than with thiopental,[9] but the amnesia is more reliable. A number of factors influence the rapidity of action of midazolam and the other benzodiazepines when used for induction of general anesthesia. These factors are dose, speed of injection, degree of premedication, age, and ASA physical status.[9,56] In a well premedicated, healthy patient, midazolam (0.2 mg/kg given in 5 to 15 seconds) will induce anesthesia in 28 seconds whereas diazepam (0.5

TABLE 9-4. Uses and Doses of Intravenous Benzodiazepines

	Midazolam	Diazepam	Lorazepam
Induction	0.1 to 0.2 mg/kg	0.3–0.5 mg/kg	0.1 mg/kg
Maintenance	0.05 mg/kg PRN 1.0 μg/kg/min	0.1 mg/kg PRN	0.02 mg/kg PRN
Sedation[a]	0.5–1 mg repeated 0.07 mg/kg IM	2 mg repeated	0.25 mg repeated

[a] Incremental doses given until desired degree of sedation obtained. PRN, as required to keep patient hypnotic and amnestic.

mg/kg given in 5 to 15 secs) produces induction in 39 seconds.[36] Elderly patients require lower doses of midazolam than younger patients,[57] possibly due to increased susceptibility of the elderly to benzodiazepines.[58] Patients older than age 55 and ASA physical status greater than III require a 20 percent or greater reduction in the induction dose of midazolam.[9]

Awakening after benzodiazepine induction is the result of the redistribution of drug from the brain to the different, less well-perfused tissues. The emergence (defined as orientation to time and place) of young, healthy volunteers who have received 10 mg IV of midazolam occurs in about 15 minutes,[29] and after an induction dose of 0.15 mg/kg in about 17 minutes.[59] Emergence time is related to dose and the administration of adjuvant anesthetic drugs.[9] The emergence from a midazolam (0.32 mg/kg)/fentanyl anesthetic is about 10 minutes longer than a thiopental (4.75 mg/kg)/fentanyl anesthetic.[60] This difference accounts for the preference of some anesthesiologists for barbiturates as induction drugs for short operations. With longer operations there is no advantage to barbiturate induction compared to midazolam.

Benzodiazepines lack analgesic properties and must be used with other anesthetic drugs to provide sufficient analgesia; however, as a maintenance anesthetic drug during general anesthesia, benzodiazepines provide hypnosis and amnesia. Double-blind studies comparing midazolam and thiopental as the hypnotic component for balanced anesthesia[60,61] have shown that midazolam is superior for this use because of better amnesia and a smoother hemodynamic course. Opioid requirements are less with midazolam. Midazolam (0.6 mg/kg) lowers the MAC of halothane 30 percent[62] and presumably other inhaled anesthetics. The question of an optimal redosing scheme after induction when midazolam is used as a maintenance hypnotic component of general anesthesia has not been answered. The amnestic period after an anesthetic dose is about 1 to 2 hours. Infusions of midazolam have been used to assure a constant and appropriate depth of anesthesia.[62] Experience indicates that a plasma level of more than 50 ng/ml when used with adjuvant opioids (e.g., fentanyl) and/or inhaled anesthetics (e.g., N_2O, volatile anesthetics) is achieved with a bolus loading dose of 0.05 to 0.15 mg/kg and a continuous infusion of 0.25 to 1 μg/kg/min.[64] This is sufficient to keep the patient asleep and amnestic but arousable at the end of surgery. Lower infusion doses may be required in some patients and with certain opioids. Midazolam as well as diazepam and lorazepam will accumulate in the blood with repeated bolus administrations or continuous infusion, just as drug levels with most intravenous anesthetics do on repeated injections. If the benzodiazepines do accumulate with repeated administrations, prolonged arousal time can be anticipated. This is less of a problem with midazolam than diazepam and lorazepam because of the greater clearance of midazolam.

Side Effects and Contraindications

Benzodiazepines are remarkably safe drugs. They have relatively high margins of safety, especially compared to barbiturates. They are also free of allergic reactions and do not suppress the adrenal gland.[65] The most significant problem with midazolam is respiratory depression when given for conscious sedation. The major side effects of lorazepam and diazepam are venous irritation and thrombophlebitis, problems related to aqueous insolubility and requisite solvents.[9] When used as sedatives or for induction and maintenance of anesthesia, benzodiazepines can produce an undesirable degree or prolonged interval of postoperative amnesia, sedation, and, rarely, respiratory depression. These residual effects can be reversed with flumazenil, the specific benzodiazepine receptor antagonist.

FLUMAZENIL

Flumazenil (Anexate) is the first benzodiazepine antagonist for clinical use. The preclinical pharmacologic studies with flumazenil revealed that flumazenil is a benzodiazepine receptor ligand with high affinity, great specificity, and minimal intrinsic effect.[27] Flumazenil, like the agonists it replaces at the benzodiazepine receptor, interacts with the receptor in a concentration-dependent manner. It is a competitive antagonist at the benzodiazepine receptor; therefore its antagonism is reversible and surmountable. Flumazenil has minimal intrinsic activity,[27,66] which means that it produces very weak benzodiazepine receptor agonist effects, significantly less than clinical agonists. Flumazenil (like all competitive antagonists at receptors) does not displace the agonist but rather will occupy the receptor when an agonist dissociates from the receptor. The half-time (or half-life) of a receptor-ligand bond is a few milliseconds to a few seconds, and new ligand receptor bonds are then immediately made. This very dynamic situation accounts for the ability of either an agonist or antagonist to readily occupy the receptor. The proportion of receptors occupied by the agonist in the presence of an antagonist obeys the law of mass action and depends on the affinities and concentrations of the two ligands.[27] Equation 1 expresses this relationship[67]:

$$\frac{[R_{Ago}]}{[R_t]} = \frac{1}{1 + \dfrac{K_{Ago}}{[Ago]}\left(1 + \dfrac{[Ant]}{K_{Ant}}\right)} \quad (1)$$

where: $[R_{Ago}]$ = receptor concentration of agonist
$[R_t]$ = total number of receptors
K_{Ago} = dissociation constant for agonist
K_{Ant} = dissociation constant for antagonist
[Ago] = concentration of agonist at the receptors
[Ant] = concentration of antagonist at the receptor

The ratio of agonist to the total receptors produces the effects of the agonist drug: The antagonist can alter this ratio, depending on its concentration and dissociation constant (Eq. 1). Thus flumazenil, which is an avid (high affinity) ligand will replace a relatively weak agonist such as diazepam as long as it is given in sufficient dose (i.e., high [Ant]). However, flumazenil is relatively rapidly cleared and the net result is that the [Ant] is reduced over time compared to [Ago]; thus the proportion of receptors occupied by agonist will increase and the potential for resedation exists (Fig. 9-8). This is less likely to happen when flumazenil is used to reverse midazolam, which has a more rapid clearance than other benzodiazepine agonists.[68] Another important concept is that when flumazenil is given in the presence of very high doses of agonist (e.g., when a mistake in dosing has occurred or suicide is attempted), flumazenil in a low dose will attenuate the deep depression of CNS (loss of consciousness, respiratory depression) by reducing the fractional receptor occupancy by the agonist: the agonist effects that occur at low fractional receptor occupancy are not diminished (drowsiness, amnesia). Conversely, high doses of flumazenil in the presence of low doses of agonist will completely reverse virtually all the agonist effects. Flumazenil can precipitate withdrawal symptoms in animals, in humans or physically dependent on a benzodiazepine receptor agonist.[69] This is not a problem when used to reverse benzodiazepine receptor agonists used for anesthesia.

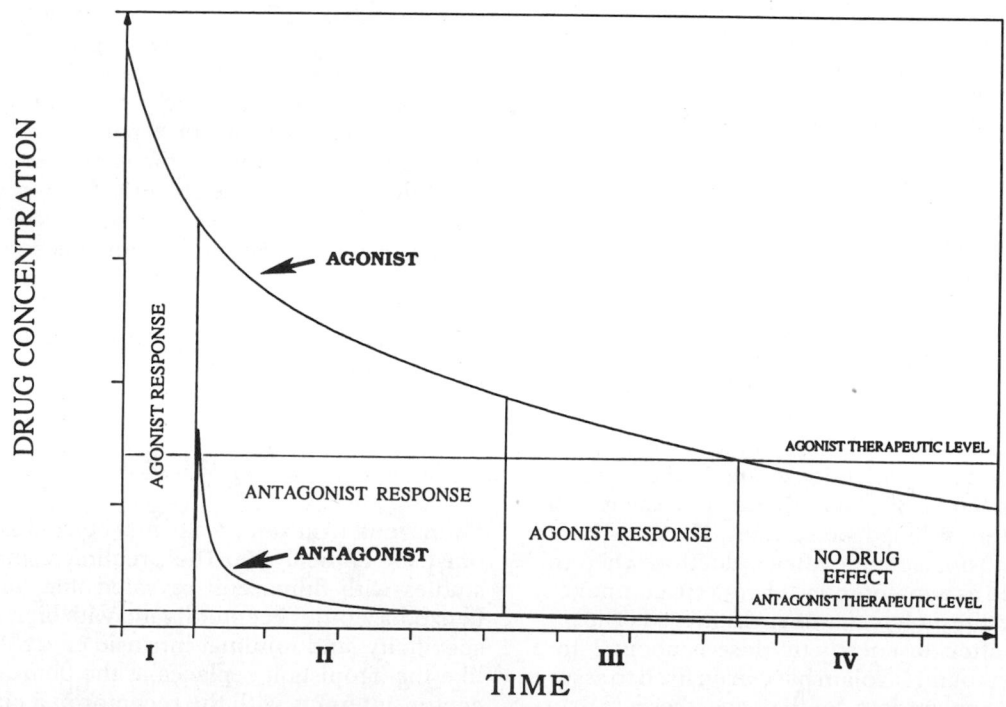

Fig. 9-8. Schematic representation of the interaction of a short-acting antagonist with a longer-acting agonist that results in resedation. Upper curve shows agonist blood level disappearance and lower curve shows antagonist plasma disappearance. There are four conditions represented: (I) agonist response; (II) antagonist response (the antagonist reverses the agonist effect); (III) agonist response (resedation or resumption of agonist response with disappearance of short-lasting antagonist); and (IV) no drug effect with disappearance of both agonist and antagonist (both drugs below therapeutic level).

Physicochemical Characteristics

Flumazenil was synthesized in 1979 and is similar to midazolam and other classic benzodiazepines except for the absence of the phenyl group, which is replaced by a carbonyl group (Fig. 9-1).[70] It forms a colorless crystalline powder with a pK of 1.7 and has weak, but sufficient water solubility to prepare in aqueous solution. The octanol/aqueous buffer partition coefficient is 14, demonstrating moderate lipid solubility at pH 7.4.[70]

Metabolism

Flumazenil, like the other benzodiazepines, is metabolized in the liver. The drug is rapidly cleared from the plasma. It has three known metabolites, *N*-desmethylflumazenil, *N*-desmethylflumazenil acid, and flumazenil acid.[71] Activity of these metabolites and their corresponding glucuronides is not known at present. The glucuronides probably are excreted in the urine. Because flumazenil is still under investigation, many details regarding the clinical metabolism of this drug have not been studied.

Pharmacokinetics

Flumazenil is a short-lived compound. The pharmacokinetics have been described in a variety of clinical settings and summary results are in Table 9-2.[71,72] Of particular note is the fact that compared to benzodiazepine receptor agonists, flumazenil has the highest clearance and shortest elimination half-life. The plasma half-life of flumazenil is about 1 hour: it is the shortest lived of all benzodiazepines used in anesthesia practice. This means that the potential exists for the antagonist to be cleared leaving concentrations of agonist at the receptor site sufficient to cause resedation.[68] To maintain a constant therapeutic blood level over a prolonged time, either repeated administrations or a continuous infusion are required. An infusion rate of 30 to 60 μg/min (0.5 to 1 μg/kg/min) has been used for this purpose.[73] The high blood clearance of flumazenil approaches hepatic blood flow, indicating that liver clearance is partially dependent on hepatic blood flow. Flumazenil, compared to other benzodiazepines, has a relatively high proportion of unbound drug. The protein binding of flumazenil is low, with the free fraction ranging from 54 to 64 percent.[71] This could contribute to the rapid onset and greater clearance, but this is unproven.

Pharmacology

When given in the absence of a benzodiazepine receptor agonist, flumazenil has little discernible CNS effects. Although intrinsic (agonist and inverse agonist) effects have been ascribed to flumazenil,[66] they are difficult to observe clinically. It is postulated that in low doses a stimulating effect can be seen and that in high doses a central depressant effect becomes more likely.[26] When administered to patients who have agonists causing CNS depression, flumazenil produces rapid and dependable reversal of unconsciousness, respiratory depression, sedation, amnesia, and psychomotor dysfunction.[26,72,74,75] Flumazenil can be given prior to, during, or after the agonist to block or reverse the CNS effects of the agonist. The usual clinical need will be to reverse the effects of agonists given prior to flumazenil. Agonists that flumazenil has successfully reversed include midazolam, diazepam, lorazepam, and flunitrazepam. The onset is very rapid; peak effect occurs in 1 to 3 minutes,[26] which coincides with the detection of ^{11}C-flumazenil in human brain.[76] Flumazenil reverses the agonist by replacing it at the benzodiazepine receptor, and its onset and duration are governed by the law of mass action (Eq. 1). A predicted therapeutic plasma level for flumazenil is 20 ng/ml[71]; however, because the relative binding characteristics of agonist and antagonist dictate in part the residual agonist benzodiazepine receptor occupation, different doses and plasma levels of flumazenil will be required to reverse particular agonists. These reactions have not been fully studied, but it is known that higher doses of flumazenil are required to reverse lorazepam than diazepam,[74] lorazepam being more potent than diazepam. Although it is premature to be certain, it does not appear that flumazenil administration after long-term benzodiazepine use produces severe withdrawal reactions.

The duration of action of flumazenil is determined by the dose, the dose of the agonist, and the specific agonist that is being reversed. The duration will be dictated by factors in Equation 1. Studies have shown that during a constant infusion of agonist the duration of flumazenil is dependent on the dose, but that 45 to 90 minutes of antagonism can be expected after a dose of 3.0 mg IV.[77] This is an artificial setting because in clinical practice flumazenil will be given after the cessation of administration of agonist.

The effects of flumazenil on the respiratory and cardiovascular system show that it is devoid of the respiratory and cardiovascular depressant effects of benzodiazepine receptor agonists. A relatively large dose of flumazenil (0.1 mg/kg) given to volunteers did not produce significant respiratory depression.[78] However, when given in the presence of an agonist, there are significant respiratory effects. Flumazenil will reverse respiratory depression caused by agonists. Given to volunteers made apneic with midazolam, flumazenil reversed the respiratory depression.[79] Clearly more data are required to optimally define the respiratory effects of flumazenil benzodiazepine receptor-agonist reversal. Incremental doses, up to 3 mg IV, in patients with ischemic heart disease have no significant effect on cardiovascular variables.[80] The administration of flumazenil to patients given agonists is remarkably free of cardiovascular effects,[26,81,82] unlike the experience of opioid reversal with naloxone. Of particular interest is the effect of flumazenil benzodiazepine receptor-agonist reversal on catecholamines, because this is the suspected mechanism of opioid reversal hyperdynamic response. Flumazenil, although it does reverse sedation, is not associated with significantly higher catecholamines than that seen in patients receiving saline,[81,83,84] but the rise in catecholamines that accompanies arousal is more rapid after flumazenil.[83]

Uses and Doses

There are relatively few uses for a benzodiazepine antagonist (Table 9-5). The uses include the diagnostic and therapeutic reversal of benzodiazepine receptor agonists. For diagnostic use, flumazenil may be given in incremental doses of 0.1 to 0.2 mg IV up to 3 mg. If there is no change in the CNS sedation, it is unlikely that CNS depression is solely on the basis of benzodiazepine overdose. More commonly in anesthesia the use of flumazenil will be to reverse the patient who remains depressed after administration of a benzodiazepine for conscious sedation or use during general anesthesia. Flumazenil will reliably reverse sedation, respiratory depression, and the amnesia of benzodiazepines. The dosage guidelines are in Table 9-5, but it must be emphasized that large-scale dosing studies have not yet been completed. The dose varies with the particular benzodiazepine being reversed, and the duration of reversal is dependent on the kinetics of both the agonist and flumazenil. Surveillance is recommended if a long-lasting benzodiazepine is reversed with a single administration of flumazenil because of the relatively short-lived effect. Flumazenil may be administered by continuous infusion to prevent resedation with longer-lasting benzodiazepine receptor agonists. It is postulated that the availability of flumazenil will extend the usefulness of benzodiazepine agonists, although it will not necessarily alter the safety of this class of drugs.

Side Effects and Contraindications

Flumazenil has been given in large oral and intravenous doses with remarkably few toxic reactions.[26] It is free of local or tissue irritant properties, and there are no known organotoxicities. Like all benzodiazepines, it appears to have a very high safety margin, probably higher than agonists because it does not produce prominent CNS depression. Unless it is found that reversal of patients who have a chronic history of benzodiazepine use causes withdrawal reactions including seizures,

TABLE 9-5. Uses and Doses of Flumazenil

Reversal of benzodiazepines[a]	0.1–0.2 mg repeated[b] up to 3.0 mg
Diagnosis in coma	0.5 mg repeated up to 1.0 mg

[a] The dose required to reverse each benzodiazepine (BZD) will depend on residual BZD and the particular BZD; i.e., higher doses are required for more potent BZDs (see text).
[b] The degree of reversal should be titrated by repeating 0.2-mg increments every 1 to 2 minutes until the desired level of reversal is achieved.

there is no current contraindication for the use of flumazenil. An important caution is that resedation could occur because of the relatively short half-life of this drug.

PHENCYCLIDINES (KETAMINE)

History

Phencyclidine was the first drug of this class to be used for anesthesia. It was synthesized by Maddox and introduced into clinical use by Greifenstein et al in 1958[85] and Johnstone et al in 1959.[86] Although phencyclidine proved useful as an anesthetic, it produced unacceptably high adverse psychological effects of hallucinations and delirium in the postanesthetic recovery period. Cyclohexamine, a congener of phencyclidine, was tried clinically in 1959 by Lear and coworkers[87] but found to be less efficacious in terms of analgesia and yet had as many adverse psychotomimetic effects as phencyclidine. Neither of these drugs is used clinically today, although phencyclidine is available for illicit recreational use. Ketamine (Ketalar) was synthesized in 1962 by Stevens and first used in humans by Corssen and Domino in 1965.[88] It was chosen from among 200 phencyclidine derivatives and proved to be the most promising in laboratory animal testing. Ketamine was released for clinical use in 1970 and still enjoys use in a variety of clinical settings. Ketamine is unique among most other anesthetic drugs because it does not depress the cardiovascular and respiratory systems.[89,90] It does possess some of the worrisome psychological adverse effects found with the other phencyclidines.

Physicochemical Characteristics

Ketamine (Fig. 9-9) has a molecular weight of 238, is partially water soluble, and forms a white crystalline salt with a pK_a of 7.5.[89,90] It has a lipid solubility 5 to 10 times that of thiopental.[91] Ketamine is prepared in a slightly acidic (pH 3.5 to 5.5) solution and comes in concentrations of 10, 50, and 100 mg ketamine base per milliliter of sodium chloride containing the preservative benzethonium chloride. The ketamine molecule contains a chiral center producing two resolvable optical isomers or enantiomers (Fig. 9-9). The commercial preparation is a racemic mixture of both isomers in equal amounts.[89]

Metabolism

Ketamine is metabolized by the hepatic microsomal enzymes responsible for most drug detoxification. The major pathway involves N-demethylation to form norketamine (metabolite I), which is then hydroxylated to form hyroxy-norketamines. These products are conjugated to water-soluble glucuronide derivatives and excreted in the urine.[89,90,92] The activity of the principal

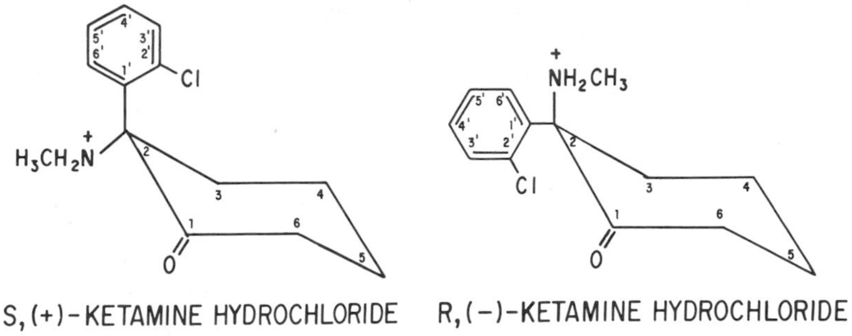

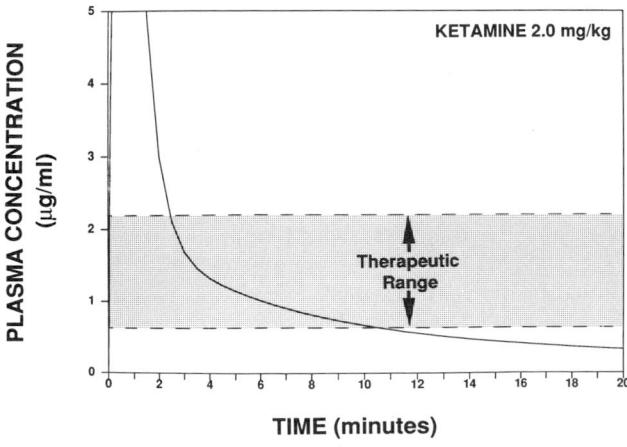

Fig. 9-9. Stereoisomers of ketamine as it is formulated.

metabolites of ketamine have not been well studied, but norketamine (metabolite I) has been shown to have significantly less (between 20 and 30 percent) activity than the parent compound.[93-95] Little is known about the activity of the other metabolites, but it is probable that ketamine is the major active drug.

Pharmacokinetics

The pharmacokinetics of ketamine have not been as well studied as many other intravenous anesthetics. Ketamine pharmacokinetics after bolus administration of anesthetizing doses (2 to 2.5 mg/kg),[96] following a subanesthetic dose (0.25 mg/kg)[96,97] and after continuous infusion (steady-state plasma level of about 2000 ng/ml),[98] has been examined. Regardless of the dose, ketamine plasma disappearance can be described by a two-compartment model. Table 9-2 contains the pharmacokinetic values from bolus-administration studies.[96] Of note is the rapid distribution reflected in the relatively brief $t\frac{1}{2}\alpha$ of 11 to 16 minutes (Fig. 9-10). The high lipid solubility is reflected in the relatively large volume of distribution of nearly 3 L/kg. Clearance is also relatively high, ranging from 890 to 1127 ml/min, which accounts for the relatively short elimination half-life of 2 to 3 hours. The mean total body clearance (1.4 L/min) is approximately equal to liver blood flow, which means that changes in liver blood flow will affect clearance. Thus the administration of a drug such as halothane that reduces hepatic blood flow will reduce ketamine clearance.[99,100]

Pharmacology

Central Nervous System Effects

Ketamine produces dose-related unconsciousness and analgesia. The anesthetized state has been termed *dissociative anesthesia* because patients who receive ketamine alone appear to be in a cataleptic state unlike other states of anesthesia that resemble normal sleep. The ketamine anesthetized patients have profound analgesia, but keep their eyes open and maintain many of the protective reflexes such as corneal, cough, and swallow. There is no recall of surgery or anesthesia, but amnesia is not as prominent with ketamine as with the benzodiazepines. Because ketamine has a small molecular weight, a pK_a near the physiologic pH, and relatively high lipid solubility, it crosses the blood-brain barrier rapidly and therefore has an onset of action within 30 seconds of administration. The maximal effect occurs in about 1 minute. After ketamine administration, pupils dilate moderately and nystagmus occurs. Lacrimation and salivation are common, as is increased skeletal muscle tone, often with coordinated, but seemingly purposeless movements of the arms, legs, trunk, and head. Although there is great interindividual variability, plasma levels of 0.6 to 2.0 mg/ml are considered the minimum concentrations for general anesthesia,[98,99,101,102] but children may require slightly higher plasma levels (0.8 μg/ml to 4.0 μg/ml).[103] The duration of ketamine anesthesia after a single administration of a general anesthetic dose (2 mg/kg IV) is 10 to 15 minutes[90] (Fig. 9-10), and full orientation to person, place, and time occurs within 15 to 30 minutes.[104] The duration of ketamine anesthesia is determined by the dose; higher doses produce more prolonged anesthesia,[105] and the concurrent use of other anesthetics will

Fig. 9-10. Simulated time course of plasma levels of ketamine following an induction dose of 2.0 mg/kg. Plasma levels required for hypnosis and amnesia during surgery are 0.7 to 2.2 μg/ml with awakening usually occurring below 0.5 μg/ml.

also prolong the time of emergence. Because there is a reasonably good correlation between blood level of ketamine and CNS effect, it appears that the reason for ketamine's relatively short duration of action is that it redistributes from the brain and blood to the other tissues in the body. Thus, the termination of effect after a single bolus administration of ketamine is caused by drug redistribution from the well-perfused tissues to the less well-perfused tissues. Analgesia occurs at considerably lower levels than loss of consciousness. The plasma level at which pain thresholds are elevated is ≥ 0.1 $\mu g/ml$.[99] This means that there is a considerable period of postoperative analgesia after ketamine general anesthesia and that subanesthetic doses can be used to produce analgesia.

The primary site of CNS action of ketamine appears to be the thalamo-neocortical projection system.[106] It selectively depresses neuronal function in parts of the cortex (especially association areas) and thalamus, while simultaneously stimulating parts of the limbic system, including the hippocampus. This creates what is termed a *functional disorganization*[90] of nonspecific pathways in midbrain and thalamic areas.[107,108] There is also evidence that ketamine depresses transmission of impulses in the medial medullary reticular formation, important to transmission of the affective-emotional components of nociception from the spinal cord to higher brain centers.[109] There is some evidence that ketamine occupies opiate receptors in the brain and spinal cord that could account for some of the analgesic effects.[89,90,110,111] Although a number of drugs have been used to antagonize ketamine, there is no specific receptor antagonist yet known that reverses all the CNS effects of ketamine.

Ketamine increases cerebral metabolism, blood flow, and intracranial pressure. Ketamine, because of its excitatory CNS effects, which can be detected by generalized EEG development of theta wave activity,[105] as well as petit-mal-seizurelike activity in the hippocampus,[112] increases $CMRO_2$. Whereas theta-wave activity signals the analgesic activity of ketamine, alpha waves indicate its absence. There is an increase in cerebral blood flow that appears higher than the increase in $CMRO_2$, which cannot be explained. With the increase in cerebral blood flow as well as the generalized increase in sympathetic nervous system response, there is an increase in intracranial pressure after ketamine.[113,114] The increase in $CMRO_2$ and cerebral blood flow can be blocked by the use of thiopental[115] or diazepam.[116] Cerebrovascular responsiveness to CO_2 appears to be preserved with ketamine; therefore, reducing $PaCO_2$ will attenuate the rise in intracranial pressure after ketamine[114] (also see Ch. 54).

Ketamine, like other phencyclidines, produces undesirable psychological reactions. These occur during the awakening from ketamine anesthesia and are termed *emergence reactions*. These reactions vary in severity and classification. The common manifestations of these reactions is vivid dreaming, extracorporeal experiences (sense of floating out of body), and illusions (the misinterpretation of a real, external sensory experience).[117] These instances of dreaming and illusion are often associated with excitement, confusion, euphoria, and fear.[90] They occur in the first hour of emergence and usually abate within one to several hours. It has been postulated[89] that the psychic emergence reactions occur secondary to ketamine-induced depression of auditory and visual relay nuclei, leading to misperception and/or misinterpretation of auditory and visual stimuli. The incidence ranges from as low as 3 to 5 percent[89,90] to as high as 100 percent,[117] and a clinically relevant range is probably 10 to 30 percent of adult patients who receive ketamine as a sole or major part of the anesthetic technique. Factors that affect the incidence are age,[118] dose,[90] gender,[119] psychological susceptibility,[120] and concurrent drugs. Pediatric patients do not report as high an incidence of unpleasant emergence reactions as adult patients, nor do men compared to women. Higher doses and rapid administration of large doses seems to predispose to a higher incidence of adverse affects.[121,122] Finally, certain personality types seem prone to the development of emergence reactions. Patients who score high in psychotism on the Eysenck Personality Inventory are prone to develop emergence reactions,[120] and people who commonly dream at home are more likely to have postoperative dreams with ketamine in the hospital.[121] A number of drugs have been used to reduce the incidence and severity of postoperative reactions to ketamine[89,90,123]; the benzodiazepines seem to be the most effective group of drugs to attenuate or treat ketamine emergence reactions. Midazolam,[89] lorazepam,[124] and diazepam[125] are useful in reducing the reactions to ketamine. The mechanism is not known, but it is probable that both the sedative and amnestic actions of the benzodiazepines make them superior to other sedative hypnotics.

Respiratory System Effects

Ketamine has minimal effects on the central respiratory drive, as reflected by an unaltered response to CO_2.[126] There can be a transient (1 to 3 minutes) decrease in minute ventilation after the bolus administration of an anesthetizing dose of ketamine (2 mg/kg IV).[105,127,128] Unusually high doses can produce apnea,[129] but this is seldom seen. Arterial blood gases are generally preserved when ketamine is used alone for anesthesia or analgesia; however, with the use of adjuvant sedatives or anesthetic drugs, respiratory depression can occur.

Ketamine is a bronchial smooth muscle relaxant. When ketamine is given to patients with reactive airway disease and bronchospasm, pulmonary compliance is improved.[130,131] Ketamine is as effective as halothane or enflurane in preventing experimentally induced bronchospasm.[132] The mechanism for this effect is probably a result of the sympathomimetic response to ketamine, but there are isolated bronchial smooth muscle studies that show that ketamine can directly antagonize the spasmogenic effects of carbachol and histamine.[133] A potential respiratory problem especially in children is the increased salivation that follows ketamine. This can produce upper airway obstruction, which can be further complicated by laryngospasm. Also, although swallow, cough, sneeze, and gag reflexes are relatively intact after ketamine, there is evidence that silent aspiration can occur during ketamine anesthesia.[134] Nevertheless, compared to other intravenous anesthetic drugs, ketamine has unique respiratory effects that clearly distinguish it from the others, which depress respiration centrally and predispose to significant respiratory depression and loss of protective reflexes.

Cardiovascular System Effects

Ketamine also has unique cardiovascular effects; it stimulates the cardiovascular system and is usually associated with increases in blood pressure, heart rate, and cardiac output (Table 9-3). Other anesthetic drugs either effect no change in hemodynamic variables or produce vasodilation with or without cardiac depression. The increase in cardiovascular function is associated with increased work and myocardial oxygen consumption. The normal heart is able to increase oxygen supply by increased cardiac output and decreased coronary vascular resistance so that coronary blood flow is appropriate for the increase in oxygen consumption.[135] The hemodynamic changes are not related to the dose of ketamine; for example, there is no difference between changes after the administration of 0.5 and 1.5 mg/kg IV.[136] It is also interesting that a second dose of ketamine produces hemodynamic effects less than or even opposite to the first dose.[137] The hemodynamic changes after anesthesia induction with ketamine tend to be the same in healthy patients and those with a variety of acquired or congenital heart disease.[128,136,138-140] In congenital heart diseased patients, there are no significant changes in shunt directions or fraction[141] or systemic oxygenation after ketamine induction of anesthesia.[142] In patients who have elevated pulmonary artery pressure (as with mitral valvular and some congenital lesions), ketamine seems to cause a more pronounced increase in pulmonary vascular resistance than in systemic vascular resistance.[140,141,143,144]

The mechanism by which ketamine stimulates the circulatory system remains enigmatic, but it appears that rather than a peripheral mechanism such as baroreflex inhibition,[145,146] it is central.[147-149] Ketamine injected directly into the central nervous system produces an immediate sympathetic nervous system hemodynamic response.[150] Ketamine also causes the sympathoneuronal release of norepinephrine, which can be detected in venous blood.[151] Blockade of this effect is possible with barbiturates, benzodiazepines, and droperidol.[149-152] Ketamine in vitro has negative inotropic effects. Myocardial depression has been demonstrated in isolated rabbit hearts,[153] intact dogs,[154] and isolated canine heart preparations.[155] The centrally mediated sympathetic responses to ketamine usually override the direct depressant effects of ketamine. Some peripheral nervous system actions of ketamine play an undetermined role in the hemodynamic effects of ketamine. Ketamine inhibits intraneuronal uptake of catecholamines in a cocaine-like effect[156,157] and inhibits extraneuronal norepinephrine uptake.[158]

Stimulation of the cardiovascular system is not always desirable, and a number of pharmacologic methods have been used to block the ketamine-induced tachycardia and systemic hypertension. Successful methods include the use of adrenergic antagonists (both α and β) as well as a variety of vasodilators.[159] However, probably the most fruitful approach has been the prior administration of benzodiazepines. Modest doses of diazepam, flunitrazepam, and midazolam all attenuate the hemodynamic effects of ketamine. It is also possible to lessen the tachycardia and hypertension of ketamine by using a continuous-infusion technique with or without a benzodiazepine.[160] Other general anesthetics, particularly the inhalation anesthetics,[161] will blunt the hemodynamic effect of ketamine. Ketamine can produce hemodynamic depression in this setting of deep anesthesia, when sympathetic responses do not accompany its administration.

Uses

The many unique features of ketamine pharmacology as well as its propensity to produce unwanted emergence reactions have placed ketamine outside the realm of routine clinical use enjoyed by the barbiturates and benzodiazepines. Nevertheless, ketamine has an important and sometimes unrivaled place in the practice of anesthesiology.

Induction and Maintenance of Anesthesia

Poor risk patients (ASA Class $\geq$ IV), those with respiratory and cardiovascular system disorders (excluding ischemic heart disease), represent the majority of candidates for ketamine induction, particularly patients with bronchospastic airway disease or patients with hemodynamic compromise based on either hypovolemia or intrinsic myocardial disease (not coronary artery disease). Ketamine bronchodilation and profound analgesia allowing the use of high oxygen concentrations make ketamine an excellent choice for the induction of patients with reactive airway disease. Healthy patients who are trauma victims whose blood loss is extensive are also candidates for rapid-sequence anesthesia induction[162] with ketamine. Use of ketamine in these patients does not obviate the need to prepare the patient preoperatively appropriately, including restoration of blood volume. Other cardiac diseases that can be optimally managed with ketamine anesthesia are cardiac tamponade and restrictive pericarditis.[163] The fact that ketamine preserves heart rate and right atrial pressure through its sympathetic stimulating effects makes ketamine an excellent anesthetic induction and maintenance drug in this setting. Ketamine is also often used in patients with congenital heart disease, especially those in whom the propensity for right to left shunting exists.

Ketamine combined with diazepam or midazolam can be given by continuous infusion to produce very satisfactory cardiac anesthesia for valvular and ischemic heart disease. The combination of the benzodiazepines with ketamine attenuates or eliminates the unwanted tachycardia and hypertension as well as postoperative psychological derangements. With this technique[160] there are minimal hemodynamic perturbations, profound analgesia, dependable amnesia, and an uneventful convalescence. The comparison of this technique with a continuous benzodiazepine with opioid has not been made.

Sedation

Ketamine is particularly suited for sedation of the pediatric patient undergoing procedures away from the operating room. Pediatric patients have less adverse emergence reactions[118] than do adults, making its use in pediatrics more versatile. Ketamine is used for sedation and/or general anesthesia for the following pediatric procedures: cardiac catheterization, radiation therapy, radiologic studies, dressing changes, and dental work. It may be given intramuscularly without the necessity for intravenous access, and it may be administered without an anesthetic machine (although caution regarding the airway must be exercised as with any sedative technique). Usually a subanesthetic dose (≤ 1.0 mg/kg IV) is used for dressing changes, which gives adequate operating conditions but rapid return to normal function including the resumption of eating, which is important in maintaining proper nutrition in burn patients.[89,90] Often ketamine is combined with premedication of a barbiturate or benzodiazepine and an antisialagogue (e.g., glycopyrrolate) to facilitate management. The premedications reduce the dose requirement for ketamine, and the antisialagogue reduces the sometimes troublesome salivation.

In adults and children ketamine can be used as a supplement or adjunct to regional anesthesia extending the usefulness of the primary (local anesthetic) form of anesthesia. In this setting ketamine can be used prior to the application of painful blocks,[164] but more commonly it is used for sedation or supplemental anesthesia during long or uncomfortable procedures. When used for supplementation of regional anesthesia, ketamine (0.5 mg/kg IV) combined with diazepam (0.15 mg/kg IV) is better accepted by patients and not associated with greater side effects than those seen in unsedated patients.[165] Ketamine in low doses can also be combined with N_2O for the supplementation of conduction or local anesthesia. These techniques of ketamine administration are used in outpatient and inpatient settings, and although patients are comfortable and cooperative, dreams and other unpleasant emergence reactions can occur.[89]

Doses and Routes of Administration

Ketamine can be administered intravenously, intramuscularly, orally, and rectally. The vast majority of clinical use involves the IV and IM routes, where the drug rapidly achieves therapeutic levels. The dose depends on the desired therapeutic effect and the route of administration. Table 9-6 contains general recommended doses for the IV and IM administration of ketamine for various therapeutic goals.[89] Most anesthetic drugs because of their side effects require that dosage by reduced in the elderly and seriously ill. Such a recommendation probably is prudent with ketamine, although data supporting this are not available. Patients who have been critically ill for a prolonged period may have exhausted their catecholamine stores and may exhibit the circulatory depressant effects of ketamine.[166] The peak action after IV administration is 30 to 60 seconds. Onset is about 5 minutes, with peak effect in about 20 minutes after IM administration. The continuous infusion of IV ketamine with or without concomitant drugs is a satisfactory method to keep blood levels in the therapeutic range. The use of concomitant drugs such as benzodiazepines permits a lower dose requirement for ketamine while enhancing the recovery by reducing emergence reactions.

Side Effects and Contraindications

The common psychological emergence reactions have been discussed previously. Contraindications to ketamine relate to specific pharmacologic actions and patient pathology. Patients with increased intracranial pressure and with intracranial mass lesions should not receive ketamine because it can increase the intracranial pressure and has been reported to cause apnea on this basis[167] (also see Ch. 54). Because ketamine has a propensity to cause hypertension and tachycardia with a commensurate increase in myocardial oxygen con-

TABLE 9-6. Uses and Doses of Ketamine

Induction of general anesthesia[a]		
0.5–2 mg/kg IV		
4–6 mg/kg IM		
Maintenance of good anesthesia		
0.5–1 mg/kg IV	PRN	with N_2O 50% in O_2
15–45 µg/kg/min IV		with N_2O 50–70% in O_2
30–90 µg/kg/min IV		without N_2O
Sedation and analgesia		
0.2–0.8 mg/kg IV		more than 2–3 min
2–4 mg/kg IM		

[a] Lower doses are used if adjuvant drugs such as midazolam or thiopental are also given.

sumption, it is contraindicated in patients with ischemic heart disease when it is used as the sole anesthetic.[139] Likewise, it is unwise to give ketamine to patients with vascular aneurysms because of the possible sudden change in arterial pressure. Patients with psychiatric diseases such as schizophrenia or history of adverse reactions to ketamine or one of its congeners also constitute a contraindication.[89]

ETOMIDATE

History

Etomidate (Amidate, Hypnomidate) was synthesized in 1964.[168] It was introduced into clinical practice in 1972.[169] Its properties include hemodynamic stability, minimal respiratory depression, cerebral protection, and pharmacokinetics enabling rapid recovery following either a single dose or a continuous infusion. In animals etomidate also provides a wider margin of safety (ED_{50}/LD_{50}) than thiopental (26.4 versus 4.6).[170] These benefits soon led to the use of etomidate for induction, for maintenance of anesthesia, and for prolonged sedation in the critically ill. This enthusiasm for widespread use, however, was tempered by reports of etomidate inhibiting steroid synthesis after single doses and infusions.[171-173] This effect, combined with other minor disadvantages, such as pain on injection, thrombophlebitis, myoclonia, and a relatively high incidence of nausea and vomiting, led to several editorials[174,175] questioning the role of etomidate in modern anesthetic practice.

Physicochemical Characteristics

Etomidate is an imidazole derivative (R-(+)-pentylethyl-1H-imidazole-5 carboxylate sulfate).[170] Its chemical structure is illustrated in Fig. 9-11. Etomidate exists at two isomers but only the (+) isomer is active as an hypnotic.[176] Its molecular weight is 342.36.[176] Etomidate is water insoluble and is unstable in a neutral solution. It therefore has been formulated with several solvents.[177] Presently it is supplied as a 2 mg/kg propylene glycol (35 percent v/v) solution with a pH of 8.1 and an osmolality of 4,640 mOsm/L.

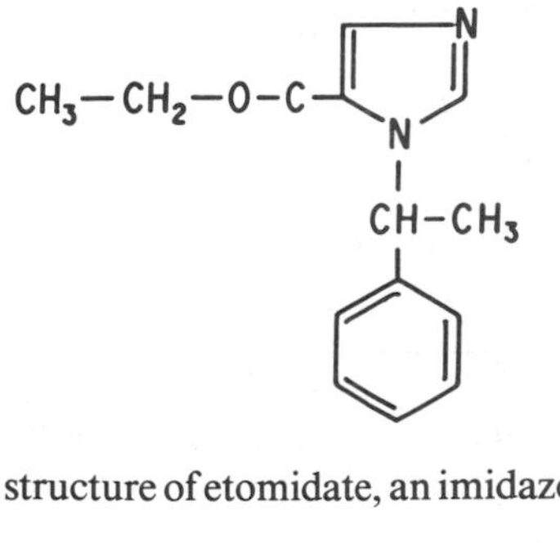

Fig. 9-11. The structure of etomidate, an imidazole derivative.

Metabolism

Etomidate is metabolized in the liver primarily by ester hydrolysis to carboxylic acid of etomidate (major metabolite) or by *n*-dealkylation.[176] The main metabolite is inactive.[177] Only 2 percent of the drug is excreted unchanged. The rest is excreted as metabolites by the kidney (85 percent) and bile (13 percent).[177]

Pharmacokinetics

The pharmacokinetics of etomidate have been calculated following single bolus doses and continuous infusion[178-182] (Table 9-2). The kinetics of etomidate are best described by an open three-compartment model.[178-180] It has an initial distribution half-life of 3 minutes and redistribution half-life of 29 minutes.[178,180] The elimination half-life varies from 2.9 to 5.3 hours.[178-182] Clearance of etomidate by the liver is high (18 to 25 ml/kg/min) with an hepatic extraction ratio of 0.5 to 0.9.[177-181] Thus drugs affecting hepatic blood flow will alter its elimination half-life. The volume of distribution at steady state is 2.5 to 4.5 L/kg.[178-182] Seventy-five percent of etomidate is protein bound.[183] Pathologic conditions altering serum proteins (e.g., hepatic or renal disease) vary the amount of the free (unbound) fraction and thus may vary its pharmacologic effect.[183]

In patients with cirrhosis, the volume of distribution is doubled while clearance is normal. This results in an elimination half-life double normal.[184] Increasing age is associated with a smaller initial volume of distribution and a decreased clearance of etomidate.[185] The relatively short elimination half-life and rapid clearance of etomidate makes it suitable for administration in a single dose, multiple doses, or as a continuous infusion.

Pharmacology

Central Nervous System Effects

The primary action of etomidate on the CNS is hypnosis. This is achieved in one arm-brain circulation following a normal induction dose (0.3 mg/kg). The duration of hypnosis is 5 to 15 minutes, but it is dose dependent.[177,186] Etomidate has no analgesic activity. Plasma levels required during the maintenance of anesthesia are of the order of 300 to 500 ng/ml, for sedation 150 to 300 ng/ml, and awakening 150 to 250 ng/ml[181,186-188] (Fig. 9-12). The mechanism by which etomidate produces hypnosis is not fully elucidated; however, it may partly be related to the GABA-ergic system as its action may be antagonized by GABA antagonists.[189]

Etomidate acutely lowers intracranial pressure (ICP) ± 30 percent in patients with already raised ICP[190] (also see Ch. 54). At a dose of 0.2 to 0.3 mg/kg it also reduces cerebral blood flow (34 percent) and $CMRO_2$ (45 percent) without altering mean arterial pressure.[191] Thus, cerebral perfusion pressure is maintained or increased and there is a net increase in the

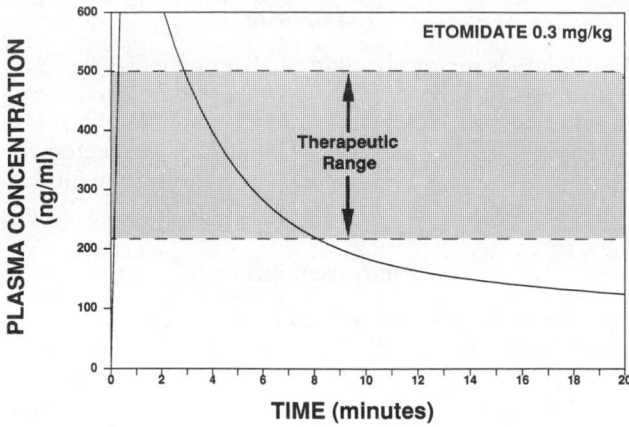

Fig. 9-12. Simulated time course of plasma levels of etomidate following an induction dose of 0.3 mg/kg. Plasma levels required for hypnosis during surgery are 300 to 500 ng/ml, with awakening usually occurring below 225 ng/ml.

cerebral oxygen supply–demand ratio.[191] Cerebral vascular reactivity is still maintained following etomidate administration.[192] In animals, etomidate has reduced brain pathology following acute ischemic insult.[193] To maintain the effects of etomidate on ICP, high infusion rates (60 μg/kg/min) are necessary.[192] Combined infusion plus bolus doses can be used to control rises in ICP, but this may be associated with a drop in mean blood pressure and therefore a reduction in perfusion pressure and loss of beneficial effect.[191] A dose of 0.3 mg/kg rapidly reduces intraocular pressure 30 to 60 percent.[194] The decrease in intraocular pressure following a single dose lasts 5 minutes, but the reduction may be maintained by an infusion of 20 μg/kg/min[194] (also see Ch. 64).

Etomidate produces changes in the EEG similar to the barbiturates.[195] There is an initial increase in alpha amplitude with sharp beta bursts followed by mixed delta-theta waves, with delta-wave activity predominating prior to the onset of periodic burst suppression.[195] The absence of beta waves in the initial phase of induction with etomidate is the major difference in EEG changes compared to thiopental.[195] Etomidate has been associated with grand mal seizures[196,197] and has been shown to produce increased epileptic EEG activity in patients having surgery to remove seizure foci.[197,198] Etomidate is also associated with a high incidence of myoclonic movement.[199,200] The myoclonia is not associated with seizurelike EEG activity.[195] It is believed that the myoclonic movement results from activity in either the brain stem or deep cerebral structures.[169]

The effect of etomidate on auditory-evoked potentials is similar to those produced by the inhaled anesthetics, with a dose-dependent increase in latency and decreasing amplitude of the early cortical components (Pa and Nb).[201] Amplitude and latency of upper limb cortical somatosensory-evoked potentials are increased following 0.4 mg/kg etomidate.[202] Brain-stem-evoked re-

sponses are unaltered following etomidate administration.[201]

Respiratory System Effects

Etomidate has minimal effect on ventilation. Ventilatory response to CO_2 is depressed by etomidate, but the ventilatory drive at any given CO_2 tension is greater than that following an equipotent dose of methohexital.[203] Similarly, the response to occlusion pressure is less depressed following etomidate as compared to an equivalent dose of methohexital.[204] Induction with etomidate produces a brief period of hyperventilation[205,206] sometimes followed by a similarly brief period of apnea.[206] This results in a slight increase in $PaCO_2$ (± 15 percent) but no change in PaO_2.[205,207] The incidence of apnea is altered by premedication.[199,206] Etomidate may result in hiccuping or coughing.[177] The incidence is similar to that following methohexital.[177] Etomidate does not induce histamine release in either normal patients or patients with reactive airways disease.[208]

Cardiovascular System Effects

The minimal effect of etomidate on cardiovascular function is one of its main advantages[205,207,209–212] (Table 9-3). An induction dose of 0.3 mg/kg of etomidate given to patients for noncardiac surgery results in less than 10 percent change in mean arterial pressure, mean pulmonary artery pressure, pulmonary capillary wedge pressure, central venous pressure, stroke volume, cardiac index, and systemic vascular resistance.[210] Heart rate is minimally increased (10 percent) and pulmonary vascular resistance is decreased (18 percent).[210] A relatively large dose of etomidate, 0.45 mg/kg (i.e., 50 percent larger than a normal induction dose)[209] also produces minimal changes in cardiovascular parameters. In patients with ischemic heart disease or valvular pathology,[207,211] etomidate (0.3 mg/kg) produces similar minimal alterations in cardiovascular parameters. Etomidate, in patients with mitral or aortic valve pathology, produces slightly greater changes in mean arterial pressure (-19 percent), systemic vascular resistance (-17 percent), and pulmonary vascular resistance ($+27$ percent)[205] than in patients without cardiac disease. Following induction (18 mg) and infusion (2.4 mg/min), etomidate produces a 50 percent decrease in myocardial blood flow and oxygen consumption and a 20 to 30 percent increase in coronary sinus blood oxygen saturation.[213] Myocardial oxygen supply–demand ratio is thus well maintained.[212,213] The addition of an opioid (fentanyl) to etomidate during induction results in a slightly greater decrease in mean arterial blood pressure (20 percent), systemic vascular resistance (14 percent), and cardiac index (12 percent).[211] However, etomidate, because of its lack of analgesic efficacy does not ablate the sympathetic response to laryngoscopy and intubation.[199,214] Thus, for a smooth hemodynamic induction-intubation sequence, an opiate or inhaled anesthetic needs to be combined with etomidate.

Endocrine Effects

A major disadvantage of etomidate is the inhibition of adrenal synthesis. This effect of etomidate was first reported by Ledingham in 1983. An increase in morbidity in patients sedated with an infusion of etomidate in the intensive care unit was noted.[172] Etomidate suppresses cortisol production following both a single dose and a continuous infusion[172,173] by a reversible and concentration-dependent block of 11-β-hydroxylase (Fig. 9-13). This results in an increase in cortisol precursors, 11-deoxycortisol, and 17-hydroxyprogesterone, as well as an increase in ACTH. The block of 11-β-hydroxylase (and to a lesser extent 17-α-hydroxylase)[215] appears related to the free imidazole radical of etomidate binding cytochrome P450.[216-218] This results in inhibition of ascorbic acid resynthesis, which is required for steroid production in humans.[216,218] Vitamin C supplementation restores cortisol levels to normal following the use of etomidate.[216] The block of the cytochrome P-450 dependent enzyme 11-β-hydroxylase also results in decreased mineralocorticoid production and an increase in intermediaries (11-deoxycorticosterone).[172,173,175] The actual impact of this reversible block of 11-β-hydroxylase on postoperative outcome when etomidate is used for induction or short maintenance periods (minutes–hours) is not established. It is only following prolonged infusions (hours–days) in compromised patients that an increase in morbidity and mortality has been reported.[171]

Other Effects

Etomidate reduces the ED_{50} of pancuronium[219] and therefore appears to enhance the neuromuscular blockade of nondepolarizing neuromuscular blockers. Hepatic function is unaltered by etomidate.[177,178] In vitro etomidate inhibits aminolivulinic acid synthetase, but it has been administered in patients with porphyria without inducing an acute attack of porphyria.[220]

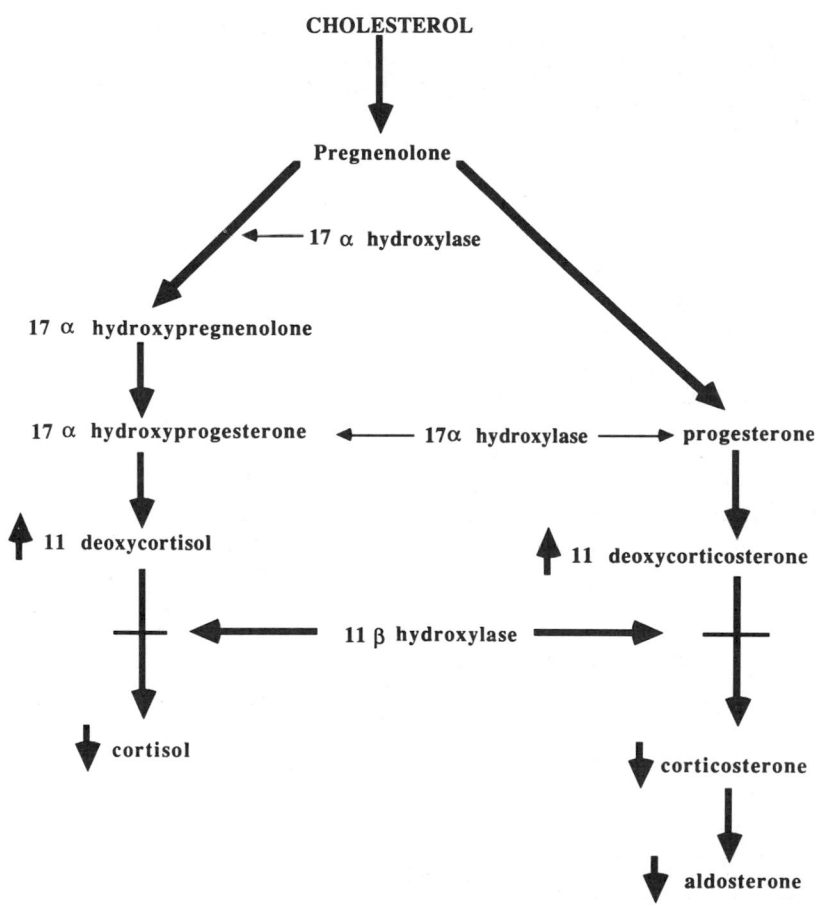

Fig. 9-13. Pathway for the biosynthesis of cortisol and aldosterone. The sites at which etomidate effects cortisol/aldosterone synthesis by its action on 11-β-hydroxylase (major site) and 17-α-hydroxylase (minor site) are illustrated.

Uses

Induction and Maintenance of Anesthesia

Etomidate has been used for both the induction and maintenance of anesthesia (Table 9-7). The induction dose of etomidate varies from 0.2 mg/kg to 0.4 mg/kg.[169,177,200] Premedication with a narcotic, benzodiazepine, or barbiturate will reduce the induction dose.[169] Onset of anesthesia following 0.3 mg/kg etomidate is rapid (one arm-brain circulation) and is equivalent to that obtained with an induction dose of thiopental or methohexital.[169,177,214] The duration of anesthesia following a single induction dose is 5 to 15 minutes[169,177,221] (Fig. 9-12). Repeat doses of etomidate, either by bolus or infusion, will prolong the duration of hypnosis. Recovery following etomidate is rapid.[169,199,200,221-224] The addition of small doses of fentanyl with etomidate for short surgical procedures reduces the required dose of etomidate and allows earlier awakening. In children, induction with rectal administration of etomidate has been obtained with 6.5 mg/kg. Hypnosis occurs in 4 minutes. At this dose hemodynamics are unaltered and recovery is still rapid.[225]

A variety of infusion schemes have been devised to utilize etomidate as a maintenance agent for the hypnotic component of anesthesia. Most schemes aim to achieve a plasma level of 300 to 500 ng/ml, which is the concentration necessary for hypnosis.[181,182,187,188] Both two- and three-stage infusions have been successfully used. These consist of an initial rapid infusion of 100 μg/kg/min for 10 minutes followed by 10 μg/kg/min thereafter,[188] or 100 μg/kg/min for 3 minutes, 20 μg/kg/min for 27 minutes, and 10 μg/kg/min thereafter.[181] Loss of consciousness with these techniques occurs after 100 to 120 seconds.[181] The infusion is usually terminated 10 minutes prior to desired awakening.[181] During an infusion, hemodynamics are well maintained and adequate spontaneous ventilation is present.[226] The incidence of pain on injection, myoclonus, and thrombophlebitis tend to be less with an infusion technique.[181,187,226] The concentrated form of etomidate used for continuous infusion is not available in the United States.

Sedation

Prolonged sedation for patients in the intensive care unit, though initially popular following the release of etomidate, is now contraindicated owing to inhibition of corticosteroid and mineralocorticoid production with subsequent increase in morbidity. Short-term sedation has not gained popularity.

Side Effects and Contraindications

Although etomidate provides stable hemodynamics and minimal respiratory depression, it is associated with several adverse effects when used for induction. These are pain on injection, myoclonic movement, and hiccuping.[169,177,199,200,221-223] Etomidate is also associated with a high incidence of nausea and vomiting[200,222,223] and thrombophlebitis of the vein used for its injection.[227] Pain on injection is less with the present propylene glycol formulation,[200,224] and is further reduced by using a large vein[169,221] or a benzodiazepine plus narcotic premedication.[199,224] Preinjection of a small dose of lidocaine (20 to 40 mg) into the vein with a partially inflated cuff, 1 to 2 minutes prior to etomidate administration, also reduces the pain on injection.[228] The incidence of pain on injection varies from 10 to 50 percent. The incidence of muscle movement (myoclonus) and hiccuping is also highly variable (10 to 70 percent). Myoclonus is reduced by premedication with either a narcotic or benzodiazepine.[224] Speed of injection, fast or slow, has also been advocated in reducing myoclonus.[221,224]

Nausea and vomiting is particularly frequent following the use of etomidate (30 to 40 percent).[199,200,223,224] This compares to an incidence of 10 to 20 percent with methohexital[177,222] or thiopental.[199,220] The addition of fentanyl to etomidate further increases the incidence of nausea and vomiting.[199,200] Nausea and vomiting are singularly the most common reason for patients to rate anesthesia with etomidate unsatisfactory.[223] The incidence of thrombophlebitis has increased with the present propylene glycol formulation (23 percent).[229] Intra-arterial injection of etomidate is not associated with local or vascular pathology.[169]

PROPOFOL

History

Propofol (Diprivan) is the most recent intravenous anesthetic to be introduced into clinical practice. Work in the early 1970s on substituted derivatives of phenol with hypnotic properties resulted in the development of 2, 6 diisopropofol.[230] The first clinical trial by Kay and Rolly, reported in 1977, confirmed the potential of propofol as an anesthetic induction agent.[231] Propofol is insoluble in water and therefore was initially prepared with Cremophor EL (BASF Aktiengesellschaft). Because of anaphylactoid reactions associated with Cremophor EL in this early formulation of propofol,[232] the drug was reformulated in an emulsion. Propofol has

TABLE 9-7. Uses and Doses of Etomidate

Induction of general anesthesia	0.2–0.3 mg/kg IV
Maintenance of general anesthesia	10 μg/kg/min IV with N_2O and an opiate
Sedation	5–8 μg/kg/min IV only for short periods of sedation due to inhibition of corticosteroid synthesis

been used for induction and maintenance of anesthesia as well as for sedation for short periods (to supplement regional anesthesia) and for longer periods (for patients in intensive care units).

Physicochemical Characteristics

Propofol is one of a group of alkylphenols that have hypnotic properties in animals.[233] The structure of propofol is illustrated in Fig. 9-14. The alkylphenols are oils at room temperature and thus are insoluble in aqueous solution but are highly lipid soluble. The present formulation consists of 1 percent (wt/vol) propofol, 10 percent soyabean oil, 2.25 percent glycerol, and 1.2 percent purified egg phosphatide. It has a pH of 7 and appears as a slightly viscous milky-white substance. Propofol will initially be released in the United States in 20-ml clear glass ampules. Propofol is stable at room temperature and is not light sensitive. If a dilute solution of propofol is required, it is compatible with 5 percent dextrose water.

Metabolism

Propofol is rapidly metabolized in the liver by conjugation to glucuronide and sulfate.[234] This produces water soluble compounds which are excreted by the kidneys.[234] Less than 1 percent propofol is excreted unchanged in urine and only 2 percent is excreted in feces.[234] The metabolites of propofol are thought not to be active. Because clearance of propofol exceeds hepatic blood flow, extrahepatic metabolism or extrarenal elimination (e.g., lungs) has been suggested.

Pharmacokinetics

The pharmacokinetics of propofol have been evaluated by numerous investigators following a wide range of doses as well as following continuous infusions[234-240] and have been described by both two- and three-compartment models (Table 9-2). Following a single bolus injection, whole-blood propofol levels decrease very rapidly owing to both redistribution and elimination (Fig. 9-15). The initial distribution half-life of propofol is 2 to 8 minutes.[234,236] In studies using a two-compartment model the elimination half-life varies from 1.0 to 3 hours.[234,235,239,240] Studies describing a three-compartment model have a redistribution phase with a half-life of 30 to 60 minutes and an elimination half-life of 4 to 7

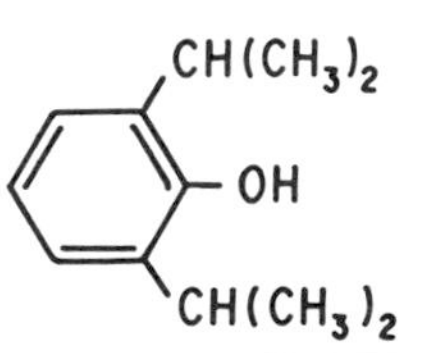

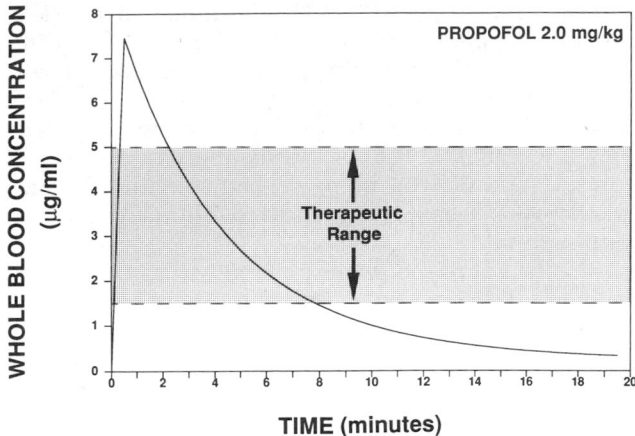

Fig. 9-15. Simulated time course of whole-blood levels of propofol following an induction dose of 2.0 mg/kg. Blood levels required for anesthesia during surgery are 2 to 5 μg/kg, with awakening usually occurring below a blood level of 1.5 μg/ml.

hours.[236-238,240] This longer elimination half-life is indicative of a deep compartment with limited perfusion that results in a slow return of propofol back to the central compartment. This may be important following prolonged infusions when accumulation may occur, preventing rapid emergence on termination of the infusion. The volume of distribution of the central compartment has been calculated as 20 to 40 L, and the volume of distribution at steady state as 150 to 700 L.[234-240] The clearance of propofol is extremely high, 1.5 to 2.1 L/min.[234-240] This exceeds hepatic blood flow.

The pharmacokinetics of propofol may be altered by a variety of factors; for example, gender, weight, pre-existing disease, age, and concomitant medication.[236,237,240-242] Women have a higher volume of distribution and higher clearance rates, but the elimination half-life is similar in males and females.[236,240] The elderly have decreased clearance rates but a smaller central compartment volume.[237,240] Hepatic disease appears to result in a larger steady state and central compartment volumes.[241] Clearance is unchanged, but the elimination half-life is slightly prolonged.[241] Fentanyl administration may reduce the clearance of propofol. Preliminary data indicate that propofol kinetics are unaltered by renal disease.[242]

Pharmacology

Central Nervous System Effects

Propofol is primarily an hypnotic. Unlike barbiturates, propofol is not antanalgesic, but it has not been established if propofol has analgesic properties.[243] The onset of hypnosis following doses of 2.5 mg/kg is rapid (one-arm brain circulation).[244,245] Propofol displays hysteresis of its hypnotic effect,[246] and therefore lower doses (1 to 1.5 mg/kg) can induce anesthesia but time to onset

Fig. 9-14. The structure of propofol, an alkylphenol derivative.

of anesthesia is longer.[244,247] The duration of hypnosis is also dose dependent but lasts 5 to 10 minutes following 2 to 2.5 mg/kg.[244,248] At subhypnotic doses propofol will provide sedation and amnesia.[249,250] Propofol alters mood following short surgical procedures less than does thiopental.[251] Propofol also tends to produce a general state of well being.[251] Hallucinations[252] and opisthotonos[253] have been reported following propofol administration.

The effect of propofol on the EEG was assessed after 2.5 mg/kg followed by an infusion. There is an initial increase in alpha-rhythm followed by shift to delta and theta frequency. High infusion rates produce burst suppression.[254] Using EEG power analysis, amplitude increases after induction but is then unaltered at propofol blood concentrations of 3 to 8 $\mu g/ml$.[246] At propofol concentrations of greater than 8 $\mu g/ml$, amplitude markedly decreases with periods of burst suppression.[246] There is a strong correlation between log blood concentration of propofol and percent delta activity content and an inverse correlation with percent beta activity content.[246]

The effect of propofol on epileptic EEG activity is controversial. Initial studies in mice indicate that propofol neither induced nor provided anticonvulsant activity.[255] In a single report propofol was used to treat epileptic seizures.[256] Propofol also results in a shorter duration of motor and EEG seizure activity following ECT compared to methohexital.[257] Interestingly, propofol has been associated with grand mal seizures and has been used for cortical mapping of epileptogenic foci.[258,259] Propofol produces a decrease in amplitude of the early components of somatosensory-evoked potentials.[260] There is a small, nonsignificant increase in latency of the P_{40} and N_{50} components.[260] Like other intravenous anesthetics, propofol does not alter brain-stem auditory-evoked potentials.[261] There is, however, a dose-dependent prolongation of latency and decrease in amplitude of cortical middle latency auditory potentials.[261]

Propofol will decrease intracranial pressure in patients with either normal or raised intracranial pressure.[262-266] In patients with normal ICP the decrease in intracranial pressure (± 30 percent) is associated with a small decrease in cerebral perfusion pressure (± 10 percent).[265] The addition of small doses of fentanyl and supplemental doses of propofol ablate the rise of intracranial pressures secondary to endotracheal intubation.[265] Normal cerebral reactivity to CO_2 is also maintained during a propofol infusion.[262] In patients with raised intracranial pressure the decrease in ICP (30 to 50 percent) is associated with significant decreases in cerebral perfusion pressure[263,267] and therefore may not be beneficial. Propofol reduces $CMRO_2$ 36 percent.[262] With a background of 0.5 percent enflurane propofol still reduces $CMRO_2$ 18 percent while lactate and glucose metabolism remain unchanged.[266] Propofol acutely reduces intraocular pressure (30 to 40 percent).[268,269] Compared to thiopental, propofol produces a greater decrease in intraocular pressure and following a small second dose is more effective in preventing the rise in intraocular pressure secondary to succinylcholine and endotracheal intubation.[269]

The propofol whole-blood concentration required to prevent movement on skin incision in 50 percent of patients [when combined with a benzodiazepine premedication (lorazepam 1 to 2 mg) and 66 percent N_2O] is 2.5 $\mu g/ml$.[270] This concentration is reduced to 1.7 $\mu g/ml$ with a morphine premedication (0.15 mg/kg).[271] The concentration of propofol (when combined with 66 percent N_2O) required during nonmajor surgery varies from 1.5 to 4.5 $\mu g/ml$[239,240] and for major surgery from 2.5 to 6 $\mu g/ml$.[275] Awakening usually occurs below a concentration of 1.6 $\mu g/ml$,[239,240,248] and orientation below 1.2 $\mu g/ml$.[239,240] Age and concomitant opiate administration will vary the propofol concentration required to provide adequate anesthesia.[240]

Respiratory System Effects

Propofol affects the respiratory system qualitatively similar to the barbiturates.[272-274] Apnea occurs after an induction dose of propofol. The incidence and duration of apnea appears dependent on the dose, speed of injection, and concomitant premedication. An induction dose of propofol results in a 25 to 30 percent incidence of apnea.[272,275] The apnea occurring with propofol, however may be prolonged (greater than 30 seconds). The incidence of prolonged apnea (greater than 30 seconds) is further increased by the addition of an opiate either as a premedication or just prior to induction.[272,275,276] The incidence of prolonged apnea with propofol is greater than that seen with other commonly used intravenous induction agents.[272,276] The onset of apnea is usually preceded by a marked reduction in tidal volume and tachypnea.[274] Following a 2.5 mg/kg induction dose of propofol, respiratory rate is significantly decreased for 2 minutes[272] and minute volume is significantly reduced up to 4 minutes, indicating a more prolonged effect of propofol on tidal volume than respiratory rate. Using inductance plethysmography, similar changes in respiratory rate and minute volume are noted as well as a reduction in forced residual capacity (± 200 ml).[273]

A maintenance infusion of propofol (100 $\mu g/kg/min$) results in a decrease in tidal volume (± 40 percent) and an increase in respiratory frequency (± 20 percent) with an unpredictable change in minute ventilation.[274] Doubling the infusion rate from 100 $\mu g/kg/min$ to 200 $\mu g/kg/min$ causes a further moderate decrease in tidal volume (455 to 380 ml) but no change in respiratory frequency.[274] The ventilatory response to CO_2 is also decreased during a maintenance infusion of propofol.[274] At 100 $\mu g/kg/min$ there is a 58 percent reduction in the slope of the CO_2 response curve.[274] This is similar to the 50 percent depression of CO_2 responsiveness measured at 1 MAC halothane[277] or a brief infusion of 3 mg/kg/min of thiopental.[278] Doubling the infusion rate (and presumably blood level) of propofol results in only minimal further decrease in CO_2 responsiveness.[274] This is in contrast to halothane, where a doubling of MAC results in a halving of the CO_2 response.[277] Propofol, 1.5 to 2.5 mg/kg, results in an acute rise in $PaCO_2$ (13 to 22 percent) and a decrease in pH.[279-281] PaO_2 does not change significantly.[279-281] These changes are similar to those seen following an induction dose of thiopental.[280,281] During a maintenance infusion of propofol (54 μg/kg/min) $PaCO_2$ is moderately increased from 39 mmHg to 52 mmHg.[282] Doubling this infusion rate does not result in a further increase in $PaCO_2$.[282] In patients whose anesthesia is maintained with either a variable-rate infusion of propofol or methohexital, $PaCO_2$ increases similarly and remains within clinically acceptable levels.[283]

Cardiovascular System Effects

The cardiovascular effects of propofol have been evaluated following its use for both induction and maintenance of anesthesia[213,279-282,284-289] (Table 9-3). The most prominent effect of propofol is a drop in arterial blood pressure during induction of anesthesia. Independent of the presence of cardiovascular disease an induction dose of 2 to 2.5 mg/kg produces a 25 to 40 percent reduction of systolic blood pressure.[280,282,287-289] Similar changes are seen in mean and diastolic pressure. The decrease in arterial pressure is associated with a decrease in cardiac output/cardiac index ($\pm$15 percent),[280,282,287-289] stroke volume index ($\pm$20 percent),[282,288,289] and systemic vascular resistance (15 to 25 percent).[280,282,287,288] Left ventricular stroke-work index is also decreased $\pm$30 percent.[288] In patients with valvular heart disease pulmonary artery and pulmonary capillary wedge pressure are also reduced, implying the resultant decrease in pressure is due to a decrease in both preload and afterload.[279] The drop in systemic pressure following an induction dose of propofol appears to be due to both vasodilation and myocardial depression. Heart rate does not change significantly after an induction dose of propofol. It has been suggested that propofol resets rather than inhibits the baroreflex.[290]

During the maintenance of anesthesia with a propofol infusion, systolic pressure remains between 20 and 30 percent below preinduction levels.[282,288] In patients allowed to breathe room air during a maintenance infusion of 100 μg/kg/min propofol, there is a significant decrease in systemic vascular resistance (30 percent), but cardiac index and stroke index are unaltered.[288] In contrast, in patients receiving a narcotic premedication and nitrous oxide with an infusion of propofol (54 and 108 mg/kg/min) for maintenance during surgery, systemic vascular resistance is not significantly decreased from baseline, but cardiac output and stroke volume are.[282] These differences in the effect of propofol on systemic vascular resistance may be due to the presence of nitrous oxide or surgical stimulation. In-

creasing the infusion rate of propofol from 54 to 108 μg/kg/min (blood concentration 2.1 to 4.2 μg/ml) produces only a slightly greater decrease in arterial blood pressure ($\pm$10 percent).[282] Heart rate has been reported to increase,[281,286] decrease,[279,285] and remain unchanged[284] when anesthesia is maintained with propofol. An infusion of propofol results in a significant reduction in both myocardial blood flow and myocardial oxygen consumption.[213,286] This would tend to imply that global myocardial oxygen supply–demand ratio is preserved. The addition of fentanyl (3 μg/kg) to propofol (2.4 mg/kg) results in a significantly greater reduction in mean arterial pressure, heart rate, and cardiac output.[289] Endotracheal intubation generally returns arterial pressure to baseline, largely due to an increase in systemic vascular resistance (SVR).[285,289]

Other Effects

Initial reports indicated that propofol in Cremaphor EL potentiated the action of nondepolarizing neuromuscular blockers.[291,292] However, subsequent studies using propofol in its new formulation failed to show any potentiating effect of propofol (as compared to thiopental) on neuromuscular blockade produced by both nondepolarizing and depolarizing neuromuscular blocking agents.[293,294] Propofol produces no effect on the evoked electromyogram or twitch tension;[293] however, good intubating conditions after propofol alone have been reported.[295]

Preliminary data indicate that propofol does not trigger malignant hyperpyrexia.[296,297] Propofol following a single dose or prolonged infusion does not affect corticosteroid synthesis or alter the normal response to ACTH stimulation. Propofol, in the emulsion formulation, does not alter hepatic, hematologic, or fibrinolytic function.[298,301-302] The initial formulation of propofol with cremaphor was associated with anaphylactoid reactions.[232] The new preparation appears free from histamine release.[303]

Uses

Induction and Maintenance of Anesthesia

Propofol is suitable for both the induction and maintenance of anesthesia (Table 9-8). The induction dose of propofol varies from 1.5 to 2.5 mg/kg.[244,304,305] The ED_{95} in unpremedicated patients is 2.25 to 2.5 mg/kg.[304,306] The present formulation of propofol appears to be slightly less potent than the original Cremaphor EL solution. Premedication (with an opiate) reduces the induction dose to 1.5 to 2.0 mg/kg.[307] Increasing age also reduces the dose of propofol required to induce anesthesia.[308,309] A dose of 1 mg/kg (with premedication) to 1.75 mg/kg (without premedication) is recommended for inducing anesthesia in patients more than 60 years old.[309]

Induction of anesthesia following propofol occurs in

TABLE 9-8. Uses and Doses of Propofol

Induction of general anesthesia	1–2.5 mg/kg IV; dose reduced with age over 50 years
Maintenance of general anesthesia	50–150 μg/kg/min IV combined with N_2O or an opiate
Sedation	25–75 μg/kg/min IV

one arm-brain circulation and is similar to that obtained with the barbiturates.[284,305] Rapid administration (5 seconds) of a 2 mg/kg dose of propofol is more successful in inducing anesthesia than giving the same dose over 60 seconds.[245] Propofol exhibits hysteresis of its hypnotic[246] effect; therefore, to obtain a rapid onset, a relative overdose is administered. The duration of anesthesia after a single induction dose of 1 mg/kg is 2.8 minutes.[305] This increases linearly with increasing doses to 8.4 minutes following 3 mg/kg.[305] Propofol has been evaluated as an induction agent in children 3 to 14 years old. Its action in children is similar to that seen in adults.[310,311]

Propofol, when used for induction of anesthesia in shorter procedures, results in a significantly quicker recovery and earlier return of psychomotor function compared to thiopental or methohexital, irrespective of the agent used for the maintenance of anesthesia.[312–314] The incidence of nausea and vomiting when propofol is used for induction is also markedly less than following the other intravenous induction agents.[306,313] It has thus been suggested that propofol may possess antiemetic properties.[315]

Propofol, because of greater ease of control of anesthetic depth and more rapid recovery, is superior to barbiturates for the maintenance of anesthesia[283,316,317] and appears equal to the inhalation agents.[247,312,318] Propofol can be given as intermittent boluses or a continuous infusion for maintenance of anesthesia.[319] Following a satisfactory induction dose, a bolus of 10 to 40 mg is needed every few minutes to maintain anesthesia. As these doses need to be given frequently, it is more suitable to administer propofol as a continuous infusion. Several infusion schemes have been used to achieve adequate plasma concentrations of propofol.[317,320] Following an induction dose, an infusion of 100 to 200 μg/kg/min of propofol is usually needed.[240,247,270,271,283,312,316,317] The infusion rate is then titrated to individual requirements and the surgical stimulus. Morphine, fentanyl, and alfentanil combined with propofol reduce the required infusion rate and dose.[270,271,321] Increasing age is also associated with a decrease in the infusion requirements of propofol.[322] The blood levels of propofol (2.5 to 6 μg/ml) required for surgery have been established.[239,240,248,270,271,318] The knowledge of these levels and of the pharmacokinetics of propofol have enabled the use of pharmacokinetic model-driven infusion systems to deliver propofol as a continuous infusion for the maintenance of anesthesia.[247,320,323,324]

For short (less than 1 hour) body-surface procedures, the advantages of a more rapid recovery and decreased nausea and vomiting are still evident.[312] However, if propofol is used for longer or more major procedures, both recovery and the incidence of nausea and vomiting are similar to that following thiopental/isoflurane anesthesia.[247,312]

Sedation

Reports of the use of propofol for sedation have been enthusiastic but limited. Propofol has been evaluated for sedation during surgical procedures[249,250,325,326] and for patients ventilated in the intensive care unit.[300,327,328] Propofol, by continuous infusion, provides a readily titratable level of sedation and a rapid recovery once infusion is terminated.[250,325,327,329] A major concern with a prolonged infusion of propofol for sedation is that accumulation of propofol occurs within the deep compartments and therefore recovery following the termination of a prolonged infusion is no longer rapid. However, in a study of patients sedated in the intensive care unit for 4 days with propofol, recovery to consciousness was rapid (± 10 minutes). Both the rate of recovery and decrease in plasma concentration were similar at 24 and 96 hours when the infusion was discontinued. Also, the plasma concentration required for sedation and for awakening were similar at 24 and 96 hours, implying that tolerance to propofol did not occur.[329] Infusion rates required for sedation to supplement regional anesthesia in healthy patients is approximately half that required for general anesthesia (i.e., 50 to 60 μg/kg/min).[249,325] In elderly patients (over 65 years) and sicker patients the necessary infusion rates are markedly reduced.[249,300,327] Thus, it is important to individually titrate the infusion to the desired effect. During the period of infusion with propofol, patients are amnestic.[325,327] In comparison to sedation maintained with midazolam, propofol sedation provides equal or better control and more rapid recovery.[250,325,327] In ventilated patients, more rapid recovery translates to more rapid extubation when sedation is terminated.[327]

Side Effects and Contraindications

Induction of anesthesia with propofol is associated with several side effects. These include pain on injection, myoclonus, apnea, a decrease in arterial blood pressure, and, very rarely, thrombophlebitis of the vein into which propofol is injected. Pain on injection is generally less than with etomidate and equal to that obtained with methohexital but greater than after thiopental.[298,311] The pain on injection is reduced by using a large vein, avoiding veins in the dorsum of the hand, and adding lidocaine to the propofol solution.[298] Myoclonus occurs more frequently following propofol than with thiopental but less frequently than following etomidate or methohexital.[311] Apnea following induction with propofol is common. The incidence of apnea may be similar to that obtained following thiopental or methohexital; however, propofol produces a greater incidence of apnea lasting longer than 30 seconds.[270,276] The addition of an opiate increases the incidence of apnea, especially prolonged apnea.[270,275]

The decrease in systemic blood pressure associated with induction of anesthesia with propofol is its most significant side effect on induction. The addition of an opiate just prior to induction of anesthesia appears to augment the decrease in arterial blood pressure.[289] Perhaps slow administration and lower doses in adequately prehydrated patients may attenuate the decrease in arterial blood pressure. Conversely, in laryngoscopy and endotracheal intubation, increase in mean arterial pressure, heart rate, and systemic vascular resistance are less following propofol than thiopental.[285,289]

DROPERIDOL

History

General anesthesia with inhaled anesthetics and barbiturates depress the entire CNS in a nonspecific manner. Laborit and Huguenard in the 1950s sought an anesthetic technique that would produce "artificial hibernation" devoid of circulatory and respiratory depression.[330,331] Their concept was to use drugs that would produce neurovegetative blockade ("multifocal inhibition") of cellular, autonomic, and endocrine mechanisms normally activated in response to stress.[332] The first attempt at developing this concept was the "lytic cocktail" containing an analgesic (meperidine), two tranquilizers (chlorpromazine and promethazine), and atropine. Although this combination of drugs did enjoy widespread use for conscious sedation, it produced respiratory depression. It was not used for general anesthesia. Janssen[333] synthesized haloperidol, the first member of the butyrophenones, which would become

the primary "neuroleptic" component in neuroleptanesthesia (NLAN). DeCastro and Mundeleer in 1959 combined haloperidol with phenoperidine (a meperidine derivative also synthesized by Janssen), the forerunner to the current practice of neuroleptanesthesia. Droperidol, a derivative of haloperidol and fentanyl, a phenoperidine cogener, both again synthesized by Janssen, was used by DeCastro and Mundeleer in a combination they reported superior to haloperidol and phenoperidine.[334] This neuroleptanesthetic combination produced more rapid onset of analgesia, less respiratory depression, and fewer extrapyramidal side effects. The fixed combination of droperidol and fentanyl, marketed as Innovar in the United States, is the current drug used for NLAN.

Droperidol is a butyrophenone, a fluorinated derivative of phenothiazines (Fig. 9-16).[332] Butyrophenones produce CNS depression characterized by marked apparent tranquility and cataleptic immobility. They are potent antiemetics. Droperidol is a very potent butyrophenone and, like the others, produces its action centrally at sites where dopamine, norepinephrine, and serotonin act. It has been postulated that butyrophenones might occupy GABA receptors on the postsynaptic membrane, thereby reducing synaptic transmission and resulting in a buildup of dopamine in the intersynaptic cleft.[332,333] An imbalance in dopamine and acetylcholine is thought to occur, which results in alteration in normal transmission of signals in the CNS. The chemoreceptor trigger zone (CTZ) is the emetic center, and "red" astrocytes transport neurolept molecules from the capillary to dopaminergic synapses in the CTZ where they occupy GABA receptors (Fig. 9-17). This is thought to be the mechanism by which droperidol exerts its antiemetic effect.[335]

Metabolism and Pharmacokinetics

Droperidol is biotransformed in the liver into two primary metabolites.[336] The plasma decay of droperidol can be described by a two-compartment model. The pharmacokinetics[337] are shown in Table 9-2. It should be noted that the clearance of droperidol is relatively large (14 ml/kg/min) and the elimination half-life is relatively short (103 to 134 minutes).[337,338] The plasma disappearance is similar to fentanyl (Fig. 9-18), yet discrepancy in duration of effect of the two has been the subject of criticism because they are formulated together in Innovar. The seemingly longer CNS action of

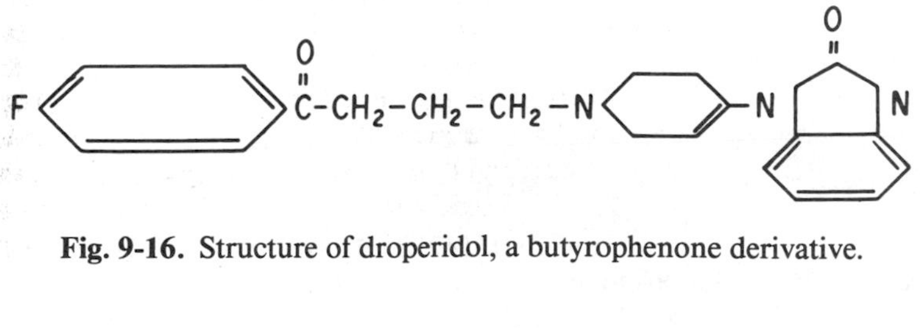

Fig. 9-16. Structure of droperidol, a butyrophenone derivative.

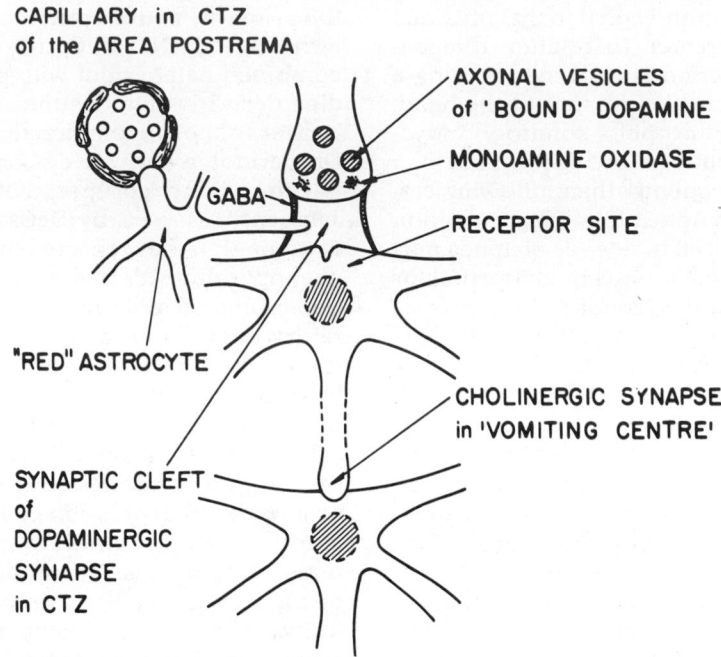

Fig. 9-17. Site of action of droperidol. Mode of action of NLAN drugs at the CTZ. (From Janssen,[371] with permission.)

droperidol has prompted some to postulate that droperidol has a propensity to occupy CNS receptors,[337] and that it has greater receptor binding than does fentanyl.

Pharmacology

Central Nervous System Effects

The effects of neuroleptics on human cerebrospinal fluid (CBF) and $CMRO_2$ have not been studied. Droperidol causes potent cerebral vasoconstriction in dogs, producing a 40 percent reduction in CBF. No significant change in $CMRO_2$ occurs during droperidol administration.[339] The EEG in conscious patients shows some reduction in the frequency in the alpha range, with occasional slowing to the theta range.[340]

Respiratory System Effects

Droperidol has little effect when used alone on the respiratory system.[341] Droperidol (0.44 mg/kg) given to surgical patients produced a slight reduction in respira-

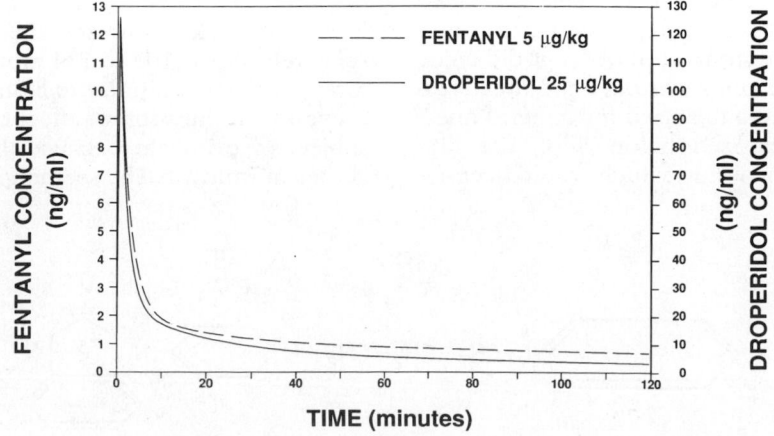

Fig. 9-18. Simulated time course of plasma levels of fentanyl and droperidol after an induction dose of fentanyl (50 μg/kg) and droperidol (250 μg/kg). Note the parallel plasma disappearance of the drugs.

tory rate.[342] Droperidol (3 mg IV) had no significant effect on tidal volume in volunteers.[343] More detailed respiratory studies are not available.

Cardiovascular System Effects

The predominant cardiovascular effect of droperidol is vasodilation with a decrease in blood pressure (Table 9-3). This is considered a result of moderate α-adrenergic blockade.[336,344,345] Importantly, the dopamine-induced increase in renal blood flow (renal artery flowmeter methodology) is not significantly impaired by the administration of droperidol.[346] Droperidol has little effect on myocardial contractility.[347] It seems to possess some antiarrhythmic effects much like those of quinidine.[347,348]

INNOVAR

Innovar is a combination of droperidol and fentanyl in a ratio of 50:1 (droperidol 2.5 mg/ml and fentanyl 50 μg/ml). Lactic acid is added for adjustment of pH to 3.5. The pharmacologic effects of Innovar are those of its two component drugs. Droperidol produces hypnosis, sedation, and antiemetic effects while fentanyl produces analgesia. There is no apparent synergistic or supra-additive effect of the two drugs, but simply an additive effect; that is, the effects of each drug add to those of the other. Recovery from NLAN produced by Innovar is usually prompt after the cessation of N_2O, and consciousness returns within 3 to 5 minutes.[332] In the recovery period, patients tend to be drowsy, detached, and free of pain, nausea, and vomiting.

Pharmacology

Respiratory System Effects

Innovar produces respiratory depression in a dose-related fashion. Respiratory effects are peripheral and central and are produced by fentanyl. The peripheral effects involve trunchal rigidity. The central respiratory depression is a result of fentanyl action at the respiratory center. Both respiratory rate and tidal volume are reduced by Innovar[343,349,351]; the contribution of droperidol to this is limited.[352] Innovar and/or the combination or droperidol with fentanyl reduces respiratory function more than droperidol alone.[342,343] Respiratory depression can be antagonized by the administration of an opioid competitive antagonist.

Cardiovascular System Effects

The primary cardiovascular effect of Innovar is a decrease in arterial blood pressure.[350] This is the droperidol component that produces α-adrenergic blockade. Heart rate decreases from the fentanyl-induced increased vagal tone.[12] Despite these changes, Innovar does not significantly reduce cardiac output in patients with adequate blood volumes. The antiarrhythmic

properties of droperidol are those present in Innovar.[353]

Uses

Neuroleptanesthesia may be induced with droperidol and fentanyl (or other opioids) separately or with the drug Innovar. Innovar should be used with caution during induction because of possible vasodilation and hypotension. It is recommended that a test dose of 1 to 2 ml be administered prior to induction of NLAN with Innovar. If the components are given separately, droperidol should be administered first in a dose of about 5 to 10 mg (5 to 15 μg/kg) and followed by incremental doses of fentanyl in 50 to 100 μg increments. The usual induction dose of Innovar is 0.1 to 0.15 ml/kg (Table 9-9) in fit adults; this is almost always administered with N_2O and a muscle relaxant. It is recommended that 200 to 300 ml of balanced salt solution be administered prior to induction and that hypotension be treated with further fluid administration. Elderly and other high-risk patients require less Innovar for induction of anesthesia. Supplementation of anesthesia during NLAN should be with fentanyl and not Innovar. The reason for this is that the prolonged duration of action of droperidol will produce postoperative somnolence if it is repeated during the operation.

Innovar in markedly reduced doses can be used for intravenous sedation during conduction anesthesia or selected diagnostic procedures performed under local anesthesia. The customary dose of Innovar for sedation is about 2 to 4 ml given in divided doses titrating to the desired level of sedation. Innovar has been used for many types of procedures and can be safely used in most. Operations that are particularly suited for Innovar are those with a high incidence of postoperative nausea and vomiting (e.g., middle ear surgery). Small doses of droperidol or Innovar may be helpful in outpatient procedures that are associated with nausea and vomiting. Innovar may also be used as a sedative/analgesic for sedation during diagnostic and surgical procedures. It does not produce reliable amnesia.

Side Effects and Contraindications

Innovar is not associated with organ toxicity or tissue or venous irritation. However, it does have several adverse effects. Muscle rigidity is a consequence of the

TABLE 9-9. Uses and Doses of Innovar

Induction of general anesthesia
0.1–0.15 ml/kg with N_2O 50–66% in O_2[a]
Maintenance of general anesthesia
Fentanyl   1–2 μg/kg PRN
Fentanyl   0.01–0.05 μg/kg/min
Sedation and analgesia
0.5–1.0 ml IV repeated and titrated to desired effect
1–2 ml IM

[a] Dose should be reduced in hypovolemic and other high risk patients. Each ml of Innovar contain droperidol 2.5 μg and fentanyl 50 μg.

fentanyl and is more of a problem if large doses are given rapidly. Treatment and prevention include giving a muscle relaxant with the Innovar. Respiratory depression is also a result of the fentanyl and can be reversed with an opioid antagonist, but this can reverse the analgesia and may precipitate hypertension. Hypotension from the droperidol component is a common side effect of Innovar that can be treated with intravascular blood-volume expansion or an α-adrenergic agonist (e.g., phenylephrine). Prolonged somnolence or detachment is a result of the droperidol and is dose related. Although this has been reversed with physostigmine (2 mg), this is not a specific antagonist and the possibility that resedation may occur is real because droperidol clearance is less than that of physostigmine. Extrapyramidal complications manifested by dyskinesia, especially of the face, neck, and pharyngeal muscles, with speech and swallowing difficulties, grimacing, trismus, oculogyric spasms, and torticollis occur in a small percentage of patients given Innovar.[354] It is the droperidol component that produces this reaction. Treatment of this may be with diphenhydramine or benztropine. Some patients have an unusual psychological reaction, particularly when Innovar is used as a premedicant, and patients have refused to have surgery after Innovar premedication. Patients report hallucinations and bizarre sensations of weightlessness and loss of body image; these reactions can be successfully treated with a benzodiazepine. A final and very rare complication of Innovar is the malignant neuroleptic syndrome.[355,356] This syndrome is characterized by hyperthermia, muscular rigidity, autonomic instability. The muscular hypertonicity is lead-pipe. Although this reaction can be distinguished from malignant hyperthermia by the temperature course (which is lower) and muscle biopsy studies, dantrolene has been successfully used to treat the syndrome.[355] Bromocriptine, a central dopamine agonist, has also been used (2.5 to 10 mg tid PO) to treat this syndrome, which is mostly encountered in patients taking butyrophenones and phenothiazines for psychiatric disturbances.

OTHER INTRAVENOUS HYPNOTICS

Propanidid, althesin, minaxolone, and gamma-hydroxybutyric acid (GABA) have been used to induce anesthesia; however, none are available in the United States. Propanidid is a eugenol derivative that is highly water insoluble. Onset of anesthesia and recovery is rapid. The rapid recovery is due to both redistribution and metabolism. The drug is metabolized by pseudocholinesterase, resulting in an elimination half-life of 10 minutes. The major disadvantage of propanidid is a high incidence of severe allergic reaction, which has prevented its release in the United States and resulted in its withdrawal in several other countries.

Althesin is a combination of two steroids, alphaxalone (primary active steroid) and alphadolone (to increase solubility). Like propanidid, althesin is highly water insoluble and is dissolved in Cremophor EL. Althesin has similar properties to other intravenous induction agents and is also useful for the maintenance of anesthesia and sedation when given by infusion. Like propanidid, a high incidence of hypersensitivity reactions (approximately 1 in 10,000) has resulted in the total withdrawal of this intravenous anesthetic.

Minaxolone is an attempt to provide a water-soluble steroid. It has only been available for investigative purposes. Patients induced with minaxolone show a relatively high incidence of excitatory phenomenon as well as prolonged recovery. It is unlikely therefore that minaxolone will reach general clinical practice. GABA is closely related to naturally occurring neuroinhibitors and is capable of producing anesthesia. However it results in significant side effects, including prolonged recovery, emergence delirium, extrapyramidal muscle movement, and venous irritation. The drug has therefore not been approved for clinical practice in the United States.

The search for an ideal intravenous hypnotic continues; however at present only the α_2-adrenergic blockers show any potential for human investigation. The α_2-adrenergic blockers have proved to be useful hypnotics in animals.[357] The cardiovascular effects (hypotension) of these drugs may be their major drawback. However they show sufficient advantages that human clinical trials are being undertaken.

SUMMARY

A great variety of intravenous drugs are available for use in the care of patients requiring general anesthesia. The selection of a particular drug must be based on the individual patients need for hypnosis, amnesia, and analgesia. Drug selection must match the physiology and/or the pathophysiology of the individual patient with the pharmacology of the particular drug. Thus, for example, a patient in shock who required anesthesia induction should receive the drug that will produce rapid onset of effect without causing further hemodynamic compromise. The knowledge of the clinical pharmacology of each of the intravenous anesthetic drugs enables the clinician to safely and effectively induce and maintain sedation and/or general anesthesia. There is no single perfect drug for any particular patient, but rather it is the informed practitioner who wisely employs the appropriate drug or drugs in the practice of good anesthesia care.

REFERENCES

1. Cohen MM, Duncan PG, Tate RB: Does anesthesia contribute to operative mortality? JAMA 260:2859, 1988
2. Greenblatt DJ, Shader RI: Benzodiazepines in Clinical Practice. Raven Press, New York, 1974
3. Randall LO, Schallek W, Heise GA, et al: The psychosedative

properties of methaminodiazepoxide. J Pharmacol Exp Ther 129:163, 1960

4. Lemere F: Toxic reactions to chlordiazepoxide. JAMA 174:893, 1960

5. Walser A, Benjamin LE, Sr., Flynn T, et al: Quinazolines and 1,4-benzodiazepines. 84, Synthesis and reactions of imidazo (1,5-a)(1,4)-benzodiazepines. J Org Chem 43:936, 1978

6. Urban BJ, Amaha K, Steen SN: Investigation of 1-4-benzodiazepine derivatives as basal anesthetic agents. Anesth Analg 45:733, 1966

7. McClish A: Diazepam as an intravenous induction agent for general anaesthesia. Can Anaesth Soc J 13:562, 1966

8. Stovner J, Endresen R: Intravenous anaesthesia with diazepam. Acta Anaesth Scand Suppl 24:223, 1966

9. Reves JG, Fragen RJ, Vinik HR, Greenblatt DJ: Midazolam: Pharmacology and uses. Anesthesiology 62:310, 1985

10. Haefely W, Hunkeler W: The story of flumazenil. Eur J Anaesthesiol 2:3, 1988

11. Barnett A, Fiore JW: Acute tolerance to diazepam in cats and its possible relationship to diazepam metabolism. Eur J Pharmacol 13:239, 1971

12. Marta JA, Davis HS, Eisele JH: Vagomimetic effects of morphine and Innovar in man. Anesth Analg 52:817, 1973

13. Squires RF, Braestrup C: Benzodiazepine receptors in rat brain. Nature 266:732, 1977

14. Greenblatt DJ, Shader RI, Abernethy DR: Medical intelligence drug therapy: Current status of benzodiazepines. New Engl J Med 309:354, 1983

15. Arendt RM, Greenblatt DJ, DeJong RH, et al: In vitro correlates of benzodiazepine cerebrospinal fluid uptake, pharmacodynamic action and peripheral distribution. J Pharmacol Exp Ther 227:98, 1983

16. Elliott HW: Metabolism of lorazepam. Br J Anaesth 48:1017, 1976

17. Blitt CD: Clinical pharmacology of lorazepam. p. 135. In Brown BR, Jr. (ed): New Pharmacologic Vistas in Anesthesia. FA Davis, Philadelphia, 1983

18. Klotz U, Reimann I: Elevation of steady-state diazepam levels by cimetidine. Clin Pharmacol Ther 30:513, 1981

19. Reves JG: Benzodiazepines. p. 157. In Prys-Roberts C, Hugg CC (eds): Pharmacokinetics of Anaesthesia. Blackwell Scientific Publications, Boston, 1984

20. Kassai A, Eichelbaum M, Klotz U: No evidence of a genetic polymorphism in the oxidative metabolism of midazolam. Clin Pharmacokinet 15:319, 1988

21. Ziegler WH, Schalch E, Leishman B, Eckert M: Comparison of the effects of intravenously administered midazolam, triazolam and their hydroxy metabolites. Br J Clin Pharmacol 16:63S, 1983

22. Greenblatt DJ, Shader RI, Harmatz JS: Benzodiazepines: A summary of pharmacokinetic properties. Br J Clin Pharmacol 11:11, 1981

23. MacLeod SM, Giles HG, Bengert B: Age- and gender-related differences in diazepam pharmacokinetics. J Clin Pharmacol 19:15, 1979

24. Greenblatt DJ, Abernethy DR, Locniskar A, et al: Effect of age, gender, and obesity on midazolam kinetics. Anesthesiology 61:27, 1984

25. Mohler H, Richards JG: The benzodiazepine receptor: A pharmacological control element of brain function. Eur J Anaesthesiol 2:15, 1988

26. Amrein R, Hetzel W, Harmann D, Lorscheid T: Clinical pharmacology of flumazenil. Eur J Anaesthesiol 2:65, 1988

27. Haefely W: The preclinical pharmacology of flumazenil. Eur J Anaesthesiol 2:25, 1988

28. Forster A, Juge O, Morel D: Effects of midazolam on cerebral blood flow in human volunteers. Anesthesiology 53:A263, 1981

29. Brown CR, Sarnquist FH, Canup CA, Pedley TA: Clinical electroencephalographic and pharmacokinetic studies of water-soluble benzodiazepine, midazolam maleate. Anesthesiology 50:467, 1979

30. de Jong RH, Bonin JD: Benzodiazepines protect mice from local anesthetic convulsions and deaths. Anesth Analg 60:385, 1981

31. Denault M, Yernault JC, DeCoster A: Double-blind comparison of the respiratory effects of parenteral lorazepam and diazepam in patients with chronic obstructive lung disease. Curr Med Res Opin 2:611, 1975

32. Forster A, Gardaz JP, Suter PM, Gemperle M: Respiratory depression by midazolam and diazepam. Anesthesiology 53:494, 1980

33. Sunzel M, Paalzow L, Berggren L, Eriksson I: Respiratory and cardiovascular effects in relation to plasma levels of midazolam and diazepam. Br J Clin Pharmacol 25:561, 1988

34. Gross JB, Zebrowski ME, Carel WD, et al: Time course of ventilatory depression after thiopental and midazolam in normal subjects and in patients with chronic obstructive pulmonary disease. Anesthesiology 58:540, 1983

35. Paulson BA, Becker LD, Way WL: The effects of intravenous lorazepam alone and with meperidine on ventilation in man. Acta Anaesthesiol Scand 27:400, 1983

36. Samuelson PN, Reves JG, Kouchoukos NT, et al: Hemodynamic responses to anesthetic induction with midazolam or diazepam in patients with ischemic heart disease. Anesth Analg 60:802, 1981

37. Rao S, Sherbaniuk RW, Prasad K, et al: Cardiopulmonary effects of diazepam. Clin Pharmacol Ther 1973; 14:182, 1973

38. Samuelson PN, Lell WA, Kouchoukos NT, et al: Hemodynamics during diazepam induction of anesthesia for coronary artery bypass grafting. South Med J 73:332, 1980

39. Cote P, Gueret P, Courassa MG: Systemic and coronary hemodynamic effects of diazepam in patients with normal and diseased coronary arteries. Circulation 50:1210, 1974

40. Reves JG, Samuelson PN, Lewis S: Midazolam maleate induction in patients with ischaemic heart disease: Haemodynamic observations. Can Anaesth Soc J 26:402, 1979

41. Reves JG, Samuelson PN, Linnan M: Effects of midazolam maleate in patients with elevated pulmonary artery occluded pressure. p. 253. In Aldrete JA, Stanley TH (eds): Trends in Intravenous Anesthesia. Year Book Medical Publishers, Chicago, 1980

42. Elliott HW, Nomof N, Navarro G, et al: Central nervous system and cardiovascular effects of lorazepam in man. Clin Pharmacol Ther 12:468, 1971

43. Ruff R, Reves JG, Croughwell ND, Brusino FG: The cardiovascular effects of benzodiazepines. p. 3. In Estafanous FG (ed): Anesthesia and the Heart Patient. Butterworths, Boston, 1989

44. Reves JG, Gelman S: Cardiovascular effects of intravenous anesthetic drugs. p. 179. In Covino BL, Fozzard HA, Rehder K, Strichartz G (eds): Effects of Anesthesia. Am Physiol Soc, Bethesda, MD, 1985

45. Marty J, Gauzit R, Lefevre P, et al: Effects of diazepam and midazolam on baroreflex control of heart rate and on sympathetic activity in humans. Anesth Analg 65:113, 1986

46. Lebowitz PW, Cote ME, Daniels AL, et al: Comparative cardiovascular effects of midazolam and thiopental in healthy patients. Anesth Analg 61:771, 1982

47. Croughwell N, Reves JG, Hawkins E: Cardiovascular

changes after midazolam in patients with aortic stenosis: Effects of nitrous oxide. Anesth Analg 67:S1, 1988

48. Tomichek RC, Rosow CE, Schneider RC, et al: Cardiovascular effects of diazepam-fentanyl anesthesia in patients with coronary artery disease. Anesth Analg 61:217, 1982

49. Heikkila H, Jalonen J, Arola M, et al: Midazolam as adjunct to high-dose fentanyl anaesthesia for coronary artery bypass grafting operation. Acta Anaesthesiol Scand 28:683, 1984

50. Benson KT, Tomlinson DL, Goto H, Arakawa K: Cardiovascular effects of lorazepam during sufentanil anesthesia. Anesth Analg 67:966, 1988

51. Windsor JPW, Sherry K, Feneck RO, Sebel PS: Sufentanil and nitrous oxide anaesthesia for cardiac surgery. Br J Anaesth 61:662, 1988

52. Reves JG, Croughwell N: Valium-fentanyl interaction. p. 356. In Reves JG, Hall KD (eds): Common Problems in Cardiac Anesthesia. Year Book Medical Publishers, Chicago, 1987

53. Cole SG, Brozinsky S, Isenberg JI: Midazolam, a new more potent benzodiazepine, compared with diazepam: A randomized, double-blind study of preendoscopic sedatives. Gastrointest Endosc 29:219, 1983

54. George KA, Dundee JW: Relative amnesic actions of diazepam, flunitrazepam and lorazepam in man. Br J Clin Pharmacol 4:45, 1977

55. Fragen RJ, Caldwell N: Lorazepam premedication: Lack of recall and relief anxiety. Anesth Analg 55:792, 1976

56. Kanto J, Sjovall S, Vuori A: Effect of different kinds of premedication on the induction properties of midazolam. Br J Anaesth 54:507, 1982

57. Gamble JAS, Kawar P, Dundee JW, Moore J, Briggs LP: Evaluation of midazolam as an intravenous induction agent. Anaesthesia 36:868, 1981

58. Greenblatt DJ, Sellers EM, Shader RI: Drug disposition in old age. N Engl J Med 306:1081, 1982

59. Forster A, Gardaz JP, Suter PM, Gemperle M: I.V. midazolam as an induction agent for anaesthesia: A study in volunteers. Br J Anaesth 52:907, 1980

60. Reves JG, Vinik R, Hirschfield AM, et al: Midazolam compared with thiopentone as a hypnotic component in balanced anaesthesia: A randomized, double-blind study. Can Anaesth Soc J 26:42, 1979

61. Crawford ME, Carl P, Andersen RS, Mikkelsen BO: Comparison between midazolam and thiopentone-based balanced anaesthesia for day-care surgery. Br J Anaesth 56:165, 1984

62. Melvin MA, Johnson BH, Quasha AL, Eger EI II: Induction of anesthesia with midazolam decreases halothane MAC in humans. Anesthesiology 57:238, 1982

63. Nilsson A, Persson MP: Total intravenous anaesthesia—is there a future for midazolam? Acta Anaesthesiol Scand 32:S87:6, 1988

64. Reves JG, Jacobs JR, Croughwell ND, et al: Computer-assisted continuous infusion of midazolam for anesthesia during cardiac surgery. R Vinik (ed): Excerpta Medica, (in press)

65. Nilsson A, Persson MP, Hartvig P, Wide L: Effect of total intravenous anaesthesia with midazolam/alfentanil on the adrenocrotical and hyperglycaemic response to abdominal surgery. Acta Anaesthesiol Scand 32:379, 1988

66. File SE, Pellow S: Intrinsic actions of the benzodiazepine receptor antagonist RO 15-1788. Psychopharmacol 88:I, 1986

67. Limbird LE: Cell Surface Receptors: A Short Course on Theory and Methods. Nijhoff, Boston, 1986

68. Lauven P, Schwilden H, Stoeckel H, Greenblatt DJ: The effect of a benzodiazepine antagonist Ro 15-1788 in the presence of stable concentrations of midazolam. Anesthesiology 63:61, 1985

69. Cumin R, Bonetti EP, Scherschlicht R, Haefely WE: Use of the specific benzodiazepine antagonist, Ro 15-1788, in studies of physiological dependence on benzodiazepines. Experientia 38:833, 1982

70. Hunkeler W: Preclinical research findings with flumazenil (Ro 15-1788, Anexate™): Chemistry. Eur J Anaesthesiol 2:37, 1988

71. Klotz U: Drug interactions and clinical pharmacokinetics of flumazenil. Eur J Anaesthesiol 2:103, 1988

72. Klotz U, Kanto J: Pharmacokinetics and clinical use of flumazenil (Ro 15-1788). Clin Pharmacokinet 14:1, 1988

73. Kleinberger G, Grimm G, Laggner A, et al: Weaning patients from mechanical ventilation by benzodiazepine antagonist RO 15-1788. Lancet 2:268, 1986

74. Dunton AW, Schwam E, Pitman V, et al: Flumazenil: US clinical pharamcology studies. Eur J Anaesthesiol 2:81, 1988

75. Forster A, Juge O, Louis M, Nahory A: Effects of a specific benzodiazepine antagonist (Ro 15-1788) on cerebral blood flow. Anesth Analg 66:309, 1987

76. Samson Y, Hantraye P, Baron JC, et al: Kinetics and displacement of (11C) Ro 15-1788, a benzodiazepine antagonist, studied in human brain in vivo by positron tomography. Eur J Pharmacol 110:247, 1985

77. Dunton AW, Schwam E, Pitman V, et al: The relationship between dose and duration of action of intravenous flumazenil in reversing sedation induced by a continuation infusion of midazolam. Eur J Anaesthesiol 2:97, 1988

78. Forster A, Crettenand G, Morel DR: Absence of ventilatory agonist or inverse agonist effects of an overdose of Ro 15-1788. A specific benzodiazepine antagonist. Anesthesiology 67:A144, 1987

79. Rouiller M, Forster A, Gemperle M: Evaluation de l'efficacite et de la tolerance d'un antagoniste des benzodiazepines (Ro 15-1788). Ann Fr Anesth Reanim 6:1, 1987

80. Croughwell ND, Reves JR, Will CJ, et al: Safety of flumazenil in patients with ischemic heart disease. Eur J Anaesthesiol 2:177, 1988

81. Duka T, Achenheil M, Noderer J, et al: Changes in noradrenaline plasma levels and behavioural responses induced by benzodiazepine agonists with the benzodiazepine antagonist Ro 15-1788. Psychopharmacology 90:351, 1986

82. Geller E, Chernilas J, Halpern P, et al: Haemodynamics following reversal of benzodiazepine sedation with Ro 15-1788 in cardiac patients. Anesthesiology 65:A49, 1986

83. Marty J, Joyon D: Haemodynamic responses following reversal of benzodiazepine-induced anaesthesia or sedation with flumazenil. Eur J Anaesthesiol 2:167, 1988

84. White PF, Shafer A, Boyle WA, Doze VA: Stress response following reversal of benzodiazepine-induced sedation. Eur J Anaesthesiol 2:173, 1988

85. Greifenstein FE, DeVault M, Yoshitake J, Gajewski JR: A study of a 1-aryl cyclo hexyl amine for anesthesia. Anesth Analg 37:283, 1958

86. Johnstone M, Evans V, Baigel S: Sernyl (CI-395) in clinical anesthesia. Br J Anaesth 31:433, 1959

87. Lear E, Suntay R, Pallin IM, Chiron AE: Cyclohexamine (CI-400): a new intravenous agent. Anesthesiology 20:330, 1959

88. Corssen G, Domino EF: Dissociative anesthesia: Further pharmacologic studies and first clinical experience with the phencyclidine derivative CI-581. Anesth Analg 45:29, 1966

89. White PF, Way WL, Trevor AJ: Ketamine — its pharmacology and therapeutic uses. Anesthesiology 56:119, 1982

90. Corssen G, Reves JG, Stanley TH (eds): Dissociative anesthesia. p. 99. In Intravenous Anesthesia and Analgesia. Lea & Febiger, Philadelphia, 1988

91. Cohen ML, Trevor AJ: On the cerebral accumulation of ketamine and the relationship between metabolism of the drug and its pharmacological effects. J Pharmacol Exp Ther 189:351, 1974

92. Chang T, Glazko AJ: Biotransformation and disposition of ketamine. Int Anesthesiol Clin 12:157, 1974

93. Chen G: The pharmacology of ketamine. In Kreuscher H (ed): Ketamine. Springer-Verlag, Berlin, 1969

94. White PF, Johnston RR, Pudwill CR: Interaction of ketamine and halothane in rats. Anesthesiology 42:179, 1975

95. Cohen ML, Chan SL, Bhargava HN, et al: Inhibition of mammalian brain acetylcholinesterase by ketamine. Biochem Pharmacol 23:1647, 1974

96. Clements JA, Nimmo WS: The pharmacokinetics and analgesic effect of ketamine in man. Br J Anaesth 53:27, 1981

97. Grant IS, Nimmo WS, Clements JA: Pharmacokinetics and analgesic effects of i.m. and oral ketamine. Br J Anaesth 53:805, 1981

98. Idvall J, Ahlgren I, Aronsen KF, Stenberg P: Ketamine infusions: Pharmacokinetics and clinical effects. Br J Anaesth 51:1167, 1979

99. Nimmo WS, Clements JA: Ketamine. p. 235. In Prys-Roberts C, Hug CC (eds): Phamacokinetics of Anesthesia. Blackwell Scientific Publications, Boston, 1984

100. White PF, Marietta MP, Pudwill CR, et al: Effects of halothane anesthesia on the biodisposition of ketamine in rats. J Pharmacol Exp Ther 196:545, 1976

101. Domino EF: Ketamine: Isomers and metabolites. p. 696. In Rugheimer, Zindler (eds): Anaesthesiology, International Congress Series 538, Excerpta Medica, Netherlands 1980

102. Little B, Chang T, Chucot L, et al: A study of ketamine as an obstetrical anaesthetic agent. Am J Obstet Gynecol 113:247, 1972

103. Grant IS, Nimmo WS, McNicol LR, Clements JA: Ketamine disposition in children and adults. Br J Anaesth 55:1107, 1983

104. Corssen G, Miyasaka M, Domino EF: Changing concepts in pain control during surgery; dissociative anesthesia with CI-581: A progress report. Anesth Analg 47:746, 1968

105. Domino EF, Chodoff P, Corssen G: Pharmacologic effects of CI-581, a new dissociative anesthetic in man. Clin Pharmacol Ther 6:279, 1965

106. Miyasaka M, Domino EF: Neuronal mechanisms of ketamine-induced anesthesia. Int J Neuropharmacol 7:557, 1968

107. Sparkes DL, Corssen G, Aizenman B, Black J: Further studies of the neural mechanisms of ketamine-induced anesthesia in the rhesus monkey. Anesth Analg 54:189, 1975

108. Massopust LC, Wolin LR, Albin MS: Electrophysiologic and behavioral responses to ketamine hydrochloride in the rhesus monkey. Anesth Analg 51:329, 1972

109. Ohtani M, Kikuchi H, Kitahata LM, et al: Effects of ketamine on nociceptive cells in the medical medullary reticular formation of the cat. Anesthesiology 51:414, 1979

110. Finck AD, Ngai SH: A possible mechanism of ketamine-induced analgesia. Anesthesiology 51:S34, 1979

111. Fratta W, Casu M, Belestrieri A, et al: Failure of ketamine to interact with opiate receptors. Eur J Pharmacol 61:389, 1980

112. Kayama Y, Iwama K: The EEG, evoked potentials, and single-unit activity during ketamine anesthesia in cats. Anesthesiology 36:316, 1972

113. Gardner AE, Dannemiller FJ, Dean D: Intracranial cerebrospinal fluid pressure in man during ketamine anesthesia. Anesth Analg 51:741, 1972

114. Shapiro HM, Wyte SR, Harris AB: Ketamine anaesthesia in patients with intracranial pathology. Br J Anaesth 44:1200, 1972

115. Dawson B, Michenfelder D, Theye A: Effects of ketamine on canine cerebral blood flow and metabolism; modification by prior administration of thiopental. Anesth Analg 50:443, 1971

116. Thorsen T, Gran L: Ketamine/diazepam infusion anaesthesia with special attention to the effect on cerebrospinal fluid pressure and arterial blood pressure. Acta Anaesth Scand 24:1, 1980

117. Garfield JM: A comparison of psychologic responses to ketamine and thiopental-nitrous oxide-halothane anesthesia. Anesthesiology 36:329, 1972

118. Sussman DR: A comparative evaluation of ketamine anesthesia in children and adults. Anesthesiology 40:459 1974

119. Dundee JW, Bovill JG, Clarke RSJ, Pandit SK: Problems with ketamine in adults. Anaesthesia 26:86, 1971

120. Khorramzadeh E, Lotfy AO: Personality predisposition and emergence phenomena with ketamine. Psychosomatics 17:94, 1976

121. Hejja P, Galloon S: A consideration of ketamine dreams. Can Anaesth Soc J 22:100, 1975

122. Wolfsohn NL: Ketamine dosage for induction based on lean body mass. Anesth Analg 51:299, 1972

123. Johnson M: The prevention of ketamine dreams. Anaesth Intens Care 1:70, 1972

124. Dundee JW, Lilburn JK: Ketamine-lorazepam: Attenuation of the psychic sequelae of ketamine by lorazepam. Anaesthesia 37:312, 1977

125. Kothary SP, Zsigmond EK: A double-blind study of the effective antihallucinatory doses of diazepam prior to ketamine anesthesia. Clin Pharmacol Ther 21:108, 1977

126. Soliman MG, Brinale GF, Kuster G: Response to hypercapnia under ketamine anaesthesia. Can Anaesth Soc J 22:486, 1975

127. Virtue RW, Alanis JM, Mori M, et al: An anesthetic agent: 2-orthochlorophenyl, 2-methylamino cyclohexanone CI-581. Anesthesiology 28:823, 1967

128. Stanley V, Hunt J, Willis KW, Stephen CR: Cardiovascular and respiratory function with CI-581. Anesth Analg 47:760, 1968

129. Dillon JB: Clinical experience with repeated ketamine administration for procedures requiring anesthesia. p. 82. In Kreuscher H (ed): Ketamine. Springer-Verlag, Berlin, 1969

130. Huber FC, Reves JG, Gutierrez J, Corssen G: Ketamine: Its effect on airway resistance in man. South Med J 65:1176, 1972

131. Corssen G, Gutierrez J, Reves JG, Huber FC: Ketamine in the anesthetic management of asthmatic patients. Anesth Analg 51:588, 1972

132. Hirshman CA: Ketamine block of bronchospasm in experimental canine asthma. Br J Anaesthesiol 51:713, 1979

133. Wanna HT, Gergis SD: Procaine, lidocaine, and ketamine inhibit histamine-induced contracture of guinea pig tracheal muscle in vitro. Anesth Analg 57:25, 1978

134. Taylor PA, Towey RM: Depression of laryngeal reflexes during ketamine anesthesia. Br Med J 2:688, 1971

135. Sonntag H, Heiss HW, Knoll D, et al: Coronary blood flow and myocardial oxygen consumption in patients during induction of anesthesia with droperidol/fentanyl or ketamine. Z Kreislaufforsch 61:1092, 1972

136. Zsigmond EK, Domino EF: Clinical pharmacology and cur-

rent uses of ketamine. p. 283. In Aldrete JA, Stanley TH (eds): Trends in Intravenous Anesthesia. Year Book Medical Publishers, Chicago, 1980

137. Savege TM, Colvin MP, Weaver EJM, et al: A comparison of some cardiorespiratory effects of althesin and ketamine when used for induction of anaesthesia in patients with cardiac disease. Br J Anaesth 48:1071, 1976

138. Gooding JM, Dimick AR, Tavakoli M, et al: A physiologic analysis of cardiopulmonary responses to ketamine anesthesia in noncardiac patients. Anesth Analg 56:813, 1977

139. Reves JG, Lell WA, McCracken LE, Jr., et al: Comparison of morphine and ketamine anesthetic techniques for coronary surgery: A randomized study. South Med J 71:33, 1978

140. Spotoff H, Korshin JD, Sorensen MB, et al: The cardiovascular effects of ketamine used for induction of anaesthesia in patients with valvular heart disease. Can Anaesth Soc J 26:463, 1979

141. Morray JP, Lynn AM, Stamm SJ, et al: Hemodynamic effects of ketamine in children with congenital heart disease. Anesth Analg 63:895, 1984

142. Greeley WJ, Bushman GA, Davis DP, Reves JG: Comparative effects of halothane and ketamine on systemic arterial oxygen saturation in children with cyanotic heart disease. Anesthesiology 65:666, 1986

143. Faithfull NS, Haider R: Ketamine for cardiac catheterization: An evaluation of its use in children. Anaesthesia 26:318, 1971

144. Hickey PR, Hansen DD, Cramolini GM, et al: Pulmonary and systemic hemodynamic responses to ketamine in infants with normal and elevated pulmonary vascular resistance. Anesthesiology 62:287, 1985

145. Slogoff S, Allen GW: The role of baroreceptors in the cardiovascular response to ketamine. Anesth Analg 53:704, 1974

146. Dowdy EG, Kaya K: Studies of the mechanism of cardiovascular responses to CI-581. Anesthesiology 29:931, 1968

147. Chodoff P: Evidence for central adrenergic action of ketamine. Anesth Analg 51:247, 1972

148. Wong DHW, Jenkins LC: An experimental study of the mechanism of action of ketamine on the central nervous system. Can Anaesth Soc J 21:57, 1974

149. Iwatsuki M, Aoba Y, Sato K, Iwatsuki N: Clinical study of CI-581, a phencyclidine derivative. Tohoku J Exp Med 93:39, 1967

150. Ivankovich AD, Miletich DJ, Reimann C, et al: Cardiovascular effects of centrally administered ketamine in goats. Anesth Analg 53:924, 1974

151. Zsigmond EK, Kothary SP, Matsuki A, et al: Diazepam for prevention of the rise in plasma catecholamines caused by ketamine. Clin Pharmacol Ther 15:223, 1974

152. Balfors E, Haggmark S, Nyhman H, et al: Droperidol inhibits the effects of intravenous ketamine on central hemodynamics and myocardial oxygen consumption in patients with generalized atherosclerotic disease. Anesth Analg 62:193, 1983

153. Miletich DJ, Ivankovich AD, Albrecht RF, et al: The effect of ketamine on catecholamine metabolism in the isolated perfused rat heart. Anesthesiology 39:271, 1973

154. Valicenti JF, Newman WH, Bagwell EE, et al: Myocardial contractility during induction and steady-state ketamine anesthesia. Anesth Analg 52:190, 1973

155. Urthaler F, Walker AA, James TN: Comparison of the inotropic action of morphine and ketamine studied in canine cardiac muscle. J Thorac Cardiovasc Surg 72:142, 1976

156. Hill GE, Wong KC, Shaw CL, et al: Interactions of ketamine with vasoactive amines at normothermia and hypothermia in the isolated rabbit heart. Anesthesiology 48:315, 1978

157. Nedergaard OA: Cocaine-like effect of ketamine on vascular adrenergic neurones. Eur J Pharmacol 23:153, 1973

158. Salt PJ, Barnes PK, Beswick FJ: Inhibition of neuronal and extraneuronal uptake of noradrenaline by ketamine in the isolated perfused rat heart. Br J Anaesth 51:835, 1979

159. Reves JG, Flezzani P, Kissin I: Pharmacology of intravenous anesthetic induction drugs. p. 125. In Kaplan JA (ed): Cardiac Anesthesia. 2nd Ed. Grune & Stratton, Orlando, FL, 1987

160. Hatano S, Keane DM, Boggs RE, et al: Diazepam-ketamine anaesthesia for open heart surgery: A "micro-mini" drip administration technique. Can Anaesth Soc J 23:648, 1976

161. Bidwal AV, Stanley TH, Graves CL, et al: The effects of ketamine on cardiovascular dynamics during halothane and enflurane anesthesia. Anesth Analg 54:588, 1975

162. Corssen G, Reves JG, Carter JR: Neuroleptanesthesia, dissociative anesthesia, and hemorrhage. Int Anesthesiol Clin 12:145, 1974

163. Kingston HG, Bretherton KW, Holloway AM, et al: A comparison between ketamine and diazepam as induction agents for pericardiectomy. Anesth Intens Care 6:66, 1978

164. Thompson GE, Moore DC: Ketamine, diazepam, and Innovar®: A computerized comparitive study. Anesth Analg 50:458, 1971

165. Korttila K, Levanen J: Untoward effects of ketamine combined with diazepam for supplementing conduction anaesthesia in young and middle-aged adults. Acta Anaesth Scand 22:640, 1978

166. Waxman K, Shoemaker WC, Lippmann M: Cardioavascular effects of anesthetic induction with ketamine. Anesth Analg 59:355, 1980

167. Shapiro HM: Intracranial hypertension: Therapeutic and anesthetic considerations. Anesthesiology 43:445, 1971

168. Godefroi EF, Jansen PAJ, Van Der Eycken CAM, et al: DL-1-(1-arylalkyl) imidazole-5 carbohydrate ester. A novel type of hypnotic agent. J Med Chem 8:222, 1965

169. Doenicke A: Etomidate a new intravenous hypnotic. Acta Anaesthesiol Belg 3(25):307, 1974

170. Janssen PAJ, Niemegeers CJE, Schellekens KHL, Lenaerts FM: Etomidate, R-(+)-ethyl (α-methyl-benzyl) imidazole-5-carboxylate (R16659) a potent, short acting and relatively atoxic intravenous hypnotic agent in rats. Arzneim-Forsch (Drug Res) 21:1234, 1971

171. Ledingham IM, Watt I: Influence of sedation on mortality in critically ill multiple trauma patients (letter). Lancet 1:1270, 1983

172. Wagner RL, White PF: Etomidate inhibits adrenocortical function in surgical patients. Anesthesiology 60:647, 1984

173. Fragen RJ, Shanks CA, Molteni A, Avram MJ: Effects of etomidate on hormonal response to surgical stress. Anesthesiology 60:652, 1984

174. Longnecker D: Stress free: To be or not to be? (editorial). Anesthesiology 61:643, 1984

175. Owen H, Spence AA: Etomidate (editorial). Br J Anaesth 56:555, 1984

176. Corssen G, Reves JG, Stanley TH: p. 285. In Intravenous Anesthesia and Analgesia. Lea & Febiger, Philadelphia, 1988

177. Nimmo WS, Miller M: Pharmacology of etomidate, Contemp Anesth Pract 7:83, 1983

178. Van Hamme MJ, Ghoneim MM, Amber JJ: Pharmacokinetics of etomidate, a new intravenous anesthetic. Anesthesiology 49:274, 1978

179. Hebron BS, Edbrooke DL, Newby DM, Mather SJ: Pharmacokinetics of etomidate associated with prolonged I.V. infusion. Br J Anaesth 58:281, 1983

180. De Ruiter G, Popescu DT, de Boer AG, et al: Pharmacoki-

netics of etomidate in surgical patients. Arch Int Pharmacodyn Ther 249:180, 1981

181. Fragen RJ, Avram MJ, Henthorn TK, Caldwell NJ: Pharmacokinetically designed etomidate infusion regimen for hypnosis. Anesth Analg 62:654, 1983

182. Schuttler J, Schwilden H, Stoeckel H: Infusion strategies to investigate the pharmacokinetics and pharmacodynamics of hypnotic drugs: Etomidate as an example. Eur J Anaesthesiol 2:133, 1985

183. Meuldermans WEG, Heykants JJP: The plasma protein binding and distribution of etomidate in dog, rat and human blood. Arch Int Pharmacodyn Ther 221:150, 1976

184. Van Beem H, Manger FW, Van Boxtel C, Van Benten N: Etomidate anaesthesia in patients with cirrhosis of the liver: Pharmacokinetic data. Anaesthesia 38:61, 1983

185. Arden JR, Holley FO, Stanski DR: Increased sensitivity to etomidate in the elderly: Initial distribution versus altered brain response. Anesthesiology 65:19, 1986

186. Doenicke A, Loffler B, Kugler J, et al: Plasma concentrations and EEG after various regimens of etomidate. Br J Anaesth 54:393, 1982

187. Schuttler J, Schwilden H, Stoekel H: Pharmacokinetics as applied to total intravenous anaesthesia. Practical implications. Anaesthesia. 38:53, 1983

188. Sear JW, Walters FJM, Wilkins DG, Willatts SM: Etomidate by infusion for neuroanaesthesia. Kinetic and dynamic interactions with nitrous oxide. Anaesthesia 39:12, 1984

189. Evans RH, Hill RG: GABA — mimetic action of etomidate. Br J Pharmacol 61:484, 1977

190. Dearden NM, McDowall DG: Comparison of etomidate and althesin in the reduction of increased intracranial pressure after head injury. Br J Anaesth, 57:361, 1985

191. Cold GE, Eskesen V, Eriksen H, et al: CBF and $CMRO_2$ during continuous etomidate infusion supplemented with N_2O and fentanyl in patients with supratentorial cerebral tumor. A dose response study. Acta Anaesthesiol Scand 29:490, 1985

192. Renou AM, Vernhiet J, Macrez P, et al: Cerebral blood flow and metabolism during etomidate anaesthesia in man. Br J Anaesth 50:1047, 1978

193. Tulleken CAF, Van Dieren A, Jonkman J, Kalend Z: Clinical and experimental experience with etomidate as a brain protective agent. J Cereb Blood Flow Metab 2(i):S92, 1982

194. Thomson MF, Brock-Utne JG, Bean P, et al: Anesthesia and intra occular pressure: A comparative study of total intravenous anesthesia using etomidate with conventional inhalational anaesthesia. Anaesthesia 37:758, 1982

195. Ghoneim MM, Yamada T: Etomidate: A clinical and electrographic comparison with thiopental. Anesth Analg 56:479, 1977

196. Lees NW, Hendry JGB: Etomidate in urological outpatient anaesthesia. Anaesthesia 32:592, 1977

197. Ebrahim ZY, Deboer GE, Luders H, et al: Effect of etomidate on the electroencephalogram of patients with epilepsy. Anesth Analg 65:1004, 1986

198. Gancher S, Laer KD, Krieger W: Activation of epileptogenic activity by etomidate. Anesthesiology, 61:616, 1984

199. Giese JL, Stockham RJ, Stanley TH, et al: Etomidate versus thiopental for induction of anesthesia. Anesth Analg 64:871, 1985

200. Fragen RJ, Caldwell N: Comparison of a new formulation of etomidate with thiopental side effects and awakening times. Anesthesiology 50:242, 1979

201. Thornton C, Heneghan CPH, Navaratnarajah M, et al: Effect of etomidate on the auditory evoked response in man. Br J Anaesth 57:554, 1985

202. McPherson RW, Sell B, Traystman RJ: Effects of thiopental,

fentanyl and etomidate on upper extremity somatosensory evoked potentials in humans. Anesthesiology 65:584, 1986

203. Choi SD, Spaulding BC, Gross JB, Apfelbaum JL: Comparison of the ventilatory effects of etomidate and methohexital. Anesthesiology 62:442, 1985

204. Kay B: The measurement of occlusion pressure during anaesthesia. A comparison of the depression of respiratory drive by methohexitone and etomidate. Anaesthesia 34:543, 1979

205. Colvin MP, Savege TM, Newland PE, et al: Cardiorespiratory changes following induction of anaesthesia with etomidate in patients with cardiac disease. Br J Anaesth 51:551, 1979

206. Morgan M, Lumley J, Whitwan JG: Respiratory effects of etomidate. Br J Anaesth 49:233, 1977

207. Gooding JM, Weng J, Smith RA, et al: Cardiovascular and pulmonary responses following etomidate induction of anesthesia in patients with demonstrated cardiac disease. Anesth Analg 58:40, 1979

208. Guldager H, Sodergaard I, Jensen FM, Cold G: Basophil histamine release in asthma patients after in vitro provocation with althesin and etomidate. Acta Anaesthesiol Scand 29:352, 1985

209. Criado A, Maseda J, Navarro E, Escarpa A, Avello F: Induction of anaesthesia with etomidate: Haemodynamic study of 36 patients. Br J Anaesth 52:803, 1980

210. Gooding J, Corssen G: Effect of etomidate on the cardiovascular system. Anesth Analg 56:717, 1977

211. Lindeburg T, Spotoft H, Sorensen MB, Skovsted P: Cardiovascular effects of etomidate used for induction and in combination with fentanyl pancuronium for maintenance of anaesthesia in patients with valvular heart disease. Acta Anaesth Scand 26:205, 1982

212. Kettler D, Sonntag H, Dontah U, et al: Hemodynamics, myocardial mechanics, oxygen requirements and oxygen consumption of the human heart during etomidate induction into anaesthesia. Anaesthetist 23:116, 1974

213. Larsen R, Rathgeber J, Bagdahn A, et al: Effects of propofol on cardiovascular dynamics and coronary blood flow in geriatric patients. A comparison with etomidate. Anaesthesia 435:25, 1988

214. Nauta J, Stanley TH, de Lange S, et al: Anaesthetic induction with alfentanil: Comparison with thiopental, midazolam and etomidate. Can Anaes Soc J 30:53, 1983

215. Allolio B, Dorr H, Stuttman R, et al: Effect of a single bolus of etomidate upon eight major corticosteroid hormones and plasma ACTH. Clin Endocrinol (Oxf) 22:281, 1985

216. Boidin MP, Erdman WE, Faithfull NS: The role of ascorbic acid in etomidate toxicity. Eur J Anaesthesiol 3:417, 1986

217. Lamberts SW, Bons EG, Bruining HA, de Jong FH: Differential effects of the imidazole derivatives etomidate, ektoconazole and miconazole and of metapyrone on the secretion of cortisol and its precursors by human adrenocorticol cells. J Pharmacol Exp Ther 240:259, 1987

218. Boiden MP: Steroid response to ACTH and to ascorbinic acid during infusion of etomidate for general surgery. Acta Anaesthesiol Belg 36:15, 1985

219. Booij LHDJ, Crul JF: The comparative influence of gamma-hydroxy butyric acid, althesin and etomidate on the neuromuscular blocking potency of pancuronium in man. Acta Anaesth Belg 30:219, 1979

220. Famewo CE: Induction of anaesthesia with etomidate in a patient with acute intermittent porphyria. Can Anaesth Soc J 32:171, 1985

221. Famewo CE, Adugbesan CO: Further experience with etomidate. Can Anaesth Soc J 25:131, 1978

222. Craig J, Cooper GM, Sear JW: Recovery from day-case anaes-

thesia. Comparison between methohexitone, althesin and etomidate. Br J Anaesth 54:447, 1982

223. Wells JKG: Comparison of ICI 35868, etomidate and methohexitone for day-care anesthesia. Br J Anaesth 57:732, 1985

224. Zacharias M, Dundee JW, Clark RS, Hegarty JE: Effect of preanesthetic medication on etomidate. Br J Anaesth 51:127, 1979

225. Linton DM, Thornington RE: Etomidate as a rectal induction agent. Part ii. A clinical study in children. S Afr Med J 64:309, 1983

226. Lees NW, Glasser J, McGroarty FJ, Miller BM: Etomidate and fentanyl for maintenance of anaesthesia. Br J Anaesth 53:959, 1981

227. Kortilla K, Aromaa U: Venous complications after intravenous injection of diazepam, thiopentone and etomidate. Acta Anaesth Scand 24:227, 1980

228. Galloway PA, Nicoll JM, Leiman BC: Pain reduction with etomidate injection (Letter) Anaesthesia 37:352, 1982

229. Zacharias M, Clark RS, Dundee JW, Johnston SB: Venous sequelae following etomidate. Br J Anaesth 51:779, 1975

230. Fragen RJ: Diprivan (Propofol): A historical perspective. Semin Anesthesia 7(1):1, 1988

231. Kay B, Rolly G: ICI 35 868, a new intravenous induction agent. Acta Anaesth Belg 28:303, 1977

232. Briggs LP, Clarke RSJ, Watkins J: An adverse reaction to the administration of disoprofol (Diprivan). Anesthesia 37:1099, 1982

233. James R, Glen JB: Synthesis, biological evaluation, and preliminary structure-activity considerations of a series of alkylphenols as intravenous anesthetic agents. J Med Chem 23:1350, 1980

234. Simons PJ, Cockshott ID, Douglas EJ, et al: Blood concentrations, metabolism and elimination after a subanesthetic intravenous dose of ^{14}C-propofol (Diprivan) to male volunteers (Abstract). Postgrad Med J 61:64, 1985

235. Adam HK, Briggs LP, Bahar M, et al: Pharmacokinetic evaluation of ICI 35 868 in man. Single induction doses with different rates of injection. Br J Anaesth 55:97, 1983

236. Kay NH, Sear JW, Upington J, et al: Disposition of propofol in patients undergoing surgery. A comparison in men and women. Br J Anaesth 58:1075, 1986

237. Kirkpatrick T, Cockshott ID, Douglas EJ, Nimmo WS: Pharmacokinetics of propofol (Diprivan) in elderly patients. Br J Anaesth 60:146, 1988

238. Gepts E, Camu F, Cockshott ID, Douglas EJ: Disposition of propofol administered as constant rate intravenous infusions in humans. Anesth Analg 66:1256, 1987

239. Schuttler J, Stoeckel H, Schwilden H: Pharmacokinetic and pharmacodynamic modelling of propofol (Diprivan) in volunteers and surgical patients. Postgrad Med J 61:53, 1985

240. Shafer A, Doze VA, Shafer SL, White PF: Pharmacokinetics and pharmacodynamics of propofol infusions during general anesthesia. Anesthesiology 69:348, 1988

241. Servin F, Desmonts JM, Farinttir, et al: Pharmacokinetics of propofol given as a continuous infusion in a cirrhotic patient. Preliminary results. Ann Fr Anesth Reanim 6:228, 1987

242. Morcos WE, Payne JP: The induction of anaesthesia with propofol (Diprivan) compared in normal and renal failure patients. Postgrad Med J 61:62, 1985

243. Briggs LP, Dundee JW, Bahar M, Clarke RSJ: Comparison of the effect of diisopropylphenol (ICI 35 868) and thiopentone on response to somatic pain. Br J Anaesth 54:307, 1982

244. Major E, Verniquet AJW, Waddell TK, et al: A study of three doses of ICI 35 868 for induction and maintenance of anaesthesia. Br J Anaesth 53:267, 1981

245. Rolly G, Versichelen L, Huyghe L, Mungroop H: Effect of speed of injection on induction of anesthesia using propofol. Br J Anaesth 57:743, 1985

246. Yate PM, Maynard DE, Major E, et al: Anaesthesia with ICI 35 868 monitored by the cerebral function analyzing monitor (CFAM). Eur J Anaesthes 3:159, 1986

247. Glass P, Ginsberg B, Hawkins ED, et al: Comparison of sodium thiopental isoflurane to propofol (delivered by means of a pharmacokinetic model-driven device) for the induction maintenance and recovery from anesthesia. Anesthesiology 69:A575, 1988

248. Adam HK, Kay B, Douglas EJ: Blood diisoprofol levels in anesthetized patients. Correlation of concentration after single or repeated doses with hypnotic activity. Anaesthesia 37:536, 1982

249. Mackenzie N, Grant IS: Propofol for intravenous sedation. Anaesthesia 42:3, 1987

250. Wilson E, Mackenzie N, Grant IS: A comparison of propofol and midazolam by infusion to provide sedation in patients who receive spinal anaesthesia. Anaesthesia 43:91, 1988

251. McDonald NJ, Mannion D, Lee P, et al: Mood evaluation and outpatient anesthesia. A comparison between propofol and thiopentone. Anaesthesia 43:68, 1988

252. Nelson VM: Hallucinations after propofol (letter). Anaesthesia 43:170, 1988

253. Cameron AE: Opisthotonis again (letter). Anaesthesia 42:1124, 1987

254. Hazeau C, Tisserant D, Vespignani H, et al: Electroencephalographic changes produced by propofol. Ann Fr Anesth Reanim 6:261, 1987

255. Glen JB, Hunter SC, Blackburn TP, Wood P: Interaction studies and other investigations of the pharmacology of propofol (Diprivan). Postgrad Med J 61:7, 1985

256. Wood PR, Browne GPR, Pugh S: Propofol infusion for the treatment of status epilepticus (Letter). Lancet 1:480, 1988

257. Dwyer R, McCaughey W, Lavery J, McCarthy G, Dundee JW: Comparison of propofol and methohexitone as anesthetic agents for electroconvulsive therapy. Anaesthesia 43:459, 1988

258. Hodkinson BP, Frith RW, Mee EW: Propofol and the electroencephalogram. Lancet 2:1518, 1987

259. Committee on Safety of Medicines: Propofol. Curr Prob 20, 1987

260. Maurette P, Simeon F, Castagnera L, et al: Propofol anaesthesia alters somatosensory evoked corticol potentials. Anaesthesia 43:44, 1988

261. Savoia G, Esposito C, Belfiore F, et al: Propofol infusion and auditory evoked potentials. Anaesthesia 43:46, 1988

262. Stephan H, Sonntag H, Schenk HD, Kohlhausen S: Effects of Disoprivan on cerebral blood flow, cerebral oxygen consumption and cerebral vascular reactivity. Anaesthetist 36:60, 1987

263. Hartung HJ: Intracranial pressure after propofol and thiopental administration in patients with severe head trauma. Anaesthetist 36:285, 1987

264. Hartung HJ: Effect of propofol (Disoprivan) on intracranial pressure. Preliminary results. Der Anesthetist 36:66, 1987

265. Ravussin P, Guinard JP, Ralley F, Thorin D: Effect of propofol on cerebrospinal fluid pressure and cerebral perfussion pressure in patients undergoing craniotomy. Anaesthesia 43:37, 1988

266. Vandesteene A, Trempont V, Engelman E, et al: Effect of propofol on cerebral blood flow and metabolism in man. Anaesthesia 43:42, 1988

267. Herregods L, Verberke J, Rolly G, Colardyn F: Effect of pro-

pofol on elevated intracranial pressure. Preliminary results. Anaesthesia 43:107, 1988

268. Mirakhur RK, Shepherd WFI: Intraocular pressure changes with propofol (Diprivan): Comparison with thiopentone. Postgrad Med J 61:41, 1985

269. Mirakhur RK, Shepherd WFI, Darrah WC: Propofol or thiopentone: Effects on intraocular pressure associated with induction of anaesthesia and tracheal intubation (facilitated with suxamethonium). Br J Anaesth 59:431, 1987

270. Turtle MJ, Cullen P, Prys-Roberts C, et al: Dose requirements of propofol by infusion during nitrous oxide anaesthesia in man. II: Patients premedicated with lorazepam. Br J Anaesth 59:283, 1987

271. Spelina KR, Coates DP, Monk CR, et al: Dose requirements of propofol by infusion during nitrous oxide anaesthesia in man. I: Patients premedicated with morphine sulphate. Br J Anaesth 58:1080, 1986

272. Taylor MB, Grounds RM, Dulrooney PD, Morgan M: Ventilatory effects of propofol during induction of anesthesia. Comparison with thiopentone. Anaesthesia 41:816, 1986

273. Grounds RM, Maxwell DL, Taylor MB, et al: Acute ventilatory changes during IV induction of anaesthesia with thiopentone or propofol in man. Studies using inductance plethyomography. Br J Anaesth 59:1098, 1987

274. Goodman NW, Black AMS, Carter JA: Some ventilatory effects of propofol as sole anesthetic agent. Br J Anaesth 59:1497, 1987

275. Sanderson JH, Blades JF: Multicentre study of propofol in day case surgery. Anaesthesia 43:70, 1988

276. Gold MI, Abraham EC, Herrington C: A controlled investigation of propofol, thiopentone and methohexitone. Can J Anaesth 34:478, 1987

277. Munson ES, Larson CP, Babad AA, et al: The effects of halothane, fluroxene and cyclopropane on ventilation: A comparative study in man. Anesthesiology 27:716, 1966

278. Knill RL, Clement JL, Gelb AW: Ventilatory responses mediated by chemoreceptors in anaesthetized man. Adv Exp Med Biol 99:67, 1978

279. Aun C, Major E: The cardiorespiratory effects of ICI 35 868 in patients with valvular heart disease. Anaesthesia 39:1096, 1984

280. Grounds RM, Twigley AJ, Carli F, et al: The haemodynamic effects of thiopentone and propofol. Anaesthesia 40:735, 1985

281. Al-Khudhairi D, Gordon G, Morgan M, Whitwam JG: Acute cardiovascular changes following disoprofol. Effects in heavily sedated patients with coronary artery disease. Anaesthesia 37:1007, 1982

282. Coates DP, Monk CR, Prys-Roberts C, Turtle M: Hemodynamic effects of infusions of the emulsion formulation of propofol during nitrous oxide anesthesia in humans. Anesth Analg 66:64, 1987

283. Doze VA, Westphal L, White P: Comparison of propofol with methohexital for outpatient anesthesia. Anesth Analg 65:1189, 1986

284. Vermeyen KM, Erpels FA, Janssen LA, et al: Propofol-fentanyl anaesthesia for coronary bypass surgery in patients with good left ventricular function. Br J Anaesth 59:1115, 1987

285. Patrick MR, Blair IJ, Feneck RO, Sebel PS: A comparison of the haemodynamic effects of propofol (Diprivan) on thiopentone in patients with coronary artery disease. Postgrad Med J 61:23, 1985

286. Stephan H, Sonntag H, Schenk HD, et al: Effects of propofol on cardiovascular dynamics, myocardial blood flow and myocardial metabolism in patients with coronary artery disease. Br J Anaesth 58:969, 1986

287. Coates DP, Prys-Roberts C, Spelina KR, et al: Propofol (Diprivan) by intravenous infusion with nitrous oxide: Dose requirements and hemodynamic effects. Postgrad Med J 61:76, 1985

288. Claeys MA, Gepts E, Camu F: Haemodynamic changes during anaesthesia induced and maintained with propofol. Br J Anaesth 60:3, 1983

289. Ban Aken H, Meinshausen E, Prien T, et al: The influence of fentanyl and tracheal intubation on the hemodynamic effects of anesthesia induction with propofol/N_2O in humans. Anesthesiology 68:157, 1988

290. Cullen PM, Turtle M, Prys-Roberts C, et al: Effect of propofol anesthesia on baroreflex activity in humans. Anesth Analg 66:1115, 1987

291. Fragen RJ, Booij LHD, Van der Pol F, et al: Interactions of diisopropylphenol (ICI 35 868) with suxamethonium, vecuronium and pancuronium in vitro. Br J Anaesth 55:433, 1983

292. Robertson EN, Fragen RJ, Booij LHDJ, et al: Some effects of diisopropylphenol (ICI 35 868) on the pharmacodynamics of atracurium and vecuronium in anaesthetized man. Br J Anaesth 55:723, 1983

293. De Grood PMRM, Van Egmond J, Van De Wetering M, et al: Lack of effects of emulsified propofol (Diprivan) on vecuronium pharmacodynamics — preliminary results in man. Postgrad Med J 61:28, 1985

294. Nightingale P, Petts NV, Healy TEJ, et al: Induction of anaesthesia with propofol (Diprivan) or thiopentone and interactions with suxamethonium, atracurium and vecuronium. Postgrad Med J 61:31, 1985

295. McKeating K, Bali IM, Dundee JW: The effects of thiopentone and propofol on upper airway integrity. Anaesthesia 43:638, 1988

296. Richardson J: Propofol infusion for coronary artery bypass surgery in a patient with suspected malignant hyperpyrexia (Letter). Anaesthesia 42:1125, 1987

297. Hopkinson KC, Denborough M: Propofol and malignant hyperpyrexia (Letter). Lancet 1:191, 1988

298. Stark RD, Binks SM, Dukka VN, et al: A review of the safety and tolerance of propofol (Diprivan). Postgrad Med J 61:152, 1985

299. Fragen RJ, Weiss HW, Molteni A: The effect of propofol on adrenocortical steroidogenesis: A comparative study with etomidate and thiopental. Anesthesiology 66:839, 1987

300. Newman LH, McDonald JC, Wallace PGM, Ledingham IMcA: Propofol infusion for sedation in intensive care. Anaesthesia 42:929, 1987

301. Robinson FP, Patterson CC: Changes in liver function tests after propofol (Diprivan). Postgrad Med J 61:160, 1985

302. Sear JW, Uppington J, Kay NH: Haemotological and biochemical changes during anaesthesia with propofol (Diprivan). Postgrad Med J 61:165, 1985

303. Doenicke A, Lorenz W, Stanworth D, et al: Effects of propofol (Diprivan) on histamine release, immunoglobulin levels and activation of complement in healthy volunteers. Postgrad Med J 61:15, 1985

304. Cummings GC, Dixon J, Kay NH, et al: Dose requirements of ICI 35, 868 (propofol, Diprivan) in a new formulation for induction of anaesthesia. Anaesthesia 39:1168, 1984

305. Kay B, Stephenson DK: Dose response relationship for disoprofol (ICI 35 868; Diprivan). Comparison with methohexitone. Anaesthesia 36:863, 1981

306. Rutter DV, Morgan M, Lumley J, Owen R: ICI 35 868 (Dipri-

van): A new intravenous induction agent. Anaesthesia 35:1188, 1980

307. Briggs LP, White M: The effects of premedication on anaesthesia with propofol (Diprivan). Postgrad Med J 61:35, 1985

308. Dundee JW, Robinson FP, McCollum JSC, Patterson CC: Sensitivity to propofol in the elderly. Anaesthesia 41:482, 1986

309. Steib A, Freys G, Curzola U, Otteni JC: Propofol in elderly high risk patients. A comparison of haemodynamic effects with thiopentone during induction of anaesthesia. Anaesthesia 43:111, 1988

310. Purcell-Jones G, Yates A, Baker JR, James IG: Comparison of the induction characteristics of thiopentone and propofol in children. Br J Anaesth 59:1431, 1987

311. Mirakhur RK: Induction characteristics of propofol in children: Comparison with thiopentone. Anaesthesia 43:593, 1988

312. Doze VA, Shafer A, White PF: Propofol-nitrous oxide versus thiopental-isoflurane-nitrous oxide for general anesthesia. Anesthesiology 69:63, 1988

313. Heath PJ, Kennedy DJ, Ogg TW, et al: Which intravenous induction agent for day surgery: A comparison of propofol, thiopentone, methohexitone and etomidate. Anaesthesia. 43:365, 1988

314. Mackenzie N, Grant IS: Comparison of the new emulsion formulation of propofol with methohexitone and thiopentone for induction of anaesthesia in day cases. Br J Anaesth 57:725, 1985

315. McCollum JSC, Milligan KR, Dundee JW: The antiemetic action of propofol. Anaesthesia 43:239, 1988

316. Kay B: Propofol and alfentanil infusion: A comparison with methohexitone and alfentanil for major surgery. Anaesthesia 41:589, 1986

317. Mackenzie N, Grant IS: Propofol (Diprivan) for continuous intravenous anaesthesia. A comparison with methohexitone. Postgrad Med J 61:70, 1985

318. Sear JW, Shaw I, Wolf A, Kay NH: Infusions of propofol to supplement nitrous-oxide-oxygen for the maintenance of anaesthesia. A comparison with halothane. Anaesthesia 43:18, 1988

319. Robinson FP: Propofol (Diprivan) by intermittent bolus with nitrous oxide in oxygen for body surface operations. Postgrad Med J 61:116, 1985

320. Roberts FL, Dixon J, Lewis GTR, et al: Induction and maintenance of propofol anaesthesia. A manual infusion scheme. Anaesthesia 43:14, 1988

321. Thomas VL, Saunders DA: The effect of fentanyl on propofol requirements for day case anesthesia. Anaesthesia 43:73, 1988

322. Hilton P, Dev VJ, Major E: Intravenous anaesthesia with propofol and alfentanil. The influence of age and weight. Anaesthesia 41:640, 1986

323. Schüttler J, Kloos S, Schwilden H, Stoeckel H: Total intravenous anaesthesia with propofol and alfentanil by computer assisted infusion. Anaesthesia 43:2, 1988

324. Tackley RM, Lewis GTR, Prys-Roberts C, et al: Open loop control of propofol infusions (Abstract). Br J Anaesth 59:935, 1987

325. Fanard L, Van Steenberge A, Demeirey A, Van Der Puyl F: Comparison between propofol and midazolam as sedative agents for surgery under regional anaesthesia. Anaesthesia 43:87, 1988

326. Gepts E, Claeys MA, Camu F, Smekens L: Infusion of propofol (Diprivan) as sedative technique for colonoscopies. Postgrad Med J 61:120, 1987

327. Grounds RM, Lalor JM, Lumley J, et al: Propofol infusion for sedation in the intensive care unit: Preliminary report. Br Med J 294:397, 1985

328. Beller JP, Pottecher T, Manigin P, et al: Long-term sedation with propofol during intensive care. Preliminary results of the study of recovery and pharmacokinetics. Ann Fr Anesth Reanim 6:334, 1987

329. Beller JP, Pottecher T, Lugnier A, et al: Prolonged sedation with propofol in ICU patients. Recovery and blood concentration changes during periodic interruptions in infusion. Br J Anaesth 61:583, 1988

330. Laborit H, Huguenard P: Practique de l'hibernotherapie en chirurgie et en medicine. Masson, Paris, 1954

331. Laborit H: Stress and cellular function. JB Lippincott, Philadelphia, 1959

332. Corssen G, Reves JG, Stanley TH: Neuroleptanalgesia and neuroleptanesthesia. p. 175. In Corssen G et al. (eds): Intravenous Anaesthesia and Analgesia. Lea & Febiger, Philadelphia, 1988

333. Janssen PAJ: The pharmacology of haloperidol. Int J Neuropsychiatr 3(Suppl 1):10, 1967

334. DeCastro J, Mundeleer P: Anesthesie sans barbituriques; la neurolept analgesie (R1406, R1625, hydergine, procain). Anesth Analg 16:1022, 1959

335. Borison HL, Wang SC: Physiology and pharmacology of vomiting. Pharmacol Rev 5:193, 1953

336. Janssen PAJ: Zur Frage des Abbaus und der Ausscheidung der bei Neuroleptanalgesie zur Anwendung kommenden Pharmaka. In Henschel WF (ed): Die Neuroleptanalgesie. Springer-Verlag, Berlin, 1966

337. Fischler M, Bonnet F, Trang H, et al: The pharmacokinetics of droperidol in anesthetized patients. Anesthesiology 64:486, 1986

338. Cressman WA, Plostnieks J, Johnson PC: Absorption, metabolism and excretion of droperidol by human subjects following intramuscular and intravenous administration. Anesthesiology 38:363, 1973

339. Michenfelder JD, Theye RA: Effects of fentanyl, droperidol, and Innovar on canine cerebral metabolism and blood flow. Br J Anaesth 43:630, 1971

340. Barker J, Harper AM, McDowall DG, et al: Cerebral blood flow, cerebrospinal fluid pressure and EEG activity during neuroleptanalgesia induced with dehydrobenzperidol and phenoperidine. Br J Anaesth 40:143, 1968

341. Prys-Roberts C, Kelman GR: The influence of drugs used in neuroleptanalgesia on cardiovascular and ventilatory function. Br J Anaesth 39:134, 1967

342. Corssen G, Domino EF, Sweet RB: Neuroleptanalgesia and anesthesia. Anesth Analg 43:748, 1964

343. Israel JS, Jansen GT, Dobkin AB: Circulatory and respiratory response to tilt with pentazocine (Win 20, 228), droperidol (R4749), droperidol-fentanyl (Innovar), and methotrimeprazine in normal healthy male subjects. Anesthesiology 26:253, 1965

344. Janssen PAJ, Niemegeers CJE, Schellekens KHL, et al: The pharmacology of dehydrobenzperidol (R4749), a new potent and short-acting neuroleptic agent chemically related to haloperidol. Arzneimittelforschung 13:205, 1963

345. Stanley TH: Cardiovascular effects of droperidol during enflurane and enflurane-nitrous oxide anaesthesia in man. Can Anaesth Soc J 25:26, 1978

346. Birch AA, Boyce WH: Effects of droperidol-dopamine interaction on renal blood flow in man. Anesthesiology 47:70, 1977

347. Yelonsky J, Katz R, Dietrich E: A study of some of the phar-

macologic actions of droperidol. Toxicol Appl Pharmacol 6:37, 1964

348. Long G, Dripps RD, Price HL: Measurements of anti-arrhythmic potency of drugs in man: Effects of dehydrobenzperidol. Anesthesiology 28:318, 1967

349. Yelnosky J, Gardocki JF: A study of some of the pharmacologic actions of fentanyl citrate and droperidol. Toxicol Appl Pharmacol 6:48, 1964

350. Stoelting RK, Gibbs PS, Creasser CW, Peterson C: Hemodynamic and ventilatory responses to fentanyl, fentanyl-droperidol and nitrous oxide in patients with acquired valvular heart disease. Anesthesiology 42:319, 1975

351. Harper MH, Hickey RF, Cromwell TH, Linwood S: The magnitude and duration of respiratory depression produced by fentanyl and fentanyl plus droperidol in man. J Pharmacol Exp Ther 199:464, 1976

352. Corssen G, DeKornfield TJ: Comparison of the respiratory depressant effects of fentanyl, fentanyl and droperidol, and morphine. Anesthesiology 27:213, 1966

353. Ivankovich AD, El-Etr AA, Janeczko GF, Maronic JP: The effect of ouabaine and of Innovar anesthesia on digitalis tolerance in dogs. Anesth Analg 54:106, 1975

354. Patton CM: Rapid induction of acute dyskinesia by droperidol. Anesthesiology 43:126, 1975

355. Guze BH, Baxter LR, Jr: Current concepts: Neuroleptic malignant syndrome. N Engl J Med 313:163, 1985

356. Parikh AM, Camara EG: Neuroleptic malignant syndrome. Am Fam Phy 37:296, 1988

357. Segal IS, Vickesy RG, Walton JK, et al: Descmedetomidate diminishes halothane anesthetic requirements in rats through a postsynaptic alpha$_2$ adrenergic receptor. Anesthesiology 69:818, 1988

358. Tweed WA, Minuck M, Mymin D: Circulatory responses to ketamine anesthesia. Anesthesiology 37:613, 1972

359. Tweed WA, Mymin D: Myocardial force-velocity relations during ketamine anesthesia at constant heart rate. Anesthesiology 41:49–52, 1974

360. Nishimura K, Kitamura Y, Hamai R, et al: Pharmacological studies of ketamine hydrochloride in the cardiovascular system. Osaka City Med J 19:17, 1973

361. Dhadphale PR, Behrendt DM, Jackson PF, et al: The effect of diazepam on contractility in the intact human heart. Abstracts of Scientific Papers, New Orleans, ASA Annual Meeting, 1977

362. Prakash R, Thurer R, Vargas A, et al: Cardiovascular effects of diazepam induction in patients for aortocoronary saphenous vein bypass grafts. Abstracts of Scientific Papers, ASA Annual Meeting, San Francisco, 1976

363. Jackson APF, Dhadphale PR, Callaghan ML, et al: Haemodynamic studies during induction of anaesthesia for open-heart surgery using diazepam and ketamine. Br J Anaesth 50:375, 1978

364. Cote P, Noble J, Bourassa MG: Systemic vasodilation following diazepam after combined sympathetic and parasympathetic blockade in patients with coronary heart disease. Cath Cardiovasc Diagn 2:369, 1976

365. Ruff R, Reves JG: Hemodynamic effects of a lorazepam-fentanyl anesthetic induction for coronary artery bypass surgery. J Cardiothoracic Anesthesia (In press)

366. Schmucker P, van Ackern K, Franke N, et al: Einwirkung von intravenos appliziertem lormetazepam auf hamodynamik und arterielle blutgase bei patienten mit koronarer herzekrankkung. Anaesthetist 31:557, 1982

367. Lebowitz PW, Cote ME, Daniels AL, et al: Cardiovascular effects of midazolam and thiopentone for induction of anesthesia in ill surgical patients. Can Anaesth Soc J 30:19, 1983

368. Marty J, Nitenberg A, Blancet F, et al: Effects of midazolam on the coronary circulation in patients with coronary artery disease. Anesthesiology 64:206, 1986

369. Kwar P, Carson IW, Clarke RSJ, et al: Haemodynamic changes during induction of anaesthesia with midazolam and diazepam (Valium) in patients undergoing coronary artery bypass surgery. Anaesthesia 40:767, 1985

370. Moffet AC (ed): Clarke's Isolation and Identification of Drugs. 2nd Ed. Pharmaceutical Press, London, 1986

371. Janssen PAJ: Pharmacological Aspects. p. 151. In Bente D, Bradley P (eds): Neuropsychopharmacology. Elsevier Science Publishing, Amsterdam, 1965

10

NARCOTIC INTRAVENOUS ANESTHETICS

Peter L. Bailey
Theodore H. Stanley

Continued

INTRODUCTION

Opioids have been administered for hundreds of years to allay anxiety and reduce the pain associated with surgery.[1] Many of these compounds are used not only for premedication and analgesia during and after anesthesia and surgery, but also as primary or sole intravenous anesthetics. Some investigators suggest that, with minor modifications, one of a number of new synthetic opioids may qualify as the "ideal intravenous anesthetic."[2] Others state that it is unrealistic to expect newer opioids to be markedly different from or more efficacious than older compounds.[3] In this chapter, we discuss the pharmacology and use of naturally occurring and synthetic intravenous opioids in contemporary anesthetic practice.

The terms *opioid, opiate, narcotic, narcotic analgesic,* and *narcotic anesthetic* are used to describe drugs that specifically bind to any of several subspecies of opioid receptors. These drugs share some of the pharmacologic properties of one or more of the naturally occurring opioids.

HISTORY

Although morphine and morphinelike alkaloids had been used for analgesia and sedation for centuries, the isolation of morphine from opium by Serturner in 1803 and the introduction of the syringe and hollow needle to clinical practice by Wood in 1853 finally permitted opioids to be administered in carefully measured doses.[1] Morphine then was frequently used intramuscularly for preoperative medication, as a supplement during ether or chloroform anesthesia, and postoperatively for analgesia. Late in the 19th century, large amounts of morphine (1 to 2 mg/kg) plus scopolamine (1 to 3 mg/70 kg) were administered in divided doses intravenously, intramuscularly, or both, as a complete anesthetic.[4,5] Although initially popular, this technique rapidly fell into disfavor because of an increase in operative morbidity and mortality.[1,6] For the next 30 to 40 years, anesthesiologists rarely used narcotic analgesics intraoperatively (also see Ch. 1).

Introduction of the ultra-short-acting barbiturates as intravenous anesthetics and popularization of the concept of "balanced anesthesia"[7] led to renewed enthusiasm for the intraoperative use of opioids. Two important events in this development were the synthesis of meperidine in 1939 and its use for anesthesia with nitrous oxide with or without *d*-tubocurarine.[8] Many variations of the nitrous oxide-narcotic technique became popular. At first, thiopental, *d*-tubocurarine (for muscle relaxation), and opioids such as morphine, meperidine, or alphaprodine were used for nitrous oxide-narcotic anesthesia. The introduction of Innovar, the combination of the tranquilizer droperidol with the short-acting narcotic fentanyl, signalled a further option.[9] Subsequently, a variety of intravenous supplements were used, including hypnotics, sedatives, tranquilizers, and additional analgesics.[10-14] These techniques were termed *balanced anesthesia,* because each intravenously administered compound was selected and used for a specific purpose, such as analgesia, amnesia, muscle relaxation, or abolition of autonomic reflexes. Currently, opioid agonists, compounds with mixed opioid agonist and antagonist properties, and sedative-hypnotics are being administered intravenously during anesthesia with low concentrations of potent inhaled anesthetics. This practice is based on the belief that the intravenous supplements reduce the concentrations of inhaled anesthetics required for anesthesia. This may result in less depression of the cardiovascular and other organ systems.[15-17]

De Castro,[18] Lowenstein et al.,[19] and Stanley and Webster[2] reintroduced the concept that high doses of opioids could produce complete anesthesia. They administered morphine or fentanyl intravenously until consciousness was lost. Ventilation was then controlled and a high inspired concentration of oxygen was administered. Morphine (0.5 to 1.0 mg/kg), administered intravenously to patients while they breathed 100 percent oxygen, did not alter the cardiovascular dynamics in those patients who did not have cardiac disease and in many cases improved the cardiovascular status of those with significant valvular disease.[19] These reports led to additional studies evaluating morphine and other opioids as the sole anesthetic for patients with poor cardiovascular reserve undergoing major operative procedures.[20-23] Unfortunately, problems with incomplete amnesia,[24,25] histamine release,[26] prolonged postoperative respiratory depression,[27,28] in-

TABLE 10-1. Lowest ED$_{50}$ Values in the Tail Withdrawal Test in Rats, LD$_{50}$ Values, Safety Margins, and Potency Ratio of Different Analgesics after Intravenous Administration

Compound	Lowest ED$_{50}$ (mg/kg)	LD$_{50}$ (mg/kg)	Therapeutic Index (Safety Margin)	Potency Ratio
Meperidine	6.0	29.0	4.8	1
Alfentanil	0.044	47.5	1,080	137
Fentanyl	0.011	3.1	277	550
Sufentanil	0.0007	17.9	25,211	8,500
Lofentanil	0.00059	0.066	112	10,200
Carfentanil	0.00034	3.4	10,000	17,800

creased blood volume requirements secondary to marked venodilation,[22] and hypotension and hypertension[21] diminished the popularity of morphine as a complete anesthetic.[24]

In contrast, the synthetic opioid fentanyl has become popular as a component of balanced anesthesia,[9,23] as a supplement when using an inhaled anesthetic,[15,16,29] and also in large doses (50 to 150 μg/kg) as a primary or complete anesthetic.[2,25,30] Unfortunately, large doses of fentanyl also cause significant postoperative respiratory depression,[2,30] which mitigated against its use in healthy patients undergoing most short elective operative procedures. Nevertheless, as with large doses of morphine, fentanyl can be used as a complete anesthetic while minimally depressing cardiovascular function. This aspect of opioid-based anesthesia makes it useful for patients who have little or no cardiovascular reserve. In addition, fentanyl-oxygen anesthesia produces less prolonged postoperative respiratory depression, greater cardiovascular stability, no histamine release, and no venodilation, as compared with morphine.[2,25–28,30,31]

More recently, sufentanil and alfentanil have been introduced into clinical practice. These and other new drugs are more potent and potentially safer than fentanyl as anesthetics (Table 10-1). Sufentanil is more "anesthetic" than fentanyl in terms of reducing the possibility of a hypertensive response when used as the sole anesthetic during cardiac surgical procedures. Alfentanil is less likely than fentanyl to provide adequate anesthesia under such circumstances. In the case of alfentanil, however, the dose required to produce plasma levels necessary to obtund responses to many surgical stimuli is well defined and readily achieved.[32] This is important, since plasma concentration differences following standard doses of opioids range up to fivefold. Similarly, the variability in therapeutic plasma levels, which effectively block a defined response to a surgical stimulus in 50 percent of test subjects (i.e., Cp$_{50}$), is also three- to fivefold.

The skin and buccal, nasal, vaginal, and rectal mucosal surfaces can serve as alternative routes for administering narcotic analgesics.[33] These approaches have resulted in transdermal fentanyl applications, sufentanil nasal sprays, fentanyl-impregnated lollipops, and a variety of rectally, vaginally, and sublingually adminis-

tered opioids. The value of these alternative routes and their applications are being explored.

CLASSIFICATION

Opioids are usually classified as naturally occurring, semisynthetic, and synthetic (Table 10-2). Morphine, codeine, and papaverine, the only naturally occurring opioids of clinical significance, are obtained from the poppy plant, *Papaver somniferum*. These compounds can be divided into two chemical classes, the phenanthrenes (morphine and codeine) and the benzylisoquinoline derivatives (papaverine). Of the naturally occurring opioids, only morphine is of importance as an intravenous analgesic or anesthetic.

The semisynthetic opioids are derivatives of morphine in which any one of several changes has been made such as etherification of one hydroxyl group (codeine), esterification of both hydroxyl groups (heroin), oxidation of the alcoholic hydroxyl to a ketone, or reduction of a double bond on the benzene ring (hydromorphone). Thebaine derivatives used clinically to provide analgesia include oxymorphone and oxycodone. Etorphine (M99), another thebaine derivative, is several thousand times more potent than morphine;

TABLE 10-2. Classification of Opioid Compounds

Naturally occurring
  Morphine
  Codeine
  Papaverine
  Thebaine

Semisynthetic
  Heroin
  Dihydromorphone/morphinone
  Thebaine derivatives (e.g., etorphine, buprenorphine)

Synthetic
  Morphinan series (e.g., levorphanol, butorphanol)
  Diphenylpropylamine series (e.g., methadone)
  Benzomorphinan series (e.g., pentazocine)
  Phenylpiperidine series (e.g., meperidine, fentanyl, sufentanil, alfentanil)

this compound has been used successfully for immobilization and anesthesia in wildlife management.[34]

The synthetic compounds resemble morphine but are usually entirely man-made. They are divided into four groups: the morphinan derivatives (levorphanol), the diphenyl or methadone derivatives (methadone or *d*-propoxyphene), the benzomorphans (phenazocine and pentazocine), and the phenylpiperidine derivatives (meperidine, fentanyl, alfentanil, and sufentanil). The general phenylpiperidine skeletal structure and the derivatives meperidine and fentanyl are illustrated in Figure 10-1. Important opiate receptor research compounds (ketocyclazocine and SKF 10,047) also belong to this group. Although many of these opioids have been used intravenously for analgesia or anesthesia experimentally, only the phenylpiperidine derivatives currently play an important role in anesthesia.

Clinicians often find the classification of opioids as agonists, partial agonists, mixed agonist-antagonists, and antagonists more useful. The pure opioid agonists are used most often in anesthesia. These drugs produce their effects primarily through interactions at the mu opiate receptor (see below). Partial agonists such as buprenorphine do not appear to produce the full spectrum or magnitude of mu-receptor-mediated effects when interacting with this receptor. Mixed agonist-antagonist compounds such as nalbuphine act as an agonist at one receptor (kappa) and an antagonist at another (mu), while the antagonist naloxone elicits little or no effects on its own at clinical doses but acts competitively to displace agonists from mu, kappa, delta, and sigma receptors, although to different degrees.

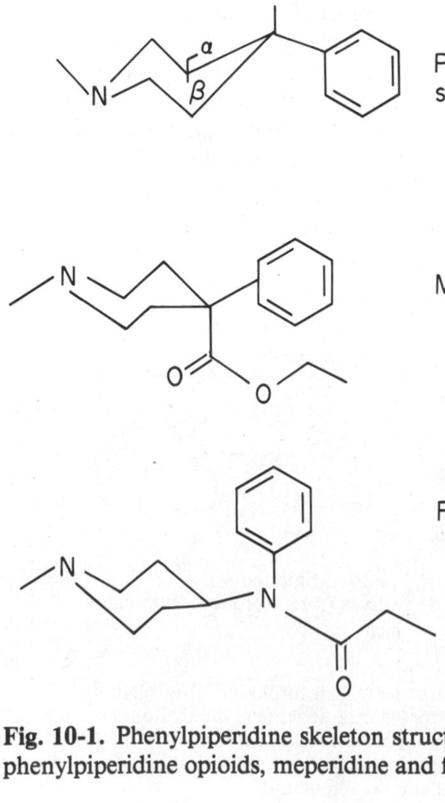

MECHANISMS OF ACTION

Structure-Activity Relationships

The structural dissimilarities among compounds displaying opiate activity almost defy a common mechanism as the basis for opioid structure-activity relationships. However, a detailed analysis of opioid stereospecificity has been used to describe a hypothetical three-dimensional model of the opiate receptor responsible for opioid activity.[35] Structurally, opioids are complex, three-dimensional compounds that usually exist as two optical isomers, that is, molecules that are mirror images of each other and identical in chemical composition but that cannot be superimposed.[36] Usually only the *l*-rotary isomer is capable of producing analgesia.

A close relationship exists between the stereochemical structure of an opioid compound and the presence or absence of analgesic activity.[37,38] Indeed, relatively minor molecular changes such as the degree of ionization produced by variations in pH may cause significant alteration in the pharmacologic activity of opioid compounds.[38]

The prototype opioid is morphine. Its rigid pentacyclic structure conforms to a T shape[35] (Fig. 10-2). Morphine demonstrates several other structural characteristics common to most opioids: a tertiary positively charged basic nitrogen, a quaternary carbon (C-13 in morphine) that is separated from the basic nitrogen by an ethane chain ($-CH_2-CH_2-$) and attached to a phenyl group, a phenolic hydroxyl group (in morphine derivatives) or ketone group (meperidine, methadone), and the presence of an aromatic ring whose center is 4.55 Å from the nitrogen atom.[35,39,40]

The morphine molecule also contains a phenylpiperidine structure (an aromatic ring attached to a six-membered ring containing five carbons and one nitrogen). This moiety is present in opioids that otherwise seem unrelated to morphine, for example, fentanyl (Fig. 10-1).[35] Short-chain alkyl group substitution at the basic amino group (the group essential for opioid activity) results in mixed opioid agonist-antagonists.[41] Additional hydroxylation of C-14 produces opioids with antagonist and no agonist properties.[42] Phenylalanine and tyrosine may be important structural elements of the endogenous opioids (enkephalins and endorphins) and other endogenous opioidlike neural transmitters and modulators.[43,44]

Site of Action: Opiate Receptors

In 1973, three independent investigators described the presence of an "opioid receptor" in nervous tissue and hypothesized that endogenous substances probably

Fig. 10-1. Phenylpiperidine skeleton structure and synthetic phenylpiperidine opioids, meperidine and fentanyl.

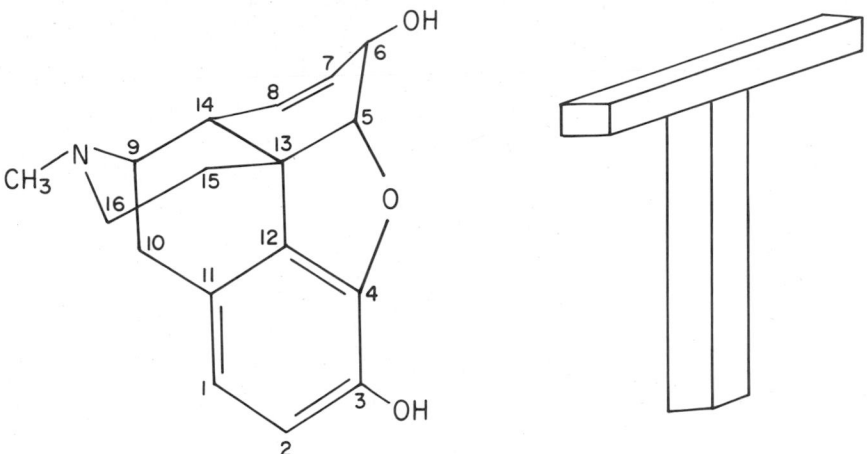

Fig. 10-2. T-shaped molecule of morphine. (From Thorpe,[35] with permission.)

stimulate this structure.[45-47] A few years later, the endogenous opiates were discovered.

The lock-and-key analogy for the receptor-opioid compound interactions, although surely an oversimplification, is mechanistically instructive. While agonist and antagonist opioids have both been described as "fitting" into the lock, only the agonist is able to "turn in the lock." Thus, pure antagonist opioids have intrinsic activities or efficacies of 0, while pure agonist opioids have intrinsic activities of 1. Some opioids (i.e., partial agonists or mixed agonist-antagonists) exhibit intermediate intrinsic activities. Figures 10-3A to D illustrate these various types of compounds and their interactions schematically.

The individual profile of a receptor is derived from the potency and the physiologic effects of a variety of agonist and agonist-antagonist interactions, the results of various bioassay and binding studies, structure-activity relationship data, and numerous other screening evaluations. For example, potency usually correlates well with receptor affinity and is described by the IC_{50} value (the concentration of an agent that lowers the specific binding of [³H]naloxone by 50 percent). The greater the affinity of a drug for the receptor, the lower the IC_{50}.[41] The more potent an agonist is, the fewer number of molecules necessary to elicit a certain level of effect.

Opioid receptor occupancy correlates with analgesia and anesthesia in rats. Increasing doses of the highly potent synthetic mu-receptor-stimulating opioid lofentanil produce increasing analgesia and finally, at 25 to 30 percent receptor occupancy, anesthesia.[48] The relationship between percent receptor occupancy and opioid effects does not occur as would be predicted by the law of mass action. That is, the biological ED_{50} for an opioid effect does not correspond to a 50 percent receptor occupancy.

Bioassay systems are used to help evaluate potency. The response to transmural electrical stimulation of a number of isolated tissues can be inhibited by opioids. This effect is most likely mediated by the presynaptic inhibition of transmitter release. The two most important of these systems are the guinea pig ileum (GPI) and mouse vas deferens (MVD). For example, morphine inhibits electrically induced contractions of the isolated GPI. Data from these systems correlate well with opioid analgesic potency[49] as determined by numerous intact animal and clinical evaluations. Biochemical characterization of the opiate receptor (synaptosomal protein and lipid), binding assays, and biochemical treatments are other tools that have been used in receptor research.[41] Although the physical isolation of opioid receptors has not yet been achieved, some physical characteristics have been delineated.[50]

Soon after the structures of some of the endogenous opioids were determined, differences were noted in their activity, particularly when they were compared with morphine in bioassay systems. For example, agonist and antagonist interactions can be quantified by the pA_2 (the negative log of the concentration of antagonist that doubles the concentration of agonist necessary to produce a particular response).[51] Numerous studies have shown that the pA_2 of naloxone for a variety of pure agonist opioids is 7. This suggests a common receptor mechanism.[52,53] In contrast, a pA_2 of 6 for [d-Ala²-d-Leu⁵]enkephalin suggests that this particular opioid acts on a different receptor.[54] In addition, the potency of various opioid agonists differs depending on the bioassay used. This differential ordering of activity across several tissue types underlies the theory of different receptor types. If only one receptor type existed, potency ratios or ordering should be constant in all bioassays. As a result, investigators suggested that separate and/or different receptors for these compounds exist, such as a mu receptor for morphine and a delta receptor for enkephalin. These proposals were supported by central nervous system (CNS) binding and autoradiographic studies.[55,56]

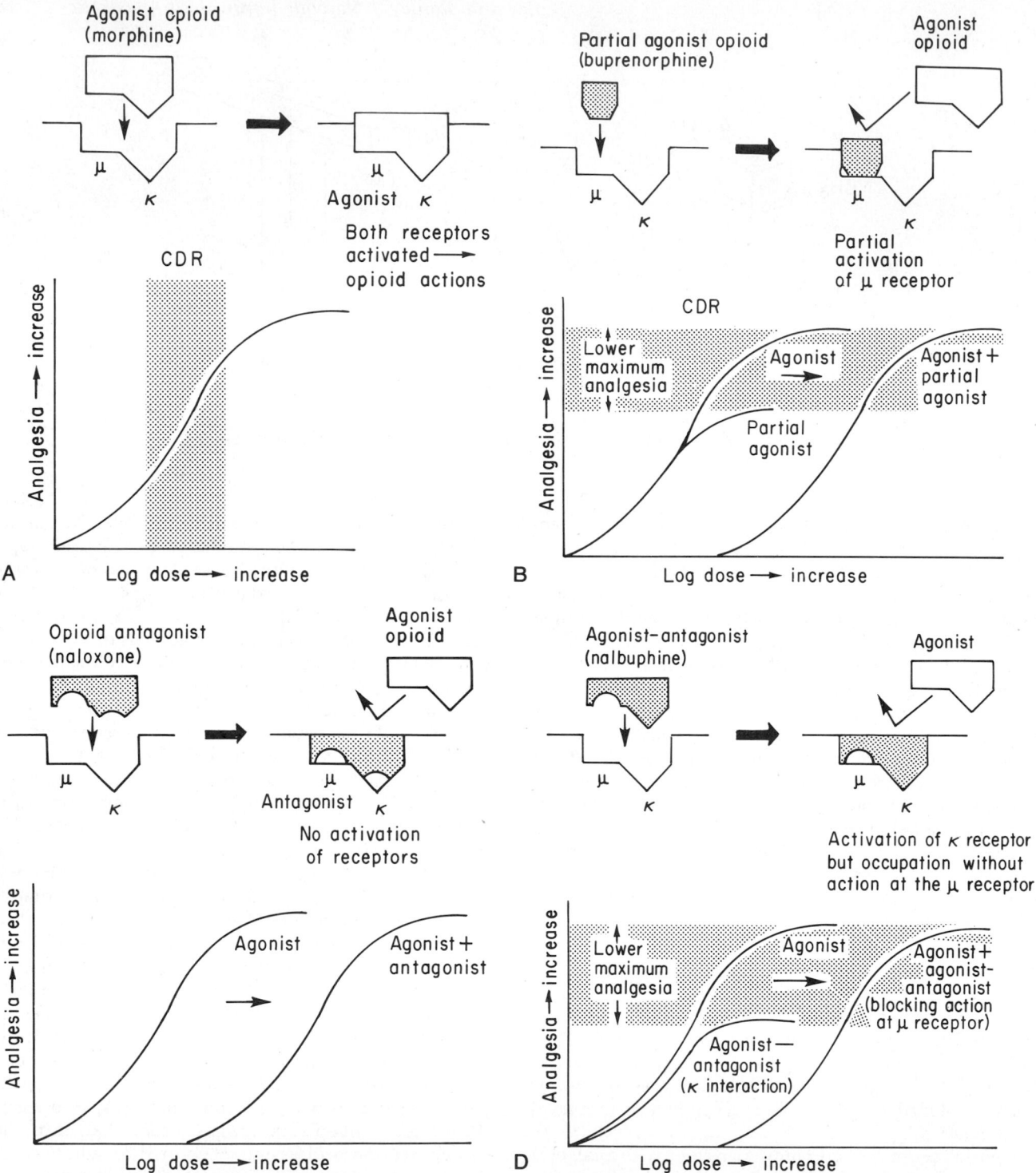

Fig. 10-3. Receptor interactions of opioids. Opioid-receptor interactions are illustrated in terms of a lock and key diagram with two receptor sites, mu (μ) and kappa (κ), and a representative dose-response (DR) curve of analgesic effects. **(A)** An opioid agonist stimulates both the μ and κ receptors. The steep portion of the DR curve is in the clinical dose range (CDR), and analgesia is unlimited. **(B)** Partial agonists such as buprenorphine combine with the μ receptor, but they have only limited activity. The DR curve is flatter, with a lower maximum effect. The partial agonist will shift the DR curve for an agonist to the right. **(C)** The opioid antagonist, naloxone, can occupy both mu and kappa receptors, but it has no intrinsic activity. The antagonist will shift the DR curve for an agonist to the right. **(D)** The agonist-antagonist opioids, such as nalbuphine, may have mixed effects at the μ and κ receptors. Analgesia occurs by kappa receptor agonist activity, while mu receptor function is blocked. This naloxonelike effect would shift the DR curve to a μ-agonist to the right. (From Hare,[922] with permission.)

TABLE 10-3. Characteristics of Opioid Receptors

Receptor	Tissue Bioassay	Agonists	Major Actions
Mu			
Mu$_1$	Guinea pig ileum	Morphine Meptazinol Phenylpiperidines	Analgesia Bradycardia Sedation
Mu$_2$	Guinea pig ileum	Morphine Phenylpiperidines	Respiratory depression Euphoria Physical dependence
Delta	Mouse vas deferens	*d*-Ala-*d*-Leu Enkephalin	Analgesia (weak) Respiratory depression
Kappa	Rabbit vas deferens	Ketocyclazocine Dynorphin Nalbuphine Butorphanol	Analgesia (weak) Respiratory depression Sedation
Sigma		SKF 10,047 Pentazocine	Dysphoria-delirium, mydriasis Hallucinations Tachycardia Hypertension
Epsilon	Rat vas deferens	β-Endorphin	Stress response Acupuncture

The picture soon became even more complex. Although enkephalins and morphine do not show cross-tolerance in bioassay systems, that is, GPI and MVD evaluations, they do in analgesic studies. Thus, it appears that analgesia is probably mediated through a number of receptors, some with high affinity for narcotic analgesics, the mu$_1$ receptors, and some with low affinity, the mu$_2$ and delta receptors.[57,58] It has been proposed that analgesia (mu$_1$) and respiratory depression (mu$_2$) are mediated by different subclasses of receptors.[59] Furthermore, the concentration and proportion of the receptor subtypes seem to change with time. For example, mu$_1$ receptors increase in number and concentration as newborn mice grow and thus provide more analgesia after a similar dose of an opioid agonist.[60] Mu$_1$ receptors also appear more prominent in supraspinal analgesia, whereas delta receptors may be more important for spinal analgesia.[61] Other opioid receptor subtypes seem to play a role in endogenous opioid neurotransmission and in the mediation of opioid effects (Table 10-3). For example, the kappa receptor agonist ethylketocyclazocine produces sedation and analgesia without causing much respiratory depression.[62] Kappa receptor activation may explain in part some of the effects (analgesia with limited respiratory depression) of some mixed agonist-antagonists such as nalbuphine.[63]

Opiate receptors are found in many areas in the CNS, including the cerebral cortex, the limbic cortex (anterior and posterior amygdala and hippocampus), hypothalamus, medial thalamus, midbrain (periaqueductal gray), extrapyramidal area (caudate, striatum, and putamen), substantia gelatinosa, and sympathetic preganglionic neurons[62,64] (Table 10-4). Gray matter has more receptors than does white matter. Structures and pathways involved with pain usually contain the highest concentrations of opiate receptors[65]; however, the presence of opioid receptors in other areas of the CNS

TABLE 10-4. Mu and Delta Opiate Receptors in Rat Brain Regions

Predominantly Mu	Predominantly Delta	Mu and Delta
Laminae I and IV of cerebral cortex	Laminae II, III, and V of cerebral cortex	Laminae VI of cerebral cortex
Streaks and clusters in corpus striatum	Diffuse grains in corpus striatum	Nucleus tractus solitarius
Thalamus (dorsomedial, ventral)	Amygdala	Vagal fibers
Hypothalamus	Nucleus accumbens	Nucleus ambiguus
Hippocampus (pyramidal cell layer)	Olfactory tubercle	Substantia gelatinosa of spinal cord
Periaqueductal gray	Pontine nuclei	Trigeminal nucleus
Interpeduncular nucleus		
Superior and inferior colliculus		
Midbrain median raphe, caudate, putamen		

(Adapted from Goodman et al.,[56] with permission.)

(e.g., basal ganglia, limbic area, cerebral cortex) suggests other roles for the endogenous opiates and their receptors.

The periaqueductal gray area is one of the few regions in the CNS in which microinjections of morphine or direct electrical stimulation produce analgesia that can be blocked with naloxone.[66-68] Stimulation of periaqueductal gray receptors with morphine, electricity, or endogenous opiatelike peptides may result in a barrage of impulses that move down the neuraxis and inhibit the transmission of nociceptive information from peripheral nerves into the spinal cord.[68] The integrity of certain neurotransmitter systems connecting the pain-inhibiting system in the brain to the spinal cord is necessary for morphine to exert its full analgesic action. Satoh and Takagi[69] found that morphine blockade of transmission of spinal cord potentials evoked by painful stimulation is inhibited by high spinal cord transection. Other sites such as the nucleus reticularis gigantocellularis demonstrate specific suppression of noxiously evoked activity by certain opioids.

Other mechanisms besides descending inhibition underlie the analgesic action of morphine. The substantia gelatinosa of the spinal cord also possesses a dense collection of opiate receptors.[36,70] Direct application of narcotics to these receptors creates intense analgesia. Undoubtedly, narcotics produce analgesia by acting at receptors both in the spinal cord and in higher centers. Opiate receptors are also localized in the substantia gelatinosa of the caudal spinal trigeminal nucleus, the nucleus receiving pain fibers from the face and hands via branches of the 5th, 7th, 9th, and 10th cranial nerves.[66] Within the brain stem, opiate receptors are highly concentrated in the solitary nuclei that receive visceral sensory fibers from the 9th and 10th cranial nerves and the area postrema. Stimulation of the solitary nuclei depresses gastric secretion and the cough reflex and causes orthostatic hypotension. Stimulation of the area postrema with its chemoreceptor trigger zone results in nausea and vomiting.

The distribution of opioid receptors in the CNS does not strictly parallel the distribution of endogenous opioids with the possible exception of kappa receptors and dynorphin in man. In addition, many pharmacologic observations, for example, bioassays, give little insight into the physiologic roles opioids really play. Thus, increased potency of an endogenous substance does not necessarily imply greater biologic importance. Nevertheless, some key observations are in order with regards to opioids and analgesia. The mu receptor appears to be the major antinociception site and is located in both the brain and spinal cord with highest concentrations in the periaqueductal gray and substantia gelatinosa, respectively. Opioid-induced analgesia at the mu receptor is dose dependent. Whether or not the pharmacologic separation of an analgesic receptor (mu_1) and a respiratory depression receptor (mu_2) will translate into a clinical reality in the future is not known. There is no selective systemic agonist available

for delta receptors, and the enkephalins are rapidly degraded. The degree of analgesia that is produced by stimulation of the delta receptor is unclear (and may be more important at the spinal cord level). Kappa receptors appear to play a role in producing mild to moderate analgesia at the spinal cord level for nonthermal painful stimuli. Sigma receptors do not appear to be associated with analgesia. The epsilon receptor is primarily activated by β-endorphin but may contribute little to opioid-induced analgesia. On the other hand, β-endorphin has been implicated in stress-induced alterations in nociception and plays more of a neuromodulating or hormonal role than a transmitter-type role. Intrathecal injection or application of β-endorphin does, however, produce analgesia in humans.

The main mechanism underlying opioid action is stimulation of stereospecific receptors on or near sodium channels in excitable cell membranes, which results in depression of active sodium conductance.[71] In addition, opioid agonists produce a local anestheticlike effect on the surface of excitable cell membranes that does not involve a stereospecific receptor. Opioids may also block neuron excitability by a mechanism involving increased membrane potassium conductance or by blocking the opening of voltage-sensitive calcium channels.[71] These changes hyperpolarize cellular membranes, make them more difficult to depolarize, and thus decrease neurotransmission. Serotonergic pathways may also in part modulate opioid-mediated analgesia.[72] Finally, some opioid effects may be elicited at γ-aminobutyric acid (GABA) receptors, which are closely associated with benzodiazepine receptors.

Receptorology has also shed some light on the phenomenon of tolerance. Tolerance in fact represents an uncoupling of the usual drug-receptor effect. This is probably achieved by down regulation of the number of receptors and/or their affinity for agonists or by an uncoupling between the receptor and the intracellular second messenger. Interestingly, there is little cross-tolerance between most receptor subtypes. In addition, the most potent opioid agonists with the largest receptor reserve (i.e., they occupy the lowest percentage of receptors to produce a given effect) appear to be least prone to producing tolerance.[73] Furthermore, studies support the concept that tolerance is surmountable by increasing dose, at least initially.

Receptorology has also helped delineate, through receptor pharmacokinetic studies, how certain drugs can have a duration of action that extends well beyond what their plasma half-lives would predict. For example, buprenorphine's dissociation from the mu receptor is much slower than fentanyl's and does not parallel plasma concentrations.[74] The high affinity of buprenorphine for mu receptors also accounts for the difficulty of reversing its effects with naloxone. Other pharmacologic phenomena have been explained by radioligand-receptor studies. A marked and widespread disappearance of mu and delta receptors has been shown to occur in the aging brain.[75] Interestingly, the opposite occurs with benzodiazepine receptors during aging, indicating that these effects are specific and not representative of a general phenomenon.

The cardiovascular system possesses opioid receptors that have been documented by radioligand studies to exist in the heart, the cardiac branches of the vagus and sympathetic nerves, the central cardiovascular regulatory centers, and the adrenal medulla.[76] Complex receptor-mediated effects are under investigation, and their description is beyond the scope of this chapter. Nevertheless, available data indicate potential roles for and implications of opioids in shock, myocardial ischemia, and other cardiovascular events.

Endogenous Opiates

The discovery of opioid receptors in the CNS led to the hypothesis, and later the discovery, of endogenous opiatelike substances. Hughes et al.[77] first described two brain pentapeptides, methionine-enkephalin and leucine-enkephalin, that shared a four-amino-acid sequence (Tyr-Gly-Gly-Phe), had potent affinities for opiate-binding sites, and whose opiate effects were reversed by naloxone. Large endogenous opioid peptides, β-endorphin[78] and dynorphin,[79] were also described.

Three distinct precursor molecules (coded for by three distinct genes) are at the origin of three families of endogenously produced opioids in man. The biosynthesis of all these endogenous opiates is complex. However, it is now known that proopiocortin, a prohormone with a molecular weight of 30,000, is cleaved to form adrenocorticotropic hormone (ACTH) and a substance called β-lipotropin (β-LPH).[41] β-LPH is devoid of opioid activity and in turn is cleaved to yield β-endorphin.[80] The enkephalins have different precursors than those of β-endorphin, although the amino acid sequence for methionine-enkephalin is contained in β-LPH (amino acid sequence 61 to 65). Proenkephalin, a peptide with a molecular weight of 30,000, is the precursor for Met-enkephalin and several other enkephalins.[81] Dynorphin, one of the more recently described endogenous opioids, is derived from a third precursor, called prodynorphin. The differential biochemical processing of endogenous opiates parallels regional differences in endogenous opiate compounds, distribution, and concentration.[41] In spite of their differences, all three families of endogenous opioids possess the common amino acid sequence Tyr-Gly-Gly-Phe.

The endogenous opiates exist in virtually all vertebrate species and in many invertebrates as well.[82] The highest concentrations of β-endorphin occur in the pituitary gland (anterior and intermediate lobes greater than posterior lobe) and in the medial, basal, and arcuate region of the hypothalamus.[83] Some long-axoned endorphin-releasing neurons synapse at upper brain stem locations implicated in recognition of nociceptive processes. Some of these synapses are located in the septum, the periaqueductal gray, and the thalamus. It is unclear whether β-endorphin exists functionally in the spinal cord. β-endorphin also exists outside the CNS, in the small intestine, placenta, and plasma.[84,85] By contrast, enkephalins are widely distributed in many areas of the CNS (amygdala, globus pallidus, striatum, hypothalamus, thalamus, brain stem, and spinal cord dorsal horn laminae I, II, and V) that receive afferent nociceptive information. Enkephalins have also been isolated in the peripheral nervous system (peripheral ganglia, autonomic nervous system, adrenal medulla), as well as the gastrointestinal tract and plasma.[41]

Dynorphin is found in the hypothalamoneurohypophyseal axis, but as with the other two families of opioids, the importance of this finding remains unclear. Dynorphin appears to be distributed in other CNS areas relevant to nociception: the periaqueductal gray, limbic system, thalamus, and laminae I and V of the dorsal horn in the spinal cord.

A functional hierarchy exists in nociception and the endogenous opioids. In peripheral sensory nerves extending to the dorsal horn of the spinal cord where primary processing of afferent nociceptive information occurs, both dynorphins and enkephalins are active. In the midbrain, brain stem, and thalamus, where key ascending and descending relay stations for nociception reside, rich concentrations of dynorphins, enkephalins, and β-endorphin innervations from the hypothalamus exist. The descending analgesic system mentioned above extends from the brain stem to the dorsal horn of the spinal cord. The midbrain periaqueductal gray sends a major projection to the raphe nuclei of the brain stem. Serotonergic projections from the raphe nuclei to the spinal cord gray can suppress the nociceptive response of spinothalamic neurons.[41] Higher brain centers involved in the affective dimension of pain (limbic system, amygdala, and cortex) contain significant populations of neurons where dynorphin, enkephalin, and β-endorphin are found.

β-Endorphin probably does not play a role in basal nociceptive thresholds but rather modulates nociception during stress, midbrain periaqueductal gray stimulation, and acupuncture. Enkephalins may play some role in acupuncture-mediated analgesia. Enkephalins may also elicit analgesia through the release of substance P in the dorsal horn. Enkephalins act as inhibitory neurotransmitters. This is consistent with their wide distribution and rapid inactivation throughout the neuraxis. Dynorphin is thought to play a more important role in nociception at the spinal cord level (through activation of the kappa receptor) than in the brain.

There have been many other roles postulated for endogenous opioids, but they are incompletely defined. For example, mu receptors can mediate an antidiuresis while kappa receptor activation elicits a free water diuresis. The physiologic importance of these phenomena is unknown. Other roles include the modulation of respiratory responses to various stimuli and drugs[86] and participation in the cardiovascular depression seen in shock.[87] Several studies demonstrate increases in endogenous opioids in patients with chronic obstructive pulmonary disease (COPD). It has been suggested that they serve a protective mechanism that lessens the stress of prolonged dyspnea and reduces excessive increases in the work of breathing.[86] This is especially true in advanced COPD where abnormal ventilation/perfusion relations do not improve with increased ventilation.[86] Conversely, naloxone may improve ventilation in certain cases of respiratory failure. The clinical implications of these and other roles for the endogenous opiates remain controversial and unclear. A detailed discussion is beyond the scope of this chapter but may be obtained in recent reviews.[76,86,88,89]

ANALGESIA-AMNESIA-ANESTHESIA

Are Opioids Anesthetics?

Although opiate narcotics have achieved prominence as principal or sole anesthetics in cardiac and other selected surgeries, whether or not opioids alone are capable of producing anesthesia is a question that continues to be vigorously debated.[3,24,90] To date, there is no study demonstrating that an opioid alone can reliably produce anesthesia in humans in the absence of all other supplements, including muscle relaxants and premedicants.

The most popular model used to examine whether or not opiate narcotics can serve as anesthetics has been to assess their ability to substitute for a potent inhaled anesthetic in dogs[91-96] and rats[97,98] subjected to tail-clamp minimum alveolar concentration (MAC) evaluations. A consistent 60 to 70 percent reduction in the MAC of enflurane or isoflurane occurs in dogs with morphine,[94] fentanyl,[95] alfentanil,[91,93] and sufentanil.[92] The fact that further increases in narcotic doses and plasma levels often resulted in no additional MAC reductions after a certain MAC reduction was achieved has led to the conclusion that maximum opioid narcotic effects reach a ceiling that is subanesthetic.[94,95]

Opioid narcotics reduce the MAC of inhaled anesthetics more in rats than in dogs: 84 percent for morphine[98] and 90 percent for sufentanil without a plateau or ceiling effect noted[97] (Fig. 10-4). In contrast to investigators using the dog model, these researchers concluded that "sufentanil is essentially a complete anesthetic."[97] Other reports demonstrating lower thiopental requirements for loss of consciousness after sufentanil than fentanyl support the greater anesthetic capabilities of sufentanil over fentanyl[99] (Fig. 10-5).

For numerous reasons, MAC reduction studies have significant limitations. Species differences, although minimal in terms of MAC determinations with inhaled anesthetics, are significant with opioids[94,98,100,101] and render extrapolation of results to humans questionable. Some authors argue that a similarity between opioids and associated cardiovascular effects in humans and dogs supports the conclusion that responses of the two species to narcotic analgesics are similar.[91,102] Others have found that dogs are not only

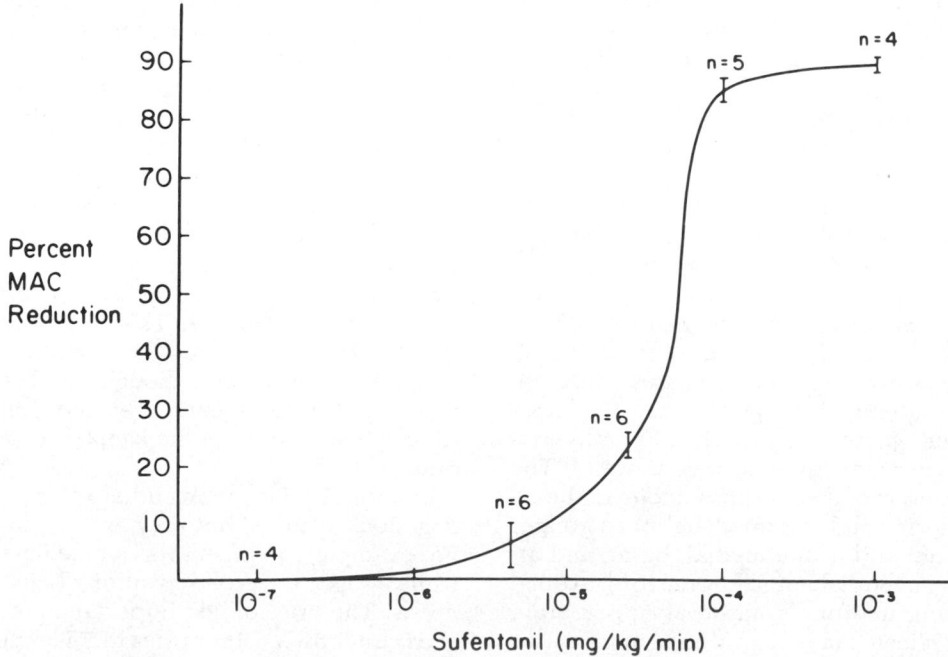

Fig. 10-4. Reduction of halothane MAC in the rat observed with progressively increased sufentanil dosage. (From Hecker et al.,[97] with permission.)

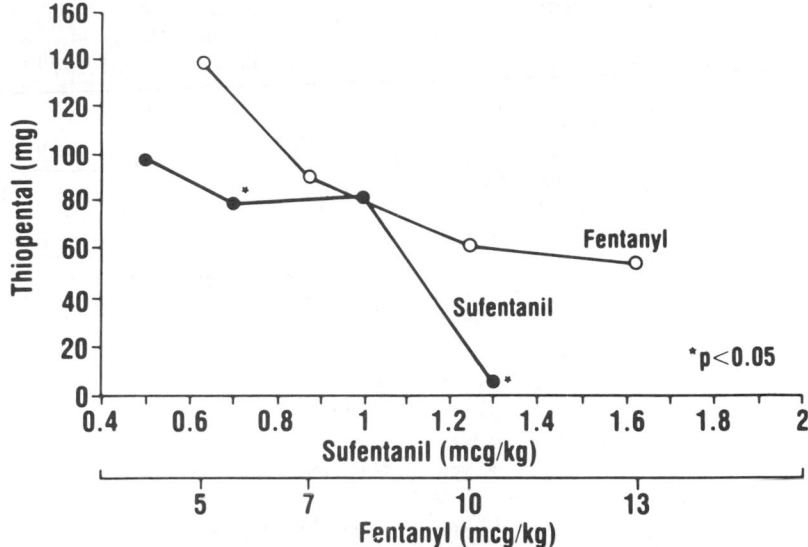

Fig. 10-5. Plot of thiopental requirement for induction of sleep versus opioid dose in surgical patients. Thiopental was administered intravenously in 25-mg increments every 30 seconds until the subject was unconscious. Sufentanil and fentanyl doses were plotted on the same scale, using a potency ratio of 1:8. The thiopental requirement was significantly smaller ($P < 0.0001$) for sufentanil (0.7 and 1.3 μg/kg) compared with equipotent doses of fentanyl (5 and 10 μg/kg, respectively). Only 1 of the 10 patients receiving sufentanil (1.3 μg/kg) required any thiopental, compared with 10 of 10 in the fentanyl (10 μg/kg) group, and 8 of 10 in the fentanyl (13 μg/kg) group ($P < 0.0001$). (From Bowdle and Ward,[99] with permission.)

more resistant to opioid narcotics but also demonstrate a markedly different profile of effects compared with humans.[100]

The method (i.e., tail clamp) used to elicit a motor response during MAC reduction studies may test for analgesia but not anesthesia. Thus, tail-clamp-induced motor responses can be totally absent in animals that have received opioid narcotics and are conscious and still present in animals rendered unconscious with barbiturates.[103] These findings raise serious questions about the validity of tail-clamp responses for determination of the presence or absence of anesthesia. Kissin and Brown[104] have also shown that reserpine dissociates the anesthetic effects of fentanyl (as manifested by the loss of the righting reflex in rats) from its analgesic effects (tail-clamp response). In addition, elimination of the motor response occurs at deeper levels of anesthesia than unconsciousness, amnesia, and analgesia.[105] Thus, the results of motor response evaluations do not necessarily indicate the anesthetic capabilities of opioids. Finally, inhaled anesthetics such as halothane may inhibit the descending pain inhibitory pathways that opioid narcotics activate. Thus, potent inhaled anesthetics may antagonize opioid effects.[106]

Nevertheless, the presumed specific mechanism by which opioid narcotics act has led to the opinion that they should not be expected to produce anesthesia.[90] In addition, the receptor occupation theory and the demonstration of a ceiling to opioid effects in MAC reduction studies in dogs have led some investigators to question whether titrating additional narcotic after an apparent ceiling is reached can produce additional CNS depression (anesthesia).[107] However, the ability of a drug to produce analgesia in subanesthetic concentrations and loss of consciousness in higher concentrations may be mediated, at least in part, by different processes (see above).[108] A dual mechanism in the anesthetic action of opioids has been proposed and requires that in addition to receptor-mediated effects, an opioid must be lipid soluble enough to function as a general anesthetic.[109] Interestingly, a biphasic response has been noted with sufentanil[97] and fentanyl[100] (Fig. 10-4).

Awareness under General Anesthesia

The problem of patient awareness under general anesthesia is as old as the specialty itself. However, it was with the introduction of muscle relaxants that the importance of the problem became fully recognized. Muscle relaxants permitted greater flexibility for the anesthesiologist and surgeon. For example, the development and clinical application of muscle relaxants permitted lighter levels of general anesthesia and simultaneously encouraged the search for and use of many other drugs as anesthetics or anesthetic adjuvants.

While opiate narcotics are often used as the primary or sole anesthetic, some authors argue that opioids do not produce unconsciousness,[90] and therefore, are not complete anesthetics.

While various definitions of *consciousness* and *awareness* have been proposed, the most practical definition is "the spontaneous recall of events occurring during general anesthesia." A key word in this definition is spontaneous, for there are numerous studies documenting that the registration or retention of mental images or information under general anesthesia commonly occurs and can be demonstrated or elicited postoperatively by hypnosis[110] and word or picture recognition tests.[111] In addition, electroencephalographic (EEG) and auditory evoked responses document that auditory functioning is left largely intact even under inhalational anesthesia.[112] Intraoperative suggestions made to fully anesthetized patients can also impact their postoperative course in such ways as decreasing the need for urinary bladder catheterization.[113] It is, therefore, not necessary or perhaps not even possible to block the registration or retention of all information in patients who undergo general anesthesia. It is rather the consolidation of such material and the recollection or recall of intraoperative events that should most concern the anesthesiologist.

Whether the use of opiate narcotics in anesthesia is associated with an increased incidence of awareness is debatable. Awareness has been reported with many anesthetic techniques.[114-119] Whether the incidence of awareness has increased because of the use of opioid narcotics is unknown.[120-122] While the reported incidence of awareness during anesthesia varies greatly (1 to 25 percent),[120] a 1 to 2 percent incidence is generally accepted as accurate.

Several measures can be taken to minimize the occurrence of awareness under general anesthesia, or the problems that can arise when a patient has such an experience. Preoperative evaluation of the patient allows the making of decisions regarding the role an opiate narcotic and its dose should play in intraoperative management. Nonetheless, predicting the appropriate drug and dose remains difficult. Generally, healthier patients with normal or high cardiac outputs prior to anesthesia require larger doses of narcotics for anesthesia than do patients who have serious metabolic disease or cardiovascular limitations, especially reduced cardiac output.[2,28,30] Older patients experience higher blood and presumably brain concentrations of opioids than do younger patients after a similar dose. This probably explains the ease with which older patients are rendered anesthetic with opioids[123] (Table 10-5). Patients' habits (e.g., smoking, alcohol consumption) may also influence anesthetic requirements.[124] Acute tolerance may also decrease intraoperative effects.[125] Undoubtedly, differences in plasma protein binding, fat solubility, hepatic metabolism, renal excretion, and regional perfusion influence requirements for opioids as well. In selected cases (cardiac anesthesia, trauma) where opiate narcotics may be the sole anesthetic, preoperative discussion of the possibility of

TABLE 10-5. Unconsciousness as a Function of Age in 72 Patients Given Fentanyl (30 μg/kg) for Induction of Anesthesia

Age (yrs)	% Rendered Unconscious
18–39	57
31–45	77
46–60	53
>60	100

$\chi^2 = 4.787$; $P = 0.0287$.
(From Bailey et al.,[123] with permission.)

awareness is recommended. Although pain does not often accompany awareness, the results of a national inquiry in Great Britain suggest that this is not always the case.[112] In that survey, 41 percent of patients felt pain during their awareness episodes.

The ability to monitor for intraoperative awareness remains limited (also see Ch. 30). Although monitoring CNS activity (EEG, sensory evoked potentials) or esophageal contractility may be of assistance in evaluating depth of anesthesia, reliably producing a level of CNS depression consistent with lack of awareness remains a clinical art. Signs suggestive of the possibility of awareness are usually limited to movement and increased autonomic activity. Hypertension, tachycardia, pupil dilation, tearing, sweating, or salivation may indicate too light a level of anesthesia. Eye lid motion, swallowing, increased spontaneous respiratory effort, and extremity or head motion are other signs often assumed to indicate inadequate amnesia. Monitoring for muscle activity as an indicator of awareness is in fact quite valuable because muscle movements usually occur before the threshold for awareness is reached. Indeed, motor signs (muscle movements) frequently occur prior to changes in hemodynamics or activation of the sympathetic nervous system.[122] Unfortunately, the use of muscle relaxants during narcotic-based anesthesia removes this important clinical sign. Limiting muscle relaxant use during nitrous narcotic anesthesia to appropriate indications (e.g., intra-abdominal or ophthalmic surgery) improves the detection of possible awareness.

The incidence of awareness can be reduced by adding one or more sedative-hypnotics during premedication, induction, and/or maintenance of anesthesia. While administration of supplements (nitrous oxide, diazepam, droperidol) or larger doses of narcotics will increase the likelihood of amnesia,[126] they do not guarantee it.[117,123] Furthermore, undesirable side effects such as prolonged postoperative respiratory depression and cardiovascular depression are frequent after administration of most supplements.[10,11,127] Many clinicians use 0.3 to 0.6 MAC or MAC-awake concentrations of potent inhaled anesthetics in the hope of ensuring amnesia. Unfortunately, the hemodynamic stability sought with a narcotic technique may be compromised with this approach as well.

In light of current understanding of awareness and

CNS function under anesthesia, intraoperative conversation, especially that which contains material meaningful to the patient, should be curtailed during anesthesia and surgery. Although potent stimuli such as laryngoscopy, tracheal intubation, skin incision, sternotomy, and aortic root dissection are considered to be the events most frequently associated with awareness, comments about a patient's size or discussion of clinical aspects of the patient's case can also cause EEG arousal and be recalled.[112] On the other hand, intraoperative therapeutic suggestion, which can be used to significantly improve patient outcome,[113] remains underutilized.

Not all cases of intraoperative awareness are reported by patients postoperatively. The absence of spontaneous recall, therefore, does not ensure a lack of awareness under anesthesia. Traumatic neurosis consisting of nightmares, anxiety, preoccupation with death, and reluctance to discuss the incident is a symptom complex often associated with awareness during surgery.[117,128] Awareness associated with anesthesia is best dealt with by informing patients of its possibility preoperatively and by frank and open discussion of such an episode after an occurrence. Direct explanation is considered to be the most helpful approach to a reluctant and fearful patient.[128]

CARDIOVASCULAR ACTIONS

Although hypotension, hypertension, bradycardia, and numerous other cardiovascular problems were reported following morphine administration, these side effects seem to occur less frequently after fentanyl.[2,19] The newer, more potent opioid, sufentanil, also produces minimal changes in cardiovascular dynamics.[129,130] Likewise, alfentanil provides superior cardiovascular stability when compared with non-opioid drugs used to induce anesthesia,[131] although some patients have significant hemodynamic fluctuations.[132]

Slow administration of morphine (1 mg/kg over 5 to 10 minutes intravenously) usually does not cause significant circulatory changes in supine patients with or without cardiac disease.[19] In patients with aortic valvular disease, stroke volume and cardiac output may be increased after morphine administration, probably because the compound does not result in myocardial depression but does decrease systemic vascular resistance, at least transiently.[19,133,134] Vasko and co-workers[135] found that morphine in dogs has a significant positive inotropic effect that is dependent on endogenous catecholamine release. Morphine increases blood and urine catecholamine concentrations in a dose-dependent manner in patients with cardiac disease.[136–138] The release of catecholamines by morphine and meperidine follows and parallels histamine release.[139,140]

Although large doses (0.5 to 30 µg/kg) of fentanyl produce significant increases in plasma catecholamines in dogs,[141] anesthetic doses of fentanyl (24 to 75 µg/kg) decrease rather than increase plasma catecholamine and cortisol concentrations in humans.[142] The effect of fentanyl on plasma catecholamines may be dose dependent. Hicks et al.[143] noted elevated plasma norepinephrine levels after 15 µg/kg of fentanyl, but normal (baseline) values after 50 µg/kg in human subjects. Similarly, anesthetic doses of sufentanil usually do not change circulating catecholamine concentrations. Most investigators have reported that fentanyl has no effect on myocardial contractility or cardiac output.[2,144,145] However, others have reported negative[143] or positive[146] inotropic effects, and still others a myocardial depression-sparing action of fentanyl during halothane and enflurane anesthesia.[15,16]

Despite the minimal cardiovascular effects of opioids, significant hypotension, hypertension, and cardiac arrhythmias have occurred after the administration of virtually all opioid narcotics.

Hypotension

Most opioids reduce sympathetic and enhance vagal and parasympathetic tone, particularly when administered in a large intravenous bolus dose. If not countered by indirect effects (e.g., catecholamine release) or the coadministration of drugs with anticholinergic or sympathetic activity (e.g., atropine or pancuronium), opioids can cause hypotension. Patients depending on high sympathetic tone or exogenous catecholamines to maintain cardiovascular function are more predisposed to hypotension after opioids. These and other specific cardiovascular effects of the opioid analgesics, for example, histamine release and venodilation, are addressed below.

Morphine

Hypotension can occur during and after administration of even small doses of morphine (5 to 10 mg intravenously).[147] With anesthetic doses (1 to 4 mg/kg intravenously), hypotension occurs more frequently and is more profound.[24,148] Indeed, Conahan et al.[148] found an incidence of hypotension (systolic blood pressure less than 70 mmHg) of 10 percent during induction of anesthesia with morphine in patients about to undergo cardiac valvular surgery. Several mechanisms may contribute to the hypotension associated with morphine (Table 10-6). Rate of morphine infusion is important in producing and/or avoiding hypotension. Hypotension is not uncommon when the infusion rate is 10 mg/min or greater but is rare when it is less than or equal to 5 mg/min.[149]

Morphine (1 mg/kg) produces marked increases in plasma histamine in some patients (Table 10-7). These changes usually result in an increase in cardiac index and decreases in arterial blood pressure and systemic

TABLE 10-6. Potential Mechanisms Underlying Morphine-Induced Hypotension

1. Histamine release
2. Centrally mediated decrease in sympathetic tone
3. Vagus-induced bradycardia
4. Direct and indirect venous and arterial vasodilation
5. Splanchnic sequestration of blood

vascular resistance.[150] Similar cardiovascular changes occur when patients are pretreated with diphenhydramine (a histamine H_1-antagonist) or cimetidine (a histamine H_2-antagonist) before morphine. However, in patients pretreated with both H_1- and H_2-antagonists, the cardiovascular responses are significantly attenuated despite comparable increases in plasma histamine concentrations. These data and other reports[139,140,151] strongly suggest that many of the hemodynamic effects of morphine are caused by histamine and indicate a possible means of their prevention.

Increases in plasma histamine after morphine cause dilation of terminal arterioles. Histamine also produces direct positive cardiac chronotropic and inotropic actions that are receptor mediated. Finally, histamine also causes sympathoadrenal activation secondary to catecholamine release. Hypotension is less frequent with high-dose fentanyl anesthesia in part because, unlike morphine, fentanyl does not produce increases in plasma histamine.[150] Likewise, sufentanil and alfentanil do not produce changes in plasma histamine.[31]

Morphine reduces venous and arterial tone both in experimental animals and in human subjects. A decrease in venous return to the heart can follow, which may contribute to hypotension.[19,22,152–158] Arterial dilation is of shorter duration than venodilation after morphine.[155,158] Venodilation after morphine is dose related and necessitates an increase in the volume of blood and/or crystalloid fluids administered to maintain adequate ventricular filling.[22,155] Patients anesthetized with morphine, as compared with halothane, have increased blood requirements during and after surgery (Table 10-8). Venodilation and increased blood requirements apparently do not occur with lower doses of morphine (less than 0.5 mg/kg) plus nitrous oxide.

Zelis and co-workers[159] found that morphine selectively impairs certain sympathetic reflexes involving peripheral veins. Their data suggest that this response is due to a CNS action of the drug with secondary withdrawal of sympathetic tone. Vasodilation after morphine may also be due to a direct effect of morphine on vascular smooth muscle.[150,152,158] At high doses, morphine inhibits the presynaptic release of norepinephrine in saphenous vein rings, resulting in a decreased contractile response to electrical stimulation.[158] This effect is not reversed by naloxone nor attenuated by histamine blockers. In dogs, hypotension after large doses of morphine (1 mg/kg) has been attributed to changes in the distribution of blood flow.[160] Although it was not associated with sustained decreases in cardiac output, blood pressure, or total peripheral resistance, Priano and Vatner[160] found that 1 and 3 mg/kg of morphine produces significant decreases in mesenteric and renal blood flow in dogs.

Hypotension after morphine is not related to myocardial depression, although in healthy volunteers morphine (2 mg/kg) does cause a prolongation of the pre-ejection period, an estimate of isovolumetric cardiac contractility.[161,162] High doses of morphine (3 mg/kg) activate the sympathoadrenal system (while producing peripheral vasodilation).[163] These changes could counteract myocardial-depressant effects of the opioid. On the other hand, increases in sympathetic activity could be detrimental in some patients. Moffitt et al.[134] showed that 1 mg/kg of morphine does not inhibit lactate production and can produce ischemia with surgical stimulation in patients undergoing coronary artery bypass operations. In summary, hypotension from morphine can be minimized or eliminated by pretreatment with both H_1- and H_2-histamine antagonists given simultaneously, by use of a slow drug infusion rate, by volume loading, and by placement of patients in Trendelenburg (head-down) position during periods of rapid drug infusion. Interestingly, these are approaches also used to minimize hypotension from *d*-tubocurarine, atracurium, and mivacurium (also see Ch. 12).

Meperidine

Meperidine, in contrast to most other opioids, decreases myocardial contractility in isolated cardiac preparations and intact animals.[164] Equianalgesic doses

TABLE 10-7. Correlations of Histamine Release and Cardiac Index, Heart Rate, Blood Pressure, and Systemic Vascular Resistance during Administration of Morphine (1 mg/kg)

Period	Blood Pressure (mmHg)	Diastolic Blood Pressure (mmHg)	Cardiac Index (L/min/m²)	Heart Rate (beats/min)	Systemic Vascular Resistance (mmHg/L/min)	Venous Histamine (pg/ml)
I. Control	88 ± 4	71 ± 3	2.4 ± 0.2	57 ± 2	15.5 ± 1	880 ± 163
II. Placebo	85 ± 3	67 ± 2	2.6 ± 0.1	57 ± 2	14.8 ± 1	657 ± 98
III. One-third of dose	79 ± 5	61 ± 4[a]	2.8 ± 0.1	58 ± 2	12.2 ± 1[a]	2.467 ± 1.208[a]
IV. 2 min after	61 ± 4[a]	45 ± 4[a]	3.0 ± 0.2	59 ± 3	9.0 ± 1[a]	7.437 ± 2.684[a]
V. 5 min after	73 ± 8	59 ± 7[a]	2.9 ± 0.3	64 ± 4	11.5 ± 1[a]	4.980 ± 1.681[a]
VI. 10 min after	74 ± 5	57 ± 5[a]	2.7 ± 0.2	59 ± 4	12.7 ± 1[a]	3.307 ± 1.090[a]

[a]$P < 0.05$ compared with control.
(From Moss and Rosow,[151] with permission.)

TABLE 10-8. Blood Requirements during Surgery (Aortic Valve Replacement or Coronary Artery Bypass Operation) and for the First Postoperative Day in 61 Patients Anesthetized with Morphine (1.0 to 4.0 mg/kg) plus Oxygen or Halothane (0.1 to 1.5%) plus 30 Percent Nitrous Oxide and Oxygen

Pathology	Anesthetic	Mean Blood Requirements (ml)	
		Intraoperative	Postoperative
Aortic valvular disease	Morphine	2.800[a]	1,652[a]
	Halothane	1,010	757
Coronary artery disease	Morphine	2,705[a]	1,417[a]
	Halothane	1,750	722

[a]$P = 0.05$ in student's paired t test when compared with halothane values.
(Modified from Stanley et al.,[155] with permission.)

of meperidine are 20 times more depressant to the contractile element of the isolated cat papillary muscle than morphine.[164] In humans, meperidine-nitrous oxide anesthesia produces greater cardiovascular depression than morphine-nitrous oxide anesthesia.[165,166] Even in relatively low doses (2 to 2.5 mg/kg), meperidine causes a decrease in arterial blood pressure, peripheral resistance, and cardiac output and an increase in heart rate.[166-171] Anesthetic doses of meperidine (10 mg/kg intravenously) are associated with marked decreases in cardiac output and frequently cause cardiac arrest in dogs[167] (Fig. 10-6).

Meperidine also causes histamine release more frequently than most other opioids, including morphine,

fentanyl, sufentanil, or alfentanil. Flacke et al.[140] found that 5 of 16 patients had increased plasma histamine concentrations after meperidine, whereas only 1 of 10 patients receiving morphine had similar changes. Increases in plasma histamine occur most often in females and are highly correlated to the magnitude of subsequent hypotension.[140]

Meperidine, in contrast to morphine, rarely results in bradycardia but can cause tachycardia. Some have attributed tachycardia after meperidine to its structural similarity to atropine. Others (G. De Castro, personal communication) believe meperidine-associated increases in heart rate are related to early manifestations of its toxic CNS effects. Meperidine's ability to increase

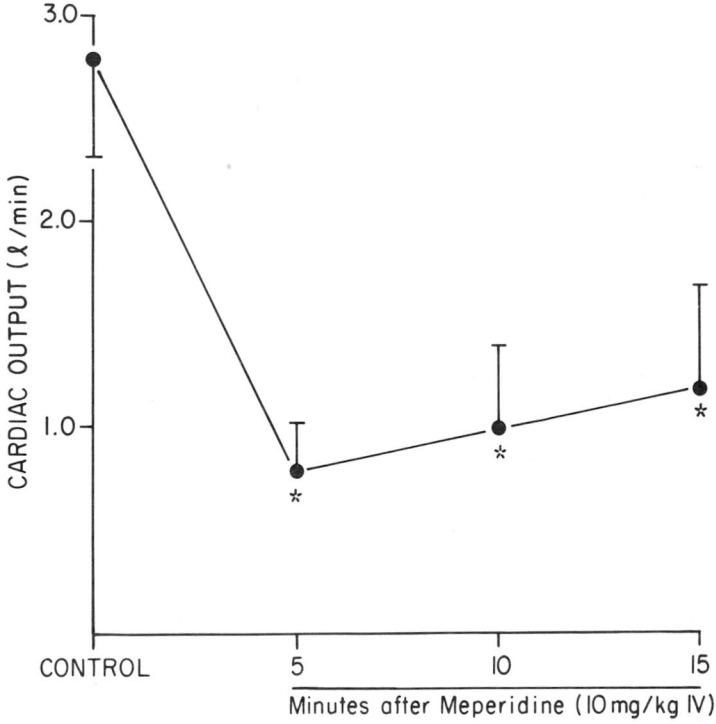

Fig. 10-6. Cardiac output (mean ± standard deviation) before and after meperidine (10 mg/kg intravenously) in nine basally anesthetized (sodium thiopental) mongrel dogs. * $P < 0.0.1$, one-way analysis of variance. (Unpublished data from T. H. Stanley.)

plasma histamine, depress myocardial contractility, and increase heart rate has reduced its popularity as an anesthetic.

Fentanyl

Fentanyl in analgesic (2 to 10 μg/kg) or anesthetic (30 to 100 μg/kg) doses seldom causes significant decreases in blood pressure when given alone, even in patients with poor left ventricular function (LVF).[2,23,143,144,172,173] Some investigators believe that absence of hypotension after fentanyl is chiefly related to its lack of effect on plasma histamine concentrations.[150]

Most evidence indicates that fentanyl produces little or no change in myocardial contractility,[2,15,144,145,174] although a few investigators have reported a small negative inotropic effect.[143,150,175] Virtually all hemodynamic variables, including heart rate, arterial blood pressure, cardiac output, systemic and pulmonary vascular resistance, and pulmonary artery occlusion or wedge pressure, remain unchanged after large (anesthetic) doses of fentanyl.[2,144,150,172,173,175]

Most recently, Miller et al.[176] compared induction of anesthesia (in patients premedicated with lorazepam scheduled for coronary artery surgery) with fentanyl (75 μg/kg), sufentanil (15 μg/kg), and alfentanil (125 μg/kg followed by 5 μg/kg/min). Induction of anesthesia with fentanyl was associated with the least change in mean arterial pressure and myocardial performance. While sufentanil did not produce hemodynamic instability, it did cause myocardial depression. Those investigators and others have suggested that fentanyl may be preferred over sufentanil in patients with poor LVF. On the other hand, other investigators have found better hemodynamic stability and less hypotension after sufentanil than fentanyl in patients undergoing valvular heart surgery.[177] In contrast, most available data suggest that alfentanil is associated with more hypotension, bradycardia, and surgically induced hypertension than either fentanyl or sufentanil.

Hypotension after fentanyl is probably most related to associated bradycardia and can be prevented or treated with anticholinergics, ephedrine, or even pancuronium.[178,179] Patients with high sympathetic tone are more likely to experience hypotension after fentanyl. Flacke et al.[180] have postulated that cardiovascular depression after fentanyl is due to inhibition of central sympathetic outflow that is apart from analgesia or other sensory-depressant effects of the narcotic. They found that naloxone reversal of fentanyl-induced cardiovascular depression is blocked by clonidine, an α_2-agonist. Thus, some central cardiovascular-regulating mechanisms are opioid sensitive. After eliminating all autonomic tone in dogs, Flacke et al.[181] found minimal hemodynamic changes after fentanyl or fentanyl plus large doses of diazepam. Thus, they concluded that hypotension induced by fentanyl was indirect in nature, that is, mediated by a decrease in CNS sympathetic vasoregulatory outflow.

Sufentanil

Sufentanil, which is 5 to 10 times more potent than fentanyl, causes hypotension with equal or greater frequency than the latter. Since sufentanil is available in similar concentrations as fentanyl (50 μg/ml) a possible cause of hypotension is relative overdose. Sufentanil does not produce increases in plasma histamine but does cause vagus-induced bradycardia.[31] Ablation of sympathetic tone and enhanced parasympathetic tone are the most likely mechanisms for sufentanil-associated hypotension. Sufentanil-induced hypotension may also be mediated by a direct depression of vascular smooth muscle.[182]

Several studies suggest that sufentanil is not only more potent than fentanyl but is also closer to a "complete anesthetic." These claims are supported by greater MAC reduction during coadministration of inhaled anesthetics in laboratory animals and less hemodynamic responses to stimuli such as intubation than fentanyl.[176] Sufentanil causes more hypotension than equipotent doses of fentanyl. Mathews et al.[183] found sufentanil (5 μg/kg) produced lower mean arterial blood pressures than fentanyl (25 μg/kg) during induction of anesthesia in patients having coronary artery surgery. Sebel and Bovill[130] also found that sufentanil (15 μg/kg, injected over 2 minutes) caused significantly lower blood pressures during induction of anesthesia in patients premedicated with lorazepam and scheduled for coronary artery surgery than equipotent doses of fentanyl. Two of these authors' patients had marked decreases in their systolic blood pressure (116 to 60 mmHg and 150 to 70 mmHg). Miller et al.[176] showed that although sufentanil (15 μg/kg) attenuated the hemodynamic response to tracheal intubation better than fentanyl (75 μg/kg), it impaired myocardial function and depressed systolic blood pressure more. On the other hand, Lake and DiFazio[177] found that sufentanil (5 μg/kg) produced more complete and reliable anesthesia and less hypotension than fentanyl (25 μg/kg). Careful titration may be even more warranted with sufentanil, in order to minimize significant hypotension, especially in patients dependent on high intrinsic sympathetic tone or with poor LVF.

Alfentanil

Alfentanil, a rapidly and particularly short-acting agent with a high therapeutic index (1,080) in rats,[184] is approximately one-fifth to one-third as potent as fentanyl. Studies in dogs have demonstrated little change in hemodynamics with moderate doses (160 μg/kg) of alfentanil and transient cardiac stimulation (increases in LV contractility, aortic blood flow velocity, and acceleration) with very large doses (5 mg/kg).[169] Heart rate, cardiac output, and pulmonary and systemic vascular resistance increased following 5 mg/kg of alfentanil. Other investigators found transient increases in myocardial contractility, mean aortic, pulmonary artery, and left and right atrial pressures, and systemic vascular resistance with lower doses (200 μg/kg) of alfentanil in dogs.[185,186]

Some authors have found that alfentanil causes similar decreases in heart rate, arterial blood pressure, and cardiac index as fentanyl,[52,114,187] while others have reported that alfentanil produces a less desirable hemodynamic profile (more hypotension as well as myocardial ischemia) than fentanyl and sufentanil in patients undergoing coronary artery grafting.[132,176,188-190] Titration to specific end point (e.g., loss of consciousness) rather than the administration of a precalculated bolus will minimize adverse cardiovascular effects.

Hypertension

Sudden increases in arterial blood pressure, especially during endotracheal intubation or profound surgical stimulation, have been a common problem associated with narcotic anesthesia and is most often attributed to light anesthesia. Wynands et al.[173] have also shown that patients with good LVF will more frequently become hypertensive than patients with poor LVF during fentanyl anesthesia for coronary artery surgery. They did not attribute this phenomenon to differences in depth of anesthesia but rather to the fact that patients with preserved myocardial function were more able to increase cardiac index in response to increases in systemic vascular resistance induced by surgical stimuli. Patients with limited myocardial reserve could not always maintain cardiac output in the face of an increased systemic vascular resistance, and thus their arterial blood pressure did not increase and might even decrease.

Two other mechanisms (sympathetic activation and cardiogenic reflexes) may underlie hypertension associated with opioid-based anesthesia. Thomson et al.[191] reported the occurrence of a hyperdynamic cardiovascular response to induction of anesthesia with high-dose fentanyl in 10 percent of patients and attributed it to central sympathetic activation. Opioids may increase catecholamine levels even without increases in plasma histamine. Fentanyl increases norepinephrine release from some sympathetic nerve endings and may also inhibit neuronal uptake of norepinephrine in dogs. Both increases and decreases in serum catecholamines have been reported in humans after fentanyl. Gaumann et al.[192] have also recently reported that sufentanil produced 6- to 20-fold increases in adrenal vein concentrations of catecholamines and parallel increases in arterial blood pressures in cats. Interestingly, sufentanil and the accompanying increase in catecholamine levels prevented the hypotension that normally occurred in these animals after a 25 percent loss of blood volume.

Aortic root dissection causes hypertension via stimulation of a specific cardiogenic reflex,[193] which is not associated with increases in plasma catecholamine concentrations or light levels of anesthesia.[114] Although

higher doses of fentanyl or sufentanil can attenuate this hypertension, no dose of any opioid reliably prevents hypertension during surgery in humans.

Morphine

Hypertension during cardiovascular surgery was also a problem in patients anesthetized with morphine.[21,194] Arens et al.[21] reported a 36 percent incidence of hypertension, defined as an increase in systolic blood pressure to greater than 200 mmHg or an increase of 60 mmHg above preoperative pressure, in patients undergoing coronary artery surgery with 1.5 to 3.0 mg/kg of morphine. Hasbrouk[194] using up to 595 mg of morphine found that arterial blood pressure increased about 15 percent above baseline and documented simultaneous increases in plasma epinephrine and norepinephrine. Conahan et al.[148] found more severe hypertension in cardiac valve surgery patients anesthetized with morphine compared with those receiving halothane anesthesia. These episodes were attributed to increases in systemic vascular resistance.

Hypertension during morphine anesthesia has been variously attributed to light or inadequate anesthesia,[27] reflex mechanisms,[24] stimulation of the renin-angiotensin mechanism,[195] and sympathoadrenal activation.[163]

Fentanyl

Although hypertension is rare before endotracheal intubation or surgical stimulation with high-dose fentanyl anesthesia during cardiac surgery, it is the most common cardiovascular disturbance during or after sternotomy and aortic root manipulation.[172,196-198] Incidences of hypertension specifically related to sternotomy range- from 0 to 100 percent in patients given fentanyl (50 to 100 μg/kg).[2,172,196-201] Possible explanations for this variability include the type of premedication, the rate of fentanyl administration, the induction and subsequent dose(s) of fentanyl, the timing of its administration, and the type, dose, and rate of administration of various muscle relaxants used for endotracheal intubation and surgical relaxation. Other factors include the degree of β-adrenergic and/or calcium channel blockade present at the time of surgery, preoperative ventricular function, volume status, patient habits, and the presence or absence of awareness.[117,124,197,198,200,201]

Although satisfactory control of hemodynamics can be achieved by increasing the dose of fentanyl,[197,200] use of extremely high doses is not always warranted considering associated side effects and the availability of alternative techniques. Doses of fentanyl of 140 μg/kg or more are likely to result in prolonged respiratory depression during the postoperative period and an increased need for vasopressor support.[200,202] Satisfactory blood pressure control can be achieved with fentanyl (50 to 120 μg/kg) plus vasodilator therapy.[196,197,199,200,203] However, with lower doses of fentanyl (less than or equal to 50 μg/kg) and no supplements, there may be an increased risk of intraoperative awareness that is virtually eliminated with doses of greater than 120 μg/kg but has occasionally been reported with lower doses.[117-119]

The total amount of fentanyl used is often limited to 100 μg/kg. When hemodynamic control is not achieved with this dose, vasodilator therapy is begun with sodium nitroprusside or nitroglycerin. Other clinicians may supplement anesthesia with a potent inhaled anesthetic and/or an intravenous sedative-hypnotic[2,117] to control episodes of hypertension. Mixing inhaled anesthetics with high doses of fentanyl can decrease stroke volume, cardiac output, and mean arterial blood pressure and increase ventricular filling pressure.[29,204] Yet fentanyl and potent inhaled anesthetics (enflurane or halothane) can be given together without decreasing myocardial contractility or arterial blood pressure, cardiac output, and stroke volume.[15,16] Furthermore, some inhaled anesthetics (halothane or isoflurane) may protect the myocardium during periods of ischemia.[205,206] On the other hand, some clinicians avoid any use of isoflurane in patients at significant risk for myocardial ischemia because of the risk of coronary artery steal. In addition, the effects of adding inhaled anesthetics to large doses of fentanyl or other opioids on the myocardial oxygen supply-demand ratio in patients with coronary artery disease are not always predictable.

Fentanyl, like other opioids, and indeed all anesthetics, is never completely predictable in terms of its ability to eliminate hemodynamic responses to painful stimuli. Indeed, some have concluded that plasma fentanyl concentrations that reliably block hypertensive responses to noxious stimuli may not exist (Fig. 10-7).[202]

Sufentanil

While some investigators find little difference between fentanyl and sufentanil when used as primary anesthetics for cardiac surgery,[183,207] many believe that sufentanil provides better control of the hemodynamic responses to endotracheal intubation,[176] sternotomy, and sternal spread.[201] They also claim that sufentanil decreases the need for vasodilators during cardiopulmonary bypass, the post-bypass period, and postoperatively.[201] While sufentanil alone is probably more effective than equipotent doses of fentanyl, it does not guarantee complete control of intraoperative arterial blood pressure.[130] Furthermore, preoperative and intraoperative use of β-adrenergic blockers, calcium entry blockers, nitrates, sedative-hypnotic premedicants, and muscle relaxants can also influence the incidence of intraoperative hemodynamic responses (see below).

Sufentanil (15 to 25 μg/kg) is usually titrated by either infusion (25 to 200 μg/min) or intermittent bolus (10 to 100 μg) for cardiac surgery. Sufentanil (5 to 10 μg) also more effectively blunts the hemodynamic response to noxious stimuli than fentanyl in infants undergoing cardiac surgery.[208] Sufentanil, like fentanyl, decreases pulmonary vascular resistance in infants.

Alfentanil

Alfentanil shares most of the cardiovascular properties of fentanyl and sufentanil at comparable doses. When administered alone to unpremedicated healthy patients, alfentanil (175 μg/kg) eliminates increases in heart rate and arterial blood pressure, while thiopental (3 to 4 mg/kg) plus lidocaine (1.5 mg/kg) does not. Others have found cardiovascular stimulation during and after induction of anesthesia with alfentanil.[209] The ED$_{50}$ for loss of consciousness of alfentanil usually lies between 100 and 125 μg/kg.[209,210] Unfortunately, alfentanil is less reliable than fentanyl and sufentanil in blocking increases in heart rate and arterial blood pressure during anesthetic induction, sternotomy, sternal spread, and aortotomy in patients with ischemic heart disease having coronary artery surgery.[211] A higher incidence of ischemia during alfentanil anesthesia than with comparable doses of fentanyl or sufentanil has also been reported.[176] Although some investigators believe alfentanil is a suitable anesthetic for cardiac surgery,[114] alfentanil will probably not supplant fentanyl or sufentanil as a sole anesthetic during cardiac surgery.

Heart Rate, Rhythm, and Baroreceptor Function

With the exception of meperidine, all mu-receptor-stimulating opioid analgesics usually produce decreases in heart rate. Fentanyl-induced bradycardia is more marked in anesthetized than conscious dogs or human subjects.[212,213] When used for induction of anesthesia, there is a higher incidence of bradycardia when patients or dogs breathe pure oxygen than when nitrous oxide is used with oxygen.[214,215] This may be due to the increase in sympathetic nervous system activity associated with nitrous oxide anesthesia.[216,217] Second and subsequent doses of fentanyl cause less bradycardia than do initial doses.[141,214] Infusions in dogs decrease heart rate after the first 50 μg/kg of fentanyl.[205] Administration of additional fentanyl (up to 2 mg/kg) is required to duplicate the initial percent decrease in heart rate.[141] The degree of bradycardia after infusion of opioids may be dose related,[205,212,218] although opioids do not always produce dose-dependent effects on heart rate.[209] An equally important factor may be the speed of injection. Although a well-controlled experimental investigation has not been published, clinical experience in human subjects and animals studies with numerous species[214,218-221] suggest that bradycardia can be minimized by slow administration of potent opioids. Premedication with atropine or glycopyrrolate attenuates bradycardia induced by morphine, fentanyl, and other highly potent opioids but does not always eliminate it.[2,30,123,141,214,219] Atropine is often effective in treating opioid-induced bradycardia, although even large doses

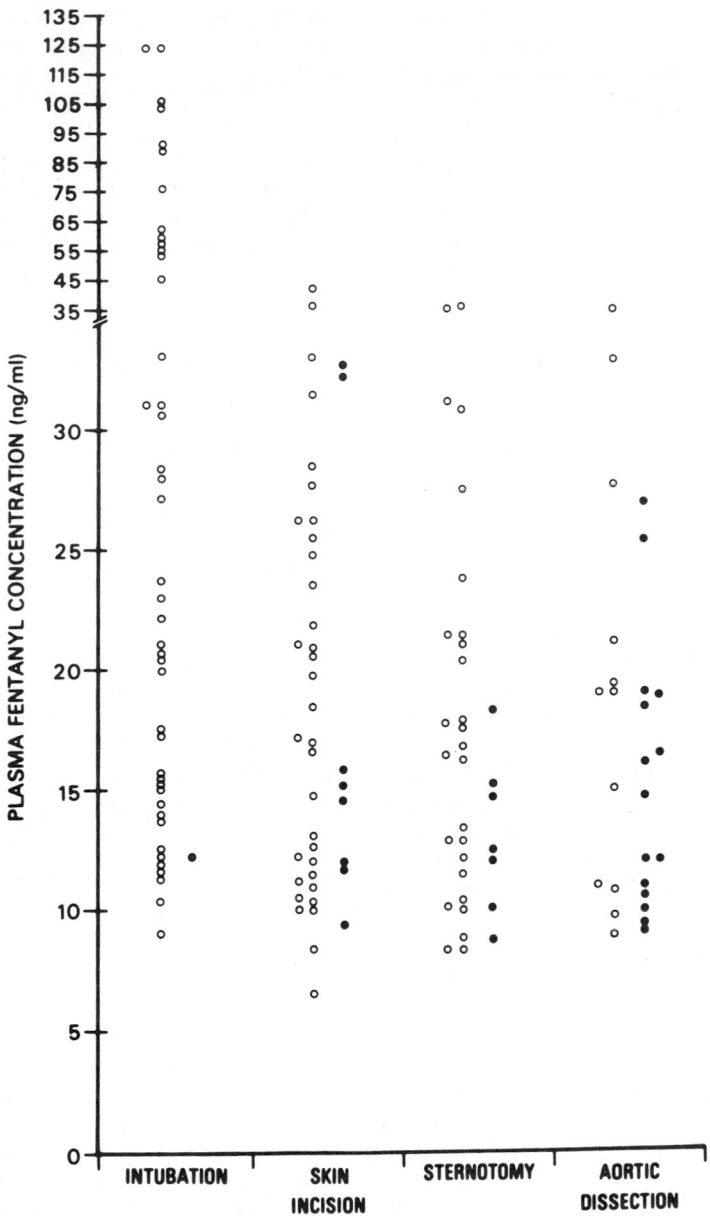

Fig. 10-7. Plasma fentanyl concentration and number of patients with a hypertensive response at each event studied. ●, hypertensive; ○, normotensive. (From Wynands et al.,[202] with permission.)

(1 to 2 mg) are occasionally ineffective. Administration of small to moderate doses of intravenous pancuronium (0.5 to 2.0 mg) prior to induction of anesthesia with fentanyl or other potent narcotics attenuates bradycardia.[219,222,223]

The mechanism of fentanyl-induced bradycardia, while not completely understood, is most likely due to stimulation of the central vagal nucleus.[212] Bradycardia is almost totally prevented by bilateral vagotomy[212] or pharmacologic vagal block with atropine.[214] Blockade of sympathetic chronotropic action may also play a minor role.[212] Similar mechanisms have been proposed for morphine.[224,225] Morphine is also thought to have

a direct effect on the sinoatrial node[226,227] and to depress atrioventricular (AV) conduction.[228] Morphine, through histamine release, can cause increases in heart rate. Histamine has positive chronotropic effects and can cause sympathoadrenal activation. Meperidine can cause a tachycardia that may be related to a vagolytic property as a result of its structural similarity to atropine. Increases in heart rate may also occur due to the release of histamine, as a reflex response to hypotension, or to accumulation of normeperidine, the principal metabolite of meperidine.

Asystole may follow opioid-induced bradycardia, and several case reports illustrate predisposing factors

(Table 10-9)[229-232] (also see Ch. 12). Sufentanil and alfentanil appear to be more likely than fentanyl to result in asystole. Opioid-induced decreases in sympathetic tone coupled with vagal stimulation may predispose certain patients to this problem. Severe bradycardia and asystole often appear before or during laryngoscopy and intubation. Laryngoscopy can relieve or exacerbate bradyarrhythmias or asystole. Asystoles of 10 to 12 seconds may resolve on their own but usually respond to atropine (0.4 to 0.8 mg intravenously). On occasion much larger doses of atropine (more than 1.0 mg), isproterenol, or a precordial thump may be required to treat severe bradycardia and asystole.

Fentanyl prolongs the P-R interval, AV node conduction, and the refractory period of the AV node.[233] Although these effects could theoretically lead to the development of arrhythmias of the re-entry type, this rarely occurs in practice. The overall effect of narcotic anesthesia may be antiarrhythmic. Although doses of epinephrine sufficient to induce arrhythmias in dogs are the same during narcotic-nitrous oxide anesthesia and halothane or enflurane plus nitrous oxide anesthesia, the incidence of malignant arrhythmias (ventricular tachycardia and ventricular fibrillation) was less with narcotics plus nitrous oxide.[234] Sufentanil prolongs action potential duration in isolated canine cardiac Purkinje fibers. This may be related to enhanced Ca^{++} entry during the plateau phase of the action potential.[234] Opioids can also prolong the QT interval. However, the risk of opioid use in patients with QT abnormalities or receiving medications such as quinidine is unknown.[235]

Supraventricular tachycardia is the most common arrhythmia, other than bradycardia, noted during narcotic anesthetic techniques.[236] Supraventricular tachycardia usually occurs during or immediately after endotracheal intubation or surgical stimulation. This suggests that inadequate anesthesia rather than a direct effect of the narcotic is responsible for these abnormalities. Increases in heart rate often parallel increases in blood pressure when narcotic dosage or anesthesia is inadequate.

Opioids are often used to prevent increases in heart rate during anesthesia, particularly during the induction-intubation sequence. The use of fentanyl (3 to 7 μg/kg), alfentanil (15 to 30 μg/kg), or sufentanil (0.2 to 0.8 μg/kg) decreases requirements for sodium thiopental and etomidate. In addition, increases in heart rate and arterial blood pressure that occur during laryngoscopy and intubation are better controlled when drugs like thiopental are used after narcotic pretreatment. Opioids also blunt or prevent increases in heart rate that accompany the administration of isoflurane[236] or other inhaled anesthetics.[237]

Low-pressure baroreceptors at the junction of the great vessels and atria are sensitive to decreases in filling pressure. Their stimulation causes reflex increases in systemic vascular resistance to maintain arterial blood pressure. Fentanyl-diazepam-nitrous oxide anesthesia does not attenuate this reflex. Anesthesia with potent inhaled anesthetics can effect this reflex.[238] Opioids may depress arterial baroreflex control of the heart rate induced by hypotension or hypertension,[239,240] but other reports suggest that this reflex is preserved under opioid anesthesia.[239,241] Infants, after receiving 10 μg/kg of fentanyl, demonstrate significant depression of baroreflex responses.[242] The significance of this phenomenon is all the more important because cardiac output is quite dependent on heart rate in infants.

Myocardial Ischemia and Coronary Blood Flow

Cardiac anesthesiologists attempt to control hemodynamics to minimize increases in myocardial oxygen consumption, maintain oxygen supply to the heart, and avoid ischemia. While opioids do not protect against ischemia in animal models,[243,244] potent inhaled anesthetics may offer some protection. In addition, some studies suggest that fentanyl and sufentanil do not provide adequate hemodynamic control in humans during coronary artery surgery,[245,246] especially when compared with potent inhaled anesthetics.[134,247,248] A major problem with many of these studies is that a fixed dose of opioid, for example, 1 mg/kg of morphine,[134] is routinely given. Lack of flexibility of such protocols is not consistent with the clinical necessity and practice of titrating narcotics to an end point. Others have found that high doses of opioids maintain myocardial perfusion and the oxygen supply/demand ratio as well as or better than inhalation-based techniques.[249,250]

Alfentanil is associated with more myocardial ischemia (as indicated by reversal of myocardial lactate extraction to production ratios and decreases in ventricular diastolic compliance) than fentanyl or sufentanil in patients having coronary artery surgery.[176] Sufentanil causes more depression of systolic function than fentanyl but also may offer greater hemodynamic control in patients with good LVF. On the other hand, fentanyl is probably easier and safer to use than sufentanil in

TABLE 10-9. Factors Predisposing Patients to Bradycardia and Asystole during Induction of Anesthesia with Large Doses of Narcotics

1. Presence of β-adrenergic and/or calcium entry blockade

2. Premedication with or concomitant use of benzodiazepines

3. Muscle relaxants with little or no vagolytic properties (vecuronium)

4. Muscle relaxants with vagotonic properties (succinylcholine)

5. Added vagal stimuli, eg., laryngoscopy

6. Rapid administration of the opioid

patients with poor LVF. Interestingly, hemodynamics are often stable and do not reliably indicate ischemia. Kleinman et al.[251] reported that hemodynamic changes were most often absent during ischemia in patients anesthetized with either fentanyl or halothane. Recent data from a prospective randomized comparison of sufentanil versus enflurane, isoflurane, and halothane for coronary artery surgery revealed no difference in new intraoperative ischemia, the incidence of postoperative myocardial infarction, or death.[252] These results occurred despite a greater (twofold) incidence of hypotension associated with the inhaled anesthetic techniques and a greater (twofold) incidence of hypertension associated with sufentanil. Tachycardia, the only hemodynamic variable significantly related to ischemia, occurred with the same frequency with all anesthetics. Slogoff and Keats[252] and others have suggested that other factors (e.g., recent infarction, presence or absence of β-adrenergic or calcium entry blockade, prolonged aortic cross-clamp time, serious preoperative arrhythmias) are significantly more important than anesthetic technique as determinants of outcome after coronary artery surgery.[253]

Opioids, or at least fentanyl, have no significant effect on coronary vasomotion and do not diminish the ability of large coronary arteries or coronary arterioles to respond to vasoactive drugs.[254,255] This lack of effect of fentanyl on coronary autoregulation compares distinctly with the potent inhaled anesthetics, which are coronary vasodilators.

Supplements

A variety of adjuvant drugs have been used as supplements in combination with opioids. Rationales for this approach include attempts to reduce awareness, control hypertension, and decrease the total dose of opioid to minimize postoperative respiratory depression. On the other hand, certain drugs, especially the benzodiazepines, may predispose patients to hypotension when high-dose opioid anesthesia is used. In addition, although some suggest a reasonable approach to controlling hemodynamics to be a combination of opioids and inhaled anesthetics,[247] supplementation of opioid anesthesia with a variety of agents, including inhaled anesthetics, often results in a loss of cardiovascular stability.

Nitrous Oxide

Nitrous oxide is probably the most common supplement used with narcotic-based anesthesia. Nitrous oxide has minimal effects on cardiovascular dynamics when administered alone in dogs[256] but can depress myocardial contractility in humans.[257] In addition, nitrous oxide in combination with opioids is associated with significant cardiovascular depression. After administration of morphine (2 mg/kg), McDermott and Stanley[258] found that nitrous oxide produced concentration-dependent decreases in stroke volume, cardiac output, and arterial blood pressure and increases in systemic vascular resistance (Table 10-10). While fentanyl alone produces no ventricular dysfunction (even in the presence of significant coronary artery stenosis), the addition of nitrous oxide can yield significant cardiovascular depression.[23] These changes occur in humans and animals with all opioids in virtually all studies.[20,23,68,168,170,214,258-260] A lower FiO_2 rather than the presence of nitrous oxide may be responsible for the changes in cardiovascular performance.[261] Myocardial ischemia and dysfunction may occur during inhalation of nitrous oxide as coronary blood flow decreases from hypotension and an increase in coronary vascular resistance.[260] Increases in systemic vascular resistance associated with nitrous oxide supplementation of opioids may in part cause the deterioration in cardiac output and function.[144,161] Myocardial dysfunction with nitrous oxide may not be evident with routine monitoring, that is, blood pressure, because of the elevated systemic vascular resistance.[262] Despite these potential problems, nitrous oxide remains a popular supplement. In children undergoing repair of congenital cardiac defects, nitrous oxide may still be valuable and safe as a supplement to opioid anesthesia.[263]

Potent Inhaled Anesthetics

In light of the potential for adverse effects of nitrous oxide in patients anesthetized with opioids, potent inhaled anesthetics may be a better alternative. Their intrinsic ability to depress the myocardium in a dose-dependent fashion often allows the titration of agents such as halothane or enflurane to control hemodynamics when high-dose opioids are inadequate.[264-266]

TABLE 10-10. Cardiovascular Effects of 0 to 50 Percent Nitrous Oxide during Morphine Anesthesia

Parameter	Percent (Mean) N_2O					
	0	10	20	30	40	50
Stroke volume (ml)	57.0	51.0[a]	50.0[a]	46.0[a]	42.0[a]	36.0[a]
Cardiac output (L/min)	5.2	4.6[a]	4.3[a]	4.0[a]	3.7[a]	2.9[a]
Systolic arterial blood pressure (mmHg)	124.0	119.0[a]	117.0[a]	109.0[a]	104.0[a]	94.0[a]
Peripheral resistance (PRU)	159.0	176.0[a]	183.0[a]	204.0[a]	259.0[a]	312.0[a]

[a]$P < 0.05$ in student's paired t test when compared with control value.
(From McDermott and Stanley,[258] with permission.)

Low concentrations of isoflurane have been safely used to treat intraoperative hypertension during high-dose sufentanil anesthesia for coronary artery surgery.[267] However, undesirable cardiovascular depression (decreases in arterial blood pressure and cardiac index) can occur during halothane supplementation of high-dose fentanyl anesthesia and may occur with other potent inhalation agents as well.[268] In addition, ongoing ischemia may not necessarily be ameliorated by such approaches despite good hemodynamic control.[268] Others have shown that adding halothane to a sufentanil (10 to 20 μg/kg) anesthetic to control increases in blood pressure may produce hemodynamic alterations (decreased blood pressure, cardiac output, pulmonary capillary wedge pressure, and systemic vascular resistance) that exacerbate regional myocardial hypoperfusion and increase lactate production.[269] Cautious titration of potent inhaled anesthetics to control increases in arterial blood pressure during a high-dose opioid anesthetic may be most successful when techniques to assess regional myocardial function are available (e.g., transesophageal echocardiography). The risk of inducing a maldistribution in the coronary circulation exists with isoflurane and enflurane as well.[270] Nevertheless, and despite the potential problems, the ease of administration and titration of potent inhaled anesthetics makes them a useful adjunct during opioid anesthesia.

Benzodiazepines

Benzodiazepines produce few significant hemodynamic alterations when administered alone. This, combined with their potent amnestic properties, makes them a desirable supplement to high-dose opioid anesthesia, in which awareness is a potential problem. Benzodiazepines enhance and may even potentiate the effects of opioids and thus decrease narcotic requirements for loss of consciousness.[2,123,271] However, combinations of benzodiazepines and narcotics, while occasionally preserving ventricular function,[271] often cause profound decreases in arterial blood pressure and cardiac index. Some investigators have found intravenous lorazepam and high-dose fentanyl anesthesia to cause less hemodynamic changes than other benzodiazepines.[272,273] These findings are encouraging but need additional clarification.

Unfortunately, most studies indicate that benzodiazepines, even administered for premedication,[2,123, 127,227,274-276] consistently lower arterial blood pressure, heart rate, cardiac output, and systemic vascular resistance with opioid-based techniques compared with benzodiazepine-free premedication (e.g., morphine-scopolamine) or no premedication. Sudden dramatic hypotension occurs with some combinations (midazolam and sufentanil).[277,278] In patients with poor LVF, this drug regimen may prove particularly hazardous.[275]

Several mechanisms underlie the cardiovascular depression produced when benzodiazepines are added to opioids. Benzodiazepines produce a transient depression of arterial baroreflex function and a sustained decrease in sympathetic tone.[279] Catecholamine levels are lower with a diazepam-morphine combination than with morphine alone.[163] Combinations of fentanyl and diazepam result in a negative inotropic effect.[280] Decreases in systemic vascular resistance are also usually noted and are probably related to diminished sympathetic tone. Aggressive administration of intravascular fluids may attenuate decreases in arterial blood pressure, ventricular filling, and cardiac output when benzodiazepines are combined with opioids.[281]

Other Types of Supplements
(Also See Ch. 14)

β-Adrenergic Blockers

Since the 1970s it has been recognized that sympathetic responses to surgery are better controlled by continuing β-adrenergic blockade therapy through the perioperative period. During high-dose opioid anesthesia for coronary artery surgery, β-blockade reduces opioid requirements and the need for supplements, improves hemodynamic stability, and decreases intraoperative and postoperative myocardial ischemia and the incidence of arrhythmias.[282-284] Esmolol, an ultra-short-acting β-blocker, is becoming increasingly popular for use during surgery.[284,285]

α₂-Adrenergic Agonists

The role of α_2-adrenergic blockers in anesthesia is just beginning to be explored.[286] Clonidine and its congeners reduce anesthetic requirements in animal models and in humans,[287,288] probably by decreasing central sympathetic outflow and nociception.[289] The need for other supplements is also decreased, although bradycardia requiring the administration of atropine may be an occasional problem. Postoperative benefits can include higher cardiac outputs, earlier extubation, reduced plasma catecholamines, and less shivering.[288] Most studies have evaluated clonidine as a premedicant, although postoperative infusion may allow continuation of its favorable effects.[289] Respiratory function is preserved when clonidine (0.2 to 0.4 mg) is combined with morphine (0.21 mg/kg) as a premedicant.[290]

Calcium Entry Blockers

While calcium entry blockers (CEBs) can significantly depress cardiac function and cause regional wall motion abnormalities during potent inhalational anesthesia, opioid-CEB interactions appear to be mild. Fentanyl and pancuronium anesthesia does not effect verapamil pharmacokinetics. Mean arterial pressure and cardiac function and conduction also do not change appreciably in dogs when opioids and verapamil are combined.[291,292] Fentanyl anesthesia causes minimal decreases in cardiac index and only modest decreases in blood pressure and systemic vascular resistance in patients receiving verapamil.[293] On the other hand, the presence of β-adrenergic blockade, the quality of LVF, and the presence of other anesthetics will influence the response to CEBs. In addition, CEBs have different profiles of effects and can result in persistent hypotension or unpredictable responses when used as an adjunct to opioid anesthesia for controlled hypotension.[294]

Nitroglycerin

Nitroglycerin (NTG) is often used with high-dose narcotic anesthesia to treat increases in arterial blood pressure and myocardial ischemia. Opinions differ as to whether or not the routine use of an NTG infusion during high-dose fentanyl anesthesia for coronary artery surgery can reduce ischemia. Thomson et al.[295] reported that 0.5 μg/kg/min of NTG did not significantly alter the incidence of ischemia (50 percent) in patients undergoing coronary artery surgery during fentanyl-pancuronium anesthesia. Coriat et al.,[296] on the other hand, reported that 1.0 but not 0.5 μg/kg/min did significantly reduce intraoperative ischemia. These or larger doses of NTG may also result in hypotension, tachycardia, and decreases in ventricular filling pressures. The optimal doses of NTG during narcotic anesthesia have not been determined.

Muscle Relaxants
(Also See Ch. 12)

A major concern of investigators evaluating the effects of muscle relaxants during opioid-based anesthesia has been to determine how best to avoid inducing or exacerbating myocardial ischemia in patients with coronary artery disease.[283,297–308] Pancuronium may provide better hemodynamics than vecuronium,[299] metocurine, or metocurine-pancuronium combinations.[303] Pancuronium's cardiac vagolytic actions tend to attenuate opioid-induced bradycardias and support blood pressure. Others, however, have found that pancuronium causes significant increases in heart rate and myocardial ischemia.[245,297,302,305,307] Indeed, Thomson and Putnins[302] recommended avoiding pancuronium in patients having coronary artery surgery because of increased ischemia associated with its use. Others believe this is too rigid a position.[309] Many factors alter the impact of pancuronium and other muscle relaxants on hemodynamics when muscle relaxants are combined with opioids. These factors include the dose, timing, and rate of administration of each relaxant, the premedication, the intravascular volume, the state of LVF, and the presence of other drugs with actions on the autonomic nervous system. For example, β-adrenergic blockade will often attenuate or eliminate significant pancuronium-induced tachycardias.[283,300,304]

Vecuronium enhances decreases in heart rate and cardiac index after fentanyl.[298] Yet, vecuronium alone has minimal cardiovascular side effects. However, combinations of vecuronium and high doses of opioids produce negative chronotropic and inotropic effects and associated decreases in heart rate, cardiac output, and arterial blood pressure sometimes requiring vasopressor support.[299,306] O'Connor et al.[308] found that compared with vecuronium (0.15 mg/kg), pancuronium (0.15 mg/kg) produced tachycardia more often (32 versus 7 percent) in patients undergoing coronary artery surgery. However, pancuronium-induced tachycardia was easily and rapidly treated and caused no differences in ischemia or perioperative myocardial infarction. Others have found more stable hemodynamics with vecuronium than pancuronium or atracurium during opioid anesthesia,[305] while still others have found no significant differences between pancuronium and vecuronium.[304]

Metocurine (0.5 mg/kg) alone has also been reported to produce less hemodynamic fluctuation[297] than pancuronium during opioid anesthesia, although high doses (greater than 0.3 mg/kg) may produce hypotension.[303,307] Combining metocurine and pancuronium has several advantages (e.g., rapidity of onset) and can help minimize tachycardia and hypotension.[305,307,310] Investigational neuromuscular blockers may offer improved hemodynamic stability in the future.[311]

RESPIRATORY ACTIONS

All mu-receptor-stimulating opioids cause dose-dependent depression of respiration,[312] primarily through a direct action on the brain stem respiratory center.[313,314] The responsiveness of the brain stem respiratory centers to CO_2 is significantly reduced by opioids. Thus, the slopes of the ventilatory and occlusion pressure responses to CO_2 are decreased, and minute ventilatory responses to increases in $PaCO_2$ are shifted to the right (Fig. 10-8). In addition, the apneic threshold ($PaCO_2$ below which spontaneous ventilation is not initiated without hypoxia) and resting end-tidal PCO_2 are increased by opioids. Opioids also decrease hypoxic ventilatory drive.[315,316] In fact, carotid body chemoreception and hypoxic drive are blunted or eliminated by low, analgesic doses of opioids. (Opioids do not, however, affect hypoxic pulmonary vasocontriction.[317]) Opioids also blunt the increase in respiratory drive normally associated with increased loads such as increased airway resistance.[316] Opioid-induced effects on the control of respiratory rhythm and pattern include decreased respiratory rate, increased pauses, delay in expiration, irregular and/or periodic breathing, and decreased, normal, or increased tidal volume.

Opioids interfere with pontine and medullary respiratory centers that regulate respiratory rhythmicity. These interactions are complex, incompletely evaluated, and usually documented in various (e.g., decerebrate) cat models. Little direct examination of the neu-

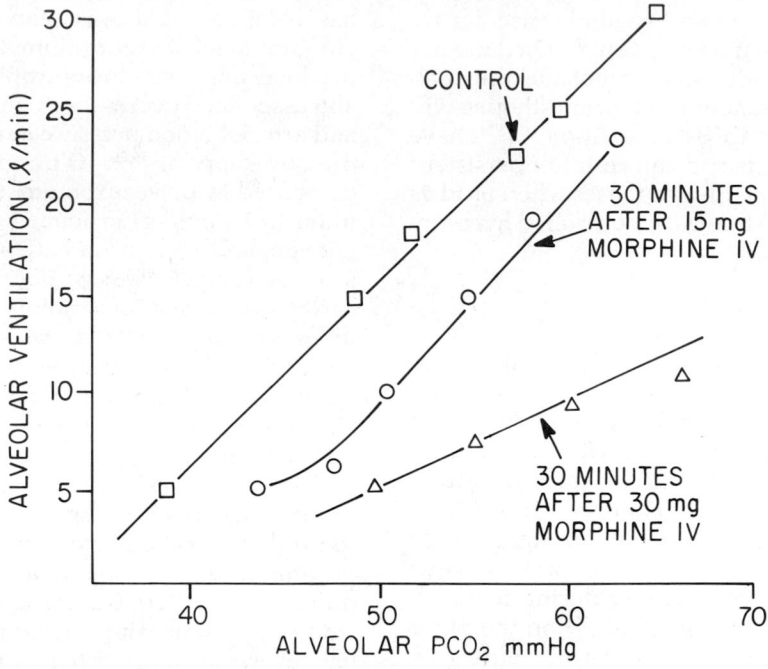

Fig. 10-8. Ventilatory response to CO_2. Control: Increases in alveolar PCO_2 produce increases in alveolar ventilation. After morphine: the response to CO_2 is shifted to the right and the slope of the response is decreased.

rophysiologic and neuropharmacologic aspects of breathing has been performed in humans. High concentrations of opiate receptors have been found in the nucleus tractus solitarius, nucleus retroambigualis, and nucleus ambiguus, areas intimately involved in the control of breathing.[318] Many reports document that specific chemosensitive brain areas mediate opioid respiratory effects.[86]

Marked depression of rib cage responses and relative stability of abdominodiaphragmatic motion occur after administration of narcotic analgesics.[319]

Fentanyl depresses respiratory drive, phase timing, and activation of respiratory muscles, whereas enflurane only decreases respiratory drive.[320] High doses of opioids totally block spontaneous respirations without necessarily producing unconsciousness.[22,30] These patients are still responsive to verbal command and usually breathe when directed to do so.

Opioids have differing effects on the distal respiratory tract. When $PaCO_2$ is allowed to increase, pulmonary dead space remains unchanged by morphine.[321] High doses of morphine (and probably other opioids) decrease bronchociliary motion.[322] Fentanyl has antimuscarinic, antihistaminergic, and antiserotonergic actions and may be superior to morphine for use in patients with asthma or other bronchospastic diseases.[323]

Many factors can change both the magnitude and duration of respiratory depression after opioid administration (Table 10-11). Patients who are sleeping are usually more sensitive to the respiratory-depressant effects of narcotics.[1] Interestingly, both sleep and morphine

relatively spare the diaphragmatic but decrease the thoracic (rib cage) component of breathing. In addition, sleep also impairs tonic and phasic upper airway muscle activity that accompanies breathing.[324] This can be worrisome when patients have a narcotic-based anes-

TABLE 10-11. Factors Increasing the Magnitude and/or Duration of Opioid-Induced Respiratory Depression

1. ↑ Dose

2. Intermittent bolus (vs. continuous infusion)

3. ↑ Brain penetration-drug delivery
   a. ↓ Distribution (↓ cardiac output)
   b. ↑ Un-ionized fraction (respiratory alkalosis)

4. ↓ Reuptake from the brain (intraoperative respiratory alkalosis)

5. ↓ Clearance (↓ hepatic blood flow, e.g., intra-abdominal surgery)

6. Secondary peaks in plasma opioid levels (reuptake of opioid from muscle, lung, fat, intestine)

7. ↑ Ionized opioid at receptor site (postoperative respiratory acidosis)

8. Sleep

9. ↑ Age

10. Metabolic alkalosis

thetic and an operation that results in little or no postoperative pain. In these patients, apparently adequate breathing can become insufficient when they fall asleep. Even small doses of narcotics markedly potentiate the normal right shift of the $PaCO_2$-alveolar ventilation curve that occurs during natural sleep.[325,326]

Older patients (over 60 years of age) are more sensitive to the anesthetic[123] and respiratory-depressant effects of opioids.[1] Older patients experience higher plasma concentrations of opioids administered on a weight basis.[327] Although older patients tend to have a lower blood volume than younger patients, the precise reason for higher plasma concentrations after similar doses is unknown. Conflicting reports argue for or against differences in pharmacokinetics (decreased clearance, increased elimination half-life) and/or pharmacodynamics (increased brain sensitivity) as the basis for the presence or absence of age-related increases in sensitivity to fentanyl[328,329] (see the section, *Pharmacokinetics*, for more details). Older patients also have more frequent apnea, periodic breathing, and upper airway obstruction after morphine compared with young adults.[330]

Morphine alone produces greater respiratory depression on a weight basis in neonates than adults. Its low lipid solubility normally limits blood-brain barrier (BBB) penetration. In neonates and infants with incomplete BBBs, morphine easily penetrates the brain. This difference is not significant with the more lipid-soluble opioids (meperidine, fentanyl, sufentanil) because their ability to penetrate the brain is not affected by BBB maturity.[331] Infants older than 3 months do not have greater fentanyl-associated ventilatory depression (assessed by resting PCO_2 and apnea) than older children and adults.[332]

The respiratory-depressant effects of opioids are increased and/or prolonged when administered with other CNS depressants, including the potent inhaled anesthetics,[333] alcohol,[1] barbiturates,[1] benzodiazepines,[334] and most of the intravenous sedatives and hypnotics. Depression of the brain stem's carbon dioxide response is the primary mechanism underlying most drug interactions producing respiratory depression. However, decreases in the hypoxic response can occur before the carbon dioxide response is affected when small doses of fentanyl (2 μg/kg) and midazolam (0.05 mg/kg)[335] are combined. Exceptions to this rule are droperidol and scopolamine, which do not enhance the respiratory-depressant effects of fentanyl or other narcotics.[336–338] Pain, particularly surgically induced pain, counteracts the respiratory-depressant effects of narcotic compounds.[333,339] It is interesting to note that tolerance to opioid-induced respiratory depression can take months to develop in patients receiving chronic methadone therapy and is usually incomplete. In addition, infants of mothers receiving methadone maintenance demonstrate impaired central chemosensitivity to carbon dioxide. They may also be at higher than normal risk for sudden infant death syndrome.

Although opioid action is usually dissipated via redistribution and hepatic metabolism rather than urinary excretion (see the section, *Pharmacokinetics*), adequacy of renal function may influence duration of narcotic activity.[28] After being anesthetized with large doses of morphine for open heart surgery, patients having higher intraoperative and postoperative urine outputs excrete more morphine in their urine and are able to sustain adequate spontaneous ventilation sooner than are patients with lower urine outputs.[28]

Hypocapnic hyperventilation enhances and prolongs postoperative respiratory depression after fentanyl (10 and 25 μg/kg).[340] Intraoperative hypercarbia produces the opposite effects.[341] Possible explanations include increased brain opioid penetration (increased un-ionized fentanyl with hypocarbia) and removal (decreased cerebral blood flow with hypocarbia). Decreased liver clearance via decreased cardiac output and hepatic blood flow may also explain this phenomenon. Also, intraoperative hyperventilation depletes carbon dioxide stores. During recovery, carbon dioxide stores are repleted, and although carbon dioxide production may be normal, carbon dioxide excretion into the blood is low, resulting in hypoventilation. In this circumstance a normal $PaCO_2$ does not necessarily indicate normal or adequate minute ventilatory volumes.

Some suggest that opioid use in anesthesia leads to increased respiratory problems.[342] While Beard et al.[342] found an increase in adverse respiratory events in the recovery room associated with the use of muscle relaxants and fentanyl, the frequency of a serious problem with fentanyl was rare (1 in 886 patients). In another study, patients receiving intravenous morphine for postoperative pain after a general anesthetic experienced more respiratory side effects than those who received regional anesthesia. Interestingly, desaturations of significance were always associated with sleep and related to obstruction, paradoxic breathing, or slow respiratory rates.[343] The analgesic dose of morphine used in the latter study was large (greater than 12 mg/70 kg intramuscularly). Again, perturbations in the pattern of breathing and timing of the phases of respiration may be more common with opioid than potent inhalational anesthesia.[320] Others have not found any correlation between postoperative desaturation and types of anesthetics used.[344]

Onset of peak respiratory depression after an analgesic dose of morphine is slower than after comparable doses of fentanyl: 30 ± 15 minutes versus 5 to 10 minutes.[312] This is due in part to the lower lipid solubility of morphine (see the section, *Pharmacokinetics*). Because of its low lipid solubility, plasma concentrations and onset of action of morphine are nearly identical after intravenous and intramuscular administration.[327] Respiratory depression induced by small doses of morphine usually lasts longer than that induced by equipotent doses of fentanyl for the same reason.[345] Downes et al.[338] found that intravenous fentanyl (100 and 200 μg/70 kg) results in a somewhat shorter period of respiratory depression than an equipotent dose of meperidine (65 to 75 mg/70 kg). These investigators also noted a faster onset and peak effect after fentanyl than meperidine.[338] Even though fentanyl has a shorter onset and quicker recovery than morphine and meperidine, small doses (2 μg/kg) produce respiratory depression for longer than is generally appreciated (more than 1 hour) in contrast to analgesia (20 to 30 minutes).[346-348] Shorter duration of analgesia than respiratory depression may only reflect the insensitivity of current methods of measuring analgesia. However, sufentanil (0.1 to 0.4 μg/kg) produces shorter-lasting respiratory depression and longer-lasting analgesia than fentanyl (1.0 to 4.0 μg/kg).[346]

Although fentanyl (10 μg/kg) given during induction of anesthesia does not usually produce troublesome postoperative respiratory depression, some investigators have found significant residual respiratory depression 5 or more hours later.[340,347,349,350] Recovery from the ventilatory effects of fentanyl closely parallels the decline of plasma levels.[351] Large doses, or repeated doses, may not permit lower plasma levels (below the threshold for significant respiratory effects) to be established by redistribution alone. Once enough drug is accumulated, termination of clinical effects is prolonged and depends on drug metabolism and elimination half-life (see the section, *Pharmacokinetics*). Thus, substantial blood levels of fentanyl (enough to result in significant respiratory depression) can persist for hours, even after small doses. Plasma fentanyl concentrations of 1.5 to 3.0 ng/ml are usually associated with significant decreases in carbon dioxide responsiveness.[340]

With higher (anesthetic) doses of fentanyl (50 to 100 μg/kg), respiratory depression can persist for many hours. Indeed, ventilation may need to be assisted or supported for 12 to 18 hours after induction of anesthesia. Some patients recover respiratory function more rapidly than do others (for unexplained reasons) and can tolerate extubation of the trachea within 6 to 8 hours of drug administration with minimal or no elevation in PaCO$_2$.[144,200] Nonetheless, when moderately large (20 to 50 μg/kg) or high doses of fentanyl are used for any kind of operation, facilities should exist for postoperative mechanical ventilation. Pharmacokinetic data predict and studies have demonstrated that both alfentanil and sufentanil allow more rapid recovery of respiratory function than fentanyl.[346,352] The pharmacodynamic effects of alfentanil and sufentanil on respiratory function are not significantly different from those of fentanyl and other opioids. Thus, significant respiratory problems can persist after anesthesia following the use of any opioid, including alfentanil.[353]

Recurrence of Respiratory Depression

Delayed or recurring respiratory depression has been reported to occur with most opioids including fentanyl,[336,350] morphine,[354] meperidine,[355] alfentanil,[353] and sufentanil.[356] Explanations for this phenomenon are not clear and are confounded by the simultaneous occurrence of numerous clinical events. These include stimulation, pain or the lack of it, supplemental analgesics and other medications, sleep, activity, hypothermia, and hemodynamic alterations. Numerous investigators have noted the occurrence of significant secondary peaks and fluctuations in plasma opioid levels during the elimination phase.[357-359] The existence of large peripheral compartments (e.g., skeletal muscle) and the variability in drug uptake from them contributes to and can augment this phenomenon. Some investigators have shown secondary peaks in fentanyl plasma levels with parallel changes in carbon dioxide sensitivity and breathing.[360,361] Interestingly, McQuay et al.[361] found a higher incidence of second peaks in plasma fentanyl levels (increases greater than or equal to 0.5 ng/ml) when an infusion technique was used compared with intermittent boluses.

The stomach can sequester up to 20 percent of an intravenous dose of fentanyl via ion trapping in its acid milieu. It has been postulated that subsequent passage into the alkaline medium of the small intestine leads to reabsorption of significant amounts of fentanyl, resulting in secondary peaks in fentanyl plasma concentrations and recurrent respiratory depression. However, this mechanism appears unlikely in view of the high hepatic extraction ratios for fentanyl and most opioids.[362] However, the importance and relative contribution of intestinal reabsorption of fentanyl and other opioids in respiratory depression is not well studied and, therefore, not clearly established. Other explanations for renarcotization include release of fentanyl trapped in the lung, which can accumulate significant amounts of fentanyl.[328]

NEUROPHYSIOLOGIC ACTIONS

In healthy, pain-free volunteers, opioids produce drowsiness, lethargy, apathy, and sleep and can cause euphoria and dysphoria. Morphine and meperidine, via histamine release, can cause a transient flushing or hot sensation. In patients, opioids, in addition to being potent analgesics and anesthetics, are cough suppressants and relieve anxiety and the distress of dyspnea.

Opioids and the EEG

The neurophysiologic state obtained by the use of large doses of opioid analgesics is not the same as the general anesthetic state resulting from inhaled anesthetics.[363] General anesthetics produce a dose-related generalized depression of the CNS, while opioid analgesics are more selective in action. Opioids probably produce anesthesia by blocking afferent input into the CNS through direct stimulation of opioid receptors.[363,364] Other, non-receptor-mediated mechanisms (e.g., local anesthetic action) have been suggested but are of unclear significance in humans.

Early studies suggested a predominant neuroexcitatory or arousal effect of opioids, including morphine and fentanyl.[365] In animals (cats), increases in cerebral oxidative metabolism have suggested an analepticlike effect. These findings differ from most general anesthetics. Species differences (opioids produce EEG seizure discharges in cats and mice) are now known to account for many of the discrepant findings in EEG results between animals and humans.

Neuroleptanalgesia with 10 to 15 mg of droperidol and fentanyl (200 to 440 μg) causes increased slow wave activity that is gradually replaced with alpha waves and patterns consistent with "surgical sleep" on the EEG.[366] Maximum effect appears to be obtained only when fentanyl is administered after droperidol, apparently owing to droperidol's brain stem (reticular activating system)-depressant properties.[366]

Small doses of fentanyl (3 μg/kg) produce minimal EEG changes,[367] while higher doses (30 to 70 μg/kg) result in high-voltage slow (delta) waves, suggesting a state consistent with anesthesia (unconsciousness, analgesia, and amnesia).[363] Absence of EEG changes in response to intubation of the trachea and surgery confirms the anesthetic effects of large doses of narcotics. Although transient isolated (usually frontotemporal) sharp wave activity can be observed after large doses of fentanyl and other narcotics, it is never generalized.

Sufentanil (0.1 μg/kg) produces EEG changes that are similar to those produced by fentanyl. These changes are greater in the elderly.[368] EEG states consistent with surgical anesthesia have been produced with doses of sufentanil as low as 2.5 μg/kg.[369] High doses of both fentanyl and sufentanil produce greater EEG changes than does morphine.[370] Opioids differ from potent inhaled anesthetics in that increasing dosage with inhaled anesthetics produces a continuum of EEG changes, eventually resulting in burst suppression and a flat EEG with overdosage. In contrast, a "ceiling effect" is reached with fentanyl, morphine, sufentanil, and other opioids. Increasing the fentanyl dosage from 50 to 150 μg/kg does not further affect the EEG.[364]

While high doses of fentanyl or sufentanil produce quite similar EEG changes,[370] the effects of alfentanil may be different.[371] Alfentanil (125 μg/kg) produces less synchronization of the EEG and less change in the relative EEG power in the delta band, suggesting a lesser depth of anesthesia.[371] In addition, EEG spindle activity is common with alfentanil and rare with fentanyl or sufentanil. The latter may represent a specific or unique effect of alfentanil. EEG data confirm that alfentanil acts more rapidly than fentanyl. Scott et al.[372] reported that the lag time between a detectable plasma concentration and change in the spectral edge is only 1 minute for alfentanil (approximately 84 μg/kg over 6 minutes) and 6 minutes for fentanyl (approximately 8.8 μg/kg over 6 minutes) (Figs. 10-9 and 10-10). Interestingly, the serum concentration ratio which resulted in similar EEG patterns in that study was 75 to 1 alfentanil/fentanyl. This contrasts with the reported intravenous dose ratio in which fentanyl is only three to five times as potent as alfentanil.

EEG analysis is useful in monitoring the depth of anesthesia.[363,370–372] Plasma narcotic levels correlate reasonably well with EEG changes,[372] and some patterns (K complexes or an increase in frequency and decrease in wave amplitude) can be used to indicate a return to awareness or light anesthesia.[371] However, problems with lead placement and signal processing as well as high cost and reliability need to be resolved before EEG analysis can be used as a routine monitor of anesthetic depth.

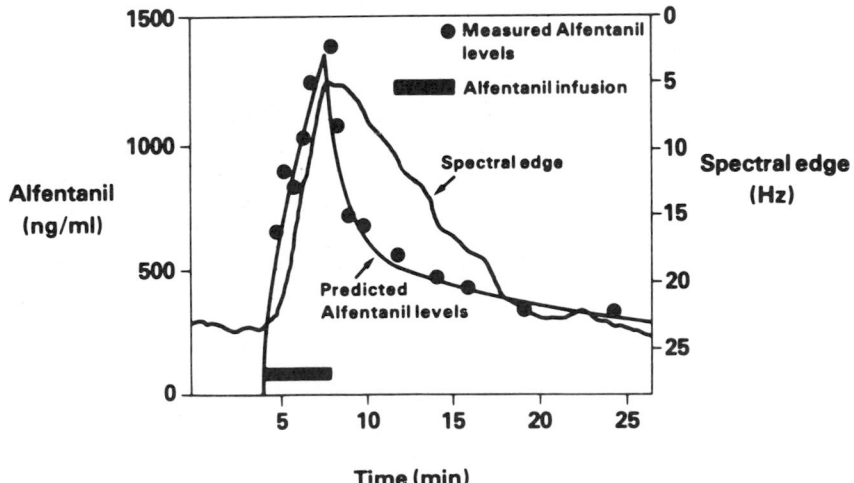

Fig. 10-9. Time course of spectral edge and serum alfentanil concentrations. Note the inverted spectral edge axis. Spectral edge changes closely parallel serum concentrations. Alfentanil infusion rate = 1,500 μg/min (solid bar). (From Scott et al.,[372] with permission.)

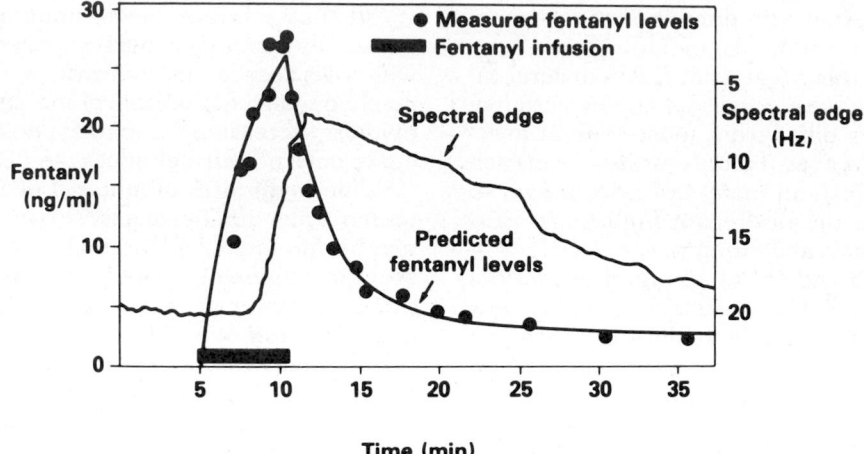

Fig. 10-10. Time course of spectral edge and serum fentanyl concentrations. Note the inverted spectral edge axis. The spectral edge changes lag behind the serum concentrations changes. Fentanyl infusion rate = 150 μg/min (solid bar). (From Scott et al.,[372] with permission.)

Opioid Action and Sensory Evoked Potentials

Numerous studies have documented that opioids do not appreciably alter somatosensory evoked potentials (SSEP) elicited at the posterior tibial or median nerve.[373-382] These studies illustrate that changes produced in SSEP latencies (increases usually less than 3 msec) and amplitudes (reductions of usually 30 to 40 percent or less) that occur after administration of opioids are compatible with successful clinical monitoring.

Although opioids do not interfere with SSEP interpretation, they do inhibit both the velocity and amplitude of transmission of nerve action potentials.[374] It follows that opioid-induced SSEP changes may occasionally be confused with neurologic injury.[378] Significant variability in opioid effects on SSEP amplitude has been reported. Amplitude has been found to decrease, increase, or remain unchanged.[374,383] Administration of opioids probably should be timed to avoid confusion with other possible causes of SSEP change.[383] Fortunately, changes induced by large doses of opioids occur rapidly and then remain stable.[381] In addition, slow intravenous infusions of opioids generally produce fewer SSEP changes than large boluses.[374] Repeated boluses produce less change than the initial injection.[375] Sebel et al.[382] did not find a significant correlation between increasing doses of fentanyl and SSEP changes. These findings confirm the stability of the SSEP signals once opioid-based anesthesia has been established. In addition, the early portions of the SSEP signal are more significant in monitoring and less affected by fentanyl than the latter parts of the SSEP.[383]

High doses of fentanyl, alfentanil, or sufentanil are compatible with reliable SSEP monitoring,[373,382] but combinations of opioids and other intravenous anesthetics may or may not be. After administration of midazolam (0.3 mg/kg), fentanyl (10 μg/kg, given as a bolus followed by an infusion of 0.2 mg/kg/h), causes little change in SSEP.[380] Thiopental (5 mg/kg bolus plus 2 mg/kg/h infusion) followed by fentanyl (10 μg/kg) will further decrease amplitudes but cause little change in latencies.[380] After etomidate (0.3 mg/kg bolus plus 2 mg/kg/h as an infusion), fentanyl (10 μg/kg) increases latency and reverses etomidate-induced increases in amplitude.[380]

Brain stem auditory evoked potentials are also minimally altered by analgesic and anesthetic doses of morphine, fentanyl, or sufentanil.[384-386]

Opioid Effects on Cerebral Blood Flow, Cerebral Metabolic Rate, and Intracranial Pressure (Also See Ch. 19)

Narcotic analgesics generally produce modest decreases (10 to 25 percent) in cerebral metabolic rate (CMR) and intracranial pressure (ICP), although these changes are influenced by the concomitant administration of other anesthetics. In contrast to volatile anesthetics, opioids cause cerebral vasoconstriction. Opioids also decrease cerebral blood flow (CBF) when combined with nitrous oxide. Morphine (1 and 3 mg/kg) with 70 percent nitrous oxide causes insignificant changes in CBF, cerebral metabolism of oxygen ($CMRO_2$), and cerebral metabolism of glucose in humans.[387] In vitro studies with morphine show a small vasoconstrictor effect on certain cerebral arteries at lower concentrations (less than 10^{-5} M), while higher concentrations (10^{-3} M) cause vasodilation.[388,389]

Fentanyl (100 μg/kg) causes dose-related reductions in CBF (maximum 50 percent) and $CMRO_2$ (maximum 35 percent) in rats receiving nitrous oxide in oxygen.[390] Fentanyl causes similar decreases in CBF and CMR in dogs,[391] lambs,[392] and humans.[393] Sufentanil also causes dose-related decreases in CBF (maximum 53 percent) and CMRO$_2$ (maximum 40 percent) in the rat.[394] Sufentanil (2 to 200 μg/kg) consistently dilated cerebral vessels producing increases in CBF and ICP with no decrease in CMR in the unanesthetized dog.[395] Fentanyl causes small increases (5 to 10 percent) in cerebral blood volume and ICP in the dog.[396,397] In addition, responses to increases in arterial CO$_2$, PaO$_2$ and arterial blood pressure remain intact with fentanyl and sufentanil.[393,398,399] Finally, fentanyl, sufentanil, and other opioids do not change cerebrospinal fluid (CSF) reabsorption and decrease CSF production.[400,401] Thus, some clinicians recommend the use of opioids in neuroanesthesia, particularly when intracranial pathology places patients at risk for elevated ICP.[396,400,401] Sufentanil and alfentanil may, however, increase CSF pressure in patients with brain tumors, whereas fentanyl does not.[397] The mechanism involved and the reason(s) for the difference with fentanyl are not known.

Muscle Rigidity

Opioids can increase muscle tone and cause severe rigidity.[402] Problems with muscular rigidity after opioid administration have been known for many years.[365,402,403–405] Corrsen et al.[402] reported an 80 percent incidence of some rigidity in patients receiving dehydrobenzperidol (0.44 mg/kg) and fentanyl (8.8 μg/kg). Grell et al.[406] found that a single intravenous dose of fentanyl (0.5 to 0.8 mg) consistently produced chest wall rigidity within 60 to 90 seconds of intravenous administration. The incidence of rigidity with opioid anesthetic techniques has varied from 0 to 100 percent.[123,144,179,210,402,404,406–408] The reasons for this variability are not completely clear but are probably related to the dose and speed of opioid administration, the concomitant use of nitrous oxide, the presence or absence of muscle relaxants, and perhaps other supplements.

Opioid-induced rigidity is characterized by increased muscle tone progressing to severe stiffness, particularly in the thoracic and abdominal muscles. Rigidity usually begins just as or after the patient loses consciousness; rigidity may rarely occur in conscious patients.[172,210] Rigidity of the thoracic muscles (wooden chest syndrome) can impair spontaneous ventilation or controlled ventilation in the nonparalyzed patient.[407] It has been suggested that glottic closure causes the difficulties with controlled ventilation during rigidity,[408] although it is not a consistent finding.[409] While the influence of dose and rate of opioid infusion on the incidence and magnitude of rigidity has not been evaluated, rapid infusions or large bolus injections seem to increase the severity of rigidity.[9,179,210,410] Rigidity is also more common in older patients and during the administration of nitrous oxide as well.[9,123,410–413] Alfentanil administered as a large rapid bolus appears to cause the highest incidence of rigidity. Rigidity occasionally occurs upon emergence from anesthesia[414] and very

rarely several hours after the last dose has been administered.[415] Delayed or postoperative rigidity may be related to a second peak in plasma fentanyl concentration. Rigidity has also been reported in a neonate whose mother was anesthetized with a narcotic.[416]

Abnormal muscle movements ranging from extremity flexion, single or multiple extremity tonic-clonic movements, to global tonic-clonic motions can also occur after the use of opioids.[123] Indeed, tonic-clonic muscle movements and/or rigidity are probably the explanation for the reports describing seizurelike movements after fentanyl and sufentanil.[417] Whether such muscle movements (including rigidity) are part of a spectrum of neuromuscular activity associated with opioids or are manifestations of subcortical seizure activity is unclear (see the section, *Neuroexcitatory Phenomena*).

The precise mechanism by which opioids cause muscle rigidity is not clearly understood. Muscle rigidity is not due to a direct action on muscle fibers, since it can be decreased or prevented by pretreatment with muscle relaxants.[123,179,418] Also, opioid-induced muscle rigidity is not associated with increases in creatinine kinase,[411] suggesting that little or no muscle damage occurs during this period. Opioids do not have significant effects on neuromuscular conduction and result in only minimal depression of monosynaptic reflexes associated with muscle stretch receptors.[411,413] Opioid-induced rigidity is probably related to a catatonic state, which can be induced by all narcotic analgesics.[419] Although some investigators have suggested that opioids produce rigidity by increasing dopamine concentrations within the striatum of the brain,[420,421] the mechanism is probably more complex. Rigidity may be the result of stimulation of mu receptors located on GABA-ergic interneurons, which can be blocked by lesions in the striatum. Striatonigral GABA pathways involved with rigidity can also be affected by both GABA agonists and antagonists.[422–424] Recent evidence indicates that the nucleus raphe pontis is an integral central site responsible for opioid-induced rigidity.[425,426] Other proposed CNS sites involved during rigidity include the periaqueductal gray area, the caudate nucleus, the nucleus accumbens, the thalamus, the posterior hypothalamus, and the superior colliculus. Some aspects of opioid-induced catatonia and rigidity (increased incidence with age, muscle movements resembling extrapyramidal side effects) are similar to Parkinson's disease and suggest a possibly similar neurochemical mechanism.

Rigidity can decrease pulmonary compliance and functional residual capacity, diminish or preclude adequate ventilation, and cause hypercarbia, hypoxia, and an elevated ICP.[179,407,408,426–428] Opioid-induced rigidity also increases pulmonary artery and central venous pressures and pulmonary vascular resistance (Table 10-12).[407,429] Transient increases in plasma fentanyl levels may be induced by rigidity.[430] Succinylcholine will reliably and rapidly terminate rigidity (provided

TABLE 10-12. Potential Problems Associated with Opioid-Induced Rigidity

Hemodynamic	↑ CVP, ↑ PAP ↑, PVR
Pulmonary	↓ Compliance, ↓ FRC, ↓ ventilation Hypercarbia Hypoxemia
Miscellaneous	↑ Oxygen consumption ↑ ICP Occluded or dislodged intravenous lines ↑ Fentanyl plasma levels

Abbreviations: CVP, central venous pressure; PAP, pulmonary artery pressure; PVR, pulmonary vascular resistance; FRC, functional residual capacity.

the intravenous infusion is not impaired by a rigid flexed extremity), eliminate associated cardiovascular changes, and usually permit controlled ventilation. Nevertheless, the unpleasant esthetics and potential risk posed by opioid-induced rigidity episodes has stimulated the search for preventive measures. Pretreatment or concomitant use of nondepolarizing muscle relaxants significantly decreases the incidence and severity of rigidity (Table 10-13).[123,179,418] Equipotent doses of metocurine may be more effective than pancuronium in both attenuating and abating rigidity, suggesting that neuromuscular blocking agents that act on prejunctional receptors are more effective in minimizing rigidity than those acting on postjunctional receptors.[418] Induction doses of sodium thiopental and less than anesthetic doses of diazepam and midazolam have also been reported to prevent, attenuate, or successfully treat rigidity. However, other reports discount the reliability of the benzodiazepines.[123,431,432] Avoidance of rigidity in clinical practice may be best achieved by using a "priming" size dose of a nondepolarizing muscle relaxant and avoiding the rapid administration of large doses of any of the opioids.

Neuroexcitatory Phenomena

Opioids as well as inhaled (diethyl ether, enflurane, isoflurane) and other intravenous (ketamine, methohexital) anesthetics can cause neuroexcitatory phenomena.[169,365,420,421,433-438] Fentanyl causes EEG seizure activity in cats (20 to 80 μg/kg),[365] rats (200 to 400 μg/kg),[419] and dogs (greater than 1,250 μg/kg).[169] Opioids have been implicated as causative in a variety of other types of neuroexcitation ranging from nystagmus and nonspecific eye movements to single extremity flexion and single- or multiple-extremity tonic or clonic-tonic activity. Global seizurelike activity consisting of myoclonic-tonic movements of the trunk and/or extremities has also been observed.[30,351,439,440] However, EEG evidence of seizure activity after fentanyl (up to 150 μg/kg), alfentanil (175 μg/kg), and sufentanil (up to 15 μg/kg) is lacking in humans.[363,370,429,441,442] Focal neuroexcitation on EEG (e.g., sharp wave activity) occasionally occurs in humans after large doses of fentanyl, sufentanil, and alfentanil.[442]

Reports of jerking movements and hyperexcitability after morphine are rare but probably similar in origin to rigidity after fentanyl.[21] Morphine produces tonic-clonic activity after epidural administration. Meperidine may also cause CNS excitability. The mechanism is unique and is related to its N-demethylated metabolite normeperidine, which is twice as likely to cause CNS excitation and convulsions as meperidine. Normeperidine has a long elimination half-life (15 to 40 hours) and is chiefly eliminated by the kidney. Normeperidine is also hydrolyzed to normeperidinic acid, which is inactive.[443] Convulsions and myoclonic jerking movements that occur after large doses of meperidine, especially in patients with decreased renal function, are most likely caused by normeperidine and are not antagonized by naloxone.[443]

Fentanyl can cause neuroexcitation ranging from delirium to grand mal seizurelike activity.[441,444-448] Animal studies demonstrate that in certain species opioids cause focal CNS excitation rather than global CNS depression.[449,450] Generally, these areas are subcortical (in particular the limbic system, which is rich in opiate receptors) and may in part explain the difficulty in documenting neuroexcitatory opioid effects by surface electroencephalography. Sufentanil (up to 50 μg/kg) can also produce neuroexcitation including tonic/clonic movements and seizurelike activity.[451-456] Inter-

TABLE 10-13. Incidence (Percent) of Patients and Degrees of Rigidity after 30 μg/kg of Fentanyl in 72 Patients

Pretreatment and Drug	No. of Subjects	Degree of Rigidity (%)[a]			
		0	1	2	3
Pancuronium					
No	37	14	3	32	51
Yes[b]	35	54	6	20	20
Diazepam					
No	38	32	8	23	37
Yes	34	35	0	30	35

[a] 0, no rigidity; 1, mild rigidity; 2, moderate rigidity; 3, severe rigidity.
[b] $P < 0.05$ compared with no pancuronium pretreatment.
(From Bailey et al.,[123] with permission.)

estingly, most reports of neuroexcitation with fentanyl or sufentanil involve the elderly, although such neuroexcitation is occasionally observed in young patients (ages 4 to 12 years).[453]

The mechanisms underlying neuroexcitatory phenomenon are not clear. Changes in central catecholamine concentrations in dopaminergic pathways have been proposed as a possible explanation.[457] Other purported mechanisms include disinhibition of pyramidal cells of the hippocampus[458] and an increase in the release of excitatory neurotransmitters, such as Met- and Leu-enkephalin, that possess epileptogenic properties.[435] Recent data suggest that at least some forms of neuroexcitation are antagonized by naloxone.[444]

Clinical circumstances do not usually allow for naloxone treatment of opioid-induced neuroexcitation following induction of anesthesia. Such therapy might preclude continuing anesthesia and surgery. The discontinuation of surgery is also not recommended because there is no known CNS morbidity associated with opioid-related neuroexcitation. Instead, if rigidity and/ or neuroexcitation occur in an unanticipated fashion, control of the airway and completion of anesthetic induction should proceed. Nevertheless, concern about the potential risk of seizures is legitimate. Neuroexcitatory phenomenon can alarm operating personnel, lead to physical harm,[445] or at least disconnect intravenous lines and make appropriate treatment difficult. Neuroexcitation is also occasionally associated with increases in heart rate and arterial blood pressure. Local increases in CBF[459] and cerebral metabolism[449] are also of theoretical concern since prolonged seizure activity, even if focal, could lead to neuronal injury and/or cellular death.[436,460,461] No neurologic deficit has been attributed to the neuroexcitatory effects of opioids.

Pupil Size and Opioid Action

Many stimuli and most anesthetics (including atropine, the ultra-short-acting barbiturates, narcotic analgesics, ephedrine, and halothane) affect pupillary diameter, probably via alterations in sympathetic and parasympathetic tone. Even such factors as eye color, age, pain, and ambient light affect the size and/or rate of change of pupillary diameter to stimuli.[462] Nevertheless, clinicians often use pupillary size to assess opioid action.

Few studies have systematically examined the response of the pupil to different anesthetic techniques. Opioids constrict the iris, and the time course of the response appears related to plasma opioid levels, even in the presence of potent inhaled anesthetics.[463,464] Opioids release cortical inhibition of the Edinger-Westphal nucleus, resulting in pupillary constriction. Direct effects on the iris are also possible.

Thermoregulation and Shivering

When decreases in body temperature reach a thermoregulatory threshold (generally 37°C), vasoconstriction occurs in an attempt to preserve core temperature. Potent inhaled anesthetics decrease the thermoregulatory threshold by about 2.5°C (to approximately 34.5°C), and although evidence is scant, it appears that nitrous oxide-fentanyl anesthesia produces similar changes.[465]

Shivering is a common phenomenon in patients recovering from anesthesia. Its physiologic purpose is to produce heat, but its occurrence in relation to anesthesia is inconsistent and incompletely understood. Nevertheless, postoperative shivering can cause several undesirable physiologic consequences including increases in oxygen consumption, carbon dioxide production, minute ventilation, and cardiac output and decreases in mixed venous oxygen saturation.[465] The severity of shivering is positively correlated with increases in oxygen consumption. Thus, an effective treatment for postoperative shivering is usually desirable.

Meperidine (25 to 50 mg/70 kg intravenously) is unique among opioids in its ability to effectively terminate or attenuate shivering in approximately 70 to 80 percent of patients.[466-470] In the presence of an opioid antagonist, higher doses may be necessary.[469] Fentanyl and morphine are apparently ineffective. Meperidine (intravenously or epidurally) is also effective in treating shivering that occurs during epidural anesthesia.[468,471]

OPIOIDS AND THE ENDOCRINE SYSTEM

Considerable interest has been expressed in the anesthetic modification of the hormonal and metabolic responses to surgical trauma. The endocrine response to surgery results in hypermetabolism and mobilization of energy supplies. Teleologically, the underlying need of the body to respond to an insult in a manner that maximizes survival is the basis of this response. The term *stress response* has been used extensively to describe the total physiologic process that occurs when patients encounter a significant insult.[222,472-476] However, the physiologic response to any insult is highly dependent on the condition and status of the individual before, during, and after the insult. Additionally, what is physically and particularly emotionally stressful and significant to one individual may have little impact on another. Plasma concentrations of the stress hormones increase during general anesthesia with most anesthetics and are further increased with surgery.[142,477,478] Surgically induced increases in most stress hormones are related to the severity of the operative trauma,[479] being much greater during intra-abdominal surgery than body surface procedures.[477,478] Increased levels of stress hormones are considered undesirable because they promote hemodynamic instability and intraoperative and postoperative metabolic catabolism.

In addition to surgical trauma, the physiologic responses of the body are triggered or altered by a host of factors including afferent nerve function from an injured area, pain, hypovolemia and hemorrhage, infection, shock, blood pH changes, CNS injury, drugs, emotion, hypoxia, starvation, temperature changes, withdrawal symptoms, and immune processes. Despite great variability in stimuli, the body's response to an insult has some common denominators among which are trophic hormones released from the hypothalamus that stimulate the pituitary to release ACTH, growth hormone (GH), prolactin, endorphin, and antidiuretic hormone (ADH). Catabolic hormones including cortisol, catecholamines, glucagon, and thyroxine are also secreted in increased amounts, and plasma concentrations of anabolic hormones such as insulin and testosterone are usually decreased.[472] Narcotic analgesics are effective in decreasing the physiologic response to stress. Multiple studies are being conducted to further define the stress response, its associated morbidity, and how these phenomena are influenced by opioids.

Mechanism

The mechanism by which large doses of opioids attenuate the endocrine and metabolic response to stress is not known. However, increasing understanding of the opiate receptors and their endogenous ligands has provided much information on the likely locations and nature of opioid effects.[480] Opioids are capable of reducing the stress response by decreasing nociceptive input, as well as by influencing centrally mediated neuroendocrine responses.

Opioid effects on nociception occur at several different levels of the neuraxis. Opioids bind to primary nociceptive afferents and produce analgesia after perineural application.[481] Multiple types of spinal cord opiate receptors are concentrated within the dorsal horn.[88,482] Additionally, distinct opiate receptors selectively act to impede pain signals arising from different forms of injury.[483-485] Descending supraspinal inhibitory neurons have been identified that originate in midbrain centers and end at the dorsal horn.[486]

Opioid effects on the central neuroendocrine response have been delineated. Studies with naloxone in narcotic-free individuals have permitted evaluation of the hormonal actions of endogenous opioids and their receptors.[487,488] Different hypothalamic opiate receptors can be stimulated by morphine and alter hormone secretion.[489] Endogenous opioid peptides seem to be important as stress hormones themselves and not just as modulators of other hormone secretion. Indirect evidence for this is drawn from the fact that β-endorphin and ACTH are cosynthesized and cosecreted during stress and are in fact derived from the same precursor, proopiomelanocortin.[490] The exogenous administration of opiates likely mimics endorphin action at receptors and as a result reduces endogenous opiate secretion through a negative feedback.

Specific Drugs

Morphine

Analysis of hormonal data from a number of studies suggests that morphine modifies hormonal responses to surgical trauma in a dose-related fashion.[491-496] Morphine, even in small doses, inhibits the release of ACTH and blocks at least part of the pituitary-adrenal response to surgical stress.[493] After morphine anesthesia (0.33 mg/kg), significant decreases in blood lactate concentrations occur but pyruvate concentrations remain unchanged.[491] Morphine anesthesia (1 mg/kg) suppresses surgically induced increases in plasma cortisol, but not human growth hormone, during major abdominal operations.[494] During cardiac surgery with morphine (4 mg/kg) anesthesia, plasma concentrations of both cortisol and human GH are not increased in the pre-bypass period but are increased during bypass.[492,494,496] Increases in plasma concentrations of these hormones continue after bypass as well as postoperatively.[492]

Morphine increases plasma levels of some hormones that normally increase during stress.[496,497] Plasma catecholamines are increased after morphine anesthesia in dogs.[497] The mechanisms underlying this effect include histamine release and subsequent catecholamine increases, adrenal medullary release mechanisms,[497,498] and catecholamine release from sympathetic nerve endings.[499] Other possibilities include reflex responses to increased carbon dioxide or hypotension (secondary to morphine-induced ventilatory depression and/or vasodilation). Morphine can also increase concentrations of catecholamines in both blood and urine in humans.[136-138] The changes in plasma norepinephrine concentrations induced by induction of anesthesia with morphine are in part related to preinduction plasma norepinephrine concentrations: patients with low preoperative plasma norepinephrine concentrations experience a small increase in arterial blood concentrations after induction of anesthesia, whereas patients with higher preoperative plasma norepinephrine concentrations experience no change or decreases in these concentrations.[136,137] Similar changes are also observed after induction of anesthesia with inhaled anesthetics.[500]

Although morphine stimulates ADH secretion in dogs and rats,[501,502] it does not appear to do so in the absence of surgical stimulus in humans.[503] Plasma ADH increases significantly during morphine (1 mg/kg) plus nitrous oxide anesthesia in humans during surgery before cardiopulmonary bypass and increases further during bypass.[503] Plasma renin activity also increases markedly in patients anesthetized with morphine (1 to 3 mg/kg) and nitrous oxide during cardiac surgery.[195] Increases in plasma renin are frequently but not always correlated with simultaneous increases in arterial pressure in these patients.[195]

Fentanyl

Fentanyl and some of its newer congeners seem to be even more effective than morphine in modifying hormonal responses to surgery. For example, fentanyl abolished the hyperglycemic response to surgery and reduced cortisol and GH responses better than halothane.[504,505]

The catecholamine response to induction of anesthesia is attenuated by fentanyl infusions in patients about to undergo coronary artery surgery,[143] especially with doses greater than 50 μg/kg.[142,143,203,506] However, increases in catecholamine concentrations during cardiopulmonary bypass are not attenuated by fentanyl[142,203] (T.H. Stanley, unpublished data). Presumably the severity of the stimulus of cardiopulmonary bypass (i.e., hemodilution, hypothermia, cardiac injury, and nonpulsatile flow) accounts for this lack of fentanyl influence. There is some evidence that vasopressin and catecholamine responses to cardiopulmonary bypass can be significantly attenuated by the use of pulsatile flow,[492] although this has not been confirmed by all investigators.[507]

Anesthesia with fentanyl (60 to 100 μg/kg) prevents increases in plasma ADH, renin, and aldosterone during the period before cardiopulmonary bypass.[30,506] This is in contrast to the significant increases of these hormones observed in similar patients anesthetized with morphine.[503] However, during bypass, plasma ADH rises significantly despite high doses (100 μg/kg) of fentanyl. High-dose fentanyl anesthesia usually prevents increases in blood glucose, plasma cortisol, and plasma GH concentrations in most patients throughout open heart operations.[142,203,506,508] However, these reductions are not consistently found in all patients, especially during and after cardiopulmonary bypass and during the postoperative period, even when fentanyl administration is continued for 12 to 18 hours after surgery.[508]

Sufentanil

Sufentanil is possibly more effective than fentanyl in modifying the endocrine and metabolic responses to cardiac surgery.[476] With the exception of prolactin, no significant increase in plasma levels of hormones or substances commonly associated with stress was found in response to induction of anesthesia, endotracheal intubation, or surgery before cardiopulmonary bypass. The response to cardiopulmonary bypass with sufentanil anesthesia is similar to that with fentanyl in that plasma ADH and catecholamine levels increase.[476,509] However, in a study in which a supplemental dose of sufentanil (10 μg/kg) was given at the initiation of cardiopulmonary bypass, catecholamine increases were attenuated, although not eliminated, compared with a single sufentanil induction dose (15 μg/kg) without similar supplementation.[475]

Alfentanil

Alfentanil, although less well studied, causes hormonal modifying effects similar to those of sufentanil.[509] Using a mean dose of 1.0 mg/kg of alfentanil, de Lange et al.[509] found no increase in plasma cortisol and catecholamines before but not during cardiopulmonary bypass. An additional study showed no increase in ADH or GH throughout coronary artery bypass surgery including cardiopulmonary bypass with 1,200 μg/kg of alfentanil.[222] Further studies need to be performed to define the role of alfentanil on the hormonal response to stress.

Clinical Significance

Fentanyl, sufentanil, and alfentanil appear to be more effective than morphine in reducing the endocrine and metabolic responses to surgery. Although higher doses are more effective, the importance of controlling these responses is still unclear. It is hoped that anesthetic techniques that minimize this stress response (i.e., elevated catecholamine levels and protein catabolism) will reduce morbidity and mortality in a variety of circumstances. There is little evidence to date supporting this theory. In addition, most reductions in metabolic responses to anesthesia and surgery are short lived.[203,505,508] With morphine, at least, there is no improvement in postoperative nitrogen balance.[492] A study in preterm infants undergoing heart surgery showed that fentanyl-nitrous oxide-curare anesthesia compared favorably to a nitrous oxide-curare technique with regard to decreases in the hormonal response to surgery, protein breakdown 2 to 3 days after surgery, and circulatory and metabolic complications.[510] Still, the hypothesis that attenuation of the neurohumoral response to surgery is beneficial in terms of postoperative morbidity and mortality is of questionable significance.

Tolerance and Opiate Abuse in the Patient

Opioid-addicted patients have multiple problems of importance to anesthesia. Common cardiopulmonary problems in opioid-addicted patients include bacterial endocarditis (particularly of the tricuspid valve), cardiac tamponade, cardiac arrhythmias, thrombophlebitis, mycotic aneurysm, septic pulmonary and systemic emboli, sepsis, pulmonary edema, bacterial pneumonia, pulmonary aspiration and abscesses, pulmonary hypertension, and talc granulomata. Restrictive lung disease and increased alveolar-arterial oxygen gradients are also not uncommon in addicted patients.[511-513] Renal disease, especially the nephrotic syndrome, is seven times more prevalent in addicted than in nonaddicted patients. Likewise, addicted patients have a higher incidence of other genitourinary problems,[511] as well as decreased erythrocyte counts and hemoglobin concentrations. Chronic morphine administration causes adrenal hypertrophy and impairs corticosteroid secretion.[1] Other problems that occur with increased incidence in opioid abusers are viral and nonviral hepatitis, human immunodeficiency syndrome, osteomyelitis, muscle weakness associated with rhabdomyolysis and myoglobinuria, and neurologic complications such as transverse myelitis, encephalitis, and cerebral abscess.

Planning anesthetic management for the addicted patient is difficult. Adequate premedication is advisable, and narcotic analgesics should not be avoided. There is no ideal anesthetic or technique to employ in the chronic addict or in the patient with an acute opiate overdose. The patient with an acute opiate overdose comes to the emergency or operating room with hypotension, bradycardia, hypoventilation, relative hypovolemia, and decreased gastrointestinal motility (see the section, *Renal and Gastrointestinal Effects*) and a stomach full of recently ingested material. Intravenous access is usually limited and difficult. Cardiovascular changes can be reversed with increments of naloxone (40 to 80 μg/70 kg every 1 to 2 minutes intravenously) until respiration is adequate. Support of the circulatory system with intravenously administered fluids and monitoring of arterial blood gases and pulmonary function can be important. It should be remembered that complete opioid reversal may turn the patient into an uncontrollable menace. Furthermore, naloxone, the usual opioid antagonist employed, has a shorter duration of action than most abused narcotics. Therefore, reappearance of narcotic effect is a potential hazard at any time.

Opioid overdose may be produced accidentally (e.g., an elderly patient with hepatic disease) or intentionally (e.g., suicide). Maximum effects will produce a comatose and apneic patient who is cyanotic with pinpoint pupils unless anoxic pupillary dilatation has supervened. If spontaneous ventilation has persisted, hypotension, bradycardia, and hypothermia are additional likely signs. Treatment of such a patient follows the basics of life support: secure and protect the airway, oxygenate and ventilate, and restore hemodynamic function.

Although some opiate addicts may be managed with local or regional anesthesia, associated psychological problems make general anesthesia easier and frequently safer. Management during surgery requires normal fluid replacement, a high oxygen concentration, frequent arterial blood gas monitoring and, on occasion, positive end-expiratory pressure. Mechanical difficulties encountered in attempting venous cannulation may occasionally necessitate femoral or central vein catheterization.

Pain relief during the postoperative period should be appropriate for the degree of pain and end with the resolution of the acute surgical condition. Methadone maintenance can be instituted for more gradual opiate withdrawal. Complete reviews of the anesthetic management of addicted patients are available.[514-516]

RENAL AND GASTROINTESTINAL EFFECTS

Renal

Morphine has significant antidiuretic properties, which may be due to a release of ADH.[403,517] Kappa agonists elicit a free water diuresis by inhibiting the secretion of or altering the response to ADH. However, in humans morphine-induced release of ADH does not occur except in unusual circumstances (i.e., when nausea and vomiting occur) or during surgical stimulation in lightly anesthetized patients.[518,519] Antidiuresis after morphine administration has been attributed to a decrease in renal blood flow and glomerular filtration rate (GFR).[405,517] Yet, in a study comparing halothane and high-dose morphine anesthetics, intraoperative and postoperative urine outputs of 61 patients undergoing similar open heart operations did not differ.[155] Furthermore, under controlled clinical conditions, morphine had no effect on GFR, urine osmolarity, or urine output.[520] However, the addition of 60 percent nitrous oxide or a more rapid administration of morphine, so that arterial blood pressure and cardiac output were reduced, markedly diminished all tests of renal function. In supine normovolemic, normocapnic dogs, morphine does reduce urine output and increases urine osmolarity despite its minimal effects on cardiovascular dynamics.[521] These data suggest that morphine increases blood levels of ADH in the dog. It appears that morphine is not an antidiuretic in supine normovolemic, normocarbic humans,[9,30] whereas it is in the dog. In the absence of surgery, morphine does not stimulate release of ADH in humans. If renal function does change during opioid anesthesia and surgery, it is probably due to secondary changes in systemic and renal hemodynamics. Giving morphine to patients whose urinary bladders are not catheterized, however, may cause a decrease in urine output via an increase in detrusor and urethral sphincter tone, resulting in retention of urine in the bladder.

Increases in urine volume and decreases in urinary sodium excretion and urine osmolality have been reported during fentanyl-oxygen anesthesia. Hunter et al.[522] reported decreases in renal plasma flow, GFR, and urine volume and increases in renovascular resistance in dogs anesthetized with nitrous oxide after 25 μg/kg of fentanyl. These changes were not altered by correction of bradyarrhythmias with atropine. Kien et al.[523] also noted a 25 percent decrease in renal cortical blood flow that paralleled changes in blood pressure, suggesting impairment of autoregulation. Unfortunately, dogs in that study were also receiving halothane. Morphine and meperidine, on the other hand, have been reported to decrease renovascular resistance.[160,524] The relevance of these animal studies is unclear in light of the presence of background anesthetics and species differences. Absence of increases in plasma ADH, renin, and aldosterone as well as hemodynamic stability indicate that fentanyl as well as sufentanil and alfentanil anesthesia most likely preserves or minimally alters renal function in humans.[222,506]

Gastrointestinal

Motility

Opioids alter lower esophageal sphincter (LES) activity, resulting in sphincter relaxation.[525] This probably accounts for the unreliability of spontaneous LES contractions as predictors of patient movement in response to skin incision when opioid-based anesthetics are used,[526] as opposed to potent inhaled anesthetics.[527]

Gastric emptying is delayed by opiates via central (vagus nerve) and peripheral (opiate receptors in the myenteric plexus and cholinergic nerve terminals) mechanisms.[528] Morphine and related opioids inhibit electrically evoked release of acetylcholine from nerves in the gastrointestinal tract. Even small doses of alfentanil (5 μg/kg) slow gastric emptying, but for a shorter period than morphine. Mixed agonist-antagonist-type drugs also delay gastric emptying.[529] Naloxone reverses opioid-induced delays in gastric emptying,[530] but metoclopromide does not.[531] The decrease in gastrointestinal motility after opioid administration explains their use as antidiarrheal agents. Whether opioid administration prior to a rapid sequence anesthetic induction increases the risk of pulmonary aspiration of gastric contents is unknown (also see Ch. 40).

Opioid effects on the intestine are complex. The ileum appears to be less sensitive to opioids than the jejunum. In fact, morphine enhances ileal propulsion before decreasing motility. As a result mouth to ileum transit time may not be significantly altered.[532] Opioid effects on the ileum are blocked by naloxone and are thus receptor mediated.[532] Opioids increase tone and decrease propulsive activity in most of the intestine (small and large). Electromyographically this is reflected by an increase in rhythmic stationary (tone) bursts and a decrease in sporadic (propagating) bursts. Some clinicians believe opioids may be indicated during surgical construction of a continent urinary reservoir because they are superior to anticholinergic drugs for terminal ileal relaxation.[533] Gastrointestinal secretions are usually increased by opioids.

Biliary Tree

All opioid agonists increase biliary duct pressure and sphincter of Oddi (choledochoduodenal sphincter) tone in a dose-dependent manner through opiate receptor-mediated mechanisms.[534–536] Duration of this action is highly correlated to plasma opioid levels (Fig. 10-11). Ultrasonic verification of morphine-induced spasm of the common bile duct exists.[537] The clinical importance of opioid-induced increases in biliary tract pressure is unknown. However, the small absolute increases in biliary pressure after opioids[538] and only a 3 percent incidence of failed intraoperative cholangiograms during fentanyl-supplemented (up to 10 μg/kg) anesthesia suggests that clinical consequences of opioid-induced increases in biliary tract pressure are minimal.[539] Opioid-induced biliary spasm rarely produces severe epigastric pain that can be confused with cholecystitis or cardiac ischemia.[540]

Meperidine has a dual effect on the biliary tract that is not receptor mediated.[541] Meperidine produces an inhibitory effect on the response of the common bile duct to electrical stimulation (antimuscarinic mechanism). Higher concentrations produce an excitatory effect and increase spontaneous contractions via direct smooth muscle stimulation. Neither of these responses is affected by naloxone. Despite these contrasting actions, meperidine increases biliary pressure in humans.

Although some reports suggest that mixed agonist-antagonist opioids like nalbuphine and butorphanol can increase biliary pressure as much as pure agonists,[538] most studies show that they produce less or little pressure change.[534,542,543] Increases in biliary pressure caused by opioids are, with the exception of meperidine, reversible with naloxone.[541,543] Glucagon (1 to 3 mg carefully titrated) also reverses opioid-induced biliary spasm.

Intestinal Circulation

The effects of opioids on intestinal circulation are complex and not completely understood. Low doses of morphine (0.5 to 1.0 mg/kg) increase intestinal blood flow (perhaps secondary to histamine release), while high doses (1 to 3 mg/kg) decrease flow.[160,544,545] Decreases in blood flow after morphine are likely related to hypotension or increases in plasma catecholamines. Fentanyl increases intestinal blood flow in a dose-dependent fashion. The increase in blood flow coupled with a substantial and dose-related decrease in intestinal oxygen uptake represents a state of "luxury perfusion" that has been hypothesized to possibly increase mesenteric and portal venous oxygen content, thereby improving hepatic oxygen supply.[544] The clinical significance of opioid-induced increases in gastrointestinal circulation is unknown.[546]

Hepatic

The effect of opioids on liver function during anesthesia and surgery is unknown. Fentanyl produces mild postanesthetic liver dysfunction in rats that is independent of the presence of cirrhosis.[547] These changes are similar to those caused by potent inhaled anesthetics (also see Ch. 6). There is evidence that fentanyl, as well as

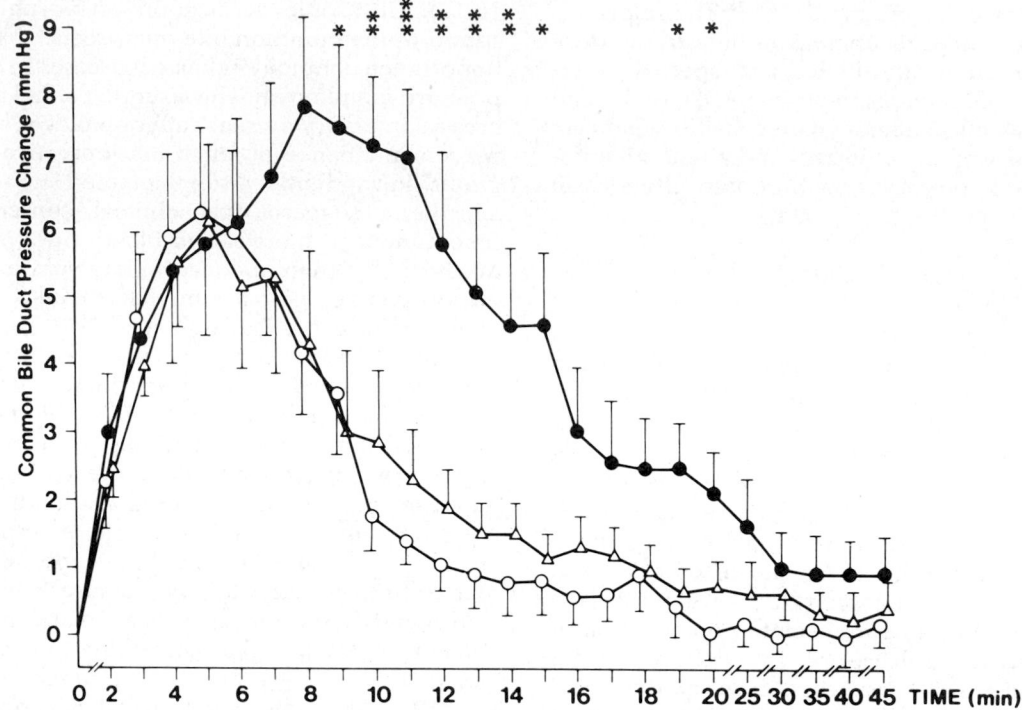

Fig. 10-11. Changes in common bile duct pressure after administration of alfentanil (7.5 [O] and 15 [Δ] μg/kg) and fentanyl (1.5 [●] μg/kg) (mean values ± standard error of the mean). Statistically significant differences in changes from baselines among the groups are indicated as follows: *, $P < 0.05$; **, $P < 0.01$; ***, $P < 0.001$. (From Hynynen et al.,[535] with permission.)

other anesthetics, can produce hepatic injury.[548] Bromosulfophthalein excretion by the liver is decreased by morphine in rats.[549] Morphine, fentanyl, and other narcotics can also increase the levels of other drugs whose elimination is limited by hepatic blood flow.[550]

Nausea and Vomiting

Narcotic analgesics usually increase the incidence of nausea and vomiting when used in the perioperative period. The physiology and prevention of nausea and

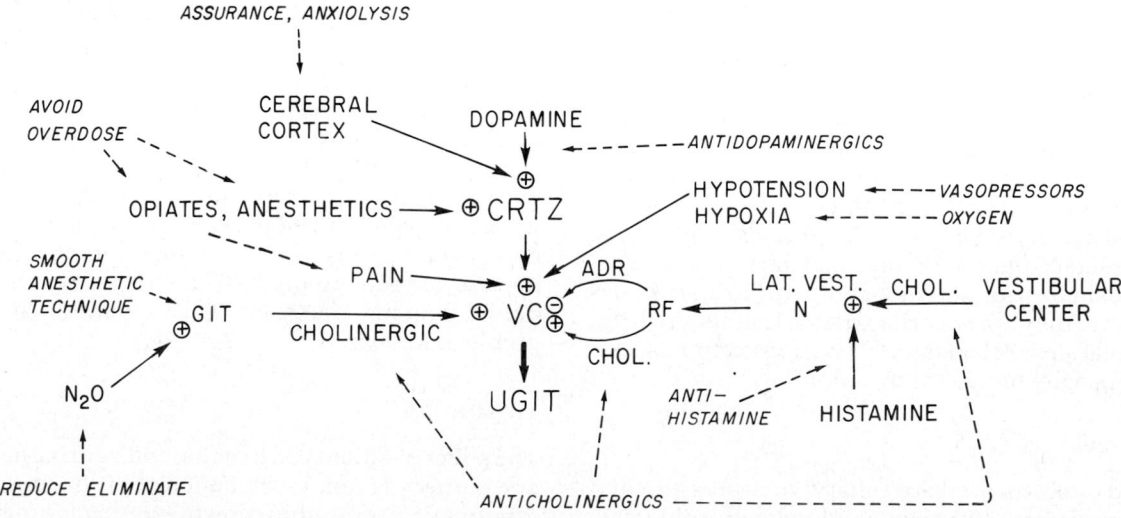

Fig. 10-12. Physiology of emesis. The chemoreceptor trigger zone (CRTZ) and the vomiting center (VC) stimulate the upper gastrointestinal tract (UGIT), resulting in emesis. Cholinergic (CHOL.) and dopaminergic pathways are integral, and a host of factors influence nausea and vomiting through these and other mechanisms. LAT. VEST. N., lateral vestibular nucleus; RF, reticular formation; ADR, adrenergic.

vomiting is summarized in Fig. 10-12. Opioids stimulate the chemoreceptor trigger zone in the area postrema of the medulla.[551] They also increase gastrointestinal secretions[515] and decrease gastrointestinal tract activity and prolong emptying times.[40] All of these actions promote nausea and vomiting. Harris[552] and colleagues postulate that opioids also have antiemetic properties and that this is related to the existence of both emetic and antiemetic brain centers possessing different opiate receptor profiles.

Some drugs can reduce the incidence of nausea and vomiting (also see Ch. 65). Some of the more efficacious agents commonly used in anesthesia are (1) drugs with anticholinergic activity, in particular scopolamine (intramuscularly, intravenously, or as a transdermal patch) and to a lesser degree atropine. Glycopyrrolate is not effective because it does not penetrate the brain. (2) Butyrophenones, in particular, droperidol (0.005 to 0.07 mg/kg intravenously), are most likely effective owing to their antidopaminergic properties. (3) Dopamine antagonists, in particular, metoclopromide (0.1 to 0.3 mg/kg intravenously), which act both centrally at the chemoreceptor trigger zone and peripherally on the gastrointestinal tract. Metoclopramide has a rapid onset but is short acting and thus more effective if administered at the end of an anesthetic. A drug with similar actions, domperidone, may be more effective, but is not currently available in the United States.

OTHER OPIOID EFFECTS
Allergic and Adverse Reactions

True allergic reactions to opioids are rare.[553] Patients often complain of being "allergic" to narcotics because of side effects, for example, pruritus. Fentanyl and meperidine have been associated with anaphylactic-type reactions[554,555] and positive intradermal skin tests. Systemic anaphylactoid reactions to opioids rarely occur. More commonly local reactions occur and are thought to be caused by preservatives or by release of histamine. Ampules of fentanyl do not contain preservatives; however, vials of fentanyl do contain methylparasept and propylparasept.

Monoamine oxidase inhibitors (MAOIs) when simultaneously administered with meperidine can cause agitation, labile arterial blood pressure, hyperpyrexia, rigidity, convulsions, respiratory depression, hypotension, and coma. The mechanism(s) of these responses may be related to increases in cerebral serotonin since meperidine blocks the neuronal uptake of serotonin. Meperidine should not be used in patients receiving MAOIs. Morphine or fentanyl are probably safer.

Reproductive and Teratogenic Effects
(Also See Ch. 6)

Fentanyl as well as sufentanil and alfentanil do not result in reproductive abnormalities or teratogenic effects in rats.[556,557] Although older studies implicate morphine, meperidine, and methadone as teratogenic drugs,[558-562] the results may have been caused by concomitant respiratory depression.[557] Fentanyl (50 to 100 μg) has no effect on uterine blood flow, uterine tone, or maternal/fetal acid-base balance in sheep.[563] Fetal plasma fentanyl concentrations peak rapidly (5 minutes) after maternal intravenous injection but do not reach maternal plasma levels.[563] Newborns of addicted mothers can exhibit narcotic withdrawal and require observation and appropriate treatment.

ANESTHETIC TECHNIQUES
(Also See Ch. 42)

Balanced Anesthesia

The concept of balanced anesthesia dates back to 1910, when George W. Crile introduced his theory of anociassociation.[564] Crile taught that psychic stimuli associated with operations could be prevented by light general anesthesia, while painful stimuli could be blocked by local analgesia. The term *balanced anesthesia* was introduced by Lundy in 1926.[7] Lundy suggested that a balance of agents and techniques (e.g., premedication, regional anesthesia, general anesthesia with one or more drugs) be used to produce the different components of anesthesia (i.e., analgesia, amnesia, muscle relaxation, and abolition of autonomic reflexes with maintenance of homeostasis)[565] (Fig. 10-13).

The introduction of *d*-tubocurarine in 1942 enabled anesthesiologists to obtain relatively controllable muscle relaxation without very deep levels of anesthesia.[566] Several techniques of balanced anesthesia were described involving induction of anesthesia with thiopental, maintenance with nitrous oxide and oxygen supple-

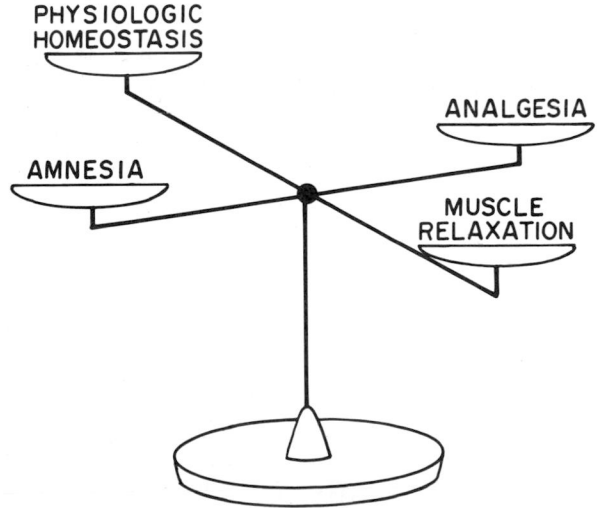

Fig. 10-13. Balanced anesthesia: addressing the four components of anesthesia.

mented with small additional doses of thiopental, and muscle relaxation with *d*-tubocurarine.[567,568] However, the combination of thiopental and nitrous oxide did not always provide sufficient analgesia for reliable prevention of unwanted sympathetic simulation during surgery. To achieve additional analgesia, Neff et al.[8] introduced meperidine as a supplement during nitrous oxide anesthesia in the United States in 1947. Two years later, a similar technique was introduced in Great Britain by Mushin and Rendell-Baker.[569] These techniques rapidly achieved widespread popularity, and many individual variations using meperidine[569,570] and other opioids were described.[571,572] Fentanyl and more recently sufentanil and alfentanil have become popular as intravenous supplements during general anesthesia with nitrous oxide and various combinations of intravenous and inhaled anesthetics.[29,334,347,573] In a double-blind comparison of fentanyl, phenoperidine, and morphine in combination with nitrous oxide for general anesthesia, little difference could be discerned among the drugs.[347] Others have found some opioids preferable over others.[574]

Although differences between opioids tend to be obscured when they are combined with other anesthetics, certain advantages may persist.[29,575] The course of anesthesia tends to be associated with less fluctuation in cardiovascular dynamics.[206] In addition, opioids decrease requirements for inhaled anesthetics[576] (presumably reducing their side effects and toxicity) and provide postoperative analgesia. Residual concentrations of potent inhaled anesthetics are poor analgesics. The use of opioids is particularly advantageous in operations involving sudden painful manipulations, such as the retraction of visceral organs during intra-abdominal surgery. Anticipation of these events and prior supplementation with a small dose of an opioid (e.g., 50 to 100 μg of fentanyl or 5 to 10 μg/kg alfentanil intravenously) will often be sufficient to prevent increases in arterial blood pressure and heart rate associated with these manipulations. Proper anticipation of a stimulus requires that any opioid be administered several minutes before that stimulus to be effective. Once the stress response is activated and catecholamines are released, opioids are much less effective in maintaining hemodynamic stability.[574] However, it is important that the timing and dose of supplemental opioid be tailored to the specific condition of the patient and the expected duration of the operation to avoid problems. The duration of action and magnitude of effect of an opioid are determined not only by its pharmacokinetic properties but by the timing, dosage, and interaction of the drug with other compounds being used as well as patient factors such as pain, cardiac and urine output, and carbon dioxide levels (see below). Giving a large dose of any opioid shortly before the end of surgery is very likely to result in postoperative respiratory depression or potentiate and prolong already existing respiratory depression.

Opioids as Supplements to the Induction of General Anesthesia

The perioperative administration of opioids provides analgesia and helps to produce a more desirable cardiovascular profile (see the section, *Cardiovascular Actions*).[577-581] Opioids can also decrease the hemodynamic response to a rapid sequence induction. The administration of fentanyl (3 to 7 μg/kg) or sufentanil (0.4 to 1.0 μg/kg)[582-584] several minutes before anesthetic induction can attenuate or eliminate changes in heart rate, blood pressure, PCWP, and other aspects of the stress response (e.g., increases plasma catecholamine concentration) that occur during laryngoscopy and intubation. Fentanyl and sufentanil also reduce the dose of thiopental required for loss of consciousness.[577,578,581] Opioids also reduce increases in heart rate associated with the use of potent inhalational anesthesia.[581] The administration of opioids prior to induction of anesthesia augments the cardiovascular-depressant effects of most induction agents, and reduced doses of these drugs are usually indicated.[580,582] In addition, timing of the administration of the opioid is important. For example, the peak effect of alfentanil occurs sooner, but is shorter lasting than that of fentanyl.

The indications for and merits of balanced anesthesia have often been questioned.[585] The factors that contribute to its popularity and the most popular techniques are reviewed below.

Important anesthetic considerations include the type and duration of surgery, the medical status of the patient, and the medications being taken. This section does not address these issues but rather attempts to define the advantages and disadvantages of narcotic analgesics in balanced anesthesia and explain how they may best be used.

Fentanyl

Fentanyl has become popular as an intravenous supplement during inhalational anesthesia. Anesthetic induction is usually achieved with a loading dose of fentanyl (2 to 8 μg/kg) followed by thiopental (1 to 4 mg/kg) and a muscle relaxant. Nitrous oxide (60 to 70 percent) in oxygen plus additional fentanyl (intermittent boluses of 25 to 50 μg every 15 to 60 minutes or a constant infusion of 0.5 to 3.0 μg/kg/h) is often used to maintain anesthesia. Shorter cases may require lower bolus doses or infusion rates.[586] Premedication with a benzodiazepine or another sedative-hypnotic reduces the need for supplements with this technique. Low concentrations of potent inhaled anesthetics (e.g., 0.2 to 0.4 percent isoflurane) are sometimes employed for short periods to avoid administering higher doses of opioids, which may increase the incidence of troublesome postoperative respiratory depression and requirements for narcotic antagonists.

Fentanyl plasma concentrations of 1.0 to 2.0 ng/ml

provide analgesia,[587] but levels of at least 2 to 3 ng/ml are usually required during surgery (at sea level) if the only inhaled anesthetic is nitrous oxide. Higher plasma opioid concentrations may be necessary at higher altitude.[588,589] Unfortunately, patient pharmacokinetics vary so much (up to fivefold) that predicting plasma levels after a given dose of an opioid is extremely difficult. Pharmacodynamic actions are equally variable; the opioid plasma concentration necessary to block increases in blood pressure and heart rate is often unpredictable.[202,587,590,591]

A balanced technique with fentanyl, titrating the opioid in anticipation of various stimuli and patient responses with pharmacokinetic guidelines in mind,* will often result in a stable hemodynamic course and rapid awakening in a pain-free patient.

Sufentanil

Sufentanil compares quite favorably to other opioids when used in a balanced anesthetic technique. In a similar fashion to fentanyl, pharmacokinetic guidelines as well as clinical experience suggest that sufentanil (0.25 to 1.0 μg/kg) plus thiopental (1 to 4 mg/kg) to produce loss of consciousness can result in a smooth induction of anesthesia. Maintenance of anesthesia is achieved with nitrous oxide (60 to 70 percent) in oxygen and further sufentanil (intermittent boluses of 0.1 to 0.25 μg/kg or constant infusion of 0.25 to 1.5 μg/kg/h). The mean sufentanil plasma concentration that is effective in blocking responses to endotracheal intubation in 50 percent of patients breathing 66 percent nitrous oxide in oxygen has been reported to be 1.08 ng/ml (range, 0.73 to 2.55 ng/ml).[592] During surgery, levels less than 0.5 ng/ml lead to an increased need for supplements.[582] Levels less than 0.25 ng/ml will often allow for adequate spontaneous ventilation.[592] Sufentanil in a balanced technique may produce greater hemodynamic stability and the need for fewer supplements than alfentanil.[593] A more rapid recovery of respiratory function also occurs with sufentanil compared to fentanyl.[594,595]

Alfentanil

Alfentanil can be used in multiple ways in balanced anesthesia. Small doses (5 to 25 μg/kg) used to supple-

ment a barbiturate induction of anesthesia help to attenuate hemodynamic responses to laryngoscopy and endotracheal intubation. Large doses (50 to 150 μg/kg) may be used with or without thiopental to induce anesthesia (Fig. 10-14). The loss of verbal response ED_{50} for alfentanil in young unpremedicated adults is 111 μg/kg.[209] Anesthesia is often maintained after such an induction with 60 to 70 percent nitrous oxide and an alfentanil infusion of 0.5 to 3.0 μg/kg/min. Intermittent boluses of alfentanil (5 to 10 μg/kg) may be used as an alternative to infusions for shorter procedures or superimposed on infusions in anticipation of the need for a higher plasma level. A bolus of 7 μg/kg will increase plasma alfentanil concentrations by 50 ng/ml (range, 20 to 100 ng/ml) if a relatively steady plasma level of alfentanil already exists. Alfentanil infusions should be terminated 15 to 30 minutes before the end of surgery[596,597] to avoid problematic residual respiratory depression. Several essential considerations when using alfentanil include the following. (1) Redistribution of the drug rapidly lowers plasma levels after an induction bolus and failure to quickly institute nitrous oxide and an alfentanil infusion may lead to inadequate anesthesia at the time of surgical incision[596] (Fig. 10-15). (2) The duration of surgery and strength of the surgical stimulus are important influences on alfentanil requirements. Ausems et al.[597] have determined the plasma concentrations of alfentanil required to supplement nitrous oxide anesthesia for several types of surgery. The Cp_{50}s (concentrations needed to adequately obtund responses to stimuli in 50 percent of patients) for several stimuli are listed in Table 10-14. The Cp_{50} for spontaneous ventilation was 223 $\pm$ 13 ng/ml. Interestingly, the more potent the stimulus, the greater the variability in

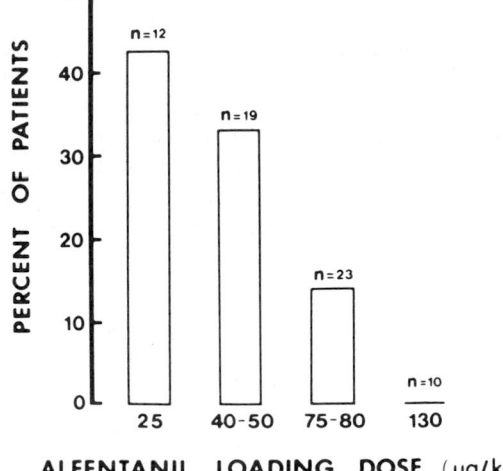

Fig. 10-14. Percentage of patients requiring additional pentothal to produce loss of consciousness after various alfentanil doses plus 2 mg/kg thiopental. (From Shafer et al.,[626] with permission.)

---

* To estimate drug requirements for a loading dose, the target concentration (e.g., plasma level) is multiplied by the volume of distribution. For example, if one wished to establish a fentanyl plasma level of 2 ng/ml (or 2 μg/L) for balanced anesthesia in a 70-kg patient, multiplication of the weight in kilograms (70) times the volume of distribution at steady state (4.0 L/kg) results in a calculated loading dose of approximately 550 μg or 11 ml. Similarly, a maintenance dose for fentanyl in the same patient could be calculated by multiplying the plasma level desired (2 ng/ml) by the clearance rate or 2 $\times$ 0.015 L/kg/min $\times$ 60 min/h or 1.8 μg/kg/h.

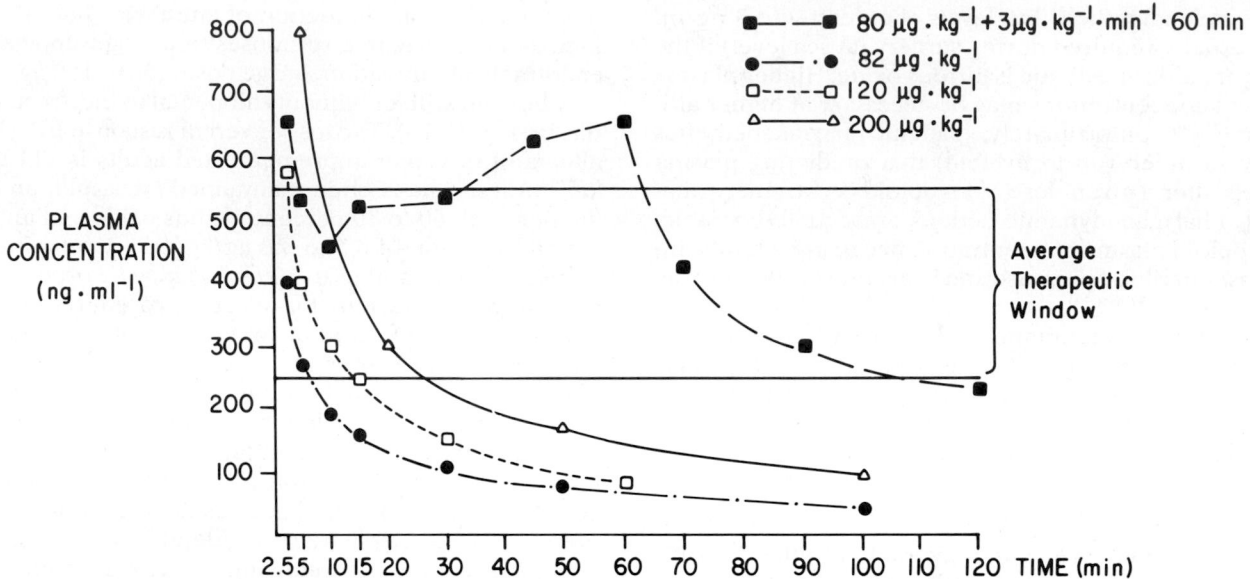

Fig. 10-15. Plasma alfentanil levels after three different bolus injections and one bolus plus continuous infusion for 1 hour.

the Cp_{50}. This is depicted in the flatter curve for upper abdominal surgery in Fig. 10-16. These numbers define target plasma concentrations. However, because of considerable variability in effective concentrations (1.6- to 3.3-fold), clinicians must still titrate both alfentanil infusions and/or the frequency and magnitude of boluses to clinical response.

Which Are the Better Opioids for Balanced Anesthesia?

Many studies have compared one opioid with another in a balanced anesthetic technique.[348,410,593,594,595,598–607] Fewer studies have compared three or more opioids in a balanced anesthetic technique.[122,347,574] Fentanyl and alfentanil have been frequently compared.[410,599,606] Some clinicians believe the rapid speed of onset with alfentanil is an attractive advantage. Intraoperative differences between fentanyl and alfentanil are few, although many clinicians are of the opinion that alfentanil produces greater decreases in heart rate and arterial blood pressure during induction of anesthe-

TABLE 10-14. Stimuli and Corresponding Cp_{50}

Stimulus	Cp_{50} (ng/ml) (mean ± SE)
Intubation	475 ± 28
Skin incision	279 ± 20
Skin closure	150 ± 23
Breast surgery	270 ± 63
Lower abdominal surgery	309 ± 44
Upper abdominal surgery	412 ± 135

(From Ausems et al.,[597] with permission.)

sia.[410,601] Although some investigators report no significant differences between these two drugs with regards to emergence,[603] most studies find alfentanil results in a more rapid recovery and a lesser need for reversal with naloxone.[410,599,601,602,605,606]

Studies comparing fentanyl and sufentanil indicate that sufentanil provides greater intraoperative hemodynamic stability,[598] more rapid emergence,[594] and less respiratory depression in the immediate postoperative period than fentanyl.[594,595] Compared with alfentanil, sufentanil may provide greater hemodynamic stability and the need for less supplementation.[593] Flacke et al.[574] compared morphine, meperidine, fentanyl, and sufentanil in a balanced anesthetic for general or orthopaedic surgery. Patients were premedicated with diazepam (5 to 10 mg) and droperidol (0.5 mg) and were anesthetized with equipotent doses of the narcotics (double blind) equivalent to 7.5 μg/kg of fentanyl plus thiopental (1 to 4 mg/kg). Anesthesia was maintained with nitrous oxide (60 to 67 percent) in oxygen and supplemental doses of opioids or thiopental as needed. Potent inhaled anesthetics were added if narcotic supplementation was inadequate. Hemodynamic and plasma catecholamine changes were greatest with morphine and meperidine and least with sufentanil. Only patients receiving sufentanil as the opioid component of their anesthetic never required supplementation with a potent inhaled anesthetic. Approximately one-third of patients in each of the other groups required such supplementation. Meperidine produced the most side effects, for example, hypotension, tachycardia, urticaria, especially during induction. Upon emergence, respiratory depression was greatest with morphine and least with fentanyl and sufentanil. While 41 percent of patients

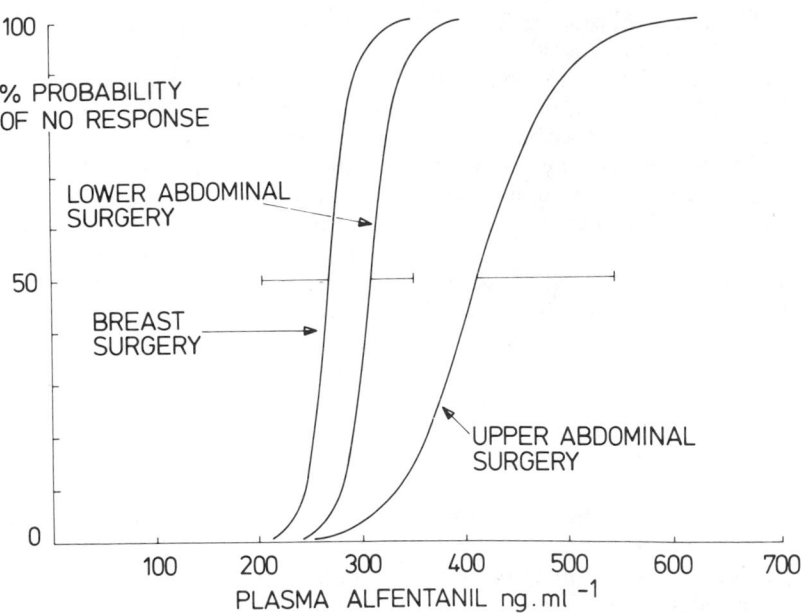

Fig. 10-16. Mean alfentanil plasma concentration-effect curves for the intraoperative period in each surgical group of patients during nitrous oxide anesthesia. The Cp_{50} and slope of these curves were determined by averaging the estimates of individual patients. Bar indicates standard deviation of Cp_{50}. (From Ausems et al.,[597] with permission.)

receiving sufentanil required naloxone, one dose (1.5 μg/kg) was always sufficient to restore adequate spontaneous ventilation. Others[122] have reported similar results in comparisons of these four opioids. These data suggest that fentanyl and sufentanil are preferable to morphine or meperidine in balanced anesthesia.[122,574]

Neuroleptanalgesia-Anesthesia

In 1949, Laborit and Huygenard[608] introduced the concept of an anesthetic technique that blocked not only cerebrocortical responses but also some cellular, endocrine, and autonomic mechanisms usually activated by surgical stimulation. This state was called *ganglioplegia* or *neuroplegia* (artificial hibernation) and was achieved by the use of a lytic cocktail consisting of chlorpromazine, promethazine, and meperidine. From this idea, De Castro and Mundeleer[575] derived the concept of neuroleptanalgesia, which involved the combination of a major tranquilizer (usually the butyrophenone droperidol) and a potent opioid analgesic (fentanyl or phenoperidine) to produce a detached, pain-free state of immobilization and insensitivity to pain. Neuroleptanalgesia is characterized by analgesia, absence of clinically apparent motor activity, suppression of autonomic reflexes, maintenance of cardiovascular stability, and amnesia in most but not all patients. The addition of an inhaled anesthetic, usually nitrous oxide, improves amnesia and analgesia and has been called neuroleptanesthesia.

Neuroleptic drugs traditionally include the phenothiazines (e.g., chlorpromazine) and the butyrophenones (e.g., haloperidol, droperidol). The phenothiazines are rarely used as an anesthetic adjuvant in the United States because of associated hypotension. Droperidol can also cause hypotension, but it is usually less severe and transient. Sedation after droperidol, especially 0.1 mg/kg or more, may last much longer than the analgesic used (e.g., fentanyl) and result in a patient who is apparently calm yet suffering from pain and mental anguish.[576] The commercial preparation of droperidol-fentanyl (Innovar) is the combination used to produce neuroleptanesthesia, although many other combinations are possible. One of Innovar's side effects includes an extrapyramidal syndrome with face and neck dyskinesia, oculogyric crisis, torticollis, agitation, and hallucinations.[576,609] Droperidol, like other butyrophenones, affects GABA receptors and alters the balance of dopamine and acetylcholine in certain brain sites. Droperidol's effects on dopamine receptors (antidopaminergic) not only account for much of its behavioral effects but for its side effects as well.[610]

Onset of effect after intravenous administration of droperidol is rapid (5 to 10 minutes). Administering droperidol alone without analgesics or other sedatives often produces feelings of discomfort or dysphoria in patients. The cardiovascular effects of droperidol are most often limited to mild hypotension that is thought to be mediated through α-adrenergic blockade.[611] Droperidol has an antiarrhythmic action that is effective during halothane anesthesia or following epinephrine-induced arrhythmias.[612-614] Droperidol may be of some benefit in patients with Wolff-Parkinson-White syndrome.[615] There is little respiratory depression induced by droperidol, although significant variability exists and occasional respiratory depression may be noted. Droperidol and other butyrophenones may enhance hypoxia-induced increases in ventilation in humans owing to their antidopaminergic effects at the carotid body.[616]

Droperidol can be used as a premedicant (0.025 to 0.075 mg/kg intramuscularly), an antiemetic (0.01 to 0.02 mg/kg intravenously), an adjunct for awake intubations (0.025 to 0.1 mg/kg intravenously), and as treatment for agitated, belligerent, or psychotic patients (0.05 to 0.2 mg/kg intravenously or intramuscularly). Neuroleptanalgesia with droperidol and a narcotic such as fentanyl is useful for monitored anesthesia care during ophthalmic surgery, endoscopic and bronchoscopic examinations, neurodiagnostic procedures, and excision of epileptogenic foci. Combining alfentanil (5 μg/kg as a bolus and/or an infusion at 1.5 μg/kg/min) with droperidol and nitrous oxide has been reported to be useful in providing patient comfort for awake craniotomies. Rapid changes in the level of sedation are easily controlled, and rigidity, apnea, and hypoxia have not been noted.[617] Supplementation with Innovar may also be of benefit during regional anesthesia.

Neuroleptanesthesia with droperidol and fentanyl has also proved useful in patients undergoing neurologic, cardiac, and general surgical procedures.[618-621] Neuroleptanesthesia has also been used effectively in neurosurgery to reduce CSF pressure in patients with and without space-occupying lesions.[622] Contraindications to neuroleptanalgesia or neuroleptanesthesia include patients receiving MAOIs, those abusing drugs or alcohol, or those with Parkinson's disease.

Continuous Infusions
(Also See Ch. 11)

Continuous infusions of fentanyl, sufentanil, and alfentanil have been evaluated as alternatives to intermittent bolus techniques in anesthesia and numerous advantages have been documented.[590,623-625] (Table 10-15). The main limitation of this approach remains the large variability in opioid requirements.[626] Some anesthesiologists prefer to administer large intravenous boluses of opioids, thus producing high plasma concentrations that are effective for nearly all stimuli. The high therapeutic index of most opioids permits this approach. In addition, in cardiac anesthesia where the application of high doses of opioids first achieved popularity, significant postoperative respiratory depression is not a problem because of mandatory postoperative mechanical ventilation. However, the use of opioids as a key component of anesthesia in many other surgical areas is most often limited by the potential for troublesome depression of ventilatory drive. For this reason, as well as others reviewed below, some anesthesiologists believe that limiting the dose of opioids, as well as optimizing their use, is better achieved by administering a loading bolus dose followed by a continuous infusion.

The principles and details of pharmacokinetics as applied to intravenous drugs are discussed in Chapters 2 and 11. Recent reviews[627] also give useful details. In essence, a loading dose (given rapidly or over several minutes) quickly establishes a target plasma level. It can be simply determined by multiplying the space to be filled (either the initial volume of distribution or the steady state volume of distribution) times the desired concentration. An infusion attempts to maintain that concentration. Various calculations can be used to maintain the ideal plasma concentration but the objective is the same: to replace the drug removed (by redistribution and metabolism) from the volume that was loaded.[628-633] Multiplying the desired plasma concentration by the clearance has been suggested to adequately estimate continuous infusion dosage. Continuous infusions are often slowed decrementally not only to seek the lowest effective concentration but also to avoid opioid accumulation when redistribution of the drug declines as the peripheral compartment is filled. The necessity or presumed benefits of invoking complicated pharmacokinetic equations have been questioned as unduly cumbersome and complicated.[634] Titration, based on a dose-response relationship with limited attention to pharmacokinetic equations or concern about ideal plasma levels, may be equally effective.

Neither morphine nor meperidine plays a significant role in modern anesthetic practice owing to their physical characteristics and higher incidences of side effects. Initial doses for fentanyl and sufentanil, when used as the primary or sole anesthetic, range from 25 to 75 μg/kg and 2 to 20 μg/kg, respectively. When loss of consciousness is ensured by simultaneous administration of other sedative-hypnotics, usually barbiturates or benzodiazepines, lower doses of opioids may be adequate. Infusion rates for fentanyl and sufentanil when used alone vary from 10 to 30 μg/kg/h and 1 to 5 μg/kg/h, respectively. The use of any inhaled anesthetic or other intravenous hypnotic, amnestic, or analgesic significantly reduces the required opioid dose and increases its effect.[635] For example, in superficial surgical procedures, fentanyl (4 to 8 μg/kg followed by a continuous infusion of 2 to 4 μg/kg/h) will often result in ade-

---

TABLE 10-15. Potential Advantages of Continuous Infusions over Intermittent Boluses of Opioids in Anesthesia

1. Decreased total dose
2. Greater hemodynamic stability
3. Decreased side effects, e.g., rigidity
4. Decreased need for supplementation
5. More rapid recovery of consciousness
6. Less respiratory depression and need for antagonists
7. Less pain in the immediate postoperative period
8. Decreased discharge time

quate plasma levels (3 to 6 ng/ml) for anesthesia when combined with nitrous oxide.

Continuous infusions of alfentanil have been extensively evaluated (see the section, *Balanced Anesthesia*). Although large variability exists with regard to the efficacy of a given plasma concentration,[626] target concentrations for numerous stimuli have been delineated (Table 10-14).[597,636] However, many factors will influence the pharmacokinetics and dynamics of alfentanil infusions too (see the section, *Factors Influencing Pharmacokinetics*). In addition, prolonged infusions may result in unpredictable recovery patterns.[637] Rarely, establishing steady state concentrations is impossible.[626] The circumstances in which alfentanil or other opioid-based anesthesia administrated by continuous infusion is appropriate or advantageous continue to be explored.

Large Doses

Morphine

Although fentanyl and sufentanil have supplanted high-dose morphine anesthesia in clinical practice, morphine will be briefly reviewed. Hypotension during induction of anesthesia with morphine (1 to 3 mg/kg) can be reduced by its slow administration over a minimum of 10 to 15 minutes. A 0.1 percent solution of morphine in either dextrose (5 percent) or dextrose-saline is infused at a rate of 5 to 10 mg/min with the patient breathing 100 percent oxygen or oxygen plus nitrous oxide until a satisfactory level of anesthesia is achieved.[20,21,22,38,638] The incidence of hypotension during induction may also be minimized by concurrent administration of a rapid infusion of intravenous fluids,[22] by placing the patient in a modified Trendelenburg position,[22] and/or by pretreatment with histamine (H_1 and H_2)-receptor blockers.[350]

Induction of anesthesia usually requires 1 to 3 mg/kg of morphine[11-13,19,21,22,194] depending on the patient's clinical condition. Larger amounts may be required in patients who have a reasonable cardiac reserve.[22] Since significant respiratory depression will occur before loss of consciousness in most patients, ventilatory assistance and then controlled ventilation are usually required. Often sedative-hypnotic compounds are added before or during administration of morphine to reduce opioid dosage and ensure amnesia.[22] Once unconsciousness has been achieved, a muscle relaxant is given, the trachea is intubated, and ventilation is continued with oxygen, an air-oxygen mixture, or nitrous oxide in oxygen.[19] Careful observation of the patient's response to laryngoscopy and intubation can provide useful information as to the adequacy of anesthesia. Increases in arterial blood pressure and heart rate, muscle or eyelid movement, and furrowing of the forehead all suggest an inadequate depth of anesthesia and are indications for additional morphine and/or intravenous or inhaled anesthetic supplementation before surgery commences. Likewise, reactions to surgical stim-uli can usually be treated by similar interventions or, if the patient is considered to be adequately anesthetized, with intravenous nitroglycerin or sodium nitroprusside or inhaled anesthetics.[12] Problems with intraoperative hemodynamic stability, the need to intervene with vasoactive agents, excessive postoperative respiratory depression, and prolonged emergence have been noted to be more frequent with morphine than with fentanyl or sufentanil.[639,640] Thus, many clinicians prefer high-dose techniques employing fentanyl or sufentanil.

Fentanyl

Many different techniques have been used by clinicians and investigators to achieve anesthesia with fentanyl.[2,117-119,141,145,179,196,197,199,202,253,301,447,460,640-643] A number of premedicants are popular, although most include morphine (0.1 to 0.14 mg/kg intramuscularly), scopolamine (0.4 mg intramuscularly) and/or a benzodiazepine. A defasciculating or priming dose of a nondepolarizing muscle relaxant (see Ch. 12) is usually administered several minutes before a large intravenous bolus of fentanyl to attenuate or prevent opioid-induced rigidity. Intubating doses of nondepolarizing muscle relaxants, usually infused concomitantly with fentanyl over 5 to 10 minutes, can also achieve reductions in rigidity. Bolus injections of fentanyl over short periods (less than 1 minute) range from 15 to 75 µg/kg. Loading doses of 20 to 40 µg/kg establish plasma fentanyl concentrations (10 to 20 ng/ml) that are often sufficient to provide stable hemodynamics throughout the induction-intubation sequence (Fig. 10-7). Some clinicians prefer to rapidly infuse a single large bolus of fentanyl (up to 150 µg/kg) to provide for both the induction and maintenance of anesthesia. Others prefer a lower loading dose of fentanyl followed by a continuous infusion ranging from 0.3 to 1.0 µg/kg/min up to or continuing through cardiopulmonary bypass (Fig. 10-17).

Although some authors suggest that inadequate anesthesia (e.g., hypertensive episodes) can be reduced or eliminated by increasing the fentanyl dose,[197] it remains difficult to predict what plasma fentanyl concentration will reliably block the hemodynamic response to the numerous stimuli that occur (Fig. 10-7).[202] Very high fentanyl doses (greater than 100 µg/kg) prolong ventilator dependency and may increase the need for postoperative vasopressors and fluids. Therefore, numerous supplements (see above) are often used to complement high-dose fentanyl anesthesia.

High-dose fentanyl anesthesia has also proved effective and safe in premature infants for repair of patent ductus arteriosus (up to 50 µg/kg)[644,645] and for pediatric heart surgery (50 to 100 µg/kg).[208,646,647]

Sufentanil

Clinicians have used high doses of sufentanil for coronary artery and cardiac valvular surgery.[201,369,476,648-652] Rigidity can occur during induction of anesthesia with

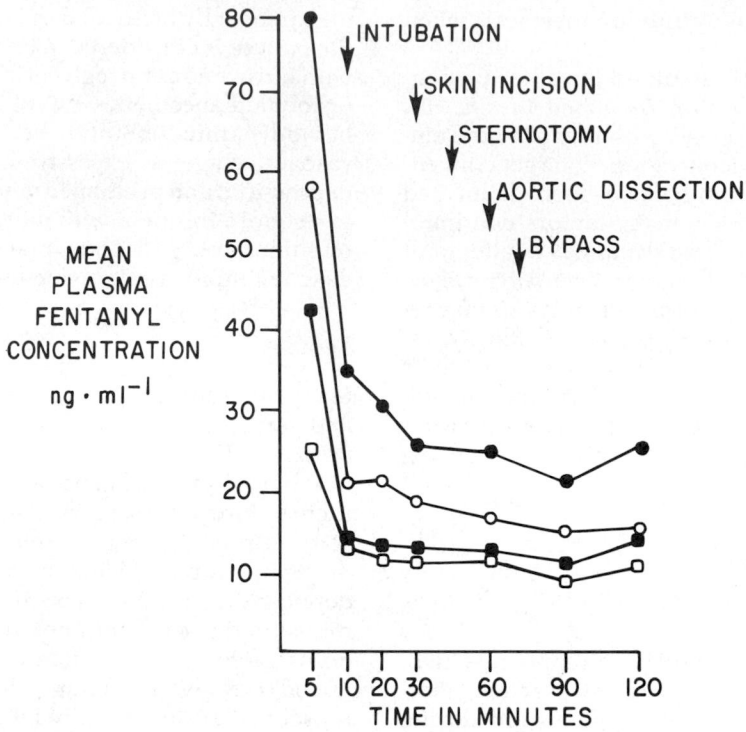

Fig. 10-17. Mean plasma fentanyl concentration (ng/ml) after fentanyl: □, 30 µg/kg followed by 0.3 µg/kg/min; ■, 40 µg/kg followed by 0.4 µg/kg/min; ○, 50 µg/kg followed by 0.5 µg/kg/min; ●, 75 µg/kg followed by 0.75 µg/kg/min. (Composite figure adapted from Wynands et al.[197] and Sprigge et al.,[642] with permission.)

sufentanil, as with fentanyl, and similar precautions are usually taken to avoid it. Induction doses of sufentanil range from 2 to 20 µg/kg administered as a bolus or infused over 2 to 10 minutes. Although larger doses are sometimes administered during or early after induction, many anesthesiologists give additional sufentanil in anticipation of provocative stimuli, that is, before skin incision and sternotomy. Total doses of sufentanil usually range from 15 to 25 µg/kg. Reports of continuous infusion techniques with sufentanil for cardiac surgery are lacking. However, Zurick et al.[369] have shown that infusions of sufentanil are useful for induction of anesthesia. They found the total dose of sufentanil needed was less and emergence was faster with infusion than with multiple bolus techniques. Nevertheless, the ease and efficacy of administering bolus injections of sufentanil for both the induction and maintenance of anesthesia has made the technique popular. On the other hand, no sufentanil technique has been described that completely eliminates hypertensive episodes, and as with fentanyl, numerous supplements are employed. High-dose sufentanil (5 to 20 µg/kg) as well as fentanyl (100 µg/kg) has also been found satisfactory in neuroanesthesia.[653]

Alfentanil

High-dose alfentanil has been less frequently applied as an anesthetic technique for cardiac surgery.[176,211,223,651] Unconsciousness is produced with 50 to 200 µg/kg. Ri-

gidity, bradycardia, and other opioid side effects occur as frequently as after sufentanil and fentanyl. Continuous infusions (2 to 12 µg/kg/min) have been used to maintain adequate plasma alfentanil concentrations (up to 2,000 ng/ml) during cardiac surgery.[223] Hemodynamic control may be more difficult with intermittent bolus techniques using alfentanil.[223]

Newer Applications of Opioids

New systems (i.e., controlled release technology) and sites for delivery (i.e., rectal, nasal and oral mucous membranes, and skin) have the potential to improve patient care by offering improved convenience, less or minimal pain on delivery, better bioavailability, heightened safety, fewer peaks and valleys in drug plasma levels, and, therefore, more effective drug action.

Transdermal Drug Delivery

Although the skin is the largest organ system in the body, until recently it was ignored as a site for systemic drug delivery. Transdermal drug delivery generally requires high solubility in both water and oil, high potency (requiring absorption of only small amounts for clinical effect), and little or no skin irritation.

Fentanyl has these properties and is the first narcotic to be evaluated in a transdermal delivery system. A typical transdermal delivery system consists of a drug reservoir and a rate-controlling membrane. The external surface of the skin-contacting membrane is coated with a drug-compatible adhesive. Advantages of delivering fentanyl transdermally in a rate-controlled fashion for perioperative analgesia include no first-pass metabolism by the liver, improved patient compliance, convenience and comfort, and consistent analgesia. Transdermal fentanyl has not yet been approved by the Food and Drug Administration, but results of clinical trials utilizing fentanyl for postoperative analgesia have been favorable.[654,655]

Because of the difficulties encountered in the passive delivery of drugs through the skin, physical and chemical methods of enhancing transdermal drug delivery are being investigated.[656,657] Iontophoresis is a technique by which passage of drug through the skin is augmented by an external electrical current. Morphine hydrochloride has been delivered iontophoretically for postoperative pain control. Patients who received morphine by iontophoresis required less additional narcotic analgesics than patients receiving a placebo after orthopaedic surgery.[657] After a short delay, plasma morphine levels are directly proportional to the electric current employed in the iontophoretic device.[657] However, electrical burns may occur with present devices because of faulty electrode contact or from current settings that are too high.

Transmucosal Drug Delivery

Although the mucosal membranes of the mouth, tongue, and nose have been utilized as a site for drug delivery (i.e., cocaine, nitroglycerin) for some time, until the past few years these sites have been overlooked as a location for narcotic delivery. Similar to transdermal drug delivery, transmucosal delivery through the oropharynx and nasopharynx eliminates hepatic first-pass metabolism, (drugs are absorbed directly into the systemic circulation) and improves patient comfort (no intramuscular injections), convenience, and compliance. The oral and nasal cavities are rich in blood vessels and lymphatics, thus transmucosal drug absorption is faster and onset of action is more rapid compared with orogastric and transdermal routes. This permits more effective titration of drug to sedative and/or analgesic end points. Possible indications for transmucosal administration include premedication, acute postoperative pain relief, and treatment of chronic pain.

Sites for transmucosal delivery in the mouth include sublingual, buccal, and gingival surfaces. While the sublingual route is easier for patients to use, increased salivary production and swallowing washes some drug down the esophagus, thus limiting its systemic availability. Since dissolution is more rapid sublingually, the buccal site is preferred for slower long-term therapy.

Buprenorphine, a potent, synthetic morphine analogue with a long half-life, is readily absorbed from sublingual mucosal tissues and has been used successfully for premedication and treatment of postoperative and cancer pain.[658-660] Sublingual buprenorphine, given 1 hour preoperatively, provides reliable preoperative sedation and postoperative analgesia similar to intramuscular morphine.[660] In two studies, sublingual buprenorphine (0.4 mg) was compared with conventional intramuscular morphine or meperidine and found to provide satisfactory postoperative analgesia. However, onset of drug effect was slow (3 hours) and thus not effective for the immediate postoperative period.[658,660] Systemic bioavailability after sublingual application is approximately 50 percent of that following intravenous administration.[659]

Initial experience with buccal morphine for postoperative analgesia has been promising. Bell et al.[661] demonstrated that buccal morphine has a 50 percent bioavailability. However, subsequent studies by Fisher et al.[662] have questioned the reliability and systemic availability of buccal morphine administration. Fisher et al.[662] showed that intramuscular morphine provided more effective premedication than a buccal tablet of morphine. Furthermore, 81 percent of patients receiving buccal morphine complained of its bitter taste, and plasma-time curves were markedly different than those reported by Bell et al. In addition, peak plasma levels after buccal morphine were lower (9.1 versus 36.0 ng/ml), time to peak levels was longer (408 versus 60 min), and bioavailability (area under the curve) was less (1.6 versus 14.8 μg-min/ml) than after intramuscular morphine.[661,662] Reasons for these markedly differing results are unclear, but those offered by Fisher et al.[662] include the wide variability in morphine absorption by the buccal route and the poor adherence and dissolution of the tablet on the buccal mucosa in patients with a dry mouth. Bioavailability was six times lower than the same dose given intramuscularly or compared with morphine nebulized to the tracheal mucosa through an endotracheal tube.[663] Morphine's low lipid solubility makes it an unlikely candidate for effective transmucosal absorption (Fig. 10-18). Opioids with a high lipid solubility, such as buprenorphine, fentanyl, and methadone, are more effectively absorbed sublingually than those with low lipid solubilities such as morphine.[664]

A novel transmucosal delivery system for fentanyl has recently been developed by incorporating the drug into a candy lozenge on a stick (lollipop). Initial studies with oral transmucosal fentanyl citrate (OTFC) in volunteers and children have shown this system to produce reliable sedation and anxiolysis when used as a premedication.[665-667] As patients suck on the lozenge, fentanyl is released and presented to the mucosal membranes of the oropharynx for absorption. Increases in plasma fentanyl and onset of clinical effect are rapid (20 to 40 minutes) after OTFC (Fig. 10-19; J. Streisand, unpublished data). Another potential advantage of OTFC is the ease of titration to a sedative or analgesic end point since the lozenge is easily removed from the mouth. This system may improve premedication, acute postoperative analgesia, and chronic pain therapy in various clinical settings.

Delivery of opioids through the nasal mucosa has also been investigated. Henderson et al.[668] administered su-

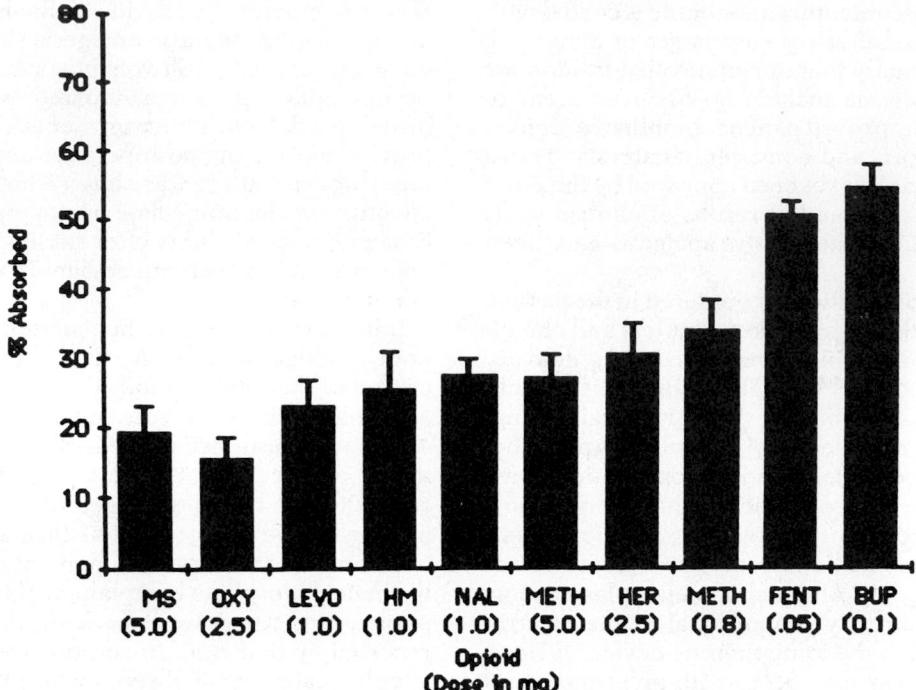

Fig. 10-18. Mean absorption (+ standard error) of various test opioids after 10 minutes in the oral cavity of normal subject (*n* = 10 for each test condition). The pH of the dosing solution was 6.5. MS, morphine sulfate; OXY, oxycodone; LEVO, levorphanol; HM, hydromorphone; NAL, naloxone; METH, methadone; HER, heroin, FENT, fentanyl; BUP, buprenorphine. (From Weinberg et al.,[664] with permission.)

fentanil (1.5, 3.0, 4.5 μg/kg) to 80 children, ranging in age from 6 months to 7 years (also see Ch. 59). Easy separation from parents was achieved in 86 percent of the children 10 minutes following administration of the premedication. Unfortunately, 61 percent of the children cried after administration and side effects included reduced ventilatory compliance (chest wall

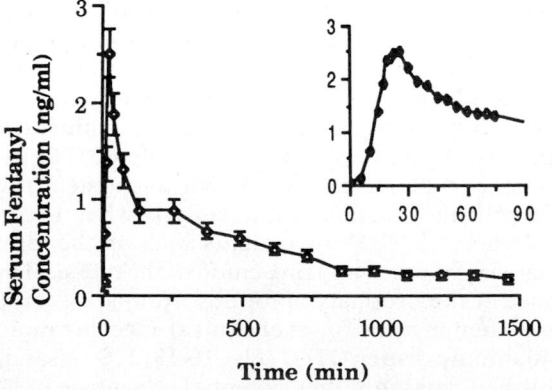

Fig. 10-19. Serum fentanyl concentrations after oral transmucosal fentanyl citrate administration (mean ± standard error of the mean). The inset shows the first 90 minutes in detail. The crosshatched bar beneath the inset shows the oral transmucosal fentanyl citrate consumption time. (Reprinted with permission from J. Streisand, unpublished data.)

rigidity) with higher doses (3.0 and 4.5 μg/kg). Nevertheless, nasal approaches may have value, especially in frightened or uncooperative children. Vercauteren et al.[669] found that a dose of only 10 μg of sufentanil induced moderate sedation without rigidity in 79 percent of healthy adults 20 to 40 minutes after nasal administration. Butorphanol has also been administered nasally. Transnasal butorphanol provides superior and more prolonged analgesia than similar doses given intravenously for postoperative pain after cesarean section.[670]

The rectal mucosa is another site for transmucosal drug delivery. While rectal methohexital is often used for premedication in young children, narcotic analgesics have not been studied until recently. Lindahl et al.[671] have shown that morphine is only poorly absorbed from the rectal mucosa of children. However, new sustained release morphine hydrogel suppositories (MHS) are promising.[672] Two suppositories have been designed. The first releases a bolus and then a smaller quantity of morphine at a constant rate to first raise and then maintain plasma levels. A second sustained-release-only suppository has also been developed to permit administration for successive 12-hour periods after administration of the first type of rectal morphine. Plasma morphine levels after MHS are lower than after intramuscular morphine,[672] but linear analog scales for pain were lower, and the incidence of nausea was reduced after rectal sustained release therapy.[672] Although rectal administration of drugs is complicated by interruption of absorption by defecation, mucosal irritation, variable systemic availability (venous drainage of the rectum is in part portal), and poor patient acceptance, further investigation of MHS seems warranted.

Oral Controlled Release Medications

Controlled, sustained release technology has not been limited to new sites for drug delivery. Despite the high first-pass metabolism seen with the narcotic analgesics, morphine has been formulated into an oral, sustained release tablet (MST) and has been evaluated for premedication,[673] for postoperative analgesia,[674,675] and for alleviating chronic cancer pain.[676] Early clinical trials have suggested that MST provides unreliable preoperative anxiolysis[673] and postoperative pain relief,[674,675] possibly because of impaired gastric emptying and delayed absorption from the small intestine. On the other hand, patients with chronic cancer pain perceived that analgesia was superior and side effects fewer with MST.[676]

OTHER OPIOID AGONISTS

Many other opioid agonists exist, but their use in surgical anesthesia is limited. Codeine (methylmorphine) is one-tenth as potent as morphine and has a high oral-parenteral potency ratio (2:3) and a plasma half-life of 2 to 3 hours. Codeine has modest analgesic but strong cough-suppressant properties after oral administration. Hepatic conversion to morphine (demethylation) probably accounts for codeine's activity.

Heroin (diacetylmorphine) is approximately twice as potent as morphine and has a 4- to 5-hour duration of action. Heroin is rapidly hydrolyzed to monacetylmorphine and then to morphine. These metabolites account for at least a portion of heroin's effects. Heroin is excreted in the urine mostly as free and conjugated morphine. Manufacture and importation of heroin is illegal in the United States.

Hydromorphone (dihydromorphinone or Dilaudid) is structurally related to morphine but is approximately 50 percent more potent. Analgesia after hydromorphone lasts 4 to 5 hours.

Oxymorphone (dehydrohydroxymorphinone or Numorphan) is also structurally related to morphine, is almost 10 times as potent, and has a similar duration of action.

Etorphine and carfentanil are opioids that are used to immobilize wild animals. Each of these compounds is several thousand times more potent than morphine.

Alphaprodine (Nisentil) is a phenylpiperidine derivative that is approximately one-fourth as potent as morphine. Alphaprodine has a rapid onset and a relatively short duration of action (2 hours). Some clinicians compare alphaprodine to meperidine but believe the former causes less less nausea and vomiting. Alphapro-

dine has been a popular analgesic for labor. Unfortunately, respiratory depression (including fetal apneic spells), fetal bradycardia, and depressed progression of labor can occur when the drug is given for analgesia during labor.

Methadone (Dolophine) has a potency and duration of effect equivalent to those of morphine, although repeated doses may produce effects through accumulation. Methadone's efficacy is reduced by 50 percent after oral administration. Its major clinical applications are in the prevention of opioid withdrawal symptoms and in the treatment of chronic pain. It can also provide postoperative pain relief.

AGONIST-ANTAGONIST OPIOIDS

The first recorded specific opioid antagonist was developed in 1914 by Pohl[677] who, in an attempt to improve the analgesic properties of codeine, synthesized N-allyl-norcodeine. He observed that this compound mildly antagonized the respiratory depression and sleep produced by morphine. However, Pohl's discovery went unnoticed for 26 years until McCawley et al.,[678] in a search for a strong analgesic with "built-in" antagonistic action, attempted to prepare N-allylmorphine (nalorphine) in 1940. Nalorphine was successfully synthesized by Weijland and Erickson[679] in 1942 and was found to be strongly antagonistic to almost all the properties of morphine.[680,681] It was also found to possess fairly strong analgesic properties in humans[682] and animals.[683,684] Unfortunately, doses of nalorphine sufficient to produce analgesia were accompanied by severe psychomimetic effects rendering it unsuitable for clinical use as an analgesic. Nalorphine was used in lower doses as an opioid antagonist.

The discovery of nalorphine provided the stimulus for the search for other drugs with combined agonist and antagonist properties. Since 1955 considerable progress has been made toward the development of potent pain-relieving drugs with less of the respiratory-depressant and addictive potential of morphine. Most of the new compounds have only minor molecular modifications of the morphine structure. The agonist-antagonists are usually produced by alkylation of the piperidine nitrogen and addition of a three-carbon side chain such a propyl, allyl, or methylallyl to morphine.[683] Changing the side chain to an amyl group restores agonist activity.

Currently there are four agonist-antagonist opioids in use in the United States: pentazocine, butorphanol, nalbuphine, and buprenorphine. All but buprenorphine are antagonists at the mu receptor and agonists at the kappa and sigma receptors. The differing degrees of interaction at the receptors contribute to the unique hemodynamic and respiratory effects of these compounds (Tables 10-16 and 10-17). Buprenorphine has high affinity but low intrinsic activity at the mu receptor, making it a partial agonist at this site. Its actions at

TABLE 10-16. Hemodynamic Effects of Agonist-Antagonist Compounds Compared with Morphine

Drug	Cardiac Workload	Blood Pressure	Heart Rate	Pulmonary Artery Pressure
Morphine	↓	↓	=↓	=↓
Buprenorphine	↓	↓	↓	?
Butorphanol	↑	=↑	=	↑
Nalbuphine	↓	=	=↓	=
Pentazocine	↑	↑	↑	↑

(From Zola and McLeod,[701] with permission.)

the kappa and sigma receptors are probably minimal. Other investigational drugs similar to buprenorphine include meptazinol, profodol, dezocine, and propiram. Agonist-antagonist opioids are less prone (but not immune) to abuse because they cause less euphoria, drug-seeking behavior, and physical dependence.

Pentazocine

Pentazocine, a benzomorphan derivative, was the first opioid agonist-antagonist to be widely used in humans.[685,686] Pentazocine is one-half to one-fourth as potent as morphine but produces similar degrees of respiratory depression in equipotent doses. Ceilings to both analgesia and respiratory depression occur after pentazocine. Although its potential for abuse is less than with morphine,[686] prolonged use of pentazocine can lead to physical dependence.[685,687–689] Pentazocine is not particularly useful in reversing the respiratory-depressant effects of fentanyl[690] but can precipitate opioid withdrawal in narcotic addicts.[691,692] Nalorphinelike dysphoric side effects are common, especially after high doses (greater than 60 mg) of pentazocine in the elderly. The dysphoric effects of pentazocine can be reversed with naloxone. While some clinicians believe the benign hemodynamic effects of morphine make it a useful analgesic for patients with myocardial infarction,[693] pentazocine depresses myocardial contractility[694] and increases arterial blood pressure, heart rate, peripheral resistance, pulmonary artery pressure, and left ventricular work index.[695,696] Pentazocine also increases blood catecholamine levels. All these changes result in an increase in myocardial oxygen demand and can exacerbate myocardial ischemia.

The plasma half-life of pentazocine is 2 to 3 hours,

while its volume of distribution is 4 to 7 L/kg and its clearance is 1.5 L/min. Hepatic biotransformation terminates pentazocine's action. Only 5 percent unchanged drug is excreted in the urine. When taken orally, pentazocine is inactivated by the liver (first-pass effect). Thus, an oral dose of pentazocine is one-fourth as potent as a parenteral dose. In Europe pentazocine (1 mg/kg) is used in a general anesthetic technique called sequential analgesic anesthesia. In this technique the drug is administered after moderate doses of fentanyl (10 to 15 μg/kg). Perioperatively, pentazocine has limited popularity in the United States because of a high incidence of postoperative nausea and vomiting, limited analgesia, antagonism of other agonists, and undesirable cardiac and psychomimetic effects.

Butorphanol

The synthesis of butorphanol (BC 2627), a phenanthrene derivative, was reported in 1973.[697] In humans butorphanol's analgesic potency is five to eight times that of morphine.[698–700] Butorphanol is only available in parenteral form. After intramuscular injection, onset of effect is rapid and peak analgesia occurs within 1 hour. While butorphanol's duration of action is similar to that of morphine, its plasma half-life is only 2 to 3 hours.[698,699] Bioavailability after oral administration is only 17 percent of a similar intravenous dose. Although butorphanol (2 mg intramuscularly) causes as much respiratory depression as 10 mg of morphine, higher doses reach a ceiling.[701,702] Side effects after butorphanol include drowsiness, sweating, nausea, and CNS stimulation. The latter are qualitatively similar but occur less frequently than those seen after pentazocine.

In healthy volunteers, butorphanol (0.03 or 0.06 mg/

TABLE 10-17. Respiratory-Depressant Effects of Agonist-Antagonists Compared with Morphine[a]

Drug	Correlation of Respiratory Depression with Dose
Morphine	Increases proportionally with dose
Buprenorphine	Ceiling effect at 0.15–1.2 mg in adults
Butorphanol	Ceiling effect at 30–60 μg/kg
Nalbuphine	Ceiling effect at 30 mg in adults
Pentazocine	Ceiling effect suggested, but difficult to study due to psychotomimetic effects

[a]Low or moderate naloxone doses readily reverse the respiratory effects produced by therapeutic doses of all drugs listed, except buprenorphine.
(From Zola and McLeod,[701] with permission.)

kg intravenously) produces no or minimal significant cardiovascular changes.[702] However, in patients with cardiac disease, butorphanol causes significant increases in cardiac index, left ventricular end-diastolic pressure, and pulmonary artery pressure.[703] These cardiovascular changes are quite similar to those produced by pentazocine.[695] Thus, butorphanol is not particularly useful in patients with congestive heart failure or a history of previous myocardial infarction.

Butorphanol provides adequate analgesia when used as a supplement in nitrous oxide-opioid-oxygen anesthetic techniques.[704,705] High doses of butorphanol (0.1 and 0.2 mg/kg/min) have been evaluated with oxygen as a complete anesthetic in dogs.[706] Seventy-five percent of dogs receiving 0.1 mg/kg/min and twenty-five percent of those receiving 0.2 mg/kg/min moved in response to a tail-clamp stimulus after 45 minutes of a butorphanol infusion. Significant cardiovascular depression occurred with both infusion rates. Still higher doses of butorphanol are not, unfortunately, more effective in preventing movement after a surgical stimulus. In another study in dogs, butorphanol decreased the MAC for enflurane by only 11 percent.[94]

As a component of nitrous oxide-opioid balanced anesthesia, butorphanol may not block tachycardia and hypertension (irrespective of dosage) with surgical stimulation,[707] although others have found butorphanol (25 mg) and morphine (127 mg) equally satisfactory as analgesic supplements in balanced anesthesia for coronary artery surgery.[708] Butorphanol (0.17 mg/kg) will result in greater immediate postoperative respiratory depression than nalbuphine (0.085 mg/kg) when used as a supplement with nitrous oxide.[709]

The antagonistic properties of butorphanol at the mu receptor are weak and do not usually interfere with the use of other opioid agonists in anesthesia.[710] However, butorphanol does partially antagonize fentanyl-induced respiratory depression.[711] Butorphanol is subject to less abuse and has less addictive potential than morphine or fentanyl but still has abuse potential.[712] Withdrawal symptoms can occur after prolonged use and usually increase in severity for several days.[713] Hepatic metabolism and urinary and a small amount of biliary excretion account for drug elimination. Acute biliary spasm can occur after butorphanol, but increases in biliary pressure are less than after equipotent doses of fentanyl or morphine.[714]

Buprenorphine

Buprenorphine is a thebaine derivative that is similar in structure but approximately 33 times as potent as morphine. Buprenorphine is a partial mu-receptor agonist. It also binds to delta and kappa receptors, but activity at the latter two sites is relatively insignificant.[74] Although burprenorphine is highly lipophilic, its opiate receptor association and dissociation is slow. Whereas fentanyl dissociates rapidly from mu receptors ($t_{1/2}$ 6.8 min-

utes), buprenorphine has a higher affinity and takes much longer ($t_{1/2}$ 166 minutes). Thus, plasma levels do not parallel central nervous system effects.[74] Buprenorphine's onset of action is slow, and its peak effect may not occur until 3 hours. Duration of effect is prolonged (up to 10 hours). Metabolism occurs in the liver with biliary excretion of most metabolites. Buprenorphine's volume of distribution is 2.8 L/kg and clearance is 20 ml/kg/min. Recommended initial analgesic doses are 0.3 to 0.4 mg.[701]

Subjective effects (e.g., euphoria) of buprenorphine are similar to those of morphine, although they occur less frequently. Nausea and vomiting are the most common side effects after buprenorphine. Buprenorphine produces respiratory depression with a ceiling after 0.15 to 1.2 mg in adults. Higher doses do not produce further respiratory depression and may actually result in increased ventilation (predominance of antagonistic actions).[715] Similar apparent reductions of respiratory depression occur with higher doses of other agonist-antagonist-type drugs. Nonetheless, at some doses respiratory depression is impressive after buprenorphine. Reversal with naloxone is limited owing to buprenorphine's high affinity for and slow dissociation from the mu opiate receptor. Very high doses of naloxone and/ or doxapram may be required for full reversal.[701]

Buprenorphine has been successfully used for premedication (0.3 mg intramuscularly),[716] as the analgesic component in balanced anesthesia (4.5 to 12 µg/kg),[717] and for postoperative pain control (0.3 mg intramuscularly).[718-720] Sublingual administration (0.4 mg) has also proved effective.[719] Buprenorphine, like the other agonist-antagonist-type compounds, is not acceptable as a sole anesthetic, and its receptor kinetic profile restricts its usefulness if other mu agonists are used concurrently. On the other hand, in high doses buprenorphine might be of particular value as an alternative to methadone for maintenance therapy in opiate addicts.

Hemodynamic effects of buprenorphine are similar to those of morphine (Table 10-16). Opioid withdrawal symptoms develop slowly (5 to 10 days) after buprenorphine is discontinued following chronic use.

Nalbuphine

Nalbuphine is an agonist-antagonist opioid that is structurally related to oxymorphone and naloxone.[721] Autoradiography studies reveal that nalbuphine binds to mu as well as kappa and delta receptors.[722] Nalbuphine acts as an antagonist at the mu receptor and an agonist at the kappa receptor. Activation of the kappa receptor yields limited analgesia, respiratory depression, and sedation.[722] Although 10 mg of nalbuphine produces similar sedation, analgesia, and respiratory depression as 10 mg of morphine, this equivalency does not persist at higher doses.[723] Maximal analgesia occurs after approximately 30 mg/70 kg of nalbuphine.[723] Nalbuphine also causes other typical opioid side effects.[723]

Nalbuphine is only available for parenteral use. Onset of effect is rapid (5 to 10 minutes) and duration is long (3 to 6 hours) owing to a long plasma elimination half-life (5 hours). Hepatic metabolism and fecal excretion account for most of the drug's elimination. Nalbuphine does not increase plasma histamine levels. Nalbuphine, (0.6 mg/kg) produces no or minimal hemodynamic changes in ASA class I and II patients or those undergoing cardiac catheterization when it is administered alone.[724,725] Premedication with nalbuphine (0.1 mg/kg) in patients scheduled for cardiac surgery results in similar sedation, relief of anxiety, and respiratory depression as morphine (0.1 mg/kg) but no significant hemodynamic changes.[726] In patients experiencing a myocardial infarction, 10 mg of nalbuphine causes small decreases in heart rate (82 to 72 beats/min), cardiac index changes (from 3.16 to 2.75 L/min/m²)and small increases in systemic vascular resistance (1,204 to 1,461 dynes · s · cm⁻⁵).[727] Changes in systemic pressure, pulmonary arterial pressure, and PCWP are not significant.[727]

Nalbuphine is occasionally used as a premedicant, as an analgesic supplement for conscious sedation or balanced anesthesia, and as a analgesic for postoperative and chronic pain problems. Conscious sedation during monitored anesthesia care has also been recommended with combinations of nalbuphine (20 to 30 mg/70 kg) and droperidol (2.5 mg)[728] or nalbuphine (0.05 to 0.2 mg/kg) and midazolam (0.05 mg/kg).[729] Apnea and/or slow respiratory rates (less than 8 breaths/min) are occasional problems with the latter drug combination.[729]

Balanced anesthesia with nalbuphine as an intravenous analgesic supplement is effective for surgical procedures unassociated with severe pain.[730] Laparoscopy with this technique results in more postoperative sedation, dreaming, and anxiety and a longer recovery room stay when nalbuphine (0.3 to 0.5 mg/kg) is compared with fentanyl (1.5 µg/kg).[730] Some claim that a combination of nalbuphine (3 mg/kg), diazepam (0.4 mg/kg), and nitrous oxide is associated with remarkable cardiovascular stability during cardiac surgery.[731] Others have found quite the opposite.[732,733] Nalbuphine's inability to decrease the MAC of potent inhaled anesthetics[94] more than 10 to 30 percent suggests that it has little or no role as a sole or primary anesthetic.

Nalbuphine provides good analgesia for mild to moderate but not severe postoperative pain.[734–736] Nalbuphine (like other agonist-antagonist compounds) interferes with the analgesia produced by pure mu agonists. Addiction, abuse, and withdrawal occur less frequently after nalbuphine than after the pure mu agonist but as frequently as after the other agonist-antagonist compounds.

Nalbuphine as an Antagonist of Opioids

Preservation of analgesia following reversal of opioid-induced respiratory depression has long been a goal of researchers and clinicians.[737] While numerous opioid antagonists have been studied in attempts to find the ideal compound (including nalorphine, levallorphan, naloxone, and numerous others), none are optimal. Nalbuphine is the latest of the hopefuls to be extensively evaluated for this purpose.[314,738–747] Nalbuphine restores normal inspiratory neuronal activity after fentanyl in cats,[314] but oxymorphone (1.5 mg)-induced respiratory depression is only partially reversed by nalbuphine in humans (0.1 mg/kg).[738] Nalbuphine (0.21 mg/kg) does not reverse and may actually increase respiratory depression after morphine (0.21 mg/kg)[745] (Fig. 10-20). In this instance nalbuphine's intrinsic respiratory depression (via kappa-receptor stimulation) replaces or is greater than morphine's mu-receptor-induced depression.

Latasch et al.[739] reported that nalbuphine (20 mg intravenously) adequately reversed respiratory depression but not analgesia in patients who had received 7 µg/kg of fentanyl and nitrous oxide for general surgery. Zsigmond et al.[747] found that nalbuphine (0.1 mg/kg) did not elicit significant cardiovascular changes or pain in patients given fentanyl-nitrous oxide anesthesia for abdominal surgery. Unfortunately, many other investigators have documented the occurrence of significant pain, hypertension, and tachycardia (often requiring pharmacologic intervention) following opioid reversal with nalbuphine.[741–744,748] Many of these reports involved patients undergoing cardiovascular procedures (abdominal vascular surgery[741] or coronary artery bypass grafting[742,743,747]). Patients at risk for myocardial ischemia or other cardiovascular problems are not good candidates for opioid reversal.

Restoration of spontaneous ventilation with small titrated doses of nalbuphine (2.5 mg every 2 to 3 minutes) results in less pain than naloxone (0.08 mg titrated similarly) after fentanyl (mean dose 25 µg/kg), isoflurane, and nitrous oxide anesthesia.[746] Renarcotization is also less frequent after nalbuphine (Table 10-18). Opioid antagonists should not be routinely used in anesthetic practice. However, cautious titration using as small a dose as possible (naloxone, 0.25 to 0.5 µg/kg, or nalbuphine, 1 to 2 mg) in appropriate patients will usually result in adequate spontaneous ventilation with some residual analgesia.[746,747]

Dezocine

Dezocine (WY 16,225) is an investigational agonist-antagonist opioid that is more potent and faster acting than morphine.[749] Side effects and duration of action are similar to those of morphine. Respiratory depression and analgesia reach a plateau after approximately 0.3 mg/kg.[749] Dezocine may prove superior to other agonist-antagonists as an anesthetic supplement because it is more effective in reducing the MAC of potent inhaled anesthetics (up to 50 percent with cyclopropane or 58 percent with enflurane) than other agonist-antagonists.[750,751] In addition, dezocine potentiates rather than antagonizes morphine and other pure mu agonist analgesics. Dezocine is a partial agonist at mu and prob-

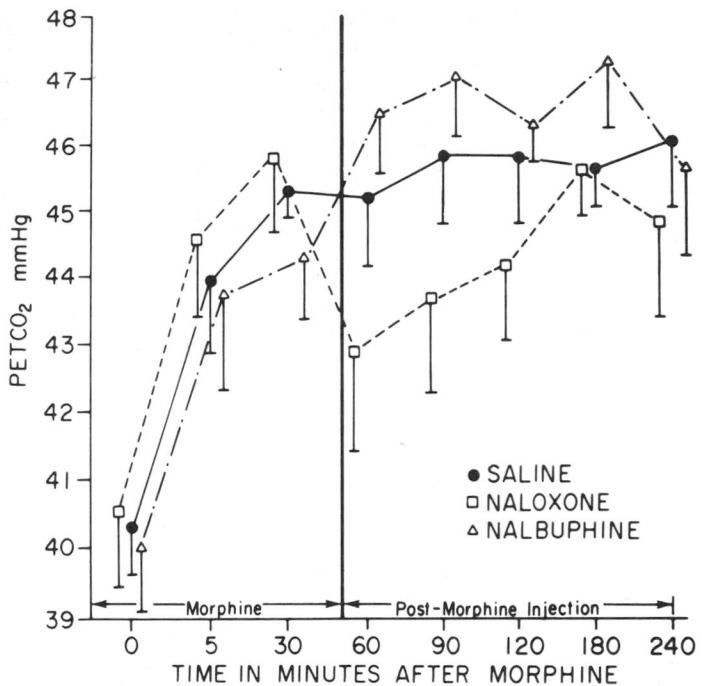

Fig. 10-20. Resting end-tidal CO_2 ($PETCO_2$) at baseline, 5 and 30 minutes after morphine (0.21 mg/kg^{-1} intravenous), and after nalbuphine (0.21 mg/kg intravenous), naloxone (0.014 mg/kg intravenous), and saline given 55 minutes after morphine. (From Bailey et al.,[745] with permission.)

ably delta receptors.[750] Dezocine does not increase plasma histamine and produces less hypotension than morphine or pentazocine in dogs.[752] Dezocine is more effective for moderate and severe pain[753] but causes myocardial depression and hypotension at high doses (20 mg/kg) in dogs.[751]

OPIOID ANTAGONISTS

Naloxone

Opioid antagonists are essential tools in scientific evaluations of opiates and opiate receptors[51] (see the section, *Mechanisms of Action*). Opioid antagonists are also used to restore spontaneous ventilation in patients who breathe inadequately after opioid overdoses or opioid anesthesia. Opioid antagonists are also useful to antagonize opioid-induced nausea and vomiting, pruritus, uri-

nary retention, and biliary spasm. Some have suggested that some "pure" mu receptor antagonists like naloxone may also be valuable as a treatment for septic and hemorrhagic shock.

Reversal of Respiratory Depression

In the early 1950s, nalorphine[754] and levallorphan[755] were evaluated as narcotic antagonists. They were often found unacceptable because of a high incidence of side effects, as well as incomplete reversal.[737] Reports of side effects (increases in heart rate and arterial blood pressure) and more serious complications (e.g., pulmonary edema) after naloxone are also numerous (Table 10-19).[756-764]

The mechanisms producing increases in arterial blood pressure and heart rate and other significant hemodynamic alterations after naloxone reversal of opioids are not well defined. Possible mechanisms in-

TABLE 10-18. Percentage of Patients Requiring Analgesics and Showing Evidence of Re-establishment of Narcosis after Nalbuphine or Naloxone Reversal of Fentanyl after Balanced Anesthesia

Group	Analgesic Required in Recovery Room	Additional Antagonists Required in Recovery Room
Naloxone	40% ($n = 12$)	16.7% ($n = 5$)
Nalbuphine	16.7% ($n = 5$)^a	7% ($n = 2$)

$^a P < 0.05$, compared with naloxone group.
(From Bailey et al.,[746] with permission.)

**TABLE 10-19. Reported Severe Complications
Following Naloxone**

Author (Ref.)	Naloxone Dose (IV, mg)	Complication
Azar (756)	0.4	HTN (270/140)
Estilo (757)	0.4	HTN (260/140); CVA
Flacke (758)	0.4	Pulmonary edema
Tanaka (759)	0.4	HTN (340/150)
Andree (760)	0.4	Cardiac arrest, death
	0.4	Cardiac arrest, death
Prough (761)	0.1	Pulmonary edema
	0.2 (+ 0.3 IM)	Pulmonary edema
Michaelis (762)	0.1	V TACH, V FIB
	0.4	V FIB
Partridge (763)	0.08	Pulmonary edema
Taff (764)	0.3	Pulmonary edema

[a]*Abbreviations:* HTN, hypertension; CVA, cardiovascular accident; V TACH, ventricular tachycardia; V FIB, ventricular fibrillation.

clude pain, rapid awakening, and sympathetic activation not necessarily due to pain. Patschke et al.[765] have shown that naloxone reversal of morphine in halothane-anesthetized dogs produces the same hemodynamic changes as it does in unanesthetized animals. Thus, pain and awakening did not cause the increases in heart rate, blood pressure, LV dP/dt, oxygen consumption, and coronary artery blood flow that were observed. They postulated that patients with coronary artery disease could be adversely effected by naloxone because of sympathetic activation. Opioids decrease sympathetic outflow through their central (brain stem and spinal) actions.[180] α-Adrenergic agonists (clonidine) and opioids decrease transmission through the same preganglionic sympathetic neurons.[64] This mechanism may explain clonidine's effectiveness in blocking hemodynamic stimulation following naloxone reversal of fentanyl.[180] Naloxone also reverses clonidine-induced decreases in potent inhaled anesthetic requirements.[766] In addition, many hypertensive patients will demonstrate reversal of the antihypertensive effects of clonidine by naloxone with concomitant elevations of their blood pressure, heart rate, peripheral vascular resistance, plasma renin activity, and plasma epinephrine and norepinephrine.[767,768] Naloxone administered by itself does not alter mean arterial pressure, heart rate, or plasma catecholamine concentrations in normotensive or hypertensive patients (not treated with clonidine) anesthetized without a narcotic.[769] Naloxone may also have a nonspecific analeptic effect through activation of a CNS arousal system.[770,771] Elevations in arterial carbon dioxide tension may also play a role in naloxone-induced hemodynamic changes during narcotic reversal.[772] Opioid reversal is perhaps best avoided in patients in whom increases in arterial blood pressure and heart rate could be detrimental. Although naloxone has been used safely in neuroanesthesia,[773] significant increases in CBF and CMRO$_2$ can occur[774] and careful titration is required. Narcotic reversal may be particularly hazardous in patients with pheochromocytoma or chromaffin tissue tumors.[775]

Onset of action after the intravenous administration of naloxone is rapid (1 to 2 minutes), and the half-life and duration of effect are short.[776,777] Naloxone is primarily metabolized in the liver via glucuronidation. Attempts to compensate for naloxone's short duration of action by increasing the dose run the risk of increasing the incidence and severity of unwanted side effects. Most often 1.0 to 2.0 μg/kg titrated in 0.5 to 1.0 μg/kg boluses every 2 to 3 minutes will restore adequate spontaneous ventilation.[746,773,778] Even smaller doses of naloxone may be adequate after alfentanil. Recurrence of respiratory depression after naloxone is due to the agent's short half-life as well as reuptake of opioid agonist from peripheral compartment tissues (e.g., muscle) and other factors (see the section, *Respiratory Actions*).

Renarcotization occurs more frequently after the use of longer-acting opioid agonists such as morphine. In these circumstances an additional intramuscular dose or continuous infusion of naloxone may be helpful. In the immediate postoperative setting, these modes of administering naloxone should not supplant good nursing care and attentive observations of respiratory function. Short-lasting opioids such as alfentanil rarely pose a danger of renarcotization, because of a rapid plasma decay curve, less chance of second plasma peaks resulting from reuptake of drug from peripheral tissues, and weak opiate receptor binding compared with fentanyl and sufentanil.[779]

While other agents (see the section, *Nalbuphine*) may be somewhat better as antagonists, a rational use of antagonists includes the following rules:

1. Use opioids in anesthesia so that reversal agents are rarely necessary.
2. Avoid inducing unnecessary intraoperative hypocapnia so that body carbon dioxide stores are not

depleted and adequate ventilatory drive remains after anesthesia and surgery.

3. Carefully titrate opioid antagonists.
4. Avoid reversal agents in patients with hypertension or cardiac or cerebrovascular disease.

Unfortunately, naloxone, although active at mu, delta, kappa, and sigma receptors, has the greatest affinity for mu receptors, through which most potent opioid effects, including respiratory depression and analgesia, are mediated. Thus, it is unlikely, with the current agents available, that analgesia can be reliably spared following reversal of respiratory depression. Careful titration of naloxone can, however, usually restore adequate spontaneous ventilation without reversal of adequate analgesia.

Some clinicians have attempted to antagonize opioids with physostigmine, a tertiary amine anticholinesterase. Although an advantage of this technique might be persistent analgesia,[780] the duration of action of physostigmine is too short (35 to 45 minutes) to be of practical value. Furthermore, the drug is unpredictable, especially when $PaCO_2$ is increased, and results in significant side effects (e.g., nausea, vomiting, bradycardia).[781,782] Therefore, reliance on more predictable and specific opioid antagonists is recommended.

Other Applications

Many other potential uses for naloxone exist. Naloxone may be useful in the treatment of *postanesthetic apnea* in infants, even when exogenous narcotics have not been administered.[783] *Primary apnea* may also be ameliorated by naloxone; however, roles for opioid antagonists in other *disorders of ventilatory control* (e.g., sudden infant death syndrome) await definition.[784] Naloxone does restore flow-resistive load compensation in patients with chronic obstructive pulmonary disease[785] and may be beneficial in other forms of respiratory failure.[786]

Although many conflicting reports and opinions exist, high doses of naloxone may reverse the effects of some nonopioid CNS depressants.[787] *Benzodiazepine* reversal has been reported after naloxone and may be related to GABA receptor effects, a nonspecific analeptic effect, or reversal of concomitantly released endogenous opiates. The advent of specific benzodiazepine antagonists (flumazenil [RO 15-1788]) will probably diminish interest in naloxone reversal of benzodiazepines. *Barbiturate* and *alcohol* reversal have also been reported after naloxone treatment. Certain metabolic products of alcohol (isoquinolines) have opioidlike actions and may account for this interaction. Opioid-GABA receptor interactions could also explain barbiturate antagonism. Naloxone may also partially antagonize *ketamine* and *nitrous oxide* analgesia. The MAC of potent *inhaled anesthetics* is uneffected by naloxone.

Naloxone increases arterial blood pressure in labora-

tory animals, primates, and some patients in *hypovolemic and septic shock*. Purported mechanisms include centrally mediated increases in sympathetic tone and decreases in parasympathetic output, and/or antagonism of endogenous opioids.[788]

Naloxone may ameliorate the neurologic deficit following an *ischemic* or *traumatic neurologic* insult in animals. Results have not been consistent, and further research is needed.[788] Naloxone may also have a therapeutic role in Alzheimer's disease, schizophrenia, intractable pruritus, and thalamic pain syndrome.

Naltrexone

Naltrexone, a new opioid receptor antagonist at mu, delta, and kappa receptors, provides two advantages when compared with naloxone. It is longer acting (plasma half-life of 8 to 12 hours versus 0.5 to 1.5 hours) and it is active orally. A single oral dose will result in a constant plasma concentration for up to 24 hours. Naltrexone is not subject to as much first-pass hepatic metabolism as naloxone. Oral naltrexone (5 to 10 mg) reduces the frequency and severity of pruritus, nausea, and vomiting associated with epidural morphine without diminishing analgesia.[789] Whether or not urinary retention or delayed respiratory depression can also be decreased or eliminated with naltrexone remains to be proved. Higher doses of naltrexone, for example, 100 mg, are used to prevent opioid activity during maintenance treatment of opioid addicts.

Nalmefene

Nalmefene is a new pure opioid antagonist structurally similar to naloxone and naltrexone. Like naloxone and naltrexone, nalmefene has a greater preference for mu than delta or kappa receptors as demonstrated by IC_{50} studies.[790] Nalmefene is long acting after oral (0.5 to 3.0 mg/kg) and parenteral (0.2 to 2.0 mg/kg) administration. It produces few or no physiologic or pharmacologic changes when administered by itself. Duration of reversal of fentanyl- and morphine-induced respiratory depression is dose dependent.[791,792] The plasma half-life of nalmefene is 8 to 10 hours. Bioavailability after oral administration is 40 to 50 percent, and peak plasma concentrations are reached in 1 to 2 hours. The drug undergoes hepatic metabolism and is excreted via the biliary and renal systems.

DRUG INTERACTIONS

The cardiovascular and respiratory effects of combining opioids with other drugs have been reviewed above. Most CNS medications including tricyclic antidepressants, phenothiazines, and MAOIs increase the magnitude and duration of all opioid effects. Although some interactions are important, the validity of past recommendations to delay surgery in patients receiving various medications, including MAOIs and similar classes of compounds, has been questioned.[793] Fentanyl and sufentanil, unlike meperidine, are probably safe in such patients. Alcohol, barbiturates, benzodiazepines, and many other CNS depressants cause greater than anticipated sedation when coadministered with opioids. Although some experimental evidence suggests that benzodiazepines and barbiturates partially antagonize opioid-induced analgesia, potentiation of opioid effects usually results when such combinations are employed clinically.

Cimetidine can prolong opioid effects by decreasing hepatic blood flow and/or diminishing hepatic metabolism. Ranitidine can also reduce hepatic blood flow but binds less to the P-450 system and has less impact on opioid metabolism than cimetidine.[794]

PHARMACOKINETICS

Specific Drugs

Morphine Sulfate

Both biexponential and triexponential equations have been used to describe the pharmacokinetics of morphine. After intravenous injection, morphine is rapidly distributed (t1/2π 1 to 2.5 minutes and t1/2α 10 to 20 minutes).[354,795-800] Reported elimination half-lives have ranged from 1.7 to 4.5 hours. In some studies, the radioimmunoassay techniques used also measure morphine metabolites and may account for high t1/2β values.[796] Morphine's volume of distribution can range from 1.25 to more than 4 L/kg in older patients. Excessive parenchymatous and skeletal muscle tissue drug uptake is probably the explanation. Morphine has a relatively low lipid solubility (fat/plasma protein partition coefficient of 0.8/1.0 versus 35/1 for fentanyl).

Morphine has a hepatic extraction ratio that is equal to or greater than hepatic blood flow, indicating a high clearance (15 to 30 ml/kg/min). Extrahepatic (renal) metabolism of morphine may account for up to 38 percent of its clearance.[801] Morphine-3-glucuronide is the major metabolite and is probably less active than morphine.[802] N-demethylation of morphine contributes to a lesser degree to its metabolism. Intramuscular as well as subcutaneous injections of morphine produce peak plasma levels in approximately 20 minutes[354] with near 100 percent bioavailability. Bioavailability of orally administered morphine is significantly lower (20 to 30 percent) than after intramuscular or subcutaneous injection.[800]

The pKa of morphine (8.0) is greater than physiologic pH and determines that after intravenous injection a only a small percentage (10 to 20 percent) is un-ionized. This, combined with its low lipid solubility (octanol/water partition coefficient of 1.4), limits the ability of morphine to penetrate tissues. While intravenous injection yields high plasma levels quickly, there is a relatively slow onset of peak CNS action. Peak spinal fluid

concentrations of morphine occur 15 to 30 minutes after intravenous injection; however, CSF morphine levels do not correlate well with ventilatory depression.[799] Penetration of morphine into and out of the brain is slow. Brain morphine levels and thus analgesia and respiratory effects are not reflected by plasma levels (Fig. 10-21). Approximately 20 to 40 percent of morphine is bound to plasma proteins, mostly albumin.[799] Elimination half-lives of morphine from the brain and the CSF are both greater than the plasma t1/2β.[799,803] The relatively more acid milieu of the brain may enhance the ionization and trapping of morphine.[803] Pharmacokinetic data for morphine and the other major opioids used in anesthesia are summarized in Table 10-20.

Meperidine

The plasma concentration versus time decay curve of meperidine is best characterized by a biexponential equation with a reported distribution half-life (t1/2α) varying from 5 to 15 minutes.[804-809] Meperidine is more highly bound to plasma proteins than morphine, principally (70 percent) to α_1-acidglycoprotein. In contrast to morphine, meperidine binds only to a minor extent to plasma albumin. Meperidine is even less un-ionized (less than 10 percent) than morphine at physiologic pH but is significantly more lipid soluble. Because of this higher lipid solubility, plasma levels of meperidine are more highly correlated with analgesia than

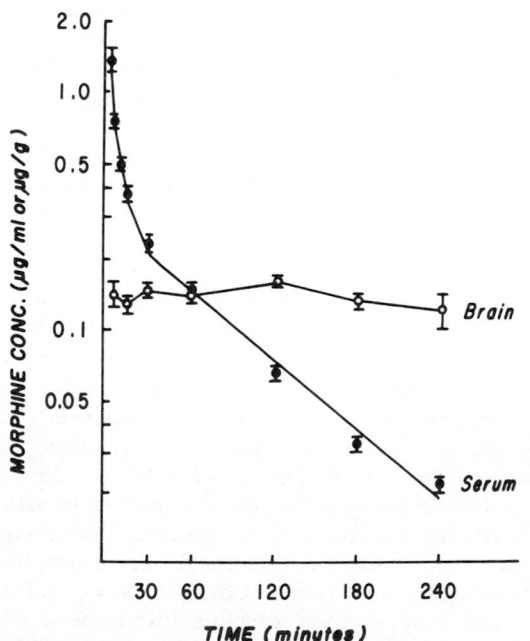

Fig. 10-21. Serum and brain decrement curves in normocarbic dogs showing relationship of brain morphine concentrations to those in serum. Note intersections of serum and brain morphine decrement curves at approximately 1 hour. Vertical bars are standard error ($n = 7$). (From Nishitateno et al.,[803] with permission.)

TABLE 10-20. Physicochemical and Pharmacokinetic Data of Commonly Used Opioid Agonists

	Morphine	Meperidine	Fentanyl	Sufentanil	Alfentanil
pKa	8.0	8.5	8.4	8.0	6.5
% un-ionized at pH 7.4	23	<10	<10	20	90
Octanol/H_2O partition coefficient	1.4	39	813	1,778	145
% Bound to Plasma Protein	20–40	70	84	93	92
t $1/2\pi$ (min)	1–2.5		1–2	1–2	1–3
t $1/2\alpha$ (min)	10–20	5–15	10–30	15–20	4–17
t $1/2\beta$ (hr)	2–4	3–5	2–4	2–3	1–2
V_{dcc} (L/kg)	0.1–0.4	1–2	0.5–1.0	0.2	0.1–0.3
V_{dss} (L/kg)	3–5	3–5	3–5	2.5–3.0	0.4–1.0
Clearance (L/min/kg)	15–30	8–18	10–20	10–15	4–9
Hepatic extration ratio	0.8–1.0	0.7–0.9	0.8–1.0	0.7–0.9	0.3–0.5

Abbreviations: t $1/2\pi$, first distribution half-life; t $1/2\alpha$, second distribution half-life; t $1/2\beta$, elimination half-life; V_{dcc}, volume of distribution at central compartment; V_{dss}, volume of distribution at steady state.

plasma levels of morphine. The volume of distribution of meperidine is similar to that of morphine (4 ± 1 L/kg),[804–808] as is its clearance (8 to 18 ml/kg/min).[804–809] Like morphine, a high hepatic extraction ratio results in biotransformation that depends on hepatic blood flow. The principal metabolic pathways of meperidine are N-demethylation and diesterification, which produce normeperidine, meperidinic acid, and normeperidinic acids as the major metabolites. Little meperidine (less than 5 percent) is excreted unchanged in the urine. Normeperidine has some opioid action and is roughly twice as potent as its parent compound in producing seizures in animals.[810] The greater epileptogenic properties of meperidine cause its therapeutic index to be less than one-tenth that of morphine (5 versus 70). The elimination half-life (t$1/2\beta$) for meperidine is approximately 4 ± 1 hours,[804–808] and excretion of its metabolites occurs predominantly via the kidney. The elimination half-life of normeperidine is considerably greater than that of meperidine, and cumulative doses can easily produce accumulation of this toxic metabolite in patients with renal and hepatic disease.[811] Intramuscular injections of meperidine result in peak plasma levels in 15 to 110 minutes.[808] Meperidine (50 to 100 mg intravenously or intramuscularly) produces variable degrees of pain relief and is not always effective in patients with severe pain.[811,812] Plasma levels of 0.5 to 0.8 μg/ml are usually necessary for relief of severe pain.[811,812] Adequate analgesia may be short lived after meperidine owing to rapid decreases in plasma levels to subtherapeutic concentrations (less than 0.1 to 0.2 μg/ml).

Fentanyl

The pharmacokinetics of fentanyl have been studied by numerous investigators.[328,357,813–817] A three-compartment model is often used to describe plasma fentanyl concentration decay.[328,357,814,815] After intravenous ad-

ministration in humans, fentanyl rapidly disappears from the plasma. More than 98 percent of an injected dose is eliminated from the plasma after 1 hour. Rapid distribution (t$1/2\pi$) of fentanyl takes 1 to 2 minutes, and a second distribution phase (t$1/2\alpha$) takes 10 to 30 minutes. Brain fentanyl levels parallel plasma levels. Spectral edge analysis of the EEG in patients receiving fentanyl (8.8 μg/kg administered over 6 minutes) suggest that the drug is best administered approximately 5 minutes before a painful stimulus.[372] (Another alternative is to administer a larger dose to rapidly saturate brain opioid receptors as well as nonreceptor storage sites.) In rats, muscle tissue is found to hold the most fentanyl after redistribution (56 percent), while maximum fat tissue content is only 17 percent.[818] The relevance of these data to humans is unknown. At steady state, fentanyl's volume of distribution (3 to 6 L/kg) and clearance (10 to 20 ml/kg/min) are both high.

Fentanyl's lipid solubility is high (Table 10-20), which explains its large volume of distribution. This large volume of distribution causes rapid uptake of fentanyl from the blood and limits hepatic access to the drug. Fentanyl must ultimately be returned to the blood to be metabolized and eliminated from the body. Hudson and Stanski[819] suggest that fentanyl's large volume of distribution results in more variability in plasma levels during the elimination phase. Such variability in plasma concentrations may be due in part to surges in muscle blood flow. Resultant fluctuations in the amount of fentanyl returned to the blood may contribute to second peaks in plasma fentanyl levels (Fig. 10-22).[357]

High hepatic clearance of fentanyl (approaching hepatic blood flow) and a high hepatic extraction ratio (approaching 1.0) minimize the contribution of enterohepatic circulation to secondary peaks in drug plasma levels.[362] On the other hand, decreases in hepatic blood flow decrease fentanyl elimination. Fentanyl is primar-

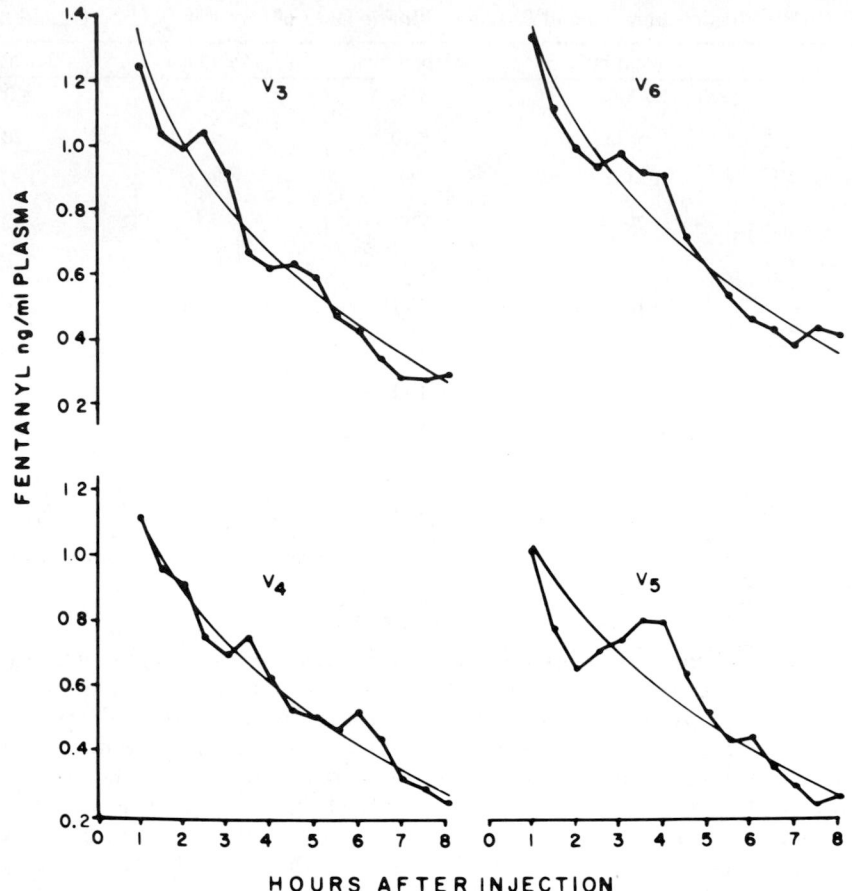

Fig. 10-22. Arithmetic plot of fentanyl level/time after a single bolus intravenous injection (3.2 or 6.4 μg/kg) in each of four subjects. The thin line represents the curve determined by nonlinear least-squares analysis of the data for each subject. Note the occurrence of second peaks. (From McClain and Hug,[357] with permission.)

ily metabolized in the liver by N-dealkylation and hydroxylation.[817] Metabolites begin to appear in the plasma as early as 1.5 minutes after injection.[818] The activity of fentanyl's metabolites is unknown but is thought to be minimal. Little fentanyl is excreted in the urine unchanged.[357]

Approximately 80 percent of fentanyl is bound to plasma proteins, and significant amounts (40 percent) are taken up by red blood cells.[820] Because the pKa of fentanyl is high (8.4) at physiologic pH, it exists mostly in the ionized form (greater than 90 percent). As noted above, fentanyl's high lipid solubility and volume of distribution contribute to variability in reported pharmacokinetic profiles.[819] Indeed, Reilly et al.[821] noted a 13-fold range of the peak plasma levels of 8.4 to 113.6 ng/ml after a 500-μg intravenous injection in adults. They also reported significant variability in other pharmacokinetic parameters. Other reasons for the large differences in reported fentanyl pharmacokinetics include small sample sizes, inadequate sampling, different fentanyl assay methods, and studies using patients on cardiopulmonary bypass.

Sufentanil

Complete investigation of the pharmacokinetics of sufentanil over a wide range of clinical doses (0.25 to 25 μg/kg) has been limited by difficulties with assay accuracy at low plasma levels (e.g., 0.3 ng/ml). Although new methods of detection have been proposed,[822] the validity of these methods is still questioned.[823] The pKa of sufentanil at physiologic pH is the same as that of morphine (8.0), and therefore, only a small amount (20 percent) exists in the un-ionized form. Sufentanil is twice as lipid soluble as fentanyl and is highly bound (93 percent) to plasma proteins including α_1-acid glycoprotein. Bovill et al.[824] have reported the most complete pharmacokinetic profile for sufentanil. In 9 of 10 patients studied, the plasma decay curves conformed to a three-compartment model. T$1/2\pi$ was 1.4 ± 0.3 minutes and t$1/2\alpha$ was 17.7 ± 2.6 minutes. After intravenous injection, the onset of sufentanil's effect was rapid and 98 percent of the dose had left the plasma within 30 minutes. Elimination half-life was 164 ± 22 minutes, and the apparent volume of the central compartment was 0.16 ± 0.02 L/kg. The apparent volume of distribution was $2.86 \pm .25$ L/kg, and hepatic clearance was high (12.7 ± 0.8 ml/kg/min). Sufentanil's hepatic extraction ratio is high (0.8), and thus changes in liver blood flow can significantly alter its elimination. A significant first-pass effect exists for orally administered sufentanil. Extensive renal tubular reabsorption leads to little unchanged sufentanil in the urine.

Sufentanil is often quoted as being 5 to 10 times as potent as fentanyl, but one potency ratio may not be adequate when comparing opioids. The potency ratio between two opioids for analgesia may differ from that for respiratory depression.[346] Thus, using a 10 to 1 potency ratio for analgesia, sufentanil results in shorter-lasting respiratory depression but longer-lasting analgesia compared with fentanyl in human volunteers.[346] Sufentanil is more tightly bound to receptors (mostly mu) than fentanyl and has only minimal nonspecific brain tissue binding.[825] These properties, along with its high degree of plasma protein binding and lower volume of distribution, are the probable explanation for sufentanil's shorter elimination half-life and duration of effect compared with fentanyl. Extensive tissue uptake of sufentanil (highly lipophilic, octanol/water partition coefficient of 1,788) and eventual return of drug from the periphery to the central circulation are the rate-limiting steps in the termination of sufentanil's effect after high doses. Pharmacokinetic variability with sufentanil is as great as with fentanyl and most other opioid agonists.

Alfentanil

The pharmacokinetics of alfentanil have been extensively evaluated[362,626,826-832] and discussed.[32,634,833-835] Following intravenous injection, alfentanil plasma concentrations fit either a two-compartment[362,626,827,828,831] or three-compartment[826,829,830] model. Distribution (range of mean $t1/2\alpha s$ reported is 4 to 17 minutes; Table 10-20) and elimination (range of mean $t1/2\beta s$ reported is 70 to 112 minutes; Table 10-20) of alfentanil are rapid. Clearance (4 to 9 ml/kg/min) is less than that of fentanyl. A small volume of distribution at steady state (0.4 to 1.0 L/kg) limits tissue drug accumulation and is largely responsible for the short elimination half-life of alfentanil despite a lower clearance than fentanyl.

Alfentanil is lipid soluble enough to permit rapid brain penetration (heptane/water partition coefficient 2.5) but significantly less so than fentanyl (heptane/water partition coefficient 9.0).[634,833] Thus, less alfentanil is taken up by and stored in nonreceptor brain tissue. This explains alfentanil's rapid decline in activity after cessation of drug administration.[372,833] At physiologic pH, alfentanil is mostly (90 percent) un-ionized owing to its relatively low pKa (6.5).[836] This, too, aids tissue (brain) penetration. Although alfentanil is largely bound to plasma proteins (90 percent),[362,829,830] binding and dissociating from plasma proteins is usually not a rate-limiting reaction.[833] Little alfentanil (less than 1 percent) appears in the urine unchanged owing to its protein binding, renal tubular reabsorption, and hepatic metabolism. Reported hepatic extraction ratios vary from 0.3 to 0.5.[362,830,837] Oxidative N-dealkylation of alfentanil produces its major metabolite, noralfentanil. Other metabolites include desmethylalfentanil, desmethylnoralfentanil, and a number of products of hydrolysis and glucuronidation.[838-840] The degradation products of alfentanil have little if any opioid activity. Patients deficient in the cytochrome P-450 form involved in debrisoquin metabolism do not have an altered disposition of alfentanil.[839,840]

The rapid onset and short duration of alfentanil, along with its other favorable properties, have led to the application of mathematical models,[835] computer-assisted devices,[841] population pharmacokinetic analysis,[842] and other techniques to improve its predictability and clinical use.[32,842] Some success has been achieved through recognition of the impact of other factors, for example, age and weight (see the section, *Factors Influencing Pharmacokinetics*) on the drug's pharmacokinetic profile.[842] However, these factors have not consistently been found to influence pharmacokinetics.[362,837] In addition, even after correcting for such variables, remaining interindividual variability in clearance remains near 50 percent.[842] Indeed, clearance rates can actually vary up to sixfold.[626] Such variability has a marked effect on plasma alfentanil concentrations.[827,841] Many investigators stress the importance of titrating alfentanil to a clinical response.[626,827,832,836,841] Using the dose-response relationship instead of dose-plasma concentration or plasma concentration-effect relationships as a guide to alfentanil use has been suggested to be more simple yet as efficacious for clinical utility.

Figure 10-15 illustrates the plasma alfentanil concentrations over time from four different studies.[827,828,830,831] Several important points are illustrated. First, bolus injections (80 to 200 μg/kg) produce initial plasma levels proportional to the dose. Second, when a maintenance infusion is not instituted, plasma levels rapidly decline and may be subtherapeutic (e.g., less than 400 ng/ml) for endotracheal intubation within a few minutes. After 50 μg/kg, plasma levels of alfentanil are less than 300 ng/ml within 3 to 5 minutes.[829] Thus, except for short procedures (less than 15 minutes), continuous infusions of alfentanil should be instituted to maintain adequate plasma concentrations. Third, increases in total dose or total time of infusion lead to a greater dependency on elimination than distribution for termination of action.[634] As illustrated in Fig. 10-15, excessive plasma levels can occur if high infusion rates are empirically employed. Fragen et al.[831] suggest 176 μg/kg of alfentanil as an induction dose followed by an infusion of 1.3 μg/kg/min as a reasonable guideline to achieve a plasma level of approximately 400 ng/ml. Terminating the alfentanil infusion 10 to 30 minutes before the end of surgery allows enough time for plasma levels to decrease from 300 to 500 ng/ml to less than 200 ng/ml.[32] Spontaneous ventilation usually resumes below 200 ng/ml while adequate analgesia persists. Several studies have also shown that when naloxone is required to restore spontaneous breathing, plasma alfentanil levels are usually greater than 200 ng/ml.[626,832]

Factors Influencing Pharmacokinetics

Dose

Changes in dose generally do not alter opioid pharmacokinetic profiles.[843-845] This suggests that biotransformation and excretion mechanisms are not easily saturated by clinical doses of opioids and that kinetics usually remain first order (drug concentration dependent). Altered alfentanil pharmacokinetics have, however, been reported with increasing doses.[846] The elimination half-life of morphine can also be prolonged when larger doses are given and sampling time is extended.[800] Dose-dependent opioid effects, for example, hypotension and decreased hepatic blood flow, may also contribute to dose-related changes in pharmacokinetics. As the dose of an opioid increases, the plasma level after drug distribution is completed also increases and can only be reduced by elimination. Small doses of fentanyl, for example, appear short acting because drug distribution rapidly lowers plasma (and brain levels) below thresholds for significant respiratory depression. After large doses, plasma levels are above the same threshold even after distribution phases are completed. Thus, apparent clinical drug action is prolonged. Further declines are slower because elimination half-lives are longer than distribution half-lives.

Acid-Base

The overall clinical impact of acid-base changes on opioid pharmacokinetics is complex, difficult to predict, and incompletely evaluated. For example, respiratory acidosis during fentanyl administration has multiple effects including increases in ionization and CBF and decreases in plasma protein binding.[803,847,848] The most lucid representation of how a change in pH can affect opioid kinetics has been described by Lüllmann et al.[849] When mechanical ventilation is abruptly terminated, respiratory acidosis rapidly decreases the pH of the extracellular (blood and interstitial) space. More fentanyl in the interstitial compartment will be ionized as determined by the Henderson-Hasselbach equation for weak bases:

$$pH = pKa + \log \frac{\text{proton acceptor (B)}}{\text{proton donor (BH}^+)}$$

More opioid receptors, on cell membranes that interact with ionized fentanyl, will be stimulated producing an enhanced opioid effect (Fig. 10-23). Additional respiratory acidosis resulting from opioid-induced depression of respiratory centers could produce a vicious cycle of ventilatory depression-acidosis-increased ionized fentanyl and increased ventilatory depression. In addition, the acidosis (and shift from free base to ionized fentanyl in the interstitial space) will draw un-ionized fentanyl out of the intracellular compartment, where fentanyl has accumulated. Finally, increased ionization will decrease the amount of fentanyl available for hepatic metabolism or renal excretion.[849] Alfentanil, with a pKa of 6.5, will not be as influenced by either pH changes or tissue accumulation.[849]

Intraoperative hyperventilation can also increase the duration of respiratory depression.[340] Brain fentanyl levels are higher with respiratory alkalosis.[341] Alkalosis also increases the lipophilicity (increased octanol/water partition coefficient) of several opioids. Serum and brain levels of morphine are elevated by 10 to 30 percent and 30 to 70 percent, respectively, in hypocapnic, alkalotic dogs.[803] Similar findings have been reported for morphine in rats subjected to alkalosis.[850] Alkalosis favors un-ionized morphine and may enhance brain penetration despite decreased CBF and increased plasma protein binding.[803] Nishitateno et al.[803] reported a decreased clearance and Schwartz et al.[851] an increased volume of distribution for sufentanil and for morphine after hyperventilation. Both changes could explain an increase in elimination half-life and duration of action. Hypercapnia also increases CNS morphine levels in the dog, although to a lesser degree. Hypercapnia also prolongs the removal of morphine from the brain, probably owing to CNS acidosis and increased morphine ionization within the brain. Thus, both intraoperative respiratory alkalosis and respiratory acidosis, especially in the immediate postoperative period, can prolong and exacerbate opioid-induced respiratory depression.

Plasma Protein Binding

Opioids are basic drugs and bind to a number of plasma proteins including α_1-acidglycoprotein, lipoproteins, and albumin. Protein binding of opioids limits drug availability at receptor sites. Fentanyl, sufentanil, and alfentanil are, respectively, 84.4, 92.5, and 92.1 percent protein bound after injection in humans.[820] Approximately 50 percent of circulating fentanyl and sufentanil are bound to albumin, while only 33 percent of alfentanil is bound to albumin. Fentanyl and sufentanil, and to a lesser extent alfentanil, are also bound to α- and β-globulins. All three opioids are bound to α_1-acidglycoprotein, but changes in α_1-acidglycoprotein concentration seem to affect unbound alfentanil the most. Increases in α_1-acidglycoprotein occur with inflammatory diseases, surgery, rheumatoid arthritis, cancer, and pneumonia and lead to an increase in opioid binding. Pregnancy and oral contraceptives decrease α_1-acidglycoprotein. Dilution of plasma proteins by one-third increases plasma free fentanyl, sufentanil, and alfentanil levels by 50, 35, and 25 percent, respectively.[820] α_1-Acidglycoprotein binds other drugs includ-

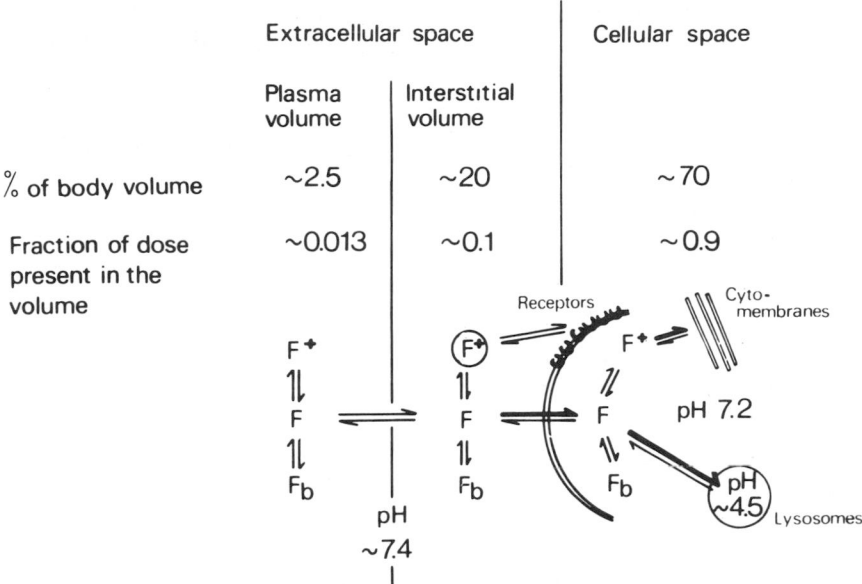

Fig. 10-23. Distribution of fentanyl within the body compartments at an extracellular pH of 7.4. The accumulation of fentanyl by the tissue is assumed to be 13-fold. In the extracellular space an equilibrium exists between the ionized fentanyl (F^+), the free base (F), and the fentanyl molecules bound to macromolecules (F_b). The concentration of ionized fentanyl within the interstitial fluid (encircled F^+) determines the pharmacological effect since the opioid receptors (∪∪) are located at the cell surface. Fentanyl as free base readily penetrates into the cells and becomes bound to cytomembranes, lysosomes, and other structures (thick arrows) and thus accumulates in the cell. A small decrease of the extracellular pH will shift the equilibrium between F and F^+ toward higher F^+ concentrations and will induce a marked release of fentanyl from the cellular compartment as a result of the decrease of the concentration of F in the interstitium. An increase of the extracellular H^+ concentration by pH 0.2 might roughly double the concentration of ionized fentanyl within the interstitial fluid and accordingly enhance its pharmacologic effect. (From Lüllmann et al.,[849] with permission.)

ing propranolol, imipramine, and lidocaine. Increases in α_1-acidglycoprotein cause increased binding of alfentanil, limit distribution, and decrease the volume of distribution (24 percent) and clearance in patients with cancer.[852] Interestingly, t1/2β is minimally altered because these two changes have opposite effects on elimination. Acid-base status also influences opioid protein binding (Table 10-21).[852]

Age
(Also See Chs. 59 & 62)

Numerous studies evaluating opioid pharmacokinetics in patients ranging from premature infants to the elderly have shown that age has a significant impact. Ex-

TABLE 10-21. Percent Changes in Plasma Protein Binding of Opioids with Acidosis and Alkalosis

Drug	pH 7.0	pH 7.8
Fentanyl	−52	+36
Sufentanil	−29	+28
Alfentanil	−6	0

(From Meuldermans et al.,[820] with permission.)

planations include increases in CNS sensitivity to morphine, fentanyl, and alfentanil at the extremes of age[329,358,853,854] and increases in percent body fat and decreases in plasma protein binding,[804] liver blood flow, and enzyme function in the aged.[855–857]

In *premature infants*, decreases in clearance and increases in elimination half-life occur after alfentanil[858] and fentanyl.[859] The likely reasons for these findings are decreased hepatic blood flow, surgery or an open ductus venosus, and immature enzyme systems, including the cytochrome P-450 system.[856] During the first week of life, *term neonates* have limited hepatic enzyme function and reduced opioid clearance. Thus, in this age group the elimination half-life of morphine is prolonged (6.8 hours). Brain penetration of morphine is also enhanced owing to an immature blood-brain barrier. Therefore, analgesic requirements are reduced in neonates.[854] While the clearance of fentanyl is normal in newborns, increases in volume of distribution can lead to prolonged elimination half-lives.[358,860] Extreme variability in fentanyl pharmacokinetics also exists in the newborn. Intraoperative fentanyl clearance can be zero or as high as 32 ml/kg/min.[861] Secondary peaks in plasma fentanyl levels have also been reported in term neonates.[358] Elimination of sufentanil is also prolonged in newborns. *Neonates* 20 to 28 days old have an active cytochrome oxidase system and better hepatic blood flow, resulting in improved opioid clearance.[862]

The pharmacokinetics of morphine in infants differ little compared to those in adults once beyond the neonatal period.[795,854] Mixed function oxidase enzymes have greater activity in *infants* than older *children*,[359] and opioids may have a shorter duration of effect in infants than in adults.[860,863-865] Thus, sufentanil undergoes greater clearance (27 ml/kg/min) and has a shorter elimination half-life (53 minutes) in infants than adults.[474]

Morphine pharmacokinetics are similar in *young children* (1 to 7 years), *older children* (7 to 15 years), and *adults*.[795] Koren et al.[863] described no change in t$1/2\alpha$, t$1/2\beta$, or clearance of fentanyl (50 μg/kg bolus plus an infusion of either 0.15 or 0.3 μg/kg/h) in young children undergoing heart surgery, although plasma levels were two to three times higher than those reported in adults. They attributed this to a decreased volume of distribution (1.4 L/kg). Johnson et al.[860] reported pharmacokinetic data for children (ages 1 to 5 years and 10 to 14 years) that were similar to adult values. Several investigators[858,864-867] have reported that the volume of distribution and elimination half-life of alfentanil are most often found to be decreased (approximately one-half of adult values) and that clearance is either normal or elevated in children. Sufentanil may also be cleared somewhat faster in children than in adults, but other pharmacokinetic parameters including elimination half-life do not differ.[474,868] Intravenous boluses of opioids in children produce higher initial plasma levels than in adults owing to decreased initial volumes of distribution. These levels, however, could decrease faster due to an increased clearance and decreased elimination half-life.

The *elderly* also dispose of opioids differently than young or middle-aged adults. Decreases in vascular volume and cardiac output lead to more drug delivery to the brain. Decreases in serum albumin that occur with age can increase free drug fraction and drug distribution. The aged are also more sensitive to the CNS effects of opioids. Intravenous morphine (10 mg/kg) transiently produces plasma concentrations in the aged that are 1.5 to 2.0 times greater than in adults for at least 5 minutes owing to a smaller initial volume of distribution.[327,869] The volume of distribution at steady state can be smaller in the elderly (1.16 versus 2.12 L/kg), and this, despite a reduced clearance, can produce a shorter elimination half-life. It must be remembered that the CNS effects of morphine do not parallel plasma morphine levels. Thus, the duration of action of morphine in the elderly can be long despite a reduced plasma half-life. Stanski et al.[354] also found a low (0.1 L/kg) initial volume of distribution for morphine in the aged (61 to 80 years). However, clearance and elimination half-life as well as other parameters were usually within the reported range for younger adults.

Chan et al.[355] studied meperidine (1.5 mg/kg) in subjects less than 30 years and greater than 70 years old. Higher plasma meperidine levels (0.7 versus 0.3 μg/ml) at 1 hour after injection were found in the older group. Plasma concentrations remained significantly elevated for at least 7 hours (Fig. 10-24[355]). They also found decreased red cell binding of meperidine in the aged. They postulated that if other tissues also bind less meperidine, drug distribution should be decreased and plasma levels higher in the first few hours after administration. Differences in metabolism of meperidine were small, but less meperidine was excreted in the urine in the elderly. This could explain the persistent elevated levels in the elderly. Others have also reported age-related increases in plasma meperidine levels and pharmacokinetics.[804]

Plasma concentrations of fentanyl (10 μg/kg) are higher in patients over 50 years old.[328] These differences become greater with time and persist for more than 10 hours. Singleton et al.[870] also found that plasma levels of fentanyl (15 μg/kg) were higher in the elderly (71 to 82 years old) than after 20 μg/kg in the young (10 to 41 years old). Bentley et al.[328] found a decreased clearance (4 versus 15 ml/kg/min) and a prolonged elimination half-life (945 versus 265 minutes) in the elderly. Volumes of distribution were not statistically significant.

Scott and Stanski,[329] using electroencephalography (power spectral analysis), showed a 50 percent reduction in the dose of fentanyl or alfentanil needed to produce a similar EEG effect as patients' ages increased from 20 to 89 years. They found no age-related differences in fentanyl pharmacokinetics. They concluded that pharmacodynamic rather than pharmacokinetic changes underlie the altered response of the aged to fentanyl.

Increases in the elimination half-life of alfentanil[329,871,872] as well as decreases in its clearance[871,872] have been reported by others to occur in the elderly. Thus, maintenance doses of alfentanil need to be decreased with age. Lemmens et al.[873] found no age-related changes in alfentanil plasma concentrations needed to block perioperative stimuli. Nevertheless, they and others[329] suggest reducing alfentanil loading dose requirements in the aged. Anticipation of a high degree of variability in the magnitude and duration of responses to all opioids in the elderly is probably the most useful approach. The overall effects of age on the volume of distribution, clearance, and elimination half-life of opioids are depicted in Fig. 10-25.

Hepatic Blood Flow and Hepatic Disease

The primary site of opioid metabolism is the liver. It follows that decreases in drug delivery (e.g., hepatic blood flow) or hepatic function could prolong opioid effects. Upper abdominal surgery that significantly decreases hepatic blood flow also decreases alfentanil clearance[874] and perhaps the elimination half-life of sufentanil.[875] However, liver disease and concomitant ab-

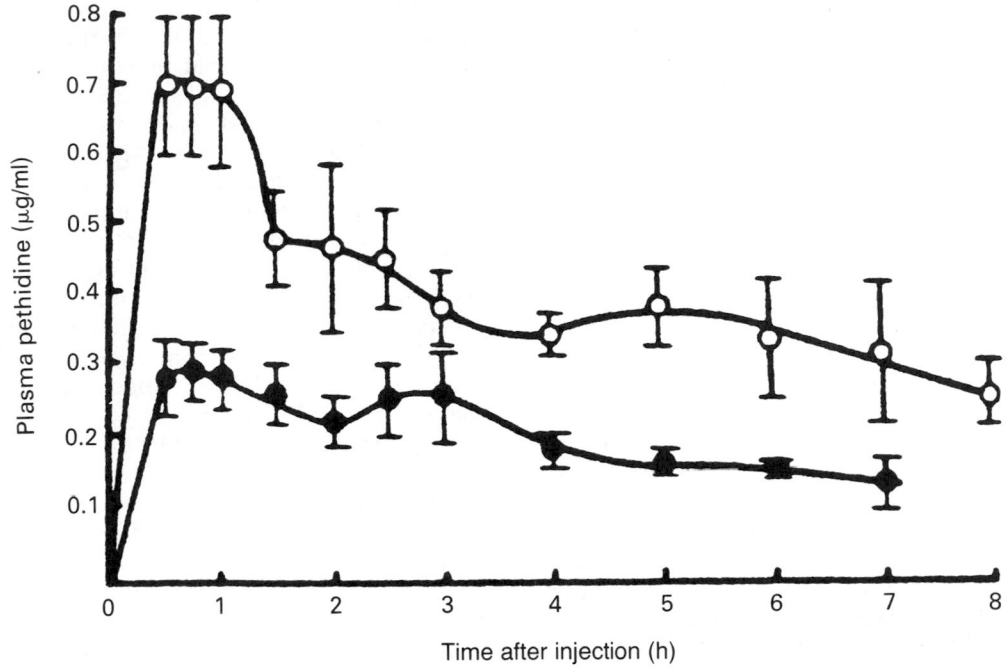

Fig. 10-24. Mean plasma pethidine (meperidine) concentrations (± standard error of mean) after an intramuscular injection (1.5 mg/kg) in a group of young (●, 16 to 40 years, *n* = 7) and a group of old (○, over 70 years, *n* = 10) subjects. (From Chan et al.,[355] with permission.)

normalities (e.g., plasma protein binding) produce a spectrum of changes. For example, Patwardhan et al.[876] found no change in the elimination half-life or clearance of morphine in six men with cirrhosis. Since indocyanine green clearance was reduced, Patwardhan et al.[876] postulated an extrahepatic site (renal and gastrointestinal) for morphine conjugation that they reasoned maintained normal elimination of morphine. Mazoit et al.,[877] on the other hand, found that morphine's elimination half-life was increased (201 versus 111 minutes)

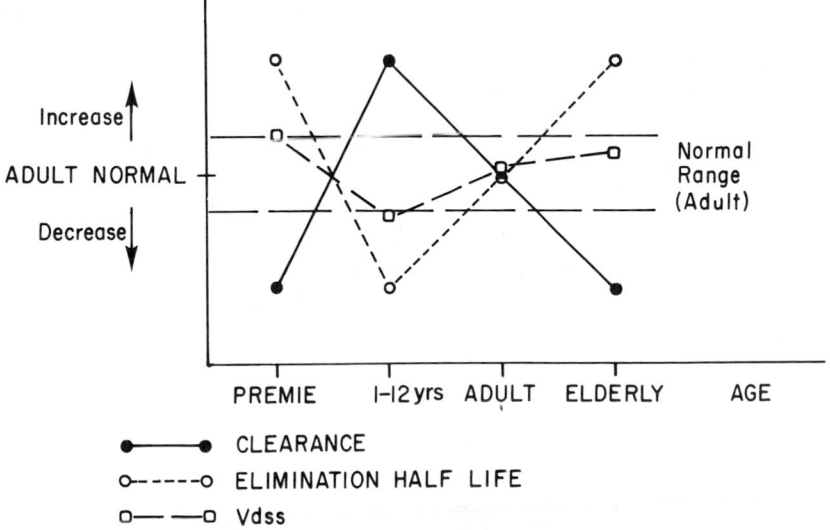

Fig. 10-25. Approximate effects of age on the clearance, volume of distribution, and elimination half-life of alfentanil. Clearance is significantly reduced at the extremes of age.

and clearance decreased (21 versus 33.5 ml/kg/min) in patients with severe cirrhosis. If uremia, hyperbilirubinemia, and hypoalbuminemia accompany liver disease, patients may also demonstrate an increased sensitivity to morphine. In this circumstance, bilirubin competes with and displaces morphine from an already reduced number of albumin-binding sites.[878] On the other hand, some authors believe that the kidneys are the primary site of morphine metabolism and that hepatic metabolism of morphine is only important with high doses.[879,880] Nevertheless, the absence of liver function results in markedly prolonged morphine and fentanyl elimination half-lives.[881,882]

Klatz et al.[883] showed that meperidine clearance was reduced (664 versus 1,316 ml/min) and elimination half-life was increased (7.0 versus 3.2 hours) in cirrhotics compared with age-matched healthy volunteers. Volumes of distribution and plasma protein binding were unchanged. Abnormalities in biochemical liver function tests did not correlate with alterations in $t1/2\beta$ or clearance. Others have also documented decreased meperidine clearance and prolonged elimination half-lives in patients with cirrhosis[884,885] and acute viral hepatitis.[886] The kinetics of meperidine are altered in patients with a history of heavy alcohol consumption.[804] An increased volume of distribution and lower initial plasma concentrations may contribute to an apparent decrease in sensitivity to meperidine in these patients.

The disposition of fentanyl is not altered in patients with cirrhosis during general anesthesia.[816] The terminal elimination half-life of fentanyl is a reflection of its slow release from tissue stores rather than hepatic elimination. Only with severe hepatic dysfunction and perhaps high doses of fentanyl will altered pharmacokinetics be observed. Decreases in hepatic blood flow may account for the prolonged elimination half-life (8.7 hours) of fentanyl (100 μg/kg) and sufentanil in patients undergoing abdominal aortic surgery.[875,887] A positive correlation exists between alcohol consumption and the need for fentanyl supplementation during nitrous oxide-oxygen-muscle relaxant anesthesia.[888] Up to 70 percent more fentanyl (6.4 versus 3.8 μg/kg/h) was needed in individuals with a mean annual consumption of 31 L of pure alcohol.

Ferrier et al.[889] evaluated the pharmacokinetics of alfentanil (50 μg/kg) in cirrhotic patients undergoing general anesthesia. Clearance was decreased and elimination half-life was prolonged (219 versus 90 minutes) compared with control patients (1.5 versus 3.1 ml/kg/min). α_1-Acidglycoprotein concentrations were not decreased, but the plasma free fraction of alfentanil was increased (18.6 versus 11.5 percent). Biochemical alteration of the sites on α_1-acidglycoprotein that bind alfentanil was thought to be responsible for the changes. Thus, an augmented and prolonged alfentanil effect can be anticipated in patients with cirrhosis. In contrast, children with cholestatic liver disease scheduled to undergo orthotopic liver transplantation showed no changes in alfentanil elimination half-life clearance and volume of distribution at steady state.[890] Patients with high alcohol consumption require higher plasma alfentanil levels than nondrinking patients. A similar difference exists in the plasma concentration at which ventilation is adequate. Decreased CNS sensitivity to opioid effects is the likely cause of these pharmacodynamic differences in alcoholics. Because alfentanil has a hepatic extraction ratio intermediate in value (0.3 to 0.5), decreases in hepatic blood flow can still decrease elimination.[837] Thus, indocyanine green clearance (a measure of hepatic blood flow) has been found to correlate with alfentanil clearance. Major intra-abdominal surgery has been shown to prolong alfentanil effects by reducing clearance from 6.8 to 2.6 ml/kg/min.[891] Sufentanil (3 μg/kg) pharmacokinetics appear to be changed in cirrhotic patients.[892] Major intra-abdominal surgery also increases the volume of distribution at steady state and the elimination half-life of sufentanil.[875] In summary, initial doses of opioids need not be decreased or increased unless CNS symptoms (encephalopathy) or heavy alcohol consumption exist in patients with liver disease. However, prolonged duration of opioid action may occur, especially in patients with severe liver disease, and maintenance doses should be decreased accordingly.

Cardiopulmonary Bypass

Cardiopulmonary bypass produces significant alterations in the pharmacokinetics of most drugs including opioids.[893] Explanations for these observations are summarized in Table 10-22. The onset of cardiopulmonary bypass initiates hemodilution and relative hypotension. Hemodilution produces a dramatic (range 30 to 80 percent) decrease in plasma levels of fentanyl,[430,894] sufentanil,[895] and alfentanil[896] (Fig. 10-26). Opioid uptake by the membrane component of the Scimed brand membrane oxygenators also contributes to the decline of plasma levels of fentanyl[863,897] and sufentanil.[898,899] Under clinical conditions membrane saturation with fentanyl proceeds slowly and reaches a maximum of 130 ng/cm².[897] Maximum uptake of sufentanil is less (11 ng/cm²).[898] Most fentanyl or sufentanil has left the plasma and is in tissue stores and receptors when cardiopulmonary bypass is started. Abrupt decreases in plasma opioid levels are thus buffered by tissue (and brain) levels of opioids. The need to administer additional opioid when cardiopulmonary bypass has been initiated has been questioned. Such a practice may actually lead to further tissue accumulation.[900] Less alfentanil is sequestered by the cardiopulmonary bypass apparatus.[901]

The hypotension that accompanies cardiopulmonary bypass alters opioid pharmacokinetics by decreasing hepatic blood flow by about 30 percent.[902] Thus, clearance of fentanyl is reduced to approximately 7 ml/kg/min.[903] Opioids with lower hepatic extraction ratios (e.g., alfentanil) will not be as affected by decreases in

TABLE 10-22. Pharmacokinetic Consequences of Cardiopulmonary Bypass

Event	Consequence
Hemodilution	50% ↓ plasma opioid level; ↑ Vdss
Decreased plasma proteins	↑ Opioid free fraction →↑ Vdss
Hypotension	—↓ Hepatic blood flow —↓ Opioid clearance —↓ Drug distribution
Membrane oxygenator	↓ Plasma opioid levels
Decreased muscle perfusion	Opioid accumulation in muscle
Lung isolation	Opioid trapping
Hypothermia	↓ Opioid potency, ↓ need for anesthesia, ↓ drug metabolism
Decreased HBF, opioid clearance and distribution	Opioid levels constant after initial decrease
Terminating cardiopulmonary bypass and improved tissue perfusion	↑ Opioid reuptake from tissues and plasma levels
Post-bypass	Prolonged t 1/2β persists

hepatic blood flow. While decreased perfusion of peripheral compartment tissues (e.g., muscle) and a decreased cardiac output[904] decrease volume of distribution at steady state, reductions in plasma protein binding and the cardiopulmonary bypass apparatus produce an apparent increase in the volume of distribution.[893] Elimination half-life for fentanyl is, therefore, increased (up to 11 hours) because of both decreased clearance and increased volume of distribution at steady state. Similar changes would be anticipated for sufentanil.

Hypothermia also decreases enzymatic hepatic activ-

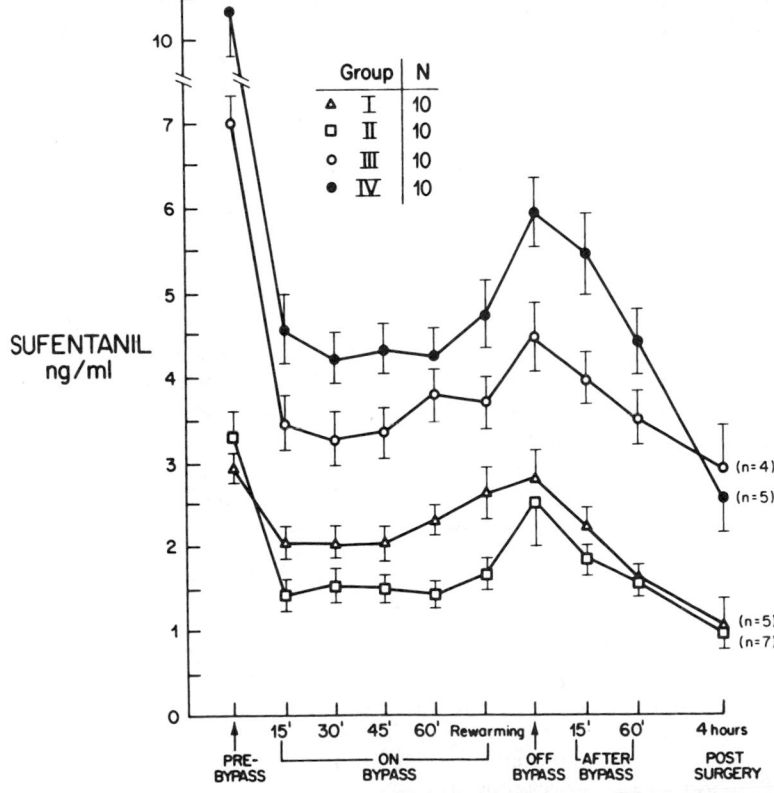

Fig. 10-26. Plasma sufentanil levels after 30 μg/kg (Δ), 10 μg/kg bolus plus 0.05 μg/kg/min infusion (□), 20 μg/kg bolus plus 0.1 μg/kg/min (○), and 40 μg/kg bolus plus 0.2 μg/kg/min infusion (●) and the influence of cardiopulmonary bypass. (From Okutani et al.,[895] with permission.)

ity and increases elimination half-life.[895] Interestingly, hypothermia decreases morphine's affinity (and potency) at mu receptors. The IC_{50} for morphine in a guinea pig ileum bioassay increases from 5.1×10^{-8} mol/L at 40°C to 41×10^{-8} mol/L at 30°C.[905] The clinical significance of cold-induced decreases in opioid potency is unknown. In addition, this effect is overridden, and probably overshadowed, by the anesthetic properties of hypothermia. After the initial decrease in plasma narcotic levels, concentrations remain stable owing to the prolonged elimination half-life.[895]

Upon termination of cardiopulmonary bypass opioid levels may actually rise and approach pre-bypass levels during fentanyl and sufentanil anesthesia (Fig. 10-26).[895] Reperfusion of organs that sequester fentanyl (muscle and lung) most likely accounts for this curious finding.[906] Pulsatile cardiopulmonary bypass, by keeping hepatic blood flow at prebypass levels and by improving deep compartment perfusion, prevents these second peaks in plasma fentanyl concentration.[907] Fentanyl plasma level decline during cardiopulmonary bypass, however, was not different when pulsatile cardiopulmonary bypass was compared to nonpulsatile cardiopulmonary bypass.

After cardiopulmonary bypass, alfentanil elimination half-life is prolonged (from 68 to 162 minutes) because decreases (by 40 percent) in α_1-acidglycoprotein levels increase alfentanil free fraction (from 5 to 14 percent) and volume of distribution (from 0.31 to 0.75 L/kg).[896] Attempts to define the pharmacokinetics of opioids over a period that includes cardiopulmonary bypass are difficult owing to the marked disruptions in plasma levels that occur.[902] Cell savers and hemoconcentration devices sequester minimal amounts of opioids (less than 0.5 percent of the injected dose) in the supernatant or ultrafiltrate. This is due to the fact that they are introduced after most of an administered opioid has left the circulation.[908]

Renal Disease

Morphine exerts a prolonged effect in patients with renal failure.[909,910] After intravenous injection, plasma morphine levels are higher in these patients than in normal individuals for 5 to 15 minutes.[911,912] Maximum differences after 0.125 mg/kg of morphine are almost twofold, 862 versus 437 ng/ml.[911] This is consistent with a reduced central volume of distribution in patients with renal disease (0.3 versus 0.8 L/kg).[912] Some investigators report significant differences in the clearance or elimination half-life of morphine in patients with renal failure.[911,912] They attribute prolonged opioid effects in this population to the accumulation of morphine-3-glucuronide, which is less potent than morphine but can produce respiratory depression and analgesia. Morphine-6-glucuronide normally represents a small fraction of morphine's metabolites, but it too can accumulate and it is more potent than morphine.

Others[879,880,913] believe that renal metabolism of morphine is important. Ball et al.[879] have shown a correlation between renal function and morphine clearance: as creatine clearance fell so did clearance of morphine. In addition, distinct plateaus in morphine plasma levels have been noted during renal transplantation.[880,913] The duration of these plateaus correlates with renal ischemic times. Morphine-glucuronide has been shown to be formed in rabbit renal tubules.[914] Whatever the mechanism of altered morphine pharmacokinetics, both loading and maintenance doses of morphine should be decreased in patients with impaired renal function. Intact renal function may be important for efficient elimination of morphine congeners (e.g., dehydrocodeine) as well.[880]

Opioid metabolites will accumulate in proportion to the degree of renal impairment. Normeperidine, a major meperidine metabolite, is normally eliminated more slowly than meperidine. It possesses twice the convulsant activity of meperidine but only one-half the analgesic potency.[914] In renal failure or in the presence of chlorpromazine[915] (which may enhance N-demethylation), normeperidine and normeperidinic acid levels may rise and produce toxic (CNS, cardiac) effects. No data are available evaluating the pharmacokinetics of meperidine in patients with impaired renal function.

Renal failure should not alter fentanyl pharmacokinetics. Fentanyl metabolites may accumulate, but they are largely inactive and nontoxic. Patients with hyperlipoproteinemia bind more fentanyl to plasma proteins but do not demonstrate a change in clinical effect.[916]

Two studies have reported alfentanil's pharmacokinetics in patients with renal failure.[917,918] Both suggested that an increased clinical effect was likely with alfentanil owing to a decreased initial volume of distribution and an increased alfentanil free fraction. Marked discrepancies exist in the results of two studies, but clearance was unchanged in both. Variations in plasma protein abnormalities (hypoproteinemia, abnormal structure, hyperlipoproteinemia, and various accumulated endogenous and exogenous substances) could possibly explain the differing results. Both reports concluded that no delay in recovery after alfentanil should be expected.

Sufentanil pharmacokinetics are not altered in any consistent fashion by kidney disease, although greater variability exists in its clearance and elimination half-life when patients have impaired renal function.[919]

Obesity

Overweight, and especially morbidly obese, individuals have many significant abnormalities in organ and system function that can alter the disposition of drugs. Lipophilic drugs should accumulate in obese individuals (because the peripheral compartment has a high percent of adipose tissue) and prolong the elimination half-life. Unfortunately, limited data are available to document this assumption. Bentley et al.[920] studied the pharmacokinetics of fentanyl (10 μg/kg) in obese and nonobese individuals. No difference was found, yet the researchers suggested administering fentanyl on a lean weight basis. Evaluations of higher doses of fentanyl could produce different findings; however, no good data exist at the present time to confirm this. The effects of obesity on alfentanil pharmacokinetics have been evaluated in only one study.[921] Interestingly, alfentanil clearance was reduced by 45 percent (321 to 179 ml/min) and elimination half-life was nearly doubled (92 to 172 minutes). If additional studies confirm these findings, it would be wise to administer alfentanil on the basis of lean body mass and maintenance doses should be decreased in anticipation of impaired clearance.

REFERENCES

1. Foldes FF, Swerdlow M, Siker ES: Narcotics and Narcotic Antagonists. Charles C Thomas, Springfield, IL, 1964

2. Stanley TH, Webster LR: Anesthetic requirements and cardiovascular effects of fentanyl-oxygen and fentanyl-diazepam-oxygen anesthesia in man. Anesth Analg 57:411, 1978

3. Lowenstein E, Philbin D: Narcotic "anesthesia" in the eighties (editorial). Anesthesiology 55:195, 1981

4. Van Hoosen B: Scopolamine-morphine anesthesia. House of Manz, Chicago, 1915

5. Smith RR: Scopolamine-morphine anesthesia, with report of two hundred and twenty-nine cases. Surg Gynecol Obstet 7:414, 1908

6. Sexton JC: Death following scopolamine-morphine injection. Lancet Clin 55:582, 1905

7. Lundy JS: Balanced anesthesia. Minn Med 9:399, 1926

8. Neff W, Mayer EC, de la Luz Perales M: Nitrous oxide and oxygen anesthesia with curare relaxation. Calif Med 66:67, 1947

9. Holderness MC, Chase PE, Dripps RD: A narcotic analgesic and a butyrophenone with nitrous oxide for general anesthesia. Anesthesiology 24:336, 1963

10. Stoelting RK: Influence of barbiturate anesthetic induction on circulatory responses to morphine. Anesth Analg 56:615, 1977

11. Stanley TH, Bennett GM, Loeser EA, et al: Cardiovascular effects of diazepam and droperidol during morphine anesthesia. Anesthesiology 44:255, 1976

12. Bennett GM, Loeser EA, Stanley TH: Cardiovascular effects of scopolamine during morphine-oxygen and morphine-nitrous oxide-oxygen anesthesia in man. Anesthesiology 46:255, 1977

13. Mannheimer WH: The use of morphine and intravenous alcohol in the anesthetic management of open heart surgery. South Med J 64:1125, 1971

14. Stanley TH: Blood pressure and pulse rate responses to ketamine during general anesthesia. Anesthesiology 39:648, 1973

15. Hamm D, Freedman B, Pellom G, et al: The maintenance of myocardial contractility by fentanyl during enflurane administration. Anesthesiology 59:A86, 1983

16. Freedman B, Hamm D, Pellom G, et al: Fentanyl-halothane anesthesia maintains myocardial contractility. Anesthesiology 59:A35, 1983

17. Cohen MM, Duncan PG, Tate RB: Does anesthesia contribute to operative mortality? JAMA 260:2859, 1988

18. De Castro J: Analgesic anesthesia based on the use of fentanyl in high doses. Anesth Vigil Subvigile 1:87, 1970

19. Lowenstein E, Hallowell P, Levin FH, et al: Cardiovascular response to large doses of intravenous morphine in man. N Engl J Med 281:1389, 1969

20. Stoelting RK, Gibbs PS: Hemodynamic effects of morphine and morphine-nitrous oxide in valvular heart disease and coronary artery disease. Anesthesiology 38:45, 1973

21. Arens JF, Benbow BP, Ochsner JL, Theard R: Morphine anesthesia for aorto-coronary bypass procedures. Anesth Analg 51:901, 1972

22. Stanley TH, Gray NJ, Staford W, Armstrong R: The effects of high-dose morphine on fluid and blood requirements in open-heart operations. Anesthesiology 38:536, 1973

23. Stoelting RK, Gibbs PS, Creasser CW, Peterson C: Hemodynamic and ventilatory response to fentanyl, fentanyl-droperidol, and nitrous oxide in patients with acquired valvular heart disease. Anesthesiology 42:319, 1975

24. Lowenstein E: Morphine "anesthesia"—a perspective. Anesthesiology 35:563, 1971

25. Hug CC: Pharmacology of anesthetic drugs. Grune & Stratton, Orlando, FL, 1979

26. Thompson WL, Walton RP: Elevation of plasma histamine levels in the dog following administration of muscle relaxants, opiates and macromolecular polymers. J Pharmacol Exp Ther 143:131, 1964

27. Bedford RF, Wollman H: Postoperative respiratory effects of morphine and halothane anesthesia: A study in patients undergoing cardiac surgery. Anesthesiology 43:1, 1975

28. Stanley TH, Lathrop GD: Urinary excretion of morphine during and after valvular and coronary-artery surgery. Anesthesiology 46:166, 1977

29. Bennett GM, Stanley TH: Cardiovascular effects of fentanyl during enflurane anesthesia in man. Anesth Analg 58:179, 1979

30. Stanley TH, Philbin DM, Coggins CH: Fentanyl-oxygen anaesthesia for coronary artery surgery: Cardiovascular and antidiuretic hormone responses. Can Anaesth Soc J 26:168, 1979

31. Rosow CE, Philbin DM, Keegan CR, Moss J: Hemodynamics and histamine release during induction with sufentanil or fentanyl. Anesthesiology 60:489, 1984

32. Stanski DR, Hug CC, Jr: Alfentanil—a kinetically predictable narcotic analgesic (editorial). Anesthesiology 57:435, 1982

33. Stanley TH: New routes of administration and new delivery systems of anesthetics. Anesthesiology 68:665, 1988

34. Woolf A: Immobilization of captive and free ranging white-tailed deer with etorphine hydrochloride. J Am Vet Med Assoc 156:636, 1970

35. Thorpe AH: Opiate structure and activity: A guide to understanding the receptor. Anesth Analg 63:143, 1984

36. Snyder SH: Opiate receptors and internal opiates. Sci Am 236:44, 1977

37. Beckett AH, Casey AF: Synthetic analgesics, stereochemical considerations. J Pharm Pharmacol 6:986, 1954

38. Beckett AH: Analgesics and their antagonists: Some steric and chemical considerations. Part I. The dissociation constants of some tertiary amines and synthetic analgesics, the conformations of methadone-type compounds. J Pharm Pharmacol 8:848, 1956

39. Braenden OJ, Eddy NB, Halback H: Synthetic substances with morphine-like effect: Relationship between chemical structure and analgesic action. Bull WHO 13:937, 1955

40. Reynolds AK, Randall LO: Morphine and allied drugs. University of Toronto Press, Toronto, 1957

41. Pasternak GW, Childers SR: Opiates, opioid peptides and their receptors. p. (F)1. In Shoemaker WM (ed): Critical Care: State of the Art. Vol. V. Society of Critical Care Medicine, Fullerton, CA, 1984

42. Osei-Gyimah P, Archer S: Some 14-beta-substituted analogues of N-(cyclopropylmethyl)nor-morphine. J Med Chem 24:212, 1981

43. Portoghese PS, Alreja BD, Larson DL: Allylprodine analogues as receptor probes. Evidence that phenolic and nonphenolic ligands interact with different subsites on identical opioid receptors. J Med Chem 24:782, 1981

44. Gorin FA, Balasubramanian TM, Cicero TJ, et al: Novel analogues of enkephalin: Identification of functional groups required for biological activity. J Med Chem 23:113, 1980

45. Pert CB, Snyder SH: Opiate receptor: Demonstration in nervous tissue. Science 179:1011, 1973

46. Terenius L: Characteristics of the "receptor" for narcotic analgesics in synaptic plasma membrane fractions from rat brain. Acta Pharmacol Toxicol 13:377, 1973

47. Simon EJ, Hiller JM, Edelman I: Sterospecific binding of the potent narcotic analgesic [^{3}H]-etorphine to rat-brain homogenate. Proc Natl Acad Sci USA 70:1947, 1973

48. Stanley TH, Leysen J, Niemegeers JE, et al: Narcotic dosage and central nervous system opiate receptor binding. Anesth Analg 62:705, 1983

49. Creese I, Snyder SH: Receptor binding and pharmacological activity of opiates in the guinea pig ileum intestine. J Pharmacol Exp Ther 194:205, 1975

50. Ueda H, Harada H, Musawa H, et al: Purified opioid μ-receptor is of a different molecular size than δ- and k-receptors. Neuro Sci Lett 75:339, 1987

51. Yaksh TL, Howe JR: Opiate receptors and their definition by antagonists. Anesthesiology 56:246, 1982

52. Takemori A: Determination of pharmacological constants: Use of narcotic antagonists to characterize analgesic receptors. Adv Biochem Psychopharmacol 8:335, 1974

53. Yaksh TL: Spinal opiate analgesia: Characteristics and principles of action. Pain 11:293, 1981

54. Tung AS, Yaksh TL: In vivo evidence for multiple opiate receptors mediating analgesia in the rat spinal cord. Brain Res 247:75, 1982

55. Chang KJ, Cuatrecasas P: Multiple opiate receptors: Enkephalins and morphine bind to receptors of different specificity. J Biol Chem 254:2610, 1979

56. Goodman RR, Snyder SH, Kuhar MJ: Differentiation of delta and mu opiate receptor localizations by light microscopic autoradiography. Proc Natl Acad Sci USA 77:6239, 1980

57. Pasternak GW, Snyder SH: Identification of novel high affinity opiate receptor binding in rat brain. Nature 253:563, 1975

58. Wolozin BL, Pasternak GW: Classification of multiple morphine and enkephalin binding sites in the central nervous system. Proc Natl Acad Sci USA 78:6181, 1981

59. Ling GSF, Spiegel K, Lockhart SH, Pasternak GW: Separation of opioid analgesia from respiratory depression: Evidence for different receptor mechanisms. J Pharmacol Exp Ther 232:149, 1985

60. Pasternak GW, Zhang AZ, Tecott L: Developmental differences between high and low affinity opiate binding sites: Their relationship to analgesia and respiratory depression. Life Sci 27:1185, 1980

61. Ling GSF, Pasternak GW: Spinal and supraspinal analgesia in the mouse: The role of subpopulations of opioid binding sites. Brain Res 271:152, 1983

62. Kuhar MJ, Pert CB, Snyder SH: Regional distribution of opiate receptor binding in monkey and human brain. Nature 245:447, 1973

63. Martin WR, Eades CG, Thompson JA, et al: The effects of morphine- and nalorphine-like drugs in the nondependent and morphine-dependent chronic spinal dog. J Pharmacol Exp Ther 197:517, 1976

64. Franz DN, Hare BD, McCloskey KL: Spinal sympathetic neurons: Possible sites of opiate withdrawal suppression by clonidine. Science 215:1643, 1982

65. Pert A, Yaksh T: Sites of morphine-induced analgesia in the primate brain: Relation to pain pathways. Brain Res 80:135, 1974

66. Goldstein A: Opiate receptors. Life Sci 14:615, 1974

67. Snyder SH: Opiate receptors in the brain. N Engl J Med 296:266, 1977

68. Mayer DJ, Wolfle TL, Akil H, et al: Analgesia from electrical stimulation in the brainstem of the rat. Science 174:1351, 1971

69. Satoh M, Takagi H: Enhancement by morphine of the central descending inhibitory influence on spinal sensory transmission. Eur J Pharmacol 14:60, 1971

70. Yaksh TL, Rudy TA: Studies on the direct spinal action of narcotics in the production of analgesia in the rat. J Pharmacol Exp Ther 202:411, 1977

71. Frank GB: Stereospecific opioid drug receptors on excitable cell membranes. Can J Physiol Pharmacol 63:1023, 1985

72. Althaus JS, Miller ED, Moscicki JC, et al: Analgetic contribution of sufentanil during halothane anesthesia: A mechanism involving serotonin. Anesth Analg 64:857, 1985

73. Christie MJ, Williams JT, North RA: Cellular mechanisms of opioid tolerance: Studies in simple brain neurons. Mol Pharmacol 32:633, 1987

74. Boas RA, Villiger JW: Clinical actions of fentanyl and buprenorphine. The significance of receptor binding. Br J Anaesth 57:192, 1985

75. Agnati LF, Fuxe K, Benfenati F, et al: Studies on aging processes (III). Acta Physiol Scand 532:45, 1984

76. Parratt JR: Opioid receptors in the cardiovascular system. p. 97. In van Zwielen PA, Schönbaum E (eds.): Progress in Pharmacology. Vol. 6/2. Gustav Fischer Verlag, Stuttgart, 1986

77. Hughes J, Smith TW, Kosterlitz HW, et al: Identification of two related pentapeptides from the brain with potent opiate agonist activity. Nature 258:577, 1975

78. Cox BM, KE Opheim, Teschemaker H, et al: A peptide-like substance from pituitary that acts like morphine. Purification and properties. Life Sci 16:1777, 1975

79. Goldstein A, Fischli W, Lowney LI, et al: Porcine pituitary dynorphin: Complete amino acid sequence of the biologically active heptadecapeptide. Proc Natl Acad Sci USA 78:7219, 1981

80. Mains RE, Eipper BA, Ling N: Common precursor to corticotropins and endorphins. Proc Natl Acad Sci USA 74:3014, 1977

81. Gubler U, Kilpatrick DL, Seeburg PH, et al: Detection and partial characterization of proenkephalin in mRNA. Proc Natl Acad Sci USA 78:5484, 1981

82. Olson GA, Olson RD, Kastin AJ, et al: Endogenous opiates: 1980. Peptides 2:349, 1981

83. Rossier J, Vargo TM, Minick S, et al: Regional dissociation of beta-endorphin and enkephalin contents in rat brain and pituitary. Proc Natl Acad Sci USA 74:5162, 1977

84. Orwall ES, Kendall JW: β-Endorphin and ACTH in extra-adrenocorticotropic pituitary sites: Gastrointestinal tract. Endocrinology 107:438, 1980

85. Houck JC, Kimball C, Chang C, et al: Placental beta-endorphin-like peptides. Science 207:78, 1980

86. Santiago TV, Edelman NH: Opioids and breathing. J Appl Physiol 59:1675, 1985

87. Tuggle DW, Horton JW: Cardiocirculatory effects of physiological doses of beta-endorphin. Circ Shock 18:215, 1986

88. Millan MJ: Multiple opioid systems and pain. Pain 27:303, 1986

89. Akil H, Watson SJ, Young E, et al: Endogenous opioids: Biology and function. Annu Rev Neurosci 7:223, 1984

90. Wong KC: Narcotics are not expected to produce unconsciousness and amnesia (editorial). Anesth Analg 62:625, 1983

91. Hall RI, Szlam F, Hug CC, Jr: The enflurane-sparing effect of alfentanil in dogs. Anesth Analg 66:1287, 1987

92. Hall RI, Murphy MR, Hug CC, Jr: The enflurane sparing effect of sufentanil in dogs. Anesthesiology 67:518, 1987

93. Hall RI, Szlam F, Hug CC: Alfentanil is not a complete anesthetic in dogs. Anesth Analg 66:S76, 1987

94. Murphy MR, Hug CC: The enflurane sparing effect of morphine, butorphanol and nalbuphine. Anesthesiology 57:489, 1982

95. Murphy MR, Hug CC: The anesthetic potency of fentanyl in terms of its reduction of enflurane MAC. Anesthesiology 57:485, 1982

96. Murphy MR, Hug CC: Efficacy of fentanyl in reducing isoflurane MAC: Antagonism by naloxone and nalbuphine. Anesthesiology 59:A338, 1983

97. Hecker BR, Lake CL, DiFazio CA, et al: The decrease of the minimum alveolar anesthetic concentration produced by sufentanil in rats. Anesth Analg 62:987, 1983

98. Lake CL, DiFazio CA, Moscicki JC, Engle JS: Reduction in halothane MAC: Comparison of morphine and alfentanil. Anesth Analg 64:807, 1985

99. Bowdle TA, Ward RJ: Anesthesia with small doses of sufentanil or fentanyl: Dose versus EEG response, speed of onset and thiopental requirement. Anesthesiology 70:26, 1989

100. Bailey PL, Port DJ, McJames S, et al: Is fentanyl an anesthetic in the dog? Anesth Analg 66:542, 1987

101. Port JD, Stanley TH, Steffey EP, et al: Intravenous carfentanil in the dog and rhesus monkey. Anesthesiology 61:A378, 1984

102. Arndt JO, Mikat M, Parasher C: Fentanyl's analgesic, respiratory, and cardiovascular actions in relation to dose and plasma concentration in unanesthetized dogs. Anesthesiology 61:355, 1984

103. Shingu K, Eger EI II, Johnson BH, et al: MAC values of thiopental and fentanyl in rats. Anesth Analg 62:51, 1983

104. Kissin I, Brown PT: Reserpine-induced changes in anesthetic action of fentanyl. Anesthesiology 62:597, 1985

105. White DC: Anaesthesia: A puration of the senses. p. 1. In Lunn JN, Rosen M (eds): Consciousness, Awareness and Pain in General Anesthesia. Butterworth, Boston, 1987

106. Kissin I, Jebeles JA: Halothane antagonizes effect of morphine on the motor reaction threshold in rats. Anesthesiology 61:671, 1984

107. Eisele JH, Jr., Steffey EP: Narcotic analgesia—ceiling effect? Anesthesiology 60:60, 1984

108. Dundee JW, Nichol RM, Black GW: Alterations in response to somatic pain associated with anesthesia. X. Further studies with inhalation agents. Br J Anaesth 34:158, 1962

109. Dodson BA, Miller KW: Evidence of a dual mechanism in the anesthetic action of an opioid peptide. Anesthesiology 62:615, 1985

110. Levinson BW: States of awareness during general anesthesia. Br J Anaesth 37:544, 1965

111. Bennett HL, Davis HS, Giamnini JA: Non-verbal response to intraoperative conversation. Br J Anaesth 57:174, 1985

112. Jones JG: Use of evokes responses in EEG to measure depth of anesthesia. p. 99. In Lunn JN, Rosen M (eds): Consciousness, Awareness and Pain in General Anesthesia. Butterworth, Boston, 1987

113. Mainord WA, Rath B, Barnett F: Anesthesia and suggestion. Paper presented at the American Psychological Association Annual Convention, Los Angeles, CA, 1983

114. Sebel PS, Bovill JG: Opiate anaesthesia: Fact or fallacy (editorial). Br J Anaesth 54:1149, 1982

115. Wilson SL, Vaughan RW, Stephen CR: Awareness, dreams and hallucinations associated with general anesthesia. Anesth Analg 54:609, 1975

116. Saucier N, Walts LF, Moreland JR: Patient awareness during nitrous oxide, oxygen and halothane anesthesia. Anesth Analg 62:239, 1983

117. Mark JB, Greenberg LM: Intraoperative awareness and hypertensive crisis during high-dose fentanyl-diazepam-oxygen anesthesia. Anesth Analg 62:698, 1983

118. Hilgenberg JC: Intraoperative awareness during high-dose fentanyl-oxygen anesthesia. Anesthesiology 54:341, 1981

119. Mummanemi N, Rao T, Montoya A: Awareness and recall with high-dose fentanyl-oxygen anesthesia. Anesth Analg 59:943, 1980

120. Crawford JS, James FM, Davies P, Crawley M: A further study of general anaesthesia for caesarean section. Br J Anaesth 48:661, 1976

121. Utting JE: Awareness: Clinical aspects. p. 171. In Lunn JN, Rosen M (eds): Consciousness, Awareness and Pain in General Anesthesia. Butterworth, Boston, 1987

122. Ghoneim MM, Dhanaraj J, Choi WW: Comparison of four opioid analgesics as supplements to nitrous oxide anesthesia. Anesth Analg 63:405, 1984

123. Bailey PL, Wilbrink J, Zwanikken P, et al: Anesthetic induction with fentanyl. Anesth Analg 64:48, 1985

124. Stanley TH, de Lange S: The influence of patient habits on dosage requirements during high dose fentanyl anesthesia. Can Anaesth Soc J 31:368, 1985

125. Shafer A, White PF, Schüttler J, Rosenthal MH: Use of a fentanyl infusion in the intensive care unit: Tolerance to its anesthetic effect. Anesthesiology 59:245, 1983

126. Silbert BS, Rosow CE, Keegan CR, et al: The effect of diazepam on induction of anesthesia with alfentanil. Anesth Analg 67:717, 1986

127. Tomichek RC, Rosow CE, Philbin DM, et al: Diazepam-fentanyl interaction: Hemodynamic and hormonal effects in coronary artery surgery. Anesth Analg 62:881, 1983

128. Blacher RS: On awakening paralyzed during surgery. A syndrome of traumatic neurosis. JAMA 234:67, 1975

129. van de Walle J, Lauwers P, Adriaensen H: Double blind comparison of fentanyl and sufentanil in anesthesia. Acta Anaesthesiol Belg 27:129, 1976

130. Sebel PS, Bovill JG: Cardiovascular effects of sufentanil anesthesia: A study in patients undergoing cardiac surgery. Anesth Analg 61:115, 1982

131. Nauta J, Stanley TH, de Lange S, et al: Anaesthetic induction with alfentanil: Comparison with thiopental, midazolam, and etomidate. Can Anaesth Soc J 30:53, 1983

132. Moldenhauer CC, Griesemer RW, Hug CC, Holbrook GW: Hemodynamic changes during rapid induction of anesthesia with alfentanil. Anesth Analg 62:276, 1983

133. Schmidt CF, Livingston AE: The action of morphine on the mammalian circulation. J Pharmacol Exp Ther 47:411, 1933

134. Moffitt EA, Sethna DH, Bussell JA, et al: Myocardial metabolism and hemodynamic responses to halothane or morphine anesthesia for coronary artery surgery. Anesth Analg 61:979, 1982

135. Vasko JS, Henney RP, Brawley RK, et al: Effects of morphine on ventricular function and myocardial contractile force. Am J Physiol 210:329, 1966

136. Stanley TH, Isern-Amaral J, Lathrop GD: Effects of morphine and halothane anaesthesia on urine norepinephrine during and after coronary artery surgery. Can Anaesth Soc J 22:478, 1975

137. Stanley TH, Isern-Amaral J, Lathrop GD: Urine norepinephrine excretion in patients undergoing mitral or aortic valve replacement with morphine anesthesia. Anesth Analg 54:509, 1975

138. Balasariswathi K, Glisson SN, El-Etr AA, et al: Serum epinephrine and norepinephrine during valve replacement and aortocoronary bypass. Can Anaesth Soc J 25:198, 1978

139. Fahmy NR, Sunder N, Soter NA: Role of histamine in the hemodynamic and plasma catecholamine responses to morphine. Clin Pharmacol Ther 33:615, 1983

140. Flacke JW, Van Etten AP, Bloor BC, et al: Histamine release by four narcotics: A double blind study in humans. Anesth Analg 66:723, 1987

141. Liu WS, Bidwai AV, Lunn JK, et al: Urine catecholamine excretion after large doses of fentanyl, fentanyl and diazepam and fentanyl, diazepam and pancuronium. Can Anaesth Soc 24:371, 1977

142. Stanley TH, Berman L, Green O, et al: Plasma catecholamine and cortisol responses to fentanyl-oxygen anesthesia for coronary-artery operations. Anesthesiology 53:250, 1980

143. Hicks HC, Mowbray AG, Yhap EO: Cardiovascular effects of and catecholamine responses to high dose fentanyl-O_2 for induction of anesthesia in patients with ischemic coronary artery disease. Anesth Analg 60:563, 1981

144. Lunn JK, Stanley TH, Webster LR, et al: High dose fentanyl anesthesia for coronary artery surgery: Plasma fentanyl concentration and influence of nitrous oxide on cardiovascular responses. Anesth Analg 58:390, 1979

145. Kentor ML, Schwalb AJ, Lieberman RW: Rapid high dose fentanyl induction for CABG. Anesthesiology 3:S95, 1980

146. Rendig SV, Amsterdam EA, Henderson GL, Mason DT: Comparative cardiac contractile actions of six narcotic analgesics: Morphine meperidine, pentazocine, fentanyl, methadone and I-α-acetylmethadol (LAAM). J Pharmacol Exp Ther 215:259, 1980

147. Drew JH, Dripps RD, Comroe JH: The effect of morphine upon the circulation of man and upon the circulatory and respiratory responses to tilting. Anesthesiology 7:44, 1946

148. Conahan TJ, Ominsky AJ, Wollman H, Stroth R: A prospective random comparison of halothane and morphine for open-heart anesthesia: One year's experience. Anesthesiology 38:528, 1973

149. Lappas DG, Geha D, Fischer JE, et al: Filling pressures of the heart and pulmonary circulation of the patient with coronary-artery disease after large intravenous doses of morphine. Anesthesiology 42:153, 1975

150. Rosow CE, Moss J, Philbin DM, Savarese JJ: Histamine release during morphine and fentanyl anesthesia. Anesthesiology 56:93, 1982

151. Moss J, Rosow CE: Histamine release by narcotics and muscle relaxants in humans. Anesthesiology 59:330, 1983

152. Lowenstein E, Whiting RB, Bittar DA, et al: Local and neurally mediated effects of morphine on skeletal muscle vascular resistance. J Pharmacol Exp Ther 180:359, 1972

153. Henney RP, Vasko JS, Brawley RK, et al: The effects of morphine on the resistance and capacitance vessels of the peripheral circulation. Heart J 72:242, 1966

154. Ward JM, McGrath RC, Weil JL: Effect of morphine on the peripheral vascular response to sympathetic stimulation. Am J Cardiol 29:659, 1972

155. Stanley TH, Gray NH, Isern-Amaral J, Patton CP: Comparison of blood requirements during morphine and halothane anesthesia for open-heart surgery. Anesthesiology 41:34, 1974

156. Greene JF, Jackman AP, Krohn KA: Mechanism of morphine induced shifts in blood volume between extracorporeal reservoir and the systemic circulation of the dog under conditions of constant blood flow and vena caval pressures. Circ Res 42:479, 1978

157. Greene JF, Jackman AP, Parsons G: The effects of morphine on the mechanical properties of the systemic circulation in the dog. Circ Res 42:474, 1978

158. Hsu HO, Hickey RF, Forbes AR: Morphine decreases peripheral vascular resistance and increases capacitance in man. Anesthesiology 50:98, 1979

159. Zelis R, Mansour EJ, Capone RJ, Mason DT: The cardiovascular effects of morphine: The peripheral capacitance and resistance vessels in human subjects. J Clin Invest 54:1247, 1974

160. Priano LL, Vatner SF: Morphine effects on cardiac output and regional blood flow distribution in conscious dogs. Anesthesiology 55:236, 1981

161. Wong KC, Martin WE, Hornbein TF, et al: The cardiovascular effects of morphine sulfate with oxygen and with nitrous oxide in man. Anesthesiology 38:542, 1973

162. Moores WY, Weiskopf RB, Baysinger M, Utley JR: Effects of halothane and morphine sulfate on myocardial compliance following total cardiopulmonary bypass. J Thorac Cardiovasc Surg 81:163, 1981

163. Hoar PF, Nelson NT, Mangano DT, et al: Adrenergic response to morphine-diazepam anesthesia for myocardial revascularization. Anesth Analg 60:406, 1981

164. Strauer BE: Contractile responses to morphine, piritramide, meperidine and fentanyl: A comparative study of effects on the isolated ventricular myocardium. Anesthesiology 37:304, 1972

165. Bennett GM, Stanley TH: Human cardiovascular responses to endotracheal intubation during morphine-N_2O and fentanyl-N_2O anesthesia. Anesthesiology 52:520, 1980

166. King BD, Elder JD, Dripps RD: The effect of the intravenous administration of meperidine upon the circulation of man and upon the circulatory response to tilt. Surg Gynecol Obstet 94:591, 1952

167. Freye E: Cardiovascular effects of high dosages of fentanyl, meperidine and naloxone in dogs. Anesth Analg 53:40, 1974

168. Stanley TH, Bidwai AV, Lunn JK, Hodges MR: Cardiovascular effects of nitrous oxide during meperidine infusion in the dog. Anesth Analg 56:836, 1977

169. De Castro J, Van de Water A, Wouters L, et al: Comparative study of cardiovascular, neurological and metabolic side effects of eight narcotics in dogs. Acta Anaesth Belg 30:5, 1979

170. Stanley TH, Liu WS: Cardiovascular effects of meperidine-N_2O anesthesia before and after pancuronium. Anesth Analg 56:669, 1977

171. Sugioka K, Boniface KJ, Davis DA: The influence of meperidine on myocardial contractility in the intact dog. Anesthesiology 18:623, 1957

172. Waller JL, Hug CC, Nagle DM, Craver JM: Hemodynamic changes during fentanyl-oxygen anesthesia for aortocoronary bypass operations. Anesthesiology 55:212, 1981

173. Wynands JE, Wong P, Whalley DG, et al: Oxygen-fentanyl anesthesia in patients with poor left ventricular function, hemodynamics and plasma fentanyl concentrations. Anesth Analg 62:476, 1983

174. Hamm D, Freedman B, Pellom G, et al: The effect of fentanyl on left ventricular function. Anesthesiology 59:A37, 1983

175. Motomura S, Kissin I, Aultman D, Reves JG: Effects of fentanyl and nitrous oxide on contractility of blood-perfused papillary muscle of the dog. Anesth Analg 63:47, 1984

176. Miller DR, Wellwood M, Teasdale SJ, et al: Effects of anaesthetic induction on myocardial function and metabolism: A comparison of fentanyl, sufentanil and alfentanil. Can J Anaesth 35:219, 1988

177. Lake CL, DiFazio CA: Sufentanil versus fentanyl: Hemodynamic effects in valvular heart disease. Anesth Analg 66:S99, 1987

178. Liu WS, Bidwai AV, Stanley TH, et al: The cardiovascular effects of diazepam and of diazepam and pancuronium during fentanyl and oxygen anaesthesia. Can Anaesth Soc J 23:395, 1976

179. Hill AB, Nahrwold ML, de Rosayro M, et al: Prevention of rigidity during fentanyl-oxygen induction of anesthesia. Anesthesiology 55:452, 1981

180. Flacke JW, Flacke WE, Bloor BC, Olewine S: Effects of fentanyl, naloxone, and clonidine on hemodynamics and plasma catecholamine levels in dogs. Anesth Analg 62:305, 1983

181. Flacke JW, David LJ, Flacke WE, et al: Effects of fentanyl and diazepam in dogs deprived of autonomic tone. Anesth Analg 64:1053, 1985

182. Starck T, Hall D, Freas W, et al: Peripheral vascular depression with sufentanil in the dog. Anesth Analg 68:S277, 1989

183. Mathews HML, Furness G, Carson IW, et al: Comparison of sufentanil-oxygen and fentanyl-oxygen anaesthesia for coronary artery bypass grafting. Br J Anaesth 60:530, 1988

184. Niemegeers CJE, Janssen PAJ: Alfentanil, a particularly short-acting intravenous narcotic analgesic. Drug Dev Res 1:83, 1981

185. Schauble JF, Chen BB, Murray PA: Marked hemodynamic effects of bolus administration of alfentanil in conscious dogs. Anesthesiology 59:A85, 1983

186. de Bruijn ND, Christian C, Fagraeus L, et al: The effects of alfentanil on global ventricular mechanics. Anesthesiology 59:A33, 1983

187. Ausems ME, Hug CC, Jr, de Lange S: Variable rate infusion of alfentanil as a supplement to nitrous oxide anesthesia for general surgery. Anesth Analg 62:982, 1983

188. Bartkowski RR, McDonnell TE: Alfentanil as an anesthetic induction agent: A comparison with thiopental-lidocaine. Anesth Analg 63:330, 1984

189. Lemmens HJM, Bovill JG, Burm AGL, Hennis PJ: Alfentanil infusion in the elderly. Anaesthesia 43:850, 1988

190. Rucquoi M, Camu F: Cardiovascular responses to large doses of alfentanil and fentanyl. Br J Anaesth 55:223, 1983

191. Thomson IR, Putnins CL, Friesen RM: Hyperdynamic cardiovascular response to anesthetic induction with high dose fentanyl. Anesth Analg 65:91, 1986

192. Gaumann DM, Yaksh TL, Tyce GM, Lucas DL: Opioids preserve the adrenal medullary response evoked by severe hemorrhage: Studies on adrenal catecholamines and Met-enkephalin secretion in halothane anesthetized cats. Anesthesiology 68:743, 1988

193. James TN, Isobe JH, Urthaler F: Analysis of components in a cardiogenic hypertensive chemoreflex. Circulation 52:179, 1975

194. Hasbrouck JD: Morphine anesthesia for open heart surgery. Ann Thorac Surg 10:364, 1970

195. Bailey DR, Miller ED, Kaplan JA, Rogers PW: The renin-angiotension-aldosterone system during cardiac surgery with morphine-nitrous oxide anesthesia. Anesthesiology 42:538, 1975

196. Quinton L, Whalley DG, Wynands JE, et al: Oxygen-high dose fentanyl-droperidol anesthesia for aortocoronary bypass surgery. Anesth Analg 60:412, 1981

197. Wynands JE, Townsend GE, Wong P, et al: Blood pressure response and plasma fentanyl concentrations during high- and very high-dose fentanyl anesthesia for coronary artery surgery. Anesth Analg 62:661, 1983

198. Edde RR: Hemodynamic changes prior to and after sternotomy in patients anesthetized with high-dose fentanyl. Anesthesiology 55:444, 1981

199. Sebel PS, Bovill JG, Boekhorst RAA, Rog P: Cardiovascular effects of high dose fentanyl anesthesia. Acta Anaesthesiol Scand 26:308, 1982

200. de Lange S, Stanley TH, Boscoe M: Comparison of anesthetic requirements and cardiovascular responses in Salt Lake City and Leiden, Holland. p. 313. Paper presented at the Seventh World Congress of Anaesthesiology. Excerpta Medica, Amsterdam, 1980

201. de Lange S, Stanley TH, Boscoe MJ, Pace NL: Comparison of sufentanil-O_2 and fentanyl-O_2 for coronary artery surgery. Anesthesiology 56:112, 1982

202. Wynands JE, Wong P, Townsend GE, et al: Narcotic requirements for intravenous anesthesia. Anesth Analg 63:101, 1983

203. Sebel PS, Bovill JG, Schellekens APM, Hawker CD: Hormonal responses of high-dose fentanyl anaesthesia: A study in patients undergoing cardiac surgery. Br J Anaesth 53:941, 1981

204. Stoelting RK, Creasser CW, Gibbs PS, Peterson C: Circulatory effects of halothane added to morphine anesthesia in patients with coronary-artery disease. Anesth Analg 53:449, 1974

205. Bland JHL, Lowenstein E: Halothane-induced decrease in experimental myocardial ischemia in the non-failing canine heart. Anesthesiology 45:287, 1976

206. Freedman B, Christian C, Hamm D, et al: Isoflurane and myocardial protection. Anesthesiology 59:A25, 1983

207. Howie MB, Reitz J, Reilley TE, et al: Does sufentanil's shorter half-life have any clinical significance? Anesthesiology 59:A146, 1983

208. Hickey PR, Hansen DD: Fentanyl- and sufentanil-oxygen-pancuronium anesthesia for cardiac surgery in infants. Anesth Analg 63:117, 1984

209. McDonnell TE, Bartkowski RR, Williams JJ: ED_{50} of alfentanil for induction of anesthesia in unpremedicated young adults. Anesthesiology 60:136, 1984

210. Nauta J, de Lange S, Koopman D, et al: Anesthetic induction with alfentanil: A new short acting narcotic analgesic. Anesth Analg 61:267, 1982

211. de Lange S, Stanley TH, Boscoe MJ: Alfentanil-oxygen anaesthesia for coronary artery surgery. Br J Anaesth 53:1291, 1981

212. Reitan JA, Stengert KB, Wymore ML, Martucci RW: Central vagal control of fentanyl-induced bradycardia during halothane anesthesia. Anesth Analg 57:31, 1978

213. Tammisto T, Takki S, Toikka P: A comparison of the circula-

tory effects in man of the analgesics fentanyl, pentazocine and pethidine. Br J Anaesth 42:317, 1970

214. Liu WS, Bidwai AV, Stanley TH, Isern-Amaral S: Cardiovascular dynamics after large doses of fentanyl and fentanyl plus N₂O in the dog. Anesth Analg 55:168, 1976

215. Prakash O, Verdouw PD, De Jong JW, et al: Haemodynamic and biochemical variables after induction of anaesthesia in patients undergoing coronary artery bypass surgery. Can Anaesth Soc J 27:223, 1980

216. Hornbein TF, Martin WE, Bonica JJ, et al: Nitrous oxide effects on the circulatory and ventilatory responses to halothane. Anesthesiology 31:250, 1969

217. Smith NT, Eger EI, Stoelting RK, et al: The cardiovascular and sympathomimetic responses to the addition of nitrous oxide to halothane in man. Anesthesiology 32:410, 1970

218. Meuleman T, Port JD, Stanley TH, Williard KF: Immobilization of elk and moose with carfentanil. J Wildl Manage 48:258, 1984

219. Reddy P, Liu WS, Port D, et al: Comparison of haemodynamic effects of anaesthetic doses of alphaprodine and sufentanil in the dog. Can Anaesth Soc J 27:345, 1980

220. Williard KF, Port JD, Stanley TH: Narcotic-oxygen anesthesia without respiratory support in the basally anesthetized dog. Anesthesiology 59:A321, 1983

221. Port JD, Stanley TH, McJames S: Topical narcotic anesthesia. Anesthesiology 59:A325, 1983

222. de Lange S, Boscoe MJ, Stanley TH, et al: Antidiuretic and growth hormone responses during coronary artery surgery with sufentanil-oxygen and alfentanil-oxygen anesthesia in man. Anesth Analg 61:434, 1982

223. de Lange S, de Bruijn N: Alfentanil-oxygen anesthesia: Plasma concentration and clinical effects during variable rate continuous infusion for coronary artery surgery. Br J Anaesth 55:S183, 1983

224. Cohn AE: The effect of morphine on the mechanism of the dog's heart after removal of one vagus nerve. Proc Soc Exp Biol Med 10:93, 1913

225. Robbins BH, Fitzhugh OG, Baxter JH, Jr: The action of morphine in slowing the pulse. J Pharmacol Exp Ther 66:216, 1939

226. Kennedy BL, West TC: Effect of morphine on electrically-induced release of autonomic mediators in the rabbit sinoatrial node. J Pharmacol Exp Ther 157:149, 1967

227. Tomichek RC, Rosow CE, Schneider RC, et al: Cardiovascular effects of diazepam-fentanyl anesthesia in patients with coronary artery disease. Anesth Analg 61:217, 1982

228. De Silva RA, Verrierm RL, Lown B: Protective effect of vagotonic action of morphine sulfate on ventricular vulnerability. Cardiovasc Res 12:167, 1978

229. Starr NJ, Sethna DH, Estafanous FG: Bradycardia and asystole following the rapid administration of sufentanil with vecuronium. Anesthesiology 64:521, 1986

230. Maryniak JK, Bishop VA: Sinus arrest after alfentanil (letter). Br J Anaesth 59:390, 1987

231. Sherman EP, Lebowitz PW, Street WC: Bradycardia following sufentanil-succinylcholine. Anesthesiology 66:106, 1987

232. Rivard JC, Lebowitz PW: Bradycardia after alfentanil-succinylcholine. Anesth Analg 67:907, 1988

233. Royster RL, Keeler DK, Haisty WK, et al: Cardiac electrophysiologic effects of fentanyl and combinations of fentanyl and combinations of fentanyl and neuromuscular relaxants in pentobarbital anesthetized dogs. Anesth Analg 67:15, 1988

234. Puerto BA, Wong KC, Puerto AX, et al: Epinephrine-induced dysrhythmias: Comparison during anaesthesia with narcotics and with halogenated agents in dogs. Can Anaesth Soc J 26:263, 1979

235. Blair JR, Pruett JK, Crumrine RS, Balser JS: Prolongation of QT interval in association with large doses of opiates. Anesthesiology 67:442, 1987

236. Bennett GM, Stanley TH: Comparison of the cardiovascular effects of morphine-N₂O and fentanyl-N₂O balanced anesthesia before and after pancuronium in man. Anesthesiology 51:S138, 1979

237. Cahalan MK, Lurz FW, Eger EI, et al: Narcotics decrease heart rate during inhalational anesthesia. Anesth Analg 66:166, 1987

238. Ebert TJ, Kotrly KJ, Madsen KE, et al: Fentanyl-diazepam anesthesia with or without N₂O does not attenuate cardiopulmonary baroreflex-mediated vasoconstrictor responses to controlled hypovolemia in humans. Anesth Analg 67:548, 1988

239. Kotrly KJ, Ebert TJ, Vucins E, et al: Baroreceptor reflex control of heart rate during isoflurane anesthesia in humans. Anesthesiology 60:173, 1984

240. Kotrly KJ, Ebert TJ, Vucins EJ, et al: Baroreceptor reflex control of heart rate during morphine sulfate, diazepam, N₂O/O₂ anesthesia in humans. Anesthesiology 61:558, 1984

241. Zimpfer M, Kotal E, Mayer N, et al: The influence of morphine on circulatory adjustments to acute progressive hemorrhage. Anaesthetist 32:259, 1983

242. Murat JM, Levron JC, Berg A, Saint-Maurice C: Effects of fentanyl on baroreceptor reflex control of heart rate in newborn infants. Anesthesiology 68:717, 1988

243. MacLeod BA, Augereau P, Walker MJA: Effects of halothane anesthesia compared with fentanyl anesthesia and no anesthesia during coronary ligation in rats. Anesthesiology 58:44, 1983

244. Frank LP, Davis RF: The effect of fentanyl on myocardial salvage in dogs after coronary artery occlusion. Anesth Analg 65:S50, 1986

245. Sonntag H, Larsen R, Hilfiker O, et al: Myocardial blood flow and oxygen consumption during high-dose fentanyl anesthesia in patients with coronary artery disease. Anesthesiology 56:417, 1982

246. Litak C, Ansley D, Wynands JE, et al: Incidence of pre-bypass ischaemia during sufentanil/O₂/pancuronium anaesthesia in patients undergoing coronary artery surgery. Can Anaesth Soc J 33:S97, 1986

247. Moffitt EA, McIntyre AJ, Barker RA, et al: Myocardial metabolism and hemodynamic responses with fentanyl-enflurane anesthesia for coronary arterial surgery. Anesth Analg 65:46, 1986

248. Heikkilä H, Jalonen J, Arola M, Laaksonen V: Haemodynamics and myocardial oxygenation during anaesthesia for coronary artery surgery: Comparison between enflurane and high-dose fentanyl anaesthesia. Acta Anaesthesiol Scand 29:457, 1985

249. Goehner P, Hollenberg M, Leung J, et al: Hemodynamic control suppresses myocardial ischemia during isoflurane or sufentanil anesthesia for CABG. Anesthesiology 69:A32, 1988

250. Skourtis CT, Nissen M, McGinnis LA, et al: The effect of high-dose fentanyl on cardiac metabolic balance and coronary circulation in patients undergoing coronary artery surgery. Anesthesiology 61:A6, 1984

251. Kleinman B, Henkin RE, Glisson SN, et al: Qualitative evaluation of coronary flow during anesthetic induction using thallium-201 perfusion scans. Anesthesiology 64:157, 1986

252. Slogoff S, Keats AS: Randomized trial of primary anesthetic agents on outcome of coronary artery bypass operations. Anesthesiology 70:179, 1989

253. Tuman KJ, Keane DM, Silins AI, et al: Effect of high dose

fentanyl on fluid and vasopressor requirements after cardiac surgery. Anesth Analg 67:S236, 1988

254. Blaise G, Sill JC, Nugent M, Vanhoutte PM: Fentanyl and responsiveness of canine coronary arterial smooth muscle. Can Anaesth Soc J 33:S104, 1986

255. Beland A, Blaise GA, Lenis SG, et al: Effect of fentanyl on the coronary circulation in an isolated heart. Can Anaesth Soc J 34:S72, 1987

256. Craythorne NWB, Darby TD: The cardiovascular effects of nitrous oxide in the dog. Br J Anaesth 37:560, 1965

257. Eisele JH, Smith NT: Cardiovascular effects of 40 percent nitrous oxide in man. Anesth Analg 51:956, 1972

258. McDermott RW, Stanley TH: Cardiovascular effects of low concentrations of nitrous oxide during morphine anesthesia. Anesthesiology 41:89, 1974

259. Bennett GM, Ready P, Liu WS, et al: Hemodynamic effects of anesthetic doses of alpha-prodine and sufentanil in dogs. Anesthesiology 51:S102, 1979

260. Moffitt EA, Scovil JE, Barker RA, et al: Myocardial metabolism and hemodynamics of nitrous oxide in fentanyl or enflurane anesthesia in coronary patients. Anesthesiology 59:A31, 1983

261. Michaels I, Barash PG: Does nitrous oxide or a reduced FiO$_2$ alter hemodynamic function during high-dose sufentanil anesthesia? Anesth Analg 62:275, 1983

262. Philbin DM, Foëx P, Drummond G, et al: Postsystolic shortening of canine left ventricle supplied by a stenotic coronary artery when nitrous oxide is added in the presence of narcotics. Anesthesiology 62:166, 1985

263. Crean P, Koren G, Goresky G, et al: Fentanyl-oxygen versus fentanyl-N$_2$O/oxygen anesthesia in children undergoing cardiac surgery. Can Anaesth Soc J 33:36, 1986

264. Moffitt EA, McIntyre AJ, Glenn JJ, et al: Myocardial metabolism and haemodynamic responses with fentanyl-halothane anaesthesia for coronary patients. Can Anaesth Soc J 32:S86, 1985

265. Hillel Z, Thys D, Goldman ME, et al: Halothane produces dose-dependent myocardial depression in man during fentanyl anesthesia. Anesth Analg 65:S71, 1986

266. Heikkilä H, Jalonen J, Arola M, et al: Low-dose enflurane as adjunct to high-dose fentanyl in patients undergoing coronary artery surgery: Stable hemodynamics and maintained myocardial oxygen balance. Anesth Analg 66:111, 1987

267. O'Young J, Mastrocostopoulas G, Hilgenberg A, et al: Myocardial circulatory and metabolic effects of isoflurane and sufentanil during coronary artery surgery. Anesthesiology 66:653, 1987

268. O'Brien DJ, Moffitt EA, McIntyre AJ, et al: Myocardial metabolism and hemodynamic responses with fentanyl-halothane anaesthesia in hypertensive patients undergoing coronary arterial surgery. Can Anaesth Soc J 33:S101, 1986

269. Mastrocostopoulos G, Athanasiadis C, Skourtis C, et al: Regional and global myocardial metabolic and coronary hemodynamic effects of halothane in cardiac patients during high dose sufentanil anesthesia. Anesth Analg 65:S93, 1986

270. Rydvall A, Häggmark S, Nyhman H, Reiz S: Effects of enflurane on coronary haemodynamics in patients with ischemic heart disease. Acta Anaesthesiol Scand 28:690, 1984

271. Dauchot PJ, van Heeckeren DW, Bastulli J, Anton AH: Sufenta requirements, plasma Sufenta and catecholamine levels after diazepam during CABG surgery. Anesth Analg 67:S45, 1988

272. Heikkilä H, Jalonen J, Laaksonen V, et al: Lorazepam and high-dose fentanyl anaesthesia: effects on haemodynamics and oxygen transportation in patients undergoing coronary revascularization. Acta Anaesthesiol Scand 28:357, 1984

273. Benson KT, Tomlinson DL, Goto H, Arakawa K: Cardiovascular effects of lorazepam during sufentanil anesthesia. Anesth Analg 67:996, 1988

274. Streisand JB, Clark NJ, Stanley TH, et al: The effects of technique and supplements on cardiovascular dynamics during anesthetic induction with alfentanil. Anesth Analg 65:S156, 1986

275. Butterworth JF, Bean VE, Royster RL: Premedication profoundly influences hemodynamics during rapid sequence induction with sufentanil-succinylcholine for aortocoronary bypass grafting. Anesthesiology 69:A65, 1988

276. Thomson IR, Bergstrom RG, Rosenbloom M, Meatherall RC: Premedication and high-dose fentanyl anesthesia for myocardial revascularization: A comparison of lorazepam versus morphine-scopolamine. Anesthesiology 68:194, 1988

277. West JM, Estrada S, Heerdt M: Sudden hypotension associated with midazolam and sufentanil (letter). Anesth Analg 66:693, 1987

278. Spiess BD, Sathoff RH, El-Ganzouri ARS, Ivankovich AD: High-dose sufentanil: Four cases of sudden hypotension on induction. Anesth Analg 65:703, 1986

279. Marty J, Gauzit R, Lefevre P, et al: Effects of diazepam and midazolam on baroreflex control of heart rate and on sympathetic activity in humans. Anesth Analg 65:113, 1986

280. Reves JG, Kissin I, Fournier SE, Smith LR: Additive negative inotropic effect of a combination of diazepam and fentanyl. Anesth Analg 63:97, 1984

281. Komatsu T, Shibutani K, Okamoto K, et al: Comparison of sufentanil-diazepam and fentanyl-diazepam anesthesia for induction. Anesth Analg 65:S82, 1986

282. Stanley TH, de Lange S, Boscoe MJ, de Bruijn N: The influence of chronic preoperative propranolol therapy on cardiovascular dynamics and narcotic requirements during operation in patients with coronary artery disease. Can Anaesth Soc J 29:319, 1982

283. Zahl K, Ellison N: Rapid induction and intubation with pancuronium or vecuronium and sufentanil for cardiac surgery. Anesthesiology 65:A519, 1986

284. Harrison L, Ralley F, Wynands JE, et al: The role of an ultra short-acting adrenergic blocker (esmolol) in patients undergoing coronary artery bypass surgery. Anesthesiology 66:413, 1987

285. Newsome LR, Roth JV, Hug CC, Jr, Nagle D: Esmolol attenuates hemodynamic responses during fentanyl-pancuronium anesthesia for aortocoronary bypass surgery. Anesth Analg 65:451, 1986

286. Hamilton WK: Fashion, Darwin and anesthetics as poisons. Anesthesiology 69:811, 1988

287. Ghignone M, Quinton L, Duke PC, et al: Effects of clonidine on narcotic requirements and hemodynamic response during induction of fentanyl anesthesia and endotracheal intubation. Anesthesiology 64:36, 1986

288. Flacke JW, Bloor BC, Flacke WE, et al: Reduced narcotic requirement by clonidine with improved hemodynamic and adrenergic stability in patients undergoing coronary bypass surgery. Anesthesiology 67:11, 1987

289. Bernard JM, Bourréli B, Pinaud M, et al: Incidence of clonidine oral premedication and postoperative IV infusion on hemodynamic and adrenergic responses during recovery from anesthesia. Anesthesiology 69:A147, 1988

290. Sperry RJ, Barley DL, Pace NL, et al: Clonidine does not depress the ventilatory response to CO$_2$ in man. Anesth Analg (in press)

291. Hill DC, Chelly JE, Dlewati A, et al: Cardiovascular effects of and interaction between calcium blocking drugs and anes-

thetics in chronically instrumented dogs. VI. Verapamil and fentanyl-pancuronium. Anesthesiology 68:874, 1988

292. Ramsay JG, Arvieux CC, Foëx P, et al: Global and regional myocardial effect of verapamil when added to fentanyl. Can Anaesth Soc J 33:S100, 1986

293. Kapur PA, Norel EJ, Dajee H, Flacke W: Haemodynamic effects of verapamil administration after large doses of fentanyl in man. Can Anaesth Soc J 33:138, 1986

294. Bernard JM, Pinaud M, Carteau S, et al: Hypotensive actions of diltiazem and nitroprusside compared during fentanyl anaesthesia for total hip arthroplasty. Can Anaesth Soc J 33:308, 1986

295. Thomson IR, Mutch AC, Culligan JD: Failure of intravenous nitroglycerin to prevent intraoperative myocardial ischemia during fentanyl-pancuronium anesthesia. Anesthesiology 61:385, 1984

296. Coriat P, Daloz M, Bousseau D, et al: Prevention of intraoperative myocardial ischemia during noncardiac surgery with intravenous nitroglycerin. Anesthesiology 61:193, 1984

297. Khoury GF, Estafanous FG, Zurick AM, Lytle B: Sufentanil/pancuronium versus sufentanil/metocurine anesthesia for coronary artery surgery. Anesthesiology 57:A47, 1982

298. Salmenperä M, Peltola K, Takkunen O, Heinonen J: Cardiovascular effects of pancuronium and vecuronium during high-dose fentanyl anesthesia. Anesth Analg 62:1059, 1983

299. Gravlee GP, Ramsey FM, Roy RC, et al: Pancuronium is hemodynamically superior to vecuronium for narcotic/relaxant induction. Anesthesiology 65:A46, 1986

300. McDonald DH, Zaidan JR: Hemodynamic effects of pancuronium and pancuronium plus metocurine in patients taking propranolol. Anesthesiology 60:359, 1984

301. Murkin JM, Moldenhauer CC, Hug CC, Jr: High-dose fentanyl for rapid induction of anaesthesia in patients with coronary artery disease. Can Anaesth Soc J 32:320, 1984

302. Thomson IR, Putnins CI: Adverse effects of pancuronium during high-dose fentanyl anesthesia for coronary artery bypass grafting. Anesthesiology 62:708, 1985

303. Hill AEG, Muller BJ: Optimum relaxant for sufentanil anesthesia. Anesthesiology 61:A393, 1984

304. Waldmann CS, Wark KJ, Sebel PS, Feneck RO: Hemodynamic effects of atracurium, vecuronium and pancuronium during sufentanil anesthesia for coronary artery bypass. Acta Anaesthesiol Scand 30:351, 1986

305. Sethna DH, Starr NJ, Estafanous FG: Cardiovascular effects of nondepolarizing neuromuscular blockers in patients with coronary artery disease. Can Anaesth Soc J 33:280, 1986

306. Heinonen J, Salmenperä M, Suomivuori M: Contribution of muscle relaxant to the haemodynamic course of high-dose fentanyl anaesthesia: A comparison of pancuronium, vecuronium and atracurium. Can Anaesth Soc J 33:597, 1986

307. Atlee JL, Laravuso RB: Muscle relaxants and high-dose fentanyl: Hemodynamics during coronary bypass surgery. Anesth Analg 63:181, 1984

308. O'Connor JP, Ramsay JG, Wynands JE, et al: The incidence of myocardial ischemia during anesthesia for coronary artery bypass surgery in patients receiving pancuronium or vecuronium. Anesthesiology 70:230, 1989

309. Savarese JJ, Lowenstein E: The name of the game: No anesthesia by cookbook. Anesthesiology 62:703, 1985

310. Lebowitz PW, Ramsey FM, Savarese JJ, et al: Combination of pancuronium and metocurine: Neuromuscular and hemodynamic advantages over pancuronium alone. Anesth Analg 60:12, 1981

311. Stoops CM, Curtis CA, Kovach DA, et al: Hemodynamic effects of doxacurium chloride in patients receiving oxygen

sufentanil anesthesia for coronary artery bypass grafting or valve replacement. Anesthesiology 69:365, 1988

312. Hickey RF, Severinghaus JW: Regulation of breathing: Drug effects. p. 1251. In Hornbein TF (ed): Lung Biology in Health and Disease. Vol. 17. Part II. Marcel Dekker, New York, 1981

313. Ngai SH: Effects of morphine and meperidine on the central respiratory mechanisms in the cat, and the action of levallorphan in antagonizing these effects. J Pharmacol Exp Ther 131:91, 1961

314. Tabatabai M, Kitahata LM, Collins JG: Disruption of the rhythmic activity of the medullary inspiratory neurons and phrenic nerve by fentanyl and reversal with nalbuphine. Anesthesiology 70:489, 1989

315. Weil JV, McCullough RE, Kline JS, Sodal IE: Diminished ventilatory response to hypoxia and hypercapnia after morphine in normal man. N Engl J Med 292:1103, 1975

316. Kryger MH, Yacoub O, Dosman J, et al: Effect of meperidine on occlusion pressure responses to hypercapnia and hypoxia with and without external inspiratory resistance. Am Rev Respir Dis 114:333, 1976

317. Bjertraes LJ: Hypoxia-induced vasoconstriction in isolated perfused lungs exposed to injectable or inhalation anesthetics. Acta Anesthesiol Scand 21:133, 1977

318. Wamsley JK: Opioid receptors: Autoradiography. Pharmacol Rev 35:69, 1983

319. Rigg JRA, Rondi P: Changes in rib cage and diaphragm contribution to ventilation after morphine. Anesthesiology 55:507, 1981

320. Drummond GB: Comparison of decreases in ventilation caused by enflurane and fentanyl during anesthesia. Br J Anaesth 55:825, 1983

321. Cooper DY, Lambertson CJ: Effect of changes in tidal volume and alveolar carbon dioxide on physiological dead space. Anesthesiology 18:106, 1957

322. Van Dongen K, Leusink H: The action of opium-alkaloids and expectorants on the ciliary movements in the air passages. Arch Int Pharmacodyn 93:261, 1953

323. Toda N, Hatano Y: Contractile responses of canine tracheal muscle during exposure to fentanyl and morphine. Anesthesiology 53:93, 1980

324. Longobardo GE, Gothe B, Goldman MD, Cherniak NS: Sleep apnea considered as a control system instability. Respir Physiol 50:311, 1982

325. Reed DJ, Kellog RH: Changes in respiratory response to CO_2 during natural sleep at sea level and at altitude. J Appl Physiol 13:325, 1958

326. Forrest WH, Bellville JW: The effect of sleep plus morphine on the respiratory response to carbon dioxide. Anesthesiology 25:137, 1964

327. Berkowitz BA, Ngai SH, Yang JC, et al: The disposition of morphine in surgical patients. Clin Pharmacol Ther 17:629, 1975

328. Bentley JB, Borel JD, Nenad RE, Jr, Gillespie TJ: Age and fentanyl pharmacokinetics. Anesth Analg 61:968, 1982

329. Scott JC, Stanski DR: Decreased fentanyl and alfentanil dose requirements with age. A simultaneous pharmacokinetic and pharmacodynamic evaluation. J Pharmacol Exp Ther 240:159, 1987

330. Arunasalam K, Davenport HT, Painter S, Jones JG: Ventilatory response to morphine in young and old subjects. Anaesthesia 38:529, 1983

331. Way WL, Costley EC, Way EL: Respiratory sensitivity of the newborn to meperidine and morphine. Clin Pharmacol Ther 6:454, 1965

332. Hertzka RE, Gauntlett IS, Fisher DM, Spellman MJ: Fen-

tanyl-induced ventilatory depression: Effects of age. Anesthesiology 70:213, 1989

333. Eckenhoff JE, Occh SR: The effects of narcotics and antagonists upon respiration and circulation in man. Clin Pharmacol Ther 1:483, 1960

334. Bailey PL, Andriano KP, Pace NL, et al: Small doses of fentanyl potentiate and prolong diazepam induced respiratory depression. Anesth Analg 63:183, 1984

335. Bailey PL, Moll JWB, Pace NL, et al: Respiratory effects of midazolam and fentanyl: Potent interaction producing hypoxemia and apnea. Anesthesiology 69:A813, 1988

336. Becker LD, Paulson BA, Miller RD, et al: Biphasic respiratory depression after fentanyl-droperidol or fentanyl alone used to supplement nitrous oxide anesthesia. Anesthesiology 44:291, 1976

337. Harper MH, Hickey RF, Cromwell TH, Linwood S: The magnitude and duration of respiratory depression produced by fentanyl and fentanyl plus droperidol in man. J Pharmacol Exp Ther 199:464, 1976

338. Downes JJ, Kemp RA, Lambertsen CJ: The magnitude and duration of respiratory depression due to fentanyl and meperidine in man. J Pharmacol Exp Ther 158:416, 1967

339. Keats AS, Girgis KZ: Respiratory depression associated with relief of pain by narcotics. Anesthesiology 29:1006, 1968

340. Cartwright P, Prys-Roberts C, Gill K, et al: Ventilatory depression related to plasma fentanyl concentrations during and after anesthesia in humans. Anesth Analg 62:966, 1983

341. Ainslie SG, Eisele JH, Corkill G: Fentanyl concentrations in brain and serum during respiratory acid-base changes in the dog. Anesthesiology 51:293, 1979

342. Beard K, Hershel J, Walker AM: Adverse respiratory events occurring in the recovery room after general anesthesia. Anesthesiology 64:269, 1986

343. Catley DM, Thornton C, Jordan C, et al: Pronounced episodic oxygen desaturation in the postoperative period: Its association with ventilatory pattern and analgesic regimen. Anesthesiology 63:20, 1985

344. Tyler IL, Tantisira B, Winter PM, Motoyama EK: Continuous monitoring of arterial oxygen saturation with pulse oximetry during transfer to the recovery room. Anesth Analg 64:1108, 1985

345. Nielsen CH, Camporesi EM, Bromage PR, et al: CO_2 sensitivity after epidural and IV morphine. Anesthesiology 55:A372, 1981

346. Bailey PL, Streisand JB, Pace NL, et al: Sufentanil produces shorter acting respiratory depression and longer lasting analgesia than equipotent doses of fentanyl in human volunteers. Anesthesiology 65:A493, 1986

347. Holmes CM: Supplementation of general anaesthesia with narcotic analgesics. Br J Anaesth 48:907, 1976

348. Kay B, Rolly G: Duration of action of analgesic supplement to anesthesia. Acta Anaesthesiol Belg 28:25, 1977

349. Rigg JRA, Goldsmith CH: Recovery of ventilatory response to carbon dioxide after thiopentone, morphine and fentanyl in man. Can Anaesth Soc J 23:370, 1976

350. Adams AP, Pybus DA: Delayed respiratory depression after use of fentanyl during anaesthesia. Br Med J 1:278, 1978

351. Hug CC, Jr, Murphy MR: Fentanyl disposition in cerebrospinal fluid and plasma and its relationship to ventilatory depression in the dog. Anesthesiology 50:342, 1979

352. Andrews CJH, Sinclair M, Prys-Roberts C, Dye A: Ventilatory effects during and after continuous infusion of fentanyl or alfentanil. Br J Anaesth 55:211, 1983

353. Mahla ME, Maj MC, Maj SEW, Moneta MD: Delayed respiratory depression after alfentanil. Anesthesiology 69:593, 1988

354. Stanski DR, Greenblatt DJ, Lowenstein E: Kinetics of intravenous and intramuscular morphine. Clin Pharmacol Ther 24:52, 1978

355. Chan K, Kendall MJ, Mitchard M, Will WDE: The effect of aging on plasma pethidine concentration. Br J Clin Pharmacol 2:297, 1975

356. Chang J, Fish KJ: Acute respiratory arrest and rigidity after anesthesia with sufentanil: A case report. Anesthesiology 63:710, 1985

357. McClain DA, Hug CC, Jr: Intravenous fentanyl kinetics. Clin Pharmacol Ther 28:106, 1980

358. Koehntop DE, Rodman JH, Brundage DM, et al: Pharmacokinetics of fentanyl in neonates. Anesth Analg 65:227, 1986

359. Singleton MA, Rosen JI, Fisher DM: Pharmacokinetics of fentanyl in infants and adults. Anesthesiology 61:A440, 1988

360. Stoeckel H, Schuttler J, Magnussen H, Hengstmann JH: Plasma fentanyl concentrations and occurrence of respiration depression in volunteers. Br J Anaesth 54:1087, 1982

361. McQuay HJ, Moore RA, Paterson GMC, Adams AP: Plasma fentanyl concentrations and clinical observations during and after operation. Br J Anaesth 51:543, 1979

362. Bower S, Hull CJ: Comparative pharmacokinetics of fentanyl and alfentanil. Br J Anaesth 54:871, 1982

363. Sebel PS, Bovill JG, Wauquier A, Rog P: Effects of high dose fentanyl anesthesia on the electroencephalogram. Anesthesiology 55:203, 1981

364. Scott JC, Stanski DR, Ponganis KV: Quantitation of fentanyl's effect on the brain using the EEG. Anesthesiology 59:A370, 1983

365. Freeman J, Ingvar DH: Effects of fentanyl on cerebral cortical blood flow and EEG in the cat. Acta Anaesthesiol Scand 11:381, 1967

366. Nilsson E, Ingvar DH: EEG findings in neuroleptanalgesia. Acta Anaesthesiol Scand 11:121, 1967

367. Ghoneim MM, Mewaldt SP, Thatcher JW: The effect of diazepam and fentanyl on mental, psychomotor and electroencephalographic functions and their rate of recovery. Psychopharmacology (Berlin) 44:61, 1975

368. Matteo RS, Ornstein E, Schwartz AE, et al: Effects of low-dose sufentanil on the EEG: Elderly vs. young. Anesthesiology 65:A553, 1986

369. Zurick AM, Khoury GF, Estafanous FG, Lytle B: Sufentanil requirement of surgical anesthesia (as determined by EEG) and its effect on awakening time. Anesth Analg 62:292, 1983

370. Smith NT, Dec-Silver H, Sanford TJ, et al: EEGs during high-dose fentanyl-, sufentanil-, or morphine-oxygen anesthesia. Anesth Analg 63:386, 1984

371. Bovill JG, Sebel PS, Wauquier A, et al: Influence of high-dose alfentanil anaesthesia on the electroencephalogram: Correlation with plasma concentrations. Br J Anaesth 55:199, 1983

372. Scott JC, Ponganis KV, Stanski DR: EEG quantitation of narcotic effect: The comparative pharmacodynamics of fentanyl and alfentanil. Anesthesiology 62:234, 1985

373. Kalkman CJ, AR Rheineck, Bovill JG: Influence of high-dose opioid anesthesia on posterior tibial nerve somatosensory cortical evoked potentials: Effects of fentanyl, sufentanil, and alfentanil. J Cardiothorac Anesth 2:758, 1988

374. Pathak KS, Brown RH, Cascorbi HF, Nash CL, Jr: Effects of fentanyl and morphine on intraoperative somatosensory cortical-evoked potentials. Anesth Analg 63:833, 1984

375. van Rheineck Leyssius AT, Kalkman CJ, Hesselink EM, Bovill JG: Effects of high dose fentanyl anesthesia on posterior tibial nerve somatosensory evoked potentials. Anesth Analg 66:S183, 1987

376. McPherson RW, Sell B, Traystman RJ: Effects of thiopental, fentanyl, and etomidate on upper extremity somatosensory evoked potentials in humans. Anesthesiology 65:584, 1986

377. McPherson RW, Mahla M, Johnson R, Traystman RJ: Effects of enflurane, isoflurane, and nitrous oxide on somatosensory evoked potentials during fentanyl anesthesia. Anesthesiology 62:626, 1985

378. Schubert A, Drummond JC, Peterson DO, Saidman LJ: The effect of high-dose fentanyl on human nerve somato-sensory-evoked responses. Can Anaesth Soc J 34:35, 1987

379. Bird J, Donegan J, Rupp S, et al: Effects of sufentanil bolus and two steady state infusions on median nerve evoked potentials. Anesthesiology 65:A341, 1986

380. Koht A, Schutz W, Schmidt G, et al: Effects of etomidate, midazolam, and thiopental on median nerve somatosensory evoked potentials and the additive effects of fentanyl and nitrous oxide. Anesth Analg 67:435, 1988

381. Koht A, Kimovec MA, Sloan TB, Carlvin AO: The effects of sufentanil on median nerve somatosensory evoked potentials. Anesth Analg 65:S81, 1986

382. Sebel PS, De Bruijn N, Jacobs J, Neville WK: Median nerve somatosensory evoked potentials during anesthesia with sufentanil or fentanyl. Anesthesiology 69:A312, 1988

383. Grundy BL: Fentanyl alters somatosensory cortical evoked potentials. Anesth Analg 59:544, 1980

384. Samra SK, Krutak-Krol H, Pohorecki R, Domino EF: Scopolamine, morphine, and brain-stem auditory evoked potentials in awake monkeys. Anesthesiology 62:437, 1985

385. Samra SK, Lilly DJ, Rush NL, Kirsh MM: Fentanyl anesthesia and human brain-stem auditory evoked potentials. Anesthesiology 61:261, 1984

386. Hyman SA, Berman ML, Bullington JC, et al: Brainstem auditory evoked potentials during balanced anesthesia with a sufentanil infusion. Anesth Analg 66:S85, 1987

387. Jober DR, Kennell EM, Bush GL, et al: Cerebral blood flow and metabolism during morphine-nitrous oxide anesthesia in man. Anesthesiology 47:16, 1977

388. Wald M: Effects of enkephalins, morphine, and naloxone on pial arterial blood flow during perivascular microapplication. J Cereb Blood Flow Metab 5:451, 1985

389. Reico L, Merin J, Reviriego J, et al: Effect of morphine on the cat middle cerebral artery. Brain Res 376:262, 1986

390. Carlsson C, Smith DS, Keykhah M, et al: The effects of high dose fentanyl on cerebral circulation and metabolism in rats. Anaesthesia 57:375, 1982

391. Michenfelder JD, Theye RA: Effects of fentanyl, droperidol, and Innovar on canine cerebral metabolism and blood flow. Br J Anaesth 43:630, 1971

392. Yaster M, Koehler RC, Traystman RJ: Effects of fentanyl on peripheral and cerebral hemodynamics in neonatal lambs. Anesthesiology 66:524, 1987

393. Vernhiet J, Renou AM, Orgogozo JM, et al: Effects of diazepam-fentanyl mixture on cerebral blood flow and oxygen consumption in man. Br J Anaesth 50:165, 1978

394. Keykhah MM, Smith DS, Carlsson C, et al: Influence of sufentanil on cerebral metabolism and circulation in the rat. Anesthesiology 63:274, 1985

395. Milde LN, Milde JR: The cerebral hemodynamic and metabolic effects of sufentanil in dogs. Anesthesiology 67:A570, 1987

396. Artru AA: Relationship between cerebral blood volume and CSF pressure during anesthesia with isoflurane or fentanyl in dogs. Anesthesiology 60:575, 1984

397. Marx W, Shah N, Long C, et al: Sufentanil, alfentanil and fentanyl: Impact on CSF pressure in patients with brain tumors. Anesthesiology 69:A627, 1988

398. Young WL, Prohovnik I, Correll JW, et al: The effect of sufentanil on cerebral hemodynamics during carotid endarterectomy. Anesthesiology 69:A591, 1988

399. McPherson RW, Traystman RJ: Fentanyl and cerebral vascular responsivity in dogs. Anesthesiology 60:180, 1984

400. Artru AA: Effects of halothane and fentanyl anesthesia on resistance to reabsorption of CSF. J Neurosurg 60:252, 1984

401. Artru AA: Effect of halothane and fentanyl on the rate of CSF production in dogs. Anesth Analg 62:581, 1983

402. Corssen G, Domino EF, Sweet RB: Neuroleptanalgesia and anesthesia. Anesth Analg 43:748, 1964

403. Hamilton WK, Cullen SC: Effect of levallorphan tartrate upon opiate induced respiratory depression. Anesthesiology 14:550, 1953

404. Janis KM: Acute rigidity with small intravenous doses of Innovar: A case report. Anesth Analg 51:375, 1972

405. Deutch S, Bastron RD, Pierce EC, Vandam LD: The effects of anaesthesia with thiopentone, nitrous oxide, narcotics and neuromuscular blocking drugs on renal function in normal man. Br J Anaesth 41:807, 1969

406. Grell FL, Koons DA, Denson JS: Fentanyl in anesthesia: A report of 500 cases. Anesth Analg 49:523, 1970

407. Comstock MK, Carter JG, Moyers JR, Stevens WC: Rigidity and hypercarbia associated with high-dose fentanyl induction of anesthesia. Anesth Analg 60:362, 1981

408. Scamman FL: Fentanyl-O_2-N_2O rigidity and pulmonary compliance. Anesth Analg 62:332, 1983

409. Arandia HY, Patil VU: Glottic closure following large doses of fentanyl. Anesthesiology 66:574, 1987

410. Coe V, Shafer A, White PF: Techniques for administering alfentanil during outpatient anesthesia — a comparison with fentanyl. Anesthesiology 59:A347, 1983

411. Gergis SD, Hoyt JL, Sokoll MD: Effects of Innovar and Innovar plus nitrous oxide on muscle tone and "H" reflex. Anesth Analg 50:743, 1971

412. Freund FG, Martin WE, Wong KC, Hornbein TF: Abdominal muscle rigidity induced by morphine and nitrous oxide. Anesthesiology 38:358, 1973

413. Sokoll MD, Hoyt JL, Gergis SD: Studies in muscle rigidity, nitrous oxide, and narcotic analgesic agents. Anesth Analg 51:1620, 1972

414. Christian CM, Waller JL, Moldenhauer CC: Postoperative rigidity following fentanyl anesthesia. Anesthesiology 58:275, 1983

415. Goldberg M, Ishak S, Garcia C, McKenna J: Postoperative rigidity following sufentanil administration. Anesthesiology 63:199, 1985

416. Jarvis AP, Arancibia CU: A case of difficult neonatal ventilation (letter). Anesth Analg 66:196, 1987

417. Sebel PS, Bovill JG: Fentanyl and convulsions. Anesth Analg 62:858, 1983

418. Jaffe TB, Ramsey FM: Attenuation of fentanyl-induced truncal rigidity. Anesthesiology 58:562, 1983

419. Mavrojammis M: L'action cataleptique de la morphine chez les rats. Contribution a la theorie toxique de la catalepsie. C R Soc Biol (Paris) 55:1092, 1903

420. Freye E, Kuschinsky K: Effects of fentanyl and droperidol on the dopamine metabolism of the rat striatum. Pharmacology 14:1, 1976

421. Jurna I, Ruzdic N, Nell T, Grossman W: The effect of alpha-methyl-p-tyrosine and substantia nigra lesions on spinal motor activity in the rat. Eur J Pharmacol 20:341, 1972

422. Havemann U, Winkler M, Kuschinsky K: Opioid receptors in the caudate nucleus can mediate EMG recorded rigidity in rats. Naunyn Schmiedebergs Arch Pharmacol 313:139, 1980

423. Havemann U, Winkler M, Gene E, Kuschinsky K: Effects of

striatal lesions with kainic acid on morphine-induced "catatonia" and increase of striatal dopamine turnover. Naunyn Schmiedebergs Arch Pharmacol 317:44, 1981

424. Havemann U, Kuschinsky K: Further characterization of opioid receptors in the striatum mediating muscular rigidity in rats. Naunyn Schmiedebergs Arch Pharmacol 317:321, 1981

425. Weinger MB, Koob GF: Further elucidation of brain sites which mediate alfentanil-induced muscle rigidity in the rat. Anesthesiology 69:A610, 1988

426. Blasco TA, Lee D, Amalric M, et al: The role of the nucleus raphe pontis and the caudate nucleus in alfentanil rigidity in the rat. Brain Res 386:280, 1986

427. Benthuysen JL, Kien ND, Quam DD: Intracranial pressure increases during alfentanil-induced rigidity. Anesthesiology 68:438, 1988

428. Kallos T, Wyche MQ, Garman JK: The effects of Innovar on functional residual capacity and total chest compliance in man. Anesthesiology 39:358, 1975

429. Benthuysen JL, Smith NT, Sanford TJ, et al: Physiology of alfentanil-induced rigidity. Anesthesiology 64:440, 1986

430. Bovill JG, Sebel PS: Pharmacokinetics of high dose fentanyl. Br J Anaesth 52:795, 1980

431. Vacanti CA, Vacanti FX: Sodium thiopental to treat fentanyl induced muscle rigidity. Anesth Analg 67:S241, 1988

432. Sanford TJ, Smith NT, Weinger MB, et al: The effect of midazolam pretreatment on alfentanil-induced muscle rigidity. Anesthesiology 69:A556, 1988

433. Carlson C, Smith DS, Keykah MM, et al: The effects of high-dose fentanyl on cerebral circulation and metabolism in rats. Anesthesiology 57:375, 1982

434. Poulton TJ, Ellingson RJ: Seizure associated with induction of anesthesia with clonidine: Effects on stress responses during general anesthesia. Anesthesiology 61:471, 1984

435. Frenk H, Urca G, Liebeskind JC: Epileptic properties of leucine and methionine-enkephalin: Comparison with morphine and reversibility by naloxone. Brain Res 147:327, 1978

436. Ingvar MK, Shaprio HM: Selective metabolic activation of the hippocampus during lidocaine-induced pre-seizure activity. Anesthesiology 54:33, 1981

437. Myers RR, Shapiro HM: Local cerebral metabolism during enflurane anesthesia: Identification of epileptogenic foci. Electroencephalogr Clin Neurophysiol 47:153, 1979

438. Crosby G, Crane AM, Sokoloff L: Local changes in cerebral glucose utilization during ketamine anesthesia. Anesthesiology 56:437, 1982

439. Hall GM: Analgesia and the metabolic response to surgery. Proc R Soc Med 3:19, 1978

440. Florence A: Attenuation of stress and haemodynamic stability. Proc R Soc Med 3:23, 1978

441. Murkin JM, Moldenhauer CC, Hug CC, Epstein CM: Absence of seizures during induction of anesthesia with high-dose fentanyl. Anesth Analg 63:489, 1984

442. Bovill JG, Sebel PS, Wauquier A, Rog P: Electroencephalographic effects of sufentanil anaesthesia in man. Br J Anaesth 54:45, 1982

443. Armstrong PJ, Bersten A: Normeperidine toxicity. Anesth Analg 65:536, 1986

444. Crawford RD, Bashoff JD: Fentanyl associated delirium in man. Anesthesiology 53:168, 1980

445. Hoien AO: Another case of grand mal seizure after fentanyl administration. Anesthesiology 60:387, 1984

446. Rao TLK, Mummanemi N, El-Etr AA: Convulsions: An unusual response to intravenous fentanyl administration. Anesth Analg 61:1020, 1982

447. Safwat AM, Daniel D: Grand-mal seizure after fentanyl administration. Anesthesiology 59:78, 1983

448. Scott JC, Sarnquist FH: Seizure-like movements during a fentanyl infusion with absence of seizure activity in a simultaneous EEG recording. Anesthesiology 62:812, 1985

449. Tommasino C, Mackawa T, Shapiro HM: Fentanyl-induced seizures activate subcortical brain metabolism. Anesthesiology 60:283, 1984

450. Young ML, Smith DS, Greenberg J, et al: Effects of sufentanil on regional cerebral glucose utilization in rats. Anesthesiology 61:564, 1984

451. Brian JE, Seifen AB: Tonic-clonic activity after sufentanil. Anesth Analg 66:481, 1987

452. Bowdle TA: Myoclonus following sufentanil without EEG seizure activity. Anesthesiology 67:593, 1987

453. Moore RA, Yang SS, McNicholas KW, et al: Hemodynamic and anesthetic effects of sufentanil as the sole anesthetic for pediatric cardiovascular surgery. Anesthesiology 62:725, 1985

454. Molbegott LP, Flashburg MH, Karasic L, Karlin BL: Probable seizures after sufentanil. Anesth Analg 66:91, 1987

455. Rosman EJ, Capan LM, Turndorf H: Another case of probable seizure after sufentanil. Anesth Analg 66:922, 1987

456. Katz RI, Eide TR, Hartman A, Poppers PJ: Two instances of seizure-like activity in the same patient associated with two different narcotics. Anesth Analg 67:289, 1988

457. Berryhill RE, Benumof JL, Janowsky DS: Morphine-induced hyperexcitability in man. Anesthesiology 50:65, 1979

458. Gloor P, Vera CL, Sperti L, Ray SN: Investigations on the mechanism of epileptic discharges in the hippocampus. Epilepsia 2:4262, 1961

459. Safo Y, Greenberg J, Young M, et al: Effects of high dose fentanyl on regional cerebral blood flow. Anesthesiology 59:A306, 1983

460. Siesjö BK: Brain Energy Metabolism. John Wiley & Sons, New York, 1978

461. Dam AM: Hippocampal neuron loss in epilepsy and after experimental seizures. Acta Neurol Scand 66:601, 1982

462. Thompson SH: The pupil. p. 326. In Moses RA (ed): Alders Physiology of the Eye. Clinical Application. CV Mosby, London, 1981

463. Ashbury AJ: Pupil response to alfentanil. A study in patients anaesthetised with halothane. Anaesthesia 41:717, 1986

464. Martin WR: Pharmacology of opioids. Pharmacol Rev 35:283, 1984

465. Sessler DI, Olofsson CI, Rubinstein EH: The thermoregulatory threshold in humans during nitrous oxide-fentanyl anesthesia. Anesthesiology 69:357, 1988

466. Kaplan JA, Griffin AV: Shivering and changes in mixed venous oxygen saturation after cardiac surgery. Anesth Analg 64:235, 1985

467. Macintyre PE, Pavlin EG, Dwersteg JF: Effect of meperidine on oxygen consumption, carbon dioxide production, and respiratory gas exchange in postanesthesia shivering. Anesth Analg 66:751, 1987

468. Casey WF, Smith CE, Katz JM, et al: Intravenous meperidine for control of shivering during caesarean section under epidural anaesthesia. Can Soc Anaesth J 35:128, 1988

469. Claybon LE, Hirsh RA: Meperidine arrests postanesthesia shivering. Anesthesiology 53:S180, 1980

470. Pauca AL, Savage RT, Simpson S, Roy RC: Effect of pethidine, fentanyl and morphine on post-operative shivering in man. Acta Anaesthesiol Scand 28:138, 1984

471. Brownridge P: Shivering related to epidural blockade with bupivicaine in labour, and the influence of epidural pethidine. Anaesth Intensive Care 14:412, 1986

472. Oyama T, Wakayama S: The endocrine responses to general anesthesia. Int Anesthesiol Clin 26:176, 1988

473. Anand KJS, Ward-Platt MP: Neonatal and pediatric stress responses to anesthesia and operation. Int Anesthesiol Clin 26:218, 1988

474. Davis PJ, Cook DR, Stiller RL, Davin-Robinson KA: Pharmacodynamics and pharmacokinetics of high-dose sufentanil in infants and children undergoing cardiac surgery. Anesth Analg 66:203, 1987

475. Samuelson PN, Reves JG, Kirklin JK, et al: Comparison of sufentanil and enflurane-nitrous oxide anesthesia for myocardial revascularization. Anesth Analg 65:217, 1986

476. Bovill JG, Sebel PS, Fiolet JW, et al: The influence of sufentanil on endocrine and metabolic responses to cardiac surgery. Anesth Analg 62:391, 1983

477. Clarke RSJ: The hyperglycaemic response to different types of surgery and anaesthesia. Br J Anaesth 42:45, 1970

478. Clarke RSJ, Johnston H, Sheridan B: The influence of anaesthesia and surgery on plasma cortisol, insulin and free fatty acids. Br J Anaesth 42:295, 1970

479. Madsen SN, Engquist A, Badwai I, Kehlet H: Cyclic AMP, glucose and cortisol in plasma during surgery. Horm Metab Res 8:483, 1976

480. Carr DB, Murphy MT: Operation, anesthesia and the endorphin system. Int Anesthesiol Clin 26:199, 1988

481. Joris JL, Dubner R, Hargreaves KM: Opioid analgesia at peripheral sites: A target for opioids during stress and inflammation? Anesth Analg 66:1277, 1987

482. Yaksh TL: Opioid receptor systems and the endorphins: A review of their spinal organization. J Neurosurg 67:157, 1987

483. Upton N, Sewell RDE, Spencer PSJ: Differentiation of potent μ- and κ-opiate agonists using heat and pressure antinociceptive profiles and combined potency analysis. Eur J Pharmacol 78:421, 1982

484. Przewlocki R, Stala L, Greczek M, et al: Analgesic effects of μ-, δ- and κ-opiate agonists and, in particular, dynorphin at the spinal level. Life Sci 33:649, 1983

485. Schmauss C, Yaksh TL: In vivo studies on spinal opiate receptor systems mediating antinociception. II. Pharmacological profiles suggesting a differential association of mu, delta and kappa receptors with visceral chemical and cutaneous thermal stimuli in the rat. J Pharmacol Exp Ther 228:1, 1984

486. Basbaum AI, Fields HL: Endogenous pain control systems: Brainstem spinal pathways and endorphin circuitry. Annu Rev Neurosci 7:309, 1984

487. Morley JE, Baranetsky NG, Wingert TD, et al: Endocrine effects of naloxone-induced opiate receptor blockade. J Clin Endocrinol Metab 50:251, 1980

488. Grossman A, Besser GM: Opiates control ACTH through a noradrenergic mechanism. Clin Endocrinol 17:287, 1982

489. Koenig JI, Mayfield MA, McCann SM, Krulich L: Differential role of the opioid μ and δ receptors in the activation of prolactin (PRL) and growth hormone (GH) secretion by morphine in the male rat. Life Sci 34:1829, 1984

490. Eipper BA, Mains RE: Structure and biosynthesis of proadrenocorticotropin/endorphin and related peptides. Endocrine Rev 1:1, 1980

491. DiFazio CA, Chen P: The influence of morphine on excess lactate production. Anesth Analg 50:211, 1971

492. Brandt MR, Korshin J, Prange Hansen A, et al: Influence of morphine anesthesia on the endocrine-metabolic response to open heart surgery. Acta Anaesthesiol Scand 22:400, 1978

493. Briggs FN, Munson PL: Studies on the mechanism of stimulation of ACTH secretion with the aid of morphine as a blocking agent. Endocrinology 57:205, 1955

494. George JM, Reier CE, Lanese RR, Rower MJ: Morphine anesthesia blocks cortisol and growth hormone response to surgical stress in humans. J Clin Endocrinol Metab 38:736, 1974

495. McDonald RK, Evans FT, Weise VK, Patrick RW: Effects of morphine and nalorphine on plasma hydrocortisone levels in man. J Pharmacol Exp Ther 125:241, 1959

496. Reier CE, George JM, Kilman JW: Cortisol and growth hormone response to surgical stress during morphine anesthesia. Anesth Analg 52:1003, 1973

497. Kayaalp SO, Kaymakcalan S: Studies on the morphine-induced release of catecholamine from the adrenal glands in the dog. Arch Int Pharmacodyn Ther 172:139, 1968

498. Fennessey MR, Ortiz A: The behavioral and cardiovascular actions of intravenously administered morphine in the conscious dog. Eur J Pharmacol 3:177, 1968

499. Klingman GI, Maynert EW: Tolerance to morphine. III. Effects on catecholamines in the heart, intestine and spleen. J Pharmacol Exp Ther 135:300, 1962

500. Roizen MF, Horrigan RW, Frazer BM: Anesthetic doses blocking adrenergic (stress) and cardiovascular responses to incision-MAC BAR. Anesthesiology 54:390, 1981

501. De Bodo RC: The antidiuretic action of morphine, and its mechanisms. J Pharmacol Exp Ther 82:74, 1944

502. Giarmann NJ, Mattie LR, Stephenson WF: Studies on the antidiuretic action of morphine. Science 117:225, 1953

503. Philbin DM, Wilson NE, Sokoloski J, Coggins C: Radioimmunoassay of antidiuretic hormone during morphine anaesthesia. Can Anaesth Soc J 23:290, 1976

504. Hall GM, Young C, Holdcroft A, Alaghband-Zadeh J: Substrate mobilisation during surgery: A comparison between halothane and fentanyl anesthesia. Anaesthesia 33:924, 1978

505. Cooper GM, Paterson JL, Ward ID, Hall GM: Fentanyl and metabolic response to gastric surgery. Anaesthesia 36:667, 1981

506. Kono K, Philbin DM, Coggins CH, et al: Renal function and stress response during halothane or fentanyl anesthesia. Anesth Analg 60:552, 1981

507. Frater RWM, Wakayama S, Oka Y, et al: Pulsatile cardiopulmonary bypass: Failure to influence hemodynamics or hormones. Circulation 62(suppl. 1):19, 1980

508. Walsh ES, Patterson JL, O'Riordan JBA, Hall GM: Effects of high dose fentanyl anaesthesia on the metabolic and endocrine response to cardiac surgery. Br J Anaesth 53:1155, 1981

509. de Lange S, Stanley TH, Boscoe MJ, et al: Catecholamine and cortisol responses to sufentanil-O_2 and alfentanil-O_2 anaesthesia during coronary artery surgery. Can Anaesth Soc J 30:248, 1983

510. Anand KJS, Sippell WG, Aynsley-Green A: Randomised trial of fentanyl anaesthesia in preterm babies undergoing surgery: Effects on the stress response. Lancet 1:243, 1987

511. Thornton WE, Thornton BP: Narcotic poisoning: A review of the literature. Am J Psychiatry 131:867, 1974

512. Cherubin CE: The medical sequelae of narcotics addiction. Ann Intern Med 67:23, 1967

513. Fracchia C: Medical complications of heroin use. Anesthetic considerations. Anesth Rev 4:45, 1977

514. Caldwell TB III: Anesthesia for patients with behavioral and environmental disorders. Anesthetic managemet of the narcotic addict. p. 681. In Katz J, Benumof JJ, Kadis LB (eds): Anesthesia and Uncommon Diseases. WB Saunders, Philadelphia, 1981

515. Giuffrida JG, Bizzarri DV, Saure AC, Sharoff RL: Anesthetic management of drug abusers. Anesth Analg 49:272, 1970

516. Jenkins LC: Anaesthetic problems due to drug abuse and dependence. Can Anaesth Soc J 19:461, 1972

517. Papper S, Papper EM: The effects of pre-anesthetic, anesthetic, and postoperative drugs on renal function. Clin Pharmacol Ther 5:205, 1964

518. Marks RM, Sachar EJ: Undertreatment of medical inpatients with narcotic analgesics. Ann Intern Med 78:173, 1973

519. Porter J, Jick H: Addiction rare in patients treated with narcotics. N Engl J Med 203:123, 1980

520. Stanley TH, Gray NH, Bidwai AV, Lordon R: The effects of high dose morphine and morphine plus nitrous oxide on urinary output in man. Can Anaesth Soc J 21:379, 1974

521. Bidwai AV, Stanley TH, Bloomer HA: Effects of anesthetic doses of morphine on renal function in the dog. Anesth Analg 54:357, 1975

522. Hunter JM, Jones RS, Utting JE: Effect of anaesthesia with nitrous oxide in oxygen and fentanyl on renal function in the artificially ventilated dog. Br J Anaesth 52:343, 1980

523. Kien ND, Reitan JA, White DA, et al: Hemodynamic responses to alfentanil in halothane-anesthetized dogs. Anesth Analg 65:765, 1986

524. Priano LL, Vatner SF: Generalized cardiovascular and regional hemodynamic effects of meperidine in conscious dogs. Anesth Analg 6:649, 1981

525. Dowlatshahi K, Evander A, Walther B, Skinner DB: Influence of morphine on the distal oesophagus and the lower oesophageal sphincter—a manometric study. Gut 26:802, 1985

526. Støen R, Sessler DI: Lower esophageal contractility does not predict movement during skin incision in patients anesthetized with alfentanil and nitrous oxide. Anesthesiology 69:A221, 1988

527. Sessler DI, Olofsson CI, Chow F: Lower esophageal contractility predicts movement during skin incisions; vecuronium does not decrease the MAC of halothane. Anesth Analg 67:S201, 1988

528. Lamki L, Sullivan S: A study of gastrointestinal opiate receptors: The role of the mu receptor on gastric emptying: Concise communication. J Nucl Med 24:689, 1983

529. Shah M, Rosen M, Vickers MD: Effect of premedication with diazepam, morphine or nalbuphine on gastrointestinal motility after surgery. Br J Anaesth 56:1235, 1984

530. Nimmo WS, Wilson J, Prescott LF: Narcotic analgesics and delayed gastric emptying during labour. Lancet 1:890, 1975

531. Frame WT, Allison RH, Moirand DD, Nimmo WS: Effect of naloxone on gastric emptying during labour. Br J Anaesth 56:263, 1984

532. Borody TJ, Quigley EEM, Phillips SF, et al: Effects of morphine and atropine on motility and transit in the human ileum. Gastroenterology 89:562, 1985

533. Thangathurai D, Oyos T, Nelson D, et al: The effect of papaverine and scopolamine on small bowel relaxation during surgery. Anesthesiology 69:A445, 1988

534. Radnay PA, Duncalf D, Novakoric M, Lesser ML: Common bile duct pressure changes after fentanyl, morphine, meperidine, butorphanol and naloxone. Anesth Analg 63:441, 1984

535. Hynynen MJ, Turanen M, Kortilla KT: Effects of alfentanil and fentanyl on common bile duct pressure. Anesth Analg 65:370, 1986

536. Vatashsky E, Haskel Y, Nissan S, Hanani M: Effect of morphine on the mechanical activity of common bile duct isolated from the guinea pig. Anesth Analg 66:245, 1987

537. Vieira ZG, Duarte B, Renigers SA, et al: Double-blind ultrasonographic demonstration of morphine-induced spasm of the common bile duct. Anesthesiology 69:A347, 1988

538. Martin DE, Joehl RJ: Butorphanol and nalbuphine cause human bile duct obstruction. Anesthesiology 59:A324, 1983

539. Jones R, Detmer M, Hill AB, et al: Incidence of choledocho-duodenal sphincter spasm during fentanyl-supplemented anesthesia. Anesth Analg 60:638, 1981

540. Maltby JR, Williams RT: Morphine-induced cardiac pain? Anesthesiology 64:527, 1986

541. Goldberg M, Vatashsky E, Haskel Y, et al: The effect of meperidine on the guinea pig extrahepatic biliary tract. Anesth Analg 66:1282, 1987

542. Vatashsky E, Haskel Y: Effect of nalbuphine on intrabiliary pressure in the early postoperative period. Can Anaesth Soc J 33:433, 1986

543. McCammon RL, Stoelting RK, Madura JA: Effects of butorphanol, nalbuphine and fentanyl on intrabiliary tract dynamics. Anesth Analg 63:139, 1984

544. Tverskoy M, Gelman S, Fowler KC, Bradley EL: Influence of fentanyl and morphine on intestinal circulation. Anesth Analg 64:577, 1985

545. Leaman DM, Levenson L, Zelis R, Shiroff R: Effect of morphine on splanchnic blood flow. Br Heart J 40:569, 1978

546. Granger DN, Richardson PDI, Kvietys PR, Mortillaro NA: Intestinal blood flow. Gastroenterology 78:837, 1980

547. Baden JM, Kundomal YR, Luttropp ME, Jr., et al: Effects of volatile anesthetics or fentanyl on hepatic function in cirrhotic rats. Anesth Analg 64:1183, 1985

548. Shingu K, Eger EI II, Johnson BH, et al: Hepatic injury induced by anesthetic agents in rats. Anesth Analg 62:140, 1983

549. Hurwitz A, Fischer HR: Effects of morphine and respiratory depression on sulfobromophthalein disposition in rats. Anesthesiology 60:537, 1984

550. Hurwitz A: Narcotic effects on phenol red disposition in mice. J Pharmacol Exp Ther 216:90, 1981

551. Wang SC, Glaviano VV: Locus of emetic action of morphine and hydergine in dogs. J Pharmacol Exp Ther 111:329, 1954

552. Harris AL: Cytotoxic therapy induced vomiting is mediated via enkephalin pathways. Lancet 1:714, 1982

553. Fisher MM: The diagnosis of acute anaphylactoid reactions to anesthetic drugs. Anaesth Intensive Care 9:234, 1981

554. Bennett MJ, Anderson LK, McMillar JC, et al: Anaphylactic reaction during anaesthesia associated with positive intradermal skin test to fentanyl. Can Anaesth Soc J 33:75, 1986

555. Levy JH, Rockoff MA: Anaphylaxis to meperidine. Anesth Analg 61:301, 1982

556. Fujinaga M, Stevenson JB, Mazze RI: Reproductive and teratogenic effects of fentanyl in Sprague-Dawley rats. Teratology 34:51, 1986

557. Fujinaga M, Mazze RI, Jackson EL, Baden JM: Reproductive and teratogenic effects of sufentanil and alfentanil in Sprague-Dawley rats. Anesth Analg 67:166, 1988

558. Harpel HS, Gautieri RF: Morphine-induced fetal malformations. J Pharm Sci 57:1590, 1968

559. Zagon IS, McLaughlin PJ: Effects of chronic morphine administration on pregnant rats and their offspring. Pharmacology 15:302, 1977

560. Hutchings DE, Hunt HF, Towey JP, et al: Methadone during pregnancy in the rat: Dose level effects on maternal and perinatal mortality and growth in the offspring. J Pharmacol Exp Ther 197:171, 1976

561. Gerber WF, Schramm LC: Congenital malformations of the central nervous system produced by narcotic and analgesics in the hamster. Am J Obstet Gynecol 123:705, 1975

562. Jurand A: Teratogenic activity of methadone hydrochloride in mouse and chick embryos. J Embryol Exp Morphol 30:449, 1973

563. Craft JB, Coaldrake LA, Bolan JC, et al: Placental passage and uterine effects of fentanyl. Anesth Analg 62:894, 1983

564. Crile GW: Phylogenetic association in relation to certain medical problems. Boston Med Surg J 163:893, 1910

565. Woodbridge PD: Changing concepts concerning depth of anesthesia. Anesthesiology 18:536, 1957

566. Griffith HR, Johnson GE: The use of curare in general anesthesia. Anesthesiology 3:418, 1942

567. Chadwick TH, Swerdlow M: Thiopentone-curare in abdominal surgery. Anaesthesia 4:76, 1949

568. Paulson JA: Thiopental sodium and ether anesthesia. JMA 150:983, 1952

569. Mushin WW, Rendell-Baker L: Pethidine as a supplement to nitrous oxide anaesthesia. Br Med J 2:472, 1949

570. Brotman M, Cullen SC: Supplementation with demerol during nitrous oxide anesthesia. Anesthesiology 10:696, 1949

571. Siker ES, Foldes FF, Pahk NM, Swerdlow M: Nisentil (1,3,dimethyl-4-phenyl-4-propionoxy piperidine): A new supplement for nitrous oxide oxygen thiopentone (pentothal sodium) anaesthesia. Br J Anaesth 26:405, 1954

572. Dundee JW, Brown SS, Hamilton RC, McDowel SA: Analgesic supplementation of light general anesthesia. A study of its advantages using sequential analysis. Anaesthesia 24:52, 1969

573. Goroszeniuk T, Whitwam JG, Morgan M: Uses of methohexitone, fentanyl and nitrous oxide for short surgical procedures. Anaesthesia 32:209, 1977

574. Flacke JW, Bloor BC, Flacke WE, et al: Comparison of morphine, meperidine, fentanyl, and sufentanil in balanced anesthesia: A double-blind study. Anesth Analg 64:897, 1985

575. De Castro J, Mundeleer R: Anesthesie sans barbituratiques: La neuroleptanalgesie. Anaesth Analg (Paris) 16:1022, 1959

576. Edmonds-Seal J, Prys-Roberts C: Pharmacology of drugs used in neuroleptanalgesia. Br J Anaesth 42:207, 1970

577. Martin DE, Rosenberg H, Aukberg SJ, et al: Low-dose fentanyl blunts circulatory responses to tracheal intubation. Anesth Analg 61:680, 1982

578. Lawes EG, Downing JW, Duncan PW, et al: Fentanyl-droperidol supplementation of rapid sequence induction in the presence of severe pregnancy-induced and pregnancy-aggravated hypertension. Br J Anaesth 59:1381, 1987

579. Cork RC, Weiss JL, Hameroff SR, Bentley J: Fentanyl preloading for rapid-sequence induction of anesthesia. Anesth Analg 63:60, 1984

580. Van Aken H, Meinshausen E, Prien T, et al: The influence of fentanyl and tracheal intubation on the hemodynamic effects of anesthesia induction with propofol/N_2O in humans. Anesthesiology 68:157, 1988

581. Cahalan MK, Lurz FW, Beaupre PN, et al: Narcotics alter the heart rate and blood pressure response to inhalation anesthetics. Anesthesiology 59:A26, 1983

582. O'Connor M, Sear JW: Sufentanil to supplement nitrous oxide in oxygen during balanced anaesthesia. Anaesthesia 43:749, 1988

583. Glenski JA, Friesen RH, Lane GA, et al: Low-dose sufentanil as a supplement to halothane/N_2O anesthesia in infants and children. Can J Anaesth 35:379, 1988

584. Murkin JM: Major surgery multicentre study group. Can Anaesth Soc J 34:S84, 1987

585. Siker ES: Analgesic supplements to nitrous oxide anaesthesia. Br Med J 2:1326, 1956

586. Griffiths G: In reply (letter). Anesthesiology 64:667, 1986

587. Gourlay GK, Kowalski SR, Plummer JL, et al: Fentanyl blood concentration-analgesic response relationship in the treatment of postoperative pain. Anesth Analg 67:329, 1988

588. Hilberman M, Hyer D: Potency of sufentanil. Anesthesiology 64:665, 1986

589. Lehmann KA, Heinrich C, van Heiss R: Balanced anesthesia and patient controlled postoperative analgesia with fentanyl: Minimum effective concentrations, accumulation and acute tolerance. Acta Anaesthesiol Belg 39:11, 1988

590. White PF: Use of continuous infusion versus intermittent bolus administration of fentanyl or ketamine during outpatient anesthesia. Anesthesiology 59:294, 1983

591. Milocco I, Schlossman D, William-Olsson G, Appelgren LK: Fentanyl-droperidol-nitrous oxide anaesthesia in patients with ischaemic heart disease and various degrees of left ventricular functional impairment. Acta Anaesthesiol Scand 29:683, 1985

592. Marty J, Couderc E, Servin F, et al: Plasma concentrations of sufentanil required to suppress hemodynamic responses to noxious stimuli during nitrous oxide anesthesia. Anesthesiology 69:A631, 1988

593. Kuperwasser B, Dahl M, McSweeney TD, Howie MB: Comparison of alfentanil and sufentanil in the ambulatory surgery procedure when used in balanced anesthesia technique. Anesth Analg 67:S122, 1988

594. Kalenda Z, Scheijground HW: Anaesthesia with sufentanilanalgesia in carotid and vertebral arteriography. A comparison with fentanyl. Anaesthetist 25:380, 1976

595. Clark NJ, Meuleman T, Liu WS, et al: Comparison of sufentanil-N_2O and fentanyl-N_2O in patients without cardiac disease undergoing general surgery. Anesthesiology 66:130, 1987

596. Ausems ME, Hug CC, Jr: Plasma concentrations of alfentanil required to supplement nitrous oxide anaesthesia for lower abdominal surgery. Br J Anaesth 55:191, 1983

597. Ausems ME, Hug CC, Jr., Stanski DR, Burm AGL: Plasma concentrations of alfentanil required to supplement nitrous oxide anesthesia for general surgery. Anesthesiology 65:362, 1986

598. van de Walle J, Lauwers P, Adriansen H: Double blind comparison of fentanyl and sufentanil in anesthesia. Acta Anaesthesiol Belg 3:129, 1976

599. Patrick M, Eagar B, Toft DF, Sebel PS: Alfentanil supplemented anesthesia for short procedures: A double blind comparison with fentanyl. Anesthesiology 59:A346, 1983

600. Rosow CE, Latta WB, Keegan CR, et al: Alfentanil and fentanyl in short surgical procedures. Anesthesiology 59:A345, 1983

601. White PF, Coe V, Shafer A, Sung ML: Comparison of alfentanil with fentanyl for outpatient anesthesia. Anesth Analg 64:99, 1986

602. Kallar SK, Keenan RL: Evaluation and comparison of recovery time from alfentanil and fentanyl for short surgical procedures. Anesthesiology 61:A379, 1984

603. Cooper GM, O'Connor M, Mark J, Harvey J: Effect of alfentanil and fentanyl on recovery from brief anaesthesia. Br J Anaesth 55:179, 1983

604. Stanley TH, Pace NL, Liu WS, et al: Alfentanil-N_2O vs fentanyl-N_2O balanced anesthesia: Comparison of plasma hormonal changes, early postoperative respiratory function, and speed of postoperative recovery. Anesth Analg 62:285, 1983

605. Kay B, Cohen AT: Intravenous anaesthesia for minor surgery. A comparison of etomidate or althesin with fentanyl and alfentanil. Br J Anaesth 55:165, 1983

606. Kestin IG, Dorje P: Anaesthesia for evacuation of retained products of conception—comparison between alfentanil

plus etomidate and fentanyl plus thiopentone. Br J Anaesth 59:364, 1987

607. McKay RD, Varner PD, Hendricks PL, et al: The evaluation of sufentanil-N_2O-O_2 anesthesia for craniotomy. Anesth Analg 63:250, 1984

608. Laborit H, Hugyenard P: Practique de L-Hibernotherapie in Chirurgie et en Medicine. Masson et Cie, Paris, 1954

609. Patton CM: Rapid induction of acute dyskinesia by droperidol. Anesthesiology 43:126, 1975

610. Janssen PAJ: Pharmacological aspects. In Bente D, Bradley P (eds): Neuropsychopharmacology. Elsevier Science Publishing, Amsterdam, 1965

611. Stanley TH: Cardiovascular effects of droperidol during enflurane and enflurane-nitrous oxide anesthesia in man. Can Anaesth Soc J 25:26, 1978

612. Long G, Dripps RD, Price HL: Measurements of anti-arrhythmic potency of drugs in man: Effects of dehydrobenzperidol. Anesthesiology 28:318, 1967

613. Bertolo L, Novakovi L, Penna M: Antiarrhythmic effects of droperidol. Anesthesiology 37:529, 1972

614. Whalley DG, Tidnam PF, Tyrell MF, Thompson DS: A comparison of the incidence of cardiac arrhythmias during two methods of anaesthesia for dental extractions. Br J Anaesth 48:1207, 1976

615. Gómez-Arnau J, Márquez-Montes J, Avello F: Fentanyl and droperidol effects on the refractoriness of the accessory pathway in the Wolff-Parkinson-White syndrome. Anesthesiology 58:307, 1983

616. Welsh MJ, Heistad DD, Abboud PM: Depression of ventilation by dopamine in man. J Clin Invest 61:708, 1978

617. Welling EC, Donegan J: Neuroleptanalgesia using alfentanil for awake craniotomy. Anesth Analg 68:57, 1989

618. Clarke AD, Tobias MA, Challen PDP: The use of neuroleptanalgesia during surgery of pheochromocytoma. Br J Anaesth 44:1093, 1972

619. Ogawa R, Fujita T: Neuroleptanaesthesia for the surgery of pheochromocytomas. Masui 21:174, 1972

620. Morgan M, Lumley J, Gillies IDS: Neuroleptanaesthesia for major surgery: Experience with 500 cases. Br J Anaesth 46:288, 1974

621. Corssen G, Chodoff P, Domino EF, Khan DR: Neuroleptanalgesia and anesthesia for open-heart surgery. J Thorac Cardiovasc Surg 49:901, 1965

622. Fitch W, Barker J, Jennett WB, McDowall DG: The influence of neuroleptanalgesic drugs on cerebrospinal fluid pressure. Br J Anaesth 41:800, 1969

623. Pathak KS, Brown RH, Nash CL, Jr, Cascorbi HF: Continuous opioid infusion for scoliosis fusion surgery. Anesth Analg 62:841, 1983

624. Alvis JM, Reves JG, Govier AV, et al: Computer assisted continuous infusions of fentanyl during cardiac anesthesia: Comparison with a manual method. Anesthesiology 63:41, 1985

625. Cork RC, Gallo JA, Weiss LB: Sufentanil infusion: Pharmacodynamics compared to bolus. Anesth Analg 67:S40, 1988

626. Shafer A, Sun ML, White PF: Pharmacokinetics and pharmacodynamics of alfentanil infusions during general anesthesia. Anesth Analg 65:1021, 1986

627. White PF: Clinical use of intravenous anesthetic and analgesic infusions. Anesth Analg 68:161, 1989

628. Wagner JG: A safe method for rapidly achieving plasma concentration plateaus. Clin Pharmacol Ther 16:691, 1974

629. Kruger-Theimer E: Continuous intravenous infusion and multicompartment accumulation. Eur J Pharmacol 4:317, 1968

630. Vaughn DP, Tucker GT: General derivation of the ideal intravenous drug input required to achieve and maintain a constant plasma drug concentration. Eur J Clin Pharmacol 10:433, 1976

631. Rigg JRA, Wong TY: A method for achieving rapidly steady-state blood concentrations of IV drugs. Br J Anaesth 53:1247, 1981

632. Schwilden H: A general method for calculating the dosage scheme in linear pharmacokinetics. Eur J Clin Pharmacol 20:379, 1981

633. Schwilden H, Schüttler J, Stoeckel H: Pharmacokinetics as applied to total intravenous anesthesia. Anaesthesia 38:51, 1983

634. Waud BE, Waud DR: Dose-response curves and pharmacokinetics. Anesthesiology 65:355, 1986

635. Desiderio DP, Thorne AC, Shah NK, et al: Alfentanil-midazolam by continuous infusion: A total intravenous anaesthetic technique for general surgery. Anesthesiology 69:A557, 1988

636. Ausems ME, Vuyk J, Hug CC, Jr, Stanski DR: Comparison of a computer-assisted infusion versus intermittent bolus administration of alfentanil as a supplement to nitrous oxide for lower abdominal surgery. Anesthesiology 68:851, 1988

637. Boerner TF, Goldberg ME, Bartkowski RR, et al: Return of cognitive function after prolonged alfentanil infusion. Anesthesiology 69:A62, 1988

638. Philbin DM, Moss J, Akins CW, et al: The use of H_1 and H_2 histamine antagonists with morphine anesthesia: A double-blind study. Anesthesiology 55:292, 1981

639. Sanford TJ, Smith NT, Dec-Silver H, Harrison WK: A comparison of morphine, fentanyl, and sufentanil anesthesia for cardiac surgery: Induction, emergence, and extubation. Anesth Analg 65:259, 1986

640. Benthuysen JL, Foltz BD, Smith T, et al: Prebypass hemodynamic stability of sufentanil-O_2, fentanyl-O_2 and morphine-O_2 anesthesia during cardiac surgery: A comparison of cardiovascular profiles. J Cardiothorac Anesth 12:749, 1988

641. Bergstrom RG, Thomson IR, Rosenbloom M, Meatherall RC: Premedication and high-dose fentanyl anaesthesia for myocardial revascularization. Can Anaesth Soc J 34:S114, 1987

642. Sprigge JS, Wynands JE, Whalley DG, et al: Fentanyl infusion anesthesia for aortocoronary bypass surgery: Plasma levels and hemodynamic response. Anesth Analg 61:972, 1982

643. Bazaral MG, Wagner R, Abi-Nader E, Estafanous FG: Comparison of effects of 15 and 60 mg/kg fentanyl used for induction of anesthesia in patients with coronary artery disease. Anesth Analg 64:312, 1985

644. Robinson S, Gregory GA: Fentanyl-air-oxygen anesthesia for ligation of patent ductus arteriosus in preterm infants. Anesth Analg 60:331, 1981

645. Walter RR, Kim YD, Macnamara TE, et al: Comparison of isoflurane vs fentanyl anesthesia in ligation of the patent ductus arteriosus in preterm infants. Anesth Analg 65:S165, 1986

646. Glenski JA, Foresen RH, Berglund NL, Henry D: Comparison of the cardiovascular effects of sufentanil, fentanyl, isoflurane and halothane during pediatric cardiac surgery. Anesthesiology 65:A438, 1986

647. Morgan P, Lynn AM, Parrot C, Morray JP: Hemodynamic and metabolic effects of two anesthetic techniques in children undergoing surgical repair of acyanotic congenital heart disease. Anesth Analg 66:1028, 1987

648. Benefiel DJ, Roizen MF, Lampe GH, et al: Morbidity after aortic surgery with sufentanil vs isoflurane anesthesia. Anesthesiology 65:A516, 1986

649. Ralley FE, Teasdale S, Wynands JE: Sufentanil for coronary

artery bypass graft surgery: The Canadian experience. Can Anaesth Soc J 34:S110, 1987

650. Howie MB, McSweeney TD, Lingam RP, Maschke SP: A comparison of fentanyl-O$_2$ and sufentanil-O$_2$ for cardiac anesthesia. Anesth Analg 64:877, 1985

651. Bovill JG, Warren PJ, Schuller JL, et al: Comparison of fentanyl, sufentanil, and alfentanil anesthesia in patients undergoing valvular heart surgery. Anesth Analg 63:1081, 1984

652. Rosow CE, Philbin DM, Moss J, et al: Sufentanil vs. fentanyl. I. Suppression of hemodynamic responses. Anesthesiology 59:A323, 1983

653. Shupak RC, Harp JR: Comparison between high-dose sufentanil-oxygen and high-dose fentanyl-oxygen for neuroanesthesia. Br J Anaesth 57:375, 1985

654. Holley FO, van Steennis C: Postoperative analgesia with fentanyl: Pharmacokinetics and pharmacodynamics of constant-rate IV and transdermal delivery. Br J Anaesth 60:608, 1988

655. Duthie DJR, Rowbotham DJ, Wyld R, et al: Plasma fentanyl concentrations during transdermal delivery of fentanyl to surgical patients. Br J Anaesth 60:614, 1988

656. Rolf D: Chemical and physical methods of enhancing transdermal drug delivery. Pharm Technol Sept:130, 1988

657. Ashburn MA, Stephen RL, Petelenz TJ, et al: Controlled iontophoretic delivery of morphine HCl for postoperative pain relief. Anesthesiology 69:A348, 1988

658. Edge WG, Cooper GM, Morgan M: Analgesic effects of sublingual buprenorphine. Anaesthesia 34:463, 1979

659. Bullingham RES, McQuay HJ, Porter EJB, et al: Sublingual buprenorphine used postoperatively: Ten hour plasma drug concentration analysis. Br J Clin Pharmacol 13:665, 1982

660. Risbo A: Sublingual buprenorphine for premedication and postoperative pain relief in orthopedic surgery. Acta Anaesthesiol Scand 29:180, 1985

661. Bell MDD, Mishra P, Weldon BD, et al: Buccal morphine—a new route for analgesia? Lancet 1:71, 1985

662. Fisher AP, Vine P, Whitlock J, Hanna M: Buccal morphine premedication. Anaesthesia 41:1104, 1986

663. Chrubasik J, Wüst H, Friedrich G, Geller E: Absorption and bioavailability of nebulized morphine. Br J Anaesth 61:228, 1988

664. Weinberg DS, Inturrisi CE, Beidenberg B, et al: Sublingual absorption of selected opioid analgesics. Clin Pharmacol Ther 44:335, 1988

665. Stanley TH, Hague BH, Mock DL, et al: Oral transmucosal fentanyl citrate (lollipop) premedication in human volunteers. Anesth Analg (in press)

666. Streisand JB, Stanley TH, Hague B, et al: Oral transmucosal fentanyl citrate premeditation in children. Anesth Analg, in press

667. Nelson P, Streisand JB, Mulder S, et al: Comparison of oral transmucosal fentanyl citrate and an oral solution of meperidine, diazepam and atropine for premedication in children. Anesthesiology 70:616, 1989

668. Henderson JM, Brodsky DA, Fisher DM, et al: Nasally administered sufentanil in children. Anesthesiology 68:671, 1988

669. Vercauteren M, Boeckx E, Hanegreefs G, et al: Intranasal sufentanil for pre-operative sedation. Anaesthesia 43:270, 1988

670. Abboud TK, et al: Transnasal analgesics: A new method for pain relief in post-cesarean section patients. Anesthesiology 69:A657, 1988

671. Lindahl S, Olsson AK, Thomson D: Rectal premedication in children. Use of diazepam, morphine and hyoscine. Anaesthesia 36:376, 1981

672. Hanning CD, Vicker AP, Smith G, et al: The morphine hydrogel suppository. Br J Anaesth 61:221, 1988

673. Simpson KH, Dearden MJ, Ellis FR, Jack TM: Premedication with slow release morphine and epidural morphine in the management of postoperative pain. Br J Anaesth 60:825, 1988

674. Banning AM, Schmidt JF, Chraemmer-Jorgensen B, Risbo A: Comparison of oral controlled release morphine and epidural morphine in the management of postoperative pain. Anesth Analg 65:385, 1986

675. Derbyshire DR, Bell A, Parry PA, Smith G: Morphine sulfate slow release, a comparison with IM morphine for postoperative analgesia. Br J Anaesth 57:858, 1985

676. Khojasteh A: Controlled-release oral morphine sulfate in the treatment of cancer pain with pharmacokinetic correlation. J Clin Oncol 5:956, 1987

677. Pohl J: Uber das *N*-allylnorecodeine, einen Antagonisten des Morphins. J Exp Pathol Ther 17:370, 1915

678. McCawley WL, Hart ER, Marsh DF: The preparation of *N*-allylnormorphine. J Am Chem Soc 63:314, 1941

679. Weijland J, Erickson AE: *N*-allylnormorphine. J Am Chem Soc 64:869, 1942

680. Unna K: Antagonistic effect of *N*-allylnormorphine upon morphine. J Pharmacol Exp Ther 79:27, 1943

681. Hart ER, McCawley EL: The pharmacology of *N*-allylnormorphine as compared with morphine. J Pharmacol Exp Ther 82:339, 1944

682. Schnider O, Hellerback J: Synthese von Morphinan. Helv Chim Acta 33:1437, 1950

683. Pearl J, Stander H, McKean DB: Effects of analgesics and other drugs on mice in phenylquinone and rotarod test. J Pharmacol Exp Ther 167:86, 1969

684. Perrin TD, Atwell L, Tice IB, et al: Analgesic activity as determined by the Nilsen method. J Pharm Sci 61:86, 1972

685. Jasinski DR, Martin WR, Hoeldtke RD: Effects of short- and long-term administration of pentazocine in man. Clin Pharmacol Ther 11:335, 1970

686. Fraser HF, Rosenberg DE: Studies on the human addiction liability of 2-hydroxy-5,9-dimethyl-2-(3,3-dimethylallyl)-6,7-benzomorphan (Win 20,228): A weak narcotic antagonist. J Pharmacol Exp Ther 143:149, 1964

687. Alarcon RD, Gelfond SD, Alarcon GS: Parenteral and oral pentazocine abuse. Johns Hopkins Med J 129:311, 1971

688. Parwatikar S, Gomez H, Knowles RR: Pentazocine dependency. Int J Addict 8:87, 1973

689. Sandoval RG, Wang RIH: Tolerance and dependence on pentazocine. N Engl J Med 230:1391, 1969

690. Kaukinen L, Kaukinen S, Eerola R, Eerola M: The antagonistic effect of pentazocine on fentanyl induced respiratory depression compared with nalorphine and naloxone. Ann Clin Res 13:396, 1981

691. Beaver WT, Wallenstein SL, Houde RW, Rogers A: A comparison of the analgesic effects of pentazocine and morphine in patients with cancer. Clin Pharmacol Ther 7:740, 1966

692. Goetz RL, Bain RV: Neonatal withdrawal symptoms associated with maternal use of pentazocine. J Pediatr 84:887, 1974

693. Leaman DM, Nellis SH, Zelis R, Field JM: Effect of morphine sulfate on human coronary blood flow. Am J Cardiol 41:324, 1978

694. Jewitt DE, Maurer RJ, Sonnenblick EJ, Shillingford JP: Pentazocine: Effect on ventricular muscle and hemodynamic changes in ischemic heart disease. Circulation 44(Suppl. II):118, 1971

695. Alderman EL, Barry WH, Graham AF: Hemodynamic effects

of morphine and pentazocine differ in cardiac patients. N Engl J Med 287:623, 1972

696. Jewitt DE, Maurer BJ, Hubner PJB: Increased pulmonary arterial pressures after pentazocine in myocardial infarction. Br Med J 1:795, 1970

697. Monkovic I, Conway TT, Wang H, et al: Total synthesis and pharmacological activities of N-substituted 3,14-dihydroxyl-morphinans. J Am Chem Soc 95:7910, 1973

698. Dobkin AB, Eamkaow S, Zak S, Caruso FS: Butorphanol: A double-blind evaluation in postoperative patients with moderate or severe pain. Can Anaesth Soc J 21:600, 1974

699. Tavakoli M, Corrsen G, Caruso FS: Butorphanol and morphine: A double-blind comparison of their parenteral analgesic activity. Anesth Analg 55:394, 1976

700. Del Pizzo A: Butorphanol, a new intravenous analgesic: Double-blind comparison with morphine sulfate in postoperative patients with moderate or severe pain. Curr Ther Res 20:221, 1976

701. Zola EM, McLeod DC: Comparative effects of analgesic efficacy of the agonist-antagonist opioids. Drug Intell Clin Pharm 17:411, 1983

702. Nagashima H, Karamanian A, Malovany R, et al: Respiratory and circulatory effects of intravenous butorphanol and morphine. Clin Pharmacol Ther 19:738, 1976

703. Popio KA, Jackson DH, Ross AM, et al: Hemodynamic and respiratory effects of morphine and butorphanol. Clin Pharmacol Ther 23:281, 1978

704. Del Pizzo A: A double-blind study of the effects of butorphanol compared with morphine in balanced anaesthesia. Can Anaesth Soc J 25:392, 1978

705. Zauder HL: Butorphanol, a new non-narcotic analgesic. p. 367. In Aldrete JA, Stanley TH (eds): Trends in Intravenous Anesthesia. Year Book Medical Publishers, Chicago, 1980

706. Sederberg J, Stanley TH, Reddy P, et al: Hemodynamic effects of butorphanol-oxygen anesthesia in dogs. Anesth Analg 60:715, 1981

707. Stanley TH, Reddy P, Tilmore S, Bennett G: The cardiovascular effects of high-dose butorphanol-nitrous oxide anaesthesia before during operation. Can Anaesth Soc J 30:337, 1983

708. Aldrete JA, de Camp T, Usubiaga LE, et al: Comparison of butorphanol and morphine as analgesics for coronary bypass surgery: A double-blind randomized study. Anesth Analg 62:78, 1983

709. Zucker JR, Neuenfeldt T, Freund PR: Respiratory effects of nalbuphine and butorphanol in anesthetized patients. Anesth Analg 66:879, 1987

710. Laffey DA, Kay NH: Premedication with butorphanol. Br J Anaesth 56:363, 1984

711. Bowdle TA, Greichen SL, Bjurstrom RL, Schoene RB: Butorphanol improves CO_2 responses and ventilation after fentanyl anesthesia. Anesth Analg 66:517, 1987

712. Vandam LD: Drug therapy: Butorphanol. N Engl J Med 302:381, 1980

713. Heel RC, Brogden RN, Speight TM, Avery GS: Butorphanol: A review of its pharmacological properties and therapeutic efficacy. Drugs 16:473, 1978

714. Dolan PF: Butorphanol and biliary spasm. Anesthesiology 63:340, 1985

715. Pedersen JE, Chraemmer-Jørgensen B, Schmidt JF, Risbo A: Naloxone — a strong analgesic in combination with high-dose buprenorphine? Br J Anaesth 57:1045, 1985

716. Sear JW, Alexander JI: Comparison of buprenorphine-hyoscine and papaveretum-hyoscine as premedicants for gynaecological surgery. Br J Anaesth 55:319, 1983

717. Obel D, Hansen LK, Hüttel MS, Andersen PK: Buprenorphine-supplemented anaesthesia. Br J Anaesth 57:271, 1985

718. Carl P, Crawford ME, Madsen NBB, et al: Pain relief after major abdominal surgery: A double-blind controlled comparison of sublingual buprenorphine, intramuscular buprenorphine, and intramuscular meperidine. Anesth Analg 66:142, 1987

719. Bullingham RES, O'Sullivan G, McQuay HJ, et al: Mandatory sublingual buprenorphine for post-operative pain. Anaesthesia 39:329, 1984

720. Maunuksela EL, Korpela R, Olkkola KT: Comparison of buprenorphine with morphine in the treatment of postoperative pain in children. Anesth Analg 67:233, 1988

721. Beaver WT, Feise GA: A comparison of the analgesic effect of intramuscular nalbuphine and morphine in patients with postoperative pain. J Pharmacol Exp Ther 204:487, 1978

722. De Souza EB, Schmidt WK, Kukor MJ: Nalbuphine: An autoradiographic opioid receptor binding profile in the central nervous system of an agonist/antagonist analgesic. J Pharmacol Exp Ther 244:391, 1988

723. Romagnoli A, Keats AS: Ceiling effect for respiratory depression by nalbuphine. Clin Pharmacol Ther 27:478, 1980

724. Fahmy NR, Sunder N, Soter NA: A comparison of histamine-releasing properties and hemodynamic effects of morphine and nalbuphine in humans. Anesth Analg 63:210, 1984

725. Romagnoli A, Keats AS: Comparative hemodynamic effects of nalbuphine and morphine in patients with coronary artery disease. Bull Tex Heart Inst 5:19, 1978

726. Lake C, Duckworth EN, DiFazio CA, Magruder MR: Cardiorespiratory effects of nalbuphine and morphine premedication in adult cardiac surgical patients. Acta Anaesthesiol Scand 28:305, 1984

727. Lee G, Low R, Amsterdam E, et al: Hemodynamic effects of morphine and nalbuphine in acute myocardial infarction. Clin Pharmacol Ther 29:576, 1981

728. Klein DS: Nalbuphine and droperidol combination for local standby sedation. Anesthesiology 58:397, 1983

729. Sury MRJ, Cole PV: Nalbuphine combined with midazolam for outpatient sedation. Anaesthesia 43:281, 1988

730. Garfield JM, Garfield FB, Philip BK, et al: A comparison of clinical and psychological effects of fentanyl and nalbuphine in ambulatory gynecologic patients. Anesth Analg 66:1303, 1987

731. Zsigmond EK, Winnie AP, Raza SMA, et al: Nalbuphine as an analgesic component in balanced anesthesia for cardiac surgery. Anesth Analg 66:1155, 1987

732. Lake CL, Duckworth EN, DiFazio CA, et al: Cardiovascular effects of nalbuphine in patients with coronary or valvular heart disease. Anesthesiology 57:498, 1982

733. Welch GW, Feldman HS: Intravenous nalbuphine. Anesth Analg 60:168, 1981

734. Krishnan A, Tolhurst-Cleaver CL, Kay B: Controlled comparison of nalbuphine and morphine for post-tonsillectomy pain. Anaesthesia 40:1178, 1985

735. Pugh GC, Drummond GB, Elton RA, MacIntyre CCA: Constant IV infusions of nalbuphine or buprenorphine for pain after abdominal surgery. Br J Anaesth 59:1364, 1987

736. Fee JPH, Brady MM, Furness G: Has nalbuphine a place in severe pain? Anesth Analg 66:S54, 1987

737. Telford J, Keats AS: Narcotic-narcotic antagonist mixtures. Anesthesiology 22:465, 1961

738. Julien RM: Effects of nalbuphine on normal and oxymorphone depressed ventilatory response to carbon dioxide challenge. Anesthesiology 57:A320, 1982

739. Latasch L, Probst S, Duziak R: Reversal by nalbuphine of

respiratory depression caused by fentanyl. Anesth Analg 63:814, 1984

740. Tran I, Durrain Z, Barabas E, et al: Hemodynamic and endocrine effects of reversal of fentanyl induced respiratory depression by nalbuphine. Anesthesiology 61:A476, 1984

741. Blaise GA, McMichan JC, Nugent M, Hollier LH: Nalbuphine produces side-effects while reversing narcotic-induced respiratory depression. Anesth Analg 65:S19, 1986

742. Ramsay JG, Wynands JE, Robbins R, Townsend GE: Early extubation after high-dose fentanyl anaesthesia for aortocoronary bypass surgery: Reversal of respiratory depression with low-dose nalbuphine. Can Anaesth Soc J 32:597, 1985

743. Moldenhauer CC, Roach GW, Finlayson DC, et al: Nalbuphine antagonism of ventilatory depression following high dose fentanyl anesthesia. Anesthesiology 62:647, 1985

744. Tabatabai M, Javadi P, Tadjziechy M, Mazloomdorst M: Effect of nalbuphine hydrochloride on fentanyl-induced respiratory depression and analgesia. Anesthesiology 61:A475, 1984

745. Bailey PL, Clark NJ, Pace NL, et al: Failure of nalbuphine to antagonize morphine. Anesth Analg 65:605, 1986

746. Bailey PL, Clark NJ, Pace NL, et al: Antagonism of postoperative opioid induced respiratory depression: Nalbuphine vs. naloxone. Anesth Analg 66:1109, 1987

747. Zsigmond EK, Durrani Z, Barabas E, et al: Endocrine and hemodynamic effects of antagonism of fentanyl-induced respiratory depression by nalbuphine. Anesth Analg 66:421, 1987

748. Jaffe RS, Moldenhauer CC, Hug CC, Jr, et al: Nalbuphine antagonism of fentanyl-induced ventilatory depression: A randomized trial. Anesthesiology 68:254, 1988

749. Gal TJ, DiFazio CA: Ventilatory and analgesic effects of dezocine in humans. Anesthesiology 61:716, 1984

750. Rowlingson JC, Moscicki JC, DiFazio C: Anesthetic potency of dezocine and its interaction with morphine in rats. Anesth Analg 62:899, 1983

751. Hall RI, Murphy MR, Szlam F, et al: Dezocine MAC reduction and evidence for myocardial depression in the presence of enflurane. Anesth Analg 66:1169, 1987

752. Lewis AJ, Kirchner A: A comparison of the cardiorespiratory effects of ciramadol, dezocine, morphine and pentazocine in the anesthetized dog. Arch Int Pharmacodyn 250:73, 1981

753. Galloway FM, Varma S: Double-blind comparison of intravenous doses of dezocine, butorphanol, and placebo for relief of postoperative pain. Anesth Analg 65:283, 1986

754. Eckenhoff JE, Elder JD, King BD: N-allyl-normorphine in the treatment of morphine or demerol narcosis. Am J Med Sci 223:191, 1952

755. Costa PJ, Bonnycastle DD: Effect of levallorphan tartrate, nalorphine HCl and WIN 7681 (1-allyl-4-pheno-4-carbethoxypiperidine) on respiratory depression and analgesia induced by some active analgesics. J Pharmacol Exp Ther 113:310, 1955

756. Azar I, Turndorf H: Severe hypertension and multiple atrial premature contractions following naloxone administration. Anesth Analg 58:524, 1979

757. Estilo AE, Cottrell JE: Naloxone, hypertension, and ruptured cerebral aneurysm. Anesthesiology 54:352, 1981

758. Flacke JW, Flacke WE, Williams GD: Acute pulmonary edema following naloxone reversal of high-dose morphine anesthesia. Anesthesiology 47:376, 1977

759. Tanaka GY: Hypertensive reaction to naloxone. JAMA 228:25, 1974

760. Andree RA: Sudden death following naloxone administration. Anesth Analg 59:782, 1980

761. Prough DS, Roy R, Bumgarner J, Shannon G: Acute pulmonary edema in healthy teenagers following conservative doses of intravenous naloxone. Anesthesiology 60:485, 1984

762. Michaelis LL, Hickey PR, Clark TA, Dixon WM: Ventricular irritability associated with the use of naloxone hydrochloride. Ann Thorac Surg 18:608, 1974

763. Partridge BL, Ward CF: Pulmonary edema following low-dose naloxone administration. Anesthesiology 65:709, 1986

764. Taff RH: Pulmonary edema following naloxone administration in a patient without heart disease. Anesthesiology 59:576, 1983

765. Patschke D, Eberlein HJ, Tarnow J, Zimmermann G: Antagonism of morphine with naloxone in dogs: Cardiovascular effects with special reference to the coronary circulation. Br J Anaesth 49:525, 1977

766. Raybould D, Bloor BC, McIntee DF, Flacke WE: Naloxone reverses the potentiation of inhalational anesthesia and hemodynamic changes induced by the acute administration of clonidine. Anesthesiology 67:A392, 1987

767. Farsang C, Kapocsi J, Vajda L, et al: Reversal by naloxone of the antihypertensive action of clonidine: Involvement of the sympathetic nervous system. Circulation 69:461, 1984

768. Levin ER, Sharp B, Drayer JIM, Weber MA: Case report: Severe hypertension induced by naloxone. Am J Med Sci 290:70, 1985

769. Estilo AE, Cottrell JE: Hemodynamic and catecholamine changes after administration of naloxone. Anesth Analg 61:349, 1982

770. Kraynack BJ, Gintautas JG: Naloxone: Analeptic action unrelated to opiate receptor antagonism? Anesthesiology 56:251, 1982

771. Aldrete JA, Goldman E: Is naloxone a nonspecific analeptic? Anesthesiology 50:270, 1979

772. Mills CA, Flacke JW, Miller JD, et al: Cardiovascular effects of fentanyl reversal by naloxone by varying arterial carbon dioxide tensions in dogs. Anesth Analg 67:730, 1988

773. Shupak RC, Harp JR, Stevenson-Smith W, et al: High-dose fentanyl for neuroanesthesia. Anesthesiology 58:579, 1983

774. Keykhah MM, Smith DS, Englebach I, Harp JR: Effects of naloxone on cerebral blood flow and metabolism. Anesthesiology 59:A309, 1983

775. Mannelli M, Maggi M, De Feo ML, et al: Naloxone administration releases catecholamines. N Engl J Med 308:654, 1982

776. Ngai SH, Berkowitz BA, Yang JC, et al: Pharmacokinetics of naloxone in rats and man. Anesthesiology 44:398, 1976

777. Kaufman RD: Relative potencies and durations of action with respect to respiratory depression of intravenous meperidine, fentanyl and alphaprodine in man. J Pharmacol Exp Ther 208:73, 1979

778. Andersen R, Dobloug I, Refstad S: Postanaesthetic use of naloxone hydrochloride after moderate doses of fentanyl. Acta Anaesthesiol Scand 20:255, 1976

779. Brown JH, Pleuvry BJ: Antagonism of the respiratory effects of alfentanil and fentanyl by naloxone in the conscious rabbit. Br J Anaesth 53:1033, 1981

780. Weinstock M, Davidson JT, Rosin AJ, Schnieden H: Effect of physostigmine on morphine-induced postoperative pain and somnolence. Br J Anaesth 54:429, 1982

781. Snir-Mor I, Weinstock M, Davidson JT, Bahar M: Physostigmine antagonizes morphine-induced respiratory depression in human subjects. Anesthesiology 59:6, 1983

782. Smith M, Ketcham TR, Nahrwold ML: Morphine, physostigmine and respiratory depression. Anesthesiology 55:A374, 1981

783. Beilin B, Vatashsky E, Aronson HB, Weinstock M: Naloxone

reversal of postoperative apnea in a premature infant. Anesthesiology 63:317, 1985

784. Chernick V: Endorphins and ventilatory control. N Engl J Med 304:122, 1981

785. Santiago TV, Remolina C, Scoles V III, Edelman NH: Endorphins and the control of breathing. N Engl J Med 304:1190, 1981

786. Williams AJ, Tarn AC, de Belder MA, Bailey AJ: Naloxone in acute respiratory failure. Lancet 2:1470, 1982

787. Jordan C, Lehane JR, Jones JG: Respiratory depression following diazepam: Reversal with high-dose naloxone. Anesthesiology 53:293, 1980

788. Smith G, Pinnock C: Naloxone — paradox or panacea? Br J Anaesth 57:547, 1985

789. Cullen M, Altstatt AH, Kwon NJ, et al: Naltrexone reversal of the side effects of epidural morphine. Anesthesiology 69:A336, 1988

790. Michel ME, Bolger G, Weisman BA: Binding of a new opiate antagonist nalmefene to rat brain membranes. Pharmacologist 26:201, 1988

791. Konieczko KM, Jones JG, Barrowcliffe MP, et al: Antagonism of morphine induced respiratory depression with nalmefene. Br J Anaesth 61:318, 1988

792. Gal TJ, DiFazio CA: Prolonged antagonism of opioid action with intravenous nalmefene in man. Anesthesiology 64:175, 1986

793. Braverman B, Ivankovich AD, McCarthy R: The effects of fentanyl and vasopressors on anesthetized dogs. Anesth Analg 63:192, 1984

794. Sedman AJ: Cimetidine — drug interactions. Am J Med 76:109, 1984

795. Dahlström B, Bolme P, Feychting H, et al: Morphine kinetics in children. Clin Pharmacol Ther 26:354, 1979

796. Stanski DR, Paalzow L, Edlund PO: Morphine pharmacokinetics: GLC assay versus radio immunoassay. J Pharm Sci 71:314, 1982

797. Murphy MR, Hug CC, Jr: Pharmacokinetics of intravenous morphine in patients anesthetized with enflurane-nitrous oxide. Anesthesiology 54:187, 1981

798. Dahlström B, Tamsen A, Paalzow L, Hartvig P: Patient controlled analgesia therapy. IV. Pharmacokinetics and analgesic plasma concentrations of morphine. Clin Pharmacokinet 7:266, 1982

799. Hug CC, Jr, Murphy MR, Rigel EP, Olson WA: Pharmacokinetics of morphine injected intravenously into the anesthetized dog. Anesthesiology 54:38, 1981

800. Berkowitz BA: The relationship of pharmacokinetics to pharmacological activity: Morphine, methadone, and naloxone. Clin Pharmacokinet 1:219, 1976

801. Mazoit JX, Sandouk P, Roche A: Extrahepatic metabolism of morphine occurs in humans. Anesthesiology 69:A456, 1988

802. Sasajima M: Analgesic effect of morphine-3-glucuronide. Keio Ogaka 47:421, 1970

803. Nishitateno K, Ngai SH, Finck AD, Berkowitz BA: Pharmacokinetics of morphine: Concentrations in the serum and brain of the dog during hyperventilation. Anesthesiology 50:520, 1979

804. Mather LE, Tucker GT, Pflug AE, et al: Meperidine kinetics in man: Intravenous injection in surgical patients and volunteers. Clin Pharmacol Ther 17:21, 1975

805. Klotz U, McHorse T, Wilkinson GR, Schenker S: The effect of cirrhosis on the disposition and elimination of meperidine in man. Clin Pharmacol Ther 16:667, 1974

806. Verbeeck RK, Branch RA, Wilkinson GR: Meperidine disposition in man: Influence of urinary pH and route of administration. Clin Pharmacol Ther 30:619, 1981

807. Stambaugh JE, Wainer IW, Sanstead J, Hemphill DM: The clinical pharmacology of meperidine: Comparison of routes of administration. J Clin Pharmacol 16:245, 1976

808. Austin KL, Stapleton JV, Mather LE: Multiple intramuscular injections: A major source of variability in analgesic response to meperidine. Pain 8:47, 1980

809. Fung DL, Asling JH, Eisele JH, et al: A comparison of alphaprodine and meperidine pharmacokinetics. J Clin Pharmacol 20:37, 1980

810. Miller JW, Anderson HH: The effect of N-demethylation on certain pharmacologic actions of morphine, codeine and meperidine in the mouse. J Pharmacol Exp Ther 112:191, 1954

811. Szeto HH, Inturrisi CE, Houde R, et al: Accumulation of normeperidine, an active metabolite of meperidine, in patients with renal failure or cancer. Ann Intern Med 86:738, 1977

812. Austin KL, Stapleton JV, Mather LE: Relationship between blood meperidine concentrations and analgesic response: A preliminary report. Anesthesiology 53:460, 1980

813. Hengstmann JH, Stockel H, Schüttler J: Infusion model for fentanyl based on pharmacokinetic analysis. Br J Anaesth 52:1021, 1980

814. Fung DL, Eisele JH: Fentanyl pharmacokinetics in awake volunteers. J Clin Pharmacol 20:652, 1980

815. Schleimer R, Benjamin E, Eisele J, Henderson G: Pharmacokinetics of fentanyl as determined by radioimmunoassay. Clin Pharmacol Ther 23:188, 1978

816. Haberer JP, Schoeffler P, Courderc E, Duvaldestin P: Fentanyl pharmacokinetics in anaesthetized patients with cirrhosis. Br J Anaesth 54:1267, 1982

817. Mather LE: Clinical pharmacokinetics of fentanyl and its newer derivatives. Clin Pharmacokinet 8:422, 1983

818. Hug CC, Murphy MR: Tissue redistribution of fentanyl and termination of its effects in rats. Anesthesiology 55:369, 1981

819. Hudson RJ, Stanski DR: Metabolism versus redistribution of fentanyl and alfentanil. Anesthesiology 59:A243, 1983

820. Meuldermans WEG, Hurkmans RMA, Heykants JJP: Plasma protein binding and distribution of fentanyl, sufentanil, alfentanil and lofentanil in blood. Arch Int Pharmacodyn Ther 257:4, 1982

821. Reilly CS, Wood AJJ, Wood M: Variability of fentanyl pharmacokinetics in man. Computer predicted plasma concentrations for three intravenous dosage regimens. Anaesthesia 40:837, 1984

822. Weldon ST, Perry DF, Cook RC, Gandolfi AJ: Detection of picogram levels of sufentanil by capillary gas chromatography. Anesthesiology 63:684, 1985

823. Avram MJ, Henthorn TK, Krejcie TC: Assay for serum sufentanil level is not sensitive. Anesthesiology 65:110, 1986

824. Bovill JG, Sebel PS, Blackburn CL, et al: The pharmacokinetics of sufentanil in surgical patients. Anesthesiology 61:502, 1984

825. Leysen JE, Gommeren W, Niemegeers CJE: [³H]sufentanil, a superior ligand for μ-opiate receptors: Binding properties and regional distribution in rat brain and spinal cord. Eur J Pharmacol 87:209, 1983

826. Bovill JG, Sebel PS, Blackburn CL, Heykants J: Kinetics of alfentanil and sufentanil: A comparison. Anesthesiology 55:A174, 1981

827. McDonnell TE, Bartkowski RR, Bonilla FA, et al: Evidence for polymorphic oxidation of alfentanil in man. Anesthesiology 57:A236, 1984

828. Schüttler J, Stoeckel H: Alfentanil (R 39209) ein neues kurwirkendes opioid. Anaesthetist 31:10, 1982

829. Bovill JG, Sebel PS, Blackburn CL, Heykants J: The pharmacokinetics of alfentanil (R39209): A new opioid analgesic. Anesthesiology 57:439, 1982

830. Camu F, Gepts E, Rucquoi M, Keykants J: Pharmacokinetics of alfentanil in man. Anesth Analg 61:657, 1982

831. Fragen RJ, Booij LHD, Braak GJJ, et al: Pharmacokinetics of the infusion of alfentanil in man. Br J Anaesth 55:1077, 1983

832. Persson MP, Nilsson A, Hartvig P: Pharmacokinetics of alfentanil in total IV anaesthesia. Br J Anaesth 60:755, 1988

833. Hug CC, Jr: Lipid solubility, pharmacokinetics, and the EEG: Are you better off today than you were four years ago? Anesthesiology 62:221, 1985

834. Grevel J, Whiting B: The relevance of pharmacokinetics to optimal intravenous anesthesia. Anesthesiology 66:1, 1987

835. Brater DC: Bayesian dosing of anesthetic agents: Esoteric or practical? Anesthesiology 69:641, 1988

836. Hull CJ: The pharmacokinetics of alfentanil in man. Br J Anaesth 55:157, 1983

837. Chauvin M, Bonnet F, Montembault C, et al: The influence of hepatic plasma flow on alfentanil plasma concentration plateaus achieved with an infusion model. Anesth Analg 65:999, 1986

838. Bovill JG, Odoom J, Heykants J: Biotransformation of alfentanil in man. Anesthesiology 69:A467, 1988

839. Lavrijsen KLM, Van Houdt JMG, Van Dyck DMJ, et al: Is the metabolism of alfentanil subject to debrisoquine polymorphism? Anesthesiology 69:535, 1988

840. Meuldermans W, van Peer A, Hendricks J, et al: Alfentanil pharmacokinetics and metabolism in humans. Anesthesiology 69:527, 1988

841. Ausems ME, Stanski DR, Hug CC, Jr: An evaluation of the accuracy of pharmacokinetic data for the computer assisted infusion of alfentanil. Br J Anaesth 57:1217, 1985

842. Maitre PO, Vozeh S, Heykants J, et al: Population pharmacokinetics of alfentanil: The average dose-plasma concentration relationship and interindividual variability in patients. Anesthesiology 66:3, 1987

843. Murphy MR, Hug CC: Dose independent pharmacokinetics of fentanyl. Anesthesiology 57:A347, 1982

844. Murphy MR, Hug CC, Jr, McClain DA: Dose independent pharmacokinetics of fentanyl. Anesthesiology 59:537, 1983

845. Koska AJ, Kramer WC, Romagnoli A, et al: Pharmacokinetics of high dose meperidine in surgical patients. Anesth Analg 60:8, 1981

846. Robbins R, Whalley DG, Donati F, et al: Altered pharmacokinetics of alfentanil. Can Anaesth Soc J 33:S103, 1986

847. Benson DW, Kaufman JJ, Koski WS: Theoretic significance of pH dependence of narcotics and narcotic antagonists in clinical anesthesia. Anesth Analg 55:253, 1976

848. Finck AD, Berkowitz BA, Hempstead J, et al: Pharmacokinetics of morphine: Effects of hypercarbia on serum and brain morphine concentrations in the dog. Anesthesiology 47:407, 1977

849. Lüllmann H, Martins BS, Peters T: pH-dependent accumulation of fentanyl, lofentanil, and alfentanil by beating guinea pig atria. Br J Anaesth 57:1012, 1985

850. Schulman DS, Kaufman JJ, Eisenstein MM, Rapoport SI: Blood pH and brain uptake of C^{14}-morphine. Anesthesiology 61:540, 1984

851. Schwartz AE, Matteo RS, Ornstein E, Thornhill M: Pharmacokinetics of sufentanil in hyperventilated patients. Anesth Analg 66:S151, 1987

852. Meistelman C, Levron JC, Barre J, et al: Effects of increased alpha-1-acid glycoprotein in cancer patients on pharmacokinetics of alfentanil. Anesthesiology 69:A602, 1988

853. Belville JW, Forrest WH, Miller E, Brown BW: Influence of age on pain relief from analgesics. A study of postoperative patients. JAMA 217:1835, 1971

854. Lynn AM, Slattery JT: Morphine pharmacokinetics in early infancy. Anesthesiology 66:136, 1987

855. Greenblatt DJ, Sellers EM, Shader RI: Drug disposition in old age. N Engl J Med 306:1081, 1982

856. Mannering FJ: Drug metabolism in the newborn. Fed Proc 44:2302, 1985

857. Liddell D, Williams F, Briant R: Phenazone (antipyrine) metabolism and distribution in young and elderly adults. Clin Exp Pharmacol Physiol 2:481, 1975

858. Davis PJ, Killian A, Stiller RL, et al: Alfentanil pharmacokinetics in premature infants and older children. Anesthesiology 69:A758, 1988

859. Collins C, Koren G, Crean P, et al: Fentanyl pharmacokinetics and hemodynamic effects in preterm infants during ligation of patent ductus arteriosus. Anesth Analg 64:1078, 1985

860. Johnson KL, Erickson JP, Holley FO, Scott JC: Fentanyl pharmacokinetics in the pediatric population. Anesthesiology 61:A441, 1984

861. Gauntlett I, Fisher DM, Hertzka RE, et al: Pharmacokinetics of fentanyl in neonatal humans and lambs: Effects of age. Anesthesiology 69:683, 1988

862. Greeley WJ, de Bruijn NP, Davis DP: Pharmacokinetics of sufentanil in pediatric patients. Anesthesiology 65:A422, 1986

863. Koren G, Goresky G, Crean P, et al: Pediatric fentanyl dosing based on pharmacokinetics during cardiac surgery. Anesth Analg 63:577, 1984

864. Sale JP, Goresky GV, Koren G, Strunin L: Pharmacokinetics of alfentanil in children. Anesth Analg 65:S129, 1986

865. Goresky GV, Koren G, Sabourin MA, et al: The pharmacokinetics of alfentanil in children. Anesthesiology 67:654, 1987

866. Roure P, Jean N, Leclerc A-C, et al: Pharmacokinetics of alfentanil in children undergoing surgery. Br J Anaesth 59:1437, 1987

867. Meistelman C, Saint-Maurice C, Lepaul M, et al: A comparison of alfentanil pharmacokinetics in children and adults. Anesthesiology 66:13, 1987

868. Greeley WJ, de Bruijn NP, Davis DP: Sufentanil pharmacokinetics in pediatric cardiovascular patients. Anesth Analg 66:1067, 1987

869. Owen JA, Sitar DS, Berger L, et al: Age-related morphine kinetics. Clin Pharmacol Ther 34:364, 1984

870. Singleton MA, Rosen JI, Fisher DM: Pharmacokinetics of fentanyl in the elderly. Br J Anaesth 60:619, 1988

871. Lemmens HJM, Bovill JG, Hennis PJ, Burm AGL: Influence of age on the pharmacokinetics of alfentanil. Anesthesiology 69:A629, 1988

872. Helmers H, van Peer A, Woestenborghs R, et al: Alfentanil kinetics in the elderly. Clin Pharmacol Ther 36:239, 1984

873. Lemmens HJM, Bovill JG, Hennis PJ, Burm GL: Age has no effect on pharmacodynamics of alfentanil. Anesth Analg 67:956, 1988

874. Gelman SI: Disturbances in hepatic blood flow during anesthesia and surgery. Arch Surg 111:881, 1976

875. Hudson RJ, Bergstrom RG, Thomson IR, et al: Pharmacokinetics of sufentanil in patients undergoing abdominal aortic surgery. Anesthesiology 70:426, 1989

876. Patwardhan RV, Johnson RF, Hoyumpa A, Jr, et al: Normal

metabolism of morphine in cirrhosis. Gastroenterology 81:1006, 1981

877. Mazoit JX, Sandouk P, Zetlaoui P, Scherrmann JM: Pharmacokinetics of unchanged morphine in normal and cirrhotic subjects. Anesth Analg 66:293, 1987

878. Olsen GD, Bennett WM, Porter GA: Morphine and phenytoin binding to plasma proteins in renal and hepatic failure. Clin Pharmacol Exp Ther 17:677, 1975

879. Ball M, Moore RA, Fischer A, et al: Renal failure and the use of morphine in intensive care. Lancet (April 6):784, 1985

880. Sear J, Moore A, Hunniset A, et al: Morphine kinetics and kidney transplantation: Morphine removal is influenced by renal ischemia. Anesth Analg 64:1065, 1985

881. Hug CC, Jr, Aldrete JA, Sampson JF, Murphy MR: Morphine anesthesia in patients with liver failure. Anesthesiology 51:S30, 1979

882. Hug CC, Jr, Murphy MR, Sampson JF, et al: Biotransformation of morphine and fentanyl in anhepatic dogs. Anesthesiology 55:A261, 1981

883. Klatz U, McHorse TS, Wilkinson GR, Schenker S: The effect of cirrhosis on the disposition and elimination of meperidine in man. Clin Pharmacol Ther 16:669, 1974

884. Neal EA, Meffin PJ, Gregory PB, et al: Enhanced bioavailability and decreased clearance of analgesics in patients with cirrhosis. Gastroenterology 77:96, 1979

885. Pond SM, Tong T, Benowitz NL, et al: Presystemic metabolism of meperidine to normeperidine in normal and cirrhotic subjects. Clin Pharmacol Ther 30:183, 1981

886. McHorse TS, Wilkinson GR, Johnson RF, Schenker S: Effect of acute viral hepatitis in man on the disposition and elimination of meperidine. Gastroenterology 68:775, 1975

887. Hudson RJ, Thomson IR, Cannon JE, et al: Pharmacokinetics of fentanyl in patients undergoing abdominal aortic surgery. Anesthesiology 64:334, 1986

888. Tammisto T, Tigerstedt I: The need for fentanyl supplementation of N_2O-O_2 relaxant anaesthesia in chronic alcoholics. Acta Anaesthesiol Scand 21:216, 1977

889. Ferrier C, Marty J, Bouffard Y, et al: Alfentanil pharmacokinetics in patients with cirrhosis. Anesthesiology 62:480, 1985

890. Davis PJ, Stiller RL, Cook DR, et al: Alfentanil pharmacokinetics in children. Anesthesiology 69:A759, 1988

891. Reitz J, MacKichan JJ, Hoffer L, et al: Reduced plasma clearance of alfentanil associated with prolonged major intra-abdominal surgery. Anesth Analg 63:265, 1984

892. Chauvin M, Ferrier C, Haberer JP, et al: Sufentanil pharmacokinetics in patients with cirrhosis. Anesth Analg 68:1, 1989

893. Holley FO, Ponganis KV, Stanski DR: Effect of cardiopulmonary bypass on the pharmacokinetics of drugs. Clin Pharmacokinet 7:234, 1982

894. Howie MB, Varma A, Sparks J, et al: Changes in plasma fentanyl levels and cardiopulmonary bypass. Abstract 722. Paper presented at the European Meeting of Anaesthesia, 1982

895. Okutani R, Philbin DM, Rosow CE, et al: Effect of hypothermic hemodilutional cardiopulmonary bypass on plasma sufentanil and catecholamine concentrations in humans. Anesth Analg 67:667, 1988

896. Hug CC, Jr, Burm AGL, de Lange S, Hermans G: Alfentanil pharmacokinetics and protein binding before and after cardiopulmonary bypass (CPB). p. 76. Paper presented at the Society of Cardiovascular Anesthesiologists, 5th Annual Meeting. San Diego, CA, 1983

897. Rosen D, Rosen K, Davidson B, Broadman L: Fentanyl uptake by the Scimed membrane oxygenator. J Cardiothorac Anesth 2:619, 1988

898. Rosen KR, Rosen DA: Absorption of sufentanil by the membrane oxygenator. Anesthesiology 65:A224, 1986

899. Durkan W, Lonergan M, Schwartz S, Fleming N: Effect of membrane oxygenators on sufentanil blood levels during cardiopulmonary bypass. Anesth Analg 67:S54, 1988

900. Flezzani P, Alvis MJ, Jacobs JR, et al: Sufentanil disposition during cardiopulmonary bypass. Can J Anaesth 34:566, 1987

901. Skacel M, Knott C, Reynold F, Aps C: Extracorporeal circuit sequestration of fentanyl and alfentanil. Br J Anaesth 58:947, 1986

902. Koska AJ III, Romagnoli A, Kramer WG: Effect of cardiopulmonary bypass on fentanyl distribution and elimination. Clin Pharmacol Ther 29:100, 1981

903. Hug CC, Jr, Moldenhauer CC: Pharmacokinetics and dynamics of fentanyl infusions in cardiac surgical patients. Anesthesiology 57:A45, 1982

904. Krejcie TC, Henthorn TK, Avram MJ: Alfentanil pharmacokinetics: Intravascular space and cardiac output. Anesthesiology 69:A466, 1988

905. Puig MM, Warner W, Tang CK, et al: Effects of temperature on the interaction of morphine with opioid receptors. Br J Anaesth 59:1459, 1987

906. Bentley JB, Cohanan TJ III, Cork RC: Fentanyl sequestration in lungs during cardiopulmonary bypass. Clin Pharmacol Ther 34:703, 1983

907. Howie MB, Mortimer W, Philip J, et al: Elimination of post bypass secondary peaks of fentanyl by pulsatile cardiopulmonary bypass. Anesthesiology 69:A60, 1988

908. Stone JG, Damask MC, Khambatta HJ: Is sufentanil removed by blood conservation devices? J Cardiothorac Anesth 2:615, 1988

909. Don HF, Dieppa RA, Taylor P: Narcotic analgesics in anuric patients. Anesthesiology 42:745, 1975

910. Mastert JW, Evers JL, Hobika GH, et al: Cardiorespiratory effects of anesthesia with morphine or fentanyl in chronic renal failure and cerebral toxicity after morphine. Br J Anaesth 43:1053, 1971

911. Aitkenhead AR, Vater M, Achola K, et al: Pharmacokinetics of single-dose i.v. morphine in normal volunteers and patients with end-stage renal failure. Br J Anaesth 56:813, 1984

912. Chauvin M, Sandouk P, Scherrmann MJ, et al: Morphine pharmacokinetics in renal failure. Anesthesiology 66:327, 1987

913. Moore A, Sear J, Baldwin D, et al: Morphine kinetics during and after renal transplantation. Clin Pharmacol Ther 35:641, 1984

914. Schali C, Roch-Ramel F: Transport and metabolism of [^{3}H] morphine in isolated nonperfused proximal tubular segments of the rabbit kidney. J Pharmacol Exp Ther 223:811, 1982

915. Stambaugh JE, Jr., Wainer IW: Drug interaction: Meperidine and chlorpromazine, a toxic combination. J Clin Pharmacol 21:140, 1981

916. Bower S: Plasma protein binding of fentanyl: The effect of hyperlipoproteinaemia and chronic renal failure. J Pharm Pharmacol 34:102, 1981

917. van Peer A, Vercauteren M, Noorduin H, et al: Alfentanil kinetics in renal insufficiency. Eur J Clin Pharmacol 30:245, 1986

918. Chauvin M, Lebrault C, Levron JC, Duvaldestin P: Pharmacokinetics of alfentanil in chronic renal failure. Anesth Analg 66:53, 1987

919. Davis PJ, Stiller RL, Cook DR, et al: Pharmacokinetics of sufentanil in adolescent patients with chronic renal failure. Anesth Analg 67:268, 1988

920. Bentley JB, Borel GD, Gillespie TJ, et al: Fentanyl pharmaco-kinetics in obese and nonobese patients. Anesthesiology 55:A177, 1981

921. Bentley JB, Finley JH, Humphrey LR, et al: Obesity and al-fentanil pharmacokinetics. Anesth Analg 62:251, 1983

922. Hare BD: The opioid analgesics: Rational selection of agents for acute and chronic pain. Hosp Formul 22:64, 1987

11

INTRAVENOUS ANESTHETIC DELIVERY

Peter S. A. Glass
James R. Jacobs
J. G. Reves

Historical Introduction
Rationale for Intravenous Drug Delivery
  Techniques
Pharmacodynamics of Intravenous Anes-
  thesia
Pharmacokinetic Basis for Continuous
  Intravenous Infusion
Manual Infusion Schemes for Intravenous
  Anesthetic Drug Administration
  Opiates

Hypnotics
Infusion Devices for Manual Delivery of
  Intravenous Anesthetics
Infusion Controllers
Positive Displacement Pumps
Commercial Pumps for Intravenous
  Anesthetic Drug Delivery
Computerized Pharmacokinetic Model-
  Driven Drug Delivery

HISTORICAL INTRODUCTION
(Also See Ch. 1)

For anesthetic drugs to be effective, they must reach their site of action within the central nervous system. In 1628, William Harvey proved in *Exercitatio Anatomica De Motu Cordis et Sanguinis In Animalibus* that venous blood was transported to the arterial circulation and thus to the organs of the body by the heart. It was recognized almost immediately that this meant that drugs given into veins could be rapidly carried to the entire body. Indeed, in 1657 Christopher Wren injected opium intravenously be means of a quill and bladder (Fig. 11-1A) in dogs and humans, rendering them un-

conscious, but Wren probably did not realize that they were "anesthetized." Sigismund Elsholtz in 1665 did give an opiate solution for the purpose of rendering subjects insensitive, but it was not until 1874 that Pierre-Cyprien Ore administered chloral hydrate intravenously for a surgical procedure. This landmark occasion followed the unsuccessful attempts by the Russian surgeon Pirogoff to administer ether intravenously in 1846, shortly after Crawford Long and William Morton had independently demonstrated the efficacy of ether insufflation for surgery.[1]

Intravenous methods of anesthetic drug delivery have depended on a steady improvement in technology. The quill and bladder first used by Wren were not signif-

A

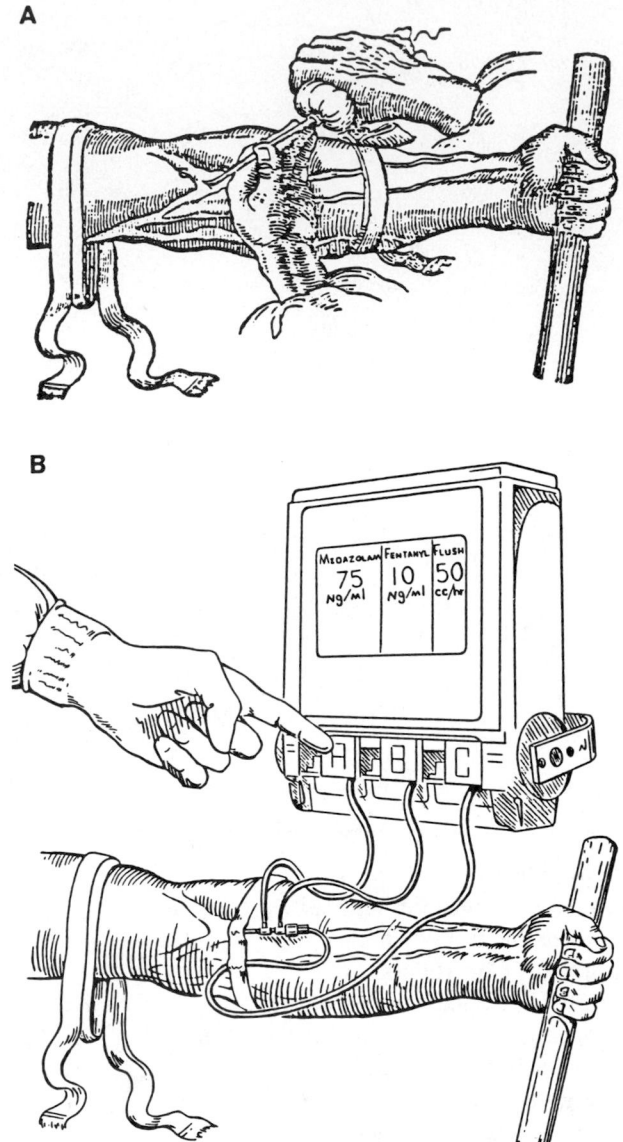

B

Fig. 11-1. Intravenous drug delivery, past and future. **(A)** Depiction of the first intravenous injection of opium, utilizing the quill and bladder. **(B)** The future of intravenous drug delivery, in which drugs are delivered with the aid of a small, sophisticated infusion pump, which permits dosing in terms of plasma drug concentration rather than amount.

icantly improved upon until Alexander Wood in 1853 employed a needle and syringe to give intravenous medications. The hollow hypodermic needle was developed by Frances Rynd, and a functional syringe was made by Charles Pravaz. Contemporary needles, catheters, and syringes are descendents of these early devices. The latest technologic development in intravenous anesthesia has been the introduction of computerized pharmacokinetic model-driven continu-

ous infusion (CACI*) (Fig. 11-1B), first published by Helmut Schwilden in 1981. He demonstrated the ability to attain desired plasma levels of an intravenous anesthetic drug by using a computer-controlled infusion pump driven by the published pharmacokinetics of the drug.[2] The ultimate development will be devices for the closed-loop administration of anesthetics, in which the desired depth of anesthesia will be maintained automatically. Unfortunately, the physiologic effects and the quantitation of anesthesia are not understood well enough, and monitoring techniques not sensitive enough for closed-loop approaches at the present time (also see Ch. 3).

With the development of more appropriate drugs and new technology, new concepts of intravenous drug administration have evolved. First, it has been realized that without the perfect sole intravenous anesthetic drug, multiple, rather than single, anesthetic drug administration is desirable. Opioids, barbiturates, and phencyclidine have at one time or another been advocated as sole anesthetics. However, because of the high doses required to achieve surgical anesthesia with these drugs, toxicity has inevitably resulted. It was George Cryle, a surgeon, who first suggested in 1901 that, rather than relying on an opioid alone for intravenous anesthesia, some supplemental drug or technique be employed. In 1959, DeCastro and Mundeleer introduced the term *neurolept anesthesia* for a combination consisting of a tranquilizer, opioid and nitrous oxide. Today, the concept and term coined by John Lundy, *balanced anesthesia,* is used to describe the administration of several anesthetic drugs simultaneously so that no single drug is given in a dosage sufficient to produce toxicity during or after surgery. A second important concept (only at present beginning to enjoy general acceptance) is that it is more rational to give intravenous anesthetic drugs continuously rather than intermittently or by high dose at the initiation of anesthesia. Ideally, just enough drug is given to achieve the therapeutic blood or plasma level, which is then maintained by continuous infusion until the end of surgery. This method of drug delivery avoids the peaks and valleys in drug levels and/or drug accumulation seen with intermittent drug administration and the overdose resulting from a large initial bolus. The availability of CACI will greatly facilitate the incorporation of continuous infusion drug delivery in daily clinical practice.

---

*CACI, which is an acronym for computer-assisted continuous infusion, is an expression coined by Dr. J. Michael Alvis.[25] In this chapter, CACI is used as a generic term for computerized pharmacokinetic model-driven drug infusion, without particular reference to the specific device developed by any one group of investigators.

RATIONALE FOR INTRAVENOUS DRUG DELIVERY TECHNIQUES

The objective of anesthetic administration (intravenous or inhalational) is to rapidly obtain and maintain anesthesia and then provide a rapid recovery following termination of administration. The use of intravenous anesthetics for these purposes has been limited by the properties of the intravenous drugs available. With the introduction of sodium thiopental in 1934, the use of an intravenous drug for induction of anesthesia was popularized, as it enabled anesthesia to be obtained rapidly. Thiopental, however, is not a suitable agent for the maintenance of anesthesia (see Ch. 8 for more details). During the last 30 years, numerous intravenous anesthetics (methohexital, 1957; propranidid, 1957; ketamine, 1966; Althesin, 1971; etomidate, 1973; propofol, 1977), hypnotics (diazepam, 1966; midazolam, 1978), and analgesics (fentanyl, 1959; sufentanil, 1979; alfentanil, 1980) have been introduced (see Chs. 8 to 10). The general trend has been to provide drugs with rapid clearance from plasma and shorter elimination half-lives. This change in the pharmacokinetics of available intravenous agents has allowed them to be utilized not only for induction but also maintenance of anesthesia.

Intravenous drugs have been used for maintenance of anesthesia by administration of a single large bolus, by intermittent bolus administration, or by continuous infusion. A single large intravenous bolus results in a concentration far in excess of the therapeutic range (Fig. 11-2). This technique, which is primarily used with the potent analgesics, results in profound respiratory depression and prolonged recovery that often necessitates postoperative mechanical ventilation. It does, however, provide excellent intraoperative hemodynamic stability. Intermittent bolus dose administration does not result in quite the same peak in drug concentration, but does produce a continuously changing plasma concentration (Fig. 11-2) and pharmacodynamic effect. To produce a stable concentration requires a continuous infusion determined by the pharmacokinetics of the drug (see below). This will theoretically result in fewer periods of poor anesthetic control, a reduction in the overall amount of drug used, and a more rapid recovery to the awake state at the termination of the infusion. These theoretical advantages have been confirmed by several investigators who have directly compared intermittent intravenous bolus administration to administration by continuous infusion.[3,4] Administration of the intravenous drug to a sin-

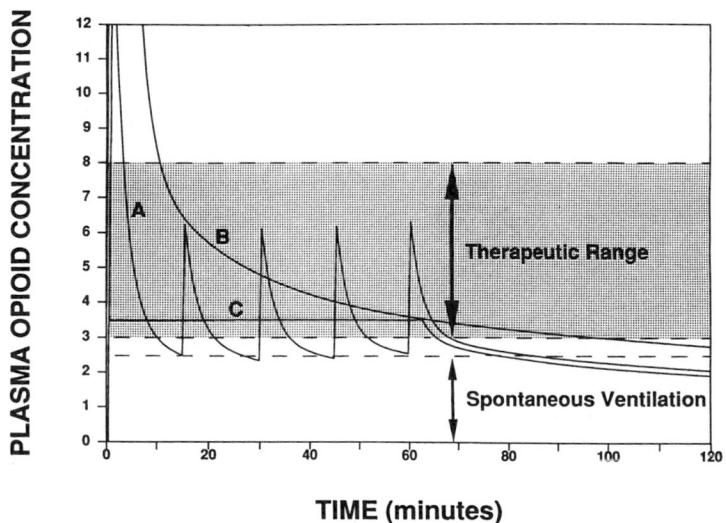

TIME (minutes)

Fig. 11-2. Simulation of plasma drug concentrations resulting from three dosing schemes for administration of a hypothetical opioid (kinetics[3] of fentanyl were used in constructing the graph) during a surgical procedure lasting 70 minutes. Curve A results from a loading bolus of 8 μg/kg followed by boluses of 1.5 μg/kg every 15 minutes. This dosing scheme results in the classic "peaks and valleys," where the plasma opioid concentration alternately swings between subtherapeutic and supratherapeutic levels. Curve B results from a single bolus of 20 μg/kg. Curve C results from a pharmacokinetic model-based continuous infusion scheme designed to maintain a constant therapeutic plasma opioid concentration. Note that at 65 minutes the plasma opioid concentration resulting from all three schemes is approximately equal but that recovery occurs most rapidly with the infusion technique, with the intermittent bolus method following close behind. When the therapeutic threshold is variable, as it is during the variable stresses of surgery, or when the surgical procedure is completed sooner than expected, a continuous infusion will be far superior to the intermittent technique both in maintaining a therapeutic concentration and in providing the potential for rapid recovery most consistently.

gle predetermined concentration is also not optimal, as the anesthetic state is varied not only by the drug concentration, but also by the degree of stimulation applied to the patient (Fig. 11-3). This variability (i.e., surgical stimuli and pharmacodynamics) necessitates that any intravenous drug administration technique must allow the clinician to titrate accurately the plasma concentration of the anesthetic drug(s) according to surgical conditions and patient response.

It may be assumed that once relative equilibration has been reached, the brain or receptor drug concentration will equal, or at least follow, a rise or fall in the concentration of drug in the blood or plasma. Therefore, pharmacokinetic information about the drug should be considered when developing dosing schemes (Fig. 11-4). The inhaled anesthetics, because of their lipid solubility and method and route of administration, rapidly approach the desired concentration set on the vaporizer (see Ch. 4). This holds true even if the inspired concentration is frequently varied. Most intravenous anesthetic drugs, however, do not rapidly achieve a stable plasma concentration if an adjustment is made only in infusion rate (Fig. 11-5). To rapidly achieve a particular plasma concentration with an intravenous drug requires both a loading dose plus an exponentially decreasing infusion. To provide a further increase of the plasma concentration requires a supplemental loading dose and an increase in infusion rate. Considering the many concentration changes that are required to titrate the depth of anesthesia appropriately, the ability to rapidly obtain and maintain particular plasma drug concentrations throughout an anesthetic procedure is beyond the realm of any manual scheme. Even though pharmacokinetically determined drug administration may be obtained manually or with CACI, to provide a means to adjust the plasma concentration continuously and conveniently for intravenous agents, a CACI device is desirable. CACI provides several theoretical advantages over manual infusion schemes. CACI is likely to be more accurate in both obtaining and varying the desired concentration and eliminates the need to calculate or even understand the complex pharmacokinetic formulas. It can also be modified for population-specific kinetics, and it can be helpful in determining when to terminate drug administration. It is likely, however, that convenience of use more than any other factor will lead to the general acceptance of CACI in clinical practice.

The ultimate success of intravenous anesthesia will depend on its ability to provide comparable outcome and advantages compared with the potent inhaled anesthetics. For example, etomidate, alfentanil, and propofol all provide a rapid onset of anesthesia, a stable maintenance phase, and rapid recovery (see Ch. 9).[1] Thus, the development of newer intravenous anesthetics and techniques of administration have allowed intravenous agents to be administered in a manner similar to that of the inhaled anesthetics. Therefore, the pharmacodynamic and pharmacokinetic principles that guide intravenous anesthesia and the devices utilized for their optimal administration must be understood.

PHARMACODYNAMICS OF INTRAVENOUS ANESTHESIA

General anesthesia is the result of drug action on the central nervous system. The state of anesthesia may be provided by a single drug or by a combination of different drugs. With the potent inhaled anesthetics, drug concentrations in the alveoli, blood, and brain reach equilibrium rapidly (see Ch. 4). This, combined with

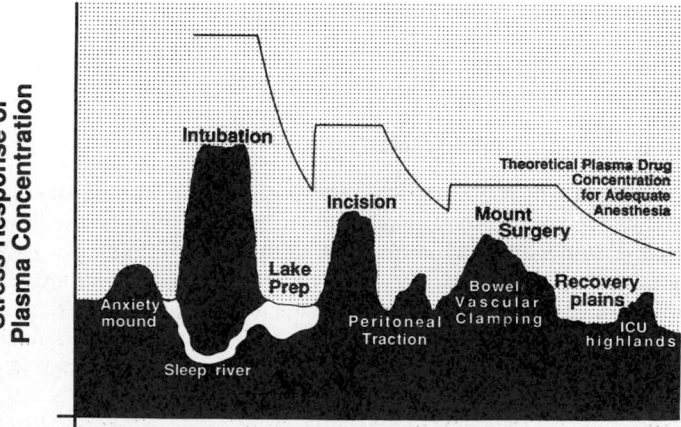

Fig. 11-3. Landscape of surgical anesthesia. The stimuli of surgery are not constant; therefore, the plasma concentration of the anesthetic drug should be titrated to match the needs of the patient.

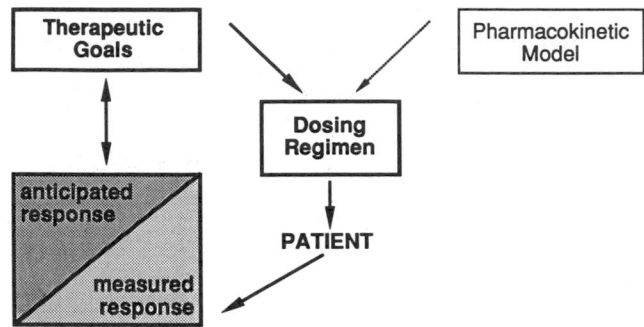

Fig. 11-4. Scheme for rational drug dosing, ideally incorporating pharmacokinetic data.

the fact that these drugs are administered according to concentration rather than dose, has allowed the establishment of minimal alveolar anesthetic concentration (MAC), an easily defined measure of anesthetic effect, for each of the potent inhaled anesthetics (see Ch. 30). Because these volatile agents act by a similar mechanism, their pharmacodynamic action is simply additive (see Ch. 3).

Quantifying the pharmacodynamic effect of intravenous anesthetic drugs is not as simple. Following a bolus dose or rapid infusion of an intravenous anesthetic, there is a time lag between peak concentration and peak effect. There may also be hysteresis in the relationship between drug concentration and offset of effect. The degree of hysteresis varies from one intravenous drug to another. Alfentanil produces minimal hysteresis for both onset and offset of electroencephalographic (EEG) effect. Fentanyl, on the other hand, has a more delayed onset, and offset of EEG effect correlates poorly with the decline of fentanyl concentration[5] (see

Ch. 10). A further difficulty in quantifying the pharmacodynamics of intravenous anesthetics is that the intravenous drugs used to provide anesthesia may be either true anesthetics (barbiturates, steroids, hindered phenols, ketamine, or imidazole derivatives), hypnotics (benzodiazepines or butyrophenones), or analgesics (opiates). The mechanism and site of action of the anesthetics, hypnotics, and analgesics are different. Therefore, because the intravenous drugs used to produce anesthesia do not all act by a unified mechanism, it cannot be assumed that their pharmacodynamics are simply additive. On the contrary, it has been demonstrated in animals and humans that certain combinations of intravenous anesthetics are synergistic rather than additive.[6,7]

An understanding of the rules governing kinetic–dynamic interaction of the intravenous anesthetics and of the techniques most appropriate to administer these drugs is still evolving; a measure of the pharmacokinetic–dynamic relationship for intravenous drugs is not yet as well defined as MAC. Notwithstanding the problems outlined above, investigators have attempted to define the concentration-effect relationship of some of the intravenous anesthetics. Early investigators used a measure of infusion rate and response to skin incision.[8] These studies defined the minimum infusion rate (MIR) necessary (when combined with 66 percent nitrous oxide) to prevent a somatic response to surgical skin incision in 50 percent of patients. The MIRs for a variety of intravenous drugs are given in Table 11-1. The MIR is not an optimum measure of the pharmacokinetic–dynamic relationship for several reasons. If only a simple constant infusion is used, it takes four elimination half-lives to reach a steady state, and therefore the measure is obtained

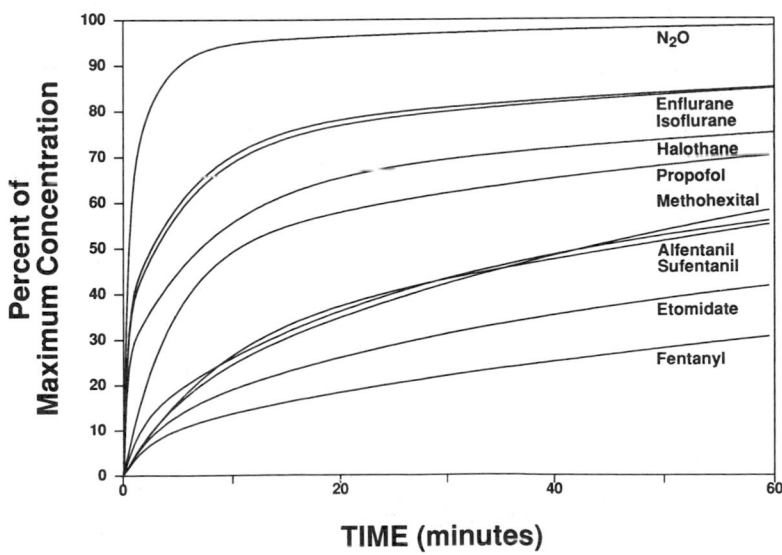

Fig. 11-5. Pharmacokinetic simulation showing the rate at which plasma drug concentrations approach their maximum value during a constant rate of administration.

TABLE 11-1. The Minimum Infusion Rate (MIR) Required (When Combined with 66% Nitrous Oxide) to Prevent a Somatic Response to Skin Incision

Drug	Premedication	$ED_{50}(MIR)$ (μg/kg/min)	ED_{95} (μg/kg/min)
Alphaxalone (Althesin)	Morphine	14	18
Alphaxalone (Althesin)	Diazepam	19	24
Methohexital	Morphine	49	76
Methohexital	Diazepam	66	81
Propofol	Morphine	54	112
Propofol	Lorazepam	130	348

prior to equilibrium being reached. The MIR was actually defined following a loading dose so that a state of equilibrium (steady state) was reached sooner. Therefore, the actual measure of the MIR is an interaction between both the loading dose and the infusion rate. The MIR also does not account for individual pharmacokinetic variability.

Since MIR did not clearly define a relationship between blood concentration and brain effect, investigators proceeded to correlate dynamic effect to plasma concentration.[9] This is obviously superior to MIR, but it is important to ensure when interpreting concentration-effect data that an equilibrium between blood and brain concentration has occurred and that hysteresis has been accounted for. The plasma concentration required to prevent a response to skin incision has been defined for alfentanil, fentanyl, sufentanil, and propofol. Average blood concentrations required for several other stimuli occurring during surgery have also been defined. These are presented in Table 11-2. For both the opiates and propofol, these values have been defined in combination with 66 percent nitrous oxide. The concentration that prevents a response to skin incision in 50 percent of subjects has been variably termed the EC_{50}, Cp_{50}, or MIC (minimum intravenous concentration). The MIC, like MAC, is a measure of potency and

will allow comparisons between the intravenous and inhalational anesthetic drugs. The MIC_{95} is a more important value as a guideline for clinical administration when using a pharmacokinetically based infusion scheme (either manual or CACI). (Also see Ch. 30).

PHARMACOKINETIC BASIS FOR CONTINUOUS INTRAVENOUS INFUSION

The medical literature is replete with articles describing pharmacokinetic models for virtually every drug administered clinically or experimentally. Practicing clinicians have found little practical value for the clinical utilization of these models, especially in short-lived circumstances such as surgical anesthesia. Most drug delivery schemes are derived empirically, without explicit consideration of the drug's pharmacokinetics. However, it is the premise of this chapter that it is desirable to be able to manipulate the plasma concentration of intravenously administered anesthetic drugs in a continuous and predictable manner, such as is common practice with the potent inhaled anesthetics. This objective requires quantitative incorporation of phar-

TABLE 11-2. Approximate Plasma Drug Levels Required for Various Stimuli (Also See Chs. 8 to 10)

Drug	Skin Incision	Major Surgery	Minor Surgery	Spontaneous Ventilation	Analgesia and/or Awakening (*)	Sedation
Alfentanil (ng/ml)	200–300	250–450	100–300	<200–250	50–100	50–200
Fentanyl (ng/ml)	3–6	4–8	2–5	<1–3	0.5–2	
Sufentanil (ng/ml)	1–3	2–5	1–3	<0.5	?	
Propofol (μg/ml)	2–6	2.5–7.5	2–6		0.8–1.8*	1–3
Methohexital (mg/ml)	5–10	5–15	5–10		1–3*	2–5
Thiopental (μg/ml)	7.5–12.5 (with N_2O) 35–45 (without N_2O)	10–20	10–20		4–8*	7.5–15
Etomidate (ng/ml)	400–600	500–1,000	300–600		200–350*	100–300
Midazolam (ng/ml)		50–250 (when combined with an opiate)	50–250 (when combined with an opiate)		150–200* (reduced to 20–70 in presence of an opiate)	40–100
Ketamine (μg/ml)	?	?	1–2		0.1–1.0	0.5–2

Drug levels are when combined with 65 to 70% N_2O unless otherwise stated. Effective plasma concentrations may differ markedly depending on premedication and intraoperative drug combinations.

macokinetic data into development of the dosing regimen.

To develop infusion schemes, a pharmacokinetic model with experimentally determined parameters (e.g., volume of distribution, clearance, k_{10}, etc.) can be exploited to derive the infusion rate profile necessary to obtain physician-specified plasma drug concentrations. Fortunately, the disposition of the intravenous anesthetic drugs presently available can be adequately described by linear pharmacokinetic models. Discussion will therefore be limited to concepts in linear pharmacokinetics. The implication of linearity is that at any point in time, the plasma drug concentration resulting from a dose of amount 2X will be twice that resulting from a dose of X. More generally, linearity implies that the system (i.e., the body acting to produce a plasma drug concentration output from a drug dosage input) behaves in accordance with the theorem of superposition. This theorem states that the response of a linear system having multiple inputs can be computed by determining the response to each individual input and then summing the individual responses to obtain the total response.

To strengthen the intuitive appeal of the concepts to be developed later in this chapter, recall that a line can be modeled as $y = mx + b$, where m and b are known constants, x is the dependent variable, and y is the independent variable. If we are interested in finding the value of x that will result in a particular value y', we need simply to compute $x = (y' - b)/m$. In other words, given a model (e.g., $y = mx + b$) of the system under consideration and the desired output of the system, it is possible to determine analytically what the input to the system must be to produce the desired output. The equations governing pharmacokinetic processes are more complex (e.g., $Cp(t) = \sum C_i e^{-\lambda_i t}$) than that of a straight line, but the same principles apply.

Several techniques are available to formulate pharmacokinetic models for drugs administered intravenously. The method used most commonly is that of measuring the plasma drug concentration at various times following an intravenous bolus injection (Fig. 11-6). Curve-fitting and statistical procedures are then used to fit concentration (Cp) versus time (t) data to models that usually take the multi-exponential form of $Cp(t) = C_1 e^{-\lambda_1 t} + C_2 e^{-\lambda_2 t}$ or $Cp(t) = C_1 e^{-\lambda_1 t} + C_2 e^{-\lambda_2 t} + C_3 e^{-\lambda_3 t}$, where t is time. The decision to use two or three exponential terms depends on which equation fits the data best from a statistical point of view. The C's and λ's are unique for each drug and characterize its disposition. Given the bolus input and the various assumptions inherent in most pharmacokinetic identification experiments, these equations may be regarded as transfer functions. As transfer functions, these equations offer a general description of the input (dosage)-output (plasma concentration) relationship of the patient or population from which they were derived and allow calculation (simulation) of the plasma drug concentration resulting from an arbitrary dosing scheme. The C's

and λ's can also be used to calculate the commonly known pharmacokinetic parameters.[10] There are model-independent techniques to obtain steady-state pharmacokinetic parameters such as clearance and volume of distribution, but knowing just these parameters permits only steady-state plasma concentrations to be computed and ignores the importance of the distribution processes.

The bi- and triexponential equations are a gross simplification of the complex and time-varying disposition of most drugs, especially recognizing that the model coefficients are usually reported as the simple average of data obtained from a very small number of volunteers or patients. Nevertheless, these equations have endured because they offer reasonably good predictive value and are usually as accurate as is possible or necessary to obtain in clinical circumstances.

Compartment models, rather than exponential equations, are frequently used to schematize the processes involved in drug disposition because they offer a much more intuitively appealing view of the pharmacokinetic phenomena. The pharmacokinetics of most of the popular intravenous anesthetic drugs have been described by a three-compartment model (Fig. 11-7). Based on similarities in blood flow and affinity for a given drug, various tissues and organs may be grouped and assigned to either the hypothetical central or peripheral compartment. The central compartment represents a distribution volume of V_1 L/kg and is usually assumed to include the blood, extracellular space, and well-perfused organs. Most significantly, it is assumed that the clinical effect of the drug is proportional to the concentration of drug in the central compartment, the blood or plasma being the only reasonable window into this compartment.

The peripheral compartments can be thought of as those tissues and organs showing a time course and extent of drug accumulation (or dissipation) different from that of the central compartment. In the three-compartment model, the two peripheral compartments may correspond roughly to fat stores and muscle tissue, respectively. However, it is important to realize that the model is merely a mathematical abstraction that describes the time course of drug concentration as a function of dosage and that no physiologic reality is implied. The sum of the compartment volumes is the apparent volume of distribution (V_d) and is simply a proportionality constant relating the drug concentration in blood or plasma to the total amount of drug in the body. The intercompartmental rate constants describe the exchange of drug between the central and peripheral compartments and are associated with the distribution phase of drug disposition. The elimination rate constant reflects all those processes acting through biotransformation or elimination to irreversibly remove or clear drug from the central compartment.

From a mathematical point of view, there is a one-to-one correspondence between bi- and triexponential equations and two- and three-compartment models, re-

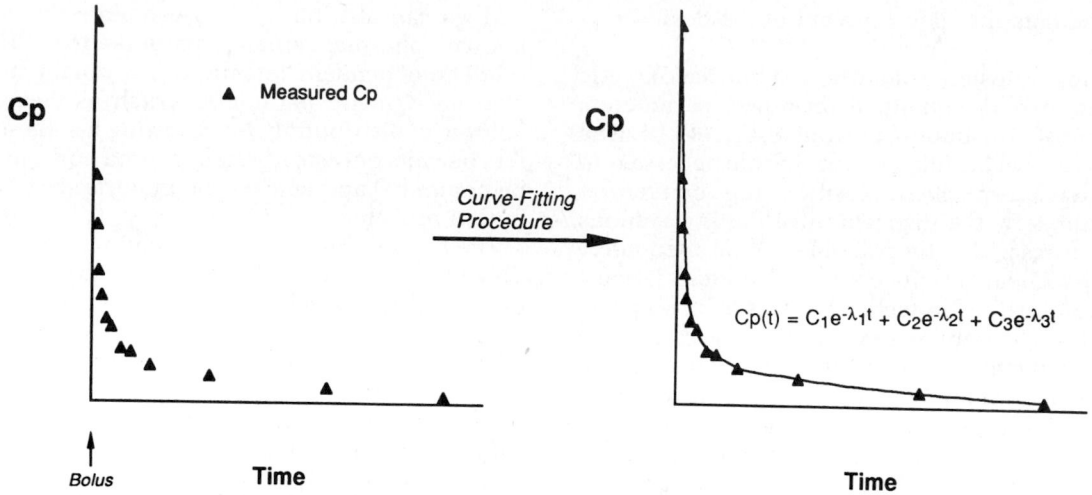

Fig. 11-6. Procedure by which pharmacokinetic parameters may be derived. The plasma drug concentration is measured at various times following a bolus dose of the drug under investigation. Curve-fitting procedures are then used to fit a multiexponential equation to the measured plasma concentrations. The coefficients of the multiexponential equation characterize the pharmacokinetics of the drug.

spectively. Once an experiment has been performed to determine the C's and λ's, the rate constants (i.e., k_{12}, k_{21}, k_{10}, etc.) and central compartment volume of the compartment model can be calculated, or vice versa.[10]

As we alluded to previously, the coefficients defining a particular pharmacokinetic model can be used to calculate the infusion rates necessary to achieve a specified concentration of drug in the central compartment or plasma. Mathematically rigorous approaches to the development of pharmacokinetically oriented manual infusion schemes for intravenous drugs have been de-

scribed by many researchers.[11,12] Most notably, the two-step infusion technique developed by Wagner[13] has been widely cited and is a classic reference in this regard. The objective has been to use the model parameters to design infusion regimens to achieve a specified plasma drug concentration, realizing that there are practical limitations to the sophistication of any infusion scheme that is to be implemented manually. Most of these theoretical treatments have resulted in schemes consisting essentially of a loading bolus or infusion followed by a maintenance infusion to achieve a

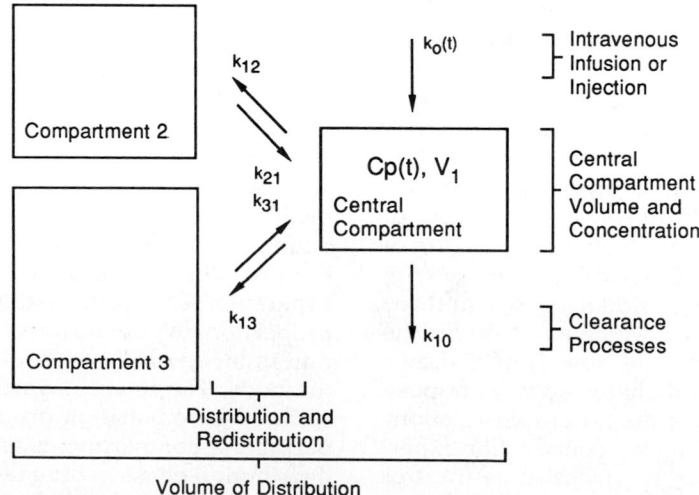

Fig. 11-7. Three-compartment model schematizing the basic pharmacokinetic processes that occur following intravenous drug administration. Explanation of symbols: V_1 (ml/kg) is the central compartment volume; $Cp(t)$ (ng/ml) is the drug concentration in the central compartment or plasma at time t; $k_o(t)$ (μg/kg/min or μg/kg) is the dosing scheme as a function of time; k_{10} (per min) is the rate constant reflecting all processes acting to irreversibly remove drug from the central compartment; and k_{ij} (per min) is the intercompartmental rate constant.

relatively stable plasma drug concentration—a practice that is well known, at least in principle, by most clinicians. The loading dose quickly raises the plasma concentration to the desired level (Cp_d), and the maintenance infusion replaces drug lost to metabolism or excretion.

Simplistically, the loading dose could be a bolus in an amount adequate to fill the entire volume of distribution

$$Bolus = Cp_d \cdot V_d$$

or just large enough to fill the central compartment

$$Bolus = Cp_d \cdot V_1$$

either of which would be followed by an infusion to replace drug lost due to clearance

$$\text{Infusion rate} = Cp_d \cdot k_{10} \cdot V_1 = Cp_d \cdot \text{clearance}$$

For a drug exhibiting one-compartment kinetics, this regimen would achieve Cp_d precisely. For drugs exhibiting multicompartment kinetics, as almost all do, the larger bolus results in plasma concentrations that are much greater than Cp_d for an extended period, while the smaller bolus results in plasma concentrations that fall below the desired level because of distribution until the infusion achieves its steady-state level (Fig. 11-8). In neither case has drug distribution been appropriately considered in designing the infusion scheme.

Although the more sophisticated approaches are mathematically elegant and do incorporate distribution, they are not readily implemented in clinical practice. There are several reasons for this, but foremost among them is the requirement to know the numerical value of all the parameters in the pharmacokinetic model and the relatively tedious calculations that must be performed with them. If the infusion regimen is designed a priori, it may not produce plasma concentrations that are adequate for the particular patient, and intraoperative adjustments will inevitably be based more on intuition than on calculations. Thus, most infusion regimens remain the empirical province of the clinician. They are in large part simple hand-me-down recipes that work well in clinical practice but that are nevertheless sufficiently unreliable in producing low plasma levels at the end of the operation and cumbersome so that continuous infusion techniques are not yet widely practiced in anesthesia.

MANUAL INFUSION SCHEMES FOR INTRAVENOUS ANESTHETIC DRUG ADMINISTRATION

Although the design of manual infusion schemes may be based on the drug's pharmacokinetics, ultimately it is the pharmacodynamic response, that is, adequate or inadequate anesthesia, that will determine the rate of

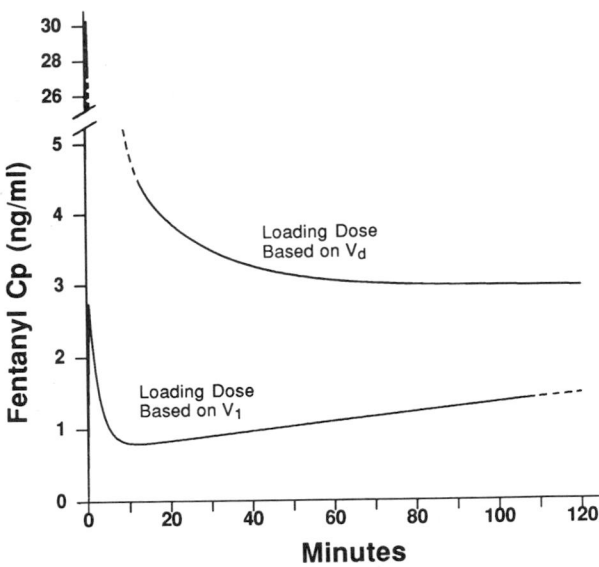

Fig. 11-8. Pharmacokinetic simulation demonstrating the limitations of infusion regimens based on simple pharmacokinetic parameters, using fentanyl as an example. These infusion schemes were designed to achieve a plasma fentanyl concentration of 3 ng/ml. The upper curve shows that a regimen with a loading dose based on the volume of distribution followed by a constant infusion based on clearance results in a transient period of extremely high plasma concentrations. If the same maintenance infusion is given but the loading dose is based on the volume of the central compartment, distribution of drug to the peripheral compartments causes the plasma concentration to fall below the desired level until the compartments reach steady-state concentrations, as shown in the lower curve.

drug administration. Average dosing schemes for administering intravenous anesthetics by infusion are given in Table 11-3. There are several important guidelines for the manual administration of intravenous anesthetics by infusion. It is essential to titrate the infusion rate continuously so that the patient is maintained just within the patient's own therapeutic level. Individuals vary markedly in their response to a given drug dose or concentration, and therefore it is essential to maintain an adequate drug level for each individual patient. The end of surgery requires lower drug levels, and therefore, by continuously titrating the infusion rate to a pharmacodynamic end point, it will provide lower drug concentrations at the end of surgery and thus facilitate a rapid recovery. If the infusion rate proves to be insufficient to maintain adequate anesthesia, then both a further loading (bolus dose) plus an increase in infusion is required to rapidly raise the drug concentration. Drug concentrations required to provide adequate anesthesia vary according to the type of surgery (e.g., surface surgery versus upper abdominal surgery). Thus, the infusion scheme should try to obtain

TABLE 11-3. Manual Infusion Schemes for Anesthesia, Sedation, or Analgesia
(Also See Chs. 8 to 10)

Drug	Anesthesia		Sedation or Analgesia	
	Loading Dose (μg/kg)	Maintenance Infusion (μg/kg/min)	Loading Dose (μg/kg)	Maintenance Infusion (μg/kg/min)
Alfentanil	50–150	0.5–3	10–25	0.25–1
Fentanyl	5–15	0.03–0.1	1–3	0.01–0.03
Sufentanil	3–10	0.01–0.05		
Ketamine	1,500–2,500	25–75	500–1,000	10–20
Propofol	1,000–2,500	50–150	250–1,000	10–50
Midazolam	50–150	0.25–1.5	25–100	0.25–1
Methohexital	1,500–2,500	50–150	250–1,000	10–50

Following the loading dose, a high infusion rate should initially be used to compensate for distribution to peripheral tissues. The infusion should then be vigilantly titrated to the lowest infusion rate that will maintain the desire end point.

higher or lower concentrations depending on the planned surgery. Various interventions also require greater drug concentrations, usually for brief periods (e.g., laryngoscopy, endotracheal intubation, skin incision) (Fig. 11-3). Therefore, the infusion scheme should be tailored to provide peak concentrations during these brief periods of intense stimulation. An adequate drug level for endotracheal intubation is often achieved by the initial loading dose, but for skin incision, etc., a further bolus dose may be necessary. When the initial loading dose is based on the central compartment volume, a high infusion rate or several repeat doses are initially required to replace drug loss resulting from redistribution.

The intravenous anesthetics can be administered (1) by infusion alone to obtain and maintain anesthesia, (2) in combination (e.g., an hypnotic plus an opiate to provide total intravenous anesthesia), or (3) to supplement inhalational anesthesia. Infusions of intravenous anesthetics may also be used to provide sedation either for brief periods (e.g., regional or topical anesthesia) or for prolonged periods (e.g., for patients on mechanical ventilators). The effect of combinations of intravenous anesthetic drugs has not been fully elucidated. Interactions between the intravenous anesthetics may result from a pharmacokinetic interaction and/or a pharmacodynamic interaction. Therefore, administration of combinations of intravenous anesthetics requires careful titration of each drug.

Opiates
(Also See Ch. 10)

Alfentanil

Several schemes have been advocated for the infusion of alfentanil. Most schemes vary in the sequence of the initial loading dose, although most provide 100 μg/kg within the first 10 minutes. Thus, the loading dose may be given as an initial rapid infusion of 50 μg/kg/min over 2 minutes or as two 50 μg/kg doses given prior to endotracheal intubation and skin incision or as a slower infusion of 10 μg/kg/min over 10 minutes. The

initial loading dose is followed by an infusion of 1 to 3 μg/kg/min. If the plasma level needs to be raised, an incremental bolus of 7 to 15 μg/kg with a 0.5 to 1 μg/kg/min increase in infusion rate is usually successful.[14] For the above infusion scheme, alfentanil is usually combined with 66 percent nitrous oxide. If a hypnotic is used with alfentanil to induce anesthesia, the dose of the hypnotic can usually be markedly reduced. Alfentanil can be infused with nitrous oxide or combined with a hypnotic for a total intravenous technique. If combined with midazolam (loading dose, 0.05 to 0.2 mg/kg, and maintenance infusion, 0.05 to 0.15 μg/kg/min) or propofol (loading dose, 1 to 2 mg/kg, and maintenance infusion, 50 to 100 μg/kg/min), the loading dose and infusion rate of alfentanil can be reduced to 10 to 50 μg/kg followed by 0.5 to 1 μg/kg/min. If alfentanil is given with a potent inhalational anesthetic at 0.25 to 0.5 MAC, both the loading dose and infusion rate can be reduced to approximately 50 percent of that used with nitrous oxide alone. The infusion of alfentanil should be discontinued approximately 20 minutes before the expected end of surgery.

For cardiac anesthesia, in the absence of adjuvant anesthetic drugs, much larger infusion rates are required. An initial infusion of 40 μg/kg/min to loss of consciousness is followed by 10 μg/kg/min until cooling. On rewarming of the patient, the infusion rate can be restarted at 2.5 μg/kg/min. If inadequate anesthesia occurs, a bolus of 30 μg/kg will usually ablate a response. Alfentanil has also been used for sedation in intensive care units. An initial loading dose of 25 μg/kg is followed by 0.5 to 1 μg/kg/min for 20 minutes and then titrated according to patient needs (0.1 to 2.0 μg/kg/min). A bolus of 3 μg/kg can be given when further supplementation is needed. Patients older than 50 years require lower infusion rates.

Fentanyl

Fentanyl by infusion has classically been used for cardiac surgery. Again, various schemes have been advocated for the loading dose, which varies from a bolus of 50 μg/kg to a rapid infusion of 4 to 5 μg/kg/min for 5 minutes or 2 to 3 μg/kg/min over 10 minutes.[15] This is followed by continuous infusion of 0.1 to 1.0 μg/kg/min. These infusion schemes are designed to obtain a plasma fentanyl level of 20 to 40 ng/ml. For noncardiac surgery, the loading dose can be reduced to 5 to 15 μg/kg followed by continuous infusion of 0.03 to 0.1 μg/kg/min to provide plasma levels of 3 to 10 ng/ml. These levels combined with 66 percent nitrous oxide provide adequate anesthesia for intra-abdominal and body surface surgery.

An analgesic level of fentanyl is obtained at a plasma concentration of 1 to 2 ng/ml. This level may be utilized intraoperatively if combined with an intravenous hypnotic or potent inhalational agent, or postoperatively for analgesia. This plasma level of fentanyl is obtained with a loading dose of 1.5 to 3 μg/kg followed by continuous infusion of 0.008 to 0.025 μg/kg/min.

Sufentanil

Sufentanil has been successfully used by infusion during cardiac anesthesia.[16] However, very little has been published about plasma levels or infusion rates of sufentanil required for noncardiac surgery. For cardiac surgery, an initial loading dose of 15 μg/kg followed by an infusion of 0.75 μg/kg/min has been used. When combined with midazolam (loading dose, 100 μg/kg, and maintenance infusion, 1.0 to 2.5 μg/kg/min), the sufentanil dose is reduced to 2 μg/kg/min for 5 minutes followed by 0.010 to 0.025 μg/kg/min thereafter. Even smaller doses of midazolam and sufentanil may be adequate for cardiac surgery.

Hypnotics
(Also See Chs. 8 and 9)

Thiopental

Thiopental is rarely used by infusion for the maintenance of surgical anesthesia. This is because the rapid recovery following a single bolus dose resulting from redistribution is lost when a prolonged infusion is used (i.e., accumulation occurs). Thiopental has been successfully used by infusion for short body surface procedures in combination with fentanyl.[17] An initial loading dose of 2 to 4 mg/kg is followed by an infusion of 200 to 300 μg/kg/min for the first 20 minutes and by 30 to 70 μg/kg/min thereafter. For sedation, an initial loading dose of 2 to 4 mg/kg is followed by an infusion of 30 to 80 μg/kg/min. When thiopental is used by infusion, its metabolism results in the formation of pentobarbital. It is uncertain whether this is of clinical significance.

Methohexital

Methohexital (unlike thiopental) can be used effectively by infusion for the maintenance of anesthesia for surgical procedures up to 2 hours duration.[8] A loading (induction) dose of 1 to 2 mg/kg is followed by an infusion of 50 to 150 μg/kg/min. Methohexital (at these in-

fusion rates) is combined with 66 percent nitrous oxide and/or an opiate. For total intravenous anesthesia, alfentanil (10 μg/kg followed by 1 μg/kg/min) can be utilized with methohexital (1.5 mg/kg followed by a variable rate of infusion of 50 to 150 μg/kg/min). Following premedication with morphine (0.15 mg/kg) or diazepam (10 mg by mouth), the MIR$_{95}$ of methohexital (combined with 66 percent nitrous oxide and after a loading dose of 1.5 mg/kg) is 80 μg/kg/min.[8] Methohexital may also be used by infusion for sedation. A loading dose of 0.5 to 1 mg/kg given over 5 to 10 minutes followed by an infusion of 15 to 25 μg/kg/min will usually provide an adequate level of sedation.

Etomidate

The use of etomidate by infusion is controversial. Most infusions with etomidate for general anesthesia are designed to provide a plasma level of etomidate of 500 ng/ml.[18] This may be achieved with either a two-stage or three-stage infusion scheme. In the two-stage scheme, etomidate is infused at 100 μg/kg/min for 10 minutes and then at 10 μg/kg/min. In the three-stage regimen, etomidate is infused at 100 μg/kg/min for 3 minutes, 20 μg/kg/min for 27 minutes, and 10 μg/kg/min thereafter. Etomidate is combined with nitrous oxide and usually an opiate given either intermittently or by continuous infusion. Etomidate plus fentanyl (loading dose, 2 to 3 μg/kg, and maintenance infusion of 0.03 to 0.06 μg/kg/min) or alfentanil (loading dose, 10 to 20 μg/kg, and maintenance infusion of 0.5 to 1 μg/kg/min) can be combined to provide a total intravenous anesthetic. The etomidate infusion can usually be terminated 10 to 15 minutes prior to the anticipated end of the surgical procedure. Etomidate has been used by infusion for cardiac surgery. An initial loading dose (used for induction) is followed by an infusion of etomidate at 20 μg/kg/min. This results in a plasma level of 550 to 900 ng/ml. The use of etomidate for prolonged sedation is contraindicated, but it may be useful for brief periods of sedation (i.e., for regional anesthesia). For sedation, a loading dose of 15 to 20 μg/kg/min for 10 minutes is followed by a maintenance infusion of 2.5 to 7.5 μg/kg/min.

Ketamine

Ketamine, although possessing both hypnotic and analgesic properties as well as suitable pharmacokinetics, is not a popular agent for the maintenance of general anesthesia owing to its psychotomimetic action. When combined with a benzodiazepine, it can provide suitable anesthesia (with or without nitrous oxide). The loading (induction) dose is 1 to 2 mg/kg followed by an infusion of 10 to 50 μg/kg/min.[19] In the absence of nitrous oxide and for more invasive surgery, higher infusion rates of 30 to 100 μg/kg/min may be necessary. Ketamine has also been used by infusion during cardiac surgery with similar infusion rates. An infusion of ketamine is also useful for analgesia and/or sedation. The loading dose can be reduced to 0.2 to 0.75 mg/kg and the infusion to 5 to 20 μg/kg/min.

Propofol

Propofol is best administered by continuous infusion. Plasma levels necessary during surgery and for awakening have been established. To obtain a plasma level of 3 to 4 μg/ml, a four-stage infusion scheme can be utilized. This consists of a loading dose of 1 mg/kg over 20 seconds followed by 170 μg/kg/min for 10 minutes, then 130 μg/kg/min for 10 minutes, and 100 μg/kg/min thereafter. More simply, a loading dose of 1 to 2 mg can be followed by an initial rapid infusion of 150 to 200 μg/kg/min, which is then titrated to about 100 μg/kg/min.[20] For short surgical procedures, generally higher average infusion rates are required, but for longer procedures, in which a steady state is achieved and redistribution contributes less, the average infusion rate is 100 to 150 μg/kg/min when combined with nitrous oxide. The addition of an opiate, either as a premedication or intraoperatively, markedly reduces the infusion rate of propofol required during surgery. When propofol is given with an opiate (rather than nitrous oxide) as part of a total intravenous anesthetic, the infusion rate of propofol remains similar to that required with nitrous oxide. Propofol has been combined with alfentanil (loading dose, 10 to 25 μg/kg, and maintenance infusion, 0.5 to 1 μg/kg/min) or fentanyl (loading dose, 2 to 5 μg/kg, and maintenance infusion, 0.025 to 0.05 μg/kg/min) for total intravenous anesthesia. The required infusion rate of propofol during anesthesia demonstrates a negative correlation with age; that is, elderly patients need lower infusion rates. For sedation during regional or topical anesthesia, an initial loading infusion of 100 to 150 μg/kg/min is given until an adequate level of sedation is achieved. This is then followed by a maintenance infusion of 25 to 75 μg/kg/min. For prolonged sedation in intensive care units, propofol has been given by infusion for several days. In critically ill patients a loading dose may not be desirable, and therefore an infusion can be started at 25 to 50 μg/kg/min. If a loading dose is desirable, 100 to 150 μg/kg/min is given until adequate sedation is achieved, which is followed by a maintenance infusion of 20 to 50 μg/kg/min.

Midazolam

Midazolam can be administered by infusion for sedation or to provide the hypnotic component of a balanced anesthetic.[21] The anesthetic effects of an opiate plus a benzodiazepine appear to be synergistic rather than additive. The loading (induction) dose of midazolam can therefore be reduced to 0.05 to 0.1 mg/kg when combined with fentanyl (2 to 5 μg/kg) or alfentanil (10 to 25 μg/kg). The midazolam maintenance infusion rate during surgical anesthesia can then be titrated between 0.25 and 1 μg/kg/min with either fentanyl (mainte-

nance infusion of 0.03 to 0.06 μg/kg/min) or alfentanil (maintenance infusion of 0.5 to 1.5 μg/kg/min). Nitrous oxide, if added to the above combinations, will further decrease the required infusion rates of both midazolam and the opiate. For cardiac surgery, similar doses of midazolam can be combined with slightly larger doses of the chosen opiate. For sedation, a midazolam loading dose of 0.05 to 0.1 mg/kg is administered. This may be given as 10 μg/kg doses until the desired level of sedation is achieved. The maintenance infusion is then titrated between 0.25 and 1 μg/kg/min. At the termination of a prolonged (days) infusion, there is a possibility of a benzodiazepine withdrawal syndrome. Therefore, the infusion might need to be slowly tapered, or a long-acting benzodiazepine may need to be given.

INFUSION DEVICES FOR MANUAL DELIVERY OF INTRAVENOUS ANESTHETICS

When administering an infusion of an intravenous anesthetic, the infusion regimen can be controlled by a variety of mechanisms. These vary from the simple CAIR clamp or Dial-a-Flo (Abbott Laboratories) to complex computer-controlled infusion pumps. Simplicity of mechanical design, however, is not necessarily correlated with ease of use. This has prompted ongoing advances in infusion device technology.

Infusion devices can be classified as either controllers or positive displacement pumps. Explicit in their title, controllers contain mechanisms that control the rate of flow produced by gravity, whereas positive displacement pumps contain active pumping mechanisms. Independent of the mechanism utilized to control flow rate, there are several features that are essential for all infusion devices used for the delivery of intravenous anesthetic drugs. These features are listed in Table 11-4.

Infusion Controllers

Infusion controllers are generally nonvolumetric pumps that rely on drop counting to calculate the volume infused. This may provide a source of error, since the volume of each drop is affected by the characteristics of the solution. Flow in infusion controllers is regulated by means of a feedback system that controls drop

TABLE 11-4. Essential Features for Infusion Devices

1. Electrical safety
2. Air detection
3. Occlusion alarm — time to alarm < 3 minutes
4. Maximum infusion pressure < 250 mmHg
5. Flow rate accuracy of ± 2%
6. Prevention of free flow
7. Continuous flow (i.e., minimal intermittent flow)
8. Function unaffected by electromagnetic fields

rate. If there is no feedback control (e.g., Dial-a-Flo), then the infusion rate also depends on the pressure difference across the valve, and any change in this pressure difference (e.g., height of fluid or venous obstruction) will alter the flow rate.

Drop rate is controlled by several mechanisms. These include (1) a pincher-anvil, which either partially occludes or intermittently pinches the administration tube such that the desired drop flow rate is maintained, (2) a rotary valve system that increases or decreases the valve radius, thus altering flow rates (i.e., flow proportional to r^{-4}), (3) a magnetically coupled steel ball-valve (this consists of a steel ball-valve that is unseated by an intermittent electromagnetic field, thus controlling the flow rate across the valve), and (4) a drip chamber diaphragm valve that occludes the drip chamber by variably occluding it with a diaphragm. The rotary valve and steel ball mechanisms prevent "run-away" on removal of the administration system from the pump. Controllers also generally contain a device to detect air in the line.

Positive Displacement Pumps

Positive displacement pumps provide a positive displacement of fluid and are capable of pumping against pressure. Because they are capable of pumping against pressure, they need to be carefully designed to prevent the infusion of air or large infiltrations. These pumps generally require special administration sets and can

be made to have extremely accurate delivery rates. Positive displacement pumps may be either nonvolumetric (drop counting) or volumetric. The pumps have either a peristaltic or piston mechanism. Peristaltic pumps utilize wobble plate, linear, or rotary mechanisms (Fig. 11-9). The wobble plate consists of a circular plate with the drive shaft off center so that as the plate rotates, it alternatively compresses and releases the tubing, forcing fluid in the required direction (this mechanism is rarely used today). Linear peristalsis consists of finger-like projections that sequentially compress the intravenous tubing against a stationary back plate, thus moving fluid within the tubing in the direction of the patient. Rotary peristaltic pumps have rollers on a wheel that compress the tubing and thus move fluid in the tube toward the patient.

Infusion pumps with a piston mechanism utilize either a to-and-fro or a screw motion to drive the piston (Fig. 11-10). The screw mechanism utilizes the rotation of the screw to drive a plunger to displace fluid. The thread of the screw and rate of rotation will determine the flow rate. Rack and pinion or belt-driven mechanisms provide a to-and-fro piston motion to pump the fluid. The piston may be within the fluid-containing cylinder (piston/cylinder cassette), or the piston may pump a flexible diaphragm. The pumping mechanism both expels and draws in fluid during the pumping cycle. The direction of flow is controlled by one-way valves or rotary valves or by alternatively occluding and releasing the inlet tube in synchrony with the pumping mechanism.

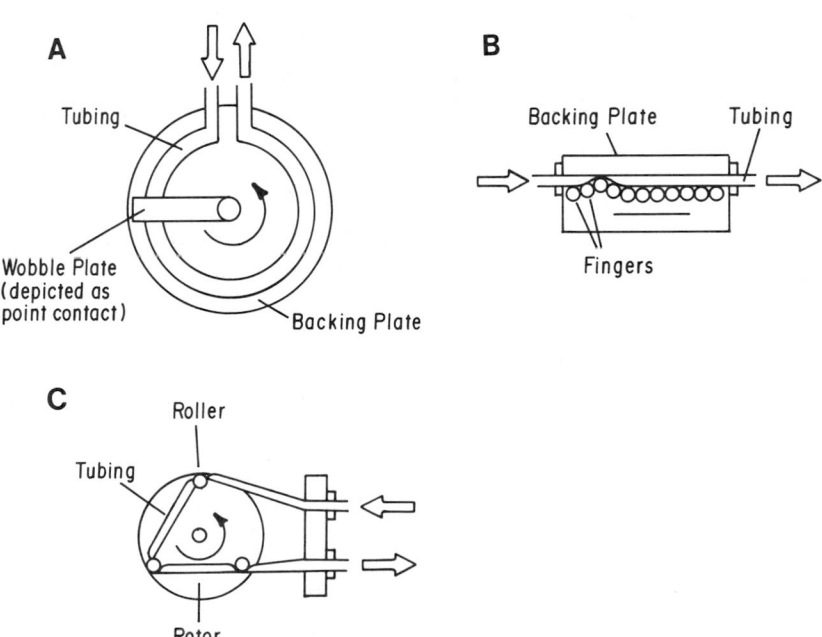

Fig. 11-9. The peristaltic mechanisms utilized for positive displacement pumps. **(A)** Wobble plate; **(B)** linear peristalsis; **(C)** rotary peristalsis.

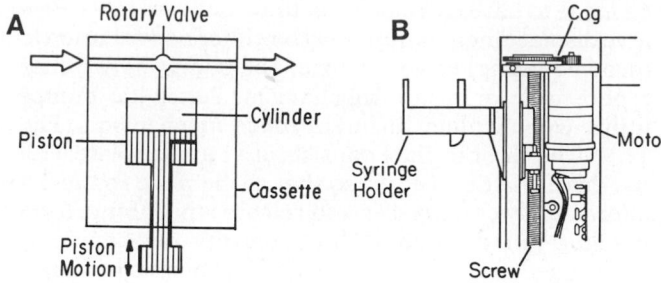

Fig. 11-10. The piston mechanisms utilized for positive displacement pumps. **(A)** To-and-fro piston; **(B)** rotating screw.

Commercial Pumps for Intravenous Anesthetic Drug Delivery

There are several specific features needed to make infusion pumps more suitable for intravenous anesthetic delivery. These features are listed in Table 11-5.

Several new pumps have attempted to provide the features necessary for more optimal intravenous anesthetic drug delivery. Recently, the first commercial pump dedicated to the delivery of an intravenous anesthetic was introduced. The pump (Bard Alfentanil Infuser; CR Bard, Inc.) is designed for the administration of the new short-acting opiate alfentanil. The pump utilizes a positive displacement screw-driven syringe. The controls of the pump are specifically modified to deliver drugs diluted to a concentration of 500 μg/ml within a 60-ml syringe. The pump has four rotary control dials. These dials are to set the infusion rate (μg/kg/min), patient weight (kg), and bolus dose (μg/kg), and there is a dial for the pump status (purge, on, off, infusion, bolus). The pump is illustrated in Figure 11-11. The pump has also been designed so that it does not exceed an infusion rate of greater than 50 μg/kg/min. This is to prevent rapid infusion of alfentanil, which

may be associated with an increased incidence of hypotension. Allowing the user to set the patient's weight and specifying the concentration of the drug to be used with the pump enables the clinician to select a bolus dose in μg/kg and/or an infusion rate of μg/kg/min. The pump thus calculates the actual volume to be delivered and therefore is the first "calculator" pump. The pump also provides a readout of μg/kg delivered while in the bolus mode, or of the total dose delivered while in the infusion mode. The infusion mechanism of the pump is linear, and therefore, although the controls are set for drugs diluted to 500 μg/ml, if the concentration is doubled, this will result in the pump delivering an infusion rate double that for which it is actually set. This has prompted the design of templates that can be utilized with the pump to deliver a variety of drugs of different concentrations. The readout of the drug dose, however, is incorrect. The manufacturers are presently developing templates that electromagnetically modify the pump and readout so that a variety of drugs of different concentrations can be used in the pump, thus increasing its versatility (Fig. 11-12). The pump senses magnets in the template that activate switches in the pump that are read by the microprocessors that then modify the pump rate and display.

A second "calculator" pump is the Auto Syringe model AS20GH (Baxter Healthcare Corporation) (Fig. 11-13). This is also a syringe pump. It requires the operator to enter the syringe size, drug concentration, and patient weight. This enables drug doses to be entered as either volume per unit time or dose per unit weight per unit time. This device is therefore a highly adaptable calculator pump that eliminates the need for the clinician to make any calculations that are both time consuming and subject to error.

Another area of pump development is in providing multiple channels in a single compact unit. Commercial pumps have successfully combined three or four channels into a unit similar in size to many presently

TABLE 11-5. Desirable Features for Infusion Pumps

1. Versatility
   Choice of bolus or infusion mode
   Internal calculator for choice of dosing scheme
   Adaptable for use with all anesthetic drugs
   Choice of infusion rate from 0–1500 ml/h with 0.1 ml/h resolution in the range 0–100 ml/h and 1 ml/h resolution in the range 100–1500 ml/h
   Choice of up to four separate channels with no opportunity for backflow or drug mixing proximal to the intravenous cannula

2. Light weight

3. Automatic priming of administration set

4. Clear display of drug being infused and infusion rate

5. Simple protocols for initiation or change of infusion rates

6. Digital interface for record keeping or external automated control

7. Automated drug recognition

8. Alarm for tubing disconnect

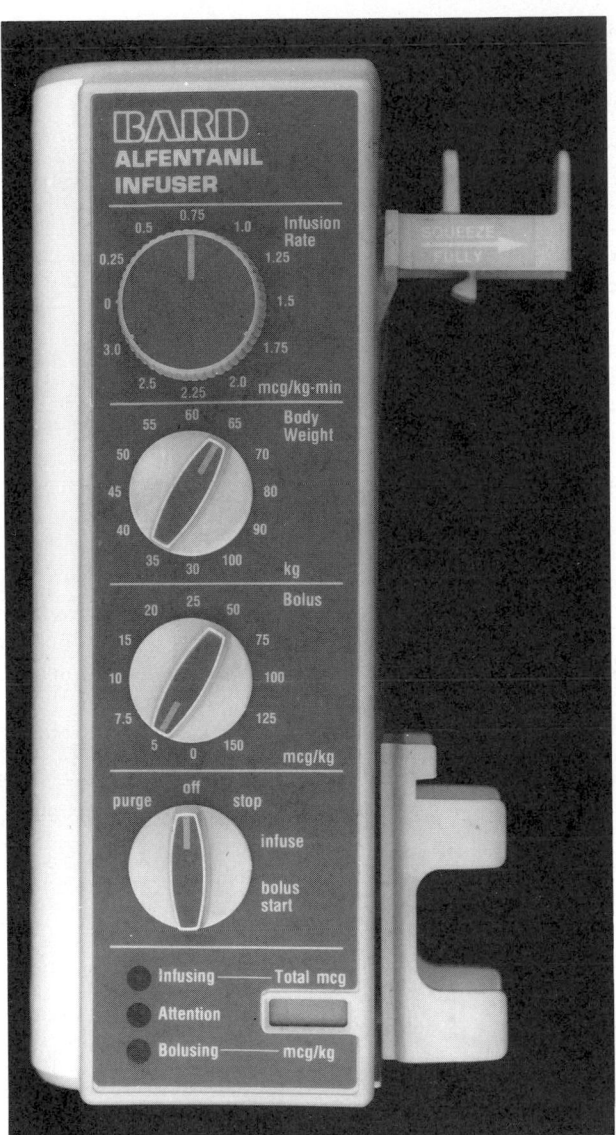

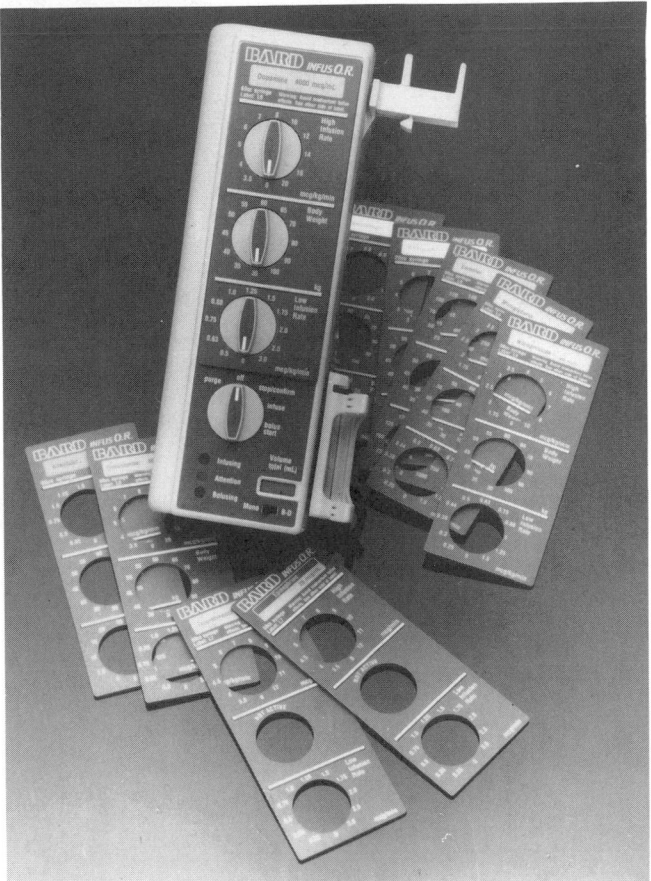

Fig. 11-12. The Bard Infus O.R. This pump is provided with drug- (and concentration)-specific templates. These templates permit the function of the pump to be automatically adjusted for the appropriate infusion of a variety of drugs.

Fig. 11-11. The Bard Alfentanil Infuser. This was the first infusion device with a calculator function dedicated to the administration of an intravenous anesthetic drug.

available single-channel pumps. At least two of these pumps have also included a calculator mode.

The Omni-Flow Operator (Omni-Flow) (Fig. 11-14) has four input channels and only a single output for drug delivery. This conformation, although providing four administration channels, has the potential for drug mixing and incompatibility. This is prevented by the pump interspacing carrier fluid between the drugs being administered. A single administration line provides tubing dead space (2 ml) that is occupied by an unknown amount of drug volume that, with highly potent agents, may have significant adverse effects. This may be prevented by attaching a stopcock to the intravenous catheter and venting the 2 ml of fluid whenever changing or discontinuing the delivery of a potent

agent. The Omni-Flow Operator has the advantage of allowing the choice of either a syringe or a bag to be used as the drug container. The pumping mechanism in the Omni-Flow is a piston diaphragm. The pump is designed to deliver drugs as ml/h, μg/h, or μg/kg/min. The display provides dosing information but does not enable the user to indicate on the display the drug used in each channel. The Omni-Flow also has a digital communication port for either record keeping or external control. The pump is compact and versatile and provides multiple channels, thus approaching an ideal infusion device for the administration of intravenous anesthetics. A second multiple-channel pump is the MiniMed III (MiniMed Technologies) (Fig. 11-15). This pump is small and compact (weight, 2.5 pounds) yet provides three separate delivery channels. The design of the software with several soft-keys enables the user to interact with the pump in several ways. This creates an extremely versatile pump, which also incorporates a port for external communications. The pumping mechanism is a reciprocating piston. The design of the pump

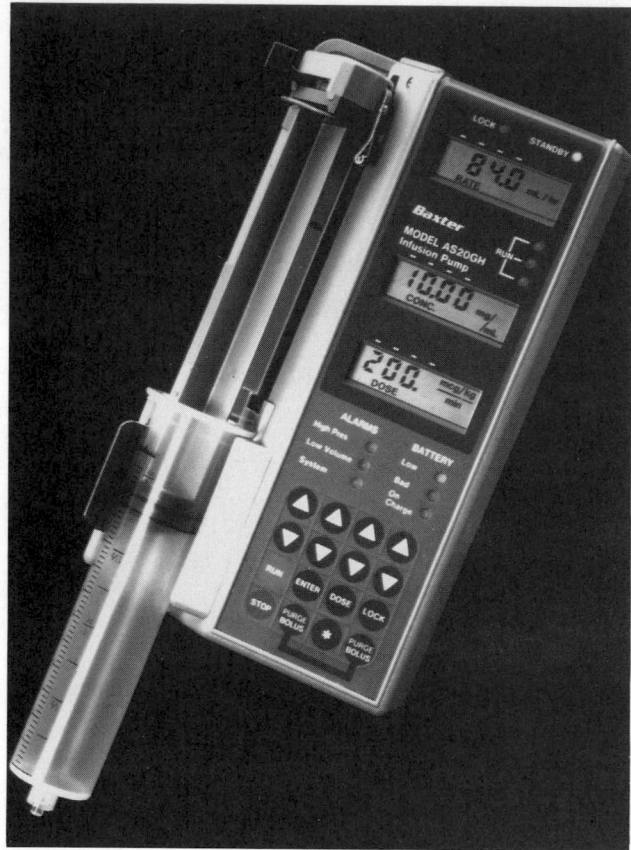

Fig. 11-13. The Baxter AS20GH infusion pump. This device incorporates a calculator function enabling administration of the selected infusate in ml/h or μg/kg/min.

allows the infusate to be delivered from either a syringe or a bag.

Major advances have been made in pump technology and design, enabling intravenous anesthetics to be conveniently delivered. However, no commercially available device for the delivery of intravenous anesthetics approaches the convenience of the present-day vaporizer. It is therefore desirable to take intravenous drug delivery systems one step further beyond a "calculator" pump to a truly "smart" pump by utilizing computerized pharmacokinetic model-driven drug delivery.

COMPUTERIZED PHARMACOKINETIC MODEL-DRIVEN DRUG DELIVERY

Kruger-Thiemer[22] described in 1968 the infusion regimen theoretically required to quickly achieve and maintain a constant plasma concentration of an intravenously administered drug whose kinetics are described by a two-compartment model. This regimen has become known as the "BET scheme." A bolus ("B") to fill the central compartment to the desired concentra-

tion is followed by a constant infusion to replace drug being eliminated ("E") from the central compartment by excretion or metabolism. Superimposed on this is an exponentially declining infusion to replace drug being transferred ("T") into the peripheral compartment. He generalized this result for multicompartment models to show, for example, that a bolus and biexponentially declining infusion superimposed on a continuous infusion are required to maintain a constant plasma concentration of a drug whose kinetics are described by a three-compartment model. Clearly, these complex dosage regimens, which require infusion rates that change continuously as a function of time until steady state is achieved, cannot be computed or implemented manually.

More than a decade after publication of Kruger-Thiemer's classic paper, as personal computers began to become commonplace, Schwilden et al.[2,23,24] interfaced a microcomputer to an infusion pump and demonstrated clinical application of the BET infusion scheme. They wrote a software program using the theorem of superposition to compute and implement BET infusion regimens in real time to obtain plasma drug concentrations specified by the anesthesiologist. The BET infusion regimen is now just one of several algorithms that have been used to effect computerized pharmacokinetic model-driven infusion (CACI) of intravenous anesthetic drugs.[25-31] All these algorithms have been derived by manipulating a pharmacokinetic model, expressed as either the multiexponential equations or compartment models described previously, to calculate the infusion rates required theoretically to obtain the desired plasma drug concentrations. In designing these algorithms, it is necessary to consider the physical limitations of the infusion device. In fact, it is not possible to implement the BET or any other analytically derived scheme precisely, since infusion pumps do not have infinite resolution; that is, pumps can infuse at 40 ml/h or at 41 ml/h but not at 40.00357 ml/h.

Each prototype CACI implementation has been somewhat different, but all are conceptually similar. Each consists of a microcomputer interfaced to a drug infusion pump, with a novel software program written by the investigators to implement the model-driven infusions. In using the device, the anesthesiologist specifies (via the computer keyboard) a desired (set point) plasma drug concentration, which is based on monitored and anticipated patient response, on the current prediction of the plasma drug concentration, and on the pharmacologic properties of the drug being administered. At frequent intervals (e.g., every 15 seconds), the software program compares the set point with the current prediction of the plasma drug concentration, which is computed, implicitly or explicitly, by real-time simulation of a pharmacokinetic model of the drug being infused. A pump control algorithm within the software program acts on any discrepancy between the predicted and desired concentrations to calculate a new infusion rate to achieve or maintain the set point.

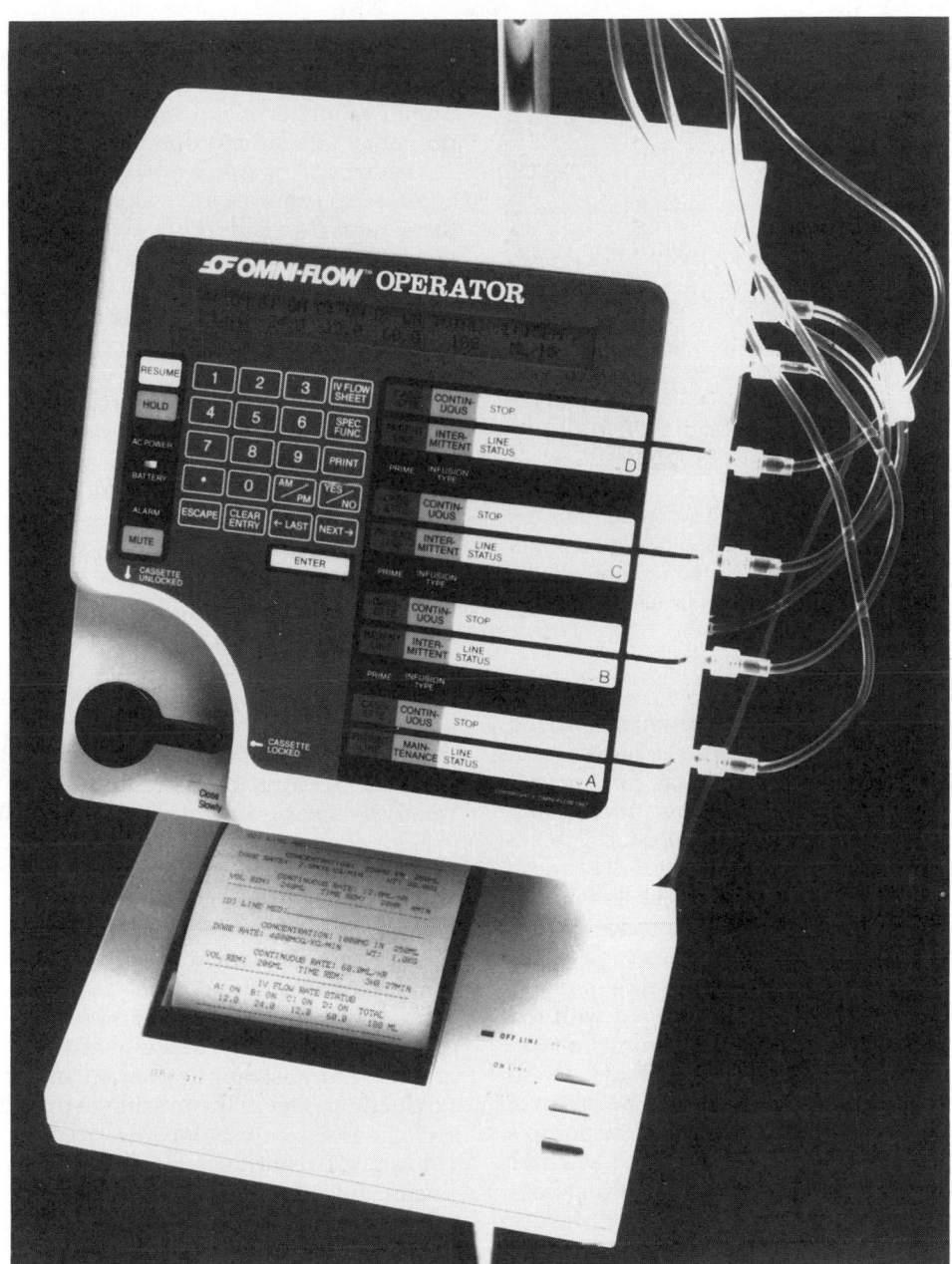

Fig. 11-14. The Omni-Flow Operator. This is a multichannel infusion device with programming and calculator functions.

The infusion rate is then transmitted electronically to the drug infusion pump, which delivers drug to the patient. The drug infusion rate is fed back into the pharmacokinetic simulation so that the next predicted plasma concentration can be computed. By communicating with the infusion device, the computer program can take into consideration, and help the user to be alerted to, error conditions, such as occlusion of the intravenous catheter. The user should be able to adjust the set point as frequently as desired. CACI cannot remove drug from the blood, but it can continuously calculate the theoretical plasma concentration and predict the time required to reach a particular level after the infusion has been decreased or terminated; this may be helpful in guiding the titration as the surgical procedure nears completion. Depending on the relevance and accuracy of the pharmacokinetic model used, CACI should be an efficient and reliable means of manipulating the concentration of drug in the plasma and thus of controlling the magnitude of the drug effect.

As a result of the increasing popularity of intravenous anesthesia and continuous infusion techniques, the in-

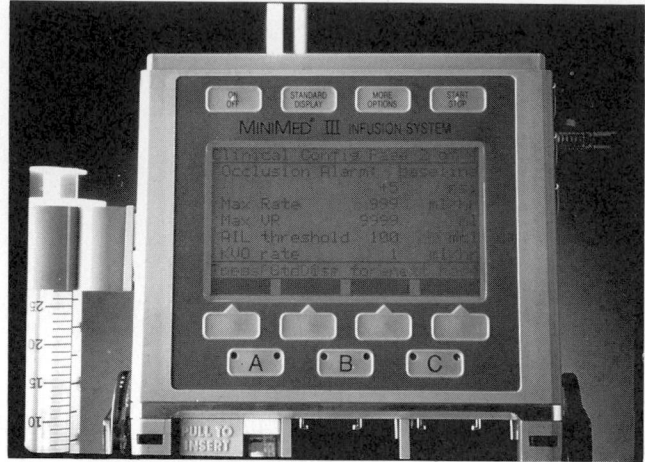

Fig. 11-15. MiniMed III. This small, multichannel infusion pump typifies the new generation of infusion devices that will permit sophisticated interaction with the computational power of the microprocessor that is already present in most of these instruments.

herent reasonableness of pharmacokinetically based drug delivery, and the promising results achieved with CACI administration of a variety of drugs by research groups around the world, CACI is now undergoing commercial development in the United States. It is expected that CACI concepts and techniques will become increasingly prevalent and that CACI devices will become generally available in clinical practice before publication of the next edition of this textbook. Standard infusion pumps, most of which already contain powerful microprocessors, will be equipped with the capability to perform pharmacokinetic model-driven infusions as a software-selectable option. Pharmacokinetic parameters for various drugs will be preprogrammed into the device. The user will use the pump's keypad to select the drug to be infused and to enter some pharmacokinetically relevant information about the patient, such as weight, age, and sex, and will ensure

that the infusion setup is primed with drug at a specified concentration. Then, the keypad will be used to enter set points in the same manner that the dial on a calibrated vaporizer is utilized in titrating the administration of an inhaled anesthetic.

Assessment of CACI administration of intravenous anesthetics requires an evaluation of both accuracy of the system (i.e., difference between the predicted and measured blood level) and outcome of patients in whom CACI has been used. The sources of inaccuracy with CACI devices include the software, the hardware, and the variability of pharmacokinetics from patient to patient (Fig. 11-16).

Inaccuracy in the software results both from the program calculating the infusion rates and from the actual pharmacokinetic parameters used for each drug. The program calculating the infusion rates can be tested against computer simulation programs and should not be a source of error.[29] Any inaccuracy owing to the infusion program or hardware can in practice be discounted, as they should be corrected prior to implementation of the device in patients. Therefore, the major cause of inaccuracy (i.e., a difference between the concentration predicted by the computer and the actual measured level) is differences between the patient's kinetics and those implemented in the computer program. Pharmacokinetics are usually defined from a relatively small population of similar age and weight. The kinetics are then calculated as the average of the group. This results in pharmacokinetic parameters that differ markedly from author to author for the same drug. This is a problem because the pharmacokinetic parameters (i.e., the rate constants and the central compartment volume) used in CACI devices are generally taken from the published literature. Thus, patient-to-patient variability, acute pharmacokinetic changes, and the many assumptions made in deriving a pharmacokinetic model in the first place preclude the possibility of consistently achieving precise accuracy when using CACI regardless of how good a particular set of coefficients are thought to be. For clinical use, however, it is not essential to have precise accuracy, but it is

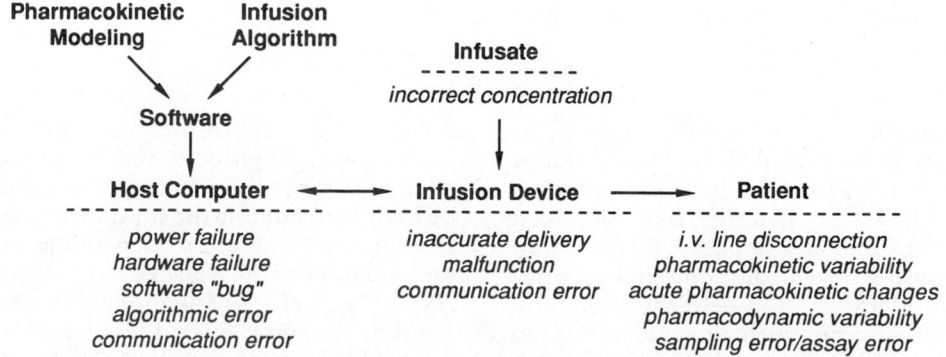

Fig. 11-16. Major sources of potential difficulty in pharmacokinetic model-driven drug delivery. In a commercial device, the computer functions would be incorporated into the infusion device itself.

necessary that CACI achieve plasma concentrations that are within a defined range. The question therefore is, do the kinetic parameters entered into the system sufficiently reflect those of the population so that the intravenous agents can be efficiently titrated to provide the optimal outcome for the patient?

Accuracy of CACI is assessed by comparing predicted blood concentration to actual measured concentration. When trying to evaluate accuracy, linear regression with calculation of the correlation coefficient has been used as a measure of accuracy. Linear regression, however, is not the correct statistical test to evaluate accuracy of a predicted to a measured value.[32] A better means of assessing accuracy of measured to predicted values is by calculating the bias and the mean absolute prediction error:

Prediction error (ng/ml) = Cp (predicted) − Cp (measured)
Prediction error (percent)

$$= \frac{Cp\ (predicted) - Cp\ (measured)}{Cp\ (predicted)} \times 100$$

Bias or mean prediction error

$$= \frac{\Sigma\ prediction\ error\ (ng/ml\ or\ \%)}{number\ of\ measurements}$$

Mean absolute prediction error (MAPE)

$$= \frac{\Sigma\ |prediction\ error|\ (ng/ml\ or\ \%)}{number\ of\ measurements}$$

When plotting the measured value against the predicted value, if the measured value equals the predicted value, then the bias is zero and all values will lie on the line of identity. Thus, the bias is a measure of the average offset from the line of identity, that is, the systematic over- or underprediction. The standard deviation of the bias is a measure of the spread of the prediction error and is called the precision. It does not, however, account for the spread that is due to both over- and underprediction. To calculate the actual size of the prediction error, the MAPE must be calculated.

The kinetic values that are responsible for the major proportion of any error are the volume of the central compartment and the elimination rate constant. A difference between the programmed volume of distribution and an individual's volume of distribution will result in a constant offset of measured to predicted values irrespective of the duration of drug administration. If, however, the elimination rate constant used in the program is different from the patient's, the error between measured and predicted values will increase with time. Thus, even though the bias ± standard deviation and mean absolute prediction error give an indication of overall performance, a time-related measure is still required to fully describe the performance of CACI.

It is desirable that CACI be as accurate as possible, and therefore, the "best" set of kinetic parameters should be utilized. The best kinetics must be the best average of the population being evaluated, and therefore the 95 percent confidence bounds of the bias must include zero.[33] It is far more difficult to give a value for the precision or MAPE. Obviously, the smaller the better, but these depend on the actual kinetic variability of the population for the individual drug. Investigators have tried to establish for various drugs the best MAPE that could be expected when utilizing CACI. This was calculated by retrospectively establishing the best pharmacokinetic values for the group studied and then recalculating the MAPE.[34] For fentanyl (with a bias of 1 percent), the MAPE with the best kinetic fit was 32 percent. Thus, for fentanyl in the general population, the optimal accuracy that can be expected is that the average measured plasma concentration is within ±32 percent of that predicted. Clinical studies with CACI fentanyl (using the pharmacokinetic parameters published by McClain and Hug[35]) produced a nonsignificant bias of −13 percent and a MAPE of 29 percent.[36] For propofol, with the best fit pharmacokinetics, the optimal performance of CACI is likely to have a precision of 36 percent.[37] CACI propofol administration[38] (using pharmacokinetic parameters derived from Gepts and Camu[39]) resulted in a nonsignificant bias and a MAPE of 32 percent. Alfentanil has been the most widely used drug administered via CACI. The estimated best performance for CACI alfentanil has not been calculated, but studies have reported a MAPE of 32 percent[33] (young females) and 23 percent[40] (elderly patients). Using an iterative approach, the best infusion rates required to obtain a single desired plasma level of either methohexital or thiopental resulted in a minimal bias and a prediction error of approximately 20 percent for both drugs.[28] It would therefore seem that when using a single set of pharmacokinetics to describe all patients, the best performance will have a precision and MAPE of 20 to 40 percent. Schüttler et al. have stated that adequate clinical performance is obtained if the bias is less than 10 to 20 percent, the MAPE is 20 to 30 percent with a maximal prediction error in any single sample of less than 50 to 60 percent.[41]

There are two methods by which the accuracy of CACI may be improved. The first (and at present the most practical) is the establishment of population pharmacokinetics. This provides pharmacokinetic values that are varied according to specified patient characteristics (e.g., age, weight, sex, pathologic disease) that are known to alter individual pharmacokinetics. A set of population pharmacokinetics has been established for alfentanil.[42] A retrospective study has confirmed that population kinetics will improve the prediction error.[43] In a prospective study employing population kinetics with CACI, the prediction error in this group of patients was 12 percent, considerably smaller than the 32 percent previously reported without population kinetics.[44] There was, however, a large bias, which, with the small prediction error, implies the central compartment volume poorly described those of the patients evaluated. There is obviously a vast amount of work still to be done to establish the value of population pharmacokinetics in improving the accuracy of CACI.

A second alternative to improve the accuracy of CACI

is to provide a closed-loop pharmacokinetic model, that is, a means by which the pharmacokinetics of each individual are measured and updated during administration of the drug. The theory of adaptive feedback control is well established. There are, however, two problems with implementing an adaptive feedback pharmacokinetic controller. First, there is no intravenous anesthetic drug that can as yet be measured on-line. The second problem is the calculation of both the central compartment volume and rate constants with data points that may be obtained during an infusion for surgical anesthesia. Samples taken early during the infusion will best describe redistribution and the central compartment volume. However, for the best estimation of elimination, samples should be taken once redistribution is near completed, that is, once steady state is obtained. This may well be too late for practical application during anesthetic procedures of only a few hours. The first problem, on-line drug concentration measurement, is an area in which technologic developments are already providing methods for a limited number of nonanesthetic drugs. The second problem has both theoretical and mathematical questions that have not yet been fully answered. A retrospective study attempted to establish whether Bayesian forecasting of individual pharmacokinetics from a single sample or from multiple samples will improve the prediction error with alfentanil administration.[45] A single sample at 60 minutes did improve overall prediction. There were, however, individuals in whom Bayesian forecasting did not improve, or actually worsened, the prediction error. In volunteers in whom individual pharmacokinetics for alfentanil had been established, subsequent administration of alfentanil with CACI provided a minimal bias and a MAPE of 20 percent.[46] These are not markedly better than the bias and MAPE obtained in studies in which published values were used for the general patient population. It is expected that as both technology and the understanding of forecasting improve, closed-loop pharmacokinetic adaptive control is likely to become a clinical tool. This is because closed-loop pharmacokinetic adaptive control is for the intravenous anesthetic agents what end-tidal monitoring is for the inhaled anesthetics.

The above reviews the accuracy of CACI. However, its performance during clinical use is of greatest importance to the practicing clinician. A degree of accuracy is essential for good clinical performance, but because of the wide difference in pharmacodynamics, absolute accuracy is not essential. As stated initially, the object of anesthesia is to rapidly obtain the anesthetic state and maintain it (with minimal effect on other physiologic parameters) and then return the patient to an awake state as soon as possible after the completion of surgery. The ability to provide this depends both on the drug utilized for anesthesia and on the administration system. The evaluation of outcome with CACI requires both a comparison between CACI and manual methods of administration with the same drug, and between CACI administration of intravenous agents and of the inhaled anesthetics. There have so far been very few comparative outcome studies with CACI.

CACI alfentanil has been compared with bolus administration.[4] CACI produced fewer incidences of muscular rigidity, hypotension, and bradycardia on induction. CACI during maintenance had also significantly fewer incidences of hemodynamic response, resulting in a greater percentage of anesthesia time within ±15 percent of the desired blood pressure and heart rate. Recovery was also associated with significantly less use of naloxone for adequate ventilation. A small study comparing manual alfentanil administration with CACI alfentanil showed no statistical differences during maintenance or recovery.[47] CACI fentanyl administration during cardiac surgery resulted in greater hemodynamic control with fewer additional drug interventions and significantly fewer episodes of either hypotension or hypertension compared with bolus dose administration.[25] CACI fentanyl administration for noncardiac surgery provides good hemodynamic stability with rapid recovery and a low incidence of naloxone requirement (12 percent) to establish adequate spontaneous ventilation.[36]

Propofol and alfentanil plus propofol have also been evaluated with CACI.[38,41,48] When the combination of alfentanil and propofol was used for a total intravenous anesthetic employing CACI, hemodynamics were unaltered during induction and intubation as well as during maintenance. Recovery was also rapid. CACI propofol compares favorably to thiopental-isoflurane anesthesia for general surgery lasting several hours.[39] Induction, maintenance, and recovery are similar between the two groups. This implies that given the appropriate means for administration, intravenous anesthesia can be equal in providing the objectives of anesthesia, that is, rapid induction and recovery with stable maintenance, when compared with inhaled anesthetics.

CACI is, in fact, for intravenous drugs what the calibrated vaporizer is to inhaled anesthetic agents, and more. Like the vaporizer, CACI facilitates drug delivery based on plasma concentration rather than on drug dosage. Just as there is variability in the uptake of volatile anesthetic drugs, there will be predicted to actual differences in the plasma concentrations obtained by using CACI. An inspired halothane concentration of 1 percent will result in an end-tidal concentration that is some fraction of 1 percent, but the physics involved ensure that the end-tidal concentration will never be higher than 1 percent. Using CACI to maintain a plasma fentanyl concentration of 3 ng/ml should result in reasonably stable plasma concentrations that hover around 3 ng/ml, but if the pharmacokinetic model being used does not adequately describe the disposition of fentanyl in the particular patient, variations in the plasma concentration may result; this is a disadvantage of CACI. To rapidly achieve the desired concentration, the CACI algorithm inherently and continuously calculates the required infusion rates. This is an advantage over both manual infusion techniques and over the analogous situation with the delivery of inhaled anesthetics by the calibrated vaporizer, in that it is not necessary to calculate a loading scheme or to use overpressurization, respectively. Finally, the time-varying stresses of surgery and variability in patient response require that the anesthesiologist titrate the administration of the potent inhaled anesthetics, using the calibrated vaporizer as a tool. These same factors, coupled with pharmacokinetic variability, likewise require that the anesthesiologist vigilantly titrate the infusion of intravenous anesthetic drugs when using CACI as a tool.

SUMMARY

In comparison with intermittent bolus administration, continuous infusion of intravenous anesthetic drugs provides greater control of anesthetic depth, thus insuring better hemodynamic control with fewer incidences of hemodynamic instability, lower total drug doses, and more rapid return to an awake state. These, with the introduction of several new intravenous anesthetic agents, have provided compelling impetus for the use of intravenous anesthesia by continuous infusion in clinical practice. The devices for the administration of intravenous anesthesia are also undergoing a rapid evolution. The introduction of pumps designed specifically for continuous intravenous anesthetic drug delivery is likely to further promote intravenous anesthesia. "Calculator" pumps enhance manual means of continuous intravenous drug administration. These pumps, although a major step forward for intravenous drug delivery, fall short of enabling the clinician to titrate drug concentration to drug effect as conveniently as is possible with the potent inhalational anesthetic drugs. Computerized pharmacokinetic model-driven drug infusions, however, provide this ability. There are several theoretical advantages of CACI over manual infusion systems, such as further improvements in hemodynamic control and a more predictable rapid awakening. The actual advantages of CACI administration of intravenous anesthetics over manual methods, or in comparison with inhalational anesthesia, are not yet well established. It also appears that present pharmacokinetic models used with CACI, though not yet optimal, are adequate for clinical use. The initial data indicate that CACI provides advantages as a system for intravenous drug delivery, but well-controlled studies with large patient populations are needed to establish its ultimate role in the clinical practice of anesthesia. Its mere convenience, however, should allow the clinician to choose the appropriate anesthetic drug for the patient based on the drug's characteristics rather than based on the convenience of the administration device.

REFERENCES

1. Corssen G, Reves JG, Stanley TH: Intravenous Anesthesia and Analgesia. Lea & Febiger, Philadelphia, 1988
2. Schwilden H: A general method for calculating the dosage scheme in linear pharmacokinetics. Eur J Clin Pharmacol 20:379, 1981
3. White PF: Use of continuous infusion versus intermittent bolus administration of fentanyl or ketamine during outpatient anesthesia. Anesthesiology 59:294, 1983
4. Ausems ME, Vuyk J, Hug CC, Jr., Stanski DR: Comparison of a computer-assisted infusion versus intermittent bolus administration of alfentanil as a supplement to nitrous oxide for lower abdominal surgery. Anesthesiology 68:851, 1988
5. Scott JC, Ponganis KV, Stanski DR: Quantitation of narcotic effect: the comparative pharmacodynamics of fentanyl and alfentanil. Anesthesiology 62:234, 1985
6. Kissin I, Brown PT, Bradley EL: Diazepam-morphine interaction in rats: a nine-fold increase in hypnotic potency (abstract). Anesth Analg 67S:114, 1988
7. Tverskoy M, Fleyshman G, Bradley EL: Midazolam-thiopental anesthetic interaction in patients. Anesth Analg 67:342, 1988
8. Prys-Roberts C, Sear JW: Non-barbiturate intravenous anaesthetics and continuous infusion anaesthesia. p. 128. In Prys-Roberts C, Hug CC Jr (eds): Pharmacokinetics of Anaesthesia. Blackwell Scientific Publications, St. Louis, 1984
9. Ausems ME, Hug CC, Jr., Stanski DR, Burm AGL: Plasma concentrations of alfentanil required to supplement nitrous oxide anesthesia for general surgery. Anesthesiology 65:362, 1986
10. Gibaldi M, Perrier P: Pharmacokinetics. 2nd Ed. Marcel Dekker, New York, 1982
11. Iliadis A, Bruno R, Cano JP: Dynamical dosage regimen calculations in linear pharmacokinetics. Comp Biomed Res 21:203, 1988
12. Schwilden H, Stoeckel H, Schuttler J, Lauven PM: Pharmacological models and their use in clinical anaesthesia. Eur J Anaesth 3:175, 1986
13. Wagner JG: A safe method for rapidly achieving plasma concentration plateaus. Clin Pharmacol Ther 16:691, 1974
14. Heykants J, Geerts P, Noorduin H, Vanden Bussche G: The pharmacokinetic basis of alfentanil infusion. Eur J Anaesth 1:17, 1987
15. Moldenhauer CC, Hug CC, Jr: Use of narcotic analgesics as anaesthetics. Clin Anaesth 2:107, 1984
16. Sebel PS, Bovill JG: Opioid analgesics in cardiac anesthesia. p. 67. In Kaplan JA (ed): Cardiac Anesthesia. 2nd Ed. Grune & Stratton, Orlando, FL, 1987
17. White PF, Dworsky WA, Horai Y, Trevor AJ: Comparison of continuous infusion fentanyl or ketamine versus thiopental —determining the mean effective serum concentrations for outpatient surgery. Anesthesiology 59:564, 1983
18. Glass PS, Leiman BC, Reves JG: Etomidate: What is its present role in anesthesia? Semin Anesth VII:143, 1988
19. White PF, Way WL, Trevor AJ: Ketamine: Its pharmacology and therapeutic uses. Anesthesiology 56:119, 1982
20. White P: Propofol: Pharmacokinetics and pharmacodynamics. Semin Anesth, VII: suppl. 1, 4–20, 1988
21. Reves JG, Glass P, Jacobs JR: Alfentanil and midazolam: New anesthetic drugs for continuous infusion and an automated method of administration. Mt Sinai Med J (in press)
22. Kruger-Thiemer E: Continuous intravenous infusion and

multicompartment accumulation. Eur J Pharmacol 4:317, 1968

23. Schwilden H, Schuttler J, Stoekel H: Pharmacokinetics as applied to total intravenous anesthesia: Theoretical considerations. Anaesthesia, suppl., 38:51–52, 1983

24. Schuttler J, Schwilden H, Stoekel H: Pharmacokinetics as applied to total intravenous anaesthesia: Practical implications. Anaesthesia, suppl., 38:53–56, 1983

25. Alvis JM, Reves JG, Govier AV, et al: Computer-assisted continuous infusions of fentanyl during cardiac anesthesia: Comparison with a manual method. Anesthesiology 63:41, 1985

26. Maitre P, Vozeh S: Computer-assisted infusions of drugs. Anesthesiology 65:344, 1986

27. Tavernier A, Coussaert E, D'Hollander A, Cantraine F: Model-based pharmacokinetic regulation in computer-assisted anesthesia: an interactive system, CARIN: Acta Anaesthesiol Belg 38:63, 1987

28. Crankshaw DP, Boyd MD, Bjorksten AR: Plasma drug efflux —a new approach to optimization of drug infusion for constant blood concentration of thiopental and methohexital. Anesthesiology 67:32, 1987

29. Shafer SL, Siegel LC, Cooke JE, Scott JC. Testing computer-controlled infusion pumps by simulation. Anesthesiology 68:261, 1988

30. Martin RW, Hill HF, Yee HC, et al: An open-loop computer-based drug infusion system. IEEE Trans Biomed Eng 34:642, 1987

31. Jacobs JR: Algorithm for optimal linear model-based control with application to pharmacokinetic model-driven drug delivery. IEEE Trans Biomed Eng (in press)

32. Sheiner LB, Beal SL: Some suggestions for measuring predictive performance. J Pharmacokinet Biopharm 9:503, 1981

33. Ausems ME, Stanski DR, Hug CC: An evaluation of the accuracy of pharmacokinetic data for the computer assisted infusion of alfentanil. Br J Anaesth 57:1217, 1985

34. Shafer SL, Varvel JR, Aziz N, Scott JC: The performance of pharmacokinetic parameters derived from a computer controlled infusion pump (abstract). Anesthesiology 69A:460, 1988

35. McClain DA, Hug CC, Jr: Intravenous fentanyl kinetics. Clin Pharmacol Ther 28:106, 1980

36. Glass P, Jacobs JR, Hawkins ED, et al: Accuracy and efficacy of a pharmacokinetic model-driven device to infuse fentanyl for anesthesia during general surgery (abstract). Anesthesiology 69A:290, 1988

37. Shafer A, Doze VA, Shafer SL, White PF: Pharmacokinetics and pharmacodynamics of propofol infusions during general anesthesia. Anesthesiology 69:348, 1988

38. Glass P, Ginsberg B, Hawkins ED, et al: Comparison of sodium thiopental/isoflurane to propofol (delivered by means of a pharmacokinetic model-driven device) for the induction, maintenance, and recovery from anesthesia (abstract). Anesthesiology 69A:575, 1988

39. Cockshott ID: Propofol ('Diprivan') pharmacokinetics and metabolism—an overview. Postgrad Med J 61: suppl. 3, 45–50, 1985

40. Lemmens HJM, Bovill JG, Burm AGL, Hennis H: Alfentanil infusion in the elderly. Anaesthesia 43:850, 1988

41. Schüttler J, Kloos S, Schwilden H, Stoeckel H: Total intravenous anaesthesia with propofol and alfentanil by computer-assisted infusion. Anaesthesia suppl., 43:2–7, 1988

42. Maitre PO, Vozeh S, Heykants J: Population pharmacokinetics of alfentanil: the average dose-plasma concentration relationship and interindividual variability in patients. Anesthesiology 66:3, 1987

43. Maitre PO, Ausems ME, Vozeh S, Stanski DR: Evaluating the accuracy of using population pharmacokinetic data to predict plasma concentrations of alfentanil. Anesthesiology 68:59, 1988

44. Raemer DB, Buschman A, Johnson MD, et al: Alfentanil pharmacokinetic model applied to ambulatory surgical patients: Does a computerized infusion improve predictability (abstract)? Anesthesiology 69A:243, 1988

45. Maitre PE, Stanski DR: Bayesian forecasting improves the prediction of intraoperative plasma concentrations of alfentanil. Anesthesiology 69:652, 1988

46. Hill HF: Pharmacokinetic tailoring of computer-controlled alfentanil infusions. p. 158. In Kroboth PD, Smith RB, Juhl RP (eds): Pharmacokinetics and Pharmacodynamics. Vol. 2. Current Problems, Potential Solutions. Harvey Whitney Books, Cincinnati, 1988

47. Glass P, Jacobs J, Alvis M, et al: Computer assisted continuous infusion of alfentanil during noncardiac anesthesia: a comparison with a manual method (abstract). Anesthesiology 65A:546, 1986

48. Tackley RM, Lewis GTR, Prys-Roberts C, et al: Computer controlled infusion of propofol. Br J Anaesth 62:46, 1989

12

PHARMACOLOGY OF MUSCLE RELAXANTS AND THEIR ANTAGONISTS

Ronald D. Miller
John J. Savarese

INTRODUCTION

In 1942 Griffith and Johnson[1] suggested that *d*-tubocurarine (dTC) was a safe drug to use during surgery to help provide good skeletal muscle relaxation. One year later, Cullen[2] reported that dTC had been given to 131 patients to produce additional skeletal muscle relaxation. In 1954 Beecher and Todd[3] published their famous report in which, by means of a multi-institutional survey, a sixfold increase in mortality rate was found for patients who received muscle relaxants versus those who did not receive muscle relaxants. This study had many faults in experimental design and thus did not deserve the publicity it received. During the subsequent years, the use of muscle relaxants has become a vitally important aspect of modern anesthesia practice.

Two philosophies govern the use of muscle relaxants. One end of the scale has been popularized by Gray and co-workers in Liverpool, England. In this approach nitrous oxide, oxygen, and large doses of muscle relaxants constitute the sole anesthetic. With this type of anesthesia, patients will usually be amnesic. However, patients occasionally recall part or all of the conversations during surgery.[4] Awareness during surgery was vividly described in an editorial.[5] A trained medical person under general anesthesia described being completely awake during a cesarean section. She specifically stated that when she moved she was given more muscle relaxant (pancuronium) rather than more anesthesia. This inappropriate practice of giving muscle relaxants, instead of analgesics or hypnotics, when a patient moves in response to pain is unfortunately a prevalent practice. Often this practice is advocated in a patient who has an unstable circulatory status. In our opinion, muscle relaxants are often inappropriately given in this situation because concentrations or doses of analgesic or hypnotic drugs are poorly adjusted to the patient's physical state. As stated by Cullen and Larson,[6] "It is, of course, true that muscle relaxants given inappropriately in these circumstances provide the surgeon with optimal conditions in a patient who does not move; unfortunately, ample evidence indicates that such misuse of muscle relaxants often means that a patient is paralyzed but not anesthetized—a state that may be satisfactory for the anesthetist and the surgeon but wholly unsatisfactory for the patient."

A further quote from Cullen and Larson[6] emulates our own philosophy concerning muscle relaxant administration: "Relaxants used to cover-up deficiencies in total anesthetic management as in the prevention or treatment of laryngospasm, movement in response to pain and hypotension due to relative overdose of analgesic or hypnotic drugs (for a particular patient) represent an inefficient and inappropriate use of these valuable adjuncts to anesthesia." Muscle relaxants should be viewed as adjuncts—not as substitutes for anesthesia. By giving them only in an anesthetized patient (e.g., no movement, hypertension, tachycardia, tearing, grimacing) and monitoring neuromuscular function, large doses of muscle relaxants can be avoided; this should decrease the incidence or prolonged paralysis and/or inadequate reversal.

This chapter discusses the clinical pharmacology and clinical use of muscle relaxants, incorporating the overall philosophy that these drugs are adjuvants, not substitutes, for anesthesia. Last, diseases of the neuromuscular system, with which the anesthesiologists are confronted, are discussed.

MONITORING NEUROMUSCULAR FUNCTION

Details of monitoring clinical neuromuscular function are described in Chapter 36. This section serves to present some general concepts before discussing the pharmacology of the specific muscle relaxants.

Peripheral Nerve Stimulation

Stimulating a peripheral nerve (usually the ulnar at the wrist or elbow) and visually observing contraction of the fingers (adductor pollicis and flexor digitorum muscles) is the most commonly advocated method of monitoring neuromuscular function clinically. This stimulation need not be restricted to the arm. Stimulating the facial or the motor nerves of a lower extremity, such as the peroneal nerve, and observing the magnitude of resultant muscular contraction can also be used for monitoring neuromuscular function.

This type of monitoring can be used to detect both magnitude and type of neuromuscular blockade. Quantitative conclusions must be guarded, however. Because of the wide margin of safety of neuromuscular function, a reduction in the contractile response to peripheral nerve stimulation is not quantitatively proportional to the action of relaxants at the receptor. For example, Waud and Waud[7] demonstrated that the twitch response of the tibialis anterior muscle of the cat in response to a single supramaximal stimulus, is not reduced unless more than 70 percent of the receptors are occupied by a nondepolarizing relaxant (Fig. 12-1). Twitch is completely eliminated when 90 percent of the receptors are occupied. Despite this limitation, the response to peripheral nerve stimulation can be extremely useful clinically. There are four especially important questions that can be partially answered by observing the response to peripheral nerve stimulation. They are as follows:

1. Is the neuromuscular blockade adequate?
2. Is the neuromuscular blockade excessive?
3. Can the neuromuscular blockade be antagonized?
4. Is the neuromuscular blockade antagonized?

Although there are many different types of peripheral nerve stimulation, as outlined in Chapter 36, the above questions can be answered with most forms of stimulation and will be discussed throughout this chapter.

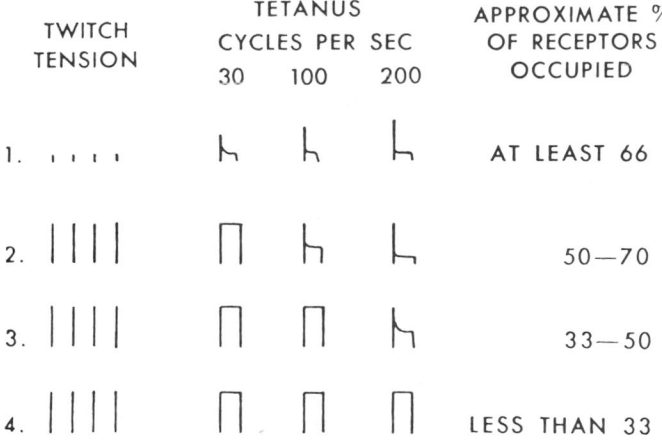

Fig. 12-1. Correlations among twitch tension, response to tetanic stimuli of varying rates of stimulation, and the fraction of receptors occupied. (Data from Waud and Waud.[7])

Whatever form of nerve stimulation is used, subtle degrees of neuromuscular blockade cannot always be detected by observing the response of a peripheral muscle. The neuromuscular junction must be stressed by a stimulus that is greater and longer in intensity than that used to elicit a single twitch. A sustained muscular contraction in response to a tetanic stimulus for 5 seconds is such a stimulus. Figure 12-1 correlates the fraction of receptors occupied with the ability to sustain contraction to varying degrees of tetanic stimuli. Unfortunately, tetanic stimuli are painful and are therefore of limited value in detecting subtle neuromuscular blockade in the unanesthetized patient, such as one in the recovery room. As reviewed in Chapter 36, there are multiple types of peripheral nerve stimulation. The specific type to use depends on the clinical purpose and which of the above questions is being answered (e.g., adequate relaxation versus adequate antagonism), as will become evident throughout this chapter.

Frequently, clinicians refer to partial reduction in twitch height in a manner that suggests that a muscle fiber can contract in a graded fashion. This simply is not true. Muscle contraction is an all-or-none phenomenon. Each fiber either contracts maximally or does not contract at all. Therefore, when twitch height (adduction of the thumb) is reduced, some fibers are contracting normally while others are still completely blocked. The stronger the response, the fewer fibers exist in a blocked state. Fade of muscular contraction in response to tetanic stimuli suggests that some fibers are more susceptible to being blocked by relaxants and need a greater release of acetylcholine (ACh) to trigger their response.

Receptor Occlusion Techniques

Work on the subject of the fraction of receptors that may be occupied during responses to various tests of neuromuscular function has been performed primarily by Waud and Waud.[7,8] While this approach is based on fundamental agonist-antagonist relationships, its main clinical value is that it allows estimation of the sensitivity of many of the tests we use clinically (Table 12-1). Although the number of receptors occupied by a relaxant cannot be counted, Waud and Waud estimated the fraction of receptors (without really knowing the absolute number of receptors) that must be unblocked by relaxant for tests of neuromuscular function to be normal. The technique estimates the fraction of receptors blocked by a nondepolarizing muscle relaxant by determining a dose-response depolarization curve from various agonist doses (succinylcholine) both in the absence and in the presence of the nondepolarizing blocker or antagonist (dTC, pancuronium). The fraction of receptors unblocked by the nondepolarizing muscle relaxant or still available for neuromuscular transmission can be estimated from the dose ratio of the agonist and blocker. For example, in the presence of dTC, 100 nmol of succinylcholine might be required to produce the same degree of depolarization produced by 10 nmol without dTC. Since ten times more succinylcholine is required with dTC, 10 percent of the receptors are still free (or 90 perent of the receptors are blocked). All other tests permit a normal response with a significant number of receptors still blocked, even at a tetanic stimulus of 200 Hz (Fig. 12-1). These results suggest that no test is available to determine whether all receptors are free of a relaxant.

TABLE 12-1. Suggested Comparison, Advantages, and Disadvantages of Tests of Neuromuscular Transmission

Test	Estimated Receptors Occupied (Percent)	Disadvantages
Tidal volume	80	Insensitive
Twitch height	75–80	Insensitive, uncomfortable, need to know twitch before relaxant administration
Sustained tetanus at 30 Hz	75–80	Insensitive, uncomfortable
Vital capacity	70–75	Insensitive, need patient cooperation
Train-of-four	70 75	Not very sensitive
Sustained tetanus at 100 Hz	50	Very painful
Inspiratory force	50	Sometimes difficult to perform without endotracheal intubation
Head lift and hand grip	33	Need patient cooperation

Respiration

Such factors as the number of receptors occupied, the presence of post-tetanic facilitation, and a sustained contraction in response to a tetanic stimulus are not really of prime importance. The presence of sustained adequate ventilation, particularly during stresses such as airway obstruction or vomiting, is our main concern as anesthesiologists. Despite the enormous number of relaxant studies in the literature, few correlate tests of neuromuscular function with adequacy of ventilation, and the conclusions are often incomplete. Walts et al.[9] concluded that sustained muscular contraction in response to tetanic stimulus (30 Hz) is a good test because it correlates with greater than 90 percent recovery of vital capacity and maximum voluntary ventilation in human volunteers. These workers concluded that the head-raising test is an unreliable index of recovery because it does not return to control when vital capacity and tetanic stimulation are within 90 percent of control. Perhaps the head-raising test is more sensitive. In fact, Johansen et al.[10] found head-lift and hand-grip strength to be 38 and 48 percent of control when both inspiratory and expiratory flow rates are greater than 90 percent of control. Furthermore, Ali et al.[11] found inspiratory force to be only 70 percent of control when vital capacity and expiratory flow rate are greater than 90 percent of control. More recently, Pavlin et al.[12] found that many of the recommended tests can return to normal, and the pharyngeal and neck muscles necessary to protect the airway can still be partially paralyzed (Fig. 12-2). As a result, they recommend that patients should be considered to be partially paralyzed until they can lift their head for 5 seconds or achieve a maximum inspiratory pressure of -35 cmH$_2$O (personal communication). From a practical point of view, patients can often sustain adequate respiration and not meet the above criteria. This means that recovery room personnel need to observe the patient closely until the above criteria are met. Obviously, the most sensitive test stresses the neuromuscular junction the most. Sensitivity depends on both the intensity and the duration of the stress applied. For example, a tetanic stimulus of 30 Hz for 10 seconds may be more stressful than one of 100 Hz for 1 second. A head-lift or hand-grip test may be insensitive when applied for 1 second or may be very sensitive when applied for 15 seconds. It obviously becomes extremely important to define tests very carefully when making comparisons.[13] In view of the scant information available, we can only recommend that there are probably several sensitive tests available that can be used to stress the neuromuscular junction in a way that includes varying both the duration and intensity of stimulation.

Clinical Conclusion

Despite the above consideration, we do not know what proportion of receptors must be available or how sensitive a test must be to ensure adequate muscle strength to overcome airway obstruction and permit effective coughing. We have concluded that the anesthesiologist should not rely on one test but should use as many tests as is practically possible (Table 12-1). For example, when the operative procedure is nearly finished and the patient is still under anesthesia, we may use a tetanic stimulus of 50 Hz or train-of-four, twitch height, tidal volume, and expiratory force to determine whether a neuromuscular blockade has been antagonized completely. Expiratory force can be determined by removing the rebreathing bag and occluding the outlet and observing the pressure on the circuit gauge (R. L. Katz, personal communication). The anesthesiologist should compare this pressure with the expiratory force determined before relaxant administration. The results of Pavlin et al.[12] and the frequent return to the recovery room of patients with partial paralysis[14] (i.e., not recognized by the anesthesiologist) emphasized the difficulty in clinically ensuring that *no* residual neuromuscular blockade exists after surgery and anesthesia.[15] It is of prime importance to use several tests and to stress the neuromuscular junction to detect possible subtle degrees of neuromuscular blockade. Later in this chapter antagonism of neuromuscular blockade is discussed in greater detail.

CHEMISTRY

Molecular Features and Physicochemical Properties

Neuromuscular blocking drugs are quaternary ammonium compounds. Positive charges at these sites in the molecules mimic the quaternary nitrogen atom of the

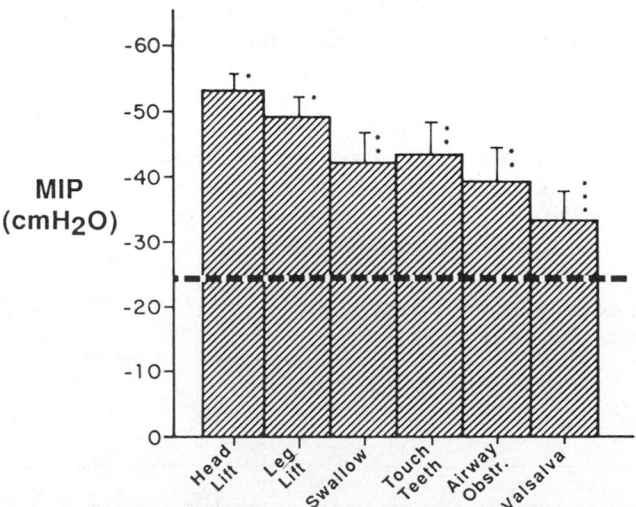

Fig. 12-2. Levels of neuromuscular blockade from dTC (as measured by maximum inspiratory pressure [MIP]) below which the indicated clinical maneuvers would not be accomplished. Obviously head lift and straight-leg raising are the most sensitive indicators of neuromuscular blockade. (From Pavlin et al.,[12] with permission.)

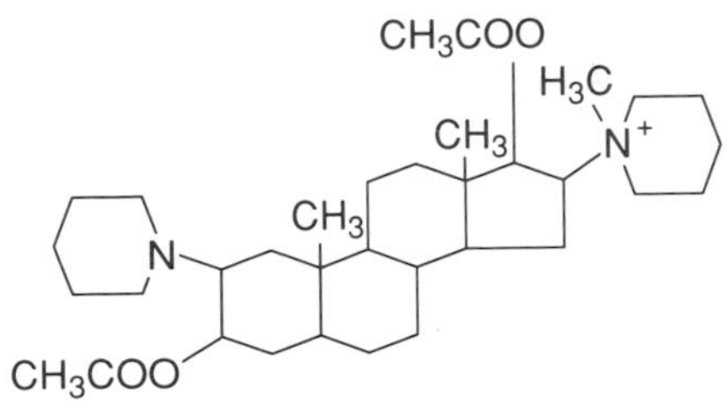

Vecuronium

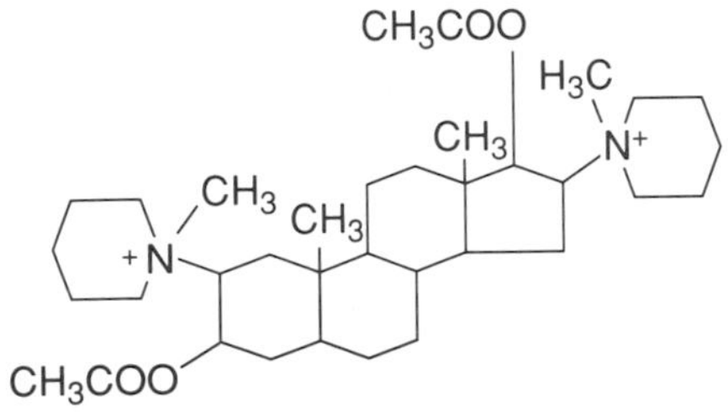

Pancuronium

Fig. 12-3. Formula for pancuronium and vecuronium. (From Miller et al.,[53] with permission.)

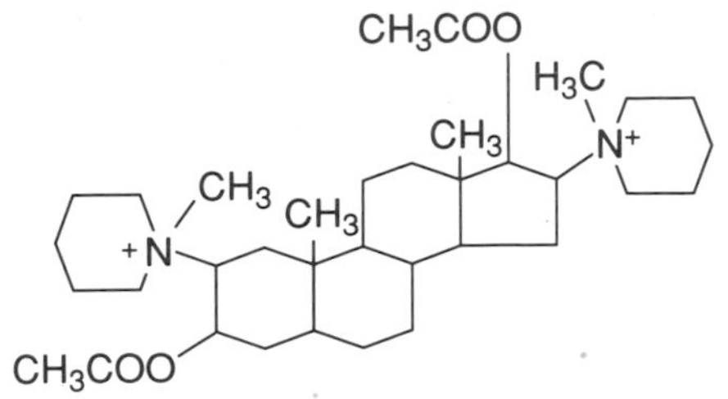

Pancuronium

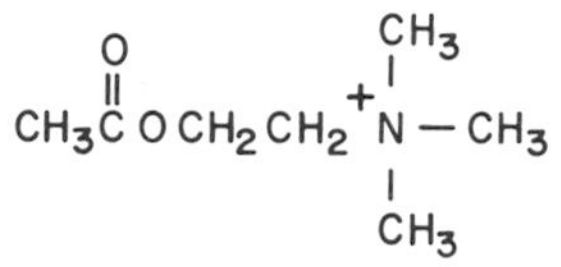

Acetylcholine

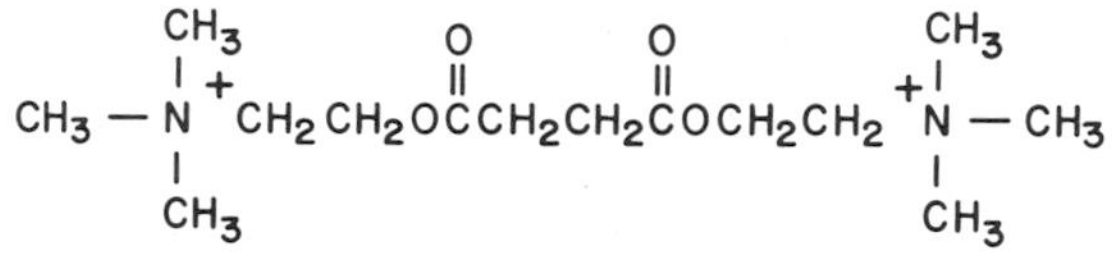

Succinylcholine
(diacetylcholine)

Fig. 12-4. Structural relationship of succinylcholine, a depolarizing agent, and pancuronium, a nondepolarizing agent, to acetylcholine, the neuromuscular transmitter. Succinylcholine, originally called diacetylcholine, is simply two molecules of acetylcholine linked through the acetate methyl groups. Like acetylcholine, succinylcholine stimulates cholinergic receptors at the neuromuscular junction and at nicotinic (ganglionic) and muscarinic autonomic sites. Pancuronium may be viewed as two acetylcholinelike fragments (outlined in dark print) properly oriented on a steroid nucleus. Pancuronium and other nondepolarizers inhibit the actions of acetylcholine at neuromuscular and autonomic cholinergic receptors.

transmitter ACh and are the principal reason for the attraction of these drugs to cholinergic receptors. These receptors are located not only at the neuromuscular junction but at other physiologic sites of action of ACh in the body as well, such as nicotinic receptors in ganglia and muscarinic receptors in the autonomic nervous system.

All relaxants are structurally related to ACh because of the quaternary groups. In some cases, such as pancuronium and vecuronium (Fig. 12-3), ACh-like structures are intentionally incorporated into the molecule. Succinylcholine is actually two molecules of ACh linked back to back through the acetate methyl groups (Fig. 12-4).

Most muscle relaxants contain two positive charges or at least two potential positive charges. These are separated by a bridging structure that is lipophilic and that varies in size. The bridging structure is different for various series of muscle relaxants and is a major determinant of potency (see the section, *Structure–Activity Relationships*).

Muscle relaxants are generally not actively metabolized by the liver, although some of the steroidal muscle relaxants are an exception. There are two reasons for this: (1) the water solubility of relaxants inhibits uptake into hepatocytes; and (2) the cytochrome P-450 oxidative enzyme system in liver microsomes requires lipophilic substrates, generally excluding the relatively hydrophilic muscle relaxants.

All muscle relaxants are highly water soluble. Their hydrophilic nature is mostly due to positive charges, which give muscle relaxants the physicochemical properties of cations in watery media such as the plasma and urine. Other chemical features of relaxants that promote either water solubility or hydrophilic properties or both are various oxygen-bearing groups. Some of these are the ester linkages of succinylcholine (Fig. 12-4) and atracurium (Fig. 12-5), the acetate groups of pancuronium and vecuronium (Fig. 12-3), the ether linkages of metocurine and dTC (Fig. 12-6), the hydroxyl groups of dTC (Fig. 12-6) and alcuronium, and the methoxy groups of dTC, metocurine, and atracurium (Figs. 12-5 and 12-6). The chemical structures of the new muscle relaxants doxacurium, pipecuronium, mivacurium, and ORG 9426 have many of the same characteristics described above and are illustrated in Figure 12-7.

Because of their water solubility, most muscle relax-

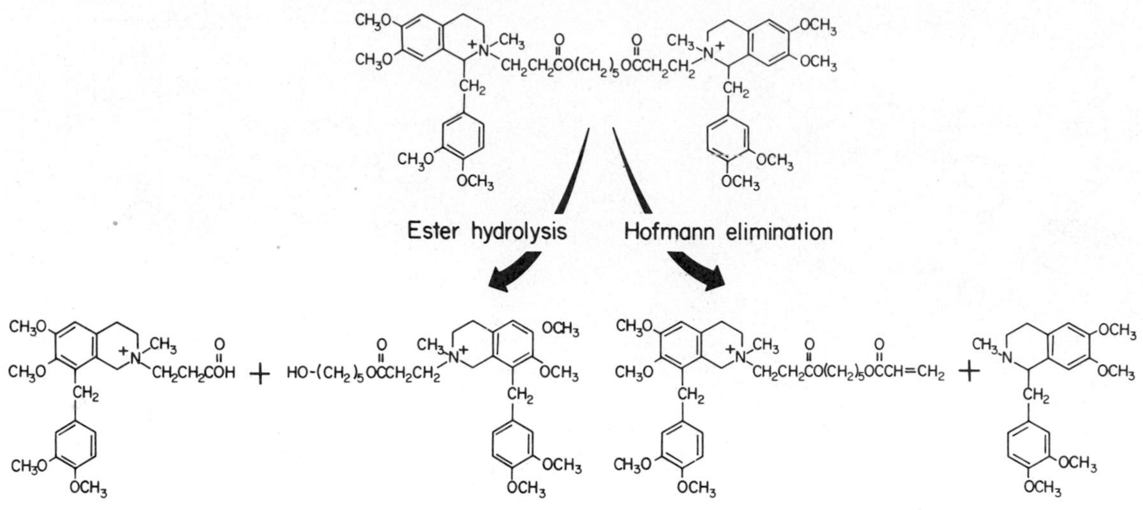

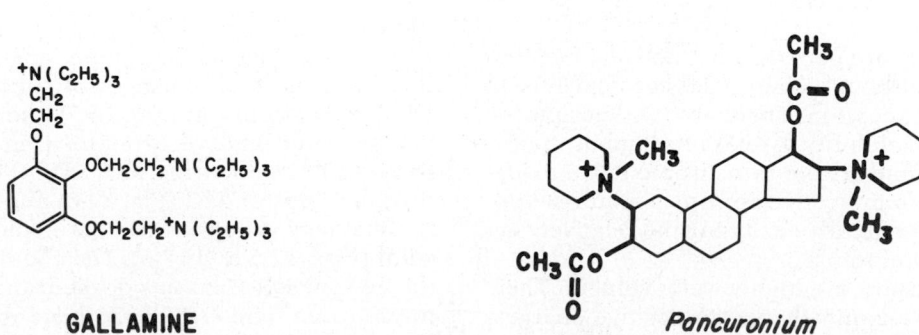

Ester hydrolysis   Hofmann elimination

Quaternary Acid   Quaternary Alcohol   Monoacrylate   Laudanosine

Fig. 12-5. Atracurium and its metabolism. (From Miller et al.,[53] with permission.)

ants, especially the long-acting muscle relaxants, are easily excreted by glomerular filtration in the urine and are generally not reabsorbed in the renal tubules. Similarly, the high water solubility generally prevents passage across lipoid membranous barriers, such as the blood-brain and placental barriers, and the lipid membranes of most cells, such as renal tubular cells, hepatocytes, and nerve and muscle cells.

Sources and Synthesis

Several relaxants are still purified from naturally occurring sources. For example, although dTC can be synthesized, it is still the least expensive to obtain from the amazonian vine *Chondodendron tomentosum*. Similarly, the intermediates for the production of metocurine and alcuronium, which are semisynthetic, are ob-

d−TUBOCURARINE

DIMETHYLTUBOCURARINE

GALLAMINE

Pancuronium

Fig. 12-6. Chemical formulas of nondepolarizing neuromuscular blocking agents available in the United States for 10 years or more.

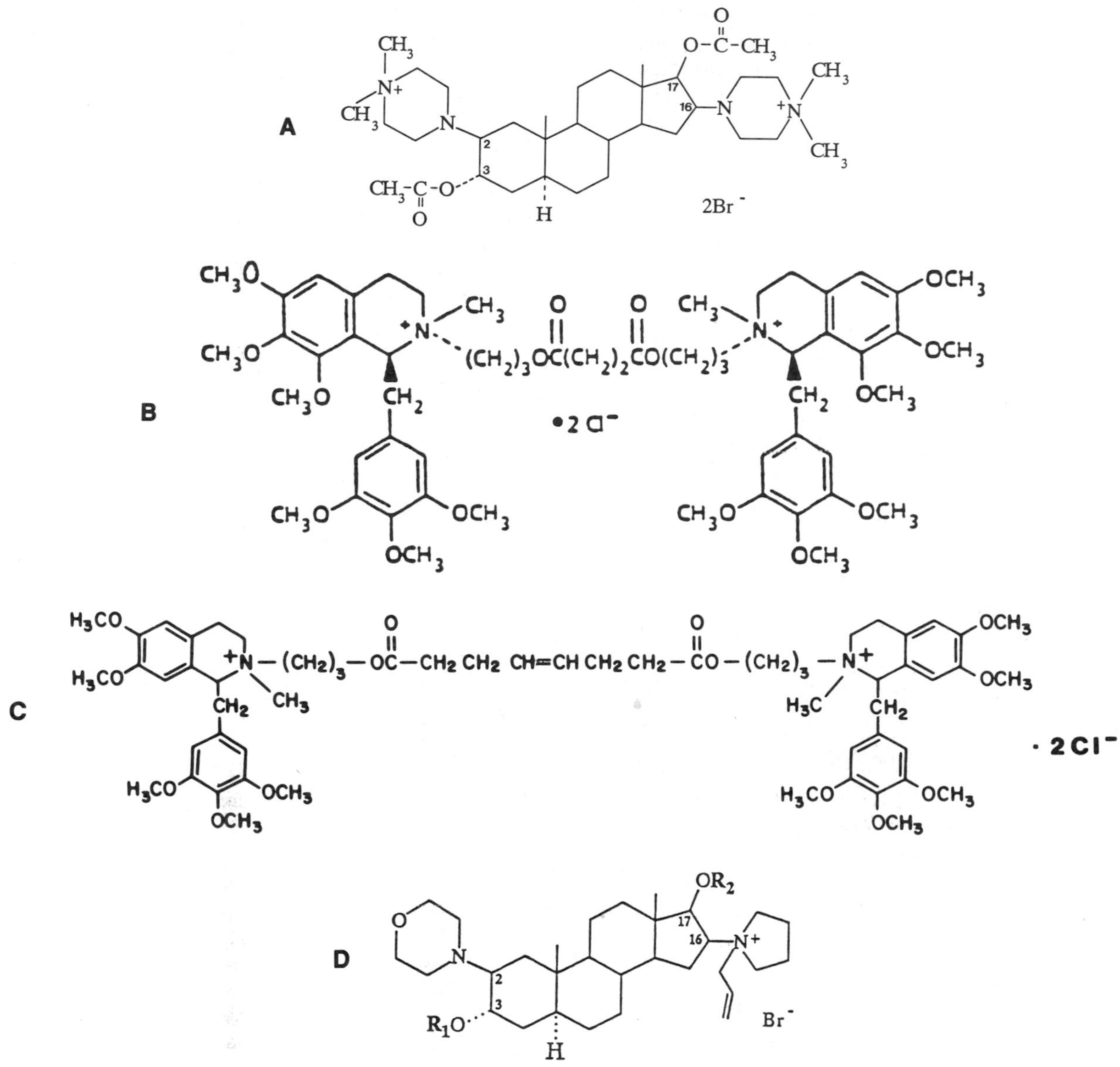

Fig. 12-7. Chemical structures of new muscle relaxants. **(A)** Pipecuronium; **(B)** doxacurium; **(C)** mivacurium; or **(D)** ORG 9436.

tained from *Chondodendron* and *Strychnos toxifera*. In fact, although pancuronium and vecuronium are entirely synthesized, their ancestor, Malouetine, the first steroidal neuromuscular blocking drug, was originally isolated from *Malouetia bequaertiana*, which grows in the jungles of the Congo.

Atracurium, succinylcholine, and gallamine are entirely synthetic. In any case, the final step in the synthesis of muscle relaxants is quaternization, which converts relatively inactive lipophilic tertiary amines into active neuromuscular blocking drugs. In one case, atracurium, this difference has been taken advantage of as a source of potential drug degradation and inactivation (see the section, *Metabolism*).

STRUCTURE–ACTIVITY
RELATIONSHIPS

There are many classic structure–activity relationships among neuromuscular blocking drugs. Bovet[16] originally noted structural differences between depolarizing muscle relaxants (leptocurares) or long, thin, flexible molecules and nondepolarizing muscle relaxants (pachycurares) or heavy, bulky, rigid molecules. As a result, an optimum interonium distance (between two quaternary nitrogen atoms) of 12 to 14 angstrom (Å) units (1.2 to 1.4 nm) was thought to be required for optimum neuromuscular blocking activity. Since 1964, however, this concept has gradually lost importance. Thus, although succinylcholine and decamethonium in their "extended" conformations may show interonium distances of 12 to 14 Å, dTC, the toxiferines (alcuronium), and the steroids (pancuronium and vecuronium) show internitrogen distances of only 10 to 11 Å (1.0 to 1.1 nm). In addition, the second nitrogen of both dTC and vecuronium is a tertiary amine that is protonated at physiologic pH. These drugs are therefore really monoquaternaries, and gallamine is a trisquaternary structure. Thus, neuromuscular blocking potency need not be associated with a bisquaternary structure. Nevertheless, fazadinium and atracurium are bisquaternaries, but their internitrogen distances are about 7.5 and 18 Å, respectively. Thus, many of the old rules obviously no longer apply as to what structures are required to impose neuromuscular blocking properties on a compound. Recent observations include several important points:

1. A fixed interonium distance of 8 Å seems to promote ganglion-blocking activity in steroidal bisquaternaries.[17] It is therefore not surprising that fazadinium shows moderate ganglion-blocking activity.[18] On the other hand, this type of side effect is minimized at 10 and 18 Å (pancuronium, vecuronium, atracurium).

2. Muscarinic blocking properties (vagolytic effect) appear prominent in trisquaternary substances (gallamine).

3. In steroidal-type neuromuscular blocking drugs, muscarinic blockade has always been a prominent side effect (pancuronium) until recently, when this side effect was bound to be entirely due to the A ring (2- to 3-position) ACh-like substitution.[19] This was corrected by Savage and colleagues[19,20] by simply removing the quaternizing methyl group in the 2-position. This eliminates the positive charge, reducing the ACh-like character, and dramatically reduces the antimuscarinic (vagolytic) property (vecuronium).[19,20]

4. Removal of both acetoxy groups from vecuronium results in a muscle relaxant of low potency, but marked affinity for cardiac muscarinic receptors. While such a compound is clinically not useful because of its cardiovascular effects, Bowman et al.[21] noted that low-potency compounds have a rapid onset of action. They concluded that a rapid onset with a nondepolarizing muscle relaxant will likely be obtained with one that has a low potency.

5. Benzylisoquinoline substances (dTC, metocurine, atracurium, and mivacurium) release histamine. In metocurine and atracurium, this tendency is reduced by the methoxy group substitutions and it is further reduced in atracurium by the electron-withdrawing effect of the carboxyl groups in the chain and by altered stereochemistry (*cis* orientation) at the 1- to 2-positions in the benzylisoquinoline structure.[22,23]

PHARMACOLOGY OF NONDEPOLARIZING MUSCLE RELAXANTS

d-Tubocurarine, pancuronium, metocurine (dimethyltubocurarine), gallamine, atracurium, and vecuronium are the nondepolarizing muscle relaxants currently available for use in the United States. In the coming years, doxacurium, pipecuronium, mivacurium, and ORG 9426 will probably become available to clinicians. Alcuronium and fazadinium are not available in the United States, but are used in other countries. The doses under various clinical situations are listed in Table 12-2. Nondepolarizing muscle relaxants can also be classified by duration of action. All nondepolarizing muscle relaxants are considered long acting with four exceptions. Vecuronium and atracurium are considered intermediate acting, mivacurium is short acting, and ORG 9426 is either short or intermediate acting. These drugs are considered together in the subsections listed below.

Pharmacokinetics and Pharmacodynamics

The rate of disappearance of muscle relaxant from blood is characterized by a rapid initial disappearance that is followed by a slower decay (Fig. 12-8). Distribution to tissues is the major cause of the initial decrease, whereas the slower decay is due to excretion. Because relaxants are highly ionized, they do not cross all membranes and have a limited volume of distribution. The volume of distribution of relaxants[24] ranges from 80 to 140 ml/kg, which is not much larger than blood volume. If the volume of distribution is reduced, then the potency of muscle relaxant may be augmented.

The development of analytic techniques to measure muscle relaxant or antagonist concentrations in blood and other body tissues is of prime importance. The plasma concentrations of all muscle relaxants and their antagonists can now be measured by mass spectrometry, gas chromatography, radioimmunoassay, fluorimetry, or high-pressure liquid chromatography.[25-32] Thus, the pharmacokinetics and pharmcodynamics of these drugs can now be studied. Why is this important clinically? Katz[33] and others emphasize the variable response of patients to muscle relaxants. We believe this variability can, in large part, be explained by differences in pharmacokinetics and pharmacodynamics: What diseases and physiologic changes alter the rate at which the relaxant leaves plasma and is eliminated (pharmacokinetics)? What diseases and physiologic changes alter sensitivity of the neuromuscular junction to muscle relaxants (pharmacodynamics)? If the answers to these questions were available, anesthesiologists could be more selective in relaxant dose and avoid much of the "variability" described by Katz[33] and others.

TABLE 12-2. Guide to Nondepolarizing Relaxant Dosage Under Different Anesthetic Techniques[a]
(Dosages in mg/kg)

| | | | After Intubation | | |
Drug	Potency Factor	Intubation	N₂O	Halothane (1 MAC)	Enflurane[b] (1 MAC)
Pancuronium	1	0.06–0.08	0.04–0.06	0.03–0.04	0.02–0.03
Metocurine	4	0.3–0.4	0.2–0.25	0.1–0.2	0.08–0.15
d-Tubocurarine	7	0.5–0.6	0.3–0.4	0.2–0.3	0.12–0.2
Gallamine	40	3.0–4.0	2.0–3.0	1.0–2.0	0.8–1.5
Alcuronium	3	0.3	0.15	0.1	0.08
Fazadinium	20	1.5	1.0	0.08	0.06
Atracurium	4	0.4–0.5	0.2–0.3	0.2	0.15
Vecuronium	0.9	0.07–0.10	0.05	0.04	0.02
Mivacurium	1.6	0.18	0.10	0.08	0.06
Pipecuronium	0.9	0.10	0.06	0.05	0.04
Doxacurium	0.4	0.06	0.04	0.03	0.02
Approximate fraction or "intubating dose"		1.0	0.7	0.5	0.3
Anesthetic potency factor			1.0	0.7	0.5

[a] Suggested dosages provide good intubating conditions under light anesthesia or satisfactory abdominal relaxation after intubation without a relaxant or with succinylcholine. Potency factors indicate the number of milligrams of other relaxants equal to 1 mg of pancuronium. Thus, pancuronium is 4, 7, 40, 3, 20, 4, and 0.9 times more potent than metocurine, *d*-tubocurarine, gallamine, alcuronium, fazadinium, atracurium, and vecuronium, respectively. Fractions indicate amount of relaxant needed under indicated condition relative to dosage required for intubation. If the "potency factors" and the "intubating dose fractions" are known, only the "intubating dose" for pancuronium need be remembered. This is intended as a guide to dosage in general. Individual relaxant requirement should be confirmed with a peripheral nerve stimulator.
[b] Probably with isoflurane also.

Size of Initial Dose

Feldman[34] holds that a strong affinity between muscle relaxant and receptor, rather than blood flow, produces the rate-limiting step in recovery from paralysis. Conse-

quently, he argues that a single large bolus of relaxant given at the start of anesthesia will produce prolonged adequate paralysis with a relatively low serum concentration of relaxant at the end of anesthesia. In contrast, Feldman suggests that frequently repeated small doses

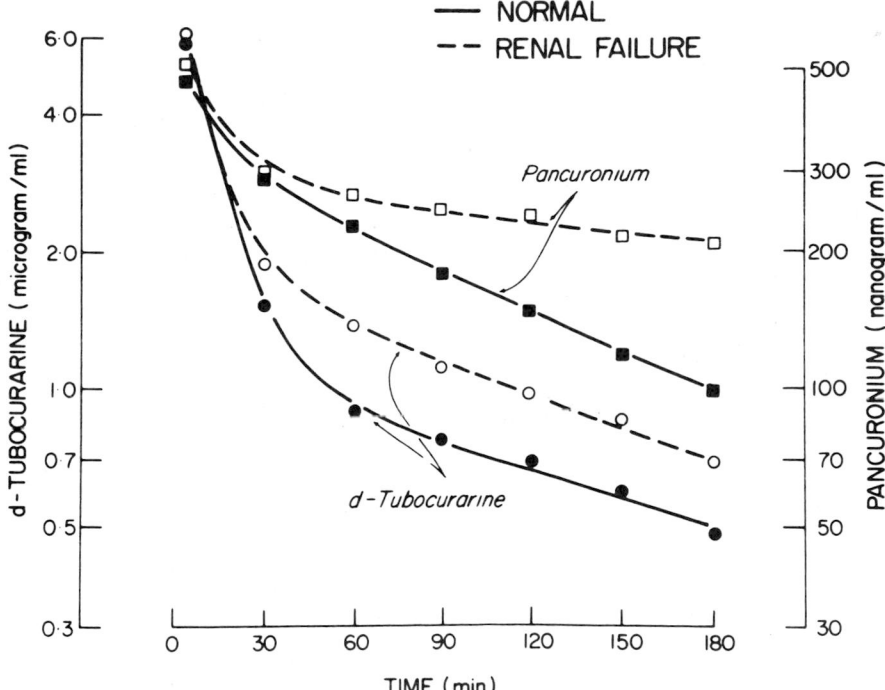

Fig. 12-8. Rates at which the plasma concentrations of *d*-tubocurarine and pancuronium decrease in patients with and without renal failure. Note that the decay rates are about the same in patients with normal renal function. However, the decay rate is much slower in patients with renal failure receiving pancuronium than those receiving *d*-tubocurarine. (Data for pancuronium from McLeod et al.[36] Those for *d*-tubocurarine from Miller et al.[24])

of relaxant that are just sufficient to produce adequate paralysis will result in higher postoperative concentrations of relaxant. He believes that the latter approach is more likely to lead to residual postoperative paralysis, with its attendant potential for respiratory complications.[34]

Certainly, initial administration of large doses of muscle relaxant has its advantages. This technique will provide excellent surgical conditions and will mitigate the necessity of precisely regulating the anesthetic dose. However, the theory that neuromuscular blockade may be easier to antagonize if a large (overdose) dose of muscle relaxant were given initially rather than small repetitive doses was tested. Ham et al.[35] found no difference in the pharmacokinetics and pharmacodynamics of dTC when given by three dosage protocols: 20 mg/m² (about 34 mg/70 kg) as a single large bolus, repeated smaller doses of 5 mg/m² (about 8 mg/70 kg), or a continuous infusion titrated to maintain a constant 90 percent depression of twitch tension. Also, no difference in neostigmine antagonism between the three dosage schedules was found. These findings do not support Feldman's prediction of a lower serum muscle relaxant concentration with a large-dose technique.[34]

Despite the lack of difference between the three dosage schedules in the Ham et al.[35] study, the use of small, frequent doses or of continuous infusion of muscle relaxant while monitoring neuromuscular function with a peripheral nerve stimulator may have advantages over the large-bolus technique. For example, the duration of neuromuscular blockade needed for a surgical procedure is not always predictable in advance; the large-dose technique may result in 100 percent blockade, which cannot always be antagonized with acetylcholinesterase (AChE) agents; with smaller doses of a continuous infusion, the extent of neuromuscular blockade can be varied more readily with changing surgical needs.

Renal Failure

Renal failure can profoundly affect the pharmacokinetics of relaxants. Gallamine, decamethonium, and probably metocurine are entirely dependent on renal excretion for their elimination (Table 12-3). Studies in humans indicate that doxacurium, pipecuronium, pancuronium, fazadinium, and alcuronium are more dependent on renal excretion than is dTC (Fig. 12-8).[24,36-45] Even though the rate at which pancuronium and dTC disappear from plasma is about the same with normal renal function, pancuronium disappears much more slowly during renal failure. However, Somogyi et al.[43] found the elimination half-life of pancuronium not to be prolonged by renal failure as much as that depicted in Figure 12-8. However, all investigators found much greater variability in patients with renal failure compared with those with normal renal function, most likely reflecting the various associated prob-

TABLE 12-3. Dependence (Percentage of Injected Dose) of Various Muscle Relaxants on the Kidney for Their Elimination[a]

Drug	Percentage of Injected Dose
Gallamine	100
Decamethonium	100
Metocurine	80–100
Doxacurium	60–90
Pipecuronium	60–90
Pancuronium	60–80
Alcuronium	70–90
Fazadinium	70–90
d-Tubocurarine	40–60
ORG 9426	10–20
Vecuronium	10–20
Atracurium	<5
Mivacurium	<10
Succinylcholine	0

[a] Determined either by measuring drug concentration in urine or more accurately by comparing plasma clearance values in patients with and without renal failure.

lems (e.g., diabetes, anemia) in patients with renal disease.

As depicted in Table 12-3, vecuronium, atracurium, and possibly mivacurium are probably the preferred muscle relaxants in patients in renal failure. Only about 10 to 20 percent of an injected dose of vecuronium appears in the urine — the remaining vecuronium is probably excreted in the bile both as the parent drug and as its 3-desacetyl metabolite.[46,47] Although vecuronium depends little on the kidney for its elimination, administration of large doses (i.e., greater than 0.1 mg/kg) or repetitive doses can result in a modestly prolonged duration of neuromuscular blockade in patients with renal failure.[48-53] Because of the metabolism of atracurium, it is not dependent on the kidney for its elimination and therefore the duration of blockade is not prolonged, although extremely large bolus doses (e.g., greater than 0.6 mg/kg) have not been tested in renal failure patients.[30,52,53]

Biliary or Liver Disease

A prolonged neuromuscular blockade results from both dTC and pancuronium since they are partly dependent on biliary excretion for their elimination. Somogyi et al.[54] found that neuromuscular blockade and elimination half-life of pancuronium were prolonged in patients with extrahepatic biliary obstruction. Duvaldestin et al.[55] found that in patients with hepatic cirrhosis, the volume of distribution is increased and the elimination half-life of pancuronium is prolonged. Because pancuronium is distributed to a larger volume in patients with cirrhosis, a larger dose of pancuronium may be required to achieve a given neuromuscular blockade. However, once that neuromuscular blockade has been achieved, it should last longer because elimination is delayed. So, even though a larger dose of pancuronium may be required initially, subsequent doses can be smaller than normally expected.

Because vecuronium is predominantly dependent on biliary excretion for its elimination,[47] initial predictions were that its duration of action would be prolonged in patients with liver disease. In fact, initial studies with large doses (0.2 mg/kg) of vecuronium did find a longer duration of action in patients with alcoholic cirrhosis.[56,57] However, when the dose of vecuronium is 0.15 mg/kg or less, the duration of neuromuscular blockade is either unchanged or actually shorter in patients with hepatic cirrhosis (Table 12-4).[57–59] From a pharmacokinetic point of view, Lebrault et al.[56] found a slower clearance with a 0.2-mg/kg dose, whereas Arden et al.[59] found no changes in clearance with a smaller dose (0.1 mg/kg) in patients with hepatic cirrhosis (Table 12-4). Whether this means that the pharmacokinetics of vecuronium are dose-dependent or there were differences in experimental design between the two studies accounting for the differing results with vecuronium in patients with cirrhosis remains to be determined. Theoretically, the neuromuscular blockade of atracurium should not be prolonged in patients with liver disease. In fact, atracurium's duration of action with doses of 0.5 mg/kg or less is either unchanged or shorter in patients with hepatic cirrhosis compared with patients with normal hepatic function.[58,60,61] There is a tendency with both vecuronium and atracurium to have a slower onset of action in patients with hepatic cirrhosis.

Also, patients with cholestatic disease tend to have a decrease in plasma clearance, presumably because the increased plasma concentrations of bile salts reduce the hepatic uptake of both vecuronium and pancuronium.[62]

Anesthesia

Inhaled anesthetics augment the neuromuscular block from nondepolarizing muscle relaxants in a dose-dependent fashion (Fig. 12-9)[63] that surprisingly does not depend on the duration of anesthesia (e.g., halothane).[64] By contrast, the ability of enflurane to enhance dTC is time dependent (as will be discussed later). Of those anesthetics studied, inhaled anesthet-

TABLE 12-4. Pharmacokinetics of Vecuronium in Patients with Normal Hepatic Functions and Those with Cirrhosis

Pharmacokinetic Variable	Normal Function (mean)	Cirrhosis (mean)
Initial distribution volume (L/kg)	0.08	0.11
Clearance (ml/kg/min)	4.50	4.40
Volume of distribution at steady state (L/kg)	0.18	0.22
Terminal elimination half-life (min)	57.70	51.40

(Data from Arden et al.[59])

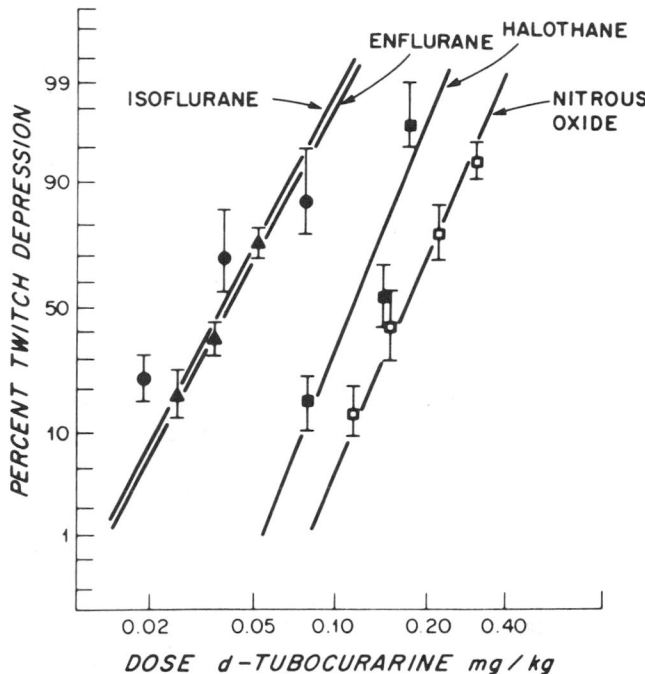

Fig. 12-9. Effect of anesthetics on a *d*-tubocurarine dose-response curve. (From Ali and Savarese,[354] with permission.)

ics augment the relaxants in decreasing order: isoflurane, desflurane, and enflurane > halothane > nitrous oxide-barbiturate-narcotic anesthesia (Figs. 12-9 and 12-10).[65,66] For reasons that have not been identified, atracurium and vecuronium are not as affected by choice of general anesthesia as are dTC and pancuronium.[53] For example, there is only an approximately 20 percent difference in the dose-response curves of these two muscle relaxants with balanced anesthesia (i.e., intravenous drugs plus nitrous oxide) compared with isoflurane anesthesia—in contrast with a 50 percent difference with dTC and pancuronium.[67] On the other hand, isoflurane and enflurane markedly reduced the infusion rate of vecuronium required to sustain a neuromuscular blockade compared with a narcotic-nitrous oxide anesthetic (Fig. 12-11).[68]

Several mechanisms have been proposed by which inhaled anesthetics produce relaxation and augment the neuromuscular blockade from muscle relaxants. The mechanisms that are probably most important are those due to the ability of inhaled anesthetics to (1) increase muscle blood flow, so that a greater fraction of the injected relaxant may reach the neuromuscular junction,[69] probably a factor only with isoflurane; (2) induce relaxation at sites proximal to the neuromuscular junction, obviously the central nervous system (CNS)[70]; (3) not decrease release of ACh from the motor nerve terminal[71]; (4) have no demonstrable effect on the cholinergic receptor[72,73]; (5) decrease the sensitivity of the postjunctional membrane to depolarization[74,75]; and (6) possibly act at a site distal to the cholin-

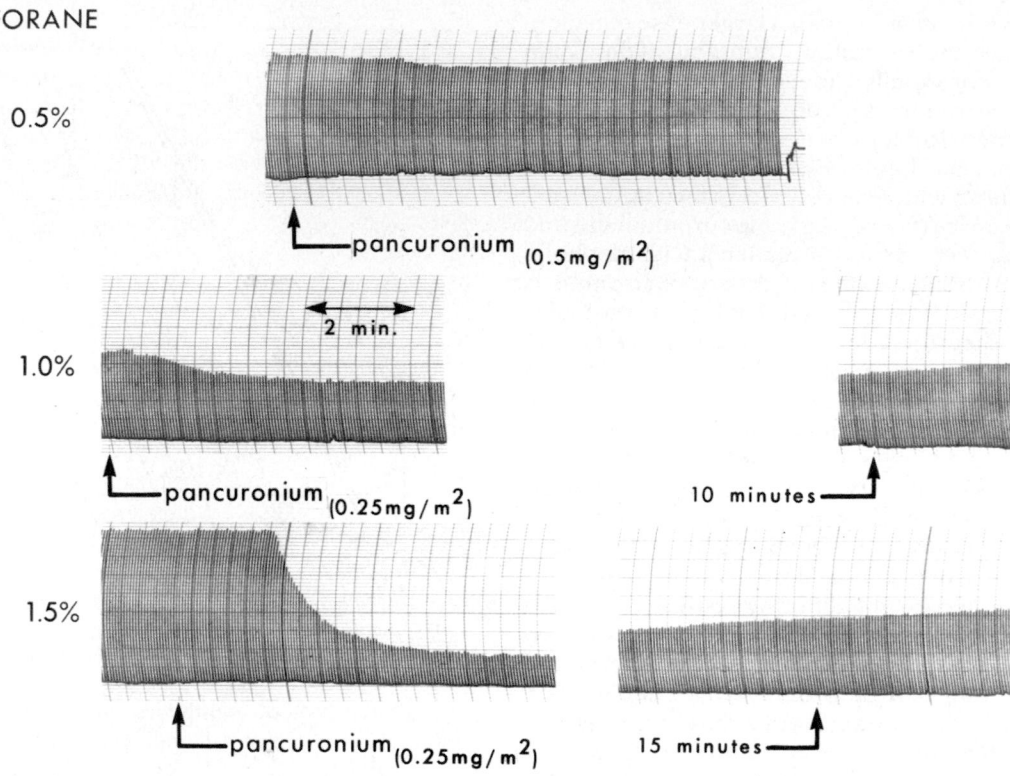

Fig. 12-10. Influence of anesthetic concentration on the magnitude of neuromuscular blockade from pancuronium. (From Miller et al.,[63] with permission.)

ergic receptor and the postjunctional membrane, such as the muscle membrane.[72,73,75]

Conceptually, although most inhaled anesthetics, such as halothane, do not decrease twitch tension, they reduce the margin of safety of neuromuscular transmission. Waud and Waud[71,72] indicate that halothane acts at a site beyond the cholinergic receptor,[71,72] perhaps with either calcium conductance or release from depolarization that may interfere with muscle contrac-

tion.[75] Yet more recent studies clearly indicate that inhaled anesthetics have specific effects on ACh receptor channels. Brett et al.,[76] using a patch clamp technique, found that isoflurane reduced the average open duration of the ACh receptor channels that remain open for activation. They then stated that the endplate current will be both reduced in amplitude (by the muscle relaxant) and have an accelerated decay (by isoflurane). Both factors will reduce the net charge transfer across

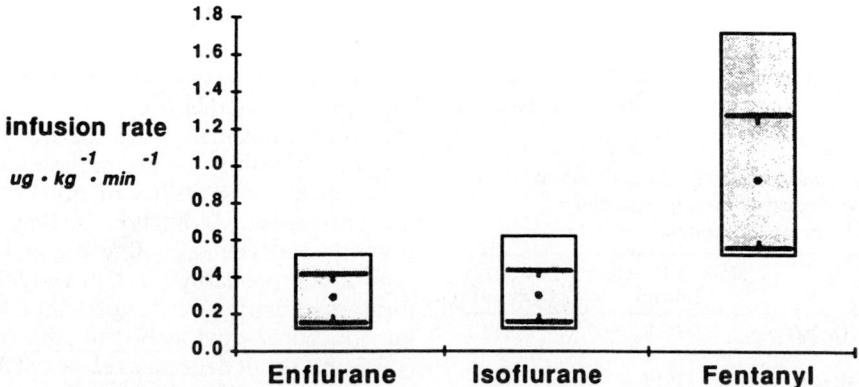

Fig. 12-11. Infusion rates of vecuronium necessry to maintain constant 90 percent depression of control twitch tension during three different anesthetics. I, standard deviation; □, range of infusion rates. (From Cannon et al.,[68] with permission.)

the endplate, which will impair neuromuscular transmission. In an excellent review by Ngai,[75] it is emphasized that inhaled anesthetics are capable of producing relaxation through their action on the CNS with minimal neuromuscular blockade. Thus, adequate surgical conditions can exist without complete neuromuscular blockade,[75] when potent anesthetic vapors are given.

Some potent anesthetics (e.g., isoflurane) increase muscle blood flow. Diversion of a larger fraction of the cardiac output to muscle may result in a proportionately greater quantity of relaxant being delivered to muscle. This mechanism has been proposed as a factor as to why the potentiating effect of isoflurane is greater than that of halothane.[69] Clearly the most important mechanism is that anesthetics inhibit motor endplate depolarization; the effect is directly related to anesthetic concentration.[77]

Despite changes in regional, renal, and hepatic blood flow, inhaled anesthetics have little or no effect on the pharmacokinetics of muscle relaxants in humans.[68,78] The ability of inhaled anesthetics to augment a nondepolarizing neuromuscular blockade is a pharmacodynamic one, that is, the blood concentration of muscle relaxants required to produce paralysis is decreased by inhaled anesthetics (Fig. 12-12).

The relationship between enflurane and dTC was demonstrated in a different way by Gencarelli et al.[79] A stepwise decrease in enflurane concentration from 2.2 to 0.5 percent during a constant infusion of dTC resulted in a reduction of neuromuscular blockade from 92 to only 8 percent twitch inhibition. This suggests that when potent inhaled anesthetics are used, a fraction of the neuromuscular blockade can be reversed by simply decreasing the anesthetic concentration and obviously does not require a drug such as neostigmine.

Unlike halothane, the ability of enflurane to enhance a dTC neuromuscular blockade is time dependent. Stanski et al.[80] found that despite a constant blood level of dTC, paralysis increased at a rate of 9 ± 4 percent/h.

They speculated that halothane achieves its maximal effect so rapidly because it acts on neural tissue (e.g., neuromuscular junction) where blood flow is high. Conversely, they speculated that in addition to the neuromuscular junction, enflurane also acts on skeletal muscle, where blood flow is less. Thus, a longer time would be required for enflurane to achieve its maximal enhancement of a nondepolarizing neuromuscular blockade.

Metabolism

Of the nondepolarizing muscle relaxants listed in Table 12-3, pancuronium, vecuronium, atracurium, and mivacurium are the only ones that are significantly metabolized. About 15 to 40 percent of an injected dose of pancuronium is deacetylated into 3-OH, 17-OH, or 3,17-OH pancuronium derivatives (Fig. 12-13). The metabolites have been studied individually in anesthetized patients.[81] The 3-OH metabolite is the most prominent in quantity and the most potent; it is one-half as potent as pancuronium (Fig. 12-14). The 3-OH metabolite has a duration of action and pharmacokinetics similar to those of pancuronium. Vecuronium is metabolized in a manner similar to that of pancuronium, with the 3-OH derivative the main metabolite. In animals, this metabolite appears to be 50 to 70 percent as potent as vecuronium.[82-84] In rats, about 15 percent of an injected dose appears in the urine and 40 percent in bile, as unchanged vecuronium.[85] An additional 30 to 40 percent of an injected dose appears in the bile as the 3-OH vecuronium.[47] Because vecuronium is excreted primarily via the bile, one might expect its 3-OH metabolite to follow the same pathway. Analysis of data obtained from renal failure patients indicates that this metabolite is cleared poorly in those patients.[86] Furthermore, extremely high levels of this metabolite appear in intensive care patients who have renal failure and have received vecuronium for several days.[87] Thus,

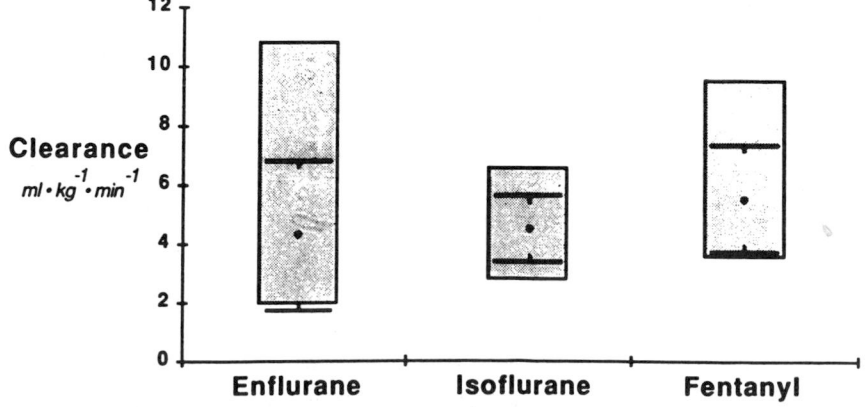

Fig. 12-12. Clearance of vecuronium calculated by dividing vecuronium infusion rates (Fig. 12-11) by the plasma concentration required for a 90 percent depression of twitch tension. ●, mean clearance; I, standard deviation; □, range. (From Cannon et al.,[68] with permission.)

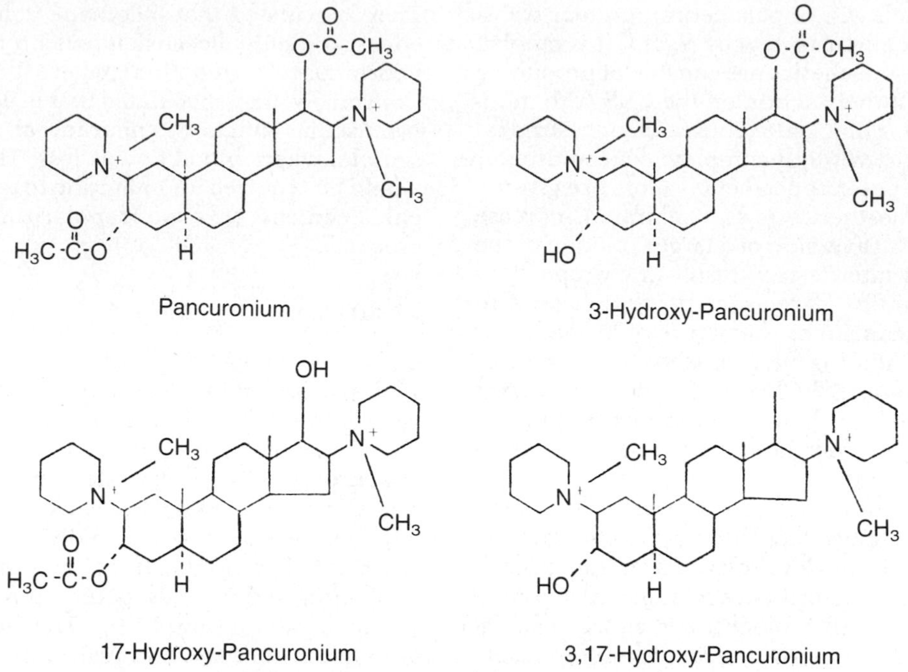

Pancuronium

3-Hydroxy-Pancuronium

17-Hydroxy-Pancuronium

3,17-Hydroxy-Pancuronium

Fig. 12-13. Formulas of pancuronium and its deacetylated metabolites.

the excretory pathway of vecuronium and its 3-OH metabolite may be different despite relatively similar structures.

Theoretically, atracurium is broken down via two pathways (Fig. 12-5). The drug undergoes Hofmann elimination, a purely chemical process that results in loss of the positive charges by molecular fragmentation to laudanosine (a tertiary amine) and a monoquater-

nary acrylate. Under the proper chemical conditions, these breakdown products may actually be used to synthesize the parent compound. They were thought to have no neuromuscular and little or no cardiovascular activity of any clinical relevance.[88] The Hofmann elimination process is nonbiologic and does not require renal, hepatic, or enzymatic function. It occurs at physiologic pH and temperature and is slowed by a fall in pH

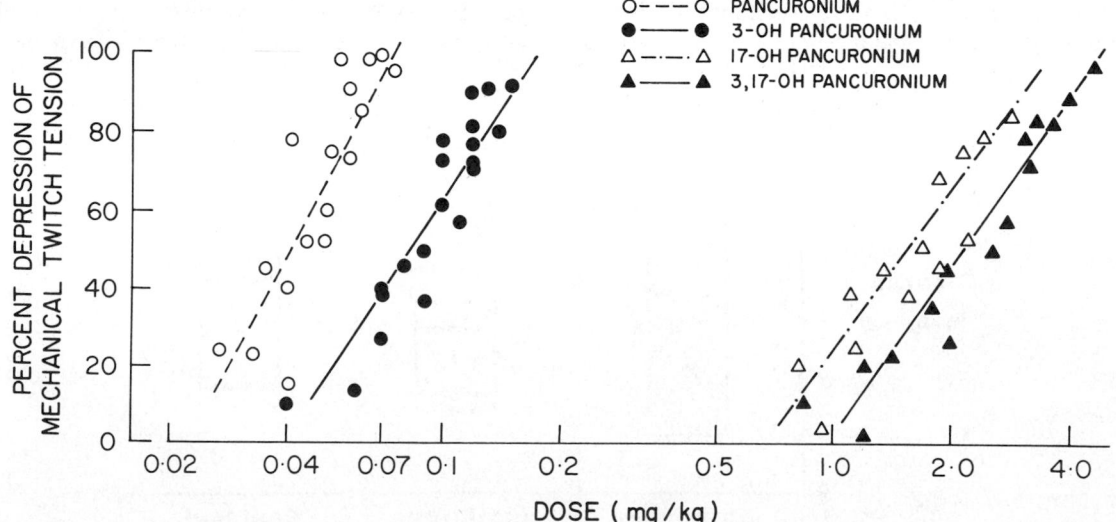

Fig. 12-14. Correlation between dose of muscle relaxant and depression of mechanical twitch tension. The lines represent analysis of linear regression. The correlation coefficients were 0.87, 0.92, 0.93, and 0.96 for pancuronium and its 3-OH, 17-OH, and 3,17-OH derivatives, respectively. (From Miller,[352] with permission.)

(i.e., acidic conditions) and especially by a decrease in temperature. In fact, atracurium's duration of action is markedly prolonged by hypothermia. (Alterations in pH within the physiologic range do not cause a clinically significant increase in the duration of action.) Thus, atracurium is relatively stable at pH 7.4 and 4°C and becomes unstable when injected into the bloodstream. Early observations on the breakdown of the drug in buffer and plasma showed a faster degradation in plasma, suggesting possible enzymatic hydrolysis of the ester groups.[89] Further recent evidence suggests that this second pathway, ester hydrolysis, is of more importance than was originally realized in the breakdown of atracurium.[90] By using a pharmacokinetic analysis, Fisher et al.[91] concluded that a significant amount of clearance of atracurium may be by routes other than ester hydrolysis and Hofmann elimination. Atracurium's metabolism is complicated and not completely resolved.[91,92]

Because of its CNS-stimulating properties, laudanosine, the main metabolite of atracurium, has received much attention and has been the subject of multiple studies, some of which are cited below. Clearly the ability of laudanosine to cause CNS stimulation depends on its blood concentration, which in turn depends on the total dose of atracurium given. Unlike atracurium, laudanosine is almost totally dependent on liver metabolism for its elimination and has a very long elimination half-life.[93,94] Not surprisingly, laudanosine concentrations are elevated in patients with liver disease[95,96] and those who have received atracurium for many hours in an intensive care unit.[97] In anesthetized humans, laudanosine levels ranging from 100 to 900 ng/ml have been measured following a single 0.5-mg/kg dose of atracurium.[30] Laudanosine freely crosses the blood-brain barrier.[93] Although much higher blood levels of laudanosine are required to cause frank seizures, a 30 percent increase in minimum anesthetic requirement (MAC)[98] and an arousal pattern on the electroencephalogram (EEG)[99] do occur at blood levels of laudanosine commonly found in anesthetized patients. Furthermore, Beemer et al.[100] found that patients awakened at a 20 percent higher arterial concentration of thiopental when atracurium had been given, which the authors attributed to the CNS stimulatory effect of laudanosine. Yet, these lower concentrations of laudanosine did not influence an animal model of epilepsy[101] or lidocaine-induced seizures.[102] In the intensive care unit, blood levels of laudanosine can be as high as 5 to 6 μg/ml. Although not known in humans, the seizure threshold in animals ranges from 3.1 μg/ml in rabbits[103] to 17 μg/ml in dogs. Thus, no adverse effects are likely to occur with atracurium's use in the operating room, but the issue is unresolved following prolonged use in the intensive care unit. Laudanosine also has cardiovascular effects. In dogs, hypotension occurs at a blood concentration of about 6.0 μg/ml,[93,104] a level found in patients in the intensive care unit. Also, laudanosine enhances stimulation-evoked release of norepineph-

rine,[105,106] which also may partly account for its CNS-stimulating effect.

Mivacurium, a new benzylisoquinoline ester, is rapidly broken down by plasma cholinesterase at a rate slightly slower than that of succinylcholine.[107] It also may be taken up by the liver and partly metabolized there.[107] Specifically, the hydrolysis rate of mivacurium is 70 percent of that of succinylcholine.[108] This mechanism of metabolism allows mivacurium to have a duration of action shorter than that of vecuronium and atracurium, but longer than that of succinylcholine.

Hypothermia

Hypothermia prolongs a dTC[109] and pancuronium[110] neuromuscular blockade. Blockades induced by both relaxants are prolonged because of delayed urinary and biliary excretion (Fig. 12-15). With pancuronium, the block is also prolonged because of decreased metabolism into inactive metabolites.[110] Therefore, hypothermia probably prolongs the block of pancuronium more than that of dTC. Hypothermia markedly prolongs the neuromuscular blockade from both vecuronium and atracurium.[111]

Age

Several years ago, Stead[112] suggested that neonates are "miniature myasthenics." Certainly development of the neuromuscular junction is not complete at birth.[113] Premature infants are more susceptible to post-tetanic exhaustion than are term infants.[114] Goudsouzian[115] found that maturation of neuromuscular transmission occurs by the first 2 months of age. Despite the apparent immaturity of the neuromuscular junction at birth, older clinical studies do not agree as to whether the newborn is more sensitive to nondepolarizing muscle relaxants.[116–122] The observed differences may be due to several factors, including the type of anesthetic and different criteria used to determine dosages, levels of relaxation, or both.

In recent years, separating the pharmacodynamics from the pharmacokinetics has allowed a more precise answer. Neonates and infants have increased sensitivity to dTC,[123] that is, a lower plasma concentration of dTC is needed to achieve a neuromuscular blockade. Nevertheless, because these young patients have a larger volume of distribution (Fig. 12-16), the dose should not differ from that used for adults. The longer elimination half-life in neonates calls for administration of subsequent doses at less frequent intervals (Table 12-5). Surprisingly, vecuronium and atracurium are quite different from the long-acting muscle relaxants. As with other muscle relaxants, infants have an increased sensitivity to vecuronium compared with adults. The marked increase in duration of action is probably because the volume of distribution decreased, while clearance did not change.[124,125] Thus, vecuronium is a long-acting muscle relaxant in the neonate.[126] In con-

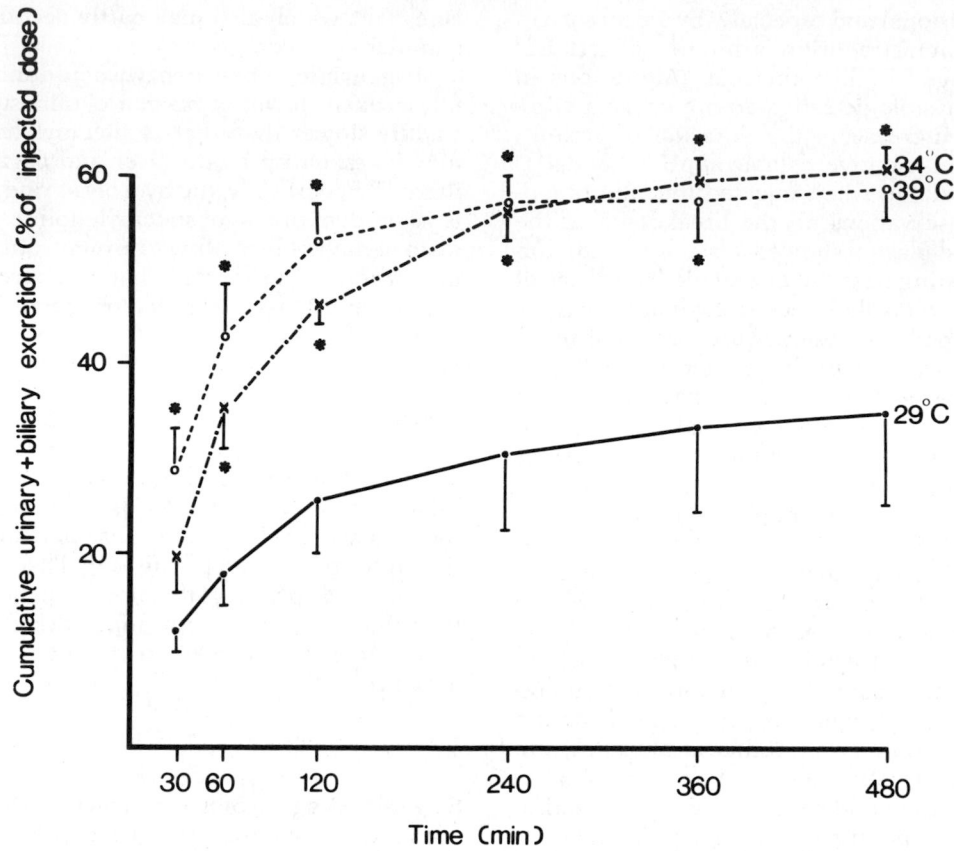

Fig. 12-15. Correlation between time after pancuronium (0.12 mg/kg) and percentage of injected dose appearing in urine and bile. (From Miller,[352] with permission.)

trast, the duration of atracurium's action is not significantly different in pediatric versus adult patients.[127-129] As with vecuronium and dTC, volume of distribution increases with atracurium in infants.[130] However, in contrast to vecuronium and dTC, total clearance in-

creased.[130] In terms of antagonism, doses of neostigmine and edrophonium used for adults are appropriate for children, although some minor dose variations have been described by Fisher et al.[131,132]

On the other end of the age scale, studies are now

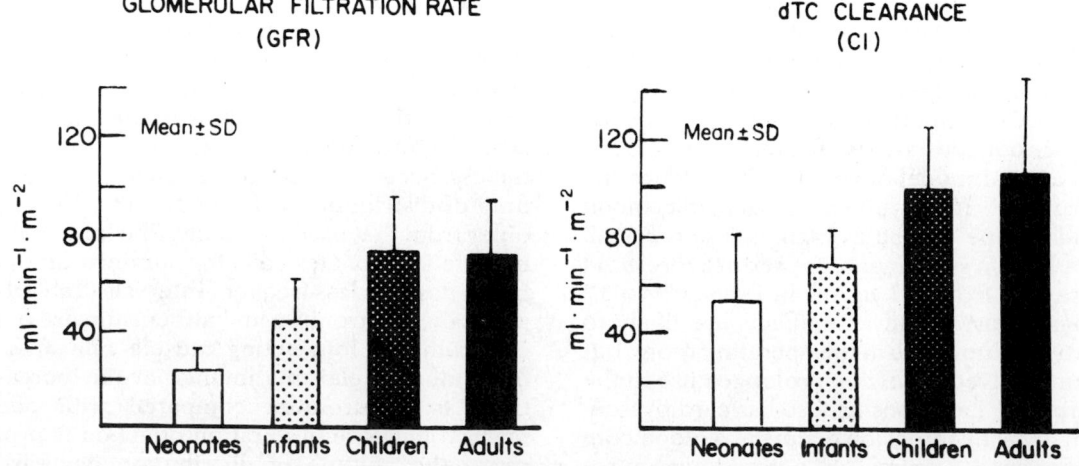

Fig. 12-16. Correlation between age, glomerular filtration, and clearance of curare. (From Fisher et al.,[123] with permission.)

TABLE 12-5. Time Course for 70 μg/kg Vecuronium (Mean ± SD)

	N	Onset (min)	Duration (min)	Recovery (min)
Infants	6	1.5 ± 0.6	73 ± 27	20 ± 8
Children	6	2.4 ± 1.4	35 ± 6	9 ± 3
Adults	6	2.9 ± 0.2	53 ± 21	13 ± 7

(From Fisher and Miller,[124] with permission.)

considering whether elderly patients (older than 60 years) may respond differently from younger patients to nondepolarizing muscle relaxants. McLeod et al.[133] found clearance of pancuronium to be inversely related to age. That is, patients in the third decade of life clear pancuronium from the plasma twice as fast as those in the ninth decade. Although neuromuscular function was not monitored, these investigators predicted a prolonged duration of neuromuscular blockade in the elderly. Also, a pharmacodynamic analysis (e.g., relationship between blood concentration of muscle relaxant and paralysis) was not performed. However, since the McLeod et al.[133] study, several investigators have examined the influence of increasing age on the pharmacokinetics and pharmacodynamics of muscle relaxants. Generally all investigators[134–136] agree that the pharmacodynamics of the muscle relaxants are not altered in the elderly. However, there is disagreement regarding the elderly and pharmacokinetics. Part of the reason for differing results is the presence of diseases associated with the elderly. Thus, separating the influence of age from disease is difficult. Rupp et al.[136] concluded that in healthy 70- to 84-year-old patients, the pharmacokinetic-pharmacodynamic response to nondepolarizing muscle relaxants does not differ markedly from their younger counterparts.

Protein Binding

Sixteen percent of dTC is bound to plasma albumin and 24 percent to gamma globulin.[137] Pancuronium was not originally thought to be bound to plasma proteins, but Thompson[138] recently demonstrated that 34 percent of pancuronium is bound to albumin and 53 percent to gamma globulin and that 13 percent is unbound. Gallamine is bound to beta and gamma globulin, although the precise extent is unknown. The clinical significance of protein binding is unclear. Theoretically, increased binding would effectively increase the volume of distribution, thereby reducing the amount of free drug available at the site of action. Increased binding might also reduce renal elimination of the drug, since only free drug is filtered at the glomerulus. Finally, the possibility of another drug displacing the muscle relaxant from the protein and releasing it as active drug must be considered. However, Thompson[138] hypothesized that the number of binding sites may remain constant as plasma protein concentration increases if the proteins combine with their own binding sites. Furthermore, bind-

ing of muscle relaxants with other sites such as cartilage and chondroitin sulfate may be qualitatively and quantitatively as important as plasma protein binding.[139] It is therefore difficult to predict the effect of altered protein binding on the pharmacokinetics of muscle relaxants. However, protein binding overall should not be of significant clinical concern. Even in patients with renal and hepatic disease—conditions that are well known to have altered protein binding to other drugs—the protein binding of dTC is not altered.[140]

Cerebrospinal Fluid and the Central Nervous System

Despite being ionized, intravenously administered nondepolarizing muscle relaxants do pass into the cerebrospinal fluid (CSF) in amounts thought to be clinically significant.[141] However, neuromuscular blockade doses of gallamine given intravenously have been found to increase the seizure threshold to lidocaine in dogs.[142] Forbes et al.[143] found intravenously administered pancuronium to reduce halothane anesthetic requirement (MAC) by 25 percent. However, more recent studies indicate that muscle relaxants do not alter anesthetic requirement.[144]

When neuromuscular blocking drugs have been given accidentally into the CSF (i.e., wrong drug given for a spinal anesthetic), myotonia, autonomic changes, and even convulsions have occurred.[145,146] Furthermore, prolonged administration of vecuronium, and probably other muscle relaxants, will result in this drug entering the CSF in critical care patients.[87] On the basis of these limited data, we conclude that small amounts of intravenously administered muscle relaxants do pass into the CSF, but the clinical significance is unclear. Also, laudanosine, a metabolite of atracurium, crosses the blood-brain barrier[93] and causes central nervous stimulation. Whether the CNS effects of muscle relaxants contribute to the morbidity and mortality of critical care patients is unknown.

Other Less-Used Muscle Relaxants

Two nondepolarizing muscle relaxants not available in the United States are described below.

Alcuronium

Although not available in the United States, alcuronium is a popular muscle relaxant in much of the world. After discovery of the extraordinary potency and very long duration of action of toxiferine, it was believed that the duration of action might be shortened, possibly at some expense to potency, if allyl groups were substituted for the methyl quaternizing groups.[147] The result was diallylbisnortoxiferine, or alcuronium, a semisynthetic substance the precursors of which are obtained from an amazonian plant, *Strychnos toxifera*.

The 95 percent effective dose (ED_{95}) under anesthesia is about 0.2 to 0.25 mg/kg.[147,148] Good intubating conditions are achieved 3 minutes after administration of 0.3 mg/kg alcuronium.[148] The duration of action is long, similar to that of dTC, so that anticholinesterases are necessary for antagonism of residual block. Although specific studies are few, alcuronium is probably potentiated to the same degree by anesthetic vapors as are other nondepolarizers, necessitating a dosage reduction of 30 to 50 percent.

One of the major advantages of alcuronium is its lack of side effects. It is a relatively weak vagolytic substance,[149] only occasionally causing a slight rise in heart rate in clinical use.[150] Alcuronium does not release histamine and is a weak ganglion blocker, making a fall in blood pressure unlikely.[151] Nevertheless, larger doses of alcuronium have been found to decrease arterial pressure,[149] particularly in patients with cardiovascular disease.[152] There is probably little or no metabolism of alcuronium, most of the drug being eliminated unchanged mainly in the urine.[38] A minor secondary pathway via the bile probably exists. The kinetic measurements of half-life (2 to 3 hours), clearance (about 100 ml/min), and distribution volume (330 ml/kg) are similar to values obtained for other, longer-acting, muscle relaxants excreted largely in the urine.[153]

Fazadinium

Original observations on fazadinium were made when a tertiary amine azo dye (an anthelminthic agent) was converted to a diquaternary compound and good neuromuscular blocking activity resulted.[154] The drug is chemically and metabolically unique in that its structure contains a tetrazine chain that can be reduced by liver enzymes in vitro.[155] Originally thought to be promising as a possible short-acting nondepolarizer,[154] its action is much longer in humans than in animals,[156] although it is somewhat shorter acting in humans than are long-acting drugs such as dTC and pancuronium.[40,157] About 0.5 to 1.0 mg/kg usually suffices for relaxation under balanced anesthesia, and 1.0 to 1.5 mg/kg is usually given for intubation of the trachea.[40,156,157] Fazadinium is potentiated by anesthetic vapors, and its action may be antagonized by anticholinesterases.

Fazadinium is strongly vagolytic[149,158] and always causes tachycardia,[159] since the dose-response curves for vagal and neuromuscular block overlap. Higher doses used for intubation also cause hypotension[159] due to a ganglion-blocking effect.[149,158] Fazadinium is probably the only nondepolarizer in clinical use that often causes hypotension because of ganglionic blockade. It is not a potent releaser of histamine. Fazadinium is reduced in vitro by an azo reductase found in the liver.[154] However, there is probably little or no metabolism in humans. The drug is probably excreted unchanged in the urine.[39,40] The half-life in one study was 76.4 minutes,[40] approximately one-half to two-thirds that of

longer-acting drugs. This finding suggests that the duration of action of fazadinium in humans is probably somewhat shorter than that of dTC but longer than the blocking action of the intermediate agents, atracurium and vecuronium. The clearance value (132 ml/min) and the volume of distribution (0.234 L/kg) are typical of a water-soluble drug excreted unchanged by the kidneys.[40,160]

Cardiovascular and Autonomic Effects

Six of the ten nondepolarizing muscle relaxants either soon to be available or already available in the United States produce cardiovascular effects. Vecuronium, doxacurium, pipecuronium, and ORG 9426 appear to be essentially devoid of cardiovascular effects. *d*-Tubocurarine and, to a much lesser extent, metocurine, atracurium, and mivacurium produce hypotension. Pancuronium and gallamine produce tachycardia and some degree of hypertension. The autonomic effects of these muscle relaxants are summarized in Table 12-6.

Autonomic Effects (General)

Interference with autonomic function by muscle relaxants produces various cardiovascular effects. Thus, one or both sides of the autonomic nervous system may be stimulated or depressed by interacting with nicotinic or muscarinic receptors at various locations called cholinoceptive sites, where ACh exerts its physiologic actions (Table 12-7). All muscle relaxants may be shown experimentally to interact with all cholinoceptive sites if large enough doses are given. In clinical practice, however, side effects are generally minor because the dose-response curves for nicotinic and muscarinic properties of relaxants are widely separated from the curves for neuromuscular blocking effects (Table 12-8). Depolarizing substances such as succinylcholine generally stimulate cholinoceptive sites, whereas non-

TABLE 12-6. Autonomic Effects of Neuromuscular Blocking Drugs

Drug	Autonomic Ganglia	Cardiac Muscarinic Receptors	Histamine Release
Succinylcholine	Stimulates	Stimulates	Slight
Decamethonium	None	None	None
d-Tubocurarine	Blocks	None	Moderate
Metocurine	Blocks weakly	None	Slight
Gallamine	None	Blocks strongly	None
Pancuronium	None	Blocks weakly	None
Alcuronium	Weak	Blocks weakly	None
Fazadinium	Moderate	Blocks strongly	None
Atracurium	None	None	Slight
Vecuronium	None	None	None
ORG 9426	None	None	None
Mivacurium	None	None	Slight
Doxacurium	None	None	None
Pipecuronium	None	None	None

TABLE 12-7. Cholinoceptive Sites That Interact with Neuromuscular Blocking Drugs

Type Receptor	Location	Function	Relaxant Interactions
Nicotinic	Neuromuscular junction— postsynaptic	Initiates depolarization in muscle endplate	Succinylcholine stimulates; nondepolarizers block
Nicotinic	Neuromuscular junction— presynaptic	Maintains ACh release during high-frequency stimulation	Succinylcholine stimulates, nondepolarizers block
Nicotinic	Autonomic ganglion; ganglion cell bodies	Initiates depolarization of ganglion cell	Succinylcholine stimulates; fazadinium and *d*-tubocurarine block
Nicotinic	Postganglionic neuron terminal; autonomic nerves	Positive feedback for transmitter release	Succinylcholine stimulates; *d*-tubocurarine and other nondepolarizers may block
Muscarinic	Sinus node of heart	Slows cardiac rate	Succinylcholine stimulates; gallamine, fazadinium, pancuronium, and alcuronium block
Muscarinic (M_i)	Autonomic ganglia; interneuron cell bodies	Inhibits depolarization by hyperpolarization	Pancuronium and gallamine block
Muscarinic (M_e)	Autonomic ganglia; ganglion cell bodies	Augments depolarization; slow, delayed depolarization	Atropine blocks; not affected by nondepolarizing muscle relaxants
Muscarinic	Postganglion neuron terminal; autonomic nerves	Negative feedback for transmitter release	Pancuronium and gallamine block
Esteratic	AChE	Hydrolysis of ACh by clinically used muscle relaxants	Not significantly affected
Esteratic	Pseudocholinesterase	Hydrolysis of ACh; weakly inhibited by vecuronium and atracurium	Inhibited by pancuronium

Abbreviations: ACh, acetylcholine; AChE, acetylcholinesterase.

depolarizers are classically blocking substances. The autonomic properties of various muscle relaxants are summarized in Table 12-6. True autonomic responses are not reduced by slower injection rates and are additive if divided doses are given. Subsequent doses of muscle relaxant, if identical to the original dose, will produce a similar response.

Another mechanism by which many muscle relaxants may produce a cardiovascular effect is histamine release. Quaternary ammonium compounds are generally weak histamine-releasing substances relative to tertiary amines such as morphine. Nevertheless, when large doses of muscle relaxants are injected rapidly by the intravenous route, some degree of erythema of the face, neck, and upper torso may develop, together with a brief fall in arterial pressure and a slight to moderate rise in heart rate. Bronchospasm is very rare. These side effects are usually of short duration (1 to 5 minutes) and are clinically insignificant in healthy patients. They may be reduced considerably by a slower injection rate. They are also prevented by prophylaxis with combinations of H_1- and H_2-blockers. If a minor degree of histamine release such as described above occurs after an initial dose of muscle relaxant, subsequent doses will usually cause no response at all, as long as they do not exceed the original dose. This is clinical evidence of tachyphylaxis, an important characteristic of histamine release.

A much more significant degree of histamine release occurs during anaphylactic or anaphylactoid reactions; these reactions are very rare. Anaphylactic reactions are mediated through immune responses. Anaphylactoid reactions probably are not immune mediated and represent an exaggerated response of a very sensitive individual.

TABLE 12-8. Approximate Autonomic Margins of Safety of Nondepolarizing Relaxants

Drug	Vagus	Sympathetic Ganglia	Histamine Release
d-Tubocurarine	0.6	2.0	1.0
Metocurine	3.0	16.0	2.0
Alcuronium	3.0	4.0	None
Pancuronium	3.0	250	None
Fazadinium	0.4	4.0	None
Atracurium	16	40	3.0
Vecuronium	20	>250	None
Gallamine	0.6	>100	None

(Data from Refs. 19, 149, 159, 172, and 353.)

Autonomic Margin of Safety

Calculation of the dose ratio (ED_{95} for neuromuscular blockade/ED_{50} for autonomic effect) for ganglion blockade, vagal (muscarinic) blockade, and histamine release can point to safety margins precluding the development of these side effects in response to clinical administration of muscle relaxants. Approximate safety ratios for nondepolarizing muscle relaxants are given in Table 12-8.

Specific Mechanisms

Ganglionic Stimulation

The depolarizing muscle relaxant succinylcholine may produce an elevation in heart rate and in arterial pressure secondary to the mechanism of ganglionic stimulation,[161,162] which is probably mediated by activation of nicotinic receptors on ganglion cells on both sides of the autonomic nervous system. In patients who have received atropine, the chief cardiovascular response is elevated heart rate and arterial pressure. In subjects not given an anticholinergic drug beforehand, the result of ganglionic stimulation may be either bradycardia and a drop in blood pressure or increased heart rate and blood pressure, depending on the patient's autonomic set at the time of administration of succinylcholine. For example, the cardiovascular response to succinylcholine in a patient who is very anxious before induction of anesthesia or who is receiving a catecholamine infusion is likely to be bradycardia with ventricular arrhythmias. In patients receiving adrenergic β-blockers, bradycardia after succinylcholine is common.

More recent studies indicate that succinylcholine produces a dose-related positive chronotropic effect through indirect stimulation of the sinoatrial node by catecholamine release from nerve endings. In contrast, succinylmonocholine causes a decrease in heart rate.[163]

Ganglionic Blockade

The ganglion-blocking effects of dTC and fazadinium occur closer to their neuromuscular blocking effects than in the case of any other muscle relaxant.[149,152] Nevertheless, the principal reason for the hypotensive property of dTC is its histamine-releasing action.[163a] Fazadinium, in large doses, causes tachycardia and hypotension.[159] Here, the decrease in blood pressure is probably due to ganglionic blockade,[158] since fazadinium is not a potent histamine releaser. Thus, the only muscle relaxant for which ganglion blockade is an important autonomic mechanism during clinical use is fazadinium.

Muscarinic Blockade

Vagal block, resulting in tachycardia, is produced by muscarinic receptor blockade at the sinus node of the heart in response to pancuronium, fazadinium, and gal-

lamine. The latter two substances are potent vagolytic drugs when this side effect occurs within and overlaps the dose range for neuromuscular blockade.[151,158] The dose-response curve for the vagolytic property of pancuronium lies slightly to the right of its neuromuscular blocking effects,[155] so that in clinical practice pancuronium is probably only partially vagolytic. The result is usually only a moderate rise in heart rate (10 to 25 beats/min) when high doses are administered.[164,165] The vagolytic effect of relaxants is limited to receptors in the sinus node. Other classic muscarinic sites in the parasympathetic nervous system, such as bowel, bladder, bronchi, and pupils, are not affected.

Muscarinic Blockade within the Sympathetic Nervous System

There are at least three sets of muscarinic receptors in the sympathetic nervous system. Two of these are blocked by neuromuscular blocking agents, such as pancuronium, gallamine, and fazadinium, that have a vagolytic property, that is, they can block muscarinic receptors in the sinus node of the heart, on the parasympathetic side of the autonomic nervous system. One mechanism, muscarinic receptor block on a dopaminergic interneuron within a pathway responsible for inhibitory input to sympathetic ganglion cells,[166] results in less modulation of augmented ganglionic traffic during periods of relatively intense stimulation; and another mechanism, muscarinic receptor blockade at adrenergic neuron terminals, results in removal of a negative feedback mechanism regulating catecholamine output.[167] Both mechanisms may not only contribute to elevations in heart rate normally seen with pancuronium but may also represent the primary mechanisms behind exaggerated responses sometimes seen in the presence of pancuronium block under light anesthesia during intense surgical stimulation (including laryngoscopy and tracheal intubation).

Inhibition of Catecholamine Reuptake

Pancuronium inhibits reuptake of norepinephrine by adrenergic nerves.[168-171] This mechanism may also contribute to exaggerated cardiovascular responses during pancuronium block.

Histamine Release

An increase of histamine levels in plasma to 200 to 300 percent of baseline levels causes a brief decrease in arterial blood pressure (1 to 5 minutes), increase in heart rate, and skin erythema about the face and neck. The benzylisoquinoline substances dTC, metocurine, and atracurium release these amounts of histamine in a dose range of 0.5 to 0.6 mg/kg for each compound. Doses in this range represent one, two, and three times the ED_{95} dose for neuromuscular blockade for each drug. Thus, the safety margin for this side effect is about three times greater for atracurium and two times greater for metocurine than for dTC. The side effect occurs well within the clinical dose range for dTC and is therefore common during its use. It is less prominent with metocurine and is uncommon with atracurium. As in the case of dTC,[163] any decrease in blood pressure that may develop during the use of these drugs is probably directly related to elevation of serum histamine levels. The amount of histamine released by any of these drugs is dose related[163,172,173] and is also related to speed of injection. Thus, cardiovascular responses to a very large dose of atracurium (0.6 mg/kg) may be prevented by slow injection or by prophylaxis with antihistamines (both H_1- and H_2-blockers are necessary).[173] Although multiple cardiovascular studies have been performed with atracurium, the most aggressive one was that of Hosking et al.[174] They gave atracurium (1.5 mg/kg) (six times the ED_{95}) as an intravenous bolus. Not surprisingly, they observed a mean decrease in mean arterial blood pressure of 30 percent and a huge increase in plasma histamine concentrations. Scott et al.[173] and Hosking et al.[174] found that combined H_1/H_2-receptor blockade attenuated these histamine-induced changes. Mivacurium also releases histamine in about the same amounts as does atracurium. When 0.15 mg/kg (two times the ED_{95}) is given over 60 seconds, only minimal cardiovascular changes occur.[175] When mivacurium is given more rapidly or in larger doses, hypotension is more likely to occur.

Specific Clinical Considerations

Hypotension

d-Tubocurarine causes hypotension, probably as a result of the liberation of histamine; in larger doses, it produces ganglionic blockade.[176-179] Dowdy et al.[179] proposed that hypotension is not caused by the dTC itself but by the preservative in which it is stored. However, in anesthetized patients, Stoelting[180,181] disproved this theory. Premedication with promethazine, an antihistamine drug, will attenuate dTC-induced hypotension.[182] Hypotension is directly related to dose of dTC and to anesthetic depth,[178] especially if the anesthetic is itself a ganglionic blocker, such as halothane. With a light level of surgical anesthesia and the use of smaller doses of dTC (15 mg/70 kg), the incidence of significant hypotension is markedly attenuated. Although hypotension can occur after administration of metocurine, the incidence and magnitude are much less than those associated with dTC. Atracurium in doses greater than 0.4 mg/kg and mivacurium in doses greater than 0.15 mg/kg occasionally cause transient hypotension due to histamine release. Histamine release can be minimized by the slow administration of these muscle relaxants.[173,175]

Tachycardia

Pancuronium causes a moderate increase in heart rate and, to a lesser extent, in cardiac output, with little or no change in systemic vascular resistance.[164,165] Although pancuronium-induced tachycardia has been attributed to a vagolytic action,[164] numerous investigators have implicated the sympathetic nervous system. Both indirect (release of norepinephrine from adrenergic nerve endings)[168,182] and direct (blockade of neuronal uptake of norepinephrine) mechanisms have been suggested.[168-170] Vercruysse et al.[171] suggested that both gallamine and pancuronium augment the release of norepinephrine in vascular tissues under vagal control. In studies in humans, Roizen et al.[183] surprisingly found a decrease in plasma norepinephrine levels after administration of either pancuronium or atropine. These workers postulated that the increase in heart rate or rate–pressure product occurs because pancuronium (or atropine) acts through baroreceptors to reduce sympathetic outflow. More specifically, the vagolytic effect of pancuronium increases heart rate and hence blood pressure, in turn influencing the baroreceptors to decrease sympathetic tone. Support for this concept is provided by the fact that prior administration of atropine will attenuate or eliminate the cardiovascular effects of pancuronium.[164] Gallamine increases heart rate by both vagolytic[184] and sympathetic stimulation.[185] Specifically, gallamine supposedly releases norepinephrine from adrenergic nerve endings in the heart by an unknown mechanism.[184] However, a positive chronotropic effect that places emphasis on the vagolytic mechanism has not been found in humans.[186] It would not be surprising to find out ultimately that gallamine and pancuronium act by similar mechanisms.

Arrhythmias

Gallamine, dTC, and succinylcholine actually reduce the incidence of epinephrine-induced arrhythmias.[187] Possibly because of enhanced atrioventricular conduction,[188] the incidence of arrhythmias from pancuronium appears to increase during halothane anesthesia.[164] Edwards et al.[189] observed a rapid tachycardia (more than 150 beats/min) that progressed to atrioventricular dissociation in two patients anesthetized with halothane. The only common factor between these two patients was that both were receiving tricyclic antidepressants. In further studies, Edwards et al.[189] found the incidence of severe ventricular arrhythmia to be common in response to administration of pancuronium to dogs receiving halothane (but not enflurane) and chronically administered tricyclic antidepressants. In conclusion, the drug interaction among tricyclic antidepressants, halothane, and pancuronium must be avoided. Use of another muscle relaxant, such as vecuronium, is probably the most convenient approach.

Bradycardia

Several case reports[190,191] have described severe bradycardia and even asystole with vecuronium administration. All of these cases were associated with narcotic administration. There can be many causes of bradycardia intraoperatively. Subsequent studies indicate that vecuronium, by itself, does not cause bradycardia.[192] When combined with other drugs (e.g., fentanyl), bradycardia may result.[193]

Clinical Management

General

Despite the wide use of muscle relaxants, little harm usually results because of the incredible safety of these drugs. In fact, it is difficult to demonstrate that one muscle relaxant is truly "safer" than another.[194-196] However, to avoid prolonged paralysis, inadequate antagonism, or both, the main goal should be to use the lowest dose possible that will still provide adequate relaxation for surgery. The rational use of muscle relaxants depends on administration by an anesthesiologist who is familiar with the operative procedure, who knows when to use muscle relaxants, who has a method for assessing the magnitude and duration of action of the specific muscle relaxant, and who understands the clinical pharmacology of the drug, including its side effects and complications. The key factor is to avoid an overdose. For example, in an adequately anesthetized patient, there is no reason to completely obliterate the twitch or train-of-four in response to peripheral nerve stimulation. Repetitive doses probably should be about one-third to one-fifth the initial dose and should not be given until some evidence of recovery from the previous dose is evident. Following these guidelines will help avoid an excessive neuromuscular blockade that cannot be antagonized.

Production of Adequate Clinical Relaxation

Several options are available to provide adequate surgical relaxation. It is important for the clinician to keep all the options in mind and to avoid relying completely on neuromuscular blockade to achieve a desired degree of relaxation. These options include adjustment of depth of general anesthesia, regional anesthesia, proper positioning of the patient on the operating table, and finally manipulation of the depth of neuromuscular blockade. The choice of one or several of these options is determined by the estimated remaining duration of surgery, the anesthetic technique, and the surgical maneuver required, as well as its estimated duration.

Control of Depth of Anesthesia

Inhaled anesthetics are commonly known to produce relaxation of skeletal muscle by multiple inhibitory influences on reflex pathways in the CNS that are responsible for maintenance of muscle tone. This action of anesthetics is dose related but usually does not cause measurable neuromuscular blockade. Very deep anesthesia with isoflurane, enflurane, and diethyl ether may cause a slight reduction of neuromuscular transmission, as measured by more sensitive indicators of clinical neuromuscular function, such as tetanus and train-of-four. It is also important to remember that, although good documentation is lacking, there is probably a relationship between relaxation and anesthetic depth during balanced anesthesia as well as during anesthesia with inhaled anesthetics. Thus, to increase relaxation by deepening anesthesia for various surgical maneuvers such as peritoneal closure, fracture or dislocation reduction, and tracheal intubation, one may not increase the inspired concentration of halothane, isoflurane, or enflurane, but may also administer a supplemental bolus of thiopental, narcotic, or lidocaine, for example. The effectiveness of neuromuscular blocking drugs increases proportionally with depth of inhalational anesthesia.[63,68]

Control of Depth of Neuromuscular Blockade

Various levels of clinical neuromuscular blockade are now demonstrable by appropriate use of a nerve stimulator (also see Ch. 36). During the use of nondepolarizing muscle relaxants, one may ascertain within narrow limits that depth of block is adequate for certain clinical maneuvers. For example, relaxation is generally inadequate for most situations if all four responses are clearly visible during train-of-four monitoring. If two or three responses are visible, relaxation should be adequate for abdominal surgery under adequate inhalational anesthesia. If only one twitch is visible, relaxation should be deep enough to permit intubation of the trachea under light anesthesia or to maintain good relaxation of the abdomen under balanced anesthesia. These general guidelines naturally assume adequate depth of general anesthesia. If anesthesia is too light, relaxation may prove inadequate, even if the indicators are well documented.

Regional Anesthesia

Regional anesthesia should always be considered alone or in combination with light general anesthesia as a means of achieving relaxation localized to the area of surgery. For example, continuous epidural or spinal anesthesia will provide good relaxation for abdominal surgery, particularly if the patient is spared the discomforts of abdominal exploration by the administration of sedative levels of inhaled anesthetics.

Patient Positioning

Adequate conditions for peritoneal closure, laryngoscopy, and other such procedures often depend considerably on suitable positioning. The operating table may be flexed slightly to make it easier to close an abdominal wound. Proper placement of the head in the sniffing position for laryngoscopy can change poor relaxation to adequate conditions for intubation.

Rapid Sequence Induction of Anesthesia and Endotracheal Intubation with Nondepolarizing Muscle Relaxants

Anesthesiologists have long considered succinylcholine the muscle relaxant of choice for this critical maneuver. There is no doubt that this is still true, since no nondepolarizer, even when given in very high doses, will permit the 60-second endotracheal intubation possible with succinylcholine. Nevertheless, a few investigators advocate large doses (0.15 to 0.2 mg/kg) of pancuronium or vecuronium (0.3 mg/kg intravenously) for rapid-sequence induction of anesthesia and endotracheal intubation (Fig. 12-17).[197-199] Actually, large doses of any nondepolarizing muscle relaxant would produce a rapid onset of neuromuscular blockade, but a corresponding long duration of blockade would result.[199]

Several recent developments suggest that our thinking regarding the rapid-sequence procedure is changing.[200] As always, the well-known side effects of succinylcholine render its use inadvisable in many situations, such as burns and extensive denervation of muscle. The newer nondepolarizing muscle relaxants, vecuronium, atracurium, and mivacurium, may be given in relatively large dosage (three times the ED_{95}) with the expectation that (1) full paralysis should last about 1 hour, (2) complete recovery should require approximately 2 hours, (3) recovery from full paralysis should have begun such that antagonism of residual block with anticholinesterase agents will be possible within about 1 hour with vecuronium and atracurium and 30 minutes with mivacurium, and (4) the cardiovascular side effects of vecuronium are absent and those of atracurium and mivacurium mild enough to permit administration of such high doses without compromising safety. Finally, several workers have recommended prior treatment with a small subparalyzing dose of the nondepolarizer a few minutes before giving a large dose for tracheal intubation.[201-204] This procedure, termed the priming principle, has been shown to accelerate the onset of block by various nondepolarizing muscle relaxants by about 30 to 60 seconds.[201-204] If the priming dose of nondepolarizing muscle relaxant is given 3 to 6 minutes before the intubating dose, tracheal intubation can be achieved about 90 seconds after injection of the second dose of muscle relaxant. For example, with vecuronium a priming dose of 0.01 mg/kg, a wait of 4 minutes, and then an intubating dose of 0.07 to 0.15 mg/kg intravenously seems to be the ideal combination.[204] The 0.07-mg/kg dose will provide adequate intubating conditions but occasional coughing. If the latter is to be prevented, the 0.1 to 0.15-mg/kg dose is recommended. Even with the priming dose, we believe that the size of the intubating dose should be as large or larger than that customarily administered under nonemergent conditions, despite the recommendations by others[201,202] that the dose be lowered after priming. Jones[205] and others believe that the disadvantages (e.g., occasional weakness with the priming dose) outweigh the advantages of the priming approach. Although larger doses and the priming principle clearly shorten the onset time of nondepolarizing muscle relaxants, the shortest onset time is still with succinylcholine.

Some may argue that endotracheal intubation within 90 seconds is not fast enough for true rapid-sequence procedure, but we consider this interval satisfactory, particularly when there is a valid contraindication to succinylcholine. We also caution that even with priming, intubating conditions at 90 seconds may not be quite as ideal as they usually are 60 seconds after succinylcholine, particularly if only small doses (3 to 4 mg/kg) of thiopental or other drugs are administered

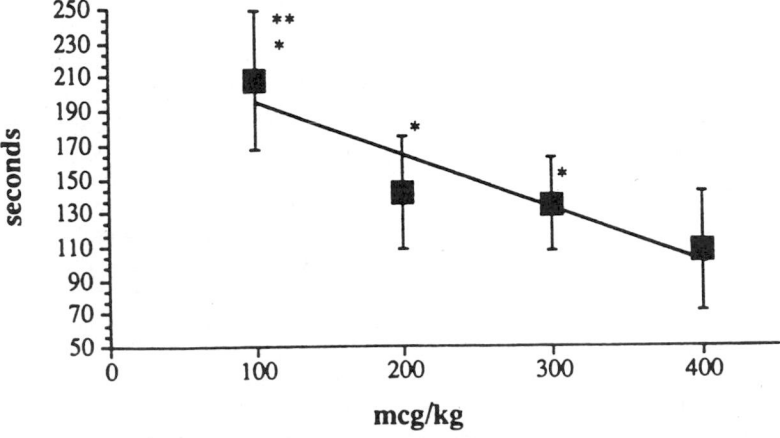

Fig. 12-17. Onset of neuromuscular blockade in seconds as defined as that time from vecuronium administration until disappearance of the response to peripheral nerve stimulation. * = 400 μg/kg is significantly different from the other doses. ** = 100 μg/kg is significantly different from the 200- and 300-μg/kg doses. (From Ginsberg et al.,[199] with permission.)

TABLE 12-9. Rapid Intubation[a] with Various Relaxants Using the Priming Technique

Drug	Priming Dose[b] (mg/kg)	Intubating Dose[c] (mg/kg)	Intubation Time[d] (sec)	Clinical Duration[e] (min)	Full Recovery[f] (min)
Succinylcholine	None	0.7	60	5–10	12–15
Succinylcholine	Nondepolarizer pretreatment	1.5	60	5–10	12–15
Mivacurium	0.02–0.03	0.16–0.3	90	25–30	40–60
Atracurium	0.06–0.08	0.6–0.8	90	45–60	60–90
Vecuronium	0.01	0.07–0.15	90	60–75	75–120
Pancuronium	0.015	0.15–0.2	90	120–150	>4 h
Metocurine	0.05	0.4–0.5	90	~150	>4 h
Pancuronium-metocurine	0.005–0.02	0.05–0.2	90	~150	>4 h

[a] For intubation with nondepolarizing muscle relaxants, the administration of adequate dosage of intravenous agents is assumed for induction of anesthesia.
[b] This dose is given as preoxygenation is begun.
[c] This dose is given 3 to 6 minutes after the priming dose. For atracurium, metocurine, and mivacurium, 30- to 60-second slow-bolus administration should be considered if it is thought desirable to avoid any cardiovascular effect. For all nondepolarizers, these dosages may be higher than recommended by the manufacturers.
[d] Conditions for intubation at this time should allow easy passage of an endotracheal tube. Conditions may not necessarily be ideal. Adequate intravenous agents for induction are mandatory.
[e] Time from injection to recovery of twitch to 25 percent of control.
[f] Time from injection to recovery of twitch to 95 percent of control.

for induction of anesthesia. Conditions for intubation depend on both depth of anesthesia and depth of paralysis. Consequently, we emphasize that, particularly in healthy young patients, larger doses of anesthetic drugs be given to ensure adequate conditions for intubation, using the priming technique, 90 seconds after the intubating dose of nondepolarizing muscle relaxant has been injected (Table 12-9). Suggested dosage regimens for various nondepolarizing muscle relaxants, using the priming technique for rapid-sequence intubation within 90 seconds, are presented in Table 12-9. Spontaneous recovery to 95 percent of control twitch height at the dosages suggested represents full recovery and spontaneous recovery to 20 to 25 percent of control twitch height represents clinical duration; at this point, facile antagonism of residual blockade with an anticholinesterase should be expected.

CLINICAL PHARMACOLOGY OF DEPOLARIZING MUSCLE RELAXANTS

Although decamethonium is available, it is rarely used. This section is devoted entirely to the clinical pharmacology of succinylcholine (see Fig. 12-4).

Pharmacokinetics and Pharmacodynamics

The extremely brief duration of action of succinylcholine is primarily due to its rapid hydrolysis by pseudocholinesterase, an enzyme of the liver and plasma. The initial metabolite, succinylmonocholine, is a much weaker neuromuscular blocker. In turn, it is metabolized to succinic acid and choline. Pseudocholinesterase has an enormous capacity to hydrolyze succinylcholine at a very rapid rate such that a small fraction of the original intravenous dose actually reaches the neuromuscular junction. Since there is little or no pseudo-

cholinesterase at the motor endplate, the neuromuscular blockade of succinylcholine is terminated by its diffusion away from the endplate into extracellular fluid. Pseudocholinesterase, therefore, influences the duration of action of succinylcholine by controlling the rate at which the latter is hydrolyzed before it reaches the endplate.

A succinylcholine neuromuscular blockade can be prolonged by a reduced quantity of normal enzyme or by an atypical form of pseudocholinesterase. Factors that have been described as lowering pseudocholinesterase levels are (1) liver disease,[206] (2) pregnancy,[207] (3) phenelzine, (4) echothiophate,[207] (5) cytotoxic drugs, (6) tetrahydroaminacrine,[208] (7) hexafluorenium,[207] (8) cancer,[209] (9) AChE inhibitors,[210,211] and metoclopramide.[212] While not all investigators agree, the most recent information indicates that cimetidine and ranitidine have no effect on succinylcholine or pseudocholinesterase activity.[213] More recently, bambuterol, a prodrug of terbutaline used for long-term treatment of asthma, has been shown to have a marked depressant effect on pseudocholinesterase activity and to prolong a succinylcholine neuromuscular blockade.[214]

Despite all the publications and effort identifying those situations in which pseudocholinesterase levels may be low, this is of little concern. In a study conducted by Foldes et al.,[206] it was found that when pseudocholinesterase was reduced to 20 percent of normal by severe liver disease, the duration of apnea after the administration of succinylcholine was increased from a normal duration of 3 minutes to almost 9 minutes. Even when eye treatment with echothiophate decreased pseudocholinesterase activity from 49 percent of control to no activity, the increase in duration of neuromuscular blockade varied from 2 to 14 minutes. In no patient did the total duration of neuromuscular blockade exceed 23 minutes.[207] In an extensive clinical study, Viby-Mogensen[215] confirmed these observations that duration of blockade from the usual clinical dose of

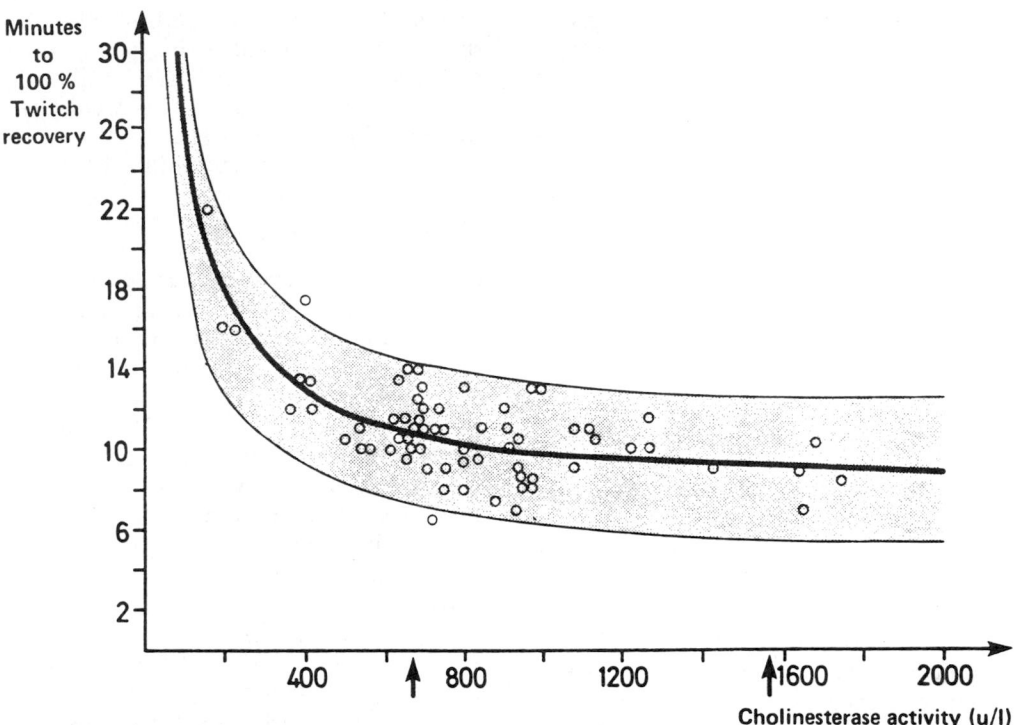

Fig. 12-18. Correlation between duration of succinylcholine neuromuscular blockade and pseudocholinesterase activity. (From Viby-Mogensen,[215] with permission.)

succinylcholine is moderately increased by low pseudocholinesterase levels (Fig. 12-18).[215] Thus, if repeated doses are given only when recovery from the previous dose of succinylcholine is evident, low pseudocholinesterase levels should slightly prolong a succinylcholine blockade, and this should present no serious problem.

A succinylcholine neuromuscular blockade can be prolonged if the patient has an abnormal genetically derived variant of pseudocholinesterase. The variant was found by Kalow and Genest[216] to respond to dibucaine differently than does normal pseudocholinesterase. Dibucaine inhibits normal pseudocholinesterase to a far greater extent than the abnormal enzyme. This observation led to the development of the dibucaine number. Under standardized test conditions, dibucaine inhibits the normal enzyme about 80 percent and an abnormal enzyme about 20 percent (Table 12-10). Subsequently, many other genetic variants of pseudocholinesterase have been identified, although the dibu-

caine-related variants are the most important. An excellent review by Pantuck and Pantuck[207] presents a more detailed assessment of this topic.

The relationship between low dibucaine numbers and low pseudocholinesterase levels is often confusing. To repeat, a patient may have a normal pseudocholinesterase level and yet, with a low dibucaine number, have a prolonged response to succinylcholine, indicating the presence of primarily atypical enzyme. Conversely, the pseudocholinesterase level may be very low, and the patient may have a normal dibucaine number, but the response to succinylcholine may be slightly prolonged[215] because of the presence of only a small total quantity of enzyme, all of which is normal. In other words, the dibucaine number does not reflect the quantity of pseudocholinesterase present, but rather the quality of the enzyme, that is, its ability to hydrolyze succinylcholine. There are other genetically abnormal pseudocholinesterases. For example, patients with a

TABLE 12-10. Relationship Between Dibucaine Number and Duration of Succinylcholine Neuromuscular Blockade

Type of Pseudocholinesterase	Frequency	Dibucaine Number[a]	Response to Succinylcholine
Homozygous typical	Normal	80	Normal
Heterozygous	1/480	50	Slightly prolonged
Homozygous atypical	1/3,200	20	Markedly prolonged

[a] The dibucaine number indicates the percentage of enzyme inhibited.

fluoride-resistant enzyme or silent enzyme can have a markedly prolonged response to succinylcholine.[217]

Two other topics deserve mention. Hexafluorenium is a nondepolarizing muscle relaxant that also inhibits pseudocholinesterase. Because of this latter effect, hexafluorenium has been used to prolong the effect of succinylcholine in an attempt to reduce the total dose. Although some clinicians have used this approach successfully, it has not proved particularly advantageous and has not gained widespread popularity.

Cardiovascular Effects

Succinylcholine-induced cardiac arrhythmias are many and varied. The drug stimulates all cholinergic autonomic receptors: nicotinic receptors in both sympathetic and parasympathetic ganglia[161] and muscarinic receptors in the sinus node of the heart. In low doses, both a negative inotropic and a chronotropic response occurs that can be attenuated by prior administration of atropine. With large doses, these effects may become positive.[162] One prominent clinical manifestation of this generalized autonomic stimulation is the development of cardiac arrhythmias. These are principally manifest as sinus bradycardia, junctional rhythms, and ventricular arrhythmias, ranging from unifocal premature ventricular contractions to ventricular fibrillation in certain special circumstances. Reports of clinical studies have noted these arrhythmias under various conditions in the presence of intense autonomic stimulus of tracheal intubation; it is not entirely clear whether the cardiac irregularities are due to the action of succinylcholine alone or to the added presence of extraneous autonomic stimulation.

Sinus Bradycardia

The autonomic mechanism involved in sinus bradycardia is stimulation of cardiac muscarinic receptors in the sinus node, particularly in nonatropinized, relatively sympathotonic subjects, such as children.[218,219] Sinus bradycardia has also been noted in adults[220] and appears more commonly after a second dose of the drug given approximately 5 minutes after the first. The bradycardia may be prevented by thiopental,[221] atropine, ganglion-blocking drugs, and nondepolarizing muscle relaxants,[221,222] the implication being that direct myocardial effects, increased muscarinic stimulation, and ganglionic stimulation may all be involved in the bradycardic response. The higher incidence of bradycardia after a second dose of succinylcholine[222] suggests that the hydrolysis products of succinylcholine (succinylmonocholine and choline) sensitize the heart.

Nodal (Junctional) Rhythms

Nodal rhythms commonly occur as bradycardias that are slower than the sinus rate measured before the administration of succinylcholine and intubation of the trachea. The mechanism probably involves relatively greater stimulation of cholinergic receptors in the sinus node, the result being suppression of the sinus mechanism and emergence of the atrioventricular node as the pacemaker. The incidence of junctional rhythm is higher after a second dose of succinylcholine but is prevented by prior administration of dTC.[221,222]

Ventricular Arrhythmias

Under stable anesthetic conditions, succinylcholine lowers the threshold of the ventricle to catecholamine-induced arrhythmias in the monkey and in the dog. Circulating catecholamine levels increase fourfold and potassium increases by one-third after succinylcholine administration in dogs.[223] Other autonomic stimuli, such as endotracheal intubation, hypoxia, hypercarbia, and operations, are probably additive to the effect of succinylcholine. To these stimuli must be added the possible influence of such drugs as digitalis, tricyclic antidepressants, monamine oxidase inhibitors, exogenous catecholamines, and anesthetic drugs such as halothane and cyclopropane, all of which may lower the ventricular threshold for ectopic activity or increase the arrhythmogenic effect of the catecholamines. The influence of digitalis has been questioned, however. Ventricular escape beats may also occur as a result of severe sinus and atrioventricular nodal slowing secondary to succinylcholine administration. The incidence of ventricular arrhythmias is further encouraged by the release of potassium from skeletal muscle as a consequence of the depolarizing action of the drug.

Complications

Hyperkalemia

Clinical reports and experimental studies have clearly shown that in patients with certain diseases or conditions an exaggerated release of potassium in response to succinylcholine may occur, occasionally of such magnitude that cardiac arrest ensues. Conditions especially susceptible to hyperkalemic response from succinylcholine are burns, trauma, nerve damage, neuromuscular disease, closed head injury, intra-abdominal infections, and renal failure.

Burns

With both denervation and burn injuries, a marked increase in receptor density occurs over the entire muscle surface. The result is hypersensitivity to depolarizing muscle relaxant (succinylcholine) and resistance to nondepolarizing muscle relaxant. Consequently, burn patients may have a significant increase in serum potassium after being given succinylcholine at levels as high as 13 mEq/L, a condition that has led to several cases of cardiac arrest. However, this susceptibility to hyperkalemia exists only between about 10 and 60 days postburn, is dose related, and varies directly with the extent of the burn.[224–226] Pretreatment with nondepolarizing muscle relaxants is not effective. Despite this evidence, our rule of thumb is that succinylcholine should not be given to a patient who has had a burn for longer than 1 week. The 60-day rule of thumb is only valid if the burn heals without infection. If infection is present, tissues are probably continuing to degenerate; in that case, the 60-day rule for delaying administration of succinylcholine should be extended.

Trauma

Birch et al.[227] studied soldiers who had undergone trauma associated with the Vietnam War and found that a significant increase in serum potassium did not occur in 59 patients until about 1 week after injury, at which time a progressive increase in the serum potassium level occurred after infusion of succinylcholine. Three weeks after injury, three of these patients with especially severe injuries showed a marked hyperkalemia (increase >3.6 mEq/L) sufficient to cause cardiac arrest. Birch and co-workers found that administration of dTC (6 mg intravenously) prevented the hyperkalemic response to succinylcholine.[227] As with burns, in the absence of infection or persistent degeneration of tissue, a patient is susceptible probably for 60 days following trauma or until adequate healing of damaged muscle has occurred.

Nerve Damage or Neuromuscular Disease

Cooperman[228] described 40 patients with neuromuscular disease, 15 of whom had an increase in serum potassium from 1 to 6 mEq/L after intravenous administration of succinylcholine (1 mg/kg). In another instance, Cooperman et al.[229] reported a hyperkalemic response, one of which was 9.05 mEq/L, in three patients with hemiplegia or paraplegia secondary to upper motor neuron lesions. These investigators concluded that the vulnerable period appears to be within the first 6 months after the onset of hemiplegia or paraplegia and within a longer period of time in patients with progressive disease such as muscular dystrophy. Cooperman and co-workers[229] speculated that in the latter instance, progressive muscle wasting or other structural change accounted for the prolonged susceptibility. They also found the degree of hyperkalemia to correlate directly with the degree and extent of muscle affected. The greatest extent of hyperkalemia was found in those patients with greater neurologic deficit and involvement of more muscle mass. For an in-depth discussion of the clinical and pathophysiologic aspects of succinylcholine-induced hyperkalemia, the reader is referred to an excellent review by Gronert and Theye.[230]

Closed Head Injury

Stevenson and Birch[231] described a well-documented case of a marked hyperkalemic response to succinylcholine in a patient with a closed head injury without peripheral paralysis. One should be hesitant in concluding that succinylcholine should not be given to a patient with a closed head injury on the basis of this single case report. However, because this case was well documented, a high degree of suspicion should exist when giving succinylcholine to this group of patients.

Intra-abdominal Infections

Kohlschütter et al.[232] found that four of nine patients with severe abdominal infections had an increase in serum potassium (2.5 to 3.1 mEq/L) from succinylcholine. These workers concluded that in the case of intra-abdominal infection persisting for longer than 1 week, the possibility of hyperkalemic response to succinylcholine should be considered.

Renal Failure

Several case reports suggest that patients with renal failure are susceptible to a hyperkalemic response to succinylcholine.[233,234] Nevertheless, more controlled studies showed patients not to be any more susceptible to an exaggerated response to succinylcholine than those with normal renal function.[235-240] Korde and Waud[238] concluded that patients with a serum potassium above 5.5 mEq/L should not only not be given succinylcholine but should not be anesthetized either. However, no data were presented to support this conclusion. In the author's (RDM's) experience in anesthetizing hundreds of patients with renal failure, succinylcholine is often the muscle relaxant of choice because of its lack of dependence on renal excretion for its elimination. One might postulate that patients who have uremic neuropathy may be susceptible to succinylcholine-induced hyperkalemia, although the evidence supporting this view is scanty.[239,240]

Increased Intraocular Pressure

Succinylcholine, given by itself, usually causes an increase in intraocular pressure (IOP). The increased IOP is manifested 1 minute after injection, peaks between the second and fourth minute, and subsides by the sixth minute.[241] The mechanism by which succinylcholine increases IOP has not been clearly defined, but it is known to involve contraction of tonic myofibrils or transient dilation of choroidal blood vessels. Apparently, sublingual administration of nifedipine will attenuate the increase in IOP from succinylcholine, which suggests a circulatory mechanism.[242] Despite this increase in IOP, use of succinylcholine for eye operations is not contraindicated unless the anterior chamber is open. Numerous investigators have found that prior administration of a subparalyzing dose of nondepolarizing muscle relaxant (e.g., gallamine, 20 mg; dTC, 3 mg; or pancuronium, 2 mg) will prevent the increase in IOP from succinylcholine.[243,244] Yet Meyers et al.[245] were unable to confirm the efficacy of this approach. Despite this discrepancy, the senior author (RDM) has successfully used this approach many times in providing anesthesia for patients with eye surgery. Furthermore, Libonati et al.[246] described the anesthetic management of 73 patients with penetrating eye injuries who also received succinylcholine; no loss of global contents resulted. Thus, despite the theoretical objections expressed by Meyers and co-workers,[245] Libonati et al.[246] and the author (RDM) conclude that use of succinylcholine in patients with penetrating eye injuries with a carefully controlled rapid-sequence induction of anesthesia (including pretreatment with a nondepolarizing muscle relaxant) is an acceptable technique. Also, the reader should consult Chapter 64. As part of the total picture, succinylcholine is only one of many factors, which includes endotracheal intubation and "bucking" on the tube, that may elevate IOP.[245] Of prime importance is ensuring that the patient is well anesthetized and is not straining. There are several approaches to accomplish this goal.

There are probably three situations in which succinylcholine should either be avoided or the above measures taken to prevent its increasing IOP: if the patient is about to undergo repair of an ocular laceration, if the patient is about to have repair of a recent surgical incision that is coming apart, and if the patient's anesthesia lightens during intraocular surgery. In the last case, succinylcholine should not be given to quiet the patient, but the surgeon should be asked to pause while anesthesia is deepened without the use of muscle relaxants.[247]

Increased Intragastric Pressure

Unlike the rather consistent increase in IOP, the increase in intragastric pressure (IGP) from succinylcholine is quite variable (Fig. 12-19). In fact, Miller and Way[248] found that 11 of 30 patients essentially had no increase in IGP. Yet 5 of 30 patients had an increase in IGP greater than 30 cmH$_2$O. The increase in IGP from succinylcholine appeared to be related to the intensity of fasciculations. Accordingly, when fasciculations were prevented by prior administration of gallamine (20 mg) or dTC (3 mg), no increase in IGP was observed.

The increase in IGP from succinylcholine is presumed to be due to fasciculation of the abdominal skeletal muscle. This is not surprising, since more coordinated abdominal skeletal muscle activity (such as straight-leg raising) may increase IGP to values as high as 120 cmH$_2$O. In addition to skeletal muscle fasciculations, the ACh-like effect of succinylcholine may be partly responsible for the observed increases in IGP. Greenan[249] observed consistent increases in IGP of 4 to 7 cmH$_2$O with direct vagal stimulation. Therefore, prior administration of vagolytic drugs may partly inhibit succinylcholine-induced increases in IGP. Thus, gallamine or pancuronium, with their vagolytic actions, should be more effective than dTC in preventing the increase in IGP. This hypothesis has not been tested, however.

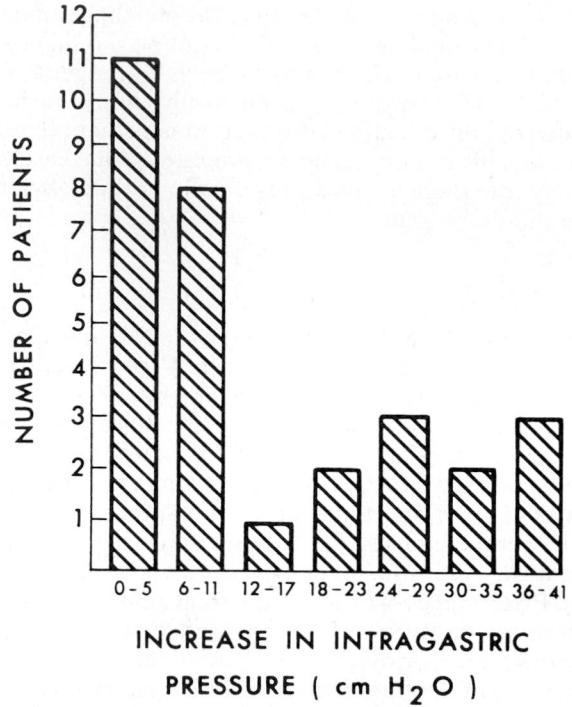

Fig. 12-19. Change in intragastric pressure from succinylcholine administration. Note that only a few patients had large increases in intragastric pressure. (From Miller and Way,[248] with permission.)

Are the increases in IGP following succinylcholine administration enough to cause incompetence of the gastroesophageal junction? Generally IGP of greater than 28 cmH$_2$O is required to overcome the competence of the gastroesophageal junction. However, when the normal oblique angle of entry of the esophagus into the stomach is altered, as may occur with pregnancy, an abdomen distended by ascites or bowel obstruction, obesity, or a hiatus hernia, the IGP required to cause incompetence of the gastroesophageal junction is frequently less than 15 cmH$_2$O.[248] Under these circumstances, regurgitation of stomach contents following succinylcholine is a distinct possibility, and precautionary measures should be taken to prevent fasciculations.

A different view of succinylcholine-induced increased IGP and its importance is expressed in Chapter 40. While there is no question that IGP increases, Gibbs and Modell (in Ch. 40) state that there is a reactive increase in esophageal pressure above the sphincter and, therefore, no net decrease in pressure across the sphincter. This leads them to conclude that there is no need for a prior small dose of nondepolarizing muscle relaxant. Because aspiration of gastric contents is not common, the efficacy of different approaches is difficult to determine. Clearly IGP does increase following succinylcholine, although the clinical importance is unknown.

Apparently succinylcholine does not increase IGP appreciably in infants and children.[250] This may be related to the minimal or absence of fasciculations from succinylcholine in these age groups.[250]

Muscle Pains

The incidence of muscle pains following administration of succinylcholine varies from 0.2 to 89 percent.[251] It occurs more frequently following minor surgery, especially in women and in ambulatory rather than bedridden patients. Waters and Mapleson[252] postulated that the pain is secondary to damage produced in muscle by the unsynchronized contraction of adjacent muscle fibers just before the onset of paralysis. That damage to muscle may occur has been substantiated by finding myoglobinemia following succinylcholine, especially in children anesthetized with halothane.[253] If this hypothesis is valid, the prevention of fasciculations should eliminate muscle pain from succinylcholine. Prior administration of a subparalyzing dose of nondepolarizing muscle relaxant clearly prevents fasciculation from succinylcholine.[254] Yet the efficacy of this approach in preventing muscle pains is questionable. Although some investigators claim that pretreatment with a subparalyzing dose of nondepolarizing muscle relaxant has no effect,[251] most believe that at least the pain from succinylcholine is attenuated.[252,254]

While the above approach emphasizes prior administration of a nondepolarizing muscle relaxant, many other approaches (too numerous to cite here) have been recommended including prior administration of aspirin.[255] The effectiveness of these approaches is difficult to quantitate when the incidence of muscle pain is so variable. In fact, Zahl and Apfelbaum[256] found that avoiding succinylcholine in favor of vecuronium did not decrease the incidence of muscle pains in women undergoing laparoscopy, placing greater emphasis on factors other than the choice of muscle relaxant.

Miller[257] believes the practice of preceding succinylcholine administration with a small dose of nondepolarizing muscle relaxant should be routine. The fasciculations certainly in no way are desirable. Furthermore, postoperative muscle pains and elevated IOP and IGP will be decreased or eliminated. Succinylcholine-induced increases in serum creatinine phosphokinase and myoglobinuria may be attenuated as well. Although the succinylcholine dose should be increased by 30 to 50 percent, this appears to present no problems[257] (Table 12-9). Occasionally patients may be very sensitive to these small doses of nondepolarizing muscle relaxants. Obviously, one should not assume that these small doses of nondepolarizing muscle relaxants will never cause a clinically significant block. Therefore, it almost goes without saying that these small, usually subparalyzing, doses of nondepolarizing muscle relaxants should not be administered in the absence of equipment for resuscitation.[258]

Intracranial Pressure (Also See Ch. 54)

Succinylcholine clearly increases intracranial pressure.[259] The mechanisms and clinical significance of this transient increase are unknown. Thus, there is no agreement as to whether succinylcholine should be given to patients in whom an increase in intracranial pressure may be harmful.

Masseter Spasm

Succinylcholine causes masseter spasm, especially in children.[260] In all likelihood, this is an exaggerated response at the neuromuscular junction and cannot be used to establish a diagnosis of malignant hyperthermia.

Interaction with Nondepolarizing Muscle Relaxants, Neostigmine, and Pyridostigmine

Nondepolarizing (atracurium, pancuronium, and vecuronium) and depolarizing (succinylcholine and decamethonium) muscle relaxants are antagonistic[261,262] or additive,[263] depending on the experimental design. Both types of relaxants are administered concomitantly in three possible situations:

1. Succinylcholine is commonly given to facilitate intubation of the trachea, and then a longer-acting nondepolarizing muscle relaxant such as vecuronium or pancuronium is administered. Presumably the block from a nondepolarizing muscle relaxant will not be altered if given after the block from succinylcholine has dissipated; however, Katz[263] reported that prior administration of succinylcholine nearly doubled the depression of twitch height from the same dose of pancuronium. A comparable increase in duration of block occurred. Yet, the duration of action of doxacurium was unaffected by prior administration of succinylcholine.[264] The reason for this difference is not clear. Also, whether this difference represents a real pharmacologic difference between pancuronium and doxacurium or whether the difference reflects experimental design is not clear.

2. A small dose of nondepolarizing agent is commonly given before administration of succinylcholine to prevent some of the adverse effects of the latter. This approach is discussed in the section on muscle pains.

3. *d*-Tubocurarine can be injected for prolonged relaxation, and then the shorter-acting succinylcholine can be given to facilitate closure of the peritoneum. The amount of succinylcholine required for adequate relaxation is directly dependent on the amount of residual dTC effect present.[261] Despite the questionable pharmacologic reasoning, concomitant administration of an antagonist and agonist in appropriate doses appears to be effective.[257] Whether it is the best way to solve the problem is the subject of much debate. Many prefer to give an additional dose of nondepolarizer that can be

easily antagonized at the end of the operation or to deepen anesthesia. The latter approach is our preference.

Another interaction with succinylcholine involves neostigmine or pyridostigmine. For example, after dTC has been used for an intra-abdominal surgery of long duration and the neuromuscular blockade has been reversed by neostigmine, the surgeon announces that another 15 minutes is needed to retrieve a remaining sponge. Should succinylcholine be given? Our experience is that succinylcholine (100 mg/70 kg, given intravenously) produces a neuromuscular blockade that normally lasts 5 to 10 minutes but will last up to 60 minutes when given soon after administration of neostigmine. Sunew and Hicks[265] found that the effect of succinylcholine (1 mg/kg) was prolonged from 11 to 35 minutes when given 5 minutes after administration of neostigmine (5 mg). This can partly be explained by inhibition of pseudocholinesterase by neostigmine and to a lesser extent by pyridostigmine.

Clinical Management

The changing characteristics of a succinylcholine neuromuscular blockade from a clinical point of view have been nicely reviewed by Lee and Katz[266] (Table 12-11).

Although the response to tetanic stimuli can be used, train-of-four stimulation has proved a very useful guide in detecting the transition from a phase I to a phase II block (Table 12-11). Clearly, both the dose and time of administration of succinylcholine are important variables, although the relative contribution of each has not been established. Practically, if the use of the drug is terminated shortly after train-of-four fade is clearly evident, rapid return of normal neuromuscular function will ensue. Also, the decision whether to attempt antagonism of a phase II block has always been controversial. However, it is now clear that if the train-of-four ratio is less than 0.4, administration of edrophonium or neostigmine results in prompt antagonism. Ramsey et al.[267] recommend that antagonism of a succinylcholine-induced phase II block with edrophonium or neostigmine be attempted after spontaneous recovery of the twitch has been observed for 20 to 30 minutes and has reached a plateau phase with further recovery proceeding slowly. These workers state that in this situation,

edrophonium and neostigmine invariably produce "dramatic" acceleration of the return of the train-of-four toward normal. According to Ramsey et al.,[267] the dosage guideline in Table 12-11 applies only to halothane or to enflurane anesthesia. With nitrous oxide intravenous anesthesia, the dosage guidelines are more variable. In any event, monitoring neuromuscular function via peripheral nerve stimulation, such as the train-of-four, will help avoid succinylcholine overdose, detect development of a phase II block, observe its rate of recovery, and assess the effect of edrophonium or neostigmine on recovery from a phase II block.

ANTAGONISM OF A NONDEPOLARIZING NEUROMUSCULAR BLOCKADE

The criteria for determining whether a block has been antagonized have been described in the section, *Monitoring Neuromuscular Function*. Neostigmine and pyridostigmine antagonize a nondepolarizing neuromuscular blockade by increasing the availability of ACh at the muscle endplate mainly by inhibition of AChE and to a much lesser extent by increased release of transmitter from the motor nerve terminals. The reader should consult Chapter 20 for more details regarding the mechanisms of action of these antagonists.

Factors That May Interfere with Antagonism

Our approach is not to give more antagonist if edrophonium (35 to 70 mg/70 kg), neostigmine (2.5 to 5.0 mg/70 kg), or pyridostigmine (10 to 20 mg/70 kg) fails to antagonize the block. These doses maximally inhibit AChE, and larger doses may cause a block themselves.[268] If these doses fail to antagonize the block, the cause of the inadequate antagonism should be sought. Some of these cases are listed below.

Intensity of Neuromuscular Blockade

The degree of neuromuscular blockade at the time that neostigmine is administered determines the speed and extent of antagonistic action by neostigmine. When twitch height is more than 20 percent of control, time

TABLE 12-11. Clinical Characteristics of a Phase I and Phase II Neuromuscular Blockade from Succinylcholine

Characteristic	Phase I	Transition	Phase II
Tetanic stimulation	No face	Slight fade	Fade
Post-tetanic facilitation	None	Slight	Yes
Train-of-four	Slight fade	Moderate fade	Marked fade
Train-of-four ratio	>0.7	0.4–0.7	<0.4
Edrophonium	Augment	Little effect	Antagonize
Recovery	Rapid	Rapid	Increasingly prolonged
Dose requirements (mg/kg)	2–3	4–5	≥6

(Adapted from Lee and Katz,[330] with permission.)

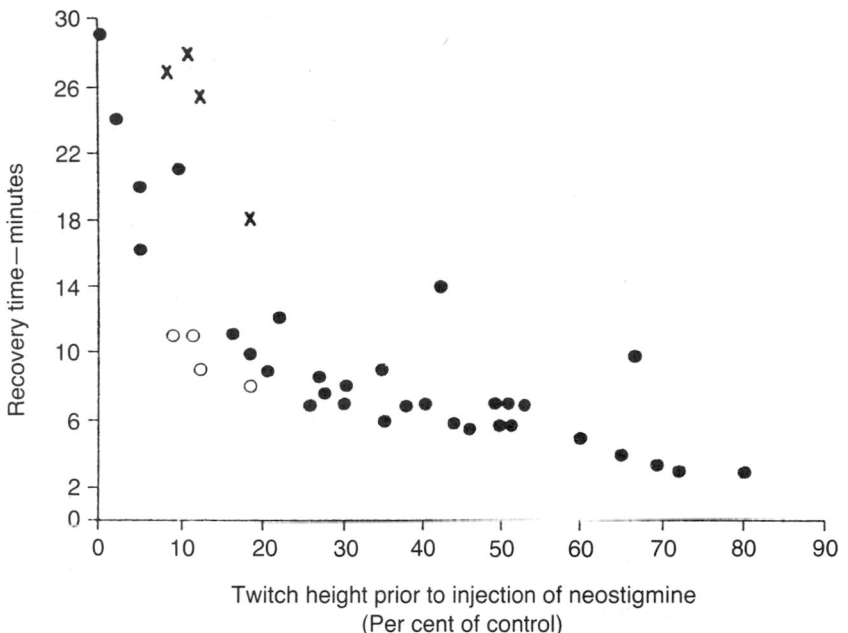

Fig. 12-20. Correlation between twitch height when a bolus of neostigmine (2.5 mg) was given intravenously and time it took for twitch height to return to its control height. (From Katz,[269] with permission.)

from neostigmine administration (2.5 mg) to attainment of control twitch height is 3 to 14 minutes. When twitch heights are less than 20 percent of control, recovery takes 8 to 29 minutes (Fig. 12-20).[269] Our observations indicate that most attempts to antagonize the block occur in the face of a 90 to 100 percent depression of twitch tension. It should not be surprising if 30 to 45 minutes is required for twitch height to return to control levels, or even longer for a sustained contraction in response to a tetanic stimulus of 50 Hz. Edrophonium has gained popularity as an antagonist because of its rapid onset and lesser atropine requirement. However, Rupp et al.[270] recently found that edrophonium is not as effective in antagonizing profound (twitch tension greater than 90 percent depression) neuromuscular blockades, especially from pancuronium and vecuronium.

When the dose of edrophonium was increased from 0.5 to 1.0 mg/kg, edrophonium was effective in antagonizing an intense neuromuscular blockade (Fig. 12-21). Whether even this dose of edrophonium is really as effective as neostigmine is controversial. Clearly, the relative potencies of edrophonium and neostigmine differ at various intensities of blockade (Fig. 12-22).[271]

Acid-Base State

Respiratory acidosis may augment a nondepolarizing neuromuscular blockade but, more importantly, limits and prevents its antagonism (Fig. 12-23).[272,273] In other words, it is impossible to antagonize a nondepolarizing neuromuscular blockade in the presence of significant respiratory acidoses ($PaCO_2$ greater than 50 mmHg). This has many clinical ramifications. For example, if a patient hypoventilates in the recovery room, attempts to antagonize a residual dTC block may fail. Administration of narcotics to relieve pain may increase the likelihood of this untoward event. Such a sequence contains an element of potential positive feedback in which respiratory depression produces more acidosis and relaxant effect, hence, more respiratory depression.

Although metabolic acidosis might also be predicted to prevent antagonism by neostigmine, this has not been substantiated.[272,273] To our surprise, metabolic alkalosis, but not metabolic acidosis, prevented neostigmine antagonism of dTC and pancuronium (Fig. 12-23).[272,273] These results suggest that extracellular hydrogen ion concentration (pH) per se may not be as important as changes in electrolytes and intracellular pH. Metabolic alkalosis produced by infusion of sodium bicarbonate will also decrease levels of extracellular potassium and calcium. We recently found that if calcium and potassium levels are not permitted to decrease, metabolic alkalosis does nothing to a pancuronium-induced neuromuscular blockade or to its antagonism by neostigmine. These findings suggest that looking at extracellular pH alone is insufficient to predict the effect of acid-base changes on neostigmine antagonism of nondepolarizing muscle relaxants. Frequently, a bolus of bicarbonate will transiently increase twitch tension. In such cases, it is concluded that meta-

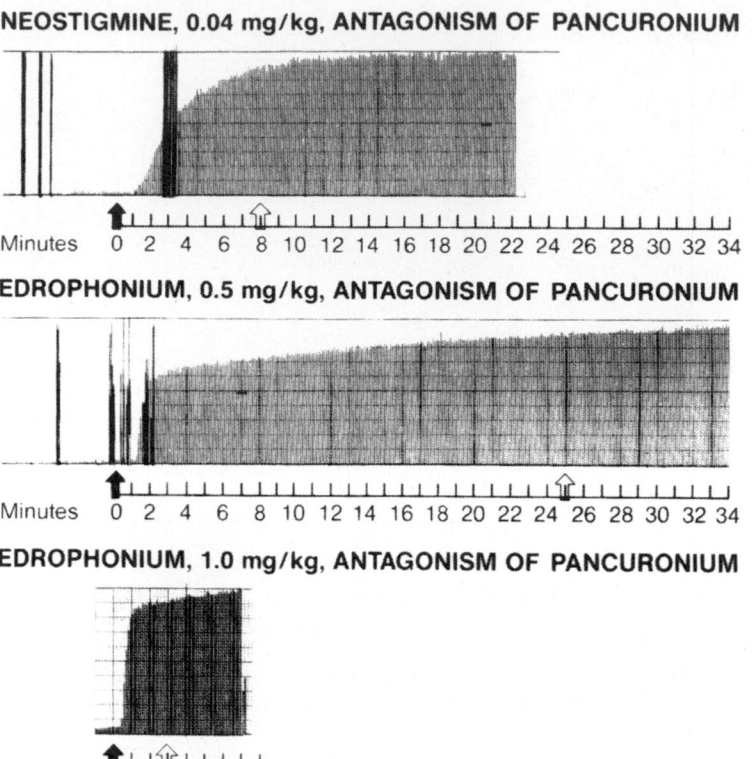

NEOSTIGMINE, 0.04 mg/kg, ANTAGONISM OF PANCURONIUM

Minutes   0 2 4 6 8 10 12 14 16 18 20 22 24 26 28 30 32 34

EDROPHONIUM, 0.5 mg/kg, ANTAGONISM OF PANCURONIUM

Minutes   0 2 4 6 8 10 12 14 16 18 20 22 24 26 28 30 32 34

EDROPHONIUM, 1.0 mg/kg, ANTAGONISM OF PANCURONIUM

Minutes   0 2 4 6 8

Fig. 12-21. Illustrations of neostigmine and edrophonium reversal of a profound (greater than 95 percent) neuromuscular blockade. While edrophonium (0.5 mg/kg) produced an immediate partial reversal, a plateau was rapidly reached (about 60 percent of control twitch tension). While neostigmine produced a slower antagonism, it was more complete. Increasing the dose of edrophonium produced a more complete antagonism, but a plateau still occurred at 85 percent of control twitch tension. (From Rupp et al.,[270] with permission.)

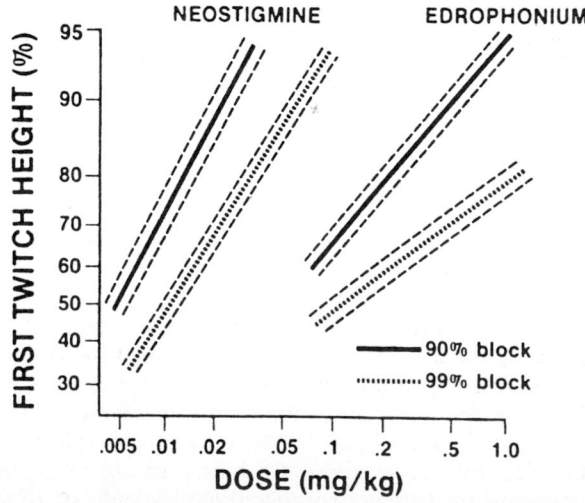

Fig. 12-22. First twitch height (logit scale) versus dose (log scale) 10 minutes after administration of neostigmine and edrophonium given at either 1 percent (99 percent block) or 10 percent (90 percent block) first twitch recovery. Thin dashed lines represent the standard error of estimate for the mean. (From Donati et al.,[271] with permission.)

bolic alkalosis antagonizes a nondepolarizing block. We submit that this type of study bears little or no relationship to the clinical situation in which metabolic alkalosis has existed for several hours or days with associated electrolyte abnormalities. What does the clinician do with such confusing information concerning metabolic acid-base changes? Because so many factors are involved, the simplest and most obvious advice is to maintain a normal acid-base state.

Electrolyte Imbalance

Although it has been the subject of several review articles,[273,274] few data are available on the effect of electrolyte imbalance on a nondepolarizing neuromuscular blockade and its antagonism by neostigmine. Low extracellular concentrations of potassium apparently enhance the block from nondepolarizing muscle relaxants and diminish the ability of neostigmine to antagonize the block. This prediction is based on the increase in endplate transmembrane potential that results from a higher ratio of intracellular to extracellular potassium. Thus, a decrease in extracellular potassium

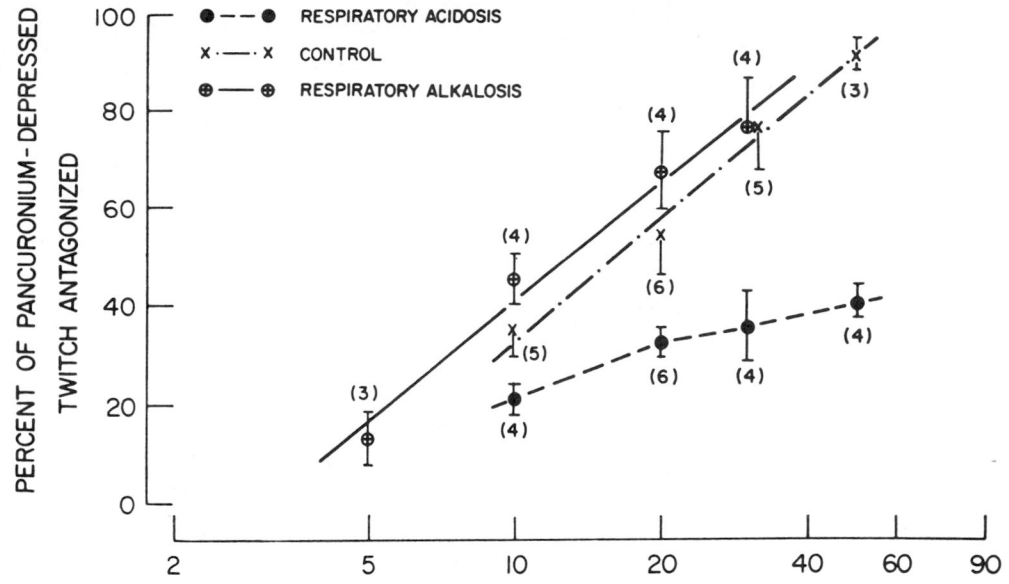

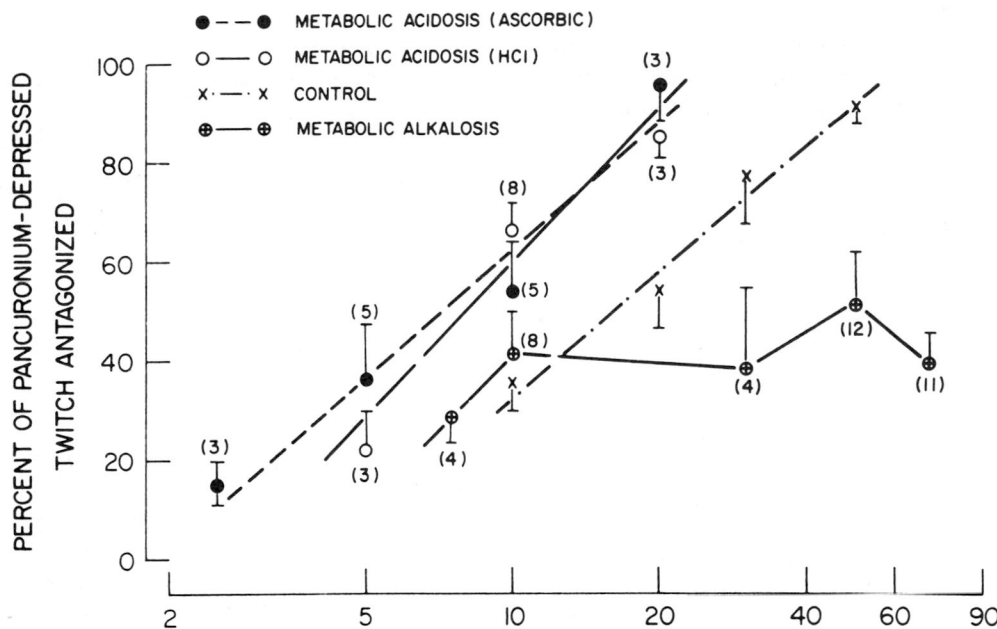

Fig. 12-23. Influence of changes in acid–base status on the ability of neostigmine to antagonize a pancuronium neuromuscular blockade. Note that with respiratory acidosis and metabolic alkalosis, neostigmine, even in large doses, does not antagonize the blood. (From Miller and Roderick,[273] with permission.)

causes hyperpolarization and increases resistance to depolarization. However, the endplate is only one aspect of the contractile mechanism, the remainder of which may be affected in a contrary fashion. For example, a low extracellular potassium level should also increase the transmembrane potential of the motor nerve terminal. Although the threshold for depolarization is increased once depolarization occurs, the nerve action potential will be larger, and this should augment ACh release and postjunctional depolarization. Which of the opposing prejunctional and postjunctional changes from hypokalemia are dominant is difficult to ascertain. Furthermore, patients with an imbalance in potassium may have other diseases or injuries that alter their response to muscle relaxants (e.g., patients with burns) (Fig. 12-24).

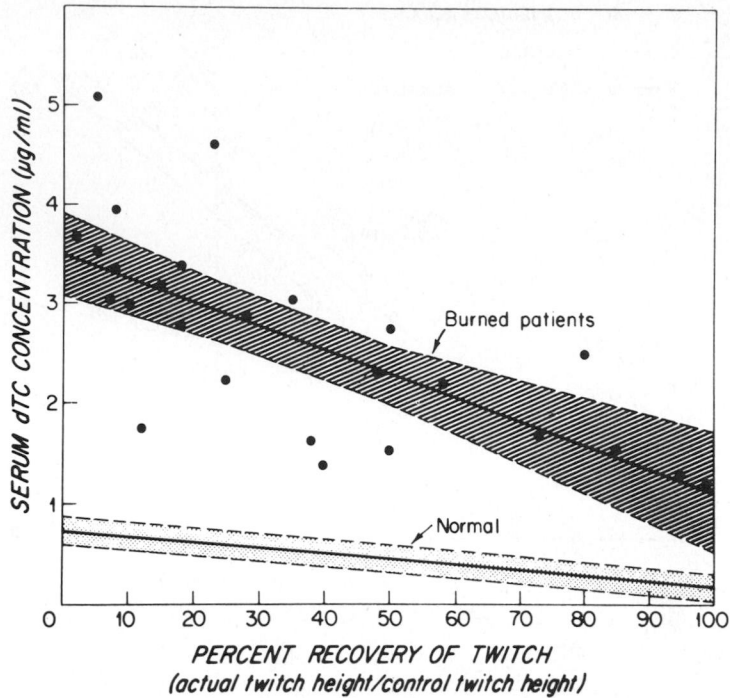

Fig. 12-24. Correlation between serum concentration of *d*-tubocurarine and percentage of depression of twitch height in patients with and without burns. Note that the burned patients appear to be relatively resistant to *d*-tubocurarine. (From Martyn et al.,[348] with permission.)

Cohen[275] and Feldman[274] speculate that, in chronic diseases, both intracellular and extracellular potassium decrease without affecting transmembrane potential. Therefore, the response to muscle relaxants and their antagonists should be normal. However, the muscle transmembrane potentials are changed in patients who are severely ill or even bedridden for a few days.[276] Also, severe dehydration should concentrate the relaxant present in plasma, thereby increasing muscle relaxant activity.

As with acid-base studies, a common error with some studies, in our opinion, is to administer a bolus of some electrolyte such as potassium and to assume that the result resembles the clinical problem of chronic hyperkalemia, which may be present in a patient for hours or days. Studies in these types of patients are difficult because many factors exist that may alter muscle relaxant action. We attempted to develop an animal model that would stimulate the type of chronic hypokalemia that anesthesiologists may observe in patients. Cats were given a diuretic without potassium supplement for 15 days. We found that less pancuronium was required for neuromuscular blockade and more neostigmine for antagonism.[277] Even though the differences were small, we were always able to antagonize the block completely. Assuming that this animal model approximates the clinical situation, changes in potassium appear to be of minor consequence.

Summary

In view of these factors and the pharmacokinetic factors discussed in the section on the pharmacology of nondepolarizing muscle relaxants, more than 70 mg/70 kg of edrophonium, 5 mg/70 kg of neostigmine, or 20 mg/70 kg of pyridostigmine should not be given unless certain questions have been answered: (1) Has enough time been allowed for the neostigmine or pyridostigmine to antagonize the block, that is, at least 15 to 30 minutes? (2) Is the neuromuscular blockade too intense to be antagonized? (3) What is the acid-base electrolyte status? (4) What is the temperature? (5) Is the patient receiving any drugs that may make antagonism difficult? (6) Has excretion of the relaxant been reduced? Quite often, answers to these questions will provide the reason for failure of neostigmine or pyridostigmine to antagonize the nondepolarizing neuromuscular blockade.

Cardiovascular Effects of Antagonism

Because only the nicotinic effects of edrophonium, neostigmine, and pyridostigmine are desired, the muscarinic effects must be blocked by atropine or glycopyrrolate. Atropine induces its vagolytic effect much more rapidly than does glycopyrrolate. To minimize cardiovascular changes, we believe atropine is better suited with the rapid-acting edrophonium and glycopyrrolate with the slower-acting neostigmine and pyridostigmine. In general, 7 µg/kg of atropine should be given with 0.5 to 1.0 mg/kg of edrophonium.[278] Glycopyrrolate (7 µg/kg) should be given with neostigmine (0.035 to 0.07 mg/kg). Giving atropine with neostigmine will induce an initial tachycardia,[279] and giving glycopyrrolate with edrophonium will induce an initial bradycardia. These are only guidelines; certainly arrhythmias can occur and doses should be readjusted accordingly.[280-282] Perhaps lower doses of neostigmine (e.g., 1.25 mg/70 kg) are equally effective as the traditional 2.5 to 5.0 mg/70 kg dose.[283] If so, perhaps the dose of vagolytic drug could be reduced and fewer arrhythmias occur.

Pharmacokinetics of Neostigmine, Pyridostigmine, and Edrophonium

The pharmacokinetics of edrophonium, neostigmine, and pyridostigmine are summarized in Table 12-12.[284-286] Several important clinical conclusions can be derived from these data.

1. The longer duration of action of pyridostigmine probably has a pharmacokinetic basis in view of the longer elimination half-life.[284,285]

2. By comparing elimination half-lives in patients with and without renal failure, we conclude that renal excretion accounts for about 50 percent of excretion of neostigmine and about 75 percent of that of pyridostigmine and edrophonium. Of prime importance clinically is that renal failure delays plasma clearance of neostigmine, pyridostigmine, and edrophonium as much as if not more than that of pancuronium and dTC. Therefore, if proper doses of anticholinesterase drugs are given and overdoses of muscle relaxants are avoided, renal failure should not be associated with "recurarization."[284,285]

3. Edrophonium has long been thought not to be a suitable antagonist because its duration of action is too short. However, when larger doses (i.e., 0.5 to 1.0 mg/kg) are used, sustained antagonism of a nondepolarizing neuromuscular blockade results.[287,288] In fact, the elimination half-life of edrophonium is similar to that of neostigmine or pyridostigmine[284] (Table 12-12). That edrophonium has a quicker onset of action and

probably fewer muscarinic side effects may justify more frequent use of this drug when antagonizing a nondepolarizing neuromuscular blockade.

DRUG INTERACTIONS

So many drugs have been shown to interact with neuromuscular blockers and/or their antagonists in animals that it is beyond the scope of this chapter to review them all. The reader is referred to older excellent reviews on drug interactions for more detailed information.[289,290] Some of the more important drug interactions are discussed below.

Antibiotics

More than 180 reports concerning enhancement of neuromuscular blockade from muscle relaxants by antibiotics have appeared in the literature. Many of the antibiotics have been shown to have a magnesiumlike depression of the evoked release of ACh (prejunctional). Yet these same antibiotics exhibit postjunctional activity.[291-294] Many investigators have attempted to classify antibiotics according to whether the prejunctional or postjunctional activity is dominant. The search for a common mechanism of antibiotic-induced neuromuscular blockade is probably futile because of several possible mechanisms inherent in the variety of antibiotics that can cause blockade. In other words, the mechanisms of neuromuscular blockade are probably different for the various antibiotics, which may account for some of the conflicting suggestions for effective remedies in the case reports (Table 12-13). Despite the intensive and excellent work of Singh et al.[292,293] attempting to elucidate the mechanisms of action of several antibiotics, they can only conclude in one of their publications[293] that

Our present results confirm that the aminoglycoside streptomycin acts primarily by a calcium-reversible prejunctional mechanism, whereas the other antibiotics tested act by different mechanisms. As the nature of the components of mixed pre- and postjunctional block produced by polymyxin B, lincomycin and clindamycin are yet unknown, reversibility of these antibiotics by standard reversal agents remains difficult to predict

TABLE 12-12. The Pharmacokinetics of Neostigmine (N), Pyridostigmine (P), and Edrophonium (E) in Patients Without and With Renal Failure

Measure	Without Renal Failure			With Renal Failure		
	N	P	E	N	P	E
Distribution half-life (min)	3.4	6.7	7.2	2.5	3.9	7.0
Elimination half-life (min)	77	113	110	181	379	304
Volume of central compartment (L/kg)	0.2	0.3	0.3	0.3	0.4	0.3
Total serum clearance (ml/kg/min)	9.1	8.6	9.5	4.8	3.1	3.9

(Data from Refs. 236–238.)

**TABLE 12-13. Interaction Among Antibiotics, Muscle Relaxants,
Neostigmine, and Calcium**

	Increase in Neuromuscular Block		Neuromuscular Block from Antibiotic-*d*Tc Antagonized by:	
Antibiotic	*d*Tc	Sch	Neostigmine	Calcium
Neomycin	Yes	Yes	Usually	Usually
Streptomycin	Yes	Yes	Usually	Usually
Gentamicin	Yes	*a*	Sometimes	Usually
Kanamycin	Yes	Yes	Sometimes	Sometimes
Paromomycin	Yes	*a*	Yes	Yes
Viomycin	Yes	*a*	Yes	Yes
Polymyxin A	Yes	*a*	No	No
Polymyxin B	Yes	Yes	No[b]	No
Colistin	Yes	Yes	No	Sometimes
Tetracycline	Yes	No	Partially	Partially
Lincomycin	Yes	*a*	Partially	Partially
Clindamycin	Yes	*a*	Partially	Partially

Abbreviations: dTC, d-tubocurarine-like drugs, which include other nondepolarizing muscle relaxants; Sch, succinylcholine.
a Not studied.
b Block is augmented by neostigmine.

and in the clinical situation it may be preferable to continue artificial ventilation until the return of spontaneous respiration.

Recently, Dupuis et al.[295] found that gentamicin and tobramycin prolonged a vecuronium but not an atracurium neuromuscular blockade. It is difficult to imagine that antibiotics would affect nondepolarizing muscle relaxants differently; this could be an important observation, and it needs to be confirmed.

Clinical experience with the antibiotics is summarized in Table 12-13. However, our approach to a prolonged neuromuscular blockade involving antibiotics is really quite straightforward. We arbitrarily administer neostigmine up to 5 mg/70 kg; more neostigmine may augment the block. When this is ineffective, ventilation should be controlled until the neuromuscular blockade terminates spontaneously. We no longer recommend the use of calcium for two reasons. First, the antagonism calcium produces usually is not sustained. Second, calcium may antagonize the antibacterial effect of the antibiotics.

Magnesium and Calcium

The effects of magnesium- and calcium-induced alterations of neuromuscular blockade have been studied in animals and in humans. Magnesium sulfate, given for treatment of preeclampsia and eclamptic toxemia, enhances the neuromuscular blocking properties of both dTC and succinylcholine.[296,297] Magnesium decreases the amount of ACh released from the motor nerve terminal, the depolarizing action of ACh on the postjunctional membrane and the excitability of the muscle fiber itself, and the amplitude of the endplate potential.[298] Thus, magnesium enhances dTC-induced blockade by reducing ACh output from the motor nerve terminal and by reducing sensitivity of the postjunctional

membrane. We cannot explain why the action of succinylcholine is enhanced, unless a desensitization block rapidly occurs with high plasma magnesium levels.

Although calcium enhances the release of ACh from the motor nerve terminal and enhances excitation-contraction coupling in muscle,[299] it also stabilizes the postjunctional membrane. This stabilization may explain why calcium only partially antagonizes magnesium-dTC-induced blockade.[297] Calcium is less effective in antagonizing magnesium-succinylcholine-induced blockade and will augment a desensitization block from succinylcholine. Again, this is probably explained by membrane stabilization.[300] A prolonged block should be anticipated when a magnesium-relaxant combination is used, since neostigmine and calcium are only partially effective antagonists.

Local Anesthetics and Antiarrhythmics

In large doses, most local anesthetics block neuromuscular transmission; and in smaller doses, they enhance the neuromuscular block from both nondepolarizing and depolarizing muscle relaxants.[301,302] Telivuo and Katz[301] found an additional decrease in twitch height and tidal volume from lidocaine, mepivacaine, prilocaine, and bupivacaine in patients partially paralyzed with nortoxiferine. Thus, local anesthetics given as antiarrhythmic agents intraoperatively or postoperatively may augment a residual neuromuscular block. The ability of neostigmine to antagonize a combined local anesthetic-relaxant neuromuscular blockade has not been studied.

In low doses, local anesthetics depress post-tetanic potentiation, and this is thought to be a neural, prejunctional effect.[303] With higher doses, local anesthetics block ACh-induced muscular contractions, and this suggests that local anesthetics have a stabilizing effect on the postjunctional membrane.[304] Also, local anesthetics have a direct effect on the muscle membrane by decreasing the strength of contraction of a curarized or denervated muscle in response to a single shock.[305] Procaine has been shown to displace calcium from the sarcolemma and thus inhibit caffeine-induced contraction of skeletal muscle.[306] Most of these mechanisms of action probably apply to all the local anesthetics. In addition, procaine inhibits plasma cholinesterase and may augment the effects of succinylcholine. In essence, local anesthetics have actions on the presynaptic, postjunctional, and muscle membranes.

Several drugs used for the treatment of arrhythmias also augment the block from muscle relaxants, particularly that of dTC.[307] For example, patients have become "recurarized" after receiving quinidine in the recovery room. These cases may represent unrecognized residual curarization that was augmented by the administration of quinidine. Quinidine potentiates the neuromuscular block from both nondepolarizing and depolarizing muscle relaxants.[308] Edrophonium was ineffective in antagonizing a nondepolarizing blockade after quinidine. In these clinical doses, quinidine appears to act at the prejunctional membrane as judged by its lack of effect on ACh-evoked twitch. However, large, nonclinical doses of quinidine given intra-arterially produce a neuromuscular blockade of the depolarizing type, augmented by edrophonium.[309]

While the preceding paragraph places emphasis on quinidine (a rarely used drug), it is not surprising that any drug that influences conduction and the electrical properties of the heart may also influence ion transport at the neuromuscular junction and, therefore, the action of muscle relaxants. Examples of such drugs include β-adrenergic blockers and calcium channel blockers. More specifically, calcium channel blockers do enhance the action of nondepolarizing muscle relaxants.[310] In an in vitro study, Bikhazi et al.[310] suggested that because calcium channel blockers are difficult to remove from muscle, long-term therapy may make reversal of neuromuscular blockade difficult. Although there can be no doubt that these cardiovascular drugs can influence the action of muscle relaxants, the clinical significance of these interactions are difficult to quantitate.

Epilepsy and Psychiatry

Any drug that can influence the CNS could influence other nervous tissue, such as the neuromuscular junction. For example, lithium has been reported to augment the neuromuscular blockade from succinylcholine and some nondepolarizing muscle relaxants.[311] Yet the clinical importance of this interaction has been challenged.[312] Phenytoin has been reported to cause resistance to neuromuscular blocking drugs[313,314]; however, acutely administered phenytoin, in large doses (10 mg/kg intravenously), augments a vecuronium neuromuscular blockade.[315] Clearly, these interactions

are difficult to predict and dictate close monitoring of neuromuscular function when muscle relaxants are given.

Hypotensive Drugs

Both hexamethonium and trimethaphan produce neuromuscular blockade alone and enhance the blockade produced by dTC.[316] However, these studies were performed in the rat diaphragm preparation with large doses of hypotensive drugs. Despite occasional clinical reports,[317] we believe that trimethaphan rarely interacts with muscle relaxants in a clinically significant manner. Nitroglycerine has been found to prolong a pancuronium neuromuscular blockade but not that from any other neuromuscular blocker.[318,319] The mechanisms for this selective action of nitroglycerine have not been elucidated.

Diuretics

In patients undergoing renal transplantation, the intensity and duration of dTC neuromuscular blockade was increased following a dose of furosemide (1 mg/kg intravenously).[320] This has been investigated further with the rat diaphragm and cat soleus preparations. In the rat diaphragm, the concentration of dTC required for neuromuscular blockade is markedly reduced at clinically relevant doses of furosemide. This diuretic has an effect on the nerve terminal (presynaptic) probably relating to the cyclic nucleotide system. Furosemide appears to inhibit the cyclic adenosine monophosphate system and to reduce the output of transmitter, resulting in enhanced dTC blockade. Clinically, this effect has been documented as significant.[320]

By contrast, mannitol appears to have no effect on a nondepolarizing neuromuscular blockade. Furthermore, increasing urine output by administration of mannitol has no effect on the rate of which dTC and presumably other muscle relaxants, are eliminated in the urine.[321] However, this lack of effect on the excretion of dTC should not be surprising. Urinary excretion of dTC depends on glomerular filtration. Mannitol is an osmotic diuretic that exerts its effect by altering the osmotic gradient within the proximal tubules so that water is retained within the tubules. Thus, an increase in urine volume in patients with adequate glomerular filtration would not be expected to increase excretion.

Azathioprine, an immunodepressant drug used in renal transplantation, has a minor antagonistic action on muscle relaxant-induced neuromuscular blockade.[322,323]

Other Nondepolarizing Muscle Relaxants

Many attempts have been made to combine nondepolarizing muscle relaxants, with the thought that they may act in an synergistic manner.[324] Perhaps this synergistic neuromuscular interaction would result in fewer adverse side effects, especially cardiovascular effects. Other studies indicate that an additive effect exists.[325,326] More recently, a synergistic interaction was found between atracurium and vecuronium.[327] Whether this interaction had any clinical benefit remains to be seen.

Dantrolene
(Also See Ch. 28)

Dantrolene, a drug used for the treatment of malignant hyperthermia, depresses skeletal muscle directly and also blocks excitation-contraction coupling. Although it does not block neuromuscular transmission, the mechanical response will be depressed without demonstrating any effect on the electromyogram.[328,329] Nondepolarizing muscle relaxants are enhanced by dantrolene.[330]

DISEASES THAT MAY ALTER MUSCLE RELAXANT ACTION

The following diseases show complex pathophysiology. Only that aspect directly relating to the use of muscle relaxants is discussed.

Myasthenia Gravis

The pathology and therapy of myasthenia gravis are superficially reviewed earlier in this chapter and in Chapter 25. Other investigators have presented excellent reviews of this topic as well.[331-334] As far as muscle relaxants are concerned, myasthenic patients respond as if already partially curarized; they are very sensitive to nondepolarizing and somewhat resistant to depolarizing muscle relaxants.[335,336] When presented with the problem of anesthetizing one of these patients, avoidance of all muscle relaxants is to be preferred. An inhaled anesthetic by itself will generally provide sufficient relaxation of skeletal muscle, including that necessary for endotracheal intubation.[337] Before administering muscle relaxants, the anesthesiologist should be sure that a profound neuromuscular blockade does not already exist; there may be other reasons for inadequate surgical exposure. The status of neuromuscular blockade should be evaluated by use of a peripheral nerve stimulator. If the twitch or train-of-four is already markedly depressed, administration of additional muscle relaxant may induce a block that is difficult to antagonize, particularly in a patient with myasthenia gravis. If additional relaxation is required, we prefer deepening anesthesia. For example, the enflurane concentration could be increased, or administration of a small dose of thiopental may be adequate. If a muscle relaxant is needed, a small dose (atracurium, 3 to 5 mg/70 kg, or vecuronium, 1 to 2 mg/70 kg) can be given, but prolonged weakness should be anticipated. Feldman[338] recommends that because of an unpredictable drug response it is probably safer to ventilate these patients electively during the postoperative period than to resort to giving large doses of anticholinesterase drugs. This recommendation is consistent with our experience and that often described in the literature[339] that surgery and anesthesia often completely alter the states of myasthenia gravis in an unpredictable manner.

Myasthenic Syndrome (Eaton-Lambert Syndrome)

Eaton-Lambert syndrome is an association between carcinomatous conditions (especially oat-cell carcinoma of the bronchus) and motor neuropathy and resembles myasthenia gravis. These patients are unusually sensitive to both nondepolarizing and depolarizing muscle relaxants.

Myotonia

The myotonic syndromes include myotonia congenita, myotonia dystrophica, and paramyotonia congenita. With the latter condition, myotonia appears only upon exposure to cold.

Myotonic dystrophy (atrophica), the most common of the three, is an inherited, autosomal dominant disease. Clinical features include weakness and wasting of the facial, cervical, and proximal limb muscles; frontal baldness; cataracts; gonadal atrophy; thyroid nodules; endocrine failure; and voluntary and percussion myotonia. Continuous, low-voltage activity with high-voltage, fibrillationlike potential bursts will be evident on the electromyogram. A mechanical stimulus will evoke a burst of rhythmic activity of 90 to 100/s, which eventually slows to low-voltage activity, the so-called divebomber effect. Cardiac conduction defects as well as myocardial failure are commonly present. Respiratory involvement is also common, secondary to weakness of skeletal muscles. While the carbon dioxide response curves are normal, mechanical ability is impaired, as reflected by a diminished vital capacity, forced vital capacity in 1 second, and maximum expiratory force. In addition, some patients have weakness of pharyngeal muscles with recurrent aspiration pneumonitis. The onset of the disease is most common in the second to fourth decade and progresses to atrophy in later years.

Anesthetic and operative mortality is increased for several reasons. The most common complication is respiratory failure postoperatively due to decreased mechanical ability, which interferes with deep breathing and coughing. Intraoperatively, cardiac conduction abnormalities may cause hemodynamic instability. Generalized myotonia may follow administration of succinylcholine in some patients. In some cases the severity of the myotonic response has precluded attempts to control ventilation. Although it is difficult to collect a large clinical experience,[340] Mitchell et al.[341] thoroughly evaluated three patients with myotonia dystrophica and their response to muscle relaxants and concluded that (1) the response to nondepolarizing muscle relaxants is normal, (2) patients with myotonia are more likely than normal patients to develop apnea after administration of sedative or anesthetic drugs, and (3) the use of depolarizing muscle relaxants is hazardous because marked generalized contracture of skeletal muscle may develop, preventing adequate airway maintenance and ventilation. Also, the use of anticholinesterases may exacerbate myotonia, although this is not well documented and was not confirmed by Mitchell et al.[341] Should myotonia develop intraoperatively, muscle blockers will not attenuate myotonia, as it is primarily a muscle membrane disease.

Myotonia may also develop in response to percussion or to shivering postoperatively. Local infiltration of the involved muscles with local anesthetics may attenuate percussion myotonia. Quinine and procainamide have been used for generalized myotonia. Although several anesthetic approaches probably are satisfactory, we have used small doses of thiopental and volatile anesthetic, avoiding all muscle relaxants. We believe the trachea should remain intubated until the patient has demonstrated adequate mechanical ventilatory ability postoperatively. Regional anesthesia may be used but will not block the myotonic response. Intravenous regional anesthesia might be useful in appropriate cases and offers the advantage of attenuating the myotonic response. A clinical series, however, has not been reported utilizing this technique.

Familial Periodic Paralysis

Familial periodic paralysis is associated with hyperkalemia, hypokalemia, or normokalemia characterized by intermittent attacks of skeletal muscle weakness and flaccid paralysis, usually sparing the bulbar musculature. With the hypokalemic type, intravenous fluids should avoid a large carbohydrate or salt load and hypokalemia. Postoperatively, if such a patient is weak, it is usually secondary to hypokalemia. Muscle relaxants should generally be avoided, although Siler and Discavage[342] noted a normal response to succinylcholine. By contrast, in hyperkalemic patients carbohydrate stores should be maintained with dextrose-rich, potassium-free intravenous solutions. Muscle relaxants, especially succinylcholine, probably should be avoided. Succinylcholine can cause myotonia in these patients.[343]

Upper and Lower Motor Neuron Disease

The potential hazards of giving succinylcholine to patients with upper or motor neuron disease is described earlier in this chapter. Their response to nondepolarizing muscle relaxants is probably greater than normal. This was well documented by Rosenbaum et al.,[344] who found that dTC (1.5 mg) given over a 30-minute period to a man with amyotrophic lateral sclerosis caused difficulty with speech and swallowing.

Yet lower motor neuron denervation results in a resistance to nondepolarizing muscle relaxants because of a proliferation of acetylcholine receptors.[345] By administering small doses of nondepolarizing muscle relaxants plus monitoring with a peripheral nerve stimulator, the anesthesiologist should be able to avoid significant problems in these patients. However, monitoring with a peripheral nerve stimulator may not be reliable in patients with an upper motor neuron lesion.[346,347] Monitoring of the unaffected limb or other confirmatory measures of neuromuscular blockade should be undertaken in these patients.

Burns

The problems with burns and succinylcholine are well documented. Martyn et al.[348] found that in patients who have sustained burns over more than 25 percent of their body surface area, both the total doses of dTC and serum concentration necessary to attain a given twitch depression are greatly increased (Fig. 12-24). This resistance has been confirmed for several other nondepolarizing muscle relaxants.[349] The mechanism has been attributed to an increase in the density of acetylcholine receptors,[350] although Marathe et al.[351] were unable to confirm this mechanism. Whatever the mechanism is, this is a pharmacodynamic rather than a pharmacokinetic response.

REFERENCES

1. Griffith HR, Johnson GE: The use of curare in general anesthesia. Anesthesiology 3:418, 1942
2. Cullen SC: The use of curare for improvement of abdominal relaxation during halothane anesthesia—report on 131 cases. Surgery 14:261, 1943
3. Beecher HK, Todd DP: A study of deaths with anesthesia and surgery. Ann Surg 140:2, 1954
4. Bogetz MS, Katz JA: Recall of surgery for major trauma. Anesthesiology 61:6, 1984
5. Editorial: On being aware. Br J Anaesth 51:711, 1979
6. Cullen SC, Larson CP, Jr: Essentials of Anesthetic Practice. Year Book Medical Publishers, Chicago, 1974
7. Waud BE, Waud DR: The relation between tetanic fade and receptor occlusion in the presence of competitive neuromuscular block. Anesthesiology 35:456, 1971
8. Waud BE, Waud DR: The relation between the response to "train-of-four" stimulation and receptor occlusion during competitive neuromuscular block. Anesthesiology 37:413, 1972
9. Walts LF, Levin N, Dillon JB: Assessment of recovery from curare. JAMA 213:1894, 1970
10. Johansen SH, Jorgensen M, Molbeck S: Effect of tubocurarine on respiratory and nonrespiratory muscle power in man. J Appl Physiol 19:990, 1964
11. Ali HH, Wilson RS, Savarese JJ, et al: The effect of tubocurarine on indirectly ilicited train-of-four muscle responses and respiratory measurements in humans. Br J Anaesth 47:570, 1975
12. Pavlin EG, Holle RH, Schoene RB: Recovery of airway pro-

tection compared with ventilation in humans after paralysis with curare. Anesthesiology 70:381, 1989

13. Miller RD: Antagonism of neuromuscular blockade. Anesthesiology 44:293, 1976

14. Viby-Mogensen J, Jorgensen BC, Ording H: Residual curarization in the recovery room. Anesthesiology 50:539, 1979

15. Miller RD: How should residual neuromuscular blockade be detected? Anesthesiology 70:379, 1989

16. Bovet D: Some aspects of the relationship between chemical constitution and curare-like activity. Ann NY Acad Sci 54:107, 1951

17. Marshall IG, Paul D, Singh H: Steroids and related studies. 22. Some actions of 4,17-dimethyl-4,17 diaza-D-homo-5-androstane dimethiodide (HS-342), a new neuromuscular blocking drug. J Pharm Pharmacol 25:441, 1973

18. Marshall IG: Ganglion blocking and vagolytic actions of 3 short-acting neuromuscular blocking drugs in the cat. J Pharm Pharmacol 25:530, 1973

19. Durant NN, Savage DS, Nelson DN, et al: The neuromuscular and autonomic blocking activities of pancuronium, ORG NC45, and other pancuronium analogues in the cat. J Pharm Pharmacol 31:831, 1979

20. Savage DS, Sleigh T, Carlyle I: The emergency of ORG NC45, 1-{(2,3,5,16,17)-3,17-bis(acetyloxy)-2-(1-piperidinyl)-androstan-16-yl}-1-methylpiperidinium bromide, from the pancuronium series. Br J Anaesth 52:3S, 1980

21. Bowman WC, Rodger IW, Houston J, et al: Structure/action relationships among some desacetoxy analogues of pancuronium and vecuronium in the anesthetized cat. Anesthesiology 69:57, 1988

22. Stenlake JB, Waigh RD, Urwin J, et al: Atracurium: Conception and inception. Br J Anaesth 55:3S, 1983

23. Basta SJ, Savarese JJ, Ali HH, et al: Histamine-releasing potencies of atracurium, dimethyl tubocurarine and tubocurarine. Br J Anaesth 55:105S, 1983

24. Miller RD, Matteo R, Benet LZ, et al: Influence of renal failure on the pharmacokinetics of d-tubocurarine in man. J Pharmacol Exp Ther 202:1, 1977

25. Furuta T, Canfell PC, Castagnoli KP, et al: Quantitation of pancuronium, 3-desacetylpancuronium, vecuronium, 3-desacetylvecuronium, pipecuronium and 3-desacetylpipecuronium in biological fluids by capillary gas chromatography by using nitrogen-sensitive detection. J Chromatogr 427:41, 1988

26. Horowitz PE, Spector S: Determination of serum d-tubocurarine concentration by radioimmunoassay. J Pharmacol Exp Ther 185:94, 1973

27. Cronnelly R, Stanski DR, Miller RD, et al: Renal function and the pharmacokinetics of neostigmine in anesthetized man. Anesthesiology 51:222, 1979

28. Kersten VW, Meijer DKF, Agoston S: Fluorimetric and chromatographic determination of pancuronium bromide and its metabolites in biological materials. Clin Chim Acta 44:59, 1973

29. Cronnelly R, Fisher DM, Miller RD, et al: Pharmacokinetics and pharmacodynamics of vecuronium (ORG NC45) and pancuronium in anesthetized man. Anesthesiology 58:405, 1984

30. Fahey MR, Rupp SM, Fisher DM, et al: Pharmacokinetics and pharmacodynamics of atracurium in patients with and without renal failure. Anesthesiology 61:699, 1984

31. Stiller RL, Cook DR: High performance liquid chromatographic (HPLC) assay for atracurium and d-tubocurarine. Anesthesiology 59:A267, 1983

32. Shinohara Y, Miller RD, Castagnoli N, Jr: Ion-pair high-per-formance liquid chromatographic assay of 4-aminopyridine in serum. J Chromatogr 230:363, 1982

33. Katz RL: Neuromuscular effects of d-tubocurarine, edrophonium and neostigmine in man. Anesthesiology 28:327, 1967

34. Feldman SA: The rational use of muscle relaxants. p. 149. In Muscle Relaxants. WB Saunders, London, 1973

35. Ham J, Miller RD, Sheiner LB, et al: Dosage-schedule independence of d-tubocurarine pharmacokinetics and pharmacodynamics and recovery of neuromuscular function. Anesthesiology 50:528, 1979

36. McLeod K, Watson MJ, Rawlings MD: Pharmacokinetics of pancuronium in patients with normal and impaired renal function. Br J Anaesth 48:341, 1976

37. Buzello W, Agoston S: Kinetics of intercompartmental disposition and excretion of tubocurarine, gallamine, alcuronium and pancuronium in patients with normal and impaired renal function. Anaesthetist 27:319, 1978

38. Raaflaub J, Frey P: Zur pharmacokinetic von diallyl-nortoxiferin bein menschen. Arzneimittelforschung 22:73, 1972

39. Blogg CE, Simpson BR, Martin LE: Metabolism of ^{3}H AH 8165 in man. Br J Anaesth 45:1233, 1973

40. Duvaldestin P, Henzel D, Demetriou M: Pharmacokinetics of fazadinium in man. Br J Anaesth 50:773, 1978

41. Brotherton WP, Matteo RS: Pharmacokinetics and pharmacodynamics of metocurine in humans with and without renal failure. Anesthesiology 55:273, 1981

42. Meijer DKF, Weitering JG, Vermeer GA, et al: Comparative pharmacokinetics of d-tubocurarine and metocurine in man. Anesthesiology 51:402, 1979

43. Somogyi AA, Shanks CA, Triggs EJ: The effect of renal failure on the disposition and neuromuscular blocking action of pancuronium bromide. Eur J Clin Pharmacol 12:23, 1977

44. Freeman JA, Cook DR, Robertson KA, et al: Pharmacokinetics of doxacurium chloride (BW A938U) in patients with organ failure. Anesth Analg 68:590, 1989

45. Caldwell JE, Canfell PC, Castagnoli KP, et al: The influence of renal failure on the pharmacokinetics and duration of action of pipecuronium bromide in patients anesthetized with halothane and nitrous oxide. Anesthesiology 70:7, 1988

46. Miller RD, Rupp SM, Fisher DM, et al: Clinical pharmacology of vecuronium and atracurium. Anesthesiology 61:444, 1984

47. Bencini AF, Mol WEM, Scaf AHJ, et al: Uptake and excretion of vecuronium bromide and pancuronium bromide in the isolated perfused rat liver. Anesthesiology 69:487, 1988

48. Bevan DR, Gyasi H: Vecuronium in renal failure. Can Anaesth Soc J 31:491, 1984

49. Starsnic MA, Goldberg ME, Ritter DE, et al: Does vecuronium accumulate in the renal transplant patient? Can J Anaesth 36:35, 1989

50. Lynam DP, Cronnelly R, Castagnoli KP, et al: The pharmacokinetics and pharmacodynamics of vecuronium in patients anesthetized with isoflurane with normal renal function or with renal failure. Anesthesiology 69:227, 1988

51. Fisher DM, Rosen JI: A pharmacokinetic explanation for increasing recovery time following larger or repeated doses of nondepolarizing muscle relaxants. Anesthesiology 65:286, 1986

52. Lepage JY, Malinge M, Cozian A, et al: Vecuronium and atracurium in patients with end-stage renal failure. Br J Anaesth 59:1004, 1987

53. Miller RD, Rupp SM, Fisher DM, et al: Clinical pharmacology of vecuronium and atracurium. Anesthesiology 61:444, 1984

54. Somogyi AA, Shanks CA, Triggs EJ: Disposition kinetics of

pancuronium bromide in patients with total biliary obstruction. Br J Anaesth 49:1103, 1977

55. Duvaldestin P, Agoston S, Henzel E, et al: Pancuronium pharmacokinetics in patients with liver cirrhosis. Br J Anaesth 50:1131, 1978

56. Lebrault C, Berger JL, D'Hollander AA, et al: Pharmacokinetics and pharmacodynamics of vecuronium (ORG NC45) in patients with cirrhosis. Anesthesiology 62:601, 1985

57. Hunter JM, Parker CJR, Jones RS, et al: The use of different doses of vecuronium in patients with liver dysfunction. Br J Anaesth 57:758, 1985

58. Bell CF, Hunter JM, Jones RS, Utting JE: Use of atracurium and vecuronium in patients with oesophageal varices. Br J Anaesth 57:160, 1985

59. Arden JR, Lynam DP, Castagnoli KP, et al: Vecuronium and alcoholic liver disease: A pharmacokinetic and pharmacodynamic analysis. Anesthesiology 68:771, 1988

60. Ward S, Neal EAM: Pharmacokinetics of atracurium in hepatic failure. Br J Anaesth 55:1169, 1983

61. Cook DR, Brandom BW, Stiller RL, et al: Pharmacokinetics of atracurium in normal and liver failure patients. Anesthesiology 61:A433, 1984

62. Lebrault C, Duvaldestin P, Henzel D, et al: Pharmacokinetics and pharmacodynamics of vecuronium in patients with cholestasis. Br J Anaesth 58:983, 1986

63. Miller RD, Way WL, Dolan WM, et al: The dependence of pancuronium and d-tubocurarine induced neuromuscular blockades on alveolar concentrations of halothane and Forane. Anesthesiology 37:573, 1972

64. Miller RD, Criqui M, Eger EI II: The influence of duration of anesthesia on a d-tubocurarine neuromuscular blockade. Anesthesiology 44:207, 1976

65. Miller RD, Way WL, Dolan MW, et al: Comparative neuromuscular effects of pancuronium, gallamine, and succinylcholine during Forane and halothane anesthesia in man. Anesthesiology 35:509, 1971

66. Fogdall RP, Miller RD: Neuromuscular effects of enflurane alone and in combination with d-tubocurarine, pancuronium, and succinylcholine in man. Anesthesiology 42:173, 1975

67. Rupp SM, Miller RD, Gencarelli PJ: Vecuronium-induced neuromuscular blockade during enflurane, isoflurane, and halothane anesthesia in humans. Anesthesiology 60:102, 1984

68. Cannon JE, Fahey MR, Castagnoli KP, et al: Continuous infusion of vecuronium: The effect of anesthetic agents. Anesthesiology 67:503, 1987

69. Vitez TS, Miller RD, Eger EI II: An in vitro comparison of halothane and isoflurane potentiation of neuromuscular blockade. Anesthesiology 41:53, 1974

70. Gergis SD, Dretchen KL, Sokoll MD, et al: Effect of anesthetics on acetylcholine release from the myoneural junction. Proc Soc Exp Biol Med 141:629, 1972

71. Waud BE, Waud DR: The effects of diethyl ether, enflurane, and isoflurane at the neuromuscular junction. Anesthesiology 42:275, 1975

72. Waud BE, Waud DR: Comparison of drug–receptor dissociation constants at the mammalian neuromuscular junction in the presence and absence of halothane. J Pharmacol Exp Ther 187:40, 1973

73. Karis JH, Gissen AJ, Nastuk WL: Mode of action of diethyl ether in blocking neuromuscular transmission. Anesthesiology 27:42, 1966

74. Gissen AJ, Karis JH, Nastuk WL: Effect of halothane on neuromuscular transmission. JAMA 197:770, 1966

75. Ngai SH: Action of general anesthetics in producing muscle relaxation: Interaction of anesthetics with relaxants. p. 279. In Katz RL (ed): Muscle Relaxants. Excerpta Medica, Amsterdam, 1975

76. Brett RS, Dilger JP, Yland KF, et al: Isoflurane causes "flickering" of the acetylcholine receptor channel: Observations using the patch clamp. Anesthesiology 69:161, 1988

77. Waud BE, Waud DR: Comparison of the effects of general anesthetics on the end-plate of skeletal muscle. Anesthesiology 43:540, 1975

78. Stanski DR, Ham J, Miller RD, et al: Pharmacokinetics and pharmacodynamics of d-tubocurarine under nitrous oxide-narcotic and halothane anesthesia. Anesthesiology 51:235, 1979

79. Gencarelli P, Miller RD, Eger EI II, et al: Decreasing enflurane concentrations and d-tubocurarine neuromuscular blockade. Anesthesiology 56:192, 1982

80. Stanski DR, Ham J, Miller RD, et al: Time dependent increase in sensitivity to dTC during enflurane anesthesia. Anesthesiology 51:S269, 1979

81. Miller RD, Agoston S, Booij LDHJ, et al: The comparative potency and pharmacokinetics of pancuronium and its metabolites in anesthetized man. Anesthesiology 207:539, 1978

82. Booij LHDJ, Vree TB, Hurkmans F, et al: Pharmacokinetics and pharmacodynamics of the muscle relaxant drug ORG NC45 and each of its metabolites in dogs. Anaesthesist 30:329, 1981

83. Marshall IG, Gibb AJ, Durant NN: Neuromuscular and vagal blocking actions of pancuronium bromide, its metabolites, and vecuronium bromide (ORG NC45) and its potential metabolites in the anesthetized cat. Br J Anaesth 55:703, 1983

84. Bencini AF, Houwertjes MC, Agoston S: Effects of hepatic uptake of vecuronium bromide and its putative metabolites on their neuromuscular blocking actions in the cat. Br J Anaesth 57:789, 1985

85. Upton RA, Nguyen TL, Miller RD, et al: Renal and biliary elimination of vecuronium (ORG NC45) and pancuronium in rats. Anesth Analg 61:313, 1982

86. Castagnoli KP, Caldwell JE, Canfell PC, et al: The pharmacokinetics of vecuronium in humans are influenced by the independent measurement of 3-desacetylvecuronium. (in press)

87. Segredo V, Matthay MA, Sharma ML, et al: Prolonged neuromuscular blockade after long-term administration of vecuronium in two critically ill patients. Anesthesiology 72, 1990

88. Chapple DJ, Clark JS: Pharmacologic action of breakdown products of atracurium and related substances. Br J Anaesth 55:115, 1983

89. Merrett RA. Thompson CW, Webb FW: *In vitro* degradation of atracurium in human plasma. Br J Anaesth 55:61, 1983

90. Stiller RL, Cook DR, Chakravorti S: *In vitro* degradation of atracurium in human plasma. Anesth Analg 64:289, 1985

91. Fisher DM, Canfell PC, Fahey MR, et al: Elimination of atracurium in humans: Contribution of Hofmann elimination and ester hydrolysis versus organ-based elimination. Anesthesiology 65:6, 1985

92. Nigrovic V, Smith MA: Inactivation of atracurium. Evidence of an additional route. Anesth Analg 66:S129, 1987

93. Hennis PJ, Fahey MR, Canfell PC, et al: Pharmacology of laudanosine in dogs. Anesthesiology 65:56, 1986

94. Canfell PC, Castagnoli N, Fahey MR, et al: The metabolic disposition of laudanosine in dog, rabbit, and man. Drug Metab Dispos 14:703, 1986

95. Parker CJR, Hunter JM: Pharmacokinetics of atracurium

and laudanosine in patients with hepatic cirrhosis. Br J Anaesth 62:177, 1989

96. Vine P, Boheimer N, Ward S, et al: Laudanosine pharmacokinetics after bolus atracurium administration in patients with hepato-biliary dysfunction. Br J Anaesth 58:1327S, 1986

97. Yate PM, Flynn PJ, Arnold RW, et al: Clinical experience and plasma laudanosine concentrations during the infusion of atracurium in the intensive therapy unit. Br J Anaesth 59:211, 1987

98. Shi WZ, Fahey MR, Fisher DM, et al: Laudanosine increases the minimum alveolar concentration (MAC) of halothane in rabbits. Anesthesiology 64:282, 1985

99. Lanier WL, Milde JH, Michenfelder JD: The cerebral effects of pancuronium and atracurium in halothane anesthetized dogs. Anesthesiology 63L:584, 1985

100. Beemer GH, Bjorksten AR, Dawson PJ, Crankshaw DP: Production of laudanosine following infusion of atracurium in man and its effect on awakening. Br J Anaesth 63:26, 1989

101. Tateishi A, Zornow MH, Scheller MS, Canfell PC: Electroencephalographic effects of laudanosine in an animal model of epilepsy. Br J Anaesth 62:548, 1989

102. Lanier WL, Sharbrough GN, Michenfelder JD: Effects of atracurium, vecuronium or pancuronium pretreatment on lignocaine seizure thresholds in cats. Br J Anaesth 60:74, 1988

103. Fahey MR, Shi W-Z, Miller RD: Inhaled anesthetics alter seizure threshold of laudanosine in rabbits. Anesthesiology 65:A115, 1986

104. Chapple DJ, Miller AA, Ward JB, Wheatly PL: Cardiovascular and neurological effects of laudanosine. Br J Anaesth 59:218, 1987

105. Kinjo M, Nagashima H, Vizi ES: Effect of atracurium and laudanosine on the release of ^{3}H-noradrenaline. Br J Anaesth 62:683, 1989

106. Pittet JF, Tassonyi E, Schopfer C, et al: Elevated plasma levels of laudanosine are associated with high plasma concentration of norepinephrine during orthotopic liver transplantation. Anesthesiology 69:A484, 1988

107. Savarese JJ, Ali HH, Basta SJ, et al: The clinical pharmacology of mivacurium chloride (BW 1090U): A short-acting ester neuromuscular blocking drug. Anesthesiology 68:723, 1988

108. Cook DR, Stiller RL, Weakly NJ: In vitro metabolism of mivacurium chloride (BW 1090) and succinylcholine. Anesth Analg 68:452, 1989

109. Ham GC, Miller RD, Benet LZ, et al: The pharmacokinetics and pharmacodynamics of d-tubocurarine during hypothermia in the cat. Anesthesiology 49:324, 1978

110. Miller RD, Agoston S, Van der Pol F, et al: Hypothermia and pharmacokinetics and pharmacodynamics of pancuronium in the cat. J Pharmacol Exp Ther 207:532, 1978

111. Buzello W, Schluermann D, Pollmaecher T, Spillner G: Unequal effects of cardiopulmonary bypass-induced hypothermia on neuromuscular blockade from constant infusion of alcuronium, d-tubocurarine, pancuronium, and vecuronium. Anesthesiology 66:842, 1987

112. Stead AL: The response of newborn infants to muscle relaxants. Br J Anaesth 27:124, 1955

113. Kelly SS, Robert DV: The effect of age on the safety factor in neuromuscular transmission in the isolated rat. Br J Anaesth 149:271, 1977

114. Kolnigsberger MR, Patten B, Lovelace RE: Studies of neuromuscular function in the newborn—a comparison of myoneural function in the full term and premature infant. Neuropediatrics 4:350, 1973

115. Goudsouzian NG: Maturation of neuromuscular transmission in the infant. Br J Anaesth 52:205, 1980

116. Bennet EJ, Ignacio A, Patel K, et al: Tubocurarine and the neonate. Br J Anaesth 48:687, 1976

117. Bush GH, Stead AL: The use of d-tubocurarine in neonatal anesthesia. Br J Anaesth 34:721, 1962

118. Churchill-Davidson HC, Wise RP: The response of the newborn infant to muscle relaxants. Can Anaesth Soc J 11:1 1964

119. Long G, Bachman L: Neuromuscular blockade by d-tubocurarine in children. Anesthesiology 28:723, 1967

120. Goudsouzian NG, Ryan JF, Savarese JJ: The neuromuscular effects of pancuronium in infants and children. Anesthesiology 41:95, 1974

121. Goudsouzian NG, Donlon JV, Savarese JJ, et al: Re-evaluation of dosage and duration of action of d-tubocurarine in the pediatric age group. Anesthesiology 43:416, 1975

122. Goudsouzian NG, Liu L, Savarese JJ: Metocurine in infants and children. Anesthesiology 49:266, 1978

123. Fisher DM, O'Keefe CO, Stanski DR, et al: Pharmacokinetics and pharmacodynamics of d-tubocurarine in infants, children and adults. Anesthesiology 57:203, 1982

124. Fisher DM, Miller RD: Neuromuscular effects of vecuronium (ORG NC45) in infants and children during N_2O, halothane anesthesia. Anesthesiology 58:519, 1983

125. Fisher DM, Castagnoli K, Miller RD: Kinetics and dynamics of vecuronium in anesthetized infants and children. Clin Pharmacol Ther 37:402, 1985

126. Meretoja OA: Is vecuronium a long acting neuromuscular blocking agent in neonates and infants? Br J Anaesth 62:184, 1989

127. Brandon BW, Woelfel SK, Cook DR, et al: Clinical pharmacology of atracurium in infants. Anesth Analg 63:309, 1984

128. Goudsouzian N, Liu LMP, Gionfriddo M, Rudd GD: Safety and efficacy of atracurium in adolescents and children anesthetized with halothane. Anesthesiology 62:75, 1985

129. Meretoja OA, Kalli I: Spontaneous recovery of neuromuscular function after atracurium in infants. Anesth Analg 65:1042, 1986

130. Fisher DM, Canfell PC, Spellman MJ, Miller RD: Pharmacokinetics and pharmacodynamics of atracurium in infants and children. Anesthesiology 72, 1990

131. Fisher DM, Cronnelly R, Sharma M, et al: Clinical pharmacology of edrophonium in infants and children. Anesthesiology 61:428, 1984

132. Fisher DM, Cronnelly R, Miller RD, et al: The neuromuscular pharmacology of neostigmine in infants and children. Anesthesiology 59:220, 1983

133. McLeod K, Hull CJ, Watson MJ: Effects of aging on the pharmacokinetics of pancuronium. Br J Anaesth 51:435, 1979

134. Matteo RS, McDaniel DD, Brotherton WP: Pharmacokinetics of d-tubocurarine in the aged. Anesthesiology 57:A271, 1982

135. Duvaldestin P, Saada J, Berger JL, et al: Pharmacokinetics, pharmacodynamics, and dose–response relationships of pancuronium in control and elderly subjects. Anesthesiology 56:36, 1982

136. Rupp SM, Castagnoli KP, Fisher DM, Miller RD: Pancuronium and vecuronium pharmacokinetics and pharmacodynamics in younger and elderly adults. Anesthesiology 67:45, 1987

137. Ghoneim MM, Pandya H: Binding of tubocurarine to specific serum protein fractions. Br J Anaesth 47:853, 1975

138. Thompson MJ: Pancuronium binding by serum proteins. Anaesthesia 31:219, 1976

139. Olsen GD, Chan EM, Riker WK: Binding of d-tubocurarine, di(methyl^{14}C) ether iodine and other amines to cartilage, chondroitin sulfate and human plasma proteins. J Pharmacol Exp Ther 195:242, 1975

140. Ghoneim MM, Kramer SE, Bannow R, et al: Binding of *d*-tubocurarine to plasma protein in normal man and in patients with hepatic or renal disease. Anesthesiology 39:410, 1973

141. Matteo RS, Pua EK, Khambatta HJ, et al: Cerebrospinal fluid levels of *d*-tubocurarine in man. Anesthesiology 46:396, 1977

142. Munson ES, Wagman IH: Elevation of lidocaine seizure threshold by gallamine. Arch Neurol 28:329, 1973

143. Forbes AR, Cohen NH, Eger EI II: Pancuronium reduces halothane requirement in man. Anesth Analg 58:497, 1979

144. Fahey MR, Sessler DI, Cannon JE, et al: Atracurium, vecuronium, and pancuronium do not alter the minimum alveolar concentration (MAC) of halothane in humans. Anesthesiology 71:53, 1989

145. Peduto VA, Gungui P, Di Martino MR, et al: Accidental subarachnoid injection of pancuronium. Anesth Analg 69:516, 1989

146. Goonewardene TW, Sentheshanmuganathan S, Kamalathan S, et al: Accidental subarachnoid injection of gallamine. Br J Anaesth 47:889, 1975

147. Foldes FF, Brown IM, Lunn JN, et al: The neuromuscular effects of diallylnortoxiferine in anesthetized subjects. Anesthesiology 42:117, 1963

148. Hunter AR: Diallyltoxiferine. Br J Anaesth 36:466, 1964

149. Hughes R, Chapple DJ: Effects of non-depolarizing neuromuscular blocking agents on autonomic mechanisms in cats. Br J Anaesth 48:59, 1976

150. Kennedy BR, Kelman GR: Cardiovascular effects of alcuronium in man. Br J Anaesth 42:625, 1970

151. Tammisto T, Welling I: The effect of alcuronium and tubocurarine on blood pressure and heart rate: A clinical comparison. Br J Anaesth 41:317, 1969

152. Harrison GA: The cardiovascular effects and some relaxant properties of four relaxants in patients about to undergo cardiac surgery. Br J Anaesth 44:485, 1972

153. Walker J, Shanks, CA, Triggs EJ: Clinical pharmacokinetics of alcuronium chloride in man. Eur J Clin Pharmacol 17:449, 1980

154. Brittain RT, Tyers MB: The pharmacology of AH 8165: A rapid-acting, short-lasting competitive neuromuscular blocking drug. Br J Anaesth 45:837, 1973

155. Bolger L, Brittain RT, Jack D, et al: Short-lasting, competitive neuromuscular blocking activity in a series of azobisarylimidazo-(1,2-a)-pyridinium dilhalides. Nature (London) 238:354, 1972

156. Arora MV, Clarke RSJ, Dundee JW, et al: Initial clinical experience with AH 8165D, a new rapidly acting non-depolarizing muscle relaxant. Anaesthesia 28:188, 1973

157. Blogg CE, Savege TM, Simpson JC, et al: A new muscle relaxant—AH 8165. Proc R Soc Med 66:1023, 1973

158. Marshall IG: The ganglion blocking and vagolytic action of three short-acting neuromuscular blocking agents in the cat. J Pharm Pharmacol 25:530, 1973

159. Savege TM, Blogg CE, Ross L: The cardiovascular effects of AH 8165. Anaesthesia 28:253, 1973

160. Hull CJ, English MJM, Sibbald A: Fazadinium and pancuronium: A pharmacodynamic study. Br J Anaesth 52:1209, 1980

161. Galindo AHF, Davis TB: Succinylcholine and cardiac excitability. Anesthesiology 23:32, 1962

162. Goat VA, Feldman SA: The dual action of suxamethonium on the isolated rabbit heart. Anaesthesia 27:149, 1972

163. Yasuda I, Hirano T, Amaha K, et al: Chronotropic effects of succinylcholine and succinylmonocholine on sinoatrial node. Anesthesiology 57:289, 1982

163a. Moss J, Rosow CE, Savarese JJ, et al: Role of histamine in the hypotensive action of *d*-tubocurarine in humans. Anesthesiology 55:19, 1981

164. Miller RD, Eger EI II, Stevens WC: Pancuronium induced tachycardia in relation to alveolar halothane, dose of pancuronium, and prior atropine. Anesthesiology 42:352, 1975

165. Stoelting RK: The hemodynamic effects of pancuronium and *d*-tubocurarine in anesthetized patients. Anesthesiology 36:612, 1972

166. Gardier RW, Tsevdos EJ, Jackson DB: Effects of gallamine and pancuronium on inhibitory transmission in cat sympathetic ganglion. J Pharmacol Exp Ther 204:46, 1978

167. Vercruysse P, Hanegreefs G, Vanhoutte PM: Influence of skeletal muscle relaxants on the prejunctional effects of acetylcholine in adrenergically-innervated blood vessels. Arch Int Pharmacodyn Ther 232:350, 1978

168. Docherty JR, McGrath JC: Sympathomimetic effects of pancuronium bromide on the cardiovascular system of the pithed rat. Br J Pharmacol 64:589, 1978

169. Quintana A: Effect of pancuronium bromide on the adrenergic reactivity of the isolated rat vas deferens. Eur J Pharmacol 46:275, 1977

170. Ivankovich AD, Milevich DJ, Albrecht RF, et al: The effect of pancuronium on myocardial contraction and catecholamine metabolism. J Pharm Pharmacol 27:837, 1975

171. Vercruysse P, Bossuyt P, Hanegreefs G, et al: Gallamine and pancuronium inhibit pre- and post-junctional muscarinic receptors in canine saphenous veins. J Pharmacol Exp Ther 209:225, 1979

172. Basta SJ, Savarese JJ, Ali HH, et al: Histamine-releasing potencies of atracurium, dimethyl-tubocurarine, and tubocurarine. Br J Anaesth 55:105S, 1983

173. Scott RPF, Savarese JJ, Ali HH, et al: Atracurium: Clinical strategies for preventing histamine release and attenuating the hemodynamic response. Anesthesiology 61:A287, 1984

174. Hosking MP, Lennon RL, Gronert GA: Combined H_1 and H_2 receptor blockade attenuates the cardiovascular effects of high-dose atracurium for rapid sequence endotracheal intubation. Anesth Analg 67:1089, 1988

175. Stoops CM, Curtis CA, Kovach DA, et al: Hemodynamic effects of mivacurium chloride administered to patients during oxygen-sufentanil anesthesia for coronary artery bypass grafting or valve replacement. Anesth Analg 68:333, 1989

176. Savarese JJ: The autonomic margins of safety of metocurine and *d*-tubocurarine in the cat. Anesthesiology 50:40, 1979

177. McCullough LS, Reier CE, Delauaois AL, et al: The effects of *d*-tubocurarine on spontaneous postganglionic sympathetic activity and histamine release. Anesthesiology 33:328, 1970

178. Munger WL, Miller RD, Stevens WC: The dependence of *d*-tubocurarine induced hypotension on the alveolar concentration of halothane, dose of *d*-tubocurarine and nitrous oxide. Anesthesiology 40:442, 1974

179. Dowdy EG, Holland WC, Yamaka I: Cardioactive properties of *d*-tubocurarine with and without preservatives. Anesthesiology 34:256, 1971

180. Stoelting RK: Blood-pressure responses to *d*-tubocurarine and its preservatives in anesthetized patients. Anesthesiology 35:315, 1971

181. Stoelting RK, Longnecker DE: Effects of promethazine on hypotension following *d*-tubocurarine use in anesthetized patients. Anesth Analg 51:509, 1972

182. Domenech JS, Garcia RC, Sasiain JMR, et al: Pancuronium bromide: An indirect sympathomimetic agent. Br J Anaesth 48:1143, 1976

183. Roizen MF, Forbes AR, Miller RD, et al: Similarity between effects of pancuronium and atropine on plasma norepinephrine levels in man. J Pharmacol Exp Ther 211:419, 1979

184. Eisele JH, Marta JA, Davis HL: Quantitative aspects of the chronotropic and neuromuscular effects of gallamine in anesthetized man. Anesthesiology 35:630, 1971

185. Brown BB, Jr, Crout JR: The sympathomimetic effect of gallamine on the heart. J Pharmacol Exp Ther 172:266, 1970

186. Reitan JA, Fraser AI, Eisele JH: Lack of cardiac inotropic effects of gallamine in anesthetized man. Anesth Analg 52:974, 1973

187. Wong KC, Wyte SR, Martin WE, et al: Antiarrhythmic effects of skeletal muscle relaxants. Anesthesiology 34:458, 1971

188. Geha DG, Cozelle BC, Raessler KL, et al: Pancuronium bromide enhances atrioventricular conduction in halothane-anesthetized dogs. Anesthesiology 46:342, 1977

189. Edwards R, Miller RD, Roizen MF, et al: Cardiac effects of imipramine and pancuronium during halothane and enflurane anesthesia. Anesthesiology 50:42, 1979

190. Clayton D: Asystole associated with vecuronium. Br J Anaesth 58:937, 1986

191. Starr NJ, Sethna DH, Estafanous FG: Bradycardia and asystole following the rapid administration of sufentanil with vecuronium. Anesthesiology 64:521, 1986

192. Cozanitis DA, Erkola O: A clinical study into the possible intrinsic bradycardic activity of vecuronium. Anaesthesia 44:648, 1989

193. Inoue K, El-Banayosy A, Stolarski L, et al: Vecuronium induced bradycardia following induction of anaesthesia with etomidate or thiopentone, with or without fentanyl. Br J Anaesth 60:10, 1988

194. Hull CJ: The safety of new drugs. Br J Anaesth 62:587, 1989

195. Jick H, Andrews EB, Tilson HH, et al: Atracurium — a post-marketing surveillance study: Methods and U.S. experience. Br J Anaesth 62:590, 1989

196. Lawson DH, Paice FM, Glavin RJ, et al: Atracurium — a post-marketing surveillance study: U.K. study and discussion. Br J Anaesth 62:596, 1989

197. Brown EM, Krishnaprasad D, Smiller B: Pancuronium for rapid induction technique for tracheal intubation. Can Anaesth Soc J 26:489, 1979

198. Bar AM, Thornley BA: Thiopentone and pancuronium crash induction. Anaesthesia 33:25, 1978

199. Ginsberg B, Glass PS, Quill T, et al: Onset and duration of neuromuscular blockade following high-dose vecuronium administration. Anesthesiology 71:201, 1989

200. Miller RD: The priming principle. Anesthesiology 62:381, 1985

201. Foldes FF: Rapid tracheal intubation with non-depolarizing neuromuscular blocking drugs: The priming principle (letter to the editor). Br J Anaesth 56:663, 1984

202. Schwarz S, Ilias W, Lackner F, et al: Rapid tracheal intubation with vecuronium: The priming principle. Anesthesiology 62:288, 1985

203. Mehta MP, Choi W, Gergis SD, et al: Rapid sequence endotracheal intubation with non-depolarizing muscle relaxants. Anesthesiology 62:392, 1985

204. Taboada JA, Rupp SM, Miller RD: Refining the priming principle for vecuronium during rapid-sequence induction of anesthesia. Anesthesiology 64:243, 1986

205. Jones RM: The priming principle: How does it work and should we be using it? Br J Anaesth 63:1, 1989

206. Foldes FF, Rendell-Baker L, Birch JH: Causes and prevention of prolonged apnea with succinylcholine. Anesth Analg 35:609, 1956

207. Pantuck EJ, Pantuck CB: Cholinesterases and anticholinesterases. p. 143. In Katz RL (ed): Muscle Relaxants. Excerpta Medica, Amsterdam, 1975

208. Lindsay PA, Tumley J: Suxamethonium apnoea mask by tetrahydroaminacrine. Anaesthesia 33:620, 1978

209. Kaniaris P, Fassoulaki A, Tiarmakopoulou K, et al: Serum cholinesterase levels in patients with cancer. Anesth Analg 58:82, 1979

210. Kopman AF, Strachovsky G, Lichtenstein L: Prolonged response to succinylcholine following physostigmine. Anesthesiology 49:142, 1978

211. Bentz EW, Stoelting RK: Prolonged response to succinylcholine following pancuronium reversal with pyridostimine. Anesthesiology 44:258, 1976

212. Kao YJ, Turner DR: Prolongation of succinylcholine block by metoclopramide. Anesthesiology 70:905, 1989

213. Woodworth GE, Sears DH, Grove TH, et al: The effect of cimetidine and ranitidine on the duration of action of succinylcholine. Anesth Analg 68:295, 1989

214. Fisher DM, Caldwell JE, Sharma M, Wiren JE: The influence of bambuterol (carbamylated terbutaline) on the duration of action of succinylcholine-induced paralysis in humans. Anesthesiology 69:757, 1988

215. Viby-Mogensen J: Correlation of succinylcholine duration of action with plasma cholinesterase activity in subjects with the genotypically normal enzyme. Anesthesiology 53:517, 1980

216. Kalow W, Genest K: A method for the detection of atypical forms of human serum cholinesterase. Determination of dibucaine numbers. Can J Biochem 35:339, 1957

217. Whittaker M: Plasma cholinesterase variants and the anesthetist. Anaesthesia 35:174, 1980

218. Craythorne NWB, Turndorf H, Dripps RD: Changes in pulse rate and rhythm associated with the use of succinylcholine in anesthetized patients. Anesthesiology 21:465, 1970

219. Leigh MD, McCoy DD, Belton KM, et al: Bradycardia following intravenous administration of succinylcholine chloride to infants and children. Anesthesiology 18:698, 1957

220. Stoelting RK, Peterson C: Heart-rate slowing and junctional rhythm following intravenous succinylcholine with and without intramuscular atropine preanesthetic medication. Anesth Analg 54:705, 1975

221. Schoenstadt DA, Whitcher CE: Observations on the mechanism of succinylcholine-induced cardiac arrhythmias. Anesthesiology 24:358, 1963

222. Mathias JA, Evans-Prosser CDG, Churchill-Davidson HC: The role of nondepolarizing drugs in the prevention of suxamethonium bradycardia. Br J Anaesth 42:609, 1970

223. Leiman BC, Katz J, Butler BD: Mechanisms of succinylcholine-induced arrhythmias in hypoxic or hypoxic:hypercarbic dogs. Anesth Analg 66:1292, 1987

224. Schaner PJ, Brown RL, Kirksey TD, et al: Succinylcholine-induced hyperkalemia in burned patients. Anesth Analg 48:764, 1969

225. Lowenstein E: Succinylcholine administration in the burned patient. Anesthesiology 27:494, 1966

226. Belin KP, Carleen CI: Cardiac arrest in the burned patient following succinylcholine administration. Anesthesiology 27:516, 1966

227. Birch AA, Mitchell GD, Playford GA, et al: Changes in serum potassium response to succinylcholine following trauma. JAMA 210:490, 1969

228. Cooperman LH: Succinylcholine-induced hyperkalemia in neuromuscular disease. JAMA 213:1867, 1970

229. Cooperman LH, Strobel GE, Jr., Kennell EM: Massive hyperkalemia after administration of succinylcholine. Anesthesiology 32:161, 1970

230. Gronert GA, Theye RA: Pathophysiology of hyperkalemia induced by succinylcholine. Anesthesiology 43:89, 1975

231. Stevenson PH, Birch AA: Succinylcholine induced hyperkalemia in a patient with a closed head injury. Anesthesiology 51:89, 1979

232. Kohlschütter B, Baur H, Roth F: Suxamethonium-induced hyperkalemia in patients with severe intra-abdominal infections. Br J Anaesth 48:557, 1976

233. Roth F, Wuthrich H: The clinical importance of hyperkalemia following suxamethonium administration. Br J Anaesth 41:311, 1969

234. Powell JN: Suxamethonium-induced hyperkalaemia in a uraemic patient. Br J Anaesth 42:806, 1970

235. Walton JD, Farman JV: Suxamethonium, potassium and renal failure. Anaesthesia 28:626, 1973

236. Miller RD, Way WL, Hamilton WK, et al: Succinylcholine-induced hyperkalemia in patients with renal failure? Anesthesiology 36:138, 1972

237. Powell R, Miller RD: The effect of repeated doses of succinylcholine on serum potassium in patients with renal failure. Anesth Analg 54:746, 1976

238. Korde M, Waud BE: Serum potassium concentrations after succinylcholine in patients with renal failure. Anesthesiology 36:142, 1972

239. Walton JD, Farman JV: Suxamethonium hyperkalemia in uremic neuropathy. Anaesthesia 28:666, 1973

240. Powell JN, Golby M: The pattern of potassium liberation following a single dose of suxamethonium in normal and uraemic rats. Br J Anaesth 43:662, 1971

241. Pandey K, Gadola RP, Dumar S: Time course of intraocular hypertension produced by suxamethonium. Br J Anaesth 44:191, 1972

242. Indu B, Batra YK, Puri GD, Singh H: Nifedipine attenuates the intraocular pressure response to intubation following succinylcholine. Can J Anaesth 36:269, 1989

243. Konchigeri HN, Lee YE, Venugopal K: Effect of pancuronium on intraocular pressure changes induced by succinylcholine. Can Anaesth Soc J 26:479, 1979

244. Miller RD, Way WL, Hickey RF: Inhibition of succinylcholine-induced increased intraocular pressure by nondepolarizing muscle relaxants. Anesthesiology 29:123, 1968

245. Meyers EF, Krupin T, Johnson M, et al: Failure of nondepolarizing neuromuscular blockers in inhibit succinylcholine-induced increased intraocular pressure, a controlled study. Anesthesiology 48:149, 1978

246. Libonati MM, Leahy JJ, Ellison N: The use of succinylcholine in penetrating eye injuries. Anesthesiology 62:637, 1985

247. Chandrashekhar J, Bruce DL: Thiopental and succinylcholine: Action on intraocular pressure. Anesth Analg 54:471, 1975

248. Miller RD, Way WL: Inhibition of succinylcholine-induced increased intragastric pressure by nondepolarizing muscle relaxants and lidocaine. Anesthesiology 34:185, 1971

249. Greenan J: The cardio-oesophageal junction. Br J Anaesth 33:432, 1961

250. Salem MR, Wong AY, Lin YH: The effect of suxamethonium on the intragastric pressure in infants and children. Br J Anaesth 44:166, 1972

251. Brodsky JB, Brock-Unte JG, Samuels SI: Pancuronium pretreatment and post-succinylcholine myalgias. Anesthesiology 51:259, 1979

252. Waters DJ, Mapleson WW: Suxamethonium pains: Hypothesis and observation. Anaesthesia 26:127, 1971

253. Ryan JF, Kagen LJ, Hyman AI: Myoglobinemia after a single dose of succinylcholine. N Engl J Med 285:824, 1971

254. Jansen EC, Hansen PH: Objective measurement of succinylcholine-induced fasciculations and the effect of pretreatment with pancuronium or gallamine. Anesthesiology 51:159, 1979

255. McLougling C, Nesbitt GA, Howe JP: Suxamethonium induced myalgia and the effect of pre-operative administration of oral aspirin. Anaesthesia 43:565, 1988

256. Zahl K, Apfelbaum JL: Muscle pain occurs after outpatient laparoscopy despite the substitution of vecuronium for succinylcholine. Anesthesiology 70:408, 1989

257. Miller RD: The advantages of giving *d*-tubocurarine before succinylcholine. Anesthesiology 37:568, 1972

258. Rogoff RC, Lippman M, Walts LF: An unusual sensitivity to *d*-tubocurarine. Anesthesiology 41:397, 1974

259. Artru AA: Muscle relaxation with succinylcholine or vecuronium does not alter the rate of CSF production or resistance to reabsorption of CSF in dogs. Anesthesiology 68:392, 1988

260. Van Der Spek AFL, Fang WB, Ashton-Miller JA, et al: Increased masticatory muscle stiffness during limb flaccidity associated with succinylcholine administration. Anesthesiology 69:11, 1988

261. Walts LF, Dillon JB: Clinical studies of the interaction between *d*-tubocurarine and succinylcholine. Anesthesiology 31:39, 1969

262. Sugai N, Hughes R, Payne JP: The effect of suxamethonium alone and its interaction with gallamine on the indirectly elicited tetanic and single twitch contractions of skeletal muscle in man during anesthesia. Br J Clin Pharmacol 2:391, 1975

263. Katz RL: Modification of the action of pancuronium by succinylcholine and halothane. Anesthesiology 35:602, 1971

264. Katz JA, Fragen RJ, Shanks CA, et al: The effects of succinylcholine on doxacurium-induced neuromuscular blockade. Anesthesiology 69:604, 1989

265. Sunew KY, Hicks RG: Effects of neostigmine and pyridostigmine on duration of succinylcholine action and pseudocholinesterase activity. Anesthesiology 49:188, 1978

266. Lee C, Katz RL: Neuromuscular pharmacology. Br J Anaesth 52:73, 1980

267. Ramsey FM, Lebowitz PW, Savarese JJ, et al: Clinical characteristics of long term succinylcholine neuromuscular blockade during balanced anesthesia. Anesth Analg 59:110, 1980

268. Payne JP, Hughes R, Azawi SA: Neuromuscular blockade by neostigmine in anaesthetized man. Br J Anaesth 52:69, 1980

269. Katz RL: Clinical neuromuscular pharmacology of pancuronium. Anesthesiology 34:550, 1971

270. Rupp SM, McChristen J, Miller RD: Neostigmine and edrophonium antagonism of varying intensity of neuromuscular blockade by atracurium, pancuronium or vecuronium. Anesthesiology 64:711, 1986

271. Donati F, Smith CE, Bevan DR: Dose-response relationships for edrophonium and neostigmine as antagonists of moderate and profound atracurium blockade. Anesth Analg 68:13, 1989

272. Miller RD, Van Nyhuis LS, Eger EI II, et al: The effect of acid–base balance on neostigmine of *d*-tubocurarine-induced neuromuscular blockade. Anesthesiology 42:377, 1975

273. Miller RD, Roderick L: The influence of acid–base changes on neostigmine antagonism of a pancuronium neuromuscular blockade. Br J Anaesth 50:317, 1978

274. Feldman SA: Effect of changes in electrolytes, hydration, and pH upon the reactions to muscle relaxants. Br J Anaesth 35:546, 1963

275. Cohen EN: Patients with altered sensitivity. Clin Anesth 2:76, 1966

276. Cunningham JN, Jr, Carter NW, Rector FC, Jr., et al: Resting

transmembrane potential difference of skeletal muscle in normal subjects and severely ill patients. J Clin Invest 50:49, 1971

277. Miller RD, Roderick LL: Diuretic-induced hypokalemia pancuronium neuromuscular blockade and its antagonism by neostigmine. Br J Anaesth 50:541, 1978

278. Cronnelly R, Morris RB, Miller RD: Edrophonium: Duration of action and atropine requirement in humans during halothane anesthesia. Anesthesiology 57:261, 1982

279. Fogdall RP, Miller RD: Antagonism of *d*-tubocurarine- and pancuronium-induced neuromuscular blockades by pyridostigmine in man. Anesthesiology 39:504, 1973

280. Glisson S, Fajardo L, El-Etr AA: Amitriptyline therapy increases electrocardiographic changes during reversal of neuromuscular blockade. Anesth Analg 57:77, 1978

281. Ramamurthy S, Shaker MH, Winnie AP: Glycopyrrolate as a substitute for atropine in neostigmine reversal of muscle relaxants. Can Anaesth Soc J 19:4, 1972

282. Tan CK, Balasaraswathi K, El-Etr AA: Neostigmine induced Wencheback phenomena. Anesthesiology Rev 7:28, 1980

283. Jones JE, Parker CJR, Hunter JM: Antagonism of blockade produced by atracurium or vecuronium with low doses of neostigmine. Br J Anaesth 61:560, 1988

284. Cronnelly R, Stanski DR, Miller RD, et al: Renal function and the pharmacokinetics of neostigmine in anesthetized patients. Anesthesiology 51:222, 1979

285. Cronnelly R, Stanski DR, Miller RD, et al: Pyridostigmine kinetics with and without renal function. Clin Pharmacol Ther 28:78, 1980

286. Morris R, Cronnelly R, Miller RD, et al: Pharmacokinetics of edrophonium and neostigmine when antagonizing a *d*-tubocurarine neuromuscular blockade in man. Anesthesiology 54:399, 1981

287. Kopman AF: Edrophonium antagonism of pancuronium-induced neuromuscular blockade in man. Anesthesiology 51:139, 1979

288. Bevan DR: Reversal of pancuronium with edrophonium. Anaesthesia 34:614, 1979

289. Argov Z, Mastaglia FL: Disorders of neuromuscular transmission caused by drugs. N Engl J Med 301:409, 1979

290. Miller RD: Factors affecting the action of muscle relaxants. p. 165. In Katz RL (ed): Muscle Relaxants. Excerpta Medica, Amsterdam, 1975

291. Lee C, de Silva AJC: Acute and subchronic neuromuscular blocking characteristics of streptomycin: A comparison with neomycin. Br J Anaesth 51:431, 1979

292. Singh YN, Harvey AL, Marshall IG: Antibiotic-induced paralysis of the mouse phrenic nerve-hemidiaphragm preparation, and reversibility by calcium and by neostigmine. Anesthesiology 48:418, 1978

293. Singh YN, Marshall IG, Harvey AL: Depression of transmitter release and postjunctional sensitivity during neuromuscular block produced by antibiotics. Br J Anaesth 51:1027, 1979

294. Sokoll MD, Gergis SD: Antibiotics and neuromuscular function. Anesthesiology 55:148, 1981

295. Dupuis JY, Martin R, Tetrault JP: Atracurium and vecuronium interaction with gentamicin and tobramycin. Can J Anaesth 36:407, 1989

296. Giesecke AH, Morris RE, Dalton MD, et al: Of magnesium, muscle relaxants, toxemic parturients, and cats. Anesth Analg 47:689, 1968

297. Ghoneim MM, Long JP: The interaction between magnesium and other neuromuscular blocking agents. Anesthesiology 32:23, 1970

298. del Castillo J, Engbek L: The nature of the neuromuscular block produced by magnesium. J Physiol (Lond) 124:370, 1954

299. Manthey AA: The effect of calcium on the desensitization of membrane receptors at the neuromuscular junction. J Gen Physiol 49:963, 1966

300. Badola RP, Chatterji S, Pandey K, et al: Effects of calcium on neuromuscular block by suxamethonium in dogs. Br J Anaesth 43:1027, 1971

301. Telivuo LL, Katz RL: The effects of modern intravenous local analgesics on respiration during partial neuromuscular block in man. Anaesthesia 25:30, 1970

302. Usubiaga JE, Wikinski JA, Morales RL: Interaction of intravenously administered procaine, lidocaine and succinylcholine in anesthetized subjects. Anesth Analg 46:39, 1967

303. Usubiaga JE, Standaert F: The effects of local anesthetics on motor nerve terminals. J Pharmacol Exp Ther 159:353, 1968

304. Kordas M: The effect of procaine on neuromuscular transmission. J Physiol (Lond) 209:689, 1970

305. Gelser RM, Matsuba M: Neuromuscular blocking actions of local anesthetics. J Pharmacol Exp Ther 103:314, 1951

306. Thorpe WR, Seeman P: The site of action of caffeine and procaine in skeletal muscle. J Pharmacol Exp Ther 179:324, 1971

307. Harrah MD, Way WL, Katzung BG: The interaction of *d*-tubocurarine with antiarrhythmic drugs. Anesthesiology 33:406, 1970

308. Miller RD, Way WL, Katzung BG: The potentiation of neuromuscular blocking agents by quinidine. Anesthesiology 28:1036, 1967

309. Miller RD, Way WL, Katzung BG: The neuromuscular effects of quinidine. Proc Soc Exp Biol Med 129:215, 1968

310. Bikhazi GB, Leung I, Flores C, et al: Potentiation of neuromuscular blocking agents by calcium channel blockers in rats. Anesth Analg 67:1, 1988

311. Hill GE, Wong KC, Hodges MR: Lithium carbonate and neuromuscular blocking agents. Anesthesiology 46:122, 1977

312. Martin BA, Kramer PM: Clinical significance of interaction between lithium and a neuromuscular blocker. Am J Psychiatry 139:1326, 1982

313. Ornstein E, Matteo RS, Young WL, Diaz J: Resistance of metocurine-induced neuromuscular blockade in patients receiving phenytoin. Anesthesiology 63:294, 1985

314. Ornstein E, Matteo RS, Schwartz AE, et al: The effect of phenytoin on the magnitude and duration of neuromuscular block following atracurium or vecuronium. Anesthesiology 67:191, 1987

315. Gray HSJ, Slater RM, Pollard BJ: The effect of acutely administered phenytoin on vecuronium-induced neuromuscular blockade. Anaesthesia 44:379, 1989

316. Deacock AR, Hargrove RL: The influence of certain ganglionic blocking agents on neuromuscular transmission. Br J Anaesth 34:357, 1962

317. Wilson SL, Miler RN, Wright C, et al: Prolonged neuromuscular blockade associated with trimethaphan. Anesth Analg 55:353, 1976

318. Glisson SN, El-Etr AA, Lim R: Prolongation of pancuronium-induced neuromuscular blockade by intravenous infusion of nitroglycerine. Anesthesiology 51:47, 1979

319. Glisson SN, Sanchez MM, El-Etr AA, et al: Nitroglycerine and the neuromuscular blockade produced by gallamine, succinylcholine, *d*-tubocurarine and pancuronium. Anesth Analg 59:117, 1980

320. Miller RD, Sohn YJ, Matteo RS: Enhancement of *d*-tubocurarine neuromuscular blockade by diuretics in man. Anesthesiology 45:442, 1976

321. Matteo RS, Nishitateno K, Pua EK, et al: Pharmacokinetics of *d*-tubocurarine in man: Effects of an osmotic diuretic on urinary excretion. Anesthesiology 52:335, 1980

322. Glidden RS, Martyn JAJ, Tomera JD: Azathioprine fails to alter the dose-response curve of *d*-tubocurarine in rats. Anesthesiology 68:595, 1988

323. Gramstad L: Atracurium, vecuronium, and pancuronium in end-stage renal failure. Br J Anaesth 59:995, 1987

324. Lebowitz PW, Ramsey FM, Savarese JJ, et al: Combination of pancuronium and metacurine. Anesth Analg 60:12, 1981

325. Ferres CJ, Mirakhus RK, Pandit SK, et al: Dose-response studies with pancuronium, vecuronium, and their combination. Br J Clin Pharmacol 18:947, 1984

326. Schuh FT: On the interaction of combinations of nondepolarizing neuromuscular blocking drugs. Anaesthetist 30:537, 1981

327. Van der Spek AFL, Zupan JT, Pollard BJ, et al: Interactions of vercuronium and atracurium in an in vitro nerve-muscle preparation. Anesth Analg 67:240, 1987

328. Nott NW, Bowman WC: Actions of dantrolene sodium on contractions of the tibialis anterior and soleus muscles of cats under chloralose anesthesia. Clin Exp Pharmacol Physiol 1:113, 1974

329. Morgan KG, Bryant SD: The mechanism of action of dantrolene sodium. J Pharmacol Exp Ther 201:138, 1977

330. Lee C, Katz RL: Neuromuscular pharmacology. A clinical update and commentary. Br J Anaesth 52:173, 1980

331. Grob D, Namba T: Characteristics and mechanisms of neuromuscular block in myasthenia gravis. Ann NY Acad Sci 274:143, 1976

332. Engel WK: Myasthenia gravis, corticosteroids, anticholinesterase. Ann NY Acad Sci 274:623, 1976

333. Gracey DR, Howard FM, Jr, Divertie B: Plasmapheresis in the treatment of ventilator-dependent myasthenia gravis. Chest 85:739, 1984

334. Seybold ME: Myasthenia gravis: A clinical and basic science review. JAMA 250:2516, 1983

335. Buzello W, Noeldge G, Krieg N, Brobmann GF: Vecuronium for muscle relaxation in patients with myasthenia gravis. Anesthesiology 64:507, 1986

336. Eisenkraft JB, Mann SM, Book WJ, Papatestas AE: Succinylcholine dose-response in myasthenia gravis. Anesthesiology 69:760, 1988

337. Nilsson E, Paloheimo M, Muller K, Heinonen J: Halothane-induced variability in the neuromuscular transmission of patients with myasthenia gravis. Acta Anaesthesiol Scand 33:395, 1989

338. Feldman SA: Muscle relaxants in pathologic states. p. 108. In Muscle Relaxants. WB Saunders, Philadelphia, 1979

339. Hedley-Whyte J, Burgess GE III, Feeley TW, et al: Respiratory management of peripheral neurologic disease. p. 245. In Applied Physiology of Respiratory Care. Little, Brown, Boston, 1976

340. Hook R, Anderson EF, Noto P: Anesthetic management of a parturient with myotonia atrophica. Anesthesiology 43:689, 1975

341. Mitchell MM, Ali HH, Savarese JJ: Myotonia and neuromuscular blocking agents. Anesthesiology 49:44, 1978

342. Siler JN, Discavage WJ: Anesthetic management of hypokalemic periodic paralysis. Anesthesiology 43:489, 1975

343. Flewellen EH, Bodensteiner JB: Anesthetic experience in a patient with hyperkalemic periodic paralysis. Anesth Rev 7:44, 1980

344. Rosenbaum KJ, Neigh JL, Strobel GE: Sensitivity to nondepolarizing muscle relaxants in amyotrophic lateral sclerosis: Report of two cases. Anesthesiology 35:638, 1971

345. Hague CW, Itani MS, Martyn JAJ: Resistance of *d*-tubocurarine in lower motor neuron injury is related to increased acetylcholine receptors at the neuromuscular junction. Anesthesiology, 1989 (in press)

346. Graham DH: Monitoring neuromuscular block may be unreliable in patients with upper-motor-neuron lesions. Anesthesiology 52:74, 1980

347. Moorthy SS, Hilgenberg JC: Resistance to nondepolarizing muscle relaxants in paretic upper extremities of patients with residual hemiplegia. Anesth Analg 59:624, 1980

348. Martyn JAJ, Szfelbein SK, Ali HH, et al: Increased *d*-tubocurarine requirement following major thermal injury. Anesthesiology 52:352, 1980

349. Diversteg JF, Pavlin EG, Heimback DM: Patients with burns are resistant to atracurium. Anesthesiology 65:517, 1986

350. Kim C, Fuke N, Martyn JAJ: Burn injury to rat increases nicotinic acetylcholine receptor in the diaphragm. Anesthesiology 68:401, 1988

351. Marathe PH, Haschke RH, Slattery JT, et al: Acetylcholine receptor density and acetylcholinesterase activity in skeletal muscle of rats following thermal injury. Anesthesiology 70:654, 1989

352. Miller RD: Recent developments with muscle relaxants and their antagonists. Can Anaesth Soc J 26:83, 1979

353. Hughes R, Chapple DJ: The pharmacology of atracurium: A new competitive neuromuscular blocking agent. Br J Anaesth 53:31, 1981

354. Ali HH, Savarese JJ: Monitoring of neuromuscular function. Anesthesiology 45:216, 1976

13
LOCAL ANESTHETICS

Gary R. Strichartz
Benjamin G. Covino

INTRODUCTION

Local anesthesia may be produced by many tertiary amine bases, certain alcohols and a variety of other drugs and toxins. However, all clinically useful agents are either aminoesters or aminoamides. These drugs, when applied in sufficient concentrations at the site of action, prevent conduction of electrical impulses by the membranes of nerve and muscle. When local anes- thetic agents are given systemically, the functions of cardiac, skeletal, and smooth muscle as well as the transmission of impulses in the peripheral and central nervous system and within the specialized conducting system of the heart may all be altered. Local anesthetics may provide analgesia in various parts of the body by topical application, injection in the vicinity of periph- eral nerve endings and major nerve trunks, or instilla- tion within the epidural or subarachnoid spaces.

BASIC PHARMACOLOGY

Chemistry

The Local Anesthetic Molecule

The typical local anesthetic molecule, exemplified by lidocaine and procaine (Fig. 13-1), is a tertiary amine separated at a distance of 6 to 9 Å from an unsaturated (aromatic) ring system (usually a benzene ring) by an intermediate chain. The tertiary amine is a base (proton acceptor). The chain always contains either an ester (—C—O) or amide (—NHC—) linkage; local anesthetics may therefore be classified as aminoester or aminoamide compounds. The amide or ester linkage contributes to anesthetic potency, since its removal results in a decrease in activity. The aromatic ring system gives a lipophilic character to its portion of the molecule, whereas the tertiary amine end is relatively hydrophilic, particularly since it is partially protonated and bears some positive charge in the physiologic pH range. Lidocaine, for example, is 65 percent protonated at pH 7.4. The structures of commonly administered local anesthetic drugs are given in Table 13-1.

Structure – Activity Relations and Physicochemical Properties

The intrinsic potency and duration of action of local anesthetics may be modified by certain changes within the molecule.

Lipophilic-Hydrophilic Balance

The lipophilic versus hydrophilic character of the local anesthetic molecule may be affected by altering the size of alkyl substitution on or near the tertiary amine or at the aromatic ring. Lipophilicity expresses the tendency of a compound to associate with membrane lipids, yet the membrane uptake of local anesthetics is rarely measured. Instead, the equilibrium partitioning into a hydrophobic solvent such as octanol is measured.[1] Such octanol/buffer partition coefficients are comparable to membrane/buffer partition coefficients for the uncharged species of local anesthetics but greatly underestimate the membrane partitioning for the charged, protonated species, octanol being a poor model for the polar regions near the membrane surface.[2] In this chapter, we use the term *hydrophobicity*, expressed by octanol/buffer partitioning, to describe a physicochemical property of local anesthetics.

Compounds with a more hydrophobic nature are obtained by increasing the size of the alkyl substitution. These agents are more potent and produce longer-lasting blocks than their less hydrophobic congeners. For example, etidocaine, which has three more carbon atoms than lidocaine in the amine end of the molecule, is four times more potent and five times longer lasting when these compounds are compared in the isolated frog sciatic nerve. Two other examples of increased potency and duration of action in the more lipophilic members of related pairs of compounds are mepivacaine-bupivacaine and procaine-tetracaine (Table 13-2); in these pairs, a butyl group is added to the tertiary amine (bupivacaine) or to the aromatic region (tetracaine). The second example illustrates the dominance of aromatic substitution, since procaine is less potent than tetracaine, even though the latter compound's tertiary amine contains three fewer methylene groups than the former's.[3-5]

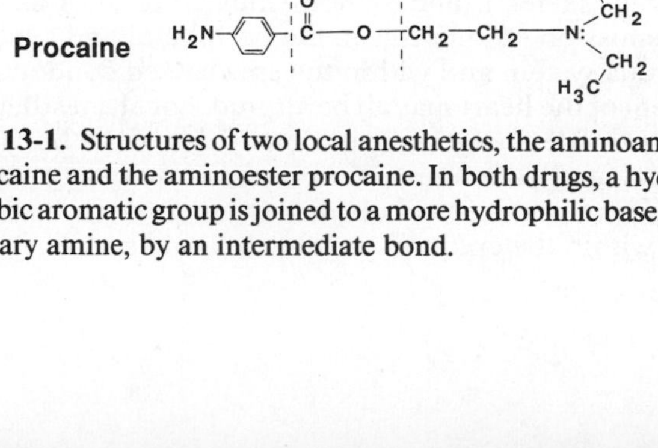

Hydrogen Ion Concentration

Local anesthetics in solution exist in a chemical equilibrium between the basic uncharged form (B) and the charged cationic form (BH$^+$). At a certain hydrogen ion concentration ($\log_{10}^{-1}[-pH]$) specific for each drug, the concentration of local anesthetic base is equal to the concentration of charged cation. This hydrogen ion concentration is identified as the pK_a. The relationship may be expressed as follows:

$$pH = pK_a - \log([BH^+]/[B])$$

The pK_a values for standard local anesthetic agents are listed in Table 13-2. The tendency to be protonated depends on environmental factors, such as temperature and ionic strength, and on the medium surrounding the drug.[1] In the relatively apolar milieu of a membrane, the average pK_a of local anesthetics is about one pH unit lower than in solution.[6] This relationship is chemically equivalent to saying that the membrane concentrates the base of the local anesthetic 10-fold more than it concentrates the protonated cations. The values of pK_a listed in Table 13-2 were measured at 37°C in physiologic salt solutions.

The pH of the surrounding medium into which the local anesthetic is injected influences drug activity by altering the relative percentage of agent present in the

Fig. 13-1. Structures of two local anesthetics, the aminoamide lidocaine and the aminoester procaine. In both drugs, a hydrophobic aromatic group is joined to a more hydrophilic base, the tertiary amine, by an intermediate bond.

TABLE 13-1. Representative Local Anesthetic Agents in Common Clinical Use

Generic[a] and Common Proprietary Name	Chemical Structure	Approximate Year of Initial Clinical Use	Main Anesthetic Utility	Representative Commercial Preperation
Cocaine	$CH_2-CH-CHCOOCH_3$ / $NCH_3-CHOOC_6H_5$ / $CH_2-CH-CH_2$	1884	Topical	Bulk powder
Benzocaine (Americaine)	$H_2N-C_6H_4-CO-OC_2H_5$	1900	Topical / Topical	20% ointment / 20% aerosol
Procaine (Novocain)	$H_2N-C_6H_4-COOCH_2CH_2N(C_2H_5)_2$	1905	Infiltration / Spinal	10 & 20 mg/ml solutions / 100 mg/ml solution
Dibucaine (Nupercaine)	quinoline, $2\text{-}OC_4H_9$, $4\text{-}CONHCH_2CH_2N(C_2H_5)_2$	1929	Spinal	0.667, 2.5, & 5 mg/ml solutions
Tetracaine (Pontocaine)	$H_9C_4(H)N-C_6H_4-COOCH_2CH_2N(CH_3)_2$	1930	Spinal / Spinal	Niphanoid crystals—20 mg/ml / 10 mg/ml solutions
Lidocaine (Xylocaine)	2,6-$(CH_3)_2C_6H_3-NHCOCH_2N(C_2H_5)_2$	1944	Infiltration / Peripheral nerve blocks / Epidural / Spinal / Topical / Topical	5 & 10 mg/ml solutions / 10, 15, & 20 mg/ml solutions / 10, 15, & 20 mg/ml solutions / 50 mg/ml solution / 2.0% jelly, viscous / 2.5%, 5.0% ointment
Chloroprocaine (Nesacaine)	H_2N-(2-Cl)$C_6H_3-COOCH_2CH_2N(C_2H_5)_2$	1955	Infiltration / Peripheral nerve blockade / Epidural	10 mg/ml solution / 10 & 20 mg/ml solutions / 20 & 30 mg/ml solutions
Mepivacaine (Carbocaine)	2,6-$(CH_3)_2C_6H_3-NHCO$-(1-CH_3-piperidine)	1957	Infiltration / Peripheral nerve blockade / Epidural	10 mg/ml solution / 10 & 20 mg/ml solutions / 10, 15, & 20 mg/ml solutions
Prilocaine (Citanest)	2-$CH_3C_6H_4-NHCOCH(CH_3)-NH-C_3H_7$	1960	Infiltration / Peripheral nerve blockade / Epidural	10 & 20 mg/ml solutions / 10, 20, & 30 mg/ml solutions / 10, 20, & 30 mg/ml solutions
Bupivacaine (Marcaine)	2,6-$(CH_3)_2C_6H_3-NHCO$-(1-C_4H_9-piperidine)	1963	Infiltration / Peripheral nerve blockade / Epidural / Spinal	2.5 mg/ml solutions / 2.5 & 5 mg/ml solutions / 2.5, 5, & 7.5 mg/ml solutions / 5 & 7.5 mg/ml solutions
Etidocaine (Duranest)	2,6-$(CH_3)_2C_6H_3-NHCOCHN(C_2H_5)$...$(C_2H_5)(C_3H_7)$	1972	Infiltration / Peripheral nerve blockade / Epidural	2.5 & 5 mg/ml solutions / 5 & 10 mg/ml solutions / 5 & 10 mg/ml solutions

[a] USP nomenclature.
(Modified from Covino and Vassallo,[106] with permission.)

TABLE 13-2. Relative In Vitro Conduction Blocking Potency and Physicochemical Properties of Local Anesthetic Drugs

Drug	Relative Conduction Blocking Potency[a]	Physicochemical Properties	
		pK_a[b]	Hydrophobicity[b]
Low potency			
Procaine	$\equiv 1$	8.9	100
Intermediate potency			
Mepivacaine	1.5	7.7	130
Prilocaine	1.8	8.0	129
Chloroprocaine	3	9.1	810
Lidocaine	2	7.8	366
High potency			
Tetracaine	8	8.4	5,822
Bupivacaine	8	8.1	3,420
Etidocaine	8	7.9	7,320

[a]Data derived from C fibers of isolated rabbit vagus and sciatic nerve.
[b]pK_a and hydrophobicity at 36°C; hydrophobicity equals octanol : buffer partition coefficient of the base; ratio of concentrations. (From Sanchez V, Arthur GR, and Strichartz GR, unpublished data).
[c]Values at 25°C.

basic or protonated form. The relationship between pK_a and the percentage of local anesthetic present in the cationic form is shown in Figure 13-2. The reasons for this pK_a effect on local anesthetic behavior are discussed in the section on mechanism of action.

Protein Binding

A strong correlation exists between local anesthetic potency, hydrophobic character, and duration of action. Also, in general, the potent, long-acting, highly hydrophobic agents (such as tetracaine, etidocaine, and bupivacaine) are bound to a greater extent to serum proteins than are their more hydrophilic counterparts

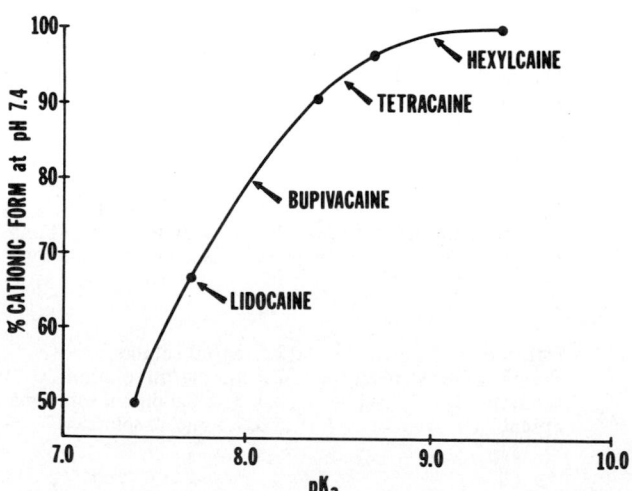

Fig. 13-2. The fraction of local anesthetic in the protonated, cationic form of aqueous solution at physiologic pH (7.4), as a function of the pK_a of the drug. (From Covino and Vassallo,[106] with permission.)

(procaine, lidocaine).[7] The correlation of potency with serum protein binding is not strong, however, and is unrelated to the mechanism of local anesthetic action. Binding and dissociation of local anesthetics at their sites of action on the ion channel are very rapid processes[8] for which equilibrium uptake by soluble serum proteins is a poor model.

ANATOMY OF THE PERIPHERAL NERVE

Each peripheral nerve axon possesses its own cell membrane, the axolemma, within which is contained the axoplasm and a variety of organelles, microtubules, and neurofilaments. Nonmyelinated nerves, such as autonomic postganglionic fibers, are further encased in a Schwann cell sheath. Most large motor and sensory fibers are enclosed in many layers of myelin, which consists of plasma membranes of specialized Schwann cells that wrap themselves around the axon during axonal outgrowth. Myelin greatly increases the speed of nerve conduction by insulating the axolemma from the surrounding conducting salt medium and forcing the action current to flow through the axoplasm to the nodes of Ranvier, which are periodic interruptions in the myelin sheath (Fig. 13-3). The ion channels that subserve impulse generation and propagation are concentrated at the nodes of Ranvier[9] but are distributed all along the axon of nonmyelinated fibers (Fig. 13-3). A classification of peripheral nerves according to fiber size and physiologic properties is presented in Table 13-3.

A typical peripheral nerve consists of several groups of axons, or fascicles. Each axon has its own connective tissue covering, the endoneurium. Each fascicle of axons is covered by a second connective tissue layer,

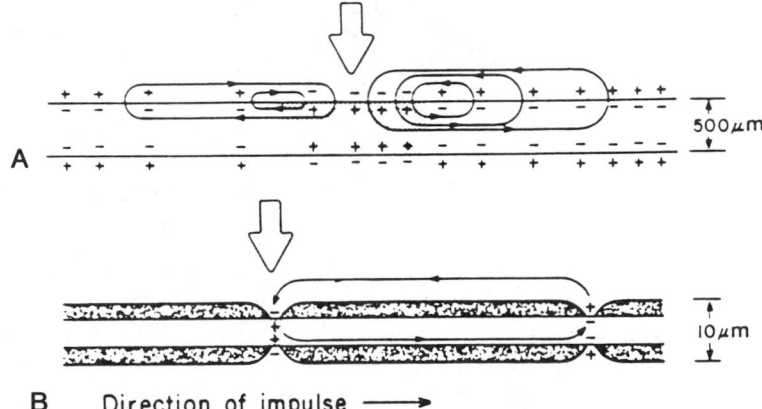

Fig. 13-3. The direction of action currents flowing in a large nonmyelinated axon (e.g., of the squid) (**A**), and in a myelinated axon (**B**). During propagation of impulses from left to right, current entering the axon at the initial rising phase of the impulse (shown by the open arrows) passes down the axoplasm (local circuit current) and depolarizes the adjacent membrane. This ionic current passes uniformly along the nonmyelinated axon but is funneled from one node of Ranvier to another in the myelinated axon.

the perineurium. The entire nerve is wrapped in an outer sheath called the epineurium (Fig. 13-4). To reach its site of action (the nerve axon), a local anesthetic molecule must traverse four or five (in the case of a myelinated nerve) connective tissues and/or lipid membranous barriers.

Structure of the Axonal Membrane

Biologic membranes consist of a bimolecular lipid layer containing proteins adsorbed to the surfaces as well as embedded or spanning the hydrocarbon core (Fig. 13-5). The bilayer character is imposed by the amphiphilic phospholipids, which have long hydrophobic fatty acyl "tails" that lie in the center of the membrane and polar hydrophilic "head groups," composed of zwitterionic (containing positive and negative charges, e.g., phosphatidylcholine, phosphatidylethanolamine) or negatively charged (phosphatidylserine, phosphatidylinositol) components, that project into the cytoplasm or the interstitial fluid. Proteins facing the exterior surface are often glycosylated with complex carbohydrates, whereas those on the intracellular surface are associated with other proteins of the cellular cytoskeleton. Within the membrane, there is lateral and rotational diffusion that allows lipids and proteins to migrate in a "fluid mosaic." Despite this general behavior, some proteins are fixed within specific regions of a membrane; sodium channels, for example, are highly localized at the nodes of Ranvier of myelinated axons.

A dynamic interaction exists between the cell's membrane and cytoplasm. Cytoplasmic enzymes may be regulated by hormone and neurotransmitter receptors in the membrane. The membrane lipids are themselves the source of certain "second messengers," and the membrane proteins, including certain ion channels, may be chemically altered and physiologically modulated by intracellular enzymes, such as kinases that specifically phosphorylate certain proteins. Although we focus here on the channel-blocking actions of local anesthetics, it is noteworthy that many other cellular activities are inhibited by this class of drugs.

TABLE 13-3. Classification of Peripheral Nerves According to Fiber Size and Physiologic Properties

Fiber Class	Subclass	Myelin	Diameter (μ)	Conduction Velocity (m/sec)	Location	Function
A	α	+	6–22	30–120	Afferent to and efferent from muscles and joints	Motor, proprioception
	β	+	6–22	30–120	Afferent to and efferent from muscles and joints	Motor, proprioception
	γ	+	3–6	15–35	Efferent to muscle spindles	Muscle tone
	δ	+	1–4	5–25	Afferent sensory nerves	Pain, temperature, touch
B		+	<3	3–15	Preganglionic sympathetic	Various autonomic functions
C	sC	−	0.3–1.3	0.7–1.3	Postganglionic sympathetic	Various autonomic functions
	dγC	−	0.4–1.2	0.1–2.0	Afferent sensory nerves	Pain, temperature, touch

(From Bonica,[170] with permission.)

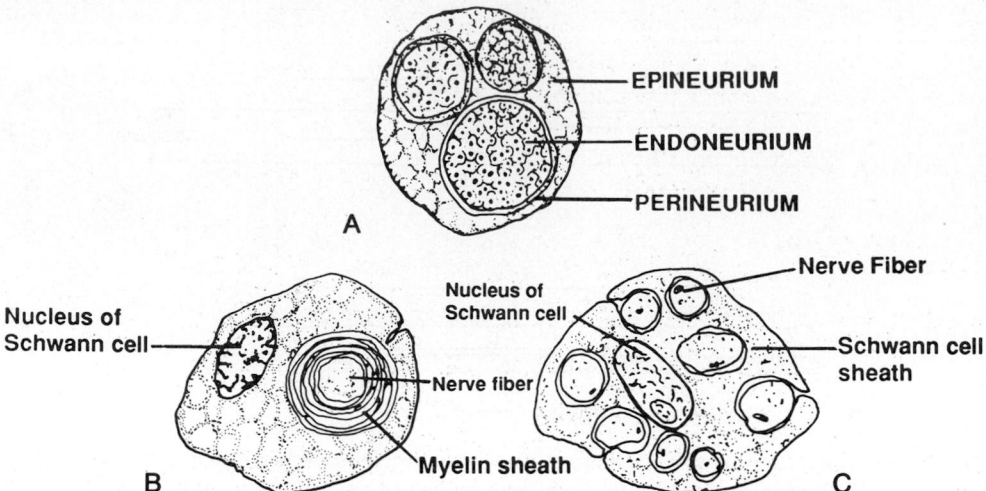

Fig. 13-4. Transverse sections of a peripheral nerve (**A**) showing the outermost epineurium, the inner perineurium that collects nerve axons in fascicles, and the endoneurium that surrounds each myelinated fiber. Each myelinated axon (**B**) is encased in the multiple membranous wrappings of myelin formed by one Schwann cell, each of which stretches longitudinally over approximately 100 times the diameter of the axon. The narrow span of axon between these myelinated segments, the node of Ranvier, contains the ion channels that support action potentials. Nonmyelinated fibers (**C**) are enclosed in bundles of 5 to 10 axons by a chain of Schwann cells that tightly embrace each axon with but one layer of membrane.

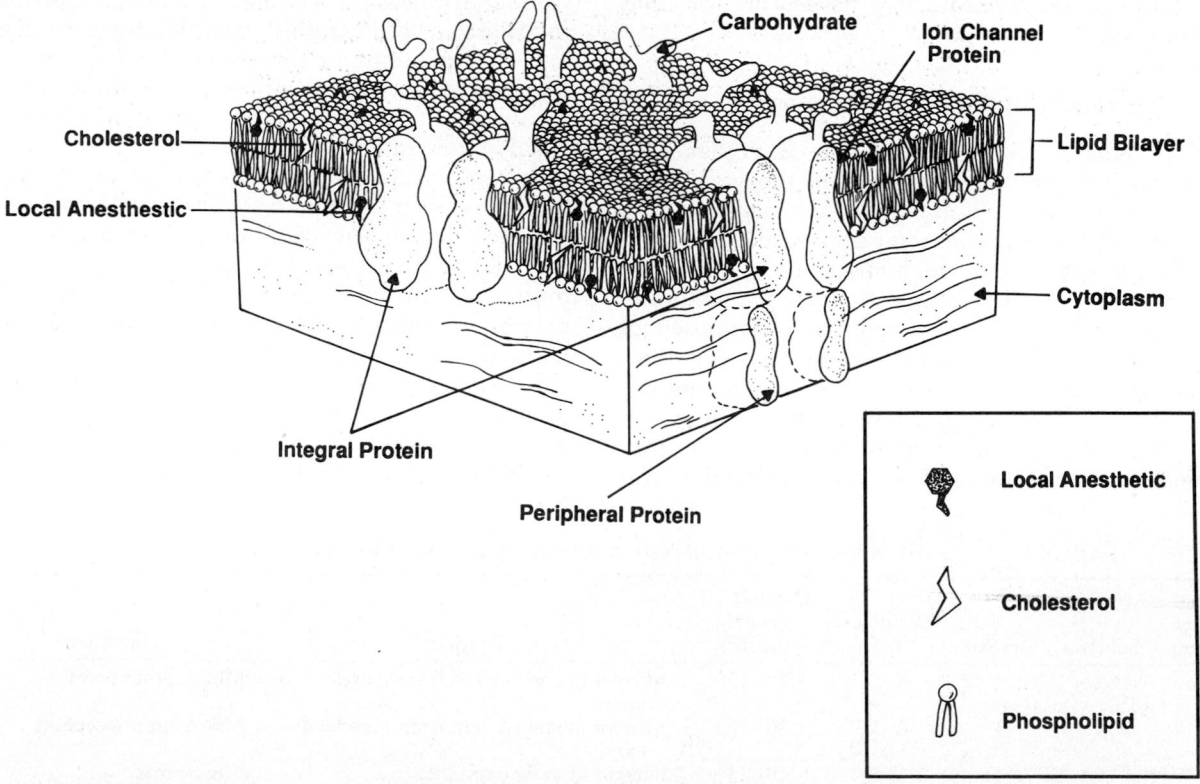

Fig. 13-5. Drawing of a typical plasma membrane showing the lipid bilayer composed of phospholipids and cholesterol molecules (in a 10:1 ratio), embedding the membrane integral proteins, and the relationship of cytoplasmic peripheral proteins and the carbohydrate moieties facing the extracellular medium. Probable locations for local anesthetics are also shown.

Physiology of Nerve Conduction

The neural membrane is able to maintain a voltage difference of 60 to 90 mV between its inner and outer aspects because at rest it is relatively impermeable to sodium ions and selectively permeable to potassium ions. An active, energy-dependent mechanism, the Na^+-K^+ pump, maintains this potential difference by constant extrusion of sodium from within the cell in exchange for a net uptake of potassium, using ATP as an energy source. Although the membrane is relatively permeable to potassium ions, an intracellular to extracellular potassium ratio of 150 to 5 mM, or 30:1, is maintained because of the active removal of potassium and because of the retentive effect of negatively charged intracellular proteins on intracellular potassium, the Donnan potential.

The nerve at rest behaves as a potassium electrode according to the Nernst equation:

$$E = \frac{-RT}{F} \ln \frac{[K^+]_i}{[K^+]_o}$$

where E = membrane potential, R = gas constant (8.315 joules/kelvin); T = temperature (kelvin); F = Faraday's constant (96,500 coulombs); and $[K^+]$ = potassium concentration inside (i) and outside (o) the cell. For potassium, therefore,

$$E = -58 \log 30, \text{ or } -85.7 \text{ mV}$$

An opposite situation exists for Na^+, which is at a higher concentration outside the cell and has a Nernst potential of about $+60$ mV. During an action potential, the nerve membrane transiently switches its selective permeability from K^+ to Na^+, thus changing the membrane potential from negative to positive and back again.[10] The progress of this potential change and the underlying events are graphed in Figure 13-6. They provide a basis for understanding local anesthetic actions.

Ion permeation through membranes occurs via special proteins called ion channels.[11] The conformations of these channels are often responsive to the membrane potential; both Na^+ and K^+ channels in nerve membranes are *activated* to an ion-permeant *(open)* conformation by membrane depolarization. Sodium channels, in addition, close to an ion-impermeant *(inactivated)* conformation following their initial activation. A small membrane depolarization, extending from an adjacent region of excited membrane for example, will begin to open both Na^+ and K^+ channels. The Na^+ channels open faster, however, and because the membrane potential is initially further from the Nernst potential for Na^+ than for K^+, the inwardly directed Na^+ current is the larger current (Fig. 13-6). Sodium ions thus entering the nerve depolarize it further, leading to the opening of more Na^+ channels and increasing the current further. This sequence of events continues in the positive feedback of the depolarizing phase until some of the Na^+ channels have inactivated and the po-

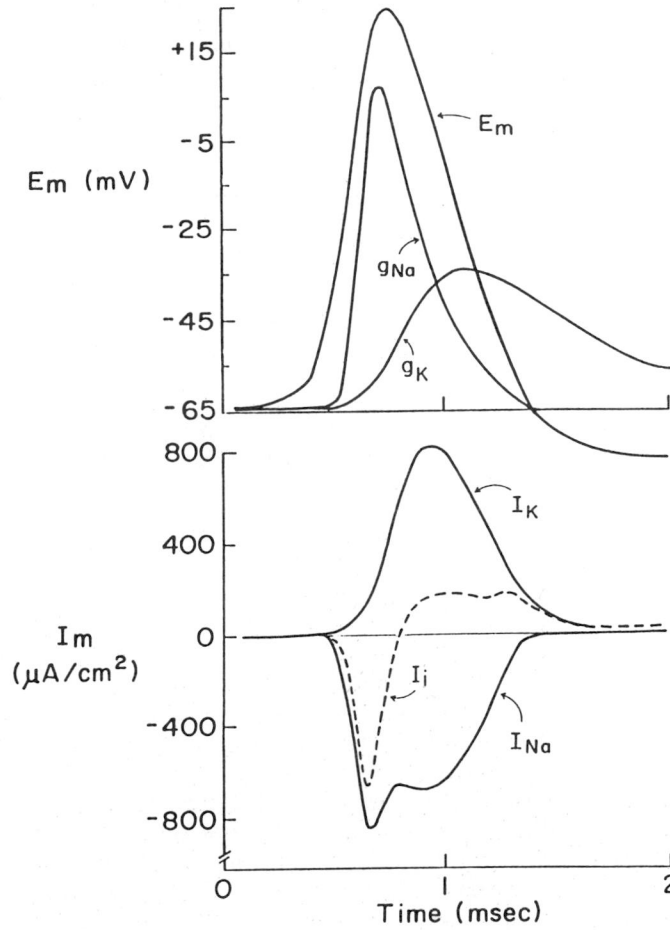

Fig. 13-6. Membrane potential (E_m), conductances of sodium (g_{Na}) and potassium (g_K), and the corresponding membrane currents (I_{Na} and I_K) that occur during a propagated action potential. Modeled from the original studies of Hodgkin and Huxley[49] on the squid giant axon, these relationships hold for almost all invertebrate and vertebrate nerve fibers. The direction of the total ionic current (I_i), which is the sum of I_{Na} and I_K, is inward (negative values) for the depolarizing phase of the action potential, outward (positive values) for the repolarizing phase.

tassium channels have opened sufficiently to change the balance of current, resulting in a net outward current that produces membrane repolarization (Fig. 13-7). The very small amount of Na^+ entering and K^+ leaving the cell as a result of this process is restored by the Na^+ — K^+ pump.[12]

Depolarizations too weak to activate enough Na^+ channels to produce a *net* inward current are below the membrane's excitability threshold. The precise value of the threshold varies among different regions of the cell and also changes in time. Directly after an impulse, when some Na^+ channels are still inactivated and some K^+ channels are still activated, the threshold is elevated

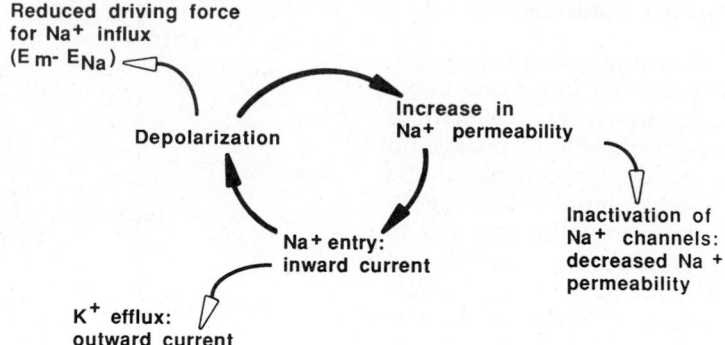

Fig. 13-7. Factors contributing to the regenerative, depolarizing phase of the action potential. Positive factors (solid arrows) increase the rate of depolarization, each element in the cycle favoring the subsequent one. Negative factors (open arrows) decrease the depolarization rate by reducing or opposing the related positive factor.

and the membrane is "refractory" to stimulation. In the repolarized membrane, as Na^+ inactivation decays and as K^+ channels return to their closed conformation, the original threshold value is restored.

The impulse is propagated along the axon by a continuous coupling between excited and nonexcited regions of membrane. Ionic current entering the axon in the excited, depolarized region (the *action current*) flows down the axoplasm and exits through the surrounding membrane, thus passively depolarizing the adjacent region (Fig. 13-3). Although this local circuit current spreads away from the excited zone in both directions, the region *behind* the impulse, having just encountered a large depolarization, is refractory, and propagation is thus unidirectional.

In a myelinated axon, the local circuit current spreads rapidly along a length composed of insulated internode (Fig. 13-3), and many nodes of Ranvier in sequence are depolarized to threshold with little intervening delay. Single impulses do not "jump" from node to node as separate, discrete events; instead, the active depolarization occurs simultaneously along several centimeters of the largest axons (see Fig. 13-11).[13] Indeed, the local circuit current is so robust that it can skip past two completely inexcitable nodes and successfully stimulate a third.[14] If nodal excitability is partially reduced, by inhibition of some of the Na^+ channels, for example, then the amplitude of impulses in successive nodes falls decrementally, a process that can continue for many centimeters.[15] This situation probably occurs during certain phases of local anesthesia, as discussed below. When the extent of inhibition of Na^+ channels is sufficient, however, the impulse is extinguished along the axon. This is the electrophysiologic event of local anesthesia.

MECHANISM OF ACTION OF LOCAL ANESTHETICS DRUGS (PHARMACODYNAMICS)

Active Form

Local anesthetic bases are poorly soluble in water but are soluble in relatively hydrophobic organic solvents. Therefore, as a matter of convenience, most of these drugs are marketed as the hydrochloride salts, which are soluble in water but insoluble in organic solvents. The pK_a of the drug and the tissue pH will determine the amount of drug that exists in solution as free base or as positively charged cation when injected into living tissue. Furthermore, the uptake of the drug by the tissue, due largely to lipophilic adsorption, will also alter its activity, both by shifting the effective pK_a downward and thereby favoring the neutral base form and by limiting the diffusion of the anesthetic away from the site of injection. Thus, moderately hydrophobic local anesthetics will act more rapidly than either slightly hydrophobic or highly hydrophobic ones delivered at the same concentration. Since the highly hydrophobic local anesthetics also have higher intrinsic potency[3] (Table 13-2), they are delivered as lower amounts and their diffusion profile is correspondingly reduced, compromising their rate of onset even further.

A lengthy debate has taken place over the issue of which form of the local anesthetic is actually responsible for prevention of impulse propagation. Early observations showed that alkaline solutions of local anesthetics more effectively blocked nerve conduction.[16] In the desheathed nerve and in the isolated single axon, the rate of inhibition by tertiary amine anesthetics also was greater at alkaline than at neutral external pH.[17,18]

From these observations it was concluded either that the neutral base in the external solution was the active species or that membrane penetration and transport, highly favored for base rather than cation species, were essential for the channel-blocking action. The second possibility is, in fact, the explanation for the alkaline acceleration of rate.[18,19] Direct control of axoplasmic pH[20] or internal perfusion with permanently charged, quaternary amine homologues shows the potency of the cationic species acting from the cytoplasmic surface.[21,22] The uncharged base also has pharmacologic activity, however, and not only molecules with tertiary amine moieties but those having hydroxyl (alcohols) or alkyl groups (e.g., benzocaine) can inhibit Na⁺ channels and block impulses.[8,19,23,24]

To obtain a clear picture of the mechanism, the inhibitory kinetics are necessary, but it is almost impossible to measure the rate of binding of local anesthetics to the receptor after their addition to a bathing solution. Drug diffusion through the unstirred layer of solution next to the membrane and the membrane itself present steps that limit the rate of receptor binding.[18,25] However, once the drug has equilibrated with membranes and solutions, it is possible to perturb the channels by depolarizing the membrane and to follow the *phasic* inhibition by local anesthetics in order to clarify the details of the binding reaction, as described in the following passage.

The Electrophysiologic Effect of Local Anesthetics

The resting membrane potential of nerve is affected little by local anesthetics.[26] As the concentration of local anesthetic applied to the nerve is increased, a decrease in the rate and degree of depolarization is produced. Inhibition of depolarization increases with time as the concentration of drug is maintained. As noted previously, local anesthetics block impulses by reducing the currents through voltage-activated Na⁺ channels.[27,28] The inhibition is not specific, however, and K⁺ currents are also reduced.[29] To the degree that local anesthetics inhibit K⁺ channels, given a constant affinity for Na⁺ channels, their potency for blocking impulses is correspondingly lowered (Fig. 13-8).[30] Furthermore, neither the reduction of amplitude nor the rate of depolarization of an action potential is proportional to the fraction of Na⁺ channels inhibited by local anesthetics, even when actions on other ion channels are excluded. Therefore, it is not possible to derive direct data on the binding of local anesthetics from measurement of nerve impulses.

By using a voltage-clamp procedure, however, Na⁺ currents and their inhibition by local anesthetics can be directly assayed (Fig. 13-9). After drug addition, the membrane is rapidly depolarized to a constant value, briefly, and the time course of currents is observed on an oscilloscope screen. Rapidly rising (activated) and subsequently declining (inactivated) Na⁺ currents are reduced for one depolarization by subclinical doses of local anesthetic (e.g., 0.2 mM lidocaine) and completely inhibited by clinical doses (e.g., 1 percent lidocaine, which equals ca. 40 mM). If the test depolarization is repetitively applied at frequencies above 5 Hz (5 pulses/s), the Na⁺ current is further reduced, incrementally for each pulse, until a new steady-state level of inhibition is reached.[22,31] This frequency-dependent inhibition, also called *phasic inhibition*, is reversed when stimulation is slowed or stopped, and currents return to the level of "tonic inhibition" observed in the resting

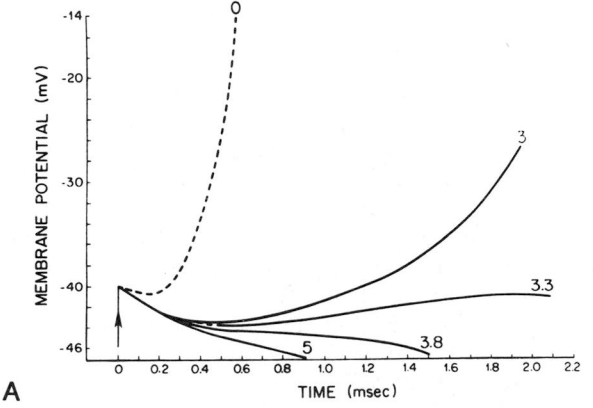
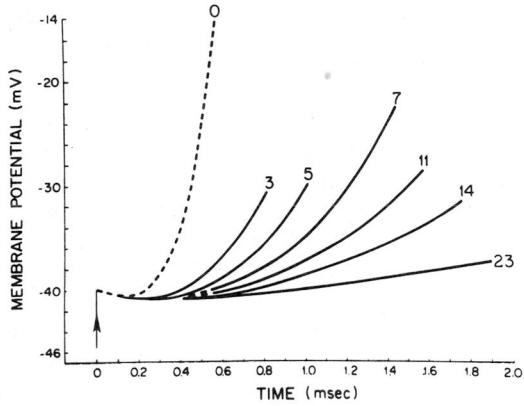

Fig. 13-8. The impulse blocking potency of local anesthetics is less if the drug inhibits potassium channels as well as sodium channels. This computer simulation shows only the initial phase of depolarization of a squid axon's action potential (see Fig. 13-6), stimulated by a 20 mV depolarization at time 0, under conditions where local anesthetic (LA) binds only to Na⁺ channels (A), or to K⁺ channels also, but with half the affinity for Na⁺ channels (B). Numbers at the ends of the traces list the drug concentration as a multiple of its equilibrium dissociation constant for Na⁺ channels, K_D. In Fig. A, impulse failure occurs when $[LA] = 3.3 \times K_D$; in Fig. B, failure occurs at seven times this concentration: $[LA] = 23 \times K_D$. (From Strichartz,[30] with permission.)

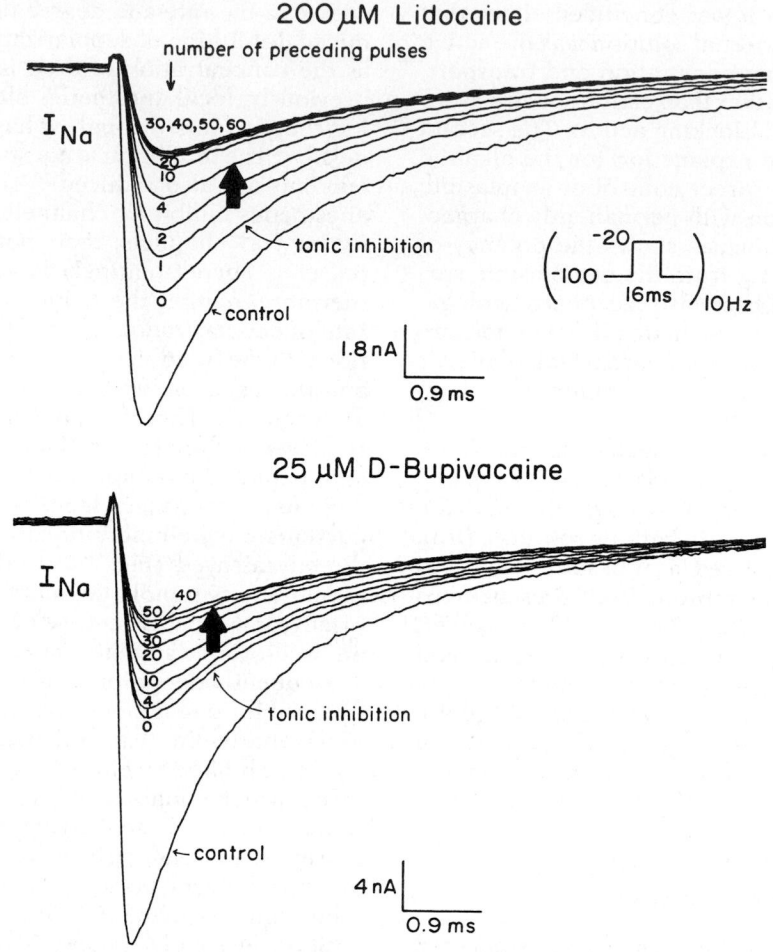

Fig. 13-9. Inhibition of Na⁺ currents in myelinated nerves exposed to lidocaine or to bupivacaine. Traces show the inward ionic currents during a 16-millisecond-long depolarization to −20 mV, before drug addition (control), for the first depolarization imposed 5 min after beginning drug exposure (0, tonic inhibition), and for the subsequent pulses in a train of depolarizations applied to 10 Hz (identified numerically by their order in the sequence; use-dependent inhibition). T = 13°C. Toad node of Ranvier. (From Chernoff,[32] with permission.)

nerve. The potency for local anesthetics to produce both tonic and phasic inhibition is related similarly to their structure, hydrophobicity, and pK_a.[32,33] There thus appears to be a single binding site for local anesthetics on the Na⁺ channel, with a *tonic* affinity at rest and an increased *phasic* affinity that occurs as a result of depolarization. The phasic blocking mode can thus be used to reveal the true kinetics of local anesthetic binding to the functional receptor.

Sodium currents are reduced by local anesthetics because the drug-bound channels fail to open. Investigations with neutral and cationic compounds show that the channel activation process is disrupted by local anesthetics.[33,34] A sodium channel inhibited by a local anesthetic is functionally similar to an inactivated channel; inactivation and anesthetic binding prevent the conformational changes that constitute the activation process by fully or partially immobilizing the channel.[35]

To some extent, blockade of the ion-conducting pore plays a part in channel inhibition, but the contribution from this mechanism seems minor.

Are inactivated channels an essential conformation for local anesthetic action? No, because when inactivation is prevented by various chemical reagents or toxins, there is little change in the tonic and phasic actions of local anesthetics.[36] Phasic channel inhibition occurs during depolarizations that are as short as neuronal impulses (1 to 5 milliseconds) because local anesthetics bind rapidly and with higher affinity to activated channels (some open, some in conformations preceding the open state) than to resting channels. During longer depolarizations, additional binding to drug-free inactivated channels can occur[19,31]; this mode of binding probably accounts for much of the therapeutic action of local anesthetic-like class I antiarrhythmics.[37]

Regardless of the channel state that binds the drug, by

its very binding the local anesthetic stabilizes that state. During phasic block, therefore, more channels become drug bound during activation, and reciprocally, less activation can occur. Overall binding of anesthetic is increased by channel activation for two reasons: more binding sites become accessible during activation (the "guarded receptor" model)[38] and drug dissocation from activated channels is slower than from resting channels (the "modulated receptor" model).[19]

The specific binding rates and affinities of local anesthetics for the different conformations of the sodium channel depend on the particular drug. When the details of this dependence are related to the physicochemical properties of the drug and to the experimental conditions, they provide insight into the nature of the local anesthetic binding site.[3,4]

The Nature of the Local Anesthetic Binding Site

Kinetic and equilibrium measurements of inhibition by diverse local anesthetics reveal much about the binding site. Like the rate of onset of tonic block, the rate of binding for phasic block is greater at a more alkaline external pH, which favors the neutral drug in the membrane and both the neutral and cationic species in the cytoplasm.[32] Curiously, cytoplasmic pH has almost no effect on phasic inhibition.[39] Drugs of greater hydrophobicity are proportionately more potent for both tonic and phasic block than less hydrophobic congeners.[3,40,41] However, at equipotent doses of two local anesthetics which differ 100-fold in hydrophobicity and in intrinsic potency (but have very similar pK_as), the rate of phasic binding is almost the same despite the 100-fold difference in their concentrations in solution. The apparent discrepancy between rates and concentrations can be reconciled by postulating that the primary blocking reaction occurs from the membrane phase, where the more potent drug is concentrated by hydrophobic uptake[19,32] (Fig. 13-10).

Dissociation of local anesthetic from the phasically activated channel depends little on hydrophobicity, size, or pK_a. This rate constant is also independent of external pH. In contrast, drug dissocation from the closed channels that exist after the membrane is repolarized depends strongly on all these factors. Dissociation is slightly faster for more hydrophobic compounds,[3] markedly faster at more alkaline than at neutral external pH,[39,42] and faster for drugs of lower pK_a.[31] One simple interpretation of these findings is that anesthetic dissociation can occur by either a hydrophobic or a hydrophilic pathway.[19] The former accommodates the uncharged base primarily and is 20 to 50 times faster than the latter, which accommodates the cationic species. There is a relatively sharp cutoff in the molecular weight dependence of dissociation of charged anesthetics from closed channels, the rate falling by 80 percent above around 250 daltons. Such behavior is consistent with a long, narrow hydrophilic escape pathway.[43] For uncharged species, a different dependence on drug size is observed; lidocaine dissociates four to five times faster than smaller or larger anesthetics, which all leave at about the same rate.[44] This anomalous behavior may reflect the unique ability of the lidocaine base to form an intramolecular bond between amine and amide groups and so increase its escape by the hydrophobic route.

Integrating these physicochemical findings resolves a dynamic picture of local anesthetic action (Fig. 13-10). The binding of tertiary amine compounds occurs primarily from the membrane phase and favors the neutral base species. Dissociation of drug involves primarily the closed conformations of the channel (excitation occurring only briefly) and is slowed by extracellular protons. In brief, hydrophobicity gets the drug to the receptor and charge keeps it there.[44]

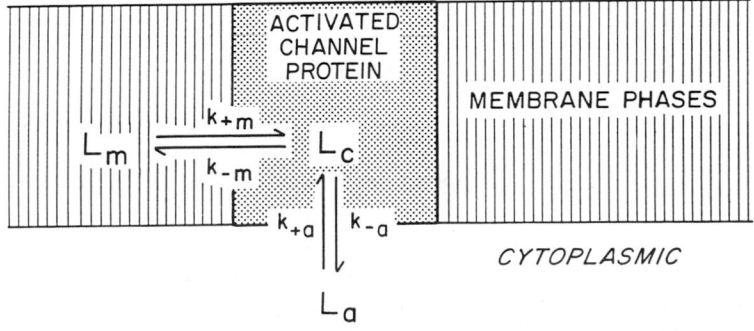

Fig. 13-10. Schematic drawing of drug access routes to a putative local anesthetic binding site on the Na^+ channel. The hydrophilic route, from the cytoplasmic phase, mediates binding of aqueous drug (L_a) directly to the receptor site. The hydrophobic route mediates binding to membrane-associated drug (L_m) to the site. The activated channel (induced by membrane depolarization) binds drug more tightly than the resting channel, but both states of the protein appear to favor the hydrophobic route.

Neurophysiologic Aspects of Phasic Inhibition

Impulse blockade is also advanced in a phasic mode. As the frequency of impulse traffic in an axon is increased, the probability of impulse blockade by local anesthetic also rises. This phenomenon develops along the length of axon exposed to drug, as shown in the panels of Figure 13-11. The first impulse to traverse the fiber, where 16 consecutive nodes have been exposed to lidocaine at a concentration that blocks 50 percent of the Na⁺ chan-

nels at rest, suffers decremental conduction along the drug-exposed region.[45] Yet the reduced impulse still provides enough current at the last anesthetized node to raise the adjacent drug-free region to threshold. Impulse propagation is thus slowed but does not fail. But the second impulse in the train encounters an exposed region of axon rendered less excitable from the residual phasic inhibition of the first impulse. Action currents at the end of the exposed region are below the margin of safety, and propagation fails.[46] The third impulse expe-

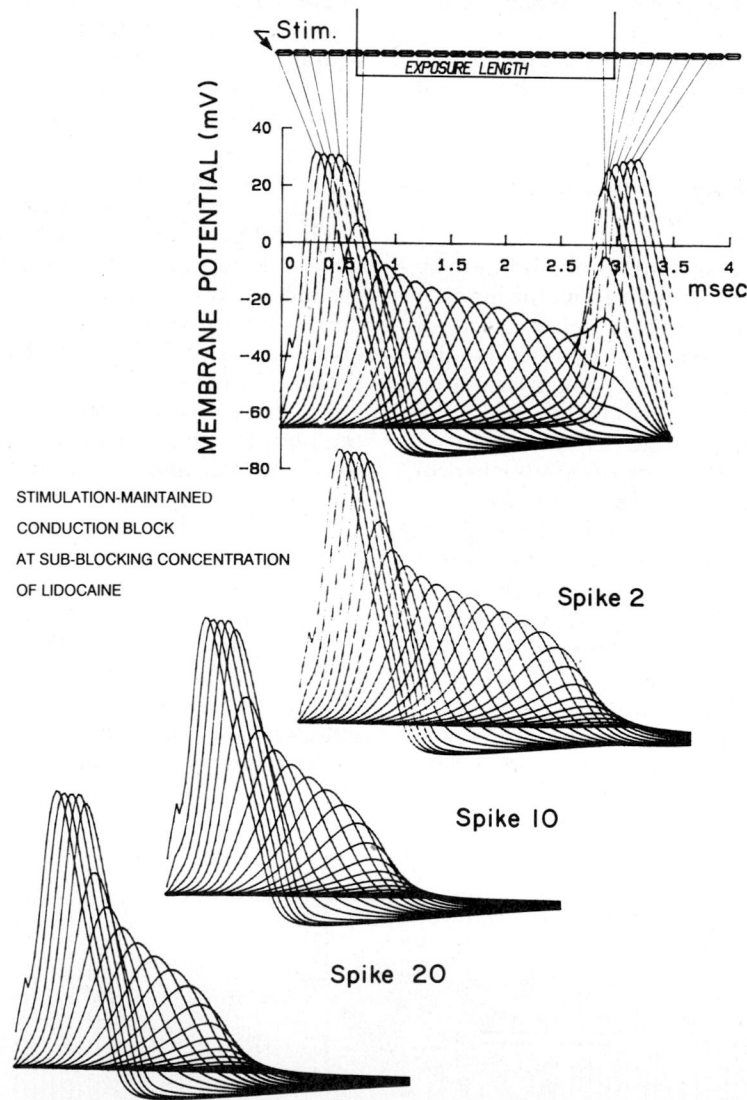

Fig. 13-11. Decremental inhibition of conducted impulses modeled in a myelinated axon shows use-dependent block. In this computer simulation, the membrane potential at each of 26 sequential nodes of Ranvier is plotted as the impulse, stimulated at the left-most node, propagating to the right. Fifteen nodes in the middle of this fiber are "exposed" to local anesthetics, which reduces both Na⁺ and K⁺ conductances to tonically inhibited levels (Fig. 13-9) for the first impulse in a train (top frame). Although this impulse's amplitude decrements continuously over the exposed length, local current at the last exposed node is still sufficient to stimulate the next, unexposed node, and conduction continues. Use-dependent drug binding during this spike lowers the Na⁺ conductance available for subsequent impulses in the train, which therefore decrement further (compare spike 2 and spike 10) and fail to sustain conduction within the exposed region. (From Raymond et al.,[46] with permission.)

riences an even greater spatial decrement. Each subsequent impulse in the train continues to fail to traverse the drugged axon; impulse activity entering the anesthetized region thus maintains its own failure.

An identical phenomenon occurs in vivo. There, the frequency of impulses encodes neuronal information; in sensory fibers, the intensity of the physiologic stimulation is encoded in the impulse discharge pattern. Local anesthetics significantly disrupt this pattern, as shown by the example of an afferent A fiber coupled to a slowly adapting mechanoreceptor in the rat footpad in Figure 13-12.[46] Application of a subclinical dose of lidocaine to the ensheathed sciatic nerve in vivo leads to a progressive reduction in the average frequency of impulses propagated by one axon, even though the mechanical stimulus intensity is increased beyond control level.

Different fiber types in the nerve will be affected differentially by local anesthetics. At the onset and during the recovery from clinical block, in particular, the longitudinal and radial diffusion of drug will produce concentration variations within and along the nerve.[47] This variation is superimposed on the dynamic use-dependent inhibition to provide variable propagation that depends on a fiber's geometry, position within the nerve, and functional as well as electrophysiologic properties.

No clear relationship has been established between the diameter of an axon and its absolute susceptibility to block by local anesthetics, although the temporal sequence of loss of various sensory and sympathetic functions during regional block is well documented.[48] For an explanation of the clinical observation, we must look beyond the strictly geometrical aspects of an axon. A consideration of fiber functions and physiologic properties may provide a future basis for these phenomena.[49]

Summary of Local Anesthetic Mechanisms

Impulse blockade by local anesthetics may be summarized by the following chronology:

1. Solutions of local anesthetic are deposited near the nerve. Diffusion of drug molecules away from this locus is a function of tissue binding, removal by the circulation, and local hydrolysis of aminoester anesthetics. The net result is penetration of the nerve sheath by remaining molecules.
2. Local anesthetic molecules then permeate the nerve's axon membranes and equilibrate there and in the axoplasm. The speed and extent of these processes depend on a particular drug's pK_a and the lipophilicity of base and cation species.

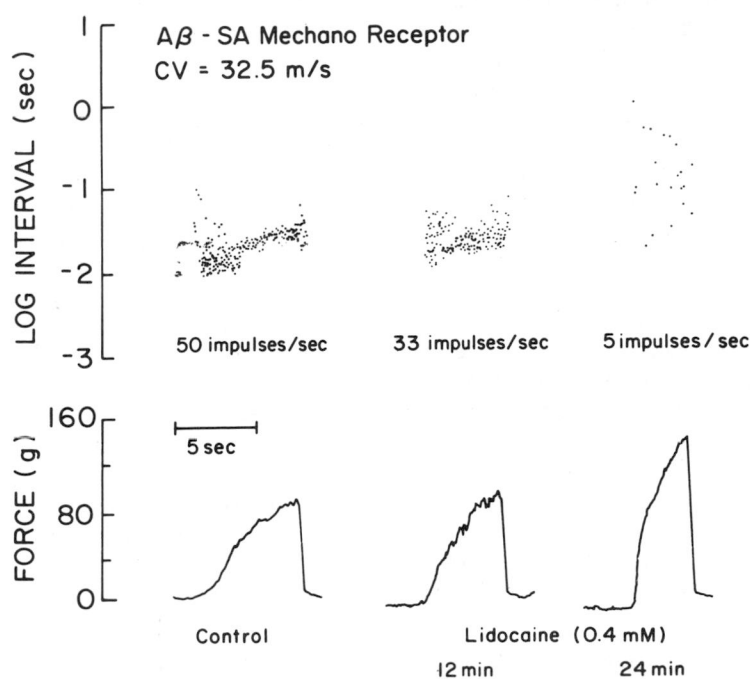

Fig. 13-12. The pattern of impulses in vivo in a cutaneous afferent of the rat is strongly modified by local anesthetic. Discharge frequency (upper traces, shown on a logarithmic scale) in response to increasing pressure on the rat's footpad (lower traces) maintains a relatively constant value (50/s, average) in this slowly adapting mechanoreceptor before drug. Bathing the ensheathed sciatic nerve with lidocaine (0.01 percent over a 2 to 3 cm length) inhibits impulse conduction through the exposed region, so that after 24 minutes of drug exposure, the average frequency has fallen by 90 percent, despite the faster and larger mechanical stimulation. (From Raymond et al.,[46] with permission.)

3. Binding of local anesthetic to sites on voltage-gated Na^+ channels prevents opening of the channels by inhibiting conformational changes that underlie channel activation.

4. During onset and recovery from local anesthesia, impulse blockade is incomplete, and "partially blocked" fibers are further inhibited by repetitive stimulation that produces an additional, "use-dependent" binding to Na^+ channels.

5. One local anesthetic binding site on the Na^+ channel may be sufficient to account for the drug's resting (tonic) and use-dependent (phasic) actions. The access to this site may potentially involve multiple pathways, but for clinical local anesthetics, the primary route is the "hydrophobic" approach from within the axon membrane.

6. The rates of onset and recovery from blockade are governed by the relatively slow diffusion of local anesthetic molecules into and out of the nerve, not by the much faster binding and dissociation to ion channels.

CLINICAL PHARMACOLOGY

The successful use of regional anesthesia requires knowledge of the pharmacologic properties of the various local anesthetic drugs, as well as technical skill in the performance of the nerve block planned. Local anesthetic requirements vary considerably depending on various factors such as type of block, surgical procedure, and physiologic status of the patient.

The clinically useful aminoester local anesthetics are procaine, chloroprocaine, and tetracaine. The amino amides consist of lidocaine, mepivacaine, prilocaine, bupivacaine, and etidocaine. The ester and amide local anesthetics differ in their chemical stability, locus of biotransformation, and allergic potential. Amides are extremely stable agents, while esters are relatively unstable in solution. The aminoesters are hydrolyzed in plasma by the cholinesterase enzymes, whereas the amide compounds undergo enzymatic degradation in the liver. *Para*- aminobenzoic acid is one of the metabolites of ester-type compounds that can induce allergic-type reactions in a small percentage of patients. The aminoamides are not metabolized to *para*-aminobenzoic acid, and reports of allergic reactions to these agents are extremely rare.

General Considerations

The clinically important properties of the various local anesthetics include potency, speed of onset, duration of anesthetic action, and differential sensory/motor blockade. As previously indicated, the profile of the individual agents is determined by their physicochemical characteristics (Table 13-2).

Anesthetic Potency

Hydrophobicity appears to be a primary determinant of intrinsic anesthetic potency,[50,51] since the anesthetic molecule must penetrate into the nerve membrane. However, clinically, the correlation between hydrophobicity and anesthetic potency is not as precise as in an isolated nerve. Lidocaine is approximately twice as potent as prilocaine in an isolated preparation,[52] but in humans little difference in anesthetic potency is apparent between these agents.[53] Similarly, etidocaine is more potent than bupivacaine in an isolated nerve, while clinically, etidocaine is actually less active than bupivacaine.[54,55] The difference between in vitro and in vivo results is related to a number of factors such as the vasodilator or tissue redistribution properties of the various local anesthetics. For example, lidocaine causes a greater degree of vasodilation than prilocaine, resulting in a more rapid vascular uptake of lidocaine such that fewer lidocaine molecules are available for neural blockade.[56] The extremely high lipid solubility of etidocaine may result in a greater uptake of this agent by adipose tissue, such as in the epidural space, which again results in fewer etidocaine molecules available for neural blockade compared with bupivacaine.

Onset of Action

The onset of conduction block in isolated nerves is related to the physicochemical properties of the individual agents. In humans, latency is also dependent on the dose or concentration of local anesthetic employed. For example, 0.25 percent bupivacaine possesses a rather slow onset of action. However, increasing the concentration to 0.75 percent results in a significant acceleration of anesthetic effect.[55] Chloroprocaine demonstrates a rapid onset of action in humans despite the facts that the pK_a of chloroprocaine is approximately 9 and that its onset of action in isolated nerves is relatively slow.[57] However, the low systemic toxicity of this agent allows the use of high concentrations (e.g., 3 percent). Therefore, the rapid onset time in vivo of chloroprocaine may be related simply to the large number of molecules placed in the vicinity of peripheral nerves. In humans, 1.5 percent lidocaine produced a more rapid onset of epidural anesthesia than 1.5 percent chloroprocaine.[58] However, 3 percent chloroprocaine resulted in a more rapid onset compared with 2.0 percent lidocaine.

Duration of Action

The duration of action of the various local anesthetics differs markedly. Procaine and chloroprocaine demonstrate a short duration of action. Lidocaine, mepivacaine, and prilocaine produce a moderate duration of anesthesia, while tetracaine, bupivacaine, and etidocaine have the longest durations of anesthesia. For example, procaine produces a duration of brachial plexus blockade of 30 to 60 minutes, while up to approximately 10 hours of anesthesia have been reported following the use of bupivacaine or etidocaine for brachial plexus blockade.[59]

In humans, the duration of anesthesia is markedly influenced by the peripheral vascular effects of the local anesthetic drugs. All local anesthetics except cocaine tend to have a biphasic effect on vascular smooth muscle. At low concentrations, these agents tend to cause vasoconstriction, whereas at clinically employed concentrations, local anesthetics cause vasodilation.[60,61] However, differences exist in the degree of vasodilator activity produced by the various drugs. For example, lidocaine is a more potent vasodilator than mepivacaine or prilocaine. Although little difference in the duration of conduction block is apparent between these agents in an isolated nerve, in vivo the duration of anesthesia produced by lidocaine is shorter than that of mepivacaine or prilocaine.

Differential Sensory/Motor Blockade

Another important clinical consideration is the ability of local anesthetic agents to cause a differential inhibition of sensory and motor activity. Bupivacaine is the most useful agent in terms of producing adequate antinociception without profound inhibition of motor activity, regardless of the regional anesthetic technique employed. Bupivacaine and etidocaine provide an interesting contrast in their differential sensory/motor blocking activity, although they are both potent long-acting anesthetic agents[56] (Fig. 13-13). Bupivacaine is widely used epidurally for obstetric procedures and relief of pain postoperatively owing to its ability to provide adequate analgesia with minimal muscle weakness or paralysis, particularly when used as an 0.125 or 0.25 percent solution. Thus, the patient in labor can be rendered painfree and still be able to move her legs, which is one of the primary reasons why this agent has enjoyed popularity for continuous epidural blockade during labor. Etidocaine, on the other hand, shows little separation between sensory and motor activities. Concentrations of etidocaine that are required to achieve adequate sensory anesthesia also cause a profound degree of local weakness. Etidocaine is a valuable agent for epidural blockade in surgical situations in which optimum muscle relaxation is desirable, but it is of limited value for obstetric analgesia and the postoperative pain relief.

Factors Influencing Anesthetic Activity in Humans

Dosage of Local Anesthetic

As the dosage of local anesthetic is increased, the probability and duration of satisfactory anesthesia will increase and the onset of block will be shortened. The

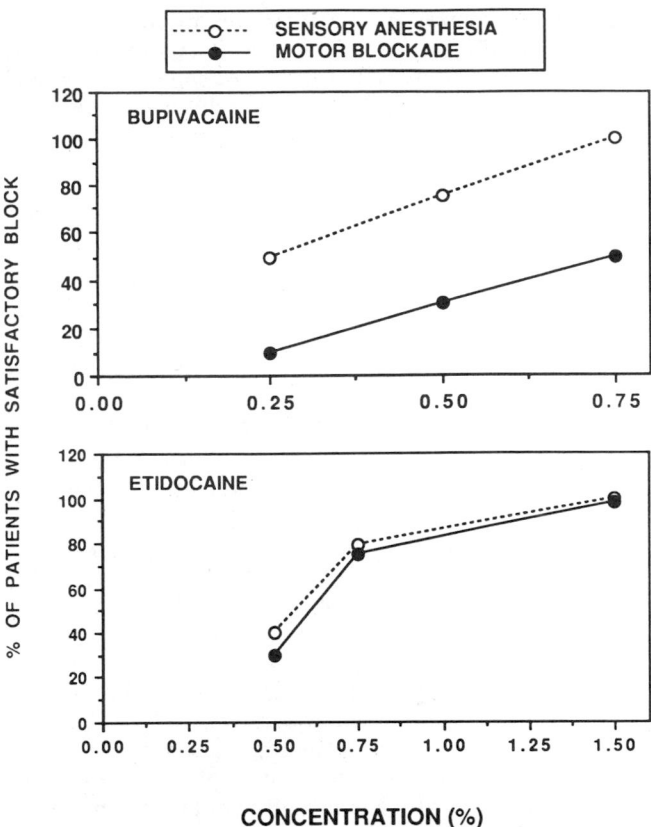

Fig. 13-13. Comparative inhibition of sensory and motor activity following the epidural administration of varying concentrations of bupivacaine and etidocaine.

dosage of local anesthetic can be increased by administering either a larger volume or a more concentrated solution. In clinical practice, an increase in dosage is usually achieved with a more concentrated solution of the specific agent. For example, increasing the concentration of epidurally administered bupivacaine from 0.125 to 0.5 percent while maintaining the same volume of injectate (10 ml) resulted in a shorter latency, improved incidence of satisfactory analgesia, and longer duration of sensory analgesia.[62] Similarly, an increase in the concentration of epidural bupivacaine in surgical patients from 0.5 to 0.75 percent with a concomitant increase in dosage from approximately 100 to 150 mg produced a more rapid onset and prolonged sensory anesthesia, a greater frequency of satisfactory sensory anesthesia, and more profound motor blockade[55] (Fig. 13-13). Prilocaine (600 mg) administered epidurally either as 30 ml of a 2 percent solution or 20 ml of a 3 percent solution showed no difference in onset, adequacy, or duration of anesthesia and onset, depth, and duration of motor blockade.[53] The volume of anesthetic solution may influence the spread of anesthesia. For example, 30 ml of 1 percent lidocaine administered into the epidural space produced a level of anesthesia that was 4.3 dermatomes higher than that achieved when 10 ml of 3 percent lidocaine was employed.[63] In summary, total dosage (volume × concentration) is probably the main determinant of the anesthetic profile of a specific agent.

Addition of Vasoconstrictors

Vasoconstrictors, usually epinephrine (5 μg/ml), are frequently included in local anesthetic solutions to decrease the rate of vascular absorption, thereby allowing more anesthetic molecules to reach the nerve membrane and so improve the depth and duration of anesthesia. Epinephrine in a concentration of 1:200,000 has been reported to provide the optimal degree of vasoconstriction when employed with lidocaine for epidural or intercostal use.[64] Other vasoconstrictor agents such as norepinephrine and phenylephrine have been used but do not appear to be superior to epinephrine. For example, equipotent concentrations of epinephrine and phenylephrine prolong the duration of spinal anesthesia produced by tetracaine to a similar extent.[65]

The ability of epinephrine to prolong the duration of anesthesia depends on the local anesthetic employed and the site of injection. Epinephrine will significantly extend the duration of both infiltration anesthesia and peripheral nerve blocks with all agents.[66,67] The duration of epidural anesthesia, however, is not markedly prolonged when epinephrine is combined with prilocaine, bupivacaine, or etidocaine.[68] The decreased vasodilator action of prilocaine compared with lidocaine may be responsible for the reduced effect of epinephrine in solutions of prilocaine. On the other hand, the high lipid solubility of bupivacaine and etidocaine results in a substantial uptake of these agents by adipose tissue in the epidural space. The subsequent slow release from adipose tissue contributes to their prolonged duration of action, which is not enhanced by epinephrine. Dilute solutions of bupivacaine may benefit from the addition of epinephrine. For example, the depth and duration of epidural analgesia in obstetric patients was improved when epinephrine 1:300:000 was added to 0.25 percent bupivacaine.[69] When 0.5 or 0.75 percent bupivacaine was used for surgical epidural blockade, the addition of epinephrine resulted in a more profound degree of motor blockade with minimal effect on the quality and duration of sensory anesthesia.[68]

Site of Injection

The most rapid onset but the shortest duration of action occurs following the intrathecal or subcutaneous administration of local anesthetics. The longest latencies and durations are observed following the performance of brachial plexus blocks. For example, intrathecal bupivacaine usually will produce anesthesia within 5 minutes that will persist for 3 to 4 hours. However, when bupivacaine is administered for brachial plexus blockade, the onset time is approximately 20 to 30 minutes, while the duration of anesthesia averages 10 hours. These differences in the onset and duration of anesthesia are due in part to the particular anatomy of the area of injection. This will influence the rate of diffusion and vascular absorption which in turn affect the amount of drug employed for various types of regional anesthesia. In the subarachnoid space, for example, the lack of a nerve sheath around the spinal cord and the deposition of the local anesthetic solution in the immediate vicinity of the spinal cord are responsible for the rapid onset of action, while the relatively small amount of drug employed for spinal anesthesia probably accounts for the short duration of conduction block.

On the other hand, the onset of brachial plexus blockade is slow since the anesthetic agent is usually deposited at some distance from the nerve roots and must diffuse through various tissue barriers before reaching the nerve membrane. The prolonged blockade is probably related to the decreased rate of vascular absorption from that site and the larger doses of drug required for this regional anesthetic technique.

Carbonation and pH Adjustment of Local Anesthetics

Carbon dioxide will enhance the diffusion of local anesthetics through the nerve sheath of an isolated nerve, resulting in a more rapid onset and a decrease in the minimum concentration (Cm) required for conduction blockade[70] (Fig. 13-14). The enhanced onset and depth of conduction blockage are due to the diffusion of carbon dioxide through the nerve membrane, thereby decreasing axoplasmic pH. The lower pH increases the rate and extent of formation of the active protonated form of the local anesthetic. In addition, the ionized local anesthetic does not readily diffuse through membranes, so that the drug remains entrapped within the axoplasm, a situation referred to as ion trapping. Moreover, carbon dioxide itself may depress neuronal excitability. Although the effect of carbon dioxide on local anesthetic activity is easily demonstrable in isolated nerve,[71] controversy exists concerning the clinical utility of carbonated local anesthetic solutions. For example, some studies have failed to demonstrate a significantly more rapid onset of action when lidocaine carbonate was compared with lidocaine hydrochloride for epidural blockade,[72] while others have reported a significant reduction in onset of epidural blockade with lidocaine carbonate.[73] Similar discrepancies existed when bupivacaine hydrochloride and bupivacaine carbonate were evaluated clinically.[74,75] Although the effect of carbon dioxide on the latency of conduction blockage may be controversial, carbonated solutions appear to improve the depth of sensory and motor blockade when administered into the epidural space.[72,73] In addition, these solutions may produce a more complete blockade of the radial, median, and

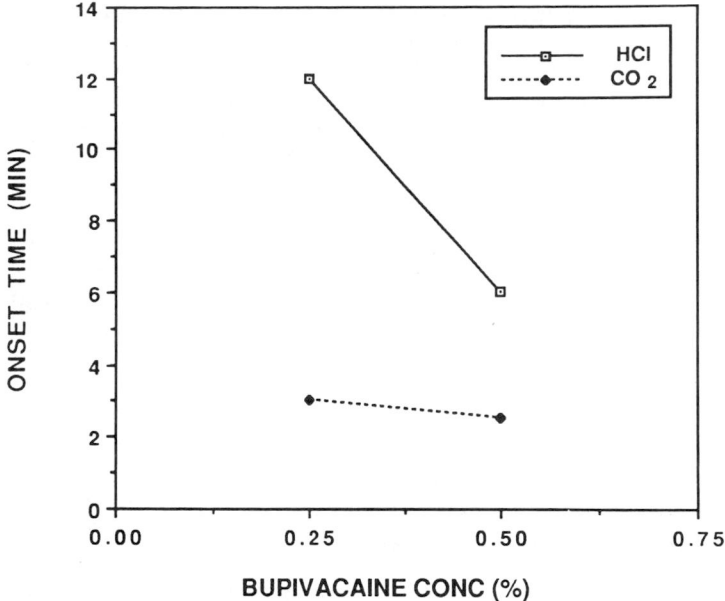

Fig. 13-14. Onset of conduction block in isolated rabbit vagus nerve exposed to 0.25 and 0.5 percent bupivacaine hydrochloride and bupivacaine carbonate.

ulnar nerves when employed for brachial plexus blockade.[27]

Addition of sodium bicarbonate to local anesthetic solutions has also been reported to decrease the onset of conduction blockade.[76,77] An increase in the pH of the local anesthetic solution will increase the amount of drug in the uncharged base form, which should enhance the rate of diffusion across the nerve sheath and nerve membrane, resulting in a more rapid onset of anesthesia. Alkalinization of solutions of bupivacaine or lidocaine reportedly did significantly decrease the latency of brachial plexus and epidural blockade.[76,77] On the other hand, at least one study failed to demonstrate an improved onset of brachial plexus blockade when the pH of bupivacaine solution was increased by the addition of sodium bicarbonate.[78]

Mixtures of Local Anesthetics

The use of mixtures of local anesthetics for regional anesthesia has become relatively popular in recent years. The basis for this practice is to compensate for the short duration of action of certain agents such as chloroprocaine or lidocaine and the long latency of other agents such as tetracaine and bupivacaine. Mixtures of chloroprocaine and bupivacaine theoretically should offer significant clinical advantages owing to the rapid onset and low systemic toxicity of chloroprocaine and the long duration of action of bupivacaine. A mixture of 3 percent chloroprocaine and 0.5 percent bupivacaine was reported to produce a short latency and prolonged duration of brachial plexus blockade.[79] However, subsequent studies indicated that the duration of epidural anesthesia produced by a mixture of

chloroprocaine and bupivacaine was significantly shorter than that obtained with bupivacaine alone, while the onset was longer than that of chloroprocaine alone.[80] Isolated nerve studies suggest that a metabolite of chloroprocaine may inhibit the binding of bupivacaine to membrane sites.[81] At present, there do not appear to be any clinically significant advantages to the use of mixtures of local anesthetic agents. Etidocaine and bupivacaine provide clinically acceptable onsets of action and prolonged durations of anesthesia. In addition, the use of catheter techniques for many forms of regional anesthesia makes it possible to indefinitely extend the duration of action of the rapidly acting agents such as chloroprocaine or lidocaine.

Pregnancy
(Also See Ch. 57)

The spread and depth of epidural and spinal anesthesia are reported to be greater in pregnant patients than in nonpregnant women.[82] This was originally attributed to mechanical factors associated with pregnancy, that is, dilated epidural veins decrease the diameter of the epidural and subarachnoid space. Hormonal alterations may also play a role in the apparent increase in local anesthetic sensitivity during pregnancy since a greater spread of epidural anesthesia occurs during the first trimester of pregnancy, preceding any gross change in vascular dimensions within the epidural or subarachnoid spaces.[83] A correlation appears to exist between progesterone levels in cerebrospinal fluid and the milligrams per segment requirement of lidocaine for spinal anesthesia in pregnant and nonpregnant patients.[84] Isolated nerve studies have shown a more rapid onset and an increased sensitivity to local anesthetic-induced conduction blockade in vagus nerves obtained from pregnant rabbits compared with nonpregnant controls.[85,86] These results suggest that hormonal changes associated with pregnancy enhance the apparent potency of local anesthetics; thus, the dosage probably should be reduced in patients during all stages of pregnancy.

CHOICE OF LOCAL ANESTHETIC FOR VARIOUS REGIONAL ANESTHETIC PROCEDURES
(Also See Chs. 44 to 46, 57, and 60)

On the basis of anatomic considerations, regional anesthesia may be divided into infiltration anesthesia, intravenous regional anesthesia, peripheral nerve blockade, central neural blockade, and topical anesthesia.

Infiltration Anesthesia

Any local anesthetic may be employed for infiltration anesthesia. Onset of action is almost immediate for all agents following intradermal or subcutaneous administration. However, duration of anesthesia varies (Table 13-4). Epinephrine will markedly prolong the duration of infiltration anesthesia by all local anesthetic drugs. This effect is most pronounced when epinephrine is added to lidocaine. Choice of a specific drug for infiltration anesthesia basically depends on the desired duration of action.

The dosage of local anesthetic required for adequate infiltration anesthesia depends on the extent of the area to be anesthetized and the expected duration of the surgical procedure. When large surface areas have to be anesthetized, large volumes of dilute anesthetic solutions should be used.

Patients frequently experience pain immediately after the subcutaneous injection of local anesthetic solutions. This is due in part to the acidic nature of these solutions.[87] In addition, certain agents such as etidocaine are associated with a greater frequency and intensity of pain, while lidocaine is perceived as less painful.[88]

Intravenous Regional Anesthesia

Intravenous regional anesthesia involves the intravenous administration of a local anesthetic agent into a tourniquet-occluded limb. The local anesthetic diffuses from the peripheral vascular bed to nonvascular tissue such as axons and nerve endings. Both the safety and efficacy of this regional anesthetic procedure depend on the interruption of blood flow to the involved limb. Intravenous regional anesthesia has been used primarily for surgical procedures on the upper limbs. Shorter procedures on the foot can also be successfully performed under intravenous regional anesthesia. Here the tourniquet should be applied just below the fibular neck to avoid pressure over the superficial peroneal nerve.

Lidocaine has been the agent utilized most frequently for intravenous regional anesthesia and is the only agent officially approved by the Food and Drug Administration for intravenous regional anesthesia in the United States. Prilocaine, mepivacaine, chloroprocaine, procaine, bupivacaine, and etidocaine have also been used successfully. However, thrombophlebitis has been reported in several patients in whom chloroprocaine was utilized.[89] Cardiovascular collapse has been reported following the use of bupivacaine for intravenous regional anesthesia, and this use of bupivacaine is not recommended in the United States.[90]

In general, approximately 3 mg/kg (40 ml of 0.5 percent solution) of preservative-free lidocaine without epinephrine is used for upper extremity procedures. For surgical procedures on the lower limbs, 50 to 100 ml of 0.25 percent lidocaine has been used.

TABLE 13-4. Infiltration Anesthesia

| Drug | Plain Solution | | Epinephrine-Containing Solution | | |
	Concentration (%)	Max Dose (mg)	Duration (min)	Max Dose (mg)	Duration (min)
Short duration					
Procaine					
Chloroprocaine	1.0–2.0	800	15–30	1,000	30–90
Moderate duration					
Lidocaine	0.5–1.0	300	30–60	500	120–360
Mepivacaine	0.5–1.0	300	45–90	500	120–360
Prilocaine	0.5–1.0	500	30–90	600	120–360
Long duration					
Bupivacaine	0.25–0.5	175	120–240	225	180–420
Etidocaine	0.5–1.0	300	120–180	400	180–420

TABLE 13-5. Minor Nerve Blocks (Also See Ch. 46)

| Drug | Usual Concentration (%) | Plain Solutions | | | Epinephrine-Containing Solutions |
		Usual Volume (ml)	Dosage (mg)	Average Duration (min)	Average Duration (min)
Procaine Chloroprocaine	2	5–20	100–400	15–30	30–60
Lidocaine Mepivacaine Prilocaine	1	5–20	50–200	60–120	120–180
Bupivacaine	0.25	5–20	12.5–50	180–360	240–480
Etidocaine	0.5	5–20	25–100	120–240	180–420

Peripheral Nerve Blockade

Regional anesthetic procedures that inhibit conduction in fibers of the peripheral nervous system can be classified together under the general category of peripheral nerve blockade. This form of regional anesthesia has been subdivided arbitrarily into minor and major nerve blocks. Minor nerve blocks are defined as procedures involving single nerve entities such as the ulnar or radial nerve. Major nerve blocks involve the blocking of two or more distinct nerves or a nerve plexus.

Most local anesthetic drugs can be used for minor nerve blocks. The onset of block is rapid with most drugs, and the choice of drug is determined primarily by the required duration of anesthesia. A classification of the various drugs according to their duration of action is shown in Table 13-5. The duration of both sensory analgesia and motor blockade is prolonged significantly when epinephrine is added to the various local anesthetic solutions.

Recently, a technique of intrapleural regional analgesia has been described as an alternative to the performance of multiple intercostal nerve blocks.[91] This procedure involves the administration of local anesthetic solution into the pleural space. An epidural needle is inserted into the pleural space, usually by way of the 4th to the 9th intercostal space. An epidural catheter is then passed into the pleural space approximately 5 cm beyond the tip of the needle. The needle is removed, and the local anesthetic is then administered through the catheter. This technique has proved useful for unilateral postoperative analgesia following cholecystectomies, mastectomies, and nephrectomies.[92,93] Its efficacy for post-thoracotomy pain is controversial.[94] Twenty to 30 ml of 0.5 percent bupivacaine with epinephrine has been employed most frequently for this technique. The duration of analgesia averages approximately 8 hours with a range of 4 to 24 hours. The advantage of this technique is the ability to administer subsequent injections of local anesthetic via the catheter to provide long-lasting analgesia without the necessity of subjecting patients to repeated multiple intercostal nerve blocks.

Brachial plexus blockade for upper limb surgery is the most common major peripheral nerve block technique. A significant difference exists between the onset of various agents when brachial plexus blocks are performed (Table 13-6). In general, the agents of intermediate potency exhibit a more rapid onset than the more potent compounds. Onset times of approximately 14 minutes for lidocaine and mepivacaine have been reported compared with mean latency values of approximately 23 minutes for bupivacaine.[95] Etidocaine may be an exception since it produces a relatively rapid onset and a long duration of block.

Epinephrine will prolong the duration of most local anesthetic agents employed for brachial plexus blockade. However, the drugs having intrinsically longer duration do not benefit as much from the addition of epinephrine. The variation in the duration of anesthesia after brachial plexus blockade is also considerably greater than that observed in other types of conduction block. For example, durations of anesthesia varying

TABLE 13-6. Major Nerve Blocks (Also See Ch. 46)

Drug w/Epinephrine 1:200,000	Usual Concentration (%)	Usual Volume (ml)	Maximal Dose (mg)	Usual Onset (min)	Usual Duration (min)
Lidocaine	1–1.5	30–50	500	10–20	120–240
Mepivacaine	1–1.5	30–50	500	10–20	180–300
Prilocaine	1–2	30–50	600	10–20	180–300
Bupivacaine	0.25–0.5	30–50	225	15–30	360–720
Etidocaine	0.5–1.0	30–50	400	10–20	360–720
Tetracaine	0.25–0.5	30–50	200	20–30	300–600

TABLE 13-7. Epidural Anesthesia (Also See Ch. 45)

Drug w/Epinephrine 1:200,000	Usual Concentration (%)	Usual Volume (ml)	Total Dose (mg)	Usual Onset (min)	Usual Duration (min)
Chloroprocaine	2–3	15–30	300–900	5–15	30–90
Lidocaine	1–2	15–30	150–500	5–15	
Mepivacaine	1–2	15–30	150–500	5–15	60–180
Prilocaine	1–3	15–30	150–600	5–15	
Bupivacaine	0.25–0.75	15–30	37.5–225	10–20	180–300
Etidocaine	1.0–1.5	15–30	150–300	5–15	

from 4 to 30 hours have been reported for bupivacaine. It would be prudent to forewarn patients about to be given a major nerve block about the possibility of prolonged sensory and motor block in the involved region, particularly when agents such as bupivacaine and etidocaine are employed.

Central Neural Blockade

Any of the local anesthetic drugs may be used for epidural anesthesia (Table 13-7). However, procaine and tetracaine are rarely used owing to their long onset times. The intermediate local anesthetic drugs will produce surgical anesthesia of 1 to 2 hours duration, whereas the long-acting drugs will usually produce 3 to 5 hours of anesthesia. The duration of short- and intermediate-acting agents is significantly prolonged by the addition of epinephrine (1:200,000), while the long-acting agents benefit little from its addition. Onset of lumbar epidural anesthesia occurs within 5 to 15 minutes following administration of chloroprocaine, lidocaine, mepivacaine, prilocaine, and etidocaine. Bupivacaine has a slower onset of action.

Bupivacaine at 0.25 and 0.5 percent produces adequate analgesia with minimal motor deficit. These solutions of bupivacaine are useful for obstetric epidural analgesia and postoperative analgesia. Bupivacaine at 0.75 percent is associated with a more profound degree of motor block, which makes this solution most suitable for major surgical procedures. Etidocaine produces adequate sensory analgesia and profound motor block and is primarily useful for surgical procedure in which muscle relaxation is required.

Agents available for subarachnoid administration are shown in Table 13-8. Tetracaine, which is the most commonly used spinal agent in the United States, is available both as niphanoid crystals and as a 1 percent solution that may be diluted with 10 percent glucose to obtain a 0.5 percent hyperbaric solution.

Hypobaric solutions of tetracaine (tetracaine in sterile water) may be utilized for specific operative situations, for example, anorectal or hip surgery. Isobaric tetracaine obtained by mixing 1 percent tetracaine with cerebrospinal fluid or normal saline is particularly useful for lower limb surgical procedures. In recent years, bupivacaine has been introduced as a spinal anesthetic agent. Bupivacaine is prepared as a hyperbaric solution at a concentration of 0.75 percent with 8.25 percent dextrose. A 0.5 percent isobaric solution of bupivacaine is also available in some countries.

Intrathecal bupivacaine possesses an anesthetic profile similar to that of tetracaine.[96,97] However, differences do exist between the two agents. Although two-segment regression of anesthesia is similar for bupivacaine and tetracaine, the total duration of sensory anesthesia is significantly longer following the sub-

TABLE 13-8. Spinal Anesthesia (Also See Ch. 45)

Drug	Usual Concentration (%)	Usual Volume (ml)	Total Dose (mg)	Baricity	Glucose Concentration (%)	Usual Duration (min)
Procaine	10.0	1–2	100–200	Hyperbaric	—	30–60
Lidocaine	1.5, 5.0	1–2	30–100	Hyperbaric	7.5	30–90
Mepivacaine	4	1–2	40–80	Hyperbaric	9.0	30–90
Tetracaine	0.25–1.0	1–4	5–20	Hyperbaric Hypobaric Isobaric	5.0	75–150
Dibucaine	0.25	1–2	2.5–5.0	Hyperbaric	5.0	75–180
	0.5	1–2	5–10	Isobaric		
	0.06	5–20	3–12	Hypobaric		
Bupivacaine	0.5	3–4	15–20	Isobaric		75–150
	0.75	2–3	15–22.5	Hyperbaric	8.25	75–150

arachnoid administration of tetracaine. The depth and duration of motor blockade are also greater with tetracaine than with bupivacaine. On the other hand, bupivacaine has been reported in some studies to be associated with less hypotension than tetracaine. In addition, the frequency of tourniquet pain in the lower limbs during certain orthopedic surgical procedures has been reported to be significantly reduced when bupivacaine instead of tetracaine is employed for spinal anesthesia.[98,99]

Lidocaine provides a short duration of spinal anesthesia, where tetracaine and bupivacaine are considered to be agents of long duration. Onset of spinal anesthesia is extremely rapid with an agent such as lidocaine. The addition of vasoconstrictor agents may prolong the duration of spinal anesthesia. The addition of 0.2 to 0.3 mg of epinephrine to tetracaine solutions will produce a 50 percent or greater increase in duration. The duration of spinal anesthesia produced by tetracaine can also be increased to a similar extent by adding 1 to 5 mg of phenylephrine. The addition of epinephrine to bupivacaine or lidocaine may not significantly prolong the duration of spinal anesthesia in thoracic segments.[100,101] However, the total duration of anesthesia, for example, in the lumbosacral roots, will be significantly increased.

Topical Anesthesia

A number of local anesthetic formulations are available for topical anesthesia (Table 13-9). Lidocaine, dibucaine, tetracaine, and benzocaine are the agents most commonly employed for topical anesthesia. In general, these preparations provide effective but relatively short durations of analgesia when applied to mucous membranes or abraded skin. In addition, lidocaine and tetracaine sprays have been employed for endotracheal anesthesia prior to intubation. Recently, a new topical anesthetic formulation (EMLA) has been evaluated for cutaneous analgesia.[102] EMLA is a eutectic mixture of 5 percent lidocaine and prilocaine base. Clinical studies have demonstrated that this preparation can decrease the pain associated with the percutaneous insertion of intravenous needles and cannulae.[103] In addition, EMLA has been successfully employed for cutaneous anesthesia in skin-grafting procedures.[104] This preparation must be applied under an occlusive bandage for 45 to 60 minutes to obtain effective cutaneous anesthesia.

PHARMACOKINETICS OF LOCAL ANESTHETIC DRUGS

The concentration of local anesthetics in blood is determined by the amounted injected, the rate of absorption from the site of injection, the rate of tissue distribution, and the rate of biotransformation and excretion of the particular drug. Specific patient-related factors such as age, cardiovascular status, and hepatic function will influence the physiologic disposition and the resultant blood concentrations of local anesthetics.

Absorption

The systemic absorption of local anesthetics is determined by the site of injection, dosage, addition of a vasoconstrictor agent, and pharmacologic profile of the agent itself. A comparison of the blood concentration of

TABLE 13-9. Various Preparations Intended for Topical Anesthesia

Anesthetic Ingredient	Concentration (%)	Pharmaceutical Application Form	Intended Area of Use
Benzocaine	1–5	Cream	Skin and mucous membrane
	20	Ointment	Skin and mucous membrane
	20	Aerosol	Skin and mucous membrane
Cocaine	4	Solution	Ear, nose, throat
Dibucaine	0.25–1	Cream	Skin
	0.25–1	Ointment	Skin
	0.25–1	Aerosol	Skin
	0.25	Solution	Ear
	2.5	Suppositories	Rectum
Cyclonine	0.5–1	Solution	Skin, oropharynx, tracheobronchial tree, urethra, rectum
Lidocaine	2–4	Solution	Oropharynx, tracheobronchial tree, nose
	2	Jelly	Urethra
	2.5–5	Ointment	Skin, mucous membrane, rectum
	2	Viscous	Oropharynx
	10	Suppositories	Rectum
	10	Aerosol	Gingival mucosa
Tetracaine	0.5–1	Ointment	Skin, rectum, mucous membrane
	0.5–1	Cream	Skin, rectum, mucous membrane
	0.25–1	Solution	Nose, tracheobronchial tree

(From Covino and Vassallo,[106] with permission.)

local anesthetics following various routes of administration reveals that the anesthetic drug level is highest after intercostal nerve blockade, followed in order of decreasing concentration by injection into the lumbar epidural space, brachial plexus site, and subcutaneous tissue[105] (Fig. 13-15). The high blood levels following intercostal administration may be related to the multiple injections required for intercostal nerve blocks, such that a local anesthetic solution is exposed to a greater vascular area, which results in a greater rate and degree of absorption. This relationship of administration site to rate of absorption is of clinical significance, since use of a fixed dose of a local anesthetic agent may be potentially toxic in one area of administration but not in others. For example, the use of 400 mg of lidocaine without epinephrine for intercostal nerve block results in an average peak venous plasma level of approximately 7 μg/ml, which is sufficiently high to cause symptoms of central nervous system toxicity in some patients.[105] This same dose of lidocaine employed for brachial plexus block yields a mean maximum blood level of approximately 3 μg/ml, which is rarely associated with signs of toxicity.[105]

The maximum blood level of local anesthetic drugs is related to the total dose of drug administered for any particular site of administration. For most drugs, there is a linear relationship between the amount of drug administered and the resultant peak anesthetic blood levels.[106] For example, the mean venous blood level of lidocaine increased from approximately 1.5 to 4 μg/ml as the total dose administered into the lumbar epidural space was increased from 200 to 600 mg. Depending on the site of administration, a peak blood level of 0.5 to 2.0 μg/ml is achieved for each 100 mg of lidocaine or mepivacaine injected.

Local anesthetic solutions frequently contain a vasoconstrictor agent, usually epinephrine, in concentrations varying from 5 to 20 μg/ml. Epinephrine decreases the rate of absorption of certain agents from various sites of administration and thus lowers their potential toxicity. A 5 μg/ml dose of epinephrine (1:200,000) significantly reduces the peak blood levels of lidocaine and mepivacaine, irrespective of the site of administration. The peak blood levels of bupivacaine and etidocaine are minimally influenced by the addition of a vasoconstrictor following injection into the lumbar epidural space.[107] However, epinephrine will significantly reduce the rate of vascular absorption of these drugs when they are used for peripheral nerve blocks such as brachial plexus blockade.[108]

Differences also exist in the rate of absorption of various local anesthetic drugs. For example, a comparison of drugs of similar anesthetic profiles reveals that lidocaine is absorbed more rapidly following brachial plexus blockade than is prilocaine, while bupivacaine is absorbed more rapidly than etidocaine.[106] Prilocaine is a less potent vasodilator than lidocaine, which accounts, in part, for the lower prilocaine blood levels. The lower peak blood levels of etidocaine compared with those of bupivacaine may be related to the greater lipid solubility of etidocaine, which results in the sequestration of this agent by adipose tissue and a decreased rate of absorption.

Distribution of Local Anesthetics

The distribution of local anesthetics can be described by a two- or three-compartment model.[109] The rapid disappearance (α) phase is believed related to uptake by rapidly equilibrating tissues, that is, tissues which have a high vascular perfusion. The slower phase of disappearance from blood (β phase) is mainly a function of distribution to slowly equilibrating tissues and the biotransformation and excretion of the compound. This secondary phase may also be subdivided into a β phase (distribution to slowly perfused tissue) and a γ phase (biotransformation and excretion). The α half-life (t1/2α) of prilocaine is shorter than that of lidocaine and mepivacaine, which indicates that prilocaine is distributed at a significantly more rapid rate from blood to tissues than the other two drugs[110] (Table 13-10). The t1/2α of lidocaine and mepivacaine are similar. In addition, the γ disappearance phase of prilocaine is more rapid than that of lidocaine and mepivacaine, suggesting a more rapid rate of biotransformation. A comparison of bupivacaine and etidocaine reveals that etidocaine has a more rapid rate of tissue redistribution and biotransformation than bupivacaine.[111]

Local anesthetic drugs are distributed throughout all body tissues, but the relative concentration in different tissues varies. In general, the more highly perfused organs show higher concentrations of local anesthetic

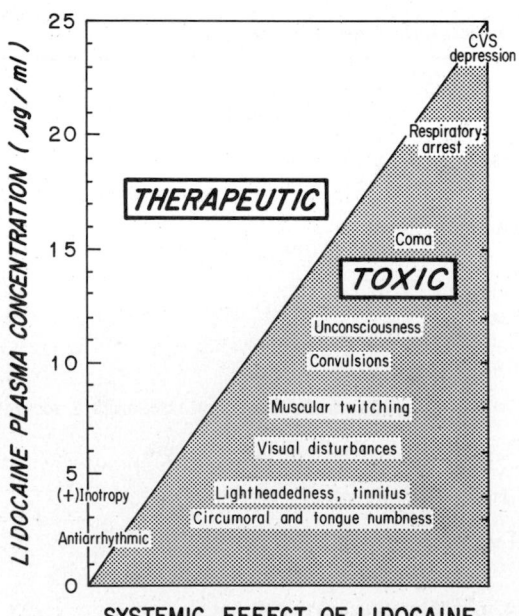

Fig. 13-15. Peak venous blood concentrations of various local anesthetics following injection into different sites. (From Covino and Vassallo,[106] with permission.)

TABLE 13-10. Pharmacokinetic Properties of Various Amide Local Anesthetics

Agent	$\tau 1/2\alpha$(min)	$\tau 1/2\beta$(min)	V_{DSS}(L)	$\tau 1/2\gamma$(hrs)	CL (L/min)
Prilocaine	0.5	5.0	261	1.5	2.84
Lidocaine	1.0	9.6	91	1.6	0.95
Mepivacaine	0.7	7.2	84	1.9	0.78
Bupivacaine	2.7	28.0	72	3.5	0.47
Etidocaine	2.2	19.0	133	2.6	1.22

Abbreviations: V_{DSS}, volume of distribution at steady state; CL, clearance.

drug than the less well perfused organs. In particular, these agents are rapidly extracted by lung tissue, so that the whole blood concentration of local anesthetics decreases markedly as they pass through the pulmonary vasculature.[112,113] The highest percentage of an injected dose of a local anesthetic agent is found in skeletal muscle. Although this tissue does not show any particular affinity for this class of drugs, the mass of skeletal muscle makes it the largest reservoir for local anesthetic drugs.

Biotransformation and Excretion

The pattern of metabolism of local anesthetic agents varies according to their chemical classification. The ester or procainelike drugs undergo hydrolysis in plasma by the pseudocholinesterase enzymes. Chloroprocaine shows the most rapid rate of hydrolysis (4.7 μmol/ml/h), compared with a rate of 1.1 μmol/ml/h for procaine and 0.3 μmol/ml/h for tetracaine.[114] Less than 2 percent of unchanged procaine is found in urine, while approximately 90 percent of *para*-aminobenzoic acid, which is a primary product of procaine hydrolysis, appears in urine. Only 33 percent of diethylaminoeth-

anol, the other hydrolysis produce of procaine, is excreted unchanged.

The aminoamide agents undergo enzymatic degradation primarily in the liver. Prilocaine undergoes the most rapid rate of hepatic metabolism, while lidocaine is metabolized somewhat more rapidly than mepivacaine.[115] In humans, the hepatic clearance of etidocaine is greater than that of bupivacaine, indicating that etidocaine is metabolized in the liver more rapidly than bupivacaine.[116] Some degradation of the amide-type compounds may take place in tissues other than liver. The formation of certain metabolites has been observed following incubation of prilocaine with kidney slices.

The biotransformation of the amide-type agents is more complex than that of the ester drugs. Although many of the metabolites of the various amide drugs have been identified, the complete transformation pathways for all the compounds in this class have not been elucidated. Most studies have been concerned with lidocaine. The main pathway of biotransformation with this agent in humans appears to involve oxidative de-ethylation of lidocaine to monethylglycinexylidide, followed by a subsequent hydrolysis of monoethylglycinexylidide to xylidine[115] (Fig. 13-16).

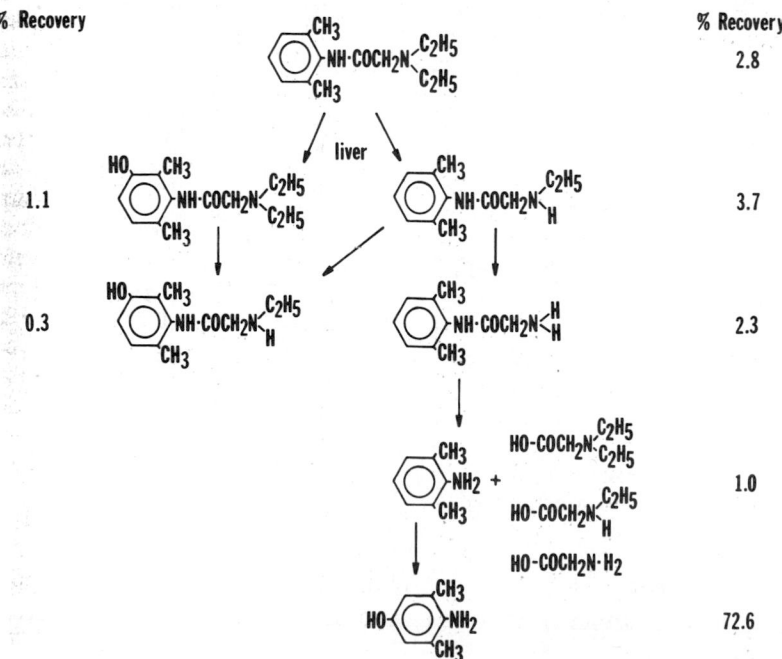

Fig. 13-16. Proposed pathway for the biotransformation of lidocaine and percent recovery of various products in urine. (From Covino and Vassallo,[106] with permission.)

The excretion of the amide-type local anesthetic drugs occurs via the kidney. Less than 5 percent of the unchanged drug is excreted via the kidney into the urine. The major portion of the injected agent appears in the urine in the form of various metabolites. The renal clearance of the amide local anesthetic drugs appears to be inversely related to their protein-binding capacity. Prilocaine, which has a lower protein-binding capacity than lidocaine, has a substantially higher clearance value than lidocaine. Renal clearance also is inversely proportional to the pH of urine, suggesting that urinary excretion of these agents occurs by non-ionic diffusion.

Pharmacokinetic Alterations by Patient Status

Patient age may influence the physiologic disposition of local anesthetics. The half-life of lidocaine following intravenous administration averaged 80 minutes in human volunteers whose ages varied from 22 to 26 years. On the other hand, volunteers 61 to 71 years of age demonstrated a significantly prolonged lidocaine half-life of 138 minutes.[117]

The rate of degradation of the amide type of local anesthetic drugs will be influenced by the hepatic status of the individual patient. In those patients in whom liver blood flow is abnormally low or in whom liver function is poor or nonexistent, significantly higher blood levels of the amide drugs occur. An average lidocaine half-life of 1.5 hours was reported in volunteers with normal hepatic function, while patients with liver disease demonstrated an average half-life of 5.0 hours.[118] The rate of lidocaine disappearance from blood has also been shown to be markedly prolonged in patients with congestive heart failure.[119] Similar rates of intravenous infusion of lidocaine result in significantly higher plasma concentrations of lidocaine in patients with cardiac failure compared with patients with normal cardiovascular function.

TOXICITY OF LOCAL ANESTHETIC DRUGS

Local anesthetic drugs are relatively free of side effects if they are administered in an appropriate dosage and in the appropriate anatomic location. However, systemic and localized toxic reactions can occur, usually owing to accidental intravascular or intrathecal injection or to the administration of an excessive dose of local anesthetic drug. In addition, specific adverse effects are associated with the use of certain drugs, such as allergic reactions to the aminoester drugs and methemoglobinemia following the use of prilocaine.

Systemic Toxicity
(Also See Chs. 44 to 46 and 57)

Systemic reactions to local anesthetics involve primarily the central nervous system and the cardiovascular system. In general, the central nervous system (CNS) is more susceptible to the systemic actions of local anesthetic agents than the cardiovascular system. The dose and blood level of local anesthetic required to produce CNS toxicity is usually lower than that which results in circulatory collapse (Fig. 13-17).

Central Nervous System Toxicity

The initial symptoms of local anesthetic-induced CNS toxicity involve feelings of lightheadedness and dizziness followed frequently by visual and auditory disturbances such as difficulty in focusing and tinnitus. Other subjective CNS symptoms include disorientation and occasional feelings of drowsiness. Objective signs of CNS toxicity are usually excitatory in nature and include shivering, muscular twitching, and tremors initially involving muscles of the face and distal parts of the extremities. Ultimately, generalized convulsions of a tonic-clonic nature occur. If a sufficiently large dose or a rapid intravenous injection of a local anesthetic is administered, the initial signs of CNS excitation are rapidly followed by a state of generalized CNS depression. Seizure activity ceases, and respiratory depression and, ultimately, respiratory arrest may occur. In some patients, CNS depression without a preceding excitatory phase is seen, particularly if other CNS depressant drugs have been administered.

CNS excitation is thought to be the result of an initial

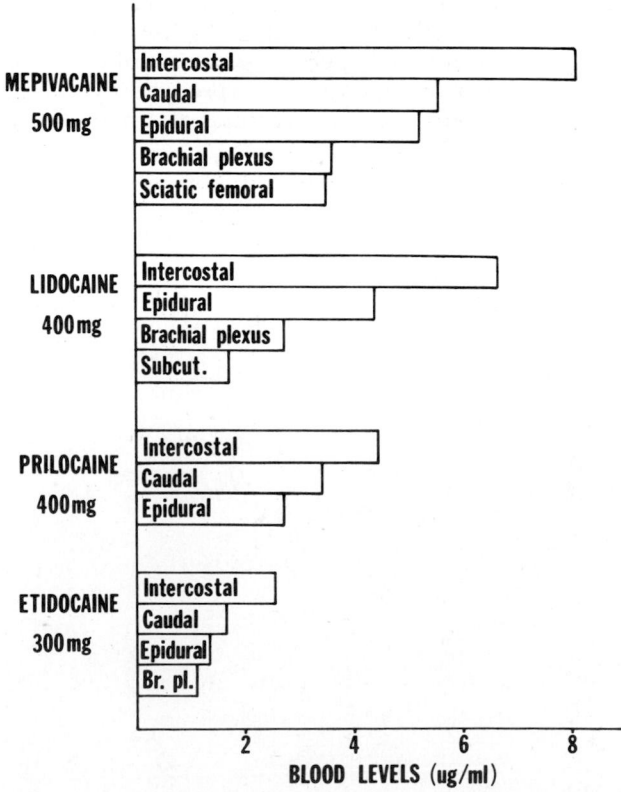

Fig. 13-17. Relationship between plasma concentration of lidocaine and various signs and symptoms of toxicity. (Modified from Mather and Cousins,[171] with permission.)

blockade of inhibitory pathways in the cerebral cortex by local anesthetic drugs.[120] The blockade of inhibitory pathways allows facilitatory neurons to function in an unopposed fashion, which results in an increase in excitatory activity leading to convulsions. An increase in the dose of local anesthetic administered leads to an inhibition of conduction on both inhibitory and facilitatory pathways, resulting in a generalized state of CNS depression.

In general, a correlation exists between the anesthetic potency and intravenous CNS toxicity of various agents[121] (Fig. 13-18). For example, in cats, the dose of intravenous procaine required to cause convulsions is approximately seven times greater than the convulsive dose of bupivacaine. However, bupivacaine is also approximately eight times more potent than procaine as a local anesthetic drug. In dogs, the relative CNS toxicity of bupivacaine, etidocaine, and lidocaine is 4:2:1, which is similar to the relative potency of these agents for the production of regional anesthesia in humans.[122] Intravenous infusion studies in human volunteers have also demonstrated an inverse relationship between the intrinsic anesthetic potency of various agents and the dosage required to induce CNS toxicity.[123,124]

The rate of injection and rapidity with which a particular blood level is achieved will alter the toxicity of local anesthetic drugs. For example, in human volunteers, an average dose of 236 mg of etidocaine and a venous blood level of 3.0 μg/ml resulted in CNS symptoms when an infusion rate of 10 mg/min was employed.[123] When the infusion rate was increased to 20 mg/min, an average of 161 mg of etidocaine, which produced a venous plasma level of approximately 2 μg/ml, caused symptoms of CNS toxicity.

The acid-base status of animals and patients can markedly affect the CNS activity of local anesthetic agents. In cats, the convulsive threshold of various local anesthetics was inversely related to the arterial PCO_2 level[121] (Fig. 13-18). An increase in $PaCO_2$ from 25 to 40 mmHg to 65 to 81 mmHg decreases the convulsive threshold of procaine, mepivacaine, prilocaine, lidocaine, and bupivacaine by approximately 50 percent. A decrease in arterial pH also will decrease the convulsive threshold of these drugs. Respiratory acidosis with a resultant increase in $PaCO_2$ and a decrease in arterial pH will consistently decrease the convulsant threshold of local anesthetic drugs. However, an elevation in both $PaCO_2$ and arterial pH as may occur during metabolic alkalosis does not increase CNS toxicity to the same degree.

An elevation of $PaCO_2$ will enhance cerebral blood flow so that more anesthetic is delivered more rapidly to the brain. In addition, diffusion of CO_2 into neuronal cells will decrease intracellular pH, which will facilitate the conversion of the base form of local anesthetic drugs to the cationic form. The cationic form does not diffuse well across the nerve membrane, so that ion trapping will occur, which will increase the apparent CNS toxicity of local anesthetics.

Hypercarbia and/or acidosis will also decrease the

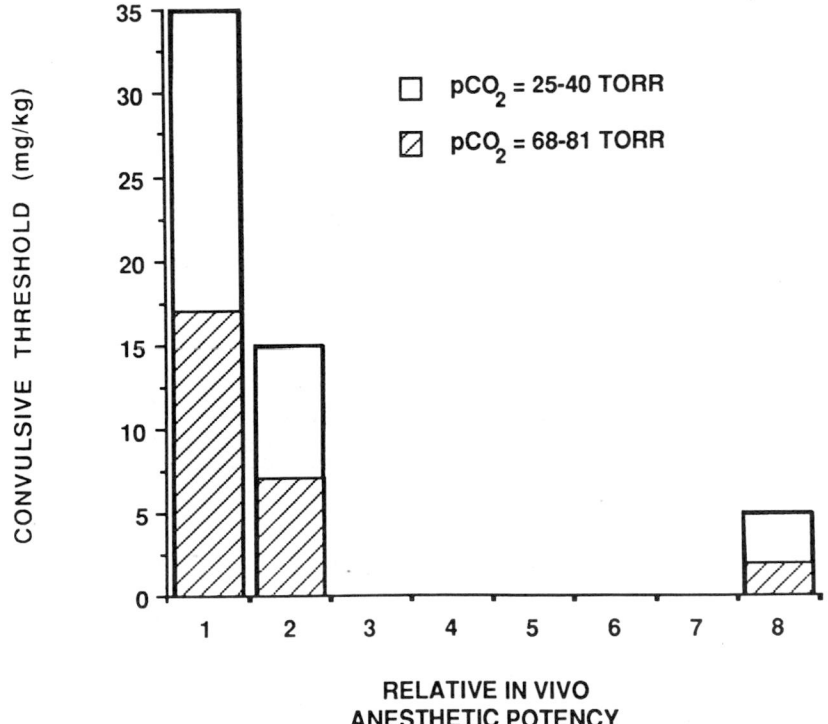

Fig. 13-18. Relationship between convulsive dose of procaine, lidocaine, and bupivacaine in cats and their relative in vivo anesthetic potency. Open bar represents convulsive dose during normocarbia and hatched bar is the convulsive dose under hypercarbic conditions.

plasma protein binding of local anesthetic agents.[125,126] Therefore, an elevation in $PaCO_2$ or a decrease in pH will increase the proportion of free drug available for diffusion into the brain. On the other hand, acidosis will increase the cationic form of the local anesthetic, which should decrease the rate of diffusion through lipoid barriers.

Cardiovascular System Toxicity

Local anesthetic agents can exert a direct action both on the heart and peripheral blood vessels.

Direct cardiac effects

The primary cardiac electrophysiologic effect of local anesthetics is a decrease in the maximum rate of depolarization in Purkinje fibers and ventricular muscle.[127–129] This reduction in the maximum rate of depolarization is believed to be due to a decrease in the availability of fast sodium channels in cardiac membranes. Action potential duration and the effective refractory period are also decreased by local anaesthetics.[129] However, the ratio of effective refractory period to action potential duration is increased both in Purkinje fibers and in ventricular muscle.

Qualitative differences may exist between the electrophysiologic effects of various agents. Bupivacaine depresses the rapid phase of depolarization (Vmax) in Purkinje fibers and ventricular muscle to a greater extent than does lidocaine.[129] In addition, the rate of recovery from a use-dependent block is slower in bupivacaine-treated papillary muscles than in lidocaine-treated muscles.[127] This slow rate of recovery results in an incomplete restoration of Vmax between action potentials, particularly at high heart rates. In contrast, recovery from lidocaine is complete, even at rapid heart rates. These differential effects of lidocaine and bupivacaine have been advanced to explain the antiarrhythmic properties of lidocaine and the arrhythmogenic potential of bupivacaine.

Electrophysiologic studies in intact dogs and in humans have shown that high blood levels of local anesthetics will prolong conduction time through various parts of the heart, as indicated in the electrocardiogram by an increase in the PR interval and QRS duration. Extremely high concentrations of local anesthetics will depress spontaneous pacemaker activity in the sinus node, resulting in sinus bradycardia and sinus arrest.

Local anesthetic drugs also exert profound effects on the mechanical activity of cardiac muscle. All local anesthetics exert a dose-dependent negative inotropic action on isolated cardiac tissue.[128,130] This depression of cardiac contractility is proportional to the conduction-blocking potency of the various agents in isolated nerves[130] (Table 13-10). The more potent agents (bupivacaine, tetracaine, and etidocaine) depress cardiac contractility at the lowest concentrations. The agents of moderate anesthetic potency, (lidocaine, mepivacaine, and prilocaine) form an intermediate group of compounds in terms of myocardial depression. Finally, procaine and chloroprocaine, which are the least potent local anesthetics, require the highest concentration to decrease cardiac contractility.

In intact dogs, a relationship exists between local anesthetic potency and myocardial depression (Table 13-11). For example, tetracaine is approximately 8 to 10 times more potent than procaine as a local anesthetic and as a myocardial depressant.[131] Hemodynamic studies in closed-chest anesthetized dogs showed that tetracaine, etidocaine, and bupivacaine caused a 50 percent decrease in cardiac output at doses of 10 to 20 mg/kg, while 30 to 40 mg/kg of lidocaine, mepivacaine, prilocaine, and chloroprocaine were required for a similar decrease in cardiac output. A dose of 100 mg/kg of procaine was needed to reduce cardiac output by 50 percent.[132,133]

Local anesthetics may depress myocardial contractility by interacting with calcium. For example, procaine has been shown to block the intracellular release of calcium in isolated sarcoplasmic reticular preparations.[134] However, in the isolated guinea pig heart, an increase in the extracellular concentration of calcium failed to reverse the negative inotropic action of bupivacaine or lidocaine.[135]

TABLE 13-11. Comparative Effect of Various Local Anesthetic Drugs on Cardiac Contractility and Cardiac Output

Drug	Relative Anesthetic Potency	Isolated Guinea Pig Atria (50% ↓) (μg/ml)	Cardiac Output In Dogs (50% ↓) (mg/kg)
Procaine	1	277	100
Chloroprocaine	1	102	30
Cocaine	2	56	—
Lidocaine	2	67	30
Prilocaine	2	42	40
Mepivacaine	2	55	40
Etidocaine	6	—	20
Bupivacaine	8	6	10
Tetracaine	8	6	20

Direct peripheral vascular effects

Local anesthetic drugs exert a biphasic effect on peripheral vascular smooth muscle. Low concentrations of lidocaine and bupivacaine produced vasoconstriction in the cremaster muscle of rats, while high concentrations increased arteriolar diameter, indicative of vasodilation.[60,61]

In vivo studies have also demonstrated that low doses of local anesthetics decrease peripheral arterial flow without any change in blood pressure, while higher doses increased blood flow.[56] Cocaine is the only local anesthetic that consistently causes vasoconstriction, owing to its ability to inhibit the uptake of norepinephrine by storage granules.[136] The excess concentration of free circulating norepinephrine is responsible for the vasoconstriction associated with the use of cocaine.

The pulmonary vasculature appears to be particularly sensitive to the stimulatory effects of local anesthetics. Procaine markedly increased pulmonary vascular resistance in a Starling heart-lung preparation.[137] Studies in intact anesthetized dogs employing pulmonary artery catheters also showed that both the ester and amide agents can cause marked increases in pulmonary artery pressure and pulmonary vascular resistance.[132,133] At doses of local anesthetics that approached lethal levels, decreases in pulmonary artery pressure and pulmonary vascular resistance were seen with both types of local anesthetic drugs.

Comparative Cardiovascular Toxicity (Also See Ch. 57)

In general, a direct relationship exists between the anesthetic potency and myocardial depression of the various drugs. In recent years, the more potent drugs, that is, bupivacaine and etidocaine, have been reported to cause rapid and profound cardiovascular depression.

The cardiotoxicity of the more potent drugs such as bupivacaine appears to differ from that of lidocaine in the following manner: (1) the ratio of the dosage required for irreversible cardiovascular collapse (CC) and the dosage which will produce CNS toxicity (convulsions), that is, the CC/CNS ratio, is lower for bupivacaine and etidocaine than for lidocaine; (2) ventricular arrhythmias and fatal ventricular fibrillation may occur following the rapid intravenous administration of a large dose of bupivacaine but not lidocaine; (3) the pregnant animal or patient may be more sensitive to the cardiotoxic effects of bupivacaine than the nonpregnant animal or patient; (4) cardiac resuscitation is more difficult following bupivacaine-induced cardiovascular collapse; (5) acidosis and hypoxia markedly potentiate the cardiotoxicity of bupivacaine.

CC/CNS Ratio

In sheep, the ratio of the dosage and blood level of bupivacaine and etidocaine associated with the development of convulsive activity and cardiovascular collapse is lower than that of lidocaine.[138] A CC/CNS dose ratio of 7.1 ± 1.1 existed for lidocaine, indicating that seven times as much drug was required to induce irreversible cardiovascular collapse as was needed for the production of convulsions (Fig. 13-19). The CC/CNS ratio for bupivacaine was 3.7 ± 0.5, and for etidocaine it was 4.4 ± 0.9. The CC/CNS blood level ratio of lidocaine was 3.6 ± 0.3 compared with values of 1.6 to 1.7 for bupivacaine and etidocaine. At the time of cardiovascular collapse, higher concentrations of bupivacaine and etidocaine were present in the myocardium compared with lidocaine, which suggests that the enhanced cardiac toxicity of these more potent agents is due to a greater myocardial uptake.

Ventricular Arrhythmias

Bupivacaine and, to a lesser degree, etidocaine may produce severe cardiac arrhythmias, including ventricular fibrillation, in various animal species[135,139–143] (Table 13-12). Ventricular arrhythmias were rarely seen with lidocaine, mepivacaine, or tetracaine. The arrhythmogenic action of bupivacaine may be related to an inhibition of the fast sodium channels in the cardiac membrane.[127–129] Bupivacaine may also block the slow calcium channels.[144] These electrophysiologic effects of bupivacaine may result in conduction abnormalities leading to a re-entrant type of arrhythmia similar to torsade de pointes arrhythmias.[140]

The cardiac arrhythmias observed in bupivacaine-treated animals are believed to be due primarily to a direct cardiac effect. Isolated guinea pig hearts perfused with bupivacaine revealed evidence of conduction block, bigeminy, and trigeminy.[135] In addition, ventricular fibrillation occurred in intact pigs in which bupivacaine was injected directly into the left anterior descending coronary artery.[145] On the other hand, injection of bupivacaine directly into certain regions of the brain resulted in the development of cardiac arrhythmias, which may indicate a relationship between the CNS and cardiotoxic effects of bupivacaine.[146,147]

Enhanced Cardiotoxicity in Pregnancy

A number of the cardiotoxic reactions reported following the use of bupivacaine occurred in pregnant patients. As a result, the 0.75 percent solution is no longer recommended for use in obstetric anesthesia in the United States. Studies in pregnant and nonpregnant sheep have shown that the CC/CNS dose ratio of bupivacaine decreased from 3.7 ± 0.5 in nonpregnant sheep to 2.7 ± 0.4 in pregnant animals.[136] However, little difference was observed in the CC/CNS blood level ratio, which varied from 1.6 ± 0.1 in nonpregnant animals to 1.4 ± 0.1 in pregnant ewes. The blood level of bupivacaine at which circulatory collapse occurred was lower in pregnant animals. No difference in the myocardial uptake of bupivacaine in pregnant and nonpregnant sheep was observed at the time of cardiovas-

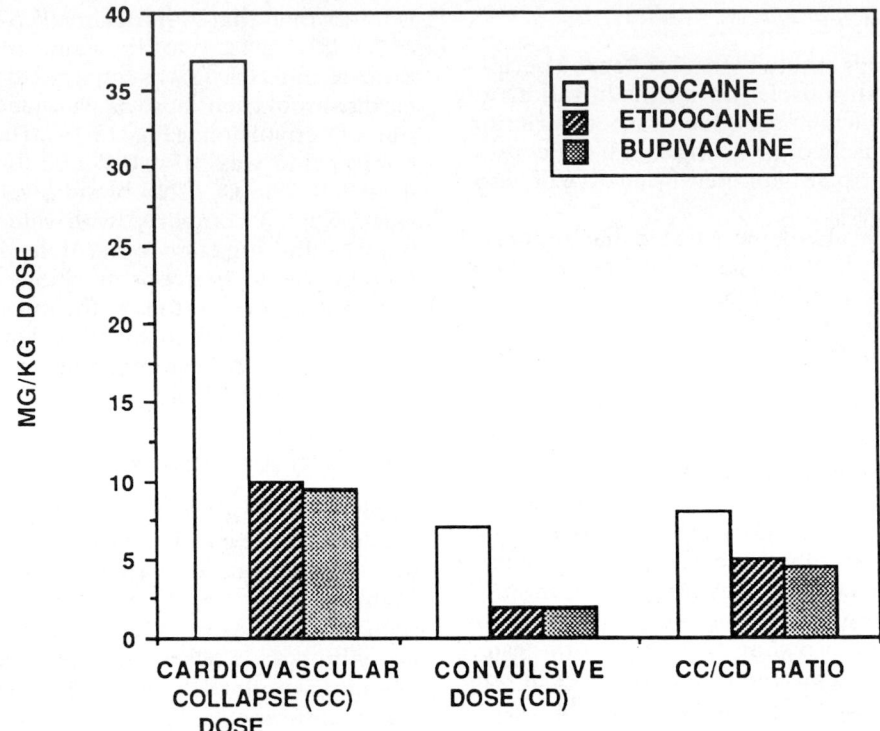

Fig. 13-19. Dose of lidocaine, bupivacaine, and etidocaine that produces convulsive activity (CD) and cardiovascular collapse (CC) in sheep.

cular collapse. Thus, if the pregnant patient is more susceptible to the cardiotoxic effects of bupivacaine, it apparently is not related to a greater myocardial uptake of drug.

Cardiac Resuscitation

Studies in acidotic and hypoxic sheep have demonstrated that cardiac resuscitation following bupivacaine-induced toxicity is difficult.[148] Studies in cats and hypoxic dogs rendered toxic with bupivacaine indicate that resuscitation is possible[149,150] if massive doses of

epinephrine and atropine are employed. In addition, bretylium but not lidocaine could raise the ventricular tachycardia threshold that was lowered by bupivacaine.[151]

Acidosis and Hypoxia

Hypercarbia, acidosis, and hypoxia will potentiate the negative chronotropic and inotropic action of lidocaine and bupivacaine in isolated cardiac tissue.[152] The combination of hypoxia and acidosis markedly poten-

TABLE 13-12. Ventricular Arrhythmias Following the Use of Lidocaine and Bupivacaine in Various Animal Preparations

| | Ventricular Arrhythmias | |
Animal Model	Lidocaine	Bupivacaine
Unanesthetized paralyzed cat	6% PVC	100% PVC
Anesthetized dog	0	0
Unanesthetized dog	0	40%—VT,VF
Unanesthetized sheep	0	80–100%–PVC,VT
Hypoxic, acidotic sheep	0	17–50%—VT,VF
Isolated guinea pig heart	0	33–50%—PVC bigeminy, trigeminy
Intracoronary injection in anesthetized pigs	VF at 64 mg	VF at 4 mg
Intracranial injections in cats	17% VT	100% VT
Intracranial injections in rats	55% VT	55% VT
	No deaths	50% deaths

Abbreviations: PVC: premature ventricular contractions; VT: ventricular tachycardia; VF: ventricular fibrillation.

tiates the cardiodepressant effects of bupivacaine. Hypoxia and acidosis also increased the frequency of cardiac arrhythmias and the mortality rate in sheep following the intravenous administration of bupivacaine.[148] Hypercarbia, acidosis, and hypoxia occur very rapidly in some patients following seizure activity owing to the rapid accidental intravascular injection of local anesthetic agents.[153] Thus, the cardiovascular depression observed in some patients following the accidental intravenous injection of bupivacaine may be related in part to the severe acid-base changes that occur during toxic reactions to this agent.

Methemoglobinemia

A unique systemic side effect associated with a specific local anesthetic agent is the formation of methemoglobinemia following the administration of large doses of prilocaine.[154] A dose-response relationship exists between the amount of prilocaine administered epidurally and the degree of methemoglobinemia. In general, doses of prilocaine of 600 mg are required for the development of clinically significant levels of methemoglobinemia. The formation of methemoglobinemia is believed to be related to the chemical structure of prilocaine. This agent has one less methyl group in the benzene ring than lidocaine. The metabolism of prilocaine in the liver results in the formation of *O*-toluidine, which is responsible for the oxidation of hemoglobin to methemoglobin.[155] The methemoglobinemia associated with the use of prilocaine is spontaneously reversible or may be treated by the intravenous administration of methylene blue.

Allergies

The aminoester agents such as procaine may produce allergic-type reactions. These agents are derivatives of *para*-aminobenzoic acid, which is known to be allergenic. The aminoamide local anesthetics are not derivatives of *para*-aminobenzoic acid, and allergic reactions to the aminoamides are extremely rare. Intradermal injections of aminoester agents in patients without a presumptive history of local anesthetic allergy resulted in positive skin reactions in 30 percent of the patients.[156] No cutaneous reactions occurred following the use of the aminoamide agents. The majority of patients with a history of alleged local anesthetic allergy showed a positive skin reaction to procaine, tetracaine, or chloroprocaine. However, no positive cutaneous response was seen following the administration of lidocaine, mepivacaine, or prilocaine. No signs of systemic anaphylaxis occurred in any of the subjects. Although the aminoamide agents appear to be relatively free from allergic-type reactions, solutions of these agents may contain a preservative, methylparaben, whose chemical structure is similar to that of *para*-aminobenzoic acid.

Local Tissue Toxicity

Local anesthetic drugs employed clinically rarely produce localized nerve damage. Concentrations of procaine, cocaine, tetracaine, and dibucaine required to produce irreversible conduction blockade in isolated frog sciatic nerves are far in excess of the concentration of these agents used clinically.[157] The intrathecal administration of tetracaine or etidocaine in rabbits resulted in histopathologic spinal cord changes following the use of 2 percent tetracaine, which exceeds the maximum concentration of 1 percent employed for spinal anesthesia in humans.[158]

In recent years, prolonged sensory and motor deficits have been reported in some patients following the epidural or subarachnoid injection of large doses of chloroprocaine.[159,160] Studies in animals have proved somewhat contradictory regarding the potential neurotoxicity of chloroprocaine[161-166] (Table 13-13). Paralysis was observed in rabbits when intrathecal chloroprocaine solutions with sodium bisulfite were employed.[165] Solutions of chloroprocaine without sodium bisulfite did not cause paralysis, whereas sodium bisulfite alone was associated with paralysis. Isolated rabbit vagus nerve studies have shown that commercial solutions of 3 percent chloroprocaine with 0.2 percent sodium bisulfite and a pH of approximately 3.0 produced irreversible conduction blockade.[166] However, a 3 percent chloroprocaine with sodium bisulfite solution buffered to a pH of 7.0 caused reversible conduction block. A 3 percent chloroprocaine solution with a pH of 3.0 but without sodium bisulfite also resulted in reversible blockade. Application of a solution of 0.2 percent sodium bisulfite alone at a pH of 3.0 resulted in irreversible conduction block, whereas a 0.2 percent sodium bisulfite solution with a pH of 7.0 caused no conduction block. The results of these studies suggest that the com-

TABLE 13-13. Animal Studies Concerning Potential Neurotoxicity of 2-Chloroprocaine and Other Local Anesthetics

Type of Study	Results
In vitro rabbit vagus nerve	Local irritation with 2-CP, but not lido and bup
In vivo rat sciatic nerve	No irritation with 2-CP and lido
In vitro rabbit vagus nerve	Irreversible block with commercial 2-CP and Na bisulfite, but not with pure 2-CP
Spinal dog	Paralysis with 2-CP, but not with bup or low pH saline
Spinal rabbit	Paralysis with commercial 2-CP and Na busulfite, but not with pure 2-CP
Spinal sheep	Minimal toxicity with 2-CP, lido, bup, and control solution
Spinal monkey	Minimal toxicity with 2-CP and bup

Abbreviations: 2-CP, 2-chloroprocaine; bup, bupivacaine; lido, lidocaine.

bination of a low pH and sodium bisulfite is responsible for the neurotoxic reactions observed following the use of large amounts of chloroprocaine solution. Chloroprocaine itself does not appear to be neurotoxic. The currently available commercial solutions of chloroprocaine do not contain sodium bisulfite.

Skeletal muscle changes have been observed following the intramuscular injection of local anesthetic agents such as lidocaine, mepivacaine, prilocaine, bupivacaine, and etidocaine.[167-169] In general, the more potent, longer-acting agents bupivacaine and etidocaine appear to cause a greater degree of localized skeletal muscle damage than the less potent, shorter-acting agents lidocaine and prilocaine. This effect on skeletal muscle is reversible, and muscle regeneration occurs rapidly and is complete within 2 weeks following injection of local anesthetic agents. These skeletal muscle changes have not been associated with overt signs of local irritation.

REFERENCES

1. Sanchez V, Arthur GR, Strichartz GR: Fundamental properties of local anesthetics. I. The dependence of lidocaine's ionization and octanol:buffer partitioning on solvent and temperature. Anesth Analg 66:159, 1987
2. Sanchez V, Ferrante FM, Cibotti N, Strichartz GR: Partitioning of tetracaine base and cation into phospholipid membranes: Relevance to anesthetic potency (abstract). Reg Anaesth, suppl., 13:81, 1988
3. Gissen A, Covino BG, Gregus J: The differential sensitivities of mammalian nerve fibers to local anesthetic agents. Anesthesiology 53:467, 1980
4. Courtney KR: Structure-activity relations for frequency-dependent sodium channel block in nerve by local anesthetics. J Pharmacol Exp Ther 213:114, 1980
5. Courtney KR, Strichartz GR: Structural elements which determine local anesthetic activity. p. 53. In Strichartz GR (ed): Handbook of Experimental Pharmacology: Local Anesthetics. Springer-Verlag, Heidelberg, 1987
6. Schreier S, Frezzatti WA Jr., Araujo PS, et al: Effect of lipid membranes on the apparent pK of the local anesthetic tetracaine: Spin label and titration studies. Biochim Biophys Acta 769:231, 1984
7. Tucker GT, Mather LE: Properties, absorption, and disposition of local anesthetic agents. p. 47. In Cousins MJ, Bridenbaugh PO (eds): Neural Blockade in Clinical Anesthesia and Management of Pain. 2nd Ed. JB Lippincott, Philadelphia, 1988
8. Ulbricht W, Stoye-Herzog M: Distinctly different rates of benzocaine action on sodium channels of Ranvier nodes kept open by chloramine-T and veratridine. Pflugers Arch 402:439, 1984
9. Ritchie JM, Rogart RB: Density of sodium channels in mammalian myelinated nerve fibers and nature of the axonal membrane under the myelin sheath. Proc Natl Acad Sci USA 74:211, 1977
10. Hodgkin AL: The Conduction of the Nervous Impulse. Charles C Thomas, Springfield, IL, 1964
11. Hille B: Ionic Channels of Excitable Membranes. Sinauer Associates, Sunderland, MA, 1984
12. Skou JC: Enzymatic basis for active transport of Na^+ and K^+ across cell membrane. Physiol Rev 45:496, 1965
13. Rushton WAH: A theory of the effects of fibre size in medullated nerve. J Physiol (Lond) 115:101, 1951
14. Tasaki I: Nervous Transmission. Charles C Thomas, Springfield, IL, 1953
15. Condouris GA, Goebel RH, Brady T: Computer simulation of local anesthetic effects using a mathematical model of myelinated nerve. J Pharmacol Exp Ther 196:737, 1976
16. Trevan JW, Boock E: The relation of hydrogen ion concentration to the action of local anaesthetics. Br J Exp Pathol 8:307, 1927
17. Ritchie JM, Ritchie B, Greengard P: The effect of the nerve sheath on the action of local anesthetics. J Pharmacol Exp Ther 150:160, 1965
18. Hille B: The pH-dependent rate of action of local anesthetics on the node of Ranvier. J Gen Physiol 69:475, 1977
19. Hille B: Local anesthetics: Hydrophilic and hydrophobic pathways for the drug-receptor reactions. J Gen Physiol 69:497, 1977
20. Narahashi T, Frazier DT, Yamada M: The site of action and active form of local anesthetics. I. Theory and pH experiments with tertiary compounds. J Pharmacol Exp Ther 171:32, 1970
21. Frazier DT, Narahashi T, Yamada M: The site of action and active form of local anesthetics. II. Experiments with quaternary compounds. J Pharmacol Exp Ther 171:45, 1970
22. Strichartz GR: The inhibition of sodium currents in myelinated nerve by quaternary derivatives of lidocaine. J Gen Physiol 62:37, 1973
23. Ritchie JM, Ritchie BR: Local anaesthetics: Effect of pH on activity. Science 162:1394, 1968
24. Chernoff DM, Strichartz GR: Tonic and phasic block of neuronal sodium currents by 5-hydroxyhexano-2',6'-xylidide, a neutral lidocaine homologue. J Gen Physiol 93:1075, 1989
25. Ulbricht W: Kinetics of drug action and equilibrium results at the node of Ranvier. Physiol Rev 61:785, 1981
26. Shanes AM, Freygang WH, Grundfest H, et al: Anesthetic and calcium action in the voltage-clamped squid giant axon. J Gen Physiol 42:793, 1959
27. Taylor RE: Effect of procaine on electrical properties of squid axon membrane. Am J Physiol 196:1071, 1959
28. Hille B: The common mode of action of three agents that decrease the transient change in sodium permeability in nerves. Nature 210:1220, 1966
29. Arhem P, Frankenhaeuser B: Local anesthetics: Effects on permeability properties of nodal membrane in myelinated nerve fibres from *Xenopus*. Potential clamp experiments. Acta Physiol Scand 91:11, 1974
30. Strichartz G: Interactions of local anesthetics with Neuronal Sodium Channels. p. 39. In Covino B, Fozzard HA, Rehder K, Strichartz G (eds): Effects of Anesthesia. Clinical Physiology Series. American Physiological Society, Bethesda, MD, 1985
31. Courtney KR, Kendig JJ, Cohen EN: The rates of interaction of local anesthetics with sodium channels in nerve. J Pharmacol Exp Ther 207:594, 1978
32. Chernoff DM: Kinetics of local anesthetic binding to sodium channels: Role of pK_a. Ph.D. dissertation. Massachusetts Institute of Technology, 1988
33. Cahalan MD, Almers W: Interactions between quaternary lidocaine, the sodium channel gates and tetrodotoxin. Biophys J 27:39, 1979
34. Neumcke B, Schwarz W, Stämpfli R: Block of Na channels in the membrane of myelinated nerve by benzocaine. Pflugers Arch 390:230, 1981

35. Bekkers JM, Greeff NG, Keynes RD, Neumcke B: The effect of local anaesthetics on the components of the asymmetry current in the squid giant axon. J Physiol (Lond) 352:653, 1984

36. Wang GK, Brodwick MS, Eaton DC, Strichartz GR: Inhibition of sodium currents by local anesthetics in chloramine-T treated squid axons: The role of Na channel activation. J Gen Physiol 89:645, 1987

37. Chernoff DM, Strichartz GR: Binding kinetics of local anesthetics to closed and open sodium channels during phasic inhibition: Relevance to anti-arrhythmic actions. In Hondeghem LM (ed): Molecular and Cellular Mechanisms of Anti-Arrhythmic Agents. Futura, Mt. Kisco, NY (in press)

38. Starmer CF, Courtney KR: Modeling ion channel blockade at guarded binding sites: Application to tertiary drugs. Am Physiol Soc H848, 1986

39. Schwarz W, Palade PT, Hille B: Local anesthetics: Effect of pH on use-dependent block of sodium channels in frog muscle. Biophys J 20:343, 1977

40. Bokesch PM, Post C, Strichartz GR: Structure-activity relationship of lidocaine homologs producing tonic and frequency-dependent impulse blockade in nerve. J Pharmacol Exp Ther 237:773, 1986

41. Yeh JZ, TenEick R: Molecular and structural basis of resting and use-dependent block of sodium current defined using disopyramide analogues. Biophys J 51:123, 1987

42. Chernoff DM, Strichartz GR: Lidocaine and bupivacaine block of sodium channels: Recovery kinetics correlate with potency for phase block (abstract). Biophys J 53:2, 537a, 1988

43. Courtney KR: Size-dependent kinetics associated with drug block of sodium current. Biophys J 45:42, 1984

44. Butterworth JF, Strichartz GR: Molecular mechanism of local anesthesia: A review. Anesthesiology (in press)

45. Raymond SA, Steffensen S, Gugino LM, Strichartz GR: The role of length of nerve exposed to local anesthetics in impulse blocking action. Anesth Analg 68:563, 1989

46. Raymond SA, Thalhammer JG, Strichartz GR: Axonal excitability: Endogenous and exogenous modulation. For Dimitrijevic (ed): Altered Sensation and Pain: Recent Achievements in Restorative Neurology 3. Karger, Basel (in press)

47. Fink BR: Mechanisms of differential axial blockade in epidural and subarachnoid anesthesia. Anesthesiology 70:851, 1989

48. Raymond SA, Gissen AJ: Mechanisms of Differential Nerve Block. p. 95. In Strichartz GR (ed): Handbook of Experimental Pharmacology: Local Anesthetics. Springer-Verlag, Heidelberg, 1987

49. Hodgkin AL, Huxley AF: A quantitative description of membrane current and its application to conduction and excitation in nerve. J Physiol (Lond) 117:500, 1952

50. Wildsmith JAW, Gissen AJ, Gregus J, Covino BG: Differential nerve blocking activity of amino-ester local anaesthetics. Br J Anaesth 57:612, 1985

51. Wildsmith JAW, Gissen AJ, Takman B, Covino BG: Differential nerve blockade: Esters vs amides and the influence of pKa. Br J Anaesth 59:379, 1987

52. Astrom A, Persson NH: Some pharmacological properties of α-methyl-αpropylamino propionanilide: a new local anesthetic. Br J Pharmacol 16:32, 1961

53. Crawford OB: Comparative evaluation in peridural anesthesia of lidocaine, mepivacaine and L-67, a new local anesthetic agent. Anesthesiology 25:321, 1964

54. Gissen AJ, Covino BG: Differential sensitivity of fast and slow fibres in mammalian nerve. III. Effect of etidocaine and bupivacaine on fast/slow fibres. Anesth Analg 61:570, 1982

55. Scott DB, McClure JH, Giasi RM, et al: Effects of concentration of local anaesthetic drugs in extradural block. Br J Anesth 52:1033, 1980

56. Blair MR: Cardiovascular pharmacology of local anesthetics. Br J Anaesth, suppl., 47:247, 1975

57. Rosenberg PH, Heinonen E, Jansson SE, Gripenberg J: Differential nerve block by bupivacaine and 2-chloroprocaine. Br J Anaesth 52:1183, 1980

58. Galindo A, Benavides O, Ortega de Munos S, et al: Comparison of anesthetic solutions used in lumbar and caudal peridural anesthesia. Anesth Analg 57:175, 1978

59. Covino BG: Pharmacology of local anaesthetic agents. Br J Anaesth 58:701, 1986

60. Johns RA, Di Fazio CA, Longnecker DE: Lidocaine constricts or dilates rat arterioles in a dose-dependent manner. Anesthesiology 62:141, 1985

61. Johns RA, Seyde WC, DiFazio CA, Longnecker DE: Dose-dependent effects of bupivacaine on rat muscle arterioles. Anesthesiology 65:186, 1986

62. Littlewood DG, Buckley P, Covino BG, et al: Comparative study of various local anaesthetic solutions in extradural block in labour. Br J Anaesth 51:475, 1979

63. Erdimir HA, Soper LE, Sweet RB: Studies of factors affecting peridural anesthesia. Anesth Analg 44:400, 1965

64. Braid DP, Scott DB: The systemic absorption of local analgesic drugs. Br J Anaesth 37:394, 1965

65. Concepcion M, Maddi R, Francis D, et al: Vasoconstrictors in spinal anesthesia with tetracaine. A comparison of epinephrine and phenylephrine. Anesth Analg 63:134, 1984

66. Swerdlow M, Jones R: The duration of action of bupivacaine, prilocaine and lignocaine. Br J Anaesth 42:335, 1970

67. Albert J, Lofstrom B: Bilateral ulnar nerve blocks for the evaluation of local anaesthetic agents. Acta Anaesthesiol Scand 9:203, 1965

68. Sinclair CJ, Scott DB: Comparison of bupivacaine and etidocaine in extradural blockade. Br J Anaesth 56:147, 1984

69. Eisenach JC, Grice SC, Dewan DM: Epinephrine enhances analgesia produced by epidural bupivacaine during labor. Anesth Analg 66:447, 1987

70. Gissen AJ, Covino BG: Differential sensitivity of fast and slow fibres in mammalian nerve. IV. Effect of carbonation of local anesthetics. Reg Anaesth 10:68, 1985

71. Bokesch PM, Raymond SA, Strichartz GR: Dependence of lidocaine potency on pH and pCO_2. Anesth Analg 66:9, 1987

72. Morrison DH: A double-blind comparison of carbonated lidocaine and lidocaine hydrochloride in epidural anaesthesia. Can Anaesth Soc J 28:387, 1981

73. Nickel PM, Bromage PR, Sherrill DL: Comparison of hydrochloride and carbonated salts of lidocaine for epidural analgesia. Reg Anaesth 11:62, 1986

74. Eckstein KL, Vincente-Eckstein A, Steiner R, Missler V: Klinische erprobung von Bupivacaine CO_2. Anaesthesist 27:1, 1978

75. McClure JH, Scott DB: Comparison of bupivacaine hydrochloride and carbonated bupivacaine in brachial plexus block by the inter-scalene technique. Br J Anaesth 53:523, 1981

76. Hilgier M: Alkalinization of bupivacaine for brachial plexus block. Reg Anaesth 10:59, 1985

77. DiFazio CA, Carron H, Grosslilght KR, et al: Comparison of pH-adjusted lidocaine solutions for epidural anesthesia. Anesth Analg 65:760, 1986

78. Bedder MD, Kozody R, Craig DB: Comparison of bupiva-

caine and alkanized bupivacaine in brachial plexus anesthesia. Anesth Analg 67:48, 1988

79. Cunningham NL, Kaplan JA: A rapid onset long acting regional anesthetic technique. Anesthesiology 41:509, 1974

80. Cohen SE, Thurlow A: Comparison of chloroprocaine-bupivacaine mixture with chloroprocaine and bupivacaine used individually for obstetric epidural analgesia. Anesthesiology 51:288, 1979

81. Corke BG, Carlson CG, Dettbarn WD: The influence of 2-chloroprocaine on the subsequent analgesic potency of bupivacaine. Anesthesiology 60:25, 1984

82. Bromage PR: Spread of analgesic solutions in the epidural space and their site of action: A statistical study. Br J Anaesth 34:161, 1962

83. Fagraeus L, Urban BJ, Bromage PR: Spread of analgesia in early pregnancy. Anesthesiology 58:184, 1983

84. Datta S, Hurley RJ, Naulty JS, et al: Plasma and cerebrospinal fluid progesterone concentrations in pregnant and nonpregnant women. Anesth Analg 65:950, 1986

85. Datta S, Lambert DH, Gregus J, et al: Differential sensitivities of mammalian nerve fibers during pregnancy. Anesth Analg 62:1070, 1983

86. Flanagan HL, Datta S, Lambert DH, et al: Effect of pregnancy on bupivacaine induced conduction blockade in the rabbit vagus nerve. Anesth Analg 66:123, 1987

87. Morris R, McKay W, Mushlin P: Comparison of pain associated with intradermal and subcutaneous infiltration with various local anesthetic solutions. Anesth Analg 66:1180, 1987

88. McKay W, Morris R, Mushlin P: Sodium bicarbonate attenuates pain on skin infiltration with lidocaine, with or without epinephrine. Anesth Analg 66:572, 1987

89. Harris WN, Slater EM, Bell HM: Regional anesthesia by the intravenous route. JAMA 194:1273, 1965

90. Albright GA: Cardiac arrest following regional anesthesia with etidocaine or bupivacaine. Anesthesiology 51:285, 1979

91. Reiestad F, Stromskag KE: Interpleural catheter in management of postoperative pain: A preliminary report. Reg Anaesth 11:89, 1986

92. Brismar B, Pettersson N, Tokics L, et al: Postoperative analgesia with intrapleural administration of bupivacaine-adrenaline. Acta Anaesthesiol Scand 31:515, 1987

93. Stromskag KE, Reiestad F, Holmquist EVO, Ogenstad S: Intrapleural administration of 0.25%, 0.375% and 0.5% bupivacaine with epinephrine after cholecystectomy. Anesth Analg 67:430, 1988

94. Rosenberg PH, Scheinin BMA, Lepantalo MJ, Lindfurs O: Continuous intrapleural infusion of bupivacaine for analgesia after thoracotomy. Anesthesiology 67:811, 1987

95. Bromage PR, Gertel M: An evaluation of two new local anaesthetics for major conduction blockade. Can Anaesth Soc J 17:557, 1970

96. Rocco AG, Mallampati SR, Boon J, et al: Double blind evaluation of intrathecal bupivacaine and tetracaine. Reg Anaesth 9:183, 1984

97. Bigler D, Hjortso NC, Edstrom H, et al: Comparative effects of intrathecal bupivacaine and tetracaine on analgesia, cardiovascular function and plasma catecholamines. Acta Anaesthesiol Scand 30:194, 1986

98. Concepcion MA, Lambert DH, Welch KA, Covino BG: Tourniquet pain during spinal anesthesia: A comparison of plain solutions of tetracaine and bupivacaine. Anesth Analg 67:828, 1988

99. Stewart A, Lambert DH, Concepcion MA, et al: Decreased incidence of tourniquet pain during spinal anesthesia with

bupivacaine: A possible explanation. Anesth Analg 67:833, 1988

100. Chambers WA, Littlewood DG, Logan MR, Scott DB: Effect of added epinephrine on spinal anesthesia with lidocaine. Anesth Analg 60:417, 1981

101. Chambers WA, Littlewood DG, Scott DB: Spinal anaesthesia with hyperbaric bupivacaine: Effect of added vasoconstrictors. Anesth Analg 61:49, 1982

102. Evers H, Von Dardel O, Juhlin L: Dermal effects of compositions based on the eutectic mixture of lignocaine and prilocaine (EMLA). Br J Anaesth 57:997, 1985

103. Hallen B, Uppfeldt A: Does lidocaine-prilocaine cream permit painfree insertion of IV catheters in children? Anesthesiology 57:340, 1982

104. Ohlsen L, Englesson S, Evers H: An anaesthetic lidocaine/prilocaine cream (EMLA) for epicutaneous application tested for split skin grafts. Scand J Plast Reconstr Surg 19:201, 1985

105. Covino BG: Pharmacokinetics of local anesthetic drugs. p. 202. In Prys-Roberts C, Hug C, Jr. (eds): Pharmacokinetics of Anesthesia. Blackwell Scientific Publications, Oxford, 1984

106. Covino BG, Vassallo HG: Local Anesthetics: Mechanisms of Action and Clinical Use. Grune & Stratton, Orlando, FL, 1976

107. Abdel-Salam AR, Vonwiller JB, Scott DB: Evaluation of etidocaine in extradural block. Br J Anaesth 47:1081, 1975

108. Wildsmith JAW, Tucker GT, Cooper S, et al: Plasma concentrations of local anaesthetics after interscalene brachial plexus block. Br J Anaesth 49:461, 1977

109. Tucker GT, Mather LE: Pharmacokinetics of local anaesthetic agents. Br J Anaesth 47:213, 1975

110. Tucker GT, Mather LE: Clinical pharmacokinetics of local anesthetics. Clin Pharmacokinet 4:241, 1979

111. Tucker GT: Pharmacokinetics of local anaesthetics. Br J Anaesth 58:717, 1986

112. Lofstrom JB, Alm BE, Bertler A, et al: Lung uptake of lidocaine. Acta Anaesth Scand 70:80, 1978

113. Lofstrom JB: Tissue distribution of local anesthetics with special reference to the lung. Int Anesthesiol Clin 16:53, 1978

114. Foldes FF, Davidson DM, Duncalf D, et al: The intravenous toxicity of local anesthetic agents in man. Clin Pharmacol Ther 6:328, 1965

115. Boyes RN: A review of the metabolism of amide local anaesthetic agents. Br J Anaesth 47:225, 1975

116. Tucker GT, Wiklund L, Berlin-Wahlen AB, Mather LE: Hepatic clearance of local anesthetics in man. J Pharmacokinet Biopharm 5:111, 1977

117. Nation RL, Triggs EJ, Selig M: Lignocaine kinetics in cardiac and aged subjects. Br J Clin Pharmacol 4:439, 1977

118. Stenson RE, Constantino RT, Harrison DC: Interrelationships of hepatic blood flow, cardiac output and blood levels of lidocaine in man. Circulation 43:205, 1971

119. Thomson PD, Melmon KL, Richardson JA, et al: Lidocaine pharmacokinetics in advanced heart failure, liver disease and renal failure in humans. Ann Intern Med 78:499, 1973

120. Wagman IH, De Jong RH, Prince DA: Effects of lidocaine on the central nervous system. Anesthesiology 28:155, 1967

121. Englesson S: The influence of acid-base changes on central nervous system toxicity of local anesthetic agents. I. An experimental study in cats. Acta Anaesthesiol Scand 18:79, 1974

122. Liu PL, Feldman HS, Giasi R, et al: Comparative CNS toxicity of lidocaine, etidocaine, bupivacaine and tetracaine in

awake dogs following rapid iv administration. Anesth Analg 62:375, 1983

123. Scott DB: Evaluation of clinical tolerance of local anaesthetic agents. Br J Anaesth 47:328, 1975

124. Arthur GR, Scott DHT, Boyes RN, Scott DB: Pharmacokinetic and clinical pharmacological studies with mepivacaine and prilocaine. Br J Anaesth 51:481, 1979

125. Burney RG, DiFazio CA, Foster JA: Effects of pH on protein binding of lidocaine. Anesth Analg 57:478, 1978

126. Apfelbaum JL, Shaw LA, Gross JB, et al: Modification of lidocaine protein binding with CO_2. Can Anaesth Soc J 32:468, 1985

127. Clarkson CW, Hohdeghem LM: Mechanisms for bupivacaine depression of cardiac conduction: Fast block of sodium channels during the action potential with slow recovery from block during diastole. Anesthesiology 62:396: 1985

128. Lynch C: Depression of myocardial contractility in vitro by bupivacaine, etidocaine and lidocaine. Anesth Analg 65:551, 1986

129. Moller RA, Covino BG: Cardiac electrophysiologic effects of lidocaine and bupivacaine. Anesth Analg 67:107, 1988

130. Block A, Covino BG: Effect of local anesthetic agents on cardiac conduction and contractility. Reg Anaesth 6:55, 1982

131. Stewart DM, Rogers WP, Mahaffrey JE, et al: Effect of local anesthetics on the cardiovascular system in the dog. Anesthesiology 24:620, 1963

132. Liu P, Feldman HS, Covino BG, et al: Acute cardiovascular toxicity of procaine, chloroprocaine and tetracaine in anesthetized ventilated dogs. Reg Anaesth 7:14, 1982

133. Liu P, Feldman HS, Covino BG, et al: Acute cardiovascular toxicity of intravenous amide local anesthetics in anesthetized ventilated dogs. Anesth Analg 61:317, 1982

134. Chamberlain B, Volpe P, Flescher S: Inhibition of calcium induced release from purified cardiac sarcoplasmic reticulum vesicles. J Br Chem 259:7547, 1984

135. Tanz RD, Heskett T, Loehning W, Fairfax CA: Comparative cardiotoxicity of bupivacaine and lidocaine in the isolated perfused mammalian heart. Anesth Analg 63:549, 1984

136. MacMillan WH: A hypothesis concerning the effect of cocaine on the action of sympathomimetic amines. Br J Pharmacol 14:385, 1959

137. Wollenberger A, Krayer O: Experimental heart failure caused by central nervous system depressants and local anesthetics. J Pharmacol Exp Ther 94:439, 1948

138. Morishima HO, Pedersen H, Finster M, et al: Bupivacaine toxicity in pregnant and nonpregnant ewes. Anesthesiology 63:134, 1985

139. Dejong R, Ronfeld R, DeRosa R: Cardiovascular effects of convulsant and supraconvulsant doses of amide local anesthetics. Anesth Analg 61:3, 1982

140. Kotelko DM, Shnider SM, Dailey PA, et al: Bupivacaine-induced cardiac arrhythmias in sheep. Anesthesiology 60:10, 1984

141. Kasten GW: High serum bupivacaine concentrations produce rhythm disturbances similar to torsades de pointes in anesthetized dogs. Reg Anaesth 11:20, 1986

142. Sage D, Feldman H, Arthur G, et al: The cardiovascular effects of convulsant doses of lidocaine and bupivacaine in the conscious dog. Reg Anaesth 10:175, 1985

143. Reiz S, Nath S: Cardiotoxicity of local anesthetic agents. Br J Anaesth 58:736, 1986

144. Coyle DE, Sperelakis N: Bupivacaine and lidocaine blockade of calcium-mediated slow action potentials in guinea pig ventricular muscle. J Pharmacol Exp Ther 242:1001, 1987

145. Nath S, Haggmark S, Johansson G, Reiz S: Differential depressant and electrophysiologic cardiotoxicity of local anesthetics: An experimental study with special reference to lidocaine and bupivacaine. Anesth Analg 65:1263, 1986

146. Heavner JE: Cardiac dysrhythmias induced by infusion of local anesthetics into the lateral cerebral ventricle of cats. Anesth Analg 65:133, 1986

147. Thomas RD, Behbehani MM, Coyle DE, Denson DD: Cardiovascular toxicity of local anesthetics: An alternative hypothesis. Anesth Analg 65:444, 1986

148. Rosen M, Thigpen J, Shnider S, et al: Bupivacaine-induced cardiotoxicity in hypoxic and acidotic sheep. Anesth Analg 64:1089, 1985

149. Chadwick HS: Toxicity and resuscitation in lidocaine or bupivacaine infused cats. Anesthesiology 63:385, 1985

150. Kasten GW, Martin ST: Successful cardiovascular resuscitation after massive intravenous bupivacaine overdosage in anesthetized dogs. Anesth Analg 64:491, 1985

151. Kasten GW, Martin ST: Bupivacaine cardiovascular toxicity: Comparison of treatment with bretylium and lidocaine. Anesth Analg 64:911, 1985

152. Sage DJ, Feldman HS, Arthur GR, et al: Influence of lidocaine and bupivacaine on isolated guinea pig atria in the presence of acidosis and hypoxia. Anesth Analg 63:1, 1984

153. Moore DC, Crawford RD, Scurlock JE: Severe hypoxia and acidosis following local anesthetic-induced convulsions. Anesthesiology 53:259, 1980

154. Lund PG, Cwik JG: Propitocaine (eitanest) and methemoglobinemia. Anesthesiology 26:569, 1965

155. Hjelm M, Holmdahl MH: Biochemical effects of aromatic amines. Acta Anaesthesiol Scand 2:99, 1965

156. Aldrete JA, Johnson DA: Evaluation of intracutaneous testing for investigation of allergy to local anesthetic agents. Anesth Analg 49:173, 1970

157. Skou JC: Local anaesthetics. II. The toxic potencies of some local anaesthetics and of butyl alcohol, determined on peripheral nerve. Acta Pharmacol Toxicol 10:292, 1954

158. Adams HJ, Mastri AR, Eicholzer AW, Kilpatrick G: Morphologic effects of intrathecal etidocaine and tetracaine on the rabbit spinal cord. Anesth Analg 53:904, 1974

159. Ravindran RS, Bond VK, Tasch MD, et al: Prolonged neural blockade following regional analgesia with 2-chloroprocaine. Anesth Analg 58:447, 1980

160. Reisner LS, Hochman BN, Plumer MH: Persistent neurologic deficit and adhesive arachnoiditis following intrathecal 2-chloroprocaine injection. Anesth Analg 58:452, 1980

161. Barsa JE, Batra M, Fink BR, Sumi SM: Prolonged neural blockade following regional analgesia with 2-chloroprocaine. Anesth Analg 61:961, 1982

162. Pizzolato D, Renegar OJ: Histopathological effects of long exposure to local anesthetics on peripheral nerves. Anesth Analg 38:138, 1959

163. Rosen MA, Baysinger CL, Shnider SM, et al: Evaluation of neurotoxicity of local anesthetics following subarachnoid injection. Anesth Analg 62:802, 1983

164. Ravindran RS, Turner MS, Miller I: Neurological effects of subarachnoid administration of 2-chloroprocaine-CE, bupivacaine and low pH normal saline in dogs. Anesth Analg 61:279, 1982

165. Wang BC, Hillman DE, Spiedholz NI, Turndorf H: Chronic neurologic deficits and Nesacaine-CE: An effect of the anesthetic, 2-chloroprocaine, or the antioxidant, sodium bisulfite? Anesth Analg 63:445, 1984

166. Gissen AJ, Datta S, Lambert D: The chloroprocaine contro-

versy. II. Is chloroprocaine neurotoxic? Reg Anaesth 9:135, 1984

167. Libelius R, Sonesson B, Stamenovic BA, Thesleff S: Denervation-like changes in skeletal muscle after treatment with a local anesthetic (Marcaine). J Anat 106:297, 1970

168. Benoit PW, Belt WD: Destruction and regeneration of skeletal muscle after treatment with a local anesthetic, bupivacaine (Marcaine). J Anat 107:547, 1970

169. Benoit PW, Belt WD: Some effects of local anesthetic agents on skeletal muscle. Exp Neurol 34:264, 1972

170. Bonica JJ: Principles and Practice of Obstetric Analgesia and Anesthesia. FA Davis, Philadelphia, 1967

171. Mather LE, Cousins MJ: Local anesthetics and their current clinical use. Drugs 18:185, 1979

14

AUTONOMIC NERVOUS SYSTEM PHARMACOLOGY

Robert G. Merin

INTRODUCTION

Autonomic pharmacology and physiology are inescapably entwined. Consequently, before presenting a detailed discussion of the drugs that act primarily through or affect the autonomic nervous system, the anatomy and physiology of the autonomic nervous system are reviewed in order to set the stage for the pharmacologic discussion. The autonomic nervous system has also been called the involuntary nervous system. It is through this series of nerves and synapses that the mammalian body attempts to regulate its ongoing physiologic functions automatically, permitting the voluntary consciousness of upper mammals, and particularly the primates, to be concerned with matters requiring even more complicated neurophysiologic circuits. Physiologically, the autonomic nervous system may be considered as having a dual function. The first function is to maintain the internal environment of the body in a state that encourages optimal function of the various organ systems. The second function is to prepare and enable the body to undertake extraordinary efforts in situations that threaten the body's well-being.

Classically, two divisions of the autonomic nervous system have been described. The parasympathetic autonomic nervous system is primarily cholinergic in function; that is, its effects on organs are mediated mostly by the neuroeffector cellular secretion of acetylcholine. The second division, the sympathetic nervous system, is primarily an adrenergic system in that the neuroeffector cellular secretory product is primarily norepinephrine (noradrenaline in the British system, hence the name of the system). In very general terms, the sympathetic nervous system is primarily stimulatory in that it excites those organ functions that prepare the body for "fight or flight." At the same time it decreases blood flow and function to organ systems that are not critical for this function. The parasympathetic nervous system can be conceived of as a restorative system that, either before or after the stress, tends to repair the body's physiologic functions and restore energy levels toward maximum. Especially as far as cardiovascular function is concerned, the sympathetic and parasympathetic nervous systems are in constant opposition, and the state of the cardiovascular system mainly depends on which system is predominant at the moment (Table 14-1). This principle is very important in understanding the action of drugs that affect the autonomic nervous system, particularly the autonomic antagonists. The physiologic result of drugs that are either adrenergic (sympathetic) or cholinergic (parasympathetic) antagonists depends to a large degree on the state of the autonomic nervous system at the time the drugs are given. This principle is further described in the discussion of the different drug classes.

In addition to the difference in the chemical receptor physiology, there are also anatomic differences in the origin and distribution of the sympathetic and parasympathetic nervous system.[1,2] The primary neurons in the

TABLE 14-1. Opposing Effects of Sympathetic and Parasympathetic Nervous System

Organ Function	SNS	PNS
Heart		
Rate	+++	———
Contractility	+++	–
Conduction	+++	——
Smooth muscle		
Vascular	+++,———	–
Bronchial	———	+++
Gastrointestinal motility	——	++
sphincter	++	——
Biliary	–	++
Uterus	++,–	+,–
Iris	——	++
Genitourinary motility	–	++
sphincter	++	——
Glands		
Respiratory	——	+++
Sweat	++	0
Salivary	±	++
Gastric	–	++

Symbols: +++, marked increase; ++, moderate increase; +, slight increase; 0, no effect; ±, slight increase or decrease; ———, marked decrease; ——, moderate decrease; –, slight decrease.

parasympathetic nervous system originate in the cranial nerve nuclei and, for the sacral component, in the S2, S3, and S4 nuclei (Fig. 14-1). These primary neurons synapse with the effector (postganglionic) neurons in the organ being innervated. Consequently, the primary neuronal (preganglionic) pathway is considerably longer than the secondary. By contrast, the primary (preganglionic) sympathetic neurons are located in the thoracic and lumbar spinal cord (Fig. 14-2). These neurons then exit the spinal cord to synapse with the secondary (postganglionic) neurons in the paravertebral sympathetic and the peripheral ganglia. Hence, the postganglionic sympathetic neuron is usually considerably longer than the preganglionic (Fig. 14-3). The primary neuron cells in the parasympathetic nervous system (except for the sacral outflow) are actually in the brain stem, hence subject directly to cortical, hypothalamic, and afferent impulses delivered to the brain stem; the sympathetic neurons must operate via another nervous relay that descends from other neurons located in the lateral portions of the reticular formation in the bulbar area of the brain stem (the vasomotor center) through the bulbospinal tract in the intermediolateral column of the spinal cord to the primary neurons of the sympathetic nervous system. Interestingly, the parasympathetic nervous system is totally cholinergic in its neurotransmission, whereas transmission in the sympathetic nervous system ganglion, the modification of that transmission, the adrenal medulla, and the

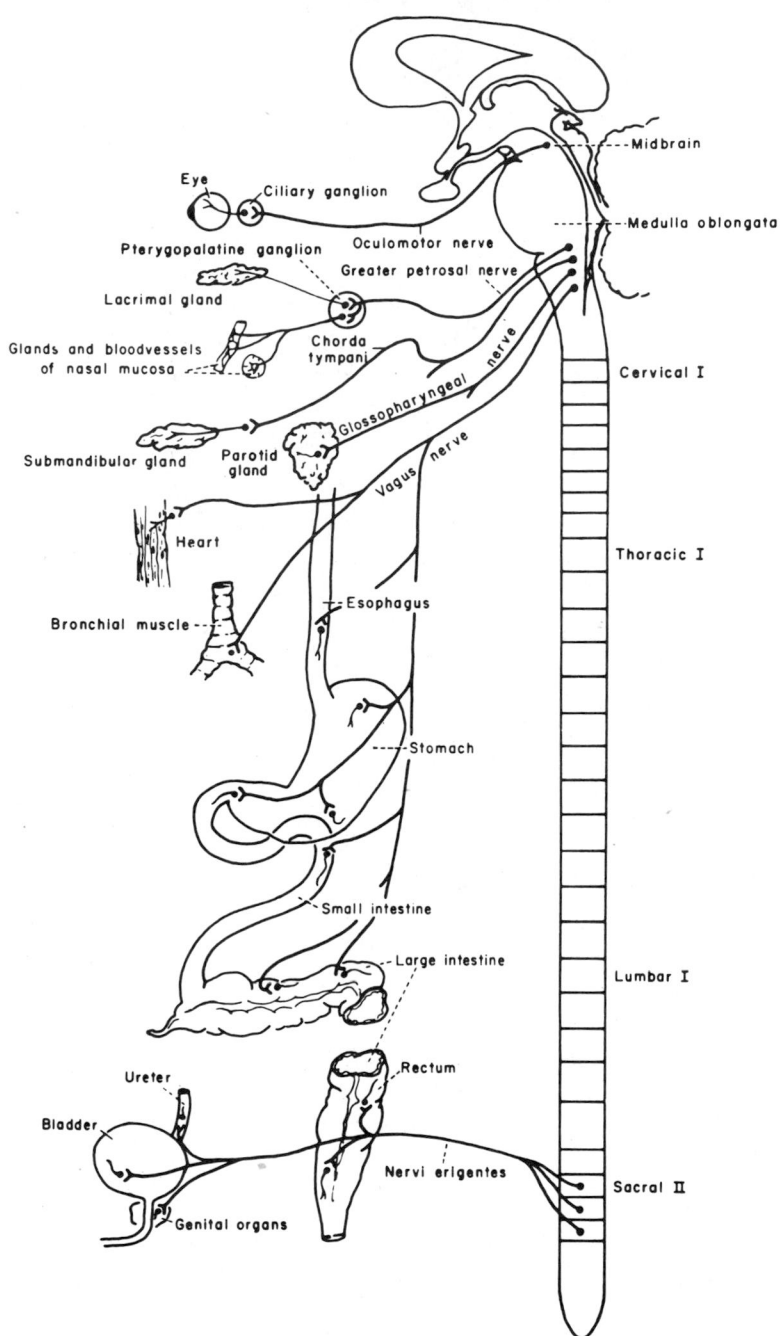

Fig. 14-1. Anatomy of the parasympathetic nervous system. (From Larsell,[130] as modified in Anson,[131] with permission.)

sweat glands are cholinergic (Fig. 14-3). Consequently, drugs that stimulate or block cholinergic receptors may also have consequences in the sympathetic nervous system, while drugs that stimulate or block adrenergic receptors usually have parasympathetic consequences only through the action of reflexes.

SYMPATHETIC NERVOUS SYSTEM

Anatomy

The preganglionic neurons of the sympathetic nervous system have cell bodies in the anterolateral gray matter of the thoracic and lumbar spinal cord from T1 through

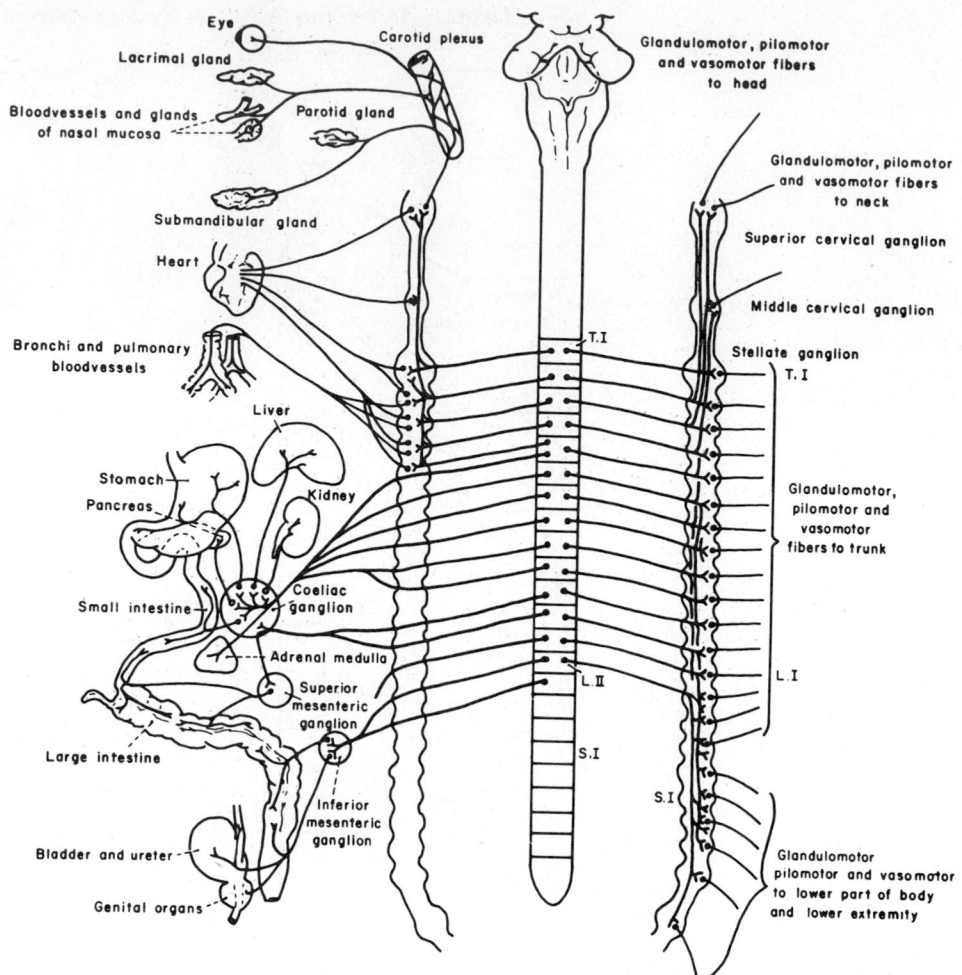

Fig. 14-2. Anatomy of the sympathetic nervous system. (From Larsell,[130] as modified in Anson,[131] with permission.)

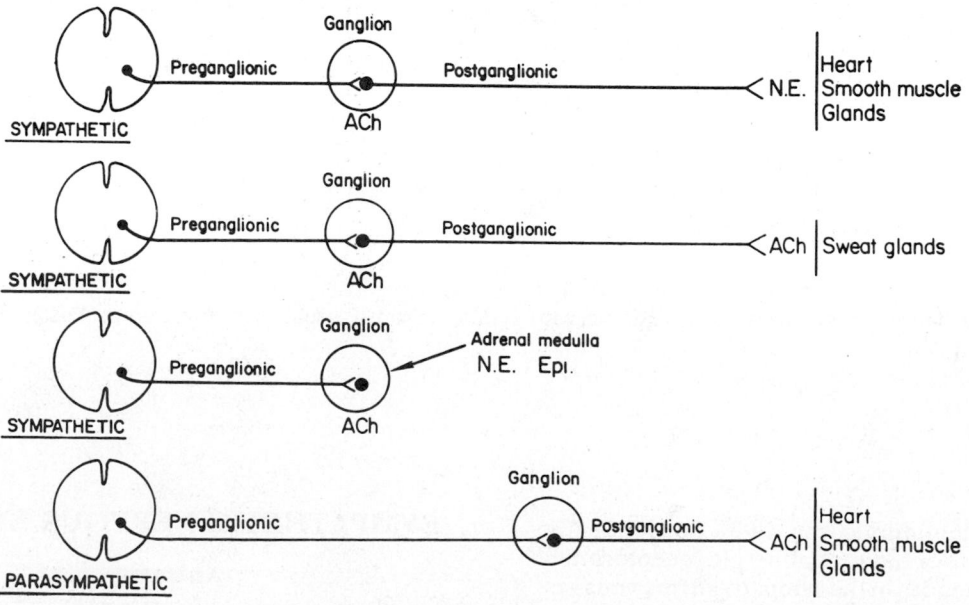

Fig. 14-3. Autonomic nervous system neurotransmission. ACh, acetylcholine; NE, norepinephrine; Epi, epinephrine.

L3 (Fig. 14-2). The preganglionic axons travel in the anterior nerve roots to the sympathetic ganglia, where they synapse with the postganglionic neurons. Most of the sympathetic ganglia lie in the paravertebral chain comprising 22 pairs situated on either side of the vertebral column. These chains are interconnected and also contain rami communicantes to the spinal nerves. The white rami carry the preganglionic axons, are myelinated, and are restricted to the aforementioned thoracolumbar outflow. The gray rami form the communication from the ganglias back to the spinal nerves and carry postganglionic fibers for distribution to the effector organs. There are also prevertebral ganglia located in the abdominal cavity but just ventral to the vertebral column (Fig. 14-2). These ganglia distribute the postganglionic axons to the visceral organs, the gastrointestinal tract, and the genitourinary tract. The celiac ganglion is innervated by T5–T12 and innervates the liver, spleen, pancreas, stomach, small bowel, proximal large bowel, and kidney. The superior mesenteric ganglion innervates the rest of the colon, whereas the inferior mesenteric ganglion is responsible for the rectum, the bladder, and the genitalia. In addition, a branch of one of the preganglionic nerves to the celiac ganglion, the greater splanchnic, innervates the adrenal medulla. The sympathetic postganglion innervation of the trunk and lower extremities is similar to that of the sensory innervation of those areas. However, there is considerable overlap, so that one sensory dermatome may receive sympathetic innervation from two to four spinal levels. The upper extremities and the head are sympathetically innervated through the three cervical ganglia (superior, middle, and inferior) and the first thoracic, which is frequently fused with the inferior cervical ganglion to form the so-called stellate ganglia. Because of these ganglionic connections, the dermatone sympathetic innervation of upper extremities is less well established. For the most part, the postganglionic fibers for the head, neck, trunk, and extremities travel with the somatic nerves.

Physiology

The effects of sympathetic nervous stimulation on the body's physiology are designed to facilitate fight or flight (Table 14-2). Ventilation is increased by both a central effect on the ventilatory centers and bronchodilation. Cardiac output is increased through increase in the contractile force of the heart as well as in the rate of contraction, and perfusion pressure for vital organs is increased by constriction of vessels to nonvital organs with little or no effect on the heart and brain. Function of both the gastrointestinal and genitourinary systems is decreased as a result of a relaxation of the smooth muscle in these organs and contraction of their sphincters. Gastrointestinal secretory activity is inhibited, and adrenal medullary output is increased. Metabolism is generally stimulated to provide more fuel for bodily function in the form of glucose and fatty acids.

TABLE 14-2 Effects of Sympathetic Nervous System Activation

	Stimulation	Inhibition
Heart	Rate, conduction, contractility	
Blood vessels	Vasoconstriction (skin, gut, liver, heart, kidney)	Vasodilation (skeletal muscle, heart, brain)
Respiration	Respiratory center	Bronchodilation
Gastrointestinal	Sphincters	Smooth muscle
Genitourinary	Sphincters	Ureteral and uterine muscle
Metabolic and endocrine	Glycogenolysis (muscle, liver) Lipolysis Gluconeogenesis Insulin release Renin release ADH release	Insulin release

Abbreviation: ADH, antidiuretic hormone or arginine vasopressin.

Other stress hormones are released. The predominant neurochemical effector for these functions is norepinephrine, which is released from the sympathetic nerve terminals. Epinephrine is the major output of the adrenal medulla and is therefore a circulating hormone rather than one that participates in end-organ sympathetic stimulation. Although attempts to categorize these effects dated from the initial observations of Dale[3] through the experiments of Cannon and Rosenbleuth,[4] the definitive classification is a result of the investigations of Ahlquist[5] and the observations of Lands et al.[6] Ahlquist[5] characterized sympathetic stimulation as being predominantly mediated through α- or β-receptor effects. Lands et al.[6] observed that β-receptor activity appeared to be divisible into at least two forms, and more recently the work of Langer[7] and others has delineated two separate α-receptor mechanisms as well. The early availability of α-receptor antagonists provided early characterization of the α-receptor. However, the β-receptor is currently better understood.[8] β-Receptor agonism appears to be primarily responsible for the effect of sympathetic nervous activation on the heart, the smooth muscle relaxation produced in the vascular and respiratory systems, the stimulation of renin secretion by the specialized cells in the kidney, and several metabolic consequences, including adipose tissue lipolysis and glycogenolysis (Table 14-3). The β_1-receptor mechanism is thought to be primarily involved in the cardiac effects[9] and release of fatty acids, whereas the β_2-receptors are primarily responsible for smooth muscle relaxation and hyperglycemia (Table 14-3). In specialized circumstances, however, β_2-receptors may also mediate cardiac activity (see below).[10] Both endogenous neurohumors, norepinephrine and epinephrine, possess α- and β-receptor agonistic activity. However,

TABLE 14-3. Adrenergic Receptor Differentiation

	Stimulation	Inhibition
Alpha		
Heart		
Blood vessels	Vasoconstriction (skin, gut, kidney, liver, heart)	
Gastrointestinal	Sphincters	
Genitourinary	Sphincters	
Metabolic and endocrine		Insulin release
Beta		
Heart	(1) Rate, conduction contractility	
Blood vessels		(2) Vasodilation (skeletal muscle, heart, brain)
Respiration	(?) Respiratory center	
Gastrointestinal		(2) Bronchodilation (2) Smooth muscle
Genitourinary		(2) Ureteral and uterine muscle
Metabolic and endocrine	(2) Glycogenolysis (muscle, liver) (1) Lipolysis (2) Gluconeogenesis (1) Insulin release (?) Renin release (?) ADH release	

Abbreviations: 1, mediated by β_1-receptors; 2, mediated by β_2-receptors; ?, controversial.

norepinephrine has minimal β_2-receptor activity, whereas epinephrine stimulates both the β_1- and β_2-receptor moieties. Thus individual tissue and organ response to sympathetic stimulation depends on (1) the receptors present, (2) the sympathetic nervous supply (i.e., how densely innervated the tissue is with terminals that contain norepinephrine), and (3) vascularity (i.e., how much epinephrine is delivered by blood vessels).

Many factors influence the density (number of) and function of the receptors. Also, the density and affinity of the receptors may vary from tissue to tissue and under different circumstances. For instance, continued β-adrenergic stimulation causes a decrease in receptor density, whereas the administration of β-receptor antagonist drugs chronically results in an increase in the number of receptors. Likewise denervation, whether chemical (6-hydroxydopamine, guanethidine) or surgical, can result in an increase in the number of receptors. The activity of the thyroid gland influences the receptor density, with hyperthyroidism increasing density and hypothyroidism decreasing density. There is some evidence that corticosteroids decrease receptor density.[9] Consequently, the reaction of the body to well-characterized sympathetic agonists may be considerably different, depending on the pathologic and environmental circumstances.[11]

β-Receptor Physiology

The membrane physiology involving β-receptor agonism is probably the best understood of any receptor mechanism. The elucidation of the role of the proteins adenylate cyclase and cyclic adenosine monophosphate (AMP) in the cellular reaction to β stimulation by Sutherland et al.[12] more than 20 years ago was the initial step in understanding this reaction. Within the past 10 years, a regulatory protein was also found in the plasma membrane, which appears to be a binding site for the guanine nucleotides (Fig. 14-4).[13,14] All three of these proteins can exist in either the inactive or active state. The initial binding of the β-agonists to the receptor converts the receptor to the active state. This allows the receptor to couple to the nucleotide regulator (N) protein. This complex then promotes the dissociation of a guanine diphosphate molecule (GDP) from its tightly bound position on the nucleotide protein. This vacated binding site now is occupied by a molecule of guanine triphosphate (GTP), which is stimulatory. The interaction of GTP with the N protein has two effects. First, it converts the receptor into its inactive state again. Second, and more importantly, it now catalyzes the inactive form of adenylate cyclase to the active form, with the resultant breakdown of adenosine triphosphate (ATP) to cyclic AMP. This leads to the stimulation of a series of protein kinases, eventually resulting in membrane phosphorylation and the final effect on the particular organ being stimulated. However, the action of a GTPase that is present on the N protein cleaves the GTP to GDP, and the N protein again assumes its inactive form. Without the GDP stimulation, the adenylate cyclase also returns to the inactive form and the receptor complex is ready for reactivation. Inasmuch as this receptor complex can exist in two forms, the inactivated free form and the activated coupled form, an equilibrium between them normally exists. A current concept of agonist and antagonist activity is that agonists possess a higher affinity for the coupled activator form of the receptor than for the inactive free form. Consequently, the presence of an agonist produces a predominance of the coupled activated complex and produces the cellular cascade resulting in organ function. On the other hand, the antagonists have affinity for both the inactive uncoupled and the active coupled form and hence stabilize this relationship so that there is no cellular activity in addition to maintaining the receptor in a relatively inactive state so that considerably more agonist is required to unbalance the equilibrium.

Thus the state of the complexes may be changed by various environmental and pathophysiologic situations. This is certainly a logical explanation for the desensitization process, which has been referred to as *tolerance* or *tachyphylaxis*. The terms used by the pharmacodynamicists to refer to these processes are *upregulation* (increased density and responsiveness) and *downregulation* (decreased density and responsiveness).

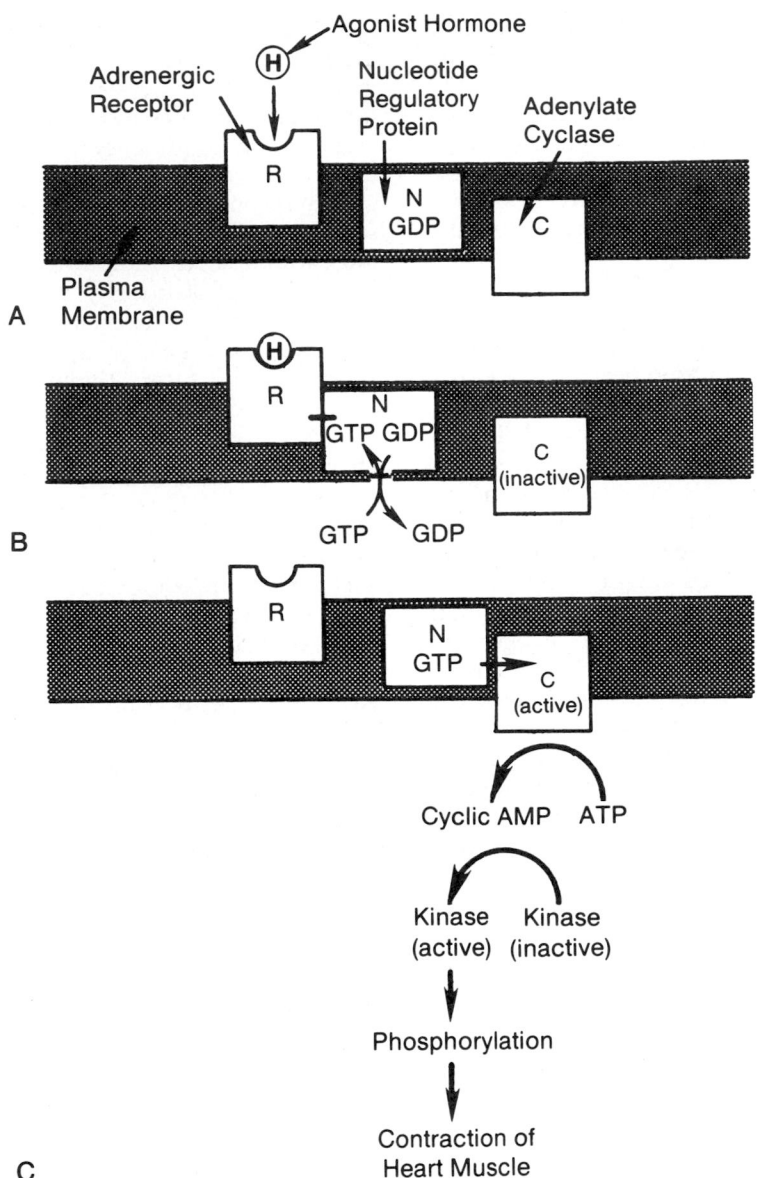

Fig. 14-4. A postulated β-receptor mechanism. **(A)** Binding of β agonist to receptor-inducing hormone (H), receptor (R), and nucleotide regulatory protein (N) complex. **(B)** Guanosine disphosphate (GDP) changed to stimulatory guanosine triphosphate (GTP). **(C)** N-GTP activates catalytic unit (C) of adenylate cyclase, leading to cyclic AMP-protein kinase-phosphorylation cascade. (Redrawn from Heinsimer and Lefkowitz,[128] with permission.)

One of the most important and best studied pathophysiologic situations where tolerance or downregulation occurs is chronic congestive heart failure. Initially, it was noted that the density of cardiac β-receptors was markedly decreased in patients with terminal heart failure.[15] Subsequently, with the demonstration that $β_1$- and $β_2$-receptors coexisted in human ventricles,[10] Bristow and coworkers using radioligand techniques documented that $β_1$-receptor density was decreased without change in the density of $β_2$-receptors in human ven-

tricles affected by congestive heart failure. Consequently, $β_2$-agonism accounted for 60 percent of the total inotropic response stimulated by isoproterenol in the failing heart, as contrasted with 40 percent in the nonfailing heart.[16]

α-Receptor Physiology

α-Receptor-mediated activity is responsible for most of the sympathetically induced smooth muscle contraction throughout the body, including the ciliary muscle of the eye, vascular smooth muscle, bronchial smooth muscle, and ureteral smooth muscle (Table 14-3).[2] In addition, the gastrointestinal (GI) and genitourinary (GU) sphincter mechanisms are also stimulated by α-adrenergic receptor function. α-Receptor agonism also controls one aspect of the metabolic control activity of the sympathetic nervous system, decreased pancreatic insulin secretion.

The need to differentiate the α-receptor into α_1 and α_2 initially revolved around a negative feedback mechanism in the sympathetic nervous system. It had been observed that the secretion of norepinephrine from the sympathetic nerve terminal was accompanied by a feedback inhibition of subsequent norepinephrine secretion (Fig. 14-5).[7] As more specific α_1-receptor antagonists were developed, these drugs were found not to block the effect of norepinephrine on the presynaptic nerve terminal. Hence, the α_2-receptor appeared to be predominantly presynaptic, mediating the decrease of norepinephrine release from the nerve terminal, whereas the major effects of α-adrenergic agonism were postsynaptic and α_1. More recently other functions for the α_2-receptors have been found. In contrast to the β-receptor whose CNS distribution and importance is still not understood, the α_2-receptor appears to be important in central nervous sympathetic mediation.[17] Specifically, α_2 agonism reduces sympathetic outflow from the central nervous system and hence acts as a sympathetic inhibitor, whereas α_2-antagonist drugs tend to have the opposite effects, that is, they tend to stimulate the CNS sympathetic nervous outflow.[18] Fur-

thermore, it is now fairly well substantiated that there are postsynaptic α_2-receptors in the periphery.[19,20] One generalization (which is still speculative) is that vascular tissue innervated by the sympathetic nervous system responds predominantly to α_1-agonists, whereas vascular tissue not innervated by the sympathetic nervous system responds primarily to α_2-agonists (which necessarily are blood-borne).[21,22] However, inasmuch as the most widely used synthetic α_1-agonist is phenylephrine (see below), obviously, this generalization breaks down. In addition, there are other studies showing that alpha$_1$ agonism can definitely be produced by blood-borne drugs.[23] Interestingly, norepinephrine appears to be a selective β_1- and α_1-agonist, whereas epinephrine appears to have both α_1- and α_2-agonist activity. These effects, however, may be dose-related, in that high doses of α-agonists primarily stimulate α_1-receptors, whereas low doses tend to stimulate α_2-receptors.[24]

The membrane biochemistry of the α-receptor has been reasonably well established, although there are still areas of controversy. It would appear that there are at least two subclasses of α_1-receptors termed α_{1a} and α_{1b}.[23] As with β-receptor activation (Fig. 14-4), a guanine nucleotide (G) protein appears to be central (Fig. 14-6). Coupling of the α_1-agonist to the α_{1a} membrane receptor triggers opening of the dihydroperidine-sensitive calcium channel and influx of extracellular calcium to raise intracellular concentration. The α_2-receptor also appears to function in this fashion. On the other hand, the α_{1b}-receptor acting also through the G protein activates phospholipase C in the inner cell

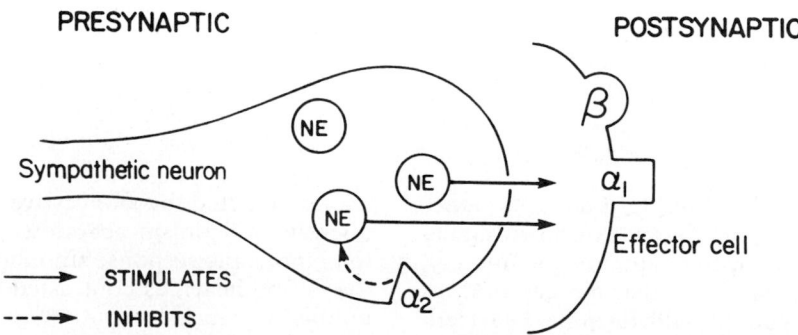

Fig. 14-5. Schematic of sympathetic end-organ synapse showing presynaptic and postsynaptic receptors. Norepinephrine (NE) stimulation of postsynaptic receptors produce classic β and α_1 effects. Stimulation of the α_2-presynaptic receptor inhibits further release of NE. (Modified Ram and Kaplan,[129] with permission.)

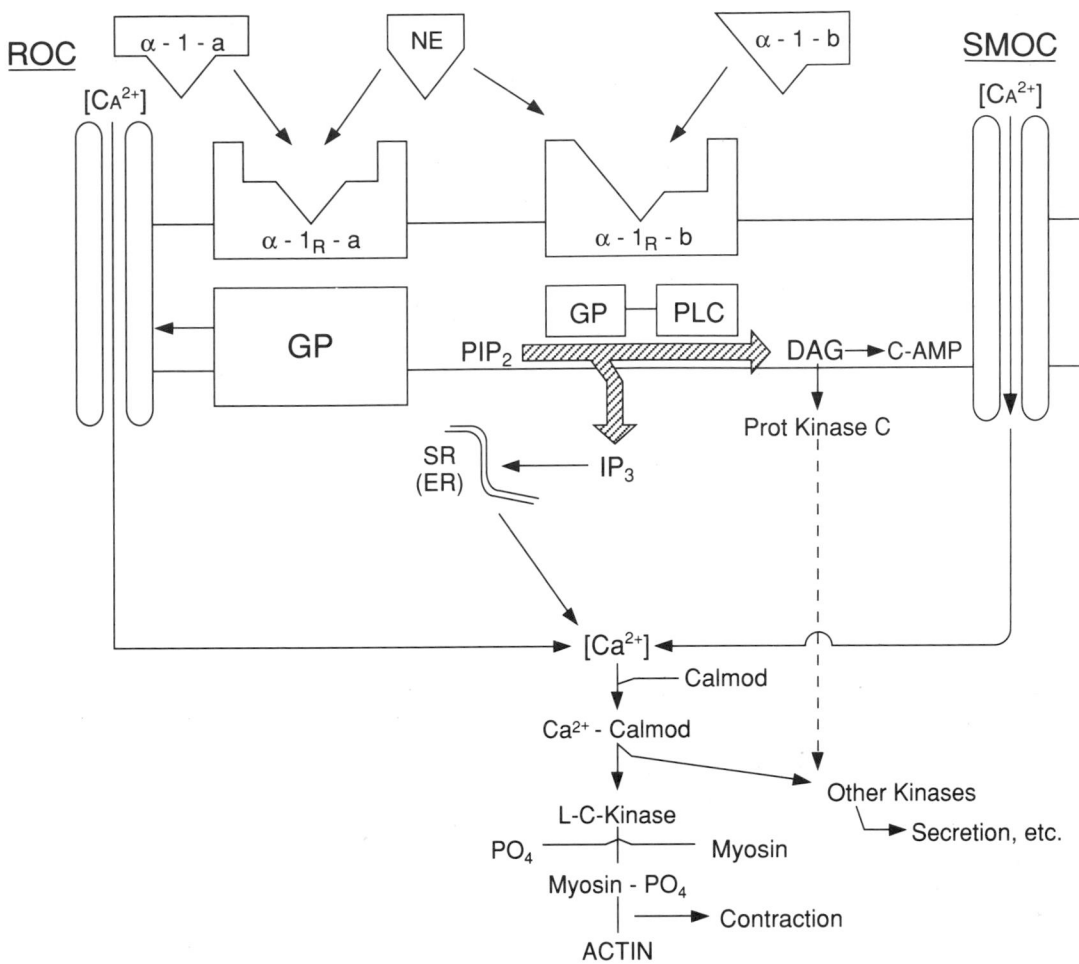

Fig. 14-6. Postulated α-receptor membrane biochemistry. Two types of α-receptors are postulated (α_{1a} and α_{1b}). The α-receptor, when stimulated by an agonist, interacts with a G protein (GP) to facilitate the opening of the receptor-operated calcium channel (ROC) and increase intracellular calcium ion concentration (Ca^{++}). The b-receptor initiates a more complicated mechanism. Receptor occupancy stimulates phospholipase C (PLC) through interaction with another GP to catalyze the breakdown of phosphoinosotol 3,4 biphosphate (PIP_2) to inositol 1,4,5 triphosphate (IP_3) and diacyl glycerol (DAG). IP_3 then stimulates release of Ca^{++} from the sarcoplasmic reticulum (SR) (or the endoplasmic reticulum [ER] in nonmuscle cells). DAG, perhaps through cyclic AMP (cAMP), facilitates opening of a second messenger operated calcium channel (SMOC) and hence also increases intracellular Ca^{++}. Norepinephrine (NE) possesses both α_{1a}- and α_{1b}-agonistic properties and can interact with both receptor mechanisms. The increased intracellular Ca^{++} then interacts with the intracellular protein calmodulin (Calmod) to activate a light-chain kinase (L-C kinase) in smooth muscle cells (or other kinases in nonmuscle cells). L-C kinase then phosphorylates myosin, allowing cross-bridge formation with actin and smooth muscle contraction. DAG also activates membrane-bound protein kinase C (Prot kinase C) to initiate a cascade of kinase activations that also may be responsible for intracellular function.

membrane, which then increases hydrolysis of the diphosphate form of phosphoinosotol (PIP_2) to the triphosphate (Ins) (1,4,5) P_3 and diacyglycerol. These two compounds then mobilize intracellular calcium stores from the sarcoplasmic reticulum and probably the subsarcolemma, resulting in a marked increase in intracellular calcium ion concentration. In addition, increasing levels of both cyclic AMP and cyclic GMP and possibly other second messengers have also been documented, also increasing calcium influx, perhaps through other calcium channels. The calcium ions bind to calmodulin. This calcium-sensitive intracellular protein then activates a myosin light chain kinase that phosphorylates the myosin light chain and facilitates the interaction between actin and myosin, resulting in the contraction of the smooth muscle. In other cells, calmodulin stimulates other kinases, resulting in effector activity (Fig. 14-6).

Dopamine Receptors

Even the mysterious (physiologically, at least) dopamine receptor has now been subdivided. Dopamine-1 (DA-1) receptors are predominantly involved in peripheral vasodilation, especially of the renal and splanchnic vessels. In addition, there is recent evidence to suggest that dopamine receptors also can inhibit sodium reabsorption, resulting in diuresis, and stimulate renin release from the kidney.[25,26] Dopamine-2 receptors (DA-2) mediate the long-recognized central neurotransmitter effects of dopamine[27] and also inhibit central sympathetic outflow and peripheral norepinephrine release at the sympathetic nerve terminal. However, there is still no agreement as to the physiologic importance of the peripheral DA-1 receptors.[28]

Synthesis and Disposition of Norepinephrine

The synthesis of the sympathetic neural transmitter norepinephrine occurs predominantly at the sympathetic nerve terminal itself (Fig. 14-7).[2,29] The essential amino acid phenylalanine is hydroxylated to tyrosine. Tyrosine is carried into the presynaptic nerve terminal cell, where it is also hydroxylated by a ubiquitous enzyme, tyrosine hydroxylase, to L-dihydroxyphenylolanine (DOPA). This is the rate-limiting step in the synthesis of norepinephrine and hence the logical locus for interference in the synthesis if such is desired. DOPA is decarboxylated by another enzyme to dopamine, which is then transported into a storage vessel where it is converted to norepinephrine by the action of still another enzyme, dopamine-β-hydroxylase. Although there are a few peripheral and central nervous system sites at which norepinephrine can then be converted to epi-

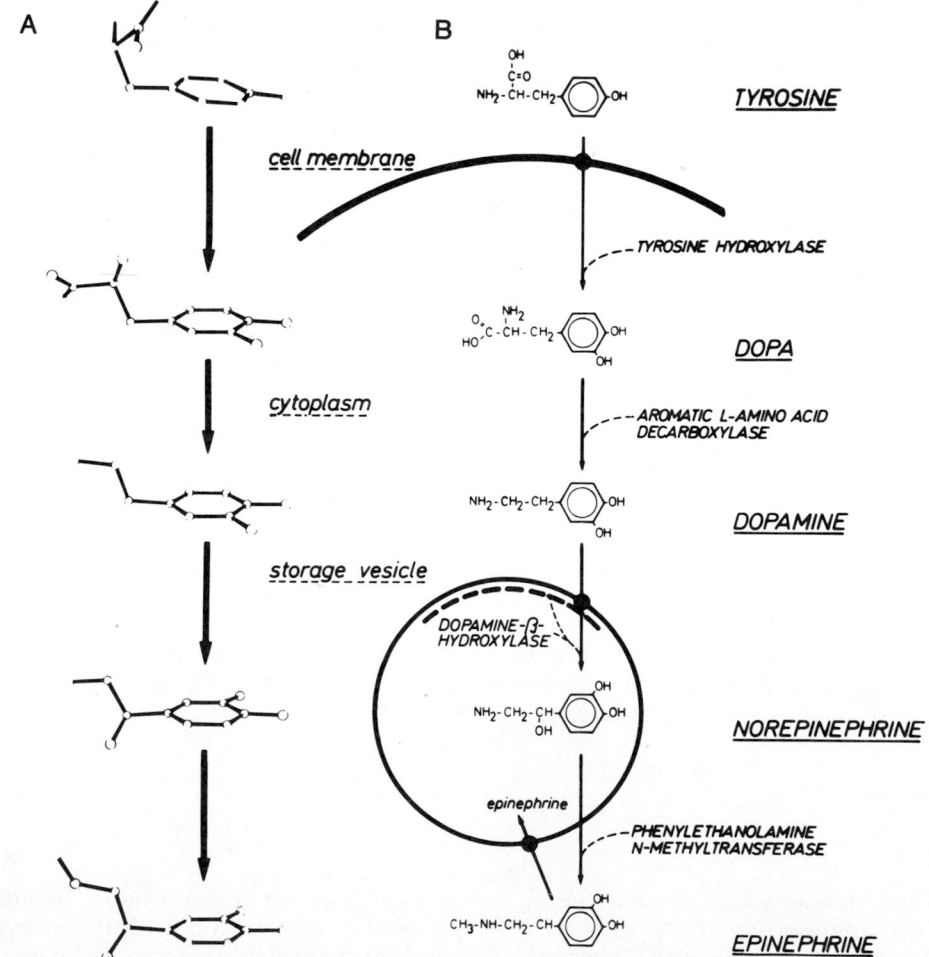

Fig. 14-7. Biosynthesis of norepinephrine and epinephrine in sympathetic nerve terminal (and adrenal medulla). **(A)** Perspective view of molecules. **(B)** Enzymatic processes. (From Shepherd and Vanhoutte,[29] with permission.)

nephrine by the action of phenylethanolamine *n*-methyltransferase (PNMT), most of the PNMT in the body is confined to the adrenal medulla, so that epinephrine is not formed in any great amount in peripheral nerve terminals.

Another interesting aspect of the synthesis of epinephrine is that the formation of PNMT is dependent on an abundant supply of glucocorticoids from the adrenal cortex.[2] The long-recognized association between adrenocortical hypofunction and sympathetic nervous function appears to be predominantly related to the role of glucocorticoids in epinephrine synthesis. The conversion of tyrosine to DOPA is the rate-limiting step in this synthetic pathway. The most important controller of tyrosine hydroxylase is the level of norepinephrine in the cells. High levels of norepinephrine inhibit tyrosine, and low levels stimulate the enzyme. Recent evidence indicates that during sympathetic nervous system stimulation, increased supply of tyrosine will also increase synthesis of norepinephrine.[30]

Once norepinephrine is synthesized and stored in the vesicles, its release is mediated through electrical depolarization of the prejunctional membrane, resulting in an influx of both sodium and calcium ions. Thus, the vesicles are stimulated to migrate to the surface and, through a process of exocytosis, release the norepinephrine into the synaptic cleft (Fig. 14-8). Not only does intracellular norepinephrine effect the synthesis of norepinephrine, but the norepinephrine in the junctional cleft also modulates subsequent release of norepinephrine by a receptor mechanism. In addition, there are other modulators of norepinephrine release at the nerve terminal (Fig. 14-9). Angiotensin II and prostacyclin are facilitators of norepinephrine release, whereas acetylcholine, histamine, and other prostaglandins are probably inhibitors of release.[29] Once released, the norepinephrine can traverse a variety of pathways (Fig. 14-10). Much of it is taken back up into the nerve terminal for recycling. Some of the norepinephrine is o-methylated by the enzyme, catechol-o-methyltransferase (COMT), or is oxidized intracellularly by another enzyme, monoamine oxidase (MAO); the resultant metabolites are eventually excreted.

PARASYMPATHETIC NERVOUS SYSTEM

Anatomy

As indicated in the Introduction, the preganglionic neurons of the parasympathetic nervous system arise from four cranial nerves and from sacral nerves S2, S3, and S4. The parasympathetic preganglionic fibers to the eye originate in the midbrain Edinger-Westphal nucleus of the third cranial nerve and synapse in the ciliary ganglion in the orbit. The nucleus of the facial nerve (cranial nerve VII) gives rise to the preganglionic fibers that form the chordae tympani, which supplies the ganglia for the sublacrimal and submandibular salivary glands, as well as the sphenopalatine ganglion, which innervates the lacrimal gland. The glossopharyngeal nucleus (cranial nerve IX) supplies the otic ganglion, which innervates the parotid gland, and finally, the most important parasympathetic nucleus is that of the vagus (cranial nerve X), which supplies the heart, tra-

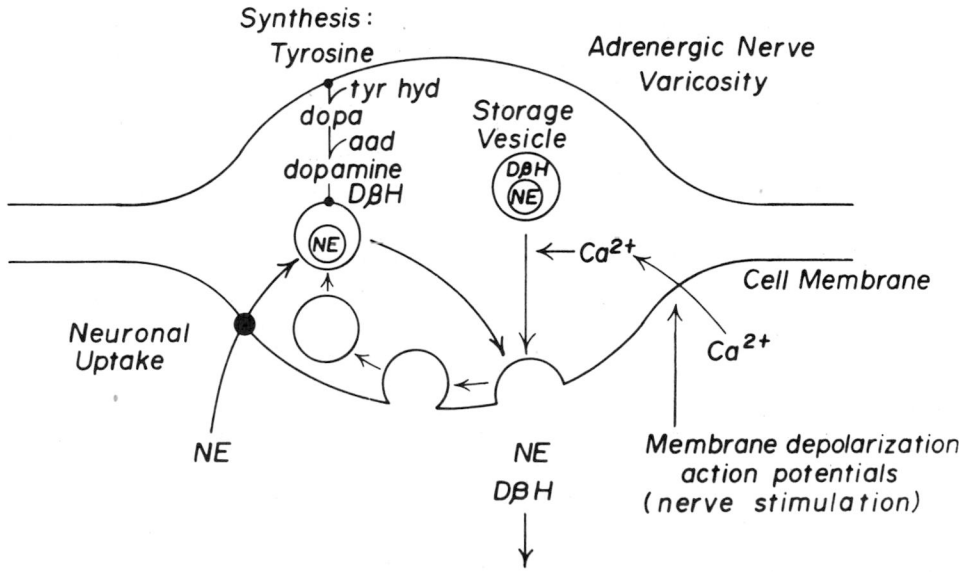

Fig. 14-8. Release and reuptake of norepinephrine at sympathetic nerve terminals. NE, norepinephrine; try hyd, tyrosine hydroxylase, aad, aromatic 1-amino decarboxylase; DβH, dopamine β-hydroxylase; ●, active carrier. (From Shepherd and Vanhoutte,[29] with permission.)

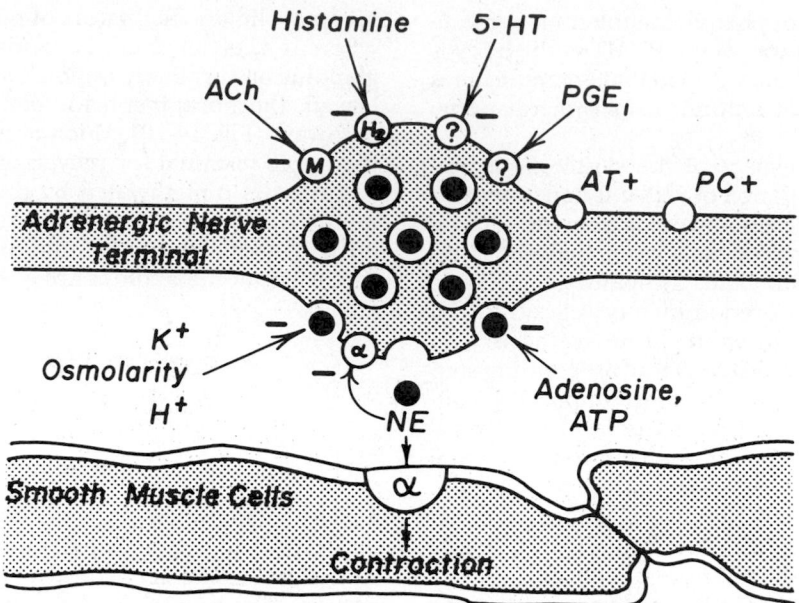

Fig. 14-9. Excitatory (+) and inhibitory (−) influences on adrenergic neurotransmission. NE, norepinephrine; M, muscarinic; ACh, acetycholine; AT, angiotensin II; PC, prostacyclin; PGE_1, prostaglandin E_1; 5-HT, 5-hydroxytyptamine; H_2, histamine receptor; α, α-adrenergic receptor; ?, unknown mechanism. (From Shephard and Vanhoutte,[29] with permission.)

cheobronchial tree, liver, spleen, kidney, and all the gastrointestinal tract except the distal colon. The sacral preganglionic outflow supplies the distal colon, urinary bladder, and genitalia.

Physiology

Acetylcholine is synthesized in the cholinergic nerve endings through the activity of an enzyme present in their mitochondria (choline acetylase). This enzyme catalyzes acetylation of choline with acetyl coenzyme A (CoA) to produce acetylcholine.[31] The release of acetylcholine at both ganglionic synapses and the parasympathetic neuroeffectors is remarkably similar to the release of norepinephrine. The release is stimulated by an action potential that results in influx of sodium and calcium into the cell. Both are necessary for the massive release of acetylcholine through a similar exocytotic process. Unlike the adrenergic nerve ending, continuous small amounts of acetylcholine are released from the cholinergic nerve ending even without nerve stimulation, resulting in random small spontaneous depolarization of the postganglionic membrane, known as miniature endplate potentials (MEPPs).[2] In contrast to norepinephrine, the released acetylcholine is rapidly hydrolyzed by an acetylcholinesterase that is present in high concentrations at all cholinergic junctions. Acetylcholine is not taken up by the prejunctional nerve terminal, so that all the released acetylcholine must be synthesized de novo, but often from intermediate precursors taken up after metabolism.

The actions of acetylcholine are almost diametrically opposed to those of norepinephrine and epinephrine (Table 14-1). The rate of cardiac contraction is markedly decreased, as is the velocity of conduction in the cardiac conduction system. There is definitely a decrease in contractility, although not as marked as the increase produced by sympathetic stimulation.[32] A number of smooth muscles are constricted, including the bronchial muscles. The effect on the gastrointestinal and genitourinary tracts is the opposite, that is, constriction of the smooth muscle in the walls and relaxation of the sphincters. Glandular secretion is generally increased by cholinergic stimulation.

The anatomic and ionic permeability characteristics of the acetylcholine receptor have been intensively investigated in skeletal muscle (also see Ch. 20). These characteristics are presumed to pertain to other cholinergic receptors. Yet, the differentiation of the receptors seen for the adrenergic receptor is not as easy to classify. The old classification suggested by Dale[33] at the turn of the century was prompted by the observation of the effects of two alkaloids, muscarine and nicotine, and the cholinergic receptors are still referred to as muscarinic and nicotinic. The nicotinic receptor is predominantly at the skeletal muscle endplate, but also occurs in autonomic ganglia. The two receptors probably are not identical, but are similar enough to be classified together. All the cholinergic neuroeffector cell receptors except skeletal muscle are known as the muscarinic receptors. The endogenous cholinergic neurotransmitter, acetylcholine, apparently has no specificity. Only through the use of specific antagonists

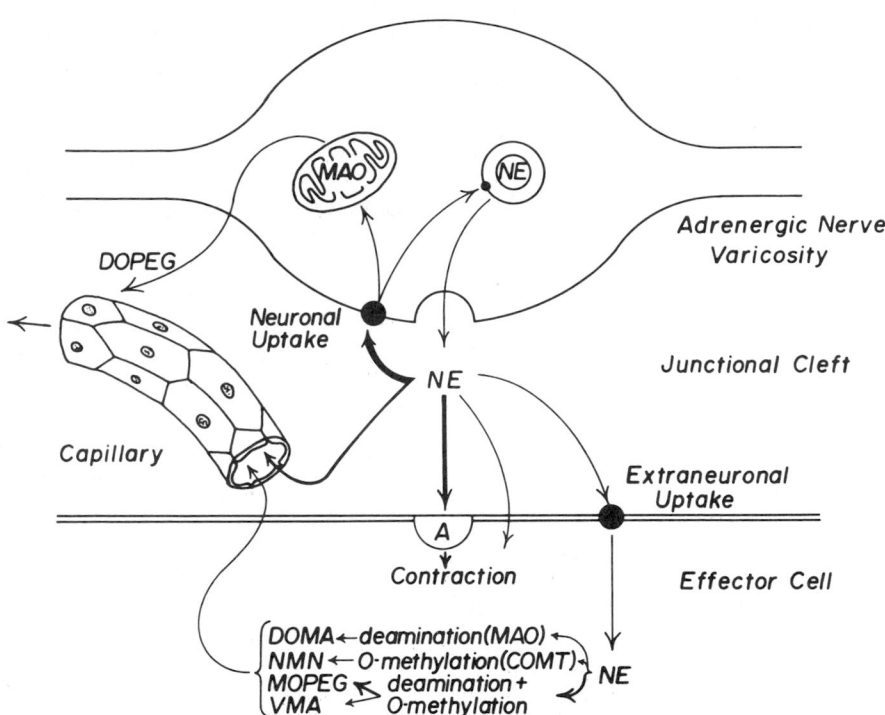

Fig. 14-10. Norepinephrine (NE) released from the adrenergic nerve varicosity enters the junctional cleft and activates the adrenergic receptors (A) on the effector cells. It is removed by (1) uptake in the nerve endings, where part of it is enzymatically degraded by the intraneuronal monoamine oxidase (MAO) to 3,4-dihydroxyphenylglycol (DOPEG), but most is recycled to the storage vesicles; (2) diffusion to the capillaries; and (3) uptake by the effector cells and enzymatic degradation by the enzymes monoamine oxidase and catechol-O-methyltransferase (COMT) to 3,4-dihydroxymandelic acid (DOMA), normetanephrine (NMN), 3-methoxy-4-dihydroxyphenylglycol (MOPEG), and 3-methoxy, 4-hydroxymandelic acid (VMA). The metabolites of norepinephrine are inactive and diffuse to the extracellular fluid and the capillaries. ●, active carrier. (From Shepherd and Vanhoutte,[29] with permission.)

can the difference between the muscarinic and nicotinic receptors be determined. As a result, structure–activity relationships have emerged. All cholinergic agonists appear to need a quaternary ammonium group as well as an atom capable of forming a hydrogen bond through an unshared pair of electrons. The distance between the two may determine whether the agonism is nicotinic or muscarinic. With muscarinic agonists, the distance appears to be about 4.4 Å, whereas for nicotinic agonists the distance is 5.9 Å. In contrast to the many drugs synthesized as adrenergic agonists, very few drugs are used as cholinergic agonists. This is because most of the cholinergic effects are not particularly desirable. The major exception to this is for pathophysiologic immobility of bowel and genitourinary tract smooth muscle.

The Autonomic Ganglia

Although the ganglia of the parasympathetic and sympathetic nervous system are anatomically distinct, physiologically they are for all intensive purposes iden-

tical.[1,2] The synapses are primarily cholinergic in nature, behaving exactly as the cholinergic synapses described in the previous section. In contrast to other cholinergic receptors, however, ganglionic transmission is probably a function of both nicotinic and muscarinic receptor activity, although the former predominates.[31] Stimulation of nicotinic receptors results in an early excitatory postsynaptic potential (EPSP).[34] There is also a late EPSP, which appears to be mediated by the muscarinic receptors and facilitates the early nicotinic EPSP. Finally, there is also a inhibitory postsynaptic potential (IPSP). As is the case with the adrenergic nerve terminal, there are also modulating effects on the ganglion nerve terminal by various endogenous substances. β-Adrenergic stimulation appears to facilitate both nicotinic and muscarinic transmission, whereas α-adrenergic stimulation inhibits this transmission. 5-hydroxytryptamine (5-HT) is mostly facilitatory but also can be inhibitory in certain areas. Dopamine may also be inhibitory through stimulation of the IPSP. It should be remembered that the adrenal medulla is a specialized ganglionic synapse and is therefore under similar influences to the autonomic ganglia.

Parasympathetic–Sympathetic Interaction

Aside from the obvious antagonistic effects of sympathetic and parasympathetic nervous stimulation on a variety of organ systems as indicated in the anatomic distribution (Fig.14-1) and general physiologic effects (Table 14-1), interaction also occurs at the cellular level. For instance, cholinergic stimulation of the heart is greatly enhanced by a high sympathetic tone. Aside from the directly opposing electrophysiologic effects, the ability of cholinergic stimulation on the adrenergic nerve terminal to decrease release of norepinephrine may be involved. However, there are also direct cellular interactions (Fig. 14-11).[35] Muscarinic cholinergic agonism inhibits adenylate cyclase activity in the heart. This may be the mechanism for the attenuation of the β-adrenergic agonist increases in intracellular cyclic AMP levels produced by muscarinic cholinergic agonism. Also, the increase in intracellular cyclic guanosine monophosphate (GMP) levels from muscarinic cholinergic receptor interaction may have a direct effect on cardiac membrane activity antagonizing the sympathetic effect. These effects on the cyclic nucleotides may also relate to receptor affinity and density mechanisms. Furthermore, cholinergic stimulation may affect the protein kinase cascade, which is ultimately responsible for end-organ adrenergic changes (Fig. 14-4). The effect of cholinergic stimulation on atrial rhythm is well documented.[32] However, cholinergic receptors in the ventricular myocardium may be important as well. For instance, a protective effect of vagal stimulation on ventricular fibrillation thresholds has been found either during sympathetic hyperactivity or in ischemia.[35] An intact parasympathetic nervous system may be protective against digitalis-induced arrhythmias. The main point of all this information is that parasympathetic–sympathetic interaction may be not only on the basis of well-known effects of the two autonomic nervous system components on the effector organ through their receptor mechanisms, but also by modification of each other's receptor-mediated effects.

AUTONOMIC PHARMACOLOGY

Ganglionic Stimulants

The prototypical ganglionic stimulant is the alkaloid nicotine. However, because this drug produces so

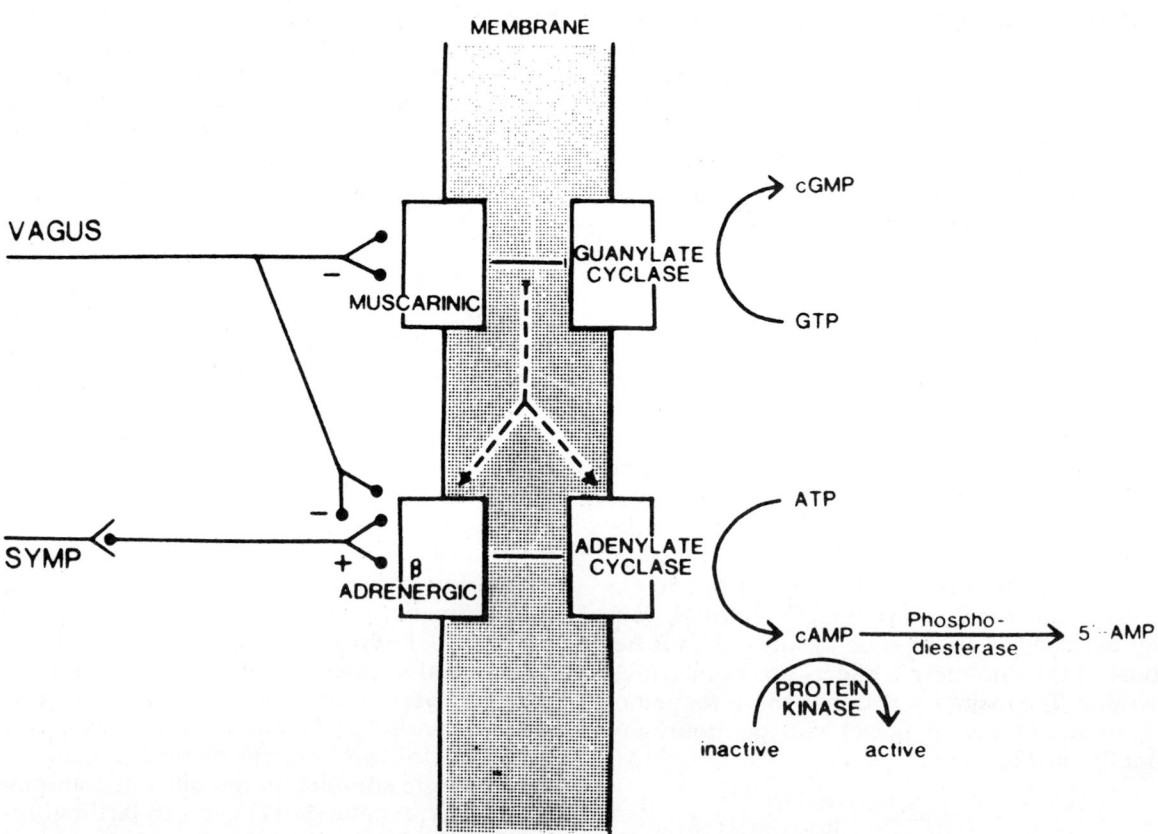

Fig. 14-11. Schematic diagram depicting possible sites of interaction between the sympathetic (SYMP) and parasympathetic (VAGUS) nervous system. Extracellular space to the left and intracellular space to the right. cGMP, cyclic guanosine monophosphate; GTP, guanosine triphosphate; cAMP, cyclic adenosine monophosphate; ATP, adenosine triphosphate. (From Reardon and Bailey,[35] with permission.)

many other adverse effects, it has been useful only as a pharmacologic tool. In addition, nicotine secondarily produces ganglionic blockade in doses similar to those that initially produce stimulation. Even when more specific ganglion stimulants such as tetramethylammonium (TMA) or dimethylphenylpiperazinium (DMPP) are used, the fact that the resulting effects are a combination of sympathetic and parasympathetic stimulation has resulted in essentially no clinical usefulness for this class of drugs.[34]

Ganglion-blocking Drugs

Before the discovery of more specific adrenergic blocking and antihypertensive drugs, the ganglion blockers were widely used as antihypertensive drugs, both chronically and acutely.[34] Unfortunately, the combined parasympathetic and sympathetic effects of ganglion blockade led to unpredictable and untoward side effects (Table 14-4). Consequently, the reasonably well-defined and investigated ganglion-blocking drugs have largely disappeared from therapeutic use. Practically the only modern use of these drugs is to induce hypotension acutely, either to treat hypertensive crisis or to intentionally induce hypotension (also see Ch. 43). The only drug still available in the United States for this purpose is trimethaphan camsylate (Arfonad), which has side effects that have markedly decreased its use. The hypotensive effect of trimethaphan is due to ganglion blockade, direct vasodilating properties, and histamine release. The last-named is more prominent in animals than in humans but still does occur. In addition, the drug is notorious for inducing tachyphylaxis (or perhaps refractoriness). In other words, the longer trimethaphan is used, the higher the dose required to produce hypotension. One of the major advantages of the drug is its short duration of action, which may be a result of hydrolysis by plasma (pseudo-) cholinesterase. The unpredictability of the systemic effects (Table 14-4) have markedly decreased the use of this drug.

PARASYMPATHETIC DRUGS

Agonists

Inasmuch as the major effect of parasympathetic stimulation is detrimental to the body during stressful situations, there has been a limited therapeutic use for these drugs. The nicotinic effects have been discussed in the previous section on the autonomic ganglia and are extensively discussed in Chapter 12. The only cholinergic agonists used clinically have been muscarinic agonists, mostly derivatives of acetylcholine (Table 14-5). The common property of the three most well-studied choline esters (methylcholine, bethanechol, and carbachol) is a marked decrease in susceptibility to hydrolysis by cholinesterase.[36] This property permits the systemic use of these drugs inasmuch as the tissue and plasma cholinesterase do not destroy them before a useful period of drug action. Both methylcholine and bethanechol are primarily muscarinic agonists, with minimal nicotinic effect, whereas carbachol has both nicotinic and muscarinic effects. None of these compounds is widely used clinically, and carbachol is limited in use for topical installation in the eye. The combination of ganglionic block and muscarinic effects results in a rapid pupillary constriction, hence the use of the drug for the treatment of glaucoma. Bethanechol (Urecholine) is the only systemically available choline ester and has been used as a stimulant for gastrointestinal and genitourinary smooth muscle. Nevertheless, its efficacy has not been impressive, and its use is generally as a last resort. Another natural alkaloid, pilocarpine, was a mainstay for the medical treatment of glaucoma until the discovery of more modern drugs. However, it may still be used topically in the eye.

If sustained systemic cholinergic agonism is neces-

TABLE 14-5 Muscarinic Actions of Acetylcholine

Heart	
Rate	——
Contractility	—
Conduction	——
Smooth muscle	
Vascular	—
Bronchial	++
Gastrointestinal motility	++
Sphincter	——
Biliary	++
Iris	++
Genitourinary motility	++
Sphincter	——
Glands	
Respiratory	+++
Sweat	++
Salivary	++
Gastrointestinal	++

Symbols: ++, marked stimulation; −, slight inhibition; ——, moderate inhibition; ———, marked inhibition.

TABLE 14-4. Effects of Ganglion Blockade

	Sympathetic Nervous System	Parasympathetic Nervous System
Cardiovascular	Vasodilation ↓ Venous return (hypotension) ↓ Cardiac output	Tachycardia
Gastrointestinal		Ileus ↓ Secretions
Genitourinary		Urinary retention
Respiratory	↓ Compliance	↓ Secretions
Eye		Mydriasis Cycloplegia
Skin	↑ Blood flow ↓ Sweating	

Symbols: ↓, decrease; ↑, increase.

sary, the most efficacious type of drugs used are the anticholinesterase drugs. These drugs are used for antagonism of nondepolarizing neuromuscular blocking drugs and the treatment of myasthenia gravis (also see Ch. 12). Although the toxicity of the organophosphate insecticides is primarily related to their anticholinesterase activity, the mechanism of this effect is different from the clinically used anticholinesterase drugs. The organophosphates produce an irreversible enzyme inhibition and have CNS effects as well.[31] Consequently, treatment of organophosphate insecticide poisoning relies on chemical compounds capable of displacing the insecticides from the enzyme and therefore of reactivating the cholinesterase activity. The most well documented of these chemicals is pradiloxime (2-PAM). An irreversible organophosphate anticholinesterase that is used clinically is echothiophate iodide, which is available as topical drops for the treatment of glaucoma. Its major advantage over other topical agents is its prolonged duration of action. Inasmuch as this chemical also inactivates plasma cholinesterase, documentation of its use in patients preoperatively is important in order to avoid prolonged action of succinylcholine (also see Ch. 12).

Antagonists

Parasympathetic (cholinergic) antagonists obviously may be primarily nicotinic or muscarinic. The nicotinic blocking drugs have been discussed in the section on autonomic ganglion drugs and in the chapters on neuromuscular blocking drugs (also see Chs. 12 and 20) and hence are not discussed further here. The cholinergic antagonists were formerly drugs of great importance in clinical medicine,[37] especially for anesthesiologists. These drugs were a mainstay in the therapy of peptic ulcer disease and various forms of "spastic bowel syndrome." They were the major ingredient in over-the-counter medications for upper respiratory illness and even for bronchial asthma. With the availability of the specific H_2 blocking drug cimetidine for peptic ulcer disease and of other antihistamines for relief of the hypersecretion seen in upper respiratory infections, these uses have markedly decreased. The topical antimuscarinic drug ipratroprium bromide has recently been released for use by aerosol in the United States. It has proved useful for certain cases of bronchial asthma, and some clinicians advocate intravenous antimuscarinic drugs as an adjuvant for treating resistant bronchospasm.[37] The drugs are still used topically for pupillary dilation in ophthalmologic practice and occasionally in the cardiac patient in whom acute bradyarrhythmias may be life-threatening. Before the introduction of the halogenated inhaled anesthetics, the use of a muscarinic anticholinergic drug in anesthetic premedication was considered mandatory to decrease secretions and prevent harmful vagal reflexes.[31] Except perhaps in children, routine use of these drugs

for premedication has decreased markedly (also see Chs. 26 and 59).

The original belladona alkaloids, atropine and scopolamine, both had notable CNS effects. Classically, atropine was considered to be stimulatory, producing excitement and delirium, whereas scopolamine was considered to be mostly sedative.[37] The combination of opiate receptor agonists, particularly morphine, and scopolamine is still widely used by cardiac anesthetists in order to sedate a patient without producing appreciable cardiorespiratory depression. The CNS effects of atropine have become apparent in recent years subsequent to relatively large doses (1 to 2 mg) given to counteract the muscarinic effect of the anticholinesterase drugs used for reversal of neuromuscular blockade reversal (also see Ch. 12). Most commonly, sedative effects were observed postoperatively, particularly in elderly patients. The most common use of atropine in clinical medicine today is probably for the aforementioned antimuscarinic effect produced by the anticholinesterases used for antagonism of neuromuscular blockade. In order to avoid the CNS effects, one of the synthetic antimuscarinic drugs, glycopyrrolate (Robinul), has gained popularity (see Table 14-6).[38,39] In contrast to atropine, this drug does not cross the blood–brain barrier. In addition, glycopyrrolate has a longer duration of action than does atropine.

In small doses, atropine produces bradycardia, which was thought to be a central effect. However, the time course as well as the fact that it occurred in vagotomized animals cast doubt on this mechanism.[31] Atropine also causes block of the inhibition of norepinephrine release produced by cholinergic effects on the adrenergic nerve terminal. Hence, this facilitation of ongoing sympathetic stimulation may enhance the effects on the sympathetic nervous system.

Atropine and scopolamine toxicity has been treated for decades by the use of the naturally occurring alkaloid physostigmine, which is an anticholinesterase that penetrates the blood–brain barrier.[37,40] Consequently, the use of this drug to treat the postoperative CNS effects of intravenous atropine has been quite successful. Also, physostigmine may reverse the CNS effects of a variety of chemical compounds, including several with known anticholinergic activity such as the tricyclic antidepressants, several major tranquilizers, and antihistamine drugs.[41] However, there is some suggestion that physostigmine may antagonize the sedative effects of the benzodiazepines as well (see also Ch. 9).[42] However, the availability of the specific benzodiazepine antago-

TABLE 14-6. Muscaranic Anticholinergic Drugs

	Duration (IV)	CNS	Gastric	Secretions
Atropine	15–30 min	++	++	++
Glycopyrrolate	2–4 h	0	+++	+++

Symbols: ++, moderate stimulation; +++, marked stimulation; 0, no effect.

nist, flumazenil, will undoubtedly supplant physostigmine for this use.[43] Although acetylcholine is undoubtedly involved in central neurotransmission, the precise role remains undetermined, as indicated by the diverse and unexplained effects of this CNS-active anticholinesterase.

SYMPATHETIC DRUGS

THE CATECHOLAMINES

The sympathetic neurotransmitter norepinephrine, the adrenal medullary vasoactive secretory product epinephrine, and dopamine are catecholamines. The nomenclature refers to the 3, 4-hydroxyl substitution on the benzene ring combined with the ethanolamine side chain (Fig. 14-12). Of the currently used sympathetic agonists, isoproterenol and dobutamine are also catecholamines. Thus most of the potent adrenergic agonist drugs are catecholamines, for the 3, 4-OH substitution on the benzene ring confers both α and β potency. The remainder of the sympathomimetic amines are non-catechol-phenylethanolamines. Substitution on the amine portion of the side chain produces increasing β-receptor activity. Less substitution favors α agonism. The two-carbon ethanolamine chain is optimal for general sympathomimetic potency. The catecholamines are metabolized by COMT; the phenylethanolamines, which have an unsubstituted α-carbon (Fig. 14-12), are metabolized by monoamine oxidase. Consequently, the noncatecholamines, which have a substituted α-carbon, tend to have a long duration of action in that they

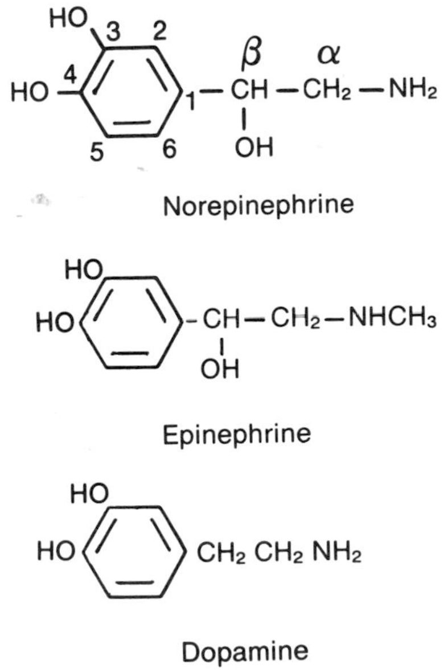

Fig. 14-12. Structure–activity relationship for endogenous catecholamines.

cannot be metabolized by either COMT or MAO.[44] Most of the potent direct-acting sympathomimetic amines have a hydroxyl group on the β-carbon, which confers asymmetry to the molecule and hence the presence of both an L- and D-isomer. The L-isomer has a much higher affinity for the peripheral adrenergic receptor, whereas the D-isomer is more specific for CNS stimulation.[44] Since the introduction of accurate and sensitive techniques for measuring plasma catecholamines, the use of such measurements has engendered controversy concerning their meaning. Inasmuch as epinephrine is a hormone secreted by the adrenal medulla delivered to the body in the blood stream, plasma concentrations of epinephrine are certainly a reasonable record of adrenal medullary activity.[45] However, several caveats need to be observed. Significant adrenal medullary secretion can occur without overall sympathetic stimulation. Also, when measuring epinephrine concentrations in blood, arterial samples might be more consistent, for venous samples may reflect the epinephrine kinetics in the organ being sampled rather than in the whole body.[46] The significance of plasma norepinephrine concentration is even more controversial.[45] Although the adrenal medulla may secrete norepinephrine, plasma norepinephrine levels probably reflect overflow from sympathetic stimulation, as most of the plasma norepinephrine released at the nerve ending is taken up again by the nerve terminal.

α-RECEPTOR DRUGS

Agonists

There are relatively few pure α-agonist drugs. Both phenylephrine and methoxamine are selective α_1-agonists, and clonidine, guanabenz, guanfacine, and dexametomidine are selective α_2-agonists. Although the α_2-agonist drugs do have some vasoconstricting properties in the intact animal, their primary effect is sympatholytic because the CNS effect predominates, resulting in a decrease in sympathetic outflow from the medullary pressor centers. Consequently, their primary use is as antihypertensive drugs. Recently, it has become apparent that clonidine and perhaps more selective α_2-agonist drugs interact with anesthetics to reduce the required anesthetic dose in several different patient populations and provide a more stable cardiovascular course. The latter appears to be a combination of the sympatholytic effect and the need for lower doses of cardioactive anesthetics.[47] The major action and usefulness of α_1-agonists are profound peripheral vasoconstriction. Phenylephrine (Neo-Synephrine) is the more useful of the two drugs for several reasons. Its duration of action, when given intravenously, is relatively short, usually in the range of 5 to 10 minutes.[44] Consequently, it is relatively easily titrated, especially by infusion. In addition, phenylephrine possesses direct cardiac stimulating activity at very high doses. In isolated ventricular muscle of various species, there can be no doubt that this positive inotropic effect is regulated through cardiac α-receptors.[48-50] Furthermore, the decreased density of β-receptors produced by chronic congestive heart failure[15,16] does not apply to α-receptors even in human myocardium.[51] Consequently, it is possible that drugs with significant α-receptor agonism may prove useful in treating severe heart failure. In any event, unintentional overdose of this drug is not as deleterious as it might be because of the cardiac-stimulating properties. In contrast, methoxamine (Vasoxyl) is a much longer-acting drug (30 to 60 minutes) and, in addition, has no cardiac-stimulating properties, even at very high doses.[44,50] In fact, at high doses the drug possesses some membrane-stabilizing properties and even β-adrenergic blocking properties. Consequently, overdoses of methoxamine are more serious than phenylephrine overdoses because of huge increases in afterload and cardiac failure, even in the healthy heart.

Antagonists

The specific effect of adrenergic blocking drugs depends on the existing sympathetic stimulation.[52] Because there is usually some baseline sympathetic tone, the major effects of α-antagonists is hypotension from vasodilation, reflex tachycardia (depending on which drug is used), pupillary constriction (depending on the level of the parasympathetic stimulation), and perhaps some gastrointestinal effects. Five major drug classes have predictable α-adrenergic blocking properties:

1. *β-Haloalkylamines.* These were the class of drugs that opened the door for adrenergic-receptor classification. The first of these drugs was dibenamine, which was shortly replaced by phenoxybenzamine (Dibenzyline). These drugs are one of the few therapeutically useful compounds that are noncompetitive irreversible antagonists. The adrenergic blockade is a result of the combination of the reactive radical of these chemicals and the α-receptor, which forms a stable nonequilibrium block.[52] The duration of *these* drugs is at least 24 hours. However, because new α-receptors (and therefore not blocked) can be synthesized, the duration of complete clinical effect of these drugs may be much shorter. These drugs appear to block both α_1- and α_2-receptors, although the α_1 block may be predominant. Phenoxybenzamine is still used to treat pheochromocytoma. The usual dose is 0.5 to 3 mg/kg/d orally.

2. *Imidazolines.* Several imidazolines have been used for adrenergic blockade.[52] The most familiar one to anesthesiologists is phentolamine (Regitine). This drug is a classic competitive blocker, so that the blockade can be overcome by an α-agonist. The drug has a very short duration of action and is usually given by intravenous infusion. In addition to the α-adrenergic blocking action, phentolamine releases endogenous norepinephrine and produces an initial sympathetic stimulation that may be undesirable. Inasmuch as phentolamine blocks both α_1- and α_2-receptors, the tachycardia seen after the establishment of α-adrenergic block with phentolamine is probably also related to the block of the α_2-receptors so that the negative feedback from norepinephrine secretion is abolished.

3. *Piperazine derivatives.* Although piperazine derivatives have been known to have α-adrenergic blocking properties for sometime, few drugs of this structure have been introduced. Prazosin (Minipress) is currently available as an oral formulation used predominantly for the treatment of hypertension, although it may be used for vasodilation in congestive heart failure and to treat pheochromocytomas.[52-54] Prazosin is a very selective α_1-receptor blocking drug. For this reason, tachycardia occurs infrequently. In addition, both the drug and its derivatives have been used as pharmacologic tools. Three analogues are currently in the testing phase. Trimazosin is a direct vasodilator as well as an α_1-antagonist. Doxazosin and tarazosin appear to be longer acting than prazosin and hence may be more clinically useful.[55]

4. *Indoles* The latest selective α_1-antagonist to be approved for clinical use in the United States is an indole, indoramin.[56,57] The pharmacology of this drug resembles prazosin very closely. However, there are some slight differences. For instance, indoramin possesses some Class III antiarrhythmic properties and in higher doses, Class I (local anesthetic) antiarrhythmic properties.[58] These direct cardiac membrane effects appear to have minimal clinical importance, however.[59]

5. *Ergot alkaloids.* These were actually the first useful drugs with α-adrenergic blocking properties.[52] However, this aspect of their pharmacology is relatively minor. They are direct vascular smooth muscle constrictors and have been useful in the management of migraine headaches and for their oxytocic properties. However, one of the synthetic derivatives, dihydroergotamine, is a potent α-adrenergic blocking drug with minor uterine and vascular stimulating properties and, like prazosin, appears to be a relatively specific α_1-blocking drug.

β-RECEPTOR DRUGS

Non-selective β-Agonists

As is the case with the α-receptor agonists, there are very few specific β-receptor agonist drugs (Table 14-7). The most well known and widely used is the prototype β-agonist isoproterenol (Isuprel) (Fig. 14-13).[44] This drug is a pure β-adrenergic agonist, has both β_1 and β_2 effects, and is the major pharmacologic tool for dissecting β-agonist activity. Isoproterenol is without doubt the most potent cardiac stimulating drug available. It markedly increases contractile force of the heart, cardiac rate, and conduction velocity. With other drugs available that are β_1-selective, the most specific indica-

TABLE 14-7. Adrenergic Agonists

	Direct	Indirect	α_1	α_2	β_1	β_2	Dose
Natural							
Norepinephrine	++++		++++	++++	++		0.05–0.3 μg/kg/min
Epinephrine	++++		++	++	++++	++++	0.05–0.2 μg/kg/min
Dopamine	++++		Dopaminergic receptor stimulation				1–5 μg/kg/min
	+++	+	+	?	+++	+++	5–15 μg/kg/min
	+++	+	+++	?	++	++	>15μg/kg/min
Synthetic							
Isoproterenol	++++				++++	++++	0.01–0.2 μg/kg/min
Mephentermine	++	+++	++	?	+++	?	0.1–0.5 mg/kg
Ephedrine	++	+++	+++	?	+++	?	0.2–1.0 mg/kg
Metaraminol	+	+++	+++	?	++	?	10–102 μg/kg
Phenylephrine	++++		++++		+		1–10 μg/kg/min
Methoxamine	++++		++++				0.05–0.2 mg/kg

Symbols: ++++, tremendous stimulation; +++, marked stimulation; ++, moderate stimulation; +, slight stimulation; ?, unknown.

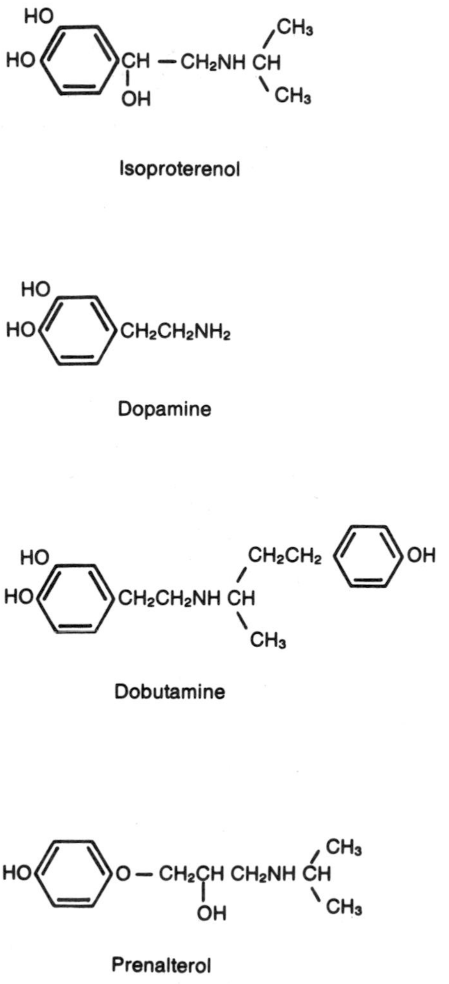

Fig. 14-13. Structure–activity relationship for β-agonist catecholamines.

tion for isoproterenol is for cardiac acceleration and in situations in which atrioventricular conduction may be decreased. Inasmuch as isoproterenol is a potent β_2-agonist, it also produces peripheral vasodilation. The resultant tachycardia and hypotension limit its use in several situations. The β_2-stimulating qualities also have made the drug useful for relieving bronchoconstriction, but the prominent β_1 effects have limited its usefulness in this situation. β_2-Selective agonists and drugs with other mechanisms of bronchodilation have essentially replaced isoproterenol as a bronchodilating drug. Isoproterenol is rapidly metabolized and has a very short duration of action. It is o-methylated by the action of COMT in the liver and other tissues. Although other catecholamines produce predominant β_1-agonist action, thus far all also possess some β_2 and/or α effects.

β_1-Selective Agonists

A major problem in modern cardiovascular intensive care is the support of the failing or ischemic heart without producing either marked tachycardia or peripheral vasodilation. For this reason, isoproterenol is currently used for only rather specific indications. Epinephrine can be used, but the prominent vasoconstriction and tachycardia often interferes with treatment of the failing heart. Dopamine is certainly the most popular drug for this purpose at the present time. However, if used in higher doses, both tachycardia and vasoconstriction can result. It was for this reason that dobutamine was synthesized and introduced (Table 14-8). Although initial reports claimed that the drug could produce profound inotropic effect without much increase in heart rate,[60] it has become apparent that dobutamine is a selective β_1 stimulant; the effects at low concentration are predominantly increased force of contraction and mild tachycardia. As higher concentrations are achieved, however, the drug becomes both a mild β_2-agonist and a mild α-agonist.[61] This α agonism is both α_1 and α_2, and stimulation of the presynaptic α_2-receptor may be one reason for the lesser degree of tachycardia seen with

TABLE 14-8. New β-Adrenergic Agonists

Drug	Mode of Action					Dose (μg/kg/min)
	α	$\beta_1 I$	$\beta_1 C$	β_2	Dopaminergic	
Dobutamine		+++	++			1–5
		+++	++	+		5–15
	+	+++	+++			>15
Prenalterol		+++	+			5–10
		+++	++	+		10–20

Symbols: I, inotropic; C, chronotropic; +++, marked stimulation; ++, moderate stimulation; +, slight stimulation.

dobutamine than with other potent sympathomimetic agents. Theoretically, a selective β_1-stimulant would result in less vasodilation and hypotension. The maintained or even increased blood pressure might also produce a decrease (or a less increase) in heart rate through the baroreceptor mechanism.

The search continues for the ideal β_1-sympathomimetic drug. One candidate that had received considerable investigation in the early 1980s was prenalterol (Table 14-8).[62] However, this drug has not been released in the United States and to my knowledge is not being widely used elsewhere. A number of other β_1-selective drugs and even some β_2-selective compounds are in investigational use for the treatment of congestive heart failure. In addition to an intravenous drug that does not produce tachycardia, obviously a drug that could be given orally to replace digitalis would be most attractive.

β-Antagonists

Without question, the most widely used group of adrenergic drugs today are the β-adrenergic receptor blocking drugs (β-blockers). From the investigative use of the early drugs dichloroisoproterenol and pronethalol, through the wide experience with the initial and approved prototype drug proranolol, and now with the multitude of drugs available for use in the United States, the β-blockers have been an extremely important class of drugs.

A curious structure–activity relationship exists in the β-adrenergic blocking drugs (Fig. 14-14). Although the initial two compounds were analogues of isoproterenol, that is, with a two-carbon ethanol side chain on the benzene ring, most of the currently available β-adrenergic blocking drugs are, in fact, propranolamines with a three-carbon side chain. The major structural change that converts these chemicals from agonists to antagonists is the substitution or loss of the hydroxyl group on the 3, 4-position of the benzene ring.[52] Like most of the β-agonists, the β-antagonists are optical isomers. The usual commercial formulation is the racemic mixture, but the L-form is the most active. The drugs are all classic, competitive antagonists, meaning that the dose–response curve is shifted to the right (Fig. 14-15). If high enough concentration of the agonist is present at the receptor site, the antagonist molecule can be displaced and the blockade overcome. The major differences between β-blockers concern the associated side effects, potency, and pharmacokinetics. The pertinent features of the currently available drugs are listed in Tables 14-9 and 14-10.

Associated Side Effects

The three major associated side effects have been termed *membrane stabilizing activity* (MSA); *intrinsic*

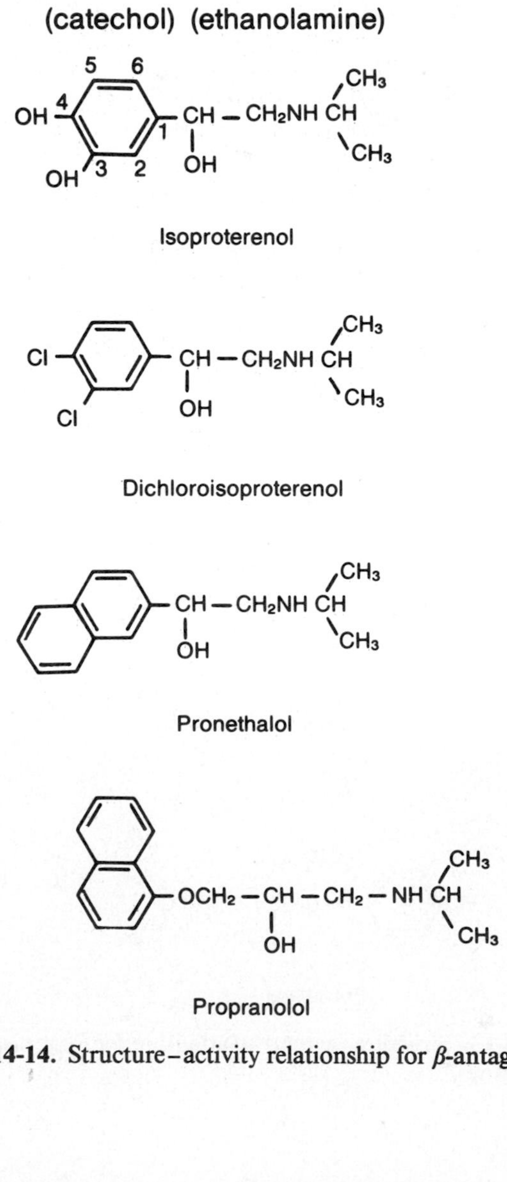

Fig. 14-14. Structure–activity relationship for β-antagonists.

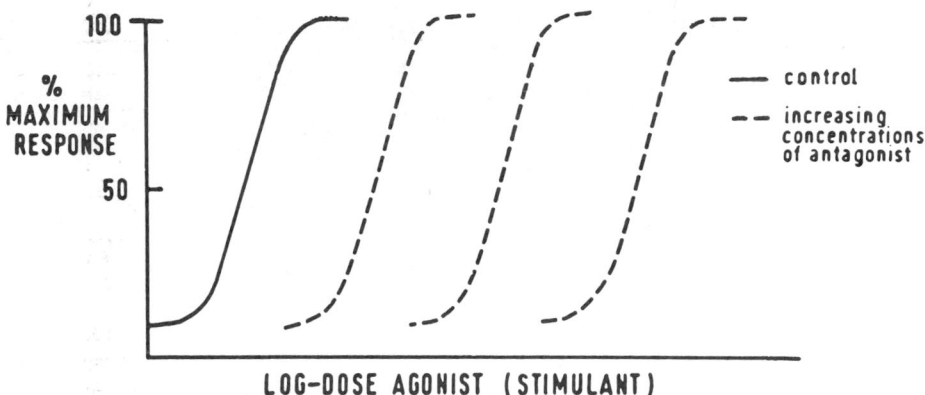

Fig. 14-15. Effect of competitive antagonist on agonist dose–response curve.

sympathomimetic activity (ISA) or *partial agonism,* and *receptor selectivity.*[63] The prototypical drug, propranolol, has MSA, which has also been called *local anesthetic activity* or *quinidinelike activity.* Initially, it was thought that this was an important component of some of the drug's action, such as its antiarrhythmic effects, but this property is apparent only at very high plasma concentrations. It would only be important, then, if the drugs were used in very large doses or immediately after a bolus dose. Consequently, this property is relatively unimportant in the clinical pharmacology of these drugs. Both of the original β-adrenergic blocking drugs, DCI and pronethalol, possessed ISA. Initially, it was thought that this was due to the release of endogenous norepinephrine, but these drugs possess partial agonist activity. This property was prominent enough in the two early drugs to interfere with their therapeutic effectiveness. However, in the two drugs in which it is currently present, pindolol and acebutolol, the partial agonist activity is less obvious. Perhaps this partial agonist activity may be advantageous in certain circumstances.[64,65] For instance, these drugs do not decrease

TABLE 14-9. Pharmacokinetics of β-Adrenergic Blocking Drugs

Drug (Trade Name)	β-half-life (h)		Dosage in renal Failure				Plasma Protein Binding (%)
	Normal	Uremia	50	35–40	15–35	<15	
				GFR (ml/min) in Renal Failure			
Propranolol (Inderal)	2–4	2–3	Normal	Slight Reduction	Slight Reduction	Slight Reduction	60–90
Timolol (Blocadren)	2–3	4	Normal	Slight Reduction	Slight Reduction	Slight Reduction	Low
Nadolol (Corgard)	16–24	45	Normal	70% dose	50% dose	30% dose	25–30
Metoprolol (Lopressor)	2.5–4.5	2.5–4.5	Normal	Normal	Normal	Normal	12
Atenolol (Tenormin)	6–9	127	Normal	Normal	50% dose	25% dose	6–16
Pindolol (Visken)	3–4	3–4	Normal	Normal	Normal	Normal	40
Oxprenolol (Trasicolor)	2–3	2–3	Normal	Normal	Normal	Normal	80
Acebutolol (Sectral)	8–10[a]	12	Normal	Normal	70% dose	50% dose	20
Labetalol (Trandate, Normodyne)	3–5	5–6	Normal	Normal	Normal	Normal	50
Esmolol (Brevibloc)	0.12	0.12	Normal	Normal	Normal	Normal	50

Abbreviation: GFR, glomerular filtration rate.
[a] Active metabolite.

TABLE 14-10. The β-Adrenergic Blocking Drugs

Drug (Trade Name)	Potency Propranolol = 1	β-Selective	Intrinsic Sympathomimetic Activity	Membrane-Stabilizing Activity	Lipid Solubility	Hepatic Metabolism (%)
Propranolol (Inderal)	1	−	−	+	High	99
Timolol (Blocadren)	6	−	−	−	Moderate	80
Nadolol (Corgard)	0.8	−	−	−	Low	27
Metoprolol (Lopressor)	1	++	−	−	Moderate	97
Atenolol (Tenormin)	1	++	−	−	Low	<10
Pindolol (Visken)	6	−	+++	+	Moderate/Low	60
Oxprenolol (Trasicolor)	1	−	++	+	Moderate	97
Acebutolol (Sectral)	0.3	+	+	+	High	80
Labetalol (Trandate, Normodyne)	0.3	−	−	−	Moderate/High	90+
Esmolol (Brevibloc)	0.5	+++	−	−	Low	0–10

heart rate as much as β-blockers without ISA, which could be advantageous. Patients with mild congestive heart failure probably tolerate the partial agonists better than the pure antagonists. In addition, patients with bronchospastic disease may benefit from the β_2 agonism from these drugs, producing some bronchodilation to offset the β_2 block. In like manner, the patient with occlusive peripheral vascular disease may also be less affected by this class of drugs. Theoretically, β_1-antagonist selectivity should also permit the use of these drugs to slow heart rate in the latter two conditions, namely bronchospasm and peripheral vascular spasm.[66] In patients with these diseases, the β_2 agonism of circulating catecholamines (and perhaps sympathetic stimulation) serve to bronchodilate and vasodilate. When a drug blocks these β_2 effects, the disease process worsens. Unfortunately, all the β_1-selective drugs at present are just that, selective. In low doses, they possess little or no β_2-blocking activity. However, for effective treatment of most of the diseases for which they are being used, high enough doses to produce some β_2 blockade are usually necessary, and development of symptoms in patients with bronchospasm and vasospasm frequently occurs.

In addition to the previously discussed documentation of the importance of β_2-receptors in mediating the adrenergically induced increase in contractile force of the heart, there is also evidence to suggest that the β_2-receptors are important in the chronotropic effect of sympathetic nervous stimulation.[67] This effect appears to be important in the demonstrated protection produced by the nonselective β-blockers propranolol and timolol given after acute myocardial infarction.[68-70] Finally, the well-known epinephrine-produced hypokalemia also seems to be moderated predominantly by β_2-receptors; hence a selective β_1-antagonist would not be as effective in preventing this effect.[71,72]

Pharmacokinetics

A physical property of this class of drugs appears to predict their metabolic fate.[73] The drugs with high or moderate lipid solubility are predominantly metabolized by the liver and tend to have a relatively short duration of action. By contrast, those agents with low lipid solubility are predominantly excreted by the kidneys and tend to be longer acting. For most of the drugs, the hepatic metabolism is accompanied by a first-pass hepatic extraction effect. This results in a relatively low bioavailability of the drugs when taken orally and a marked difference in plasma levels between oral and parenteral doses. Although most of the drugs are well absorbed by the gastrointestinal tract, the hepatic extraction is unpredictable and leads to marked interpatient variation in bioavailability. Renal function has little effect on the disposition of these highly lipid-soluble drugs but needs to be considered when using the less lipid-soluble β-blockers (Table 14-10). Another property of the drugs that may influence their effectiveness is the plasma protein binding. Again, this varies widely, with propranolol and oxprenolol being highly bound and metoprolol and timolol being poorly bound (Table 14-9).

Specific Drugs

Propranolol

For more than 10 years, propranolol was the only β-blocker available for use in the United States. Consequently, tremendous experience with propranolol has accrued and it is the standard by which the other drugs are judged. It has no ISA and is, for practical purposes, not receptor selective, but it does have MSA. It is highly lipid soluble and hence is almost totally metabolized and avidly extracted by the liver. It is also very highly protein bound, so that small changes in plasma protein, or displacement by other drugs that are protein bound can make a difference in the free drug available in the blood. Because of all these factors, the oral dose of propranolol necessary for a therapeutic effect is extremely variable. Doses from 10 mg to more than 1 g of propranolol per day have been used to produce desired effects. Propranolol is one of the few parental β-blocking formulations available for use in the United States. Because of the variability in oral dosing, it is difficult to know what dose to give intravenously; however, two different investigations have documented that infusion rates of 2 to 3 mg/h (1 mg/kg/d) of propranolol will usually produce therapeutic plasma concentrations within 3 or 4 hours.[74,75] However, these levels can be achieved by a rapid infusion (10 minutes) of 0.2 mg/kg at the beginning of the infusion.[76] With an elimination half-life of about 4 hours, it may take 20 hours for a constant infusion to reach steady-state plasma levels and even longer in patients with reduced liver function and circulatory insufficiency. For bolus administration, usually doses of 0.1 mg/kg are adequate, although most practitioners will initiate therapy with much smaller doses, particularly during anesthesia, and titrate to effect.

Timolol

Timolol was used for years topically in the eye for treatment of glaucoma. It was approved for systemic use in the United States primarily as the result of a study demonstrating decreased mortality following myocardial infarction in a group of European patients.[69] It is devoid of any of the associated side effects (Table 14-10). Although it is moderately lipid soluble and metabolized by the liver, the hepatic extraction is much less extensive than with propranolol, hence its greater bioavailability and lower variability (Table 14-9). This is the predominant advantage of timolol over propranolol.

Nadolol

As with timolol, nadolol has no associated side effects (Table 14-10). Its major difference from and advantage over propranolol appear to be in its metabolism and pharmacokinetics (Table 14-9).[73] As it is relatively lipid insoluble, its disposition is primarily renal, and it has the longest elimination half-life of any of the approved β-blocking drugs. Consequently, nadolol can be given in once-a-day dosage. Obviously, dosage must be markedly adjusted in patients with renal disease (Table 14-9).

Metoprolol

Equally potent as propranolol, metoprolol possesses β_1-selective properties and is therefore perhaps a better drug for patients with bronchospasm and vasospasm (Table 14-10). Metoprolol is mostly metabolized by the liver, in line with its moderate lipid solubility, and is highly extracted (Table 14-9). The low plasma protein binding, however, leads to more consistent dosage effects. It is another parenteral preparation available in the United States.

Atenolol

The major differences between atenolol and metoprolol, both of which have β_1-selective properties (Table 14-10), lie in the low lipid solubility of atenolol and the resultant longer half-life and dependence on the kidney for excretion (Table 14-9). As with other drugs that have a relative lack of hepatic extraction and the low plasma protein binding, oral dosing is more predictable. Of interest is the fact that atenolol is the only currently available β-adrenergic blocking drug that is an ethanolamine.

Pindolol

Although pindolol is considerably more potent than propranolol, the major therapeutic difference is its ISA (Table 14-10). For the reasons noted above, it may prove a better therapeutic agent in certain groups of patients. Basically metabolized by the liver, but not avidly extracted, oral dosing of pindolol is more predictable. However, it does not depend on the kidneys for disposition and can therefore be used in usual doses in patients with renal disease (Table 14-10).

Oxprenolol

Another approved β-blocker in the United States is similar to pindolol in many respects (Tables 14-9 and 14-10). As a result, the pharmaceutical company has decided not to market the drug at the present time.

Labetalol

This nonselective β-blocker with no ISA or MSA is one of the two newer drugs with a relatively unique property (Fig. 14-16). In addition to being a competitive β-adrenergic blocking drug, labetalol also possesses α-adrenergic blocking properties.[78-80] Depending on the species, the β blockade is 3 to 10 times more potent than the α blockade, with the potency differential perhaps 7

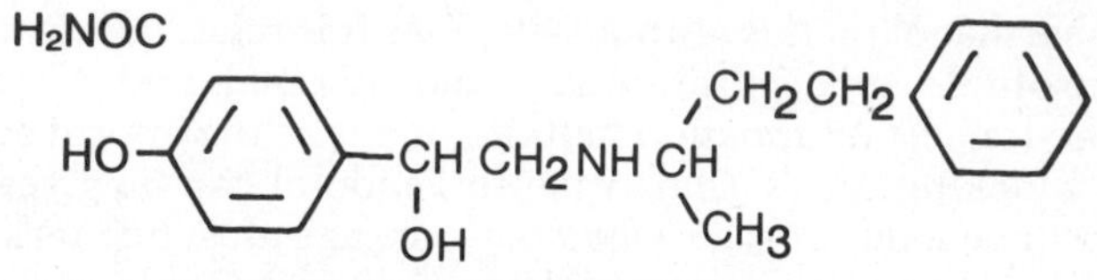

Fig. 14-16. Labetalol.

in humans. The α blockade is α_1-selective, which, as indicated above, may be an advantage for pure α-agonists. However, because labetalol is primarily a β-blocker, reflex tachycardia is certainly not a problem. The major clinical use for labetalol is in circumstances where such tachycardia is not desirable. In fact, the lack of α_2-blocking properties may be the reason why labetalol has not been as effective as a hypotensive agent as was initially hoped.

Acebutolol

As can be seen from Table 14-9, acebutolol is the only β-blocker that possesses all three associated pharmacologic properties. However, all are relatively weak, and the major difference between acebutolol and the other β-blockers is the fact that it is metabolized to an active metabolite, diacetol, which has a long elimination half-life, and hence confers a much longer duration of action for the drug than would be expected from the intermediate elimination half-life of acebutolol itself (Table 14-9).[73]

Esmolol

Esmolol is the anesthesiologist's β-adrenergic-receptor blocking drug. It is truly unique in that the drug is hydrolyzed by nonspecific esterases in the blood to produce an elimination half-life of only 9 to 10 minutes.[81] Therefore, the drug has a pharmacokinetic profile not dissimilar to the familiar thiopental and succinylcholine. In addition, the drug is β_1-selective. For both these reasons, one of the uses of this drug is in clinical circumstances where β-receptor blockade may be desirable, but perhaps relatively contraindicated because of bronchospasm and/or vasospasm. The β_1-selectivity of esmolol makes smooth muscle spasm less likely (see below), and the short duration of action means that even if it does occur, it will be short-lived. The other major usefulness for the drug is in situations where only a short duration of β-receptor blockade is desired, such as for tracheal intubations. Although the drug was originally marketed to be given by continuous infusion, inasmuch as it is essentially a short-duration metopolol (Table 14-10), it is more logical to switch to that longer duration drug (which is available intravenously) if longer duration is desirable and the possibility of adverse β-receptor or blocking effects (congestive heart failure and/or bronchospasm) is remote.

Clinical Uses

Although the response of the sympathetic nervous system enhances survival in times of stress, there are numerous circumstances in which sympathetic nervous activity proves harmful to body function. Inasmuch as the β-adrenergic receptor system is predominantly concerned with cardiac function, it is not surprising that most of the clinical uses for β-adrenergic blockade involve some aspect of cardiac pathophysiology. However, there are also areas of clinical usefulness in which the heart is not the major therapeutic target.

Cardiac Arrhythmias
(Also See Ch. 32)

The first approved use in the United States for β-adrenergic blocking drugs was in the treatment of cardiac arrhythmias. Propranolol has been particularly effective in acute and chronic therapy of superventricular tachycardia, as classic antiarrhythmic drugs such as lidocaine and quinidine have been relatively ineffective in controlling such arrhythmias.[82] The annoying arrhythmias associated with digitalis toxicity have also been effectively treated with relatively small doses of propranolol. Of course, any situation in which the arrhythmias are due to sympathetic stimulation such as pheochromocytoma or the arrhythmias associated with myocardial infarction are particularly amenable to therapy with propranolol. Another area in which this drug class may be particularly useful is in some of the arrhythmias associated with anesthesia.[83]

Ischemic Heart Disease

One of the most widespread uses of β-adrenergic blocking drugs on an outpatient basis is for the treatment of angina pectoris.[84] There can be little question that β-adrenergic blocking drugs are very effective in improving the cardiac oxygen supply–demand ratio. The predominant effect in this regard is in reducing or preventing heart rate increases associated with both increased oxygen demand and decreased supply, particularly to the subendocardium. There are now at least three large-scale epidemiologic studies that show chronic therapy with β-adrenergic blocking drugs to decrease the morbidity and mortality associated with acute myocardial infarction, especially in men.[69,70,85] Consequently, many patients with relatively few symptoms after myocardial infarction may be expected to be treated with these drugs in the future. In patients with angina pectoris, however, the calcium-channel blocking drugs have become increasingly used by physicians for symptomatic treatment. The resultant decrease in the number of patients coming to anesthesia and surgery, particularly for coronary artery bypass, being treated with β-blockers has increased the risk of tachycardia and ischemia during anesthesia.[86,87] Consequently, it may be that anesthesiologists will have to initiate therapy with β-blockers immediately before surgery and anesthesia.[88]

Hypertensive Cardiovascular Disease
(Also See Ch. 25)

As with many other types of therapy, there was an initial flurry of enthusiasm for the use of β-adrenergic blocking drugs alone for the treatment of hypertensive cardiovascular disease.[89] In the class of patients in whom hypertension is associated with a high plasma renin activity, β-adrenergic blocking drugs are the most important aspect of therapy. However, this group does not make up the majority of patients with essential hypertension. Experience in Europe in the 1970s indicated that most patients with low renin hypertension can show therapeutic improvement with huge doses of β-adrenergic blocking drugs. However, many physicians use much smaller doses of these drugs together with diuretics and peripheral vasodilators in patients without high renin hypertension.[90] The combination of β-adrenergic blocking drugs with diuretics and/or peripheral vasodilators is associated with a better quality of life and less annoying side effects (postural hypotension and impotence) and continues to be an area of widespread use. Angiotensin-converting inhibitors also appear to hold the promise of improving the quality of life for patients who need treatment for hypertension (see Ch. 25). The mechanism for the beneficial effect of β blockers in hypertension is still unclear.[89] Aside from lowering plasma renin activity in patients with high plasma renin, β blockers initially decrease cardiac output, but eventually it returns to control levels while the antihypertensive effect is still maintained. There appear to be effects on the central nervous system cardiovascular control mechanisms in long-term therapy.

Thyrotoxicosis
(Also See Ch. 25)

Many of the distressing clinical features of thyrotoxicosis appear to be mediated through β-adrenergic stimulation. Consequently, it was natural that β-adrenergic blocking drugs should be tried as therapy in such cases. The first applications were in treating patients with thyroid storm and in patients in whom conventional antithyroid drugs produced undesirable side effects. However, in recent years there has been a great deal of enthusiasm in the surgical community for preparing patients for thyroidectomy with propranolol.[91] There have now been several reasonable series for which excellent success rates have been reported, and there can be little doubt that this modality of treating hyperthyroidism, β-blockade preparation for thyroidectomy, is relatively safe and effective. However, the use of the drugs alone to treat the thyrotoxic patient is still unsound medical practice.

Obstructive Cardiomyopathy

Even before propranolol was synthesized and tested, β-adrenergic blockade (using pronethalol) was clearly effective in relieving some of the symptoms of idiopathic hypertrophic subaortic stenosis (asymmetric septal hypertrophy). Patients with other types of obstructive cardiomyopathy such as tetralogy of Fallot showed improvement as well. It has become apparent over the past decade that many patients with these diseases will eventually need surgical treatment. As pharmacologic therapy proceeds, therapeutic benefits appear to decrease, until many patients become refractory. However, there are individuals who can be maintained for long periods with relatively few side effects on β-adrenergic blocking drugs. In addition, for patients who will be surgically treated, the drugs are used for preoperative preparation.

Pheochromocytoma
(Also see Ch. 25)

This rare but challenging disease is certainly a natural setting for the use of β-adrenergic blocking drugs.[89] One of the most distressing aspects of the disease is the tachyarrhythmias, and β-adrenergic blocking drugs are specific for these arrhythmias, inasmuch as they are mediated sometimes through β-adrenergic stimulation (many arrhythmias disappear concomitant with treatment with α-adrenergic blockade alone). However, if only the β-receptors are blocked, α-receptor agonism will be intensified and the hypertension, which is also a feature of the disease, may be exaggerated. Consequently, the use of β-blocking drugs alone in the management of pheochromocytoma is contraindicated.[54] There has been some enthusiasm for the routine preoperative management of the patients with β-blockers. In most instances chronic α blockade will suffice and, unless there are tachyarrhythmias, I believe that β-blockade management of pheochromocytoma should be reserved for intraoperative tachyarrhythmias.

Miscellaneous Disorders

There are several noncardiac diseases in which therapeutic response to β-blocking drugs has been reported. There can be little doubt that small doses of propranolol have been markedly effective in reducing the incidence of certain types of hereditary tremors. Migraine headaches appear to respond spectacularly to β-blockers as far as prophylaxis is concerned. However, they are not effective for treating a developed headache. Various anxiety states, schizophrenia, and drug addiction have also been purported to respond to β-adrenergic treatment, although such therapy is not approved in the United States.

Problems Associated with β-Antagonists

Bronchoconstrictive Disease

Perhaps the β_1-selective metopolol acebutolol and atenolol or the ISA drugs pindolol and acebutolol may be used in patients with mild bronchospastic disease. However, in patients with established bronchospasm, the β-adrenergic blocking drugs may be contraindicated.[92] If bronchospasm occurs during β blockade, a β-agonist will be effective in very high doses. Under these circumstances, it is logical to use one of the selective β_2-agonists in an effort to maintain the desired cardiovascular effects of the β blockade (see Ch. 25).

Cardiac Failure

In many patients with congestive heart failure the sympathetic nervous system has been mobilized for support of their inefficient myocardium. Consequently, β-adrenergic blocking drugs may worsen the disease.[93] Perhaps the ISA drugs may be less deleterious, but the evidence is not yet conclusive.[64] Again, β-agonists can overcome the effect if used in high enough doses. It is possible to use nonadrenergic inotropic drugs such as calcium ion. However, this drug may produce more constriction than inotropy.

Peripheral Vascular Insufficiency

Again, theoretically, β_1-selective drugs and the ISA drugs may be more useful in treating peripheral vascular insufficiency. However, with well-developed peripheral vascular insufficiency, the drugs might be avoided or used only in low doses, unless better choices are not available or are judged more risky.

Hypoglycemia

Troublesome hypoglycemia may be a problem in patients on long-acting insulin preparations in whom prolongation of the hypoglycemic effect may occur along with the decrease in signs and symptoms of hypoglycemia.[94,95] Some patients may have a decrease in glucose tolerance during long-term therapy inasmuch as β stimulation does play a role in insulin release from the pancreas. If liver glycogen stores are deficient, as in patients who have been starved, hypoglycemia may be a problem intraoperatively, and all such patients should be treated with intravenous glucose.

Drug Interactions

The drug interactions with β-blockers can be divided into two categories. The first involves drug metabolism. The β-blockers that are highly hepatically metabolized (Table 14-9) will be affected by drugs that affect both liver function and blood flow, such as the antibiotic rifampin, chlorpromazine, and cimetidine. Obviously, the β-blockers that do not depend on the liver for metabolism will not be affected by these drugs. In addition, β-blockers also will decrease metabolism of other drugs because of their effect predominantly on liver blood flow, so that any drug that is metabolized by the liver may be expected to have a longer elimination half-life when given in combination with β-blockers.[72,73] The other type of drug interaction is basically cardiovascular, and the most important class of drugs that interact with the β-blockers in this manner are the calcium channel blocking drugs.[96] This effect should come as no surprise inasmuch as many of the actions of the two classes of drugs are similar, including prolonged atrioventricular conduction and decreased cardiac contractility. It is these areas where interactions can prove troublesome. In fact, a combination of various calcium channel and β-blocking drugs has proved efficacious for the treatment of ischemic heart disease and obstructive cardiomyopathy in particular.[97] The two categories of drugs when given chronically orally appear to have less deleterious interaction than when given intravenously. In particular, great caution should be exerted in administering both drugs intravenously to the same patient or given one of the drugs intravenously in a patient who is chronically receiving the other drug. The same precautions, especially as regards A-V block, are true for most of the Class I antiarrhythmics (quinidine, lidocaine, procaineamide, etc.) and digitalis. On the other hand, β-blockade has proved to be particularly efficacious for treating digitalis toxicity.

α- AND β-AGONISTS

Most of the sympathomimetic drugs in use today have mixed α- and β-stimulating properties (Table 14-7).[44] Only the β-agonist isoproterenol and the α-agonists phenylephrine and methoxamine are relatively pure drugs. The endogenous catecholamines are a perfect example. All three have mixed direct activities (Table 14-7). Although norepinephrine has a more prominent α effect, obviously the β effect is important, as it is responsible for the sympathetic nervous activation of the heart. In addition, norepinephrine is a selective β_1-agonist that exhibits very little β_2 activity. On the other hand it possesses both α_1 and α_2 activity. Epinephrine is a somewhat more prominent β-agonist than α-agonist and stimulates both β_1- and β_2-receptors and α_1- and α_2-receptors.

The third endogenous catecholamine, dopamine, has α-, β-, and dopamine receptor-mediated effects (Table 14-7).[60] The dopamine receptors are specifically activated by low doses of dopamine. Higher doses of dopamine agonize first β-receptors and then, at higher doses still, α-receptors. There is a mixed effect of dopamine with both direct agonism from the compound occurring as well as release of endogenous norepinephrine (Table 14-7). Several more specific dopamine receptor agonists are in the developmental stage. Probably the most advanced is fenoldopam, which is a selective dopamine-1 agonist receptor producing hypotension, natriuresis, diuresis, and renal vasodilation.[98] The other sympathomimetic amines all have mixed actions in two respects. In the first place, they have both a direct action on the receptor as well as the effect noted for dopamine of releasing endogenous norepinephrine.[44] The three most commonly used synthetic sympathomimetics, mephentermine (Wyamine), ephedrine, and metaraminol (Aramine), all have prominent indirect effects, although the first two agents are also direct-acting drugs. As a consequence of their norepinephrine release, the drugs have both α and β effects. Although all sympathomimetic amines are capably of producing tolerance or tachyphylaxis, the mechanism has been identified with metaraminol. Metaraminol is taken up into the sympathetic nerve ending, displacing norepinephrine and producing the sympathomimetic effect. However, after a period of time, the drug now acts as a false transmitter and subsequent sympathetic nerve stimulation results in much less effect. Consequently, the drug probably should not be used widely when other, more effective drugs are available. If α-adrenergic stimulation is desired, there are several drugs with prominent α effects that can be used. Norepinephrine has received a bad name because of its indiscriminant use without proper monitoring. The potent α-agonist properties often lead to profound vasoconstriction if inappropriately high doses are used. If the major problem is vasodilation, then certainly norepinephrine can be used by infusion as long as direct arterial pressure and cardiac output are being measured. Direct arterial pressure measurements might aid in making norepinephrine a safer drug when used for its α effects.

β_2-Selective Agonists

As soon as it became apparent that it was possible to separate β_1- and β_2-agonists chemically, the search for selective β_2-agonists for use in bronchospastic disease began. A number of drugs have been synthesized and are available clinically for this purpose.[44] The most widely used drugs include metaproterenol (Alupent, Metaprel), terbutaline (Brethine, Bricanyl), albuterol (Proventil, Ventolin), and isoetharine (Brokosol). As is the case with β-receptor antagonists, these drugs are only β_2 selective, however. In situations wherein relatively mild to moderate bronchodilation is desired, the drugs are effective with minimal β_1 side effects. However, in severe bronchospasm, therapeutic doses produce tachycardia, and sometimes arrhythmias. When used as aerosols in the tracheobronchial tree, the bronchodilating property is even more predominant, with a lower incidence of β_1 side effects. Another use for this category of β-agonists is for the tocolytic effect in pre-

mature labor.[99] Another drug, ritodrine (Yutopar), has been marketed for this purpose. As with the other β_2-selective blockers, β_1 side effects are common, including tachycardia and cytotoxic or an "overstimulation" cardiomyopathy, particularly when the drugs are used intravenously. The other β_2-selective drugs have also been used as tocolytics, and all have been associated with significant β_1 side effects as well as the occasional incidence of pulmonary edema.[100] The cause of the pulmonary edema remains obscure, but may relate to the specific intravascular fluid balance situation in the pregnant patient. Finally, the vasodilating effect and the mild cardiostimulatory properties of the β_2-selective agonists may be useful in patients with congestive heart failure.[101]

OTHER DRUGS THAT INTERACT WITH THE SYMPATHETIC NERVOUS SYSTEM
(Also See Ch. 25)

Other than the receptor-blocking drugs, the major category of therapeutic agents that interact with the sympathetic nervous system are those used to treat hypertensive cardiovascular disease. Two major classes of drugs in this category, the diuretics and the direct vasodilators, interact only insofar as their effects excite compensatory reflexes that are mediated through the sympathetic nervous system.[102] For instance, the diuretics both by a direct vasodilating effect and by a decrease in circulating blood volume stimulate sympathetic effector systems. Likewise, the direct-acting vasodilators excite the baroreflexes, resulting in increased cardiac output and heart rate, which may not only be deleterious to the therapeutic aims, but may also prevent or blunt the hypotensive effect.

Two other categories of antihypertensive drugs interact more directly with the sympathetic nervous system.

Catecholamine-Depleting Drugs

Among the earliest categories of drugs to be effectively used for treating essential hypertension were the central and peripheral catecholamine-depleting compounds.[52] The raowulfia alkaloids were used initially for treatment of psychoses but soon became widely used for the treatment of hypertension. As these drugs deplete both central and peripheral catecholamines, they have a wide spectrum of side effects other than hypotension. In particular, disorientation, confusion, and sedation were prominent side effects that mandated the discontinuance of these drugs as sole methods of treatment. They are used today primarily in small doses along with other drugs.

Guanethidine does not cross the blood–brain barrier and therefore only depletes peripheral catecholamine stores. Consequently, the CNS side effects are practically absent with this and similar drugs. They are still being used, particularly the second-generation compounds such as bethanidine, but postural hypotension and fluid retention remain a problem with these drugs. The most recently approved drug of this category is guanadrel, which has a dynamic profile entirely similar to the guanethidine drugs. However, guanadrel is better absorbed by oral administration, much faster in onset (1 to 2 hours versus 2 to 3 days), and much shorter acting ($t\frac{1}{2}\beta$ of 10 hours versus 200 hours).[103] Initially it was thought that catecholamine depletion would result in cardiovascular collapse during anesthesia. However, in the doses now being used, this has not been substantiated; these drugs should be continued until the time of surgery with the realization that sympathetic nervous system response to stress may be blunted.[102]

Drugs Affecting the Renin– Angiotensin System

The renin–angiotensin system functions to aid in maintaining body blood pressure and water homeostasis.[104] The major end product of the system, angiotensin II, is both a potent vasoconstrictor and a stimulant of the release of aldosterone from the adrenal cortex. Aldosterone causes salt and water retention by the kidney. The mechanism by which angiotensin is produced is as follows. The juxtaglomerular cells of the renal cortex secrete a proteolytic enzyme called renin, which cleaves a protein produced in the liver known as angiotensinogen to the decapeptide angiotensin I. Although this peptide has properties that stimulate CNS and peripheral sympathetic nervous activity, these effects are relatively mild compared with those produced by angiotensin II. Angiotensin I is converted almost immediately to angiotensin II by the activity of the angiotensin-converting enzyme (ACE). This enzyme is located predominantly in the endothelial tissue of the lung, and 95 percent of angiotensin I is converted to angiotensin II in one circulation time. In addition to its direct vasoconstrictive activity, angiotensin II also facilitates the prejunctional release of norepinephrine at the sympathetic nerve terminal as well as increasing efferent sympathetic nerve activity. Angiotensin II also has effects on sodium and water homeostasis. It directly decreases tubular reabsorption of sodium, increases ADH and ACTH secretion, and also stimulates the secretion of aldosterone. A minority of patients with hypertensive vascular disease have high circulating plasma renin levels, and any drugs that interfere with the formation or activity of angiotensin II will decrease blood pressure. Three drugs are presently available with this activity. The older drug is captopril (Capoten) and the newer ACE inhibitors are enalapril (Vasotec) and lisinopril (Prinivil).[105] Enalapril is effective primarily because it is hydrolyzed to the ethyl ester or enalaprilat. As a conse-

quence of this mechanism of action, the pharmacokinetics are relatively unpredictable, but generally, onset of effect is considerably slower than with captopril. Lisinopril is not a prodrug (does not need to be metabolized for its effect) but is relatively slow in onset like enalapril. Hopefully, the two new drugs may have less disturbing side effects than captopril. However, these drugs are not only effective in high renin hypertension but also in normal and low renin states as well. In addition, enalapril and captopril have also been effective in treating cardiac failure, particularly where there is an abnormally high systemic vascular resistance.[106] Consequently, there is good evidence that a conversion of angiotensin I to angiotensin II occurs not only intravascularly and in the pulmonary endothelium but also in blood vessel walls of other organ systems, so that ACE inhibitors decrease vascular responsiveness to endogenous vasoconstrictors.[107]

A number of drugs are specific angiotensin II antagonists. The most widely known of these drugs is saralasin, but it is still considered investigational only. Part of the reason is that it must be given parenterally, because it is deactivated by gastrointestinal enzymes. In addition, it is effective mostly in high-renin hypertension, unlike captopril.[104] Consequently, saralasin has been most useful as a research tool.

Drugs That Interfere with Norepinephrine Biosynthesis

One of the early efforts in synthesizing antihypertensive drugs was to find a chemical that would replace norepinephrine with a much less potent false transmitter in the nerve terminal of the sympathetic nervous system. Metaraminol has already been mentioned as one of these drugs. However, the most widely used of this type of drug is α-methyl DOPA (AMD) (Aldomet). α-Methyl DOPA enters the biosynthetic pathway for norepinephrine (Fig. 14-6) replacing DOPA. It is then decarboxylated to α-methylnorepinephrine. Initially, this chemical was thought to be a false transmitter in the peripheral sympathetic nervous system. However, in fact, the most recent concept of AMD action is that AMD is further metabolized to α-methylepinephrine in the central nervous system.[108] This chemical is a potent α_2-agonist.[109] The resulting hypotensive effect of AMD is thus from the decreased CNS sympathetic outflow produced by α_2 agonism like clonidine (see above).

Another chemical that acts in the synthetic pathway is methylparatyrosine (metyrosine). This drug is a potent inhibitor of tyrosine hydroxylase, which catalyzes the formation of DOPA from tyrosine (Fig. 14-6). Inasmuch as this is the rate-limiting step in the biosynthesis of norepinephrine, the drug decreases the amount of norepinephrine stored in the nerve terminal. It has been useful in treating resistant or malignant pheochromocytomas.[110]

GUIDELINES FOR PERIOPERATIVE MANAGEMENT OF PATIENTS RECEIVING SYMPATHETIC NERVOUS SYSTEM DRUGS
(Also See Ch. 25)

Agonists

Any patient coming into the operating room under treatment with a sympathetic nervous system agonist (with the exception of the α_2-agonists) can be considered to be seriously ill. Hence, the problems will not be those of chronic therapy, but rather of treating the cardiovascular or respiratory disease that mandates the use of these drugs. Also patients receiving long-term therapy with an adrenergic agonist may well have an abnormality of their receptor function. So-called downregulation means that the end organs will be less responsive to receptor agonism, whether because of the decrease in density of the receptor or because of a decrease in the active form of the receptor protein. Consequently, the practitioner would be well advised to have nonadrenergic drugs available for management of the problem being presented (such as methylxanthines for the treatment of bronchospasm, digitalis for the treatment of heart failure, and perhaps, when available, angiotensin or vasopressin for peripheral vasoconstriction). In the future, patients may come to the operating room with long-term β-agonist therapy such as prenalterol. The therapeutic implications of long-term therapy with this type of compound are unknown at this point.

The interaction between the α_2-agonists (at the present meaning clonidine) and anesthetics are most interesting.[47] Indeed, it would appear that administration of this class of drugs may be most advantageous for the well-being of the patient with cardiovascular disease during the perioperative period. Ghignone and colleagues have shown that premedication of hypertensive[111] and elderly patients for ophthalmologic surgery[112] reduces the need for potent anesthetic drugs and makes the intraoperative course more stable hemodynamically. Flacke and co-workers demonstrated the same effects for patients undergoing coronary artery bypass surgery.[113] The availability of more specific α_2-agonists may allow both safer anesthetics and better understanding of the basic pharmacologic mechanisms of anesthesia.[114]

Antagonists

Most patients being treated chronically with adrenergic antagonist drugs have cardiovascular disease. The most common types will be ischemic heart disease, with the β-adrenergic blocking drugs being used, and hypertensive vascular disease, for which β-blocking drugs, α_1-an-

tagonists, α_2-agonists, renin–angiotensin active drugs, direct vasodilators, and diuretics may be used. There is a common thread in the management of all these patients. If the drugs are effective in treating the disease, they should not be discontinued and should even be administered right up until the time of surgery. In some instances, it may be necessary to continue these drugs through the operative period and certainly into the postoperative period, as there have been a number of catastrophic events in which these drugs were discontinued suddenly.[115,116] The anesthesiologist should be able to manage the patient continued on these drugs during the perioperative period, realizing that the patient will not be able to respond to stress with the normal sympathetic nervous system responses. Consequently, it will be important to monitor the intravascular volume status of these patients, for they may behave as though they are hypovolemic because of the vasodilation (or at least lack of reflex vasoconstriction). In patients in whom volume replacement is not effective or contraindicated, the appropriate agonist drugs can be used. If a patient is receiving a drug that has depleted the level of endogenous norepinephrine, obviously drugs that rely on release of norepinephrine should not be used. In some instances, patients may show hypersensitivity to the direct adrenergic agonist. This is "upregulation," wherein either the density or the activity of the receptor proteins is increased by chronic antagonist therapy. Consequently, the use of agonist drugs should be carefully titrated in these patients. Except for patients with pheochromocytomas who have been treated with phenoxybenzamine, all the adrenergic antagonist drugs in use today are reversible competitive inhibitors (and even phenoxybenzamine's effects can be overcome due to availability of receptors not affected by phenoxybenzamine). Consequently, although large doses may be required, their effects can be overcome with agonist drugs.

MAO Inhibitors

Many anesthesiologists, including the author, have regarded the patient on long-term therapy with MAO inhibitors as being at particular risk for serious drug interactions during anesthesia. As recently as the second edition of this text, discontinuance of MAO inhibitors for at least 2 weeks before elective surgery was recommended. "Anesthetic management for a patient given an MAO inhibitor can be chaotic; emergency surgery on patients given MAO inhibitors can be punctuated by hemodynamic instability; case reports of hyperpyrexic coma following administration of most narcotics exists in humans and animal studies document a 10 to 50 percent incidence of hyperpyrexic coma in animals treated with MAO inhibitors that were given a variety of narcotics."[117] In addition, of course, MAO inhibition can result in intracellular neuronal build-up of norepinephrine with resultant increase in sympathomimetic effects of the mixed agonists, which release norepinephrine as their mechanism of action (see above). The sympathomimetic effects of direct-acting α- and β-agonists can also be exaggerated owing to a denervation-type hypersensitivity. However, a clinical study[118] and two recent reviews[119,120] suggest that as long as certain drugs are avoided and careful attention to patient monitoring is carried out, elective surgery may be performed safely in patients taking MAO inhibitors. Both reviews point out that oftentimes patients on this form of drug have had severe depressive illnesses and run a major risk of suicide. Consequently, discontinuance of the drugs may prove more hazardous to their life than continuance. Wells and Bjorksten[120] suggest that preoperatively the patient should have liver function studies because of the possibility of drug-induced abnormalities; that premedication should be generous to alleviate anxiety and accompanying sympathetic discharge, specifically with benzodiazepines; that monitoring probably should include beat-to-beat heart rate and blood pressure monitoring either by indirect or direct means; that the anesthetic technique should try to avoid sympathetic stimulation; that, in particular, meperidine should not be used as there is reasonable documentation of deleterious drug interactions between MAO inhibitors and meperidine; that indirect acting sympathomimetic amines such as ephedrine, metamphetamine, and mephentermine should be avoided and direct-acting mixed α- and β-agonists should be titrated carefully; and finally, that if topical anesthesia is necessary, cocaine should not be used.[120] With these modifications, current evidence suggests that MAO inhibitors may also be continued through the perioperative period.

PERIOPERATIVE USES OF SYMPATHETIC NERVOUS SYSTEM DRUGS
(Also See Ch. 25)

For the average practitioner, the major perioperative use for drugs active in the sympathetic nervous system is to treat or prevent tachycardia and arrhythmias, hypotension, or hypertension. As will be indicated, more precise definition of the cause of the blood pressure changes is necessary for logical use of these drugs, but this information may not be available in many situations.

Tachycardia and Arrhythmias

Of course, the major therapy for tachycardia during anesthesia is to address the source, which most commonly may be surgical stimulation with inadequate CNS depression or hypovolemia. In some circumstances, however, especially in patients with organic heart disease, the time necessary to correct these abnormalities may be excessive and specific pharmaco-

logic therapy is indicated. If there is not undue concern about decreased ventricular function or bronchospasm, then without question the logical choice for treating tachycardias in the perioperative period is β-adrenergic blocking drugs. As with the acute use of any potent category of drugs, careful titration is the secret to safety. Consequently, the addition of the rapid onset, short duration β_1-selective blocking drug esmolol adds a valuable tool to the armamentarium of the anesthesiologist. Several reports have documented the usefulness and relative safety of this drug.[121-123] In addition to the advantage of rapid onset, a short duration of action allows the use of the drug in situations where β blockade may be relatively contraindicated, such as compromised ventricular function, bronchospasm, or vasospasm. Although classically a β_1 blocker was thought to be advantageous for treating tachycardia, the recent evidence that β_2-receptors are also involved in regulation of heart rate may dictate that nonselective β-blockers would be more effective in treating resistant or profound tachycardias.

The β-adrenergic blocking drugs may also be effective in treating certain types of arrhythmias such as supraventricular tachycardias, atrial flutter and fibrillation, and some ventricular ectopy, particularly if there is suspicion of sympathetic nervous system origin for the last named. In addition, β-blockers are useful for treating the ventricular ectopy of digitalis toxicity. However, for other arrhythmias, noncentral nervous system drugs such as the calcium channel blocking drugs (paroxysmal supraventricular tachycardias) and classic antiarrhythmic drugs may be more useful.[102]

Hypotension

As suggested previously, treatment of hypotension logically depends on determining the cause, and precise determination of the cause necessitates measurement of cardiac output and calculation of systemic vascular resistance. However, there are circumstances where knowledge of the pathophysiology or pharmacology involved let the practitioner rationally decide on therapy without such measurements. For example, the hypotension produced by major regional anesthesia (spinal and epidural) is a combination of decreased systemic vascular resistance and venous return. Although formerly treatment concentrated on the vascular resistance using an α-sympathomimetic drug such as phenylephrine or methoxamine, recent evidence suggests that in fact for treating venous return, a β-adrenergic component is advantageous.[124] In fact, most practitioners will use a mixed agonist of the synthetic variety (e.g., ephedrine). In other circumstances, however, measurement of cardiac output and systemic vascular resistance may provide a much more logical base for therapy. If the major cause of the hypotension is decreased systemic vascular resistance, then obviously an α-agonist, particularly phenylephrine for reasons noted previously, might be used. If decrease in cardiac output is documented, again the reason for this decrease should also be sought. If there is decreased preload, then obviously fluids and probably a mixed sympathetic agonist for venoconstriction would be the logical choice. If the cardiac output is decreased because of a decrease in heart rate, then an anticholinergic muscarinic drug (atropine or glycopyrolate) or perhaps isoproterenol would be the drugs of choice. If the reason is deemed to be decrease in the contractile function of the heart, then a relatively β-selective agent such as dobutamine might be the first choice, although in view of the demonstration of the importance of β_2-receptors in failing hearts, perhaps some β_2-agonism is desirable as well. If cardiac output is compromised because of increased afterload (SVR), then vasodilation is the therapy of choice. Of course, α-adrenergic antagonist drugs would be a logical choice, but with the exception of phentolamine, we currently have no intravenous rapid onset, short duration drugs of this category. As mentioned earlier, one possible approach is drugs that combine vasodilation and a positive inotropic effect and, of course, nonselective β-agonists and even selective β_2-agonists are being used for this purpose. In addition, the nonsympathetic nervous system drugs such as the phosphodiesterase inhibitors, amrinone, milrinone, and even methyl xanthines are being tried for this purpose.[125]

Hypertension

As a rule, the treatment of hypertension is directed at decreasing systemic vascular resistance using vasodilators. As indicated earlier, we have no rapid onset, short duration intravenous α-adrenergic blocking drugs except for phentolamine, which, because of its α_2-blocking properties, results in tachycardia and perhaps tachyphylaxis. Consequently, although a ganglionic blocking drug such as trimethaphan could be used, its associated tachycardia and parasympathetic effects, as well as tachyphylaxis, have made this choice unpopular. The combined α- and β-blocking drug labetalol has been used with some success for treating hypertension in the perioperative period. However, because the drug is predominantly a β-blocker, the results have been less than satisfactory thus far.[126] In fact, although esmolol is primarily effective on the heart, this drug has been more successful in controlling blood pressure in the perioperative period.[121-123] However, most anesthesiologists choose the nonsympathetic rapid onset, short duration vasodilators. If the patient has significant coronary artery disease, frequently the first choice will be intravenous nitroglycerin, although because of its predominant venodilating properties it is not always successful.[102] The most widely used vasodilator in the perioperative period is still sodium nitroprusside, although the tachycardia and rebound hypertension associated with this drug can pose a problem. Both these effects can be avoided by combining β blockade with sodium nitroprusside, and the combined use of a short-acting β-blocker (esmolol) and nitroprusside is rapidly gaining favor.

As the saying goes, an ounce of prevention is worth a pound of cure. Many anesthesiologists are now trying to prevent hypertension and tachycardia in the perioperative period by pretreating patients.[127] Both approaches have already been noted. Either the use of a β-adrenergic blocking drug preoperatively[85] or, perhaps more effectively, pretreatment with α_2-agonists (presently meaning clonidine[111-113]) have proved successful in preventing marked hemodynamic changes in the perioperative period particularly intraoperatively, although the postoperative course thus far has not been well studied. A particular problem in the past with patients receiving antihypertensive medication has been rebound hypertension postoperatively. This problem has been best documented for clonidine and propranolol but can occur with any of the drugs, particularly the centrally acting drugs such as clonidine and methyldopa. One approach to this problem is the use of intravenous α-methyldopa in the early intraoperative period. Although the drug is available for intravenous use, the onset is prolonged with peak effects not occurring for 2 to 4 hours after intravenous injection. However, if the drug is given at the beginning of an anesthetic in a patient on prolonged therapy with an antihypertensive drug not available for parenteral use, the postoperative rebound hypertension may be avoided.

REFERENCES

1. Carrier O: Pharmacology of the Peripheral Autonomic Nervous System. Year Book Medical Publishers, Chicago, 1972
2. Weiner N, Taylor P: Neurohumoral transmission and the autonomic and somatic nervous system, p. 66. In Gilman AG, Goodman LS, Rall TW, Murad F (eds): Goodman and Gilman's Pharmacologic Basis of Therapeutics, 7th Ed. Macmillan, New York, 1985
3. Dale HH: On some physiologic actions of ergot. J Physiol (Lond) 35:163, 1906
4. Cannon WB, Rosenbleuth A: Studies on conditions of activity in endocrine organs: Sympathin E and sympathin I. Am J Physiol 104:557, 1933
5. Ahlquist RP: A study of the adrenotropic receptors. Am J Physiol 153:586, 1948
6. Lands AM, Arnold A, McAuliff IJ, et al: Differentiation of receptor systems activated by sympathomimetic amines. Nature 214:597, 1967
7. Langer SZ: Presynaptic regulation of catecholamine release. Biochem Pharmacol 23:1793, 1974
8. Heinsimer JA, Lefkowitz RJ: Adrenergic receptors: Biochemistry, regulation, molecular mechanisms and clinical indications. J Lab Clin Med 100:641, 1982
9. Hoffman BB, Lefkowitz RJ: Adrenergic receptors in the heart. Annu Rev Physiol 44:475, 1982
10. Hedberg A, Kemp FF, Josephson ME, Molinoff PB: Co-existence of beta$_1$ and beta$_2$-adrenergic receptors in the human heart. Effects of treatment with receptor antagonists or calcium entry blockers. J Pharmacol 234:561, 1985

11. Hedberg A: Adrenergic receptors. Methods of determination and mechanisms of regulation. Acta Med Scand (suppl.) 672:7, 1983

12. Sutherland EW, Robison GA, Butcher RW: Some aspects of the biological role of adenosine 3,5-monophosphate (cyclic AMP). Circulation 37:279, 1968

13. Lefkowitz R, Michel T: Plasma membrane receptors. J Clin Invest 72:1185, 1983

14. Weiss ER, Kelleher DJ, Woon CW, et al: Receptor activation of G proteins. FASEB J 2:2841, 1988

15. Bristow MR, Ginsburg R, Minobe W, et al: Decreased catecholamine sensitivity and beta-adrenergic receptor density in failing human hearts. N Engl J Med 307:205, 1982

16. Bristow RM, Ginsburg R, Umans V, et al: Beta$_1$ and beta$_2$-adrenergic receptor subpopulations in non-failing and failing human ventricular myocardium: Coupling of both receptor subtypes to muscle contraction and selective beta$_1$ receptor down-regulation in heart failure. Circ Res 59:297, 1986

17. Gross F: Central alpha-adrenoreceptors in cardiovascular regulation. Chest (suppl.) 83(2):293, 1983

18. Bousquet P, Schwartz J: Alpha-adrenergic drugs. Pharmacologic tools for the study of central vasomotor control. Biochem Pharmacol 32:1459, 1983

19. Kiowski W, Hulthen UL, Ritz R, Buhler FR: Alpha 2 adrenoreceptor mediated vasoconstriction of arteries. Clin Pharmacol Ther 34:565, 1983

20. Jie K, van Brummelen P, Vermey P, et al: Identification of vascular post-synaptic alpha 1 and alpha 2 adrenoreceptors in man. Circ Res 54:447, 1984

21. Goldberg MR, Robertson D: Yohimbine. A pharmacological probe for the study of alpha 2 adrenoreceptors. Pharmacol Rev 35:143, 1983

22. Reid JL, Hamilton CA, Hannah JAM: Peripheral alpha 1 and alpha 2 adrenoreceptor mechanisms in blood pressure control. Chest (suppl.) 83(2):302, 1983

23. Minneman KP: Alpha$_1$-adrenergic receptor subtypes, inositol phosphates and sources of cell Ca^{++}. Pharmacol Rev 40:87, 1988

24. McGrath JC: The variety of vascular alpha adrenoreceptors. Trends Pharmacol Sci 4:13, 1983

25. Lokhandwala MF, De Feo ML, Cavero I: Physiological and pharmacological significance of dopamine receptors in the cardiovascular system. p. 115. In Saito H, et al (eds): Progress in Hypertension. Vol. 1. VNU Science, Zeist, The Netherlands, 1988

26. Lokhandwala MF: Cardiovascular and renal effects of dopamine receptor agonists. ISI Atlas of Science: Pharmacology 262, 1988

27. Leff SE, Creese I: Dopamine receptors re-explained. Trends Pharmacol Sci 4:463, 1983

28. Berkowitz BA: Dopamine and dopamine receptors as target sites for cardiovascular drug action. Fed Proc 42:3019, 1983

29. Shephard JT, Vanhoutte PM: Neurohumoral regulation. p. 107. The Human Cardiovascular System. New York, Raven Press, 1979

30. Wurtman RJ, Hefti F, Melamed G: Precursor control of neurotransmitter synthesis. Pharmacol Rev 32:315, 1981

31. Flacke WE, Flacke JE: Cholinergic and anticholinergic agents. p. 160. In Smith NT, Corbascio A (eds): Drug Interactions in Anesthesia, 2nd Ed. Lea & Febiger, Philadelphia, 1986

32. Higgins CB, Vatner SF, Braunwald E: Parasympathetic control of the heart. Pharmacol Rev 25:119, 1973

33. Dale HH: The action of certain esters and ethers of choline and their relation to muscarine. J Pharmacol 6:147, 1914

34. Taylor P: Ganglionic stimulating and blocking agents. p. 215. In Gilman AG, Goodman LS, Rall TW, Murad F (eds): Goodman and Gilman's Pharmacological Basis of Therapeutics. 7th Ed., Macmillan, New York, 1985

35. Rardon DP, Bailey JC: Parasympathetic effects on electrophysiologic properties of cardiac ventricular tissue. J Am Coll Cardiol 2:1200, 1983

36. Taylor P: Cholinergic agonists. p. 100. In Gilman AG, Goodman LS, Rall TW, Murad F (eds): Goodman and Gilman's Pharmacological Basis of Therapeutics. 7th Ed. Macmillan, New York, 1985

37. Weiner N: Atropine, scopolamine and related antimuscarinic drugs. p. 130. In Gilman AG, Goodman LS, Rall TW, Murad F (eds): Goodman and Gilman's Pharmacological Basis of Therapeutics. 7th Ed. Macmillan, New York, 1985

38. Mirakhur RK, Dundee JW, Clarke RSJ: Glycopyrrolate–neostigmine mixture for antagonism of neuromuscular block: Comparison with atropine–neostigmine mixture. Br J Anaesth 49:825, 1977

39. Baraka A, Yared J-P, Karam A-M, Winnie A: Glycopyrrolate–neostigmine and atropine–neostigmine mixtures affect post-anesthetic arousal times differently. Anesth Analg 59:431, 1980

40. Cromwell EB, Ketchum JS: The treatment of scopolamine-induced delirium with physostigmine. Clin Pharmacol Ther 8:409, 1967

41. Heiser JF, Wilbert DE: Reversal of delirium induced by tricyclic antidepressant drugs with physostigmine. Am J Psychiatry 131:1275, 1974

42. Bidwai AV, Stanley TH, Rogers C, et al: Reversal of diazepam-induced post-anesthetic somnolence with physostigmine. Anesthesiology 51:256, 1979

43. Vickers MD (ed): Proceedings of International Symposium on Flumazenil. Eur J Anesthesiol (Suppl 2), 1988

44. Weiner N: Norepinephrine, epinephrine and the sympathomimetic amines. p. 145. In Gilman AG, Goodman LS, Rall TW, Murad F (eds): Goodman and Gilman's Pharmacological Basis of Therapeutics. 7th Ed. Macmillan, New York, 1985

45. Thomas J, Fouad FM, Tarazi RC, et al: Evaluation of plasma catecholamines in humans. Correlation of resting levels with cardiac responses to beta-blocking and sympatholytic drugs. Hypertension 5:858, 1983

46. Best JD, Halter JB: Release and clearance rates of epinephrine in man: Importance of arterial measurements. J Clin Endocrinol Metab 55:263, 1982

47. Longnecker DE: Alpine anesthesia: Can pretreatment with clonidine decrease the peaks and valleys? Anesthesiology 67:1, 1987

48. Benfey BG: Cardiac adrenoceptors at low temperature and the adrenoceptor interconversion hypothesis. Br J Pharmacol 61:167, 1977

49. Osnes J-B, Refsum H, Skomedal T, et al: Qualitative differences between beta-adrenergic and alpha-adrenergic inotropic effects in rat heart muscle. Acta Pharmacol Toxicol 42:235, 1978

50. Shibata S, Seriguchi DG, Iwadare S, et al: The regional and species differences on the activation of myocardial alpha-adrenoreceptors by phenylephrine and methoxamine. Gen Pharmacol 11:173, 1980

51. Bohm M Diet F, Feiler G, et al: Alpha-adrenoceptors and alpha-adrenoceptor-mediated positive inotropic effects in failing human myocardium. J Cardiovasc Pharmacol 12:357, 1988

52. Weiner N: Drugs that inhibit adrenergic nerves and block

adrenergic receptors. p. 181. In Gilman AG, Goodman LS, Rall TW, Murad F (eds): Goodman and Gilman's Pharmacological Basis of Therapeutics. 7th Ed. Macmillan, New York, 1985

53. Stanaszek WF, Kellerman D, Brogden RN, et al: Prazosin update. A review of its pharmacological properties and therapeutic use in hypertension and congestive heart failure. Drugs 25:339, 1983

54. Modlinger RS, Ertel NH, Hauptman JV: Adrenergic blockade in pheochromocytoma. Arch Intern Med 143:2245, 1983

55. Graham RM: Selective alpha 1-adrenergic antagonists: Therapeutically relevant antihypertensive agents. Am J Cardiol 53:16A, 1984

56. Shanks RG: The clinical pharmacology of indoramin. J Cardiovasc Pharmacol 8:suppl. 2, S8, 1986

57. Archibald JL: Recent developments in the pharmacology and pharmacokinetics of indoramin. J Cardiovasc Pharmacol 8(suppl. 2):S20, 1986

58. Harron DWG: Experimental evidence for the antiarrhythmic action of indoramin. J Cardiovasc Pharmacol 8(suppl. 2):S131, 1986

59. Butrous GS, Camma J: Clinical cardiac electrophysiological assessment of indoramin. J Cardiovasc Pharmacol 8(suppl. 2):S137, 1986

60. Goldberg LI, Hsieh Y-Y, Resnekov L: Newer catecholamines for treatment of heart failure and shock: An update on dopamine and a first look at dobutamine. Prog Cardiovasc Dis 19:327, 1977

61. Leier CV, Unverferth DV: Dobutamine. Ann Intern Med 99:490, 1983

62. Jennings G, Bobik A, Oddie C, et al: Cardioselectivity of prenalterol and isoprotenerol. Clin Pharmacol Ther 34:749, 1983

63. Shand DG: State of the art: Comparative pharmacology of the beta adrenoreceptor blocking drugs. Drugs 25(suppl. 2):92, 1983

64. Heikkila J, Nieminen MS: Cardiac safety of acute beta blockade: Intrinsic sympathomimetic activity is superior to beta-1 selectivity. Am Heart J 104:464, 1982

65. McDevitt DG: Beta adrenoreceptor blocking drugs and partial agonist activity. Is it clinically relevant? Drugs 25:331, 1983

66. McDevitt DG: Clinical significance of cardioselectivity. State of the art. Drugs 25(suppl. 2):219, 1983

67. Leenen FHH, Chany K, Smith DL, Reeves RA: Epinephrine and left ventricular function in humans: Effect of beta-1 vs non-selective beta-blockade. Clin Pharmacol 43:519, 1988

68. Kjekshus JK: Importance of heart rate in determining beta-blocker efficacy in acute and long-term acute myocardial infarction intervention trials. Am J Cardiol 57:43F, 1986

69. International Collaborative Study Group: Acute myocardial infarct size reduction by timolol administration. Am J Cardiol 57:28F, 1986

70. Rude RE, Buja LM, Willerson JT (MILIS Study Group): Propranolol in acute myocardial infarction: the MILIS experience. Am J Cardiol 57:38F, 1986

71. Reid JL, Whyte KF, Struthers AD: Epinephrine-induced hypokalemia: The role of beta-adrenoreceptors. Am J Cardiol 57:23F, 1986

72. Frishman WH: Clinical differences between beta-adrenergic blocking agents: Implications for therapeutic substitution. Am Heart J 113:1190, 1987

73. Riddell JG, Harron DWG, Shanks RG: Clinical pharmacokinetics of beta-adrenoreceptor antagonists and update. Clin Pharmacokinet 12:305, 1987

74. Smulyan H, Weinberg SE, Howanitz PJ: Continuous propranolol infusion following abdominal surgery. JAMA 247:2539, 1982

75. Hug CC, McDonald DH, Kaplan JA: Propranolol infusion after abdominal surgery (letter). JAMA 249:22, 1983

76. Villers D, Pinaud MLJ, Bourin M, et al: Propranolol postoperative maintenance by continuous intravenous infusion. Anesthesiology 60:594, 1984

77. Benfield P, Clissold SP, Verogden RN: Metoprolol: An updated review of its pharmacodynamic and pharmacokinetic properties, etc. Drugs 31:376,1986

78. Carter BL: Labetalol. Drug Intell Clin Pharm 17:704, 1983

79. Wallin JD, O'Neill WM: Labetalol. Current research and therapeutic status. Arch Intern Med 143:485, 1983

80. Michelson EL, Frishman WH: Labetalol: An alpha and beta adrenoreceptor blocking drug. Ann Intern Med 99:553, 1983

81. Benfield P, Sorkin EM: Esmolol: A preliminary review of its pharmacodynamic and pharmacokinetic properties and therapeutic efficacy. Drugs 33:392, 1987

82. Singh BN, Jewett DE: Beta adrenergic receptor blocking drugs in cardiac arrhythmias. Drugs 7:426, 1974

83. Ikezono E, Yasuda K, Hattori Y: Effects of propranolol on epinephrine-induced arrhythmias during halothane anesthesia in man and cats. Anesth Analg 48:598, 1969

84. Scheidt S: Beta blockade for angina and arrhythmias. Present status. Drugs 25(suppl. 2):153, 1983

85. Kahn AK: Beta adrenorecptor blocking agents. Their role in reducing chances of recurrent infarction and death. Arch Intern Med 143:1759, 1983

86. Slogoff S, Keats AS: Does chronic treatment with calcium entry blocking drugs reduce peri-operative myocardial ischemia? Anesthesiology 68:676, 1988

87. Chung F, Huston PL, Cheng DCH, et al: Calcium channel blockade does not offer adequate protection from peri-operative myocardial ischemia. Anesthesiology 69:343, 1988

88. Stone JG, Foex P, Sear JW, et al: Myocardial ischemia in untreated hypertensive patients: Effect of a single small oral dose of a beta-adrenergic blocking agent. Anesthesiology 68:495, 1988

89. McDevitt DG: Adrenoreceptor blocking drugs: Clinical pharmacology and therapeutic use. Drugs 17:267, 1979

90. Kincaid-Smith P: Beta-adrenergic receptor blocking drugs in hypertension. With special reference to their use as initial therapy. Am J Cardiol 53:12A, 1984

91. Lee TC, Coffey RJ, Currier BM, et al: Propranolol and thyroidectomy in the treatment of thyrotoxicosis. Ann Surg 195:766, 1982

92. Tattersfield AE, Harrison RN: Effect of beta blocker therapy on airway function. Drugs 25(suppl. 2):227, 1983

93. Cohn JN: Hemodynamic effects of beta blockers. Drugs 25(suppl. 2):100, 1983

94. Hansten PD: Beta blocking agents and antidiabetic drugs. Drug Intell Clin Pharm 14:46, 1980

95. Rizza RA, Cryer PE, Haymond MW, et al: Adrenergic mechanisms of catecholamine action on glucose homeostasis in man. Metabolism 29:1155, 1980

96. Lewis JG: Adverse reactions to calcium antagonists. Drugs 25:196, 1983

97. Oesterle SN, Schroeder JS: Editorial: Calcium-entry blockade, beta-adrenergic blockade and the reflex control of circulation. Circulation 65:669, 1982

98. Lokhandwala MF: Pre-clinical and clinical studies on the cardiovascular and renal effects of fenoldopam: A DA-1 receptor agonist. Drug Devel Res 10:123, 1987

99. Caritis SN, Edelstone DI, Mueller-Heubach E: Pharmaco-

logic inhibition of preterm labor. Am J Obstet Gynecol 133:557, 1979

100. Wagner JM, Morton MJ, Johnson KA, et al: Terbutaline and maternal cardiac function. JAMA 246:2697, 1981

101. Wang RYC, Lee PK, Yu DYC, et al: Terbutaline infusion in cardiogenic shock: Acute hemodynamic effects and clinical response. J Clin Pharmacol 23:355, 1983

102. Merin RG, Tonnesen AS: Cardiovascular effects of drug interactions between anesthetics and cardiovascular medications. p. 224. In Altura BM, Halevy S (eds): Cardiovascular Actions of Anesthetics and Drugs Used in Anesthesia 1. Basic Aspects. S Karger, Basel, 1986

103. Finnerty FA, Brogben RN: guanadrel: A review of its pharmacodynamic and pharmacokinetic properties in therapeutic use in hypertension. Drugs 30:21, 1985

104. Miller ED: New concepts of blood pressure control and treatment. p. 379. In Kaplan JA (ed): Cardiac Anesthesia. Vol 2: Cardiovascular Pharmacology. Grune & Stratton, New York, 1983

105. Robertson JIS, Tillman DM: Converting enzyme inhibitors in the treatment of hypertension. J Cardiovasc Pharmacol 10(suppl. 7):S43, 1987

106. Packer M: Converting enzyme-inhibition in the management of severe chronic congestive heart failure: Physiologic concepts. J Cardiovasc Pharmacol 10(suppl. 7):S83, 1987

107. Dzau BJ: Vascular angiotensin pathways: A new therapeutic target. J Cardiovasc Pharmacol 10(suppl. 7):S9, 1987

108. Beart PM, Rowe PR, Louis WJ: Alphamethyl adrenaline is a central metabolite of alpha methyldopa. J Pharm Pharmacol 35:519, 1980

109. Tung C-S, Goldberg MR, Hollister AS, et al: Central and peripheral cardiovascular effects of alpha methyl epinephrine. J Pharmacol 227:484, 1983

110. Triner L, Baer L, Gallagher R, et al: Use of metyrosine in the anesthetic management of patients with catecholamine-secreting tumors. Br J Anaesth 54:1333, 1982

111. Ghignone M, Calvillo O, Quintin L: Anesthesia and hypertension: The effects of clonidine on peri-operative hemodynamics and isoflurane requirements. Anesthesiology 67:3, 1987

112. Ghignone M, Noe C, Calvillo O, Quintin L: Anesthesia for ophthalmic surgery in the elderly: The effects of clonidine on intraocular pressure, peri-operative hemodynamics and anesthetic requirements. Anesthesiology 68:707, 1988

113. Flacke JW, Bloor BC, Flacke WE, et al: Reduced narcotic requirement by clonidine with improved hemodynamic and adrenergic stability in patients undergoing coronary bypass surgery. Anesthesiology 67:11, 1987

114. Maze M, Vickery RG, Merlone SC, Gaba DM: Anesthetic and hemodynamic effects of the alpha$_2$-adrenergic agonist Aze-

pexole in isoflurane-anesthetized dogs. Anesthesiology 68:689, 1988

115. Ragno RE: Propranolol withdrawal—Practical consideration. Arch Intern Med 141:161, 1981

116. Houston MC: Abrupt cessation of treatment in hypertension: Consideration of clinical features, mechanisms, prevention and management of the discontinuation syndrome. Am Heart J 102:415, 1981

117. Roizen MF: Anesthetic implications of concurrent diseases: Patients given drug therapy for chronic and acute medical conditions. p. 331. In Miller RD (ed.): Anesthesia. 2nd Ed. Churchill Livingstone, New York, 1986

118. El-Ganzouri AR, Ivankovich AD, Braverman B, McCarthy R: Monamine oxidase inhibitors: Should they be discontinued preoperatively? Anesth Analg 64:592, 1985

119. Stack CG, Rogers P, Linters PK: Monamine oxidase inhibitors in anesthesia. A review. Br J Anaesth 60:222, 1988

120. Wells DG, Bjorksten AR: Monamine oxidase inhibitors revisited. Can J Anaesth 36:64, 1989

121. Harrison L, Ralley FE, Wynands JE, et al: The role of an ultrashort-acting adrenergic blocker (esmolol) in patients undergoing coronary artery bypass surgery. Anesthesiology 66:413, 1987

122. Girard D, Shulman BJ, Thys DM, et al: The safety and efficacy of esmolol during myocardial revascularization. Anesthesiology 65:157, 1986

123. Newsome LR, Roth JV, Hug CC, Nagle D: Esmolol attenuates hemodynamic responses during fentanyl-pancuronium anesthesia for aortocoronary bypass surgery. Anesth Analg 65:451, 1986

124. Butterworth JF, Piccione W, Berrizbeitia LD, et al: Augmentation of venous return by adrenergic agonists during spinal anesthesia. Anesth Analg 65:612, 1986

125. Colucci WS, Wright RF, Braunwald E: New positive inotropic agents in the treatment of congestive heart failure. Part II. N Engl J Med 314:349, 1986

126. Leslie JB, Kalaygian RW, Sirgo MA, et al: Intravenous labetalol for treatment of postoperative hypertension. Anesthesiology 67:413, 1987

127. Roizen MF: Should we all have a sympathectomy at birth? Or at least preoperatively? Anesthesiology 68:482, 1988

128. Heinsimer J, Lefkowitz KJ: Hosp Pract, 18(11):115, 1983

129. Ram CVS, Kaplan NM: Alpha- and beta-receptor blocking drugs in the treatment of hypertension. Cur Probl Cardiol, 1979

130. Larsell O: Anatomy of the Nervous System. 2nd Ed. Appleton-Century-Crofts, East Norwalk, CT, 1951

131. Anson BJ (ed): Morris' Human Anatomy. McGraw Hill, New York, 1966

15
RESPIRATORY PHYSIOLOGY AND RESPIRATORY FUNCTION DURING ANESTHESIA

Jonathan L. Benumof

RESPIRATORY PHYSIOLOGY

Introduction

Understanding normal respiratory physiology is a prerequisite to understanding mechanisms of impaired gas exchange during anesthesia and surgery. Toward this end, the normal (gravity-determined) distribution of perfusion and ventilation, the major nongravitational determinants of resistance to perfusion and ventilation, the transport of the respiratory gases, and the pulmonary reflexes and special functions are presented first in this chapter. These processes and concepts are then discussed in regard to the general mechanisms of impaired gas exchange during anesthesia and surgery.

Normal (Gravity-Determined) Distribution of Perfusion, Ventilation, and the Ventilation/ Perfusion Ratio

Distribution of Pulmonary Perfusion

Contraction of the right ventricle imparts kinetic energy to the blood in the main pulmonary artery. As the kinetic energy in the main pulmonary artery is dissipated in climbing a vertical hydrostatic gradient, the absolute pressure in the pulmonary artery (Ppa) decreases 1 cmH$_2$O per cm of vertical distance up the lung (Fig. 15-1). At some height above the heart, Ppa becomes zero (atmospheric), and still higher in the lung, the Ppa becomes negative.[1] In this region, alveolar pressure (PA) then exceeds Ppa and pulmonary venous pressure (Ppv), which is very negative at this vertical height. Since the pressure outside the vessels is greater than the pressure inside the vessels, the vessels in this

region of the lung are collapsed and there is no blood flow (zone 1, PA > Ppa > Ppv). Since there is no blood flow, no gas exchange is possible, and the region functions as alveolar dead space or "wasted" ventilation. Little or no zone 1 exists in the lung under normal conditions, but the amount of zone 1 lung may be greatly increased if Ppa is reduced, as in oligemic shock, or if PA is increased, as in positive-pressure ventilation.

Further down the lung, absolute Ppa becomes positive, and blood flow will begin when Ppa exceeds PA (zone 2, Ppa > PA > Ppv). At this vertical level in the lung, PA exceeds Ppv, and blood flow is determined by the mean Ppa − PA difference rather than the more conventional Ppa − Ppv difference (see below).[2] The zone 2 blood flow–alveolar pressure relationship has the same physical characteristics as a river waterfall flowing over a dam. The height of the upstream river (before reaching the dam) is equivalent to Ppa, and the height of the dam is equivalent to PA. The rate of water flow over the dam is only proportional to the difference between the height of the upstream river and the dam (Ppa − PA), and it does not matter how far below the dam the downstream river bed (Ppv) is. This phenome-

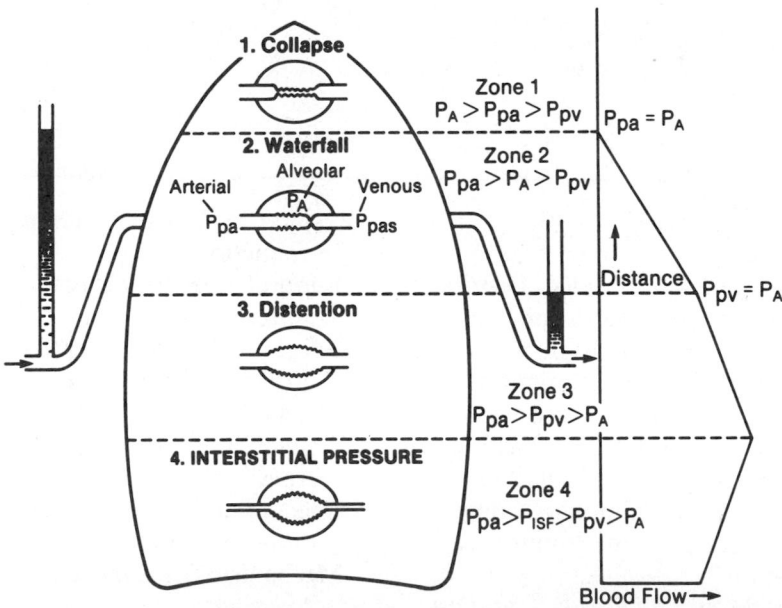

The Four Zones of the Lung

Fig. 15-1. Schematic diagram showing distribution of blood flow in the upright lung. In zone 1, alveolar pressure (PA) exceeds pulmonary artery pressure (Ppa) and no flow occurs because the intra-alveolar vessels are collapsed by the compressing alveolar pressure. In zone 2, arterial pressure exceeds alveolar pressure, but alveolar pressure exceeds venous pressure (Ppv). Flow in zone 2 is determined by the arterial-alveolar pressure difference (Ppa − PA) and has been likened to an upstream river waterfall over a dam. Since Ppa increases down zone 2 and PA remains constant, the perfusion pressure increases, and flow steadily increases down the zone. In zone 3, pulmonary venous pressure exceeds alveolar pressure, and flow is determined by the arterial-venous pressure difference (Ppa − Ppv), which is constant down this portion of the lung. However, the transmural pressure across the wall of the vessel increases down this zone so that the caliber of the vessels increases (resistance decreases) and therefore flow increases. Finally, in zone 4, pulmonary interstitial pressure becomes positive and exceeds both pulmonary venous pressure and alveolar pressure. Consequently, flow in zone 4 is determined by the arterial-interstitial pressure difference (Ppa − PISF). (Modified from West,[11] with permission.)

non has various names, including the waterfall, Starling resistor, weir (dam made by beavers), and "sluice" effect. Since mean Ppa increases down this region of the lung but mean PA is relatively constant, the mean driving pressure (Ppa − PA) increases linearly, and therefore mean blood flow increases linearly. However, respiration and pulmonary blood flow are cyclic phenomena. Therefore, absolute instantaneous Ppa, Ppv, and PA are changing all the time and the relationships between Ppa, Ppv, and PA are dynamically determined by the phase lags between the cardiac and respiratory cycles. Consequently, a given point in zone 2 may actually be in either a zone 1 or zone 3 condition at a given moment depending on whether the patient is in respiratory systole or diastole or in cardiac systole or diastole.

Still lower in the lung there is a vertical level where Ppv becomes positive and also exceeds PA. In this region, blood flow is governed by the pulmonary arteriovenous pressure difference (Ppa − Ppv) (zone 3, Ppa > Ppv > PA), for in this zone, both of these vascular pressures exceed the PA and the capillary systems are thus permanently open and blood flow is continuous. In descending zone 3, gravity causes both absolute Ppa and Ppv to increase at the same rate so that the perfusion pressure (Ppa − Ppv) is unchanged. However, the pressure outside the vessels, namely, pleural pressure (Ppl), increases less than Ppa and Ppv so that the transmural distending pressures (Ppa − Ppl and Ppv − Ppl) increase down zone 3, the vessel radii increase, vascular resistance decreases, and blood flow therefore increases further.

Finally, whenever pulmonary vascular pressures are extremely high, as they would be in a severely volume-overloaded patient, in a severely restricted and constricted pulmonary vascular bed, in an extremely dependent lung (far below the vertical level of the left atrium), and in patients with pulmonary embolism and mitral stenosis, fluid may transudate out of the pulmonary vessels into the pulmonary interstitial compartment. Transudated pulmonary interstitial fluid may significantly alter the distribution of pulmonary blood flow.

When the flow of fluid into the interstitial space is excessive and cannot be cleared adequately by lymphatics, it will accumulate in the interstitial connective tissue compartment around the large vessels and airways, forming peribronchial and periarteriolar edema fluid cuffs. The transudated pulmonary interstitial fluid fills the pulmonary interstitial space and may eliminate the normally present negative and radially expanding interstitial tension on the extra-alveolar pulmonary vessels. The expansion of the pulmonary interstitial space by fluid causes pulmonary interstitial pressure (PISF) to become positive and exceed Ppv (zone 4, Ppa > PISF > Ppv > PA).[3,4] In addition, the vascular resistance of extra-alveolar vessels may be increased at a very low lung volume (i.e., the residual volume), at which the tethering action of the pulmonary tissue on

the vessels is also lost, causing PISF to increase positively (see lung volume discussion below).[5,6] Consequently, zone 4 blood flow is governed by the arteriointerstitial pressure difference (Ppa − PISF), which is less than the Ppa − Ppv difference, and therefore zone 4 blood flow is less than zone 3 blood flow. In summary, zone 4 is a region of the lung that has transudated a large amount of fluid into the pulmonary interstitial compartment or is possibly at a very low lung volume. Both these circumstances produce a positive interstitial pressure, causing extra-alveolar vessel compression, increased extra-alveolar vascular resistance, and decreased regional blood flow.

It should be evident that as Ppa and Ppv increase, three important changes take place in the pulmonary circulation, namely, recruitment or opening of previously unperfused vessels, distention or widening of previously perfused vessels, and transudation of fluid from very distended vessels.[7,8] Thus, as mean Ppa increases, zone 1 arteries may become zone 2 arteries, and as mean Ppv increases, zone 2 veins may become zone 3 veins. The increase in both mean Ppa and Ppv distends zone 3 vessels according to their compliance and decreases the resistance to flow through them. Zone 3 vessels may become so distended that they leak fluid and become converted to zone 4 vessels. In general, recruitment is the principal change as Ppa and Ppv increase from low to moderate levels; distention is the principal change as Ppa and Ppv increase from moderate to high levels of vascular pressure; and finally, transudation is the principal change when Ppa and Ppv increase from high to very high levels.

Distribution of Ventilation

Gravity also causes vertical Ppl differences that cause, in turn, regional alveolar volume, compliance, and ventilation differences. The vertical gradient of Ppl can be best understood by imagining the lung as a plastic bag filled with semifluid contents; in other words, it is a viscoelastic structure. Without the presence of a supporting chest wall, the effect of gravity on the contents of the bag would cause the bag to bulge outward at the bottom and inward at the top (it would assume a globular shape). With the lung inside the supporting chest wall, the lung cannot assume a globular shape. However, gravity still exerts a force on the lung to assume a globular shape; the force creates a relatively more negative pressure at the top of the pleural space (where the lung pulls away from the chest wall) and a relatively more positive pressure at the bottom of the lung (where the lung is compressed against the chest wall) (Fig. 15-2). The magnitude of this pressure gradient is determined by the density of the lung. Since the lung is about one-fourth of the density of water, the gradient of Ppl (in cmH_2O) will be about one-fourth of the height of the upright lung (30 cm). Thus, Ppl increases positively by $30/4 = 7.5$ cmH_2O from the top to the bottom of the lung.[9]

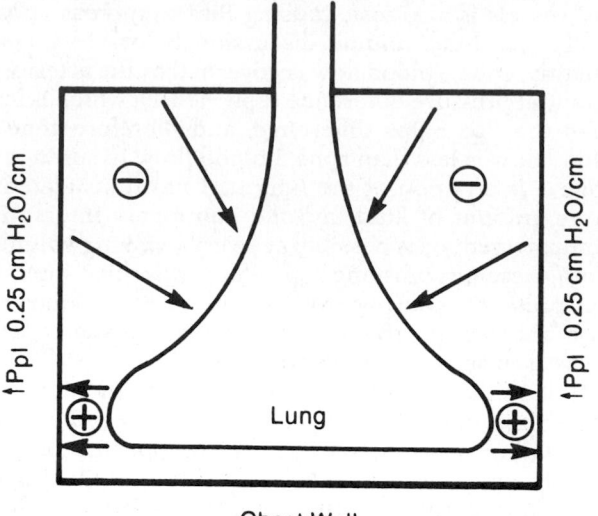

Fig. 15-2. Schematic diagram of the lung within the chest wall showing the tendency of the lung to assume a globular shape owing to the lung's viscoelastic nature. The tendency of the top of the lung to collapse inward creates a relatively negative pressure at the apex of the lung, and the tendency of the bottom of the lung to spread outward creates a relatively positive pressure at the base of the lung. Thus, pleural pressure increases by 0.25 cm H_2O per centimeter of lung dependency.

Since P_A is the same throughout the lung, the Ppl gradient causes regional differences in transpulmonary distending pressures ($P_A - Ppl$). Since Ppl is most positive (least negative) in the dependent basilar lung regions, alveoli in these regions are more compressed and therefore considerably smaller than superior, relatively noncompressed apical alveoli (there is an approximately fourfold volume difference).[10] If the regional differences in alveolar volume are translated over to a pressure–volume curve for normal lung (Fig. 15-3), the dependent small alveoli are on the mid-portion and the nondependent large alveoli are on the upper portion of the S-shaped pressure–volume curve. Since the different regional slopes of the composite curve are equal to the different regional lung compliances, dependent alveoli are relatively compliant (steep slope) and nondependent alveoli are relatively noncompliant (flat slope). Thus, most of the tidal volume is preferentially distributed to dependent alveoli, since they expand more per unit pressure change than nondependent alveoli.

Distribution of the Ventilation/Perfusion Ratio

Both blood flow and ventilation (both on the left-hand vertical axis of Fig. 15-4) increase linearly with distance down the normal upright lung (horizontal axis, reverse polarity).[11] Since blood flow increases from a very low value and more rapidly than ventilation with distance down the lung, the ventilation/perfusion ($\dot{V}_A/\dot{Q}$) ratio

(right-hand vertical axis) decreases rapidly at first and then more slowly.

The $\dot{V}_A/\dot{Q}$ ratio best expresses the amount of ventilation relative to perfusion in any given lung region. Thus, alveoli at the base of the lung are somewhat overperfused in relation to their ventilation ($\dot{V}_A/\dot{Q} < 1$). Figure 15-5 shows the calculated ventilation ($\dot{V}_A$) and blood flow ($\dot{Q}$) in liters per minute, the $\dot{V}_A/\dot{Q}$ ratio, and the alveolar PO_2 (P_AO_2) and PCO_2 (P_ACO_2) in mmHg for horizontal slices from the top (7 percent of lung volume), middle (11 percent of lung volume), and bottom (13 percent of lung volume) of the lung.[12] The P_AO_2 increases by more than 40 mmHg from 89 mmHg at the base to 132 mmHg at the apex, while PCO_2 decreases by 14 mmHg from 42 mmHg at the bottom to 28 mmHg at the top. Thus, in keeping with the regional $\dot{V}_A/\dot{Q}$, the bottom of the lung is relatively hypoxic and hypercarbic compared with the top of the lung.

Ventilation to perfusion inequalities have different effects on $PaCO_2$ compared with PaO_2. Blood passing through underventilated alveoli tends to retain its CO_2 and does not take up enough O_2; blood traversing overventilated alveoli gives off an excessive amount of CO_2 but cannot take up a proportionately increased amount of O_2 owing to the flatness of the oxyhemoglobin dissociation curve in this region (see Fig. 15-25). Hence, a lung with uneven ventilation to perfusion relationships can eliminate CO_2 from the overventilated alveoli to compensate for the underventilated alveoli. Thus, with uneven ventilation to perfusion relationships, P_ACO_2 to $PaCO_2$ gradients are small and P_AO_2 to PaO_2 gradients are usually large.

Recently, Wagner and colleagues[13] described a method of determining the continuous distribution of $\dot{V}_A/\dot{Q}$ ratios within the lung based on the pattern of elimination of a series of intravenously infused inert gases. Gases of differing solubility are dissolved in physiologic saline solution and infused into a peripheral vein until a steady state is achieved (20 minutes). Toward the end of the infusion period, samples of arterial and mixed expired gas are collected, and total ventilation and cardiac output are measured. For each gas, the ratio of arterial to mixed venous concentration (retention) and the ratio of expired to mixed venous concentration (excretion) are calculated, and retention-solubility and excretion-solubility curves are drawn. The retention- and excretion-solubility curves can be regarded as fingerprints of the particular distribution of ventilation/perfusion ratios that give rise to them.

Figure 15-6 shows the type of distributions found in young normal subjects breathing air in the semirecumbent position.[14] The distributions of both ventilation and blood flow are relatively narrow. The upper and lower 95 percent limits shown (vertical interrupted lines) correspond to $\dot{V}_A/\dot{Q}$ ratios of 0.3 and 2.1, respectively. Note that these young normal subjects had no blood flow perfusing areas with very low $\dot{V}_A/\dot{Q}$ ratios nor did they have any flood flow to unventilated or shunted areas ($\dot{V}_A/\dot{Q} = 0$) or unperfused areas ($\dot{V}_A/\dot{Q} =$

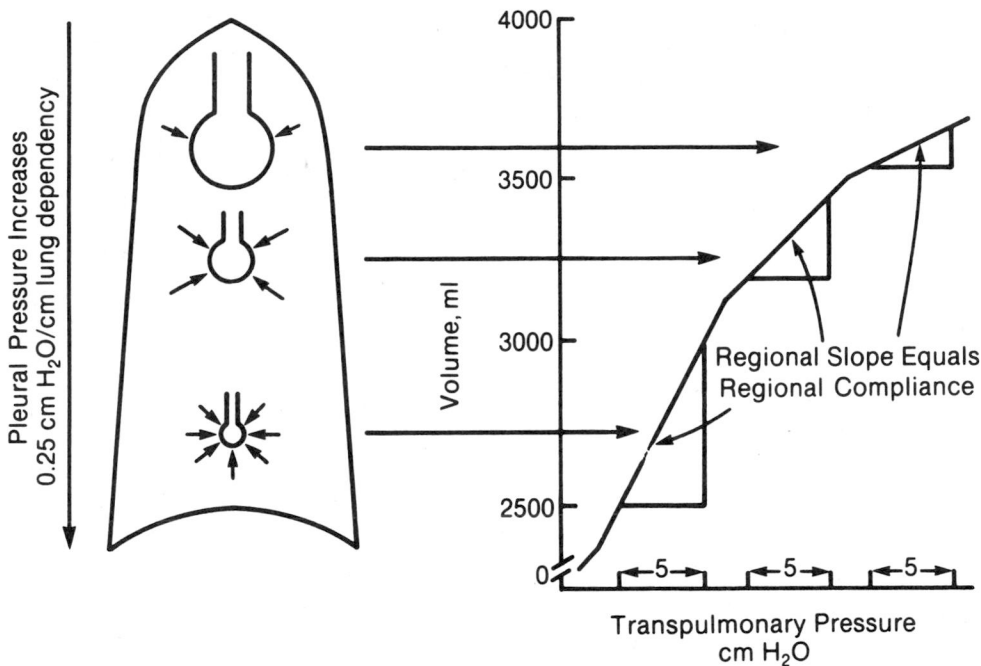

Fig. 15-3. Pleural pressure increases 0.25 cmH$_2$O every centimeter down the lung. The increase in pleural pressure causes a fourfold decrease in alveolar volume. The caliber of the air passages also decreases as lung volume decreases. When regional alveolar volume is translated over to a regional transpulmonary pressure-alveolar volume curve, small alveoli are on a steep (large slope) portion of the curve, and large alveoli are on a flat (small slope) portion of the curve. Since the regional slope equals regional compliance, the dependent small alveoli normally receive the largest share of the tidal volume. Over the normal tidal volume range (lung volume increases by 500 ml from 2,500 ml [normal FRC] to 3,000 ml), the pressure-volume relationship is linear. Lung volume values in this diagram relate to the upright position.

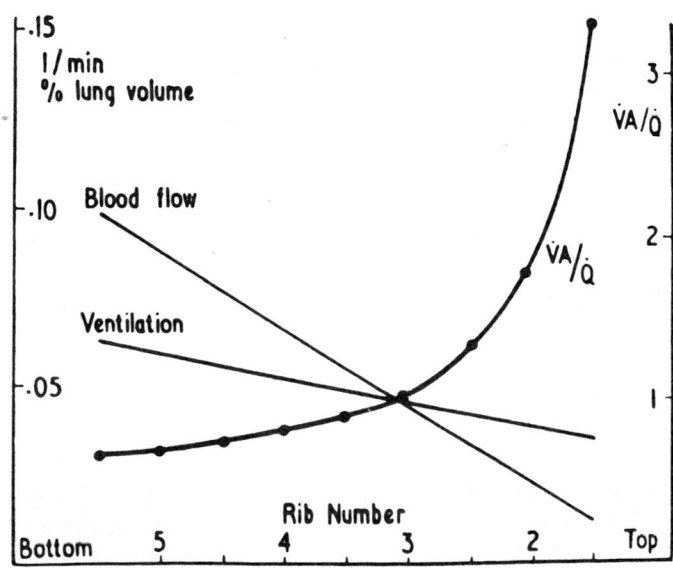

Fig. 15-4. Distribution of ventilation and blood flow (left-hand vertical axis) and the ventilation/perfusion ratio (right-hand vertical axis) in normal upright lung. Both blood flow and ventilation are expressed in L/min/percent alveolar volume and have been drawn as smoothed-out linear functions of vertical height. The closed circles mark the ventilation/perfusion ratios of horizontal lung slices (three of which are shown in Fig. 15-5). A cardiac output of 6 L/min and a total minute ventilation of 5.1 L/min was assumed. (From West,[11] with permission.)

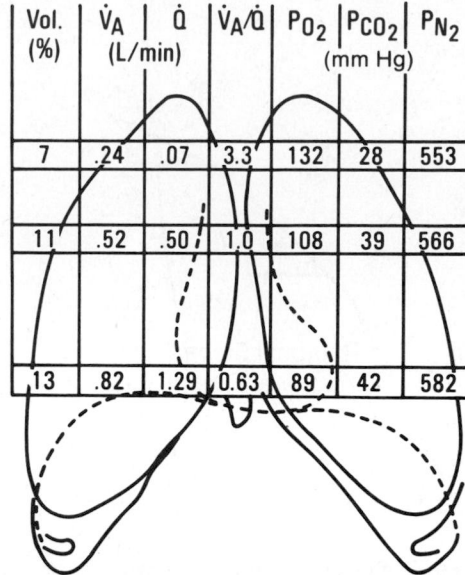

Vol. (%)	$\dot{V}_A$ (L/min)	$\dot{Q}$	$\dot{V}_A/\dot{Q}$	P_{O_2}	P_{CO_2} (mm Hg)	P_{N_2}
7	.24	.07	3.3	132	28	553
11	.52	.50	1.0	108	39	566
13	.82	1.29	0.63	89	42	582

Fig. 15-5. The ventilation/perfusion ratio ($\dot{V}_A/\dot{Q}$) and the regional composition of alveolar gas. Values for the regional flow ($\dot{Q}$), ventilation ($\dot{V}_A$), P_{O_2}, and P_{CO_2} were derived from Figure 15-4. P_{N_2} was obtained by what remains from the total gas pressure (which, including water vapor, equals 760 mmHg). The volumes [Vol. (%)] of the three lung slices are also shown. Compared with the top of the lung, the bottom of the lung has a low ventilation/perfusion ratio and is relatively hypoxic and hypercarbic. (From West,[12] with permission.)

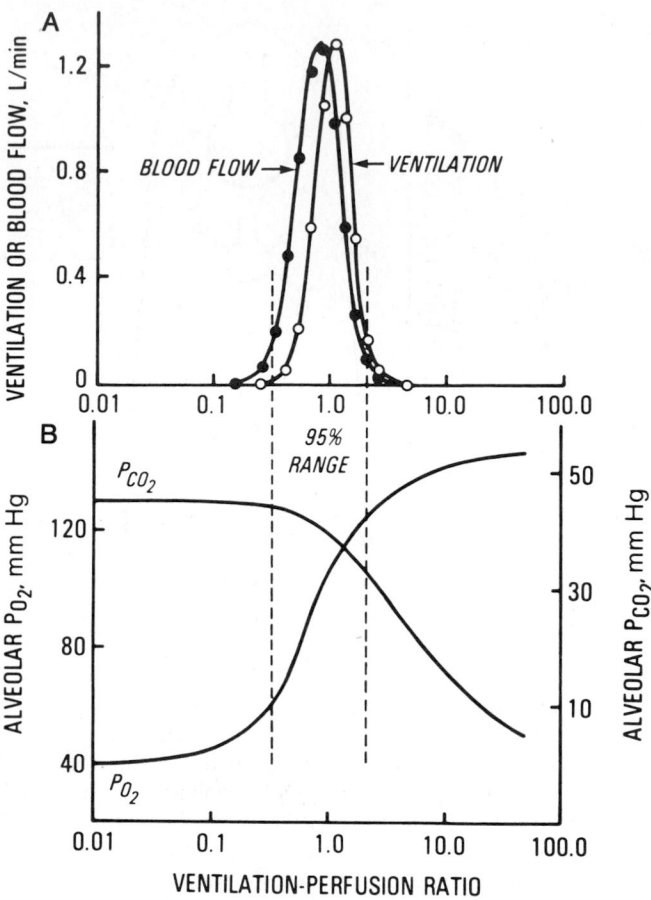

Fig. 15-6. **(A)** The average distribution of ventilation/perfusion ratios in young semirecumbent normal subjects. The 95 percent range covers ventilation/perfusion ratios from 0.3 to 2.1 (between dashed lines). **(B)** The corresponding variations of P_{O_2} and P_{CO_2} in the alveolar gas. (From West,[14] with permission.)

∞). Figure 15-6 also shows P_{AO_2} and P_{ACO_2} in respiratory units having different $\dot{V}_A/\dot{Q}$ ratios. Within the 95 percent range of $\dot{V}_A/\dot{Q}$ ratios (0.3 to 2.1), the P_{O_2} ranges from 60 to 123 mmHg while the corresponding P_{CO_2} range is 44 to 33 mmHg.

Other (Nongravitational) Important Determinants of Pulmonary Vascular Resistance and Blood Flow Distribution

Cardiac Output

As cardiac output ($\dot{Q}_t$) increases, pulmonary vascular pressures increase (Fig. 15-7).[15] Since the pulmonary vasculature is distensible, an increase in Ppa increases the radius of the pulmonary vessels, causing pulmonary vascular resistance to decrease. Exactly the opposite effect applies to the passive effect of a decrease in $\dot{Q}_T$ on the pulmonary circulation. As $\dot{Q}_T$ decreases, pulmonary vascular pressures decrease. The decrease in pulmonary vascular pressure reduces the radii of the pulmonary vessels, causing pulmonary vascular resistance to increase.

Understanding the relationship among Ppa, pulmonary vascular resistance, and cardiac output during passive events is a prerequisite to recognition of active vasomotion in the pulmonary circulation. Active vasoconstriction occurs whenever cardiac output decreases and Ppa either remains constant or increases.

Increased Ppa and pulmonary vascular resistance have been found to be "a universal feature of acute respiratory failure."[16] Active pulmonary vasoconstriction can increase Ppa and Ppv, thereby contributing to the formation of pulmonary edema, and in that way has a role in the genesis of the adult respiratory distress syndrome. Active vasodilation occurs any time cardiac output increases and Ppa either remains constant or decreases. When deliberate hypotension is achieved with sodium nitroprusside, cardiac output often remains constant or increases, but Ppa decreases and, therefore, so does pulmonary vascular resistance.

Alveolar Hypoxia

Alveolar or environmental hypoxia of in vivo and in vitro whole lung, unilateral lung, lobe, or lobule of lung causes localized pulmonary vasoconstriction. This phenomenon is called hypoxic pulmonary vasoconstriction (HPV) and is present in all mammalian species.

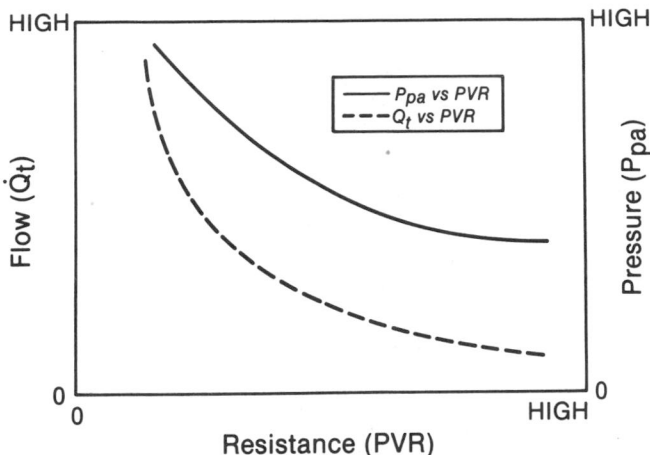

Fig. 15-7. Passive changes in pulmonary vascular resistance (PVR) as a function of pulmonary artery pressure (Ppa) and pulmonary blood flow ($\dot{Q}T$) (PVR = Ppa/$\dot{Q}T$). As flow increases, pulmonary artery pressure also increases but to a lesser extent, so that resistance decreases. As flow decreases, pulmonary artery pressure also decreases but to a lesser extent, so that resistance increases. (From Fishman,[15] with permission.)

The HPV response occurs primarily in the pulmonary arterioles of about 200-μm diameter. These vessels are advantageously situated anatomically in very close relation to the small bronchioles and alveoli, which permits rapid and direct detection of alveolar hypoxia. Indeed, blood may actually become oxygenated in small pulmonary arteries owing to the ability of oxygen to diffuse directly across the small distance between the contiguous air spaces and vessels.[17] This direct access that gas in the airways has to small arteries makes possible a very rapid and localized vascular response to changes in gas composition.

There are two major theories how alveolar hypoxia may cause pulmonary vasoconstriction.[18-22] First, alveolar hypoxia may cause the release of vasoconstrictor substance(s) into the pulmonary interstitial compartment where the substance(s) may then cause vasoconstriction. In the past 10 years, many vasoactive substances have been proposed as the mediators of HPV (e.g., leukotrienes, prostaglandins, catecholamines, serotonin, histamine, angiotensin, and bradykinin), but none has been proved to be involved primarily in the process.

Although the precise mediator of HPV is not known, it is certain that the prostaglandin products of arachidonic acid metabolism can inhibit the HPV response, and it is very possible that the leukotriene products of arachidonic acid metabolism mediate, or are at least required for, the HPV response. The general scheme of arachidonic acid metabolism is shown in Figure 15-8. Upon an appropriate stimulus, such as alveolar hypoxia, phospholipase A_2 converts the phospholipid in the cell membrane (possible in all 40 lung cell types)[23] to arachidonic acid. The released arachidonic acid can be metabolized in two ways. First, the enzyme cyclo-ox-

ygenase can convert arachidonic acid to prostaglandins; the major prostaglandin is prostaglandin I_2(prostacyclin).[24,25] Prostacyclin is a potent pulmonary vasodilator that can abolish HPV.[24,25] The cyclo-oxygenase pathway can also produce thromboxane; this product is not shown in Figure 15-8 because it is thought not to be important with regard to HPV.[26,27] Second, the enzyme lipoxygenase can convert arachidonic acid to leukotrienes. All the leukotrienes are potent pulmonary vasoconstrictors and can enhance HPV; indeed, the leukotrienes have received considerable attention as the mediator of HPV.[27] The amount of pulmonary vasoconstriction caused by hypoxia is regulated by a balance between leukotriene agonist and prostaglandin antagonist effects.

There are many experimental data that support and are consistent with the above relationship between the products of arachidonic acid metabolism and HPV (Fig. 15-8). Blockage of cyclo-oxygenase with acetylsalicylic acid,[25,28-30] indomethacin,[28-31] meclofenamate,[32,33] or ibuprofen[34,35] results in increased HPV (predominence of leukotrienes). Infusion of prostaglandins[36] and prostacyclin[37] during regional HPV and prostacyclin during regional pneumonia[28,31,38,39] decreases HPV (predominance of prostaglandins). Blockage of lipoxygenase results in decreased HPV (predominance of prostaglandins).[40-42] Blockage of leukotriene receptors with FPL 55713 causes decreased HPV (predominance of prostaglandins).[25,43,44] If both the cyclo-oxygenase-prostaglandin and the lipoxygenase-leukotriene systems were inhibited (as with BW755C), but the cyclo-oxygenase-prostaglandin system was inhibited to a greater extent (resulting in predominence of leukotrienes), then HPV was increased.[45] If cyclo-oxygenase is already blocked by ibuprofen, then the addition of BW755C relatively selectively blocks lipoxygenase (rel-

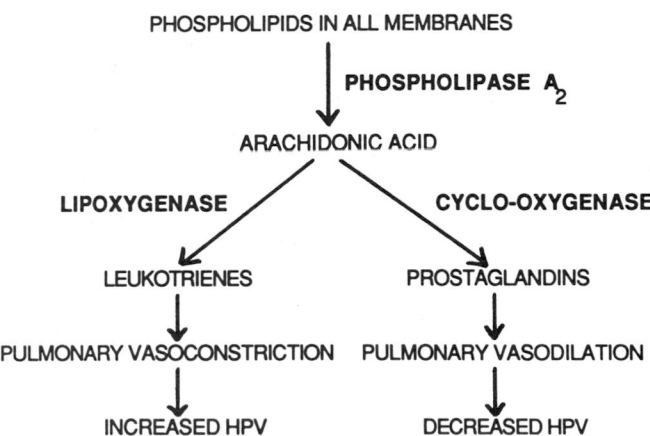

Fig. 15-8. The leukotriene products of arachidonic acid metabolism can increase hypoxic pulmonary vasoconstriction (HPV), and the prostaglandin products of arachidonic acid metabolism can decrease HPV. The amount of HPV is determined by a balance between these agonist and antagonist effects of the leukotrienes and prostaglandins, respectively.

ative increase in the cyclo-oxygenase-prostaglandin system), and HPV is relatively decreased.[34] Thus, maneuvers that promote the use of the cyclo-oxygenase-prostaglandin pathway decrease HPV, and maneuvers that promote the use of the lipoxygenase-leukotriene pathway increase HPV.

Second and/or alternatively, hypoxia also appears to directly stimulate metabolic activity of pulmonary vascular smooth muscle and to accelerate production of adenosine triphosphate (ATP) whereas in systemic vascular beds, the action of hypoxia on metabolism is depressant. Low oxygen tension also maintains the membrane of pulmonary vascular smooth muscle cells in a state of partial depolarization and influences the role of calcium in excitation-contraction coupling.[22] Thus, alveolar hypoxia may directly cause ion fluxes that cause or contribute to the vasoconstriction. In this way, elements of the vascular wall could serve both as sensor and effector of vasoconstriction.[27] In summary, HPV may be due to either a direct action of alveolar hypoxia on pulmonary vasculature or an alveolar hypoxia-induced release of a vasoactive substance(s). These two mechanisms for the production of HPV are not necessarily mutually exclusive.

There are three ways in which HPV operates in humans. First, life at high altitude or whole-lung respiration of a low inspired concentration of O_2 (FIO_2) increases Ppa. This is true for newcomers to high altitude, for the acclimatized, and for natives.[22] The vasoconstriction is considerable, and in normal people breathing 10 percent O_2, Ppa doubles while pulmonary wedge pressure remains constant.[46] The increased Ppa increases perfusion of the apices of the lung (recruitment of previously unused vessels) and results in gas exchange in a region of lung not normally utilized (i.e., zone 1). Thus, with a low FIO_2, the PaO_2 is greater and the alveolar–arterial O_2 tension difference and dead space/tidal volume ratio are less than would be expected or predicted on the basis of a normal (sea level) distribution of ventilation and blood flow. High-altitude pulmonary hypertension is an important component in the development of mountain sickness subacutely (hours to days) and cor pulmonale chronically (weeks).[47] In fact, there is now good evidence that in patients with chronic obstructive pulmonary disease, even nocturnal episodes of arterial oxygen desaturation (caused by episodic hypoventilation) are accompanied by elevations in Ppa and may account for or lead to sustained pulmonary hypertension and cor pulmonale.[48] Second, hypoventilation (low $\dot{V}A/\dot{Q}$), atelectasis, or nitrogen ventilation of any region of the lung (one lung, lobe, lobule) generally causes a diversion of blood flow away from the hypoxic to the nonhypoxic lung (40 to 50 percent, 50 to 60 percent, 60 to 70 percent, respectively) (Fig. 15-9).[49,50] The regional vasoconstriction and blood flow diversion are of great importance in minimizing transpulmonary shunt and normalizing regional $\dot{V}A/\dot{Q}$ ratios during disease of one lung, one-lung anesthesia (see Ch. 50), and inadvertent intubation of a

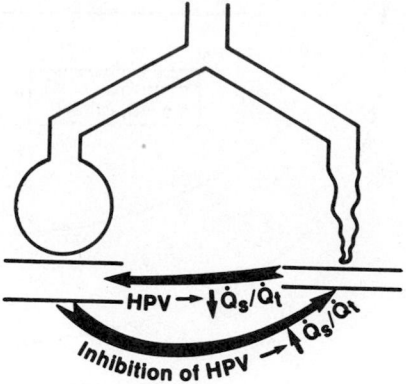

Fig. 15-9. Schematic drawing of regional hypoxic pulmonary vasoconstriction (HPV); one-lung ventilation is a common clinical example of regional HPV. HPV in the hypoxic atelectatic lung causes a redistribution of blood flow away from the hypoxic lung to the normoxic lung, thereby diminishing the amount of shunt flow ($\dot{Q}s/\dot{Q}T$) that can occur through the hypoxic lung. Inhibition of hypoxic lung HPV causes an increase in the amount of shunt flow through the hypoxic lung, thereby decreasing PaO_2.

main stem bronchus. Third, in patients with chronic obstructive pulmonary disease, asthma, pneumonia, and mitral stenosis, who do not have bronchospasm, administration of pulmonary vasodilator drugs such as isoproterenol, sodium nitroprusside, and nitroglycerin causes a decrease in PaO_2 and pulmonary vascular resistance and an increase in right-to-left transpulmonary shunt.[51] The mechanism for these changes is thought to be deleterious inhibition of pre-existing and, in some of the lesions, geographically widespread HPV without a concomitant and beneficial bronchodilation.[51] In accordance with the latter two lines of evidence (one-lung or regional hypoxia and vasodilator drug effects on whole-lung or generalized disease), HPV is thought to divert blood flow away from hypoxic regions of the lung, thereby serving as an autoregulatory mechanism that protects PaO_2 by favorably adjusting regional $\dot{V}A/\dot{Q}$ ratios. Factors that inhibit regional HPV are extensively discussed elsewhere.[52]

Lung Volume

The functional residual capacity (FRC) is the volume of lung that exists at the end of a normal exhalation after a normal tidal volume and when there is no muscle activity or pressure difference between alveoli and atmosphere. Total pulmonary vascular resistance is increased when lung volume is either increased or decreased from FRC (Fig. 15-10).[53-55] The increase in total pulmonary vascular resistance above FRC is due to alveolar compression of small intra-alveolar vessels, which results in an increase in small vessel pulmonary vascular resistance (i.e., creation of zone 1 or zone 2).[56] As a relatively small mitigating or counterbalancing ef-

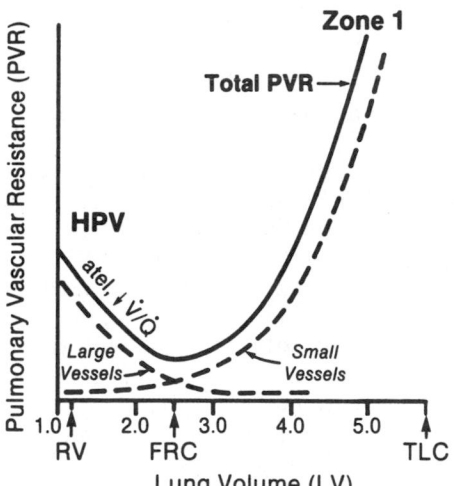

Fig. 15-10. An asymmetrical U-shaped curve relates total pulmonary vascular resistance to lung volume. The trough of the curve occurs when lung volume equals functional residual capacity (FRC). Total pulmonary resistance is the sum of resistance in small vessels (increased by increasing lung volume) and the resistance in large vessels (increased by decreasing lung volume). The end point for increasing lung volume (toward total lung capacity [TLC]) is the creation of zone 1 conditions, and the end point for decreasing lung volume (toward residual volume [RV]) is the creation of low $\dot{V}_A/\dot{Q}$ and atelectatic (atel) areas that have hypoxic pulmonary vasoconstriction (HPV). (The curve represents a composite of data from Benumof,[52] Simmons et al.,[53] and Burton and Patel.[54])

fect to the small vessel compression, the large extra-alveolar vessels may be expanded by the increased negativity of the perivascular pressure at high FRC. The increase in total pulmonary vascular resistance below FRC is due to an increase in pulmonary vascular resistance of large extra-alveolar vessels. The increase in large vessel pulmonary vascular resistance was previously thought to be due to a mechanical tortuosity or kinking of these vessels. However, small or grossly atelectic lungs are hypoxic, and it has recently been shown that the mechanism of increased large vessel pulmonary vascular resistance in these lungs is due entirely to hypoxic pulmonary vasoconstriction.[57] This conclusion has been found to be true whether the chest is open or closed and whether ventilation is by positive pressure or spontaneous.[58]

Alternate (Nonalveolar) Pathways of Blood Flow Through the Lung

There are several possible pathways for blood to travel from the right side of the heart to the left side of the heart without being fully oxygenated or oxygenated at all. Blood flow through poorly ventilated alveoli (low $\dot{V}_A/\dot{Q}$ regions at $FIO_2 < 0.3$ have a right-to-left shunt effect on oxygenation) and through nonventilated alveoli (atelectatic or consolidated regions) ($\dot{V}_A/\dot{Q} = 0$ at all

FIO_2) are sources of right-to-left shunt. Low $\dot{V}_A/\dot{Q}$ and atelectatic lung units occur in conditions in which the FRC is less than the closing capacity (OC) of the lung (see the section, *Lung Volumes, the Functional Residual Capacity, and the Closing Capacity*).

There are several right-to-left blood flow pathways through the lungs and heart that do not pass by or involve alveoli at all. The bronchial and pleural circulations originate from systemic arteries and empty into the left side of the heart without being oxygenated, constituting the 1 to 3 percent true right-to-left shunt normally present. With chronic bronchitis, the bronchial circulation may carry 10 percent of the cardiac output, and with pleuritis, the pleural circulation may carry 5 percent of the cardiac output. Consequently, there may be as much as a 10 percent and 5 percent obligatory right-to-left shunt present, respectively, under these conditions. Intrapulmonary arteriovenous anastomoses are normally closed, but in the face of acute pulmonary hypertension, such as may be caused by a pulmonary embolus, they may open and cause a direct increase in right-to-left shunt. The foramen ovale is patent in 20 to 30 percent of individuals but normally remains functionally closed because left atrial pressure exceeds right atrial pressure. However, any condition that results in right atrial pressure being greater than left atrial pressure may produce a right-to-left shunt with resultant hypoxemia and possible paradoxical embolization. Such conditions include the use of high levels of positive end-expiratory pressure (PEEP), pulmonary embolization, pulmonary hypertension, chronic obstructive pulmonary disease, pulmonary valvular stenosis, congestive heart failure, and postpneumonectomy states.[59] Esophageal to mediastinal to bronchial to pulmonary vein pathways have been described and may explain in part the hypoxemia associated with portal hypertension and cirrhosis. There are no known conditions that selectively increase thebesian channel blood flow (thebesian vessels nourish the left heart myocardium and originate and empty into the left side of the heart.)

Other (Nongravitational) Important Determinants of Pulmonary Compliance, Resistance, Lung Volume, and Ventilation

Pulmonary Compliance

For air to flow into the lungs, a pressure gradient must be developed to overcome the elastic resistance of the lungs and chest wall to expansion. These structures are arranged concentrically, and their elastic resistances are therefore additive. The relationship between the pressure gradient (ΔP) and the resultant volume increase (ΔV) of the lungs and thorax is independent of time and is known as total compliance (C_T), as expressed below:

$$C_T \ (L/cmH_2O) = \Delta V \ (L)/\Delta P \ (cmH_2O) \qquad (1)$$

The C_T of lung plus chest wall is related to the individual compliances of lungs (C_L) and chest wall (C_{cw}) according to the following expression:

$$1/C_T = 1/C_L + 1/C_{cw}$$
$$[\text{or } C_T = (C_L)(C_{cw})/C_L + C_{cw}] \qquad (2)$$

Normally, C_L and C_{cw} each equal 0.2 L/cmH$_2$O; thus $C_T = 0.1$ L/cmH$_2$O. To determine C_L, ΔV and the *transpulmonary pressure gradient* (Palveolar − Ppleural, the ΔP for the lung) must be known; to determine C_{cw}, ΔV and the *transmural pressure gradient* (Ppleural − Pambient, the ΔP for the chest wall) must be known; to determine C_T, ΔV and the *transthoracic pressure gradient* (Palveolar − Pambient, the ΔP for the lung and chest wall together) must be known. In clinical practice, only C_T is measured, which can be done dynamically or statically depending on whether a peak or plateau inspiratory pressure gradient (respectively) is used for the C_T calculation.

During a positive or negative pressure inspiration of sufficient duration, the transthoracic pressure gradient first increases to a peak value and then decreases to a somewhat lower plateau value. The peak transthoracic pressure value is due to pressure required to overcome both elastic and airway resistance (see the section, *Airway Resistance*). The transthoracic pressure decreases to a plateau value following the peak value, because, with time, gas redistributes from stiff alveoli (which expand only slightly and therefore have only a very short inspiratory period) into more compliant alveoli (which expand a great deal and therefore have a long inspiratory period). Since the gas redistributes into more compliant alveoli, less pressure is required to contain the same amount of gas, and this explains why the pressure decreases. In practical terms, dynamic compliance is the volume change divided by the peak inspiratory transthoracic pressure; static compliance is the volume change divided by the plateau inspiratory transthoracic pressure. Therefore, static C_T is usually greater than dynamic C_T, since the former calculation uses a smaller denominator (lower pressure) than the latter calculation.

The pressure in an alveolus (Palveolar) deserves special comment. The alveoli are lined with a layer of liquid. The lining of a curved surface (sphere or cylinder, as are the alveoli, bronchioles, and bronchi) with liquid creates a surface tension that tends to make the surface area that is exposed to the atmosphere as small as possible. Simply stated, water molecules crowd much closer together on the surface of a curved layer of water than elsewhere in the fluid. As lung or alveolus size decreases, the degree of curvature and the retractive surface tension force increase.

According to the Laplace equation, the pressure in an alveolus (P, in dyn/cm^2) is above ambient pressure by an amount depending on the surface tension of the lining liquid (T, in dyn/cm) and the radius of curvature of the alveolus (R, in cm). This is expressed in the following equation:

$$P = 2T/R \qquad (3)$$

Although surface tension contributes to the elastic resistance and retractive forces of the lung, two difficulties must be resolved. First, the pressure inside small alveoli should be higher than that inside large alveoli, a conclusion that stems directly from the Laplace equation (R in the denominator). From this reasoning, one would expect a progressive discharge of each small alveolus into a larger one, until eventually only one gigantic alveolus would be left (Fig. 15-11A). The second problem concerns the relationship between lung volume and the transpulmonary pressure gradient (Palveolar − Ppleural). Theoretically, the retractive forces of the lung should increase as the lung volume decreases. If this were true, lung volume should decrease in a vicious cycle, with the tendency to collapse increasing progressively as the lung volume diminished.

These two problems are resolved by the fact that the surface tension of the fluid lining the alveoli is variable and decreases as its surface area is reduced. The surface tension of alveolar fluid can reach levels that are well below the normal range for body fluids such as water and plasma. When an alveolus decreases in size, the surface tension of the lining fluid falls to a greater extent than the corresponding reduction of radius, so that the transmural pressure gradient (= 2T/R) diminishes. This explains why small alveoli do not discharge their contents into large alveoli (Fig. 15-11B) and why the elastic recoil of small alveoli is less than that of large alveoli.

The substance responsible for the reduction (and variability) of alveolar surface tension is secreted by the intra-alveolar type II pneumocyte and is a lipoprotein called surfactant that floats as a 50-Å thick film on the surface of the fluid lining the alveoli. When the surface film is reduced in area and the concentration of surfactant at the surface is increased, there is an increased surface-reducing pressure that counteracts the surface tension of the fluid lining the alveoli.

Airway Resistance

For air to flow into the lungs, a pressure gradient must also be developed to overcome the nonelastic airway resistance of the lungs to air flow. The relationship between the pressure gradient (ΔP) and the rate of air flow ($\dot{V}$) is known as airway resistance (R):

$$R\ (\text{cmH}_2\text{O/L/s}) = \frac{\Delta P\ (\text{cmH}_2\text{O})}{\Delta \dot{V}\ (\text{L/s})} \qquad (4)$$

The pressure gradient (ΔP) along the airway depends on the caliber of the airway and the rate and pattern of airflow. There are three main patterns of airflow. Laminar flow occurs when the gas passes down parallel-sided tubes at less than a certain critical velocity. With

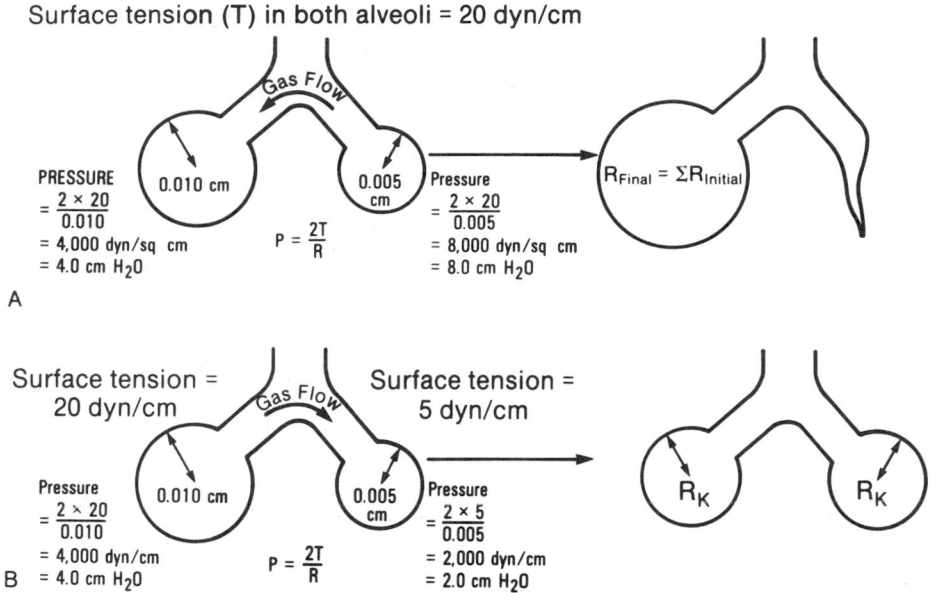

Fig. 15-11. Relationship between surface tension (T), alveolar radius (R), and alveolar transmural pressure (P). **(A)** The pressure relationship in two alveoli of different size but with the same surface tension in their lining fluids. The direction of gas flow will be from the higher pressure small alveolus to the lower pressure large alveolus, and the result is one large alveolus (Rfinal = ΣRinitial). **(B)** The pressure relationships of two alveoli of different size when allowance is made for the expected changes in surface tension (less tension in smaller alveolus). The direction of gas flow is from the larger alveolus to the smaller alveolus until the two alveoli are of equal size and are volume stable (R_K). ΣR, sum of all individual radii; K, constant.

laminar flow, the pressure drop down the tube is proportional to the flow rate and may be calculated from the equation derived by Poiseuille: $P = \dot{V} \times 8L \times u/\pi r^4 \times 980$, where P = pressure drop (in cmH$_2$O); $\dot{V}$ = volume flow rate (in ml/s); L = length of tube (in cm); r = radius of tube (in cm); and u = viscosity (in poises).

When flow exceeds the critical velocity, it becomes turbulent. The significant feature of turbulent flow is that the pressure drop along the airway is no longer directly proportional to flow rate but is proportional to the square of flow rate according to the equation $P = \dot{V}^2 pfL/4\pi^2 r^5$, where p is a gas or fluid density term and f is a friction factor that depends on the roughness of the tube wall.[60] Thus, with increases in turbulent flow (and/or orifice flow, see immediately below), P increases much more than $\dot{V}$, and therefore R increases [see eq. (4)].

Orifice flow occurs at severe constrictions such as a nearly closed larynx. In these situations, the pressure drop is also proportional to the square of the flow rate, but density replaces viscosity as the important factor in the numerator. This explains why low-density gas such as helium diminishes the resistance to flow (by threefold compared with air) in severe obstruction of the upper airway.

Since the total cross-sectional area of the airways increases as branching occurs, the velocity of airflow decreases; laminar flow is therefore chiefly confined to the airways below the main bronchi. Orifice flow occurs at the larynx, and flow in the trachea is turbulent during most of the respiratory cycle. Viewing the components that constitute each of the preceding airway pressure equations, one can see that many factors obviously may affect the pressure drop down the airways during respiration. However, variations in diameter of the smaller bronchi and bronchioles are particularly critical (bronchoconstriction may convert laminar flow to turbulent flow), and the pressure drop along the airways may become much more related to flow rate.

Different Regional Lung Time Constants

So far, the compliance and airway resistance properties of the chest have been discussed separately. In the following analysis, the pressure at the mouth is assumed to increase suddenly to a fixed positive value (Fig. 15-12)[61] that overcomes both elastic and airway resistance and is maintained at this value during inflation of the lungs. The pressure gradient required to overcome nonelastic airway resistance is the difference between the fixed mouth pressure and the instantaneous height of the dashed line in Figure 15-12 and is proportional to the flow rate during most of the respiratory cycle. Thus, the pressure gradient required to overcome nonelastic airway resistance is maximal initially but then decreases

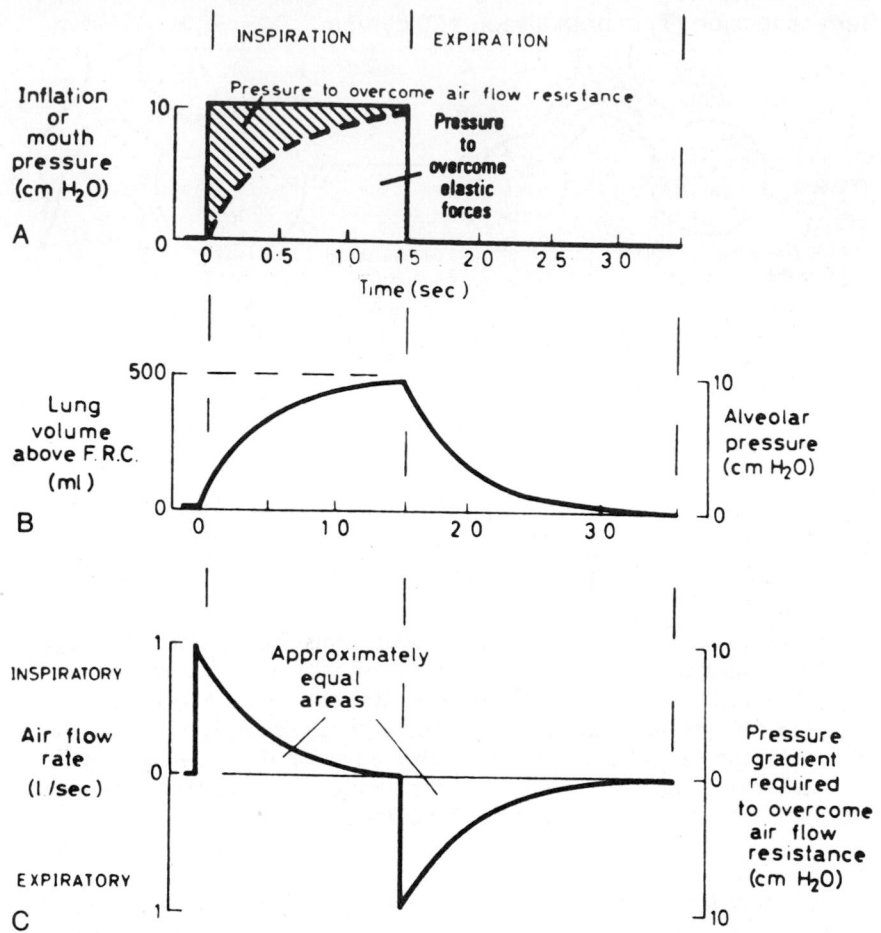

Fig. 15-12. Artificial ventilation by intermittent application of a constant pressure (square wave). Expiration is passive. The pressure required to overcome airway resistance (hatched lines, panel **A**) and airflow rate ($\dot{V}$ of equation 4, see panel **C**), which are proportional to one another, decreases exponentially. The pressure required to overcome elastic resistance (height of dashed line, panel **A**) and lung volume (see panel **B**), which are proportional to one another, increases exponentially. Values shown are typical for an anesthetized supine paralyzed patient: total dynamic compliance, 50 ml/cmH$_2$O; pulmonary resistance, 3 cmH$_2$O/L/s; apparatus resistance, 7 cmH$_2$O/L/s; total resistance, 10 cmH$_2$O/L/s; time constant, 0.5 second. (From Nunn,[61] with permission.)

exponentially (Fig. 15-12A, hatched lines). The rate of filling, therefore, also declines in an approximately exponential manner. The remainder of the pressure gradient overcomes the elastic resistance (the instantaneous height of the dashed line in Fig. 15-12A) and is proportional to the change in lung volume. Thus, the pressure gradient required to overcome elastic resistance is minimal initially but then increases exponentially (as does lung volume). Alveolar filling ceases (lung volume remains constant) when the pressure resulting from the retractive elastic forces balances the applied (mouth) pressure (Fig. 15-12A, dashed line).

Since there is only a finite time available for alveolar filling, and since alveolar filling occurs in an exponential manner, the degree of filling obviously depends on the duration of the inspiration. The rapidity of change in an exponential curve can be described by its time constant tau (τ). Tau (τ) is the time required to complete 63 percent of an exponentially changing function if the total time allowed for the function change is unlimited ($2\tau = 87$ percent, $3\tau = 95$ percent, and $4\tau = 99$ percent). For lung inflation, $\tau = C\tau \times R$; normally, $C\tau = 0.1$ L/cmH$_2$O, $R = 2.0$ cmH$_2$O/L/s, and $\tau = 0.2$ second and $3\tau = 0.6$ second.

When this equation is applied to individual alveolar units, the time taken to fill such a unit clearly increases as airway resistance increases. The time to fill an alveolar unit also increases as compliance increases, since a greater volume of air will be transferred into a more compliant alveolus before the retractive force equals the applied pressure. The compliance of individual alveoli differs from top to bottom of the lung, and the resistance of individual airways will vary widely depending on their length and caliber. Therefore, a variety of time constants for inflation exist throughout the lung.

Pathways of Collateral Ventilation

Collateral ventilation is another nongravitational determinant of the distribution of ventilation. There are four known pathways of collateral ventilation. First, interalveolar communications (pores of Kohn) exist in most species; they may range from 8 to 50 per alveolus and may increase with age and with the development of obstructive lung disease. Their precise role has not been defined, but they probably function to prevent hypoxia in neighboring, but obstructed, lung units. Second, distal bronchiolar to alveolar communications are known to exist (channels of Lambert), but their function in vivo is speculative (may be similar to pores of Kohn). Third, respiratory bronchiole to terminal bronchiole connections have been found in adjacent lung segments (channels of Martin) in healthy dogs and in humans with lung disease. Fourth, there are interlobar connections; the functional characteristics of interlobar collateral ventilation through these connections have recently been described in dogs[62] and have been observed in humans as well.[63]

The Work of Breathing

The pressure–volume characteristics of the lung also determine the work of breathing. Since

$$Work = Force \times Distance$$
$$Force = Pressure \times Area$$
$$Distance = Volume/Area \qquad (5)$$
$$Work = (Pressure \times Area)(Volume/Area)$$
$$= Pressure \times Volume$$

and ventilatory work may be analyzed by plotting pressure against volume.[64]

Two different pressure-volume diagrams are shown in Figure 15-13. During normal inspiration (left graph), transpulmonary pressure increases from 0 to 5 cmH$_2$O while 500 ml of air is drawn into the lung. Potential energy is stored by the lung during inspiration and expended during expiration; as a consequence, the entire expiratory cycle is passive. The hatched area plus the triangular area ABC represents pressure multiplied by volume and is the work of breathing. Line AB is the lower section of the pressure-volume curve of Figure 15-13. The triangular area ABC is the work required to overcome elastic forces (C$_T$), whereas the hatched area is the work required to overcome airflow or frictional resistances (R). The graph on the right shows an anesthetized patient with diffuse obstructive airway disease resulting from the accumulation of mucous secretions. There is a marked increase in both the elastic (triangle AB′C) and airway (hatched area) resistive components of respiratory work. During expiration, only 250 ml of

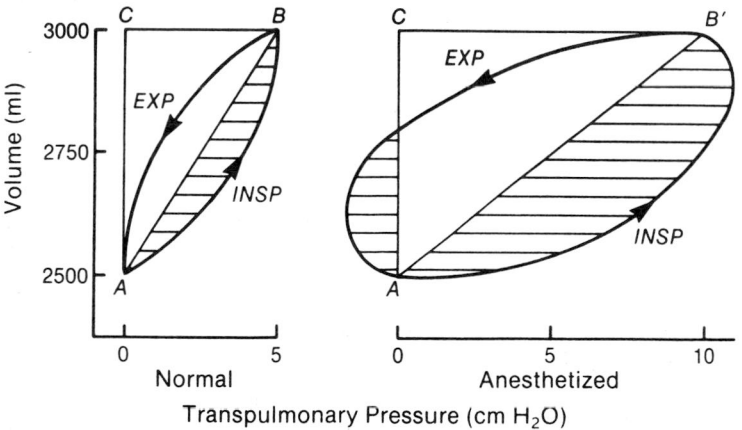

Fig. 15-13. Lung volume plotted against transpulmonary pressure in a pressure–volume diagram for an awake (normal) and an anesthetized patient. The lung compliance of the awake patient (slope of line AB = 100 ml/cmH$_2$O) equals that shown for the small dependent alveoli in Figure 15-3. The lung compliance of the anesthetized patient (slope of line AB′ = 50 ml/cmH$_2$O) equals that shown for the medium mid-lung alveoli in Figure 15-3 and for the anesthetized patient in Figure 15-12. The total area within the oval and triangles has the dimensions of pressure multiplied by volume and represents the total work of breathing. The hatched area to the right of lines AB and AB′ represents active inspiratory work necessary to overcome resistance to airflow during inspiration (INSP). The hatched area to the left of the triangle AB′C represents active expiratory work necessary to overcome resistance to airflow during expiration (EXP). Expiration is passive in the normal subject because sufficient potential energy is stored during inspiration to produce expiratory airflow. The fraction of total inspiratory work necessary to overcome elastic resistance is shown by the triangles ABC and AB′C. The anesthetized patient has a decreased compliance and increased elastic resistance work (triangle AB′C) compared with the normal patient's compliance and elastic resistance work (triangle ABC). The anesthetized patient shown in this figure has an increased airway resistance to both inspiratory and expiratory work.

air leaves the lungs during the passive phase when intrathoracic pressure reaches the equilibrium value of 0 cmH_2O. Active effort-producing work is required to force out the remaining 250 ml of air, and intrathoracic pressure actually becomes positive.

For a constant minute volume, the work done against elastic resistance is increased when breathing is deep and slow. On the other hand, the work done against airflow resistance is increased when breathing is rapid and shallow. If the two components are summated and the total work is plotted against the respiratory frequency, there is an optimal respiratory frequency at which the total work of breathing is minimal (Fig. 15-14).[65] In patients with diseased lungs in which elastic resistance is high (pulmonary fibrosis, pulmonary edema, infants), the optimum frequency is increased and rapid shallow breaths are favored. When airway resistance is high (asthma, obstructive lung disease), the optimum frequency is decreased and slow deep breaths are favored.

Lung Volumes, the Functional Residual Capacity, and the Closing Capacity

Lung Volumes and the Functional Residual Capacity

The FRC is defined as the volume of gas in the lung that exists at the end of a normal expiration when there is no airflow and alveolar pressure equals the ambient pressure. Under these conditions, expansive chest wall elastic forces are exactly balanced by retractive lung tissue elastic forces (Fig. 15-15).[66]

The expiratory reserve volume is part of the FRC; it is that additional gas beyond the end-tidal volume that can be consciously exhaled, resulting in the minimum volume of lung possible, known as the residual volume. Thus, the FRC equals the residual volume plus the expiratory reserve volume (Fig. 15-16). With regard to the other lung volumes shown in Figure 15-16, tidal volume, vital capacity, inspiratory capacity, inspiratory reserve volume, and expiratory reserve volume can all be measured by simple spirometry. Total lung volume, FRC, and residual volume all contain a fraction (the residual volume) that cannot be measured by simple spirometry. However, if one of these three volumes is measured, the others can be easily derived because the other lung volumes, which relate these three volumes to one another, can be measured by simple spirometry.

FRC can be measured by one of three techniques. The first method is to wash the nitrogen out of the lungs by several minutes of oxygen breathing with measurement of the total quantity of nitrogen eliminated. Thus, if 2 L of nitrogen is eliminated and the initial alveolar nitrogen concentration was 80 percent, the initial volume of the lung was 2.5 L. The second method uses the washin of a tracer gas such as helium. If 50 ml of helium is introduced into the lungs and, after equilibration, the helium concentration is then found to be 1 percent, the volume of the lung is 5 L. The third method of measurement of FRC uses Boyle's law, that is, $PV = K$, where P = pressure, V = volume, and K = a constant. The subject is confined within a gas-tight box (plethysmograph), so that changes in the volume of the body may be readily determined as a change in pressure within the box. Disparity between FRC as measured in the body plethysmograph and by the helium method is often used as a way of detecting large, nonventilating air-trapped blebs.[67] Obviously, there are difficulties in

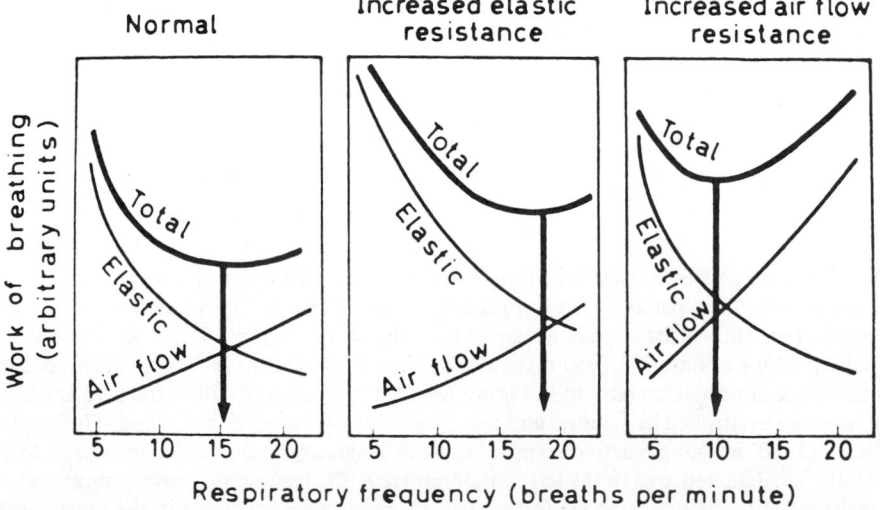

Fig. 15-14. The diagrams show the work done against elastic and airflow resistance separately and summated to indicate the total work of breathing at different respiratory frequencies. The total work of breathing has a minimum value at about 15 breaths/min under normal circumstances. For the same minute volume, minimum work is performed at higher frequencies with stiff (less compliant) lungs and at lower frequencies when the airflow resistance is increased. (From Nunn,[65] with permission.)

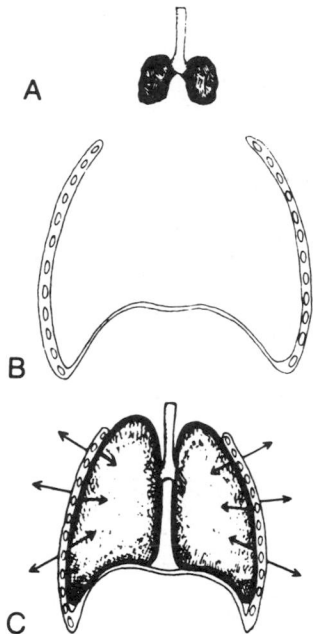

Fig. 15-15. (A) The resting state of normal lungs when they are removed from the chest cavity; that is, elastic recoil causes total collapse. (B) The resting state of a normal chest wall and diaphragm when the thoracic apex is open to the atmosphere and the thoracic contents are removed. (C) The lung volume that exists at the end of expiration—the functional residual capacity. At functional residual capacity the elastic forces of lung and chest walls are equal and in opposite directions. The pleural surfaces link these two opposing forces. (From Shapiro et al.,[66] with permission.)

applying the body plethysmograph to anesthetized patients.

Airway Closure and Closing Capacity

As discussed above in the section on the distribution of ventilation, pleural pressure increases from the top to the bottom of the lung and determines regional alveolar size, compliance, and ventilation. Of even greater importance to the anesthesiologist is the recognition that these gradients in pleural pressure may lead to airway closure and collapse of alveoli.

Airway Closure in Patients with Normal Lungs. Figure 15-17A illustrates the normal resting end-expiratory (FRC) position of the lung-chest wall combination. The distending transpulmonary and the intrathoracic air passage transmural pressure gradients are 5 cmH_2O, and the airways remain patent. During the middle of a normal inspiration (Fig. 15-17B), there is an increase in the transmural pressure gradient (to 6.8 cmH_2O), which encourages distention of intrathoracic air passages. During the middle of a normal expiration (Fig. 15-17C), expiration is passive; alveolar pressure is attributable only to the elastic recoil of the lung (2 cmH_2O), and there is a decrease (to 5.2 cmH_2O) but still a favorable (distending) intraluminal transmural pressure gradient. During the middle of a severe forced expiration (Fig. 15-17D), pleural pressure increases far above atmospheric pressure and is communicated to the alveoli, which have a pressure that is higher still owing to the elastic recoil of the alveolar septa (an additional 2 cmH_2O). At high gas flow rates, the pressure drop down the air passage is increased, and there will be a point at which intraluminal pressure equals either surrounding parenchymal or pleural pressure; that point is termed the equal pressure point (EPP). If the EPP occurs in small intrathoracic air passages (distal to the eleventh generation the airways have no cartilage

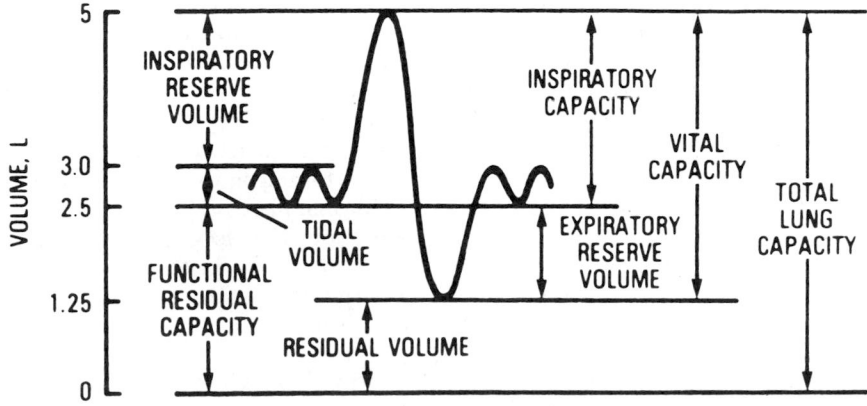

Fig. 15-16. The dynamic lung volumes that can be measured by simple spirometry are the tidal volume, inspiratory reserve volume, expiratory reserve volume, inspiratory capacity, and vital capacity. The static lung volumes are the residual volume, functional residual capacity, and total lung capacity. The static lung volumes cannot be measured by observation of a spirometer trace and require separate methods of measurement.

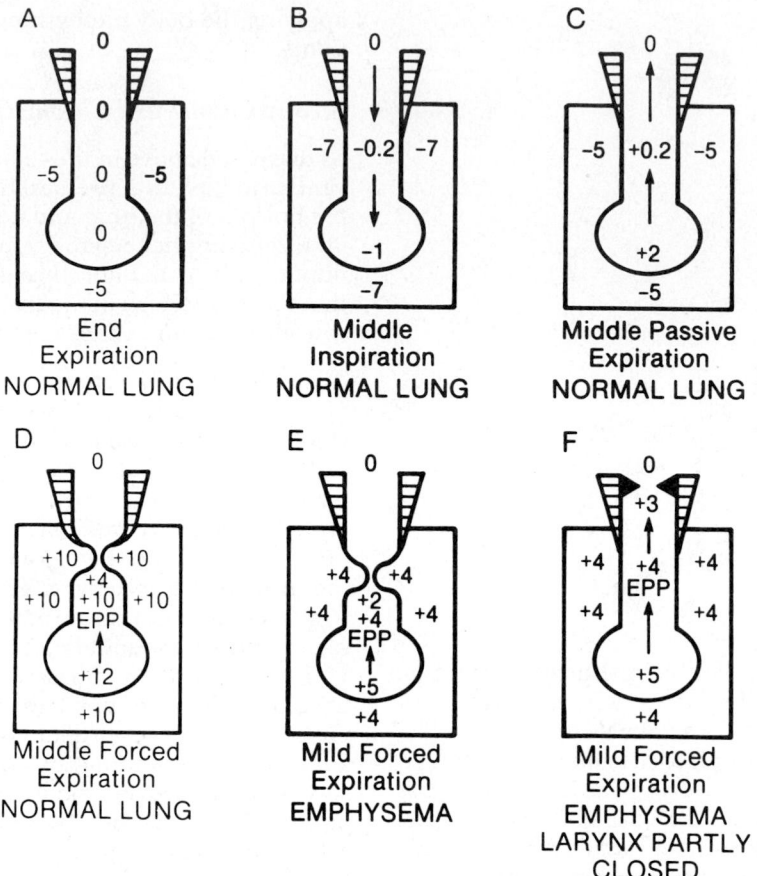

Fig. 15-17. Pressure gradients across the airways. The airways consist of a thin-walled intrathoracic portion (near the alveoli) and a more rigid (cartilaginous) intrathoracic and extrathoracic portion. During expiration, the pressure due to elastic recoil is assumed to be $+2$ cmH$_2$O in normal lungs (**A–D**) and $+1$ cmH$_2$O in abnormal lungs (**E & F**). The total pressure inside the alveolus is pleural pressure plus the elastic recoil. The arrows indicate direction of airflow. EPP, equal pressure point. See text for explanation. (From Benumof,[168] with permission.)

and are called bronchioles), they may be held open at that particular point by the tethering effect of the elastic recoil of the immediately adjacent or surrounding lung parenchyma. If the EPP occurs in large extrathoracic air passages (proximal to the eleventh generation the airways have cartilage and are called bronchi), they may be held open at that particular point by their cartilage. Downstream of the EPP (in either small or large airways), the transmural pressure gradient is reversed (-6 cmH$_2$O) and will result in airway closure. Thus, the patency of airways distal to the eleventh generation is a function of lung volume, and the patency of airways proximal to the eleventh generation is a function of intrathoracic (pleural) pressure. In extrathoracic bronchi with cartilage, the posterior membranous sheath appears to give first by invaginating into the lumen.[68] If lung volume were abnormally decreased (for example, owing to splinting) and expiration were still forced, the caliber of the airways would be relatively reduced at all times, causing the EPP and point of collapse to move progressively from larger to smaller air passages (closer to the alveolus).

In patients with normal lungs, airway closure may still occur even if exhalation is not forced, provided residual volume is approached closely enough. Even in patients with normal lungs, as lung volume decreases during expiration toward residual volume, the small airways (0.5 to 0.9 mm in diameter) will show a progressive tendency to close, whereas larger airways remain patent.[69,70] Airway closure occurs first in the dependent lung regions (as recently directly observed by computed tomography [CT]),[71] since the distending transpulmonary pressure is less and the volume change during expiration is greater. The airway closure is most likely to occur in the dependent regions of the lung whether the patient is in the supine or lateral decubitus position.[71]

Airway Closure in Patients with Abnormal Lungs. Airway closure occurs with milder active expiration, lower gas flow rates, and higher lung volumes and occurs closer to the alveolus in patients with emphysema, bronchitis, asthma, and pulmonary interstitial edema. In all four conditions, airway resistance is increased, causing a larger pressure decrease from the alveoli to the larger bronchi, thereby creating the potential for negative intrathoracic transmural pressure gradients and narrowed and collapsed airways. In addition, the structural integrity of the conducting airways may be diminished owing to inflammation and scarring, and therefore, these airways may close more readily for any given lung volume or transluminal pressure gradient.

In emphysema, the elastic recoil of the lung is reduced (to 1 cmH$_2$O in Fig. 15-17E), the air passages are poorly supported by the lung parenchyma, the point of airway resistance is close to the alveolus, and the transmural pressure gradient can become negative quickly. Therefore, during only a *mild* forced expiration in an emphysematous patient, the EPP and the point of collapse are near the alveolus (Fig. 15-17E). Use of pursed lip or grunting expiration (the equivalents of partly closing the larynx during expiration), PEEP, and a continuous positive airway pressure in an emphysematous patient restores a favorable (distending) intrathoracic transmural air pressure gradient (Fig. 15-17F). In bronchitis, the airways are structurally weakened and may close when only a small negative transmural pressure gradient is present (as with a mild forced expiration). In asthma, the middle-size airways are narrowed by bron-

chospasm, and if expiration is forced, they are further narrowed by a negative transmural pressure gradient. Finally, with pulmonary interstitial edema, perialveolar interstitial edema compresses alveoli and acutely decreases FRC; the peribronchial edema fluid cuffs (within the connective tissue sheaths around the larger arteries and bronchi) compress the bronchi and acutely increase closing volume.[72-74]

The Measurement of Closing Capacity. Closing capacity (CC) is a sensitive test of early small-airway disease and is performed by having the patient exhale to residual volume (Fig. 15-18).[75] An inhalation from residual volume toward total lung capacity is begun, and at the beginning of the inhalation, a bolus of tracer gas (^{133}Xe, helium) is injected into the inspired gas. During the initial part of this inhalation from residual volume, the first gas to enter the alveolus is the dead space gas and the tracer bolus. The tracer gas will only enter alveoli that are already open (presumably the apices of the lung; hatched lines, Fig. 15-18) and does not enter alveoli that are already closed (presumably the bases of the lung; no hatched lines, Fig. 15-18). As the inhalation continues, apical alveoli complete filling and basilar

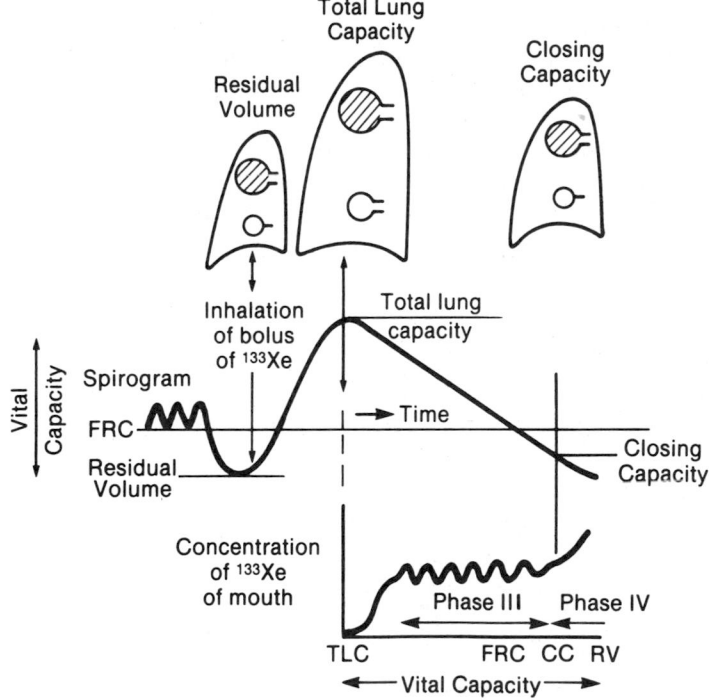

Fig. 15-18. Measurement of closing capacity by the use of a tracer gas such as xenon 133 (^{133}Xe). The bolus of tracer gas is inhaled near residual volume and, owing to airway closure in the dependent lung, is distributed *only* to those nondependent alveoli whose air passages are still open (shown crosshatched in diagram). During expiration, the concentration of the tracer gas becomes constant after the dead space is washed out. This plateau (phase III) gives way to a rising concentration of tracer gas (phase IV) when there is once again closure of the dependent airways because the only contribution made to the expired gas is by the nondependent alveoli with a high ^{133}Xe concentration. (From Nunn,[75] with permission.)

alveoli begin to open and fill, but with gas that does not contain any tracer gas.

A differential tracer gas concentration is thus established; the gas in the apices has a higher tracer concentration (Fig. 15-18 hatched lines) than that in the bases (Fig. 15-18, no hatched lines). As the subject exhales and the diaphragm ascends, a point is reached at which the small airways just above the diaphragm start to close, limiting airflow from these areas. The airflow now comes more from the upper lung fields, where the alveolar gas has a much higher tracer concentration, thus resulting in a sudden increase in the tracer gas concentration toward the end of exhalation (phase IV).

The closing volume (CV) is the difference between the onset of phase IV and residual volume; since it represents part of a vital capacity maneuver, it is expressed as a percentage of the vital lung capacity. The CV plus the residual volume is known as the CC and is expressed as a percentage of total lung capacity. Smoking, obesity, aging, and the supine position increase the CC.[76] In healthy individuals at a mean age of 44 years, CC = FRC in the supine position, and at a mean age of 66 years, CC = FRC in the upright position.[77]

The Relationship Between the Functional Residual Capacity and the Closing Capacity

The relationship between FRC and CC is far more important than consideration of the FRC or CC alone because it is this relationship that determines whether a given respiratory unit is normal, atelectatic, or has a low $\dot{V}_A/\dot{Q}$ ratio. The relationship between FRC and CC is as follows. When the volume of lung at which some airways close is greater than the whole of the tidal volume, lung volume never increases enough during tidal inspiration to open any of these airways. Thus, these airways stay closed during the entire tidal respiration. Airways that are closed all the time are equivalent to atelectasis (Fig. 15-19). If the CV of some airways lies within the tidal volume, then as lung volume increases during inspiration, some previously closed airways will open for a short time until lung volume recedes once again below the CV of these airways. Since these opening and closing airways are open for a shorter time than normal airways, they have less chance or time to participate in fresh gas exchange, a circumstance equivalent to a low ventilation to perfusion region. If the CV of the lung is below the whole of tidal respiration, no airways are closed at any time during tidal respiration; this is a normal circumstance. Anything that decreases FRC relative to CC or increases CC relative to FRC will convert normal areas to low $\dot{V}_A/\dot{Q}$ and atelectatic areas.[78] Development of low $\dot{V}_A/\dot{Q}$ and atelectatic areas will cause hypoxemia.

Mechanical intermittent positive-pressure breathing (IPPB) may be efficacious because it can take a previously spontaneously breathing patient with a low ventilation to perfusion relationship (in which CC is greater than FRC but still within the tidal volume, as depicted in Fig. 15-20, right panel) and increase the amount of inspiratory time that some previously closed (at end-exhalation) airways spend in fresh gas exchange and thereby increase the ventilation to perfusion relationship (Fig. 15-20, middle panel). However, if PEEP is added to the IPPB, the PEEP increases FRC above or to a lung volume greater than CC, thereby restoring a normal FRC to CC relationship, so that no airways are closed at any time during the tidal respiration depicted in Figure 15-20 (left panel) (IPPB + PEEP). Thus, anesthesia-induced atelectasis (CT scan shows crescent-shaped densities) in the dependent regions of patients' lungs has not been reversed with IPPB alone but has been reversed with IPPB plus PEEP (5 to 10 cmH$_2$O).[71]

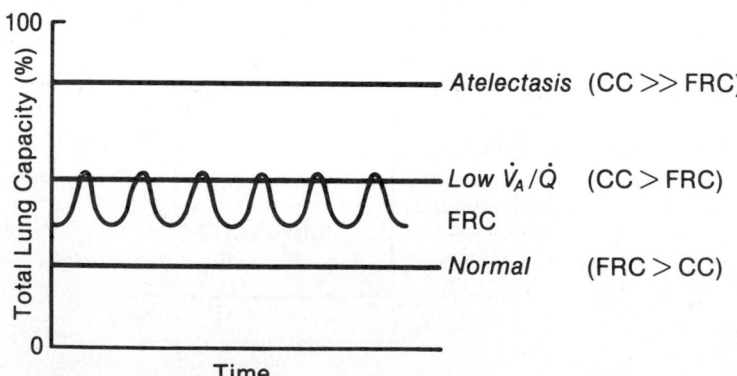

Fig. 15-19. Relationship between the functional residual capacity (FRC) (which is the percentage of total lung capacity that exists at the end of exhalation), shown by the level of each trough of the sine wave tidal volume, and the closing capacity (CC) of the lung (three different closing capacities are indicated by the three different straight lines). See text for explanation of why the three different FRC to CC relationships depicted result in normal or low ventilation to perfusion relationships ($\dot{V}_A/\dot{Q}$) or atelectasis. The abscissa is time. (From Benumof,[167] with permission.)

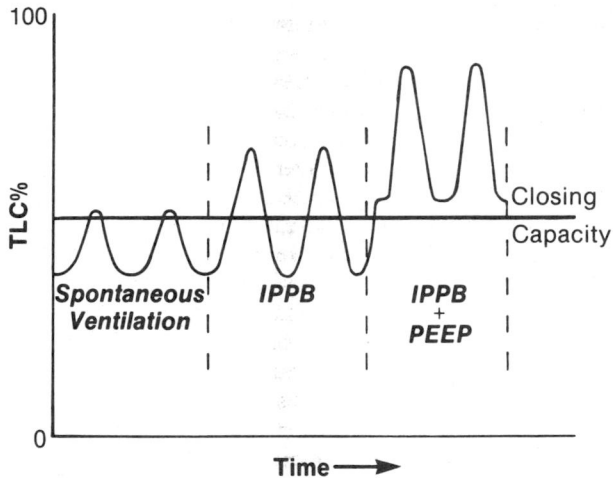

Fig. 15-20. The functional residual capacity to closing capacity relationship during spontaneous ventilation (SPON), intermittent positive-pressure breathing (IPPB), and intermittent positive-pressure breathing and positive end-expiratory pressure (IPPB + PEEP). See text for explanation of the effect of the two ventilatory maneuvers (IPPB and PEEP) on the functional residual capacity to closing capacity relationship. TLC, total lung capacity.

Oxygen and Carbon Dioxide Transport

Alveolar and Dead Space Ventilation and Alveolar Gas Tensions

In patients with normal lungs, approximately two-thirds of each breath reaches perfused alveoli to take part in gas exchange. This constitutes the effective or alveolar ventilation. The remaining one-third of each breath takes no part in gas exchange and is therefore termed the total (or effective or physiologic) dead space ventilation. The total dead space ventilation may be divided into two components: a volume of gas that ventilates the conducting airways (the anatomic dead space ventilation) and a volume of gas that ventilates unperfused alveoli (e.g., as in zone 1, pulmonary embolus, and destroyed alveolar septae) and therefore does not take part in gas exchange (the alveolar dead space ventilation). Figure 15-21 shows a two-compartment model of the lung in which the anatomic and alveolar dead space compartments have been combined into the total (physiologic) dead space compartment; the other compartment is the alveolar ventilation ($\dot{V}_A$) compartment, whose idealized ventilation/perfusion ratio is 1.0.*

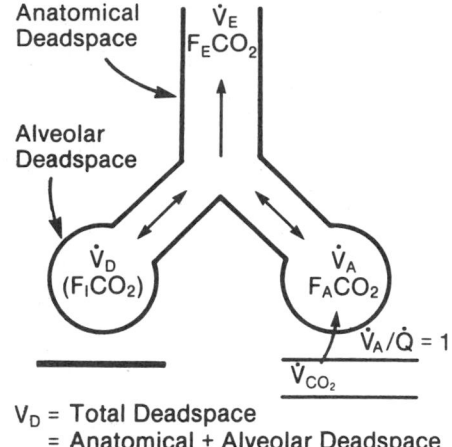

V_D = Total Deadspace
= Anatomical + Alveolar Deadspace

Fig. 15-21. Two-compartment model of lung in which the anatomic and alveolar dead space compartments have been combined into the total (physiologic) dead space (V_D). $\dot{V}_A$, alveolar ventilation; $\dot{V}_E$, expired minute ventilation; $\dot{V}_{CO_2}$, carbon dioxide production; F_ICO_2, inspired carbon dioxide fraction; F_ACO_2, alveolar carbon dioxide fraction; $\overline{F}_ECO_2$, mixed expired carbon dioxide fraction; $\dot{V}_A/\dot{Q} = 1$, equal ventilation and perfusion in L/min. Normally, the amount of CO_2 eliminated at the airway ($\dot{V}_E \cdot \overline{F}_ECO_2$) equals the amount of CO_2 removed by alveolar ventilation ($\dot{V}_A \cdot F_ACO_2$) since there is no CO_2 elimination from alveolar dead space ($F_ICO_2 = 0$).

The anatomic dead space varies with lung size and is approximately 2 ml/kg of body weight. In the normal patient lying supine, the anatomic and total dead spaces are approximately equal to each other because alveolar dead space is minimal. In the erect posture, the uppermost alveoli may not be perfused (zone 1) and alveolar dead space may increase from a negligible amount to 60 to 80 ml.

In severe lung disease, the physiologic dead space to tidal volume ratio $\dot{V}_D/\dot{V}_T$ provides a useful expression of the inefficiency of ventilation. In the normal patient, this ratio is usually less than 30 percent; that is, ventilation is more than 70 percent efficient. In the patient with obstructive airway disease, $\dot{V}_D/\dot{V}_T$ may increase to 60 to 70 percent. Under these conditions, ventilation is obviously grossly inefficient. Figure 15-22 shows the relationship between minute ventilation ($\dot{V}_E$) and $PaCO_2$ for several $\dot{V}_D/\dot{V}_T$ values. As $\dot{V}_E$ decreases, $PaCO_2$ increases for all $\dot{V}_D/\dot{V}_T$. As $\dot{V}_D/\dot{V}_T$ increases, a given decrease in $\dot{V}_E$ causes a much greater increase in $PaCO_2$. If $PaCO_2$ is to remain constant while $\dot{V}_D/\dot{V}_T$ increases, then $\dot{V}_E$ must increase.

The alveolar concentration of a gas is equal to the

---

* Figure 15-21 indicates that in a steady state, the volume of CO_2 entering the alveoli ($\dot{V}_{CO_2}$) must equal the volume of CO_2 eliminated in the expired gas ($\dot{V}_E$) ($\overline{F}_ECO_2$). Thus $\dot{V}_{CO_2} = (\dot{V}_E)(\overline{F}_ECO_2)$. But the expired gas volume consists of alveolar gas ($\dot{V}_A$)(F_ACO_2) and dead space gas ($\dot{V}_D$)(F_ICO_2). Thus $\dot{V}_{CO_2} = (\dot{V}_A)(F_ACO_2) + (\dot{V}_D)(F_ICO_2)$. Setting the first equation equal to the second equa-

tion and using the relationship $\dot{V}_E = \dot{V}_A + \dot{V}_D$, subsequent algebraic manipulation (including setting $PACO_2 = PaCO_2$) results in the physiologic dead space equation:

$$\dot{V}_D/\dot{V}_T = (PaCO_2 - \overline{P}_ECO_2)/PaCO_2 \qquad (6)$$

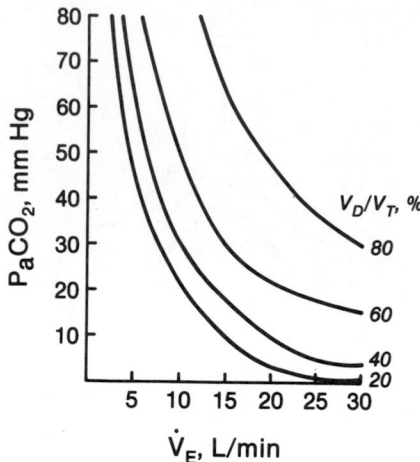

Fig. 15-22. Relationship between the minute ventilation ($\dot{V}_E$, L/min) and $PaCO_2$ for a family of total dead space to tidal volume ratios (V_D/V_T). These curves are hyperbolic [see following eq. (7)] and rise steeply at low $\dot{V}_E$ values.

difference between the inspired concentration of a gas and the ratio of the output (or uptake) of the gas to the $\dot{V}_A$. Thus, for gas X during dry conditions, $P_AX = (Pdry\ atm)(F_IX) \pm \dot{V}X$ (output or uptake)$/\dot{V}_A$, where $P_AX =$ alveolar partial pressure of gas X; $F_IX =$ inspired concentration of gas X; $Pdry\ atm =$ dry atmospheric pressure $= Pwet\ atm - PH_2O = 760 - 47 = 713$ mmHg; $\dot{V}X =$ output or uptake of gas X; $\dot{V}_A =$ alveolar ventilation. For CO_2, $P_ACO_2 = 713(F_ICO_2 + \dot{V}CO_2/\dot{V}_A)$. Since $F_ICO_2 = 0$ and using standard conversion factors,

$$P_ACO_2 = 713[\dot{V}CO_2\ (ml/min\ STPD)/\dot{V}_A\ (L/min/BTPS)(0.863)] \quad (7)$$

For example, 36 mmHg = (713)(200/4,000).

For O_2,

$$P_AO_2 = 713[F_IO_2 - \dot{V}O_2\ (ml/min)/\dot{V}_A\ (ml/min)] \quad (8)$$

For example, 100 mmHg = 713(0.21 − 225/3,200).

Figure 15-23 shows the hyperbolic relationships expressed in equations seven and eight between P_ACO_2 and $\dot{V}_A$ (and Fig. 15-22) and between P_AO_2 and $\dot{V}_A$ for different levels of $\dot{V}CO_2$ and $\dot{V}O_2$, respectively. P_ACO_2 is substituted for $PaCO_2$, since P_ACO_2 to $PaCO_2$ gradients are small (as opposed to P_AO_2 to PaO_2 gradients, which can be large). Note that as $\dot{V}_A$ increases, the second term of the right-hand side of equations (7) and (8) approaches zero and the composition of the alveolar gas approaches that of the inspired gas. In addition, it should be noted from Figure 15-24 that since anesthesia is usually administered with an oxygen-enriched gas mixture, hypercarbia is a more common result of hypoventilation than hypoxemia.

Oxygen Transport

The Oxygen-Hemoglobin Dissociation Curve

As a red blood cell (RBC) passes by the alveolus, oxygen diffuses into the plasma, increasing the partial pressure

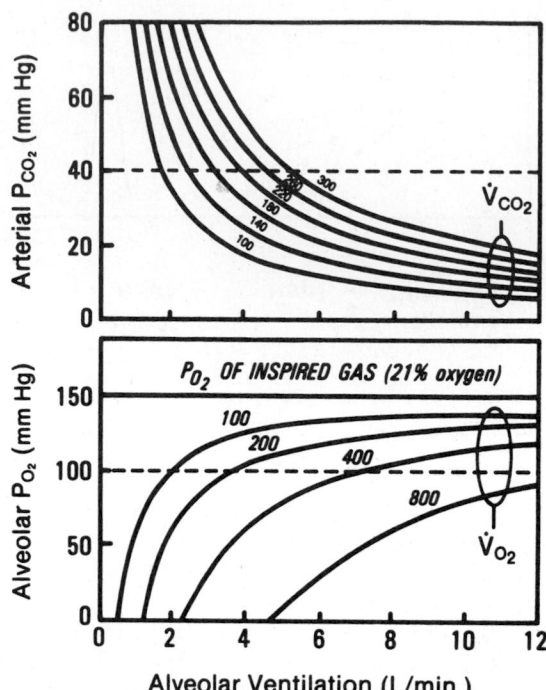

Fig. 15-23. Relationship between alveolar ventilation and P_AO_2 and PaO_2 for a family of different O_2 consumption ($\dot{V}O_2$) and CO_2 production ($\dot{V}CO_2$) is derived from equations (7) and (8) in the text and is hyperbolic. As alveolar ventilation increases, the P_AO_2 and $PaCO_2$ approach inspired concentrations. Decreases in alveolar ventilation below 4 L/min are accompanied by precipitous decreases in P_AO_2 and increases in $PaCO_2$. (From Nunn,[82] with permission.)

of oxygen (PaO_2). As PaO_2 increases, oxygen diffuses into the RBC and combines with hemoglobin (Hb). Each Hb molecule consists of four heme molecules attached to a globin molecule. Each heme molecule consists of glycine, α-ketoglutaric acid, and iron (Fe) in the ferrous (Fe^{2+}) form. Each ferrous ion has the capacity to bind with one oxygen molecule in a loose reversible combination. As the ferrous ions bind to oxygen, the Hb molecule begins to become saturated.

The oxygen-hemoglobin dissociation (oxy-Hb) curve relates the saturation of hemoglobin (y axis most right in Fig. 15-25) to the PaO_2. Hb is fully saturated (100 percent) by a PO_2 of about 700 mmHg. The normal arterial point on the right side and flat part of the oxy-Hb curve in Figure 15-25 is 95 to 98 percent saturation by a PaO_2 of about 90 to 100 mmHg. When the PO_2 is less than 60 mmHg (90 percent saturation), the saturation falls steeply, so that the amount of Hb uncombined with O_2 increases greatly for a given decrease in PO_2. Mixed venous blood has a PO_2 ($P\bar{v}O_2$) of about 40 mmHg and is approximately 75 percent saturated; this is indicated by the middle of the three points on the oxy-Hb curve in Figure 15-25.

The oxy-Hb curve can also relate the O_2 content (Co_2) (volume percent, ml of $O_2/0.1$ L of blood; y axis second most right in Fig. 15-25) to the PO_2. Oxygen is carried in

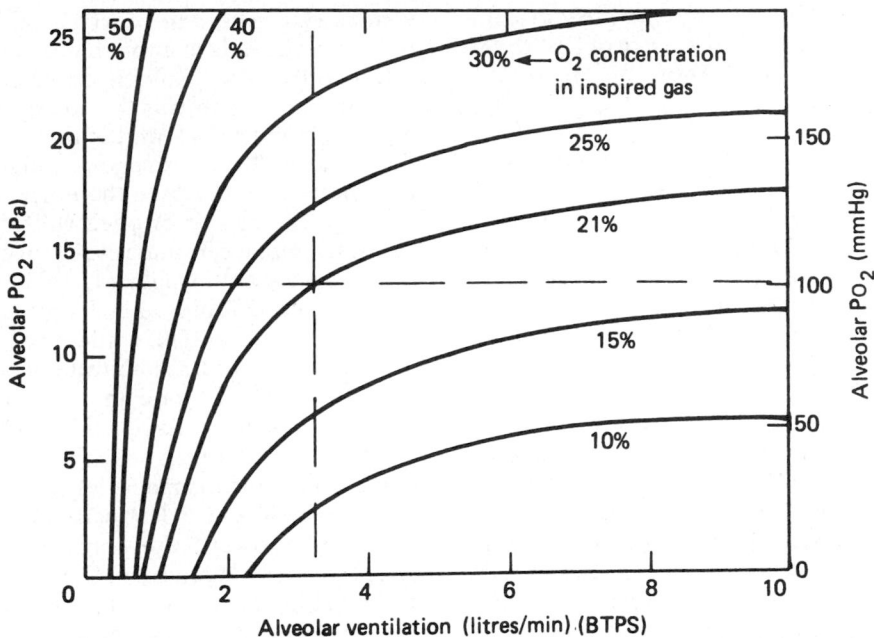

Fig. 15-24. For any given O_2 concentration in the inspired gas, the relationship between alveolar ventilation and P_AO_2 is hyperbolic. As the inspired O_2 concentration is increased, the amount that alveolar ventilation must decrease to produce hypoxemia is greatly increased.

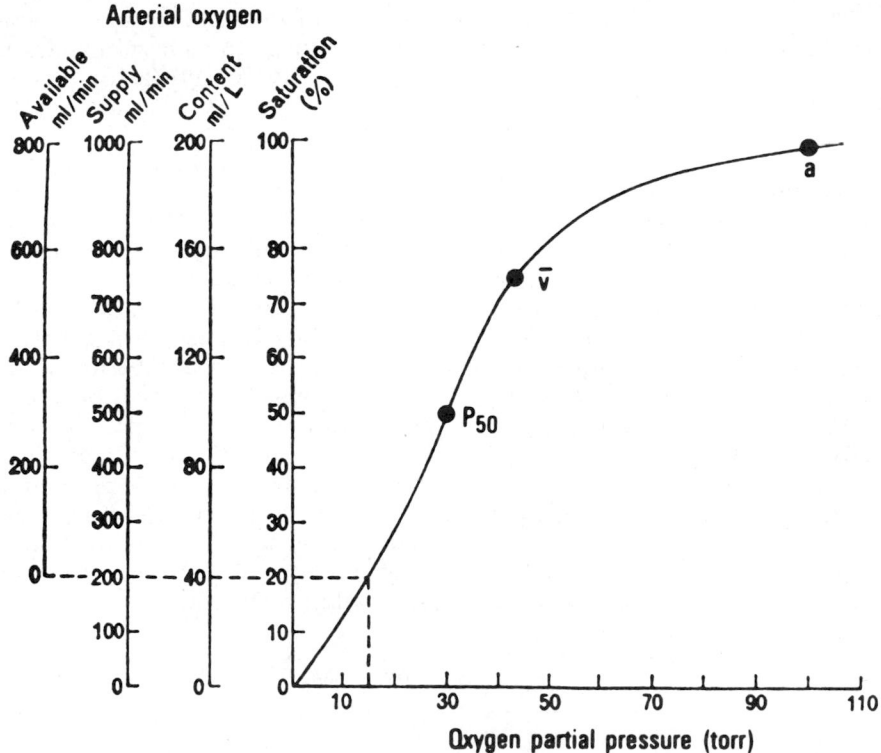

Fig. 15-25. The oxygen-hemoglobin dissociation curve. Four different ordinates are shown as a function of oxygen partial pressure (the abscissa). In order from right to left, they are: saturation (%), O_2 content (ml of O_2/0.1 L) of blood; O_2 supply to the peripheral tissues (ml/min); and O_2 available to the peripheral tissues (ml/min), which is O_2 supply minus approximately 200 ml/min that cannot be extracted below a partial pressure of 20 mmHg. Three points are shown on the curve: *a*, normal arterial; $\overline{v}$, normal mixed venous; and P_{50}, the partial pressure (27 mmHg) at which hemoglobin is 50 percent saturated.

solution in the plasma, 0.003 ml of O_2/mmHg PO_2/0.1 L, and combined with Hb, 1.39 ml of O_2/g of Hb* to the extent (percent) Hb is saturated. Thus

$$Co_2 = (1.39)(Hb)(\text{percent saturation}) + 0.003(PO_2) \quad (9)$$

For a patient with a Hb of 15 g/0.1 L, PaO_2 of 100 mmHg, and $P\bar{v}O_2$ of 40 mmHg, $CaO_2 = (1.39)(15)(1) + (0.003)(100) = 20.9 + 0.3 = 21.2$ ml of O_2/0.1 L; $C\bar{v}O_2 = (1.39)(15)(0.75) - (0.003)(40) = 15.6 + 0.1 = 15.2$ ml of O_2/0.1 L. Thus, the normal arteriovenous O_2 content difference is approximately 5.5 ml/0.1 L.

The oxy-Hb curve can also relate the O_2 transport (L/min) to the peripheral tissues (y axis third most right in Fig. 15-25) to the PO_2. This is obtained by multiplying O_2 content by the cardiac output ($\dot{Q}T$) (O_2 transport = $\dot{Q}T \times CaO_2$). To do this multiplication, one must convert the content unit of ml/0.1 L to ml/L by multiplying the usual O_2 content by 10 (results in ml of O_2/L of blood); subsequent multiplication of ml/L against $\dot{Q}T$ in L/min yields ml/min. Thus, if $\dot{Q}T = 5$ L/min and $CaO_2 = 20.4$ ml of O_2/0.1 L, then the arterial point corresponds to 1,060 ml/min going to the periphery and the venous point corresponds to 785 ml/min returning to the lungs, with $\dot{V}O_2 = 275$ ml/min.

The oxy-Hb curve can also relate the O_2 actually available to the tissues (y axis most left in Fig. 15-25) as a function of PO_2. Of the 1,000 ml/min of O_2 normally going to the periphery, 200 ml/min of O_2 cannot be extracted because it would lower the PO_2 below the level (rectangular dashed line in Fig. 15-25) at which organs such as the brain can survive; the O_2 available to the tissues is therefore 800 ml/min. This is approximately three to four times the normal resting $\dot{V}O_2$. When $\dot{Q}T = 5$ L/min and the arterial saturation is less than 40 percent, the total flow of O_2 to the periphery is reduced to 400 ml/min, so that the available O_2 is now 200 ml/min and O_2 supply just equals O_2 demand. Consequently, with low arterial saturation, tissue demand can only be met by an increase in cardiac output or, in the longer term, by an increase in Hb concentration.

The position of the oxy-Hb curve is best described by the PO_2 level at which Hb is 50 percent saturated (P_{50}). The normal adult P_{50} (the point on the left side and steep portion of the oxy-Hb curve in Fig. 15-24) is 26.7 mmHg.

The effect of a shift in the position of the oxy-Hb curve on Hb saturation depends greatly on the PO_2. In the region of the normal PaO_2 (75 to 100 mmHg), the curve is relatively horizontal, so that shifts of the curve have little effect on saturation. In the region of the mixed venous PO_2, where the curve is relatively steep, a shift of the curve leads to a much greater difference in saturation. A P_{50} of < 27 mmHg describes a left-shifted oxy-Hb curve, which means that at any given PO_2, Hb has a higher affinity for O_2 and is therefore more saturated than normal. This may require a higher tissue perfusion than normal to produce the normal amount of O_2 unloading. The causes of a left-shifted oxy-Hb curve are alkalosis (metabolic and respiratory — the Bohr effect), hypothermia, abnormal and fetal Hb, carboxyhemoglobin, methemoglobin, and decreased RBC 2,3-diphosphoglycerate (2,3-DPG) content (which may occur with transfusion of old acid-citrate-dextrose [ACD]-stored blood; storage of blood in citrate-phosphate-dextrose [CPD] minimizes changes in 2,3-DPG with time).

A P_{50} of > 27 mmHg describes a right-shifted oxy-Hb curve, which means that at any given PO_2, Hb has a low affinity for O_2 and is less saturated than normal. This may allow a lower tissue perfusion than normal to produce the normal amount of O_2 unloading. The causes of a right-shifted oxy-Hb curve are acidosis (metabolic and respiratory — the Bohr effect), hyperthermia, abnormal Hb, and increased RBC 2,3-DPG content.

Abnormalities in acid-base balance result in alteration of 2,3-DPG metabolism to shift the oxy-Hb curve to its normal position. This compensatory change in 2,3-DPG requires between 24 and 48 hours. Thus, with acute acid-base abnormalities, oxygen affinity and the position of the oxy-Hb curve change. However, with more prolonged acid-base changes, the altered levels of 2,3-DPG shift the oxy-Hb curve and, therefore, oxygen affinity back toward normal.

The Effect of $\dot{Q}s/\dot{Q}T$ on the PaO_2

Figure 15-26[82] shows the relationship between FIO_2 and PaO_2 for a family of right-to-left transpulmonary shunts ($\dot{Q}s/\dot{Q}T$); the calculations assume a constant and normal cardiac output and $PaCO_2$. With no $\dot{Q}s/\dot{Q}T$, a linear increase in FIO_2 results in a linear increase in PaO_2 (solid straight line). As the shunt is increased, the $\dot{Q}s/\dot{Q}T$ lines relating FIO_2 to PaO_2 become progressively flatter.[83] With a shunt of 50 percent of the cardiac output, an increase in FIO_2 results in almost no increase in PaO_2. The solution to the problem of hypoxemia secondary to a large shunt is not increasing the FIO_2, but rather causing a reduction in the shunt (fiberoptic bronchoscopy, PEEP, patient positioning, antibiotics, suctioning, diuretics).

The Effect of $\dot{Q}T$ and $\dot{V}O_2$ on CaO_2

In addition to an increased $\dot{Q}s/\dot{Q}T$, the CaO_2 is decreased by a decreased $\dot{Q}T$ (for a constant $\dot{V}O_2$) and by an increased $\dot{V}O_2$ (for a constant $\dot{Q}T$). In either case (decreased $\dot{Q}T$ or increased $\dot{V}O_2$), along with a constant right-to-left shunt, the tissues must extract more O_2 from the blood per unit blood volume, and therefore, the O_2 content of mixed venous blood ($C\bar{v}O_2$) must pri-

---

* Controversy exists over the magnitude of this number. Originally, 1.34 had been used,[79] but with the determination of the molecular weight of hemoglobin (64,458), the theoretical value of 1.39 has become popular.[80] Following extensive human studies, Gregory[81] observed in 1974 that the applicable value was 1.306 ml/g% in human adults. Most of the literature still, however, utilizes 1.39.

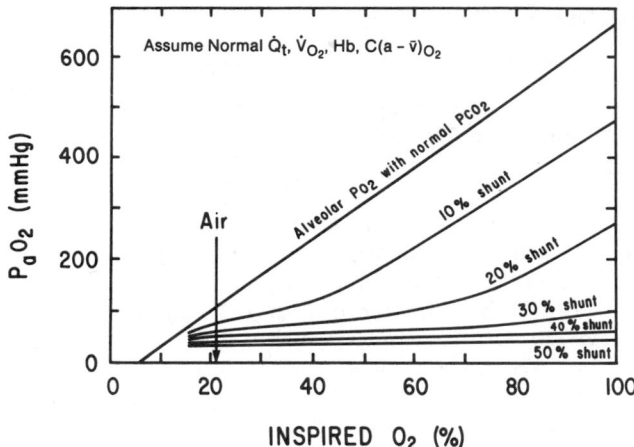

Fig. 15-26. Effect of changes in inspired oxygen concentration on PaO_2 for various right to left transpulmonary shunts. Cardiac output ($\dot{Q}T$), hemoglobin (Hb), oxygen consumption ($\dot{V}O_2$), and arteriovenous oxygen content differences [C(a − v)O_2] were assumed to be normal. (From Nunn,[82] with permission.)

marily decrease (Fig. 15-27). When the blood with lower $C\bar{v}O_2$ passes through whatever shunt that exists in the lung and remains unchanged in its O_2 composition, it must inevitably mix with oxygenated end-pulmonary capillary blood (c′ flow) and secondarily decrease the

CaO_2 (Fig. 15-27).* The larger the intrapulmonary shunt, the greater is the decrease in CaO_2 because more venous blood with lower $C\bar{v}O_2$ can admix with end-pulmonary capillary blood (see also Fig. 15-37).[84,85] Thus, the $P(A − a)O_2$ is a function of both the size of the $\dot{Q}s/\dot{Q}T$ and what is flowing through the $\dot{Q}s/\dot{Q}T$, namely, $C\bar{v}O_2$, and $C\bar{v}O_2$ is a primary function of $\dot{Q}T$ and $\dot{V}O_2$.

Figure 15-28 shows an example of a patient with a 50 percent shunt, a normal $C\bar{v}O_2$ of 15 vol percent, and a moderately low CaO_2 of 17.5 vol percent. Decreasing $\dot{Q}T$ and/or increasing $\dot{V}O_2$ causes a larger primary decrease in $C\bar{v}O_2$ to 10 vol percent and a smaller, but still significant, secondary decrease in CaO_2 to 15 vol percent; the ratio of change in $C\bar{v}O_2$ to CaO_2 in this example of 50 percent $\dot{Q}s/\dot{Q}T$ is 2 : 1.

If a decrease in $\dot{Q}T$ or an increase in $\dot{V}O_2$ is accompa-

---

* The amount of O_2 flowing through any given channel per minute in Figure 15-27 is a product of the blood flow times the O_2 content. Thus, from Figure 15-27:

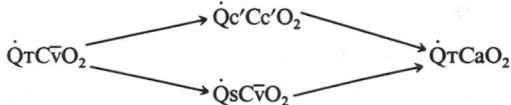

$\dot{Q}TCaO_2 = \dot{Q}c'Cc'O_2 + \dot{Q}sC\bar{v}O_2$. With $\dot{Q}c' = \dot{Q}T − \dot{Q}s$ and further algebraic manipulation[86]

$$\dot{Q}s/\dot{Q}T = Cc'O_2 − CaO_2/Cc'O_2 − C\bar{v}O_2 \qquad (10)$$

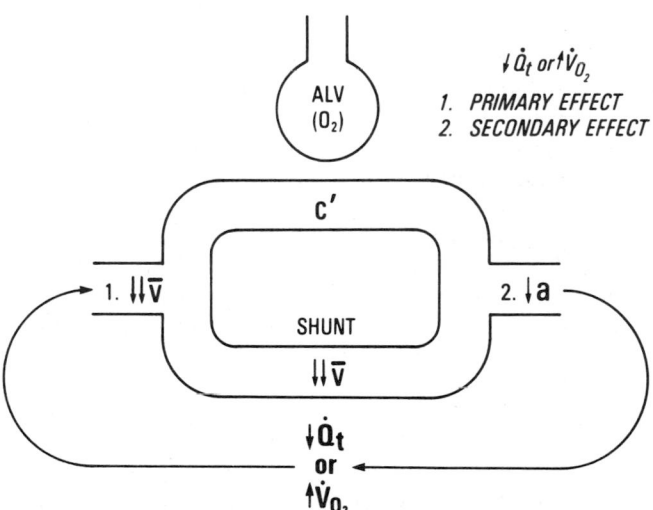

Fig. 15-27. Effect of a decrease in cardiac output or an increase in oxygen consumption on mixed venous and arterial oxygen contents. Mixed venous blood ($\bar{v}$) perfuses either ventilated alveolar (ALV O_2) capillaries and becomes oxygenated end-pulmonary capillary blood (c′) or perfuses whatever true shunt pathways exist and remains the same in composition (desaturated). These two pathways must ultimately join together to form mixed arterial (a) blood. If the cardiac output ($\dot{Q}T$) decreases and/or the oxygen consumption ($\dot{V}O_2$) increases, the tissues must extract more oxygen per unit volume of blood than under normal conditions. Thus, the primary effect of a decrease in $\dot{Q}T$ or an increase in $\dot{V}O_2$ is a decrease in mixed venous oxygen content. The mixed venous blood with a decreased oxygen content must flow through the shunt pathway as before (which may remain constant in size) and lower the arterial content of oxygen. Thus, the secondary effect of a decrease in $\dot{Q}T$ or an increase in $\dot{V}O_2$ is a decrease in arterial oxygen content.

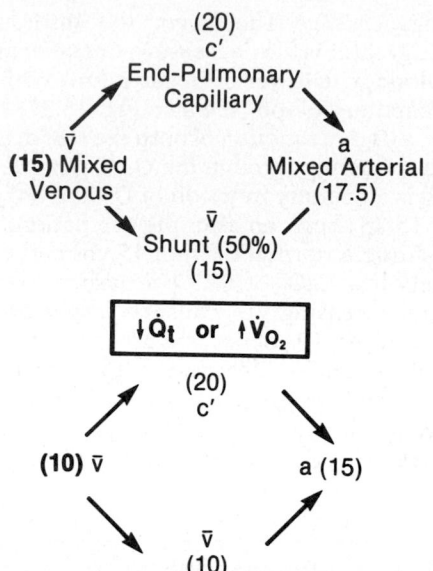

Fig. 15-28. The equivalent circuit of the pulmonary circulation in a patient with a 50 percent right-to-left shunt. Oxygen content is in ml/100 ml of blood (vol percent). A decrease in cardiac output ($\dot{Q}_T$) or an increase in O_2 consumption ($\dot{V}O_2$) can cause a decrease in mixed venous oxygen content (from 15 to 10 vol percent in this example), which in turn will cause a decrease in the arterial content of oxygen (from 17.5 to 15.0 vol percent). In this 50 percent shunt example, the decrease in mixed venous oxygen content was twice the decrease in arterial oxygen content.

nied by a decrease in $\dot{Q}s/\dot{Q}_T$, then there may be no change in PaO_2 (a decreasing effect on PaO_2 is offset by an increasing effect on PaO_2) (Table 15-1). These changes sometimes occur in diffuse lung disease. If a decrease in $\dot{Q}_T$ or an increase in $\dot{V}O_2$ is accompanied by an increase in $\dot{Q}s/\dot{Q}_T$, then PaO_2 may be greatly decreased (a decreasing effect on PaO_2 is compounded by another decreasing effect on PaO_2) (Table 15-1). These changes sometimes occur in regional adult respiratory distress syndrome (ARDS) and atelectasis.[87]

The Fick Principle

The Fick principle allows calculation of $\dot{V}O_2$ and states that the amount of O_2 consumed by the body ($\dot{V}O_2$) is equal to the amount of O_2 leaving the lungs ($\dot{Q}_T$)(CaO_2) minus the amount of O_2 returning to the lungs

($\dot{Q}_T$)($C\bar{v}O_2$). Thus

$$\dot{V}O_2 = (\dot{Q}_T)(CaO_2) - (\dot{Q}_T)(C\bar{v}O_2) = \dot{Q}_T(CaO_2 - C\bar{v}O_2);$$

Condensing the content symbols yields the usual expression of the Fick equation:

$$\dot{V}O_2 = (\dot{Q}_T)[C(a - v)O_2] \tag{11}$$

This equation states that oxygen consumption is equal to the cardiac output times the arteriovenous O_2 content difference. Normally (5 L/min)(5.5 ml)/0.1 L = 0.27 L/min (see the section, *The Oxygen-Hemoglobin Dissociation Curve*).

Similarly, the amount of O_2 consumed by the body ($\dot{V}O_2$) is equal to the amount of O_2 brought into the lungs by ventilation ($\dot{V}I$)(FIO_2) minus the amount of O_2 leaving the lungs by ventilation ($\dot{V}E$)($F\bar{E}O_2$). Thus, $\dot{V}O_2 = (\dot{V}I)(FIO_2) - (\dot{V}E)(F\bar{E}O_2)$. Since the difference between $\dot{V}I$ and $\dot{V}E$ is due to the difference between $\dot{V}O_2$ (normally, 270 ml/min) and $\dot{V}CO_2$ (normally, 200 ml/min) and is only 70 ml/min (see below), $\dot{V}I$ essentially equals $\dot{V}E$; substituting $\dot{V}E$ for $\dot{V}I$:

$$\dot{V}O_2 = \dot{V}E(FIO_2) - \dot{V}E(F\bar{E}O_2) = \dot{V}E(FIO_2 - F\bar{E}O_2) \tag{12}$$

Normally, $\dot{V}O_2 = 5.0$ L/min $(0.21 - 0.16) = 0.25$ L/min. In determining $\dot{V}O_2$ in this way, $\dot{V}E$ can be measured with a spirometer, FIO_2 can be measured with an O_2 analyzer or from known fresh gas flows, and $F\bar{E}O_2$ can be measured by collecting expired gas in a bag for a few minutes. A sample of the mixed expired gas is used to measure $P\bar{E}O_2$. To convert $P\bar{E}O_2$ to $F\bar{E}O_2$, simply divide $P\bar{E}O_2$ by dry atmospheric pressure: $P\bar{E}O_2/713 = F\bar{E}O_2$.

Additionally, the Fick equation is useful in understanding the impact of changes in $\dot{Q}_T$ on PaO_2 and $P\bar{v}O_2$. If $\dot{V}O_2$ remains constant (K) and $\dot{Q}_T$ decreases ($\downarrow$), then the arteriovenous O_2 content difference has to increase ($\uparrow$):

$$\dot{V}O_2 = K = (\downarrow)\dot{Q}_T \times (\uparrow)C(a - \bar{v})O_2.$$

The $C(a - \bar{v})O_2$ difference increases because a decrease in $\dot{Q}_T$ causes a much larger and primary decrease in $C\bar{v}O_2$ compared with a smaller and secondary decrease in CaO_2:

$$(\uparrow)C(a - \bar{v})O_2 = C(\downarrow a - \downarrow\downarrow\bar{v})O_2[84]$$

Thus, the $C\bar{v}O_2$ (and $P\bar{v}O_2$) are much more sensitive indicators of $\dot{Q}_T$, since they change more with the changes in $\dot{Q}_T$ than does CaO_2 (and PaO_2) (see also Figs. 15-27 and 15-37).

TABLE 15-1. Cardiac Output ($\dot{Q}_T$), Shunt ($\dot{Q}s/\dot{Q}_T$), Venous ($P\bar{v}O_2$), and Arterial (PaO_2) Oxygenation

Changes in $\dot{Q}_T$, $\dot{Q}s/\dot{Q}_T$, $P\bar{v}O_2$, PaO_2	Clinical Situation
If $\dot{Q}_T\downarrow \rightarrow \downarrow P\bar{v}O_2$ and $\dot{Q}s/\dot{Q}_T = K \rightarrow PaO_2\downarrow$	Classic theory, normal lung
If $\dot{Q}_T\downarrow \rightarrow \downarrow P\bar{v}O_2$ and $\dot{Q}s/\dot{Q}_T \rightarrow PaO_2 = K$	Diffuse lung disease
If $\dot{Q}_T\downarrow \rightarrow \downarrow P\bar{v}O_2$ and $\dot{Q}s/\dot{Q}_T\uparrow \rightarrow PaO_2\downarrow\downarrow$	Regional ARDS and atelectasis

Symbols: K, constant; $\downarrow$, decrease; $\uparrow$, increase.

Carbon Dioxide Transport

The amount of CO_2 circulating in the body is a function of both CO_2 elimination and production. Elimination of CO_2 depends on pulmonary blood flow and alveolar ventilation. Production of CO_2 parallels O_2 consumption according to the respiratory quotient (R):

$$R = \frac{\text{rate of } CO_2 \text{ output}}{\text{rate of } O_2 \text{ uptake}} \qquad (13)$$

Under normal resting conditions, R is 0.8; that is, only 80 percent as much CO_2 is produced as O_2 is consumed. However, this value changes as the nature of the metabolic substrate changes. If only carbohydrate is utilized, the respiratory quotient is 1.0. Conversely, with the sole use of fat, more O_2 combines with hydrogen to produce water and the R value drops to 0.7.

Carbon dioxide is transported from the mitochondria to the alveolus in a number of forms. In plasma, CO_2 exists in physical solution, hydrated to carbonic acid (H_2CO_3) and as bicarbonate (HCO_3^-). In the erythrocyte, CO_2 combines with Hb as carbaminohemoglobin ($Hb-CO_2$). The approximate relative values of H_2CO_3 ($H_2O + CO_2$), HCO_3^-, and $Hb-CO_2$ to the total CO_2 transported are 7, 80, and 13 percent, respectively.

In plasma, CO_2 exists both in physical solution and as H_2CO_3:

$$H_2O + CO_2 \rightleftharpoons H_2CO_3 \qquad (14)$$

The CO_2 in solution can be related to PCO_2 by use of Henry's law[88]:

$$PCO_2 \times \alpha = [CO_2] \text{ in solution} \qquad (15)$$

where α is the solubility coefficient of CO_2 in plasma (0.03 mmol/L/mmHg at 37°C). However, the major fraction of CO_2 produced passes into the erythrocyte. As in plasma, CO_2 combines with water to produce carbonic acid. However, unlike in plasma where the reaction is slow and most of the equilibrium is to the left, the reaction in the erythrocyte is catalyzed by the enzyme carbonic anhydrase. This zinc-containing enzyme moves the reaction to the right at a rate 1,000 times faster than in plasma. Further, nearly 99.9 percent of the carbonic acid dissociates to the bicarbonate and hydrogen ions:

$$H_2O + CO_2 \xrightarrow{\text{carbonic anhydrase}} H_2CO_3$$
$$H_2CO_3 \longrightarrow H^+ + HCO_3^- \qquad (16)$$

The hydrogen ion produced from H_2CO_3 in the production of HCO_3^- is buffered by Hb ($H^+ + Hb \rightleftharpoons HHb$). The HCO_3^- produced passes out of the erythrocyte into the plasma to perform its function as a buffer. To maintain electrical neutrality within the erythrocyte, chloride ion moves in as HCO_3^- moves out (chloride shift). Finally, CO_2 can combine with Hb in the erythrocyte (to produce $Hb-CO_2$). Again, as in the HCO_3^- release, an H^+ is formed in the reaction of CO_2 and hemoglobin. This H^+ is also buffered by Hb.

The Bohr and Haldane Effects

Just as the percent saturation of Hb with O_2 is related to PO_2, so is the total CO_2 in blood related to PCO_2. The Bohr effect is the dependence of the position of the oxy-Hb curve on PCO_2 and pH; hypercapnia and acidosis shift the curve to the right, and hypocapnia and alkalosis shift the curve to the left. The Haldane effect is the shift in the relationship of PCO_2 to total CO_2 (i.e., the CO_2 dissociation curve) caused by altered levels of O_2. Low PO_2 shifts the CO_2 dissociation curve to the left so that the blood is able to pick up more CO_2.

The Pulmonary Microcirculation, The Pulmonary Interstitial Space, and Pulmonary Interstitial Fluid Kinetics (Pulmonary Edema)

The ultrastructural appearance of an alveolar septum is schematically depicted in Figure 15-29.[89] Capillary blood is separated from alveolar gas by a series of anatomic layers: capillary endothelium, endothelial basement membrane, interstitial space, epithelial basement membrane, and alveolar epithelium (of the type I pneumocyte).

On one side of the alveolar septum (the thick, upper [Fig. 15-29], fluid- and gas-exchanging side), the epithelial and endothelial basement membranes are separated by a space of variable thickness containing connective tissue fibrils, elastic fibers, fibroblasts, and macrophages. This connective tissue is the backbone of the lung parenchyma; it forms a continuum with the connective tissue sheaths around the conducting airways and blood vessels. Thus, the pericapillary perialveolar interstitial space is continuous with the interstitial tissue space that surrounds terminal bronchioles and vessels, and both spaces constitute the connective tissue space of the lung. There are no lymphatics in the interstitial space of the alveolar septum. Instead, lymphatic capillaries first appear in the interstitial space surrounding terminal bronchioles, small arteries, and veins.

The opposite side of the alveolar septum (the thin, down [Fig. 15-29], gas-exchanging-only side) contains only fused epithelial and endothelial basement membranes. The interstitial space is thus greatly restricted on this side owing to fusion of the basement membranes. Interstitial fluid cannot separate the endothelial and epithelial cells from one another, and as a result, the space and distance barrier to fluid movement from the capillary to alveolar compartment is reduced and is composed only of the two cell linings with their associated basement membranes.[90,91]

Between the individual endothelial and epithelial cells are holes or junctions that provide a potential pathway for fluid to move from the intravascular space to the interstitial space and finally from the interstitial space to the alveolar space. The junctions between endothelial cells are relatively large and are therefore termed *loose;* the junctions between epithelial cells are

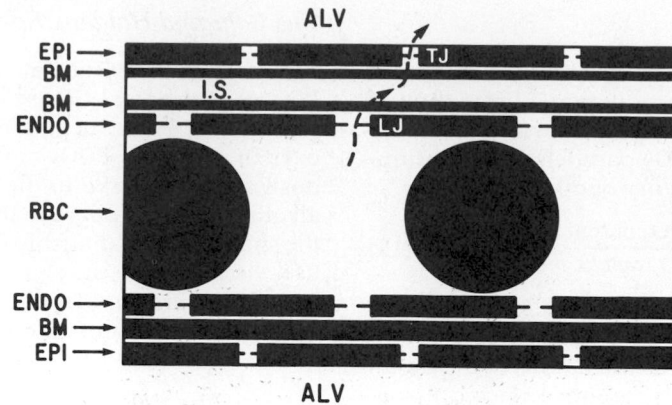

Fig. 15-29. Schematic summary of the ultrastructure of the pulmonary capillary. RBC, red blood cell; ENDO, endothelium; BM, basement membrane; IS, interstitial space; EPI, epithelium; L J, loose junction; TJ, tight junction; ALV, alveolus. The upper side of the capillary has the endothelial and epithelial basement membranes separated by an interstitial space, whereas the lower side of the capillary contains only fused endothelial and epithelial basement membranes. The dashed arrows indicate a potential pathway for fluid to move from the intravascular space to the interstitial space (through loose junctions in the endothelium) and from the interstitial space to the alveolar space (through tight junctions in the epithelium). (From Fishman,[89] with permission.)

relatively small and therefore termed *tight*. Pulmonary capillary permeability (K) is a direct function of and essentially equivalent to the size of the holes in the endothelial and epithelial linings.

To understand how pulmonary interstitial fluid is formed, stored, and cleared, it is necessary to first develop the concepts that the pulmonary interstitial space is a continuous space between a periarteriolar and peribronchial connective tissue sheath and the space between the endothelial and epithelial basement membranes in the alveolar septum, and that the space has a progressively negative distal to proximal pressure gradient.

The concepts of a continuous connective tissue sheath-alveolar septum interstitial space and a negative interstitial space pressure gradient are prerequisite to understanding interstitial fluid kinetics (Fig. 15-30). After entering the lung parenchyma, both the bronchi and arteries run within a connective tissue sheath that is formed by an invagination of the pleura at the hilum and which ends at the level of the bronchioles (Fig. 15-30A). Thus, there is a potential perivascular and peribronchial space, respectively, between the arteries and the bronchi and the connective tissue sheath. The negative pressure in the pulmonary tissues surrounding the perivascular connective tissue sheath exerts a radial outward traction force on the sheath. The radial traction creates a negative pressure within the sheath that is transmitted to the bronchi and arteries, tending to hold them open and increase their diameters (Fig. 15-30).[2] The alveolar septum interstitial space is the space between the capillaries and alveoli (or more precisely, the space between the endothelial and epithelial basement membranes) and is continuous with the interstitial tissue space that surrounds the larger arteries

and bronchi (Fig. 15-30A). Studies indicate that the alveolar interstitial pressure is also uniquely negative but not as much as the negative interstitial space pressure around the larger arteries and bronchi.[92]

The forces governing net transcapillary-interstitial space fluid movement are as follows. The net transcapillary flow of fluid (F) out of pulmonary capillaries is equal to the difference between pulmonary capillary hydrostatic pressure (Pinside) and the interstitial fluid hydrostatic pressure (Poutside) and to the difference between the capillary colloid oncotic pressure (πinside) and the interstitial colloid oncotic pressure (πoutside). These four forces will produce a steady-state fluid flow (F) during a constant capillary permeability (K).

$$F = K[(Pinside - Poutside) - (\pi inside - \pi outside)] \quad (17)$$

K is a capillary filtration coefficient expressed in ml/min/mmHg/100 g. The filtration coefficient is the product of the effective capillary surface area in a given mass of tissue and the permeability per unit surface area of the capillary wall to filter the fluid. Under normal circumstances, and at a vertical height in the lung that is at the junction of zones 2 and 3, the intravascular colloid oncotic pressure (about 26 mmHg) acts to keep water in the capillary lumen, and working against this force, the pulmonary capillary hydrostatic pressure (about 10 mmHg) acts to force water across the loose endothelial junctions into the interstitial space. If these were the only operative forces, the interstitial space, and consequently the alveolar surfaces, would be constantly dry and there would be no lymph flow. In fact, alveolar surfaces are moist, and lymphatic flow from the interstitial compartment is constant (approximately 500 ml/d). This can be explained in part by the πoutside (8 mmHg) and in part by the negative Poutside (approxi-

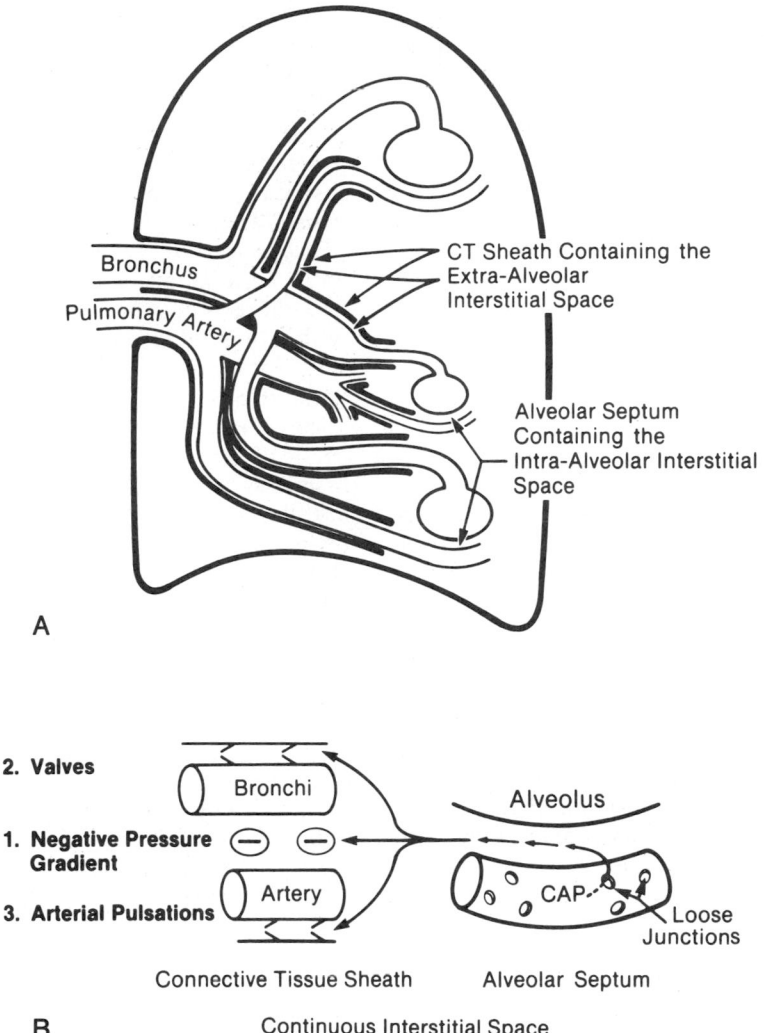

Fig. 15-30. **(A)** Schematic diagram of the concept of a continuous connective tissue sheath-alveolar septum interstitial space. The entry of the main stem bronchi and pulmonary artery into the lung parenchyma invaginates the pleura at the hilum, forming a surrounding connective tissue sheath (heavy black line). The connective tissue sheath ends at the level of the bronchioles. The space between the pulmonary arteries and bronchi and the interstitial space is continuous with the alveolar septum interstitial space. The alveolar septum interstitial space is contained within the endothelial and epithelial basement membranes of the capillaries and alveoli, respectively. **(B)** Schematic diagram showing how interstitial fluid moves from the alveolar septum interstitial space to the connective tissue interstitial space. The mechanisms are a negative pressure gradient (sump), the presence of one-way valves in the lymphatics, and the massaging action of arterial pulsations. (From Benumof,[168] with permission.)

mately 8 mmHg). Negative (subatmospheric) interstitial space pressure would promote, by suction, a slow loss of fluid across the endothelial holes.[93] Indeed, extremely negative pleural (and perivascular hydrostatic) pressure, such as might occur in a vigorously spontaneously breathing patient with an obstructed airway, can cause pulmonary interstitial edema.[94] Relative to the vertical level of the junction of zones 2 and 3, as lung height decreases (lung dependency), absolute Pinside increases, and fluid has a propensity to transudate; as lung height increases (lung nondependency), absolute

Pinside decreases, and fluid has a propensity to be reabsorbed. However, fluid transudation induced by an increase in Pinside is limited by a concomitant dilution of proteins in the interstitial space and therefore a decrease in πoutside.[95] Any change in the size of the endothelial junctions, even if the above four forces remain constant, will change the magnitude and perhaps even the direction of fluid movement; increased size of endothelial junctions (increased permeability) promotes transudation, and decreased size of endothelial junctions (decreased permeability) promotes reabsorption.

There are no lymphatics in the interstitial space of the alveolar septum. Instead, lymphatic capillaries first appear in the interstitial space sheath surrounding terminal bronchioles and small arteries. Interstitial fluid is normally removed from the alveolar interstitial space into the lymphatics by a sump (pressure gradient) mechanism, which is caused by the presence of the more negative pressure surrounding the larger arteries and bronchi.[96,97] The sump mechanism is aided by the presence of valves in the lymph vessels. In addition, since the lymphatics run in the same sheath as the pulmonary arteries, they are exposed to the massaging action of the arterial pulsations. The differential negative pressure, the lymphatic valves, and the arterial pulsations all help to propel the lymph proximally toward the hilum through the lymph nodes (pulmonary to bronchopulmonary to tracheobronchial to paratracheal to scalene and cervical nodes) to the central venous circulation depot (Fig. 15-30B). An increase in central venous pressure, which is the back pressure for lymph to flow out of the lung, would decrease lung lymph flow and, perhaps, promote pulmonary interstitial edema.

If the rate of entry of fluid into the pulmonary interstitial space exceeds the capability of the pulmonary interstitial space to clear the fluid, then the pulmonary interstitial space will fill with fluid; the fluid, now under an increased and positive driving force (P_{ISF}), will cross the relatively impermeable epithelial wall holes and the alveolar space will fill. Intra-alveolar edema fluid will additionally cause alveolar collapse and atelectasis, thereby promoting further fluid accumulation.

RESPIRATORY FUNCTION DURING ANESTHESIA

Introduction

The effect of a given anesthetic on respiratory function will depend on the depth of general anesthesia, the patient's preoperative respiratory condition, and the presence of special intraoperative anesthetic and surgical conditions.

Effect of Anesthetic Depth on Respiratory Pattern

The respiratory pattern is altered by the induction and deepening of anesthesia.[98] When the depth of anesthesia is inadequate (less than minimum alveolar concentration [MAC]), the respiratory pattern may vary from excessive hyperventilation and vocalization to breath-holding. As anesthetic depth approaches or equals MAC (light anesthesia), irregular respiration progresses to a more regular pattern, which is associated with a larger than normal tidal volume. However, during light but deepening anesthesia, the approach to a more regular respiratory pattern may be interrupted by a pause at the end of inspiration (a sort of hitch in the inspiration), followed by a relatively prolonged and active expiration in which the patient seems to exhale forcefully, rather than passively. As anesthesia deepens to moderate levels, respiration becomes faster, more regular, but more shallow. The respiratory pattern is a sine wave losing the inspiratory hitch and lengthened expiratory pause. There is little or no inspiratory or expiratory pause, and the inspiratory and expiratory periods are equivalent. Intercostal muscle activity is still present, and there is normal movement of the thoracic cage with lifting of the chest during inspiration. The respiratory rate is generally slower and the tidal volume larger with nitrous oxide–narcotic anesthesia compared with anesthesia with halogenated drugs. During deep anesthesia with halogenated drugs, increasing depression of respiration is manifested by even more rapid, shallow breathing (panting). On the other hand, with deep nitrous oxide–narcotic anesthesia, respirations become slower but may remain deep. With very deep anesthesia with all drugs, respirations are jerky or gasping in character and irregular in pattern. This results from loss of active intercostal muscle contribution to inspiration. As a result, a rocking boat movement occurs in which there is an out-of-phase depression of the chest wall during inspiration, a flaring of the lower chest margins, and a billowing of the abdomen. The reason for this type of movement is that inspiration is dependent solely on diaphragmatic effort. Independent of anesthetic depth, similar chest movements may be simulated by upper and lower airway obstruction and by partial paralysis.

Effect of Anesthetic Depth on Spontaneous Minute Ventilation

Despite the variable changes in respiratory pattern and rate as anesthesia deepens, overall spontaneous minute ventilation progressively decreases. The normal awake response to breathing CO_2 (the x axis in Fig. 15-31 shows increasing end-tidal concentration of CO_2) causes a linear increase in minute ventilation (y axis Fig. 15-31). In Figure 15-31 the slope of the line relating minute ventilation to end-tidal CO_2 concentration is 2L/min/mmHg. Figure 15-31 also shows that increasing halothane concentration displaces the end-tidal CO_2 concentration PCO_2-ventilation response curve progressively to the right (meaning that at any CO_2 concentration ventilation is less than before), decreases the slope of the curve, and shifts the apneic threshold to a higher end-tidal CO_2 concentration level.[99] Similar alterations are observed with other halogenated anesthetics and narcotics. Figures 15-22 to 15-24 show that decreases in minute ventilation will cause increases in $PaCO_2$ and decreases in PaO_2. In healthy unstimulated spontaneously breathing male volunteers, 1 MAC halothane, isoflurane, and enflurane causes a $PaCO_2$ of approximately 46, 48, and 62 mmHg, respectively.

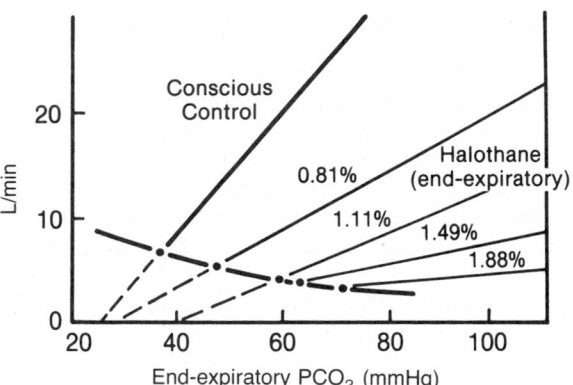

Fig. 15-31. In conscious controls (heavy solid line), increasing end-expiratory PCO_2 increases pulmonary minute volume. The dashed line is an extrapolation of the CO_2–response curve to zero ventilation and represents the apneic threshold. An increase in anesthetic (halothane) concentration (end-expiratory concentration) progressively diminishes the slope of the CO_2-response curve and shifts the apneic threshold to a higher PCO_2. The heavy line interrupted by dots shows the decrease in minute ventilation and the increase in PCO_2 that occur with increasing depth of anesthesia. (From Munson et al.,[99] with permission.)

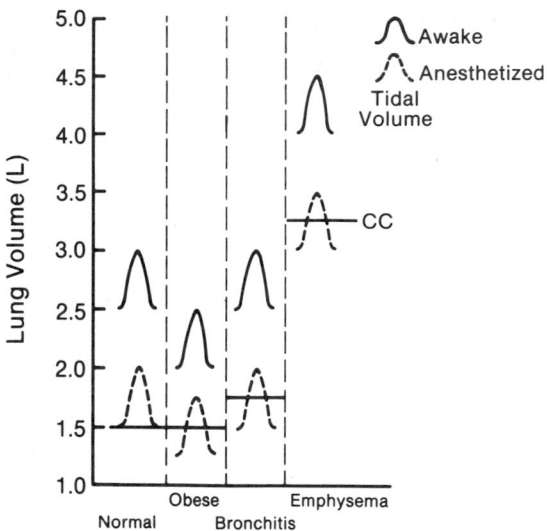

Fig. 15-32. The lung volume (ordinate) at which the tidal volume is breathed decreases (by 1 L) from the awake state to the anesthetized state. The functional residual capacity, which is the volume of lung existing at the end of the tidal volume, therefore also decreases (by 1 L) from the awake to the anesthetized state. In the normal, obese, bronchitic, and emphysematous patients, the awake functional residual capacity considerably exceeds the closing capacity (CC). In the obese, bronchitic, and emphysematous patients, the anesthetized state causes functional residual capacity to be less than closing capacity. In the normal patient, anesthesia causes the functional residual capacity to equal the closing capacity.

Effect of Pre-existing Respiratory Dysfunction on the Respiratory Effects of Anesthesia

Among the patients that anesthesiologists are frequently required to care for are (1) patients with acute chest disease (pulmonary infection, atelectasis) or systemic diseases (sepsis, cardiac and renal failure, or multiple trauma) that require emergency operations; (2) heavy smokers with subtle pathologic airway and parenchymal conditions and hyperreactive airways; (3) patients with classic emphysematous and bronchitic problems; (4) obese people prone to decreases in FRC during anesthesia;[100,101] (5) patients with chest deformities; and (6) very old patients.

The nature and magnitude of these pre-existing respiratory conditions will determine, in part, the effect of a given standard anesthetic on respiratory function. For example, in Figure 15-32 the FRC-CC relationship is depicted for normal, obese, bronchitic, and emphysematous patients. In the normal patient, FRC exceeds CC by approximately 1 L. In the latter three respiratory conditions, CC is 0.5 to 0.75 L less than FRC. If anesthesia causes a 1-L decrease in FRC, then the normal patient will have no change in the qualitative relationship between FRC and CC. In the patients with special respiratory conditions, a 1-L decrease in FRC will cause CC to exceed FRC and change the previously marginally normal FRC-CC relationship to either a grossly low $\dot{V}A/\dot{Q}$ or an atelectatic FRC-CC relationship. Similarly, patients with chronic bronchitis, who have copious airway secretions, may suffer more from an anesthetic-in-

duced decrease in mucous velocity flow than other patients. Finally, if an anesthetic drug inhibits HPV, the drug may increase shunting more in patients with pre-existing HPV than in those without pre-existing HPV. Thus, the effect of a standard anesthetic can be expected to produce varying degrees of respiratory change among patients who have different degrees of pre-existing respiratory dysfunction.

Effect of Special Intraoperative Conditions on the Respiratory Effects of Anesthesia

Some special intraoperative conditions (such as surgical position, massive blood loss, and surgical retraction on the lung), may cause impaired gas exchange. For example, some of the surgical positions (i.e., the lithotomy, jackknife, and kidney rest positions) and surgical exposure requirements may decrease cardiac output, cause hypoventilation in a spontaneously breathing patient, and reduce the FRC. The respiratory depressant effects of any anesthetic will be magnified by the type and severity of pre-existing respiratory dysfunction as well as by the number and severity of special intraoperative conditions that can embarrass respiratory function.

Mechanisms of Hypoxemia During Anesthesia

Malfunction of Equipment

Mechanical Failure of Anesthesia Apparatus to Deliver Oxygen to the Patient

Hypoxemia resulting from mechanical failure of the oxygen supply system or the anesthesia machine is a recognized hazard of anesthesia. Disconnection of the patient from the oxygen supply system (usually at the juncture of the endotracheal tube and elbow connector) is by far the most common cause of mechanical failure to deliver oxygen to the patient. Other reported causes of oxygen supply failure during anesthesia include an empty or depleted oxygen cylinder, substitution of a nonoxygen cylinder at the oxygen yoke because of absence or failure of the pin index, an erroneously filled oxygen cylinder, insufficient opening of the oxygen cylinder (which hinders a free flow of gas as pressure decreases), failure of gas pressure in a piped oxygen system, faulty locking of the piped oxygen system to the anesthesia machine, inadvertent switching of the Schrader adapters on piped lines, crossing of piped lines during construction, failure of a reducing valve or gas manifold, inadvertent disturbance of the setting of the oxygen flowmeter, employment of the fine oxygen flowmeter instead of the coarse flowmeter, fractured or sticking flowmeters, transposition of rotameter tubes, erroneous filling of a liquid oxygen reservoir with nitrogen, and fresh gas line disconnection from machine to in-line hosing.[102-106]

Mechanical Failure of Endotracheal Tube: Main Stem Bronchus Intubation

Esophageal intubation results in almost no ventilation. Virtually all other mechanical problems (except disconnect) with endotracheal tubes (such as kinking, secretion blockage, and herniated or ruptured cuffs) cause an increase in airway resistance and may result in hypoventilation. Intubation of a main stem bronchus results in the absence of ventilation of the contralateral lung. Although potentially minimized by HPV, some perfusion to the contralateral lung will always remain and shunting will increase and PaO_2 will decrease. A tube previously well positioned in the trachea may enter a bronchus after the patient or the head of a patient is turned or moved into a new position.[107] Flexion of the head causes caudad movement and extension of the head causes cephalad movement of an endotracheal tube.[107] A high incidence of main stem bronchial intubation following institution of a 30-degree Trendelenburg position has been reported.[108] Cephalad shift of the carina during the Trendelenburg position caused the previously "fixed" endotracheal tube to become located in a main stem bronchus.

Hypoventilation (Decreased Tidal Volume)

Patients under general anesthesia may have a reduced spontaneous tidal volume for two reasons. First, it may be more difficult to breathe during general anesthesia because of increased airway resistance and decreased lung compliance. Airway resistance may be increased because of reduced FRC, endotracheal intubation, the presence of external breathing apparatus and circuitry, and possible airway obstruction in patients whose tracheas are not intubated.[109] Lung compliance is reduced owing to some (or all) of the factors that can decrease FRC.[110] Second, the patients may be less willing to breathe spontaneously during general anesthesia (decreased chemical control of breathing) (Fig. 15-31).

There are two ways a decreased tidal volume may cause hypoxemia. First, shallow breathing may promote atelectasis and cause a decrease in FRC (see the section, *Ventilation History*).[111,112] Second, decreased minute ventilation decreases the overall $\dot{V}A/\dot{Q}$ ratio of the lung, which will decrease PaO_2 (Figs. 15-23 and 15-24). This is likely to occur with spontaneous ventilation during moderate to deep levels of anesthesia in which the chemical control of breathing is significantly altered.

Hyperventilation

Hypocapnic alkalosis (hyperventilation) may result in a decreased PaO_2 via several mechanisms. These mechanisms are decreased cardiac output,[84,85] and increased oxygen consumption[113,114] (see the section, *Decreased Cardiac Output and Increased Oxygen Consumption*), a left-shifted oxy-Hb curve (see the section, *The Oxygen-Hemoglobin Dissociation Curve*), decreased HPV[115] (see the section, *Inhibition of Hypoxic Pulmonary Vasoconstriction*), and/or increased airway resistance and decreased compliance[116] (see the section, *Increased Airway Resistance*).

Decrease in Functional Residual Capacity

Induction of general anesthesia is consistently accompanied by a significant (15 to 20 percent) decrease in FRC,[71,78,117] which usually causes a decrease in compliance.[110] The maximum decrease in FRC appears to occur within the first few minutes of anesthesia[71,118-120] and, in the absence of any other complicating factor, does not seem to decrease progressively during anesthesia. During anesthesia, the reduction in FRC is of the same order of magnitude whether ventilation is spontaneous or controlled. Conversely, in awake patients, FRC is only slightly reduced during controlled ventilation.[120] The reduction of FRC continues into the postoperative period.[121] For individual patients, the reduction in FRC correlates well with an increase in the alveolar-arterial PO_2 gradient during anesthesia with spontaneous breathing,[122] during anesthesia with artificial ventilation,[119] and in the postoperative period.[121] The reduced FRC may be restored to normal or above normal by the application of PEEP.[71,123] The following discussion considers all possible causes of reduced FRC.

Supine Position

Anesthesia and surgery are usually performed with the patient in the supine position. In changing from the upright to the supine position, FRC decreases by 0.5 to 1.0 L[71,78,117] because of a 4-cm cephalad displacement of the diaphragm by the abdominal viscera (Fig. 15-33). Pulmonary vascular congestion may also contribute to the decrease in FRC in the supine position, particularly in patients who experienced orthopnea preoperatively.

Induction of General Anesthesia—Change in Thoracic Cage Muscle Tone

At the end of a normal (awake) exhalation, there is slight tension in the inspiratory muscles and no tension in the expiratory muscles. Thus, at the end of a normal exhalation, there is a force tending to maintain lung volume and no force decreasing lung volume. After the induction of general anesthesia, there is a loss of the inspiratory tone and an appearance of end-expiratory tone in the abdominal expiratory muscles at the end of exhalation. The end-expiratory tone in the abdominal expiratory muscles increases intra-abdominal pressure, forces the diaphragm cephalad, and decreases FRC (Fig. 15-33).[118,124] Thus, after the induction of general anesthesia, there is loss of a force tending to maintain lung volume and gain of a force tending to decrease lung volume. Indeed, Innovar (droperidol and fentanyl

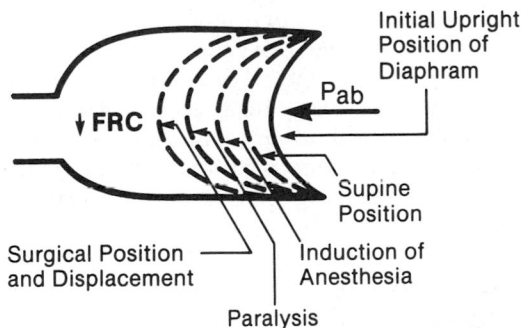

Fig. 15-33. Anesthesia and surgery may cause a progressive cephalad displacement of the diaphragm. The sequence of events involves assuming the supine position, induction of anesthesia, causation of paralysis, the assumption of several surgical positions, and displacement by retractors and packs. The cephalad displacement of the diaphragm results in a decreased functional residual capacity ($\downarrow$ FRC). P_{ab}, pressure of the abdominal contents. (From Benumof,[168] with permission.)

citrate) may increase tone in expiratory muscles to such an extent that the reduction in FRC with Innovar anesthesia alone is greater than that with Innovar plus paralysis induced by succinylcholine.[124,125]

With emphysema, exhalation may be accompanied by pursing the lips or grunting (partially closed larynx). The emphysematous patient exhales in either of these ways because both these maneuvers cause an expiratory retard that produces PEEP in the intrathoracic air passage and decreases the possibility of airway closure and a decrease in FRC (Fig. 15-17F). Endotracheal intubation bypasses the lips and glottis and may abolish normally present pursed-lip or grunting exhalation and in that way contribute to airway closure and a loss in FRC in some spontaneously breathing patients.

Paralysis

In the upright subject, the FRC and the position of the diaphragm are determined by the balance between the lung elastic recoil pulling the diaphragm cephalad and the weight of the abdominal contents pulling it caudad.[126] There is no transdiaphragmatic pressure gradient.

The situation is more complex in the supine position. The diaphragm separates two compartments of markedly different hydrostatic gradients. On the thoracic side, pressure increases approximately 0.25 cmH$_2$O/cm of lung height,[3,4] and on the abdominal side, 1.0 cmH$_2$O/cm of abdominal height.[126] This means that in horizontal postures, progressively higher transdiaphragmatic pressures must be generated toward dependent parts of the diaphragm to keep the abdominal contents out of the thorax. In the unparalyzed patient, this tension is developed by either passive stretch and shape changes of the diaphragm (causing an increased contractile force) or by neurally mediated active tension. With acute muscle paralysis, neither of these two mechanisms can operate and a shift of the diaphragm to a more cephalad position occurs (Fig. 15-33).[127] The latter position must express the true balance of forces on the diaphragm, unmodified by any passive or active muscle activity.

The cephalad shift in the FRC position of the diaphragm owing to expiratory muscle tone during general anesthesia is equal to the shift observed during paralysis (awake or anesthetized patients).[118,128] The equal shift suggests that the pressure on the diaphragm caused by an increase in expiratory muscle tone during general anesthesia is equal to the pressure on the diaphragm caused by the weight of the abdominal contents during paralysis. It is quite probable that the magnitude of these changes in FRC due to paralysis also depends on the body habitus.

Light or Inadequate Anesthesia and Active Expiration

The induction of general anesthesia can result in increased expiratory muscle tone,[124] but the increased expiratory muscle tone is not coordinated and does not contribute to the exhaled volume of gas. In contrast, spontaneous ventilation during light general anesthesia usually results in a coordinated and moderately forceful active exhalation and larger exhaled volumes. Excessively inadequate anesthesia (relative to a given stimulus) results in very forceful active exhalation, which may produce exhaled volumes of gas equal to an awake expiratory vital capacity.

As during an awake expiratory vital capacity maneuver, a forced expiration during anesthesia raises the intrathoracic and alveolar pressures considerably above atmospheric pressure (Fig. 15-17). This results in a rapid outflow of gas, and since part of the expiratory resistance lies in the smaller air passages, a pressure drop will occur between the alveoli and the main bronchi. Under these circumstances, the intrathoracic pressure rises considerably above the pressure within the main bronchi. Collapse will occur if this reversed pressure gradient is sufficiently high to overcome the tethering effect of the surrounding parenchyma on the small intrathoracic bronchioles or the structural rigidity of cartilage in the large extrathoracic bronchi. Such collapse occurs in the normal subject during a maximal forced expiration and is responsible for the associated wheeze in both awake and anesthetized patients.[129]

In the paralyzed anesthetized patient, the use of a subatmospheric expiratory pressure phase is analogous to a forced expiration in the conscious subject; the negative phase may set up the same adverse pressure gradients, which can cause airway closure, gas trapping, and a decrease in FRC. An excessively rapidly descending bellows of a ventilator during expiration has caused a subatmospheric expiratory pressure and has resulted in wheezing.[130]

Increased Airway Resistance

The overall reduction in all components of lung volume during anesthesia results in a reduced caliber of airway, which increases airway resistance and any tendency toward airway collapse (Fig. 15-34). The relationship between airway resistance and lung volume is well established (Fig. 15-35). The decreases in FRC caused by the supine position (about 0.8 L) and the induction of anesthesia (about 0.4 L) are often sufficient to explain the increased resistance seen in the healthy anesthetized patient.[109]

In addition to this expected increase in airway resistance in anesthetized patients, there are a number of additional special potential sites of increased airway resistance. These consist of the endotracheal tube (if present), the upper and lower airway passages, and the external anesthesia apparatus. Endotracheal intubation reduces the size of the trachea, usually by 30 to 50 percent (Fig. 15-34). Pharyngeal obstruction, which can be considered to be a normal feature of unconsciousness, is most common. A minor degree of this type of obstruction occurs in snoring. Laryngospasm

and obstructed endotracheal tubes (secretions, kinking, herniated cuffs) are not uncommon and may be life threatening.

Respiratory apparatus often causes resistance that is considerably higher than the resistance in the normal human respiratory tract (Fig. 15-34).[75] When a number of resistors such as those shown in Figure 15-34 are joined in a series to form an anesthetic gas circuit, they generally summate to produce a larger resistance (as with resistances in an electrical circuit).

The Supine Position, Immobility, and Excessive Intravenous Fluid Administration

Patients undergoing anesthesia and surgery are often kept supine and immobile for long periods of time. Thus, some of the lung may be continually dependent and below the left atrium, and therefore in zone 3 or 4 condition. Being in a dependent position, the lung is predisposed to fluid accumulation. Coupled with excessive fluid administration, conditions sufficient to promote transudation of fluid into the lung are present and will result in pulmonary edema and a decreased FRC. When mongrel dogs are placed in a lateral decubitus position and are anesthetized for several hours (Fig. 15-36, bottom horizontal axis), expansion of the extracellular space with fluid (top horizontal axis) causes the PO_2 (left-hand axis) of blood draining the dependent lung (closed circles) to decrease precipitously to mixed venous levels (no O_2 uptake).[131] Blood draining the nondependent lung maintains its PO_2 for a period of time but in the face of the extracellular fluid expansion also suffers a decline in its PO_2 after 5 hours. Transpulmonary shunt (right-hand axis) progressively increased. If the animals were turned every hour (and received the same fluid challenge), only the dependent lung, at the end of each hour period, suffered a decrease in oxygenation. If the animals were turned every half hour and received the same fluid challenge, neither lung suffered a decrease in oxygenation. In patients undergoing surgery in the lateral decubitus position (such as pulmonary resection [and therefore have, or will have, a restricted pulmonary vascular bed]) who receive excessive intravenous fluids, the risk of the dependent lung becoming edematous is certainly increased.

High Inspired Oxygen Concentration and Absorption Atelectasis

General anesthesia is usually administered with an increased FIO_2. In patients who have areas of moderately low $\dot{V}A/\dot{Q}$ ratios (0.1 to 0.01), the administration of FIO_2 greater than 0.3 adds enough oxygen into the alveolar space in these areas to eliminate the shuntlike effect that they have, and total measured right-to-left shunt decreases. However, when patients with a significant amount of blood flow perfusing lung units with very low $\dot{V}A/\dot{Q}$ ratios (0.01 to 0.0001) have a change in FIO_2

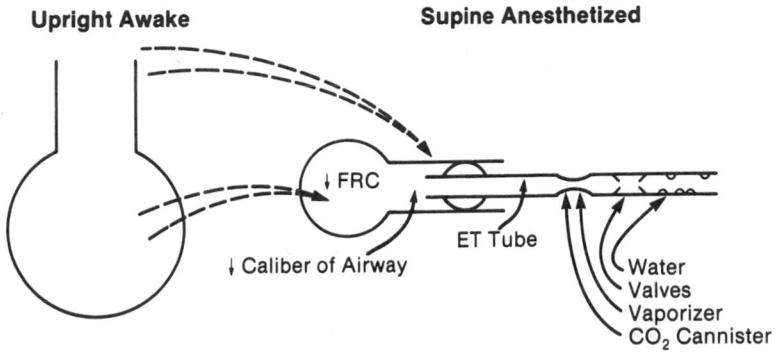

Fig. 15-34. The anesthetized patient in the supine position has an increased airway resistance owing to decreased functional residual capacity, decreased caliber of the airways, endotracheal intubation, and connection of the endotracheal tube to external breathing apparatus and circuitry. (From Benumof,[168] with permission.)

from room air to 1.0, the very low $\dot{V}_A/\dot{Q}$ units virtually disappear and a moderately large right-to-left shunt appears.[13,14,132] In these studies, the increase in shunting was equal to the amount of blood flow previously perfusing the areas with low $\dot{V}_A/\dot{Q}$ ratios during the breathing of air. Thus, in these studies the effect of breathing O_2 was to convert units that had low $\dot{V}_A/\dot{Q}$ ratios into shunt units. The pathologic basis for this data is the conversion of low $\dot{V}_A/\dot{Q}$ units into atelectatic units.

The cause of the atelectatic shunting during O_2 breathing is presumably a large increase in O_2 uptake by lung units with low $\dot{V}_A/\dot{Q}$ ratios.[132,133] A unit that has a low $\dot{V}_A/\dot{Q}$ ratio during breathing of air will have a low P_{AO_2}. When an enriched O_2 mixture is inspired, P_{AO_2} will rise, causing the rate at which O_2 moves from the alveolar gas to the capillary blood to increase greatly. The O_2 flux may increase so much that the net flow of gas into the blood exceeds the inspired flow of gas, and

the lung unit will become progressively smaller. Collapse is most likely to occur if the FiO_2 is high, the $\dot{V}_A/\dot{Q}$ ratio is low, the time of exposure of the unit with low $\dot{V}_A/\dot{Q}$ to high FiO_2 is long, and the content of O_2 in the mixed venous blood is low. Thus, given the right $\dot{V}_A/\dot{Q}$ ratio and time of administration, an FiO_2 as low as 50 percent can produce absorption atelectasis.[132,133] This phenomenon is of considerable significance in the clinical situation for two reasons. First, enriched O_2 mixtures are often used therapeutically, and it is important to know whether this therapy is causing atelectasis. Second, the amount of shunt is often estimated during breathing of 100 percent O_2, and if this maneuver results in additional shunt, the measurement will be hard to interpret.

Surgical Position

In the supine position, the abdominal contents force the diaphragm cephalad and reduce FRC.[78,118,124,128] The Trendelenburg position allows the abdominal contents to push the diaphragm further cephalad, so that the diaphragm not only must ventilate the lungs but also must lift the abdominal contents out of the thorax. The result is a predisposition to decreased FRC and atelectasis.[134] Increased pulmonary blood volume and gravitational force on the mediastinal structures are additional factors that may decrease pulmonary compliance and FRC. In the steep Trendelenburg position, most of the lung may be below the left atrium and therefore in a zone 3 or 4 condition. As such, the lung may be susceptible to the development of pulmonary interstitial edema. Thus, patients with elevated pulmonary artery pressure, such as those with mitral stenosis, do not tolerate the Trendelenburg position well.[135]

In the lateral decubitus position, the dependent lung experiences a moderate decrease in FRC and is predisposed to atelectasis, whereas the nondependent lung may have an increased FRC. The kidney and lithotomy positions also cause small decreases in FRC above that

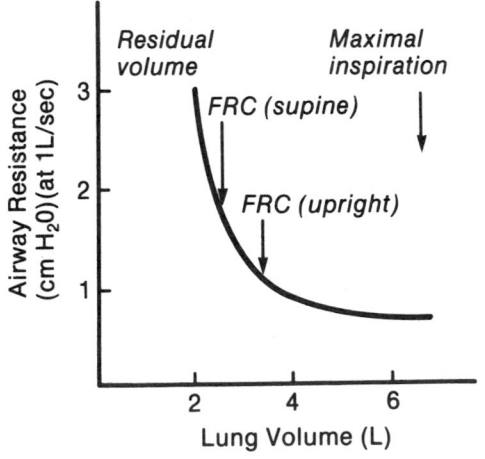

Fig. 15-35. Airway resistance is an increasing hyperbolic function of decreasing lung volume. Functional residual capacity (FRC) decreases in changing from the upright to the supine position. (From Nunn,[75] with permission.)

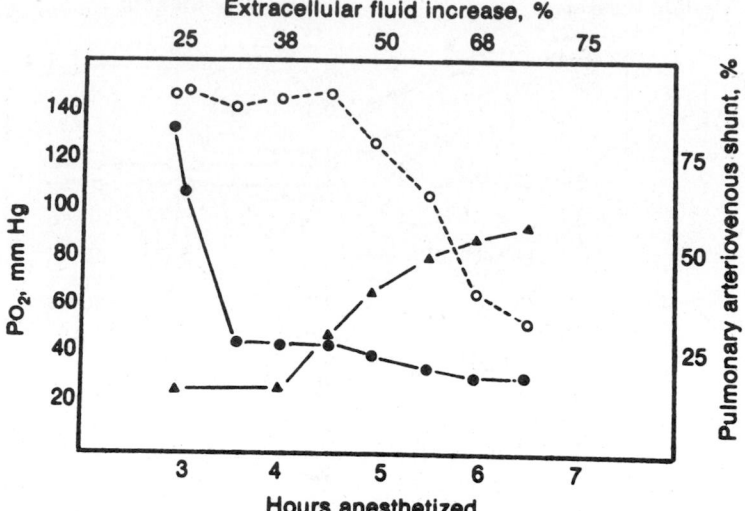

Fig. 15-36. Mongrel dogs anesthetized with pentobarbital (bottom axis), placed in a lateral decubitus position, and subjected to progressive extracellular fluid expansion (top axis) have a marked decrease in the PO_2 (left vertical axis) of blood draining the dependent lung (solid circles) and a smaller, much slower decrease in PO_2 of blood draining the nondependent lung (open circles). The pulmonary arteriovenous shunt (right vertical axis) rises progressively (triangles). (From Ray et al.,[131] with permission.)

caused by the supine position. The prone position may increase FRC.

Ventilation History (Rapid Shallow Breathing)

Rapid shallow breathing is often a regular feature of anesthesia. Monotonous shallow breathing may cause a decrease in FRC, promote atelectasis, and decrease compliance.[111,112] Initially, these changes may cause hypoxemia with normocarbia and may be reversed by periodic large inspirations and/or PEEP.

Decreased Removal of Secretions (Decreased Mucociliary Flow)

Tracheobronchial mucous glands and goblet cells produce mucus, which is swept by cilia up to the larynx where it is swallowed or expectorated. This process clears inhaled organisms and particles from the lungs. The secreted mucus consists of a surface gel layer, which lies on top of a more liquid sol layer in which the cilia beat. The tips of the cilia propel the gel layer toward the larynx (upward) during the forward stroke. As the mucus streams upward and the total cross-sectional area of the airways diminishes, absorption takes place from the sol layer to maintain a constant depth of 5 mm.[136]

Poor systemic hydration and low inspired humidity reduce mucociliary flow by increasing the viscosity of secretions and by slowing the ciliary beat.[137-139] Mucociliary flow varies directly with body or mucosal temperature (low inspired temperature) over a range of 32° to 42°C.[140,141] A high FIO_2 decreases mucociliary

flow.[142] Inflation of an endotracheal tube cuff suppresses tracheal mucous velocity,[143] which occurs within 1 hour, and apparently it does not matter whether a low- or high-compliance cuff is used. Passage of an uncuffed tube through the vocal cords that is kept in situ for several hours does not affect tracheal mucous velocity.[143]

The mechanism for endotracheal tube cuff suppression of mucociliary clearance is speculative. In the report of Sackner et al.[143] mucous velocity was decreased in the distal trachea, whereas the cuff was inflated in the proximal portion. Thus, the phenomenon cannot be attributed solely to damming of mucus at the cuff site. One possibility is that the endotracheal tube cuff caused a critical increase in the thickness of the layer of mucus proceeding distally from the cuff. Another possibility is that mechanical distention of the trachea by the endotracheal tube cuff initiated a neurogenic reflex arc that altered mucous secretions or frequency of ciliary beating.

Other investigators recently showed that when all the above-mentioned factors are controlled, halothane reversibly and progressively decreases, but does not stop, mucous flow over an inspired concentration of 1 to 3 MAC.[144] The halothane-induced depression of mucociliary clearance was likely due to depression of the ciliary beat, an effect that caused slow clearance of mucus from the distal and peripheral airways. In support of this hypothesis is the fact that cilia are morphologically similar throughout the animal kingdom, and in clinical dosages, inhaled anesthetics, including halothane, have been found to cause reversible depression of the ciliary beat of protozoa.[145]

Decreased Cardiac Output and Increased Oxygen Consumption

A decreased cardiac output ($\dot{Q}_T$) in the presence of a constant O_2 consumption ($\dot{V}O_2$), or an increased $\dot{V}O_2$ in the presence of a constant $\dot{Q}_T$, or a decreased $\dot{Q}_T$ and an increased $\dot{V}O_2$ must all result in a lower mixed venous O_2 content ($C\bar{v}O_2$). The lowered $C\bar{v}O_2$ will then flow through whichever shunt pathways exist, mix with the oxygenated end-pulmonary capillary blood, and lower the O_2 content of the arterial blood (CaO_2) (Figs. 15-27 and 15-28). Figure 15-37 shows these relationships quantitatively for several different intrapulmonary shunts.[84,85] The larger the intrapulmonary shunt, the greater the decrease in CaO_2 because more venous blood with lower $C\bar{v}O_2$ can admix with end-pulmonary capillary blood. Decreased $\dot{Q}_T$ may occur with myocardial failure and hypovolemia; the specific causes of these two conditions are beyond the scope of this chapter. Increased $\dot{V}O_2$ may occur with excessive sympathetic nervous system stimulation, hyperthermia, or shivering and can further contribute to impaired oxygenation of arterial blood.[146]

Inhibition of Hypoxic Pulmonary Vasoconstriction

Decreased regional P_AO_2 causes regional pulmonary vasoconstriction, which diverts blood flow away from hypoxic regions of the lung to better ventilated normoxic regions of the lung. The diversion of blood flow minimizes venous admixture from the underventilated or nonventilated lung regions. Inhibition of regional HPV might impair arterial oxygenation by permitting increased venous admixture from hypoxic or atelectatic areas of the lung (Fig. 15-9).

Since the pulmonary circulation is poorly endowed with smooth muscle, any condition that increases the pressure against which the vessels must constrict (i.e., the Ppa) will decrease HPV. There are numerous clinical conditions that can increase Ppa and therefore decrease HPV. Mitral stenosis,[147] volume overload,[147] low (but above room air) F_IO_2 in nondiseased lung,[148] a progressive increase in the amount of diseased lung,[148] thromboembolism,[148] hypothermia,[149] and vasoactive drugs[150] can all increase Ppa. Direct vasodilating drugs (such as isoproterenol, nitroglycerin, and sodium nitroprusside),[51,150] inhaled anesthetics,[151] and hypocapnia[115,150] can directly decrease HPV. The selective application of PEEP to only the nondiseased lung can selectively increase nondiseased lung pulmonary vascular resistance and divert blood flow back into the diseased lung.[152]

Paralysis

In the supine position, the weight of the abdominal contents pressing against the diaphragm is greatest in the dependent or posterior part of the diaphragm and least in the nondependent or anterior part of the diaphragm. In the awake patient breathing spontaneously, the active tension in the diaphragm is capable of overcoming the weight of the abdominal contents, and the diaphragm moves the most in the posterior portion (because the posterior diaphragm is stretched higher into the chest it has the smallest radius of curvature and therefore it contracts most effectively) and least in the anterior portion. This is a healthy circumstance because the greatest amount of ventilation occurs where there is the most perfusion (posteriorly or dependently), and the least amount of ventilation occurs where there is the least perfusion (anteriorly or nondependently). During paralysis and positive-pressure breathing, the passive diaphragm is displaced by the positive pressure preferentially in the anterior nondependent portion (where there is the least resistance to diaphragmatic movement) and is displaced minimally in the posterior dependent portion (where there is the most resistance to diaphragmatic movement). This is an unhealthy circumstance because the greatest amount of ventilation now occurs where there is the least perfusion, and the least amount of ventilation now occurs where there is the most perfusion.[128]

Involvement of Mechanisms of Hypoxemia in Specific Diseases

In any given pulmonary disease, many of the mechanisms of hypoxemia listed above may be involved in producing hypoxemia. Pulmonary embolism (air, fat, thrombi) (Fig. 15-38) and the evolution of the adult respiratory distress syndrome (ARDS) (Fig. 15-39) will be

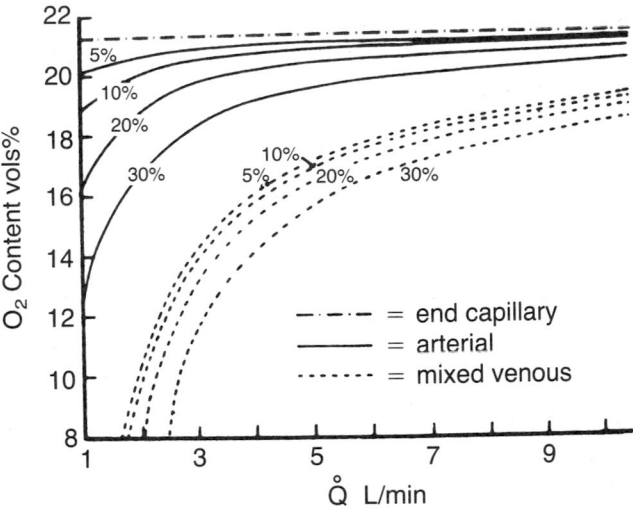

Fig. 15-37. Effects of changes in cardiac output ($\dot{Q}$) on the O_2 content of end-pulmonary capillary, arterial, and mixed venous blood for a family of different transpulmonary right-to-left shunts. The magnitude of the right-to-left shunt is indicated by the various numbered percent symbols for arterial (solid line) and mixed venous (dashed line) blood; the oxygen content of end-capillary blood is unaffected by the degree of shunting. Note that a decrease in $\dot{Q}$ results in a greater decrease in the arterial content of O_2, the larger the shunt. (From Kelman et al.,[84] with permission.)

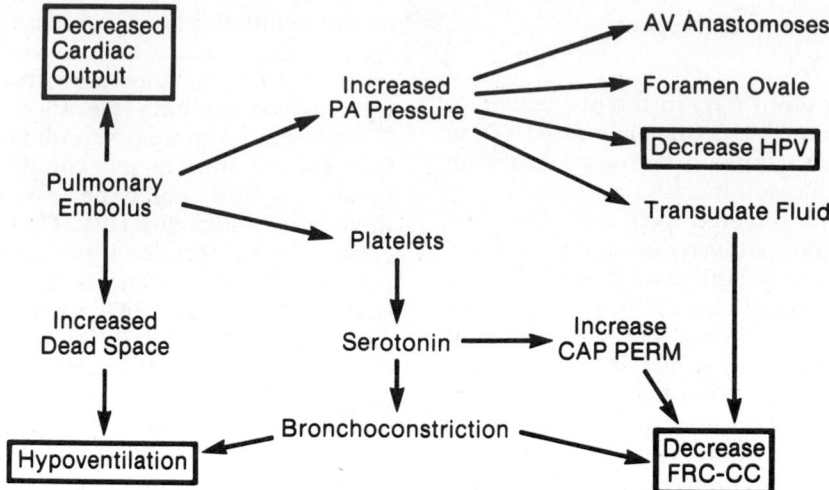

Fig. 15-38. Mechanisms of hypoxemia during pulmonary embolism. See text for explanation of pathophysiologic flow diagram. CAP PERM, capillary permeability; AV, arteriovenous; HPV, hypoxic pulmonary vasoconstriction; PA, pulmonary artery; FRC, functional residual capacity; CC, closing capacity. (From Benumof,[168] with permission.)

used to illustrate this point. A significant pulmonary embolus can cause severe increases in pulmonary artery pressure, and these increases can cause right-to-left transpulmonary shunting through opened arteriovenous anastomoses and the foramen ovale (possible in 20 percent of patients), pulmonary edema in nonembolized regions of the lung, and inhibition of HPV. The embolus may cause hypoventilation via increased dead space ventilation. If the embolus contains platelets, serotonin may be released, and this release can cause hypoventilation via bronchoconstriction and pulmonary edema via increased pulmonary capillary permeability. Finally, the pulmonary embolus can increase pulmonary vascular resistance and decrease the cardiac output.

After major hypotension, shock, or blood loss, respiratory failure often ensues, and this syndrome has been called adult respiratory distress syndrome (ARDS). The syndrome can evolve during and after anesthesia and has the hallmark characteristics of decreased FRC and compliance and hypoxemia. Following shock and trauma, plasma levels of serotonin, histamine, plasmakinins, lysozymes, superoxides, fibrin degradation products, products of complement metabolism, and fatty acids increase. Sepsis and endotoxemia may be present. Increased levels of activated complement activate neutrophils into chemotaxis in patients with trauma and pancreatitis; activated neutrophils can damage endothelial cells. These factors, along with pulmonary contusion (if it occurs), may individually or

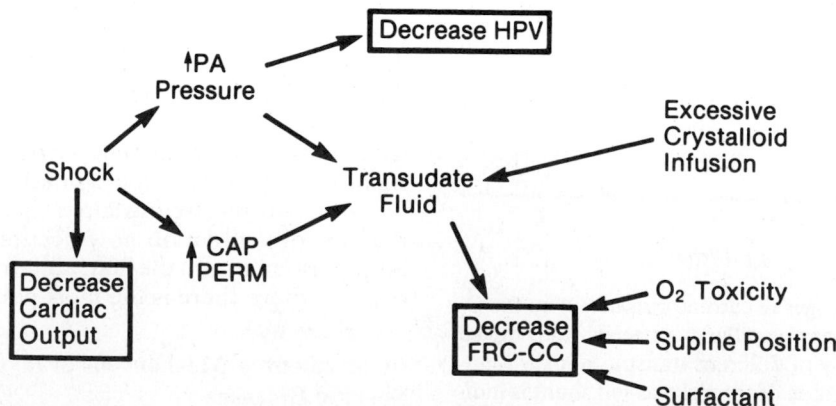

Fig. 15-39. Mechanisms of hypoxemia during the adult respiratory stress syndrome (ARDS). See text for explanation of pathophysiologic flow diagram. PA, pulmonary artery; CAP PERM, capillary permeability; HPV, hypoxic pulmonary vasoconstriction; FRC, functional residual capacity; CC, closing capacity. (From Benumof,[168] with permission.)

collectively increase pulmonary capillary permeability. After shock, acidosis, increased circulating catecholamines and sympathetic nervous system activity, leukotriene and prostaglandin release, histamine release, microembolism (with serotonin release), increased intracranial pressure (with head injury), and alveolar hypoxia may occur and may individually or collectively, particularly postresuscitation, cause a moderate increase in pulmonary artery pressure. After shock, the normal compensatory response to hypovolemia is movement of a protein-free fluid from the interstitial space into the vascular space to restore vascular volume. The dilution of vascular proteins by protein-free interstitial fluid can cause a decreased capillary colloid oncotic pressure. Increased pulmonary capillary permeability and pulmonary artery pressure along with decreased capillary colloid oncotic pressure will cause fluid transudation and pulmonary edema. Additionally, a decreased cardiac output, inhibition of HPV, immobility, supine position, excessive fluid administration, and an excessively high FIO_2 can contribute to the development of ARDS.

Mechanisms of Hypercapnia and Hypocapnia During Anesthesia

Hypercapnia

The following factors can all cause hypercapnia (Fig. 15-40).

Hypoventilation

Patients spontaneously hypoventilate during anesthesia because it is more difficult to breathe (abnormal surgical position, increased airway resistance, decreased compliance) and they are less willing to breathe (decreased respiratory drive due to anesthetics). Hypoventilation will result in hypercapnia (Figs. 15-22 and 15-23).

Increased Dead Space Ventilation

A *decrease* in pulmonary artery pressure, as during deliberate hypotension,[153] may cause an increase in zone 1 and alveolar dead space ventilation.

An *increase* in *airway pressure* (as with PEEP) may cause an increase in zone 1 and alveolar dead space ventilation.

Pulmonary embolus, thrombosis, and *vascular obliteration* (kinking, clamping, blocking of pulmonary artery during surgery) may increase the amount of lung that is ventilated but unperfused. Vascular obliteration may be responsible for the increase in dead space ventilation with age ($VD/VT = 33 + age/3$).

Rapid short inspirations may be distributed preferentially to noncompliant (short time constant for inflation) and badly perfused alveoli, while a slow inspiration allows time for distribution to more compliant (long time constant for inflation) and better perfused

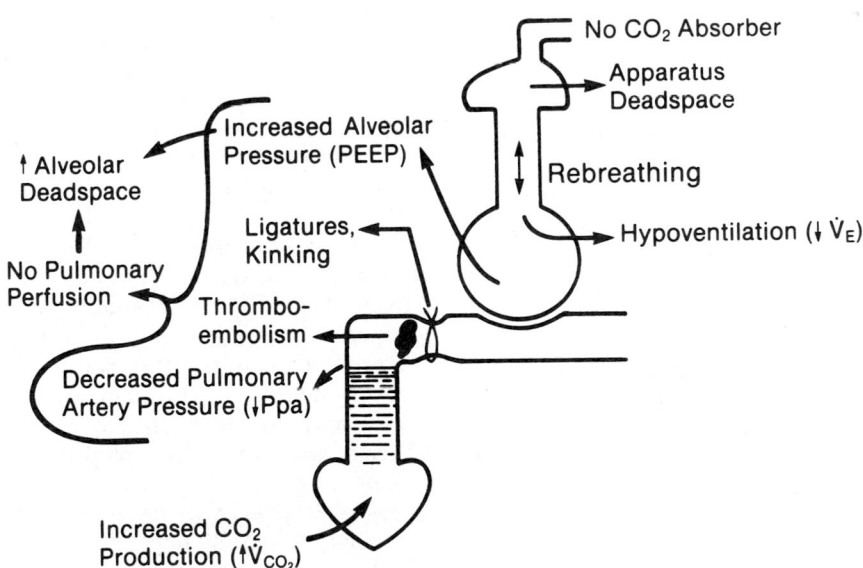

Fig. 15-40. Schematic diagram of the causes of hypercapnia during anesthesia. An increase in carbon dioxide production ($\dot{V}CO_2$) will increase $PaCO_2$ with a constant minute ventilation ($\dot{V}E$). There are several events that can increase alveolar dead space, and they consist of a decrease in pulmonary artery pressure (Ppa), the application of PEEP, thromboembolism, and mechanical interference with pulmonary arterial flow (ligatures and kinking of vessels). A decrease in minute ventilation ($\dot{V}E$) will cause an increase in $PaCO_2$ with a constant $\dot{V}CO_2$. It is possible for some anesthesia systems to cause rebreathing of CO_2. Finally, the anesthesia apparatus may increase the anatomic dead space, and inadvertent switching off of a CO_2 absorber in the presence of low fresh gas flows can increase $PaCO_2$. (From Benumof,[168] with permission.)

alveoli. Thus, rapid short inspirations may have a dead space ventilation effect.

The *anesthesia apparatus* increases total dead space (V_D/V_T) for two reasons. First, the apparatus simply increases the anatomic dead space. Inclusion of normal apparatus dead space increases the total V_D/V_T ratio from 33 percent to about 46 percent in intubated patients and to about 64 percent in patients breathing via a mask.[154] Second, anesthesia circuits cause rebreathing of expired gases, which is equivalent to dead space ventilation. The rebreathing classification by Mapleson is widely accepted.[155] The order of increasing rebreathing (decreasing clinical merit) with spontaneous ventilation with Mapleson circuits is A (Magill), D, C, and B. The order of increasing rebreathing (decreasing clinical merit) with controlled ventilation is D, B, C, and A. There will be no rebreathing in system E (Ayre T-piece) if the patient's respiratory diastole is long enough to permit washout with a given fresh gas flow (common event) or if the fresh gas flow is greater than the peak inspiratory flow rate (uncommon event).

The effects of an increase in dead space can usually be counteracted by a corresponding increase in the respiratory minute volume. If, for example, the minute volume is 10 L/min and the V_D/V_T ratio is 30 percent, the alveolar ventilation will be 7 L/min. If a pulmonary embolism occurred resulting in an increase of the V_D/V_T ratio to 50 percent, the minute volume would need to be increased to 14 L/min to maintain an alveolar ventilation of 7 L/min (14 L/min × 0.5).

Increased Carbon Dioxide Production

All the causes of increased oxygen consumption will also increase carbon dioxide production — hyperthermia, shivering, catecholamine release (light anesthesia), hypertension, and thyroid storm. If minute ventilation, total dead space, and ventilation to perfusion relationships are constant, an increase in carbon dioxide production will result in hypercapnia.

Inadvertant Switching Off of a Carbon Dioxide Absorber

Many factors, such as patient ventilatory responsiveness to carbon dioxide accumulation, fresh gas flow, circle system design, and carbon dioxide production, determine whether hypercapnia will result from inadvertant switching off or using up of a circle carbon dioxide absorber. However, high fresh gas flows (>5 L/min) minimize the problem with almost all systems for almost all patients.

Hypocapnia

The mechanisms of hypocapnia are the reverse of those that produce hypercapnia. Thus, with all other factors being equal, hyperventilation (spontaneous or controlled ventilation), decreased dead space ventilation (change from mask airway to endotracheal tube airway, decreased PEEP, increased pulmonary artery pressure, or decreased rebreathing), and decreased carbon dioxide production (hypothermia, deep anesthesia, hypotension) will lead to hypocapnia. By far the most common mechanism of hypocapnia is passive hyperventilation by mechanical means.

Physiologic Effects of Abnormalities in the Respiratory Gases

Hypoxia

The end products of aerobic metabolism (oxidative phosphorylation) are carbon dioxide and water, both of which are easily diffusible and lost from the body. The essential feature of hypoxia is the cessation of oxidative phosphorylation when mitochoncrial PO_2 falls below a critical level. Anaerobic pathways, which produce energy (adenosine triphosphate [ATP]) inefficiently, are then utilized. The main anaerobic metabolites are hydrogen and lactate ions, which are not easily excreted. They accumulate in the circulation, where they may be quantified in terms of the base deficit and the lactate/pyruvate ratio.

Since the various organs have different blood flow and oxygen consumption rates, the presentation and clinical diagnosis of hypoxia is usually related to symptoms arising from the most vulnerable organ. This is usually the brain in an awake patient and the heart in the anesthetized patient (see below), but in special circumstances it may be the spinal cord (aortic surgery), kidney (acute tubular necrosis), liver (hepatitis), or limb (claudication, gangrene).

The cardiovascular response to hypoxemia[156,157] is a product of both reflex (neural and humoral) and direct effects (Table 15-2). The reflex effects occur first and are excitory and vasoconstrictive. The neuroreflex effects result from aortic and carotid chemoreceptor, baroreceptor, and central cerebral stimulation, and the humoral reflex effects result from catecholamine and renin–angiotensin release. The direct local vascular effects of hypoxia are inhibitory and vasodilatory and occur late. The net response to hypoxia in a subject depends on the severity of the hypoxia; the severity of hypoxia determines the magnitude of and balance between the inhibitory and excitory components; the balance may vary according to the type and depth of anesthesia and the degree of pre-existing cardiovascular disease.

Mild arterial hypoxemia (arterial saturation less than normal but still 80 percent or higher) causes a general activation of the sympathetic nervous system and release of catecholamines. Consequently, heart rate, stroke volume, cardiac output, and myocardial contractility (as measured by a shortened pre-ejection period [PEP], left ventricular ejection time [LVET], and a decreased PEP/LVET ratio) are increased. Changes in systemic vascular resistance are usually slight. However, in patients under anesthesia with β-blockers, hypoxia (and hypercapnia when present) may cause circulating catecholamines to have only an α-receptor

TABLE 15-2. Cardiovascular Response to Hypoxemia

O_2 Saturation	Hemodynamic Variable					Predominant Response
	HR	BP	SV	CO	SVR	
>80	↑	↑	↑	↑	No change	Reflex, excitatory
60–80	↑baroreceptor	↓	No change	No change	↓	Local depressant > Reflex, excitatory
<60	↓	↓	↓	↓	↓	Local, depressant

Abbreviations and symbols: HR, heart rate; BP, systemic blood pressure; SV, stroke volume; CO, cardiac output; SVR, systemic vascular resistance; ↑, increase; ↓, decrease.

effect and the heart may be unstimulated (even depressed by a local hypoxia effect), and systemic vascular resistance may be increased. Consequently, cardiac output may be decreased in these patients. With moderate hypoxemia (arterial oxygen saturation 60 to 80 percent), local vasodilatation begins to predominate and systemic vascular resistance and blood pressure decrease, but heart rate may continue to be increased owing to a systemic hypotension-induced stimulation of baroreceptors. Finally, with severe hypoxemia (arterial saturation less than 60 percent), local depressant effects dominate and blood pressure falls rapidly, the pulse slows, shock develops, and the heart either fibrillates or becomes asystolic. Significant pre-existing hypotension will convert a mild hypoxemia-hemodynamic profile into a moderate hypoxemia-hemodynamic profile, and a moderate hypoxemia-hemodynamic profile into a severe hypoxemia-hemodynamic profile. Similarly, in well-anesthetized and/or sedated patients, early sympathetic nervous system reactivity to hypoxemia may be reduced and the effects of hypoxemia may be expressed only as bradycardia with severe hypotension and, ultimately, circulatory collapse.

Hypoxemia may also cause cardiac arrhythmias that may in turn potentiate the already mentioned deleterious cardiovascular effects. Hypoxemia-induced arrhythmias may be caused by multiple mechanisms; the mechanisms are interrelated because they all cause a decrease in the myocardial oxygen supply/demand ratio, which in turn increases myocardial irritability. First, arterial hypoxemia may directly decrease myocardial oxygen supply. Second, early tachycardia may cause an increased myocardial oxygen consumption and a decreased diastolic filling time may cause a decreased myocardial oxygen supply. Third, early increased systemic blood pressure may cause an increased afterload on the left ventricle that increases left ventricular oxygen demand. Fourth, late systemic hypotension may decrease myocardial oxygen supply owing to decreased diastolic perfusion pressure. The level of hypoxemia that will cause cardiac arrhythmias cannot be predicted with certainty because the myocardial oxygen supply and demand relationship in a given patient is not known (i.e., the degree of coronary artery atherosclerosis may not be known). However, if a myocardial area (or areas) become hypoxic and/or ischemic, unifocal or multifocal premature ventricular contractions, ventricular tachycardia, and ventricular fibrillation may occur.

The cardiovascular response to hypoxia includes a number of other important effects. Cerebral blood flow increases (even if hypocapnic hyperventilation is present). Ventilation will be stimulated no matter why hypoxia exists. The pulmonary distribution of blood flow is more homogeneous owing to an increased pulmonary artery pressure. Chronic hypoxia will cause an increased hemoglobin concentration and a right-shifted oxy-Hb curve (due to either an increase in 2,3-DPG or acidosis), which tends to raise tissue PO_2.

Hyperoxia (Oxygen Toxicity)

The dangers associated with the inhalation of excessive oxygen are multiple. Exposure to a high oxygen tension clearly causes pulmonary damage in healthy individuals.[158,159] A dose-time toxicity curve for humans is available from a number of studies.[158] Since the lungs of normal human volunteers cannot be directly examined to determine the rate of onset and course of toxicity, indirect measures such as the onset of symptom formation have been employed to construct the dose-time toxicity curves. Examination of the curve indicates that 100 percent oxygen should not be administered for more than 12 hours, 80 percent oxygen should not be administered for more than 24 hours, and 60 percent oxygen should not be administered for more than 36 hours. No measurable changes in pulmonary function or blood–gas exchange occur in humans during exposures to less than 50 percent oxygen even for long periods.

The dominant symptom of oxygen toxicity in human volunteers is substernal distress, which begins as a mild irritation in the area of the carina and may be accompanied by occasional coughing. As exposure continues, pain becomes more intense, and the urge to cough and to deep breathe also becomes more intense. These symptoms will progress to severe dyspnea, paroxysmal coughing, and decreased vital capacity when the FIO_2 has been 1.0 for greater than 12 hours. As toxicity progresses, other pulmonary function studies such as compliance and blood gases deteriorate. Pathologically, in animals, the lesion progresses from a tracheobronchitis (exposure for 12 hours to a few days), to involvement of the alveolar septae with pulmonary interstitial edema (exposure for a few days to 1 week), to pulmonary fibrosis of the edema (exposure greater than 1 week).[160]

Ventilatory depression may occur in those patients who, by reason of drugs or disease, have been ventilating in response to a hypoxic drive. By definition, ventilatory depression resulting from removal of a hypoxic drive by increasing the inspired oxygen concentration will cause hypercapnia but does not necessarily produce hypoxia (owing to the increased FIO_2).

Absorption atelectasis has been previously discussed (see the section, *High Inspired Oxygen Concentration and Absorption Atelectasis*). Retrolental fibroplasia, an abnormal proliferation of the immature retinal vasculature of the prematurely born infant, can occur after exposure to hyperoxia. Very premature infants are most susceptible to retrolental fibroplasia (i.e., those of less than 1.0 kg birth weight and 28 weeks' gestation). The risk of retrolental fibroplasia exists whenever an FIO_2 causes PaO_2 to be >80 mmHg for more than 3 hours in an infant whose gestational age plus life age combined is less than 44 weeks. If the ductus arteriosus is patent, arterial blood samples should be drawn from the right radial artery (umbilical or lower extremity PaO_2 is lower than the PaO_2 that the eyes are exposed to owing to ductal shunting of unoxygenated blood).

The mode of action of toxicity of oxygen in tissues is complex, but interference with metabolism seems to be widespread. Most importantly, there is inactivation of many enzymes, particularly those with sulfhydryl groups. The most acute toxic enzyme effect of oxygen in humans is a convulsive effect that occurs during exposure to pressures in excess of 2 atm absolute.

High inspired oxygen concentrations can be of use therapeutically. Clearance of gas loculi in the body may be greatly accelerated by inhalation of 100 percent oxygen. Inhalation of 100 percent oxygen creates a large nitrogen gradient from the gas space to the perfusing blood. As a result, nitrogen leaves the gas space and the space diminishes in size. The use of oxygen to remove gas may be used to ease intestinal gas pressure in patients with intestinal obstruction, to hasten recovery from pneumoencephalography, to decrease the size of an air embolus, and to aid in absorption of pneumoperitoneum and pneumothorax.

Hypercapnia

The effects of carbon dioxide on the cardiovascular system are as complex as they are for hypoxia. As with hypoxemia, hypercapnia appears to cause direct depression of both the cardiac muscle and vascular smooth muscle, but at the same time, it causes reflex stimulation of the sympathoadrenal system, which compensates to a greater or lesser extent for the primary cardiovascular depression. Even in patients under halothane anesthesia, plasma catecholamine levels increase in response to increased carbon dioxide levels in much the same way as conscious subjects. Thus, hypercapnia, like hypoxemia, may cause increased myocardial oxygen demand (tachycardia, early hypertension) and decreased myocardial oxygen supply (tachycardia, late hypotension).

Table 15-3 summarizes the interaction of anesthesia with hypercapnia in humans; increased cardiac output and decreased systemic vascular resistance should be emphasized.[161] The increase in cardiac output is most marked during anesthesia with drugs that enhance sympathetic activity and least marked with halothane and nitrous oxide. The decrease in systemic vascular resistance is most marked during enflurane anesthesia and hypercapnia. Hypercapnia is a potent pulmonary vasoconstrictor even after inhalation of 3 percent isoflurane for 5 minutes.[162]

Arrhythmias have been reported in unanesthetized humans during acute hypercapnia but have seldom been of serious import. A high $PaCO_2$ level is, however, more dangerous during general anesthesia. With halothane anesthesia, arrhythmias will frequently occur above a $PaCO_2$ arrhythmic threshold that is often constant for a particular patient.

The maximal stimulant respiratory effect is attained by a $PaCO_2$ of about 100 mmHg. With a higher $PaCO_2$, stimulation is reduced, and at very high levels respiration is depressed and later ceases altogether. The PCO_2–ventilation response curve is generally displaced to the right, and its slope is reduced by anesthetics and other depressant drugs.[163] With profound anesthesia the response curve may be flat, or even sloping downward, and CO_2 then acts as a respiratory depressant. In patients with ventilatory failure, CO_2 narcosis occurs when the $PaCO_2$ rises above 90 to 120 mmHg. Thirty percent carbon dioxide is sufficient for the production of anesthesia, and this concentration causes total but reversible flattening of the electroencephalogram.[164]

Quite apart from the effect of CO_2 upon ventilation, it exerts two other important effects that influence the oxygenation of the blood. First, if the concentration of N_2 (or other inert gas) remains constant, the concentration of CO_2 in the alveolar gas can only increase at the expense of O_2, which must be displaced. Thus, PAO_2 and PaO_2 may decrease. Second, hypercapnia shifts the oxy-Hb curve to the right, facilitating tissue oxygenation.

Chronic hypercapnia results in increased resorption of bicarbonate by the kidneys, further raising the plasma bicarbonate level and constituting a secondary or compensatory metabolic alkalosis. Chronic hypocapnia decreases renal bicarbonate resorption, resulting in further fall of plasma bicarbonate and producing a secondary or compensatory metabolic acidosis. In each case arterial pH returns toward the normal value, but the bicarbonate ion concentration departs even further from normal.

TABLE 15-3. Cardiovascular Responses to Hypercapnia (PaCO$_2$ = 60 to 83 mmHg) during Various Types of Anesthesia (1 MAC Equivalent Except for Nitrous Oxide)[a]

Anesthesia	Heart Rate	Contractility	Cardiac Output	Systemic Vascular Resistance
Conscious	++	++	+++	−
Nitrous oxide	0	+	++	− −
Fluroxene	+	+++	+++	−
Halothane	0	+	+	−
Enflurane	+	+	++	− − −
Isoflurane	++	+++	+++	−

Abbreviations and symbols: +, < 10% increase; ++, 10 to 25% increase; +++, > 25% increase; 0, no change; −, < 10% decrease; − −, 10 to 25% decrease; − − −, > 25% decrease; MAC, minimum alveolar concentration for adequate anesthesia in 50% of subjects.
[a] The increase in PaCO$_2$ in the conscious subjects was 11.5 mmHg from a normal level of 38 mmHg.

Hypercapnia is accompanied by a leakage of potassium from the cells into the plasma. A good deal of the potassium comes from the liver, probably from glucose release and mobilization, which occurs in response to the rise in plasma catecholamine levels.[165] Since the plasma potassium level takes an appreciable time to return to normal, repeated bouts of hypercapnia at short intervals result in a stepwise rise in plasma potassium.

Hypocapnia

In this section, hypocapnia is considered to be produced by passive hyperventilation (by the anesthesiologist or ventilator). Hypocapnia may cause a decrease in the cardiac output by three separate mechanisms. First, if present, an increase in intrathoracic pressure will decrease the cardiac output. Second, hypocapnia is associated with a withdrawal of sympathetic nervous system activity, and this can decrease the ionotropic state of the heart. Third, hypocapnia can increase pH, which can in turn decrease ionized Ca^{2+}, which may in turn decrease the ionotropic state of the heart. Hypocapnia with an alkalosis will also shift the oxy-Hb curve to the left, which increases the hemoglobin affinity for oxygen, impairing oxygen unloading at the tissue level. The decrease in peripheral flow and impaired ability to unload oxygen to the tissues is compounded by an increase in whole body oxygen consumption caused by an increased pH-mediated uncoupling of oxidation from phosphorylation;[166] PaCO$_2$ of 20 mmHg will increase tissue oxygen consumption by 30 percent. Consequently, hypocapnia may simultaneously increase tissue oxygen demand and decrease tissue oxygen supply. Thus, to have the same amount of oxygen delivery to the tissues, cardiac output or tissue perfusion has to increase at a time it may not be possible to do so. The cerebral effects of hypocapnia may be related to a state of cerebral acidosis and hypoxia, since hypocapnia may cause a selective reduction in the cerebral blood flow and also shifts the oxy-Hb curve to the left.

Hypocapnia may cause $\dot{V}A/\dot{Q}$ abnormalities by inhibiting HPV or by causing bronchoconstriction and a decreased lung compliance. Finally, passive hypocapnia will produce apnea.

REFERENCES

1. West JB, Dollery CT, Naimark A: Distribution of blood flow in isolated lung: Relation to vascular and alveolar pressures. J Appl Physiol 19:713, 1964
2. Permutt S, Bromberger-Barnea B, Bane HN: Alveolar pressure, pulmonary venous pressure and the vascular waterfall. Med Thorac 19:239, 1962
3. West JB, Dollery CT, Heard BE: Increased pulmonary vascular resistance in the dependent zone of the isolated dog lung caused by perivascular edema. Circ Res 17:191, 1965
4. West JB (ed): Regional Differences in the Lung. Academic Press, Orlando, FL, 1977
5. Hughes JMB, Glazier JB, Maloney JE, et al: Effect of lung volume on the distribution of pulmonary blood flow in man. Respir Physiol 4:58, 1968
6. Hughes JM, Glazier JB, Maloney JE, et al: Effect of extra-alveolar vessels on the distribution of pulmonary blood flow in the dog. J Appl Physiol 25:701, 1968
7. Permutt S, Caldini P, Maseri A, et al: Recruitment versus distensibility in the pulmonary vascular bed. p. 375. In Fishman AP, Hecht H (eds): The Pulmonary Circulation and Interstitial Space. University of Chicago Press, Chicago, 1969
8. Maseri A, Caldini P, Harward P, et al: Determinants of pulmonary vascular volume. Recruitment versus distensibility. Circ Res 31:218, 1972
9. Hoppin FG, Jr., Green ID, Mead J: Distribution of pleural surface pressure. J Appl Physiol 27:863, 1969
10. Milic-Emili J, Henderson JAM, Dolovich MB, et al: Regional distribution of inspired gas in the lung. J Appl Physiol 21:749, 1966
11. West JB: Ventilation/Blood Flow and Gas Exchange. 4th Ed. Blackwell Scientific Publications, Oxford, 1970
12. West JB: Regional differences in gas exchange in the lung of erect man. J Appl Physiol 17:893, 1962
13. Wagner PD, Saltzman HA, West JB: Measurement of continuous distributions of ventilation-perfusion ratios: Theory. J Appl Physiol 36:588, 1974
14. West JB: Blood flow to the lung and gas exchange. Anesthesiology 41:124, 1974

15. Fishman AP: Dynamics of the pulmonary circulation. p. 1667. In Hamilton WF (ed): Handbook of Physiology. Section 2. Circulation. Vol. 2. Williams & Wilkins, Baltimore, 1963

16. Zapol WM, Snider MT: Pulmonary hypertension in severe acute respiratory failure. N Engl J Med 296:476, 1977

17. Reid L: Structural and functional reappraisal of the pulmonary arterial system. In The Scientific Basis of Medicine Annual Reviews. Athlone Press, London, 1968

18. Benumof JL, Mathers JM, Wahrenbrock EA: The pulmonary interstitial compartment and the mediator of hypoxic pulmonary vasoconstriction. Microvasc Res 15:69, 1978

19. Bohr D: The pulmonary hypoxic response. Chest, suppl., 71:244, 1977

20. Bergofsky EH: Ions and membrane permeability in the regulation of the pulmonary circulation. p. 269. In Fishman AP, Hecht H (eds): The Pulmonary Circulation and Interstitial Space. University of Chicago Press, Chicago, 1969

21. Bergofsky EH: Mechanisms underlying vasomotor regulation of regional pulmonary blood flow in normal and disease states. Am J Med 57:378, 1974

22. Fishman AP: Hypoxia on the pulmonary circulation—how and where it works. Circ Res 38:221, 1976

23. Hanley SP: Prostaglandins and the lung. Lung 164:65, 1986

24. Gerber JG, Voelkel N, Nies AS, et al: Moderation of hypoxic vasoconstriction by infused arachidonic acid: Role of PGI. J Appl Physiol 49:107, 1980

25. Leeman M, Naeije R, Lejeune P, Melot C: Influence of cyclooxygenase inhibition and of leukotriene receptor blockade on pulmonary vascular pressure/cardiac index relationships in hyperoxic and in hypoxic dogs. Clin Sci 72:717, 1987

26. Weir EK, McMurtry IF, Tucker A, et al: Prostaglandin synthetase inhibitors do not decrease hypoxic pulmonary vasoconstriction. J Appl Physiol 41:714, 1976

27. Voelkel NF: Mechanisms of hypoxic pulmonary vasoconstriction. Am Rev Respir Dis 133:1186, 1986

28. Light RB: Indomethacin and ASA reduce intrapulmonary shunt in experimental pneumococcal pneumonia. Am Rev Respir Dis 134:520, 1986

29. Hales CA, Rouse E, Slate JL: Influence of aspirin and indomethacin on variability of alveolar hypoxic vasoconstriction. J Appl Physiol 45:33, 1978

30. Kadowitz PJ, Chapnick BM, Joiner PD: Influence of inhibitors of prostaglandin synthesis on the canine pulmonary vascular bed. Am J Physiol 229:941, 1975

31. Hanley PJ, Roberts D, Dobson K, Light RB: Effect of indomethacin on arterial oxygenation in critically ill patients with severe bacterial pneumonia. Lancet 1:351, 1987

32. Schulman LL, Lennon PF, Ratner SJ, Enson Y: Meclofenamate enhances blood oxygenation in acute oleic acid injury. J Appl Physiol 64:710, 1988

33. Garrett RC, Thomas HM, III: Meclofenamate uniformly decreases shunt fraction in dogs with lobar atelectasis. J Appl Physiol 54:284, 1983

34. Marshall C, Kim SD, Marshall BE: The actions of halothane, ibuprofen and BW755C on hypoxic pulmonary vasoconstriction. Anesthesiology 66:537, 1987

35. Hallemans R, Naeji R, Melot C, et al: Do cyclo-oxygenase products mediate hypoxic pulmonary vasoconstriction in man? Am Rev Respir Dis 129A:341, 1984

36. Wagner WW, Jr., Lathan LP, Capen RL: Capillary recruitment during airway hypoxia: Role of pulmonary artery pressure. J Appl Physiol 47:383, 1979

37. Sprague RS, Stephenson AH, Lonigro AJ: Prostaglandin I_2 supports blood flow to hypoxic alveoli in anesthetized dogs. J Appl Physiol 56:1246, 1984

38. Hanly P, Sienko A, Light RB: Effect of indomethacin on gas exchange, pulmonary perfusion and hemodynamics in experimental pseudomonas pneumonia. Am Rev Respir Dis 133A:282, 1986

39. Hanly P, Sienko A, Light RB: Role of endogenous prostaglandins in the hemodynamic changes during acute experimental pseudomonas pneumonia with bacteremia. Am Rev Respir Dis 133A:77, 1986

40. Kobayashi T, Newman JH, Zadoff AD, Brigham KL: Diethylcarbamazine attenuates hypoxic vasoconstriction but not the pressor response to endotoxin or PGH_2 analog in awake sheep. Am Rev Respir Dis 131A:400, 1985

41. Morganroth ML, Stenmark KR, Zirrolli JA, et al: Leukotriene C_4 production during hypoxic pulmonary vasoconstriction in isolated rat lungs. Prostaglandins 28:867, 1984

42. Morganroth ML, Reeves JT, Murphy RC, Voelkel NF: Leukotriene synthesis and receptor blockers block hypoxic pulmonary vasoconstriction. J Appl Physiol 56:1340, 1984

43. Ahmed T, Oliver W: Does slow-reacting substance of anaphylaxis mediate hypoxic pulmonary vasoconstriction? Am Rev Respir Dis 127:566, 1983

44. Ahmed T, Oliver W, Frank BL, et al: Hypoxic pulmonary vasoconstriction in conscious sheep: Role of mast cell degranulation. Am Rev Respir Dis 126:291, 1982

45. Garrett RC, Foster S, Thomas HM, III: Lipoxygenase and cyclooxygenase blockade by BW755C enhances pulmonary hypoxic vasoconstriction. J Appl Physiol 62:129, 1987

46. Doyle JT, Wilson JS, Warren JV: The pulmonary vascular responses to short-term hypoxia in human subjects. Circulation 5:263, 1952

47. Fishman AP: State of the art. Chronic cor pulmonale. Am Rev Respir Dis 114:775, 1976

48. Boysen PG, Block AJ, Wynne JW, et al: Nocturnal pulmonary hypertension in patients with chronic obstructive pulmonary disease. Chest 76:536, 1979

49. Zasslow MA, Benumof JL, Trousdale FR: Hypoxic pulmonary vasoconstriction and the size of the hypoxic compartment. J Appl Physiol 53:626, 1982

50. Marshall BE, Marshall C: Continuity of response to hypoxic pulmonary vasoconstriction. J Appl Physiol 49:189, 1980

51. Benumof JL: Hypoxic pulmonary vasoconstriction and sodium nitroprusside perfusion. Anesthesiology 50:481, 1979

52. Benumof JL: Anesthesia for Thoracic Surgery. Ch. 4 and 8. WB Saunders, Philadelphia, 1987

53. Simmons DH, Linde CM, Miller JH, et al: Relation of lung volume and pulmonary vascular resistance. Circ Res 9:465, 1961

54. Burton AC, Patel DJ: Effect on pulmonary vascular resistance of inflation of the rabbit lungs. J Appl Physiol 12:239, 1958

55. Wittenberger JL, McGregor M, Berglund E, et al: Influence of state of inflation of the lung on pulmonary vascular resistance. J Appl Physiol 15:878, 1960

56. Benumof JL, Rogers SN, Moyce PR, et al: Hypoxic pulmonary vasoconstriction and regional and whole lung PEEP in the dog. Anesthesiology 52:503, 1979

57. Benumof JL: Mechanism of decreased blood flow to the atelectatic lung. J Appl Physiol 46:1047, 1978

58. Pirlo AF, Benumof JL, Trousdale FR: Atelectatic lobe blood flow: Open vs. closed chest, positive pressure vs. spontaneous ventilation. J Appl Physiol 50:1022, 1981

59. Hagen PT, Scholz DG, Edwards WD: Incidence and size of patent foramen ovale during the first ten decades of life: An autopsy study of 965 normal hearts. Mayo Clin Proc 59:17, 1984

60. Sykes MK: The mechanics of ventilation. p. 174. In Scurr C,

Feldman S (eds): Scientific Foundations of Anesthesia. FA Davis, Philadelphia, 1970

61. Nunn JF: Mechanisms of pulmonary ventilation. p. 64. Applied Respiratory Physiology. 3rd Ed. Butterworths, London, 1987

62. Scanlon TS, Benumof JL: Demonstration of interlobar collateral ventilation. J Appl Physiol 46:658, 1979

63. Kent EM, Blades B: The surgical anatomy of the pulmonary lobes. J Thorac Surg 12:18, 1941

64. Peters RM: Work of breathing following trauma. J Trauma 8:915, 1968

65. Nunn JF: The minute volume of pulmonary ventilation. p. 65. Applied Respiratory Physiology. 3rd Ed. Butterworths, London, 1987

66. Shapiro BA, Harrison RA, Trout CA: The mechanics of ventilation. p. 57. Clinical Application of Respiratory Care. 2nd Ed. Year Book Medical Publishers, Chicago, 1979

67. Comroe JH, Forster RE, Dubois AB, et al: The Lung. 2nd Ed. Year Book Medical Publishers, Chicago, 1962

68. Macklem PT, Fraser RG, Bates DV: Bronchial pressures and dimensions in health and obstructive airway disease. J Appl Physiol 18:699, 1983

69. Craig DB, Wahba WM, Don HF, et al: "Closing volume" and its relationship to gas exchange in seated and supine positions. J Appl Physiol 31:717, 1971

70. Burger EJ, Jr., Macklem P: Airway closure: Demonstration by breathing 100% O_2 at low lung volumes and by N_2 washout. J Appl Physiol 25:139, 1968

71. Brismer B, Hedenstierna G, Lundquist H, et al: Pulmonary densities during anesthesia with muscular relaxation—a proposal of atelectasis. Anesthesiology 62:422, 1985

72. Hales CA, Kazemi H: Small airways function in myocardial infarction. N Engl J Med 290:761, 1974

73. Harken AH, O'Connor NE: The influence of clinically undetectable edema on small airway closure in the dog. Ann Surg 184:183, 1976

74. Biddle TL, Yu PN, Hodges M, et al: Hypoxemia and lung water in acute myocardial infarction. Am Heart J 92:692, 1976

75. Nunn JF: Resistance to gas flow. p. 397. Applied Respiratory Physiology. 3rd Ed. Butterworths, London, 1987

76. Rehder K, Marsh HM, Rodarte JR, et al: Airway closure. Anesthesiology 47:40, 1977

77. Leblanc P, Ruff F, Milic-Emili J: Effects of age and body position on "airway closure" in man. J Appl Physiol 28:448, 1970

78. Craig DB, Wahba WM, Don HF, et al: "Closing volume" and its relationship to gas exchange in seated and supine positions. J Appl Physiol 31:717, 1971

79. Foex P, Prys-Roberts C, Hahn CEW, et al: Comparison of oxygen content of blood measured directly with values derived from measurement of oxygen tension. Br J Anaesth 42:803, 1970

80. Sykes MK, Adams AP, Finley WEI, et al: The cardiorespiratory effects of hemorrhage and overtransfusion in dogs. Br J Anaesth 42:573, 1970

81. Gregory IC: The oxygen and carbon monoxide capacities of foetal and adult blood. J Physiol 236:625, 1974

82. Nunn JF: Oxygen. p. 109. Applied Respiratory Physiology. 3rd Ed. Butterworths, London, 1987

83. Lawler PGP, Nunn JF: A re-assessment of the validity of the iso-shunt graph. Br J Anaesth 56:1325, 1984

84. Kelman GF, Nunn JF, Prys-Roberts C, et al: The influence of the cardiac output on arterial oxygenation: A theoretical study. Br J Anaesth 39:450, 1967

85. Philbin DM, Sullivan SF, Bowman FO, et al: Post-operative hypoxemia: Contribution of the cardiac output. Anesthesiology 32:136, 1970

86. Berggren SM: The oxygen deficit of arterial blood caused by non-ventilating parts of the lung. Acta Physiol Scand, 4:suppl. 11, 1, 1942

87. Cheney FW, Colley PS: The effect of cardiac output on arterial blood oxygenation. Anesthesiology 52:496, 1980

88. Henry W: Experiments on the quantity of gases absorbed by water at different temperatures and under different pressures. Philos Trans R Soc 93:29, 1803

89. Fishman AP: Pulmonary edema: The water-exchanging function of the lung. Circulation 46:390, 1972

90. Low FN: Lung interstitium, development, morphology, fluid content. p. 17. In Staub NC (ed): Lung Water and Solute Exchange. Marcel Dekker, New York, 1978

91. Weibel ER: Morphological basis of alveolar-capillary gas exchange. Physiol Rev 53:419, 1973

92. Guyton AC: A concept of negative interstitial pressure based on pressures in implanted perforated capsules. Circ Res 12:399, 1963

93. Smith-Erichsen N, Bo G: Airway closure and fluid filtration in the lung. Br J Anaesth 51:475, 1979

94. Oswalt CE, Gates GA, Holmstrom EMG: Pulmonary edema as a complication of acute airway obstruction. Rev Surg 34:364, 1977

95. Staub NC: Pulmonary edema: Physiologic approaches to management. Chest 74:559, 1978

96. Permutt S: Effect of interstitial pressure of the lung on pulmonary circulation. Med Thorac 22:118, 1965

97. Staub NC: "State of the art" review. Pathogenesis of pulmonary edema. Am Rev Respir Dis 109:358, 1974

98. Benumof JL: Monitoring respiratory function during anesthesia. p. 31. In Saidman LJ, Smith NT (eds): Monitoring in Anesthesia. John Wiley & Sons, New York, 1978

99. Munson ES, Larson CP, Jr., Babad AA, et al: The effects of halothane, fluroxene and cyclopropane on ventilation: A comparative study in man. Anesthesiology 27:716, 1966

100. Couture J, Picken J, Trop D, et al: Airway closure in normal, obese, and anesthetized supine subjects. Fed Proc 29:269, 1970

101. Don HF, Craig DB, Wahba WM, et al: The measurement of gas trapped in the lungs at functional residual capacity and the effects of posture. Anesthesiology 35:582, 1971

102. Ward CS: The prevention of accidents associated with anesthetic apparatus. Br J Anaesth 40:692, 1968

103. Mazze RI: Therapeutic misadventures with oxygen delivery systems: The need for continuous in-line oxygen monitors. Anesth Analg 51:787, 1972

104. Epstein RM, Rackow H, Lee ASJ, et al: Prevention of accidental breathing of anoxic gas mixture during anesthesia. Anesthesiology 23:1, 1962

105. Sprague DH, Archer GW: Intraoperative hypoxia from an erroneously filled liquid oxygen reservoir. Anesthesiology 42:360, 1975

106. Eger EI II, Epstein RM: Hazards of anesthetic equipment. Anesthesiology 25:490, 1964

107. Martin JT: Positioning in Anesthesia and Surgery. WB Saunders, Philadelphia, 1978

108. Heinonen J, Takki S, Tammisto T: Effect of the Trendelenburg tilt and other procedures on the position of endotracheal tubes. Lancet 1:850, 1969

109. Mead J, Agostoni E: Dynamics of breathing. p. 411. In Fenn WO, Rahn H (eds.): Handbook of Physiology. Section 3. Respiration. Vol. 1. Williams & Wilkins, Baltimore, 1964

110. Don HF, Robson JG: The mechanics of the respiratory system during anesthesia. Anesthesiology 26:168, 1965

111. Bendixen HH, Hedley-Whyte J, Chir B, et al: Impaired oxygenation in surgical patients during general anesthesia with controlled ventilation. N Engl J Med 269:991, 1963

112. Bendixen HH, Bullwinkel B, Hedley-Whyte J, et al: Atelectasis and shunting during spontaneous ventilation in anesthetized patients. Anesthesiology 25:297, 1964

113. Cain SM: Increased oxygen uptake with passive hyperventilation of dogs. J Appl Physiol 28:4, 1970

114. Karetzky MS, Cain SM: Effect of carbon dioxide on oxygen uptake during hyperventilation in normal man. J Appl Physiol 28:8, 1970

115. Benumof JL, Mathers JM, Wahrenbrock EA: Cyclic hypoxic pulmonary vasoconstriction induced by concomitant carbon dioxide changes. J Appl Physiol 41:466, 1976

116. Cutillo A, Omboni E, Perondi R, et al: Effect of hypocapnia on pulmonary mechanics in normal subjects and in patients with chronic obstructive lung disease. Am Rev Respir Dis 110:25, 1974

117. Don H: The mechanical properties of the respiratory system during anesthesia. p. 113. In Kafer ER (ed): International Anesthesiology Clinics. Vol. 15. Anesthesia and Respiratory Function. Little Brown, Boston, 1977

118. Don HF, Wahba M, Cuadrado L, et al: The effects of anesthesia and 100 percent oxygen on the functional residual capacity of the lungs. Anesthesiology 32:521, 1970

119. Hewlett AM, Hulands GH, Nunn JF, et al: Functional residual capacity during anaesthesia. III. Artificial ventilation. Br J Anaesth 46:495, 1974

120. Westbrook PR, Stubbs SE, Sessler AD, et al: Effects of anesthesia and muscle paralysis on respiratory mechanics in normal man. J Appl Physiol 34:81, 1973

121. Alexander JI, Spence AA, Parikh RK, et al: The role of airway closure in postoperative hypoxemia. Br J Anaesth 45:34, 1973

122. Hickey RF, Visick W, Fairley HB, et al: Effects of halothane anesthesia on functional residual capacity and alveolar-arterial oxygen tension difference. Anesthesiology 38:20, 1973

123. Wyche MQ, Teichner RL, Kallos T, et al: Effects of continuous positive-pressure breathing on functional residual capacity and arterial oxygenation during intra-abdominal operation. Anesthesiology 38:68, 1973

124. Freund F, Roos A, Dodd RB: Expiratory activity of the abdominal muscles in man during general anesthesia. J Appl Physiol 19:693, 1964

125. Kallos T, Wyche MQ, Garman JK: The effect of Innovar on functional residual capacity and total chest compliance. Anesthesiology 39:558, 1973

126. Campbell EJM, Agostini E, David JN: The Respiratory Muscles: Mechanics and Neural Control. 2nd Ed. WB Saunders, Philadelphia, 1970

127. Milic-emili J, Mead J, Tanner JM: Topography of esophageal pressure as a function of posture in man. J Appl Physiol 19:212, 1964

128. Froese AB, Bryan CA: Effects of anesthesia and paralysis on diaphragmatic mechanics in man. Anesthesiology 41:242, 1974

129. Dekker E, Defares JG, Heemstra H: Direct measurement of intrabronchial pressure. Its application to the location of the check-value mechanism. J Appl Physiol 13:35, 1958

130. Ward CF, Gagnon RL, Benumof JL: Wheezing after induction of general anesthesia: Negative expiratory pressure revisited. Anesth Analg 58:49, 1979

131. Ray JF, Yost L, Moallem S, et al: Immobility, hypoxemia, and pulmonary arteriovenous shunting. Arch Surg 109:537, 1974

132. Wagner PD, Laravuso RB, Uhl RR, et al: Continuous distributions of ventilation-perfusion ratios in normal subjects breathing air and 100% O_2. J Clin Invest 54:54, 1974

133. Briscoe WA, Cree EM, Filler, et al: Lung volume, alveolar ventilation and perfusion interrelationships in chronic pulmonary emphysema. J Appl Physiol 15:785, 1960

134. Slocum HC, Hoeflich EA, Allen CR: Circulatory and respiratory distress from extreme positions on the operating table. Surg Gynecol Obstet 84:1065, 1947

135. Laver MB, Hallowell P, Goldblatt A: Pulmonary dysfunction secondary to heart disease: Aspects relevant to anesthesia and surgery. Anesthesiology 33:161, 1970

136. Yeaker H: Tracheobronchial secretions. Am J Med 50:493, 1971

137. Forbes AR: Humidification and mucous flow in the intubated trachea. Br J Anaesth 45:874, 1973

138. Bang BG, Bang FB: Effect of water deprivation on nasal mucous flow. Proc Soc Exp Biol Med 106:516, 1961

139. Hirsch JA, Tokayer JL, Robinson MJ, et al: Effects of dry air and subsequent humidification on tracheal mucous velocity in dogs. J Appl Physiol 39:242, 1975

140. Dalhamn T: Mucous flow and ciliary activity in the tracheas of rats exposed to respiratory irritant gases. Acta Physiol Scand, 36:suppl. 123, 1, 1956

141. Hill L: The ciliary movement of tne trachea studies in vitro. Lancet 2:802, 1928

142. Sackner MA, Landa J, Hirsch J, et al: Pulmonary effects of oxygen breathing. Ann Intern Med 82:40, 1975

143. Sackner MA, Hirsch J, Epstein S: Effect of cuffed endotracheal tubes on tracheal mucous velocity. Chest 68:774, 1975

144. Forbes AR: Halothane depresses mucociliary flow in the trachea. Anesthesiology 45:59, 1976

145. Nunn JF, Sturrock JE, Wills EJ, et al: The effect of inhalation anaesthetics on the swimming velocity of Tetrahymena pyriformis. J Cell Sci 15:537, 1974

146. Prys-Roberts C: The metabolic regulation of circulatory transport. p. 87. In Scurr C, Feldman S (eds): Scientific Foundation of Anesthesia. FA Davis, Philadelphia, 1970

147. Benumof JL, Wahrenbrock EA: Blunted hypoxic pulmonary vasoconstriction by increased lung vascular pressures. J Appl Physiol 38:846, 1975

148. Scanlon TS, Benumof JL, Wahrenbrock EA, et al: Hypoxic pulmonary vasoconstriction and the ratio of hypoxic lung to perfused normoxic lung. Anesthesiology 49:177, 1978

149. Benumof JL, Wahrenbrock EA: Dependency of hypoxic pulmonary vasoconstriction on temperature. J Appl Physiol 42:56, 1977

150. Benumof JL: Anesthesia for Thoracic Surgery. Ch. 4. WB Saunders, Philadelphia, 1987

151. Benumof JL: Anesthesia for Thoracic Surgery. Ch. 8. WB Saunders, Philadelphia, 1987

152. Benumof JL: One lung ventilation: Which lung should be PEEPed? Anesthesiology 56:161, 1982

153. Eckenhoff JE, Enderby GEH, Larson A, et al: Pulmonary gas exchange during deliberate hypotension. Br J Anaesth 35:750, 1963

154. Kain ML, Panday J, Nunn JF: The effect of intubation on the dead space during halothane anaesthesia. Br J Anaesth 41:94, 1969

155. Conway CM: Anesthetic circuits. p. 509. In Scurr C, Feldman S (eds): Scientific Foundations of Anesthesia. 2nd Ed. William Heinemann Medical Books, London, 1974

156. Heistad DD, Abboud FM: Circulatory adjustments to hypoxia. Dickinson W. Richards Lecture. Circulation 61:463, 1980

157. Roberts JG: The effect of hypoxia on the systemic circulation

during anaesthesia. p. 311. In Prys-Roberts E (ed): The Circulation in Anaesthesia: Applied Physiology and Pharmacology. Blackwell Scientific Publications, Oxford, 1980

158. Winter PM, Smith G: The toxicity of oxygen. Anesthesiology 37:210, 1972

159. Lambertsen CJ: Effects of oxygen at high partial pressure. p. 1027. In Fenn WO, Rahn H (eds): Handbook of Physiology. Section 3. Respiration. Vol. 2. Williams & Wilkins, Baltimore, 1965

160. Nash G, Blennerhasset JB, Pontoppidan H: Pulmonary lesions associated with oxygen therapy and artificial ventilation. N Engl J Med 276:368, 1967

161. Prys-Roberts C: Hypercapnia. p. 435. In Gray TC, Nunn JF, Utting JE (eds): General Anaesthesia. 4th Ed. Butterworth, London, 1980

162. Wattwil LMT, Olsson JG: Circulatory effects of isoflurane during hypercapnia. Anesth Analg 66:1234, 1987

163. Severinghaus JW, Larson CP: Respiration in anesthesia. p. 1219. In Fenn WO, Rahn H (eds): Handbook of Physiology. Section 3. Respiration. Vol. 2. Williams & Wilkins, Baltimore, 1965

164. Clowes GHA, Hopkins AL, Simeone FA: A comparison of the physiological effects of hypercapnia and hypoxia in the production of cardiac arrest. Ann Surg 142:446, 1955

165. Fenn WO, Asano T: Effects of carbon dioxide inhalation on potassium liberation from the liver. Am J Physiol 185:567, 1956

166. Patterson RW: Effect of $PaCO_2$ on O_2 consumption during cardiopulmonary bypass in man. Anesth Analg 55:269, 1976

167. Benumof JL: The pulmonary circulation. Ch. 7. In Kaplan JA (ed): Thoracic Anesthesia. Churchill Livingstone, New York, 1983

168. Benumof JL: Anesthesia for Thoracic Surgery. WB Saunders, Philadelphia, 1987

16

CARDIOVASCULAR PHYSIOLOGY

Daniel M. Thys
Joel A. Kaplan

INTRODUCTION

In this chapter, cardiac physiology is emphasized. The physiology of the peripheral vasculature and regulation of blood flow to specific organs are discussed in other chapters (e.g., cerebral blood flow in Ch. 19 and renal blood flow in Ch. 18). Therefore, the purposes of this chapter are as follows:

1. To review concepts of cardiac physiology as they apply to anesthesia
2. To clarify the language of cardiac physiology
3. To indicate new, as well as old, techniques used to measure cardiac function
4. To review where these techniques have been applied to anesthetic agents

Under normal conditions, the heart acts as a servant by varying the cardiac output in accordance with total tissue needs.[1] Tissue needs may change secondary to exercise, infection, heart disease, trauma, surgery, or administration of drugs or anesthetics. Although the heart receives much of the emphasis, the needs of peripheral tissues are actually regulating circulatory requirements. The heart serves only as the limiting factor in many patients with severe cardiac disease. In this regard, there are three definitions that are often confused and which should be clearly separated.[2]

Circulatory function is the function of the entire circulatory system, including the heart, blood vessels, and blood volume. Failure of any one of these can lead to significant circulatory dysfunction. For example, hypovolemia can lead to circulatory failure or shock in the presence of normal blood vessels and a normal heart.

Cardiac function includes the function of the myocardium valves, conduction tissue, and supporting structures. Dysfunction of any of these can lead to cardiac and circulatory failure. The myocardium can be entirely normal, but with insufficient valves the heart can fail.

551

Myocardial function depends on the cardiac muscle itself and its blood supply. There can be myocardial failure based on actual muscle damage or based on myocardial ischemia and inadequate muscle function. Certainly, myocardial dysfunction will then produce cardiac dysfunction and circulatory problems.

The primary function of the heart is to deliver sufficient oxygenated blood to meet the metabolic requirements of the peripheral tissues. One definition of heart failure is that the heart is unable to pump blood at a rate sufficient to meet these requirements. Therefore, the cardiac output is usually considered the key test of cardiac function. However, cardiac output and myocardial function or contractility cannot be related in a simple, straightforward manner. The contractile state of the myocardium is only one of several determinants of the heart's ability to eject an adequate cardiac output.[3]

For the purpose of this chapter, cardiac physiology is discussed in a stepwise fashion. First, the events occurring during a single cardiac contraction are described. Thereafter, the importance of stroke volume, as the mechanical product of such a contraction, and its determinants are reviewed. Subsequently, the relationship between cardiac output and the peripheral circulation is analyzed by studying ventricular function curves. Finally, a brief overview of the coronary circulation is provided.

THE CARDIAC CYCLE

During the cardiac contraction, temporal changes in ventricular pressure and volume can be observed. A record of these changes can be displayed over time for each of these variables (Fig. 16-1). On such a recording, systolic events are indicated by increasing ventricular pressure (Fig. 16-1, *A–C*) followed by decreasing ventricular volume (Fig. 16-1, *C–D*), while in diastole an initial decrease in ventricular pressure (Fig. 16-1, *G–H*) is followed by an increasing volume (Fig. 16-1, *H–I*). In a different approach, changes in pressure and volume are analyzed simultaneously within the framework of a pressure–volume diagram. On such a diagram, volume is depicted on the horizontal axis, while pressure is shown on the vertical axis. A single contraction will result in a pressure–volume loop consisting of four phases (Fig. 16-2). The first phase begins at end-diastole. It represents the *isovolumic contraction phase* and is marked by a rapid increase in ventricular pressure in the absence of a volume change. As soon as the ventricular pressure exceeds the aortic pressure, the aortic valve opens and the second phase or *ejection phase* begins. During the ejection phase, ventricular volume decreases while an initial increase in ventricular pressure is usually followed by a decrease. When equilibrium is reached between ventricular and aortic pressures and volumes, ejection ceases and the aortic valve closes. At this point, the end-systolic point, the ventricular volume has reached its smallest size. After closure of

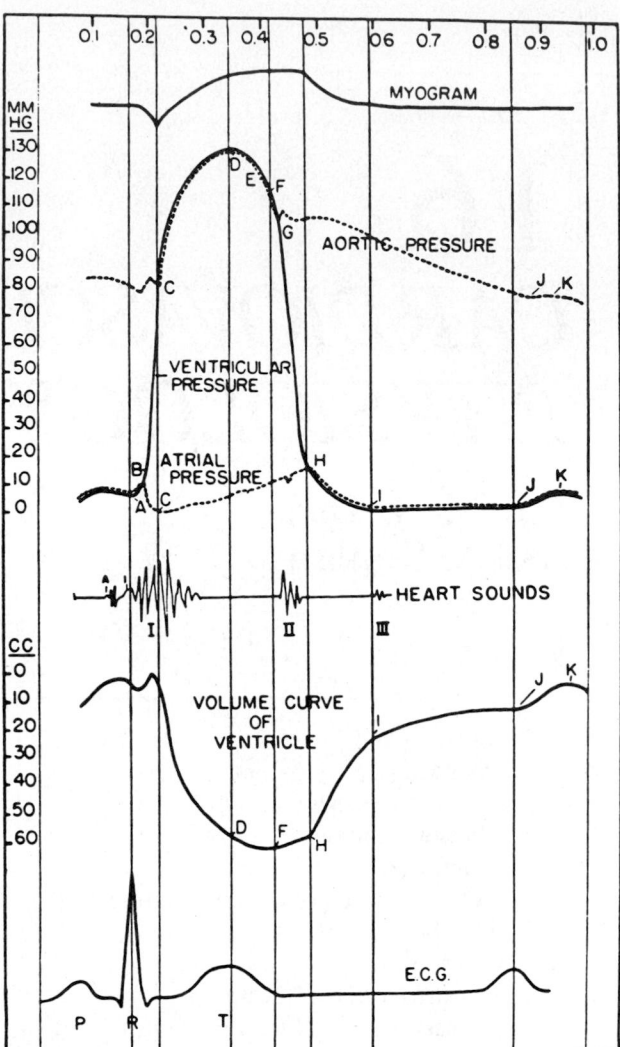

Fig. 16-1. Display, over time, of various cardiac variables for a single cardiac cycle. (See text for details.) (From Wiggens,[126] with permission.)

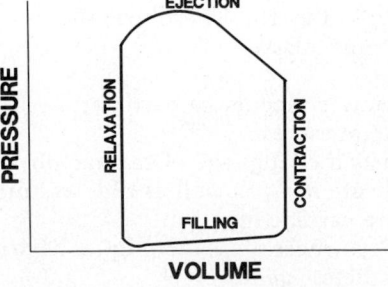

Fig. 16-2. Display of a cardiac cycle as a pressure–volume loop. The various phases of the cycle are identified. (See text for details.)

the aortic valve, the ventricular *relaxation phase* begins. It is marked by a rapid decrease in ventricular pressure with little change in ventricular volume.

While the ventricular pressure decreases, the left atrium is being filled from the pulmonary veins. This filling is manifested by increasing atrial pressure and volume. The last phase of the contraction begins when the atrial pressure exceeds the ventricular pressure, the mitral valve opens, and the filling of the ventricle starts. During the *ventricular filling phase*, the ventricular volume increases markedly, while under normal circumstances, the increase in ventricular pressure is more gradual and of limited extent. It proceeds until a new ventricular depolarization leads to the next ventricular contraction. In recent years, the pressure–volume framework has been found exceptionally useful for the study of cardiac performance because it allows one to assess, within a single model, systolic and diastolic ventricular properties, arterial and venous vascular properties, ventriculovascular interactions, and myocardial energetics.[4]

Cardiac Phases

Isovolumic Contraction Phase

Since the early work of Frank,[5] it has been known that the tension (T) developed by cardiac muscle is determined by the initial length (L) or stretch of the muscle. In isolated muscles, maximal tension is achieved at an optimal length known as L_{max}. For muscle lengths below or above L_{max}, the developed tension is less than maximal (Fig. 16-3). As a result of advances in laboratory techniques, it is now known that the primary determinant of developed tension is not the muscle length per se, but the sarcomere length (SL).[6,7] While the SL-T relation is fairly similar to the L-T relation, some differences, such as the absence of a descending limb, are present.[8]

In intact hearts, the equivalent of the length-tension relation is the pressure–volume relation measured during the isovolumic phase of the contraction (the Frank relation).[9] The pressure developed during the isovolumic contraction is determined by Laplace's law, which states that

$$P \approx \frac{(2hT)}{r}$$

where P = the developed pressure, T = the wall tension, h = the wall thickness, and r = the radius of the ventricle. According to the Laplace equation, the radius (r) rather than the ventricular volume (πr^3) determines pressure. As a result, the effects of changes in end-diastolic volume on developed pressure will be attenuated by the three-dimensional nature of volume. When end-diastolic volume increases by 50 percent (from 100 to 150 ml), the radius only increases by 14 percent (from 3.17 to 3.63 cm). If such a small change in muscle or sarcomere length is to lead to a change in developed

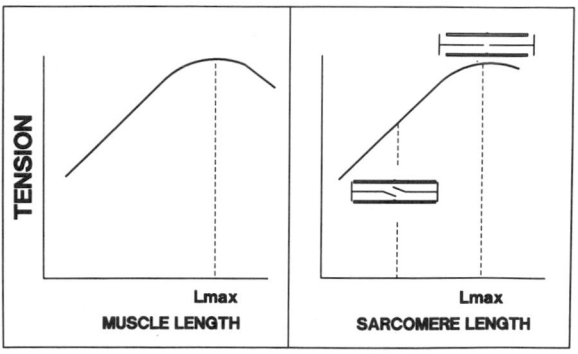

Fig. 16-3. (A) Length-tension diagram for an isolated cardiac muscle. (B) Sarcomere length-tension diagram. At L_{max}, the thick and thin filaments overlap perfectly.

pressure, the wall tension must be very sensitive to changes in sarcomere length. Indeed, the SL-T relation for cardiac muscle is very steep, and for an increase in SL from 1.6 to 2.3 μm, the wall tension increases from zero to maximum. With increases in contractility, the slope of the SL-T relation is shifted to the left so that, for any given sarcomere length, the developed tension and pressure will be higher. The same is true for maximal changes in tension over time (dT/dt) and pressure over time (dP/dt).[10]

Ejection Phase

Nearly 20 years after Frank had published his observations on the L-T relation, Paterson and Starling[11] reported the results of their observations in ejecting mammalian hearts. They noted that, at constant aortic pressure, an increase in end-diastolic volume produces an increase in stroke volume (the Starling relation). The Starling relation differs from the Frank relation in that it not only depends on the SL-T relation but also on the interaction between muscle force, velocity, and length. In isolated muscle, the force-velocity-length relationship has been extensively studied.[12,13] Multiple data points are obtained by studying the contraction of isolated muscles at various preloads (initial muscle length) and afterloads (developed force) (Fig. 16-4). This relationship is often represented as a three-dimensional plot in which force, length, and velocity are the axes (Fig. 16-5).

When individual points along the three axes are connected, a surface is generated that represents the contractility of the isolated muscle. With increases in contractility, the surface is shifted upward, while a decrease in contractility produces a downward shift.

The force-velocity-length concept cannot readily be applied in the clinical setting because the appropriate measurements are difficult to obtain in the intact heart.[14,15] In clinical practice, these measurement difficulties are often circumvented by limiting the studies of the ejection phase to its beginning (end-diastolic vol-

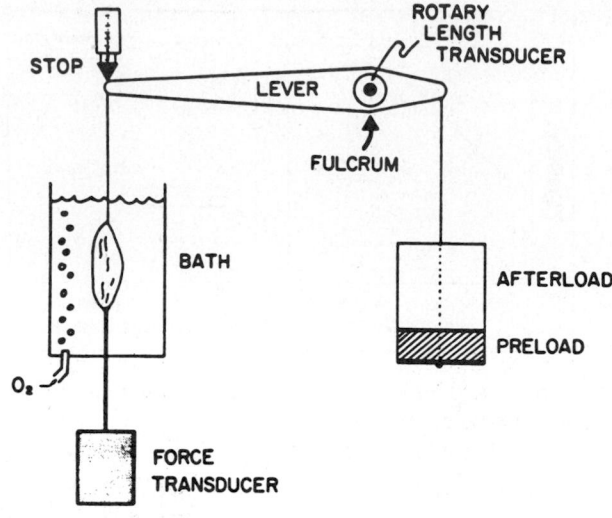

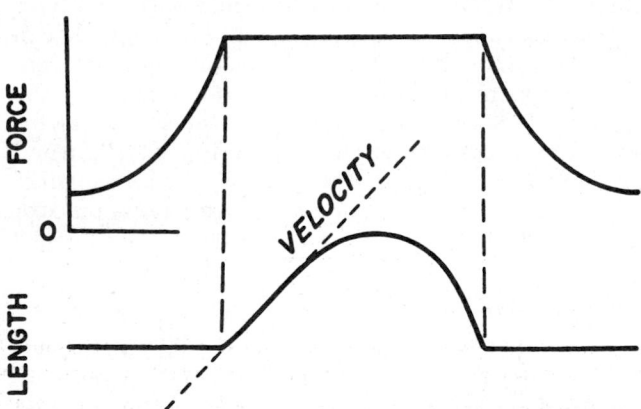

Fig. 16-4. Schematic of an isolated muscle preparation and the force-velocity-length developed during a single contraction.

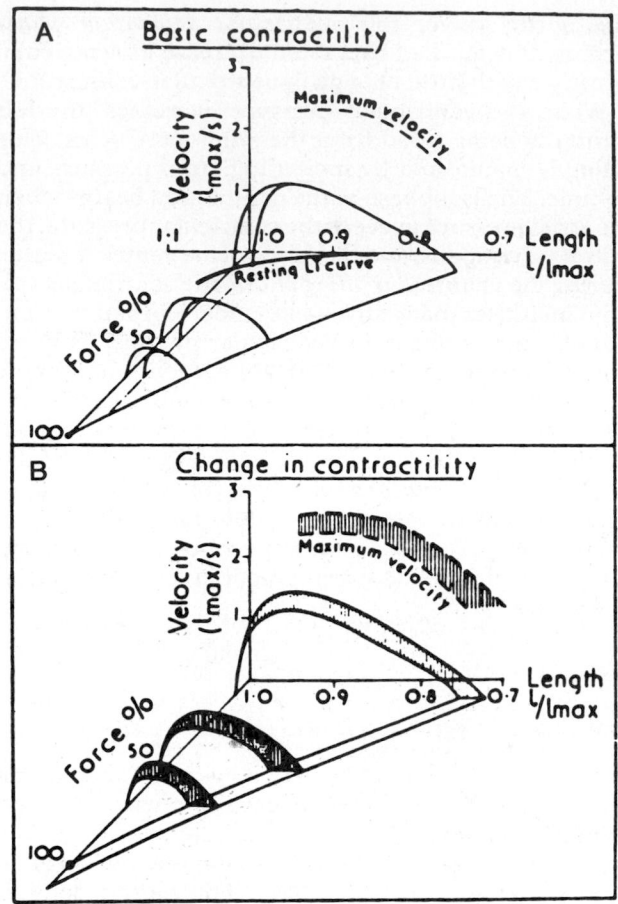

Fig. 16-5. Three-dimensional relationship between force, velocity, and length in a series of isotonic contractions in cardiac muscle. The surface so created represents the level of basic contractile state (**A**). With an increase in contractility, the lines and surface are shifted upward (**B**). (From Brutsaert,[127] with permission.)

ume or EDV) and end point (end-systolic volume or ESV) (Fig. 16-6). The difference between EDV and ESV is the stroke volume (SV), and contractility is commonly expressed as the ejection fraction (EF):

$$EF = \frac{SV}{EDV}$$

For each contraction, the end-systolic volume is the smallest volume to which the heart is able to contract. It will be determined by the contractile state of the ventricle and the properties of the vascular system.

Relaxation Phase

After the end-systolic volume has been reached, the pressure in the ventricle decreases rapidly. This phase of the contraction is known as the *relaxation phase* and

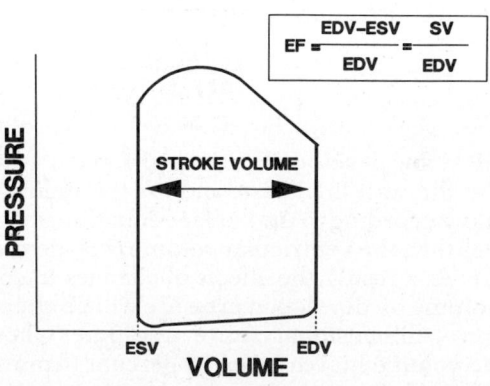

Fig. 16-6. Pressure–volume diagram indicating end-diastolic volume (EDV), end-systolic volume (ESV), stroke volume, and the equation to calculate ejection fraction (EF).

TABLE 16-1. Determinants of Relaxation in the Intact Heart

Loading
Internal restoring forces (cardiac fiber)
External restoring forces (intact heart)
  Configurational loading: end-ejection pressure–volume relation

Hemodynamic loading (cardiocirculatory system)
  Arterial impedance
  Transmission of pressure wave in coronary circulation
  Laplace relationship during rapid filling phase, pericardium,
    right ventricular hemodynamics

Inactivation
Metabolic control: coronary circulation
Neurohumoral control: catecholamines
Drugs

Nonuniformity
Spatial and temporal distribution of force and loading inactivation

represents the process by which the heart returns to its precontractile configuration.[16] It has received much attention in recent years because abnormalities of relaxation have been noted in several cardiac disorders. In both the isolated cardiac muscle and the intact heart, relaxation is controlled by a triple control mechanism.[17] The three interacting determinants of relaxation are (1) the prevailing load, (2) inactivation (the processes regulating the detachment of actin-myosin cross-bridges), and (3) the nonuniform distribution of load and inactivation in space and time (Table 16-1). Because relaxation is intimately related to the previous contraction phase (activation or cross-bridge formation) and is an energy-requiring process, some have proposed that it be considered as an integral part of ventricular systole[18] (Fig. 16-7).

Filling Phase

When left atrial pressure exceeds left ventricular pressure (the pressure crossover point), the mitral valve opens and filling of the left ventricle begins. It consists of an early, rapid filling phase and an atrial phase, occurring as a result of the atrial contraction. Flow across the mitral valve is primarily determined by the pressure gradient between the left atrium and left ventricle. During filling, the ventricle distends and both its pressure and volume increase. The diastolic pressure–volume relation, or distensibility, is often represented by a pressure–volume curve that is complex and influenced by many factors. These include (1) factors extrinsic to the left ventricle, (2) the physical properties of the left ventricle, and (3) the three determinants of myocardial relaxation (Table 16-2).

STROKE VOLUME

Definition

The stroke volume is the amount of blood ejected by the ventricle with each single contraction. Within the pressure–volume framework, stroke volume is readily

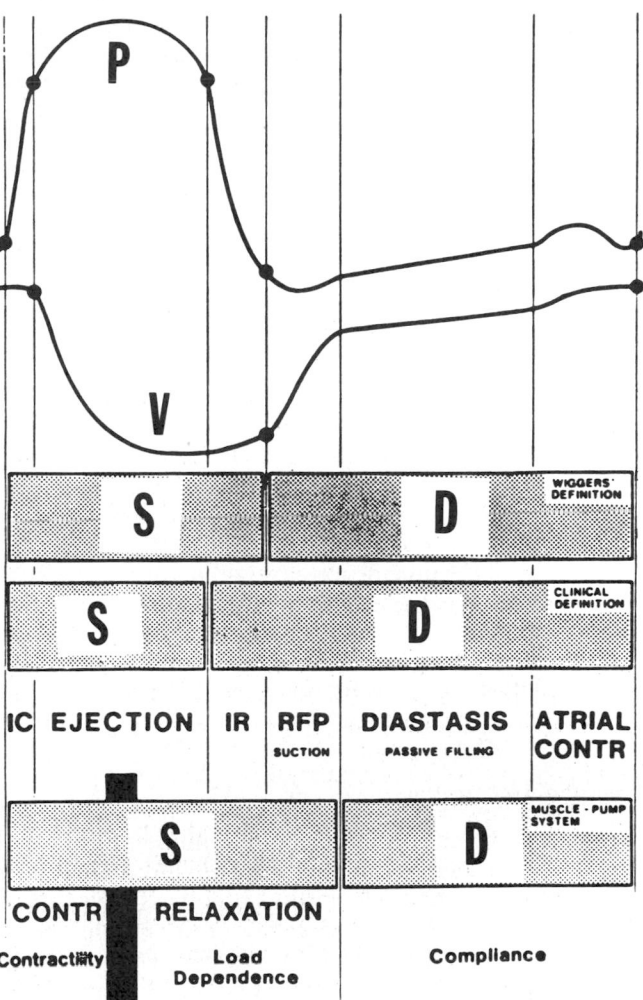

Fig. 16-7. Brutsaert's proposal for a new definition of the systole (S) and diastole (D). P, ventricular pressure; V, ventricular volume; IC, isovolumic contraction phase; IR, isovolumic relaxation phase; RFP, rapid filling phase; Contr, contraction. The heavy black line indicates peak ventricular pressure. (From Brutsaert et al.,[17] with permission.)

TABLE 16-2. Determinants of Left Ventricular Distensibility

Extrinsic factors
Pericardium
Right ventricle
Intrapleural and mediastinal pressure
Coronary vascular volume

Physical properties of the left ventricle
Ventricular geometry
  Volume
  Wall thickness
Composition of ventricular wall (scar, amyloid)

Myocardial relaxation
Load
Inactivation
Spatial and temporal nonuniformity

recognized as the difference between the end-diastolic and end-systolic volume (Fig. 16-6). The conventional determinants of stroke volume are analogous to those of force-velocity-length measurements in isolated muscle preparations: the preload, the afterload, and the contractility. While these variables are clearly defined and understood for isolated muscles, their meaning is much more ambiguous in the intact heart.

Determinants of Stroke Volume

Preload

In the isolated muscle, the preload represents the load imposed on the muscle before contraction and is obtained by hanging a small weight at the end of the resting muscle (Fig. 16-4A). The end-diastolic length is thus assumed to determine the force generated in the next systole. Some recent evidence suggests, however, that the history of the muscle length changes occurring during the entire diastole is also an important determinant of this force.[19]

In the intact heart, end-diastolic volume is generally accepted as the most valid measure of ventricular preload.

Preload Measurement

The left ventricular end-diastolic volume (LVEDV) is difficult to measure clinically, and measurement is only beginning to be possible with techniques such as echocardiography, ventriculography, radionuclide scans, and conductance, all of which can be used both in the operating room and in the intensive care unit. Recently, transesophageal echocardiography has been extensively used to measure the left ventricular end-diastolic area as an approximation of left ventricular volume; however, it is limited by its two-dimensionality and therefore is not a totally adequate measure of the true LVEDV. Despite this limitation, we were recently able to demonstrate that in surgical patients, EDV derived from a single-plane echocardiogram was a significant determinant of stroke volume.[20]

Left ventricular end-diastolic pressure (LVEDP) is usually measured clinically as an approximation of the LVEDV (preload) of the left heart[21] (Fig. 16-8).

This assumes that left ventricular compliance is entirely normal, which is not a valid assumption in many patients with cardiac disease (Fig. 16-9). With ischemic heart disease or aortic stenosis, the left ventricular compliance curve is frequently shifted to the left, where small increases in volume can produce large increases in left ventricular filling pressure (decreased compliance). With aortic insufficiency or relief of myocardial ischemia with vasodilator drugs, compliance increases and large volumes can be placed in the left ventricle with minimal increases in pressure. Therefore, LVEDP is not always a good reflection of LVEDV.[22] The LVEDP can be measured with a catheter in the left ventricle,

but this is usually done only at cardiac catheterization and not during surgery, because a high incidence of ventricular arrhythmias exists with this technique.

During cardiac surgery, the preload of the left heart is frequently measured by inserting a catheter into the left atrium and measuring left atrial pressure (LAP), which gives a good approximation of the LVEDP, as long as there is a normal mitral valve.[23] The Swan-Ganz flow-directed pulmonary arterial catheter is now being used most often to ascertain the left ventricular filling pressure.[24] The pulmonary capillary wedge pressure (PCWP) or pulmonary artery occluded pressure (PAOP) is usually a good reflection of the LAP.[25] Marked alterations in airway pressure, such as occurs during the use of high levels of positive end-expiratory pressure, may disturb the relationship between the PCWP and left atrial pressure.[26] Depending on the compliance of the pulmonary parenchyma, either part or all of the airway pressure may be transmitted to the pulmonary arterial catheter. This must be considered when evaluating left ventricular filling pressure with the Swan-Ganz catheter in patients receiving mechanical ventilation and positive end-expiratory pressure. Also, the location of the tip of the catheter in relation to the left atrium must be ascertained. If the catheter tip is in zone 1 of the lung, it will reflect airway pressure instead of LAP.[27] When the catheter cannot be placed in the wedge position, the pulmonary artery diastolic pressure (PADP) may be used to estimate the LAP and is usually quite accurate.[25] However, if the pulmonary vascular resistance is markedly elevated, a large disparity between the PADP and the LAP will exist.

The central venous pressure (CVP) is the poorest approximation of LVEDP but is often used to estimate the LVEDP in patients with good function of both the right and left ventricles. However, when cardiac disease is characterized by disparate right and left ventricular function, the CVP may be misleading when quantitating left ventricular filling pressure.[28] An important concept to remember is that left ventricular and right ventricular preloads and function curves are not always equal or even parallel.[29] The CVP can be higher or lower than the LVEDP, depending on the underlying pathology. However, the CVP is a reasonably good reflection of right ventricular preload. It accurately reflects right ventricular end-diastolic volume in most cases, unless a change in right ventricular compliance occurs with events such as a right ventricular infarction.

Factors affecting the preload of the heart include the total blood volume, body position, intrathoracic pressure, intrapericardial pressure, venous tone, pumping action of skeletal muscles, and the atrial contribution to ventricular filling.[30] Large increases in heart rate decrease the duration of diastole and hence can lower preload. Synchronous atrial contraction makes a significant contribution to left ventricular preload. This is best seen when a patient develops a nodal rhythm. There is often a 10 to 30 percent decrease in blood

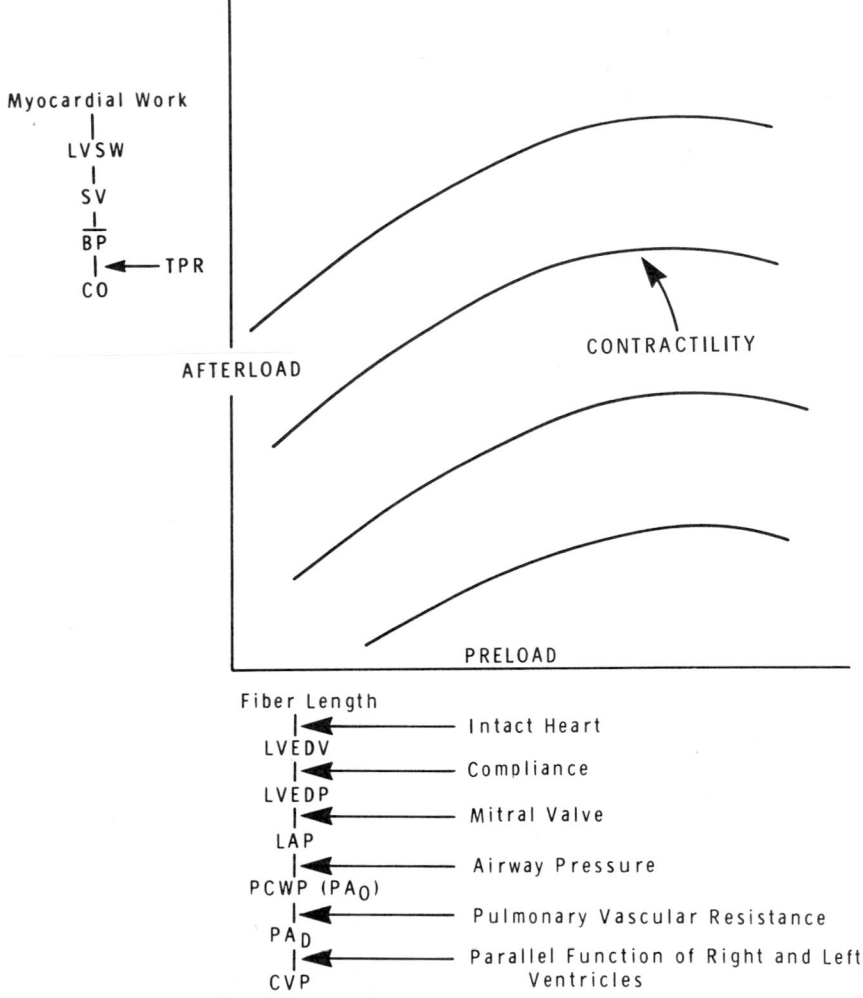

Fig. 16-8. The Frank-Starling family of curves is demonstrated. The horizontal axis represents the preload of the heart, and the various factors used to estimate preload are shown. The vertical axis represents the myocardial work, and the various factors used to represent this are shown. The vertical axis is also affected by the afterload of the heart. (See the text for details.) LVSW, left ventricular stroke work, SV, stroke volume, BP, mean blood pressure; TPR, total peripheral resistance; CO, cardiac output; LVEDV, left ventricular end-diastolic volume; LVEDP, left ventricular end-diastolic pressure; LAP, left atrial pressure; PCWP, pulmonary capillary wedge pressure; PA_O, pulmonary artery occluded pressure; PA_D, pulmonary artery diastolic pressure; CVP, central venous pressure. (Modified from Bonner,[128] with permission.)

pressure and cardiac output with loss of atrial contraction. The hemodynamic effect of loss of this contribution to preload is most severe in patients with decreased left ventricular compliance (aortic stenosis or idiopathic hypertrophic subaortic stenosis).

The vertical or work axis on the Starling curve shown in Figure 16-8 would ideally reflect myocardial work, but this value cannot be derived clinically. Variables often placed on this axis instead of work are blood pressure (BP), cardiac output (CO), stroke volume (SV), and left ventricular stroke work (LVSW) derived from the cardiac output, all of which can be obtained clini-

cally with hemodynamic monitors, including the Swan-Ganz catheter and thermal dilution cardiac outputs. The afterload, as expressed by total peripheral resistance (TPR) or systemic vascular resistance (SVR), also has an effect on this axis. Bolooki[31] has modified the curve to include an axis for TPR (Fig. 16-10).

According to Starling's law, increases on the filling pressure axis should lead to increases in work. Sarnoff and Berglund[29] described a series of curves that fit on this diagram (Figs. 16-8 and 16-11). Curves moving up and toward the left show an increase in myocardial contractility when more work is done at a lower filling

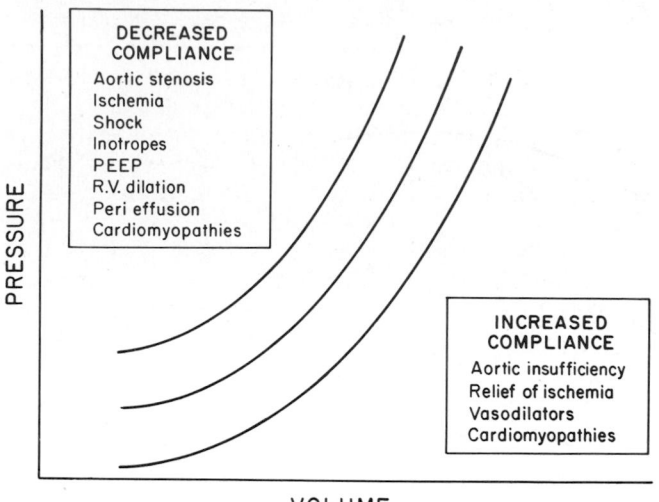

Fig. 16-9. The left ventricular compliance is the relationship between the LVEDP and the LVEDV. An increased compliance shifts the curve down and to the right, while a decreased compliance shifts it up and to the left. Examples of increased and decreased compliance are shown in the boxes.

pressure. Curves moving down and to the right show decreased work at higher filling pressures.

Afterload

While there is broad agreement on the definition of preload, afterload is considerably more difficult to de-

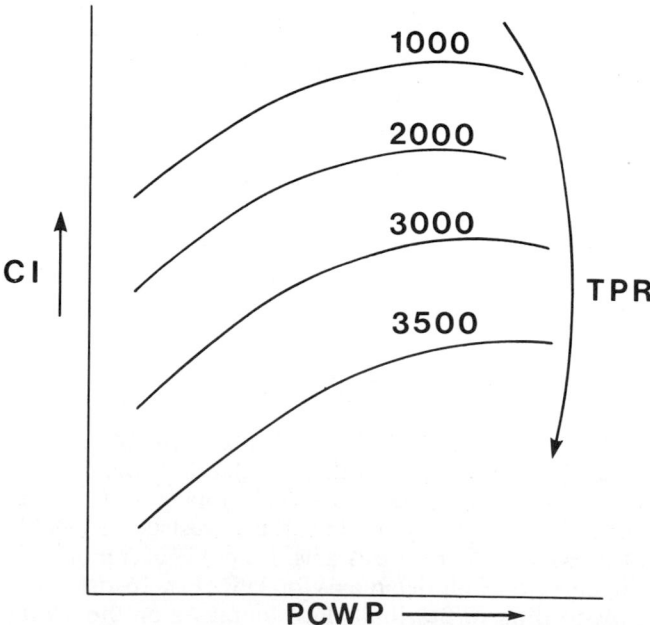

Fig. 16-10. The family of Frank-Starling curves is demonstrated with the cardiac index (CI) on the vertical axis and the pulmonary capillary wedge pressure (PCWP) on the horizontal axis. As total peripheral resistance (TPR) is increased from 1,000 toward 3,500 dynes·s·cm^{-5}, the curves are shifted down and to the right.

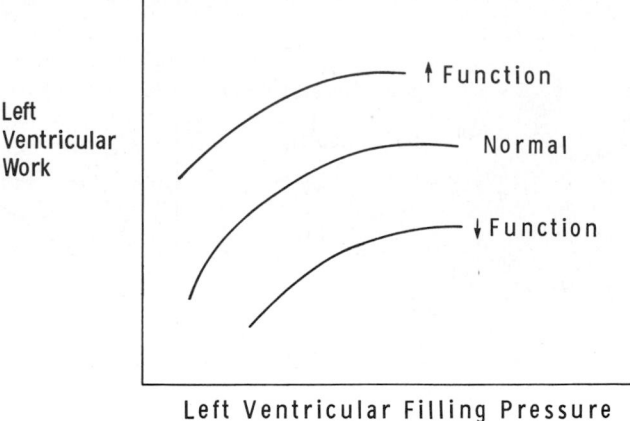

Fig. 16-11. The Frank-Starling family of curves is demonstrated, with increasing left ventricular function moving the curve up and to the left and decreasing left ventricular function moving the curve down and to the right.

fine, and various schools of thought provide different interpretations for its meaning. In the isolated muscle, afterload is defined by the force, beyond the preload, that the muscle needs to develop before it is allowed to shorten (Fig. 16-4). The muscle's total load is equal to the sum of preload and afterload.

For the intact ejecting ventricle, some have proposed definitions of afterload that are analogous to the one developed for isolated muscle. They incorporate ventricular pressure, volume, and wall stress. To some extent they are inadequate, however, because the developed force, and thus the afterload, changes continuously throughout ejection.[32] In addition, these variables are difficult to measure, and wall stress, in particular, is unevenly distributed across the ventricular cavity. In a simplified approach, wall stress measured at end-systole has also been proposed as a measure of afterload.[33] It represents the force that limits additional muscle shortening and is inversely related to the overall extent and mean velocity of fiber shortening.[34]

An alternative approach to the determination of afterload has been proposed by Milnor[35] and others. It involves the measurement of arterial input impedance as an expression of the arterial system's response to the pulsatile flow injected into the aorta. It requires the instantaneous derivation of pressure and flow at the root of the aorta and a complex frequency analysis of these two signals.

The systemic vascular resistance is a highly simplified version of arterial impedance. It ignores the pulsatile component of the ventricular ejection and is proportional to the ratio of mean pressure over mean flow.

Finally, investigators who have been intensely involved with the study of cardiac performance within the pressure–volume framework have proposed yet another definition of afterload.[36] It is based on the observation that for any bolus of blood (stroke volume) ejected into the arterial system, a pressure will be generated. If the stroke volume is larger, the pressure will be higher. When various values of stroke volume versus end-systolic pressure (P_{es}) are plotted, a linear relation is obtained. This relation is called *effective arterial elastance* (Ea) and is for any given contraction approximately equal to the end-systolic pressure (P_{es}) over stroke volume (Fig. 16-12).

Afterload Measurement

The measurement of end-systolic wall stress (σ_{es}), as an index of afterload, requires the determination of end-systolic ventricular pressure (P_{es}), dimension (D_{es}), and wall thickness (h_{es}). Ventricular pressure is preferably measured by intraventricular micromanometry, although a peripheral dicrotic notch pressure could be utilized. Ventricular dimensions and wall thickness can be obtained by either ventriculography or echocardiography. Wall stress is calculated by a modification of the standard Laplace equation:

$$\sigma_{es} \approx \frac{(P_{es} \cdot D_{es})}{h_{es}}$$

For the measurement of arterial impedance, instantaneous flow and pressure must be accurately measured in the ascending aorta. In humans, the instantaneous measurement of flow presents a considerable challenge and is usually performed with electromagnetic or Doppler flow tip catheters.[37] The frequency components of both the flow and the pressure signal are then analyzed by Fourier transform. In this process, both the pressure wave and flow wave are decomposed into a series of sine waves with a variety of frequencies and phases. At each frequency, the amplitude ratio of the pressure wave to the corresponding frequency component of the flow wave must be calculated. These

amplitude ratios are called the impedance moduli ($dynes \cdot s \cdot cm^{-5}$) and are plotted as a function of the frequency (Fig. 16-13). The phase shift between the pressure wave and the flow wave is also calculated and plotted at each frequency. The impedance modulus at zero frequency is equivalent to the systemic vascular resistance. It ignores the pulsatile component of flow and pressure.

The systemic vascular resistance (SVR) is more commonly measured by the determination of central venous pressure (CVP), mean arterial pressure (MAP) and cardiac output (CO). Its value is calculated by the formula

$$SVR = 80 \times \frac{(MAP - CVP)}{CO}$$

and is expressed in units of $dynes \cdot s \cdot cm^{-5}$. Mean arterial pressure, by itself, is not a good indicator of afterload.

Afterload reduction has become a mainstay of the modern therapy of left or right ventricular failure.[38] The failing left or right ventricle cannot pump against increased peripheral or pulmonary resistance, respectively, and therefore modern therapeutic interventions using vasodilators to reduce arterial afterload have become extremely useful. Figure 16-14 demonstrates how a normal left ventricle maintains normal function or even increases stroke volume with increased TPR (Anrep effect); however, a failing ventricle is severely compromised by increased resistance.

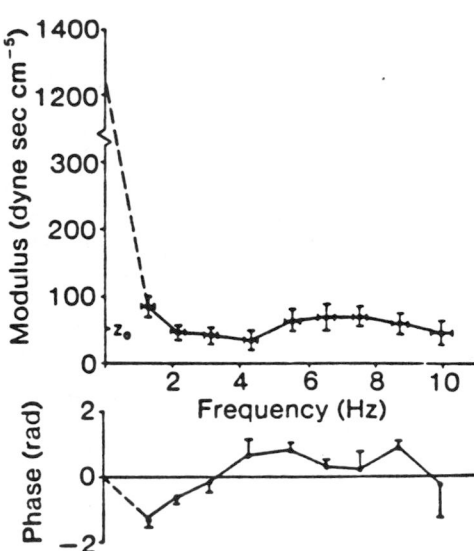

Fig. 16-13. Aortic input impedance determined by Fourier analysis in humans. Data represent mean plus or minus standard errors averaged from five normal subjects. Z_O denotes the estimated level of characteristic impedance, which is about 4 percent of total arterial resistance. (From Nichols et al.,[37] with permission.)

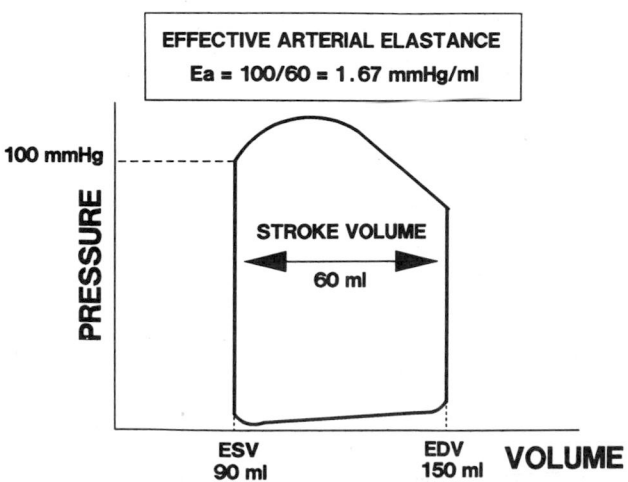

Fig. 16-12. Example of how effective arterial elastance is calculated from end-systolic pressure over stroke volume.

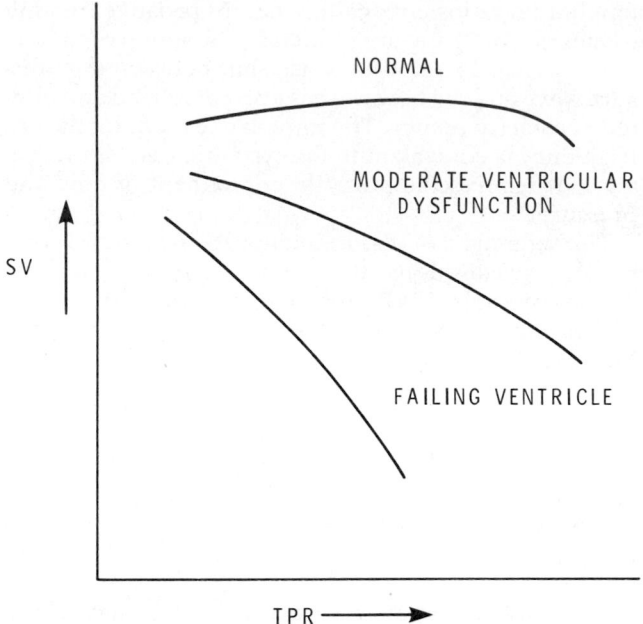

Fig. 16-14. The relationship of stroke volume (SV) to total peripheral resistance (TPR) is demonstrated in normal and failing ventricles. (Modified from Cohn and Franciosa,[129] with permission.)

Contractility

The third determinant of stroke volume is contractility. Contractility is an intrinsic property of the cardiac cell. It defines the amount of work that the heart can perform at a given load. Contractility is primarily deter-

mined by the availability of intracellular Ca^{++}. With depolarization of the cardiac cell a small amount of Ca^{++} enters the cell and triggers the release of additional Ca^{++} from intracellular storage sites (sarcoplasmic reticulum). The Ca^{++} binds to troponin, tropomyosin is displaced from the active binding site on actin, and actin-myosin cross-bridges are formed (Fig. 16-15). If the intracellular Ca^{++} concentration is higher, a larger number of actin-myosin cross-bridges are formed. All agents with positive inotropic properties, such as the catecholamines, have in common that they increase intracellular Ca^{++}, while negative inotropes have the opposite effect (Table 16-3).

Contractility Measurement

Over the years, a large number of methods have been suggested to measure contractility. This wide variety of techniques suggests that contractility is difficult to measure. One approach to the classification of indices of contractility is to divide them according to the phase of the cardiac cycle during which the measurement is obtained.

Isovolumic Contraction Phase Indices. As indicated by their name, isovolumic phase indices are obtained during the isovolumic phase of the contraction, before the aortic valve opens. The prototype for these indices is dP/dt. It is obtained by placing a catheter with a micromanometer at its tip in the left ventricle. The left ventricular pressure is continuously sampled while an electronic differentiator calculates the first derivative of pressure or dP/dt (mmHg/s). The highest value of dP/dt, or peak dP/dt, is considered proportional to con-

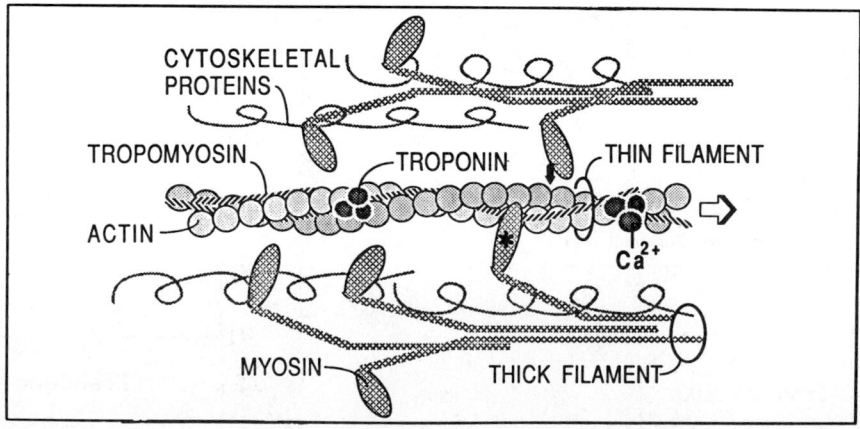

Fig. 16-15. Components of a unit of contractile behavior of the heart. Regulatory proteins overlay the actin monomers on the thin filaments. Sites for force generation are made available as calcium binding results in displacement of tropomyosin on actin, which could be enhanced (small arrow) by pre-existing cross-bridges (asterisk). Filamentous cytoskeletal proteins, which extend from the Z band to the M zone or the backbone of the thick filament, constitute compliant elements that position the thick filament and resist sarcomere lengthening. Their imposition between the thick and thin filaments suggests that steric interaction between contractile and parallel elements occurs, which might affect activation. The broad arrow points to the center of the A band. (From Krueger,[130] with permission.)

TABLE 16-3. Factors Affecting Contractility

Factors increasing contractility

Sympathetic stimulation—direct increases of force of contraction, as well as indirect increases owing to increased heart rate (rate treppe effect, or Bowditch phenomenon)

Parasympathetic inhibition producing increased heart rate

Administration of positive inotropic drugs such as digitalis

Factors decreasing contractility

Parasympathetic stimulation—decreased rate effect

Sympathetic inhibition—via withdrawal of catecholamines or blockade of adrenergic receptors

Administration of β-adrenergic blocking drugs, slow calcium channel blockers, or other myocardial depressants

Myocardial ischemia and infarction

Intrinsic myocardial diseases such as cardiomyopathies

Hypoxia or acidosis

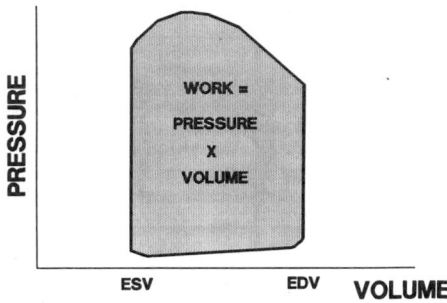

Fig. 16-16. Mechanical work is equal to the product of pressure and volume.

tractility. It should be obvious from our earlier description of this phase of the contraction that the developed pressure and dP/dt will be very much determined by the initial length of the cardiac muscle. In other words, peak dP/dt is preload dependent. If the end-diastolic volume can be measured, for instance with echocardiography, a preload correction can be applied

$$\frac{(peak\ dP/dt)}{LVEDV}$$

Ejection Phase Indices. With the increasing availability of noninvasive cardiac imaging techniques (echocardiography and radionuclides), ejection phase indices are widely utilized in clinical practice. The standard ejection phase index is the ejection fraction (EF)

$$EF = \frac{SV}{EDV}$$

Its derivation requires the measurement of end-systolic and end-diastolic volumes. Stroke volume is calculated as the difference between EDV and ESV. Because ventricular emptying is, in part, determined by the properties of the vascular system, EF is afterload dependent. Within the framework of the pressure–volume diagram, the effects of afterload or ejection fraction can easily be recognized. As stated earlier, contractility is defined as the heart's ability to perform work. In the pressure–volume diagram, mechanical work is equal to the area (work = pressure × volume) within the pressure–volume loop of a cardiac cycle (Fig. 16-16). At equal preloads (EDV) but different afterloads (effective arterial elastance = P_{es}/SV), two ventricles can have identical ejection fractions while performing widely different amounts of work (Fig. 16-17).

Load-Independent Indices. Because traditional indices of contractility are so load dependent, different approaches to the quantitation of the contractile proper-

ties of the heart have been explored. In one such approach, Suga, Sagawa, and colleagues[39,40] have studied instantaneous pressure and volume in isolated canine hearts. The ratio of ventricular pressure over volume is the ventricular elastance, which varies throughout the cardiac cycle *(time-varying elastance)*. For each cardiac cycle, Suga et al.[39] defined the maximal value of this ratio as the end-systolic elastance (E_{es}) and the point at which it was reached as the end-systolic point. They further noted that with rapid decreases in preload, all consecutive end-systolic points were positioned on single straight line, known as the end-systolic pressure–volume relation (ESPVR) (Fig. 16-18). The slope of this line (E_{es}) is proportional to contractility: it is steeper at higher contractility and flatter at lower contractility (Fig. 16-19). A change in preload is part of the measure-

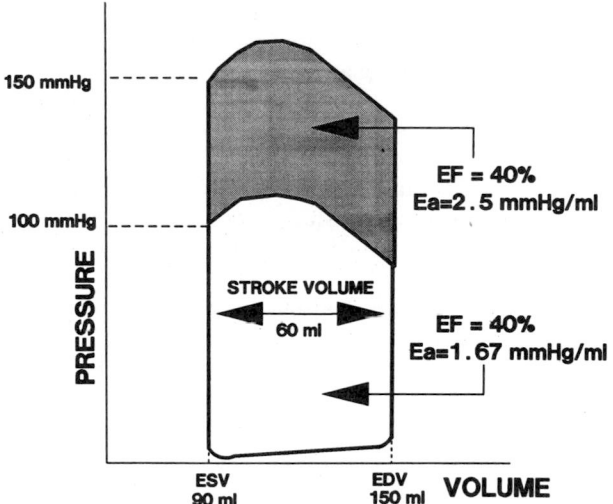

Fig. 16-17. Two pressure–volume loops representing contractions with identical ejection fractions (40 percent) and stroke volumes (60 ml) but markedly different mechanical work. Since more mechanical work was performed during the contraction with the higher afterload (Ea), the contractility of the ventricle that generated this pressure–volume loop was greater than the contractility of the other ventricle, despite the identical ejection fractions.

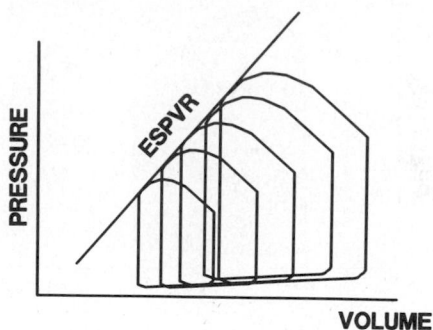

Fig. 16-18. The ESPVR is obtained by connecting all the end-systolic points measured during a rapid decrease in preload.

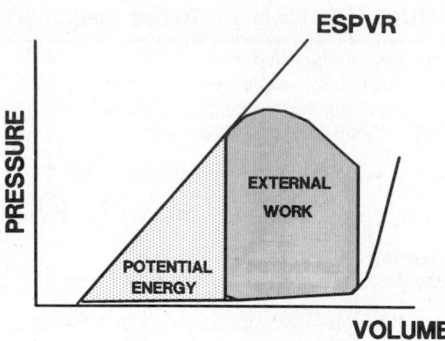

Fig. 16-20. The total oxygen consumption of the heart is equal to the sum of the oxygen required for mechanical work and the end-systolic elastic potential energy.

ment, while afterload has little effect on the ESPVR slope.

Although the clinical application of the ESPVR concept has been hampered by the difficulty of measuring instantaneous ventricular volumes, it provides such a useful framework for analysis of ventricular function that it warrants extensive discussion.[41] In addition, with the introduction of new technology, such as echocardiography and conductance catheters, the ability to measure ventricular volumes continuously is rapidly becoming a reality.[42,43]

In addition to the measurement of contractility, the ESPVR allows the study of myocardial energetics and of the interaction between the ventricle and the vascular system. Myocardial oxygen consumption can be divided into two components: oxygen is required (1) for the heart's mechanical work, and (2) for its basal metabolism and activation (excitation-contraction coupling). Using the ESPVR concept, Suga et al.[44] were able to demonstrate that the amount of oxygen consumed by the heart for mechanical work is proportional to the area within the pressure–volume loop (remember that work = pressure × volume) (Fig. 16-20). They further showed that the triangular area enclosed by the ESPVR, the diastolic pressure–volume relation, and the relax-

ation limb of the pressure–volume loop is proportional to the oxygen consumed for the maintenance of basal metabolism and activation. With this approach to myocardial energetics, it is easy to understand why the administration of positive inotropes results in increased oxygen consumption beyond the increase due to greater mechanical work[45] (Fig. 16-21).

Another useful aspect of the ESPVR concept is that it allows the simultaneous study of ventricular function and the coupling of the ventricle to the vascular system. While ventricular contractility is defined by the slope of the ESPVR (E_{es} or end-systolic ventricular elastance), the vascular response to ventricular emptying is defined by the effective arterial elastance (see above). Both are expressed as a ratio of pressure over volume and can be plotted in a pressure–volume diagram (Fig. 16-22). If the arterial elastance slope is rearranged so that it intersects the volume axis at the end-diastolic volume, it will cross the ESPVR at the end-systolic point. Thus, if end-diastolic volume (preload), Ea (afterload), and E_{es} (contractility) are known, stroke volume can be predicted. This was confirmed experimentally by Sunagawa et al.[46] (Fig. 16-23).

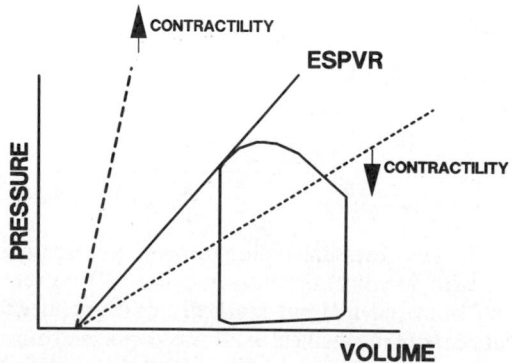

Fig. 16-19. The slope of the ESPVR is proportional to contractility—it is steeper at higher contractility and flatter at lower contractility.

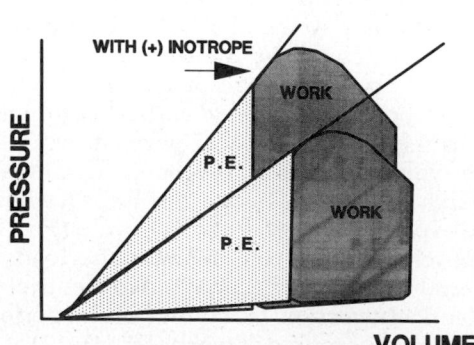

Fig. 16-21. The administration of a positive inotrope results not only in increased mechanical work, but also in increased potential energy (P.E.)

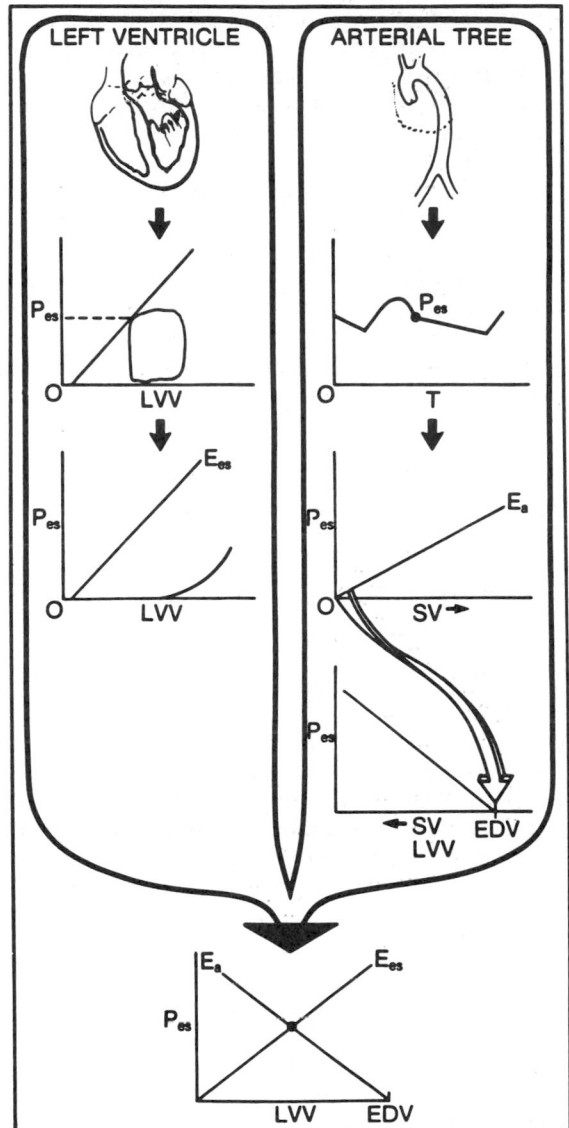

Fig. 16-22. Illustration of the cardiovascular coupling concept proposed by Sunagawa et al.[46] The left ventricular system is on the left, while the arterial system is on the right. By rearranging the effective arterial elastance (Ea) slope, so that its origin lies at end-diastolic volume (EDV), the Ea slope and the ESPVR slope intersect. Stroke volume (SV) is equal to the horizontal distance between EDV and the intersection of the two slopes. LVV, left ventricular volume; P_{es}, end-systolic pressure; E_{es}, end-systolic elastance; T, time. (From Sunagawa et al.,[46] with permission.)

CARDIAC OUTPUT

Definition

The cardiac output is the amount of blood pumped to the peripheral circulation per minute. It is a measurement reflecting the status of the entire circulatory sys-

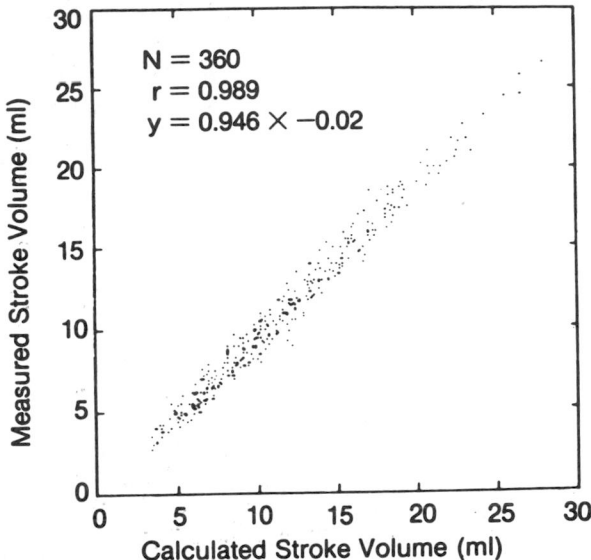

Fig. 16-23. Comparison in the isolated dog heart of the relation between directly measured stroke volume and the stroke volume predicted on the basis of the coupling of Ea and ESPVR. (From Maughan,[131] with permission.)

tem, not only that of the heart, and is governed by autoregulation in the tissues.[47] Although affected by a number of peripheral factors, cardiac output may not be able to change much in the presence of severe cardiac dysfunction. The cardiac output (CO) equals the stroke volume (SV) per beat times the heart rate (HR) per minute

$$CO = SV \times HR$$

Normal average values are a cardiac output of 5 to 6 L/min in a 70-kg man, with a stroke volume of 60 to 90 ml/beat and a heart rate of 80 beats/min. To compare patients with different body sizes, cardiac output may be corrected in relation to body surface area and is then called the cardiac index (CI), which equals the cardiac output divided by the body surface area (BSA)

$$CI = CO/BSA$$

The normal value for a 70-kg man is 2.5 to 3.5 L/min/m². A normal person has a tremendous reserve capacity to increase cardiac output to as much as 25 to 30 L/min. Factors controlling the cardiac output include venous return to the heart, peripheral vascular resistance, peripheral tissue oxygen needs, blood volume, body position, pattern and type of respiration, heart rate, and myocardial contractility.

The two main determinants of cardiac output are heart rate and stroke volume. Heart rate depends on the intrinsic rhythmicity of the sinoatrial node and is further affected by extrinsic neural or humoral factors. The neural input to the cardiac conduction system is via both the sympathetic and parasympathetic nervous systems. These changes can lead to increases or decreases in the heart rate and therefore the cardiac output. The cardiac output can also be affected by changes in stroke volume caused by alterations in myocardial fiber shortening. The four factors affecting the stroke volume through this mechanism are preload, afterload, contractility, and wall motion abnormalities. The resultant cardiac output is then distributed throughout the various vascular beds of the body, including the central nervous system, myocardium, renal and splanchnic beds, skeletal muscle, and skin. The peripheral vasculature is affected by a number of intrinsic factors, such as metabolic demand, and extrinsic factors, such as neural and humoral stimuli, all of which produce the appropriate distribution of the cardiac output.[48]

The cardiac output may be increased by increases in heart rate, increases in left ventricular volume (preload) produced by an increased venous return, decreases in afterload such as that which occurs with peripheral vasodilatation or in the presence of an arteriovenous fistula, or increases in myocardial function such as occurs with increased endogenous or exogenous catecholamine stimulation.

Decreases in cardiac output can be produced by parasympathetic stimulation, producing a decrease in heart rate; a decrease in preload; an increase in afterload; or intrinsic myocardial disease or drugs limiting myocardial contractility.

An example of the tremendous increase possible in cardiac output is seen in young patients (<40 years) during extreme exercise (Table 16-4).

Control of Heart Rate

At constant stroke volume, cardiac output is a linear function of heart rate. The heart rate is primarily determined by the rhythmicity of the sinoatrial node resulting from the spontaneous phase IV depolarization of its pacemaker cells. The sinoatrial node's intrinsic control of heart rate is affected by extrinsic neural and humoral factors. The neural factors stimulating the heart via the autonomic nervous system are of great importance in altering the heart rate. Humoral factors such as circulating catecholamines are of less importance in most situations. Sympathetic stimulation of the heart increases heart rate by increasing the slope of phase IV depolarization, whereas parasympathetic stimulation decreases phase IV depolarization and results in a slowing of the heart rate. Sympathetic neural influences on the heart travel through the cervical (superior, middle, and inferior) ganglia and the thoracic cardiac accelerator nerves (T1 to T4) and affect the sinoatrial node, the

atrioventricular node, and the ventricular muscle and conduction system. Parasympathetic neural influences on the heart travel via the vagus nerves to the sinoatrial and atrioventricular nodes with minimal influence on the ventricular conduction system. Vagal influences produce a decreased heart rate, decreased atrial force of contraction, and delayed atrioventricular conduction. Studies by Higgins et al.[49] have shown the relative dominance of the parasympathetic nervous system in the control of normal heart rate. They found that the normal baroreceptor-induced slowing of heart rate is mediated largely by the parasympathetic system. In patients with heart disease, both a depletion of cardiac catecholamine stores and a markedly abnormal baroreceptor reflex mechanism produce gross alterations in autonomic control of cardiac rate.[49]

Measurement of Cardiac Output and Stroke Volume

Cardiac output is increasingly being monitored during and after surgery (also see Ch. 31). Serial measurements can be used to assess the general status of the circulation and to determine the appropriate hemodynamic therapy and estimate its efficacy. However, equally useful are the variables that may be determined once the cardiac output is known.[50] These variables include the peripheral and pulmonary vascular resistances, stroke volumes, and stroke work. Formulas for these parameters are shown in Table 16-5.

Cardiac output can be measured by several techniques. The thermodilution method utilizing the Swan-Ganz catheter is the clinical method of choice. With this technique, multiple outputs can be obtained at frequent intervals, along with measures of both right and left ventricular filling pressure. In 1970, Swan and co-workers[24] introduced this catheter for thermodilution cardiac output measurements and found that thermodilution-measured flow was accurate to within 2 percent of the known pump flow in vitro. In 20 patients, they showed that the standard deviation of triplicate measurements was 4.6 percent in the range of 2 to 8 L/min of cardiac output.[51] Other investigators have shown excellent correlation between dye and thermodilution cardiac outputs in patients after cardiac surgery.[52] The thermodilution method may be even more accurate than the dye dilution method at low cardiac outputs, since there is no recirculation of the indicator in the thermodilution technique.

To provide a high rate of reproducibility, the technique of thermodilution cardiac output measurements should be standardized. The injectate temperature and

TABLE 16-4. Cardiac Output Values

	Heart Rate (beats/min)	×	Stroke Volume (ml/beat)	=	Cardiac Output (ml/min)
At rest	70		80		5,600
Moderate exercise	130		130		16,900
Extreme exercise	200		150		30,000

TABLE 16-5. Formulas for Variables That Can Be Determined from the Cardiac Output[a]

Formula	Range of Values
$SV = \dfrac{CO}{HR} \times 100$	60–90 ml
$SI = \dfrac{SV}{BSA}$	40–60 ml/m^2
$LVSWI = 1.36 \times \dfrac{(MAP - PCWP) \times SI}{100}$	45–60 g-m/m^2
$RVSWI = 1.36 \times \dfrac{(PAP - CVP) \times SI}{100}$	5–10 g-m/m^2
$SVR = \dfrac{(MAP - CVP) \times 80}{CO}$	900–1,500 dynes·s·cm^{-5}
$PVR = \dfrac{(PAP - PCWP) \times 80}{CO}$	50–150 dynes·s·cm^{-5}

[a] All these parameters are rapidly derived in both the operating room and intensive care unit by using programmable portable calculators now available.
Abbreviations: SV, stroke volume; CO, cardiac output; HR, heart rate; BSA, body surface area; LVSWI, left ventricular stroke work index; MAP, mean arterial pressure; PCWP, mean pulmonary capillary wedge pressure; RVSWI, right ventricular stroke work index; PAP, mean pulmonary artery pressure; CVP, mean central venous pressure; SVR, systemic vascular resistance; SI, stroke index.

volume, as well as the speed of injection, should be carefully controlled and duplicated. Reproducibile results have been obtained by using injections of 10 ml of either cold (1 to 2°C) or room temperature 5 percent dextrose in water. All measurements should be made in duplicate or triplicate. Some investigators believe that all measurements should be made in expiration, while others think that they should be made throughout the respiratory cycle and averaged. Necessary equipment includes a sterile system for maintaining the injectate, a cardiac output computer, and instruments to obtain precise temperature measurements of the injectate and of the patient. Additional equipment that may be used are a mechanical injector for greater injection speed and reproducibility and a recorder for observation and hand calculation of the curves.

The usual pulmonary arterial thermodilution cardiac output catheter contains two fine wires that extend the length of the catheter and terminate in a thermistor embedded in the catheter wall just proximal to the balloon. The principle of measurement is similar to the dye dilution method of cardiac outputs, except that a cold solution acts as the indicator.[53] A known change in the temperature is induced at one point in the circulation, and the resulting change in temperature is detected at a point downstream. The baseline pulmonary artery body temperature is recorded in the computer, the cold solution is then injected via the proximal port into the right atrium, and the resulting temperature change is detected by the thermistor in the pulmonary artery. The newest thermodilution catheters automatically measure the body temperature and the injectate temperature. The thermistor acts as a variable resistor in a Wheatstone bridge, with a linear relationship between temperature and electrical resistance. The change in temperature alters the resistance and thus the output from the bridge, which is amplified and recorded, and the cardiac output is calculated by the computer.

The thermal dilution technique measures right-sided cardiac outputs. This is very important because the technique cannot be used for patients with intracardiac shunts—totally erroneous data will be obtained.[54] For example, a patient with a ventricular septal defect and a left-to-right shunt will have a falsely elevated cardiac output measured by this technique. The technique appears so simple that errors are frequently introduced in clinical practice. Erroneous cardiac outputs can be obtained by injecting the wrong volume of solution, injecting too slowly or irregularly, or injecting while large volumes of fluid are being administered to the right heart (e.g., from the cardiopulmonary bypass pump or rapidly through a large-bore intravenous catheter).

Early in the development of the thermodilution method, attempts were made to provide a continuous thermal signal and therefore a continuous cardiac output determination. The initial experiments focused on the use of intravascular heating devices.[55,56] However, because heating blood is more dangerous than cooling it, the use of heating devices was inherently more risky. As a result, very low amplitude heat signals needed to be used and separation of the introduced heat signal from background thermal variations became a major problem. More recently, Philip et al.[57] have again explored the possibility of a continuous thermal signal. However, they used a very low power (5 W) sinusoidal thermal signal. With this system, the average increase in blood temperature was only of the order of 0.02°C at typical flows. They tested the system both in vitro and in vivo and obtained satisfactory correlations with conventional thermodilution over a wide range of cardiac outputs.

Other methods to measure cardiac output include the standard Fick and dye dilution techniques, as well as direct flowmeter techniques, including Doppler and aortic pulse contour measurements.[58] The Fick technique is the standard for steady-state measurements of cardiac output and is said to be accurate within ±10 percent. The technique is complex and cumbersome, however, involving both the collection of expired gases and right heart catheterization to obtain mixed venous blood. Davis et al.[59] have shown that cardiac output measurements by the Fick technique can also be employed by using carbon dioxide in a rebreathing system instead of the standard oxygen Fick method.

A continuous monitor of mixed venous oxygen saturation ($S\bar{v}O_2$) has recently been introduced as an index of cardiac output and overall tissue perfusion. The catheter oximeter system consists of a special pulmonary arterial catheter containing two fiberoptic filaments that permit continuous monitoring of $S\bar{v}O_2$ by a companion oximeter. A drop in $S\bar{v}O_2$ can be due to reduced cardiac output, increased oxygen demand, or decreased oxygen supply, and it is a useful monitor of the development of inadequate tissue perfusions.[60] The physiologic principle of this technique is based on a decrease in cardiac output in the face of a constant oxygen consumption, leading to an increase in oxygen extraction from the blood and therefore a reduction in $S\bar{v}O_2$. However, arterial oxygenation and oxygen consumption must not change for $S\bar{v}O_2$ to be correlated with cardiac output. During surgery and anesthesia, when oxygenation and oxygen consumption are fairly constant, changes in $S\bar{v}O_2$ equal to or greater than 5 percent are correlated with changes in cardiac index. There is an 80 percent probability that an $S\bar{v}O_2$ decrease equal to or greater than 5 percent reflects a significant decrease in cardiac index in this setting.[61] However, in the presence of pronounced changes in PaO_2 such as those seen during thoracic anesthesia, the $S\bar{v}O_2$ reflects PaO_2 rather than cardiac index.[62] In the postoperative period, when shivering is common, a decrease in $S\bar{v}O_2$ is frequently due to an increase in oxygen consumption rather than a decrease in cardiac output. This relationship can best be understood by looking at the Fick equation in its standard form

$$CO = \frac{\dot{V}O_2}{CaO_2 - C\bar{v}O_2}$$

CaO_2 = arterial O_2 content
$C\bar{v}O_2$ = mixed venous O_2 content
$\dot{V}O_2$ = oxygen consumption

or, when arranged in terms of saturation,

$$S\bar{v}O_2 = SaO_2 - \frac{\dot{V}O_2}{CO \times Hb \times 1.34}$$

Hb = hemoglobin

With the widespread availability of mass spectrometry, interest in the intraoperative application of the direct Fick principle has again risen. Heneghan et al.[63] have designed a system to measure metabolic gas exchange during general anesthesia. It uses a mass spectrometer, a mixing box, and two inert gases. They obtained measurements in patients undergoing cardiac surgery and demonstrated that the variations in inspired and expired minute volumes were within 2 percent, while they were within 10 percent for oxygen consumption, carbon dioxide output, and respiratory quotient.[63] These investigators also utilized this gas-measuring system to determine cardiac output during anesthesia and observed that the cardiac output values obtained with the two inert gases were reproducible but lower than those obtained with the direct Fick principle.[64]

Recently, Davies et al.[65] have also attempted to measure cardiac output continuously by means of the Fick principle. To measure oxygen consumption and carbon dioxide production, they used a self-contained instrument (MGM II, Utah Medical Products, Midvale, UT) that collects expired gas in a mixing chamber and measures expired ventilation with an ultrasonic flow transducer. Inspired and expired gas samples were alternatively conducted to an infrared CO_2 analyzer and a zirconium oxide CO_2 analyzer. In pigs, continuous SaO_2 values were obtained with a fiberoptic catheter placed in the carotid artery, while continuous SvO_2 values were measured with a second flow-directed pulmonary artery fiberoptic catheter. They compared the continuous Fick principle cardiac outputs with simultaneous thermodilution cardiac outputs, as well as with continuous pulmonary artery electromagnetic flow measurements. Good correlations were obtained between the continuous Fick principle and the two other methods. In humans, SaO_2 values were measured by pulse oximetry.[66] The investigators obtained a total of 237 simultaneous Fick and thermodilution cardiac output measurements in 21 ventilated, postcardiac surgery patients. Although the correlation between the two techniques was good (r = 0.86), they noted that the Fick results were consistently lower than the thermodilution measurements. Cardiac output has recently also been measured, in humans, by a Fick method that utilizes a computerized system for measuring oxygen consumption and carbon dioxide production.[67] Cardiac output values determined with this system were compared with thermodilution measurements in intubated patients. A good correlation (r = 0.92) was observed between the two systems, indicating that the accuracy of the Fick technique was high. More noteworthy was that the Fick measurements were more reproducible than the thermodilution measurements (the average standard deviation was 195 ml/min for Fick, versus 1,020 ml/min for thermodilution).

The indicator dye dilution method with indocyanine green dye had been the most popular technique of cardiac output measurements prior to the thermodilution method. This technique consists of a rapid injection of a precise amount of dye into the venous circulation, where the indicator mixes with blood, passes rapidly through the heart and lungs into the arterial circulation, and is detected by sampling arterial blood and passing it through a densitometer. Complex mathematical formulas are necessary to calculate the cardiac output by this method, since there is a significant amount of recirculation. This technique is still useful when intracardiac shunts are present and, in fact, may be used to confirm their presence.

In recent years, an earpiece densitometer has been developed for the measurement of cardiac output by dye dilution.[68] The earpiece alleviates the need for arterial blood sampling and therefore greatly simplifies the measurement technique. The earpiece contains a light source, an inflatable rubber diaphragm, and two phototransistors (805 and 900 nm). The dye concentration in the blood is computed from the change in light absorption, measured with the phototransistors. The results obtained with this technique have been compared with conventional dye dilution and thermodilution results.[69-71] Some investigators have found excellent correlation, while others were not as successful. The reproducibility of the earpiece method has been found comparable to that of thermodilution. The quality of the results appears to be determined by patient selection, the judicious rejection of unsuitable curves, and the site of indicator injection. Another recent design consists of a fiberoptic catheter for the determination of oxygen saturation, as well as dye concentration. The catheter appears most useful in children who have undergone surgical correction of congenital heart disease. It is placed in the pulmonary artery at the time of surgery and allows continuous monitoring of mixed venous saturation, with intermittent measurements of dye cardiac outputs, without arterial blood sampling.

Another method of cardiac output measurement utilizing computers is the Warner aortic pulse contour analysis technique. This allows on-line measurement of stroke volume after insertion of a central aortic catheter. However, this technique makes assumptions concerning a constant compliance of the systemic vascular bed that are not valid with certain therapeutic interventions or anesthetic techniques. Therefore, this technique has been questioned by some and has not gained great popularity. Recently, English and colleagues[72] compared pulse contour and thermodilution cardiac output measurements. The pulse contour method was found to be inaccurate in any situation in which systemic vascular resistance changed by 30 percent or more. Patients with frequent marked changes in cardiovascular dynamics, as occur in the operating room and intensive care unit, should not have their cardiac outputs measured by this technique. Pharmacologic studies in which peripheral resistance may change (e.g., studies of anesthetic induction with narcotics or neuroleptanesthetic drugs) should also be performed with a more reliable technique of cardiac output measurement.

Doppler

Cardiac output can also be determined by imaging (M-mode, two-dimensional [2-D]) and Doppler echocardiography. For M-mode and 2-D echocardiographic determinations, linear or area measurements are converted to volumes and cardiac output is computed as the product of heart rate and stroke volume (end-diastolic volume — end-systolic volume). When M-mode transesophageal echocardiography was used to measure the left ventricular systolic and diastolic volumes, correlations between cardiac output measured by dye or thermodilution and by echocardiography varied markedly ($r = 0.72$ to $r = 0.97$).[73-75] A good correlation between thermodilution and echo-derived cardiac output was observed when 2-D echocardiography was used to determine left ventricular size ($r = 0.8$).[20]

The determination of stroke volume by Doppler echocardiography is based on the measurement of blood flow velocities across cardiac valves or in the aorta.[76] To calculate stroke volume, the duration of flow, the flow velocity integral, and the cross-sectional area of the conduit through which flow occurs must be known. The ascending aorta is frequently selected for Doppler velocity measurements because parallel alignment of the ultrasound beam and the aortic flow can readily be obtained by placement of a transducer in the suprasternal notch. Although the best location for the measurement of aortic cross-sectional area is still being debated, it is commonly accepted that the aortic root is nearly circular and that its size changes minimally during ventricular ejection.

Numerous investigators found good correlation between the cardiac output measured by combined Doppler echocardiography and thermodilution or Fick cardiac output.[77-80] Recently, a dedicated continuous wave Doppler device has been introduced for the intraoperative measurement of cardiac output. The Doppler transducers are mounted on a 24-French esophageal stethoscope, which continuously measures blood flow velocities in the descending aorta. A single measurement of ascending aortic flow is obtained by suprasternal sampling, after the aortic diameter has been measured by echocardiography or calculated by an algorithm. The relationship between ascending and descending aortic flow is assumed constant. In two recent studies, a fairly good correlation was observed between esophageal Doppler and thermodilution cardiac output determinations.[81,82]

Although the shape of the mitral valve changes during diastolic flow, velocity measurements across the mitral valve have also been utilized for cardiac output determinations. Using a transesophageal pulsed Doppler probe, Roewer and co-workers[83] found that thermodilution and mitral valve cardiac output values correlated well ($r = 0.95$). They also observed good correlation between thermodilution cardiac output and pulmonary artery blood flow velocity.

The first attempts at measuring cardiac output by thoracic electrical impedance date to 1966, when Kubicek et al.[84] presented an empiric equation for the calculation of left ventricular stroke volume. Electrical impedance (Z) is the resistance to alternating or sinusoidal current flow. It is a complex, frequency dependent, parameter which is governed by Ohm's law:

$$Z = E/I$$

where Z = impedance in Øhms (Ω), E = voltage, and I = current in amperes.

To measure thoracic electrical impedance, an alternating current of low amplitude and high frequency is introduced and simultaneously sensed by two sets of electrodes placed around the neck and lower thorax. Changes in thoracic impedance are induced by ventilation and pulsatile blood flow. For the measurement of cardiac output, only the cardiac-induced pulsatile component is analyzed (δZ). Experimental work suggests that 70 to 80 percent of δZ originates from the thoracic aorta.

Donovan et al.[85] recently compared cardiac output measurements obtained by transthoracic impedance and by thermodilution in 27 critically ill patients, using the standard Kubicek equation. They did not find a satisfactory correlation between the two cardiac output methods. Bernstein[86,87] has recently modified the Kubicek equation and has compared 94 simultaneous thoracic electrical impedance and thermodilution cardiac outputs in critically ill patients. The overall correlation between the two techniques was good (r = 0.88), and 85 percent of the data points fell within the 20 percent confidence limits. The greatest disparity between the two techniques was observed at very low flows (<2 L/min).

Appel et al.[88] using a device that incorporates the Bernstein modifications, also compared cardiac output by thoracic electrical impedance and thermodilution in 16 critically ill patients. They compared 391 pairs of simultaneous cardiac outputs and found an r value of 0.83. The Bernstein modification thus appears to improve the accuracy of the bioimpedance method, but additional studies will be required to identify and quantitate the limitations of the technique.

VENTRICULAR FUNCTION AND CURVES

Systolic Function

Multiple measurements of cardiac output and its derivatives, along with ventricular filling pressure, allow the construction of Frank-Starling ventricular function curves.[89] The Frank-Starling mechanism of the heart relates the filling volume of the heart (preload) to the stroke volume of the corresponding ventricle. A Starling diagram showing both right and left ventricular function curves is shown in Figure 16-24. Measurements of left ventricular function should have the

PCWP or another measurement of left ventricular filling pressure on the horizontal axis, and the left ventricular stroke work index (LVSWI) on the vertical axis. To measure right ventricular function, these could be replaced by the CVP on the horizontal axis and the RVSWI on the vertical axis. It is not accurate, however, to mix one measurement from each side of the heart, for example, CVP and LVSWI. Interventions that increase contractility shift the curves up and to the left. Disease states or drugs that depress the heart shift the curves down and to the right. These ventricular function curves can be used for the following:

1. To assess the hemodynamic effects of anesthetic drugs
2. To guide cardiovascular therapy during anesthesia or in the postoperative period
3. To aid in the treatment of heart failure patients with inotrope or vasodilator therapy
4. To guide therapeutic decisions when terminating cardiopulmonary bypass
5. To guide therapy in patients requiring the intra-aortic balloon

A number of therapeutic interventions can be performed on the patient with a low output syndrome.[90] The proper choice depends on an understanding of the underlying cardiac physiology and the use of the Starling curve. The first step in the treatment of a patient who is hypotensive with a low filling pressure and low cardiac output is to increase the patient's filling volume or preload by the administration of a volume infusion. This is done in an effort to move the patient up on the Starling curve to a maximum point of function with a PCWP of about 10 to 15 mmHg. The infusion is usually given in increments of 100 ml while monitoring the filling pressure and the resultant change in blood pressure, stroke volume, or cardiac output. With hypovolemia alone, volume infusion should improve the hemodynamic variables and be the only therapy necessary. With heart failure or low output syndromes, further therapeutic interventions will be necessary, and these can be seen in Figure 16-25, where the patient starts with a high filling pressure and a low cardiac output at point 1. Further volume administration at this point would be fruitless and, in fact, possibly dangerous because it would take the patient over the hump of the Starling curve and overdistend the ventricle even further. A number of therapeutic interventions such as inotropes, vasodilators, diuretics, or the intra-aortic balloon could be used in this patient, and they would have different effects on the cardiovascular system. Most physicians would choose an inotropic drug such as dopamine in the patient with a low output syndrome and a low blood pressure. A dose of 5 μg/kg/min of dopamine might move the patient from point 1 on the curve to a higher Starling curve up and toward the left at point 2. Other inotropic drugs such as calcium chloride, digitalis, dobutamine, and epinephrine would have similar effects. A diuretic, such as furosemide, administered to

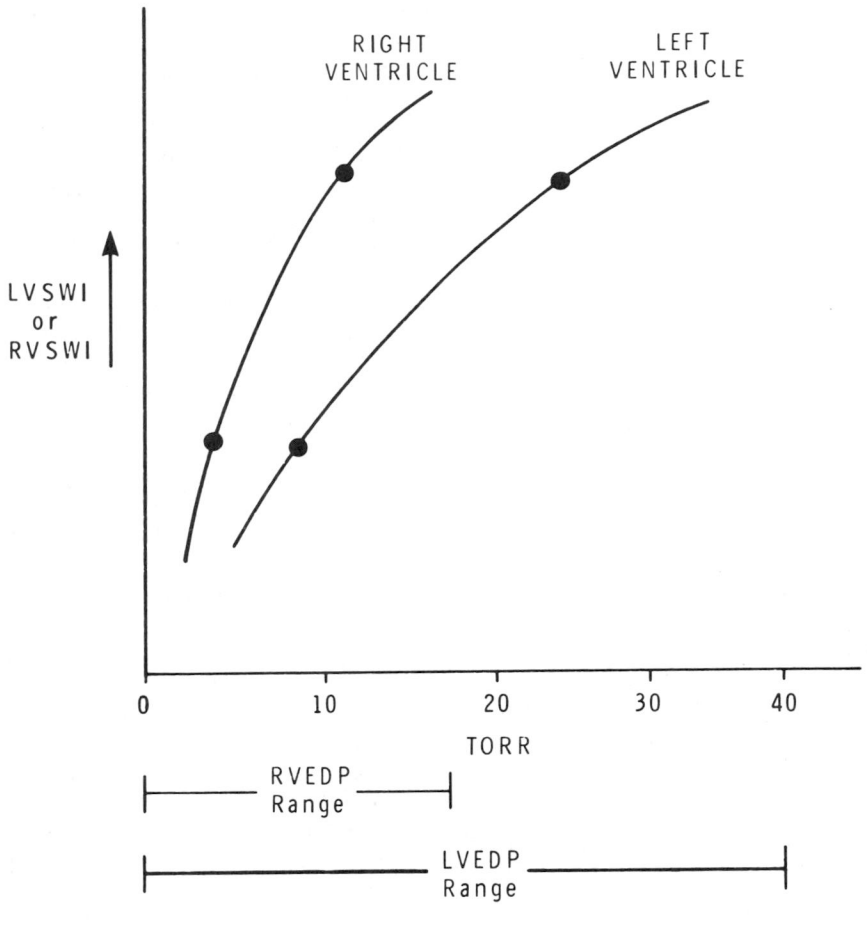

Fig. 16-24. The Frank-Starling diagram of both the right and left ventricles is demonstrated. Notice that the curves are not parallel and cover different ventricular filling pressure ranges.

the patient at point 1 may move the patient to point 6 by reducing left ventricular filling pressure and not augment stroke volume, cardiac output, or blood pressure. It would serve only to reduce signs of congestive heart failure such as pulmonary edema. This would also be true of other venodilators, such as morphine, given at this point.

The therapeutic intervention of impedance reduction or afterload reduction can be used to move the patient from point 1 up to point 3.[38] An arteriolar dilator such as phentolamine or a low dose of sodium nitroprusside would tend to reduce the impedance to ejection and allow the patient to move up and to the left on the Starling curve, similar to what occurs with positive inotropic drugs (Figs. 16-10 and 16-25). The advantage of using a vasodilator instead of a positive inotropic drug is that there is no increase in myocardial oxygen demand required by the vasodilator. However, administering a vasodilator to a patient with heart failure is a tricky therapeutic undertaking. Excessive administration of the vasodilator can move the patient from point

1 to point 4, where extra volume infusions may be necessary to maintain the preload. In fact, often an attempt to maximally reduce the afterload is made by administering a large dose of an arterial vasodilator and then augmenting the preload by additional volume infusion to bring the patient from point 1 to point 4 and then back to point 3. An approach of minimizing the afterload while maximizing the preload is a very good clinical tool.[91] Not all the vasodilators have similar hemodynamic effects. Figure 16-26 shows the difference between an arterial dilator such as phentolamine (A) and a venodilator such as nitroglycerin (V). An arterial dilator will reduce afterload and allow the patient to move up and to the left on the Starling curve from point 1 to point 3 in Figure 16-25. A venodilator such as a low dose of nitroglycerin will simply reduce preload, and not afterload, and move the patient from point 1 to point 6 to the Starling curve in Figure 16-25. A drug such as sodium nitroprusside (A + V), which has effects on both preload and afterload, is probably best in this situation, because it will reduce afterload, allow an in-

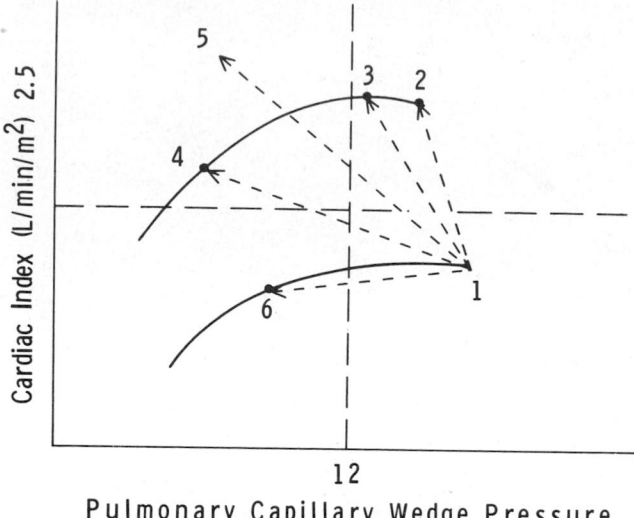

Pulmonary Capillary Wedge Pressure (torr)

Fig. 16-25. The figure demonstrates a patient at point 1 on a hypofunctioning Starling curve. Five therapeutic interventions are made, and the results are demonstrated on the Starling curve showing increased function. These therapeutic interventions are labeled 2 to 6. (See text for a full explanation.)

creased stroke volume and cardiac output, and, at the same time, reduce the symptoms of pulmonary congestion by its venodilating properties.[92] Combinations of inotropes, like dopamine, and mixed arterial, and venous vasodilators, like sodium nitroprusside, have become extremely popular and tend to give the largest

increase in cardiac index and largest decrease in filling pressure, as shown by point 5 in Figure 16-25. Mechanical interventions such as the intra-aortic balloon pump tend to reduce preload and afterload while augmenting coronary blood flow and increasing contractility, and thus also shift the curve up and to the left, similar to combinations of inotropes and vasodilators at point 5 (Fig. 16-27).

By utilizing direct measurements of preload (e.g., PCWP), indirect measurements of afterload (e.g., systemic vascular resistance), and ventricular function curves to assess myocardial contractility, the clinician can think about the cardiovascular system in specific terms and apply rational therapeutic interventions to clinical situation (Fig. 16-28). Alterations of preload, afterload, and contractility can then be specifically corrected. For example, if the preload is decreased, volume can be infused with crystalloid, colloid, or whole blood, depending on the patient's hematocrit.[93] If necessary, while the preload is being augmented, systemic vascular resistance can be increased with a small dose of an α-adrenergic vasoconstrictor. This latter step would only be a very temporary measure while the preload was being augmented by volume infusion. If the problem is that the preload is too high—for example, a PCWP over 18 mmHg—then administration of a diuretic, such as furosemide, or a venodilator, such as nitroglycerin, would correct the hemodynamic abnormality. If the wedge pressure is elevated owing to heart failure, it may even be necessary to intervene with an inotropic agent. In some situations, it may be that the afterload is the abnormal hemodynamic parameter. If the systemic vascular resistance and mean arterial blood pressure are found to be very low, then fluids can

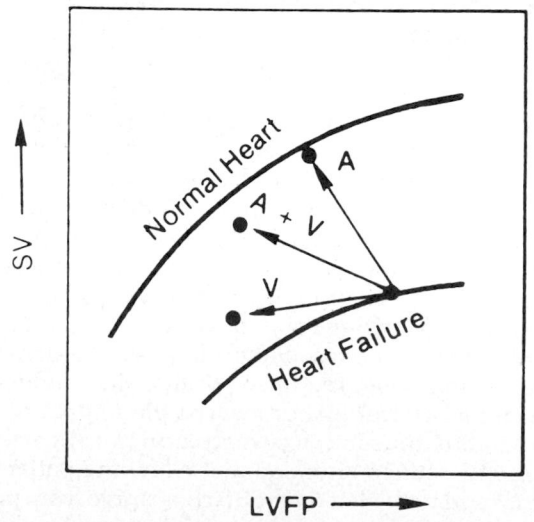

Fig. 16-26. Frank-Starling ventricular function curves of a normal heart and a heart in failure are demonstrated. The effects of three different types of vasodilators are demonstrated. An arterial dilator (A), a venodilator (V), and a mixed arterial dilator and venodilator (A + V) are shown. (See the text for details.) (From Mehta,[92] with permission.)

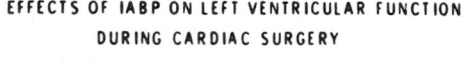

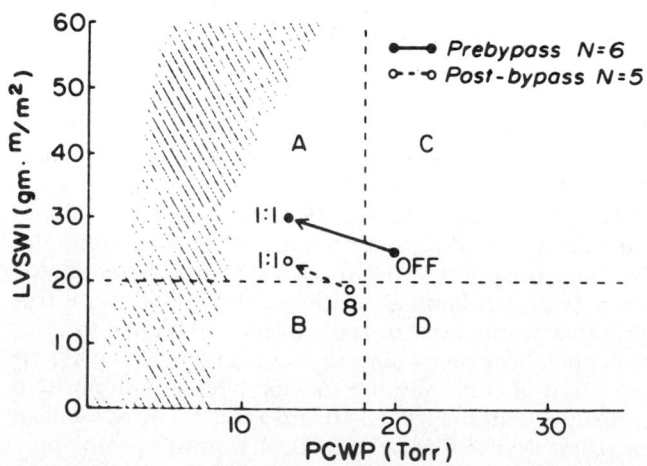

Fig. 16-27. Left ventricular function diagram with the normal range shaded dark. Intra-aortic counterpulsation moved patients, in both the pre-bypass and post-bypass groups, up and to the left on the curves. (From Kaplan et al.,[132] with permission.)

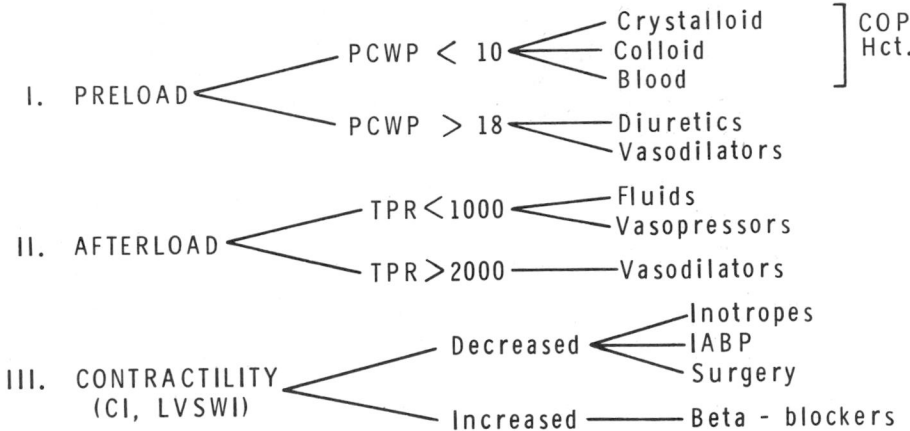

Fig. 16-28. Rational cardiovascular therapy for specific hemodynamic abnormalities is demonstrated. CI, cardiac index; LVSWI, left ventricular stroke work index; PCWP, pulmonary capillary wedge pressure; TPR, total peripheral resistance; IABP, intra-aortic balloon pump; COP, colloid oncotic pressure; Hct, hematocrit.

be infused and α-adrenergic vasoconstrictors administered. If the afterload is very high and impedance to left ventricular ejection is altering left ventricular function, then an arterial vasodilator such as sodium nitroprusside or phentolamine could be used to augment stroke volume and cardiac output, which probably would cause little change in blood pressure. If contractility is the primary abnormality, administration of inotropic drugs or the use of the intra-aortic balloon may provide effective therapy. In the rare situation in which contractility is markedly elevated and this is the hemodynamic abnormality, direct myocardial depressants such as halogenated anesthetic agents or intravenous propranolol could be administered.

Diastolic Function

In the last 10 years, it has been clearly recognized that in some patients the signs and symptoms of congestive heart failure are primarily due to diastolic dysfunction.[94-96] In these patients, various degrees of congestive heart failure are observed in the presence of normal or even increased left ventricular systolic function (Fig. 16-29).

In the evaluation of these patients, various investigators have focused their attention either on the isovolumic relaxation phase or on the ventricular filling phase. The filling phase itself can be further divided into an early and late component.

Isovolumic Relaxation Phase

As stated above, ventricular relaxation is an energy-requiring process. It has, therefore, been postulated that myocardial ischemia may result in impaired ventricular relaxation, and efforts have been aimed at clinical measurements of relaxation. In the technique most commonly utilized to assess relaxation, ventricular pressure is measured continuously by a catheter with a micromanometer at its tip. The decrease in ventricular pressure is assumed to be exponential, and the time constant of the pressure decay (τ or tau) is used as the index of relaxation.[97] In patients undergoing coronary artery bypass surgery, Humphrey et al.[98] recently measured the time constant of relaxation before and after cardiopulmonary bypass. They noted that immediately after coronary bypass, ventricular relaxation was enhanced, probably owing to relief of ischemia.[98]

Ventricular Filling Phase

Early Filling

Early filling is most frequently assessed by measuring the peak ventricular filling rate with radionuclides or the peak flow velocity with Doppler echocardiography. Recent animal and human studies have extensively investigated the determinants of peak early flow velocity. Variables that have been clearly recognized as determinants of peak early velocity include the left atrial V-wave pressure, the left ventricular relaxation rate, and the systemic arterial pressure. The peak early flow velocity varies directly with increasing left atrial pressure and inversely with increases in the rate of relaxation or systemic arterial pressure.[99] Other factors that have not been directly associated with the peak early velocity but are nonetheless important for the onset of diastolic flow are the ventricular suction effect and mitral ring recoil. The manner in which all these factors influence peak early velocity is complex and interrelated. Some studies suggest that changes in left atrial pressure have more pronounced effects than changes in left ventricular rate of relaxation. Interpretation of diastolic peak velocity will be further confounded by changes in heart rate.

When myocardial ischemia is produced by transient occlusion of a coronary artery, as during angioplasty, the rapid observation of a reduced peak early velocity is

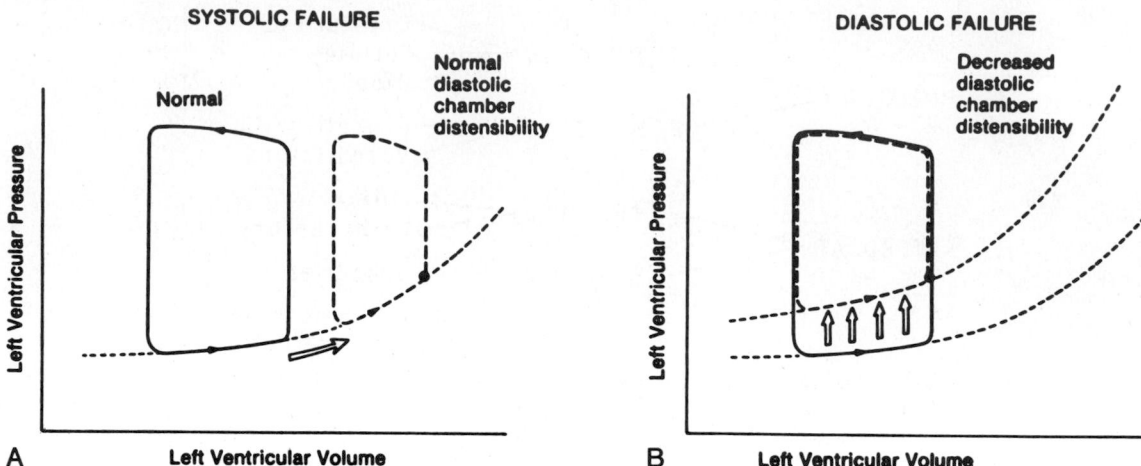

Fig. 16-29. (A) A schematized left ventricular pressure–volume loop from a patient with primary systolic failure. A normal left ventricular pressure–volume loop (solid loop) is shown on the left portion of the curve, whereas the transition to systolic failure (dashed loop) is shown on the right portion of the curve. Systolic failure is manifest as an increase in left ventricular end-systolic volume and as a reduction in the extent of shortening (stroke volume). Left ventricular end-diastolic pressure is increased because left ventricular volume is increased. As indicated by the arrow, the diastolic portion of the pressure–volume loop has simply shifted to the right along the same diastolic pressure–volume relation. No change in the distensibility of the left ventricle has occurred. (B) A left ventricular pressure–volume loop from a patient with primary diastolic failure (dashed loop). Note that the LVEDP is the same as that in the patient with primary systolic failure, as denoted by the dot (·) on the pressure–volume loops in both figures. However, in Fig. B, this is related to an upward shift of the left ventricular diastolic pressure–volume relation (arrows). This indicates a decrease in left ventricular diastolic distensibility such that a higher diastolic pressure is required to achieve the same diastolic volume. In this patient, no change in end-diastolic volume or systolic shortening has occurred. (From Lorell,[133] with permission.)

suggestive or impaired relaxation. In one study, diastolic left ventricular dysfunction was the earliest change noted after coronary occlusion and it often preceded the development of abnormal systolic function.[100] In another study, it was observed that acute ischemia not only altered early ventricular filling but also produced marked abnormalities in late ventricular filling.[101]

Late Filling

The late filling of the ventricle is predominantly determined by ventricular distensibility. The factors that influence distensibility have been reviewed in an earlier section of this chapter (see Table 16-1). They include extrinsic factors, the physical properties of the ventricle, and myocardial relaxation. Late filling is often evaluated by simultaneously measuring ventricular diastolic pressures and volumes. On a pressure–volume diagram, they describe a curvilinear relation. The slope of a tangent to the curve (dP/dV) defines chamber stiffness at a given filling pressure (Fig. 16-30). Acute changes in left ventricular chamber stiffness have been observed during angina and acute coronary occlusion (Fig. 16-31).

PHYSIOLOGY OF THE CORONARY CIRCULATION

The right and left coronary arteries, which begin at the root of the aorta, provide the entire blood supply to the myocardium. The right coronary artery principally supplies the right atrium and ventricle, while the left main coronary artery divides into the left anterior descending and circumflex arteries, which principally supply the left atrium and ventricle, respectively. There are many variations of the usual coronary anatomy, and significant overlap exists between the different vessels and the areas of the heart they supply. In humans, the right coronary artery supplies the sinus node in about 55 percent of individuals, while the left circumflex artery supplies the sinus node in the other 45 percent. Blood supply to the atrioventricular node is provided by the right coronary artery in 90 percent of individuals and by the circumflex branch of the left coronary artery in the remaining 10 percent. The papillary muscles of the left ventricle are of vital functional significance. The anterior papillary muscle is almost always supplied by branches of the left coronary artery, while the posterior muscle usually receives blood flow from both the

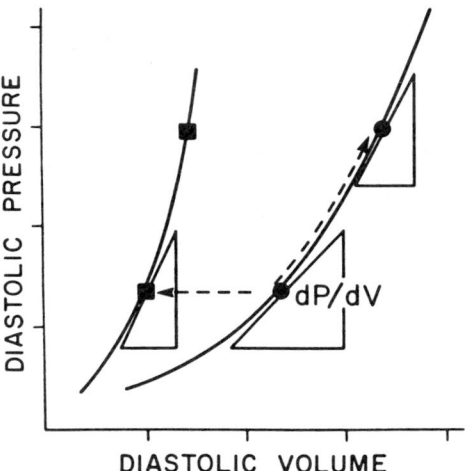

Fig. 16-30. Diastolic pressure–volume diagram. The slope of a tangent to the pressure–volume curve (dP/dV) represents chamber stiffness at a given diastolic pressure: with a progressive increase in volume, stiffness progressively increases (preload-dependent change in stiffness). A leftward shift of the pressure–volume curve also increases chamber stiffness. (From Gaasch et al.,[134] with permission.)

left and right coronary artery branches. In both instances, the collateral supply is usually good.[102]

After passage of the blood through the coronary capillary beds, most of the venous return occurs via the coronary sinus into the right atrium. However, there are also vascular communications directly between the vessels and the cardiac chambers. These include arteriosinusoidal communications, arterioluminal communications, and the thebesian vessels. The thebesian vessels are small veins that connect the capillary beds directly with the cardiac chambers and also communicate with other cardiac veins and thebesian veins. Thus, intercommunication exists among all the minute ves-

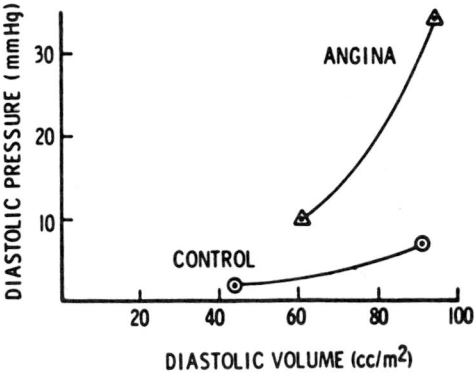

Fig. 16-31. Left ventricular diastolic pressure–volume relations during angina pectoris. The marked increase in diastolic pressure that occurred during angina was due to an upward shift of the diastolic pressure-volume curve. (From Gaasch et al.,[134] with permission.)

sels of the myocardium in the form of an extensive plexus of subendocardial vessels.

Normal Coronary Blood Flow

The resting coronary blood flow in the typical 70-kg man is approximately 225 ml/min, which is about 4 to 5 percent of the total cardiac output. When a normal person exercises vigorously, there is a proportional increase in both the cardiac output and coronary blood flow. A number of factors affect the regulation of coronary blood flow as outlined below.[103]

Aortic Blood Pressure

Changes in aortic diastolic pressure generally evoke parallel changes in coronary blood flow. The normal coronary circulation demonstrates autoregulation of its blood flow in the intermediate coronary perfusion pressure range of 60 to 150 mmHg.[104] However, under normal conditions, the blood pressure is kept within relatively narrow limits, so that changes in coronary blood pressure are primarily caused by caliber changes in the coronary resistance vessels in response to metabolic demands of the heart.

Most coronary blood flow to the left ventricle occurs during diastole. The reason for this is that as the cardiac muscle contracts, it compresses the myocardial vasculature and thereby impairs blood flow during systole. During diastole, the compression on the myocardial vasculature by ventricular muscle relaxes and coronary blood flow driven by the aortic diastolic blood pressure increases. The intramural systolic force is so great during early ventricular systole that blood flow, as measured in large coronary arteries supplying the left ventricle, is briefly reversed. The maximum left coronary inflow occurs in early diastole when the ventricles have relaxed and extravascular compression of the coronary vessels is absent. This flow pattern is observed in the phasic coronary blood flow curve for the left coronary artery seen in Figure 16-32.[103] After initial reversal in early systole, left coronary blood flow follows aortic pressure until early diastole, when it rises abruptly and then declines slowly as aortic pressure falls during the remainder of diastole. Blood flow in the right coronary artery shows a similar pattern, but because of the lower pressure developed during systole by the thin right ventricle, reversal of blood flow does not occur in early systole and systolic blood flow constitutes a much greater proportion of the coronary inflow than it does in the left coronary artery. In fact, in the right coronary artery, blood flow occurs relatively freely throughout both systole and diastole.

During systole a gradient of myocardial pressures occurs, with the greatest pressure development being in the subendocardium and the least pressure development being in the epicardium.[105] This pressure gradient is important because the left ventricular muscle compresses the subendocardial vasculature much more

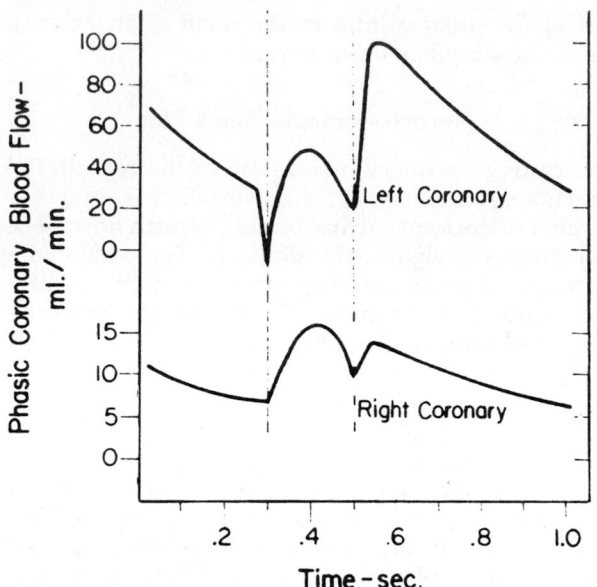

Fig. 16-32. Comparison of phasic coronary blood flow of the left and right coronary arteries. (See text for details.) (From Berne and Levy,[103] with permission.)

dium of the left ventricle, the pressure development during systole is less than in the subendocardium, and in the subepicardium the pressure development is even less. However, under normal conditions this pressure gradient does not result in subendocardial ischemia, since greater diastolic flow in the subendocardium compensates for the reduced systolic flow.[106] Radioactive microsphere studies have shown that blood flow to the epicardial and endocardial halves of the left ventricle is approximately equal under normal circumstances.[107] This is probably due to the fact that the tone of the subendocardial resistance vessels is less than that of the subepicardial vessels. Under abnormal conditions, such as severe hypotension, the ratio of endocardial to epicardial blood flow falls below 1.0. This indicates that the blood flow through the endocardial region is more severely impaired than that through the epicardial region of the ventricle during hypotension.[108]

than it does the subepicardial vessels. Thus, reduced blood flow to the subendocardium of the left ventricle places this area of the myocardium at the greatest risk. It can be seen from Figure 16-33 that during systole the pressure in the subendocardium of the left ventricle approximates that in the left ventricular cavity. No blood will flow through the subendocardial region of the left ventricle during systole. In the mid-myocar-

Left Ventricular End-Diastolic Pressure

The coronary perfusion pressure (CPP) is usually defined as the aortic diastolic blood pressure (DBP) minus the left ventricular end-diastolic pressure (LVEDP):

$$CPP = DBP - LVEDP$$

Elevation of the LVEDP will decrease the gradient of blood flow to the vulnerable subendocardial tissue during diastole as much as will a decrease in the diastolic

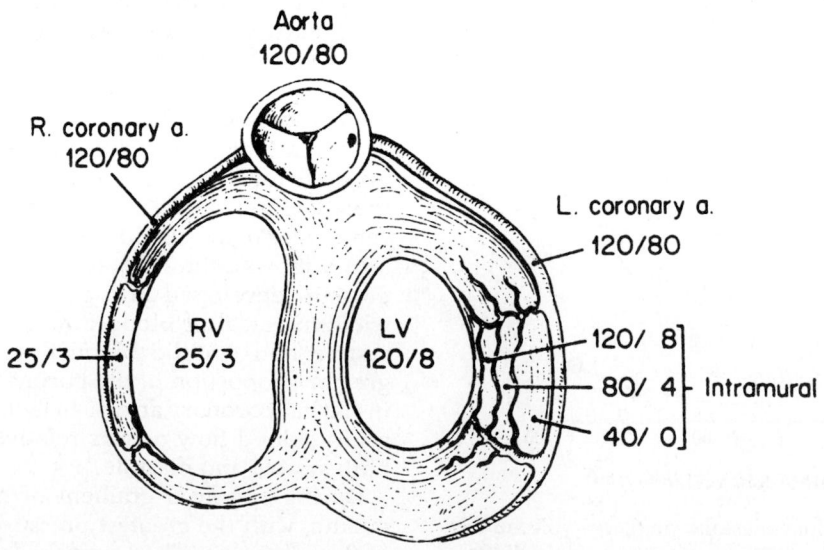

Fig. 16-33. Diagrammatic cross-section of the heart to indicate intramyocardial compressive forces in different parts of the myocardium. RV, right ventricle; LV, left ventricle. (From Hoffman and Buckberg,[135] with permission.)

blood pressure.[109] This relationship can be seen below:

CPP	=	DBP		LVEDP
70	=	80	−	10
50	=	60	−	10
50	=	80	−	30

If coronary artery disease is present (Fig. 16-34), significant stenosis will decrease the coronary artery diastolic pressure well below the aortic diastolic pressure, and elevation of LVEDP can seriously jeopardize the subendocardium as seen below.[100]

Aortic BP		Distal Coronary BP	−	LVEDP	=	CPP
80	→	50	−	4	=	46
80	→	50	−	30	=	20

In fact, a vicious cycle of myocardial ischemia can be produced in patients with coronary artery disease by increases in LVEDP (Fig. 16-35). THe LVEDP elevation can produce subendocardial ischemia, which will then lead to both ventricular dysfunction and the production of ventricular arrhythmias. However, remember that myocardial ischemia itself can produce left ventricular dysfunction and elevations in LVEDP.[109]

Hoffman and Buckberg[108] have described a relationship called the endocardial viability ratio (EVR), or diastolic pressure-time index (DPTI) over tension-time index (TTI), which describes the ratio of the myocardial oxygen supply to the myocardial oxygen demand.[110] This ratio is used to estimate subendocardial blood flow. To assess the oxygen supply the DPTI is used, and for the oxygen demand the TTI is used. The

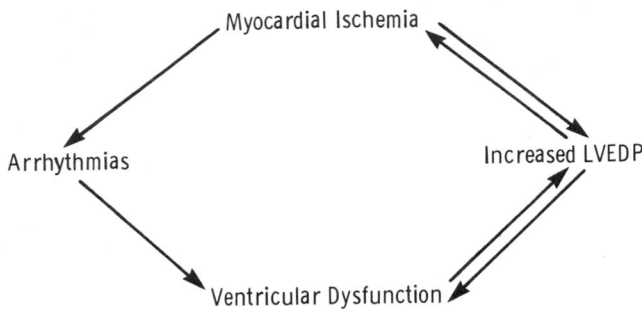

Fig. 16-35. The vicious cycle of myocardial ischemia that can be precipitated by elevations in the left ventricular filling pressure.

formula described by Hoffman and Buckberg is

$$EVR = \frac{DPTI}{TTI} = \frac{(DBP - LAP) \times d}{SP \times s} = \frac{oxygen\ supply}{oxygen\ demand}$$

where DBP = the mean aortic diastolic pressure, LAP = the mean left atrial pressure (or LVEDP), SP = the mean systemic arterial pressure, d = the diastolic time, and s = the systolic time.

A normal EVR is 1.0 or above when the DPTI equals or exceeds the TTI. When the EVR is less than 0.7, Hoffman and Buckberg[111] found that the left ventricular endocardial blood flow fell in proportion to the epicardial flow (decreased endocardial/epicardial ratio), which indicates subendocardial ischemia. The endocardial/epicardial ratio fell whether the decreased EVR was secondary to decreased aortic diastolic pressure, increased left atrial pressure, or increased heart rate. Figure 16-36 shows the effect the intra-aortic balloon has on increasing the EVR.[31]

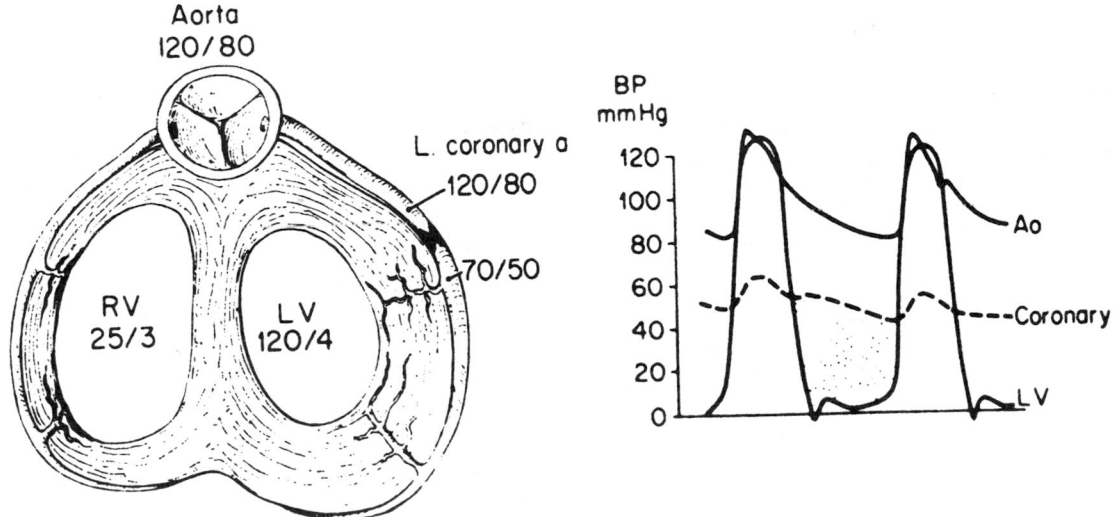

Fig. 16-34. Diagrammatic cross-section of the heart to indicate coronary arterial pressure beyond a severe obstructive arterial lesion. On the left are shown the aortic, distal coronary, and left ventricular pressures. The stippled area indicates the diastolic pressure-time area for the region of the heart supplied by the partially obstructed coronary artery. (From Hoffman and Buckberg,[135] with permission.)

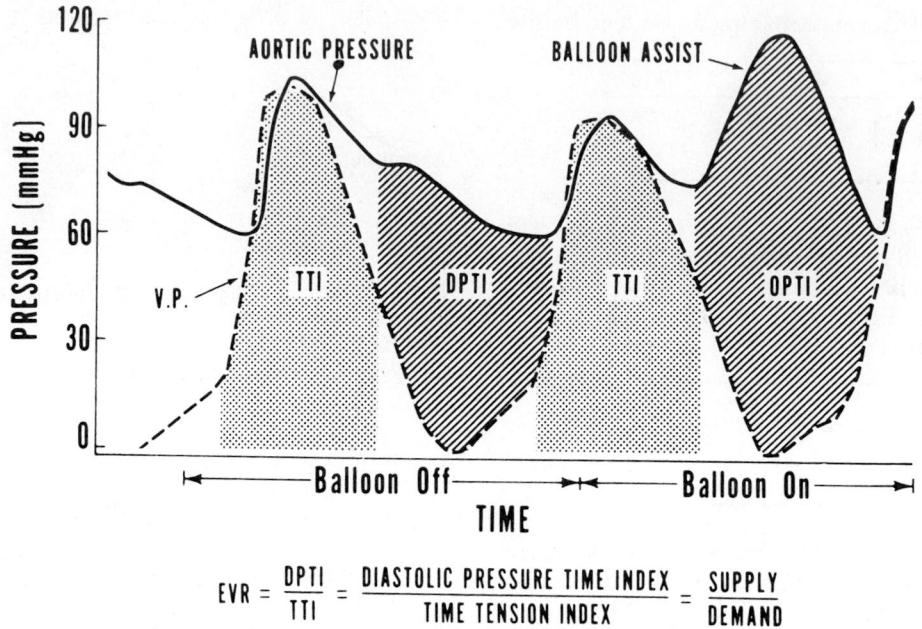

$$EVR = \frac{DPTI}{TTI} = \frac{DIASTOLIC\ PRESSURE\ TIME\ INDEX}{TIME\ TENSION\ INDEX} = \frac{SUPPLY}{DEMAND}$$

Fig. 16-36. The diastolic pressure-time index (DPTI) and tension-time index, (TTI) areas are shown. From these the endocardial viability ratio is calculated. The effect of the intra-aortic balloon pump on the endocardial viability ratio is demonstrated. There is a marked increase in DPTI compared with TTI. (From Bolooki,[31] with permission.)

Alterations in Heart Rate

A change in the heart rate is accomplished chiefly by shortening or lengthening diastole. Approximately 70 percent of the coronary blood flow in humans occurs during diastole.[112] With tachycardia, the proportion of time spent in diastole decreases and therefore the coronary blood flow is directly reduced. With bradycardia, the opposite is true, and coronary blood flow increases. This relationship can be seen in the endocardial viability ratio formula above. Diastolic time does not vary linearly with heart rate. Two factors determine the duration of diastole: (1) heart rate and (2) duration of systole. Owing to the nonlinear relationship between heart rate and the percentage of diastole, small changes in heart rate, especially at slower rates, produce dramatic changes in the percentage of diastole (Fig. 16-37).[113] As shown in Figure 16-37, an increase in heart rate from 50 to 70 beats/min produces a reduction of the diastolic percentage from 75 to 50 percent, whereas a change in heart rate from 70 to 90 beats/min only reduces diastolic time from 50 to 45 percent.

Local Metabolic Factors

There is a close relationship between the level of myocardial activity and the magnitude of the coronary blood flow. Blood flow through the coronary vasculature to the myocardium is regulated by the need of the cardiac muscle for oxygen. Thus, hypoxia probably dilates the coronary arterial resistance vessels. The pre-

cise mechanism by which hypoxia dilates the coronary arterioles is not known, but it is postulated that either decreased oxygen tension directly causes relaxation of the coronary arterioles or hypoxia causes release of vasodilator substances (e.g., adenosine) that relax the resistance vessels within the myocardium. According to the adenosine hypothesis, a reduction in myocardial oxygen tension produced by reduced coronary blood flow, hypoxemia, or increased metabolic activity of the heart leads to the breakdown of adenosine nucleotides to adenosine, which diffuses out of the cardiac cells and induces dilatation of the coronary resistance vessels.[114] This dilatation results in an increase in coronary blood flow that enhances the washout of adenosine and reduces its formation by raising myocardial oxygen tension toward control levels. Under normal resting conditions, only small amounts of adenosine are released by the heart, and thus adenosine exerts a minimal dilating effect.

Neural and Neurohumoral Factors

The automatic nervous system affects coronary blood flow in two ways. There is a direct effect of released neurotransmitters on the coronary vessels themselves. Both α- and β-adrenergic receptors are known to exist in the coronary vasculature.[115] The epicardial coronary vessels have a preponderance of α-receptors, and the intramuscular and subendocardial coronary arteries have a preponderance of β-receptors. The usual effect of sympathetic stimulation is a lowering of coronary

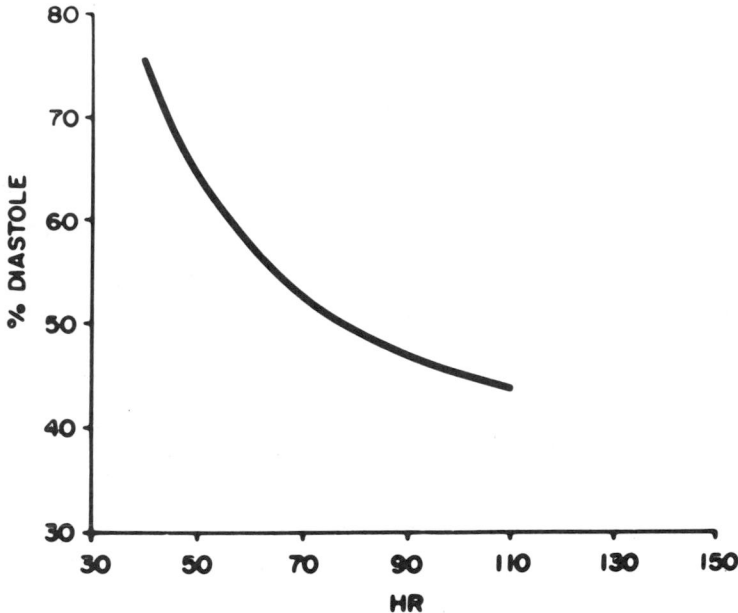

Fig. 16-37. Relationship between heart rate (HR) and percent diastole. Small changes in HR produce dramatic changes in the percent diastole at slower HRs. (Modified from Boudoulas et al,[113] with permission.)

vascular resistance, since most of the resistance to blood flow occurs in the intramuscular coronary arterioles, which are stimulated by β-receptors. However, on occasion, it is believed that α-adrenergic-mediated constriction of the epicardial arteries can predominate, producing myocardial ischemia, as is seen in Prinzmetal's angina.[116] There also appears to be some parasympathetic nervous system innervation of the coronary vessels, and this may produce a slight vasodilatory effect.[117] The indirect mechanism by which the autonomic nervous system exerts control over coronary blood flow is through myocardial stimulation resulting from released catecholamines. For example, epinephrine produces an increase in heart rate and myocardial contractility that leads to a secondary increase in coronary blood flow to meet the increased oxygen demand. This indirect effect appears to be more important than the direct effect on the vessels themselves.

Myocardial Oxygen Balance

The delicate balance between the myocardial oxygen supply and the myocardial oxygen demand is the overall controlling factor in the coronary circulation. In humans, blood flow through the coronary circulation is regulated primarily in proportion to the myocardium's demand for oxygen. The heart extracts approximately 65 percent of the oxygen from the arterial blood as the blood passes through it. This represents a near maximum extraction of oxygen, and the heart is able to remove little in the way of additional oxygen from blood as the demand for oxygen by the ventricles increases.

Thus, when the heart requires extra oxygen, it must increase its coronary blood flow.

Figure 16-38 shows the detrimental changes that can occur in the myocardial oxygen balance. A decreased myocardial oxygen supply can be caused by a number of factors. Decreased coronary blood flow will be produced by tachycardia, because this will limit the diastolic filling time to the left ventricle. The coronary perfusion pressure gradient can be decreased by either a decrease in the aortic diastolic blood pressure or an increase in LVEDP. This is extremely important in patients with coronary artery disease. The increase in the LVEDP acts as a back-pressure and tends to limit the subendocardial blood flow.[106] Subendocardial ischemia is easily produced by increases in LVEDP and is rapidly reversed by decreasing the LVEDP with drugs such as nitroglycerin. Hyperventilation to a $PaCO_2$ of 20 to 25 mmHg will decrease coronary blood flow, shift the oxygen-hemoglobin dissociation curve to the left, and decrease 2,3-diphosphoglycerate. These factors will interfere with the delivery of oxygen to the myocardium. Decreased oxygen delivery will also be present when severe anemia or hypoxemia exists.

Coronary artery spasm is becoming recognized as a more important cause of decreased myocardial blood flow than had previously been believed. Disease states such as Prinzmetal's angina are primarily based on coronary artery spasm, but there may be a degree of coronary artery disease.[118] This may be due to autonomic innervation of the coronary vessels, since in some patients the administration of an α-adrenergic constricting drug can produce coronary spasm and reduce coro-

DECREASED MYOCARDIAL
OXYGEN SUPPLY

1. Decreased coronary blood flow
    a. Tachycardia
    b. Diastolic hypotension
    c. Increased preload
    d. Hypocapnia
    e. Coronary spasm
2. Decreased oxygen delivery
    a. Anemia
    b. Hypoxia
    c. Decreased 2,3 DPG

INCREASED MYOCARDIAL
OXYGEN DEMAND

1. Tachycardia
2. Increased wall tension
    a. Increased preload
    b. Increased afterload
3. Increased contractility

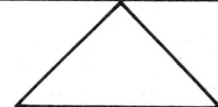

Fig. 16-38. Detrimental changes that can occur in the myocardial balance. Tachycardia and increased preload are marked to stand out, since they appear on both sides of the balance.

nary blood flow to the epicardial vessels. In other situations, it may be due to withdrawal of drugs such as nitrates or slow-channel calcium blockers or to administration of calcium.[119,120]

Since oxygen demand by the heart determines coronary blood flow, it is important to know the major hemodynamic alterations that will increase the myocardial oxygen demand. An increased heart rate is very detrimental in the presence of coronary artery disease, since diastolic filling time (oxygen supply) is decreased and oxygen demand increased; therefore, perfusion of the myocardium suffers and ischemia frequently results.[121,122]

Increases in left ventricular wall tension produced by an increased LVEDP or an increased blood pressure (afterload) will also increase myocardial oxygen demand. The pressure that the left ventricle develops during systole is directly correlated with the demand for myocardial oxygen. This area under the systemic arterial blood pressure curve during systole was first called the tension-time index by Sarnoff and co-workers[123] and is one of the indirect indices of myocardial oxygen demand used by some.[124] Thus, systolic hypertension is accompanied by the left ventricle is also proportional to the LVEDP. A large, dilated, or distended left ventricle will have an increased oxygen demand. Thus, both tachycardia and an increase in left ventricular filling pressure will decrease myocardial oxygen supply as well as increase myocardial oxygen demand.

The last factor that increases myocardial oxygen demand is increased myocardial contractility. The velocity of myocardial contraction is directly proportional to the myocardial oxygen demand. Braunwald[112] has

clearly shown that an increase in myocardial contractility results in a substantial increase in myocardial oxygen demand at any given level of developed tension. A positive inotropic drug administered to an individual with a normal ventricle will produce an increase in contractility and myocardial oxygen demand. If, however, the positive inotropic agent is administered to a patient with an overdistended failing left ventricle, there may be a net decrease in myocardial oxygen demand, as shown for digitalis administration (Fig. 16-39). Thus, there is a difference when a positive inotropic drug is administered to either a normal or a failing left ventricle in relation to myocardial oxygen demand. In fact, an inotrope may be beneficial if the ventricle is overdistended, as long as it does not reduce

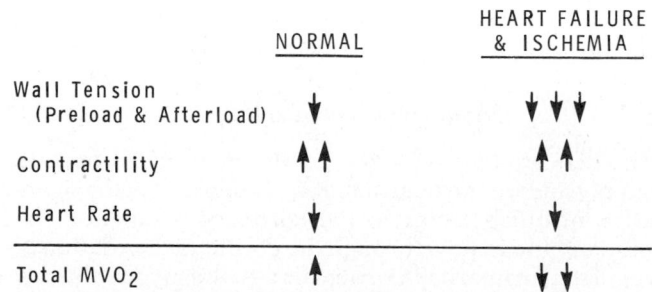

Fig. 16-39. Effects of an inotropic drug such as digitalis on the myocardial oxygen demand of a normal and a failing ventricle. There is an overall increase in myocardial oxygen demand in the normal heart and a marked decrease in the failing, or ischemic, heart. (From Mason,[124] with permission.)

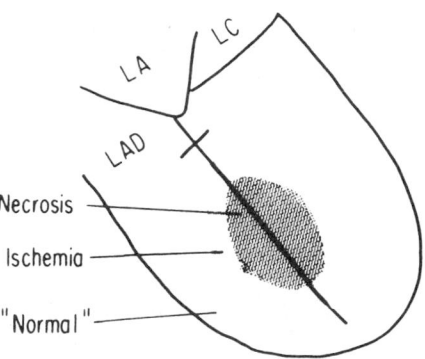

Fig. 16-40. Different zones of myocardial tissue following coronary artery occlusion are shown. These are the central necrotic dead zone, the surrounding peri-infarction zone of ischemia with potentially viable tissue, and the zone of nonischemic normal tissue. (From Mueller et al.,[136] with permission.)

diastolic blood pressure or increase heart rate too much.[124]

Changes in cardiac output alone do not increase myocardial oxygen demand. For example, if cardiac output is increased by decreasing total peripheral resistance, even though the heart will have an increased stroke volume and stroke work, there will be little change in myocardial oxygen demand. If, however, the cardiac output is increased by a significant increase in heart rate or if there is a significant increase in arterial blood pressure, then there will be an increase in myocardial oxygen demand. Thus, if the arterial pressure and heart rate are kept constant, stroke volume can be increased with little accompanying increase in myocardial oxygen demand. This may be one of the significant beneficial effects of the use of vasodilators.

The myocardial oxygen balance represents a dynamic rather than a static process. In severe ischemia or infarction, the damaged area is not totally defined at the time of the insult but can be made better or worse by interventions or events.[125] Figure 16-40 shows an area of necrosis surrounded by the peri-infarction zone of ischemia. This ischemic "twilight zone" can be salvaged or destroyed by appropriate or inappropriate interventions. Increases or decreases in the amount of ischemic tissue progressing to necrosis can be demonstrated by enzyme measurements and the electrocardiogram (Fig. 16-41). Myocardial ischemia will be decreased by reducing the myocardial oxygen demand (e.g., correcting hypoxemia) or possibly by improving the myocardial metabolic environment (e.g., glucose-insulin-potassium infusion). Myocardial ischemia may be worsened by increasing the oxygen demand (e.g., as in tachycardia) or decreasing the oxygen supply (e.g., as in severe hypotension).[110]

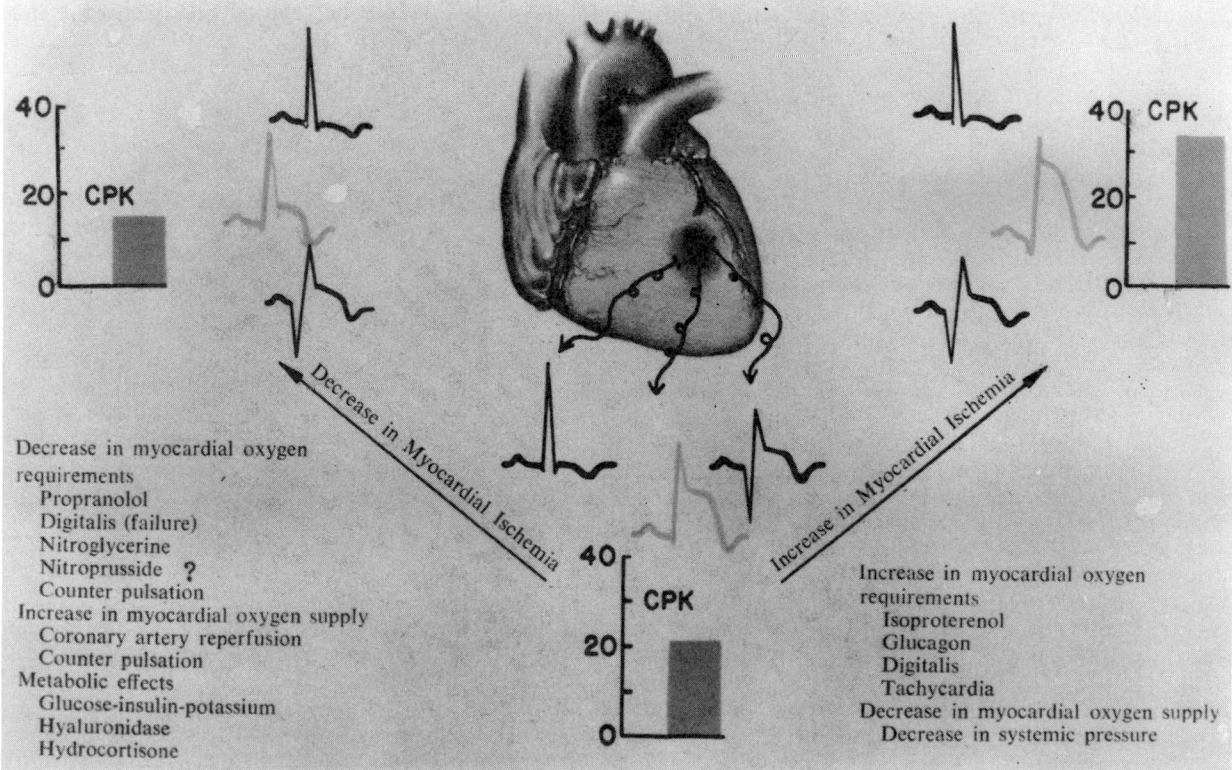

Fig. 16-41. Potential modifications of myocardial ischemia. (From Parker,[137] with permission.)

REFERENCES

1. Guyton AC: Regulation of cardiac output. N Engl J Med 227:805, 1967
2. Braunwald E: Determinates and assessment of cardiac function. N Engl J Med 296:86, 1977
3. Braunwald E: On the difference between the heart's output and its contractile state. Circulation 43:171, 1971
4. Sagawa K, Maughan L, Suga H, et al: Cardiac contraction and the pressure-volume relationship. Oxford University Press, New York, 1988
5. Frank O: Zur dynamik des herzmuskels. Z Biol 32:370, 1895
6. Ter Keurs HEDJ, Rijnsburger WH, van Heuningen R, et al: Tension development and sarcomere length in rat cardiac trabeculae. Evidence of length-dependent activation. Circ Res 46:703, 1980
7. Kentish JC, ter Keurs HEDJ, Ricciardi L, et al: Comparison between the sarcomere length-force relations of intact and skinned trabeculae from rat right ventricle. Circ Res 58:755, 1986
8. Jewell BR: A reexamination of the influence of muscle length on myocardial performance. Circ Res 40:221, 1977
9. Kentish JC: The length-tension relation in the myocardium and its cellular basis. Heart Failure 4:125, 1988
10. Lakatta EG, Jewell BR: Length-dependent activation; its effects on the length-tension relation in cat ventricular muscle. Circ Res 40:251, 1977
11. Paterson S, Starling EH: On the mechanical factors which determine the output of the ventricles. J Physiol 48:357, 1914
12. Brutsaert DL, Sonnenblick EH: Force-velocity-length relations in the contractile elements in heart muscle of the cat. Circ Res 24:137, 1969
13. Forman R, Ford LE, Sonnenblick EH: Effect of muscle length on the force-velocity relationship of tetanized cardiac muscle. Circ Res 31:195, 1972
14. Parmley WW: Mechanics of ventricular muscle. p. 53. In Levine HJ, Gaasch WH (eds): The Ventricle. Martinus Nijhoff Publishing, Boston, 1985
15. Peterson KL, Uther JH, Shabetai R, et al: Assessment of left ventricular performance in man. Instantaneous tension-velocity-length relations obtained with the aid of an electromagnetic velocity catheter in the ascending aorta. Circulation 47:924, 1973
16. Brutsaert DL, Housmans PR, Goethals MA: Dual control of relaxation. Its role in the ventricular function in the mammalian heart. Circ Res 47:637, 1980
17. Brutsaert DL, Rademakers, FE, Sys SU: Triple control of relaxation: Implications in cardiac disease. Circulation 69:190, 1984
18. Brutsaert DL, Rademakers FE, Sys SU, et al: Analysis of relaxation in the evaluation of ventricular function of the heart. Prog Cardiovasc Dis 28:143, 1985
19. Nichols WW: The influence of diastolic length on the contractility of isolated cat papillary muscle. J Physiol (Lond) 361:269, 1985
20. Thys DM, Hillel Z, Goldman ME, et al: A comparison of hemodynamic indices derived by invasive monitoring and two-dimensional echocardiography. Anesthesiology 67:630, 1987
21. Kaplan JA (ed): Cardiac Anesthesia. Grune & Stratton, Orlando, FL, 1979
22. Kaplan JA, Wells PH: Early diagnosis of myocardial ischemia using the pulmonary arterial catheter. Anesth Analg 60:789, 1981
23. Humphrey CB, Oury JH, Virgill RW, et al: An analysis of direct and indirect measurement of left atrial filling pressures. J Thorac Cardiovasc Surg 41:643, 1976
24. Swan HJC, Ganz W, Forrester JS, et al: Catheterization of the heart in man with the use of a flow directed balloon-tip catheter. N Engl J Med 283:447, 1970
25. Lappas D, Lell WA, Gabel JC, et al: Indirect measurement of left atrial pressure in surgical patients—pulmonary capillary wedge pressure and pulmonary artery diastolic pressure compared with left atrial pressure. Anesthesiology 38:384, 1973
26. Lorzman J, Powers SR, Older T, et al: Correlation of pulmonary wedge and left atrial pressure: A study in the patient receiving positive end-expiratory pressure ventilation. Arch Surg 109:270, 1974
27. Pace NL: A critique of flow directed pulmonary artery catheterization. Anesthesiology 47:455, 1977
28. Civetta JM, Cagel JC, Laver MB: Disparate ventricular function in surgical patients. Surg Forum 22:136, 1971
29. Sarnoff SJ, Berglund E: Ventricular function. I. Starling's law of the heart studied by means of simultaneous right and left ventricular function curves in the dog. Circulation 9:706, 1954
30. Ross J, Sobel BE: Regulation of cardiac contraction. Annu Rev Physiol 34:47, 1972
31. Bolooki H: Clinical Applications of the Intraaortic Balloon Pump. Futura, Mount Kisco, NY, 1977
32. Sagawa K, Maughan L, Suga H, et al: Cardiac contraction and the pressure-volume relationship. p. 28. Oxford University Press, New York, 1988
33. Weber KT, Janicki JS, Hunter WC, et al: The contractile behavior of the heart and its functional coupling to the circulation. Prog Cardiovasc Dis 24:375, 1982
34. Lang RM, Borow KM, Neumann A, et al: Systemic vascular resistance: An unreliable index of left ventricular afterload. Circulation 74:1114, 1986
35. Milnor WR: Arterial impedance as ventricular afterload. Circ Res 36:565, 1975
36. Sunagawa K, Maughan WL, Burkhoff D, et al: Left ventricular interaction with arterial load studied in isolated canine ventricle. Am J Physiol 245:H773, 1983
37. Nichols WW, Conti CR, Walker WE, et al: Input impedance of the systemic circulation in man. Circ Res 40:451, 1977
38. Kaplan JA: Vasodilators and combined inotrope and vasodilator therapy for the low output syndrome. In Kaplan JA (ed): Cardiac Anesthesia: Cardiovascular Pharmacology. Grune & Stratton, Orlando, FL, 1983
39. Suga H, Sagawa K, Shoukas AA: Load independence of the instantaneous pressure-volume ratio of the canine left ventricle and effects of epinephrine and heart ratio on the ratio. Circ Res 32:314, 1973
40. Suga H, Sagawa K: Instantaneous pressure-volume relationships and their ratio in the excised, supported canine left ventricle. Circ Res 35:117, 1974
41. Kass DA, Maughan WL: From "Emax" to pressure-volume relations: A broader view. Circulation 77:1203, 1988
42. Kass DA, Yamazaki T, Burkhoff D, et al: Determination of left ventricular end-systolic pressure-volume relationships by conductance (volume) catheter technique. Circulation 73:586, 1986
43. Martin RW, Graham MM, Kao R, Basheim G: Measurement of left ventricular ejection fraction with three-dimensional reconstructed transesophageal scans: Comparison to radionuclide and thermal dilution measurements. J Cardiothorac Anesth 3:260, 1989

44. Suga H, Hayashi T, Shirahata M: Ventricular systolic pressure-volume area as predictor of cardiac oxygen consumption. Am J Physiol 240:H39, 1981

45. Nozawa T, Yasumura Y, Futaki S, et al: Efficiency of energy transfer from pressure-volume area to external mechanical work increases with contractile state and decreases with afterload in the left ventricle of the anesthetized closed-chest dog. Circulation 77:1116, 1988

46. Sunagawa K, Maughan WL, Burkhoff D, et al: Left ventricular interaction with arterial load studied in isolated canine ventricle. Am J Physiol 245:H773, 1983

47. Guyton AC, Coleman TG, Granger HJ: Circulation: Overall regulation. Annu Rev Physiol 34:13, 1972

48. Braunwald E: Regulation of the circulation. N Engl J Med 290:1124, 1974

49. Higgins CB, Vatner SF, Braunwald E: Parasympathetic control of the heart. Pharmacol Rev 25:119, 1973

50. Gorlin R: Practical cardiac hemodynamics. N Engl J Med 296:203, 1977

51. Ganz W, Donoso R, Marcus AS, et al: A new technique for measurement of cardiac output by thermodilution in man. Am J Cardiol 27:392, 1971

52. Kohanna SH, Cunningham JN: Monitoring of cardiac output by thermodilution after open heart surgery. J Thorac Cardiovasc Surg 73:451, 1977

53. Ganz W, Swan JHC: Measurement of blood flow by thermodilution. Am J Cardiol 29:241, 1972

54. Kahan F, Profeta J, Thys, DM: High cardiac output measurements in a patient with congestive heart failure. J Cardiothoracic Anesthesiol 1:234, 1987

55. Barankay T, Jansco T, Nagay S, et al: Cardiac output estimation by a thermodilution method involving intravascular heating and thermistor recording. Acta Physiol Acad Sci Hung 38:167, 1970

56. Khalil HH, Richardson TQ, Guyton AC: Measurement of cardiac output by thermal dilution and direct Fick methods in dogs. J Appl Physiol 21:1131, 1966

57. Philip JH, Long MC, Quinn MD, et al: Continuous thermal measurement of cardiac output. IEEE Trans Biomed Eng 31:393, 1984

58. Guyton AC, Jones EC, Hallman TG: Circulatory Physiology: Cardiac Output and Its Regulation. 2nd Ed. WB Saunders, Philadelphia, 1973

59. Davis CC, Jones NL, Sealey BJ: Measurements of cardiac output in seriously ill patients using a CO_2 rebreathing method. Chest 73:167, 1978

60. McMickan JC: Continuous monitoring of mixed venous oxygen saturation in clinical practice. Mt Sinai J Med 51:569, 1984

61. Waller JC, Kaplan JA, Bauman DI, Craver JM: Clinical evaluation of a new fiberoptic catheter oximeter during cardiac surgery. Anesth Analg 61:676, 1982

62. Thys DM, Cohen E, Eisenkraft JB: Mixed venous oxygen saturation during thoracic anesthesia. Anesthesiology 69:1005, 1988

63. Heneghan CPH, Gillbe CE, Brantwaithe MA: Measurement of metabolic gas exchange during anesthesia. Br J Anaesth 53:73, 1981

64. Heneghan CPH, Brantwaithe MA: Non-invasive measurement of cardiac output during anaesthesia. Br J Anaesth 53:351, 1981

65. Davies G, Hess D, Jebson P: Continuous Fick cardiac output compared to continuous pulmonary artery electromagnetic flow measurements in pigs. Anesthesiology 66:805, 1987

66. Davies G, Jebson PJR, Glasgow BM, Hess DR: Continuous Fick cardiac output compared to thermodilution cardiac output. Crit Care Med 14:881, 1986

67. Carpenter JP, Nair S, Staw I: Cardiac output determination: Thermodilution versus a new computerized Fick method. Crit Care Med 13:576, 1985

68. Robinson PS, Crowther A, Jenkins BS, et al: A computerized dichromatic earpiece densitometer for the measurement of cardiac output. Cardiovasc Res 13:420, 1979

69. Grasberg RC, Yeston NS: Less-invasive cardiac output monitoring by earpiece densitometry. Crit Care Med 14:577, 1986

70. Powner DJ, Dahl D, Shucker L: Ear densitometer cardiac outputs versus thermodilution outputs. Crit Care Med 12:148, 1984

71. Tanner G, Barash PG: Cardiac output measured by earpiece densitometry vs. thermodilution. Crit Care Med 12:1082, 1984

72. English JB, Hodges MR, Sentker C, et al: Comparison of aortic pulse-wave contour analysis and thermodilution methods of measuring cardiac output during anesthesia in the dog. Anesthesiology 52:56, 1980

73. Matsumoto M, Oka Y, Strom J, et al: Application of transesophageal echocardiography to continuous intraoperative monitoring of left ventricular performance. Am J Cardiol 46:95, 1980

74. Terai C, Vensihi M, Sugimoto H, et al: Transesophageal echocardiographic dimensional analysis of four cardiac chambers during positive end-expiratory pressure. Anesthesiology 63:640, 1985

75. Kronik G, Slany J, Moslacher H: Comparative value of 8 M-mode echocardiographic formulas for determining left ventricular stroke volume. A correlative study with thermodilution and left ventricular single-plane cineangiography. Circulation 60:1308, 1979

76. Skjaerpe T, Hegrenaes L, Ihlen H: Cardiac output. p. 306. In Hatle L, Angelsen B (eds): Doppler Ultrasound in Cardiology. 2nd Ed. Lea & Febiger, Philadelphia, 1985

77. Leoppky JA, Greene ER, Hockenga DE, et al: Beat-by-beat stroke volume assessment by pulsed Doppler in upright and supine exercise. J Appl Physiol 50:1174, 1981

78. Goldberg SJ, Sahn DJ, Allen HD, et al: Evaluation of pulmonary and systemic blood flow by 2-dimensional Doppler echocardiography using fast Fourier transform spectral analysis. Am J Cardiol 50:1394, 1982

79. Fisher DC, Sahn DJ, Friedman MJ, et al: The effect of variations of pulsed Doppler sampling site on calculation of cardiac output: An experimental study in open-chest dogs. Circulation 67:370, 1983

80. Magnin PA, Stewart JA, Myers S, et al: Combined Doppler and phased-array echocardiographic estimation of cardiac output. Circulation 63:388, 1981

81. Mark JB, Steinbrook RA, Gugino LD, et al: Continuous non-invasive monitoring of cardiac output with esophageal Doppler ultrasound during cardiac surgery. Anesth Analg 65:1013, 1986

82. Freund PR: Modification in the transesophageal Doppler: Comparision with thermodilution measurement during cardiac output in anesthetized man (abstract). Anesthesiology 65A:144, 1986

83. Roewer N, Bednarz F, Driadha A, et al: Intraoperative cardiac output determination from transmitral and pulmonary blood flow measurements using transesophageal pulsed Doppler echocardiography. Anesthesiology 65A:639, 1987

84. Kubicek WG, Karegis JN, Patterson RP, et al: Development and evaluation of an impedance cardiac output system. Aerospace Med 37:1208, 1966

85. Donovan KD, Dobb GJ, Woods WPD, et al: Comparison of transthoracic electrical impedance and thermodilution methods for measuring cardiac output. Crit Care Med 14:1038, 1986

86. Bernstein DP: A new stroke volume equation for thoracic electrical bioimpedance: Theory and rationale. Crit Care Med 14:904, 1986

87. Bernstein DP: Continuous non-invasive real-time monitoring of stroke volume and cardiac output by thoracic electrical bioimpedance. Crit Care Med 14:898, 1986

88. Appel PL, Kram HB, Mackabee J, et al: Comparison of measurements of cardiac output by bioimpedance and thermodilution in severely ill surgical patients. Crit Care Med 14:933, 1986

89. Sarnoff SJ: Myocardial contractility as described by ventricular function curves: Observation on Starling's law of the heart. Physiol Rev 35:107, 1955

90. Kaplan JA: Cardiac Anesthesia: Cardiovascular Pharmacology. Grune & Stratton, Orlando, FL, 1983

91. Ross J: Afterload mismatch and preload reserve: A conceptual framework for the analysis of ventricular function. Prog Cardiovasc Dis 18:255, 1976

92. Mehta J: Vasodilators in the treatment of heart failure. JAMA 238:2534, 1977

93. Raphael LD, Mantle JA, Moraski RE, et al: Quantitative assessment of ventricular performance in unstable ischemic heart disease by dextran function curves. Circulation 55:858, 1977

94. Dodek A, Kassenbaum DG, Bristow JD: Pulmonary edema in coronary artery disease without cardiomegaly. N Engl J Med 25:1347, 1972

95. Dougherty AM, Naccarelli CV, Gray EL, et al: Congestive heart failure with normal systolic function. Am J Cardiol 54:778, 1984

96. Topol EJ, Traill TA, Fortuin NJ: Hypertensive hypertrophic cardiomyopathy of the elderly. N Engl J Med 312:277, 1985

97. Raff GL, Glantz SA: Volume loading slows left ventricular isovolumic relaxation rate. Circ Res 48:813, 1981

98. Humphrey LS, Topol EJ, Rosenfeld GI, et al: Immediate enhancement of left ventricular relaxation by coronary bypass grafting: Intraoperative assessment. Circulation 77:886, 1988

99. Choong CY, Abascal V, Thomas JD, et al: Combined influence of ventricular loading and relaxation on the transmitral flow velocity profile in dogs measured by Doppler echocardiography. Circulation 78:672, 1988

100. Labovitz AJ, Lewen MK, Kern M, et al: Evaluation of left ventricular systolic and diastolic dysfunction during transient myocardial ischemia produced by angioplasty. J Am Coll Cardiol 10:748, 1987

101. Bowman LK, Cleman MW, Cabin HS, et al: Dynamics of early and late left ventricular filling determined by Doppler two-dimensional echocardiography during percutaneous transluminal coronary angioplasty. Am J Cardiol 61:541, 1988

102. James TN: Anatomy of the coronary arteries and veins. p. 32. In Hurst JW (ed): The Heart. 4th Ed. McGraw-Hill, New York, 1978

103. Berne RM, Levy MN: Coronary circulation and cardiac metabolism. In Cardiovascular Physiology. 4th Ed. CV Mosby, St. Louis, 1981

104. Hoffman JIE: Determinates and prediction of transmural myocardial perfusion. Circulation 58:381, 1978

105. Hoffman JIE, Buckberg GD: Regional myocardial ischemia — causes, prediction and prevention. Vasc Surg 8:115, 1974

106. Klocke FJ, Ellis AK, Orlick AE: Sympathetic influences on coronary perfusion and evolving concepts of driving pressure, resistance, and transmural flow regulation. Anesthesiology 52:1, 1980

107. Schwartz PJ, Stone HL: Tonic influence of the sympathetic nervous system on myocardial reactive hyperemia and on coronary blood flow distribution in dogs. Circ Res 41:51, 1977

108. Hoffman JIE, Buckberg GD: Pathophysiology of subendocardial ischemia. Br Med J 1:76, 1975

109. Gamble WJ, LaFarge CG, Fyler DC, et al: Regional coronary venous oxygen saturation and myocardial oxygen tension following abrupt changes in ventricular pressure in the isolated dog heart. Circ Res 34:672, 1974

110. Hillis LD, Braunwald E: Myocardial ischemia. N Engl J Med 296:971, 1034, 1093, 1977

111. Hoffman JIE, Buckberg GD: Transmural variations in myocardial perfusion. p. 37. In Yu PN, Goodwin JF (eds): Progress in Cardiology. Lea & Febiger, Philadelphia, 1976

112. Braunwald E: Control of myocardial oxygen consumption: Physiologic and clinical considerations. Am J Cardiol 27:416, 1971

113. Boudoulas H, Rittgers SV, Lewis RP, et al: Changes in diastolic time with various pharmacologic agents. Circulation 60:164, 1979

114. Rubio R, Bene RM: Release of adenosine by the normal myocardium in dogs and its relationship to regulation of coronary resistance. Circ Res 25:407, 1969

115. Feigl EO: Sympathetic control of coronary circulation. Circ Res 20:262, 1967

116. Mudge GH, Grossman W, Mills RM, et al: Reflex increase in coronary vascular resistance in patients with ischemic heart disease. N Engl J Med 295:1333, 1976

117. Feigl EO: Parasympathetic control of coronary blood flow in dogs. Circ Res 25:509, 1969

118. Deanfield JE, Maseri A, Selwyn AP, et al: Myocardial ischemia during daily life in patients with stable angina: Its relation to symptoms and heart rate changes. Lancet 2:753, 1983

119. Cohen DJ, Foley RW, Ryan JM: Intraoperative coronary artery spasm successfully treated with nitroglycerin and nifedipine. Ann Thorac Surg 36:97, 1983

120. Engelman RM, Hadji-Rousou I, Breyer RH, et al: Rebound vasospasm after coronary revascularization in association with calcium antagonist withdrawal. Ann Thorac Surg 37:469, 1984

121. Boulanger M, Maille JG, Pelletier GB, et al: Vasospastic angina after calcium injection. Anesth Analg 63:1124, 1984

122. Gobel FL, Nordstrom LA, Nelson RR, et al: The rate pressure product as an index of myocardial oxygen consumption during exercise in patients with angina pectoris. Circulation 57:549, 1978

123. Sarnoff SJ, Braunwald E, Welsh GH, et al: Hemodynamic determinates of oxygen consumption of the heart with special reference to the tension-time index. Am J Physiol 192:148, 1958

124. Mason DT: Regulation of cardiac performance in clinical heart disease. In Mason DT (ed): Congestive Heart Failure. Yorke Medical Books, New York, 1976

125. Kones RJ, Phillips JH: Reduction in myocardial infarct size: Prevention of heart cell death. South Med J 69:442, 1976

126. Wiggens CJ: Dynamics of ventricular contraction under abnormal conditions (the Henry Jackson Memorial Lecture). Circulation 5:321, 1952

127. Brutsaert DL: The force-velocity-length-time interrelation of

cardiac muscle. In The Physiological Basis of Starling's Law of the Heart. Ciba Foundation Symposium 24. Elsevier/ North-Holland, Amsterdam, 1974

128. Bonner J: Clinical use of pulmonary artery (Swan-Ganz) catheter. Anesthesiol Rev July:26, 1977

129. Cohn JN, Franciosa JA: Vasodilator therapy of cardiac failure. N Engl J Med 297:27, 1977

130. Krueger JW: Fundamental mechanisms that govern cardiac function: A short review of sarcomere mechanics. Heart Failure 4:137, 1988

131. Maughan WL: Ventricular pressure-volume relations in heart failure: Ventriculo-vascular coupling. Heart Failure 4:224, 1988

132. Kaplan JA, Craver JM, Jones EL, et al: The role of the intraaortic balloon in cardiac anesthesia and surgery. Am Heart J 98:580, 1979

133. Lorell BH: Left ventricular diastolic pressure-volume relations: Understanding and managing congestive heart failure. Heart Failure 4:206, 1988

134. Gaasch WH, Apstein CS, Levine HJ: Diastolic properties of the left ventricle. p. 143. In Levine HJ, Gaasch WH (eds): The Ventricle. Martinus Nijhoff Publishing, Boston, 1985

135. Hoffman JIE, Buckberg GD: Regional myocardial ischemia —causes, prediction and prevention. Vasc Surg 8:115, 1974

136. Mueller H, Ayres SM, Grace WJ: Principle defects which account for shock following acute myocardial infarction in man: Implications for treatment. Crit Care Med 1:27, 1973

137. Parker JO: Myocardial infarction: Ways to reduce the damage. Resident Staff Physician May:63, 1976

17
HEPATIC PHYSIOLOGY

Mervyn Maze

LIVER BLOOD FLOW

Anatomic Considerations

The liver receives its major blood supply from the portal vein and the hepatic artery. The portal vein is a valveless afferent nutrient vessel of the liver carrying blood from the entire capillary system of the digestive tract, spleen, pancreas, and gallbladder. The hepatic artery is a branch of the celiac axis and at its origin is called the common hepatic artery. The sinusoids are the hepatic capillaries formed by the total merging of the hepatic arterial and portal streams and are the principal blood flow conduit in the liver parenchyma[1] (Fig. 17-1). These vessels are lined by thin endothelial cells, large Kupffer cells, and fat-storing Ito cells. Fenestrations of the endothelium facilitate passage of blood constituents into the space of Disse, thereby gaining access to the hepatic parenchymal cells. Blood flows along the sinusoids to the central vein of the hepatic veins that drain the liver and empty into the inferior vena cava.

The total liver blood flow is between 800 and 1,200 ml/min, of which roughly one-third is supplied by the hepatic artery, with the portal vein supplying the remainder. This represents a total flow of approximately 100 ml/100 g of liver weight.

Measurement of Hepatic Blood Flow

The unique capacity of the liver to remove materials from the circulation means that clearance techniques can be used to measure hepatic blood flow. Clearance is a measure of the overall efficiency of hepatic extraction and is dependent on both the flow and the hepatic cellular function.

If a substance is cleared from the circulation exclusively by the liver, the Fick principle can be used to derive total hepatic blood flow. This clearance technique does not differentiate between blood perfusing the parenchyma and blood flowing through hepatic shunts but represents the sum of both. The most satisfactory substance for this technique has proved to be indocyanine green.[2]

Indicator dilution methods for assessing hepatic blood flow have the advantage over clearance methods in that hepatic function is not a dependent variable.

585

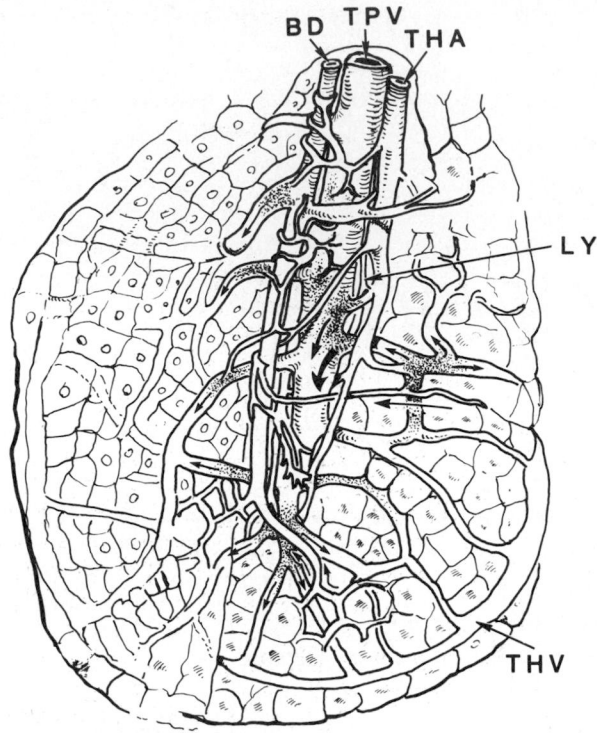

Fig. 17-1. Microcirculatory hepatic unit. The unit consists of the terminal portal venule (TPV), with the sinusoids branching off it and forming a glomus; and the hepatic arteriole (THA), lacing with its branches a plexus around the terminal bile ductule (BD). The arterioles empty (S) into the sinusoids and TPV. The sinusoids run along the outside of cell plates and cords, inside of which are the capillaries of the secretory and excretory systems of the liver. The glomus of sinusoids is drained by at least two terminal hepatic venules (THV). Ly, lymphatics. (Modified from Rappaport,[1] with permission.)

Radiolabeled marker substances, especially iodinated serum albumin, are injected intrasplenically; the flow through the liver is then estimated from indicator dilution curves obtained either by continuous sampling from one hepatic vein or by external γ scintillation counting.[3] This technique is valid when the marker substance is not metabolized by the liver and when there is uniform mixing. Furthermore, allowance for recirculation must be made.[4]

In the single-injection technique, the change in plasma concentration over time is computed after the intravenous injection of a single dose of a test substance that is cleared exclusively by the liver. An elimination curve is then obtained from which the parameter of blood flow is derived in a manner similar to that performed in pharmacokinetic analysis. Radioactive particulate matter such as [198]Au is very efficiently phagocytosed by the reticuloendothelial cells in the liver; the area under the initial curve is used as a measure of blood flow assuming a normally functioning reticuloendothelial system. This estimate of hepatic blood flow most closely approximates the values obtained by the direct electromagnetic method.[5]

The square-wave electromagnetic flow probes are the most reliable direct method for the measurement of hepatic artery and portal vein blood flow.[6] This does require invasive techniques for implantation, which can perturb the system. However, once implanted, these probes can be left in situ, and measurements can then be made in the unanesthetized patient by telemetry. Rarely performed measurements of hemodynamic pressure include percutaneous splenic puncture or intrahepatic parenchymal puncture for portal venous pressure, while intrahepatic arterial pressure is usually reflected by the systemic arterial pressure.

Regulation of Liver Blood Flow

Intrinsic

Pressure-flow autoregulation in the hepatic arterial system exists in the metabolically active (postprandial) but not in the unstimulated (fasted) liver.[7] The basal tone of the resistance vessels is minimal at 80 mmHg and increases as arterial pressure rises, maintaining a fairly stable flow over the physiologic pressure range.[8] Since surgery is most often performed in the fasted stage, it is likely that pressure-flow autoregulation does not exist to any great degree during anesthesia and surgery. In the portal venous vascular bed, there is a linear pressure-flow relationship. This reflects the fact that the portal venous inflow is principally determined by the outflow from the intestine and the spleen. The portal venous pressure is the more likely regulated variable, and this remains constant over a wide range in flow in the healthy liver.[9] This state of affairs prevents an extreme rise in portal venous pressure that would otherwise impair venous drainage from the spleen and the gastrointestinal tract. Changes in hepatic venous pressure may affect pressure-flow autoregulation. For example, in congestive cardiac failure, elevation in hepatic venous pressure will induce constriction of the hepatic arterioles and a decrease flow through the hepatic arterial vasculature.[10] Conversely, such elevations in hepatic venous pressure will decrease inflow resistance in the portal circuit.[11]

A semi-reciprocal relationship exists between the hepatic artery and the portal vein such that an increase in blood flow through one circuit leads to an increased inflow resistance in the other circuit that tends to maintain the total liver blood flow constant.[12] Thus, when portal venous flow decreases, hepatic arterial resistance decreases and hepatic arterial flow increases. When portal blood flow increases, hepatic arterial resistance increases, producing a decrease in hepatic arterial flow. However, a reduction in hepatic arterial flow is not associated with an increase in portal venous blood flow. Conversely, total occlusion of one inflow circuit reduces the vascular resistance of the other circuit by up to 20 percent.[13] These hemodynamic interactions are quantitatively too small to compensate completely for total deprivation of one inflow circuit. Total hepatic arterial occlusion, which was employed as a putative treatment for portal hypertension, is ineffective unless rearterialization of the liver occurs from the anastomoses of the phrenic arteries.[14] Neither systemic venous nor arterial blood is a substitute for total deprivation of portal inflow, and hepatic necrosis may occur.[15]

Changes in the composition of the portal venous and systemic blood composition will have a profound effect on liver blood flow. Arterial hypoxemia (below a PaO_2 of 30 mmHg) doubles hepatic arterial vascular resistance and produces an initial fall in estimated hepatic blood flow, while systemic hyperoxia is without direct effect.[16] Systemic hypercarbia and associated acidosis increase both the hepatic arterial and portal venous blood flows by a direct effect.[17] Systemic hypocarbia and alkalosis produce the opposite response, with reductions in both portal venous and hepatic arterial blood flow.[18] A decrease in the portal oxygen tension and pH together with an increase in PaO_2 occur during digestion and absorption, resulting in an increase in hepatic arterial blood flow. Postprandial hyperosmolarity increases both hepatic arterial and portal venous blood flow by about 10 percent.[19]

Extrinsic

Stimulation of the outflow of the sympathetic nervous system reduces liver blood flow and blood volume abruptly, and 80 percent of the hepatic blood can be expelled within 20 seconds.[20] The liver in this way represents a major reservoir of whole blood that can be rapidly distributed in a precise and controlled manner in response to the activity of its autonomic innervation. Functional vagal innervation does exist in the dog, but rather than affecting total liver blood flow, it affects regional distribution within the liver by exerting effects on presinusoidal sphincters.[21]

Of the systemic hormones, epinephrine is the most likely to attain vasoactive concentrations physiologically. Both α- and β-adrenoceptors have been pharmacologically demonstrated in the hepatic arterial bed, whereas in the portal vasculature only α-adrenoceptors exist.[22] Thus, epinephrine injected directly into the hepatic artery will initially induce vasoconstriction via the α-adrenoceptors, followed by vasodilation mediated by the β-adrenoceptors; the portal bed will only vasoconstrict in response to intraportal epinephrine. Any action of dopamine on the liver circulation is of little physiologic significance, since any vascular effect it possesses alone would be overwhelmed by the concomitant presence of epinephrine, norepinephrine, and sympathetic activation.[18]

Glucagon causes a graded and long-lasting hepatic arterial vasodilation and can antagonize the hepatic arterial vasoconstrictor responses to a wide range of physiologic stimuli including stressed-induced sympathoadrenal outflow.[23] Vasoactive intestinal polypeptide, secretin, and pentagastrin all cause vasodilation when injected intra-arterially in nanomolar concentrations. No effect is seen on the portal venous response to intraportal injections of these gastrointestinal hormones.[24] Bradykinin, 5-hydroxytryptamine, histamine, and prostaglandins of the E type are present in hepatic blood, but the concentrations necessary to elicit vasoactive effects are not normally attained.[24] Angiotensin II evokes profound vasoconstriction of both hepatic arterial and portal beds together with a significant reduction in mesenteric outflow, and this translates into a substantial reduction in total liver blood flow.[25] Whether administered by the intra-arterial, intraportal, or intravenous routes, vasopressin induces marked splanchnic vasoconstriction; consequently, reduction in venous outflow into the portal system and a reduction in inflow resistance in the portal vasculature seen after vasopressin administration make this hormone very effective in alleviating portal hypertension.[26]

Effects of Anesthesia on Liver Blood Flow

Apart from the specific effects of the individual anesthetics on liver blood flow, one needs to consider the ancillary influences, including surgery[27] and the mode of ventilation. During upper abdominal surgery, total hepatic blood flow can be decreased by up to 60 percent by surgery alone; this is considerably greater than any alteration produced by anesthetics. When ventilation is controlled, portal venous blood flow decreases because of an increase in splanchnic vascular resistance.[28] The application of positive end-expiratory pressure (PEEP) will decrease hepatic blood flow even further by increasing the hepatic venous pressure.[29]

All anesthetics and techniques that decrease cardiac output will produce at least proportional decrements in total hepatic blood flow. In addition, some anesthetics have more specific effects or hepatic blood flow to either mitigate or accentuate these changes. Halothane anesthesia may decrease hepatic blood flow to a greater extent by increasing hepatic arterial resistance.[30] In one study, the effect of enflurane on liver blood flow was similar to that for halothane at equipotent concentrations,[31] while in another study, enflurane was shown to have a more favorable effect than halothane.[32] Isoflurane increases hepatic artery blood flow at both 1 and 2 minimum alveolar concentration (MAC) in contradistinction to halothane (Fig. 17-2).[33] Recently, isoflurane increases in total hepatic blood flow in humans were measured by pulsed Doppler method.[34]

The accumulation of CO_2 during spontaneous ventilation with the volatile anesthetics may induce a paradoxic effect. Since hypercarbia increases sympathetic nervous activity, the indirect effect will be sympathetic vasoconstriction. However, the functional splanchnic denervation caused by the ganglion-blocking properties of halothane will result in the direct effect of hyper-

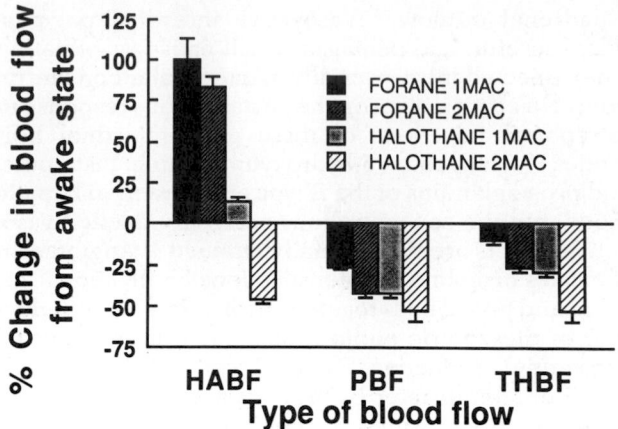

Fig. 17-2. Comparative effects of halothane, 1 MAC (▦), halothane, 2 MAC (▨), forane, 1 MAC (■), and forane, 2 MAC (▨) on hepatic arterial (HABF), portal (PBF), and total hepatic (THBF) blood flows in chronically instrumented dogs. (Modified from Gelman et al.,[33] with permission.)

carbia predominating, resulting in splanchnic vasodilation.[35]

When hepatic blood flow is surgically interrupted by ligation of the hepatic artery, the ensuing histologic liver damage in rats was noted to be much more severe after 1 MAC halothane for 2 hours than was produced by equipotent anesthesia with either enflurane or isoflurane.[36] These animals were pretreated with pentobarbital to effect enzyme induction, a manipulation that can profoundly affect hepatic blood flow.[37] Of the intravenous anesthetics, thiopental, nitrous oxide, and *d*-tubocurarine together with hyperventilation will decrease hepatic blood flow by approximately 30 percent.[28] Neuroleptanesthesia has a similar effect on hepatic blood flow, as does enflurane.[38] Morphine and scopolamine used in premedicant doses were found to exert little effect on liver blood flow.[39] Regional anesthesia will also decrease hepatic blood flow. The extent to which subarachnoid block will decrease hepatic blood flow will depend on the level of the block, and a T4 level of anesthesia will result in a 20 percent reduction in liver blood flow, which closely parallels the drop in systemic blood pressure.[40] The effects of induced hypotension on liver blood flow have also been examined. When the mean arterial blood pressure is decreased by 40 percent with a sodium nitroprusside infusion, there is no net change in liver blood flow, although there is an inversion in the contributions from the portal and hepatic vascular beds.[41] However, when more profound hypotension is induced with trimethaphan to levels of ±20 mmHg, ischemic injury does ensue.[42] Although all forms of anesthesia do decrease liver blood flow, there is also a decrease in oxygen requirements by the liver such that anoxic metabolism does not routinely occur.[43]

DRUG BIOTRANSFORMATION

Most xenobiotics contain lipophilic functional groups to facilitate penetration of membrane barriers, thereby expediting intestinal absorption. Excretion of these compound in the underivatized state would occur quite slowly owing to a high degree of protein binding and because of renal tubular reabsorption. Thus, a function of drug biotransformation is to render molecules more polar so that the products can be efficiently eliminated. Drug metabolism is primarily a hepatic event, although this also occurs in the kidney and to a lesser extent in the intestine, lung, and skin. The dominant role of the liver in metabolism relates to its location, which facilitates access to compounds absorbed from the intestine. By converting lipophilic substances to excretable metabolites, hepatic enzymes detoxify drugs by terminating their pharmacologic activity. Unfortunately, reactive intermediates, which themselves are responsible for some toxic effects, may be formed during metabolism.

Enzymatic Reactions

The enzymatic reactions involved in hepatic drug metabolism may be divided into functionalization reactions[44] (phase I) and conjugation or synthetic reactions (phase II). Phase I reactions often generate reactive species because they introduce carboxyl, epoxide, or hydroxyl groups into the parent compound. Phase II reactions are catalyzed by transferase enzymes in which the chemical groups generated by phase I reactions serve as receptors of polar substances such as acetate, amino acids, sulfate, glucuronic acid, and glutathione[45] (Table 17-1). The products of phase II reactions are usually less toxic and less biologically active than those of the parent compound. Furthermore, the water solubility of the phase II products is enhanced beyond that achieved by phase I reactions alone.

Phase I Reactions

Oxidation is the most common form of drug biotransformation, accounting for more than 90 percent of all reactions. It is catalyzed by the cytochrome P-450 system and to a lesser extent by the mixed function oxidases; for the latter, substrate specificity is limited to nitrogen- and sulfur-containing compounds. The P-450 oxidation system is an electron transport chain with a final cytochromal receptor associated primarily with membranes of the endoplasmic reticulum. The cytochromes, which are heme-containing proteins, are termed either P-450 or P-448, depending on the wavelength of the maximal absorption spectrum after carbon monoxide binding.[46] The net effect of oxidation by the P-450 system is that the oxygen molecule is split, one atom is reduced to water, and the second is incorporated into the product.[47] Many of the reductive path-

TABLE 17-1. Major Routes of Drug Metabolism

Functionalization Reactions	Examples
Oxidations	
Aliphatic hydroxylation $R \cdot CH_2R' \longrightarrow R \cdot CHOH \cdot R'$ (alcohol)	Thiopentone, methohexitone, pentazocine, pethidine, glutethionine, doxapram
Aromatic hydroxylation $R \cdot C_6H_5 \longrightarrow R \cdot C_6H_4 \cdot OH$ (phenol)	Chlorpromazine, lignocaine, bupivacaine, mepivacaine, pethidine, phenobarbitone, glutethimide
O-Dealkylation $R \cdot O \cdot CH_2R' \longrightarrow [R \cdot O \cdot CHOH \cdot R'] \longrightarrow R \cdot OH + R' \cdot CHO$ (ether) (alcohol) (aldehyde)	Phenacetin, codeine, metnoxyflurane, fluoroxene
N-Dealkylation $R \cdot NHCH_2R' \longrightarrow [R \cdot NHCHOH \cdot R'] \longrightarrow R \cdot NH_2 + R' \cdot CHO$ (2° amine) (1° amine) (aldehyde) $R_2N \cdot CH_2R' \longrightarrow [R_2N \cdot CHOH \cdot R'] \longrightarrow R_2NH + R' \cdot CHO$ (3° amine) (2° amine) (aldehyde)	Ephedrine, isoprenaline Lignocaine, mepivacaine, bupivacaine, etidocaine, pethidine, chlorpromazine, pethidine, ketamine, fentanyl, morphine, codeine, atropine, methadone, propoxyphene, diazepam (ring amide)
S-Dealkylation $R \cdot S \cdot CH_2R' \longrightarrow [R \cdot S \cdot CHOH \cdot R'] \longrightarrow R \cdot SH + R' \cdot CHO$ (sulfide) (thiol) (aldehyde)	Methitural
N-Oxidation $R \cdot NH_2 \longrightarrow R \cdot NHOH$ (1° amine) (hydroxylamine) $R_3 \cdot N \longrightarrow R_3N \longrightarrow O$ (3° amine)(amine oxide)	Norpethidine Chlorpromazine, tetracaine, morphine, pethidine
S-Oxidation $R \cdot S \cdot R' \longrightarrow R \cdot \overset{\overset{\displaystyle O}{\|}}{S} \cdot R'$ (sulfide) (sulfoxide)	Chlorpromazine

Deamination (equivalent to N-dealkylation)
$R_2CH \cdot NHR' \longrightarrow [R_2CHOH \cdot NHR'] \longrightarrow R_2CO + R' \cdot NH_2$
(amine)   (carbinolamine)   (aldehyde (amine or
                                  or ketone) ammonia)
             $R_2C{=}NOH$
             (oxime)
	Amphetamine

Desulfuration $R \cdot \overset{\overset{\displaystyle S}{\|}}{C} \cdot R' \longrightarrow \left[R \cdot \overset{\overset{\displaystyle S \cdot OH}{\|}}{C} \cdot R' \right] \longrightarrow R \cdot \overset{\overset{\displaystyle O}{\|}}{C} \cdot R'$ (thioketone) (ketone)	Thiobarbiturates
Dehalogenation (X = Cl or Br) $R \cdot CH(X)_2 \longrightarrow \left[R \cdot \overset{\overset{\displaystyle OH}{\|}}{C}(X)_2 \right] \longrightarrow R \cdot COOH$ (alkylidene halide) (carboxylic acid)	Halothane, methoxyflurane, enflurane
Reductions	
Azo reduction $R \cdot N{=}N \cdot R' \longrightarrow R \cdot NH_2 + R' \cdot NH_2$ (1° amines)	Fazadinium
Nitro reduction $R \cdot NO_2 \longrightarrow R \cdot NH_2$ (1° amine)	Nitrazepam
Carbonyl reduction $R \cdot CO \cdot R' \longrightarrow R \cdot CHOH \cdot R'$ (ketone) (alcohol)	Prednisone
Alcohol dehydrogenase $R \cdot CH_2OH \longrightarrow R \cdot CHO$ (aldehyde) $R \cdot CH(OH)_2 \longrightarrow R \cdot CH_2OH$ (alcohol)	Ethanol Chloral hydrate

Continued

TABLE 17-1. *(continued)*

Functionalization Reactions	Examples

Hydrolyses

Ester hydrolysis $R \cdot COOR' \longrightarrow R \cdot COOH + R'OH$
(carboxylic acid) (alcohol)

Examples: Acetylsalicylic acid, procaine, chloroprocaine, tetracaine, cocaine, suxamethonium, propanidid, pethidine, etomidate, pancuronium[a]

Amide hydrolysis $R \cdot CONHR' \longrightarrow R \cdot COOH + R'NH_2$
(carboxylic acid) (amine)

Examples: Prilocaine, lignocaine, etidocaine, fentanyl

Glucuronide conjugation

O-Glucuronides

$\left.\begin{array}{l} R \cdot OH \text{ (alcohol)} \\ R \cdot C_6H_4OH \text{ (phenol)} \end{array}\right\} + UDPGA \xrightarrow{\text{UDP-glucuronyltransferase}} \left\{\begin{array}{l} R \cdot Ogluc. \\ R \cdot C_6H_4Ogluc. \end{array}\right.$ $+ UDP$

Examples: Oxazepam, paracetamol, morphine, codeine, nalorphine, naloxone

N-Glucuronides

$\left.\begin{array}{l} R \cdot C_6H_4 \cdot NH_2 \text{ (amine)} \\ R \cdot SO_2NH \cdot R' \text{ (sulfonamide)} \end{array}\right\} + UDPGA \xrightarrow{\text{UDP-glucuronyltransferase}} \left\{\begin{array}{l} R \cdot C_6H_4NHgluc. \\ R \cdot SO_2NR' \\ \quad\quad\quad | \\ \quad\quad\quad gluc. \end{array}\right.$ $+ UDP$

Sulfate conjugation

$\left.\begin{array}{l} R \cdot OH \text{ (alcohol)} \\ R \cdot C_6H_4OH \text{ (phenol)} \end{array}\right\} + PAPS \xrightarrow{\text{sulfokinase}} \left\{\begin{array}{l} R \cdot OSO_3H \\ R \cdot C_6H_4O \cdot SO_3H \end{array}\right.$ $+ ADP$

Examples: Paracetamol, morphine, isoprenaline

Acetylation

$\left.\begin{array}{l} R \cdot C_6H_4 \cdot NH_2 \text{ (amine)} \\ R \cdot SO_2NHR' \text{ (sulfonamide)} \end{array}\right\} \xrightarrow{\text{ATP/CoA}} \left\{\begin{array}{l} R \cdot C_6H_4 \cdot NHCOCH_3 \\ R \cdot SO_2 \cdot NR' \\ \quad\quad\quad | \\ \quad\quad\quad COCH_3 \end{array}\right.$

Examples: Procainamide

Methylation

$\left.\begin{array}{l} R \cdot C_6H_4OH \text{ (phenol)} \\ R \cdot NH_2 \text{ (amine)} \end{array}\right\} + SAM \xrightarrow{\text{methyltransferase}} \left\{\begin{array}{l} R \cdot C_6H_4OCH_3 \\ R \cdot NHCH_3 \end{array}\right.$

Examples: Morphine; Norepinephrine

Conjugation with amino acids

$R \cdot C_6H_4 \cdot COOH + glycine \longrightarrow R \cdot C_6H_4 \cdot CONHCH_2COOH$
(carboxylic acid)   (hippuric acid)

Examples: Salicylic acid

Conjugation with glutathione

$R \cdot C_6H_5 + GSH \longrightarrow R \cdot C_6H_4 \cdot S \cdot CH_2CH(COOH) \cdot NHCOCH_3$
(mercapturic acid)

Examples: Paracetamol

[a] Equivalent to deacetylation.
Cofactors: UDPGA, uridine diphosphate glucuronic acid; PAPS, adenosine-3'-phosphate-5'-phosphosulfate; GSH, glutathione; SAM, S-adenosylmethionine; ATP/CoA, adenosine triphosphate/acetylcoenzyme A.
(Modified from Tucker,[45] with permission.)

ways in the liver are also catalyzed by cytochrome P-450, including those for epoxide reduction, reductive dehalogenation, nitro reduction, and microsomal azo reduction.[48] The reduction of aldehydes and ketones is catalyzed by a family of pyridine[49] nucleotide-dependent dehydrogenases found in the cellular cytosolic fraction. Two classes of enzymes that catalyze the hydrolytic reactions include the esterases and the epoxide hydrolases. Hydrolysis is an uncommon drug biotransformation reaction that is usually catalyzed by esterases that are synthesized in the liver but often effect hydrolysis in the plasma (e.g., plasma cholinesterases). The products of ester hydrolysis, an acid and an alcohol, are more water soluble than the parent ester and are easily capable of undergoing phase II reactions. Epoxides formed during oxidative metabolism of aromatic and olefinic compounds are relatively reactive compounds capable of binding covalently to proteins and nucleic acids. These epoxides may be detoxified by microsomal hydrolases as well as by conjugation with glutathione.

Phase II Reactions

Frequently, the final step in the metabolism of a foreign compound involves conjugation with a water-soluble metabolite. The most common conjugate encountered is the glucuronic acid adduct catalyzed by UDP-glucuronyltransferase, which is localized to the endoplasmic reticulum. Glutathione, a cysteine-containing tripeptide, is conjugated to xenobiotics by its free thiol group. This reaction is catalyzed by glutathione-*s*-transferase but can occur, albeit at a slower rate, in its absence. Glutathione is able to attach at electrophilic intermediates; occasionally these electrophilic intermediates are able to react spontaneously with thiol groups on proteins and with amine centers on nucleic acids. The glutathione-*s*-transferases ensure that highly reactive molecules are rapidly conjugated with glutathione, thus preventing toxic reactions. Under adverse conditions (e.g., starvation), the available gluthione substrate may be rapidly depleted,[50] so that potentially toxic compounds accumulate. Administration of cysteamine (mercaptoethylamine) or *N*-acetylcysteine (glutathione precursors) enhances the rate of synthesis of glutathione and is effective in combatting the toxicity of certain electrophilic compounds. Cytosolic sulfotransferases catalyze the sulfation reaction of alcohols, bile acids, and a wide range of phenolic compounds.

The cystolic enzyme catechol-*o*-methyltransferase is the prototype of enzymes catalyzing methylation reaction. Methylation reactions actually decrease water solubility, although they do detoxify the compounds. Acetylation of amine-containing drugs is another example of a phase II reaction that results in a less soluble metabolite. Acetylating capacity in human liver reveals polymorphism with both slow and rapid acetylators.[51] Amino acid conjugation, primarily of aromatic carboxylic acids, differs in two important respects. This reaction is catalyzed in the mitochondria and before the conjugation can occur, the xenobiotic must be activated to the coenzyme A-thiol adduct.

Perfusion Model of Hepatic Drug Elimination

During the last 10 years, perfusion models of hepatic drug elimination have been advanced to focus attention on the physiologic variables that can influence hepatic drug elimination.[52] Not only does this model address the important determinants of hepatic drug disposition such as hepatic blood flow, intrinsic hepatic clearance, and protein binding,[53] but it weighs the importance of a specific variable depending on whether the drug is efficiently or poorly extracted by the liver. Thus, elimination of a drug that has a high extraction ratio will be influenced more directly by changes in hepatic blood flow than by changes in intrinsic hepatic clearance or protein binding. While elimination may not be affected by changes in protein binding, it is important to remember that changes in protein binding of highly extracted drugs may alter their pharmacologic effect. The disposition of poorly extracted drugs is more sensitive to changes in the intrinsic ability of the liver to eliminate a drug and in binding of the drug to blood constituents than it is to hepatic blood flow. A compilation of

TABLE 17-2. Drugs That Are Efficiently or Poorly Extracted from the Blood by the Liver

Efficiently Extracted Drugs	Poorly Extracted Drugs
Lidocaine	Acetaminophen
Meperidine	Amobarbital
Morphine	Antipyrine
Nortriptyline	Chloramphenical
Pentazocine	Chlordiazepoxide
Propoxyphene	Chlorpromazine
Popranolol	Clindamycin
	Diazepam
	Digitoxin
	Hexobarbital
	Phenytoin
	Quinidine
	Theophyline
	Tolbutamide
	Warfarin

(Modified from Williams and Bonet,[54] with permission.)

frequently employed drugs with high and low extraction ratios are tabulated in Table 17-2.[54]

Factors Affecting Hepatic Drug Metabolism

More than 300 compounds, including drugs, insecticides, organic solvents, carcinogens, and other environmental contaminants, are known to stimulate some type of microsomal xenobiotic-metabolizing activity.[55] These enzyme-inducing compounds result in an increase in the cellular amount of ribonucleic acid (RNA) coding for the appropriate enzyme in the cell. Clinical effects of enzyme induction only become apparent when the rate-controlling step in detoxification or elimination is affected. However, induction may have major effects in enhancing the metabolism of xenobiotics to toxic intermediates. For example, isoniazid will enhance defluorination of enflurane, thereby increasing the risk of fluoride nephrotoxicity. The rate and manner in which an individual metabolizes drugs are determined in part by genetic factors,[56] but these are rarely apparent unless they result in toxicity. For example, decreased rates of isoniazid metabolism through differences in *N*-acetyltransferase activity (slow acetylators) in the liver may result in peripheral neuropathies.

Delayed development of xenobiotic metabolism in fetal liver, which extends into the newborn period, has a protective role. Polar compounds that would otherwise be the product of xenobiotic metabolic reactions in the liver would accumulate in the fetus because of lack of transfer across the fetoplacental barrier. The cytochrome P-450 content in the liver of newborns is only 28 percent of what is normally present. Phase II reaction rates are exceedingly slow, as reflected by the development of neonatal hyperbilirubinemia because of delayed development of bilirubin-UDP-glucuronyltransferase. At the other end of the life cycle there appear to be decreased metabolic rates for meperidine[57] and amylobarbital.[58] More often the cause of increased plasma half-lives of drugs in geriatric patients is due to changes in drug distribution rather than in metabolism.[59]

A number of factors in the perioperative period are known to decrease hepatic drug-metabolizing activity, including inflammation,[60] fever,[61] and the infusion of nitrogen-free[62] and nitrogen-rich[63] solutions. On the other hand, in the recumbent position hepatic blood flow will increase by up to 50 percent, thereby increasing clearance of flow-dependent drugs.

Effects of Anesthesia on Drug Metabolism

Ketamine is capable of inducing its own metabolism, which may account for the rapid development of tolerance to this agent.[64] Diazepam has been reported to both increase and decrease its own metabolism.[65]

Anesthetics capable of decreasing hepatic blood flow will influence the clearance of perfusion-dependent drugs with high extraction ratios. More important, the volatile anesthetics, especially halothane, inhibit drug biotransformation by direct effects on the cytochrome P-450 and glucuronyltransferase systems. Halothane impairs the metabolism of phenytoin,[66] warfarin,[67] and ketamine.[68] Halothane anesthesia also decreases the metabolism of enflurane in rats, possibly by competing for the same drug-metabolizing sites on microsomal enzymes.[69] However, a noncompetitive inhibitory role for halothane in drug metabolism has also been advanced.[70] Fentanyl clearance is also decreased by concomitant halothane administration, possibly by its effect on hepatic blood flow,[71] and similar findings have been noted with verapamil[72] and propranolol clearance during halothane anesthesia.[73] In isolated rat hepatocytes, halothane and enflurane were both found to inhibit the metabolism of acetaminophen, antipyrine, and sulfanilamide in a dose-dependent manner over a clinically relevant range.[74] However, in a study involving chronic exposure of humans to trace anesthetic concentrations of halothane, Duvaldestin et al.[75] demonstrated a 29 percent increase in antipyrine metabolism, which is highly suggestive of enzyme induction. Subsequent animal data suggest that it is the cytochrome c reductase activity that is most likely to be altered by chronic low-level exposure.[76]

METABOLIC FUNCTION

Protein

The liver is the major site of amino acid metabolism. It involves two different reactions: (1) breakdown of amino acids to form substrates for the carbohydrate and fat metabolic pathways, and (2) synthesis of a large number of biologically essential proteins.

Albumin, the major protein in human serum, accounts for 15 percent of the total hepatic protein synthesis. Albumin synthesis ranges from 120 to 300 mg/kg/d. The higher figure is noted in the neonatal liver, and there is a progressive decline in the synthetic rate with age.[77] Factors that regulate albumin synthesis include dietary availability of amino acids,[78] hormonal balance, and plasma oncotic pressure.[79] Intravascular albumin accounts for about 40 percent of the exchangeable albumin pool, and in this location it exerts its principal function—maintenance of normal oncotic pressure. A variety of substances bind to albumin in the serum, and as such albumin is an important transport vehicle for drugs, hormones, metals, and metabolites. The half-life of albumin is approximately 20 days, so that a decrease in serum albumin is unlikely to occur within a short period of acute liver injury. In patients with ascites and chronic liver disease, the total exchangeable pool of albumin may be normal, but the serum level is often low.[80]

The vitamin K-dependent coagulation factors II, VII, IX, and X are synthesized in the liver together with factors V, XI, XII, XIII and fibrinogen, which are not dependent on vitamin K for synthesis. If the fat-soluble vitamin K is deficient, as in obstructive jaundice, or is antagonized by one of the coumadin anticoagulants, then the coagulation factors are synthesized at the normal rate, but they lack the γ-carboxylglutamic acid residues, which are attached as a post-translational event under the influence of vitamin K. Thus, immunologically similar but functionally inactive proteins appear in the plasma of subjects deficient in vitamin K or treated with one of the coumadin anticoagulants.[81] The half-lives of the coagulation factors are relatively short; thus, abnormalities in coagulation quickly become apparent in acute liver damage. The actual level of clotting factors in the plasma represents a balance between synthesis and catabolism, and since the liver also synthesizes inhibitors of both coagulation and fibrinolysis, a combination of decreased synthesis and increased removal may arise in acute liver disease. Thus, prothrombin time (deficiency of factors II, V, VII, and X) is prolonged in parenchymal liver disease. Used as a liver function test, the prothrombin time has proved of some value in predicting the outcome of patients suffering from acute liver cell failure after hepatotoxin ingestion.[82]

Ceruloplasmin, the copper-containing α-globulin, is synthesized in the liver. The plasma level is increased in biliary cirrhosis, Hodgkin's disease, pregnancy, and myocardial infarction, and as such it is considered an acute-phase reactant protein.[83] Decreased levels of ceruloplasmin are found in Wilson's disease, while there is a nonselective diminution of this protein together with other proteins in acute liver failure and in the nephrotic syndrome. The major function for ceruloplasmin is the transport of copper. Additionally, it can also function as a monoamine oxidase, and in this role may exert an effect on the degradation of circulating biogenic amines such as norepinephrine and 5-hydroxytryptamine.

The liver is also the principal site for haptoglobin synthesis. The major function of this glycoprotein is to form a strong, stable complex with hemoglobin that has been released from senescent erythrocytes. In this way haptoglobin fosters recycling and conservation of heme iron. Haptoglobin is not considered a true transport protein, since the entire haptoglobin-hemoglobin complex is extracted and metabolized by the liver. Changes in haptoglobin levels are not uniform in liver disease, since the levels rise in inflammatory liver disease and in obstructive jaundice, while low values are seen in severe liver disease. In hemolytic crises, the extraction of the haptoglobin-hemoglobin complex is more rapid than the maximal rate of haptoglobin synthesis, so that the circulating level of haptoglobin falls.

Other proteins synthesized by the liver include α-antitrypsin, which is responsible for 90 percent of the antitrypsin activity of serum; α-macroglobulin, which is a protease inhibitor; antithrombin III, which inhibits all the proteases of the intrinsic coagulation system and whose activity is greatly enhanced by heparin; and α-acidglycoprotein, C-reactive protein, and transferrin, the iron transport protein. Disturbances in liver function can significantly affect the production of these proteins, but deficiencies in synthesis alone rarely cause appreciable clinical problems.

Breakdown of amino acids by transamination and oxidative deamination leads to the formation of keto acids, ammonia, and glutamine within the liver. The Krebs-Henseleit urea cycle converts the ammonia and most of the other nitrogen excretory products into urea. Both severe acute and chronic liver disease are characterized by a failure to synthesize urea, as a result of which its blood concentration is significantly reduced. There is also an excessive accumulation of ammonia that in some way contributes to the encephalopathy often noted in hepatic failure.[84]

Carbohydrates

The liver is especially important for maintaining a normal blood glucose in the circulation, especially after a carbohydrate meal, and also for releasing glucose into the bloodstream during a diurnal fast or sustained exercise.[85] The rate of uptake or release of glucose by the liver is proportional to the degree of hypoglycemia or hyperglycemia, and thus the blood glucose concentration determines whether the liver is a glucose-producing or glucose-using organ.

The liver responds to conditioning of carbohydrate deprivation by increasing the rate of glucose production from endogenous sources. Liver glycogen is degraded to provide glucose, which is then released into the blood. Glycogen metabolism within the liver is regulated by two rate-limiting enzymes: (1) glycogen synthase, which synthesizes chains of glucose residues from UDP-glucose units, and (2) glycogen phosphorylase, which degrades glycogen, one glucose residue at a time, to glucose 1-phosphate[86] (Fig. 17-2). The activity of these two enzymes depends on whether they exist in the phosphorylated or dephosphorylated form, which itself is a function of the activity of cyclic adenosine monophosphate (cAMP)-dependent protein kinase. Glucagon will also increase the gluconeogenic rate by facilitating transport of both alanine across the liver cell membrane and pyruvate across the inner mitochondrial membrane. Catecholamines probably stimulate the rate of gluconeogenesis via cAMP-dependent (β-mimetic) and cAMP-independent (α-mimetic) mechanisms.[87] Insulin antagonizes the action of both glucagon and catecholamines on hepatic gluconeogenesis. After glycogen stores in the liver have been exhausted by starvation (± 24 hours) or prolonged exercise, the only remaining endogenous source of glucose is by gluconeogenesis using lactate, glycerol, and certain amino acids (especially alanine and glutamine) as precursors. The action of glucagon and catechlomines on the gluconeogenic pathway is mediated by an increase in the cAMP concentration and therefore an increase in the activity of cAMP-dependent protein kinase.[88]

Fat

Lipid reaches the liver via the lymph and the blood in the form of chylomicrons, where it is broken down by stepwise degradation to acetylcoenzyme A (acetyl-CoA). This is a key molecule in a number of metabolic processes involving fat in the tricarboxylic acid cycle or the synthesis of triglyceride, phospholipid, cholesterol, and lipoproteins. Glucose calories in excess of those needed to saturate hepatic glycogen stores as well as the other pathways for its disposition are converted very efficiently to fatty acids in the liver. Acetyl-CoA carboxylase is the rate-limiting fatty acid-synthesizing enzyme.[89] In addition to the dynamic regulation of the enzyme, the supply of its substrate is shut off by the same conditions that lead to a decrease in its activity, such as fasting. The two pathways available for the metabolic disposal of fatty acids in the liver are esterification and oxidation[90] (Fig. 17-3). Oxidation occurs in the fasted state when the hepatic concentration of malonyl-CoA falls.[91] Glucagon markedly stimulates the rate of fatty acid oxidation in liver, whereas insulin inhibits this. The β-oxidation of fatty acids proceeds to acetyl-CoA in the mitochondria, where the acetyl-CoA is further oxidized in the tricarboxylic acid cycle to CO_2 and H_2O or is converted to ketone bodies. However, the liver lacks the enzyme required for oxidation of ketones, which is present in abundance in most other tissues. The amount of ketosis in the fasted state is self-limited, since ketones stimulate insulin secretion from the pancreas,[92] limiting lipolysis in adipose tissue and thus liver availability and oxidation of fatty acids. This fail-

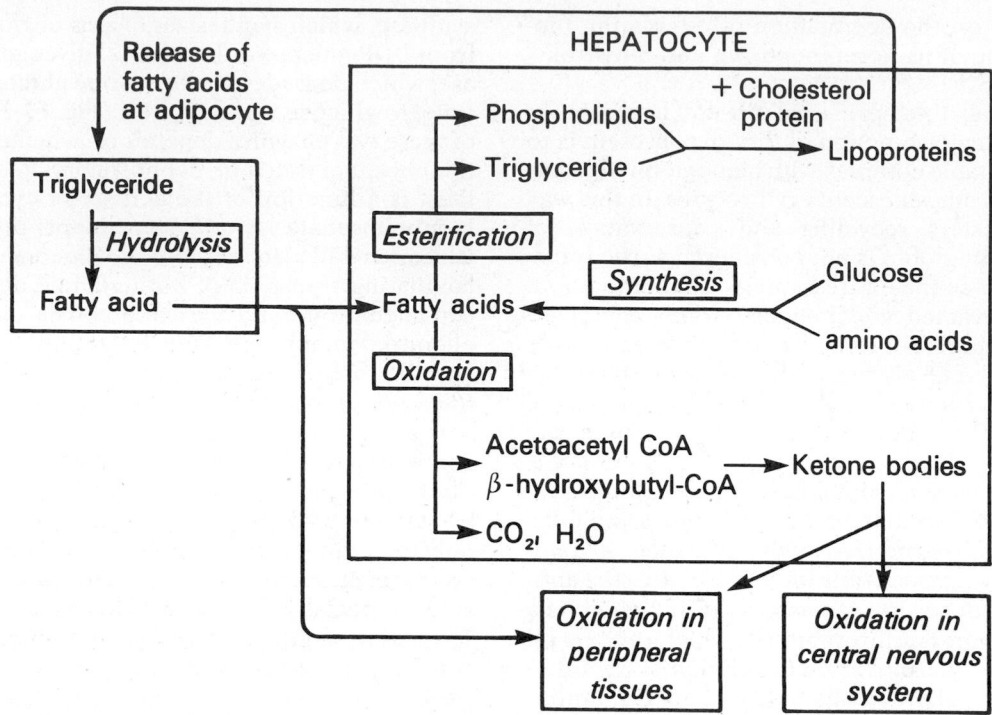

Fig. 17-3. Liver-adipose cycle for the storage and metabolism of fatty acids. (Modified from Zakim,[90] with permission.)

safe mechanism is obviously lacking in states of insulin deficiency.

Fatty acids are esterified in the liver with glycerol to form triglycerides, which are then incorporated into lipoproteins, principally very low density lipoprotein (VLDL), which are secreted by the liver. The principal factor affecting VLDL production is the amount of free fatty acids reaching the liver. Secretion of VLDL is also stimulated by insulin[93] and estrogens.[94]

The liver is the most active site of cholesterol biosynthesis, although virtually every mammalian cell can synthesize cholesterol at some point in its life cycle.[95] The step that is usually rate determining in cholesterol biosynthesis occurs when the CoA is cleaved from β-hydroxy-β-methylglutaryl-coenzyme A (HMG-CoA). This reaction is catalyzed by HMG-CoA reductase. Factors that have been reported to affect hepatic cholesterol synthesis are tabulated[95] (Table 17-3). Cholesterol is secreted in the form of lipoproteins, and extrahepatically it is a substrate for hormone and membrane synthesis. Two other processes important in cholesterol metabolism and unique to the liver are its catabolism to bile acids and the elimination of the native compound by secretion into the bile. The rate-limiting step in formation of bile acid is cholesterol's conversion to the 7 α-hydroxylated derivative, reaction catalyzed by 7 α-hydroxylase. The bile acids are then conjugated to either taurine or glycine in the liver to form salts and are excreted in the bile, where the bile salts facilitate intes-

tinal fat absorption through their emulsifying properties.

Bilirubin

About 300 mg of bilirubin is formed daily, mostly from the destruction of senescent erythrocytes. The heme part of the myoglobin molecule is converted to bilirubin and is carried to the liver tightly bound to albumin. Within the liver cell bilirubin is conjugated with glucuronic acid. Unlike unconjugated bilirubin, the conjugated form is nontoxic, and the pigment is now readily

TABLE 17-3. Factors Reported to Affect Hepatic Cholesterol Synthesis

Increase	Decrease
Bile fistula	Cholesterol feeding
Cholestyramine	Bile acid feeding
Ileal resection	Oxygenated sterols
Fat feeding	Fasting
Fatty acid infusion	Protein synthesis inhibitors
Thyroid hormone	Clofibrate
Corticosteroids	Nicotinic acid
Adrenergic agents	Masculine gender
Glucagon	Aging
Triton WR1339	
X-irradiation	
Nephrosis	

(Modified from Cooper,[95] with permission.)

secreted by the liver into the bile and thence alimentary tract. A small portion of the conjugated bilirubin formed by the hepatic cells returns to the plasma, either directly into the liver sinusoids or indirectly by absorption into the blood from the bile ducts or lymphatics. Appreciable amounts of conjugated bilirubins in plasma virtually always reflect defective hepatic secretion, which in the presence of minor liver damage may occur without increasing the plasma level of total bilirubins to more than 1 mg/dl.[96]

Effects of Anesthesia on Hepatic Metabolism

In response to fasting and surgical trauma, there is an increase in the circulating concentrations of catabolic hormones such as catecholamines, glucagon, and cortisol and a concomitant decrease in plasma concentrations of the anabolic hormones insulin and testosterone. These endocrine changes result in substrate mobilization and ultimately produce a catabolic state with negative nitrogen balance. There is an increase in protein degradation with a concomitant rise in urea production and excretion and a decrease in protein synthesis from surgical trauma.[97] The severity of these changes largely depends on the extent of the surgery and the initial status.[98] Hypoglycemia is a ubiquitous associant of surgery, but whether this is due to increased hepatic glycogenolysis is in dispute. Hepatic fat metabolism is little affected by surgery. Inasmuch as anesthetic agents can affect the release of these stress hormones they will alter hepatic metabolism. If the afferent neurogenic impulses from the area of surgical trauma are blocked by extradural analgesia, these endocrine-metabolic responses can be greatly attenuated, resulting in improved nitrogen balance. This can be most effectively accomplished with extradural analgesia,[99] with lesser effects noted with halothane,[100] enflurane,[101] morphine,[102] and either thiopental[103] or fentanyl[104] supplementation of nitrous oxide anesthesia.

Few studies have been conducted to determine the direct effects of anesthetics on intermediary metabolism, and those studies that have been done are largely confined to experiments involving halothane. Halothane inhibits the consumption of oxygen, urea synthesis, and gluconeogenesis in the isolated perfused liver.[105] This effect can be abolished when the fatty acid oleate is added to the perfusing medium.[106] Since the major pathways for clearing lactate from the plasma are also inhibited by halothane, there is an increase in lactate levels over and above that normally observed after the addition of fructose to the medium of the isolated perfused liver.[107] More recently, the effect of halothane on protein metabolism has been addressed. Recent studies reveal that exposure to halothane inhibits the peptide chain initiation step in protein synthesis within 15 minutes,[108] while the process of protein secretion is unaffected. In isolated rat hepatocytes, halothane and enflurane, from 0.5 to 2.0 mM, both inhibited protein synthesis in a dose-dependent manner.[74]

TABLE 17-4. Composition of Bile

	Liver Bile	Gallbladder Bile
Water	97.5 g%	95 g%
Bile salts	1.1 g%	6 g%
Bilirubin	0.04 g%	0.3 g%
Cholesterol	0.1 g%	0.3 to 0.9 g%
Fatty Acids	0.12 g%	0.3 to 1.2 g%
Lecithin	0.04 g%	0.3 g%
Na^+	145 mEq/L	130 mEq/L

BILE FORMATION

Bile eliminates many endogenous and exogenous substances (Table 17-4) from the liver while at the same time fulfilling an important function as a digestive fluid.[109] The bile is primarily formed by the hepatocyte (canalicular bile) and is then modified downstream in the ductules, ducts, and gallbladder mucosa by reabsorption and secretion of electrolytes and water. By this process, constituents such as bile salts, cholesterol, and phospholipids become highly concentrated in the gallbladder bile. The capacity of bile to keep cholesterol in solution is limited by the concentration of phospholipids and bile acids, and this can be expressed by a triangular phase diagram[110] (Fig. 17-4). The range of cholesterol concentrations in which the micellar phase is preserved is narrow; relatively small changes in concentration in one of the three compounds can result in supersaturated bile and gallstone formation.

Narcotic agents cause spasms in the Oddi sphincter and a rise in the pressure in the common bile duct.[111] This effect can be largely attenuated by halothane and, to a lesser extent, by enflurane.[112]

HEMATOLOGIC FUNCTION

Erythropoietic activity is largely confined to the liver from the 9th to the 24th week of gestation and continues to be an important site for hematopoiesis until approximately 2 months after birth. However, with the development of the bone marrow, recognizable hematopoietic cells completely disappear from the liver and only persist in the setting of congenital hemolytic anemias. Those cells may reappear in response to bone marrow failure or in the presence of myeloproliferative disorders. Heme is synthesized predominantly in the bone marrow and the liver by way of porphyrin metabolites. Patients with acute hepatic porphyrias have a defect in hepatic heme synthesis and may have their illness exacerbated by many anesthetic agents including barbiturates, benzodiazepines, ketamine, pentazocine, and halothane.[113]

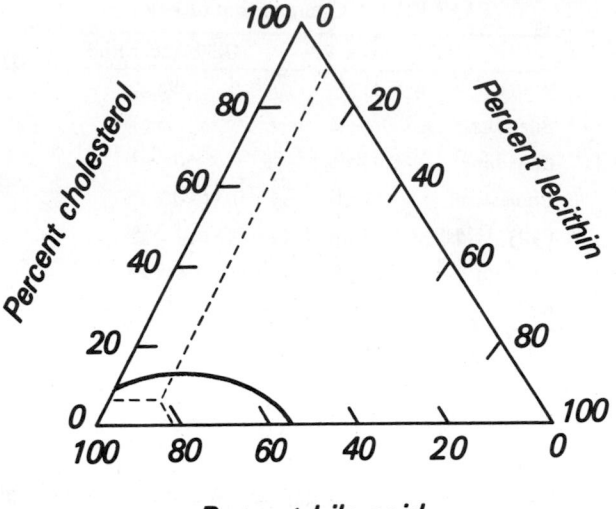

Fig. 17-4. Triangular coordinates used to plot the composition of bile in terms of its content of cholesterol, lecithin (phospholipid), and bile salts. The point joined by the dotted lines represents a mixture of 5 percent cholesterol, 15 percent lecithin, and 80 percent bile salts. A bile sample with this composition lies in the micellar zone and is undersaturated with cholesterol. Bile samples above the curved line are supersaturated and contain crystals. (Modified from Admirand and Small,[110] with permission.)

HUMORAL FUNCTION

The liver plays a vital role in the biotransformation of many hormones. The liver is the major site for degradation of insulin, and fully 50 percent of insulin secreted by the pancreas is degraded by the liver in a single passage and never reaches the systemic circulation.[114] Thyroxine (T_4), the major secretary product of the thyroid gland, is actively taken up by the liver, where it is further activated by its conversion to triiodothyronine (T_3) and can also be inactivated. In addition, the liver synthesizes the plasma proteins that bind the thyroid hormones. Thus, the liver can influence the distribution of the thyroid hormones between the intracellular and extracellular compartments. Aldosterone, estrogens, androgens, and antidiuretic hormone (ADH) are all inactivated by the liver; thus, the presence of liver disease will result in profound endocrine abnormalities.

IMMUNOLOGIC FUNCTION

The liver is the largest organ in the reticuloendothelial system, for as much as 10 percent of the liver weight is derived from the Kupffer cell mass. Teleologically, the importance of this system relates to its ability to phagocytose antigens absorbed from the gastrointestinal tract, acting as a filter for the systemic circulation.

EVALUATION OF LIVER FUNCTION

Clinical Tests

The clinical evaluation of the liver and biliary tract should include a complete history and physical examination with appropriate laboratory tests to identify subclinical abnormalities and to define the disease process at a higher level of resolution. Particular attention in the history should be devoted to information regarding drug and alcohol intake: exposure to chemicals, toxic agents, and jaundiced persons; receipt of injections and transfusions; family history of liver or biliary tract disease; itch, jaundice, abdominal pain, and indigestion; and alteration in stool or urine color. Physical examination should concentrate on establishing the size and texture of the liver and spleen, detection of jaundice, ascites, collateral portal circulation, spider angiomata, hepatic encephalopathy, and fetor hepaticus.

Laboratory Tests

The plasma activity of the *S*-aminotransferases is due to the release of intracellular protein from injured cells from a variety of organs, especially the liver, heart, skeletal muscle, adipose tissue, brain, and kidney. Because of the ubiquity of the aminotransferases, the use of the serum level of these enzymes has been questioned. Liver-specific enzymes, such as ornithine carbamyl dehydrogenase and alcohol dehydrogenase, have been used experimentally but are not widely available for clinical application. Serum glutamic oxaloacetic transaminase (SGOT) is also referred to as aspartate aminotransferase (AsT), while serum glutamic pyruvic transaminase (SGPT) is also referred to as alanine aminotransferase (AlT). The enzymatic activity is reported in international units (IU), which is the number of micromoles of substrate transformed per minute. Elevations of serum aminotransferase activity occur with minor cell injury, but there appears to be no dependable correlation between peak enzyme levels reached in an individual and the severity or prognosis of the disease and hence they are not truly tests of liver function. Acute parenchymal lesions are associated with much higher values than are chronic lesions. For example, acute viral hepatitis A or B often produces peak elevations in serial values within the range of 500 to 5,000 IU/L.[115] Nonhepatic diseases such as myocardial infarction, neuromuscular disorders, acute pancreatitis, infarction of the kidney, brain, lung, or limb, and hemolytic anemias as well as the postoperative state may cause modest elevations, usually of the SGOT, with little change in SGPT except in certain rare neuromuscular disorders.

Serum albumin is a good indicator of hepatocyte function, but abnormal distribution, increased plasma volume, and possibly abnormal degradation may also contribute to hypoalbuminemia in liver disease. Serum albumin concentration is a useful index of the severity of cellular dysfunction in chronic liver disease. Changes in synthetic rate only lead to changes in concentration after an appreciable time lag, and therefore the use of this variable for assessing acute liver disease is questionable. Unlike albumin, which has a half-life of approximately 20 days, the half-lives of the liver-derived coagulation factors are very short, ranging from 4 days for fibrinogen to a few hours for factor VII. Thus, a decrease in hepatic synthesis caused by liver damage is quickly reflected in a decrease in the plasma levels of these coagulation factors, which is best tested by an estimation of the prothrombin time. Abnormalities of the prothrombin time indicate impaired hepatic synthesis of some or all of the clotting factors I, II, V, VII, and X. Failure to readily correct this abnormality by administration of vitamin K indicates that severe hepatocellular disease is present and that the impaired absorption of the fat-soluble vitamin from the gastrointestinal tract may be only partially responsible for the clotting abnormality. In acute liver failure, prothrombin time correlates with the degree of encephalopathy.

Dye removal tests with Bromsulfalein, indocyanine green, or rose bengal have been used to test the function of the liver with respect to blood flow, uptake, intracellular binding, metabolic transformation, and biliary excretion. If any of these physiologic functions is disordered, systemic retention of dye will occur. For quantitative assessment of specific functions of the hepatocyte, more complicated techniques can be employed, including galactose elimination and bile acid disappearance tests.

The functional status of the excretory apparatus of the liver is best assessed by measuring the bilirubin in the serum, which in the majority of the normal population will not exceed 1 mg percent. However, as many as 10 percent of otherwise normal persons have mildly elevated values for serum total bilirubin that are entirely accounted for by an increase in unconjugated bilirubin. These subjects have Gilbert syndrome (benign unconjugated hyperbilirubinemia) and probably represent the lowermost pole of the normal distribution of hepatic bilirubin UDP-glucuronyltransferase in the population. When the serum bilirubin is above 4 mg percent, this abnormality may be detected clinically as a yellow discoloration of body tissues, which is best appreciated in the sclerae by the use of natural light. Conjugated bilirubin in serum indicates dysfunction of either the liver parenchyma or bile ducts. Even in unconjugated hyperbilirubinemia from acute hemolysis there may be an increase in the conjugated fraction. An increase in urine bilirubin indicates the presence of conjugated bilirubin in the serum since unconjugated bilirubin is not excreted by the kidney.

Disturbances in the transport function of the hepatocyte, particularly in regard to the excretion of conjugated bile acids or mechanical obstruction of the biliary tree, cause increased amounts of alkaline phosphase to enter plasma. Since the placenta, bone, and intestines also contribute to alkaline phosphatase activity in the plasma, it is important to identify the tissue of origin when elevated concentrations occur. Procedures available to differentiate the sources of the increased enzyme include simultaneous determination of 5'-nucleotidase or leucine aminopeptidase and/or γ-glutamyl transpeptidase. Despite the fact that 5'-nucleotides can also be found in other tissues such as the placenta, bone, and the aorta, its activity in the serum does not rise during normal pregnancy, during the period of normal bone growth, or in diseases of the bone. In known hepatobiliary diseases, elevations in alkaline phosphatase and 5'-nucleotidase tend to parallel each other, and for these reasons estimates of levels of 5'-nucleotidase in serum are most useful in distinguishing between hepatic and nonhepatic causes of an increase in alkaline phosphatase activity.

Radiologic techniques for demonstrating the biliary tract include percutaneous and endoscopic cholangiography. Percutaneous transhepatic cholangiography is especially of value when dilated bile ducts are present. This technique can safely be used if the biliary system is explored within 4 hours of puncture to a dilated duct or if a drainage system is left in situ. Endoscopic cholangiography is useful in localizing the site of biliary tract disease before surgery. Furthermore, papillotomy via the endoscope can obviate the need for surgical treatment of common bile duct stones. Esophagogastroscopy is a reliable and simple method for detecting submucosal varices in the upper digestive tract. Hepatic venous pressure and measurements are useful in defining the level of block in patients with portal hypertension, while splenoportography delineates the splenic and portal veins. Radionuclide and ultrasonic scanning are useful for detecting space-occupying lesions of the hepatobiliary system. For evaluation of the immunologic status of the patient with suspected liver disease, the presence of high serum gamma globulin is a strong indicator of significant chronic liver disease.

Antinuclear antibody is present in 75 percent of patients with chronic active hepatitis, and the antimitochondrial antibody is present in nearly all cases of primary biliary cirrhosis. α-Fetoprotein is a marker of primary liver cell cancer. Infection with the virus of types A and B hepatitis is associated with the appearance of specific antigens and antibodies in serum.

REFERENCES

1. Rappaport AM: Hepatic blood flow. p. 1. In Javitt NB (ed): Liver and Biliary Test Physiology. University Park Press, Baltimore, 1980
2. Caesar J, Sheldon S, Chiandussi L, et al: The use of indocyanine green in the measurement of hepatic blood flow and as a test of hepatic function. Clin Sci 21:43, 1961
3. Reichman S, Davis WE, Storaasli JP, et al: Measurement of hepatic blood flow by indicator dilution techniques. J Clin Invest 37:1848, 1958
4. Huet P-M, Lavoie P, Viallet A: Simultaneous estimation of

hepatic and portal flows by an indicator dilution technique. J Lab Clin Med 82:836, 1973

5. Szabo G, Benyo I, Sandor J, et al: Estimation of hepatic blood flow in the dog with the Xe and hydrogen washout, Au-colloid uptake techniques and with the electromagnetic flowmeter. Res Exp Med 169:69, 1976

6. Hopkinson BR, Schenk WG: The electromagnetic measurement of liver blood flow and cardiac output in conscious dogs during feeding and exercise. Surgery 63:970, 1968

7. Norris CP, Barnes GE, Smith EE, et al: Autoregulation of superior mesenteric blood flow in fasted and fed dogs. Am J Physiol 237:H174, 1979

8. Greenway CV, Lawson AE, Mellander S: The effects of stimulation of the hepatic nerves, infusions of noradrenaline and occlusion of the carotid artery on liver blood flow in the anaesthetized cat. J Physiol (Lond) 192:21, 1967

9. Richardson PDI, Withrington PG: Liver blood flow. Pflugers Arch 299:311, 1968

10. Lutz J, Peiper U, Bauereisen E: Appearance and size of venovasometer reactions in the liver circulation. Gastroenterology 81:159, 1981

11. Hanson KM, Johnson PC: Local control of hepatic arterial and portal venous flow in the dog. Am J Physiol 211:712, 1966

12. Lautt WW: Mechanism and role of intrinsic regulation of hepatic arterial blood flow. Hepatic arterial buffer response. Am J Physiol 249:6549, 1988

13. Richardson PDI, Withrington PG: Pressure flow relationships and the effects of noradrenaline and isoprenaline on the simultaneously perfused hepatic arterial and portal venous vascular beds of the dog. J Physiol (Lond) 282:451, 1978

14. Kim DK, Kinne DE, Fortner JG: Occlusion of the hepatic artery in man. Surg Gynecol Obstet 136:966, 1973

15. Marchorio TL, Porter KA, Brown BA: The effect of partial portacaval transposition on the canine liver. Surgery 61:723, 1967

16. Hughes RL, Mathie RT, Campbell D: Systemic hypoxia and hyperoxia and liver blood flow in the greyhound. Pflugers Arch 381:151, 1979

17. Scholtholt J, Shiraishi T: The reaction of liver and intestinal blood flow to a generalized hypoxia, hypocapnia in the anesthetized dog. Pflugers Arch 318:185, 1979

18. Richardson PDI, Withrington PG: Physiologic regulation of the hepatic circulation. Annu Rev Physiol 44:57, 1982

19. Richardson PDI, Withrington PG: Effects of intraportal infusions of hypertonic solutions on hepatic hemodynamics in the dog. J Physiol (Lond) 301:82, 1980

20. Carneiro JJ, Donald DE: Changes in liver blood flow and blood content in dogs during direct nerve activity. Circ Res 40:150, 1977

21. Rappaport AM, Schneiderman JH: The function of the hepatic artery. Rev Physiol Biochem Pharmacol 76:130, 1976

22. Richardson PDI, Withrington PG: The role of beta receptors in the responses of the hepatic arterial bed of the dog to phenylephrine, isoprenaline, noradrenaline and adrenaline. Br J Pharmacol 60:239, 1977

23. Richardson PDI, Withrington PG: Glucagon inhibition of hepatic arterial responses to hepatic nerve stimulation. Am J Physiol 233:H647, 1977

24. Richardson PDI, Withrington PG: Physiologic regulation of the hepatic circulation. Fed Proc 41:2111, 1982

25. Cohen MM, Sitar DS, McNeil JR, et al: Vasopressin and angiotensin and resistance vessels of spleen, intestine and liver. Am J Physiol 218:1704, 1970

26. Richardson PDI, Withrington PG: Effects of intra-arterial and intraportal injections of vasopressin on the hepatic arterial and portal venous vascular beds of the dog. Circ Res 43:496, 1978

27. Gelman SI: Disturbances in hepatic blood flow during anesthesia and surgery. Arch Surg 111:881, 1976

28. Cooperman LH, Warden JC, Price HL: Splanchnic circulation during N_2O anesthesia and hypocarbia in normal man. Anesthesiology 29:254, 1968

29. Johnson EE, Hedley-Whyte J: Continuing positive-pressure ventilation and choledochoduodenal flow resistance. J Appl Physiol 39:937, 1975

30. Therlin L, Andreen M, Inestedt L: Effect of controlled halothane anesthesia on splanchnic blood flow and cardiac output in the dog. Acta Anaesthesiol Scand 19:146, 1975

31. Hughes RL, Campbell D, Fitch W: Effects of enflurane and halothane on liver blood flow and oxygen consumption in the greyhound. Br J Anaesth 52:1079, 1980

32. Instedt L, Andreen M: Effects of enflurane on hemodynamics and oxygen consumption in the dog with special reference to the liver and preportal tissue. Acta Anaesthesiol Scand 23:1, 1979

33. Gelman S, Fowler KC, Smith LR: Liver circulation and function during isoflurane and halothane anesthesia. Anesthesiology 61:726, 1984

34. Payen D, Gatecel C, Dupuy P, et al: Effects of isoflurane vs. halothane on human arterial hepatic blood flow (AHBF) and portal vein blood flow (PVBF) after surgical stress. Anesthesiology 69A:77, 1988

35. Epstein RM, Deutsch S, Cooperman LH, et al: Splanchnic circulation during halothane anesthesia and hypercapnia in normal man. Anesthesiology 27:654, 1966

36. Harper MH, Collins P, Johnson BH, et al: Postanesthetic hepatic injury in rats: Influence of alterations in hepatic blood flow, surgery and anesthesia time. Anesth Anal 61:79, 1982

37. Yates MS, Hiley CR, Roberts PJ: Differential effects of hepatic microsomal enzyme inducing agents on liver blood flow. Biochem Pharmacol 27:2617, 1978

38. Andreen M: Inhalation versus intravenous anesthesia. Effects on hepatic and splanchnic circulation. Acta Anaesthesiol Scand (Suppl) 75:25, 1982

39. Epstein RM, Wheeler HO, Frumin MJ, et al: The effect of hypercapnia on estimated hepatic blood flow, circulating splanchnic blood volume, and hepatic sulfobromophthalein clearance during general anesthesia in man. J Clin Invest 40:592, 1961

40. Kennedy WF, Everett GB, Cobb LA, et al: Simultaneous systemic and hepatic hemodynamic measurements during high spinal anesthesia in normal man. Anesth Analg 49:1016, 1970

41. Gelman S, Ernest EA: Hepatic circulation during sodium nitroprusside infusion in the dog. Anesthesiology 49:182, 1978

42. Dong WK, Bledsoe SW, Eng DY, et al: Profound arterial hypotension in dogs. Anesthesiology 58:61, 1983

43. Price HL, Davidson IA, Clement AF, et al: Can general anesthetics produce splanchnic visceral hypoxia by reducing regional blood flow. Anesthesiology 27:24, 1966

44. Testa B, Jenner P: Novel drug metabolites produced by functionalization reactions: Chemistry and toxicology. Drug Metab Rev 7:325, 1978

45. Tucker GR: Drug metabolism. Br J Anaesth 51:603, 1979

46. Omura T, Sato E, Cooper DY, et al: Functional cytochrome P-450 of microsomes. Fed Proc 24:1181, 1965

47. White RE, Coon MJ: Oxygen activation by cytochrome P-450. Annu Rev Biochem 49:315, 1980

48. Bentley P, Oesch F: Foreign compound metabolism in the liver. p. 157. In Popper H, Schaffner F (eds): Progress in Liver Disease. Grune & Stratton, Orlando, FL, 1982

49. Bachur NR: Cytoplasmic aldo-keto reductases: A class of metabolizing enzymes. Science 193:595, 1976

50. Chasseaud LF: Conjugation with glutathione and mercaptopuric acid excretion. p. 77. In Arias IM, Jakoby WB (eds): Glutathione: Metabolism and Function. Raven Press, New York, 1976

51. Evans DAP, White TA: Humans acetylation polymorphine. J Lab Clin Med 63:394, 1964

52. Wilkinson GR, Shand DG: A physiological approach to hepatic drug clearance. Clin Pharmacol Ther 18:377, 1976

53. Williams RL: Drug administration in hepatic disease. N Engl J Med 309:1616, 1983

54. Williams RL, Bonet LZ: Hepatic function and pharmacokinetics. p. 230. In Zakim D, Boyer TD (eds): Hepatology: A Textbook of Liver Disease. WB Saunders, Philadelphia, 1982

55. Conney A: Pharmacological implications of microsomal enzyme induction. Pharmacol Rev 19:317, 1967

56. Smith RE, Rawlins MD: Variability in Human Drug Response. Butterworths, London, 1973

57. Chan K, Kendall MJ, Mitchard M, et al: The effect of ageing on plasma pethidine concentrations. Br J Clin Pharmacol 2:297, 1975

58. Irvine RE, Grove J, Toseland PA, et al: The effect of age on the hydroxylation of amylobarbitone sodium in man. Br J Clin Pharmacol 1:41, 1974

59. Nation RL, Triggs EJ, Selig M: Lignocaine kinetics in cardiac patients and aged subjects. Br J Clin Pharmacol 4:439, 1977

60. Whitehouse MW, Beck FJ: Impaired drug metabolism in rats with adjuvant-induced arthritis. Drug Metab Disp 1:251, 1973

61. Elin RJ, Vesell ES, Wolff SM: Effects of etiocholanolone-induced fever on plasma antipyrine half-lives and metabolic clearance. Clin Pharmacol Ther 17:337, 1975

62. Alvares AP, Anderson GE, Conney AH, et al: Interactions between nutritional factors and drug biotransformation in man. Proc Natl Acad Sci USA 73:2501, 1976

63. Pantuck EJ, Pantuck CB, Weissman C, et al: Effects of parental nutritional regimens on oxidative drug metabolism. Anesthesiology 60:534, 1984

64. Livingstone A, Waterman AE: The development of tolerance to ketamine in rats and the significance of hepatic metabolism. Br J Pharmacol 64:63, 1978

65. Kanto J, Lisalo E, Lehtinen V, et al: Concentration of diazepam after an acute and chronic administration. Psychopharmcologica 36:123, 1974

66. Karlin JM, Kutt H: Acute diphenylhydantoin intoxication following halothane anesthesia. J Pediatr 76:941, 1970

67. Ghoneim MM, Delle M, Wilson WR, et al: Alteration of warfarin kinetics in man associated with exposure to an operating room environment. Anesthesiology 43:333, 1975

68. White PF, Johnstone RR, Pudwill CR: Interaction of ketamine and halothane in rats. Anesthesiology 42:179, 1975

69. Fish KJ, Rice SA: Halothane inhibits metabolism of enflurane in Fischer 344 rats. Anesthesiology 59:417, 1983

70. Brown B: The diphasic action of halothane on the oxidative metabolism of drugs by the liver. Anesthesiology 35:241, 1971

71. Borel JD, Bently JB, Nenad RE, et al: Influence of halothane on fentanyl pharmacokinetics. Anesthesiology 57A:239, 1982

72. Rogers K, Chelly J, Merin RG, et al: Verapamil halothane interaction in the chronically instrumented dog. Anesth Analg 63:268, 1984

73. Reilly CS, Wood AJJ, Kashakjn RP, et al: The effect of halothane on drug disposition: Contribution of changes in intrinsic drug metabolizing capacity and hepatic blood flow. Anesthesiology 63:70, 1985

74. Aune H, Bessesen A, Olsen H, et al: Acute effects of halothane and enflurane on drug metabolism and protein synthesis in isolated rat hepatocytes. Acta Pharmacol Toxicol 53:363, 1983

75. Duvaldestin P, Mazze RI, Nivoche Y, et al: Occupational exposure to halothane results in enzyme induction in anesthesia. Anesthesiology 54:57, 1981

76. Dale O, Nielsen K, Westgaord G, et al: Drug metabolizing enzymes in the rat after inhalation of halothane and enflurane. Br J Anesth 55:1217, 1983

77. Rothschild MA, Oratz M, Schreiber SS: Albumin synthesis. N Engl J Med 286:748, 1975

78. Kirsch R, Frith L, Black E, et al: Regulation of albumin synthesis by alteration of dietary protein. Nature 217:578, 1968

79. Schreiber G, Urban J: Synthesis and secretion of albumin. Rev Physiol Biochem Pharmacol 82:27, 1978

80. Rothschild MA, Oratz M, Zimmon D, et al: Albumin synthesis in cirrhotic subjects with ascites studied with carbonate-^{14}C. Clin Invest 8:344, 1969

81. Hemker HC, Veltkamp JJ, Hensen A, et al: Nature of prothrombin biosynthesis: Pre-prothrombinaemia in vitamin K deficiency. Nature 200:589, 1963

82. Clarke R, Rake MO, Flute PT, et al: Coagulation abnormalities in acute liver failure: Pathogenic and therapeutic implications. Scand J Gastroenterol, 8:suppl. 19, 63, 1973

83. Laurie SH, Mohammed ES: Ceruloplasmin: The enigmatic copper protein. Coord Chem Rev 33:279, 1980

84. Zieve L: Amino acids in liver failure. Gastroenterology 76:219, 1979

85. Cahill GF, Ashmore J, Renold AE, et al: Blood glucose and the liver. Am J Med 26:264, 1959

86. Stanley JC: The regulation of glucose production. Br J Anaesth 53:137, 1981

87. Hems DA, Whitton PD: Control of hepatic glycogenolysis. Physiol Rev 60:1, 1980

88. Pilkis SJ, Park CR, Clans TH: Hormonal control of hepatic gluconeogenesis. Vitam Horm 36:383, 1978

89. Black K, Vance D: Control mechanisms in the synthesis of saturated fatty acids. Annu Rev Biochem 46:263, 1977

90. Zakim D: Metabolism of glucose and fatty acids by the liver. p. 77. In Zakim D, Boyer TD (eds): Hepatology: A Textbook of Liver Disease. WB Saunders, Philadelphia, 1982

91. Mayes PA, Felts JM: Regulation of fat metabolism in the liver. Nature 215:716, 1967

92. Williamson DH, Hems R: Metabolism and function of ketone bodies. p. 275. In Bartley W, Kornherb HL, Quayle JR (eds): Essays in Cell Metabolism. Wiley Interscience, London, 1970

93. Olesky JM, Farquahr JW, Reaven GM: Reappraisal of the role of insulin in hypertriglyceridemia. Am J Med 57:551, 1974

94. Chan L, Jackson RL, O'Malley BW, et al: Synthesis of very low density lipoprotein in the cockerel: Effects of estrogen. J Clin Invest 58:368, 1976

95. Cooper AD: Hepatic lipoprotein and cholestrol metabolism. p. 109. In Zakim D, Boyer TD (eds): Hepatology: A Textbook of Liver Disease. WB Saunders, Philadelphia, 1982

96. Schmid R: Bilirubin metabolism: State of the art. Gastroenterology 74:1307, 1978

97. Traynor C, Hall GM: Endocrine and metabolic changes during surgery: Anaesthetic implication. Br J Anaesth 53:153, 1981

98. Flack A: Protein metabolism after surgery. Proc Nutr Soc 39:125, 1981

99. Brandt MR, Fernandez A, Morhorst R, et al: Epidural analgesia improves postoperative negative nitrogen balance. Br Med J Anesth 1:1106, 1978

100. Oyama T, Takazawa T: Effects of halothane anesthesia and surgery on growth hormone and insulin levels in plasma. Br J Anesth 23:179, 1972

101. Oyama T, Matsuki A, Kudo M: Effects of enflurane anesthesia and surgery on carbohydrate and fat metabolism in man. Anaesthesia 27:179, 1972

102. Brandt MR, Korshin J, Prange-Hansen J, et al: Influence of morphine anesthesia on the endocrine-metabolic response to open-heart surgery. Acta Anaesthesiol Scand 22:400, 1978

103. Clarke RSJ: The hyperglycemic response to different types of surgery and anesthesia. Br J Anaesth 42:45, 1970

104. Hall GM, Young C, Holdcroft A, et al: Substrate mobilization action during surgery. Anaesthesia 33:924, 1978

105. Biebuyck JF, Lund P, Krebs HA: The effects of halothane on glycolysis and biosynthetic processes of the isolated perfused rat liver. Biochem J 128:711, 1972

106. Biebuyck JF, Lund P, Krebs HA: The protective effect of oleate on metabolic changes produced by halothane in rat liver. Biochem J 128:721, 1972

107. Biebuyck JF: Effects of anesthetic agents on metabolic pathways. Br J Anaesth 45:263, 1973

108. Rannels DE, Flaim KE, Jefferson LS: Halothane inhibits synthesis of retained and secreted proteins in perfused rat liver. Anesthesiology 57A:231, 1982

109. Guyton AC: Textbook of Medical Physiology. 6th Ed. p. 871. WB Saunders, Philadelphia, 1982

110. Admirand WH, Small DM: The physicochemical basis of cholesterol gallstone formation in man. J Clin Invest 47:1043, 1968

111. Radnay PA, Duncalf D, Novakovic M, et al: Common bile duct pressure changes after fentanyl, morphine, meperidine, butorphanol and nalaxone. Anesth Analg 63:441, 1984

112. Zylanoff PL, Mark-Savage P, Martucci RW, et al: Common bile duct responses to anesthetic agents in dogs. Anesthesiology 51:S32, 1979

113. Bonkowsky HL: Porphyrin and heme metabolism and the porphyrias. p. 351. In Zakim D, Boyer TD (eds): Hepatology: A Textbook of Liver Disease. WB Saunders, Philadelphia, 1982

114. Rojdmarke S, Bloom G, Chou MCY, et al: Hepatic extraction of exogenous insulin and glucagon in the dog. Endocrinology 102:806, 1978

115. Leevy CM, Popper H, Sherlock S: Diseases of the Liver and Biliary Tract. p. 115. DHEW Publication No. NIH 76-725, 1976

18
RENAL PHYSIOLOGY

Richard I. Mazze

RENAL PHYSIOLOGY

The kidneys are paired organs that lie retroperitoneally on either side of the vertebral column against the posterior abdominal wall. When incised, three separate anatomic zones are apparent: the cortex, outer medulla, and inner medulla. Each kidney is composed of approximately one million functional units, or nephrons, classified as either superficial or juxtamedullary according to the location and length of some of their tubular structures. Both types of nephrons originate in the cortex, beginning as a glomerular capillary network surrounded by Bowman's capsule. This capsule leads into a proximal tubule, which is convoluted in its cortical course, and becomes straight limbed as it descends into the outer medulla, where it is designated the loop of Henle. Henle's loop of superficial nephrons descends just to the junction of the inner and outer medulla; there it makes a hairpin turn, becomes thick limbed, and ascends to the cortex. The ascending limb returns to the glomerulus of the nephron from which it originated and touches it with a group of cells called the macula densa; it then forms a distal convoluted tubule. Within the cortex the distal convoluted tubules fuse forming collecting tubules. These, in turn, join together in the inner medulla forming collecting ducts, which ultimately may carry glomerular filtrate from as many as 3,000 to 5,000 nephrons. In humans, approximately 85 percent of nephrons are located superficially in the cortex and have short loops of Henle. The renal corpus-

cles of the remaining 15 percent of nephrons are located in the juxtamedullary area and have long loops of Henle that dip deep into the renal papilla; this configuration makes them suitable for conservation of water.

The renal corpuscles and the proximal and distal convoluted tubules are confined to the cortical portion of the kidneys; they are surrounded by a vascular system that receives approximately 80 percent of the blood reaching the kidney. Henle's loop and the major portion of each collecting duct are in the renal medulla; their blood supply comes from the vasa recta, derived from the efferent arterioles of the juxtamedullary nephrons.

The fundamental operations performed by the kidney are filtration, reabsorption, and secretion. These are integrated in such a fashion that the kidney is able to carry out a number of functions:

1. Regulation of volume and composition of body fluids (i.e., conservation of water and essential substances and maintenance of acid-base balance)
2. Detoxification and excretion of nonessential materials
3. Participation in extrarenal regulatory mechanisms; for example, the kidney elaborates renin, a proteolytic enzyme involved in the formation of angiotensin, which, in turn, contributes to the regulation of aldosterone secretion
4. Endocrine functions; for example, the kidney elaborates erythropoietin, a hormone that regulates red cell production

601

Renal Hemodynamics

Kidney function and the renal circulation are so closely linked that it would be difficult to consider the former without knowledge of the latter. Thus, renal blood flow (RBF) will be given initial consideration.

Renal Blood Flow

Measurement of Renal Blood Flow

Together the kidneys weigh approximately 300 g, or 0.4 percent of total body weight; they receive 20 to 25 percent of cardiac output. Total RBF is most commonly measured by determining the clearance of *p*-aminohippurate (PAH) by the kidneys. PAH is filtered by the glomerulus and secreted by renal tubular cells so at plasma levels below the maximum secretory capacity of the tubules PAH is completely cleared from the blood in a single passage through the kidneys. PAH clearance (C_{PAH}) is therefore equal to renal plasma flow (RPF) and is calculated the standard by clearance formula

$$C_{PAH} = \frac{U_{PAH}V}{P_{PAH}}$$

where U_{PAH} is the urinary PAH concentration in milligrams per 100 ml, V is the urinary flow rate in milliliters per minute, and P_{PAH} is the plasma PAH concentration in milligrams per 100 ml. The formula for renal blood flow is as follows:

$$RBF = \frac{RPF}{1 - Hct}$$

Using these formulas, it has been determined that in the patient of average size (1.73 m²) RBF is approximately 1,200 ml/min and RPF is 650 ml/min.

The PAH clearance method of measuring RBF is based on a simplification of the Fick principle and makes the assumption that renal venous PAH concentration is negligible. Actually, PAH extraction (E_{PAH}) averages 0.90 for the entire kidney, with E_{PAH} equal to 0.95 for the outer cortex and 0.82 for the inner cortex and medulla.[1] Also, E_{PAH} varies in disease states, such as oliguric renal failure, when it may decrease to zero, or during intravascular fluid administration with lactated Ringer's solution, mannitol, or plasma, when it may decrease by as much as 20 percent.[2] Determinations of E_{PAH} during anesthesia have not been reported; thus, the major assumption underlying the measurement of RBF in anesthetized patients is open to question.

Intrarenal blood flow has been measured by indirect methods.[3,4] Dye dilution techniques have demonstrated rapid blood flow within the renal cortex and much slower flow within the medulla. Isotope washout techniques employing ⁸⁵Kr and ¹³³Xe have permitted identification of four regions, each having a distinct pattern of blood flow: cortex, outer medulla, inner medulla, and hilar and perirenal fat[4] (Fig. 18-1). Isotope techniques have an advantage over conventional clearance techniques of measuring RBF independent of urinary flow rate.

The blood flow to each zone of the kidney has a distinct relationship to the function of the zone. In humans, approximately 80 percent of RBF goes to the renal cortex[3,4]; this is equal to about 400 to 500 ml/100 g/min. High cortical blood flow is necessary to carry out the excretory and regulatory functions that occur in this zone. More deeply within the kidney, the outer medulla receives approximately 15 percent of total renal blood flow, while the inner medulla is relatively poorly perfused and receives only 1 to 3 percent of total RBF. Increasing medullary hypertonicity is essential to the urinary concentrating function of the kidney, the osmolality of the medulla varying from 300 mOsm/kg at the corticomedullary junction to 1,200 mOsm/kg at the tip of the inner medulla. The countercurrent arrangement of renal tubules and blood vessels in the medulla and the low inner medullary blood flow (<15 ml/100 g/min) is essential for the establishment and maintenance of this osmotic gradient. Higher medullary blood flow would result in washout of solute and abolition of the osmotic gradient.

Results of studies of renal hemodynamics during oliguric and anuric states suggest that the common pathogenic feature of acute renal failure of diverse etiologies is a major (70 percent) reduction in total RBF with a shift of remaining flow from cortical to juxtamedullary and medullary regions.[5]

Control of Renal Blood Flow

Renal blood flow is subject to two types of regulation: (1) extrinsic nervous and hormonal regulation, and (2) intrinsic autoregulation.

Extrinsic Nervous Regulation. The blood vessels of the kidney are richly supplied with sympathetic constrictor fibers derived from the T4 to L1 spinal cord segments distributed through the celiac and renal plexuses. There is no sympathetic dilator or parasympathetic innervation of the kidney. Renal blood flow appears to be regulated to maintain glomerular filtration rate (GFR). At rest, in the supine position, and in an environment of neutral temperature, there is little tonic sympathetic control of RBF.[6] When minimal or moderate stress is present, RBF falls slightly but GFR is maintained, suggesting that there is efferent arteriolar constriction. During severe stress, induced by such diverse stimuli as general anesthesia, hypoxia, syncope, strenuous exercise, pain, and hemorrhage, there are large decreases in both RBF and GFR. The major changes in renal hemodynamics associated with severe stress are thought to be mediated via stimulation of the sympathetic nervous system.

Extrinsic Hormonal Regulation. The catecholamines, epinephrine and norepinephrine, are the neurohumoral transmitter substances of the sympathetic nervous system. In humans, about 10 times more epineph-

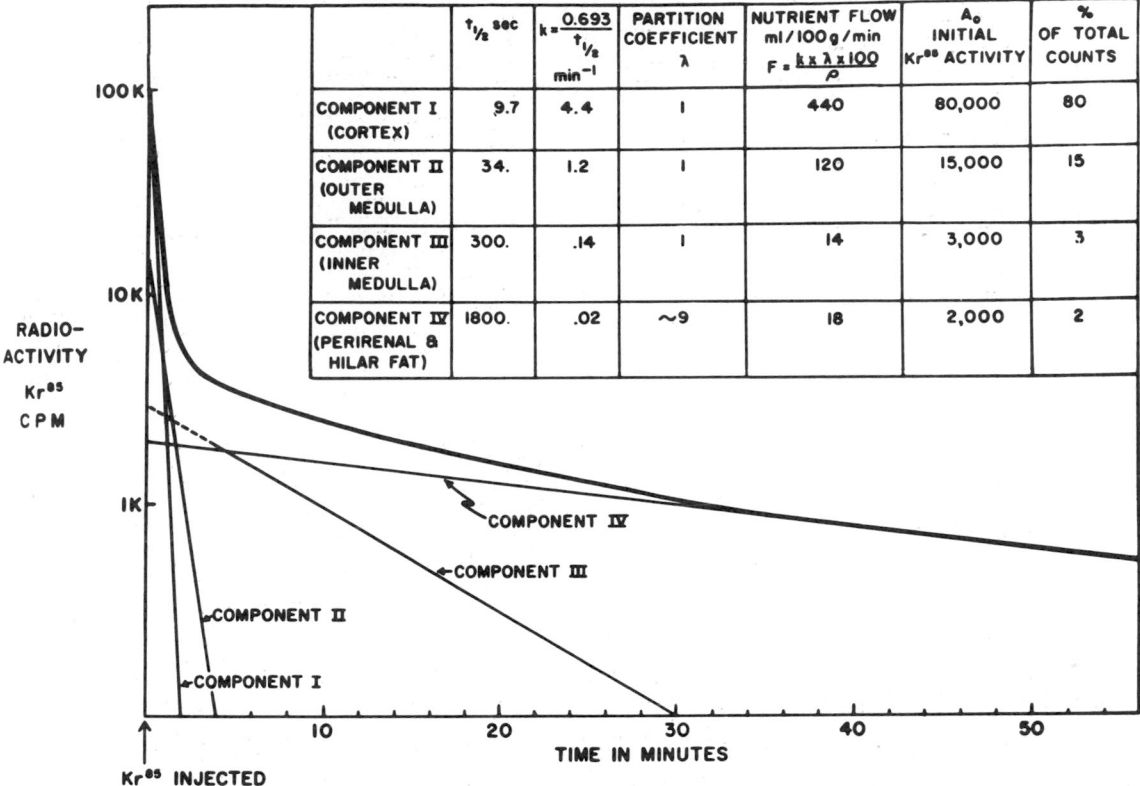

	$t_{1/2}$ sec	$k = \dfrac{0.693}{t_{1/2}}$ min^{-1}	PARTITION COEFFICIENT λ	NUTRIENT FLOW ml/100 g/min $F = \dfrac{k \times \lambda \times 100}{\rho}$	A_o INITIAL Kr^{85} ACTIVITY	% OF TOTAL COUNTS
COMPONENT I (CORTEX)	9.7	4.4	1	440	80,000	80
COMPONENT II (OUTER MEDULLA)	34.	1.2	1	120	15,000	15
COMPONENT III (INNER MEDULLA)	300.	.14	1	14	3,000	3
COMPONENT IV (PERIRENAL & HILAR FAT)	1800.	.02	~9	18	2,000	2

Fig. 18-1. Typical ^{85}Kr disappearance curve (heavy black line) after injection of the isotope into the renal artery. Graphic representation of the resultant exponentials is shown by the thinner lines. The accompanying table presents pertinent data and values derived from such a curve. (From Thorburn et al.,[4] with permission.)

rine than norepinephrine is found in the adrenal glands, while norepinephrine is the predominant neurotransmitter substance in the sympathetic nerves and is the adrenergic mediator liberated by their stimulation.[7] Administration of epinephrine and norepinephrine in low concentrations results in an increase in systemic blood pressure accompanied by a decrease in total RBF and no change in GFR; this suggests that constriction of afferent and efferent glomerular arterioles is approximately equal. However, epinephrine and norepinephrine, when administered in high concentrations and particularly when infused intravenously, cause a marked fall in both RBF and GFR. Selective renal arteriograms and studies with ^{85}Xe have demonstrated that most of the change in RBF following epinephrine infusion is due to abolition of superficial cortical blood flow, with little or no change in medullary flow.[8]

Dopamine is the immediate metabolic precursor of norepinephrine and epinephrine. It also is the predominant neurotransmitter of the mammalian extrapyramidal system and has intrinsic pharmacologic properties as well.[9] At very low doses, 1 to 3 μg/kg/min, dopamine reduces renal and mesenteric vascular resistance, apparently acting by stimulating specific dopaminergic receptors in these vascular beds. There is an associated increase in RBF, GFR, and sodium excretion secondary

to intracortical redistribution of blood flow. When infused intravenously at low doses, 1 to 10 μg/kg/min, dopamine acts as a β_1-adrenergic agonist; it increases systolic and pulse pressures with little effect on diastolic blood pressure and total peripheral resistance. At doses greater than 10 μg/kg/min dopamine acts as an α-adrenergic agonist, causing marked sympathomimetic responses.[10,11] There is considerable overlap in these responses to exogenously administered dopamine. It has not been determined whether endogenously secreted dopamine acting at α- or β-adrenergic or dopaminergic receptors is involved in the normal physiologic (or the pathophysiologic) control of RBF, GFR, and electrolyte excretion. The physiologic responses to catecholamine secretion and to renin release (see below) are much greater than those to dopamine, so it is likely that the latter is not a usual modulator of renal hemodynamics and function.

The renin-angiotensin hormonal pathway affects RBF (Fig. 18-2). Renin is a proteolytic enzyme produced by the juxtaglomerular cells, which are formed from the tunica media of the afferent arteriole. Renin acts enzymatically on its substrate, angiotensinogen, a circulating plasma α_2-globulin, to release the decapeptide angiotensin I. Like renin and angiotensinogen, angiotensin I has no known physiologic actions. However, it is rapidly hydrolyzed by converting enzymes,

ANGIOTENSIN FORMATION

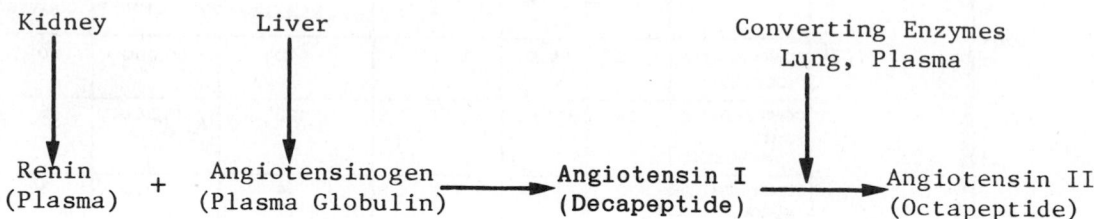

ANGIOTENSIN DESTRUCTION AND REMOVAL

(A)   Angiotensin II   =   Receptor Tissue Binding

(B)   Angiotensin II   +   Angiotensinases = Inactive Products

ACTIONS OF ANGIOTENSIN II

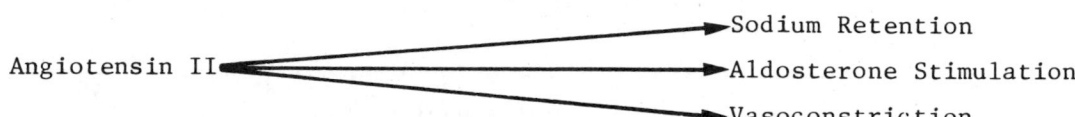

Fig. 18-2. Components of the renin-angiotensin system illustrating formation, destruction or removal, and actions of angiotensin II. (From Laragh and Sealey,[13] with permission.)

present primarily in lung but also in plasma, to form the octapeptide angiotensin II, a strongly pressor and renal vasoconstricting substance. Angiotensin II activity is one of the major factors governing the release of aldosterone. The immediate stimulus for the renal release of renin is unknown, but several factors affected by administration of anesthetics are involved. These include sodium content of tubular fluid, catecholamine levels, sympathetic nerve impulses, and intraluminal pressure of afferent arterioles.[12] Figure 18-3 diagrams the renin-angiotensin-aldosterone feedback loop for regulating sodium balance and arterial pressure. Within the kidney, low concentrations of angiotensin II reduce RBF without altering GFR. High concentrations result in a fall of both RBF and GFR with a redistribution of intrarenal blood flow similar to that which occurs following epinephrine infusion. Reduced RBF during hemorrhagic hypotension is due to increased concentrations of circulating catecholamines and angiotensin as well as to increased sympathetic nervous system activity.[13] These hormonal factors are probably involved in the changes in total RBF and intrarenal distribution of flow that occur during other forms of severe stress.

The prostaglandins may be involved in the physiologic regulation of intrarenal blood flow. Prostaglandins are fatty acids found in many tissues, including seminal vesicle, lung, brain, pancreas, and renal medulla. They have potent vasodepressor and antihyper-

tensive activity, acting directly on peripheral arterioles. Infusion of prostaglandin results in increased sodium excretion independent of changes in GFR, as well as increased cortical blood flow and decreased medullary blood flow.[14] This response is consistent with the observation that increased blood flow to outer cortical nephrons, with their short loops of Henle, results in diuresis and enhanced sodium excretion, while increased blood flow to juxtamedullary nephrons, with their long loops of Henle, results in sodium retention.

Currently, there is no evidence that other vasoactive hormonal substances in physiologic concentration, such as vasopressin or serotonin, affect total RBF or cause alterations in distribution of intrarenal blood flow.

Autoregulation of Renal Blood Flow. Autoregulation of RBF refers to the maintenance of relatively constant RBF despite changes in mean arterial blood pressure within the range of 80 to 180 mmHg. Constant RBF is preserved in innervated, denervated, and isolated kidneys and during α-adrenergic blockade of intrarenal ganglia with phentolamine and phenoxybenzamine, suggesting that changes in resistance are controlled entirely by the kidney.[15] Not only is RBF autoregulated, but GFR appears to be autoregulated as well, indicating that the resistance elements are located in the preglomerular vascular segments. Several theories have been

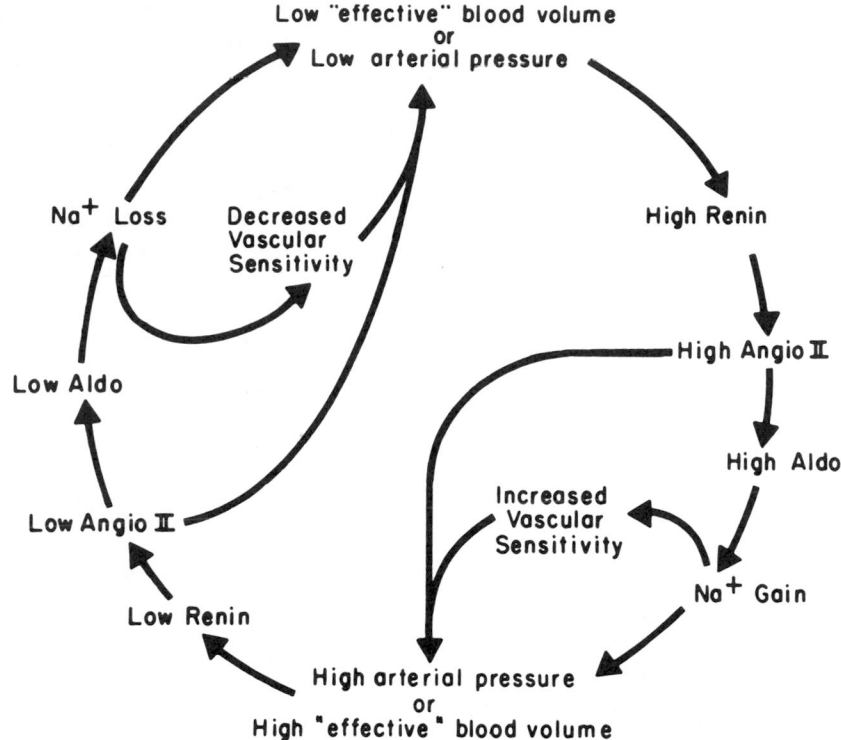

Fig. 18-3. The renin-angiotensin-aldosterone feedback loop for regulation of sodium balance and arterial blood pressure. (From Laragh and Sealey,[13] with permission.)

proposed to explain autoregulation of RBF.[15] These include (1) regulation by alteration in intrarenal tissue pressure; (2) regulation by accumulation of metabolites having vasoactive properties; (3) regulation by changes in tangential wall tension of the arteriole (myogenic theory); and (4) regulation by a feedback mechanism between the distal tubular lumen and the afferent arteriole via the macula densa. No known single mechanism explains the phenomenon of autoregulation during all the physiologic circumstances in which it has been shown to exist.

The implications of autoregulation of RBF are that glomerular capillaries are protected from large increases in systemic pressure and that renal function may be maintained during hypotension. However, there may be significant changes in RBF and GFR despite maintenance of systemic blood pressure in the 80 to 180 mmHg range due to the alterations in extrinsic nervous and hormonal factors controlling blood flow.

Medullary Blood Flow

The blood supply of the medulla is primarily derived from the straight limbs of the vasa recta. These vessels originate from the efferent arterioles of the juxtamedullary glomeruli and are arranged in bundles in the outer zone of the medulla. There is also a secondary system, consisting of a rich capillary plexus continuous throughout the cortex and medulla. Blood flow to the outer and inner medulla, per unit of tissue weight, is much lower than to the cortex, accounting for no more than 20 percent of total RBF. Of this, the inner medulla receives only 1 to 3 percent of total RBF and has the lowest flow in the kidney. Low medullary flow is probably due to the high resistance that occurs as a result of the extraordinary length of the vasa recta, increased plasma protein content of the medullary vessels, and crenation of red cells in the hypertonic environment.

The medullary circulation plays an integral role in the urinary concentrating mechanism, controlling the rate of solute removal from the interstitium and thereby regulating medullary osmolality. The vasa recta participate in this process, functioning as a countercurrent exchanger. That is, the hairpin arrangement of the vasa recta as they descend into the inner medulla favors the passive exchange of solute and water across vessel walls. Water leaves the descending limb of the vasa recta and enters the more hypertonic ascending limb, bypassing the inner medulla. At the same time, medullary solute travels in the opposite direction, going from the hypertonic ascending limb of the vasa recta to the interstitium and then entering the relatively less concentrated descending limb. This anatomic arrangement favors the maintenance of an osmotic gradient in which osmolality at the tip of the renal papilla may reach 1,200 mOsm/kg.

Renal Oxygen Consumption

The average renal arteriovenous (a–v) oxygen difference is 1.7 ml/100 ml. When RBF increases, at blood pressures greater than 60 mmHg, oxygen consumption per 100 ml of blood flow remains relatively constant, so that total renal oxygen consumption increases. This contrasts with the situation in most other organs in which the average a–v oxygen difference is 4 to 5 ml/100 ml and there is an inverse relationship between a–v oxygen difference and blood flow. The direct relationship between RBF and renal oxygen consumption is explained by the fact that GFR varies directly with RBF and that tubular reabsorption of sodium increases with increasing GFR. Since 75 to 80 percent of the energy expended by the kidney is involved in active sodium transport, the seemingly anomalous relationship between RBF and renal oxygen consumption is actually appropriate. Renal oxygen consumption is decreased in those situations in which RBF is maintained or increased and sodium transport is decreased, as during ureteral occlusion, osmotic diuresis, or decreased GFR. When blood pressure decreases below 60 mmHg and glomerular filtration ceases, an inverse relationship exists between RBF and renal oxygen consumption. In that case, renal oxygen consumption is relatively constant, at approximately 0.2 mmol/min/100 g, and is primarily for renal nutrient purposes.

Glomerular Filtration

Approximately 180 L of glomerular fluid is produced each day by the process of filtration through the glomerular capillary membrane. This process does not involve expenditure of metabolic energy; rather, filtration depends on hydrostatic pressure produced by contraction of the heart. In the glomerulus, hydrostatic pressure in the afferent arteriole is approximately 75 mmHg. This is opposed by a plasma oncotic pressure of approximately 30 mmHg and an intraglomerular pressure in Bowman's capsule of 10 mmHg. Adjustment of afferent and efferent arteriolar size prevents variations in blood pressure from effecting large changes in filtration pressure. However, GFR is reduced by extremes in exercise and emotion, either by direct autonomic control of vascular tone or by release of circulating vasoactive catecholamines or polypeptides, such as angiotensin. Changes in vascular resistance may alter intrarenal distribution of blood flow, shifting blood flow from cortical to juxtamedullary nephrons, thereby affecting GFR.

The process by which some substances are filtered and others are not is still not completely understood. Present theory has it that the glomerular capillary membrane, which has approximately 1 m² of total filtration area, contains pores that are negatively charged. These pores are freely permeable to water, ions, and small negatively charged molecules less than 30 to 40 Å in diameter. Molecules of 40 to 80 Å are variably filtered, the extent of filtration being dependent on molecular charge. Thus, albumin, which is negatively charged and has a diameter of about 60 Å, usually is not filtered, whereas neutral dextran of the same diameter has a filtration index of about 0.5. Molecules greater than 80 Å in diameter will not pass through the membrane at all. This results in complete filtration of unbound substances with a molecular weight of 15,000 or less, reduced filtration of substances with a molecular weight in the range of 35,000, and insignificant filtration of substances with a molecular weight of 70,000 or more. Another theory proposes that the glomerular membrane, rather than containing pores, acts as a hydrated gel. Still another theory postulates that the membrane is not a fixed structure but contains aqueous channels between loosely bonded protein and lipid components. Both types of membranes would permit the passage, by diffusion, of water and low-molecular-weight solutes.[16-18]

Measurement of GFR is usually made indirectly by determining the clearance of inulin, a fructose polysaccharide with a molecular weight of 5,000. Inulin is completely filtered by the glomerulus and is not reabsorbed or secreted by the renal tubules. Glomerular filtration rate is equal to the number of milliliters of plasma completely cleared of inulin (C_{in}) per minute, expressed by the formula,

$$C_{in} = \frac{U_{in} V}{P_{in}}$$

where U_{in} is the urinary inulin concentration, V is the urinary flow rate in milliliters per minute, and P_{in} is the plasma inulin concentration. Using this method it has been determined that GFR in a patient of average size is approximately 125 ml/min. However, measurement of C_{in} is not always practical, since a constant infusion of inulin must be maintained; therefore, measurement of 24-hour endogenous creatinine clearance is most often used for clinical measurement of glomerular filtration rate. This results in values approximately 10 percent higher than those calculated from C_{in} because creatinine is secreted by the renal tubules. For clinical purposes, especially for measuring long-term changes in GFR, 24-hour endogenous creatinine clearance is satisfactory. Twenty-four-hour endogenous urea clearance also has been used in measuring GFR; however, urea is reabsorbed from renal tubular cells in a variable manner, so that urea clearance is unreliable as a measure of GFR.

Tubular Transport

The renal tubules function not only to reduce the large quantity of glomerular filtrate from 180 L to approximately 1 L/d, but also to alter the composition of the tubular fluid by the processes of reabsorption and secretion. Tubular transport processes are of two types, passive and active. Transport is said to be passive if it can be attributed to physical forces, which in biologic systems are most commonly due to differences in concentration or electrical potential that create gradients across membranes. An example of this occurs when urine becomes concentrated; water leaves the collecting duct because of the greater salt concentration in the surrounding medullary interstitium. Movement of water occurs because of the osmotic gradient. Transport is passive because only physical forces are involved.

Active transport is defined as the net movement of a particle against an electrochemical potential gradient at the cost of metabolic energy. A specific example of this is the establishment of the high salt concentration in the medullary interstitium. Sodium chloride is pumped from the ascending limb of Henle's loop, an area in which its concentration is relatively low, to the medullary interstitium, an area in which its concentration is relatively high. In general, a property of cell membranes is the ability to transport sodium from the cell interior, a region of low sodium concentration, to the cell exterior, a region of high sodium concentration. The energy source for the process, ATP, is hydrolyzed by an enzyme in cell membranes, Na^+-K^+-ATPase, that requires sodium and potassium to function. During the process of ATP hydrolysis, sodium is extruded from the cell and potassium is accumulated in the cell. If one of the steps does not occur because the appropriate substrate or enzyme is not present, the system will be deprived of energy and the net movement of actively transported substances against their electrochemical potential gradients will be diminished or abolished. Such inhibition of active transport is commonly seen if a system is cooled, deprived of oxygen, or exposed to specific metabolic inhibitors, such as dinitrophenol or inorganic fluoride.

Tubular Reabsorption

Water and many solutes are reabsorbed from the tubular lumen into the peritubular interstitial fluid and then into the blood. The term reabsorption refers to the direction of transport, that is, out of the tubular lumen. It is used whether transport is active or passive. Tubular reabsorption permits the conservation of substances essential to normal function, such as water, glucose, amino acids, and electrolytes. Micropuncture studies have been invaluable in determining the function of specific areas of the nephron, demonstrating that some substances, such as water and sodium, are reabsorbed throughout the nephron, whereas others, such as glucose, amino acids, and bicarbonate, are reabsorbed primarily in one area (the proximal tubule). Many substances, such as glucose and phosphate, are completely reabsorbed at low plasma concentrations. However, for some substances the amount reabsorbed reaches a maximum value; thereafter, regardless of the plasma concentration, the excess of filtered material is excreted. This maximum value is known as the transport maximum, or T_m. Not only glucose and phosphate but other sugars, sulfate, many amino acids, uric acid, and probably albumin each have a T_m. The T_m phenomenon apparently is not due to exhaustion of the energy supply of the tubular cell but more likely is due to saturation of the carrier for a particular substance. There also appears to be competitive inhibition of the reabsorption of some substances, for example, fructose infusion will diminish or abolish the tubular reabsorption of glucose.

Tubular Secretion

Secretion also refers to the direction of movement, that is, from peritubular blood, renal interstitium, or tubular cell into the tubular lumen, regardless of whether the transport is passive or active. A great number of substances are secreted, many of which are either weak acids or weak bases, such as the sulfonic acids, carboxylic acid, and the amines. Tubular secretion is also the major route for elimination of toxic metabolic products and foreign substances, including drugs. Many drugs are not filtered at the glomerulus because they are bound to plasma proteins. These are eliminated by tubular secretion, which in some cases is so efficient that all the bound material is removed in a single passage through the kidney. Various antibiotics and the iodinated compounds used in radiography are excreted in this fashion. Tubular secretion is also the means by which the inorganic ions potassium, hydrogen, and ammonium enter the urine. There is a separate secretory system for anions and another for cations. Neither system is highly specific, as each transports a wide variety of inorganic compounds with the appropriate electrical charge. However, there appears to be competition among the ions that are transported. The efficiency of the tubular secretory system for transporting certain organic acids, such as PAH, from peritubular blood to the tubular lumen is the basis for the measurement of RBF. As with tubular reabsorptive mechanisms, there is a T_m for secretion of many substances.

Bidirectional Transport

When a substance is said to be reabsorbed, its net flux is from the tubular lumen to the blood. This does not exclude the possibility that the substance is simultaneously secreted. In fact, for most substances, net tubular reabsorption is the algebraic sum of fluxes in both directions. The mode of transport in any one direction may be passive or active or a combination of the two. For example, sodium ion undergoes net reabsorption, being actively reabsorbed and passively secreted. Potassium ion is reabsorbed in the proximal tubules and loops of Henle, secreted in the distal tubules, and reabsorbed in the collecting ducts. Other substances, such as urea and uric acid, are also handled by tubular transport processes involving both reabsorption and secretion.

Urine Concentration and Dilution

The ability to form concentrated urine is associated with the presence of loops of Henle interposed between proximal and distal segments of renal tubules. Only mammals and birds can form urine hypertonic to plasma, and only these two classes possess loops of Henle. Since the greater the length of Henle's loop the greater the concentrating power of the kidney, it had been incorrectly assumed that antidiuretic hormone (ADH) stimulates reabsorption of water by the loop of Henle and that formation of hypertonic urine occurs in these loops. Micropuncture studies of rat kidney tubules failed to confirm this hypothesis, for if it were true, fluid collected from the distal tubules would have been as hypertonic as ureteral urine. In fact, distal tubular fluid is either hypotonic or isotonic to the final urine but never hypertonic. The site of the final concentration of urine must therefore be the collecting ducts.

Initially, the mechanism of concentration was thought to involve the active reabsorption of water. However, the formation of concentrated urine by active reabsorption of water requires an excessive amount of energy, whereas the reabsorption of ions and the osmotic equilibration of water is more efficient. For example, the reabsorption of 1.0 ml of isotonic saline by a mechanism that actively pumps sodium and permits the osmotic equilibration of water would require approximately 10^{20} successive combinations and dissociations of sodium with its carrier. Reabsorption by a mechanism that actively pumps water and permits passive diffusion of sodium would require 300 times that number of successive combinations and dissociations of water and carrier. The energy required for concentrating urine by the latter process is far in excess of that which is available to the kidney. The process by which final urinary osmolality may reach 1,200 mOsm/kg in humans and in species such as the kangaroo rat, 5,000 mOsm/kg, through passive reabsorption of water is known as countercurrent multiplication of concentration.[19]

The Urinary Concentrating and Diluting Mechanisms

Each day, approximately 180 L of water, 27,000 mEq of sodium, and 20,000 mEq of chloride are filtered through the glomeruli of normal humans. The driving force for filtration is the hydrostatic pressure of plasma in the capillaries; filtration is opposed by the pressure in Bowman's capsule and the oncotic pressure exerted by plasma proteins. The filtrate flows past proximal tubule cells that are highly permeable to sodium chloride and are adjoined at relatively impermeable tight junctions. Sodium passively enters tubular cells down the concentration gradient from the sodium-rich tubular fluid to the sodium-poor intracellular fluid and down the electrical gradient from the electrically positive tubular lumen to the electrically negative cell. Chloride follows to maintain electrochemical neutrality and

water follows in response to the osmotic gradient created by the movement of sodium and chloride. The intracellular Na^+-K^+-ATPase energy-driven sodium pump extrudes sodium from the cell into the interstitium of the cortex in exchange for potassium. Chloride and water passively follow. Most of the ions and water deposited in the interstitium are carried away by the peritubular capillaries, although some leak back across the relatively impermeable tight junctions into the tubular lumen. This process serves to reduce the volume of fluid in the proximal tubule by approximately 75 percent with no change in osmotic activity.

As tubular fluid progresses down the thin descending limb of Henle's loop, water diffuses into the hypertonic interstitium of the medulla and papilla (Fig. 18-4). This

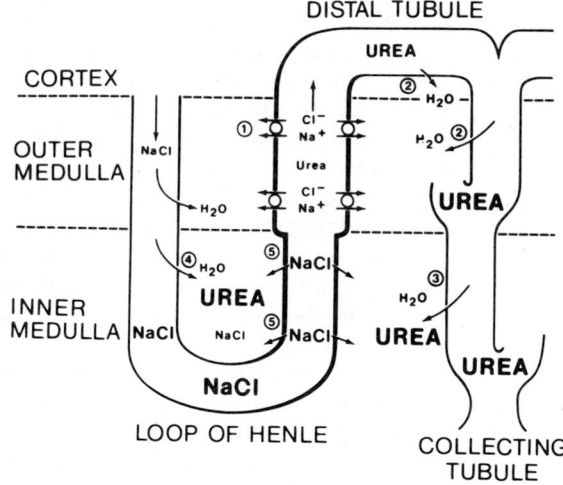

Fig. 18-4. Schematic representation of the inner medullary concentrating mechanism. The thin ascending limb, the thick ascending limb, and the first part of the distal tubule are impermeable to water, as indicated by the thickened lines. In the thick ascending limb, active chloride reabsorption, accompanied by passive sodium movement (1), renders the tubular fluid dilute and the outer medullary interstitium hyperosmotic. In the last part of the distal tubule and in the collecting tubule in the cortex and outer medulla, water is reabsorbed along its osmotic gradient (2), increasing the concentration of urea that remains behind. In the inner medulla both water and urea are reabsorbed from the collecting duct (3). Some urea reenters the loop of Henle (not shown). This medullary recycling of urea, in addition to trapping urea by countercurrent exchange in the vasa recta (not shown), causes urea to accumulate in large quantities in the medullary interstitium (indicated by the large type), where it osmotically extracts water from the descending limb (4) and thereby concentrates sodium chloride in descending-limb fluid. When the fluid rich in NaCl enters the NaCl-permeable (but water-impermeable) thin ascending limb, NaCl moves passively down its concentration gradient (5), rendering the tubular fluid relatively hypo-osmotic to the surrounding interstitium. (From Jamison and Maffly,[20] with permission.)

section is poorly permeable to sodium and incapable of active transport so little reabsorption occurs at this site. The net effect is that volume decreases and osmotic pressure increases progressively to the point of reversal of flow. The thin ascending limb of Henle's loop is water impermeable but permits diffusion and some active transport of sodium and chloride. The thick ascending limb also is water impermeable, but chloride is actively transported and sodium follows passively.[21,22] In fact, chloride transport in this segment is of critical importance, as it is the driving force for both urinary dilution and concentration. At each level, a gradient of about 200 mOsm/L is established between tubular contents and interstitium as the concentration within the lumen decreases and that of the interstitium increases. The proximity of the descending limb and the hypertonicity of the interstitium facilitate osmotic diffusion of water from the descending limb and concentration of its contents.

Regardless of whether the final urine is concentrated or dilute, the fluid that enters the distal convoluted tubules is always hypotonic to the surrounding cortical interstitial fluid and its volume is approximately 15 percent that of the original glomerular filtrate.[23] When the level of circulating ADH is high, the epithelial cells of the distal tubules and the cortical collecting ducts are freely permeable to water but are impermeable to urea. Thus, urea concentration increases and tubular fluid becomes isotonic with cortical interstitial fluid by the middle of the distal segment. The active reabsorption of sodium and the passive osmotic diffusion of water continue in the distal tubule, reducing volume to about 5 to 8 percent that of the original glomerular filtrate. In the medulla, ADH increases collecting duct permeability to water and urea so that during antidiuresis urea accounts for 50 percent of medullary osmolality. Thus, collecting duct fluid, initially isosmotic, becomes progressively concentrated as it gives up water to the hypertonic medullary interstitium. The final urine enters the renal pelvis at a rate less than 0.5 percent that of GFR and as concentrated as the interstitial tissue at the tip of the papilla.

Some of the water, sodium, and urea that have diffused out of the descending limb of Henle's loop and the collecting ducts may reenter Henle's loop. Most of the solute, however, enters the capillaries that make up the vasa recta of the medulla and papilla. These vessels serve as countercurrent exchangers to reduce excessive loss of osmotically active solute from the medulla and the papilla. Nevertheless, some solute returns to the systemic circulation. The return of urea explains why its clearance is less than that of true GFR, particularly during antidiuresis, and why urea clearance is dependent on urinary flow rate.

When the level of circulating ADH is low, the epithelium of the distal tubules and collecting ducts are impermeable to water. The hypotonicity of tubular fluid leaving the loop of Henle is maintained throughout the remainder of the nephron and, indeed, it may be re-duced to a final value as low as 30 mOsm/kg by the continued active extrusion of solute.

Action of Diuretics

The kidney normally maintains the salt content of the extracellular compartment within narrow limits. The accumulation of sodium and subsequent formation of edema are extensions of the normal physiologic mechanisms that maintain this balance and seek to conserve salt and water during hypovolemia. With the exception of osmotic diuretics, all diuretic agents alter this delicate balance by interfering with the ability of the kidney to conserve sodium.

The specific sites of action of diuretics have been established by micropuncture studies, by assessing the effects of the agents on the urinary concentrating and diluting mechanisms, by observing their effect on potassium excretion, and by ultrastructural examinations.[24] For example, a diuretic that acts by decreasing sodium and water reabsorption in the proximal tubule (acetazolamide) may not exert a significant effect on net sodium and water excretion, since most of the increased amounts of water and solute delivered from the proximal tubule to the remainder of the nephron will be reabsorbed, primarily in the loop of Henle. To the contrary, diuretics acting in the loop of Henle will cause large increases in urinary salt and water excretion, since the more distal nephron cannot reabsorb large amounts of sodium. For the kidney to form concentrated urine, chloride reabsorption in the medullary portion of the ascending limb of the loop of Henle must be intact, while the ability to form dilute urine is dependent on normal function of the chloride reabsorption mechanisms of both the medullary and cortical portions of the ascending limb. Thus, the loop diuretics ethacrynic acid and furosemide, by virtue of their inhibition of chloride reabsorption in the medullary ascending limb, interfere with urinary dilution and concentration.[25] Thiazide diuretics, acting primarily in the cortical portion of the ascending limb, only impair diluting ability. Urinary potassium excretion occurs largely as a result of potassium secretion in the distal cortical nephron. There it is electrochemically linked to sodium excretion, which is influenced by aldosterone, and is directly proportional to the rate of flow of tubular fluid. Diuretics that act proximal to the site of potassium secretion increase distal tubular flow rate and, therefore, potassium excretion. To the contrary, an agent such as spironolactone, which inhibits sodium reabsorption at this distal site, decreases potassium secretion and excretion. The next section reviews the pharmacology of the specific categories of diuretics.

Diuretic Drugs

There are six major categories of diuretics; their characteristics are noted in Table 18-1 and their sites of action in Figure 18-5.[26] Diuretics are classified as mercur-

TABLE 18-1. Characteristics of Diuretic Drugs

Type of Diuretic	Generic Name	Usual Dosage Schedule	Onset of Effect	Peak Effect	Duration of Action
Carbonic anhydrase inhibitors	Acetazolamide	250–375 mg/d	2 h	6 h	24 h
Benzothiazide derivatives	Chlorothiazide	500–1,000 mg/d, oral	1 h	4 h	6–12 h
	Hydrochlorothiazide	50–100 mg/d, oral	2 h	4 h	24–36 h
	Trichlormethiazide	4–8 mg/d, oral	2 h	6 h	24 h
	Chlorthalidone	100 mg/d, oral	2 h	6 h	12–24 h
	Metolazone	2.5–10 mg/d, oral	1 h	2 h	12–24 h
Potassium-sparing diuretics	Triamterene	100–300 mg/d, oral	2 h	6–8 h	12–16 h
	Spironolactone	25 mg, oral, 4 times/d	Gradual onset	2–3 days after beginning therapy	2–3 days after ending therapy
Loop diuretics	Furosemide	40–120 mg/d	Oral, 1 h; IV, 5 min	1–2 h; 30 min	6 h; 2 h
	Ethacrynic acid	50–100 mg/d	Oral, 30 min; IV, 15 min	2 h; 45 min	6–8 h; 3 h
	Bumetanide	0.125–1.0 mg/d, oral	30–60 min	1–2 h	3 h
Osmotic agents	Mannitol	12–60 g/d, IV	5 min	30–45 min	2–3 h

(Modified from Frazier and Yager,[24] with permission.)

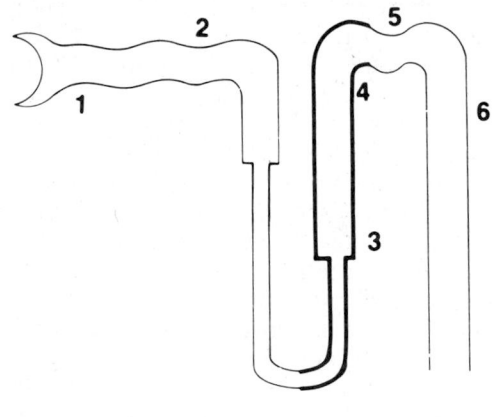

Diuretic	Site 1	2	3	4	5	6
Mannitol	(+)		+	(+)	(+)	
Acetazolamide		+			(+)	
Mercurial Diuretics	(+)		+	(+)		(+)
Thiazide Diuretics		(+)		+	(+)	
Ethacrynic acid	(+)		+	(+)	(+)	
Furosemide	(+)	(+)	+	(+)	(+)	
Spironolactone						+
Triamterene					+	
Amiloride					+	

+ = major   (+) = minor actions

Fig. 18-5. Sites of action of diuretic drugs. (From Merin and Bastron,[26] with permission.)

ials, carbonic anhydrase inhibitors, benzothiazide derivatives, potassium-sparing diuretics, loop diuretics, and osmotic agents.

Mercurials

Mercurial diuretics act primarily in the thick ascending limb of the loop of Henle by interfering with chloride transport.[27] Their administration is accompanied by moderate chloride loss with only minimal loss of potassium and bicarbonate. Therefore, treatment usually results in a metabolic alkalosis that limits the diuretic response to chronic dosage. Responsiveness can be restored by ammonium chloride therapy. Mercurial diuretics have fallen into disuse because of the need to administer them parenterally, their delayed onset of action, and the occasional toxic reactions associated with their administration. The latter have included sudden death, presumably due to inadvertent intravenous injection, and renal failure and hemorrhagic colitis, thought to be a consequence of heavy metal poisoning.

Carbonic Anhydrase Inhibitors

These drugs are of interest because they were the first orally effective agents. Also, they are derived from the antibacterial sulfonamides and are therefore the forerunners of the modern-day thiazide group of diuretics. Carbonic anhydrase inhibitors are rarely used today except during ophthalmologic surgery, where they are preferred because of their ability to reduce intraocular pressure. They act primarily in the proximal tubule delaying the dehydration of carbonic acid, thus interfering with the generation of H^+ from CO_2 and H_2O.[28] They also directly impair NA^+–H^+ exchange in the proximal tubule and throughout the nephron. Inhibition of renal H^+ secretion results in sodium bicarbonate diuresis with enhanced Na^+-K^+ exchange in the distal nephron. Hyperchloremic acidosis with hypokalemia follows their administration, ultimately limiting their diuretic action. Acetazolamide is the most commonly used drug in this category.

Benzothiazide Derivatives

These diuretics were developed by alteration of the basic sulfonamide structure. Their primary action is to inhibit sodium reabsorption in the cortical diluting segment, that is, between the ascending limb of the loop of Henle and the portion of the distal tubule where sodium reabsorption is regulated by aldosterone.[29] Thus, thiazide diuretics interfere with the ability to dilute but not to concentrate urine. Following thiazide administration, Na^+-K^+ exchange in the distal nephron is accelerated, leading to hypokalemia and alkalosis in addition to hyponatremia. Extracellular fluid volume depletion, hyperglycemia, and hyperuricemia are seen as well. Potassium depletion may result in life-threatening cardiac arrhythmias, particularly in patients receiving digitalis therapy. Thus, dietary potassium supplementation should be prescribed in conjunction with thiazide treatment. The thiazides cause a moderate increase in renal vascular resistance and, as a consequence of volume contraction, depression of GFR. Therefore, they may be ineffective in patients with reduced renal function. Metolazone, alone or in combination with furosemide, may be effective in patients with GFR less than 20 ml/min. The thiazide derivatives are moderately potent, so that despite their drawbacks they possess a favorable therapeutic risk–benefit ratio. They are the most widely used of the oral diuretics.

Potassium-Sparing Diuretics

These agents are antikaliuretic and moderately natriuretic. Spironolactone has a steroidal structure and is a specific aldosterone antagonist.[30] Triamterene and amiloride are organic bases and do not depend on aldosterone for their effect.[30,31] Aldosterone acts in the distal nephron by causing an increase in the tubular reabsorption of sodium and an increase in the exchange of sodium for potassium and H^+. Spironolactone is a true competitive inhibitor of aldosterone having no effect in the adrenalectomized subject. Triamterene and amiloride not only antagonize the renal tubular effects of aldosterone but also produce natriuresis and interfere with potassium and H^+ excretion, even in the absence of functioning adrenal tissue. All three drugs interfere with urinary dilution but have little effect on concentrating ability. Since aldosterone-mediated tubular reabsorption of sodium constitutes only a small fraction of total sodium reabsorption, the acute diuresis resulting from administration of these agents is small. However, their cumulative effects may be great, especially in patients with high aldosterone levels. Aldosterone antagonists are usually administered as a supplement to diuretics that block sodium reabsorption more proximally in the nephron in order to prevent or treat the potassium loss produced by these agents.

Loop Diuretics

Although chemically quite different from each other, furosemide (a sulfonamide derivative) and ethacrynic acid (a derivative of phenoxyacetic acid) act in a similar manner. A third loop diuretic, bumetanide, similar in structure and action to furosemide but with a higher milligram potency, has recently become available in the United States. At the tubular level, both act primarily by inhibiting active chloride transport in the thick ascending limb of Henle's loop.[32,33] This is the crucial step in the countercurrent multiplication mechanism so that both urinary concentration and dilution are impaired by the loop diuretics. Since 15 to 30 percent of filtered sodium is usually reabsorbed in the ascending limb, a massive diuresis of isosmotic or slightly dilute urine may occur following their administration. In addition, since large amounts of sodium are presented to distal tubule aldosterone-sensitive cation exchange sites, there may be massive potassium loss. Furosemide and ethacrynic acid also cause renal vasodilation apparently due to increased prostaglandin production and decreased prostaglandin degradation. Renal vasodilation appears to be important to the action of the loop diuretics as prostaglandin synthetase inhibitors, for example, indomethacin, abolish the vasodilation and blunt the diuresis produced by these agents.[34] The loop diuretics are so potent that they are also thought to upset the homeostatic processes responsible for regulation of body fluid tonicity and volume. The most serious complication associated with their administration has been sudden and severe contraction of intravascular fluid volume, which has led to hypotension, circulatory collapse, and death. After large doses of furosemide and ethacrynic acid, there may be carbohydrate intolerance, hyperuricemia, or permanent hearing loss. Hepatic decompensation has been reported in patients with cirrhosis. Thus, great caution must be exercised when loop diuretics are used.

The use of massive doses of furosemide (600 to 3,200 mg) and ethacrynic acid in the treatment of acute oliguric states has been advocated as a method of distinguishing functional from parenchymal renal failure and as a means of preventing the latter condition.[35,36] Although there is little doubt that urinary output and sodium excretion often are increased after treatment with these agents, except in the case of prerenal failure due to circulatory overload, there is significant disagreement whether the course of the underlying disease process is altered.[37] Similar arguments have been raised both for and against the use of hypertonic mannitol for the diagnosis and prevention of acute oliguric renal failure. Whether or not the basic disease process is modified, the management of patients with nonoliguric or high output renal failure is less complicated and carries a lower mortality rate than does that of oliguric renal failure.[38] Therefore, it would appear reasonable to administer a diuretic agent, initially mannitol, and if there is no response to it, furosemide, to patients with markedly reduced urinary output. However, this treatment should only be carried out in conjunction with etiologically oriented therapy, that is, correction of blood volume and fluid–electrolyte disturbances.

Osmotic Diuretics
(Also See Ch. 54)

Mannitol and urea are the two agents in this category that are used clinically. They are freely filtered at the glomerulus but are not significantly reabsorbed. Mannitol is the more effective because of its greater impermeability to cells; it has also been studied more widely.[39,40] Intravenous infusion of a hypertonic (20 to 25 percent) solution acutely increases intravascular osmolality so that cellular water is brought into the extracellular space in an attempt to restore osmotic homeostasis. Mannitol also has a vasodilatory effect on afferent renal arterioles, thus causing an increase in RBF and dissipation of medullary hyperosmolality. Since osmotic diuretics are not reabsorbed, they hold on to the intravascular water they have obligated and, secondarily, to some sodium. However, because transport processes in the thick ascending limb and the more distal nephron remain intact, the major diuresis is of water with a lesser loss of salt.

Osmotic diuretics have a limited ability to increase salt excretion, so they are not useful in the treatment of edematous states. However, hypertonic mannitol has been administered for the prevention and treatment of acute oliguric renal failure. Its effect on the underlying disease process is disputed. If it does have a beneficial effect, it is probably because mannitol, in addition to osmotically obligating excretion of water, produces renal arteriolar dilation with a subsequent increase in RBF and GFR. A drawback to the use of mannitol is that it can precipitate pulmonary edema in patients with early congestive heart failure or with limited cardiac reserve. Also, in some patients, translocation of cellular water to the intravascular space results in hyponatremia. This is a particular problem in those patients who truly have acute renal failure and are unable to excrete the infused mannitol load.

Treatment with diuretics is obviously not without its hazards. The most common complications are intravascular volume and electrolyte depletion that, at times, are so severe as to be life threatening. Therefore, diuretics should be used only after a diagnosis has been made and etiologically directed therapy has been instituted, and if the therapeutic risk–benefit ratio is favorable.

EFFECTS OF ANESTHETICS ON RENAL FUNCTION

In 1905, Pringle et al.[41] reported the effects of surgery with ether anesthesia on water and nonprotein nitrogen excretion in eight patients. Urine flow, which averaged 50 ml/h on the day prior to surgery, increased during the induction of anesthesia, decreased progressively to 1.2 ml/h during the surgery, and returned toward normal postoperatively. Average urine output in the 24 hours following operation was 17 ml/h, or about 408 ml for the day. Changes in nonprotein nitrogen excretion paralleled those in urinary flow rate but were less marked. Patients with the smallest postoperative urinary output had received the smallest quantities of fluid or had vomited excessively on the day of surgery.

Since Pringle's report, many investigators have measured renal function during anesthesia and surgery. After general anesthesia, the pattern of response is one of temporary depression of all measured function: urinary flow rate, GFR, RBF, and electrolyte excretion (Table 18-2). After spinal and epidural anesthesia, there are similar decrements in renal function with the magnitude of the change tending to parallel the degree of sympathetic blockade.[53] Generally, changes are only one-third to one-half as great as those seen after general anesthesia. The consistent and generalized depression of renal function that has been observed during and after surgery has been attributed to a number of factors, including the type and duration of the surgical procedure; the physical status of the patient, especially that of the cardiovascular and renal systems; preoperative and intraoperative blood volume, fluid and electrolyte balance; depth of anesthesia; and the choice of anesthetic agent. Only the broadest comparisons of anesthetic agents can be made from the data in Table 18-2 because of differences among the studies in premedication, depth of anesthesia, fluid regimens, and other aspects of the experimental protocol.

In most cases, the changes in renal function associated with anesthesia and surgery are completely reversible. At the termination of short uncomplicated procedures, RBF and GFR usually return to normal within a few hours. When surgery is more extensive and anesthesia is prolonged, secondary effects related to the endocrine system may be manifested by impaired ability to promptly excrete a water load or to elaborate concentrated urine.[54,55] These abnormalities may persist for several days. The depression in renal function specifically caused by anesthetic agents is probably due to several factors: indirect effects on the circulatory, sympathetic nervous, and endocrine systems and direct effects on tubular transport. Generally, the indirect effects, as described below, are more profound and are thought to be most important. However, methoxyflurane causes direct depression of renal tubular function,

TABLE 18-2. Effects of Anesthesia on Renal Function

Agent	Depth	Premedication	% of Control					Remarks
			RBF	GFR	Filtration Fraction	Urine Flow	Na Excretion	
Cyclopropane[42]	2nd plane	Meperidine Atropine	31	45	156	32	16	250 ml/h 5% dextrose or normal saline
Cyclopropane[43]	Light Deep	Atropine Atropine	72 34	74 45	109 150	— —	— —	No fluid administration
Cyclopropane[44]	2nd plane	None	58	61	114	35	33	Hydrated with 1 L of 4% fructose, nonoperated
Ether Diethyl[42]	2nd plane	Atropine Meperidine	48	61	132	42	37	250 ml/h of 5% dextrose or normal saline
Ether Diethyl[43]	Light Deep	Atropine Atropine	65 42	78 57	124 142	— —	— —	No fluid administration
Enflurane[44]	1.4%	Morphine Scopolamine	77	79	111	67	—	Hydrated with 15 ml/kg of isotonic glucose–saline
Halothane[46]	0.5–1.0%	Morphine Scopolamine	39	52	134	43	43	No fluids during operation
Halothane[46]	1.2–3.0%	Morphine Scopolamine	31	42	126	36	36	No fluids during operation
Halothane[47]	0.5–1.0%	Morphine Scopolamine	88	92	104	—	—	Hydrated during and before operation with 15 ml/kg of isotonic glucose—saline
Halothane[47]	1.2–3.0%	Morphine Scopolamine	53	60	110	—	—	Hydrated during and before operation with 15 ml/kg of isotonic glucose–saline
Halothane[48]	2nd plane	None	62	81	139	37	36	Hydrated with 1 L of 4% fructose, nonoperated
Isoflurane[49]	0.7–1.3%	Morphine	51	63	119	34	—	Hydrated with 15 ml/kg of isotonic glucose–saline nonoperated
Methoxyflurane[50]	0.6–0.8%	Atropine	70	79	111	46	—	No fluid information
Neurolept analgesia[51]	2nd plane	None	97	97	100	58	66	No fluids during operation
Thiopental[52]	2nd plane	Meperidine Atropine	70	68	97	48	30	250 ml/h of 5% dextrose or normal saline
Thiopental nitrous oxide[52]	Light	Morphine Atropine	64	73	122	41	39	Hydrated with 1 L of 4% fructose, nonoperated

Abbreviations: GFR, glomerula filtration rate; RBF, renal blood flow.
References are superscript numbers.

probably due to inorganic fluoride inhibition of chloride transport in the medullary descending limb of Henle's loop.

Indirect Effects of Anesthetics

Circulatory System

Profound disturbances in the circulation may accompany anesthesia and surgery and can be expected to result in equally profound disturbances in renal hemodynamics and tubular function. During general anesthesia, RBF may be depressed as a consequence of hypotension, renal vasoconstriction, or a combination of both. All anesthetic agents are myocardial depressants. Whether or not hypotension occurs depends on the depth of anesthesia and whether there is compensatory peripheral vasoconstriction. One type of response is produced by the anesthetic agents cyclopropane and diethyl ether, formerly widely used in clinical practice. Administration of these drugs results in increased blood levels of catecholamines and, as a consequence, peripheral vasoconstriction.[56] Blood pressure is maintained but at the price of a marked increase in renal vascular resistance,[44] decreased RBF, and a marked depression of renal function. Halothane, enflurane, isoflurane, and thiopental, although not provoking a catecholamine response, probably cause a mild to moderate increase in renal vascular resistance[45,46,48,49,52] to compensate for hypotension. Renal blood flow and GFR fall, but the depression in renal function with these agents is considerably less than with catecholamine release. In a third category are central nervous system depressant drugs with α-adrenergic blocking activity, such as droperidol, which are administered in combination with narcotics to produce general anesthesia.[51] α-Adrenergic blocking agents prevent redistribution of intrarenal blood flow including the marked reduction in cortical perfusion that occurs as a consequence of catecholamine release.[57] Thus, anesthesia with agents such as droperidol may result in the smallest changes in renal hemodynamics.[51]

Sympathetic Nervous System

The role of the sympathetic nervous system in mediating the renal effects of anesthetic agents was first demonstrated by Berne[58] in dogs with one normal and one denervated kidney. Before induction of pentobarbital or chloralose anesthesia, RBF and GFR of the denervated and normally innervated kidneys were the same. However, after induction of anesthesia, RBF and GFR of the normally innervated side decreased, while no changes were seen in the denervated side. It was postulated that the changes in the normally innervated kidney were due to increased vasoconstrictor tone secondary to anesthetic administration. Extrapolation of these results to clinical practice suggests that spinal or epidural anesthesia results in only minimal alterations in renal function or reverses the deleterious effects on renal hemodynamics caused by manuvers such as aortic cross-clamping. However, Gamulin et al.[59] showed that this was not the case when they administered epidural plus light general anesthesia to well-hydrated patients undergoing infrarenal cross-clamping of the aorta and were not able to prevent intraoperative decreases in renal hemodynamics or postoperative decreases in creatinine clearance. Humoral factors, such as those mediated by the renin-angiotensin system, renal prostaglandins, and kallikrein, no doubt were operative in this circumstance.

Studies of autoregulation of RBF (RBF maintained constant at systemic blood pressures of 80 to 100 mmHg) during anesthesia with the inhalation agents have yielded conflicting results. In one study, Leighton et al.[60] showed that methoxyflurane administration to dogs resulted in a 35 percent decrease in RBF, while mean blood pressure decreased from 125 mmHg to only 102 mmHg, an observation consistent with impaired autoregulation. In another study, however, the same investigators[61] demonstrated that halothane did not interfere with autoregulation, a result similar to that reported by Bastron et al.[62] using the isolated perfused kidney model. In the clinical investigations cited in Table 18-2, RBF decreased as much as 30 to 70 percent after administration of the various anesthetic agents, although arterial blood pressure rarely decreased below 80 to 90 mmHg. These repairs suggest that autoregulation is impaired. Other nonanesthetic drugs that paralyze smooth muscle, such as potassium cyanide and papaverine, also abolish autoregulation, suggesting that autoregulatory resistance changes are of myogenic rather than of sympathetic nervous system origin.

Endocrine System

The kidney both acts as an endocrine organ and is acted on by several hormones. For example, growth hormone and thyroid hormone increase GFR, while parathyroid hormone and ADH influence tubular function. The kidney produces several hormones, some of which act within the kidney (renin), while others, such as vitamin D and erythropoietin, act peripherally. Endocrine effects on renal function during anesthesia are of great importance and are closely tied to the circulatory effects discussed above. Most important in regulating urine volume is antidiuretic hormone (ADH). Renin-angiotensin, aldosterone, epinephrine, and norepinephrine also play crucial roles in electrolyte excretion and regulation of renal blood flow.

Antidiuretic Hormone

Much is known about ADH, an octapeptide formed in cells of the supraoptic and paraventricular nuclei of the hypothalamus.[63] It is transported to the posterior lobe of the pituitary gland by the axons that make up the supraopticohypophyseal tracts. ADH release is primarily controlled by two signals: variations in plasma osmolality and blood volume. Osmoreceptor cells in the carotid body and the pituitary are sensitive to osmolality changes of approximately 2 percent.[64] An increase in osmolality (hemoconcentration) will cause release of ADH and production of concentrated urine. A decrease in osmolality (hemodilution) will produce the opposite effect. Blood volume changes are sensed by stretch receptors in the walls of the atria. In response to the appropriate stimuli they alter their rate of firing, thereby modulating ADH release. Hemorrhage, positive pressure ventilation, and the upright position are thought to increase ADH secretion, whereas distention of a balloon in the left atrium, negative pressure ventilation, and immersion in water up to the neck will result in decreased ADH release. A fall in arterial blood pressure, as sensed by arterial baroreceptors, also can stimulate ADH release. Of the various stimuli, change of osmolality is normally the more important. Atrial stretch receptors and arterial baroreceptors are relatively unimportant until significant changes in blood volume have occurred.

General anesthesia and narcotics are thought to be

minor stimuli to the release of ADH; however, results of studies in this area have been inconsistent.[65-67] In support of the role of these agents in regulating ADH release, Duke et al.[65] showed that 4 to 32 μg of morphine injected into the supraoptic nuclei of dogs undergoing water diuresis resulted in a rapid fall in urine flow with the degree and duration of change proportional to the dose of morphine.[65] There was no change in systemic blood pressure, RBF, or GFR. Control injection of the same volume of saline into the supraoptic nuclei produced only a fleeting change in the rate of urinary flow. Duke and associates[65] concluded that the inhibitory action of morphine on urinary flow rate was due to the liberation of ADH.

The principal evidence against narcotic- and general anesthetic-induced ADH responses comes from studies in which morphine, 2.5 mg/kg, ether, and cyclopropane caused an antidiuretic effect both in normal dogs undergoing water diuresis and in dogs with diabetes insipidus.[65] Clearly, the latter finding argues against an ADH-mediated effect. In clinical studies, Moran et al.[68] showed that induction of anesthesia with thiopental, N$_2$O, and halothane did not elicit a significant ADH response, whereas blood loss and traction on abdominal viscera resulted in a large increase in blood levels of ADH. Changes in urinary output and free-water clearance could be correlated with changes in ADH level. Using cardiopulmonary bypass with halothane or morphine anesthesia, Philbin and Coggins[69] reported similar findings in patients undergoing cardiac operations. ADH levels did not change after induction of anesthesia, but they did increase significantly in groups of patients anesthetized with 0.5 percent halothane or 1 mg/kg morphine. There was no change in ADH levels in a third group of patients administered 2 mg/kg morphine, suggesting that the increases in the other two groups represented a stress response that could be attenuated by deeper anesthesia.

A study by Korinek et al.[70] in surgical patients supports this conclusion. They assessed the effect of extradural morphine on ADH secretion for 6 hours after surgery in a group of patients administered extradural bupivacaine, a group administered extradural morphine, and a group administered extradural morphine plus bupivacaine for intraoperative anesthesia and postoperative pain control; similar degrees of analgesia prevailed in all three groups. Plasma ADH levels were unchanged in the patients treated only with bupivacaine, whereas they increased in both other groups. Korinek et al.[70] concluded that extradural morphine induced ADH secretion, perhaps as a consequence of migration of morphine to the brainstem. A study by Bormann et al.[71] showed that epidural fentanyl administered for postoperative pain control also was associated with increased ADH levels, however, less so than intramuscularly administered narcotics.

To establish beyond a doubt that general anesthetics and narcotics cause ADH release, it would be necessary to demonstrate that their administration results in a decrease in urinary flow rate, a reciprocal increase in urinary solute excretion, no change in renal hemodynamics, and an increase in circulating ADH.[67] Because of the multiple systemic effects produced by anesthesia and operation, these conditions are difficult to meet. In the absence of such evidence, it seems reasonable to assume that both altered renal hemodynamics and ADH secretion are responsible for the decrease in urinary flow rate associated with the administration of narcotics and general anesthetic agents. From a practical viewpoint, the reduction in urinary flow rate, RBF, and GFR produced by overnight dehydration and narcotic premedication can be prevented by the preanesthetic administration of 10 to 15 ml/kg of body weight of isotonic glucose–saline solution.[47,72]

Epinephrine and Norepinephrine

Both epinephrine and norepinephrine produce marked renal vasoconstriction with a shift of blood flow away from cortical nephrons. This results in a decrease in RBF and, to a lesser extent, in GFR.[57] Sodium, chloride, and potassium excretion are reduced, probably due to the decrease in the filtered load of these ions with subsequent increased reabsorption from the tubules. Antidiuresis also may occur. It is difficult to determine how much of the renal effects of anesthetic agents, such as ether and cyclopropane,[42,43] are due to the increase in catecholamine secretion they provoke and how much are due to their other systemic effects.

Renin-Angiotensin

The development of a radioimmunoassay technique for renin has facilitated precise measurement of this hormone. However, results of the studies and their interpretation differ. Pettinger[73] has reported large increases (as much as 20-fold) in the renin activity of rats after administration of diethyl ether, cyclopropane, methoxyflurane, halothane, pentobarbital, morphine, and ketamine. Miller et al.[74,75] could not demonstrate increased plasma renin activity in rats anesthetized with fluroxene, halothane, enflurane, or ketamine or in patients anesthetized with ketamine. They suggested that the former studies may have been carried out before a steady state was achieved and that the experimental animals were excited. In patients undergoing thyroid or parathyroid surgery with isoflurane anesthesia, Udelsman et al.[76] demonstrated only small increases in plasma renin activity. The role of renin-angiotensin in the renal effects of anesthetic agents awaits further clarification.

Aldosterone

Aldosterone, the hormone responsible for the precise control of sodium excretion, is formed in the zona glomerulosa of the adrenal cortex. Aldosterone acts on several epithelial tissues: distal tubule, cortical collecting duct, salivary gland duct, sweat gland duct, epididymis, and small and large intestines. In all cases, it stimulates reabsorption of sodium from the lumen back into the blood. It also promotes potassium secretion in the distal tubule and salivary gland duct.[77] Four factors are known to cause an increase in aldosterone secretion level: (1) increased plasma potassium concentration; (2) increased adrenocorticotropic hormone (ACTH) level; (3) low-sodium diet; and (4) increased plasma angiotensin II concentration.[78] It is not known whether anesthetic agents act directly on the adrenal gland to cause aldosterone release. They probably act indirectly by (1) causing ADH release, which in turn stimulates secretion of ACTH; (2) stimulating the sympathetic nervous system, causing renal vasoconstriction, which leads to renin and ultimately to angiotensin II formation; or (3) causing peripheral vasodilation, after which the expanded vascular compartment is interpreted by baroreceptors as a decrease in functional extracellular fluid volume. Again, this leads to formation of angiotensin II and then to release of aldosterone.

Despite the fact that administration of anesthesia leads to aldosterone release, it is well known that serum sodium concentration falls after general anesthesia and surgery. Hyponatremia has been ascribed to dominance of ADH effect, liberation of endogenous sodium-free water from oxidation of fat, and overabundant administration of sodium-free fluids. Indeed, the postoperative patient was once thought to be intolerant to sodium administration, leading to the development of the practice of infusing small volumes of sodium-free fluid during the 1940s. The reversal of this view during the 1960s and subsequent modifications in the concepts of perioperative fluid therapy are discussed in Chapter 47.

Direct Effects of Anesthetics

The direct effects of anesthetic agents on renal function probably are obscured by the more marked indirect effects that occur not only in response to administration of anesthesia but in response to various other stresses present throughout the perioperative period. Nevertheless, there are reports that demonstrate that anesthetic agents alter active sodium transport in experimental preparations, such as kidney cortex slices, toad bladder, frog skin, and squid giant axon. Using rabbit cortex slices, Bastron et al.[79] demonstrated that 2 to 8 MAC concentrations of methoxyflurane and halothane depressed organic acid (PAH) transport. In the isolated toad bladder, Andersen[80] reported that treatment with cyclopropane and nitrous oxide gave rise to dose-dependent stimulation of active sodium transport, whereas treatment with halothane and methoxyflurane resulted in dose-dependent inhibition of active sodium transport. Diethyl ether produced a biphasic response: initial stimulation followed by inhibition of ion transport both in the toad bladder and in the squid giant axon.

In an effort to elucidate the mechanism of the above responses, and because epinephrine is known to stimulate sodium transport in frog skin, Andersen[81] performed additional experiments in bladders from toads previously treated with reserpine, with α- and β-adrenergic blocking agents, and with epinephrine. Cyclopropane was used as the test gas. In untreated bladders, cyclopropane produced dose-dependent stimulation of sodium transport, while in bladders treated with reserpine and those treated with the α-adrenergic blocking agents phenoxybenzamine and phentolamine, cyclopropane produced dose-dependent inhibition of sodium transport. β-blocking agents had no effect on the bladder response to cyclopropane. Andersen[80,81] also reported that stimulation of sodium transport after simultaneous administration of epinephrine and cyclopropane far exceeded the estimated additive effect of the two drugs. He concluded that the synergism of cyclopropane and epinephrine on sodium transport in toad bladder was mediated by an α-adrenergic receptor. Furthermore, he suggested that the enhancement of sodium transport brought about by diethyl ether and nitrous oxide may occur through a similar interaction with epinephrine, whereas inhibition of sodium transport by anesthetic agents may be a direct effect.

Extrapolation of the results of these studies to intact animals suggests that direct effects of anesthetic agents also occur in the renal tubule. However, it is likely that the direct effects of anesthetic agents on the renal function of surgical patients are minor compared with the major indirect effects of anesthesia and surgery.

Delayed Effects of Anesthetics: Direct Nephrotoxicity

The kidney is particularly susceptible to damage from drugs or toxins because of its rich blood supply and the increased concentration of excreted compounds that occurs in renal tubular cells during reabsorption or secretion. Additionally, medullary hypertonicity is associated with the concentration of compounds to a degree not possible in other interstitial tissues of the body. The amount of damage produced by nephrotoxins depends on many factors, such as the concentration of toxin in the target area, the duration of exposure, the susceptibility of the tissue to the toxin, the degree of toxin binding to plasma proteins and to renal and nonrenal tissues, and the rapidity of renal and extrarenal elimination. Toxic damage to the kidney may be either acute or chronic; it may predominantly affect glomerular function or cause generalized renal damage. Toxicity can be manifested by anuria, oliguria, or polyuria with urinary volume usually inversely proportional to the severity of the lesion.

Among the anesthetic drugs, only methoxyflurane causes nephrotoxicity[82-84]; this occurs as a consequence of its biotransformation to fluoride ion.[84] Fluoride is a potent inhibitor of metabolic processes. The fact that urinary dilution as well as concentration is

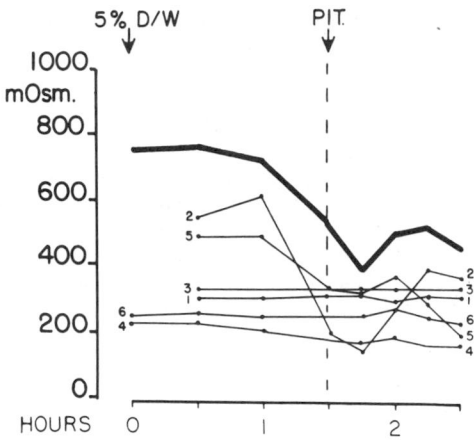

URINE OSMOLALITY CHALLENGE TEST

Fig. 18-6. Patients were administered 1 L of 5 percent dextrose in water, after which they received 0.57 mU/kg of vasopressin. Patients 1, 3, 4, and 6 were not able to dilute or concentrate their urine in response to these treatments. (From Crandell et al.,[82] with permission.)

affected (Fig. 18-6) suggests that fluoride is interfering with active chloride transport in the medullary portion of the loop of Henle and perhaps in the cortical diluting segment. In addition, by acting as a vasodilator, fluoride may cause increased vasa recta blood flow and washout of medullary solute.[85] It is also likely that proximal tubular swelling and necrosis, the morphologic lesion most commonly associated with methoxyflurane nephrotoxicity, contributes to the clinical syndrome.[86] Interference with isosmotic reabsorption of glomerular filtrate would result in presentation of an excessive load of salt and water to the more distal nephron. This would prevent development of maximum osmolality in the loop of Henle and medulla and would lead to a concentrating defect. All the above mechanisms probably contribute to fluoride-induced nephrotoxicity with interference with chloride transport in the ascending limb of the loop of Henle probably the most important. Clinical aspects of the syndrome of anesthetic nephrotoxicity are discussed in Chapter 26.

REFERENCES

1. Nissen OI: The extraction fraction of p-aminohippurate in the superficial and deep venous drainage area of the cat kidney. Acta Physiol Scand 73:329, 1968
2. Nissen OI: Changes in the filtration fractions in the superficial and deep venous drainage area of the cat kidney due to fluid loading. Acta Physiol Scand 73:320, 1968
3. Ladefoged J, Pedersen F: Renal blood flow, circulation times and vascular volume in normal man measured by the intrarenal arterial injection—external counting technique. Acta Physiol Scand 69:220, 1967
4. Thorburn GD, Kopald HH, Herd JA, et al: Intrarenal distribution of nutrient blood flow determined with krypton[85] in the unanesthetized dog. Circ Res 13:290, 1963
5. Hollenberg NK, Adams DF, Oken DE, et al: Acute renal failure due to nephrotoxins: Renal hemodynamic and angiographic studies in man. N Engl J Med 282:1329, 1970
6. Smith HW: Physiology of the renal circulation. Harvey Lect 35:166, 1939–1940
7. Von Euler US: III. Epinephrine and norepinephrine. Adrenaline and noradrenaline. Distribution and action. Pharmacol Rev 6:15, 1954
8. Hollenberg NK, Epstein M, Rosen SM, et al: Acute oliguric renal failure in man: Evidence for preferential renal cortical ischemia. Medicine (Baltimore) 47:455, 1968
9. Goldberg LI: Cardiovascular and renal actions of dopamine: Potential clinical applications. Pharmacol Rev 24:12, 1972
10. Hardaker WT, Wechsler AS: Redistribution of renal intracortical blood flow during dopamine infusion in dogs. Circ Res 33:437, 1973
11. Goldberg LI: Dopamine: Clinical uses of an endogenous catecholamine. N Engl J Med 291:707, 1974
12. Vander AJ: Control of renin release. Physiol Rev 37:359, 1967
13. Laragh JF, Sealey JE: The renin-angiotensin-aldosterone hormonal system and regulation of sodium, potassium and blood pressure homeostasis. p. 831. In Orloff J. Berliner RW (eds): Handbook of Physiology. Section 8. Renal Physiology. American Physiologic Society, Washington, DC, 1973
14. Stein JH: The renal circulation. p. 215. In Brenner BM, Rector FC, Jr. (eds): The Kidney. WB Saunders, Philadelphia, 1976
15. Thurau K: Nature of autoregulation of renal blood flow. p. 174. In Shreiner GE (ed): Proceedings of the Third Congress of Nephrology, Washington. S Karger, Basel, 1967
16. Brenner BM, Humes HD: Mechanics of glomerular ultrafiltration. N Engl J Med 297:148, 1977
17. Brenner BM, Hostetter HT: Molecular basis of proteinuria of glomerular origin. N Engl J Med 298:826, 1978
18. Marsh DJ: Renal Physiology. Raven Press, New York, 1983
19. Wirz H, Hargitay B, Kuhn W: Lokalisation des Konzentrierungsprosesses in der Niere durch direkte Kryoskopie. Helv Physiol Pharmacol Acta 9:196, 1951
20. Jamison RL, Maffly RH: The urinary concentrating mechanism. N Engl J Med 295:1059, 1976
21. Burg MB, Green N: Function of thick ascending limb of Henle's loop. Am J Physiol 224:659, 1973
22. Rocha AS, Kokko JB: Sodium chloride and water transport in the medullary thick ascending limb of Henle. J Clin Invest 52:612, 1973
23. Gottschalk CW, Mylle M: Micropuncture study of the mammalian urinary concentrating mechanism: Evidence for the counter current hypothesis. Am J Physiol 196:927, 1959
24. Frazier HS, Yager H: The clinical use of diuretics. N Engl J Med 288:246, 455, 1973
25. Burg MB: Tubular chloride transport and the mode of action of some diuretics. Kidney Int 9:189, 1976
26. Merin RG, Bastron RD: Diuretics. p. 145. In Smith NT, Miller RD, Corbascio AN (eds): Drug Interactions in Anesthesia. Lea & Febiger, Philadelphia, 1981
27. Burg MB, Green N: Effects of mersalyl on the thick ascending limb of Henle's loop. Kidney Int 4:245, 1973
28. Maren TH: Carbonic anhydrase: Chemistry, physiology and inhibition. Physiol Rev 47:595, 1967
29. Earley LE, Kahn M, Orloff J: The effects of infusions of chlorothiazide derivatives on urinary dilution and concentration in the dog. J Clin Invest 40:857, 1961
30. Liddle GW: Aldosterone antagonists and triamterene. Ann NY Acad Sci 139:466, 1966

31. Jacobson HR, Kokko JP: Diuretics: Sites and mechanisms of action. Annu Rev Pharmacol Toxicol 16:201, 1976

32. Burg MB, Green N: Effect of ethacrynic acid on the thick ascending limb of Henle's loop. Kidney Int 4:301, 1973

33. Burg MB, Stoner J, Green N: Furosemide effect on isolated perfused tubules. Am J Physiol 255:119, 1973

34. Hook JB, Bailie MD: Release of vasoactive materials from the kidney by diuretics. J Clin Pharmacol 17:673, 1977

35. Cantarovich F, Locatelli A, Fernandez JC, et al: Furosemide in high doses in the treatment of acute renal failure. Postgrad Med J, suppl., 47:13, 1971

36. Stahl WM, Stone AM: Prophylactic diuresis with ethacrynic acid for prevention of postoperative renal failure. Ann Surg 172:361, 1970

37. Kleinknecht D, Ganeval D, Gonzales-Duque LA, et al: Furosemide in acute oliguric renal failure. A controlled trial. Nephron 17:51, 1976

38. Lordon RE: Acute renal failure following battle injury—mortality, complications and treatment. p. 109. In Friedman EA, Eliahou HE (eds) Proceedings of the Conference on Acute Renal Failure. DHEW Publication No. (NIH) 74-608 U.S. Government Printing Office, Washington, DC, 1973

39. Barry KG, Malloy JP: Oliguric renal failure. Evaluation and therapy by the intravenous infusion of mannitol. JAMA 179:510, 1962

40. Nissenson AR, Weston RE, Kleeman CR: Mannitol. West J Med 131:277, 1979

41. Pringle H, Maunsell RCB, Pringle S: Clinical effects of ether anaesthesia on renal activity. Br Med J 2:542, 1905

42. Burnett CH, Bloomberg EL, Shortz G, et al: A comparison of the effects of ether and cyclopropane anesthesia on the renal function of man. J Pharmacol Exp Ther 96:380, 1949

43. Habif DV, Papper EM, Fitpatrick HF, et al: The renal and hepatic blood flow, glomerular filtration rate, and urinary output of electrolytes during cyclopropane, ether and thiopental anesthesia, operation, and the immediate postoperative period. Surgery 30:241, 1951

44. Miles BE, de Wardener HF, Churchill-Davidson HC, et al: The effect on the renal circulation of pentamenthonium bromide during anesthesia. Clin Sci 11:73, 1952

45. Cousins MJ, Greenstein LR, Hitt BA, et al: Metabolism and renal effects of enflurane in man. Anesthesiology 44:44, 1976

46. Mazze RI, Schwartz FD, Slocum HC, et al: Renal function during anesthesia and surgery. I. The effects of halothane anesthesia. Anesthesiology 24:279, 1963

47. Barry KG, Mazze RI, Schwartz FD: Prevention of surgical oliguria and renal haemodynamic suppression by sustained hydration. N Engl J Med 270:1371, 1964

48. Deutsch S, Goldberg M, Stephen GW, et al: Effects of halothane anesthesia on renal function in normal man. Anesthesiology 27:793, 1966

49. Mazze RI, Cousins MJ, Barr GA: Renal effects and metabolism of isoflurane in man. Anesthesiology 40:536, 1974

50. Auberger H, Heinrich J: Methoxyflurane und nierefuncktion. Anaesthesist 14:202, 1965

51. Gorman HM, Craythorne MWB: The effects of a new neurolept-analgesic agent (Innovar) on renal function in man. Acta Anaesthesiol Scand, suppl., 24:111, 1966

52. Deutsch S, Bastron RD, Pierce EC Jr, et al: The effects of anaesthesia with thiopentone, nitrous oxide, narcotics and neuromuscular blocking drugs on renal function in normal man. Br J Anaesth 41:807, 1969

53. Kennedy WF, Sawyer TK, Gerbershagen HU, et al: Systematic cardiovascular and renal hemodynamic alterations during peridural anesthesia in normal man. Anesthesiology 31:414, 1969

54. Gullick HD, Raisz LG: Changes in renal concentrating ability associated with major surgical procedures. N Engl J Med 262:1309, 1960

55. Hayes MA, Goldenberg IS: Renal effects of anesthesia and operation mediated by endocrines. Anesthesiology 24:487, 1963

56. Price HL, Linde HW, Jone RE, et al: Sympathoadrenal responses to general anesthesia in man and their relation to hemodynamics. Anesthesiology 20:563, 1959

57. Hollenberg NK, Epstein M, Rosen SM, et al: Acute oliguric renal failure in man. Evidence for preferential renal cortical ischemia. Medicine (Baltimore) 47:455, 1968

58. Berne RM: Hemodynamics and sodium excretion of denervated kidney in anesthetized and unanesthetized dog. Am J Physiol 171:148, 1952

59. Gamulin Z, Forster A, Simonet F, et al: Effects of renal sympathetic blockade on renal hemodynamics in patients undergoing major aortic abdominal surgery. Anesthesiology 65:688, 1986

60. Leighton KM, Koth B, Wenkstern BM: Autoregulation of renal blood flow: Alteration by methoxyflurane. Can Anaesth Soc J 20:173, 1973

61. Leighton KM, Bruce C: Distribution of kidney blood flow: A comparison of methoxyflurane and halothane effects as measured by heated thermocouple. Can Anaesth Soc J 22:125, 1975

62. Bastron RD, Perkins FM, Pyne JL: Autoregulation of renal blood flow during halothane anesthesia. Anesthesiology 46:142, 1977

63. Jamison RL, Kriz W: Urinary Concentrating Mechanism: Structure and Function. p. 13. Oxford University Press, New York, 1982

64. Verney EB: The antidiuretic hormone and the factors which determine its release. Proc R Soc Lond [Biol] 135:25, 1947

65. Duke HN, Pickford M, Watt JA: The antidiuretic action of morphine; its site and mode of action in the hypothalamus of the dog. Q J Exp Physiol 36:149, 1951

66. Bachman L: The antidiuretic effects of anesthetic agents. Anesthesiology 16:939, 1951

67. Papper S, Saxon L, Burg MB, et al: The effect of morphine sulphate upon the renal excretion of water and solute in man. J Lab Clin Med 50:692, 1957

68. Moran WH, Jr, Mittenberger FW, Shuayb WA, et al: Relationship of antidiuretic hormone section to surgical stress. Surgery 56:99, 1964

69. Philbin D, Coggins CH: Plasma antidiuretic hormone levels in cardiac surgical patients during morphine and halothane anesthesia. Anesthesiology 49:95, 1978

70. Korinek AM, Languille M, Bonnet F, et al: Effect of postoperative extradural morphine on ADH secretion. Br J Anaesth 57:407, 1985

71. Bormann B, Weidler B, Dennhardt R, et al: Influence of epidural fentanyl on stress-induced elevation of plasma vasopressin (ADH) after surgery. Anesth Analg 62:727, 1983

72. Mazze RI, Barry KG: Prevention of functional renal failure during anesthesia and surgery by sustained hydration and mannitol infusion. Anesth Analg 46:61, 1967

73. Pettinger WA: Anesthetics and the renin-angiotensin-aldosterone axis (editorial). Anesthesiology 48:393, 1978

74. Miller ED Jr, Baily D, Kaplan J, et al: The effect of ketamine on the renin-angiotensin system. Anesthesiology 42:503, 1975

75. Miller ED Jr, Longnecker DE, Peach MJ: The regulatory func-

tion of the renin-angiotensin system during general anesthesia. Anesthesiology 48:399, 1978

76. Udelsman R, Norton JA, Jelenich SE, et al: Responses of the hypothalamic-pituitary-adrenal and renin-angiotensin axes and the sympathetic system during controlled surgical and anesthetic stress. J Clin Endocrinol Metab 64:986, 1987

77. Barger AC, Berlin RD, Tulenko JF: Infusion of aldosterone, 9-α-fluorohydrocortisone and antidiuretic hormone into the renal artery of normal and adrenalectomized unanesthetized dogs: Effect on electrolyte and water excretions. Endocrinology 62:804, 1958

78. Sharp GWG, Leaf A: Effects of aldosterone and its mechanism of action on sodium transport. p. 803. In Orloff J, Berliner RW (eds): Handbook of Physiology. Section 8. Renal Physiology. American Physiologic Society, Washington, DC, 1973

79. Bastron RD, Perkins FM, Kaloyanides GJ: In vitro inhibition of PAH transport by halogenated anesthetics. J Pharmacol Exp Ther 200:75, 1977

80. Andersen NB: Effect of general anesthetics on sodium transport in the isolated toad bladder. Anesthesiology 27:304, 1966

81. Andersen NB: Synergistic effect of cyclopropane and epinephrine on sodium transport in toad bladder. Anesthesiology 28:438, 1967

82. Crandell WB, Pappas SG, Macdonald A: Nephrotoxicity associated with methoxyflurane anesthesia. Anesthesiology 27:591, 1966

83. Mazze RI, Shue GL, Jackson SH: Renal dysfunction associated with methoxyflurane anesthesia: A randomized prospective clinical evaluation. JAMA 216:278, 1971

84. Mazze RI, Trudell JR, Cousins MJ: Methoxyflurane metabolism and renal dysfunction: Clinical correlation in man. Anesthesiology 35:247, 1971

85. Whitford GM, Taves DR: Fluoride induced diuresis: Renal–tissue solute concentrations, functional, hemodynamic and histologic correlates in the rat. Anesthesiology 39:416, 1973

86. Kosek JC, Mazze RI, Cousins MJ: The morphology and pathogenesis of nephrotoxicity following methoxyflurane (Penthrane) anesthesia. Lab Invest 27:575, 1972

19

CEREBRAL PHYSIOLOGY

John C. Drummond
Harvey M. Shapiro

INTRODUCTION

The effects of anesthetic drugs and techniques on cerebral physiology, and, in particular, their effects on cerebral blood flow and metabolism are described in this chapter. The pathophysiology of cerebral ischemia and cerebral protection are briefly discussed. Information of immediate relevance to the rationale for the anesthetic and intensive care management of patients with intracranial pathology is emphasized. Chapter 54 presents the clinical management of these patients in detail. The effects of anesthetics on the electroencephalogram and evoked responses are reviewed in Chapter 35.

The final section of this chapter provides a brief description of the methods used in many of the investigations of cerebral physiology from which the information in this chapter is derived. Readers who are unfamiliar with the various measurement techniques and their limitations may wish to review that section first. Table 19-1 lists the abbreviations used frequently in this chapter.

TABLE 19-1. Frequently Used Abbreviations

BBB	Blood-brain barrier
CBF	Cerebral blood flow
CBV	Cerebral blood volume
CMR	Cerebral metabolic rate
CMRg	Cerebral metabolic rate for glucose
$CMRO_2$	Cerebral metabolic rate for oxygen
CPP	Cerebral perfusion pressure
CSF	Cerebrospinal fluid
CSFP	Cerebrospinal fluid pressure
CVP	Central venous pressure
CVR	Cerebrovascular resistance
ECF	Extracellular fluid
EEG	Electroencephalogram
ICP	Intracranial pressure
l-CBF	Local cerebral blood flow
MAC	Minimal alveolar concentration
MAP	Mean arterial pressure
MRI	Magnetic resonance imaging
MRS	Magnetic resonance spectroscopy
PET	Positron emission tomography
rCBF	Regional cerebral blood flow
SPECT	Single proton emission computed tomography
Xe/CT	Xenon-enhanced computed tomography

TABLE 19-2. Normal Cerebral Physiologic Values

Parameter	Value
CBF	
Global	45–55 ml/100 g/min
Cortical CBF (mostly gray matter)	75–80 ml/100 g/min
Subcortical CBF (mostly white matter)	~20 ml/100 g/min
$CMRO_2$	3–3.5 ml/100 g/min
CVR	1.5–2.1 mmHg · 100 g · min/ml
Cerebral venous PO_2	35–40 mmHg
ICP (supine)	8–12 mmHg

REGULATION OF CEREBRAL BLOOD FLOW

Anesthetics cause dose-related and reversible alterations in central nervous system (CNS) function that result in unconsciousness and analgesia. These anesthetic-induced changes in brain function are accompanied by alterations in many aspects of cerebral physiology including cerebral blood flow (CBF), cerebral metabolic rate (CMR), and electrophysiologic function (electroencephalogram [EEG], evoked responses). The changes in CBF and CMR can be of clinical importance in patients with neurosurgical diseases. Certain anesthetic drugs and techniques have the potential to adversely affect the diseased brain and the conduct of the neurosurgical procedure. However, in certain instances, the effects of general anesthesia on CBF and CMR can be manipulated to improve both the operative course and the clinical outcome of patients with neurologic disorders.

The adult human brain weighs approximately 1,350 g and therefore represents about 2 percent of total body weight. However, it receives 12 to 15 percent of cardiac output. This high flow rate is a reflection of the brain's high metabolic rate. At rest, the brain consumes oxygen at an average rate of approximately 3.5 ml of oxygen per 100 g of brain tissue per min. Whole brain oxygen consumption ($13.5 \times 3.5 = 47$ ml/min) represents about 20 percent of total body oxygen utilization. Normal values for CBF, CMR, and other physiologic variables are provided in Table 19-2.

A large proportion of the brain's energy consumption, approximately 60 percent,[1] is used to support electrophysiologic function. The depolarization-repolarization activity that occurs and that is reflected in the EEG requires energy expenditure for the maintenance and restoration of ionic gradients and for the synthesis, transport, and reuptake of neurotransmitters. The remainder of the energy consumed by the brain is involved in cellular homeostatic activities that include maintenance of the neuron's relatively large membrane mass. Local CBF (l-CBF) and l-CMR within the brain are very heterogeneous, and both are approximately four times greater in gray matter than in white matter. The cell population of the brain is also heterogeneous in its oxygen requirements. Glial cells make up about one-half of the brain's volume and require less energy than neurons. Besides providing a physically supportive latticework for the brain, the glial cells are important in the reuptake of neurotransmitters and in the delivery and removal of metabolic substrates and wastes.

The brain's substantial demand for substrate must be met by adequate delivery of oxygen and glucose by blood flow. However, the space constraints imposed by the noncompliant cranium and meninges require that blood flow not be excessive. Not surprisingly, there are elaborate mechanisms for the regulation of CBF. These mechanisms, which include chemical, myogenic, and neurogenic factors, are listed in Table 19-3.

Chemical Regulation of CBF

Several factors cause changes in the cerebral biochemical environment that result in adjustments of CBF. These include changes in CMR, $PaCO_2$, and PaO_2.

Cerebral Metabolic Rate

Increased neuronal activity results in increased local brain metabolism, and this increase in l-CMR is associated with a well-matched, proportional change in l-CBF.[2] Regional CBF (rCBF) and rCMR measurements performed in humans during maneuvers designed to activate specific brain regions provide evidence of the strict local coupling of CMR and CBF. During hand movements, both rCBF and $rCMRO_2$ increase rapidly and simultaneously in the appropriate contralateral cortical area.[3] Other studies have demonstrated similar changes in rCBF distribution during both psychologi-

TABLE 19-3. Factors Influencing CBF

Factor	Comment
Chemical/metabolic/humoral	
CMR	CMR influence assumes
Anesthetics	intact flow-metabolism
Temperature	coupling, the mechanism
Arousal and seizures	of which is not understood
$PaCO_2$	
PaO_2	
Vasoactive drugs	
Anesthetics	
Vasodilators	
Pressors	
Myogenic	
Autoregulation and MAP	The autoregulation mechanism is fragile and in many pathologic states CBF is pressure passive (Fig. 19-5).
Rheologic	
Blood viscosity	
Neurogenic	Contribution and clinical
Extracranial sympathetic pathways	significance poorly
Intracranial pathways	defined

cal tasks and sensory stimulation.[4,5] The adjustments in l-CBF are thought to occur as a result of the opening and closing of sphincterlike vasomotor mechanisms in response to local alterations in cerebral metabolism.[6] While it is clear that local metabolic factors play a major role in these adjustments in CBF, the precise mechanism of flow-metabolism coupling remains unknown. A variety of metabolic by-products and epiphenomena have been considered as the intermediaries. These include hydrogen ion concentration, extracellular potassium and/or calcium ion concentration, the products of membrane phospholipid metabo-

lism (thromboxane and certain prostaglandins), and adenosine.[7] However, there are weaknesses in the data supporting each of the potential metabolic mediators that has been evaluated, and the mechanisms of coupling must be viewed as undetermined.[7]

CMR is influenced by several phenomena in the neurosurgical environment including the functional state of the nervous system, anesthetics, and temperature.

Functional State

CMR decreases during sleep and increases during sensory stimulation, mental tasks, or arousal from any cause. During epileptoid activity CMR increases may be extreme.

Anesthetic Drugs

The effect of individual anesthetics on CMR is presented in greater detail in a later section. In general, anesthetics suppress CMR, with ketamine the notable exception. It appears that the component of cerebral metabolism on which anesthetics act is predominately that associated with electrophysiologic function.[1] With several agents, for example, barbiturates,[1] isoflurane,[8] and etomidate,[9] increasing plasma concentrations cause progressive suppression of EEG activity and a concomitant reduction in CMR. However, increasing the plasma level beyond that required to first achieve isoelectricity of the EEG results in no further depression of CMR. The component of CMR required for the maintenance of cellular integrity, the "housekeeping" component, is apparently unaltered by anesthetics (Fig. 19-1). There are data to suggest that lidocaine in large doses (160 mg/kg in the dog) is a possible exception.[10] This may arise because the membrane-stabilizing effect of lidocaine reduces the energy requirement for the maintenance of membrane integrity.

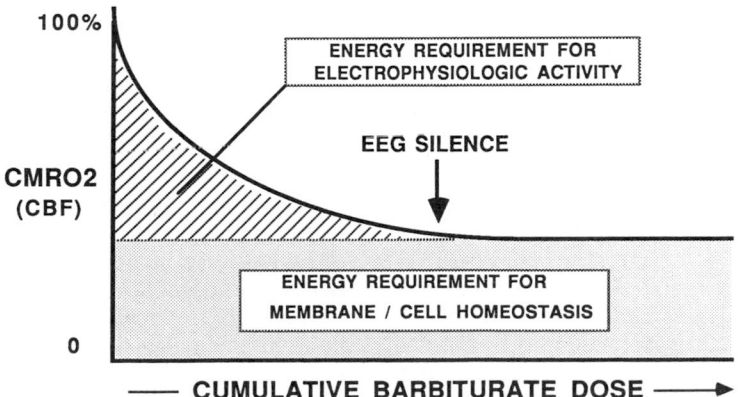

Fig. 19-1. Interdependency[1] of cerebral electrophysiologic function and CMR. Administration of various anesthetics[1,8,9] including barbiturates results in a dose-related reduction in $CMRO_2$ and CBF. The maximum reduction occurs with the dose that results in electrocerebral silence. At this point energy utilization associated with electrophysiologic activity has been reduced to zero but energy utilization for cellular homeostasis persists unchanged. Additional barbiturate causes no further decrease in CBF or $CMRO_2$.

The $CMRO_2$ values observed when isoelectricity is established with different anesthetics are very similar. The inference that anesthetic-induced EEG isoelectricity represents a single physiologic state no matter what agent is employed easily follows. However, the latter is by no means proved. In fact, there is evidence to the contrary. When barbiturates are administered to the point of isoelectricity, a uniform depression of CBF and CMR occurs throughout the brain. When isoelectricity occurs during isoflurane administration, the relative suppression of CMR and CBF is greater in the neocortex than in other portions of the cerebrum.[11,12] Cortical somatosensory evoked responses to median nerve stimulation can be recorded readily at doses of pentothal far in excess of those required to cause isoelectricity[13] but are difficult to elicit[14] at concentrations of isoflurane associated with a burst suppression pattern, for example, 1.5 minimal alveolar concentration (MAC) or the onset of isoelectricity[15] (Fig. 19-2). These differences

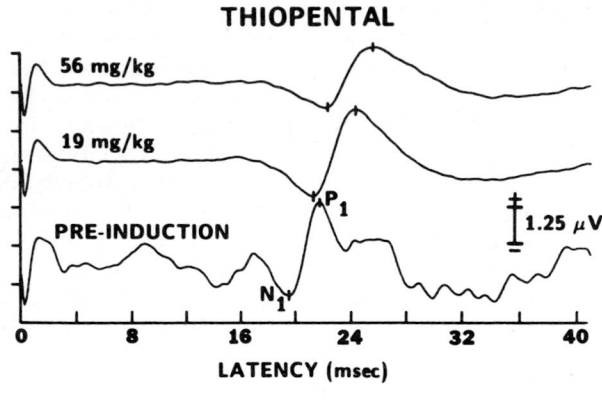

THIOPENTAL

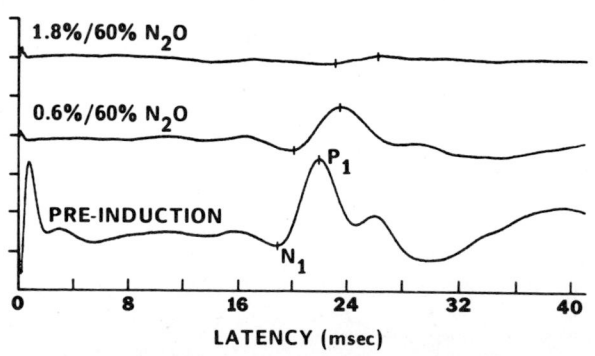

ISOFLURANE

Fig. 19-2. Cortical somatosensory evoked responses to median nerve stimulation in humans preinduction and during anesthesia with thiopental and isoflurane-N_2O. Despite an equivalent or greater degree of probable CMR reduction with thiopental, cortical evoked responses are better preserved than during anesthesia with isoflurane. This suggests that the EEG isoelectricity achieved with different anesthetics should not be assumed to be equivalent electrophysiologic states. The cumulative thiopental doses and expired concentrations of isoflurane and N_2O are indicated.

may be of some relevance to discussions of differences in the protective potential of agents that can produce isoelectricity.

Temperature

The effects of hypothermia of the brain are reviewed in detail by Michenfelder.[16] CMR decreases by 6 to 7 percent per Celsius degree of temperature reduction.[16] As is the case with some anesthetics, hypothermia can also cause isoelectricity of the EEG (at about 20°C). However, in contrast to anesthetics, temperature reduction beyond that at which isoelectricity first occurs *does* produce a further decrease in CMR (Fig. 19-3). This occurs because, while anesthetics reduce only the component of CMR associated with neuronal function, hypothermia causes proportional decreases in the rate of energy utilization associated with both electrophysiologic function and the maintenance of cellular integrity. $CMRO_2$ at 18°C is less than 10 percent of normothermic control values, and this accounts for the brain's tolerance for moderate periods of circulatory arrest at these and lower temperatures.

Hyperthermia has an opposite influence on cerebral physiology. Between 37 and 42°C, CBF and CMR increase. However, above 42°C a dramatic reduction in cerebral oxygen consumption occurs, an indication of a threshold for a toxic effect of hyperthermia that may occur as a result of protein (enzyme) degradation.

$PaCO_2$

CBF varies directly with $PaCO_2$ (Fig. 19-4). The effect is greatest within the range of physiologic $PaCO_2$ variation. CBF changes 1 to 2 ml/100 g/min for each 1 mmHg change in $PaCO_2$ around normal $PaCO_2$ values.[17] This response is attenuated below a $PaCO_2$ of 25 mmHg.[17] Under normal circumstances CBF sensitivity to changes in $PaCO_2$ ($\Delta CBF/\Delta PaCO_2$) appears to be positively correlated with resting levels of CBF.[18] Accordingly, anesthetics that alter resting CBF cause changes in the CO_2 response of the cerebral circulation. However, CO_2 responsiveness has been observed in normal brain during anesthesia with all of the numerous anesthetics that have been studied.[17,19-21]

The changes in CBF caused by $PaCO_2$ depend on pH alterations in the extracellular fluid (ECF) of the brain.[22] The changes in ECF pH and CBF occur rapidly after $PaCO_2$ adjustments because CO_2 diffuses freely across the cerebrovascular endothelium. Note that in contrast to a *respiratory* acidosis, acute systemic *metabolic* acidosis has little immediate effect on CBF because the blood-brain barrier (BBB) excludes the hydrogen ion (H^+) from the perivascular space. Although the CBF changes in response to a $PaCO_2$ alteration occur rapidly, they are not sustained. CBF returns to normal over 6 to 8 hours[23,24] because CSF pH gradually normalizes as a result of the extrusion of bicarbonate. Numerous investigations have sought to deter-

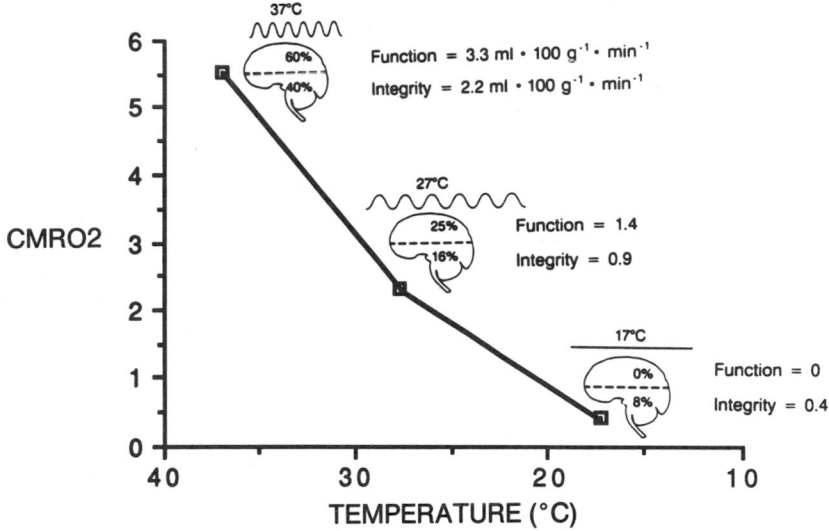

Fig. 19-3. Effect of temperature reduction on $CMRO_2$. Hypothermia reduces *both* of the components of cerebral metabolic activity identified in Figure 19-1: that associated with neuronal electrophysiologic activity (Function) and that associated with the maintenance of cellular homeostasis (Integrity). This is in contrast to anesthetics that alter only the function component. (Modified from Michenfelder,[16] with permission.)

mine whether hyperventilation can cause cerebral ischemia.[25-33] The data indicate that, in normal subjects, ischemia will not occur at $PaCO_2$ greater than 20 mmHg, and this generalization appears also to apply during induced hypotension.[34-36] However, physiologic alterations, as evidenced by both metabolic and electroencephalographic abnormalities, have been observed in human volunteers[28,30] and in normal animals[25,29,32] at extreme hypocapnia ($PaCO_2 < 15$ mmHg), and in dogs submitted to the combination of severe hypocapnia ($PaCO_2 = 10$ mmHg) and severe anemia (hemoglobin of 5 g/dl).[27] In one of these studies,[30] EEG abnormalities and paresthesiae occurred in volunteers hyperventilating to $PaCO_2$ values less than 20 mmHg, and these effects were reversed by hyperbaric oxygenation, suggesting that they were truly

caused by ischemia. In two separate investigations in cats, at $PaCO_2$ levels of 10 to 12 mmHg[25,32] modest reductions in brain phosphocreatine levels with increased brain lactate but normal ATP levels were observed. It has been suggested[32] that the observed changes may in part reflect pH-related alterations in enzyme function (specifically, an increase in the activity of phosphofructokinase causing increased lactate formation) rather than ischemia. Nonetheless, given that there is very little additional benefit in terms of compliance improvement below a $PaCO_2$ level of 20 to 25 mmHg, it seems prudent to limit acute $PaCO_2$ reduction to 20 to 25 mmHg in previously normocarbic individuals.

The patient who has had a chronic alteration of $PaCO_2$ deserves special consideration. Cerebrospinal fluid (CSF) bicarbonate adaptation occurs with a half-life (t1/2) of about 6 hours during prolonged hypocapnia or hypercapnia, and CSF pH gradually returns to normal despite a sustained alteration of arterial pH.[37] Thereafter, the acute normalization of $PaCO_2$ will result in a significant CSF acidosis (after hypocapnia) or alkalosis (after hypercapnia). The former will result in increased CBF with a concomitant intracranial pressure (ICP) increase that will depend on the prevailing intracranial compliance. The latter conveys the theoretical risk of ischemia.

PaO_2

Changes in PaO_2 from 60 to over 300 mmHg have little influence on CBF. Below a PaO_2 of 60 mmHg, CBF increases rapidly (Fig. 19-4). The mechanisms mediating the cerebral vasodilation during hypoxia are not fully

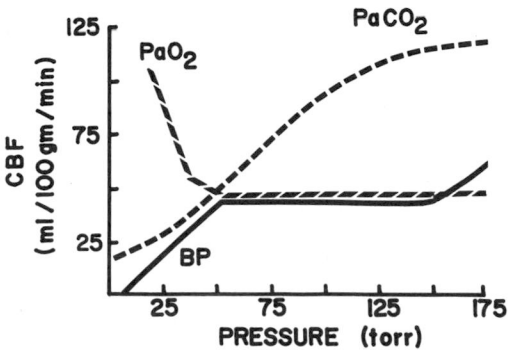

Fig. 19-4. Changes in CBF caused by independent alterations in $PaCO_2$ (dashed line), PaO_2 (parallelogram dashes), and blood pressure (solid line).

understood but may include neurogenic influences initiated by peripheral chemoreceptors and direct vascular hypoxic effects mediated by lactic acidosis. At high PaO_2 values CBF decreases modestly. At 1 atmosphere of oxygen, CBF is reduced by 15 percent.

Myogenic Regulation (Autoregulation) of CBF

Autoregulation refers to the intrinsic capacity of the cerebral circulation to adjust its resistance to maintain CBF constant over a wide range of mean arterial pressures (MAPs). In normal subjects, the limits of autoregulation are approximately 50 and 150 mmHg (Fig. 19-4). Above and below this range, CBF is pressure dependent (pressure passive) and varies linearly with cerebral perfusion pressure (CPP). Autoregulation is influenced by various pathologic processes and, in addition, by the time course over which CPP changes occur. Even within the range over which autoregulation normally occurs, a rapid change in arterial pressure will result in a transient (3 to 4 minutes) alteration of CBF.[38]

The precise mechanism by which autoregulation is accomplished is not known. It appears to be an intrinsic characteristic of cerebral vascular smooth muscle (i.e., it is myogenic) since it can be demonstrated in isolated vessels.[39] Autoregulation is easily impaired. It is modified by numerous cerebral disease processes (Fig. 19-5) and by cerebral vasodilators including volatile anesthetics (Fig. 19-6). Neurogenic influences and vasoactive agents also affect the CBF response to changing CPP. These are discussed in subsequent sections.

Many investigations of the effects of anesthetics on autoregulation suffer from important methodologic limitations. Commonly, CBF measurements are performed while MAP is manipulated during or after administration of the anesthetic of interest. Difficulty arises because the method of MAP manipulation may itself influence autoregulation and/or have an independent dose-related influence on CBF via direct effects on the cerebral vascular smooth muscle (e.g., vasodilation, vasoconstriction). In these situations the results may not accurately reflect the effect of the agent of interest on the status of the intrinsic myogenic response (autoregulation) to changing CPP, but rather the effects of the CPP manipulation technique. An investigation of "autoregulation" during halothane anesthesia is a useful example.[40] MAP elevation was accomplished in dogs with either angiotensin or norepinephrine. Higher CBF values were observed when angiotensin was employed. It was concluded that halothane impairs autoregulation (probably true) and that norepinephrine "restores" it. In fact, it is probable that norepinephrine has no effect at all on autoregulation, and that, in the circumstances of the experiment, it was directly causing cerebral vasoconstriction. To many this will be little more than a semantic issue because the study data should accurately represent the behavior of the cerebral circulation in the circumstances of the study. However, this imprecise use of the term autoregulation can lead to inappropriate extrapolation of the experimental data to other situations. Investigations of autoregulation should be reviewed carefully.

Neurogenic Regulation of CBF

There is considerable evidence of extensive innervation of the cerebral vasculature. The density of innervation declines with vessel size, and the greatest neurogenic influence appears to be exerted upon larger cerebral arteries.[41] It is therefore likely that neurogenic control is more important in the CBF regulation of large brain areas than in precise local CBF modulation. This innervation includes cholinergic,[42] adrenergic (sympathetic and nonsympathetic),[43] and serotonergic[44,45] systems of extracranial and intracranial origin. It is certain that in animals there is an extracranial sympathetic influence via the superior cervical ganglion.[46-50] The intracranial pathways are much less certain, although there is considerable evidence of innervation arising from several nuclei in animals including the locus ceruleus[51] and the dorsal raphe nucleus.[45] The clearest evidence of the functional significance of neurogenic influences emerges from studies of CBF autoregulation.[52,53] Hemorrhagic shock, a high sympathetic tone state, results in a lower CBF at a given arterial

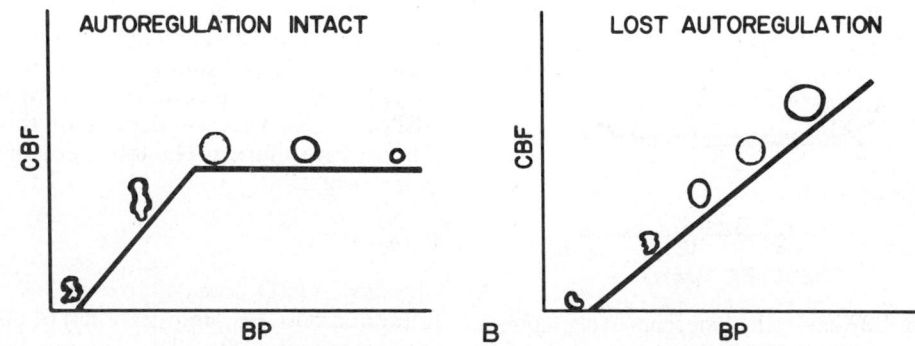

Fig. 19-5. Effect of blood pressure on CBF and vascular diameter when autoregulation is intact (**A**) or absent (**B**). In the latter situation CBF is pressure passive.

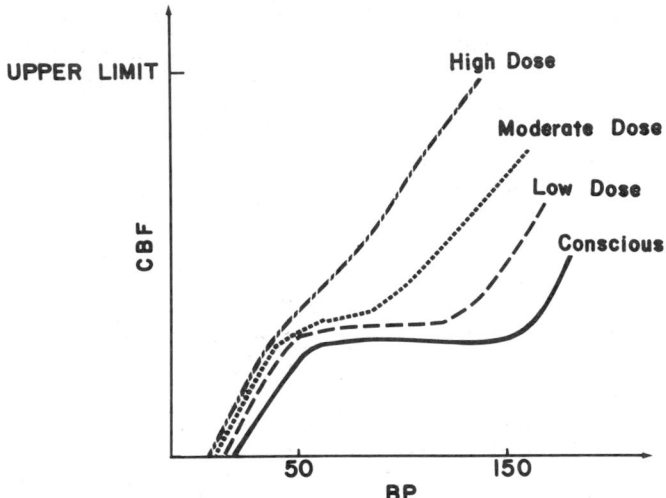

Fig. 19-6. Schematic representation of the effect of increasing concentrations of a typical volatile anesthetic on CBF autoregulation. Both the upper and lower thresholds are shifted to the left.

pressure than that observed when hypotension is produced with sympatholytic drugs. This is presumably because, during shock, a sympathetically mediated vasoconstrictive effect shifts the lower end of the autoregulatory plateau (Fig. 19-4) to the right. It is not clear what the relative contributions of humoral and neural mechanisms are to this phenomenon; however, there is certainly a neurogenic component in some species because sympathetic denervation increases CBF during hemorrhagic shock in the baboon.[52] Activation of cerebral sympathetic innervation also shifts the upper limit of autoregulation to the right and offers some protection against hypertensive breakthrough of the BBB.[54]

Viscosity Effects on CBF

Blood viscosity can influence CBF. Hematocrit is the single most important determinant of blood viscosity.[55] In healthy subjects, hematocrit variation within the normal range (33 to 45 percent) probably results in only trivial alteration of CBF. Beyond this range changes may be more obvious. In polycythemia vera, a marked increase in cerebrovascular resistance (CVR) resulting from increased blood viscosity can reduce CBF to one-half of normal values.[56] In anemia, CVR is reduced and CBF increases. However, this may result not only from reduction in viscosity but also in response to reduced oxygen-carrying capacity of blood. The effect of viscosity reduction on CBF is more obvious in the setting of focal cerebral ischemia when vasodilation in response to impaired oxygen delivery is probably already maximal. In this setting, viscosity reduction accomplished by hemodilution results in increases in CBF in the ischemic territory.[57-59] The best available information suggests that in the setting of focal cerebral ischemia, a hematocrit of 30 to 34 percent will result in optimal oxygen delivery.[60]

Vasoactive Agents

A large number of agents with intrinsic vascular effects are employed in contemporary anesthetic practice. These include both anesthetics and numerous vasoactive drugs used specifically for hemodynamic manipulation. This section deals with the latter. The actions of anesthetics are discussed in a later section.

Systemic Vasodilators

The majority of the drugs used to induce hypotension (including sodium nitroprusside, nitroglycerin, hydralazine, adenosine, calcium channel blockers) also cause cerebral vasodilation. As a result, CBF either increases or is maintained at prehypotensive levels. In addition, CBF is maintained at lower MAPs when hypotension is induced with a cerebral vasodilator than with either hemorrhage or a noncerebral vasodilator, for example, the ganglionic blocker trimethaphan.[61] The ICP effects of the vasodilators are empirically less dramatic when hypotension is induced slowly.[62] This probably reflects the more effective interplay of compensatory mechanisms (CSF and venous blood shifts) when changes occur more slowly.

Catecholamine Agonists and Antagonists

Numerous drugs with agonist and antagonist activity at catecholamine receptors (α_1, α_2, β, and dopamine) are in common use. The data regarding the effects of these agents on cerebral physiology contain numerous apparent inconsistencies. In part, these arise because of differences between species,[49] because of differences in the receptor populations on different vessels (e.g., intraparenchymal versus extraparenchymal) within a given species,[49] and because of model differences (e.g., in vivo versus in vitro). However, other variables have probably contributed. These include the magnitude of the systemic blood pressure changes that occurred as a result of administration of the agent of interest, the status of the autoregulation mechanism (as determined by the anesthetics employed and/or damage inherent to the preparation), and the status of the BBB. Those who intend to review this literature should also appreciate that the effects of pressors are reported by various authors in terms of effects on either CBF or CVR. An increase in CVR is occasionally presented as prima facie evidence that the agent in question is a cerebral vasoconstrictor. Recall, however, that the normal autoregulatory response to a rising MAP entails cerebral vasoconstriction (an increase in CVR) to maintain a constant CBF. Accordingly, an increase in CVR may indicate that the agent has a direct effect on the cerebral vasculature, but alternatively it may indicate the absence of a direct effect and preservation of autoregulation. It is probably most practical to think in terms of changes in CBF rather than changes in CVR because CBF is the variable that is most important to the clinician. The information below and in Table 19-4 emphasizes data obtained in investigations of pressor agents in intact preparations and gives greatest weight to results obtained in humans and higher primates.

α_1-Agonists

Agents with a predominant α_1-agonist effect, for example, Neo-Synephrine (phenylephrine) and norepinephrine, appear to have a species-dependent cerebral vasoconstrictor effect. In both dogs and goats, norepinephrine infusion at rates resulting in a moderate elevation of MAP (ca. 30 mmHg) is associated with a reduction in CBF that can be blocked by α_1-antagonists.[63-67] By contrast, moderate doses of α_1-agonists do not appear to cause cerebral vasoconstriction

TABLE 19-4. Best Estimates of the Influence of Pure Catecholamine Receptor Agonists and Specific Pressor Substances on CBF and CMR[a]

Agonist	CBF	CMR
Pure		
α_1	−	0
α_2	−−	0
β	0	0
β (BBB open)	+++	+++
Dopamine	++	−
Dopamine (high dose)	?−	?0
Mixed		
Norepinephrine	−	0
Norepinephrine (BBB open)	++	++
Epinephrine	−	0
Epinephrine (BBB open)	+++	+++

[a] When species differences occurred, data from primates were given preference.
Symbols: +, increase; −, decrease (the number of symbols indicates the magnitude of the effect); 0, no effect.

in rats.[68-70] The response in higher primates including humans may be intermediate between the extremes represented by dogs and rats. Intracarotid infusions of norepinephrine in doses that caused minimal increases in MAP resulted in no change in CBF in humans[71] and baboons.[72] A larger intravenous dose of norepinephrine administered by King et al.[73] (average MAP increased from 91 to 117 mmHg) cause a modest 9 percent reduction in global CBF.

The CBF increase attributed to noradrenaline in some studies may be the result of BBB abnormalities. There are data to suggest that β-mimetic agents (norepinephrine has some β activity) cause activation of cerebral metabolism with a parallel coupled increase in CBF when they gain access to the brain parenchyma via a defective BBB[69,72,74] (see the section, *Epinephrine*).

In summary, it seems likely that circulating α_1-agonists will have a small to moderate vasoconstrictor influence in normal humans with the exception that norepinephrine may cause vasodilation when the BBB is defective.

Epinephrine

It is difficult to reconcile all the available information. It appears likely that epinephrine in moderate doses has little direct effect on the cerebral vasculature but that β-receptor activation results in an increase in CMR with accompanying increases in CBF. The latter effect occurs at high doses, and it is not certain whether it can occur in the normal cerebral circulation or whether a deficiency of the BBB must occur to permit catecholamine access to the brain.

There have been two investigations of the effect of epinephrine on CBF in awake humans. Olesen[71] observed no change in CBF in response to an intracarotid infusion of approximately 6 μg/min of epinephrine, a dose that caused no change in MAP. King et al.[73] administered intravenous epinephrine in doses sufficient to increase MAP from 91 to 109 mmHg. CBF and $CMRO_2$ increased by 22 and 24 percent, respectively.

Evidence that a BBB defect is necessary for the effect on CMR to occur comes from investigations by MacKenzie et al.[72] and Artru et al.[74] MacKenzie et al.[72] observed no effect of intracarotid norepinephrine on CBF and CMR in normal baboons. However, when they disrupted the BBB by the intracarotid injection of hypertonic urea, norepinephrine caused increases in CBF and CMR. Artru et al.[74] demonstrated that epinephrine caused $CMRO_2$ elevation in dogs but only when BBB permeability to Evans blue was present. The subjects of King et al. (see above) in whom CMR increased should have had an intact BBB. However, they experienced subjective symptoms, for example, palpitations, apprehension, excitement, and the CBF and $CMRO_2$ changes may have been a secondary arousal phenomenon. Berntman et al.[69] in an investigation in N_2O-sedated rats, obtained results that paralleled those of Olesen,[71] and King et al.[73] They observed no change in CBF or CMRO$_2$ during intravenous infusion of a dose of epinephrine (2 μg/kg/min) that resulted in no change in MAP. However, the administration of 8 μg/kg/min caused an increase in MAP, CBF, and CMRO$_2$. The rats in this investigation were normal, but MAP was transiently very high (180 mmHg) and such transients can open the BBB.[75] In an investigation in normal dogs, Bunegin et al.[76] observed no change in CBF in response to esmolol administration. There have been no investigations of the effect of β-blockers in the presence of an abnormal BBB.

It appears probable that epinephrine, like norepinephrine, will have little effect on CBF and CMR unless the BBB is opened by disease processes, anesthetics, or extreme and/or sudden MAP elevation. When the BBB is open, epinephrine will cause increases in CBF and CMR and these effects will be greater than those seen with norepinephrine.

Dopamine

Dopamine is widely employed in the treatment of hemodynamic dysfunction. In addition, it is commonly used to augment the function of the normal cardiovascular system when MAP elevation is desired as an adjunct to the treatment of focal cerebral ischemia, especially in the setting of vasospasm. Nonetheless, there are few data regarding its effects on CBF and CMR. The majority of the data are provided by von Essen and colleagues,[64,77,78] who measured CBF in dogs. His reports indicate a triphasic effect with CBF reduction occurring at both low ($<$ 2 μg/kg/min) and moderate to high (7 to 20 μg/kg/min) doses and increases occurring at intermediate (2 to 6 μg/kg/min) doses. There were no changes in CMRO$_2$.[64] The CBF reduction in both dose ranges was blocked by phentolamine and was therefore attributed to an α-agonist effect of dopamine. The CBF increase was blocked by dopamine receptor antagonists (haloperidol, pimozide).[78] Tuor et al.[70] studied dopamine in rats. Large doses of dopamine (200 μg/kg/min) were required to induce moderate hypertension (MAP of 150 mmHg). A substantial increase in CBF occurred, that is, the vasoconstriction seen in the dog was not apparent. The CMR for glucose (CMRg) was subtley reduced during dopamine infusion. Taken together, these data suggest that the predominant effect of dopamine in the normal cerebral vasculature will probably be vasodilation with minimal CMR change. It is unclear whether dopamine will cause cerebral vasoconstriction when used in high doses in humans. An overview of the literature regarding the CBF effects of pressors suggests that the dog is more susceptible to the vasoconstrictor effects of α-agonists than are primates and that the results of von Essen should not be assumed to apply to humans. However, an in vitro investigation of human cerebral arteries[79] revealed that while the initial effect of dopamine was relaxation, high concentrations caused contraction that was attenuated by α-

antagonists. Therefore, dopamine, in fact, may cause α-mediated vasoconstriction in humans in vivo. However, undefined concentrations of dopamine that are high enough to cause substantial α-activity are probably required.

α_2-Agonists

There is considerable current interest in α_2-agonists because of their apparent analgesic and sedative effects. However, their role in anesthetic practice is not yet well defined and to date there have been few investigations of their effects on CBF and CMR. An investigation of the highly specific α_2-agonist dexmedetomidine performed by Zornow et al.[80] in isoflurane-anesthetized dogs revealed a potent cerebral vasoconstrictive effect with no influence on CMRO$_2$. There are no other studies regarding CMR effects. However, there are additional data to support the likely occurrence of CBF reduction by this class of agents. An investigation of CBF during hemorrhagic hypotension[81] revealed preservation of CBF at lower MAP levels in cats treated with the α_2-antagonist yohimbine. Investigations of clonidine, a less specific and less potent α_2-agonist, have also revealed reductions in CBF in both humans[82] and cats[83] following intravenous administration, and a decrease in spinal cord blood flow following intrathecal administration in the rat.[84] CBF reduction is not the response to α_2-agonists that might initially be anticipated from first principles. α_2-Agonists are most commonly thought to act via a presynaptically mediated inhibition of norepinephrine release. Given that topical norepinephrine applied to cerebral vessels causes vasoconstriction,[50] an *increase* in CBF with α_2-agonists would seem the more likely response. Accordingly, other mechanisms of action must be considered. These include the possible contribution of postsynaptic α_2-receptors causing vasoconstriction[85] and/or the action of α_2-agonists at a central site, for example, the locus ceruleus, involved in the neurogenic control of the cerebral circulation.[51]

Age

Aging, from childhood to late adulthood, is associated with progressive reduction of CBF and CMRO$_2$.[86,87] This flow reduction is probably not secondary to progressive arterial stenosis, because cerebral circulatory responses to arterial blood pressure and PaCO$_2$ alterations persist.[88] It may reflect the progressive neuronal loss that occurs with age.

EFFECTS OF ANESTHETIC DRUGS ON CBF AND CMR

This section deals with the effect of anesthetics on CBF and CMR. It includes limited mention of influences on autoregulation, CO$_2$ responsiveness, and cerebral blood volume (CBV). Discussions of effects on CSF dynamics, the BBB, and epileptogenesis are in the section, *Cerebral Physiology in Pathologic States.*

In neuroanesthesia, considerable emphasis is placed on the manner in which anesthetic drugs and techniques influence CBF. The rationale is twofold. First, the delivery of energy substrates is dependent on CBF, and in the setting of ischemia, modest alterations in CBF can substantially influence neuronal outcome (see below). Second, the control and manipulation of CBF is central to the management of ICP because of the effect of CBF on CBV. In normal brain, over a $PaCO_2$ range of approximately 20 to 80 mmHg, CBV changes by about 0.04 ml/100 g of brain for each 1 mmHg change in $PaCO_2$.[89] In an adult brain weighing about 1,400 g, this can amount to a 17-ml change in total CBV for a $PaCO_2$ range of 25 to 55 mmHg. Autoregulation normally serves to prevent MAP-related increases in CBV, but when it is impaired or its limit (ca. 150 mmHg) is exceeded, CBF and CBV increase in proportion to arterial blood pressure, as shown in Figures 19-4 and 19-5. In normal subjects, the initial increases in CBV do not result in significant ICP elevation because there is latitude for compensatory adjustments by other intracranial compartments (e.g., translocation of venous blood and CSF to extracerebral vessels and the spinal CSF space, respectively). When intracranial compliance* is reduced, a CBV increase can cause herniation or reduce CPP sufficiently to cause ischemia. While CBV and CBF usually vary in parallel, there are exceptions. CBV increases during cerebral ischemia[90,91] and after a sudden, substantial reduction in MAP because of cerebral vasodilation. There have been several investigations of the effects of anesthetics on CBV. In general, the observed effects confirm a parallel relationship between CBF and CBV.[92-94]

The importance of blood volume on the venous side of the cerebral circulation should also not be overlooked. Engorgement of these vessels as a result of the head down posture, compression of the jugular venous system, or high intrathoracic pressure can have dramatic effects on ICP (Fig. 19-7). While the intracranial veins are a largely passive compartment, there is evidence that, in some species, there is some active control of venous caliber by either neurogenic or humoral mechanisms.[47,49,95] However, there is no evidence that these effects have clinical significance.

Intravenous Anesthetics

The general pattern of the effect of intravenous anesthetics is one of parallel alterations in CMR and CBF. The vast majority of intravenous agents cause a decrease in both. Ketamine, which causes an increase in

---

* Note a well entrenched misuse of terminology. The "compliance" curve that is commonly drawn to describe the intracranial pressure-volume relationship (Fig. 54-9) actually depicts the relationship $\Delta P/\Delta V$ (elastance) and not $\Delta V/\Delta P$ (compliance).

CMR and CBF, is the exception. The effects of selected intravenous anesthetics on human CBF are compared in Figure 19-8.

It is probable that intravenous anesthetic-induced changes in CBF are largely the result of effects on CMR with parallel (coupled) changes in CBF. If this were the entire explanation, the CBF/CMR ratio would be the same for all agents. It is not. It is therefore likely that there are also direct effects on cerebral vascular smooth muscle (e.g., vasoconstriction, vasodilation, alteration of autoregulatory function) that make contributions to the net effect. For instance, barbiturates, which are generally thought of as cerebral vasoconstrictors, actually cause relaxation of cerebral vascular smooth muscle in isolated vessel preparations.[96] However, in vivo a substantial reduction in CMR occurs and the net effect at the point of EEG isoelectricity is vasoconstriction and a substantial decrease in CBF.[1,97] When additional barbiturate is administered beyond isoelectricity, results on cerebral vascular tone and CBF are conflicting.[1,98] It appears that, in general, autoregulation and CO_2 responsiveness are preserved during administration of intravenous anesthetics.

Barbiturates

A dose-dependent reduction in CBF and CMR occurs with barbiturates. With the onset of anesthesia, CBF and $CMRO_2$ are reduced by about 30 percent.[99,100] When large doses of thiopental cause EEG suppression to the isoelectric point, CBF and CMR are reduced by about 50 percent.[1,97] Further increases in dose have no additional effect.[1] These observations suggest that the major effect of nontoxic doses of depressant anesthetics is a reduction in the component of cerebral metabolism that is linked to brain function (e.g., neurophysiologic activity), with only minimal effects on the second component, that related to cellular homeostasis (e.g., maintenance of cell membrane integrity, ion transport) (Fig. 19-1). Recall (see above) that, by contrast, hypothermia suppresses both components of metabolic rate. Temperature reduction to 28°C is associated with a reduction in CBF and CMR comparable to that which occurs at normothermia during pentobarbital-induced isoelectricity (i.e., about 50 percent). However, temperature-dependent depression of CMR and CBF continues beyond the point of isoelectricity to very low temperatures (Fig. 19-3).[16]

Tolerance to the CBF and CMR effects of barbiturates may develop quickly.[101] In patients with severe head injury in whom barbiturate coma was maintained for 72 hours, the thiamylal blood concentration required to maintain EEG burst suppression was observed to be increased by the end of the first 24 hours and continued to increase over the next 48 hours.[102] Dogs maintained in deep barbiturate anesthesia, characterized by extreme EEG suppression, for 24 hours experienced a gradual increase in $CMRO_2$ and CBF.[103] During deep

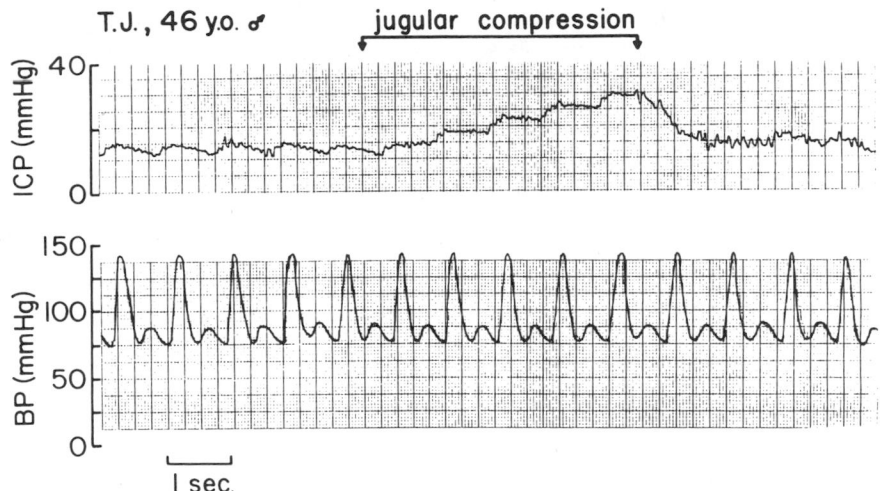

Fig. 19-7. Effect of cerebral venous outflow obstruction on ICP in a patient with an intracerebral hematoma. Bilateral jugular compression was applied briefly to verify the function of a newly placed ventriculostomy. The ICP response illustrates the importance of maintaining free cerebral venous drainage.

pentobarbital anesthesia autoregulation is maintained to arterial pressures as low as 60 mmHg.[56] CO_2 responsiveness also persists.[19]

Narcotics

There are inconsistencies in the available information, but it is likely that narcotics have very little effect on CBF and CMR in the normal, unstimulated nervous sys-

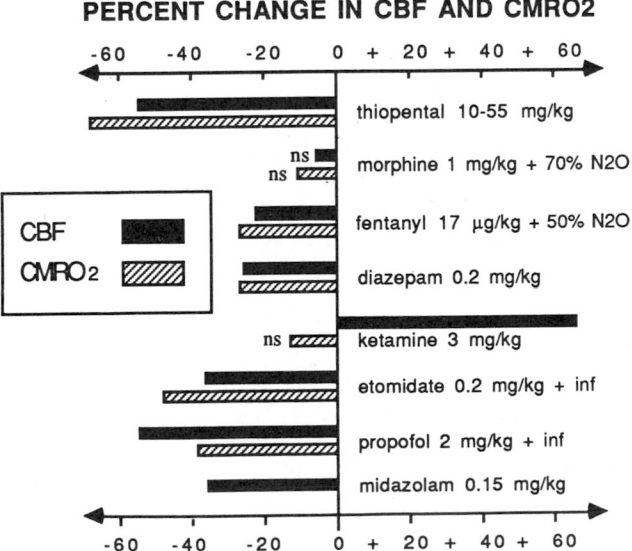

Fig. 19-8. Changes in CBF and $CMRO_2$ caused by intravenous anesthetics. The data are derived from human investigations and are presented as percent change from unanesthetized control values. No data for the $CMRO_2$ effects of midazolam are available. (See text for details.) ns, not statistically significant. (Data from refs. 97, 105, 108, 123, 125, 136, 143, and 152.)

tem. When changes occur, the general pattern is one of modest reductions in both CBF and CMR. The inconsistencies in the literature probably arise largely because, in many studies, the control state entailed paralysis and nominal sedation, often with nitrous oxide alone. In these studies, in which substantial reductions of CBF and CMR were frequently observed, the effect of the narcotic was probably a combination of the inherent effect of the drug plus a substantial component due to reduction of arousal. Comparable effects related to reduction of arousal may occur and be important clinically. However, they should be viewed as nonspecific effects of sedation and/or pain control rather than as specific properties of narcotics. The following discussion emphasizes investigations in which control measurements were unlikely to have been markedly influenced by arousal phenomena.

Morphine

When morphine (ca. 1 mg/kg) was administered as the sole agent in humans, Moyer et al.[104] observed no effect on global CBF and a 41 percent decrease in $CMRO_2$. The latter is a substantial reduction and the absence of a simultaneous CBF adjustment is surprising. There have been no other investigations of morphine alone in humans. Jobes et al.[105] gave morphine (1 and 3 mg/kg) with 70 percent N_2O to patients and observed no significant change in CBF or CMR. The N_2O that was used might be expected to have caused a tendency toward increases in CBF and CMR. The relative absence of *net* changes in these variables from the awake control measurements suggests a small to moderate depressive effect of morphine on CBF and CMR at this large dose. Takeshita et al.[106] gave morphine (3 mg/kg) to dogs sedated with 70 percent N_2O (approximately 0.6 MAC).

They observed reductions of global CBF and $CMRO_2$ of approximately 60 and 17 percent, respectively. These data cannot be completely reconciled, and the data of Jobes et al.[105] are probably relevant to the most common clinical situations. Autoregulation was observed to be intact between MAPs of 60 and 120 mmHg in human volunteers anesthetized with morphine (2 mg/kg) and 70 percent N_2O.[107]

Fentanyl

Limited human data are available. Vernhiet et al.[108] measured CBF and $CMRO_2$ before and during anesthesia with 12 to 30 (mean, 16) $\mu g/kg$ of fentanyl with 50 percent N_2O in patients about to undergo cerebral angiography. Atropine and pancuronium were the only other drugs administered. Neither mean CBF nor mean $CMRO_2$ changed significantly from awake control values in their group of six subjects. However, one of the patients (an epileptic) had dramatic and unexplained increases in both CBF and $CMRO_2$. For the remaining five, CBF and $CMRO_2$ decreased by 21 and 26 percent, respectively ($P < 0.05$). The data for fentanyl-N_2O presented in Figure 19-8 are derived from these five patients who received an average of 17 $\mu g/kg$ of fentanyl. Murkin et al.[109] measured CBF before and after induction of anesthesia with high-dose fentanyl (100 $\mu g/kg$) and diazepam (0.4 mg/kg). CBF fell by 25 percent, although part of this effect may well have been the result of the benzodiazepine (see below) rather than fentanyl. There are additional data derived from animal experiments. McPherson and Traystman[110] administered fentanyl (25 $\mu g/kg$) to pentobarbital-anesthetized dogs and observed no effect on CBF and CMR. CO_2 responsiveness and autoregulation were unaffected, and the hyperemic CBF response to hypoxia also remained intact. Several investigations in lightly anesthetized animals[111-113] have demonstrated much larger fentanyl-induced reductions in CBF and/or CMR than those observed in humans. These data taken together suggest that fentanyl will cause a moderate reduction in CBF and CMR in the normal quiescent brain and will, like morphine, cause larger reductions when administered during arousal.

Alfentanil

There have been no studies of the CBF and $CMRO_2$ effects of alfentanil in humans. McPherson et al.[114] administered alfentanil (320 $\mu g/kg$) to pentobarbital-anesthetized dogs. The results were similar to those of their earlier investigation of fentanyl (see above), that is, no changes in CBF, CMR, CO_2 responsiveness, autoregulation, or the CBF response to hypoxia.

Sufentanil

There have been three investigations of the CBF and CMR effects of sufentanil in humans. Murkin et al.[115] induced anesthesia with 10 $\mu g/kg$ of sufentanil in mor-

phine-lorazepam premedicated subjects. They observed a 25 percent reduction of CBF and a 21 percent reduction in $CMRO_2$. Young et al.[116] measured CBF and CMR during anesthesia with sufentanil (1.5 to 2.0 $\mu g/kg$ followed by infusion of 0.1 to 0.3 $\mu g/kg/h$) and N_2O and compared the values with those obtained during anesthesia with 0.75 percent isoflurane and N_2O. CBF and CMR were, respectively, 31 and 44 percent less during sufentanil anesthesia. These latter results cannot be interpreted quantitatively but are consistent with a moderate reduction of global CBF and CMR by sufentanil in humans. Vernhiet et al.,[108] in the same investigation mentioned above in connection with fentanyl, measured CBF and $CMRO_2$ before and during anesthesia with 2 $\mu g/kg$ of sufentanil with 50 percent N_2O in six neurologically intact patients about to undergo cerebral angiography. For the six patients, average global CBF increased by 36 percent, which was not statistically significant ($P < 0.10$). The response was quite variable. CBF decreased in two patients (range 5 to 12 percent) and increased in the remaining four (range 26 to 100 percent). $CMRO_2$ was unchanged. In rats, sufentanil caused dose-related reductions in global CBF and $CMRO_2$ to a maximum of 53 and 40 percent, respectively, despite the occurrence of brief epileptoid activity.[117]

The data from the foregoing studies, with the exception of those from the small population of Vernhiet et al.,[108] lead to the anticipation of no change or a reduction in ICP as a result of administration of either sufentanil or alfentanil. The available data do not bear out this prediction. Marx et al.[118] reported lumbar CSF pressure (L-CSFP) and calculated "cerebral" perfusion pressure (CPP = MAP − L-CSFP) before and after administration of sufentanil (1 $\mu g/kg$), alfentanil (50 $\mu g/kg$) and fentanyl (5 $\mu g/kg$) in thiopental-N_2O-vecuronium-anesthetized, normocapnic patients about to undergo supratentorial tumor resection. The mean prenarcotic L-CSFPs were 11, 13, and 9 mmHg in the three groups, suggesting, at worst, a moderate initial impairment of the compliance of the CSF space. In the 10 minutes following narcotic administration, average maximum changes (± standard error) in L-CSFP were as follows: sufentanil, +89 ±5 percent ($P < 0.05$); alfentanil, +22 ±5 percent ($P < 0.05$); fentanyl, −8 ±7 percent (not significant). All three narcotics caused a reduction in MAP, and the changes in CPP were greater with alfentanil (−37 ±3 percent) than with sufentanil (−25 ±5 percent) or fentanyl (−14 ±3 percent). The increases in L-CSFP were readily overcome by subsequent induction of hypocapnia. Because acute CPP reduction per se might have caused a reduction in CBF and thereby influenced the results (because of acute cerebral vasodilation in response to a sudden reduction in MAP), these investigators repeated their study using phenylephrine to support MAP. They observed substantial L-CSFP increases with *both* sufentanil and alfentanil and, again, no appreciable effect with fentanyl (R. Bedford, personal communication). These data, at least with respect to sufentanil, appear inconsistent with some of the human CBF data mentioned above. However, in experiments in dogs (venous outflow model), Milde and Milde[119,120] observed increases in CBF and ICP following sufentanil administration. These increases occurred in the absence of changes in $CMRO_2$. The latter leads to the suspicion of an intrinsic vasodilating effect by sufentanil that would make it (and perhaps alfentanil) unique among narcotics. The time course of the response in the studies of Marx et al.,[118] and Milde and Milde[119,120] was sufficiently short that a similar transient vasodilating effect could have occurred and waned before the CBF measurements that were made in the patients studied by Murkin et al.[115] and Young et al.[116]

This issue will no doubt undergo further investigation, and it is currently difficult to draw a firm clinical conclusion. Note that the L-CSFP increases observed by Marx et al.[118] occurred at normocapnia and were easily overcome by hyperventilation. In addition, From et al. performed an investigation in which patients undergoing supratentorial craniotomies were anesthetized with fentanyl, sufentanil, or alfentanil with N_2O and hypocapnia was maintained. The neurosurgeon, who was blinded to the anesthetic, evaluated conditions in the operative field, and there were no between-group differences (R. From, University of Iowa, personal communication). Shupak and Harp[121] and Bristow et al.[122] also found no adverse effects on conditions in the surgical field when sufentanil was administered during craniotomies. These drugs should therefore probably not be viewed as in any way contraindicated, although they should be used in conjunction with hypocapnia.

Benzodiazepines

Benzodiazepines cause parallel reductions in CBF and CMR in humans and monkeys. CBF and $CMRO_2$ decreased by 25 percent when 15 mg of diazepam was given to head-injured patients.[123] Lorazepam given to monkeys in doses sufficient to cause sedation reduced CBF by 24 percent and $CMRO_2$ by 21 percent.[124] The effects of midazolam on CBF (but not CMR) have also been studied in humans. Forster et al.[125,126] observed a 30 to 34 percent reduction in CBF after administration of 0.15 mg/kg of midazolam to awake healthy human volunteers. CO_2 responsiveness was preserved.[21] The foregoing studies indicate that benzodiazepines should cause moderate reduction of CBF in humans and suggest that the effect may be metabolically coupled.

The extent of the CBF-CMR reduction produced by benzodiazepines is probably intermediate between the decreases caused by narcotics (minimal) and barbiturates (substantial). Using the canine venous outflow model, Michenfelder[1] observed a minimum $CMRO_2$ of 2.2 ml/100 g/min during administration of very large doses of thiopental. In two separate studies in the same laboratory, Fleischer et al.[127] and Nugent et al.[128] identified 4.0 and 2.9 ml/100 g/min, respectively, as the minimum $CMRO_2$ attainable with midazolam.

Benzodiazepines should be safe to administer to pa-

tients with intracranial hypertension provided that respiratory depression and an increase $PaCO_2$ do not occur.

Flumazenil

Flumazenil (initially identified as RO 15-1788) is a highly specific, competitive benzodiazepine receptor antagonist. It had no effect on CBF when administered to unanesthetized human volunteers,[126] and CBF, CMR, and ICP were all unchanged after administration of flumazenil to isoflurane-N_2O-anesthetized dogs that had not received a benzodiazepine.[129] In two investigations in dogs with normal intracranial compliance,[127,129] flumazenil resulted in reversal of the CBF, CMR, and ICP lowering effects of midazolam. However, in addition, it caused a substantial but short-lived overshoot above premidazolam levels in both CBF (by 44 to 56 percent) and ICP (by 180 to 217 percent). CMR did not rise above control levels in either study, indicating that the CBF increase was not metabolically coupled. The effect is unexplained but may be a neurogenically mediated arousal phenomenon. Pending further information and, in particular, human clinical experience, this drug should probably be used cautiously in the reversal of benzodiazepine-induced sedation in patients with impaired intracranial compliance.

Droperidol

There have been no human investigations of the CBF-CMR effects of droperidol alone. Sari et al.[130] studied a droperidol (0.25 mg/kg)-fentanyl (5 μg/kg) combination in humans. Alcuronium was given to prevent rigidity. Normocapnia was maintained by mask ventilation and the patients were otherwise unstimulated. CBF, $CMRO_2$, and jugular bulb pressure were unchanged, although CPP decreased by 16 percent. Misfeldt et al.[131] gave 7.5 to 12.5 mg of droperidol to patients with supratentorial tumors during anesthesia with N_2O and gallamine. Mean ICP, which was 24 mmHg (i.e., poor compliance) preinjection, was unchanged by droperidol. However, ICP increases that were readily controlled by hyperventilation occurred in individual patients. MAP fell such that CPP decreased by 24 percent. Miller et al.[132] observed no change in ICP and "a small fall" in MAP after 5 to 10 mg of droperidol. These and other data[113,133] taken together suggest that droperidol is not a cerebral vasodilator and probably has little effect on CBF and CMR in humans. The occasional ICP increases observed by Misfeldt et al.[131] may have reflected a normal autoregulation-mediated vasodilation in response to an abrupt fall in MAP.

Ketamine

Among the intravenous anesthetics, ketamine is unique in its ability to activate cerebral function (i.e., increase CMR) during anesthesia. CBF also increases, and this may be the result of a combination of direct cerebral vasodilating effects[134] and a coupled effect caused by the increased CMR.[135] CBF increases have been observed in two studies in humans.[136,137] In other reports,[138,139] the occurrence of the anticipated ICP correlate of the CBF increase has been confirmed. Animal studies indicate that the changes in CMR are regionally variable. In rats, substantial increases in CMR occur in limbic system structures simultaneously with modest changes or small decreases in cortical structures.[135,140] Depth electrode studies of ketamine-induced convulsive phenomena suggest that similar preferential activation of thalamic and limbic structures also occurs in humans.[141] The CMR increases that have been repeatedly demonstrated in animals,[135,140,142] however, have not been verified in humans. In the only investigation of CMR effects in humans, Takeshita et al.[136] observed a 62 percent increase in CBF and no change in CMR, and the explanation for this discrepancy is unclear.

Autoregulation during ketamine administration has not been directly tested. CO_2 responsiveness persists intact, since hyperventilation can reduce the ICP elevation caused by ketamine.[139]

Etomidate

The effects of etomidate on CBF and CMR are superficially similar to those of barbiturates. Roughly parallel reductions in CBF and CMR occur in humans[143,144] and are in general accompanied by progressive suppression of the EEG.[145] The CBF/CMR changes are substantial. Renou et al.[143] gave approximately 0.2 mg/kg of etomidate to adults and observed mean reductions in CBF and CMR of 34 and 45 percent respectively. In dogs, as is the case with barbiturates, no further reduction of CMR occurs when additional drug is administered beyond a dose sufficient to produce isoelectricity.[9] This latter phenomenon has not been demonstrated in humans. However, Bingham et al.[146] observed that etomidate lowered ICP (probably because of metabolically coupled reduction of CBF) when administered to severely head injured patients with well-preserved EEG activity but was ineffective when there was substantial antecedent EEG suppression. Canine data reviewed by Milde et al.[9] suggest that, while substantial, the global CMR suppression attainable with etomidate is slightly less profound than that achieved with isoflurane and barbiturates. This is consistent with the observations of Davis et al.[147] that, unlike barbiturates, which cause CMR suppression throughout the brain, the CMR suppression caused by etomidate is regionally variable and occurs predominately in forebrain structures.

Etomidate has been shown to be effective in reducing ICP without causing reduction of CPP in head-injured patients.[148] However, concerns regarding the occurrence of adrenocortical suppression will probably limit its use in this setting. Reactivity to CO_2 is preserved in humans during etomidate administration.[143,144] Autoregulation has not been evaluated.

Althesin

Althesin is a combination of two steroids. It is not currently available in the United States because of the sporadic occurrence of anaphylactoid phenomena. Althesin has effects on CBF and CMR that are similar to those of etomidate. Reduction of both CBF and CMR with simultaneous EEG suppression occurs.[149] In the rat, the CMR suppression is also most apparent in forebrain structures.[150] Althesin is similar to etomidate in its capacity to reduce ICP with reasonable maintenance of CPP in head-injured patients.[148]

Propofol

Propofol (2,6-diisopropylphenol) has undergone limited investigation. Two studies in humans revealed reductions in CBF and CMR after propofol administration.[151,152] In one, Stephan et al.[152] administered propofol by bolus plus infusion (2 mg/kg and 0.2 mg/kg/min, respectively) and observed average CBF and CMR decreases of 51 and 36 percent, respectively. ICP was not measured in that investigation, but in a separate study, Ravussin et al.[153] measured lumbar CSF pressure during induction of anesthesia by slow bolus administration of propofol (1.5 mg/kg over 30 seconds) in patients scheduled for craniotomy. They observed maximum average reductions in L-CSFP and CPP of 32 and 10 percent, respectively.

Lidocaine

Lidocaine produces a dose-related reduction of $CMRO_2$ in experimental animals.[154] In dogs, 3 mg/kg lowered $CMRO_2$ by 10 percent, and 15 mg/kg reduced it by 27 percent. When very large doses (160 mg/kg) were given to dogs, the reduction in $CMRO_2$ was at least as great as that seen with high-dose barbiturates.[155] Bedford et al.[156] compared the effectiveness of bolus doses of pentothal (3 mg/kg) and lidocaine (1.5 mg/kg) in controlling the acute increase in ICP that occurred following application of a pin head holder or skin incision in craniotomy patients. The two regimens were equally effective in causing ICP reduction. However, the MAP decrease was greater with pentothal. Accordingly, a bolus dose of lidocaine is a reasonable adjunct to the prevention or treatment of acute ICP elevation and has been recommended for use in the prevention of ICP increases associated with endotracheal suctioning.[157] Note that large doses of lidocaine can produce seizures in humans and in some experimental animals.[158] Lidocaine-induced seizures have not been reported in anesthetized humans. None the less, it seems appropriate to restrict lidocaine doses to amounts that achieve serum levels less than the seizure threshold (>5 to 10 $\mu g/ml$) in awake humans.[159] Viegas and Stoelting[160] reported peak serum concentrations of 6.6 to 8.5 $\mu g/ml$ after a 2 mg/kg intratracheal bolus of lidocaine. Bolus doses of 1.5 to 2.0 mg/kg therefore seem appropriate.

Inhaled Anesthetics

Volatile Anesthetics

The important clinical consequences of volatile anesthetic administration are derived from the increases in CBF and CBV, and consequently ICP, that can occur. Of the commonly employed volatile anesthetics, the order of vasodilating potency is approximately halothane >> enflurane > isoflurane.[161-163] There is less available information regarding the newer agents sevoflurane and desflurane (see below); however, it appears likely that their effects on the cerebral vasculature are similar to those of isoflurane. In this section, halothane, enflurane, and isoflurane are discussed together under a series of subheadings dealing with their effects on various aspects of cerebral physiology. The effects of the three common volatile anesthetics on global CBF in humans are presented in Figure 19-9.

The pattern of volatile anesthetic influence on cerebral physiology is a striking departure from that observed with the intravenous anesthetics, which cause generally parallel changes in CMR and CBF. All the volatile anesthetics produce a dose-related reduction in CMR while simultaneously causing an increase in CBF.[8,164-166] As a consequence of this pattern it has been said that volatile anesthetics cause "uncoupling" of flow and metabolism. However, there is evidence that coupling (CBF adjustments paralleling changes in CMR) persists during volatile agent anesthesia.[165,167,168] The clearest evidence was the demonstration of dramatic parallel increases in CBF and CMR when seizures occurred in hypocapnic enflurane-anesthetized dogs.[165] In addition, when noxious stimuli after the EEG pattern during halothane anesthesia, CBF increases occur in association with increases in CMRO$_2$.[168] Accordingly, it is probably more accurate to say that the CBF/CMR ratio is altered (increased) by volatile anesthetics. This alteration is apparently dose related because under steady state conditions there is a positive correlation between MAC multiples and the CBF/CMRO$_2$ ratio for all volatile anesthetics (Fig. 19-10).

CBF-CMR Effects

Volatile anesthetics depress cardiovascular function and modify autoregulation. Accordingly, their effects on CBF and ICP can only be compared when arterial pressure is supported to a common level. In humans, when MAP is maintained at 80 mmHg, equipotent (1.1 MAC) levels of halothane, enflurane, and isoflurane cause CBF increases (Kety-Schmidt method) of 191, 37, and 18 percent, respectively (Fig. 19-9).[161] A similar potency scale was observed in a study that compared the degree of brain surface protrusion through a craniectomy in cats.[169] Enflurane at 1.0 and 1.5 MAC and isoflu-

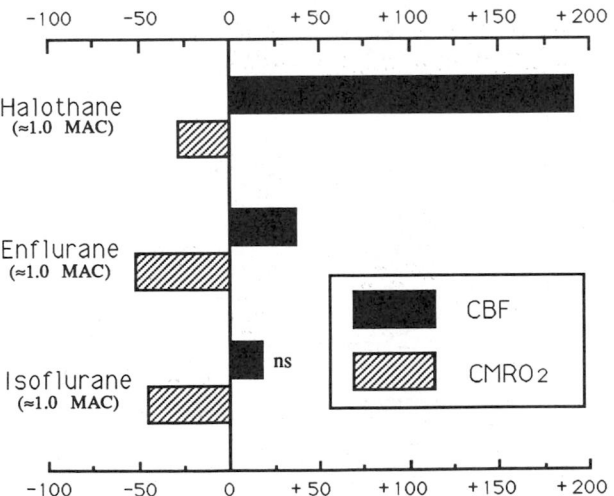

Fig. 19-9. Percent changes in CBF and CMRO$_2$ caused by volatile anesthetics. The CBF data were obtained during 1.1 MAC anesthesia (with blood pressure support) in humans[161] and are expressed as percent change from awake control values. The CMRO$_2$ data were obtained in the cat,[162,166] and are expressed as percent change from N$_2$O-sedated control values. ns, not statistically significant. (Data from Murphy et al.,[161] Todd et al.,[162] and Todd and Drummond.[166])

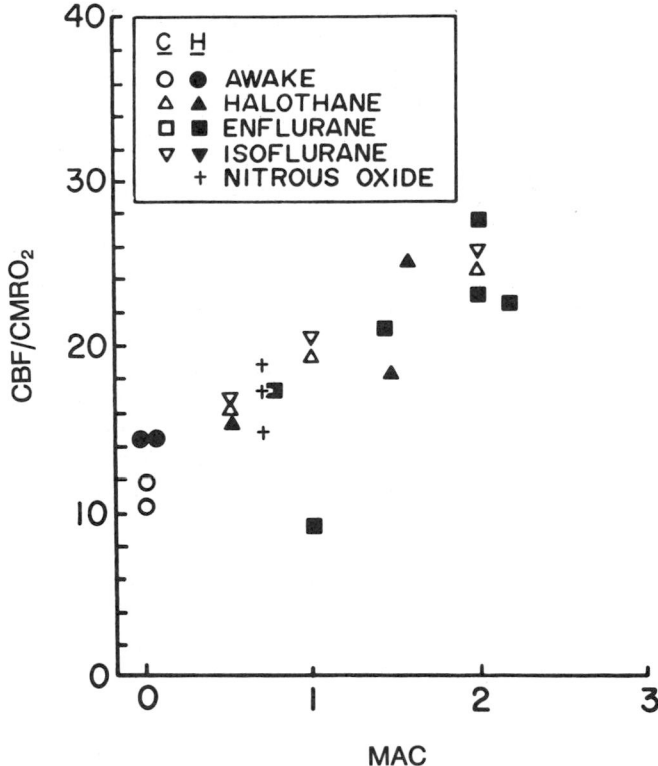

Fig. 19-10. Effect of anesthetic depth (MAC) of the volatile anesthetics and nitrous oxide on the CBF/CMRO$_2$ ratio in humans (H) (shaded symbols) and cats (C) (unshaded symbols). (Data from Smith and Wollman,[17] Sakabe et al.,[203] and Todd and Drummond.[166])

rane at all MAC levels caused less brain protrusion than did halothane at comparable dose levels.

There is some nonlinearity in the CBF and CMR dose-response relationships for volatile anesthetics. The initial appearance of an EEG pattern associated with the onset of anesthesia with halothane, enflurane, and isoflurane is accompanied by a precipitous decline in $CMRO_2$.[99] Thereafter, $CMRO_2$ declines in a slower dose-dependent manner. Other studies during anesthetic induction with halothane found marked increases in CBF prior to any alteration in CMR.[100] This may indicate that the direct effect of halothane on smooth muscle develops more rapidly than influences related to depression of CMR.

The degree of $CMRO_2$ reduction that occurs at a given MAC level is greater with isoflurane and enflurane than with halothane (Fig. 19-9). No direct comparisons of the three anesthetics have been performed in humans. The administration of 1.0 MAC of each anesthetic to N_2O-sedated cats resulted in approximate $CMRO_2$ reductions of 25 percent with halothane and 50 percent with isoflurane and enflurane.[162,166] The $CMRO_2$ reduction is dose related. However, with isoflurane, maximum suppression is attained simultaneously with the occurrence of EEG isoelectricity.[8] This occurs at clinically relevant concentrations of isoflurane, that is, less than 2.0 MAC in humans.[15] In dogs, additional isoflurane up to 6.0 percent end-tidal results in no further CMR reduction and no indication of metabolic toxicity.[8] Halothane presents a contrast to this pattern. Halothane concentrations in excess of 4.0 MAC are required to achieve EEG isoelectricity in dogs, and additional halothane causes further reduction of $CMRO_2$ in concert with alterations in energy charge. The latter changes, which are reversible, suggest interference with oxidative phosphorylation.[164] These data indicate that, unlike isoflurane, halothane can produce reversible toxicity when administered in very high concentrations.

The effect of volatile anesthetics on CBF is probably the sum of several influences. These include a tendency toward CBF reduction caused by a depression of CMR, and vasodilation caused by a substantial direct effect on vascular smooth muscle.[167] The latter apparently predominates, and the net effect of the volatile anesthetics is an increase in CBF. The suppression of CMR caused by equi-MAC concentrations of the volatile agents differs (isoflurane and enflurane > halothane) (Fig. 19-9), and it is probable, although unproved, that this is the basis of the difference in the magnitude of the CBF increases they cause (halothane > enflurane and isoflurane). The CMR nadir that occurs with isoflurane at the onset of EEG isoelectricity may have implications with respect to ICP. If isoflurane has a substantial direct vasodilating effect on the cerebral vasculature that is offset by an opposing metabolically mediated vasoconstricting influence, it might be surmised that when near maximal reduction of CMR has occurred additional isoflurane will have a predominately vasodilating effect.

There are data to support this prediction. Murphy et al.[161] observed no increase in CBF (versus awake control measurements) during anesthesia with 0.6 and 1.1 MAC isoflurane (with blood pressure support), but at 1.6 MAC CBF had increased by 100 percent. Maekawa et al.[11] measured CBF and l-CMRg in rats both awake and during anesthesia with increasing concentrations of isoflurane. One MAC isoflurane resulted in an average CMRg decrease in five cortical areas of 54 percent of the awake control value and no change in average CBF. An additional 1.0 MAC (i.e., a total of 2.0 MAC) caused a further CMRg reduction of only 20 percent of the control value and CBF simultaneously increased by 70 percent (Fig. 19-11). Sainz et al.[170] recorded ICP during administration of isoflurane to hypocapnic patients with intracranial tumors. Isoflurane in concentrations of 1.0 and 1.5 percent caused no change in ICP, but ICP increased with the administration of 2.0 percent isoflurane. Newburg et al.[8] also recorded CBF up to and beyond the concentration of isoflurane necessary to produce EEG suppression in the dog. $CMRO_2$ and CBF were both unchanged when isoflurane was increased from 3 to 6 percent, which is a pattern different from that observed in the three previous studies. However, MAP was decreased and a large dose of phenylephrine (which their data indicate is a cerebral vasoconstrictor in the dog) was being administered with the higher dose of isoflurane. These data together suggest that isoflurane is a significant cerebral vasodilator when administered in concentrations at and above those associated with near maximal CMR suppression or, perhaps, when

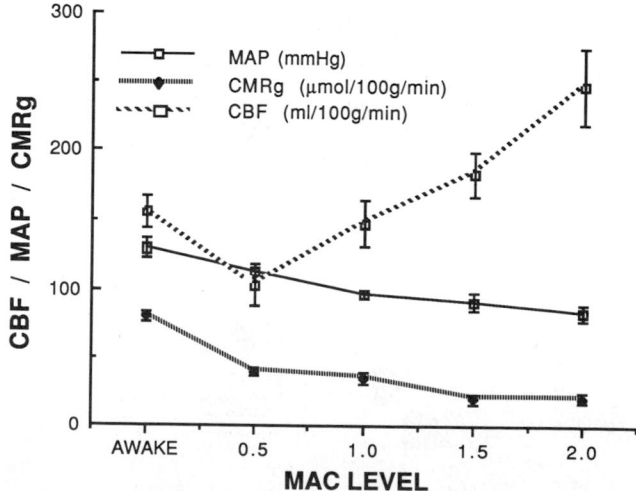

Fig. 19-11. Relationship between changes in l-CMRg and l-CBF in the motor-sensory cortex in rats during isoflurane anesthesia. The majority of the CMR suppression caused by isoflurane has occurred by 1.0 MAC and in this concentration range CBF is not increased. Thereafter, additional isoflurane causes little further CMR reduction and cerebral vasodilation occurs. These data (±standard deviation) suggest the importance of metabolic coupling determining the CBF effects of isoflurane. (Data from Maekawa et al.[11])

administered in situations were the component of CMR that is associated with electrophysiologic function is already suppressed by other drugs[167] or pathologic processes.

Distribution of CBF/CMR Changes

The regional distribution in anesthetic-induced changes in CBF and CMR differs markedly with halothane and isoflurane. Halothane produces relatively homogeneous changes throughout the brain. CBF is globally increased and CMR is globally depressed. The changes caused by isoflurane are more heterogeneous. CBF increases are greater in subcortical areas and hindbrain structures than in the neocortex (Fig. 19-12).[12,171] For CMR the converse is true, with greater reduction in the neocortex than in the subcortex.[11] These distribution differences may explain certain apparent contradictions in the existing literature. Todd and Drummond[166] compared the CBF effects of halothane and isoflurane in the cat. They observed smaller increases in CBF with isoflurane but equivalent increase in ICP. The ICP changes may have been influenced by CBF effects in the subcortex and hindbrain that were not reflected by their CBF technique, xenon 133 and external gamma counters, a method that emphasizes cortical flow phenomena. There are also apparent contradictions within human investigations. Eintrei et al.[163] reported no increase in CBF when isoflurane was administered to patients undergoing craniotomy, yet both Adams et al.[172] and Campkin and Flinn[173] have reported that administration of isoflurane to normocapnic subjects with intracranial pathology can result in increases in CSF pressure. The CBF methodology used by Eintrei et al.[163] measured cortical flow exclusively, and accordingly, these results of the three investigations are again consistent with a pattern of minimal vasodilation in the cortex with greater increases in CBF subcortically. In the studies of Adams et al.[172] and Campkin and Flinn,[173] the increases in CSFP were usually readily prevented or reversed by the in-

duction of hypocapnia. However, there have been reports of apparent isoflurane-induced increases of ICP despite the induction of hypocapnia.[174] This information taken in sum indicates that while isoflurane may have little cerebral vasodilating effect in the cortex, it nontheless causes net cerebral vasodilation in a dose-dependent fashion. When used in the setting of impaired intracranial compliance it should be used with discretion and with attention to the other important determinants of ICP, in particular carbon dioxide tension. The net vasodilating effect of equi-MAC concentrations of isoflurane is less in humans than that of halothane, and the former is probably therefore preferable if a volatile anesthetic is to be used in the setting of impaired intracranial compliance. That is not to say that halothane is contraindicated in these circumstances. It has been clearly demonstrated that when hypocapnia is established prior to the introduction of halothane, the increases in ICP that might otherwise occur in a normocapnic patient with poor intracranial compliance can be prevented or greatly attenuated.[175] Nonetheless, many clinicians will prefer isoflurane because the margin for error is probably wider than with halothane. In addition, it has been demonstrated that avoidance of major ICP elevation can be accomplished by the induction of hypocapnia *simultaneously* with the introduction of isoflurane,[172] whereas CO_2 reduction should be instituted *before* exposure to halothane[175] if ICP increases are to be prevented in a patient population at risk.

Time Dependency of CBF Effects

The effect of volatile anesthetics on CBF is time dependent. After an initial increase, CBF falls substantially. Studies performed in dogs[171,176] and goats[23] suggest that recovery to pre-volatile anesthetic levels occurs between 2.5 and 5 hours after exposure. In dogs, a steady state CBF was achieved 3 hours after introduction of 1.3 MAC isoflurane and 5 hours after introduction of 1.7 MAC halothane.[171] In that study, 1.7 MAC isoflurane

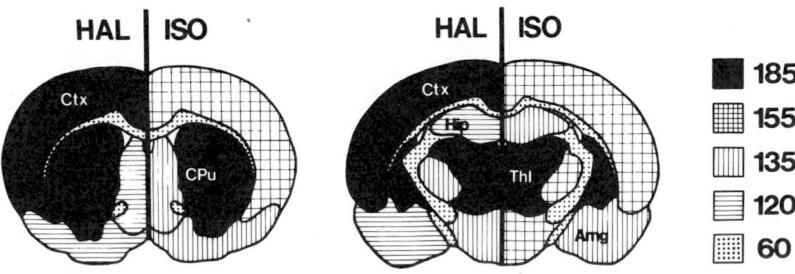

Fig. 19-12. Regional differences in the CBF effects of isoflurane (ISO) and halothane (HAL).[12] The figure is a schematic representation of CBF in a coronal autoradiographic image of rat brain. The key indicates the approximate CBF (ml/100 g/min). In cortex, CBF is less during anesthesia with isoflurane than with halothane. In the subcortex, CBF is similar during anesthesia with the two anesthetics in some structures, and in others is greater with isoflurane. Average hemispheric CBF with the two agents is very similar. Ctx, cortex; CPu, caudate-putamen; Hip, hippocampus; Thl, thalamus; Amg, amygdala. (From Hansen et al.,[12] with permission.)

produced a larger initial increase in CBF and a more prolonged (5 hours) recovery to a final steady state CBF. The data suggest that the time course depends on the magnitude of the initial CBF elevation. The mechanism of this effect is not understood, although it has been determined that it is not related to time-dependent changes in the status of autoregulation[23] or CSF pH.[176]

Cerebral Blood Volume

CBF influences ICP because of the positive correlation between CBF and CBV. CBV has been shown to increase with the administration of both N_2O and isoflurane in humans. In addition, CBV has been shown to increase and to be accompanied by parallel changes in CSFP when halothane, enflurane, and isoflurane are administered to dogs.[92,93] Fentanyl, by contrast, causes a reduction in CBF in N_2O-sedated dogs[113] and has been shown to reduce CBV and CSFP.[92] Artru[92] reported that while the CBV alterations lasted for greater than 3 hours with all four drugs, CSFP normalized after approximately 20 minutes during anesthesia with isoflurane and fentanyl. He attributed these discrepancies in time course to differences in the effects of the four anesthetics on CSF dynamics, that is, the rate of CSF secretion and absorption (see discussion below). Note that Artru's observation of a sustained (> 3 h) increase in CBV during administration of 1.4 percent isoflurane dogs requires reconciliation with the observations (see above) of Boarini et al.,[171] who reported a substantial decline in CBF at the end of 3 hours of anesthesia with 1.5 percent isoflurane in dogs. It is an unexplored possibility that anesthetics have an effect on the volume of the intracranial venous compartment that is separate from effects on CBF. It must suffice to say that while CBF influences are probably the major mechanism of volatile anesthetic effects on ICP, other factors may contribute in as yet poorly defined ways. Note also that, to the clinician, it is most likely to be the acute CBF effects of anesthetics that are the most important. Difficulties with intracranial compliance are most likely to arise early in the anesthesia when acute anesthetic effects can compound other difficulties that may arise with induction and initial surgical stimulation, for example, arousal, hypertension, hypercapnia, coughing, and straining. Accordingly, the slowly evolving delayed effects of anesthetics (on CBF, CBV, and CSF dynamics) are likely to be much less important clinically. This will be particularly true of potential effects on CSF dynamics, which will be moot in situations in which the CSF space is opened, for example, in the vast majority of craniotomies and in any patient with a ventriculostomy in place.

CO_2 Responsiveness and Autoregulation

CO_2 responsiveness is well maintained during anesthesia with all the volatile anesthetics.[17,20,177] By contrast, autoregulation of CBF in response to rising arterial pressure is impaired. This impairment appears to be most apparent with the anesthetics that cause the greatest cerebral vasodilation[161,166] and is dose related (Fig. 19-6).[178]

Epileptogenesis

Enflurane and isoflurane are very similar in terms of their effects on most elements of cerebral physiology including CBF, CMR, and ICP. However, enflurane is unique among the commonly used inhaled anesthetics in that it is potentially epileptogenic in the clinical setting. Of particular relevance to neuroanesthesia is the observation that hypocapnia potentiates seizure-type discharges during enflurane anesthesia.[179] A systematic study of epileptogenicity in dogs during hypocapnia revealed that enflurane caused noise-activated seizures, that isoflurane elicited spikes without seizures, and that no epileptoid activity occurred with halothane.[180] Enflurane-induced seizure activity is associated with substantial increases in CBF and $CMRO_2$. When epileptoid activity was elicited in the dog with the combination of 1.5 MAC enflurane, hypocapnia, and a noise stimulus, the EEG change was accompanied by a 40 to 50 percent increase in both $CMRO_2$ and CBF.[165] A 50 percent decrease in $CMRO_2$ was noted in human volunteers anesthetized with 3 percent enflurane, but with the onset of seizure activity $CMRO_2$ returned to normal.[181] In animal investigations, enflurane-induced increases in CMRg during EEG spiking have been demonstrated in several subcortical structures including the hippocampus and other limbic system structures[182] and in corticothalamic pathways. These regions are assumed to be the origin of seizure activity. There is no evidence that this type of EEG activity is deleterious when oxygen delivery is maintained during the event. However, since seizure activity can elevate brain metabolism by as much as 400 percent, the use of enflurane, especially in high doses and with hypocapnia, should be limited in patients predisposed to seizures and/or with occlusive cerebrovascular disease. Note also that amitriptyline and ketamine[183] have been reported to reduce the seizure threshold for enflurane.

The EEG-activating property of enflurane has been used intraoperatively to activate and identify seizure foci that are to be surgically resected, and in this situation spike activity not present preoperatively has been observed to persist after surgery.[184] There have also been two reports of seizures in the immediate postoperative period following enflurane anesthesia in both predisposed[185] and nonpredisposed individuals.[186] There have been no apparent permanent sequelae from these events, and, in fact, this association is not a rigorously proven one. At worst, such occurrences are extremely uncommon.

Isoflurane can cause EEG spiking and myoclonus but in the experimental setting has not been associated with the frank epileptoid activity induced by enflurane. The clinical experience with isoflurane is very large, and unexplained "seizurelike activity" has been reported in only two patients. One occurrence was intraoperative[187] and the other was immediately postoperative.[188] It therefore appears that epileptogenesis is not a clinical concern with isoflurane. In fact, isoflurane has been successfully used to control EEG seizure activity in refractory status epilepticus.[189]

Brain Glucose Concentration

Kofke et al.[190] compared the brain concentrations of glucose and several other intermediary metabolites during administration of halothane, enflurane, and isoflurane in rats. Brain glucose was greater with isoflurane than with halothane and enflurane, but there were no differences in any of the other markers. Plasma glucose concentration was also increased in the isoflurane group, and the plasma/brain glucose ratio did not differ among the three anesthetics. There have been no evaluations of brain glucose concentration in humans; however, an increased plasma glucose concentration (versus halothane) has been reported to occur during isoflurane anesthesia.[191] The concern is that increased glucose availability has been shown in both clinical and experimental circumstances to worsen outcome following an episode of cerebral ischemia. However, the clinical significance of this effect of isoflurane is completely unknown, and at present, the issue should be viewed as a matter of laboratory interest only.

Sevoflurane

Sevoflurane is a halogenated ether. It is relatively insoluble (blood/gas partition coefficient of 0.60), and rapid induction and emergence can therefore be achieved. Some fluoride ion release occurs in vivo,[192] and it is unstable in the presence of soda lime, yielding metabolites whose toxicities have not been evaluated.[193] It is in clinical use in Japan but, to date, has not been released in North America. Scheller et al.[194] compared the effects of sevoflurane and isoflurane in normal rabbits. Sevoflurane was indistinguishable from isoflurane in terms of its effects on CBF, $CMRO_2$, ICP, and EEG.

Desflurane (I653)

Desflurane (I653) is also a new, relatively insoluble (blood/gas partition coefficient of 0.42) halogenated ether. It requires delivery systems different from those used with the other volatile anesthetics because it is a gas at room temperature. There have, as yet, been no investigations of the CBF, $CMRO_2$, and ICP effects of desflurane. Rampil et al.[195] compared the dose-related effects of desflurane, isoflurane, and enflurane on the EEG in the pig. The EEG patterns observed with desflurane and isoflurane were very similar. When hypocapnia was induced during 1.2 MAC anesthesia, seizures occurred with enflurane but not with desflurane or isoflurane.

Nitrous Oxide

The available data indicate unequivocally that N_2O can cause increases in CBF and ICP. The magnitude of the effect is less certain and probably varies from situation to situation. The apparent discrepancies between the numerous investigations may reflect the intrusion of (1) second-stage arousal phenomena in studies in which N_2O was the sole anesthetic administered, (2) the effect of decreased arousal owing to the provision of analgesia or loss of awareness after the superimposition of N_2O on a stressful control state, and (3) the occurrence of drug interactions. The most dramatic reported increases in ICP or CBF in humans[196,197] and experimental animals[198,199] have occurred when N_2O was administered alone or with minimal background anesthesia. For instance, Henriksen and Jorgensen[196] recorded ICP before and during spontaneous breathing of 66 percent N_2O by patients with intracranial tumors. Mean ICP rose from 13 to 40 mmHg. However, it appears that when N_2O is administered in conjunction with certain other anesthetics, its CBF effect may be considerably reduced. In an investigation of patients with intracranial tumors and poor intracranial compliance (mean preinduction ICP of 27 mmHg),[200] when 50 percent N_2O was introduced during barbiturate anesthesia and after the induction of hypocapnia the effect on ICP was negligible. Phirman and Shapiro[201] observed that a reproducible increase in ICP that had occurred in response to 70 percent N_2O administration to a comatose patient was prevented by prior administration of a combination of pentothal and diazepam despite no change in baseline ICP. There is other information that indicates that barbiturates and benzodiazepines individually blunt the CBF response to N_2O.[201,202] Narcotics appear to have a similar effect. Jobes et al.[105] reported that anesthesia with 1 mg/kg of morphine plus 70 percent N_2O resulted in no change in CBF from awake control values. While their study did not attempt to evaluate the effect of N_2O per se, the data suggest that N_2O (administered with morphine) did not cause substantial cerebral vasodilation.

The interaction of N_2O with volatile anesthetics appears to be different from that observed with fixed anesthetics. While the data set is incomplete, the available information suggests that when N_2O is added to an established anesthetic with a volatile anesthetic, CBF increases will occur. In all the investigations, including one in humans, in which N_2O has been added to an anesthetic of 1.0 MAC or greater, substantial CBF increases have been recorded.[203-209] The results of two investigations indicate that the effect may be positively correlated with inhaled anesthetic concentration. The data of Drummond et al. (rabbits)[207] and Manohar and Parks (pigs)[206] suggest that the CBF increase caused by N_2O is exaggerated at higher concentrations of both halothane and isoflurane. There are, however, two other investigations performed in dogs in which N_2O caused smaller CBF increments as the expired concentration of halothane increased.[199,210] These investigations involved sub-MAC concentrations of halothane, and the results may have reflected a combination of the effects of N_2O per se plus the effect of the elimination of pain or awareness.

There is not uniform agreement as to the effect of N_2O on CMR. Parallel changes in CBF and CMR,[198] CBF increases without alteration of CMR,[209] and CMR alteration occurring without changes in CBF[211] have all been reported. This is doubtless the product of differences in species, methods, depth of background anesthesia, and interactions with simultaneously administered agents. There are few data obtained in humans. Wollman et al.[211] reported that 70 percent N_2O caused a 15 percent reduction in $CMRO_2$ in human volunteers. However, both premedication and induction of anesthesia were accomplished with barbiturates and the control group was nonconcurrent. From animal experimentation it appears likely that, at least in some circumstances, N_2O causes increases in CMR. The "cleanest" investigation is that of Pelligrino et al.,[198] who measured cortical CBF and CMR in awake goats that received N_2O without premedication or other supplements. After 60 minutes of N_2O inhalation, cortical $CMRO_2$ was increased to 170 percent of control and global CBF was increased to 143 percent of control. The goats showed no evidence of an excitement stage. They became lethargic and experienced a fall in plasma epinephrine levels suggesting the absence of stress.

The CBF response to CO_2 is preserved during administration of N_2O.[207,209,211] Despite the inconsistencies that are evident, the data indicate that the vasodilatory action of N_2O can be clinically significant in neurosurgical patients with reduced intracranial compliance. However, it appears that N_2O-induced cerebral vasodilation can be considerably blunted by the simultaneous administration of fixed anesthetics, although not all anesthetics have been evaluated and the dose-response relationships are not well defined. N_2O has been widely used in neurosurgery and banishing it is inconsistent with the accumulated experience. Nonetheless, in circumstances in which ICP is persistently elevated or the surgical field is persistently tight, N_2O should be viewed as a potential contributing factor.

Muscle Relaxants

Nondepolarizing Muscle Relaxants

The only recognized direct effect of nondepolarizing muscle relaxants on the cerebral vasculature occurs via the release of histamine. Histamine can result in a reduction in CPP because of the simultaneous increase in ICP (caused by cerebral vasodilation) and decrease in MAP that can occur.[212] It is not entirely clear when the BBB is intact whether histamine can directly cause cerebral vasodilation or whether it is a secondary (autoregulatory) response to a reduction in MAP. d-Tubocurarine is the most potent histamine releaser among available muscle relaxants. Metocurine and atracurium also release histamine in lesser quantities.[213]

However, for atracurium, and probably metocurine, the effect is clinically inconsequential. The indirect actions of muscle relaxants may also have significant effects on cerebral physiology. Muscle relaxants that cause an increase in arterial pressure (e.g., pancuronium) may elevate ICP when the MAP increase is abrupt and/or when CBF autoregulation has been modified by disease processes. Muscle relaxants may reduce ICP because coughing and straining are prevented and this results in a lowering of central venous pressure (CVP) with a concomitant reduction in cerebral venous outflow impedance.

Vecuronium and atracurium are the two most recently introduced nondepolarizing muscle relaxants. The administration of vecuronium (0.1 to 0.14 mg/kg) to patients with intracranial tumors resulted in modest reduction of ICP and MAP with no significant change in CPP.[214,215] Rosa et al.[216] gave atracurium (0.6 mg/kg) to patients with space-occupying intracranial lesions during anesthesia with pentothal, N_2O, and fentanyl. They observed no changes in ICP, MAP, or CVP. A similar absence of effect has been observed after administration of atracurium to both monkeys[217] and cats[218] with experimental intracranial hypertension. A metabolite of atracurium, laudanosine, may be epileptogenic. However, while large doses of atracurium caused an EEG arousal pattern in dogs, CBF, CMR, and ICP were unaltered.[219] In cats, the seizure threshold for lidocaine-induced seizures was not different during paralysis with atracurium, vecuronium, or pancuronium.[220] In rabbits, laudanosine administration did not increase the severity of the epileptoid activity caused by direct application of a cephalosporin to the cortical surface.[221] It appears highly unlikely that epiletogenesis will occur in humans with atracurium.[222,223]

In summary, vecuronium, atracurium, and pancuronium (if acute MAP elevation is prevented with the latter) are all reasonable muscle relaxants for use in the patient with or at risk for intracranial hypertension. Curare is best administered slowly and in small divided doses to avoid substantial histamine release.

Succinylcholine

Succinylcholine can produce elevation of ICP in lightly anesthetized subjects. Minton et al.[224] studied patients with intracranial tumors. Their subjects received morphine (0.1 mg/kg) 1 hour prior to induction of anesthesia. The latter was accomplished with thiopental (6 mg/kg). The patients were ventilated by mask with 70 percent N_2O to maintain normocapnia and then received succinylcholine (1 mg/kg). ICP increased from 15 ± 1 (standard error) to a maximum of 20 ± 2 mmHg after 1 to 3 minutes and returned to baseline in 8 to 10 minutes. The effect appears to be the result of cerebral activation (as evidenced by EEG changes and CBF increases) caused by afferent activity from the muscle spindle apparatus.[225] Note, however, that there is a poor correlation between the occurrence of visible muscle fasiculations and an increase in ICP. As might be expected with what appears to be an arousal phenomenon, deep anesthesia has been observed to prevent succinylcholine-induced ICP increases in the dog.[225] In humans, the ICP increase is also blocked by paralysis with vecuronium[224] and by "defasciculation" with metocurine (0.03 mg/kg).[226] The efficacy of other defasciculating agents has not been examined in humans. However, defasciculation with pancuronium did not prevent ICP increases in the dog.[227]

Although succinylcholine *can* produce ICP increases, it need not be viewed as contraindicated in circumstances in which its use for rapid attainment of paralysis is otherwise seen as appropriate. As with many drugs the concern should be not whether it is used but how it is used. If administered with proper attention to the control of CO_2 tension, blood pressure, and depth of anesthesia, and following defasciculation, preferably with metocurine pending additional information, little hazard should attend its use.

OTHER EFFECTS OF ANESTHETICS ON CEREBRAL PHYSIOLOGY

CSF Dynamics

There are approximately 150 ml of CSF in the adult human, half within the cranium and half in the spinal CSF space. The CSF, which is formed in the choroid plexuses and to a lesser extent by transependymal diffusion from the brain interstitium into the ventricular system, is replaced about three times per day.[228] It functions both as a cushion for the CNS and as an excretory pathway. Anesthetics have been shown to influence both the rate of formation and the rate of reabsorption of CSF. Table 19-5 provides nonquantitative information as to the direction of the influences of common anesthetics. All the information has been derived from dogs,[229-233] and these processes have not been examined in humans. The time course of these effects is slow. In clinical situations in which the CSF space is to be opened (most craniotomies) or in which a ventriculostomy is in place, they are probably clinically irrelevant. There may be relevance when a prolonged closed cranium procedure is to be performed in a patient with poor intracranial compliance. The most deleterious potential combination of effects in the setting of poor

intracranial compliance is one of increased CSF production and decreased reabsorption. In the dog, this pattern occurs with enflurane, and this is perhaps another reason (in addition to the potential for epileptogenesis in the presence of cerebral injury and hypocapnia) for omission of enflurane in this circumstance. With this exception, anesthetic selection should be made on the basis of other physiologic properties.

Blood-Brain Barrier

In the majority of the body's capillary beds, there are fenestrations approximately 65 Å in diameter between endothelial cells. In the brain, with the exception of the choroid plexus, the pituitary, and the area postrema, tight junctions reduce this pore size to approximately 8 Å. As a result, large molecules and most ions are prevented from entering the brain interstitium. There is little evidence that anesthetics alter the function of this BBB in most circumstances. However, it has been repeatedly demonstrated that acute hypertension can breach the barrier[234,235] and that certain anesthetics facilitate this phenomenon.[236] Forster et al.[75] observed that Evans blue extravasation into rabbit brain was greater when acute hypertension occurred during anesthesia with halothane than with thiopental. It is probable that the effect is the nonspecific result of cerebral vasodilation[237] rather than a specific effect of halothane. These results were obtained in the setting of extreme, abrupt hypertension in animals with an initially normal BBB. There is also evidence that anesthetics may influence the leakiness of an abnormal BBB at normotension. Smith and Marque[238] submitted dogs to 5 hours of anesthesia following a freeze lesion (which causes an opening of the BBB). Cerebral water accumulation at 24 hours was less in animals anesthetized with pentobarbital or fentanyl-droperidol-N_2O than with halothane, enflurane, or isoflurane. To our knowledge, only a single investigation has attempted a comparison of anesthetic effects on BBB function during anesthesia in humans. Pashayan et al.[239] studied children undergoing ventriculoperitoneal shunt placement. They reported that albumin entered the CSF in greater quantities during anesthesia with halothane than with a thiopental-sufentanil combination. The clinical significance of this phenomenon is unknown.

Epileptogenesis

Several commonly employed anesthetics have some epileptogenic potential, particularly in predisposed individuals. A concern is that seizure activity may go unrecognized in an anesthetized and paralyzed patient and result in neuronal injury if substrate demand (CMR) exceeds supply for a prolonged period. A second concern is that the epileptogenic effect will persist in the postanesthesia period when seizures may occur in less well controlled circumstances than exist in the operating room. In practice, it appears that spontaneous seizures during or after anesthesia have been ex-

TABLE 19-5. Effects of Anesthetic on Rate of CSF Secretion and Absorption[a]

	Halothane	Enflurane	Isoflurane	Fentanyl	Ketamine	N_2O
Secretion	↓	↑	0	0	0	0
Absorption	↓	↓	↑	↑	↓	0

[a] Upward arrows indicate an increase in the rate of CSF absorption or secretion, and downward arrows indicate a decrease. The information is presented nonquantitatively and effects may vary with dose. The data are derived from various studies by Artru (see text).

tremely rare events. Nonetheless, in patients with processes that might predispose to seizures, it seems prudent to avoid the use of potentially epileptogenic agents in situations in which there are reasonable alternatives.

Enflurane

The epileptogenic properties of enflurane are discussed above in the section, *Volatile Anesthetics*.

Methohexital

Myoclonic activity is sometimes observed with methohexital, and this drug has been used to activate seizure foci during cortical mapping.[240,241] One clinical report[242] describes the occurrence of seizures in two pediatric patients after induction doses of methohexital administered rectally in one and intramuscularly in the other. Both of these patients had temporal lobe lesions and had had previous seizures. It appears that it is specifically patients with seizures of temporal lobe origin, typically of the psychomotor variety, that are at risk for seizure activation by methohexital.[242,243] It may be noteworthy that recurrent spontaneous seizures after methohexital anesthesia for electroconvulsive therapy have never been reported.

Ketamine

Depth electrode recordings in epileptic patients revealed the occurrence of isolated subcortical seizure activity originating in limbic and thalamic areas during ketamine anesthesia and demonstrated that this subcortical activation may not be reflected in surface EEG recordings.[244] The sporadic occurrence of seizures following ketamine anesthesia in nonpredisposed patients has also been reported.[245] Ketamine has also been reported to precipitate severe myoclonus in an infant with myoclonic encephalopathy.[246]

Etomidate

Etomidate has been shown to be effective in activating seizure foci intraoperatively[247-249] and has been reported to cause "epileptiform" EEG activity in normal subjects during anesthesia.[249] Etomidate also causes myoclonus, and a single instance of severe, sustained myoclonus immediately following anesthesia with etomidate by infusion has been reported.[250]

Narcotics

Seizures can be elicited readily in some animals with narcotics,[117,251-253] but humans do not have a clinically significant susceptibility to this effect. Several publications, unaccompanied by EEG recordings, report that grand mal convulsions have occurred in patients who received both high[254] and low doses of fentanyl.[255,256] However, systematic investigations of EEG changes during administration of relatively large doses of fentanyl, sufentanil, and alfentanil in humans have *not* documented neuroexcitatory activity,[257-259] and the seizures may have been an exaggerated rigidity phenomenon. Note that untreated rigidity may itself also have important CNS consequences. ICP elevation was observed when alfentanil-induced rigidity occurred in rats during controlled ventilation.[260] The effect probably arose because the associated increase in CVP caused cerebral venous congestion. In the absence of ventilatory support, both hypercapnia and hypoxemia may also occur.

Atracurium

See the discussion regarding the atracurium metabolite, laudanosine, in the section, *Nondepolarizing Muscle Relaxants*.

CEREBRAL PHYSIOLOGY IN PATHOLOGIC STATES

Cerebral Ischemia

Pathophysiology

The brain has a high rate of energy utilization and a very limited energy storage capacity. It is therefore extremely vulnerable in the event of interruption of substrate (oxygen, glucose) supply. Only a simplified overview of the pathophysiology of ischemic neuronal injury is presented here. Calcium is probably central to this complex process.[261] Calcium is present in the cytosol of normal neurons where it performs important functions (e.g., second messenger, coenzyme). It gains access to the cytosol in several ways (Fig. 19-13A). It enters via both neurotransmitter (e.g., glutamate)-gated and voltage-dependent channels (e.g., calcium channels). It is also released from intracellular storage sites in the mitochondria and endoplasmic reticulum, for example, through the actions of second messengers such as inosotol triphosphate (IP3), that have been generated by the action of agonists at metabolotrophic cell surface receptors. Calcium's normal concentration range is tightly regulated by energy-consuming processes that serve to extrude it from the cell, to resequester it in the mitochondria and endoplasmic reticulum, and to inactivate the factors, such as IP3, that liberate calcium from storage sties.

In the event of cerebral ischemia there are two simultaneous impacts on these processes. There is excess release into the synapse of the neurotransmitters that activate the various calcium influx processes, and shortly thereafter, there is a failure of the supply of ATP that is necessary to clear the calcium from the cytosol (Fig. 19-13B). Among calcium's normal intracellular functions is the activation of various kinases, lipases, and proteases. The sustained activation of these enzymes by elevated cytosolic calcium during ischemia

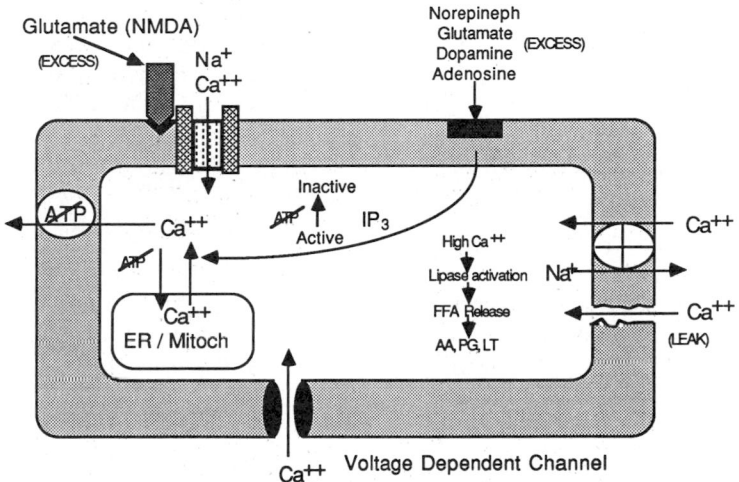

A. Normal

Glutamate (NMDA)

Na⁺
Ca⁺⁺

Norepineph
Glutamate
Dopamine
Adenosine

ATP

Ca⁺⁺

Inactive

ATP   IP₃
Active

Ca⁺⁺

Ca⁺⁺

ATP

Na⁺

Ca⁺⁺

ER / Mitoch

Ca⁺⁺   Voltage Dependent Channel

B. Hypoxia / Ischemia

Glutamate (NMDA)

(EXCESS)

Na⁺
Ca⁺⁺

Norepineph
Glutamate (EXCESS)
Dopamine
Adenosine

ATP

Ca⁺⁺

Inactive

ATP   IP₃
Active

High Ca⁺⁺

Lipase activation   Na⁺

ATP

FFA Release

Ca⁺⁺

AA, PG, LT

Ca⁺⁺

(LEAK)

ER / Mitoch

Ca⁺⁺   Voltage Dependent Channel

Fig. 19-13. Cytosolic calcium homeostasis. **(A)** Normal Ca⁺⁺ homeostasis. Ca⁺⁺ enters the cytosol via voltage-dependent or agonist (e.g., glutamate)-gated channels, or from the endoplasmic reticulum (ER) and mitochondria (Mitoch). The latter release is initiated in part by second messengers such as inositol triphosphate (IP3) generated by the action of various agonists at cell surface receptors. Removal of Ca⁺⁺ from the cytosol is accomplished by ATP-consuming pumps that extrude Ca⁺⁺ from the cell or resequester it in the ER/Mitoch. Some Ca⁺⁺ may be eliminated by a nonenergy-consuming electrostatic exchange pump. **(B)** Ischemic and hypoxic conditions. The agonists that initiate Ca⁺⁺ entry are present in excess. ATP deficiency leads to failure of the Ca⁺⁺ extrusion pumps and to reduced degradation of IP3 (an energy-requiring process). High intracellular Na+ may cause reversal of the function of the electrostatic pump. The high cytosolic Ca⁺⁺ leads to activation of enzymes including lipases that result in free fatty acid (FFA) release from membranes and eicosanoid generation. AA, arachadonic acid; PG, prostaglandins; LT, leukotrienes.

results, among other things, in the liberation of fatty acids from membranes. Chemically reactive free radicals that are generated during the reperfusion process further contribute to the degradation of membrane lipids. The latter are the substrates for the generation of arachidonic acid and various prostaglandins and leukotrienes. These "eicosanoids" have numerous effects in-

cluding vasoconstriction, vasodilation, leukotaxis, and alteration of membrane permeability, all of which can contribute to the evolution of the ischemic neuronal insult.

Lactate formation is an additional element of the pathophysiologic process. Lactic acid is formed as a result of the anaerobic glycolysis that takes place after the failure of the supply of oxygen. The associated pH decline contributes to the deterioration of the intracellular environment. An elevated preischemic serum glucose level may accelerate this process by providing additional substrate for anaerobic glycolysis.[262-265]

Much has been made of the difference between complete cerebral ischemia, as occurs during cardiac arrest, and incomplete cerebral ischemia, as may occur during occlusion of a major cerebral vessel or severe hypotension. However, it is unlikely that the pathophysiologic processes are materially different. The important difference is that the residual blood flow may result in enough oxygen delivery to allow for some generation of adenosine triphosphate (ATP) and thereby to stave off the catastrophic irreversible membrane failure that occurs within minutes during normothermic complete cerebral ischemia. This difference in the rate of failure of energy supply[266,267] (Fig. 19-14) can result in a much greater apparent tolerance for focal or incomplete ischemia than for complete global ischemia, for example, during cardiac arrest. The difference is in reality a matter of severity rather than of the actual pathophysiology of the insult with the exception that limited residual perfusion may potentially be detrimental in the event of hyperglycemia.

Critical CBF Levels and the Ischemic Penumbra Concept

In the face of a declining oxygen supply, neuronal function deteriorates progressively rather than in an all or none fashion (Fig. 19-15). There is a substantial reserve below normal CBF levels (> 50 ml/100 g/min). It is not until CBF has fallen to approximately 22 ml/100 g/min that EEG evidence of ischemia begins to appear. At a CBF level of approximately 15 ml/100 g/min, the cortical EEG is isoelectric. However, it is not until CBF is reduced to about 6 ml/100 g/min that indications of potentially irreversible membrane failure (elevated extracellular potassium[268]) are rapidly evident. As CBF decreases in the flow range between 15 and 6 ml/100 g/min, a progressive deterioration of energy supply occurs, leading eventually, with a time course that may encompass hours[269] rather than minutes, to membrane failure and neuronal death. The brain regions falling within this CBF range are referred to as the *ischemic penumbra* — a region within which the neuronal dysfunction is temporarily reversible but within which neuronal death will occur if flow is not restored.[268] It is the ischemic penumbra phenomenon that accounts for instances (e.g., carotid endarterectomy) in which neurologic recovery occurs in situations where the EEG was flat for periods longer than those normally associated with neurologic injury. The studies defining this progression have been performed principally in the cerebral cortex of baboons[268,270] and monkeys,[269] and the actual CBF levels at which the various decrements in function occur may vary with both anesthetic[271] and species. However, in humans anesthetized with halothane and N_2O, the CBF threshold for the initial EEG change[272] is similar to that observed in the animal investigations.

Cerebral Protection

As outlined above, cerebral ischemic injury involves a process by which energy supply falls short of energy demand, in which the intracellular environment deteriorates (increased Ca^{++}, decreased pH), membrane damage occurs, and secondary processes (eicosanoids,

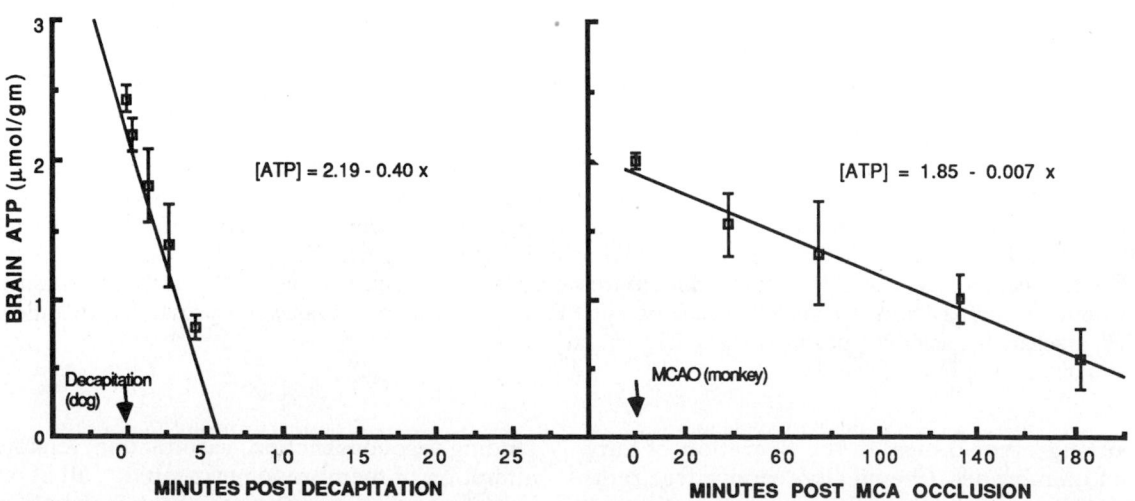

Fig. 19-14. Comparison of the rates of failure of energy supply (ATP) in complete global ischemia (produced by decapitation in dogs)[267] and in complete focal ischemia (middle cerebral artery occlusion in monkeys).[266] In the presence of residual CBF, energy supply failure is substantially delayed. (Data from Michenfelder and Theye[267] and Michenfelder and Sundt.[266])

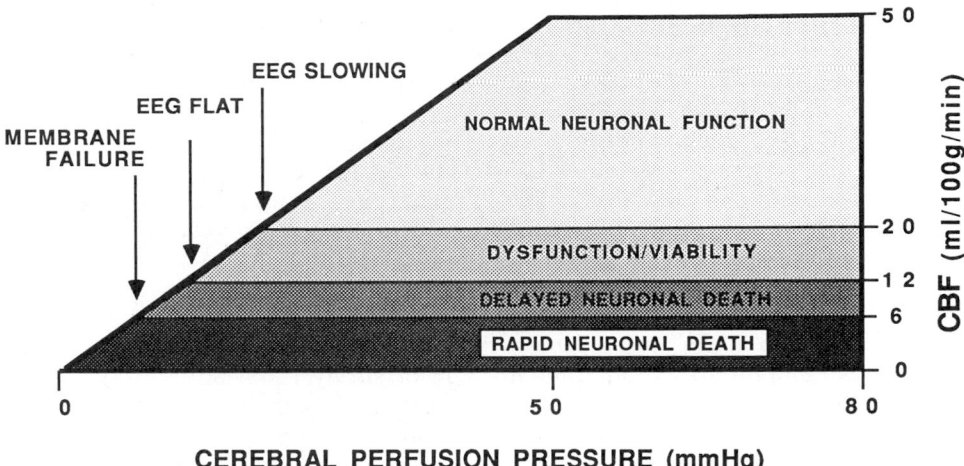

CEREBRAL PERFUSION PRESSURE (mmHg)

Fig. 19-15. Relationships between cerebral perfusion, CBF, the EEG, and the functional status and viability of neurons. In the approximate CBF range of 6 to 12 ml/100 g/min, the energy supply is insufficient to support electrophysiologic activity (i.e., EEG flat) but can prevent complete membrane failure and neuronal death for extended periods (see Fig. 19-14). These areas are referred to as the ischemic penumbra.[268] The data are derived from studies in the cerebral cortex of barbiturate-anesthetized baboons.[268,270] and unanesthetized monkeys.[269] The thresholds may vary with anesthetic and species.[271] (Data from Astrup et al.,[268] Branston et al.,[270] and Jones et al.[269])

free radicals) that aggravate the injury are initiated. The numerous brain protection strategies that have been studied in both the laboratory and the clinic can be classified according to the phase of this sequence that each addresses. They are listed in Table 19-6. Brain protection regimens will logically be most effective when instituted before the onset of ischemia. However, it is reasonable to anticipate some efficacy of certain therapies initiated after the beginning of the insult because many of the insult processes will be on-going in the ischemia and reperfusion phases. The literature dealing with cerebral protection and resuscitation is enormous and cannot be thoroughly reviewed here. Reviews of brain protection are available.[261,273-275] Of the many

TABLE 19-6. Ischemic Neuronal Injury: Pathogenetic Sequence and Related Protection Strategies[a]

Insult Mechanism	Protection Strategy	Therapy Example
Failure of energy supply	Decrease energy demand, i.e., CMR	Barbiturates* Hypothermia*
	Increase energy supply, i.e., CBF	Induced hypertension* Hemodilution*
	Prevent supranormal energy demand	Seizure prophylaxis and control*
Intracellular lactic acidosis	Avoid excess glucose supply	Omit glucose solutions*
Increased cytosolic Ca++	Block Ca++ access to neuron	Ca++ blockers* Glutamate antagonists
Membrane damage	Antioxidants and antilipolytics Inhibit free radical formation	Aminosteroids Iron chelators (e.g., deferoxamine)[298] Xanthine oxidase inhibitors (e.g., allopurinol)[299]
	Scavenge free radicals	Superoxide dismutase Catalase[300]
Fatty acid metabolite-mediated damage	Inhibit formation of prostaglandins and leukotrienes	Inhibitors of lipoxygenase,[301] cyclo-oxygenase,[302] and thromboxane synthetase[303]

[a] While each of the therapy examples has shown efficacy in at least one laboratory investigation, only those designated * have been proved or are accepted as clinically applicable. For items not discussed in the text, a single recent reference is provided.

promising protection and resuscitation strategies, only a limited number (discussed below) have reached the stage of human application. Some (presented first below) are relevant to ischemia of any type, and others are of greater relevance in focal ischemia in which energy supply failure may be more gradual and in which there is potential for manipulation of collateral flow.

Hypothermia is routinely used in anticipation of circulatory arrest. It is not widely used in anticipation of possible focal ischemic events, for example, aneurysm surgery, although animal data indicate that even modest temperature reduction (2 to 3°C)[276] has a demonstrable protective effect, and moderate hypothermia in this setting may again become fashionable.

The withholding of glucose-containing solutions in situations in which cerebral ischemia may occur is now an established practice. The inevitable questions of whether and how quickly immediate prerisk treatment with insulin of an elevated plasma glucose reduces risk to normoglycemic levels have not been answered. At this time, insulin administration (with its attendant risks) in patients with modest glucose elevation, for example, 175 to 250 mg/dl, is not justified.

Normalization of systemic pH, the prevention and treatment of seizures, which dramatically increase CMR, and control of ICP and CPP are all, while mundane and lacking in the appeal of the pharmacologic silver bullet, important elements of brain protection and resuscitation.

Isoflurane is also a potent suppressant of CMR in cerebral cortex, and EEG evidence suggestive of a protective effect in humans[271] has been reported. The available laboratory data, however, provide less consistent support for a protective effect of isoflurane than is the case for barbiturates.[277-282]

The calcium channel blocker nimodipine has been shown to reduce the severity of neurologic injury when given for a prolonged period after aneurysmal subarachnoid hemorrhage.[283] Additional calcium-blocking drugs and the use of these drugs in other settings will no doubt evolve rapidly although there has, as yet, been no convincing demonstration of efficacy in humans in any setting other than subarachnoid hemorrhage. Note that these drugs are cerebral vasodilators. ICP elevation may therefore occur, and they should be used with caution in patients with intracranial hypertension.[284]

Focal (Incomplete) Ischemia

There have been numerous demonstrations of the protective efficacy of barbiturates in focal cerebral ischemia. The effect has been attributed principally to suppression of CMR, although flow redistribution effects and free radical scavenging[285] have been suggested to contribute. There has been a single demonstration of effectiveness in humans in the setting of focal incomplete ischemia.[286] Barbiturate suppression of CMR to the point of EEG isoelectricity may be logical therapy when it can be applied before or early in the course of a period of temporary focal ischemia, for example, temporary occlusion during aneurysm surgery. Its appropriateness will be determined by the anticipated risk of the occlusive event, by the patient's cardiovascular status, by the physician's willingness to accept the possible prolongation of arousal, and other factors.

Measures designed to augment CBF (an important determinant of energy supply) are also important. In the ischemic penumbra (described above) small improvements in CBF have the potential to prolong neuronal survival substantially. The maintenance of a high normal CPP can augment collateral flow[68] and improve neurologic function.[91,287] However, this practice carries the inadequately explored risks of increased edema and hemorrhagic infarction if used as support during more than brief periods of ischemia.

Normocapnia should be maintained. Hypercapnia has the potential to cause an intracerebral steal and may worsen intracellular pH. Hypocapnia, despite some support for the occurrence of a favorable so-called Robin Hood or inverse steal,[288,289] has not generally proved effective in either laboratory or clinical settings.[290-294] However, several of these investigations examined prolonged ischemia and hypocapnia, and their results may not be relevant to the shorter episodes that would more commonly arise in the operating room. Nonetheless, pending further information, normocapnia remains the standard practice.

Although hemodilution has not proved effective in studies of human stroke, both laboratory and human data (the latter derived from patients with subarachoid hemorrhage) support the practice, and it is an established part of the management of the ischemia associated with vasospasm. However, the data do not currently justify routine hemodilution (a hematocrit of 30 to 35 percent is the theoretical optimum) in patients in whom focal ischemia *might* occur in the operating room. However, the potentially deleterious effects of hemoconcentration should help to further suppress the out of date notion that neurosurgical patients should be "run dry." An elevated hematocrit, because of viscosity effects, reduces CBF.[56] It is our unsubstantiated opinion that in anticipation of a procedure in which incomplete ischemia might occur, for example, carotid endarterectomy, a hematocrit in excess of 50 to 55 percent should be lowered by preoperative phlebotomy.

The risks of extension of cerebral infarction in the event of subsequent anesthesia and surgery have not been formally studied. In patients who have suffered a stroke, CBF undergoes marked changes, and areas of both high and low CBF have been observed and normal vasomotor responses may be lost. Approximately 4 to 6 weeks are required for these changes to stabilize.[295] Therefore, pending other information, it seems reasonable to defer elective surgery for this period after an occlusive vascular accident to minimize the risk of recurrent stroke.

Cardiac Arrest

Maintenance of adequate perfusion pressures after a cardiac arrest is of considerable importance. Hypotension developing after resuscitation from cardiac arrest may aggravate microcirculatory and vasospastic processes occurring at this time and increase brain damage.[304] Intracranial hypertension occurs in two phases after resuscitation from cardiac arrest. The first phase, which is usually transient, is due to increased CBV during reactive hyperemia and cellular hydration as a consequence of cytotoxic cerebral edema. While this phase is usually self-limiting, reduction in CPP due to elevated ICP may reduce the effective CPP and impede reflow. Some investigators suggest early aggressive use of osmotic diuretics to avoid this problem.[305] A late phase of intracranial hypertension may occur and is due to the development of extensive vasogenic cerebral edema associated with brain necrosis. Attempts to control this type of intracranial hypertension with osmotherapy usually fail. ICP monitoring is not generally employed because the patients who developed these delayed ICP increases have sustained massive tissue damage. Both barbiturate and calcium channel blockers have been administered after cardiac arrest. The former is ineffective.[306-308] The calcium channel blocker nimodipine improved neurologic outcome when administered after complete global ischemia in a primate model[309] but was ineffective after complete global ischemia in the cat[310] and the dog.[311] In a small human patient cohort, nimodipine was shown to improve CBF but not neurologic outcome after cardiac arrest.[312] However, its effect on neurologic outcome has not yet been fully evaluated.

Chronic Arterial Hypertension

In chronic hypertension, both the upper and lower limits of autoregulation are shifted to the right. A recurrent concern is that of acceptable levels of hypotension in the chronically hypertensive patient. Strict quantitative guidelines are not available to guide the anesthesiologist in defining permissible blood pressure decreases in individual patients. In the absence of recognized cerebrovascular disease or transient ischemic attacks, a mean blood pressure decrease of not more than 50 mmHg from baseline values will likely be tolerated without adverse neurologic sequelae. This suggestion is predicated upon the fact that the hypertensive autoregulatory curve appears to be shifted to the right without distortion and that normally at least a 50 mmHg decline in arterial pressure is tolerated.

Intracranial Hypertension

Intracranial hypertension is discussed in detail in Chapter 54 and the material here is intended only as an overview. Therapy is aimed at controlling the volume of the contents of the intracranial compartment. The four compartments (blood, CSF, intracellular and extracellular fluid, and cells) and the various techniques for manipulating their volumes are presented in Table 19-7. Note that it is the blood compartment with which the anesthesiologist will be most greatly concerned because it is mobile and easily subject to manipulation. A theme that unites many aspects of ICP management is the necessity to avoid drugs and techniques that cause cerebral vasodilation (with the attendant increases in CBF and CBV) and to select those that cause cerebral vasoconstriction. Recall also that both autoregulation and CO_2 responsiveness may be impaired. Autoregulation is particularly vulnerable and at least some portion of the cerebral circulation should be assumed to be pressure passive in the face of most disorders that cause elevated ICP. CO_2 responsiveness is more robust and its absence is, in general, indicative of a severe brain injury.

Brain Tumors

There are few data regarding the physiology of intracranial tumors. Arbit et al.[313] measured CBF in cerebral tumors using laser-Doppler technology. They found that CO_2 responsiveness was usually present and that autoregulation was occasionally apparent. In general the tumors had a lower CBF than normal brain. There is often considerable edema in association with intracranial tumors. Bedford et al.[314] showed that the radiologic extent of the edema (which presumably represents the extent of abnormal vessel leakiness) correlated with the severity of the ICP elevation that occurred in association with intubation-related hypertension. Empirically, the edema associated with tumors is improved by steroids, and it has been shown in patients with intracranial tumors[315] that, over a time course as short as 6 hours, BBB function is improved by administration of dexamethasone.

TABLE 19-7. Intracranial Compartments and Techniques for Manipulation of Their Volume

Compartment	Volume Control Methods
Cells (including neurons, glia, tumors, and extravasated blood)	Surgical removal
Fluid (intracellular and extracellular)	Diuretics
	Steroids (principally tumors)
CSF	Drainage
Blood	
Arterial side	Decrease CBF
Venous side	Improve cerebral venous drainage

Coma and Epilepsy

Coma, regardless of its etiology, is associated with reductions in brain metabolism. In the case of lesions occurring in the reticular activating system of the brain stem, the reduction in CMR probably represents a normal physiologic adjustment to reduced functional activity. Patients with isolated brain stem lesions and normal cerebral hemispheres have been shown to have an 80 percent reduction in CBF and CMR.[316] During generalized seizure activity, CMR and CBF may increase dramatically. The intensive motor and brain activity accompanying generalized seizures leads to the development of systemic and cerebral acidosis, accompanied by a reduction in arterial oxygenation, an increase in $PaCO_2$, and peripheral lactic acidosis. If generalized seizure activity continues unabated, arterial hypotension and death supervene. With muscular relaxation and measures ensuring adequate oxygenation and ventilation, the systemic acidosis and hypotension can be avoided and the severity of cerebral acidosis diminished. The corrective effects of oxygenation and ventilation represent a cardiovascular protective effect rather than one directly affecting the brain. The mechanism of cerebral acidosis during seizures is unknown. It can develop with evidence of cerebral hyperfusion, as shown by cerebral venous hyperoxia and the absence of depletion of high-energy phosphates. This points to a maldistribution in CBF during seizure activity and/or to utilization of metabolic pathways not immediately related to aerobic metabolism. During relatively brief episodes of continuous seizures, the brain seems able to meet the high metabolic demands. When the seizures are allowed to continue for a prolonged period, they can be self-perpetuating and lead to the development of irreversible neuronal damage.[317] Therapy aimed at interrupting the seizure and restoring a normal balance between cerebral metabolic demands and blood flow is indicated. Barbiturates, benzodiazepines, or other potent anticonvulsants are appropriate. Adequate ventilation, oxygenation, and maintenance of blood pressure are important adjunctive measures. Muscle relaxants must be viewed as purely symptomatic therapy, because they do not alter the abnormal cerebral electrical activity. The potentially injurious nature of seizures justifies attention to prevention. Practices vary. However, patients who have sustained a severe head injury or a subarachnoid hemorrhage and any patient in whom a substantial cortical incision is planned are at risk and prophylactic anticonvulsants should be considered.

MEASUREMENT OF CBF AND CMR

In the clinical practice of anesthesiology, measurements of CBF and CMR are almost never made. Nonetheless, anesthesiologists make daily use of information derived from such measurements. Accordingly, it is appropriate to have a general understanding of how these measurements are made and, above all, to appreciate the limitations of the various techniques.

The available techniques may be classified as providing information that is global (entire brain), regional, or local. Global CBF measurements allow predictions about overall CBF effects. These may be very relevant in predicting ICP responses. However, they may fail to represent the status of focally abnormal areas, especially if these areas are relatively small or receive little tracer because of low flow. This limitation may be obviated by techniques (described below) that provide a greater degree of spatial resolution, for example, PET, Xe/CT, SPECT, ^{133}Xe washout with external gamma detection, and hydrogen clearance. The resolution of these regional techniques varies considerably, from a few cubic millimeters with hydrogen clearance to several cubic centimeters for the various xenon washout methods. The designation "local" is generally reserved for autoradiographic techniques that entail histologic sectioning of the brain after administration of radiolabeled tracers and permit evaluation of brain regions of less than 1 mm^2. Table 19-8 provides a listing of methods that have been used in humans or that are in common use in the laboratory.

The majority of CBF techniques are applications of the Fick principle. The first to be used in humans was the global flow method of Kety and Schmidt.[318] It is still in use. Arterial and cerebral venous blood, the latter taken from a catheter in the jugular bulb, are sampled intermittently during the washin (or washout) of a relatively insoluble, freely diffusible, inert tracer substance such as xenon 133, krypton 85, or N_2O. The concentration of the tracer in cerebral venous blood is assumed to represent brain tissue concentration. The time required for equilibration of arterial blood and venous blood is inversely proportional to flow, and when the blood/brain partition coefficient of the tracer is known, a quantitative determination of global CBF can be made. The method assumes steady state conditions for the duration of the sampling period (10 to 20 minutes). The intra-arterial, intravenous, and inhaled ^{133}Xe methods, hydrogen clearance, thermal clearance, autoradiography, positron emission tomography (PET), and xenon-enhanced computed tomography (Xe/CT) are also applications of the Fick principle. In each instance, the brian concentration of the tracer is identified by some means other than the sampling of the cerebral venous effluent. For instance, the ^{133}Xe techniques employ external counting of the emitted gamma radiation and brain concentrations can be derived by reference to the established blood/brain partition coefficient for xenon.

CMR can be determined if the cerebral arteriovenous content difference for a substrate (oxygen or glucose) is measured simultaneously with the determination of CBF. For instance, $CMRO_2$ is the product of the O_2 content difference between arterial and venous blood × CBF. The net rate of production of metabolites (e.g., lactate) can also be derived by a similar calculation.

TABLE 19-8. Methods for the Measurement of CBF

Technique	Regional Specificity	Human Use
Kety-Schmidt	Global	Yes
Venous outflow	Global	No
Extracerebral flow probe (electromagnetic)	Global	Yes
Xenon washout	Regional	Yes
PET	Regional	Yes
SPECT	Regional	Yes
Xe/CT	Regional	Yes
Thermal clearance	Regional	Yes
Hydrogen clearance	Regional	No
Microspheres	Regional	No
Autoradiography	Local	No
Laser-Doppler	Local	Yes

Note that the accuracy of a CMR determination is not ensured unless the venous effluent sampled comes from precisely the same compartment in which the CBF is measured. This may not be the case if, for instance, rCBF is measured by external gamma counters and the CMR determination is based on a sample from the jugular bulb. Note also that CMR as determined in this fashion is also a global measure and may fail to represent the status of focally abnormal areas. In normal awake adult humans, $CMRO_2$ is 3.0 to 3.5 ml of $O_2/100$ g of brain tissue/min.

Xenon Washout

Of the methods that provide regional CBF information, it is ^{133}Xe washout utilizing external gamma radiation detectors that is most readily applied in the surgical environment. The ^{133}Xe can be administered intra-arterially, intravenously, or by inhalation. However, the method suffers from the limitation that abnormalities in regional flow may be obscured by the look-through phenomenon. This occurs when an area of very low flow is surrounded by an area of relatively high flow and is seen as normal by the extracranially positioned gamma detectors.[319] This problem is obviated by methods that use CT techniques to measure local tracer concentrations.

Positron Emission Tomography

PET is an extremely powerful tool for investigations of cerebral physiology.[320] Nuclear decay by positron emission results in the generation of two high-energy annihilation photons. The photons are emitted on trajectories 180 degrees apart. Thus, an array of paired detectors that register only coincident events permits very precise determination of the photons' plane of origin. This eliminates the problem of radiation scatter that reduces the resolution of other emission tomographic techniques. In addition, the high energy of these photons minimizes tissue attenuation. There are

positron-emitting isotopes of several of the most common elements in biologic systems (e.g., carbon, nitrogen, oxygen, fluorine), and a wide spectrum of physiologic compounds can be labeled. PET can noninvasively provide two- or three-dimensional maps of several parameters including CBF, CMR, CBV, BBB function, and drug pharmokinetics. The disadvantage is that the method is cumbersome and expensive, in large part because of the cyclotron that must be immediately at hand to generate the short-lived positron-emitting radionuclides (^{15}O, ^{18}F, ^{11}C, and ^{13}N) that are required. However, because of the short half-lives it is possible to perform serial measurements of complementary physiologic phenomena (e.g., CBF, $CMRO_2$, and CBV).

Xenon-Enhanced Computed Tomography (Xe/CT)

Nonradioactive xenon alters the radiodensity of CT brain images in a concentration-related manner. The local brain concentration is CBF dependent and because the blood/brain partition coefficient for Xe is known, a quantitative measure of CBF can be derived.[321-322] The method has been applied clinically[323]; however, its validity has been challenged because xenon itself has been reported to cause increases in CBF.[324]

Single Proton Emission Computed Tomography

Single proton emission computed tomography (SPECT) employs rotating, collimated gamma counters to obtain tomographic brain images. The tracers are labeled with longer-lived gamma-emitting isotopes, most often technetium 99m, and therefore a cyclotron with its inherent cost and inconvenience is not required. The majority of systems provide only relative CBF information. Absolute values can be obtained by scaling the SPECT image against some other measure of CBF, for example, ^{133}Xe clearance.[325]

Magnetic Resonance Techniques

Atoms that have nuclei with angular momentum oscillate when disturbed by a radiofrequency (RF) pulse. While oscillating they in turn emit an RF signal corresponding to their inherent resonant frequency. Hydrogen and phosphorus have suitable nuclei and occur in sufficient quantity in biologic systems to permit detection of their emitted RF signal. Magnetic resonance imaging (MRI) instruments characteristically employ RF detectors tuned to the resonant frequencies of the hydrogen nucleus (a proton). Multiple detectors and emission tomographic software are used to generate two-dimensional images that in large part depend on the varying concentrations of water in different tissues.[326,327] MRI techniques for the assessment of CBF are under investigation[328] but are not yet established.

While imaging is the common clinical application of magnetic resonance principles, it is magnetic resonance spectroscopy (MRS)[329] that has been most relevant to investigations of cerebral physiology. Phosphorus 31 is the tracer of principle interest because of its involvement in bioenergetic processes. The resonant frequency of ^{31}P varies slightly according to the molecule to which it is attached. As a result, discrete signals are emitted by phosphocreatine (PCr), ATP, ADP, and free inorganic phosphate (P_i). Signal intensities provide a measure of the changing relative concentrations of these molecules, and accordingly, changes in energy charge can be assessed. In addition, the relationship between P_i and PCr can be used to derive intracellular pH. These measurements can be performed quickly (ca. 4 minutes) and repeatedly during the evolution and resolution of a physiologic disturbance. A potential limitation is that the current tissue resolution of MRS is limited to 60 mm³.

Electromagnetic Flow Probes and Doppler Techniques

Electromagnetic flow probes and Doppler techniques provide a direct assessment of flow within relatively large vessels. Both suffer from the limitation that they do not truly measure tissue perfusion in that there may be uncertainty as to the distribution of flow past the measurement point. Electromagnetic probes have been used principally in the animal laboratory[198] and, on occasion, to provide an on-line measure of shunt function during carotid endarterectomy.[330] Doppler techniques can be applied to both intracranial and extracranial cerebral vessels. Note that Doppler methodology allows determination of velocity, that is, the speed at which the blood is moving, but that blood *flow* (i.e., the volume of blood per unit time) cannot be derived unless vessel diameter is measured simultaneously. For intracranial vessels in adults the available technique, transcranial Doppler,[331,332] provides only velocity information. While in general a decrease in flow velocity will be observed when CBF decreases, there

will be exceptions. For instance, with the onset of vasospasm (and the associated decrease in CBF) velocity through the affected vessel, for example, the middle cerebral artery, will *increase*,[333] presumably because the blood accelerates as it is forced through the narrowed artery. A second Doppler technique has been employed recently.[313] Laser-Doppler flowmetry can provide CBF information for regions as small as 1 mm³ and is therefore a local CBF technique. The method uses a monochromatic laser source to illuminate tissue regions of probe-dependent size. Flow velocity information is obtained by examining the Doppler shifting of the returning light. Some insight into not only blood velocity but also flow can be obtained by determining the percentage of the returning light that is Doppler shifted. For the time being, however, this technique should be viewed as nonquantitative.

Hydrogen Clearance

Hydrogen clearance involves the placement of a platinum electrode in the tissue of interest with a second electrode, for example, silver-silver chloride, in a remote location. Hydrogen is administered in low concentration. Molecular hydrogen is oxidized to hydrogen ion at the platinum electrode and a current proportional to the hydrogen concentration in the adjacent tissue is generated between the two electrodes. When inspired hydrogen gas is eliminated, tissue hydrogen concentration and the derived current decrease in a flow-dependent fashion. A quantitative measure of flow can be derived. The method has been extensively used in investigations of cerebral physiology. However, some doubt has recently been cast on this technique because of the demonstration that the physical presence of the electrode in otherwise normal brain results in a prolonged (approximately 6 hour) reduction in regional CBF in the gerbil.[334]

Clinical Applications

The intraoperative use of the CBF-CMR techniques reviewed above has generally been restricted to research applications. In a limited number of centers, xenon clearance techniques have been used during carotid endarterectomy to assess the need for a temporary shunt during vascular occlusion.[271] Regional CBF studies performed in these instances have revealed a good correlation between CBF and the EEG pattern, and the latter accordingly provides a very acceptable alternative. The transcranial Doppler has been used recently in intensive care settings to provide an early indication of the onset of vasospasm.[333]

REFERENCES

1. Michenfelder JD: The interdependency of cerebral function and metabolic effects following massive doses of thiopental in the dog. Anesthesiology 41:231, 1974

2. Leniger-Follert E, Hossman KA: Micro-flow and evoked potentials in the somato-motor cortex of the cat brain during specific sensory activation. Acta Neurol Scand, 60:suppl. 72, 10, 1979

3. Olesen J: Contralateral local increase in cerebral blood flow in man during arm work. Brain 94:635, 1971

4. Miyaoka M, Shinohara M, Batipps M, et al: The relationship between the intensity of the stimulus and the metabolic response in the visual system of the rat. Acta Neurol Scand, 60:suppl. 72, 16, 1979

5. Greenberg J, Hand P, Sylverstro A, et al: Localized metabolic flow couple during functional activity. Acta Neurol Scand, 60:suppl. 72, 12, 1979

6. Nakai K, Imni H, Kamei I, et al: Microarchitecture of rat parietal cortex with special reference to vascular "sphincters." Scanning electron microscopic and dark field microscopic study. Stroke 12:653, 1981

7. Lou HC, Edvinsson L, MacKenzie ET: The concept of coupling blood flow to brain function: Revision required? Ann Neurol 22:289, 1987

8. Newburg LA, Milde JH, Michenfelder JD: The cerebral metabolic effects of isoflurane at and above concentrations that suppress cortical electrical activity. Anesthesiology 59:23, 1983

9. Milde LN, Milde JH, Michenfelder JD: Cerebral functional, metabolic and hemodynamic effects of etomidate in dogs. Anesthesiology 63:371, 1985

10. Astrup J, Sorensen PM, Sorensen HR: Inhibition of cerebral oxygen and glucose consumption in the dog by hypothermia, pentobarbital and lidocaine. Anesthesiology 55:263, 1981

11. Maekawa T, Tommasino C, Shapiro HM, et al: Local cerebral blood flow and glucose utilization during isoflurane anesthesia in the rat. Anesthesiology 65:144, 1986

12. Hansen TD, Warner DS, Todd MM, et al: Distribution of cerebral blood flow during halothane versus isoflurane anesthesia in rats. Anesthesiology 69:332, 1988

13. Drummond JC, Todd MM, U HS: The effect of high dose sodium thiopental on brain stem auditory and median nerve somatosensory evoked responses in humans. Anesthesiology 63:249, 1985

14. Peterson DO, Drummond JC, Todd MM: The effects of halothane, enflurane, isoflurane, and nitrous oxide upon somatosensory evoked potentials in man. Anesthesiology 65:35, 1986

15. Eger EI, Stevens WC, Cromwell TH: The electroencephalogram in man anesthetized with forane. Anesthesiology 35:504, 1971

16. Michenfelder JD: Anesthesia and the Brain: Clinical, Functional, Metabolic, and Vascular Correlates. Churchill Livingstone, New York, 1988

17. Smith AL, Wollman H: Cerebral blood flow and metabolism: Effects of anesthetic drugs and techniques. Anesthesiology 36:378, 1972

18. Sato M, Pawlik G, Heiss WD: Comparative studies of regional CNS blood flow autoregulation and responses to CO_2 in the cat. Stroke 15:91, 1984

19. Kassel NF, Hitchson PW, Gerk MK, et al: Influence of changes in arterial PCO_2 on cerebral blood flow and metabolism during high-dose barbiturate therapy in dogs. J Neurosurg 54:615, 1981

20. Drummond JC, Todd MM: The response of the feline cerebral circulation to $PaCO_2$ during anesthesia with isoflurane and halothane and during sedation with nitrous oxide. Anesthesiology 62:268, 1985

21. Forster A, Juge O, Morel D: Effects of midazolam on cerebral hemodynamics and cerebral vasomotor responsiveness to carbon dioxide. J Cereb Blood Flow Metab 3:246, 1983

22. Koehler RC, Traystman RJ: Bicarbonate ion modulation of cerebral blood flow during hypoxia and hypercapnia. Am J Physiol 243:H33, 1982

23. Albrecht RF, Miletich DJ, Madala LR: Normalization of cerebral blood flow during prolonged halothane anesthesia. Anesthesiology 58:26, 1983

24. Raichle ME, Posner JB, Plum F: Cerebral blood flow during and after hyperventilation. Arch Neurol 23:394, 1970

25. Grote J, Zimmer K, Schubert R: Effects of severe arterial hypocapnia on regional blood flow regulation, tissue PO_2 and metabolism in the brain cortex of cats. Eur J Physiol 391:195, 1981

26. Stoyka WW, Schutz H: Cerebral response to hypocapnia in normal and brain-injured dogs. Can Anaesth Soc J 21:205, 1974

27. Michenfelder JD, Theye RA: The effects of profound hypocapnia and dilutional anemia on canine cerebral metabolism and blood flow. Anesthesiology 31:449, 1969

28. Alexander SC, Smith TC, Stroebel G, et al: Cerebral carbohydrate metabolism of man during respiratory and metabolic alkalosis. J Appl Physiol 24:66, 1968

29. Hansen NB, Nowicki PT, Miller RR, et al: Alterations in cerebral blood flow and oxygen consumption during prolonged hypocarbia. Pediatr Res 20:147, 1986

30. Reivich M, Cohen PJ, Greenbaum L: Alterations in the electroencephalogram of awake man produced by hyperventilation: Effects of 100% oxygen at 3 atmospheres (absolute) pressure. Neurology 16:304, 1966

31. Hagerdal M, Harp JR, Siesjö BK: Influence of changes in arterial PCO_2 on cerebral blood flow and cerebral energy state during hypothermia in the rat. Acta Anaesthesiol Scand, suppl., 57:25, 1975

32. Bruce DA: Effects of hyperventilation on cerebral blood flow and metabolism. Clin Perinatol 11:673, 1984

33. Hilberman M, Nioka S, Subramanian H, et al: Brain pH during respiratory acidosis and alkalosis, a ^{31}P NMR study. Anesthesiology 61:A317, 1984

34. Artru AA: Cerebral vascular responses to hypocapnia during nitroglycerin-induced hypotension. Neurosurgery 16:468, 1985

35. Artru AA, Katz RA, Colley PS: Autoregulation of cerebral blood flow during normocapnia and hypocapnia in dogs. Anesthesiology 70:288, 1989

36. Boarini DJ, Kassell NF, Sprowell JA, et al: Cerebrovascular effects of hypocapnia during adenosine-induced arterial hypotension. J Neurosurg 63:937, 1985

37. Plum F, Siesjö BK: Recent advances in CSF physiology. Anesthesiology 42:708, 1975

38. Greenfield JC, Rembert JC, Tindall GT: Transient changes in cerebral vascular resistance during the Valsalva maneuver in man. Stroke 15:76, 1984

39. Vinall PE, Simeone FA: Cerebral autoregulation: An *in vitro* study. Stroke 12:640, 1981

40. Chikovani O, Corkill G, McLeish I, et al: Effect on canine cerebral blood flow of two common pressor agents during prolonged halothane anesthesia. Surg Neurol 9:211, 1978

41. Dahl E: The innervation of the cerebral arteries. J Anat 115:53, 1973

42. Hara H, Jansen I, Ekman R, et al: Acetylcholine and vasoactive intestinal peptide in cerebral blood vessels: Effect of extirpation of the sphenopalatine ganglion. J Cereb Blood Flow Metabol 9:204, 1989

43. Edvinsson L, Lindvall M, Nielsen KC, Owman CH: Are brain

vessels innervated also by central (non-sympathetic) adrenergic neurones? Brain Res 63:496, 1973

44. Edvinsson L, Dequeurce A, Duverger D, et al: Central serotonergic nerves project to the pial vessels of the brain. Nature 306:55, 1983

45. Bonvento G, Lacombe P, Seylaz J: Effects of electrical stimulation of the dorsal raphe nucleus on local cerebral blood flow in the rat. J Cereb Blood Flow Metab 9:251, 1989

46. Busija DW: Sympathetic nerves reduce cerebral blood flow during hypoxia in awake rabbits. Am J Physiol 247:H446, 1984

47. Auer LM, Edvinsson L, Johansson BB: Effect of sympathetic nerve stimulation and adrenoceptor blockade on pial arterial and venous calibre and on intracranial pressure in the cat. Acta Physiol Scand 119:213, 1983

48. MacKenzie ET, McGeorge AD, Graham DT, et al: Effects of increasing arterial pressure on cerebral blood flow in the baboon: influence of the sympathetic nervous system. Pflugers Arch 378:189, 1979

49. Bevan JA: Autonomic pharmacologist's guide to the cerebral circulation. Trends Pharmacol Sci June:234, 1984

50. Wei EP, Raper AJ, Kontos HA, Patterson JL: Determinants of response of pial arteries to norepinephrine and sympathetic nerve stimulation. Stroke 6:654, 1975

51. Reddy RSV, Yaksh TL, Anderson RE, Sundt TM: Effect in cat of locus coeruleus lesions on the response of cerebral blood flow and cardiac output to altered $PaCO_2$. Brain Res 365:278, 1986

52. Fitch W, MacKenzie ET, Harper AM: Effects of decreasing arterial blood pressure on cerebral blood flow in the baboon, influence of the sympathetic nervous system. Circ Res 37:550, 1975

53. Bill A, Linder J, Linder M: Sympathetic effect on cerebral blood vessels in acute arterial hypertension. Acta Physiol Scand 96:114, 1976

54. Johansson BB, Auer LM: Neurogenic modification of the vulnerability of the blood-brain-barrier during acute hypertension in conscious rats. Acta Physiol Scand 117:507, 1983

55. Harrison MJG: Influence of haematocrit in the cerebral circulation. Cerebrovasc Brain Metab Rev 1:55, 1989

56. Reivich M: Regulation of the cerebral circulation. Clin Neurosurg 1:378, 1969

57. Cole DJ, Drummond JC, Shapiro HM, et al: The effect of hypervolemic-hemodilution with and without hypertension on cerebral blood flow following middle cerebral artery occlusion in the rat. Anesthesiology 71:580, 1989

58. Heros RC, Korosue K: Hemodilution for cerebral ischemia. Stroke 20:423, 1989

59. Korosue K, Ishida K, Matsuoka H, et al: Clinical, hemodynamic, and hemorheological effects of isovolemic hemodilution in acute cerebral infarction. Neurosurgery 23:148, 1988

60. Kee DB, Wood JH: Rheology of the cerebral circulation. Neurosurgery 15:125, 1984

61. Maekawa T, McDowall DG, Okuda Y: Brain-surface oxygen tension and cerebral cortical blood flow during hemorrhagic and drug-induced hypotension in the cat. Anesthesiology 51:313, 1979

62. Marsh ML, Shapiro HM, Smith RW, et al: Changes in neurologic status and intracranial pressure associated with sodium nitroprusside administration. Anesthesiology 51:336, 1979

63. Ekström-Jodal B, von Essen C, Haggendal E: Effects of noradrenaline on the cerebral blood flow in the dog. Acta Neurol Scand 50:11, 1974

64. von Essen C: Effects of dopamine, noradrenaline and 5-hydroxytryptamine on the cerebral blood flow in the dog. J Pharm Pharmacol 24:G68, 1972

65. Oberdorster G, Lang R, Zimmer R: Direct effects of α- and β-sympathomimetic amines on the cerebral circulation of the dog. Pflugers Arch 340:145, 1973

66. Lluch S, Reimann C, Glick G: Evidence for the direct effect of adrenergic drugs on the cerebral vascular bed of the unanesthetized goat. Stroke 4:50, 1973

67. Haggendal E: Effects of some vasoactive drugs on the vessels of cerebral grey matter in the dog. Acta Physiol Scand, suppl., 66:55, 1965

68. Drummond JC, Oh YS, Cole DJ, et al: Phenylephrine-induced hypertension decreases the area of ischemia following middle cerebral artery occlusion in the rat. Stroke 20:1538, 1989

69. Berntman L, Dahlgren N, Siesjö BK: Influence of intravenously administered catecholamines on cerebral oxygen consumption and blood flow in the rat. Acta Physiol Scand 104:101, 1978

70. Tuor UI, Edvinsson L, McCulloch J: Catecholamines and the relationship between cerebral blood flow and glucose use. Am Physiol Soc 251:H824, 1986

71. Olesen J: The effect of intracarotid epinephrine, norepinephrine, and angiotensin on the regional cerebral blood flow in man. Neurology 22:978, 1972

72. MacKenzie ET, McCullock J, O'Keane M, et al: Cerebral circulation and norepinephrine: Relevance of the blood-brain barrier. Am J Physiol 231:483, 1976

73. King BD, Sokoloff L, Wechsler RL: The effects of l-epinephrine and l-norepinephrine upon cerebral circulation and metabolism in man. J Clin Invest 31:273, 1952

74. Artru AA, Nugent M, Michenfelder JD: Anesthetics affect the cerebral metabolic response to circulatory catecholamines. J Neurochem 36:1941, 1981

75. Forster A, Van Horn K, Marshall LF, et al: Anesthetic effects of blood-brain barrier function during acute arterial hypertension. Anesthesiology 49:26, 1978

76. Bunegin L, Albin MS, Gelineau EF: Effect of esmolol on cerebral blood flow during intracranial hypertension and hemorrhagic hypovolemia. Anesthesiology 67:A424, 1987

77. von Essen C, Zervas NT, Brown DR, et al: Local cerebral blood flow in the dog during intravenous infusion of dopamine. Surg Neurol 13:181, 1980

78. von Essen C: Effects of dopamine on the cerebral blood flow in the dog. Acta Neurol Scand 50:39, 1974

79. Toda N: Dopamine vasodilates human cerebral artery. Experientia 39:1131, 1983

80. Zornow MH, Fleischer JE, Nakakimura K, Drummond JC: Cerebral effects of the alpha-2 agonist, dexmedetomidine. Anesthesiology 71:A612, 1989

81. Edvinsson L, MacKenzie ET, Robert JP, et al: Cerebrovascular responses to haemorrhagic hypotension in anaesthetized cats. Effects of alpha-adrenoceptor antagonists. Acta Physiol Scand 123:317, 1985

82. James IM, Larbi E, Zaimis E: The effect of acute intravenous administration of clonidine on cerebral blood flow in man. Br J Pharmacol 39:198P, 1970

83. Kanawati IS, Yaksh TL, Anderson RE, Marsh RW: Effects of clonidine on cerebral blood flow and the response to arterial CO_2. J Cereb Blood Flow Metab 6:358, 1986

84. Crosby G, Russo M: The spinal blood flow effect of subarachnoid clonidine. Anesthesiology 67:A417, 1987

85. Busija DW, Leffler CW: Exogenous norepinephrine constricts cerebral arterioles via alpha-2 adrenoceptors in newborn pigs. J Cereb Blood Flow Metab 7:184, 1987

86. Lassen NA, Feinberg I, Lane MH: Bilateral studies of cere-

bral oxygen uptake in young and aged normal subjects and in patients with organic dementia. J Clin Invest 39:491, 1960

87. Michenfelder JD, Theye RA: The relationship of age to canine cerebral metabolic rate. J Surg Res 9:645, 1969

88. Simard D, Olesen J, Paulson OB, et al: Regional cerebral blood flow and its regulation in dementia. Brain 94:273, 1971

89. Grubb RL, Raichle ME, Eichling JO, et al: The effects of changes in PaCO$_2$ on cerebral blood volume, blood flow, and vascular mean transit time. Stroke 5:630, 1974

90. Gibbs JM, Wise RJS, Leenders KL, et al: Evaluation of cerebral perfusion reserve in patients with carotid-artery occlusion. Lancet 1:310, 1984

91. Montgomery EB, Grubb L, Raichle ME: Cerebral hemodynamics and metabolism in postoperative cerebral vasospasm and treatment with hypertensive therapy. Ann Neurol 9:502, 1981

92. Artru A: Relationship between cerebral blood volume and CSF pressure during anesthesia with isoflurane or fentanyl in dogs. Anesthesiology 60:575, 1984

93. Artru A: Relationship between cerebral blood volume and CSF pressure during anesthesia with halothane or enflurane in dogs. Anesthesiology 58:533, 1983

94. Archer DP, Labrecque P, Tyler JL, et al: Cerebral blood volume is increased in dogs during administration of nitrous oxide or isoflurane. Anesthesiology 67:642, 1987

95. Ulrich K, Kuschinsky W: In vivo effects of alpha-adrenoceptor agonists and antagonists on pial veins of cats. Stroke 16:880, 1985

96. Marin J, Lobato RD, Rico ML, et al: Effect of pentobarbital on the reactivity of isolated human cerebral arteries. J Neurosurg 54:521, 1981

97. Pierce EC, Lambertsen CJ, Deutch S, et al: Cerebral circulation and metabolism during thiopental anesthesia and hyperventilation in man. J Clin Invest 41:1664, 1962

98. Scheller MS, Smith RC, Drummond JC: Isoflurane influences the effects of barbiturates on cerebral blood flow in rabbits. Anesthesiology 67:A406, 1987

99. Stulken EH, Milde JH, Michenfelder JD, et al: The non-linear response of cerebral metabolism to low concentrations of halothane, enflurane, isoflurane and thiopental. Anesthesiology 46:28, 1977

100. Albrecht RF, Miletich DJ, Rosenberg R, et al: Cerebral blood flow and metabolic changes from induction to onset of anesthesia with halothane or pentobarbital. Anesthesiology 47:252, 1977

101. Altenburg BM, Michenfelder JD, Theye RA: Acute tolerance to thiopental in canine cerebral oxygen consumption studies. Anesthesiology 31:433, 1969

102. Sawada Y, Sugimoto H, Kobayashi H, et al: Acute tolerance to high-dose barbiturate in patients with severe head injuries. Anesthesiology 56:53, 1982

103. Gronert GA, Michenfelder JD, Sharbrough FW, et al: Canine cerebral metabolic tolerance during 24 hours deep pentobarbital anesthesia. Anesthesiology 55:110, 1981

104. Moyer JH, Pontius R, Morris G, Hirshberger R: Effect of morphine and *N*-allylnormorphine on cerebral hemodynamics and oxygen metabolism. Circulation 15:379, 1957

105. Jobes DR, Kennell EM, Bush GL, et al: Cerebral blood flow and metabolism during morphine-nitrous oxide anesthesia in man. Anesthesiology 47:16, 1977

106. Takeshita H, Michenfelder JD, Theye RA: The effect of morphine and *N*-allynormorphine on canine cerebral metabolism and circulation. Anesthesiology 37:605, 1972

107. Jobes DR, Kennell EM, Bitner R, et al: Effects of morphine-

108. Vernhiet J, Marcez P, Renou AM, et al: Effets des fortes doses de morphinomimetiques (fentanyl et fentathienyl) sur la circulation cerebrale du sujet normal. Ann Anesthesiol Fr 18:803, 1977

109. Murkin JM, Farrar JK, Tweed WA, et al: Relationship between cerebral blood flow and O$_2$ consumption during high dose narcotic anesthesia for cardiac surgery. Anesthesiology 63:A44, 1985

110. McPherson RW, Traystman RJ: Fentanyl and cerebral vascular responsivity in dogs. Anesthesiology 60:180, 1984

111. Baughman VL, Hoffman WE, Albrecht RF, et al: Cerebral vascular and metabolic effects of fentanyl and midazolam in young and aged rats. Anesthesiology 67:314, 1987

112. Safo Y, Young ML, Smith DS, et al: Effects of fentanyl on local cerebral blood flow in the rat. Acta Anaesthesiol Scand 29:594, 1985

113. Michenfelder JD, Theye RA: Effects of fentany, droperidol and Innovar on canine cerebral metabolism and blood flow. Br J Anaesth 43:630, 1971

114. McPherson RW, Krempasanka E, Eimerl D, et al: Effects of alfentanil on cerebral vascular reactivity in dogs. Br J Anaesth 57:1232, 1985

115. Murkin JM, Farrar JK, Tweed WA: Sufentanil anaesthesia reduces cerebral blood flow and cerebral oxygen consumption. Can J Anaesth 35:S131, 1988

116. Young WL, Prohovnik I, Correll JW, et al: The effect of sufentanil on cerebral hemodynamics during carotid endarterectomy. Anesthesiology 69:A591, 1988

117. Keykhah MM, Smith DS, Carlsson C, et al: Influence of sufentanil on cerebral metabolism and circulation in the rat. Anesthesiology 63:274, 1985

118. Marx W, Shah N, Long C, et al: Sufentanil, alfentanil and fentanyl: Impact on cerebrospinal fluid pressure in patients with brain tumors. J Neurosurg Anesth 1:3, 1989

119. Milde LN, Milde JH: The cerebral hemodynamic and metabolic effects of sufentanil in dogs. Anesthesiology 67:A570, 1987

120. Milde LN, Milde JH: Cerebral effects of sufentanil in dogs with reduced intracranial compliance. Anesth Analg 68:S196, 1989

121. Shupak RC, Harp JR: Comparison between high-dose sufentanil-oxygen and high-dose fentanyl-oxygen for neuroanesthesia. Br J Anaesth 57:375, 1985

122. Bristow A, Shalev D, Rice B, et al: Low-dose synthetic narcotic infusions for cerebral relaxation during craniotomies. Anesth Analg 66:413, 1987

123. Cotev S, Shalit MN: Effects of diazepam on cerebral blood flow and oxygen uptake after head injury. Anesthesiology 43:117, 1975

124. Rockoff MA, Naughton KVH, Ingvar M, et al: Cerebral circulatory and metabolic responses to intravenously administered lorazepam. Anesthesiology 53:215, 1980

125. Forster A, Juge O, Morel D: Effects of midazolam on cerebral blood flow. Anesthesiology 56:453, 1982

126. Forster A, Juge O, Louis M, et al: Effects of a specific benzodiazepine antagonist (RO 15-1788) on cerebral blood flow. Anesth Analg 66:309, 1987

127. Fleischer JE, Milde JH, Moyer TP, et al: Cerebral effects of high-dose midazolam and subsequent reversal with RO 15-1788 in dogs. Anesthesiology 68:234, 1988

128. Nugent M, Artru AA, Michenfelder JD: Cerebral metabolic, vascular and protective effects of midazolam maleate. Anesthesiology 56:172, 1982

129. Artru AA: Flumazenil reversal of midazolam in dogs: Dose-

related changes in cerebral blood flow, metabolism, EEG, and CSF pressure. J Neurosurg Anesth 1:46, 1989

130. Sari A, Okuda Y, Takeshita H: The effects of thalamonal on cerebral circulation and oxygen consumption in man. Br J Anaesth 44:330, 1972

131. Misfeldt BB, Jorgensen PB, Spotoft H, Ronde F: The effects of droperidol and fentanyl on intracranial pressure and cerebral perfusion pressure in neurosurgical patients. Br J Anaesth 48:963, 1976

132. Miller R, Tausk HC, Stark DCC: Effect of Innovar, fentanyl and droperidol on the cerebrospinal fluid pressure in neurosurgical patients. Can Anaesth Soc J 22:502, 1975

133. Fitch W, Barker FJ, Jennet WB, McDowall DG: The influence of neuroleptanalgesic drugs on cerebrospinal fluid pressure. Br J Anaesth 41:800, 1969

134. Fukuda S, Murakawa T, Takeshita H, et al: Direct effects of ketamine on isolated canine cerebral and mesentric arteries. Anaesth Analg 62:553, 1983

135. Cavazutti M, Porro CA, Biral GP, et al: Ketamine effects on local cerebral blood flow and metabolism in the rat. J Cereb Blood Flow Metab 7:806, 1987

136. Takeshita H, Okuda Y, Sari A: The effects of ketamine on cerebral circulation and metabolism in man. Anesthesiology 36:69, 1972

137. Hougaard K, Hansen A, Brodersen P: The effect of ketamine on regional cerebral blood flow in man. Anesthesiology 41:562, 1974

138. Belopavlovic M, Buchthal A: Modification of ketamine-induced intracranial hypertension in neurosurgical patients by pretreatment with midazolam. Acta Anaesthesiol Scand 26:458, 1982

139. Shapiro HM, Wyte SR, Harris AB: Ketamine anesthesia in patients with intracranial pathology. Br J Anaesth 44:1200, 1972

140. Crosby G, Crane AM, Sokoloff L: Local changes in cerebral glucose utilization during ketamine anesthesia. Anesthesiology 56:437, 1982

141. Ferrer-Allado T, Brechner VL, Dymond A, et al: Ketamine-induced electroconvulsive phenomena in the human limbic and thalamic regions. Anesthesiology 38:333, 1973

142. Davis DW, Mans AM, Biebuyck JF, Hawkins RA: The influence of ketamine on regional brain glucose use. Anesthesiology 69:199, 1988

143. Renou AM, Vernhiet J, Macrez P, et al: Cerebral blood flow and metabolism during etomidate anaesthesia in man. Br J Anaesth 50:1047, 1978

144. Cold GE, Eskesen V, Eriksen H, et al: CBF and CMRO$_2$ during continuous etomidate infusion supplemented with N$_2$O and fentanyl in patients with supratentorial cerebral tumour. A dose-response study. Acta Anaesthesiol Scand 29:490, 1985

145. Cold GE, Eskesen V, Eriksen H, et al: Changes in CMRO$_2$, EEG and concentration of etomidate in serum and brain tissue during craniotomy with continuous etomidate supplemented with N$_2$O and fentanyl. Acta Anaesthesiol Scand 30:159, 1986

146. Bingham RM, Propcaccio F, Prior PF, et al: Cerebral electrical activity influences the effects of etomidate on cerebral perfusion pressure in traumatic coma. Br J Anaesth 57:843, 1985

147. Davis DW, Mans AM, Biebuyck JF, et al: Regional brain glucose utilization in rats during etomidate anesthesia. Anesthesiology 64:751, 1986

148. Dearden NM, McDowall DG: Comparison of etomidate and althesin in the reduction of increased intracranial pressure after head injury. Br J Anaesth 57:361, 1985

149. Bendsten A, Kruse A, Madsen JB, et al: Use of a continuous infusion of althesin in neuroanaesthesia. Br J Anaesth 57:369, 1985

150. Davis DW, Hawkins RA, Mans AM, et al: Regional cerebral glucose utilization during althesin anesthesia. Anesthesiology 61:362, 1984

151. Vandesteene A, Trempont V, Engleman E, et al: Effect of propofol on cerebral blood flow and metabolism in man. Anaesthesia 43:42, 1988

152. Stephan H, Sonntag H, Schenk HD, et al: Effects of Disoprivan on cerebral blood flow, cerebral oxygen consumption and cerebral vascular reactivity. Anaesthetist 36:60, 1987

153. Ravussin P, Guinard JP, Ralley F, et al: Effect of propofol on cerebrospinal fluid pressure and cerebral perfusion pressure in patients undergoing craniotomy. Anaesthesia 43:37, 1988

154. Sakabe T, Maekawa T, Ishikawa T, Takeshita H: The effects of lidocaine on canine cerebral metabolism and circulation related to the electroencephalogram. Anesthesiology 40:433, 1974

155. Astrup J, Sorensen PM, Sorensen HR: Inhibition of cerebral oxygen and glucose consumption in the dog by hypothermia, pentobarbital and lidocaine. Anesthesiology 55:263, 1981

156. Bedford RF, Persing JA, Pobereskin L, et al: Lidocaine or thiopental for rapid control of intracranial hypertension. Anesth Analg 59:435, 1980

157. Donegan MF, Bedford RF: Intravenously administered lidocaine prevents intracranial hypertension during endotracheal suctioning. Anesthesiology 52:516, 1980

158. Tommasino C, Maekawa T, Shapiro HM: Local cerebral blood flow during lidocaine-induced seizures in rats. Anesthesiology 64:771, 1986

159. Stoelting RK: Pharmacology and Physiology in Anesthetic Practice. JB Lippincott, New York, 1987

160. Viegas O, Stoelting RK: Lidocaine in arterial blood after laryngotracheal administration. Anesthesiology 43:491, 1975

161. Murphy FL, Kennell EM, Johnstone RE, et al: The effects of enflurane, isoflurane and halothane on cerebral blood flow and metabolism in man. p. 61. Abstracts of Scientific Papers, 1974 ASA Meeting

162. Todd MM, Drummond JC, Shapiro HM: Comparative cerebrovascular and metabolic effects of halothane, enflurane, and isoflurane. Anesthesiology 57:A332, 1982

163. Eintrei C, Leszniewski W, Carlsson C: Local application of xenon for measurement of regional cerebral blood flow (rCBF) during halothane, enflurane, and isoflurane anesthesia in humans. Anesthesiology 63:391, 1985

164. Michenfelder JD, Theye RA: In vivo toxic effects of halothane on canine cerebral metabolism pathways. Am J Physiol 229:1050, 1975

165. Michenfelder JD, Cucchiara RF: Canine cerebral oxygen consumption during enflurane anesthesia and its modification during induced seizures. Anesthesiology 40:575, 1974

166. Todd MM, Drummond JC: A comparison of the cerebrovascular and metabolic effects of halothane and isoflurane in the cat. Anesthesiology 60:276, 1984

167. Drummond JC, Todd MM, Scheller MS, Shapiro HM: A comparison of the direct cerebral vasodilating potencies of halothane and isoflurane in the New Zealand White rabbit. Anesthesiology 65:462, 1986

168. Kuramoto T, Oshita S, Takeshita H, et al: Modification of the relationship between cerebral metabolism, blood flow and electroencephalogram by stimulation during anesthesia in the dog. Anesthesiology 51:211, 1979

169. Drummond JC, Todd MM, Toutant SM, et al: Brain surface

protrusion during enflurane, halothane, and isoflurane anesthesia in cats. Anesthesiology 59:288, 1983

170. Sainz JJG, Camiruaga JAE, Cano FF, De La Herran JL: Effects of isoflurane on intraventricular pressure in neurosurgical patients. Br J Anaesth 61:347, 1988

171. Boarini DJ, Kassel NF, Coester HC, et al: Comparison of systemic and cerebrovascular effects of isoflurane and halothane. Neurosurgery 15:400, 1984

172. Adams RW, Cucchiara RF, Gronet GA, et al: Isoflurane and cerebrospinal fluid pressure in neurosurgical patients. Anesthesiology 54:97, 1981

173. Campkin TV, Finn RM: Isoflurane and cerebrospinal fluid pressure—a study in neurosurgical patients undergoing intracranial shunt procedures. Anaesthesia 44:50, 1989

174. Grosslight K, Foster R, Colohan AR, Bedford RF: Isoflurane for neuroanesthesia: Risk factors for increases in intracranial pressure. Anesthesiology 63:533, 1985

175. Adams RW, Gronert GA, Sundt TM, et al: Halothane, hypocapnia, and cerebrospinal fluid pressure in neurosurgery. Anesthesiology 37:510, 1972

176. Warner DS, Boarini DJ, Kassell NF: Cerebrovascular adaptation to prolonged halothane anesthesia is not related to cerebrospinal fluid pH. Anesthesiology 63:243, 1985

177. Madsen JB, Cold GE, Hansen ES, Bardrum B: Cerebral blood flow, cerebral metabolic rate of oxygen and relative CO_2-reactivity during craniotomy for supratentorial cerebral tumors in halothane anaesthesia. A dose-response study. Acta Anaesthesiol Scand 31:454, 1987

178. Morita H, Bleyaert AL, Stezoski SW, et al: The effect of halothane anesthesia on cerebral blood flow, autoregulation and cerebral metabolism of oxygen and glucose. p. 63. Abstracts of Scientific Papers. 1974 ASA Meeting

179. Neigh JL, Garman JK, Harp JR: The electroencephalographic pattern during anesthesia with ethrane. Anesthesiology 35:482, 1971

180. Joas TC, Stevens WC, Eger EI II: Electroencephalographic seizure activity in dogs during anesthesia. Br J Anaesth 43:739, 1971

181. Wollman H, Smith AL, Hoffman JC: Cerebral blood flow and oxygen consumption in man during electroencephalographic seizure patterns induced by anesthesia with ethrane (abstract). Fed Proc 28:356, 1967

182. Myers RR, Shapiro HM: Local cerebral metabolism during enflurane anesthesia: Identification of epiloptogenic foci. Electroencephogr Clin Neurophysiol 47:153, 1979

183. Sprague DH, Wolf S: Enflurane seizures in patients taking amitriptyline. Anesth Analg 61:67, 1982

184. Fleming DC, Fitzpatrick J, Fariell RG, et al: Diagnostic activation of epileptogenic foci by enflurane. Anesthesiology 52:431, 1980

185. Opitz A, Brecht S, Stenyel E: Enflurane anesthesia in epilepticus. Anaesthetist 26:329, 1977

186. Kruczek M, Albin MS, Wolf S, Bertoni JM: Postoperative seizure activity following enflurane anesthesia. Anesthesiology 53:175, 1980

187. Hymes JA: Seizure activity during isoflurane anesthesia. Anesth Analg 64:367, 1985

188. Harrison JL: Postoperative seizures after isoflurane anesthesia. Anesth Analg 65:1235, 1986

189. Kofke WA, Snider MT, O'Connel BK, et al: Isoflurane stops refractory seizures. Anesthesiology 67:A400, 1987

190. Kofke WA, Hawkins RA, Davis DW, Biebuyck JF: Comparison of the effects of volatile anesthetics on brain glucose metabolism in rats. Anesthesiology 66:810, 1987

191. Stevens WC, Eger EI, Joas TA, et al: Comparative toxicity of isoflurane, halothane, fluroxene, and diethyl ether in human volunteers. Can Anaesth Soc J 20:357, 1973

192. Martis L, Lynch S, Napoli MD, Woods EF: Biotransformation of sevoflurane in dogs and rats. Anesth Analg 60:301, 1981

193. Strum DP, Johnson H, Eger EI: Stability of sevoflurane in soda lime. Anesthesiology 67:779, 1987

194. Scheller MS, Tateishi A, Drummond JC, Zornow MH: The effects of sevoflurane on cerebral blood flow, cerebral metabolic rate for oxygen, intracranial pressure, and the electroencephalogram are similar to those of isoflurane in the rabbit. Anesthesiology 68:548, 1988

195. Rampil IJ, Weiskopf RB, Brown JG, et al: 1653 and isoflurane produce similar dose-related changes in the electroencephalogram of pigs. Anesthesiology 69:298, 1988

196. Henriksen HT, Jorgensen PB: The effect of nitrous oxide on intracranial pressure in patients with intracranial disorders. Br J Anaesth 45:486, 1973

197. Moss E, McDowall DG: ICP increases with 50% nitrous oxide in oxygen in severe head injuries during controlled ventilation. Br J Anaesth 51:757, 1979

198. Pelligrino DA, Miletich DJ, Hoffman WE, et al: Nitrous oxide markedly increases cerebral cortical metabolic rate and blood flow in the goat. Anesthesiology 60:405, 1984

199. Theye RA, Michenfelder JD: Effect of nitrous oxide on canine cerebral metabolism. Anesthesiology 29:1119, 1968

200. Misfeldt BB, Jorgensen PB, Rishoj M: The effect of nitrous oxide and halothane upon the intracranial pressure in hypocapnic patients with intracranial disorders. Br J Anaesth 46:853, 1974

201. Phirman JR, Shapiro HM: Modification of nitrous oxide induced intracranial hypertension by prior induction of anesthesia. Anesthesiology 46:150, 1977

202. Hoffman WE, Miletich DJ, Albrecht RF: The effects of midazolam on cerebral blood flow and oxygen consumption and its interaction with nitrous oxide. Anesth Analg 65:729, 1986

203. Sakabe T, Kuramoto T, Kumagae S, et al: Cerebral responses to the addition of nitrous oxide to halothane in man. Br J Anaesth 48:957, 1976

204. Manohar M, Parks C: Porcine regional brain and myocardial blood flows during halothane-O_2 and halothane-nitrous oxide anesthesia: Comparisons with equipotent isoflurane anesthesia. Am J Vet Res 45:465, 1984

205. Manohar M, Parks C: Porcine brain and myocardial perfusion during enflurane anesthesia without and with nitrous oxide. J Cardiovasc Pharmacol 6:1092, 1984

206. Manohar M, Parks C: Regional distribution of brain and myocardial perfusion in swine while awake and during 1.0 and 1.5 MAC isoflurane anaesthesia produced without or with 50% nitrous oxide. Cardiovasc Res 18:344, 1984

207. Drummond JC, Scheller MS, Todd MM: The effect of nitrous oxide on cortical cerebral blood flow during anesthesia with halothane and isoflurane, with and without morphine, in the rabbit. Anesth Analg 66:1083, 1987

208. Todd MM: The effects of $PaCO_2$ on the cerebrovascular response to nitrous oxide in the halothane-anesthetized rabbit. Anesth Analg 66:1090, 1987

209. Kaieda R, Todd MM, Warner DS: The effects of anesthetics and $PaCO_2$ on the cerebrovascular, metabolic, and electroencephalographic responses to nitrous oxide in the rabbit. Anesth Analg 68:135, 1989

210. Sakabe T, Kuramoto T, Kumagae S, et al: Cerebral effects of nitrous oxide in the dog. Anesthesiology 48:195, 1978

211. Wollman H, Aleander CS, Cohen PJ, et al: Cerebral circulation during general anesthesia and hyperventilation in man. Anesthesiology 26:329, 1965

212. Tarkkanen L, Laitinen L, Johansson G: Effects of *d*-tubocurarine on intracranial pressure and thalamic electrical impedance. Anesthesiology 40:247, 1974

213. Basta SJ, Savarese JJ, Ali HH, et al: Histamine-releasing potencies of atracurium, dimethyl tubocurarine and tubocurarine. Br J Anaesth 55:105S, 1983

214. Rosa G, Sanfilippo M, Vilardi V, et al: Effects of vecuronium bromide on intracranial pressure and cerebral perfusion pressure. Br J Anaesth 58:437, 1986

215. Stirt JA, Maggio W, Haworth C, et al: Vecuronium: Effect on intracranial pressure and hemodynamics in neurosurgical patients. Anesthesiology 67:570, 1987

216. Rosa G, Orfei P, Sanfilippo M, et al: The effects of atracurium besylate (Tracrium) on intracranial pressure and cerebral perfusion pressure. Anesth Analg 65:381, 1986

217. Haigh JD, Nemoto EM, DeWolf AM, et al: Comparison of the effects of succinylcholine and atracurium on intracranial pressure in monkeys with intracranial hypertension. Can Anaesth Soc J 33:421, 1986

218. Griffin JP, Litwak B, Cottrell JE, et al: Intracranial pressure, mean arterial pressure and heart rate after rapid paralysis with atracurium in cats. Can Anaesth Soc J 32:618, 1985

219. Lanier WL, Milde JH, Michenfelder JD: The cerebral effects of pancuronium and atracurium in halothane-anesthetized dogs. Anesthesiology 63:589, 1985

220. Lanier WL, Sharbrough F, Michenfelder JD: Effects of atracurium, vecuronium or pancuronium pretreatment on lignocaine seizure thresholds in cats. Br J Anaesth 60:74, 1988

221. Tateishi A, Zornow MH, Scheller MS, et al: Electroencephalographic effects of laudanosine in an animal model of epilepsy. Br J Anaesth 62:548,1989

222. Chapple DJ, Miller A, Ward JB, et al: Cardiovascular and neurological effects of laudanosine. Br J Anaesth 59:218, 1987

223. Standaert FG: Magic bullets, science and medicine. Anesthesiology 63:577, 1985

224. Minton MD, Grosslight K, Stirt JA, et al: Increases in intracranial pressure from succinylcholine: Prevention by prior nondepolarizing blockade. Anesthesiology 65:165, 1986

225. Lanier WL, Milde JH, Michenfelder JD: Cerebral stimulation following succinylcholine in dogs. Anesthesiology 64:551, 1986

226. Stirt JA, Grosslight KR, Bedford RF, et al: Defasciculation with metocurine prevents succinylcholine-induced increases in intracranial pressure. Anesthesiology 67:50, 1987

227. Lanier WL, Iaizzo PA, Milde JH: Cerebral function and muscle afferent activity following i.v. succinylcholine in dogs: The effects of pretreatment with defasciculating doses of pancuronium. Anesthesiology 71:87–95, 1989

228. Cutler RWP, Spertell RB: Cerebrospinal fluid: A selective review. Ann Neurol 11:1, 1982

229. Artru AA: Effects of halothane and fentanyl on the rate of CSF production in dogs. Anesth Analg 62:581, 1983

230. Artru AA: Effects of halothane and fentanyl anesthesia on resistance to absorption of CSF. J Neurosurg 60:252, 1984

231. Artru AA: Isoflurane does not increase the rate of CSF production in the dog. Anesthesiology 60:193, 1984

232. Artru AA: Effects of enflurane and isoflurane on resistance to reabsorption of cerebrospinal fluid in dogs. Anesthesiology 61:529, 1984

233. Artru AA, Nugent M, Michenfelder JD: Enflurane causes a prolonged and reversible increase in the rate of CSF production in the dog. Anesthesiology 57:255, 1982

234. Johansson B, Li CL, Olsson Y, Klatzo I: The effect of acute arterial hypertension on the blood-brain barrier to protein tracers. Acta Neuropathol 16:117, 1970

235. Hatashita S, Hoff JT, Ishi S: Focal brain edema associated with acute arterial hypertension. J Neurosurg 64:643, 1986

236. Johansson B, Linder LE: Do nitrous oxide and lidocaine modify the blood-brain-barrier in acute hypertension in the rat? Acta Anaesthesiol Scand 24:65, 1980

237. Johansson B: Blood-brain barrier dysfunction in acute arterial hypertension after papaverine-induced vasodilation. Acta Neurol Scand 50:573, 1974

238. Smith AL, Marque JJ: Anesthetics and cerebral edema. Anesthesiology 45:64, 1976

239. Pashayan AG, Mickle JP, Vetter TR, et al: Blood-CSF barrier function during general anesthesia in children undergoing ventriculoperitoneal shunt placement. Anesthesiology 69:A626, 1988

240. Archer DP, McKenna JMA, Morin L, et al: Conscious sedation analgesia during craniotomy for intractable epilepsy: A review of 354 consecutive cases. Can J Anaesth 35:338, 1988

241. Ford EW, Morrell F, Whisler WW: Methohexital anesthesia in the surgical treatment of uncontrollable epilepsy. Anesth Analg 61:997, 1982

242. Rockoff MA, Goudsouzian NG: Seizures induced by methohexital. Anesthesiology 54:333, 1981

243. Musella L, Wilder BJ, Schmidt RP: Electroencephalographic activation with intravenous methohexital in psychomotor epilepsy. Neurology 21:594, 1971

244. Ferrer-Allado T, Brechner VL, Dymond A, et al: Ketamine induced electroconvulsive phenomena in human limbic and thalamic regions. Anesthesiology 38:333, 1973

245. Steen P, Michenfelder JD: Neurotoxicity of anesthetics. Anesthesiology 50:437, 1979

246. Burrows FA, Seeman RG: Ketamine and myoclonic encephalopathy of infants (Kinsborne syndrome). Anesth Analg 61:873, 1982

247. Ebrahim ZY, DeBoer GE, Lüders H, et al: Effect of etomidate on the electroencephalogram of patients with epilepsy. Anesth Analg 65:1004, 1986

248. Gancher S, Laxer KD, Krieger W: Activation of epileptogenic activity by etomidate. Anesthesiology 61:616, 1984

249. Krieger W, Copperman J, Laxer DL: Seizures with etomidate anesthesia. Anesth Analg 64:1226, 1985

250. Laughlin TP, Newberg LA: Prolonged myoclonus after etomidate anesthesia. Anesth Analg 64:80, 1985

251. Maewaka T, Tommasino C, Shapiro HM: Local cerebral blood flow with fentanyl-induced seizures. J Cereb Blood Flow Metab 4:88, 1984

252. De Castro J, Van De Water A, Wouters L, et al: Comparative study of cardiovascular neurological and metabolic side-effects of eight narcotics in dogs. Acta Anaesthesiol Belg 30:5, 1979

253. Young ML, Smith DS, Greenberg J, et al: Effects of sufentanil on regional cerebral glucose utilization in rats. Anesthesiology 61:564, 1984

254. Rao TLK, Mummaneni N, El-Etr AA: Convulsions: An unusual response to intravenous fentanyl administration. Anesth Analg 61:1020, 1982

255. Safwat AM, Danile D: Grand mal seizure after fentanyl administration. Anesthesiology 59:78, 1983

256. Hoien A: Another case of grand mal seizure after fentanyl administration. Anesthesiology 60:387, 1984

257. Murkin JM, Moldenhauer CC, Hug CC, et al: Absence of seizures during induction of anesthesia with high dose fentanyl. Anesth Analg 63:489, 1984

258. Smith NT, Westover CJ, Quinn M, et al: An electroencephalographic comparison of alfentanil with other narcotics and with thiopental. J Clin Monitor 1:236, 1985

259. Smith NT, Dec-Silver H, Sanford TJ, et al: EEGs during high-

dose fentayl-, sufentanil-, or morphine-oxygen anesthesia. Anesth Analg 63:386, 1984

260. Benthuysen JL, Kien ND, Quam DD: Intracranial pressure increases during alfentanil-induced rigidity. Anesthesiology 68:438, 1988

261. Siesjö BK, Bengtsson F: Calcium fluxes, calcium antagonists, and calcium-related pathology in brain ischemia, hypoglycemia, and spreading depression: A unifying hypothesis. J Cereb Blood Flow Metab 9:127, 1989

262. Pulsinelli WA, Waldman S, Rawlinson D, et al: Moderate hyperglycemia augments ischemic brain damage: A neuropathologic study in the rat. Neurology 32:1239, 1982

263. Nakakimura K, Fleischer JE, Drummond JC, et al: Glucose administration prior to cardiac arrest worsens neurologic outcome in cats. Anesthesiology (in press)

264. Lanier WL, Stangland KJ, Scheithauer BW, et al: The effects of dextrose infusion and head position on neurologic outcome after complete cerebral ischemia in primates: Examination of a model. Anesthesiology 66:39, 1987

265. Drummond JC, Moore SS: The influence of dextrose administration on neurologic outcome after temporary spinal cord ischemia in the rabbit. Anesthesiology 70:64, 1989

266. Michenfelder JD, Sundt TM: Cerebral ATP and lactate levels in the squirrel monkey following occlusion of the middle cerebral artery. Stroke 2:319, 1971

267. Michenfelder JD, Theye RA: The effects of anesthesia and hypothermia on canine cerebral ATP and lactate during anoxia produced by decapitation. Anesthesiology 33:430, 1970

268. Astrup J, Symon L, Branston NM, et al: Cortical evoked potential and extracellular potassium and hydrogen at critical levels of brain ischemia. Stroke 8:51, 1977

269. Jones TH, Morawetz RB, Crowell RM, et al: Thresholds of focal cerebral ischemia in awake monkeys. J Neurosurg 54:773, 1981

270. Branston NM, Symon L, Crockard HA, et al: Relationship between the cortical evoked potential and local cortical blood flow following acute middle cerebral artery occlusion in the baboon. Exp Neurol 45:195, 1974

271. Michenfelder JD, Sundt TM, Fode N, et al: Isoflurane when compared to enflurane and halothane decreases the frequency of cerebral ischemia during carotid endarterectomy. Anesthesiology 67:336, 1987

272. Sundt TM, Sharbrough FW, Piepgras DG, et al: Correlation of cerebral blood flow and electroencephalographic changes during carotid endarterectomy with results of surgery and hemodynamics of cerebral ischemia. Mayo Clin Proc 56:533, 1981

273. Steen PA, Gisvold SE: Drug therapy in brain ischemia. Br J Anaesth 57:96, 1985

274. Shapiro HM: Brain protection: Fact or fancy. In Shoemaker WC (ed): Critical Care State of the Art. Vol. 6. The Society of Critical Care Medicine, Fullerton, Cal., 1985

275. Safar P: Resuscitation from clinical death: Pathophysiologic limits and therapeutic potentials. Crit Care Med 16:923, 1988

276. Busto R, Dietrich WD, Globus MYT, et al: Small differences in intraischemic brain temperature critically determine the extent of ischemic neuronal injury. J Cereb Blood Flow Metab 7:729, 1987

277. Warner DS, Deshpande JK, Wieloch T: The effect of isoflurane on neuronal necrosis following near-complete forebrain ischemia in the rat. Anesthesiology 64:19, 1986

278. Nehls DG, Todd MM, Spetzler RF, et al: A comparison of the cerebral protective effects of isoflurane and barbiturates during temporary focal ischemia in primates. Anesthesiology 66:453, 1987

279. Baughman VL, Hoffman WE, Miletich DJ, et al: Neurologic outcome in rats following incomplete cerebral ischemia during halothane, isoflurane, or N$_2$O. Anesthesiology 69:192, 1988

280. Milde LN, Milde JH, Lanier WL, et al: Comparison of the effects of isoflurane and thiopental on neurologic outcome and neuropathology after temporary focal cerebral ischemia in primates. Anesthesiology 69:905, 1988

281. Gelb AW, Boisvert DP, Tang C, et al: Primate brain tolerance to temporary focal cerebral ischemia during isoflurane- or sodium nitroprusside-induced hypotension. Anesthesiology 70:678, 1989

282. Baughman VL, Hoffman WE, Thomas C, et al: The interaction of nitrous oxide and isoflurane with incomplete cerebral ischemia in the rat. Anesthesiology 70:767, 1989

283. Pickard JD, Murray GD, Illingworth R, et al: Effect of oral nimodipine on cerebral infarction and outcome after subarachnoid haemorrhage: British aneurysm nimodipine trial. Br J Med 298:638, 1989

284. Bedford RF, Dacey R, Winn HR, et al: Adverse impact of calcium entry blocker (verapamil) on intracranial pressure in patients with tumors. J Neurosurg 59:800, 1983

285. Shapiro HM: Barbiturates in brain ischemia. Br J Anaesth 57:82, 1985

286. Nussmeier NA, Arlund C, Slogoff S: Neuropsychiatric complication after cardiopulmonary bypass: Cerebral protection by a barbiturate. Anesthesiology 64:165, 1986

287. Wise G, Sutter R, Burkholder J: The treatment of brain ischemia with vasopressor drugs. Stroke 3:135, 1972

288. Soloway M, Nadel W, Albin MS, et al: The effect of hyperventilation on subsequent cerebral infarction. Anesthesiology 29:975, 1968

289. Artru AA, Merriman HG: Hypocapnia added to hypertension to reverse EEG changes during carotid endarterectomy. Anesthesiology 70:1016, 1989

290. Michenfelder JD, Sundt TM: The effect of PaCO$_2$ on the metabolism of ischemic brain in squirrel monkeys. Anesthesiology 38:445, 1973

291. Michenfelder JD, Milde JH: Failure of prolonged hypocapnia, hypothermia, or hypertension to favorably alter acute stroke in primates. Stroke 8:87, 1977

292. Waltz AG, Sundt TM, Michenfelder JD: Cerebral blood flow during carotid endarterectomy. Circulation 65:1091, 1972

293. Christensen MS, Paulson OB, Olesen J, et al: Cerebral apoplexy (stroke) treated with or without prolonged artificial hyperventilation. 1. Cerebral circulation, clinical course, and cause of death. Stroke 4:568, 1973

294. Ruta TS, Drummond JC, Cole DG, et al: The effect of hypocapnia on cerebral blood flow during middle cerebral artery occlusion in the rat. Anesthesiology 71:A604, 1989

295. Paulson OB: Cerebral apoplexy (stroke): Pathogenesis, pathophysiology and therapy as illustrated by regional blood flow measurement in the brain. Stroke 2:327, 1971

296. Albers GW, Goldberg MP, Choi DW: N-Methyl-D-aspartate antagonists: Ready for clinical trial in brain ischemia? Ann Neurol 25:398, 1989

297. Natale JE, Schott RJ, Hall ED, et al: Effect of the aminosteroid U74006F after cardiopulmonary arrest in dogs. Stroke 19:1371, 1988

298. Kompala SD, Babbs CF, Blako KE: Effect of deferoxamine on late deaths following CPR in rats. Ann Emerg Med 15:405, 1986

299. Martz D, Rayos G, Schielke GP, et al: Allopurinol and dimethylthiourea reduce brain infarction following middle cerebral artery occlusion in rats. Stroke 20:488, 1989

300. Liu TH, Beckman JS, Freeman BA, et al: Polyethylene gly-

col-conjugated superoxide dismutase and catalase reduce ischemic brain injury. Am J Physiol 256:H589, 1989

301. Minamisawa H, Terashi A, Katayama Y, et al: Brain eicosanoid levels in spontaneously hypertensive rats after ischemia with reperfusion: Leukotriene C4 as a possible cause of cerebral edema. Stroke 19:372, 1988

302. Stevens MK, Yaksh TL: Time course of release in vivo of PGE2, PGF2, 6-keto PGF-1δ and TxB2 into the brain extracellular space after 15 min of incomplete global ischemia in the presence and absence of cyclooxygenase inhibition. J Cereb Blood Flow Metab 8:790, 1988

303. Pettigrew LC, Grotta JC, Rhoades HM, et al: Effect of thromboxane synthase inhibition on eiscosanoid levels and blood flow in ischemic rat brain. Stroke 20:627, 1989

304. Cantu RC, Ames A III, DiGiancanto G, et al: Hypotension: A major factor limiting recovery from cerebral ischemia. J Surg Res 9:525, 1969

305. Hossmann KA: Treatment of experimental cerebral ischemia. J Cereb Blood Flow Metab 2:275, 1982

306. Abramson NS, Safar P, Detre KM, et al: Randomized clinical study of thiopental loading in comatose survivors of cardiac arrest. N Engl J Med 314:397, 1986

307. Todd MM, Chadwich HC, Shapiro HM, et al: The neurologic effects of thiopental therapy following cardiac arrest in cats. Anesthesiology 57:76, 1982

308. Gisvold SE, Safar P, Hendrix HHL, et al: Thiopental treatment after global ischemia in pig-tailed monkeys. Anesthesiology 60:88, 1984

309. Steen PA, Gisvold SE, Milde JH, et al: Nimodipine improves outcome when given after complete cerebral ischemia in primates. Anesthesiology 62:406, 1985

310. Tateishi A, Fleischer JE, Drummond JC, et al: Effect of nimodipine upon neurologic outcome when administered following fourteen minutes of cardiac arrest in the cat. Stroke 20:1044, 1989

311. Steen PA, Newberg LA, Milde JH, et al: Cerebral blood flow and neurologic outcome when nimodipine is given after complete cerebral ischemia in the dog. J Cereb Blood Flow Metab 4:82, 1984

312. Forsman M, Aarseth HP, Nordby HK, et al: Effects of nimodipine on cerebral blood flow and cerebrospinal fluid pressure after cardiac arrest: Correlation with neurologic outcome. Anesth Analg 68:436, 1989

313. Arbit E, DiResta GR, Bedford RF, et al: Intraoperative measurement of cerebral and tumor blood flow with laser-Doppler flowmetry. Neurosurgery 24:166, 1989

314. Bedford RF, Morris L, Jane JA: Intracranial hypertension during surgery for supratentorial tumor: correlation with preoperative computed tomography scans. Anesth Analg 61:430, 1982

315. Jarden JO, Dhawan V, Moeller JR, et al: The time course of steroid action on blood-to-brain and blood-to-tumor transport of 82 RB: A positron emission tomographic study. Ann Neurol 25:239, 1989

316. Ingvar DH: Cerebral blood flow and metabolism in complete apallic syndromes, states of severe dementia, and in akinetic mutism. Acta Neurol Scand 49:233, 1973

317. Westerlain CG: Mortality and morbidity from serial seizures: An experimental study. Epilepsia 15:155, 1974

318. Kety S, Schmidt CF: The determination of cerebral blood flow in man by the use of nitrous oxide in low concentrations. Am J Physiol 143:53, 1945

319. Ingvar DH, Lassen NA: Atraumatic two-dimensional rCBF measurements using stationary detectors and inhalation or intravenous administration of 133-xenon. J Cereb Blood Flow Metab 2:271, 1982

320. Raichle ME: Positron emission tomography. Ann Rev Neurosci 6:249, 1983

321. Kishore PR, Rao GU, Fernandez RE, et al: Regional cerebral blood flow measurements using stable xenon enhanced computed tomography: A theoretical and experimental evaluation. J Comput Assist Tomogr 8:619, 1984

322. Gur D, Yonas H, Good WF: Local cerebral blood flow by xenon-enhanced CT: Current status, potential improvements and future directions. Cerebrovasc Brain Metab Rev 1:68, 1989

323. Yonas H, Sekhar L, Johnson DW, et al: Determination of irreversible ischemia by xenon-enhanced computed tomographic monitoring of cerebral blood flow in patients with symptomatic vasospasm. Neurosurgery 24:368, 1989

324. Junck L, Dhawan V, Thaler HT, et al: Effects of xenon and krypton on regional cerebral blood flow in the rat. J Cereb Blood Flow Metab 5:126, 1985

325. Inugami A, Kanno I, Uemura K, et al: Linearization correction of 99m-TC-labeled hexamethyl-propylene amine oxime (HM-PAO) image in terms of regional CBF distribution: Comparison to $C^{15}O_2$ inhalation steady-state method measured by positron emission tomography. J Cereb Blood Flow Metab 8:S52, 1988

326. Kramer DM: Basic principles of magnetic resonance imaging. Radiol Clin North Am 22:765, 1984

327. Bydder GM, Steiner RE: NMR imaging of the brain. Neuroradiology 23:231, 1982

328. Young IR, Hall AS, Bryant DJ, et al: Assessment of brain perfusion with MR imaging. J Comput Assist Tomogr 12:721, 1988

329. Hilberman M, Subramanian VH, Haselgrove J, et al: In vivo time-resolved brain phosphorus nuclear magnetic resonance. J Cereb Blood Flow Metab 4:334, 1984

330. Lindsey RL: A simple solution for determining shunt flow during carotid endarterectomy. Anesthesiology 61:215, 1984

331. DeWitt LD, Wechsler LR: Transcranial Doppler. Stroke 19:915, 1988

332. Kontos HA: Validity of cerebral arterial blood flow calculations from velocity measurements. Stroke 20:1, 1989

333. Sekhar LN, Wechsler LR, Yonas H, et al: Value of transcranial Doppler examination in the diagnosis of cerebral vasospasm after subarachnoid hemorrhage. Neurosurgery 22:813, 1988

334. Tomida S, Wagner HG, Klatzo I, et al: Effect of acute electrode placement on regional CBF in the gerbil: A comparison of blood flow measured by hydrogen clearance, [^{3}H] nicotine, and [^{14}C]iodoantipyrine techniques. J Cereb Blood Flow Metab 9:79, 1989

20
NEUROMUSCULAR PHYSIOLOGY

Frank G. Standaert

INTRODUCTION

Claude Bernard's study of the effects of curare on neuromuscular transmission demonstrated the special sensitivity to drugs of the junction between nerve and muscle and opened the whole field of synaptic pharmacology and physiology. The neuromuscular junction became a model in which to study the mechanism of communication between cells and, 150 years later, is a focal point of very intensive research that has implications for every aspect of neuroscience, including the use of drugs in anesthesia.

The notion that acetylcholine is released from the nerve and detected by special substances, receptors, in the muscle arose very early in research on the junction but was not widely accepted as the most likely method of transmission until the mid-20th century. Today there are disagreements about the details of the process but very little about the major outlines.

At the most straightforward level, the classical model of nerve signalling to muscle via acetylcholine can be used to understand the broad picture. At another level, there is the addition of new, more detailed information on processes within the classical scheme. At still another, there are insights into how muscle relaxants act in ways that are not encompassed by the classical scheme. Although this broadening scope makes the situation seem more complex, the information also brings experimentally derived knowledge much closer to clinical observations. As a result, we can understand certain phenomena that were beyond our ken a few years ago.

Some of the new insights, particularly those that arise from the study of receptors, are described below. However, there are other areas of research. For example, important current work is concerned with the manner in which the nerve ending regulates the synthesis and release of transmitter and how these processes are influenced by drugs, particularly relaxants. A part of this work challenges a major tenant of classical theory: it asks whether acetylcholine really is contained in and released from vesicles in the nerve ending. Also, there is intensive research to learn how the synthesis of receptors is regulated and how receptors are moved to and anchored in the endplate. Equally vital is work seeking to learn the role of postjunctional processes, especially phosphorylation of critical proteins, on receptor function. There is great interest in the materials,

659

besides acetylcholine, and particularly trophic factors, that carry messages between nerve and muscle. The information about acetylcholinesterase is growing explosively. The work being done in these areas is of great importance, but the confluence of theoretical and practical knowledge is not yet complete. Several reviews have been published and should be consulted.[1-9]

NEUROMUSCULAR TRANSMISSION

An Overview

Neuromuscular transmission is easily described. The nerve synthesizes and stores acetylcholine in small, uniformly sized packages called vesicles. Stimulation of the nerve causes these vesicles to migrate to the surface of the nerve, rupture, and discharge acetylcholine into the cleft separating nerve from muscle. Receptors in the endplate of the muscle respond to the acetylcholine by opening channels for ions to move across the muscle membrane and depolarize it. This movement of ions produces an endplate potential that triggers the adjacent muscle membrane into initiating a contraction. The acetylcholine detached from the receptor reacts with an enzyme, acetylcholinesterase, which also is in the cleft, and is destroyed. Drugs, notably depolarizing relaxants, can act on the receptors to mimic the effect of acetylcholine and cause depolarization of the endplate. Conversely, nondepolarizing relaxants also act on the receptors, but they prevent acetylcholine from reacting, so they prevent depolarization. Other compounds, sometimes called reversing agents, inhibit acetylcholinesterase and, by delaying the hydrolysis of acetylcholine, allow it to antagonize the effects of nondepolarizing relaxants.

The neuromuscular junction is specialized, both on the nerve side and on the muscle side, to transmit and receive chemical messages. Each motoneuron runs without interruption from the ventral horn of the spinal cord to the neuromuscular junction as a large myelinated axon. As it approaches the muscle, it branches repeatedly to contact many muscle cells and to gather them into a functional group known as a motor unit. Since all the muscle cells in a unit are excited by a single neuron, stimulation of the nerve, either electrically or by a depolarizing compound such as succinylcholine, causes all muscle cells in the motor unit to contract synchronously. The synchronous contraction of the cells in a motor unit is a fasciculation and often is vigorous enough to be observed through the skin.

The axon of the motor nerve carries not only electrical signals from the spinal cord to the muscles but also all the biochemical apparatus needed to let the nerve ending transform the electrical signal into a chemical one. All the enzymes and other proteins, macromolecules, and membrane components needed by the nerve ending to synthesize, store, and release acetylcholine are made in the cell body and are transported distally by axonal transport. Only small molecules, such as the choline and acetate used to synthesize transmitter, are obtained locally by the nerve ending.

The ending of the nerve is very different from the rest of the cell (Fig. 20-1). It is covered by a Schwann cell, but it is not myelinated. It is small, but it is filled with mitochondria and the materials of chemical transmission. The nerve endings of frogs are straight, thin, and long, which is why this species is used so often by those studying the junction with microelectrodes, whereas those of mammals are complex multibranching structures arranged in complicated arrays on a tiny area of the muscle surface (Fig. 20-2). The nerve endings on fast muscles are larger and more complicated than those on slow muscles. The shape of the nerve ending probably relates to the contractile speed of the muscle, but the nature of the relationship is unknown. The difference in the nerve endings, and in the muscle surfaces related to them, are probably responsible for the differences in the response to muscle relaxants of fast and slow muscles, but the nature of these relationships, too, is unknown.

The nerve is separated from the surface of the muscle by a gap of about 20 nm, the junctional cleft. The muscle surface is heavily corrugated, with deep invaginations of the junctional cleft, the secondary clefts, between the many folds in the muscle membrane. The total surface area is very large, and the membrane is separated from the contractile elements by a zone that is rich in mitochondria and other materials apparently specialized to receive transmission from the nerve and transduce it into muscle contractions. The exact appearance of the muscular part to the junction corresponds with that of the nerve ending and like the latter varies from species to species and with the function of the muscle (fast or slow). A capillary invariable runs close to each neuromuscular junction (Fig. 20-2).

Adult human muscles have only one neuromuscular junction per cell, with the important exception of some of the cells in the extraocular muscles. These are *tonic* muscles and, unlike other striated muscles, they are multiply innervated, with several neuromuscular junctions strung along the surface of each muscle cell. These muscles do not contract and relax quickly, as other striated muscles do, but contract and relax slowly; indeed, they can maintain a steady contraction, or contracture, whose strength is proportional to the stimulus received. Physiologically, this apparently is a specialization that holds the eye steadily in position. These muscles are important to an anesthetist because depolarizing relaxants affect them differently from most skeletal muscles. Instead of causing a brief contraction that is followed by paralysis, the drugs cause extraocular muscles to go into long-lasting contractures that pull the eye against the orbit and contribute to a rise in the pressure of the intraocular fluid.[10]

Although the demarcation between the membrane of the junction and the membrane of the rest of the muscle

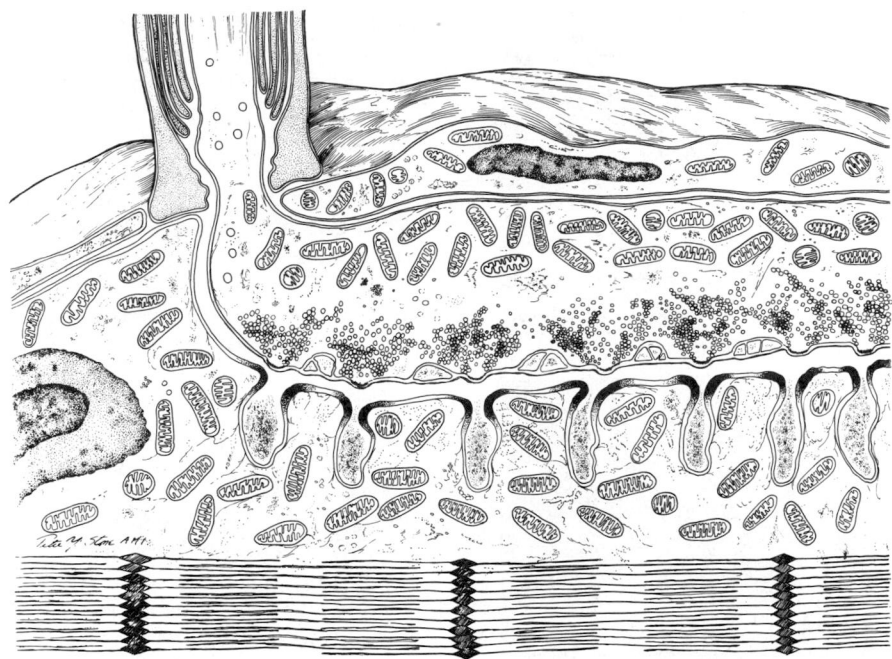

Fig. 20-1. Longitudinal section of frog neuromuscular junction. The myelinated axon ends in a nerve terminal that is covered with a Schwann cell (top). The nerve terminal (center) has vesicles clustered about membrane thickenings, the active zones, toward its synaptic side, and mitochondria and microtubules toward its other side. A synaptic gutter, made up of a primary and many secondary junctional clefts, separates the nerve from the muscle (bottom). The muscle surface is corrugated, and dense areas on the shoulders of each fold contain receptors. (Sketch adapted from Heuser,[41] with permission.)

cell looks very sharp, there is a narrow transition zone, the perijunctional area, between the two. This area is critical to the function of the neuromuscular junction, because it is here that the potential developed at the endplate is converted to an action potential that sweeps the muscle to initiate contraction. The perijunctional area is just beginning to be investigated, but apparently it is a transitional zone in which the membrane contains a mixture of the receptors ordinarily found in the junction and of the sodium channels ordinarily found in the muscle membrane proper. It is much richer in sodium channels than more distal parts of the muscle membrane, which enhances its capacity to respond to an endplate potential and trigger a wave of depolarization along the muscle.[11]

The zone is close enough to the nerve ending to be influenced by transmitter released from it and also is connected closely enough to the muscle proper to be influenced by electrical activity in it. Consequently, it participates actively in the modulation of neuromuscular transmission and in an individual's response to muscle relaxants. Moreover, special variants of receptors and sodium channels can appear in this area at different stages of life and in response to abnormal increases or decreases in nerve activity. This variability seems to contribute to the quantitative differences in response to relaxants seen in patients with different clinical statuses and of different ages.

Quantal Theory

The presently accepted description of the mechanism of neuromuscular transmission arose in the mid-1960s with the observation of small, spontaneous depolarizing potentials at neuromuscular junctions. These potentials are only 1/100th the amplitude of the endplate potential evoked when the motor nerve is stimulated, but, except for size, they resemble the endplate potential in time course and in the ways they are affected by drugs. Therefore they are called miniature endplate potentials (MEPP). Statistical analysis led to the conclusion that they are unitary responses; that is, there is a minimum size for the MEPP, and all MEPP are either of this size or a multiple of it. Since MEPP are too big to be produced by a single molecule of acetylcholine, it was deduced that they are produced by uniformly sized packages, or quanta, of transmitter. Further analysis suggested that the endplate potential evoked by nerve stimulation is produced by 200 to 300 quanta released simultaneously.

At about the same time that MEPP were discovered, electron microscopy of neuromuscular junctions showed the nerve endings to be rich in small, round, electron-transparent structures called vesicles. Because these are uniform in size and are congregated near the synaptic surface of the nerve endings, it was logical to postulate that they are anatomic correlates of

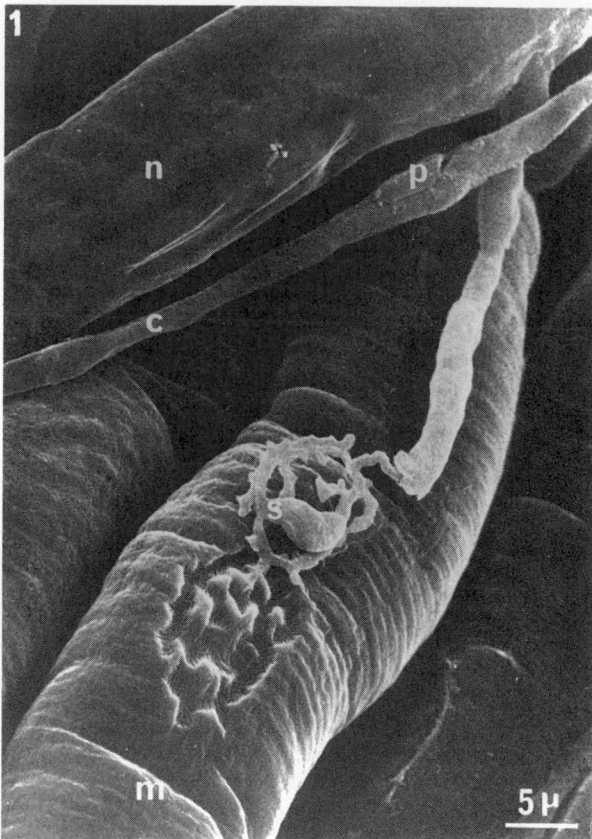

Fig. 20-2. Scanning electron micrograph of a neuromuscular junction in hamster peroneus longus muscle. The preparation has been treated with HCl and the nerve ending separated form the endplate to show its structure, that of the synaptic gutter, and the sharp demarcation between the endplate and the main muscle membrane. *m*, muscle; *n*, nerve; *s*, Schwann cell; *c*, capillary; *p*, perictye. (From Matsuda et al.,[42] with permission.)

MEPP, that is, each vesicle holds one quantum of transmitter. Thus, release of transmitter from motor nerves was believed to be quantized; the stimulus-evoked endplate potential is the summated depolarization produced by the synchronous discharge of quanta from several hundred vesicles. As a result, the vision of neuromuscular transmission that emerges from physiologic studies is almost universally described with reference to the vesicles seen via the electron microscope.[12]

The neuromuscular junction appears to be ideally developed to transmit by this mechanism. Modern electron micrographs provide remarkable pictures of nerve endings and the vesicles in them. The contents of the ending are obviously not homogeneous. As illustrated in Figure 20-1, the vesicles are congregated in the portion toward the junctional surface, and microtubules, mitochondria, and other support structures are toward the opposite side. More pertinent is the arrangement of the vesicles. They are ordered in a repeating pattern of triangular arrays, with the apex of each triangle enclosing a small, electron-dense, thickened patch of membrane referred to as an active zone. This thickened area is a cross-section of a band that runs across the width of the synaptic surface of the nerve ending and that is believed to be the structure to which vesicles attach before they rupture into the junctional cleft. The exact sites of attachment lie on the sides of the active zone, rather than in the center of it. Very highly magnified electron micrographs reveal small particles arranged alongside the active zone, between vesicles. These are postulated to be special proteins that form channels through the membrane and allow calcium to enter the nerve and cause the release of vesicles.[13]

On the muscle side of the junction, the membrane is very convoluted and exposes a very large area to the junctional cleft. The surface is highly organized and is rich with receptors; there are about 5,000,000 of them in each junction. The top of each fold runs exactly between two active zones in the nerve ending (Fig. 20-1). More importantly, the shoulders of each fold are aligned with the vesicle release sites at the sides of the active zones. Elegant electron micrographs show that the nerve and muscle are held in tight alignment by protein filaments that span the cleft from nerve to endplate. Receptors are concentrated on the shoulders of the folds, almost completely covering the surface. Their numbers diminish as the distance from the shoulder increases, so that they are sparse deep in the cleft between two folds.

The propagation of an action potential from the axon into the nerve ending allows calcium to enter the ending, and this causes vesicles to migrate to the active zone, fuse with the neural membrane, and empty their contents of acetylcholine into the junctional cleft. Since the release sites are along the sides of the active zones and immediately opposite the receptors on the postjunctional surface, little transmitter is wasted and the response of the muscle is coupled very directly with the signal from the nerve. The amount of acetylcholine released by each nerve impulse is large, at least 200 quanta of about 5,000 molecules each, and the number of receptors activated by the transmitter released by a nerve impulse also is large, about 500,000. The ions that flow through the activated receptor/channels cause a maximum depolarization of the endplate. The depolarization in turn causes an endplate potential that is greater than the threshold for stimulation of the muscle.

This is a very vigorous system. The signal is carried by more molecules of transmitter than need be, and these evoke a response that is greater than need be. At the same time, only a small fraction of the available vesicles and receptor/channels are used to send each signal. So, transmission has a substantial margin of safety, and at the same time, the system has a substantial capacity in reserve.

THE NEUROMUSCULAR JUNCTION

Motor Nerve Endings

Neuromuscular transmission starts in the nerve ending, and its completeness depends on the integrity and function of this structure and the effects of drugs on it. A nerve action potential is the normal activator of the system that releases transmitter but is not, per se, the trigger. That function belongs to a calcium flux initiated by the action potential. Neither sodium flux nor depolarization will produce release of transmitter if calcium is not present, and the introduction of calcium into a nerve ending, by microinjection of the ion or by insertion of exogenous calcium ionophores into the membrane, will release transmitter even if the nerve is not depolarized. Moreover, the number of quanta released by a stimulated nerve is greatly influenced by the concentration of ionized calcium in the extracellular fluid. There are data that show that the change in quantal content of an endplate potential is proportional to the fourth power of the change in calcium concentration; that is, doubling the extracellular calcium results in a 16-fold increase in the quantal content of an endplate potential.

It is not only the concentration of calcium that influences the number of quanta of transmitter released but also the length of time during which the calcium flows into the nerve ending; that is, the quantal content of the endplate potential is a function of the total number of calcium ions in the ending after a nerve is stimulated. The calcium current begins about the time the action potential approaches its maximum and persists until the membrane potential is returned to normal by outward fluxes of potassium. Because the calcium current normally is stopped by the flow of potassium that occurs at the end of an action potential, the flow of calcium can be prolonged by drugs, such as 4-aminopyridine, that slow or prevent potassium flux. The increase in quantal content produced in this way can reach astounding proportions. For example, an endplate potential in frog muscle normally is produced by no more than 400 quanta, but in the presence of the potassium antagonists 3,4-diaminopyridine and tetraethylammonium, an action potential may release as many as 80,000 quanta.[14]

Calcium is presumed to enter the nerve via special proteins that form channels through the nerve membrane, possibly along the active zones. The channels are opened by the voltage change accompanying the action potential. At least two kinds of calcium channels are involved, a *fast* one and a *slow* one. The fast channel is the one of primary concern because it is the one usually involved in the release of transmitter. It is voltage dependent and responds quickly to depolarization of the nerve ending by an action potential. Tiny concentrations of divalent inorganic cations, for example, Mg^{++}, Cd^{++}, Mn^{++}, block calcium entry through this channel and profoundly impair neuromuscular transmission. In contrast, this channel is not affected by organic drugs that block calcium entry, such as verapamil, diltiazem, and nifedipine, that have profound effects on the cardiovascular system. As a result, organic drugs that block calcium entry have no significant effect on the normal release of acetylcholine or on the strength of neuromuscular transmission.

Calcium entry-blocking drugs may increase the blockage of neuromuscular transmission induced by nondepolarizing relaxants, but the effect is small and not everyone has been able to observe it. The explanation may be in the fact that there is also a slow calcium channel in the nerve ending and that the slow one is quite unlike the fast one. For instance, the former is opened later and stays open longer (hence, the name "slow"), and it is easily blocked by organic blocking drugs (e.g., verapamil, diltiazem) but not by inorganic cations. Also, unlike the fast channel, it is activated by cAMP, and the flux of calcium initiated by increased cyclic adenosine monophosphate (cAMP) can be blocked by low concentrations of the organic blocking drugs. Since adenylate cyclase, the enzyme that forms cAMP, is activated by epinephrine and by endorphins, the activity of the slow channel may be accentuated by these hormones and prolong calcium flow and strengthen transmission in an individual under stress. This late calcium flux would be sensitive to reduction by calcium entry-blocking drugs; accordingly, an interaction between organic drugs that block calcium entry and muscle relaxants may be seen in certain individuals and at certain times.

The exact mechanism by which calcium causes release of transmitter is not yet known, but recent work with highly specific antibodies has identified a group of specialized proteins, including synaptophysin and synapsin I, that seem to be involved in the process. The presence of calcium in the cytoplasm activates these proteins, sometimes directly and sometimes by reacting first with other proteins, such as calmodulin or calcitonin gene-related peptide. The process is far from known, but it seems possible that vesicles that are anchored to the nerve's cytoskeleton are moved into position along the active zone by contractile proteins. Although put immediately adjacent to the nerve membrane, the vesicles are screened from it by a shell of protein. The entry of calcium into the cell somehow disrupts the screen and allows the vesicle membrane to fuse with the cell membrane and discharge vesicle contents into the synaptic cleft. The sequence of protein actions is tightly coordinated but complex and takes appreciable time, about 1 ms, to be carried out. This time accounts for the delay between the depolarization of the nerve ending and that of the endplate, the synaptic delay.[9,15,16]

The vesicular membrane fuses with that of the nerve and becomes incorporated into it, but only temporarily. The patch of membrane that originated from a vesicle is marked with special proteins that allow it to be recovered and returned as a rudimentary vesicle into the cytoplasm of the ending. In the ending it is filled with acetylcholine actively transported into it from the cytoplasm and is moved into position for release. Early in the recovery cycle, the new vesicle is surrounded by an electron-dense coating presumably made of protein, but this disappears when the recycling process is completed. Some data suggest that there are two very closely related classes of vesicles. One, called VP2, is a dynamic group close to the active zones that is actively engaged in transmission and that recycles and refills with acetylcholine quickly. The other, VP1, functions similarly but more slowly and seems to be more distant from the active zones. The more numerous VP1s seem to serve as a form of reserve and/or to replenish VP2s.[7]

Repeated stimulation requires the nerve ending to replenish its stores of releasable transmitter by a process known as mobilization. Strictly speaking, mobilization is a mathematic parameter derived from statistical analysis of endplate potentials and so has no physiologic correlates or mechanistic implications, but the term commonly is applied to the aggregate of all steps involved in maintaining the nerve ending's capacity to release transmitter — everything from the acquisition of choline and the synthesis of acetate to the movement of vesicles to the release sites. The dynamics of the individual steps are difficult to study, and despite the obvious importance of the subject, little is known about them. Sodium flux seems to be an important factor in the overall process and in many of the intermediate steps. It is this ion that causes the depolarization of

the nerve ending, and the voltage change, per se, may have intracellular effects. Also, the uptake of choline, which probably is a rate-limiting step, seems to be linked to the simultaneous entry of sodium, and so does the activity of choline acetyltransferase, the enzyme that synthesizes acetylcholine, and of mitochondria. It is not known whether all the effects of sodium are direct or if some or all of them are mediated through the depolarization of the membrane, through sodium-induced translocation of intracellular calcium, or via the activity of one or more adenosine triphosphatase (ATPase)-based transport systems.[17]

In summary, the observations behind the quantal theory, together with the results of biochemical studies, lead to the scheme sketched in Figure 20-3. The complex molecules used in the synthesis and storage of acetylcholine, such as the enzymes, the transport proteins, and new membrane for vesicles, are made in the cell body and transported through the axon to the nerve terminal. The simple molecules choline and acetate are obtained from the environment of the nerve ending, the former by a special system that transports it from the extracellular fluid to the cytoplasm and the latter in the form of acetylcoenzyme A from mitochondria. The two substrates react on the enzyme choline acetyltransferase to form acetylcholine. The newly made acetylcholine is stored in cytoplasm until it is transported into vesicles, which are moved into position for release. The nerve action potential causes sodium to flow across the membrane, and the resulting depolarization initiates the entry of calcium into the nerve and the release of acetylcholine.

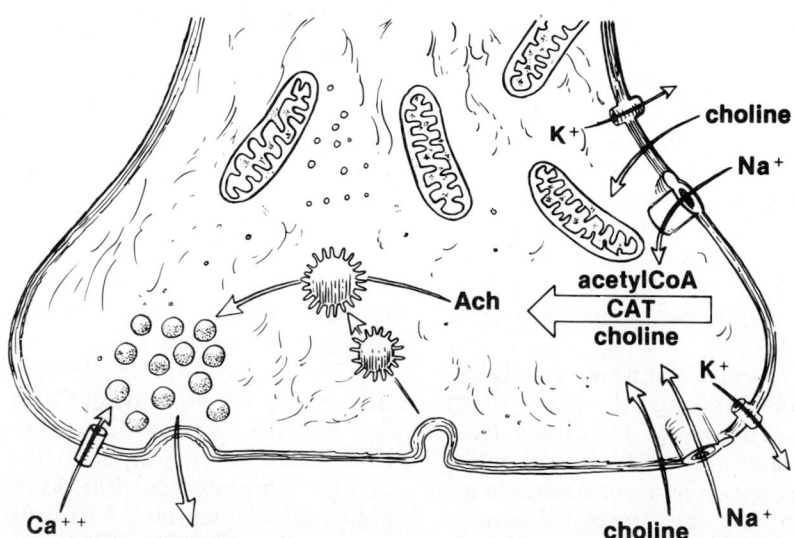

Fig. 20-3. Scheme of the motor nerve ending that includes some apparatus for transmitter synthesis, storage, and release. Large intraterminal structures are mitochondria. Acetylcholine, synthesized from choline and acetylcoenzyme A, is transported into coated vesicles that are moved to release sites. The entry of calcium causes vesicles to fuse with the membrane and discharge transmitter. Membrane from the vesicle is extracted from the nerve membrane and recycled as coated vesicles. Ach, acetylcholine; CAT, choline acetyltransferase; acetylCoA, acetylcoenzyme A.

Cholinesterase

The acetylcholine released from the nerve diffuses across the junctional cleft and reacts with specialized proteins, receptors, in the endplate membrane to initiate the muscle part of neuromuscular transmission. Transmitter molecules that do not react immediately with a receptor or that are released from the binding site on a receptor are destroyed almost instantly by the acetylcholinesterase in the junctional cleft. In the cleft, acetylcholinesterase is an asymmetric protein attached to the basement membrane of the muscle by thin stalks of collagen.[1,4] Schematically, it is like bundles of balloons attached by strings to the muscle (Fig. 20-4). Most of the molecules of acetylcholine released from the nerve initially pass by these enzymes and reach the postjunctional receptors; but as they are released from the receptors, they invariably encounter acetylcholinesterase and are destroyed. Under normal circumstances, a molecule of acetylcholine reacts with only one receptor before it is hydrolyzed. Acetylcholine is a potent messenger, but it is very short-lived; it is destroyed less than 1 ms after it is released.

Postjunctional Receptors

The receptors of the endplate are remarkable in that they seem to have arisen early in evolution; there seem to be only minor differences between the endplate receptors of human beings, frogs, electric fish, and other organisms.[18] This continuity through evolutionary lines greatly facilitates research; while the ultimate object of inquiry may be the receptors of human beings, research

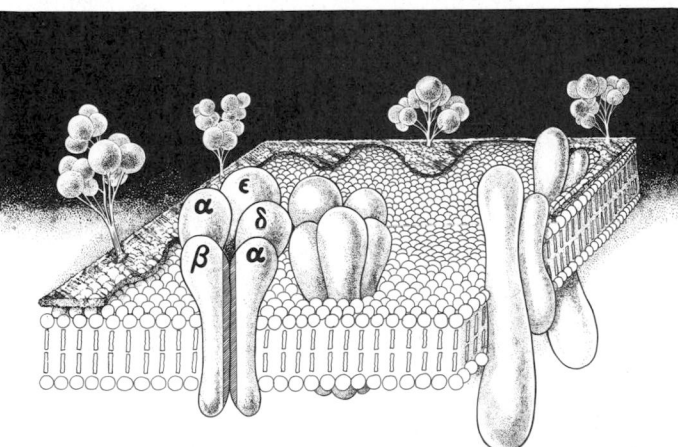

Fig. 20-4. Sketch of the postjunctional membrane. The two structures in the center represent receptors. Each member of the pair is made of five subunits arranged in a circle around a channel. The structure at the right represents Na-K-ATPase, another molecule that crosses from one side of the membrane to the other. The balloonlike structures at the periphery represent acetylcholinesterase.

is far more readily carried out on lower species or on cells grown in culture.

Some of the most valuable of the original work was done on materials derived from electric fish of the *Torpedo* family. These fish have such enormous numbers of acetylcholine receptors in their electric organs that it is practical to isolate receptors chemically and to study their morphologic and biochemical properties in the laboratory. More recently, the messenger ribonucleic acid (mRNA) that controls the synthesis of receptors has been isolated. When this is injected into the oocytes of frogs, the cells manufacture large numbers of receptors, making these available for study. Also, the techniques of molecular engineering can modify the mRNA and so cause the oocytes to produce receptors with special characteristics. In this way, a great deal has been learned about the correlation between chemical composition and biologic function. Preparations of purified receptors from frog eggs and from higher organisms, including human beings, are used to study in exquisite detail the mechanisms that underlie physiologic and pharmacologic responses to acetylcholine and related agonists and antagonists.[19-21]

As one result of the precision of current research, two variants of postjunctional neuromuscular nicotinic receptors have been described.[22] These differ from each other only in detail, rather than in major ways, and the differences are not so great as to affect our understanding of the role of receptors in neuromuscular transmission. Hence they can be neglected in a general discussion. However, small as the differences are, they can cause significant variations among the responses of individual patients to a drug and apparently are responsible for some of the anomalous results that may be observed when administering relaxants to particular individuals. Some of these effects and their causes are described below.

Receptors are synthesized in muscle cells, which make a series of protein subunits and assemble them into cylinders. These are inserted into the membrane and held rigidly in place in such a way that each cylinder crosses from one side of the muscle cell membrane to the other. Normally these are closed, but if acetylcholine reacts with specific sites on the extracellular end, then the proteins undergo a change in conformation that opens a tube in the center of the cylinder to form a channel that allows cations to move along their concentration gradients. When the channel is open, sodium and calcium flow from the outside of the cell to the inside, and potassium flows from the inside to the outside. The net current is depolarizing and creates the endplate potential that stimulates the muscle to contract. The channel in the tube is large enough to accommodate many cations and electrically neutral molecules, but it excludes anions, for instance, chloride.

Receptors from neuromuscular junctions have been isolated and purified, and their structure is known in detail.[23] Also, the mRNAs controlling receptor synthesis have been analyzed, and thus the amino acid sequences in the molecule are known. The key features are sketched in Figure 20-4. Receptors almost always are found in pairs. Each of the pair is a protein with a molecular weight of about 250,000 d, that is, it is made up of about 1,000 amino acids and has five subunits, which are designated α, β, δ, and ϵ. There are two α-subunits and one of each of the others. The receptor complex is about 11 nm in length, one-half of which protrudes from the extracellular surface of the membrane. The protein passes entirely through the membrane but extends only about 2 nm into the cytoplasm.

The acetylcholine-binding areas are on the 40,000 d α-subunits, and these are the sites of competition between cholinergic agonists and antagonists. Both agonists and antagonists are attracted to the site and either may occupy it. When both α-subunit sites are occupied by an agonist, the protein molecule undergoes the conformation change that forms a channel for ions to flow (Fig. 20-5). The current carried by the ions depolarizes adjacent membrane. Both α-subunits must be occupied simultaneously by agonist; if only one of them is occupied, the channel remains closed. This is the basis for the prevention of depolarization by antagonists. Drugs such as tubocurarine act because they bind to either or both α-subunits and in so doing prevent acetylcholine from binding and opening the channel. This interaction between agonists and antagonists is competitive, and the outcome, transmission or blockade, depends on the relative concentrations and binding characteristics of the drugs involved.

Just as individual receptors can be seen with electron microscopes or isolated and analyzed biochemically, so it is possible to measure their electrical function. The most direct method is patch clamping, in which a glass micropipette is used to probe the membrane surface until a single functional receptor is encompassed. The tip of the pipette is pressed into the lipid of the membrane and the electronic apparatus is arranged to clamp the membrane potential and measure the current that flows through the channel of the receptor. The solution in the pipette can contain acetylcholine, tubocurarine, another drug, or a mixture of drugs. The arrangement is sketched in Figure 20-6.

Figure 20-7A illustrates the mechanism of the classical action of acetylcholine on endplate receptors. The figure sketches a section of membrane in which some receptors have bound two molecules of acetylcholine. Current flows through these channels, while other channels remain closed because the receptor does not have two molecules of agonist on it. The sketch also contains a representation of acetylcholinesterase, which destroys acetylcholine by hydrolyzing it to acetate and choline.

Figure 20-7B is a schematic example of a record that may be obtained with a patch clamp when an agonist is in the pipette and can react with acetylcholine recognition sites on a receptor to open the channel. In this situation, randomly occurring downward-going (depolarizing) rectangular pulses are recorded. Each of these pulses is caused by current flowing across the membrane while two agonist molecules are attached to a receptor, activating it and opening the channel. The pulse stops when the channel closes and one or both agonist molecules detach from the receptor. The current that passes through each open channel is minuscule, only a few picoamperes (about 10^4 ions/ms), but each neuromuscular junction contains about 5 million receptor/channels, and the current that flows when many are opened at once (as, for example, through the 500,000 that are activated in response to a burst of acetylcholine from the nerve ending) is substantial, more than enough to depolarize the entire region and create the endplate potential that triggers muscle contraction.

The receptor and its channel make a powerful amplifier; the current carried by two ions of acetylcholine

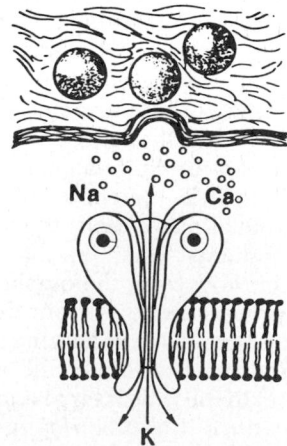

Fig. 20-5. Acetylcholine receptor in the open conformation. The binding of acetylcholine (dots) to both α-subunits triggers a conformational change that opens the channel and allows ions to flow across the postsynaptic membrane.

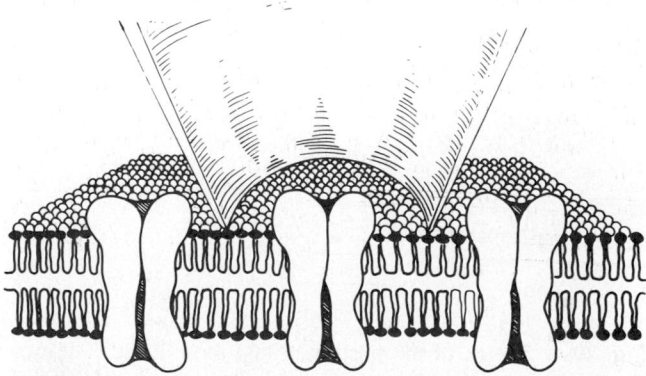

Fig. 20-6. Patch clamp technique. Micropipette encloses a single functional acetylcholine receptor in a patch of postsynaptic membrane. Electronics are arranged so that current passing through the ion channel can be measured. Pipette may contain any combination of agonist, antagonist, and/or drug.

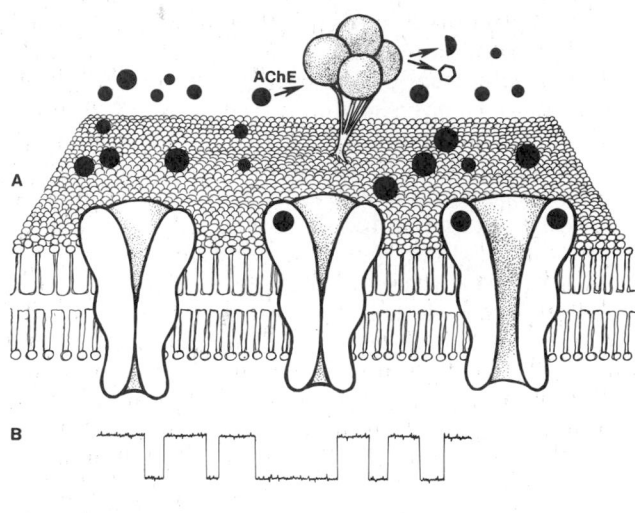

Acetylcholine ●
Choline ◗
Acetate ○

Fig. 20-7. (A) The classical action of acetylcholine on endplate receptors. The ion channel is not opened unless acetylcholine is on recognition sites of both α-subunits simultaneously. AChE, acetylcholinesterase. (B) Pulses of current flowing through a single patch-clamped channel when only an agonist is present in the pipette. Each downward-going square wave is caused by 20 to 30 pS of current and lasts for 1 to 3 ms.

from the nerve is converted by a receptor/channel into a current carried by tens of thousands of ions of sodium, calcium, and potassium. The receptor also is a switch. It is closed and off until acetylcholine binds; then it snaps open and passes current. When acetylcholine leaves, the channel snaps shut and cuts off the current.

The opening of a channel is the basic event in the reception of neuromuscular transmission; it causes the conversion of chemical signals from a nerve into current flows and potentials in a muscle. The event is simple conceptually, but it is capable of many variations, which accounts for the capacity of drugs of many kinds to influence neuromuscular transmission. There are several million receptors at the neuromuscular junction of each muscle cell, and the current carried by the individual channels is additive; the total current is nothing more than a summation of events occurring at individual channels. We are used to thinking of the final event, the endplate potential, as a graded phenomenon that, for example, may be reduced in magnitude or extended in time by certain drugs, but in reality, the endplate potential is a result of many all-or-nothing events occurring simultaneously at a myriad of individual ion channels, and it is these tiny events that are affected by drugs.

Individual channels are capable of a wide variety of actions.[24,25] They may open or stay closed, thus affecting total current flow across the membrane. They may open for a longer or shorter time than normal, open or close more gradually than usual, open briefly and re-

peatedly (chatter), or pass fewer or more ions per opening than they usually do. Also, their function is influenced by drugs; changes in the fluidity of the membrane; temperature; the electrolyte balance in the milieu; and other physical and chemical factors.[26] Thus, receptor/channels are dynamic structures that are capable of a wide variety of interactions with drugs and of entering a wide variety of current-passing states. Because the receptor/channel is the basic unit of transmission, transmission itself is subject to influence by many of the drugs and circumstances encountered in an anesthetized patient. Since whatever happens to an individual channel is multiplied several hundred thousand times to cause a change in the endplate potential, all the influences on channel activity ultimately are reflected in the strength, or weakness, of neuromuscular transmission and the contraction of a muscle.

DRUG EFFECTS ON POSTJUNCTIONAL RECEPTORS

Classical Actions

Nondepolarizing Relaxants

The nondepolarizing relaxants prevent depolarization of the endplate because they are attracted to the acetylcholine recognition sites of the α-subunits and, while there, prevent acetylcholine from binding and causing the ion channel to open. The reaction is a competition between acetylcholine and the relaxant, which means that the outcome depends on the relative concentrations of the chemicals and their comparative affinities for the receptor. From this follow all the customary descriptions of the effects of nondepolarizing agents on neuromuscular transmission.

Figure 20-8A shows a sketch of a system exposed to a modest concentration of tubocurarine, for example, one that might cause a 10 to 20 percent reduction in the strength of an evoked twitch. Some receptors attract two acetylcholine molecules and open the channel to depolarize that segment of membrane. Others attract one acetylcholine and one tubocurarine molecule; these channels will not open, and no current will flow. The third receptor is particularly interesting because, as sketched, it has acetylcholine on one α-subunit and nothing on the other. What will happen depends on which of the molecules above it wins the competition for the vacant site. If acetylcholine wins, the channel will open and the membrane will be depolarized; if tubocurarine wins, the channel will stay closed and the membrane will not be depolarized.

Figure 20-8B contains a sketch of the electrical activity recorded in a patch clamp experiment in which both acetylcholine and tubocurarine are in the pipette. When two agonists bind to the receptor, the receptor activates and opens its channel to permit ions to flow; a downward-going pulse is recorded. At other times, one or two tubocurarine molecules may attach to the recep-

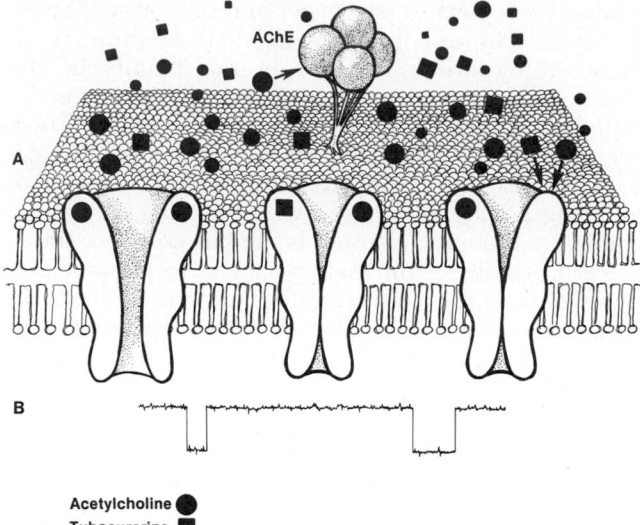

Acetylcholine ●
Tubocurarine ■

Fig. 20-8. (A) The classical action of antagonists of acetylcholine on endplate receptors with tubocurarine as the example. Acetylcholine is in competition with tubocurarine for the receptor's recognition site (right receptor), but may also react with acetylcholinesterase (AChE). Inhibiting the enzyme increases the lifetime of acetylcholine and the probability that it will react with a receptor. (B) Sketch of a patch clamp record of current flowing through a channel when both agonist and antagonist are in the pipette. Since current does not flow when antagonist is on the recognition site, channels open less often than when only agonist is present (compare with Fig. 20-7B).

tor, in which case the receptor is not available to agonists; so the channel stays closed until the tubocurarine leaves. Since the channel is not opened, no current flows and no pulse is recorded. The result is a record of apparently normal agonist-induced pulses of current, but there are fewer pulses per unit of time than if there were no tubocurarine. Because current flows through each channel less often, the amount flowing through the entire endplate at any instant is reduced from normal. This results in a smaller endplate potential and, if carried far enough, a blockade of transmission. This is a molecular description of the classical competitive interaction between acetylcholine and tubocurarine at the neuromuscular junction.

Figure 20-8A illustrates the role of cholinesterase inhibitors. Normally, acetylcholinesterase destroys acetylcholine and removes it from the competition for a receptor, so normally tubocurarine wins the competition and transmission is blocked. If, however, an inhibitor such as neostigmine is added, the cholinesterase cannot destroy acetylcholine. This lets the concentration of agonist in the cleft remain high, and this high concentration tips the competition between acetylcholine and tubocurarine to favor the former. This improves the chances of two acetylcholines binding to a receptor, even though tubocurarine is still in the environment. In this way, cholinesterase inhibitors can

overcome a neuromuscular block produced by nondepolarizing relaxants.

While these descriptions are valid qualitatively, the competition is not simple quantitatively. Since the channel will not open unless acetylcholine is attached to both of the recognition sites, it follows that two molecules of acetylcholine are required to produce an effect, while a single molecule of antagonist is adequate to prevent the effect. This modifies the competition by biasing it strongly toward the antagonist. Mathematically, the bias is logarithmic. For example, if the concentration of tubocurarine in the area is doubled, the concentration of acetylcholine must be increased fourfold if it is to remain competitive. In practical terms, this means that blockades produced by high concentrations of antagonist are more difficult to reverse than those produced by low concentrations. Moreover, since the concentration of acetylcholine is increased only indirectly, by inhibiting acetylcholinesterase, blockades produced by large doses of nondepolarizing relaxants may be impossible to reverse by this means.

Depolarizing Relaxants

At the molecular level, the depolarizing relaxants mimic the effect of acetylcholine. Figure 20-9A illustrates the process and sketches the immediate effects of a modest dose of depolarizing relaxant. If two molecules of agonist (acetylcholine and/or a depolarizing relaxant) attach to the acetylcholine recognition sites of the receptor, the channel will open and pass current that causes the endplate to depolarize. The agonists attach only briefly to the receptor, so each opening of a single channel is very short, about 1 ms or less. In this sense, there is little difference between acetylcholine and a depolarizing relaxant either in effect or in duration of effect.

However, this similarity is difficult to appreciate from the clinical effects of these drugs. From the clinician's point of view, the response to acetylcholine is over in seconds while that to a depolarizing relaxant lasts minutes to hours. Moreover, depolarizing relaxants characteristically have a biphasic action on muscle, initially causing it to contract and then causing it to relax.

The time differences are due to the different ways in which the body rids itself of the compounds. Acetylcholine from the nerve is rapidly destroyed by the acetylcholinesterase in the junction. Thus, the cleft is cleared of transmitter and resets to a resting state long before another nerve impulse arrives. In contrast, neither succinylcholine nor decamethonium is susceptible to hydrolysis by acetylcholinesterase. The drugs are not eliminated from the junctional cleft until they are eliminated from the plasma, and so the time it takes to clear the drug from the body as a whole is the principal determinant of how long the drug lasts. Whole-body clearance of a muscle relaxant is very slow compared with the destruction of acetylcholine by junctional acetyl-

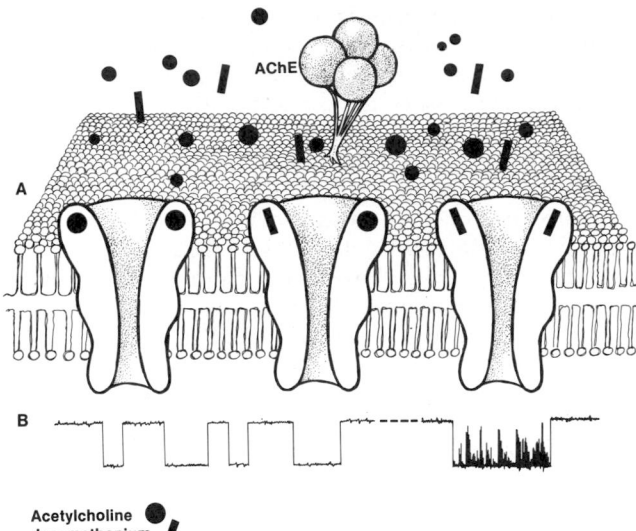

Fig. 20-9. (A) The classical action of agonists on endplate receptors with acetylcholine and decamethonium as examples. Any combination of two agonist molecules causes the channel to open. Different agonists cause pulses of different durations to be recorded by a patch clamp, depending on the agonist's binding to the receptor. AChE, acetylcholinesterase. **(B)** Sketch of a patch clamp record of pulses of current flowing through a channel when decamethonium is in pipette. Left four pulses: Drug acting only as an agonist, causing channel to open and current to flow. Right pulse: Pulse recorded during channel blockade. Agents that rapidly hop into and out of the open channel cause interruption of the current and flickering of the pulse as drug molecules enter and leave the opened channel. (See text for details.)

channel, is a cylindrical protein that can form a tube across the membrane for sodium ions to flow through. However, unlike the acetylcholine receptor/channel, it is not responsive to chemicals. Only a sharply changing electrical field can cause it to open its tube. Moreover, two parts of its structure act as gates that allow or stop the flow of sodium ions.[27] Both gates must be open if sodium is to flow through the channel; the closing of either cuts off the flow. Because these two gates act sequentially, a sodium channel has three functional conformation states (Fig. 20-10). It must move progressively from one state to another (counterclockwise in Fig. 20-10).

When the sodium channel is in its resting state, one gate is open (the lower one in Fig. 20-10) but the other is closed and so ions cannot pass. When the molecule is subject to a sudden change in voltage by depolarization of adjacent membrane, the top gate (called a voltage-dependent gate) opens, and since the bottom gate is still open, sodium flows through the channel. The voltage-dependent gate stays open as long as the molecule is subject to a depolarizing influence on its membrane; it will not close until the depolarization disappears. However, shortly after the voltage-dependent gate opens, the bottom gate (the inactivation gate, a time-dependent gate) closes and again cuts off the flow of ions. This gate closes spontaneously, even though the molecule is still exposed to a depolarized membrane. It cannot open again until the voltage-dependent gate closes.

Normally, acetylcholine is hydrolyzed quickly, and the depolarization of the endplate is brief. The flow of ions through the receptor/channels of the endplate causes the endplate to depolarize, and the electrical

cholinesterase, even when the plasma cholinesterase that hydrolyzes succinylcholine is normal. Since muscle relaxant molecules are not cleared from the cleft quickly, they react repeatedly with receptors, attaching to another almost as soon as they come off of a first one. In this way, they repeatedly open channels and continuously depolarize the endplate.

The quick shift from excitation of muscle contraction to blockade of transmission occurs even though—indeed, because—the endplate is continuously depolarized. This comes about because of the juxtaposition at the edge of the endplate of two different kinds of membrane, that of the endplate and that of the muscle, each of which has a different kind of ion channel. The membrane of the endplate contains receptor/channels that open when they bind acetylcholine or a similar chemical. The membrane of the muscle contains sodium channels that do not respond to chemicals but open when they are exposed to a transmembrane voltage change. Thus, the channels in the two parts of the membrane respond to different stimuli, chemical and electrical.

The sodium channel, like the acetylcholine receptor/

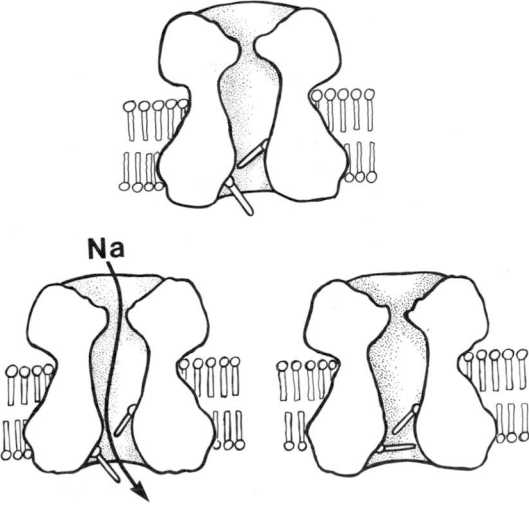

Fig. 20-10. Sketch of sodium channel. The bars represent parts of the molecule that act as gates. The upper one is voltage dependent; the lower one is time dependent. The top drawing represents the resting state. Once activated by a voltage change, the molecule and its gates progress as illustrated, but only in the counterclockwise direction.

effects of the depolarization extend to and influence the sodium channels in the adjacent perijunctional membrane. These open and depolarize the membrane. The depolarization spreads from one sodium channel to the next so that a wave of depolarization spreads along the muscle and triggers muscle contraction. Upon the hydrolysis of acetylcholine, ion flow across the endplate stops, the endplate membrane repolarizes, and the system resets itself. The sodium channels quickly complete their cycles and return to their resting state.

When a depolarizing muscle relaxant is administered, the initial response is like that to acetylcholine, but since the relaxant is not hydrolyzed, depolarization of the endplate is not brief. The sequence of molecular events is sketched in Figure 20-11. The depolarization of the endplate by the muscle relaxant initially causes the voltage gate in adjacent sodium channels to open,

and so a wave of depolarization sweeps along the muscle and it contracts. Shortly after the voltage-dependent gate opens, the time-dependent inactivation gate closes. Since the muscle relaxant is not removed from the cleft, the endplate continues to be depolarized. The sodium channel molecules immediately adjacent to the endplate are influenced by the depolarization of the endplate; their voltage gates continue to stay open, and their inactivation gates stay closed. This state persists until the voltage gate closes and the molecule can complete its cycle, that is, until the time when the endplate is no longer depolarized. Since sodium cannot flow through these channels, this segment of perijunctional membrane does not depolarize. The sodium channel molecules distal to the endplate are influenced by the voltage across the perijunctional zone, not that in the endplate. When the flow of ions through the sodium

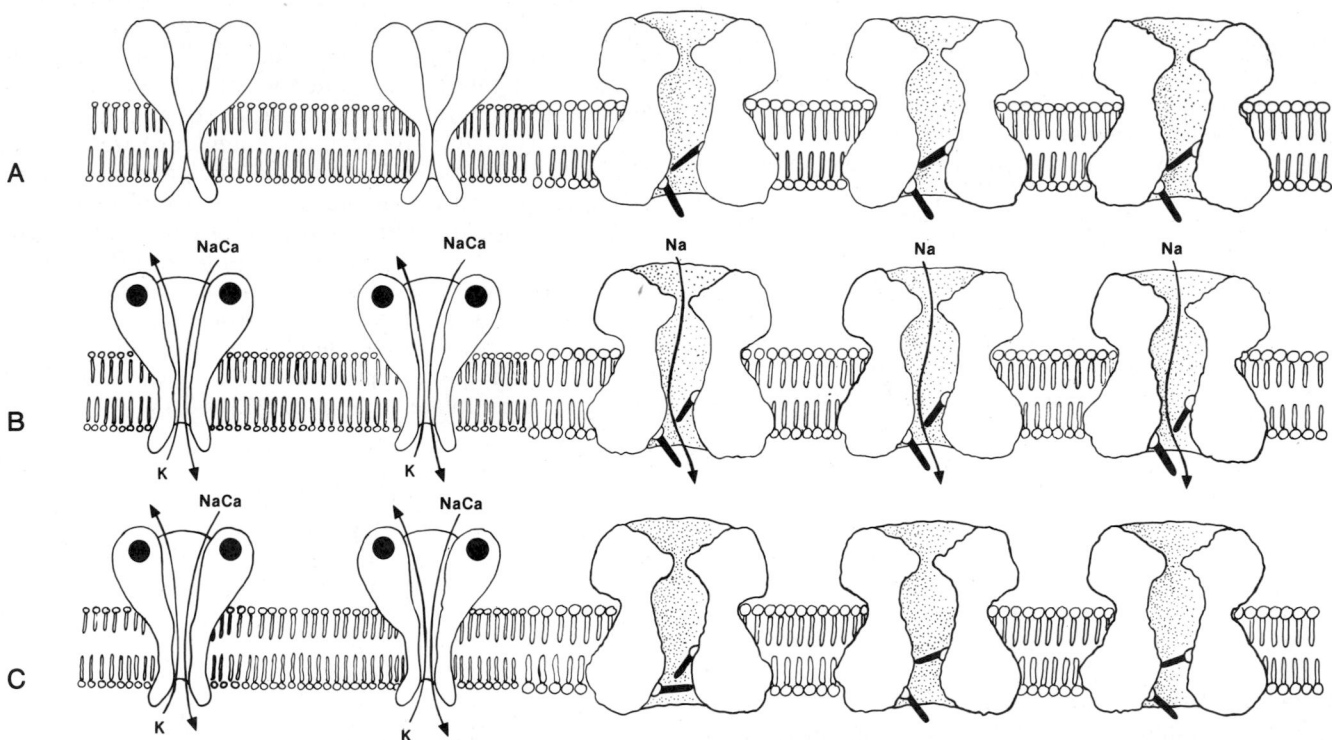

Fig. 20-11. Accommodation blockade. Molecules in the left two vertical columns represent receptors in the endplate that are chemically sensitive, voltage insensitive. Molecules in right three columns represent sodium channels in muscle membrane that are voltage sensitive, chemically insensitive. Appendages within sodium channels represent gates; the top one is normally closed, but opens and is held open when a voltage is applied across the membrane. The bottom gate is the inactivation gate; normally it is open, but it closes spontaneously soon after the voltage-dependent gate opens. Both gates must be open simultaneously if sodium is to flow through channel. (A) Resting membrane, no current flow through any channel. (B) Agonist applied to endplate receptors; voltage developed by current flow through receptor/channel causes gates in adjacent sodium channels to open. Current flow through left sodium channel causes voltage change that opens next sodium channel, etc., and a wave of depolarization propagates along muscle. (C) Endplate still depolarized, so voltage-dependent gate in sodium channel next to endplate remains open and the inactivation gate closes. Since no ions flow through it, there is no voltage change across the membrane around that channel, and the gates in the next two sodium channels return to their resting positions. The inability of the left-most sodium channel (in the perijunctional zone) to pass sodium current in response to depolarization of endplate causes blockade of neuromuscular transmission.

channels in the perijunctional zone stops, because the inactivation gates have closed, the channels downstream are freed of depolarizing influence. In effect, the perijunctional zone becomes a buffer that shields the rest of the muscle from events at the endplate. Shielded from the depolarized endplate, sodium channels in the muscle complete their cycles and return to the resting state. The result is that the membrane is separated into three zones: the endplate, which is depolarized by succinylcholine; the perijunctional muscle membrane in which the sodium channels are frozen in an inactivated state; and the rest of the membrane in which the sodium channels are in the resting state. Since a burst of acetylcholine from the nerve cannot overcome the inactivated sodium channels in the perijunctional zone, neuromuscular transmission is blocked.

This reaction to the prolonged effects of a depolarizing drug, sometimes called accommodation, is due to the juxtaposition of a chemically excitable membrane and an electrically excitable membrane and so occurs in most skeletal muscles. However, the extraocular muscles contain tonic muscle, which is multiply innervated and chemically excitable along its whole surface. Accommodation does not occur, and these muscles can undergo a sustained contracture in the presence of succinylcholine. The tension so developed forces the eye against the orbit and accounts for part of the rise in intraocular pressure produced by depolarizing relaxants. There is also evidence that the extraocular muscles contain a special type of receptor that does not desensitize (see below) in the continued presence of acetylcholine or other agonists[28] (also see Ch. 64).

Nonclassical Actions

Many drugs can react with the neuromuscular receptor to change its function and to impair transmission, but they are not competitive with acetylcholine. Hence, they do not fit the classical model and are not antagonized by increasing levels of acetylcholine with cholinesterase inhibitors. Such drugs are involved in two clinically important reactions, receptor desensitization and channel blockade. The former occurs in the receptor molecule, while the latter occurs in the ion channel.

Desensitization

The sketches of Figures 20-4 and 20-5 suggest that the receptor is rigid and fixed in shape, but this is not the case. The receptor is a macromolecule set in the lipid of the muscle membrane and, because of its flexibility and the fluidity of the lipid around it, is capable of existing in a number of states.[26] Several states with practical importance are sketched in Figure 20-12. The three illustrated in the top row are the traditional ones that are important to neuromuscular transmission. The resting receptor at the left is free of agonist, so its channel is closed and ions cannot flow through it to depolarize the

membrane. The center sketch depicts the receptor immediately after the second molecule of agonist attaches; the recognition sites are occupied, but the channel is not yet opened. The sketch at the right represents the situation an instant later. The receptor has undergone the conformation change that opens the channel and allows ions to flow. The sketch shows that the system reverses as agonists dissociate from the receptor. These reactions are the bases of normal neuromuscular transmission.

The structures sketched in the bottom row depict another situation: receptors that bind agonists but that do not undergo the conformation change that opens the channel. Receptors in these states are termed desensitized; that is, they are not sensitive to the channel-opening actions of agonists. They bind agonists, usually with exceptional avidity, but the binding does not result in the opening of the channel. Receptor molecules constantly undergo spontaneous changes in conformation, including transformation into and out of desensitized states.

Desensitization has practical consequences, because desensitized receptors are not able to participate in neuromuscular transmission. Since the total number of receptors is finite, the presence of desensitized receptors means that fewer than usual receptor/channels are available to carry transmembrane current. Therefore, the production of desensitized receptors decreases the intensity of neuromuscular transmission. If so many receptors are desensitized that there are not enough normal ones left to depolarize the motor endplate, then neuromuscular transmission will not occur. Even if only some receptors are desensitized, neuromuscular transmission will be impaired and the system will be more susceptible to blockade by conventional antagonists, such as tubocurarine or pancuronium.

It is common knowledge that agonists induce desensitization, but that is only part of the story. Receptors are in a constant state of transition between resting and desensitized states, whether or not agonists are present. Agonists promote the transition to a desensitized state or, because they bind very tightly to desensitized receptors, trap a receptor in a desensitized state. So can many other drugs. For example, antagonists bind tightly to desensitized receptors and can trap molecules in these states. This action of antagonists is not competitive with acetylcholine; in fact, it may be augmented by acetylcholine, if the latter promotes the change to a desensitized state.

Just as importantly, many other drugs used by anesthetists may promote the shift of receptors from a normal state to a desensitized state, or may react with desensitized molecules to prevent them from returning to normal.[29,30] These drugs, some of which are listed in Figure 20-13, can weaken neuromuscular transmission or, by reducing the margin of safety that normally exists at the neuromuscular junction, can cause an apparent increase in the capacity of nondepolarizing agents to block transmission. Again, these actions are not based

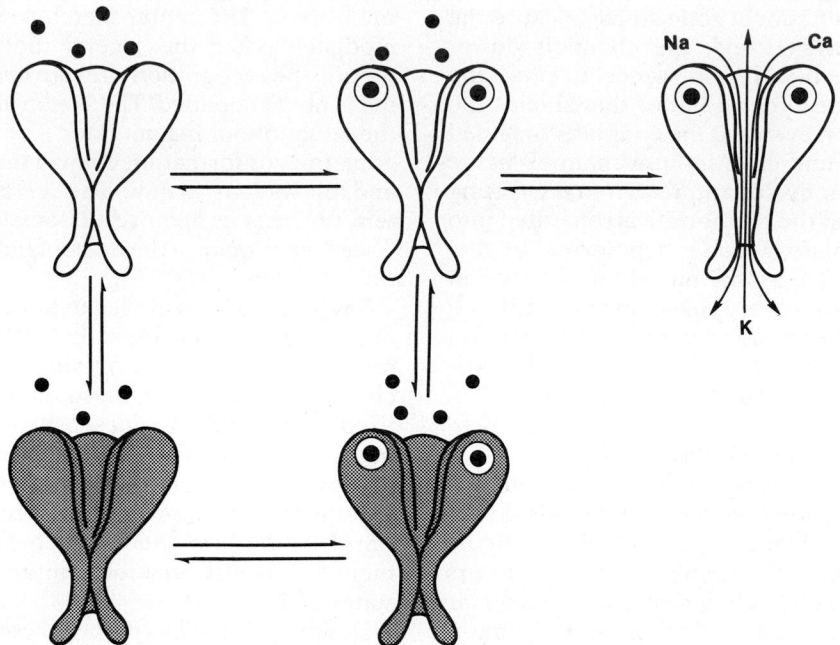

Fig. 20-12. Several states of endplate receptors. Upper row (left to right): resting; resting with agonist bound to recognition sites but channel not yet opened; active with open channel conducting ions. Lower row (left to right): desensitized without agonist; desensitized with agonist bound to recognition sites. All but one are nonconducting. (From Standaert,[30] with permission.)

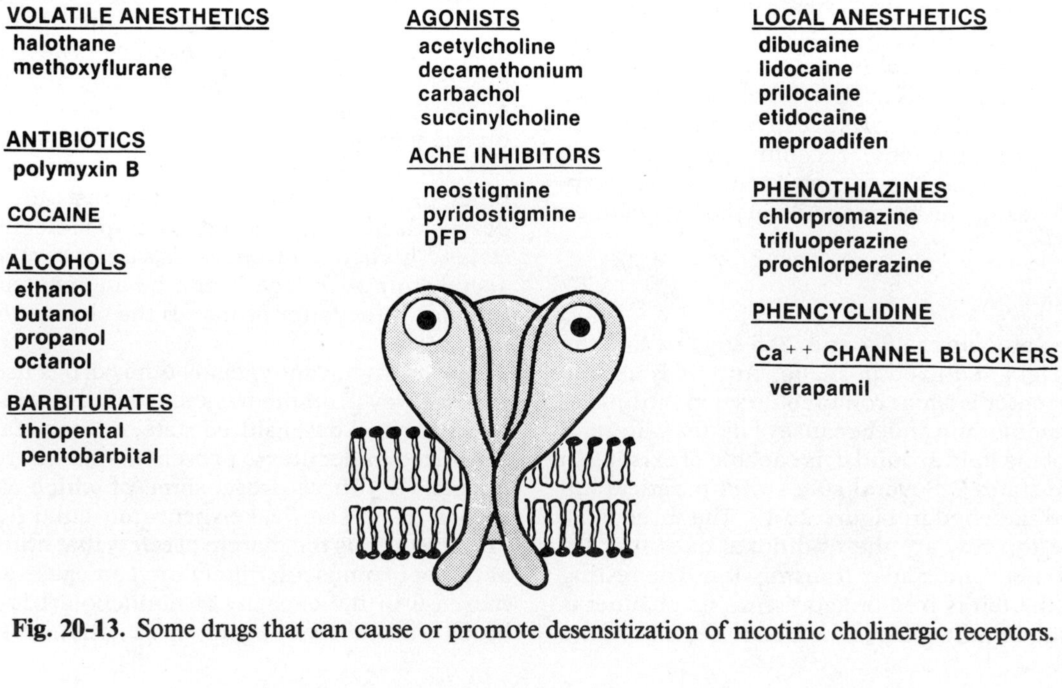

VOLATILE ANESTHETICS
halothane
methoxyflurane

ANTIBIOTICS
polymyxin B

COCAINE

ALCOHOLS
ethanol
butanol
propanol
octanol

BARBITURATES
thiopental
pentobarbital

AGONISTS
acetylcholine
decamethonium
carbachol
succinylcholine

AChE INHIBITORS
neostigmine
pyridostigmine
DFP

LOCAL ANESTHETICS
dibucaine
lidocaine
prilocaine
etidocaine
meproadifen

PHENOTHIAZINES
chlorpromazine
trifluoperazine
prochlorperazine

PHENCYCLIDINE

Ca^{++} **CHANNEL BLOCKERS**
verapamil

Fig. 20-13. Some drugs that can cause or promote desensitization of nicotinic cholinergic receptors.

on a competition between the drug and acetylcholine and so do not fit the classical competitive model.

The mechanisms by which desensitization occurs are not known. The receptor is a large molecule, 1,000 times larger by weight than most drugs or gases, and the protein provides many places where the smaller molecules may act. Also, the receptor is in the lipid of the endplate membrane, and the interface between lipid and protein provides additional potential sites of reaction. Several different conformations of the protein are known, and because acetylcholine cannot cause the ion channel to open in any of them, they all are included in the functional term desensitization. Recently obtained evidence suggests that desensitization is accompanied by phosphorylation of tyrosine in the receptor protein.[31] There are several different phosphorylation processes, and phosphorylation can occur at several sites in the subunits of the receptor, so many variants are possible. Except for knowing that some of the phosphorylation reactions are stimulated by cAMP while others are not, there is still little knowledge of the processes involved or of their physiologic functions.

The several molecular conformations of desensitized receptors probably underlie the several varieties of desensitization that are observed in the laboratory and in the operating room. One variety occurs very rapidly, within a few milliseconds after application of an agonist, and soon enough to affect the response to neural stimuli at physiologic frequencies. It may contribute to the tetanic fade seen after the administration of a nondepolarizing relaxant. Other varieties develop much more slowly and last longer. Their physiologic relevance is not known, but they occur regularly in experimental and clinical situations and can lead to significant misinterpretations of data; the preparation seems to be normal but is less responsive to agonists than usual.

There also is the phenomenon caused by depolarizing relaxants and known as phase II block. This frequently is referred to as a desensitization block but should not be, because desensitization of receptors is only one of many phenomena that contribute to the process. Phase II block is discussed more fully below.

Channel Blockade

Interference with the flow of ions through transmembrane channels is a feature of the action of many drugs. It is well known, for instance, that local anesthetics block the sodium channels in nerves and that calcium entry blockers block the calcium channels in the heart and blood vessels. Channel blockade is an important feature of drugs that act at the neuromuscular junction. It occurs with concentrations of drugs used clinically and may contribute to some of the phenomena and drug interactions that are observed in anesthetized patients.

Two major types of channel blockade can occur, open channel blockade and closed channel blockade (Fig. 20-14).[32,33] Closed channel blockade is difficult to study experimentally, so little is known about it, but there are drugs that can react around the mouth of the channel and by their presence prevent physiologic ions from passing through the channel and depolarizing the endplate. Since the reaction is around the mouth of the channel, the process can take place whether or not the channel is opened. This type of blockade is believed to be part of the neuromuscular pharmacology of, for example, some antibiotics; cocaine; quinidine; piperocaine; tricyclic antidepressants; naltrexone; naloxone; and histrionicotoxin.

Much more is known about open channel blockade. In it, a drug molecule enters a channel that has been opened by reaction with acetylcholine, but does not penetrate all the way through. When in the channel, the drug impedes the flow of physiologic ions and thus prevents depolarization of the endplate. Many of these drugs exhibit two characteristics. (1) They are use dependent, which means that they can enter the channel only when it is open, and so the intensity of their effect depends on how often the channel is opened or used; and (2) they are driven into the channel by the electrical interaction between the potential across the membrane and the charge inherent in the drug's molecular structure. In this case, the intensity of effect varies with the potential across the endplate membrane. Channel blockade is not limited to electrically charged mole-

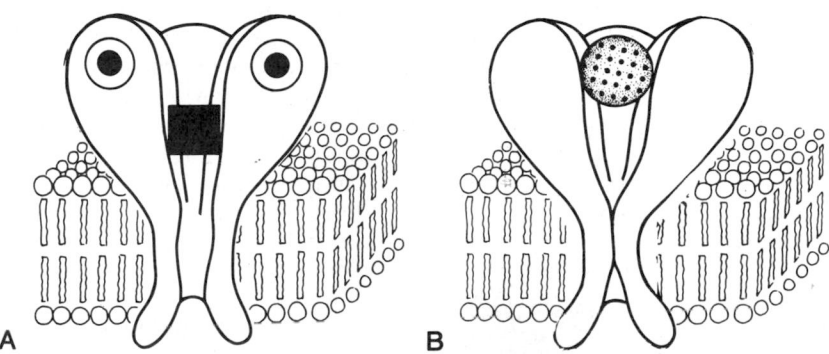

Fig. 20-14. Channel blockade. **(A)** Open; **(B)** closed.

cules; however, and many that are neutral at physiologic pH can enter and block the channel.

The duration of the blockade also may vary with the characteristics of the molecule. Some drugs that penetrate the opened channel leave quickly. They transiently block the current flow and cause the downward-going current pulse recorded in a patch clamp to flicker (Fig. 20-9). Others bind to some point on the wall of the channel and cause a longer-lasting blockade of transmitter current. Sometimes the latter are trapped in the channel when it closes and severely alter channel-opening kinetics. Others, including theophylline, interfere with channel closing. In this case, the current through the channel, while reduced from normal in amplitude, is prolonged.

Open channel blockade occurs because the extracellular end of the ion channel is much larger than the segment of the protein that crosses the membrane (Fig. 20-14). Big molecules can enter the mouth of the channel but go no farther; some of them stay for only a short time, but others bind to the walls. Since a drug in the channel impedes or prevents the normal flow of ions through it, these drugs prevent depolarization of the endplate and weaken or block neuromuscular transmission. However, since the action is not at the acetylcholine-binding site, it is not a competitive antagonism of acetylcholine and is not relieved by administering acetylcholine. Indeed, increasing the concentration of acetylcholine may cause the channels to open more often and thereby become more susceptible to blockade by use-dependent compounds. For similar reasons, cholinesterase inhibitors are not useful as antagonists of channel blockades. In addition, there is evidence that neostigmine and related cholinesterase inhibitors themselves can act as channel-blocking drugs.

The muscle relaxants are among the more interesting channel blockers. All can enter the opened channel. Even though all may act at both the acetylcholine recognition site of the receptor and in the channel, a given drug may act preferentially at one or the other site. For instance, pancuronium preferentially binds to the recognition site; there is a substantial difference in the concentration that blocks recognition sites and causes a competitive blockade and that needed to cause channel blockade. On the other hand, gallamine seems to act equally at the two sites. Tubocurarine is in between; at low doses, those that produce minimal blockage of transmission clinically, the drug is essentially a pure antagonist at the recognition site, while at larger doses, those that produce complete or near complete blockade, it also enters and blocks channels.

Decamethonium and succinylcholine are particularly interesting, because as agonists they open channels, but as slim molecules they also enter and block them. In fact, decamethonium and some other long, thin molecules can go all the way through the open channel and enter the muscle cytoplasm.

The effects of desensitization and of channel blockade are summarized in Figure 20-15, which sketches

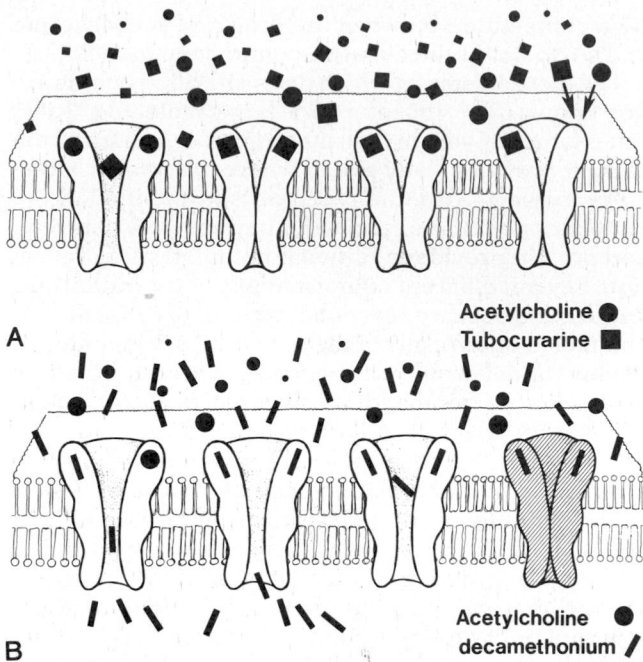

Fig. 20-15. Some effects of exposure to high concentrations of drugs for a long time. **(A)** Antagonists. Three receptors at the right have recognition site blockade; the one at the left has an open channel blockade. **(B)** Agonists. Receptor on right is desensitized. Receptor to right of center has an open channel blockade. At left: Decamethonium has penetrated open channel and entered cytoplasm.

the results of exposure to high and prolonged concentrations of muscle relaxants. The top sketch represents tubocurarine. In this case, the concentration of relaxant is much greater than that in Figure 20-8, and the molecular situation is very different from the one in that sketch. The center receptor has two tubocurarine molecules and is closed. The channel in the left one has been opened by acetylcholine, but a tubocurarine molecule in the channel prevents current from flowing through it. The receptor at the right already has bound one tubocurarine, so it makes no difference whether acetylcholine or tubocurarine binds to the other site; the channel cannot open in either case. It is apparent why the administration of a cholinesterase inhibitor will not be as beneficial as it is against low concentrations of the muscle relaxant.

The sketch at the bottom of Figure 20-15 depicts some results of a prolonged exposure to a high concentration of a depolarizing muscle relaxant, for example, decamethonium. Decamethonium and acetylcholine are both agonists; when two molecules of either, or a combination of the two, bind to the receptor, it opens its channel and allows ions to flow to depolarize the membrane. However, decamethonium molecules can enter the channel and block current flow and depolarization of this membrane segment. Some receptors, like those at the far right, have desensitized in the presence of decamethonium; their channels cannot be opened. Also, decamethonium is a slim molecule that can pass through opened ion channels and enter the muscle cytoplasm. In this situation the neuromuscular block is complex. Some drug molecules cause depolarization, while others cause channel blockade, promote desensitization of the receptor, or interfere with intracellular processes.

Phase II Blockade

Phase II blockade is a strange phenomenon that slowly occurs at junctions continuously exposed to depolarizing agents. The junction is depolarized by the initial application of a depolarizing muscle relaxant, but then the membrane potential gradually recovers toward normal, even though the junction is still exposed to drug. Neuromuscular transmission usually remains blocked throughout the exposure.

Several things seem to be involved. All the events depicted in Figure 20-15 contribute. In addition, the repeated opening of channels allows a continuous efflux of potassium and influx of sodium, and the resulting abnormal electrolyte balance distorts the function of the junctional membrane. Calcium entering the muscle via the opened channels can cause disruption of subendplate elements and of the receptors themselves. On the other hand, the activity of a sodium-potassium ATPase pump in the membrane (Fig. 20-4) increases as intracellular sodium rises and, by pumping sodium out of the cell and potassium into it, works to restore the ionic balance to normal. Since the ratio of intracellular/extracellular potassium determines the membrane potential, the return of the ratio toward normal restores the membrane potential toward normal, even though channels remain open and ion flux through them remains high.[34]

The relative effects of the several phenomena depend on the duration of exposure to drug, the particular drug used and its concentration, and even the type of muscle, fast or slow. Interactions with anesthetics and other agents also affect the process, and so do the characteristics of individual patients. Similar and other phenomena occur prejunctionally to affect the rate and amount of transmitter release and mobilization. With so many variables involved in the interference with neuromuscular transmission, Phase II block is a complex and ever-changing phenomenon. It is difficult to predict what will happen in any given circumstance, or to understand why it happened.

In light of the complexity, it is not surprising that it is not possible to predict the response of the blockade to the administration of cholinesterase inhibitors. Usually, the blockade is refractory to reversal early and late in the course of the process, but it may be responsive during the midperiod. The reason is not known, but one possibility is that as the activity of the sodium-potassium ATPase pump restores the junctional membrane potential toward normal, the electrical influence on the sodium channels in the perijunctional zone wanes and the sodium channels complete their cycle and return to a resting state. Removal of the accommodation block may allow signals from the nerve, enhanced in the presence of a cholinesterase inhibitor, to be transferred to the muscle and trigger contractions.

Miscellaneous Noncompetitive Actions

Anything physiologic or pharmacologic that interferes with the receptor, directly or via its lipid environment, may cause a change in transmission. Several kinds of reactions cause drug-induced changes in the dynamics of the receptor so that, instead of opening and closing sharply, the modified channels are sluggish. They open more slowly and stay open longer and/or they close slowly and in several steps. These effects on channels cause corresponding changes in the flow of ions and distortions of the endplate currents. The clinical effect depends on the molecular event. For examples, procaine, ketamine, inhaled anesthetics, or other drugs that dissolve in the membrane lipid may change the opening or closing characteristics of the channel. By interfering with its switching function, they modify current flow and transmission. If the channel is prevented from opening, transmission is weakened. If, on the other hand, the channel is prevented from or slowed in closing, transmission is prolonged and may be enhanced enough to overcome a blockade produced by nondepolarizing agents. Prolongation of the open time of channels, for instance, seems to be the mechanisms by which procaine can antagonize the blockade of transmission produced by tubocurarine.

ATYPICAL RECEPTORS

Extrajunctional Receptors

The receptors just discussed are those in the neuromuscular junctions of normal, active adults. Another type is made in muscle cells that have no innervation; for example, after avulsion of a nerve in an adult or before innervation in a fetus. Originally, it was thought that these were two distinct proteins, one, an extrajunctional receptor, that was produced after a muscle was denervated and another, a fetal receptor, that was formed only during fetal life. Now, however, the two are recognized to be the same and both are referred to as extrajunctional receptors.

Junctional and extrajunctional receptors differ in several major aspects. The names imply one difference: location. Junctional receptors are confined to the endplate region of the muscle membrane, but extrajunctional ones are not (Fig. 20-16A). They tend to be concentrated in the area of the neuromuscular junction, but they may be inserted anywhere in the muscle membrane. Despite the name, they are not excluded from the endplate, and junctional and extrajunctional recep-

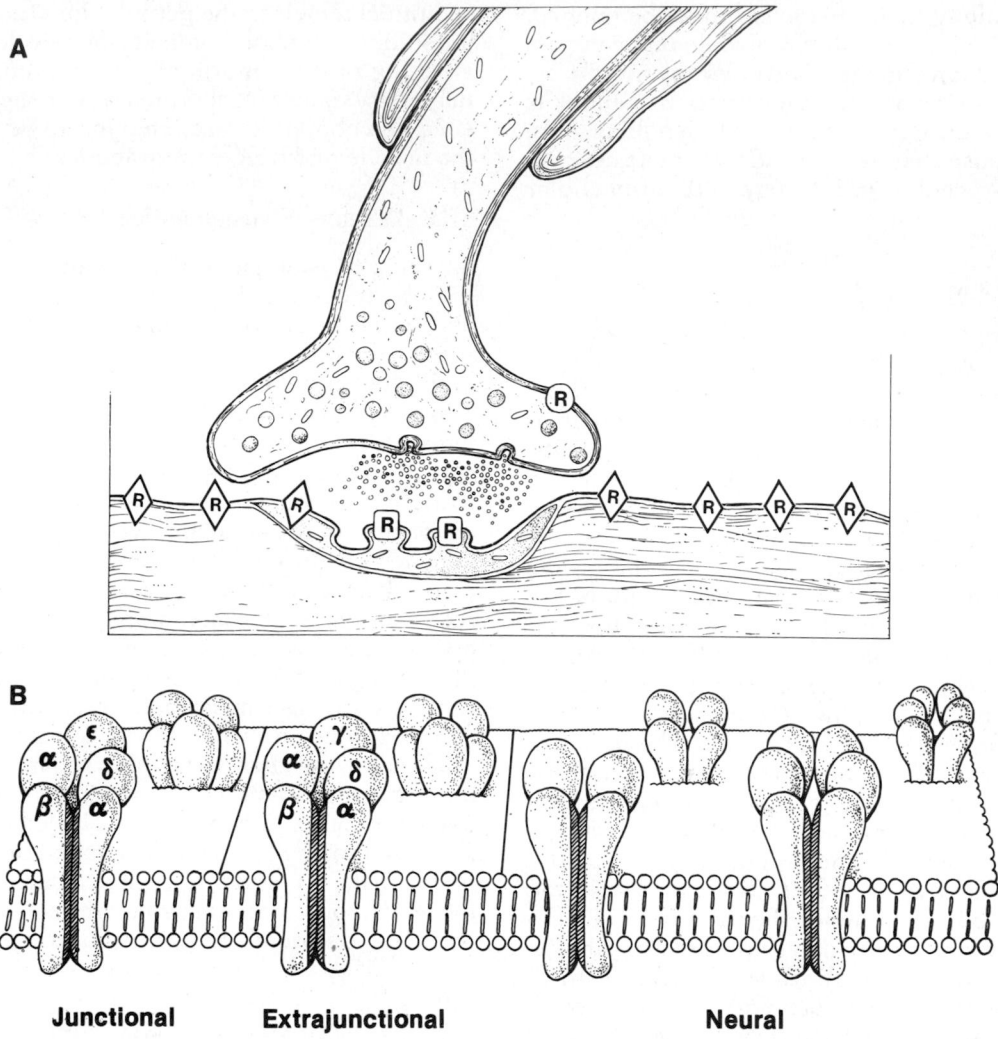

A

B

Junctional   **Extrajunctional**   **Neural**

Fig. 20-16. **(A)** Sketch of neuromuscular junction with deficient neural activity. Muscle membrane contains extrajunctional receptors (⬦R⬦). Endplate membrane contains both junctional ([R]) and extrajunctional receptors. The nerve ending contains nicotinic cholinoreceptors (Ⓡ). **(B)** Artist's renditions of the structures of junctional, extrajunctional, and neural receptors. The structure of the neural receptors is not fully known, but they contain an even number of subunits (e.g., four or six).

tors often coexist in this part of the muscle membrane. At the molecular level, the two types of receptors differ in only one of five subunits (Fig. 20-16B). In the extrajunctional receptor, the ϵ-subunit of the junctional receptor is replaced by a one called γ.[35,36] The ϵ- and γ-subunits differ from each other very little, but the differences are great enough to affect the physiology and pharmacology of the receptor and its ion channel.

The mechanisms that determine whether junctional or extrajunctional receptors will be synthesized are not known, but the control systems clearly are associated with nerve activity.[37,38] All muscle cells have the genetic material needed to synthesize both types of receptor, but in the normal adult only the systems for the manufacture of junctional receptors are expressed. The synthesis of extrajunctional receptors is repressed by

neural influence(s), and these receptors usually are not made. However, the systems for the synthesis of extrajunctional receptors are only dormant, and they are activated whenever the influence of the nerve is diminished or abolished.

The change in receptor pattern with nerve activity is most cleanly seen in the developing embryo. Before they are innervated, the muscle cells of a fetus synthesize only extrajunctional receptors. These are made in the interior of the muscle cell and transported in groups to the surface where they are inserted into the membrane over the length and width of the cell. As the fetus develops and the muscles become innervated, muscle cells begin to manufacture junctional receptors also. These are inserted into the developing endplate. Innervation progresses slowly during fetal life and infancy, and a child is usually about 2 years old before the neuromuscular contacts are mature. Before then, both types of receptors are produced. The number of extrajunctional receptors, and the part of muscle surface they cover, is graded with the degree of neural influence, and these receptors diminish in concentration and disappear from the peripheral part of the muscle as the nerve-muscle contact matures. The muscle cell does not stop making extrajunctional receptors until the nerve-muscle contact is fully mature and active. Before then, junctional and extrajunctional receptors coexist in the endplate.

The adult pattern is stabilized by trophic influences from the nerve, and the synthesis of extrajunctional receptors may be accelerated any time neural activity is impaired or removed. For instance, extrajunctional receptors are made in the muscles of individuals who have had strokes, or spinal cord injuries, or those who have become bedridden. They may even be produced in the muscles of a limb immobilized in a cast. In these circumstances, in which nerve activity is reduced but not abolished, extrajunctional receptors are inserted into the muscle membrane in and around the endplate. The muscle continues to make junctional receptors, and the two kinds coexist in the endplate. If denervation of the muscle is complete and prolonged, for instance, after avulsion of the nerve or in amyotrophic lateral sclerosis, then extrajunctional receptors are inserted all over the surface of the muscle and the cell may stop making junctional receptors.

The functional difference between the two kinds of receptors that is most pertinent for this discussion is the difference in responsiveness to muscle relaxants. Extrajunctional receptors are activated by lower concentrations of agonists, for example, acetylcholine and succinylcholine, than junctional receptors and the channels stay open longer and allow more ions to flow each time a receptor is activated. In contrast, extrajunctional receptors are less sensitive than junctional receptors to antagonists, for example, the nondepolarizing muscle relaxants.

It is well known that serious complications can occur if a depolarizing muscle relaxant, for example, succinylcholine, is administered to a patient in whom one or more muscles are denervated. In these people, numerous extrajunctional receptors are scattered over a large surface of the muscle, and the receptors are especially sensitive to succinylcholine. The channels opened by the agonist allow potassium to escape from the muscle and enter the blood. A large part of the muscle surface is involved and there are many channels, each of which stays open for a long time. Consequently, the amount of potassium that moves from muscle to blood can be very large, and the resulting hyperpotassemia can cause dangerous disturbances in cardiac rhythm. Moreover, it is difficult to prevent the hyperpotassemia. Extrajunctional receptors are not very sensitive to blockade by nondepolarizing relaxants; and so while the rise in blood potassium induced by the administration of a de-

polarizing muscle relaxant may be blunted, it is not prevented by the prior administration of a nondepolarizing muscle relaxant.

The consequences of differential sensitivity to relaxants are more subtle in those individuals who have had only a moderate reduction of nerve activity. Only a small portion of the muscle membrane contains extrajunctional receptors, and the amount of potassium lost through these usually is inconsequential. However, if neural activity is deficient, extrajunctional receptors are inserted into the membrane of the endplate. In this position, they are influenced by acetylcholine released from the nerve and contribute to neuromuscular transmission. Since they are not as easily blocked by a nondepolarizing muscle relaxant as junctional receptors are, it is more difficult than usual to block neuromuscular transmission, and these individuals may have to be given more than the usual amount of nondepolarizing muscle relaxant before they can be fully paralyzed. The differential sensitivity may occur in only certain parts of the body or certain muscles, if only some muscles are affected by the diminution of nerve activity, for example, after a stroke. It may occur very quickly. The processes that synthesize receptors are very dynamic, and extrajunctional receptors appear in the membrane only a few hours after nerve activity slows or stops. A patient's receptor mixture, and sensitivity to muscle relaxants, can begin to change within a day or two after an injury or hospitalization.

Similar phenomena probably contribute to the poorly predictable response of neonates and infants to muscle relaxants.[39] Until the neuromuscular junction is mature, it contains a mixture of junctional and extrajunctional receptors. The mixture varies less with the chronologic age of the child than it does with activity at the neuromuscular junction. Since nerve-muscle systems do not all mature at the same rate, the mixture of receptors may vary, not only from one individual to another, but also from one limb or muscle to another. Moreover, it can vary with the health and vigor of the child; the more active and mobile individuals have the relatively more mature neuromuscular junctions. Since junctional and extrajunctional receptors differ significantly in their sensitivity to nondepolarizing muscle relaxants, the amount of relaxant needed to produce muscle paralysis will differ from one individual to another in poorly predictable ways.

The situation is even more complex with regard to depolarizing muscle relaxants. Extrajunctional receptors are more sensitive to these drugs than junctional receptors are, and therefore, it might be expected that a smaller than usual dose would produce paralysis in a neonate or infant. However, depolarization of the endplate is not the immediate cause of the neuromuscular blockade produced by this class of drugs. Rather, it is the functional insulation of the endplate from the muscle membrane by a ring of sodium channels in the perijunctional zone that have accommodated to the depolarization of the endplate. This insulating ring is produced best when there is a sharp demarcation between the chemically sensitive junctional channels and the electrically sensitive sodium channels. Since the demarcation may be blurred at immature junctions, in which chemically sensitive extrajunctional receptors are present in both the endplate and in the perijunctional zone, the response of a neonate or an infant to the administration of a depolarizing muscle relaxant may not be the same as that of an adult.

Prejunctional Receptors

The nerve ending is the least well understood part of the neuromuscular junction. Obviously, it is essential to the accomplishment of neuromuscular transmission, and it is probable that many drugs affect its capacity to carry out its functions. While it is a tiny structure, it is an extraordinarily complex one with an abundance of potential targets for drug action. However, the ending is so small that it is frustratingly difficult to study, and we know little of its normal functions, let alone the ways in which these are modified by drugs.

One of the main thrusts of current investigations is to learn whether or not there are receptors in the nerve ending and, if there are, what they do. The presence of prejunctional nicotinic cholinergic receptors (nicotinic cholinoceptors) has been postulated for decades, largely because of the many known instances of interactions between cholinergic agonists and antagonists on prejunctional phenomena. Years ago, this belief was bolstered by electron micrographs which showed that bungarotoxin, a polypeptide derived from snake venom that causes neuromuscular blockade, binds to prejunctional membranes, much as it does to receptors in the postjunctional membrane. However, later studies showed that bungarotoxin can be washed away from receptors in the nerve ending, whereas it binds irreversibly to endplate receptors.

This difference in reversibility of binding suggests that the receptors in the nerve ending are more like those in the central nervous system, ganglia, and other parts of the nervous system than like those in muscles. Our knowledge of nicotinic cholinoceptors in the nervous system lags far behind that of those in muscle, but the available evidence suggests that while the two classes are related, they are not the same. Like postjunctional receptors, those in the nervous system seem to be cylindrical assemblages of protein subunits that span the cell membrane and, when activated, allow the passage of ions. Further, the subunits seem to be close relatives of the α- and β-subunits of the muscle receptor. However, neural receptors seem to be composed of only two kinds of subunits and do not include the several others found in muscle receptors. Moreover, neural receptors seem to be composed of an even number of subunits, for example, four or six, instead of the five that compose postjunctional receptors. Several variants of each the α- and β-subunits have been found and several combinations of the variants are known, so that a greater variety of receptors and pharmacologic specificities may exist in the nervous system than in muscles.[18,22]

To date, prejunctional nicotinic cholinoceptors have neither been isolated nor recorded from, and we have no knowledge of their composition or function. However, given the differences between nerve and muscle types, it is very likely that the binding characteristics of those in the nerve are very different from those in the endplate. For instance, tubocurarine and hexamethonium bind very poorly to the recognition sites of ganglionic nicotinic cholinoceptors and are not effective competitive antagonists of acetylcholine at this site. Instead, they block the opened channels of these receptors and owe their ability to block ganglionic transmission to this property. The functional characteristics of the receptor channels also may be different. For example, the depolarization of the nerve ending initiated by the administration of acetylcholine can be prevented by tetrodotoxin, a specific blocker of sodium flux that has no effect on the endplate.

Vigorous attempts are being made to learn of the links between prejunctional nicotinic receptors and three phenomena observed daily in the operating room: (1) the fade in strength of tetanic muscle contractions produced in patients given nondepolarizing relaxants; (2) the occurrence of fasciculations in patients given succinylcholine; (3) the brief enhancement of contraction strength that occurs after the administration of succinylcholine and before blockade ensues. All these are neural phenomena. Fade occurs because the amount of transmitter released from the nerve diminishes with time during high-frequency stimulation. Fasciculations occur when all the muscle cells in a motor unit contract synchronously. Since only the nerve supplying these cells can synchronize them, the initiating event must be in the nerve. The brief enhancement of muscle strength is due to the generation in the nerve ending of a short series of action potentials that follows the stimulus evoked potential. This stimulus-bound repetitive activity is transmitted to the muscle and causes it to undergo a brief, forceful, tetanic contraction.[17]

The connection between prejunctional receptors and transmitter release has been pursued vigorously, but the work is difficult to do and progress has been disappointingly slow. The processes seem to be different in nerves that are stimulated slowly, for example, 1 Hz or less, and those that are stimulated rapidly, for example, 50 Hz. With regard to the former, it has been postulated that a prejunctional nicotinic cholinoceptor that can be blocked by tubocurarine may exert inhibitory control over the amount of transmitter released by a single nerve stimulus. That is, acetylcholine that leaks spontaneously into the junctional cleft activates the receptor and decreases the amount of acetylcholine released by a nerve impulse. Blocking this receptor with tubocurarine releases the inhibitory control, and thus a nerve impulse releases more transmitter than usual. Tubocurarine has been shown to increase transmitter release as postulated, but the mechanism by which this occurs is not known. It must be subtle and/or indirect; acetylcholine itself has no measurable effect on the spontaneous or stimulated release of transmitter. Nor does tubocurarine; it does not affect the entry of calcium into the nerve ending or the release of acetylcholine from vesicles. It does seem to affect, by slowing slightly, the reactions that occur in the nerve between the entry of calcium and the release of transmitter; that is, it causes a slight increase in the synaptic delay, but the relevance of this action to the control of transmitter release is obscure.

The mechanisms that underlie the effects of tubocurarine on release of transmitter during high-frequency stimulation are similarly unknown. It is postulated[40] that a nicotinic cholinoceptor in the nerve ending senses the amount of transmitter in the cleft and adjusts the mobilization of transmitter from reserves so that the ending will always have what it needs to maintain transmission. Fade occurs when transmitter output declines because the nondepolarizing muscle relaxant blocks this receptor and impairs mobilization. In this circumstance, the transmitter available for immediate release is not replenished quickly enough to meet the demand imposed by a high-frequency stimulus. Whether or not these are the same receptors as those that modulate the quantal content of single stimuli is not known. Similarly, the mechanisms by which a receptor might modulate any of the many steps involved in mobilization are not known. Several of the steps are known to need sodium, but whether or not nondepolarizing relaxants slow sodium movement through the receptor/channel in the nerve ending is not known.

A prejunctional nicotinic cholinoceptor probably contributes to the fasciculations produced by the rapid administration of succinylcholine by causing depolarization of the nerve and, hence, firing of its action potential. The depolarization need not be entirely at the motor nerve ending; the stretch receptor systems in muscle spindles that sense muscle tension are also cholinergic, and depolarizing compounds can act on them to stimulate motor nerves reflexly and produce fasciculations. Because depolarization of motor nerve endings would cause a burst of transmitter to be released, this effect probably also causes part of the initial burst of muscle contractions. Perhaps this flood of acetylcholine may add with the initial flow of succinylcholine into the neuromuscular junction to cause the rapid onset of neuromuscular blockade that is characteristic of this drug.

Unlike the previous phenomena, prejunctional cholinoceptors probably are not involved in the generation of stimulus-bound repetitive activity and the enhancement (potentiation) of muscle contraction strength caused by succinylcholine and many other drugs. Stimulus-bound repetitive activity was noticed and established to be neural almost 50 years ago. Since then a large number of drugs of many different clinical and pharmacologic classes have been shown to generate stimulus-bound repetitive activity, or to prevent its generation. Even though it has been observed for so long and is known to be produced or abolished by so many drugs, the mechanism of generation is not yet established beyond controversy. Although stimulus-bound repetitive activity and potentiation of muscle contraction strength are readily produced in the laboratory, they are not easily produced in the operating room because they are suppressed by muscle relaxants and most inhaled anesthetics.

An early idea that has persisted to this date is that, under certain conditions, acetylcholine released from the ending refluxes onto prejunctional cholinoceptors to depolarize the nerve and cause the generation of the additional action potentials. This notion may seem plausible with, for instance, drugs that inhibit acetylcholinesterase, but it is inadequate to explain the actions of all the different drugs and processes that cause stimulus-bound repetitive activity, many of which have no effect on the amount of transmitter released or on the transmitter's duration of action in the junctional cleft. Nor does it explain the facile abolition of the phenomenon by compounds such as the inhaled anesthetics, barbiturates, or phenytoin that have no effect on cholinergic receptors. It does not explain why stimulus-bound repetitive activity is generated in some motor nerves, but not in others. And, it does not explain how the repetitive activity generated by some drugs, for example, the anticholinesterases, can be abolished by the organic calcium entry blockers such as verapamil that have no effect on the prejunctional actions of acetylcholine.

A much more likely mechanism for the production of the repetitive activity is an electrical interaction between the nerve ending and an adjacent node of Ranvier in the nerve trunk. It is known that many drugs can prolong the afterpotential of the nerve ending while not affecting that of the nerve trunk, either because the former is unmyelinated, or because it has ion channels that are absent from the node of Ranvier, for example, calcium and potassium channels. For instance, the afterpotential in the nerve ending may be prolonged by blocking the potassium current that normally ends it, by prolonging the depolarizing flux of sodium ions, by enhancing the depolarizing flux of calcium ions, or by merely slowing conduction velocity in the membrane of the nerve ending. Regardless of the mechanism, if the prolongation were adequate and the geometry of the nerve and its ending appropriate, then the afternegativity in the ending would stimulate the nearest node of Ranvier in the nerve to generate multiple action potentials. The phenomenon would be prevented or abolished by any drug that attenuated the afterpotential in the nerve ending or that raised the firing threshold of the node of Ranvier.

Besides nicotinic cholinoceptors, motor nerve endings probably have several other kinds of receptors. Several investigators have postulated that the ending has muscarinic cholinoceptors that modulate the release of transmitter. The data offered in support of this notion are weak and cannot be reproduced consistently, so the idea is not generally accepted at this time. Far better grounds exist for thinking that the ending has an adrenergic receptor. More than 50 years ago, it was shown that epinephrine can antagonize a blockade of transmission produced by tubocurarine. This effect is mediated through a receptor of the α class that is connected to adenylate cyclase. When activated, the cyclase generates cAMP, which facilitates the flux of calcium into the nerve ending, probably through the slow calcium channel. This in turn increases the release of transmitter and prolongs the time during which it is released, the two conditions favoring the antagonism of tubocurarine. Despite the knowledge of this receptor, and of the mechanism by which it influences transmitter release, we know nothing of its physiologic role and, as with so many prejunctional systems, we know almost nothing about the consequences of drug actions on the adrenergic system in the nerve ending.

The nerve ending is known or suspected to bear several other receptor systems, such as opiate receptors, dopaminergic receptors, adenosine receptors, purinergic receptors, and receptors for various neuropeptides that are suspected of being cotransmitters or hormones, but again almost nothing is known of them, their functions, or their responses to the drugs anesthetists use. The situation is most frustrating. Intuitively, we believe that a structure as vital and as complex as the nerve ending must be the substrate for important drug effects, but the nerve ending is so tiny and so difficult to investigate that the growth in our knowledge is painfully slow.

ANTAGONISM OF NEUROMUSCULAR BLOCKADE

Since the nondepolarizing muscle relaxants block neuromuscular transmission predominantly by competitive antagonism of acetylcholine at the postjunctional receptor, the most straightforward way to attempt to overcome their effects is to increase the competitive position of acetylcholine. Two factors are important. First, the concentration of acetylcholine is important. Increasing the number of molecules of acetylcholine in the junctional cleft changes the agonist/antagonist ratio and increases the probability that agonist molecules will occupy the recognition sites of the receptor. It also increases the probability that an unoccupied receptor will become occupied. Normally only about 500,000 of the 5,000,000 available receptors are activated by a single nerve impulse, and so a large number of receptors are in reserve and could be occupied by an agonist. Second, the length of time acetylcholine is in the cleft before it is destroyed is important. Acetylcholine cannot displace a molecule of antagonist from a receptor; it must wait for the antagonist to dissociate spontaneously before it can compete for the freed site.

The nondepolarizing muscle relaxants bind to the receptor for less than a millisecond, which is longer than the normal lifetime of acetylcholine in the junctional cleft. Put another way, the destruction of acetylcholine normally takes place so quickly that most of it is destroyed before any significant number of antagonist molecules have dissociated. The agonist has no chance to activate a receptor, and so neuromuscular transmission is blocked. Prolonging the time during which acetylcholine is in the junction allows time for dissociation of the antagonist and for receptors to be freed and available to acetylcholine. Also, it allows molecules of the agonist to diffuse farther and increases the probability that they will encounter and react with reserve receptors.

These factors are exploited clinically by two classes of drugs: potassium-blocking agents and inhibitors of acetylcholinesterase. The best known of the potassium-blocking agents is 4-aminopyridine. The actions of this drug are predominantly prejunctional: it impedes the efflux of potassium from the nerve ending. Since the efflux of potassium is the event that normally ends the action potential of the nerve ending, this action prolongs the depolarization of the nerve. Because the flux of calcium into the nerve continues for as long as the depolarization lasts, drugs of this class indirectly increase the flux of calcium into the nerve ending. Since the release of acetylcholine is proportional to the influx of calcium, the nerve ending releases more acetylcholine and releases it for a longer time than usual. Both of the conditions in the preceding paragraph are present, and drugs of this class are very effective antagonists of nondepolarizing muscle relaxants. Because these drugs act prejunctionally, they can antagonize a blockade produced by certain antibiotics, notably the polymyxins, that act on the nerve ending.

Although 4-aminopyridine, and drugs like it, are used clinically, their use is severely handicapped because they are not specific; they affect the release of transmitters by all nerve endings, whether these endings are on motor nerves, on autonomic nerves, or in the central nervous system. Accordingly, their use is accompanied by a variety of undesirable effects. These effects can be attenuated by manipulating the dose or by concomitant therapy, but the practical use of potassium-blocking agents is limited to special circumstances. Several investigators are seeking more specific analogues, but to date the search has not had dramatic success.

The commonly used antagonists, for example, neostigmine, pyridostigmine, and edrophonium, all inhibit acetylcholinesterase. When the enzyme is inhibited, acetylcholine is not destroyed in the junctional cleft and is present long enough to compete for the receptors from which a nondepolarizing agent dissociates. The extra time also permits acetylcholine to diffuse in the cleft and bind to and act as an agonist on reserve receptors.

The mechanisms by which these compounds inhibit acetylcholinesterase are similar, but not identical.

Neostigmine and pyridostigmine are attracted to the enzyme by electrostatic interaction between the positively charged nitrogens in them and the negatively charged catalytic site of the enzyme. Once on the enzyme, they react chemically with it and are hydrolyzed by it. In the hydrolytic process, a shift of intramolecular bonds occurs and the carbamate from the inhibitor binds via a covalent bond to the catalytic site of the enzyme. This produces a carbamylated enzyme that is not capable of further action; that is, the enzyme is inhibited. The chemical sequence is much like the one in the hydrolysis of acetylcholine, except in the latter case the product is an acetylated enzyme. Both the acetylated and the carbamylated enzymes are subject to attack by water, which cleaves the covalent bond and restores the enzyme to its initial, active state, but cleavage of the acetylated enzyme is accomplished in nanoseconds, so there is no perceptible inhibition of the enzyme's catalytic activity, while the carbamate-enzyme bond remains intact for many minutes and the enzyme is inactivated for a substantial time.

Edrophonium has neither an ester nor a carbamate group, so there is nothing to be hydrolyzed. It is attracted and bound to the catalytic site of the enzyme by the electrostatic attraction between the positively charged nitrogen in the drug and the negatively charged site of the enzyme. Access of other molecules to the catalytic site is prevented by the presence of edrophonium, so the enzyme is inhibited, but the blockade is very short lived; the edrophonium departs the enzyme in milliseconds. The shortness of the molecular blockade has been known for a long time, and for decades edrophonium was considered to have too short an action to be useful in anesthesia. However, it is now realized that the duration of the molecular reaction does not determine the duration of action of this drug in a patient. Rather, it is the duration of the drug in the body as a whole, and this depends on renal clearance, not events at the neuromuscular junction (also see Ch. 12). Individual molecules of edrophonium may reside on the enzyme for a very short time; but as one leaves, it is almost instantly replaced by another, so that the practical inhibition of the enzyme continues for as long as there is drug in the body. Since the rate at which the body rids itself of edrophonium is about the same as that for neostigmine or pyridostigmine, the period during which acetylcholinesterase is inhibited and the reversal of a blockade induced by a nondepolarizing muscle relaxant lasts is about the same for all three drugs.

The cholinesterase inhibitors act preferentially at the neuromuscular junction, but the degree of preference is not great and acetylcholinesterase in other synapses is also inhibited. It frequently is desirable to administer an atropine like drug along with the cholinesterase inhibitor to cancel the effects of acetylcholine that accumulates in the muscarinic synapses of the gut, bronchi, or cardiovascular system.

The three drugs discussed above do not affect synapses in the central nervous system because all are quaternary ammonium ions that do not easily penetrate the blood-brain barrier. Other cholinesterase inhibitors, notably physostigmine and tetrahydroaminoacridine (THA) are not quaternary ammonium compounds, and they have profound effects in the central nervous system. These may be antagonized by atropine but not by one of its quaternary ammonium derivatives, such as glycopyrrolate. Unlike the other cholinesterase inhibitors, physostigmine and THA are also potent inhibitors of the enzyme phosphodiesterase, which plays an important role in the regulation of transmitter release at many synapses in the central nervous system. This action may be related to the reported unique efficacy of these two materials in the treatment of Alzheimer's dementia.

The actions of cholinesterase inhibitors at the neuromuscular junction are not limited to the reactions with the enzyme. Postjunctionally, those compounds that contain several methyl groups on a positively charged nitrogen can act as agonists on the receptor/channels and thus initiate ion flow and enhance neuromuscular transmission. All the drugs of this class also act in or on receptors to influence the kinetics of the open-close cycle and to block the ion channel.[32,33] The contributions of these effects to the clinical activity of the drugs are not known. These drugs also have prejunctional actions. It has been known for almost 50 years that they cause the nerve ending to respond to a single stimulus by generating a brief train of stimulus-bound repetitive potentials that are transmitted to the muscle and cause the latter to contract more strongly than normal. The mechanisms by which these actions may be produced are discussed above.

These drugs may also increase the release of transmitter from the nerve ending, apparently by increasing the flux of calcium into the nerve ending. Neostigmine, physostigmine, and certain organophosphates can increase the frequency of MEPP and increase the quantal content of endplate potentials, apparently by increasing the duration of the nerve action potential and thus the time during which calcium may enter the nerve ending. The neural actions of these drugs are prevented by organic calcium entry antagonists, such as verapamil, even though the antagonists have no effect on the main stimulus-induced release of transmitter. Also, continuous exposure to the carbamate- or organophosphate-containing inhibitors causes degeneration of prejunctional and postjunctional structures, apparently because these accumulate toxic amounts of calcium.

SUMMARY

We intuitively recognize that no drug has only one site or one mechanism of action and that the muscle relaxants are not exceptions to this rule. The neuromuscular junction provides a rich array of substrates for drug action, and every drug works at several sites. The major

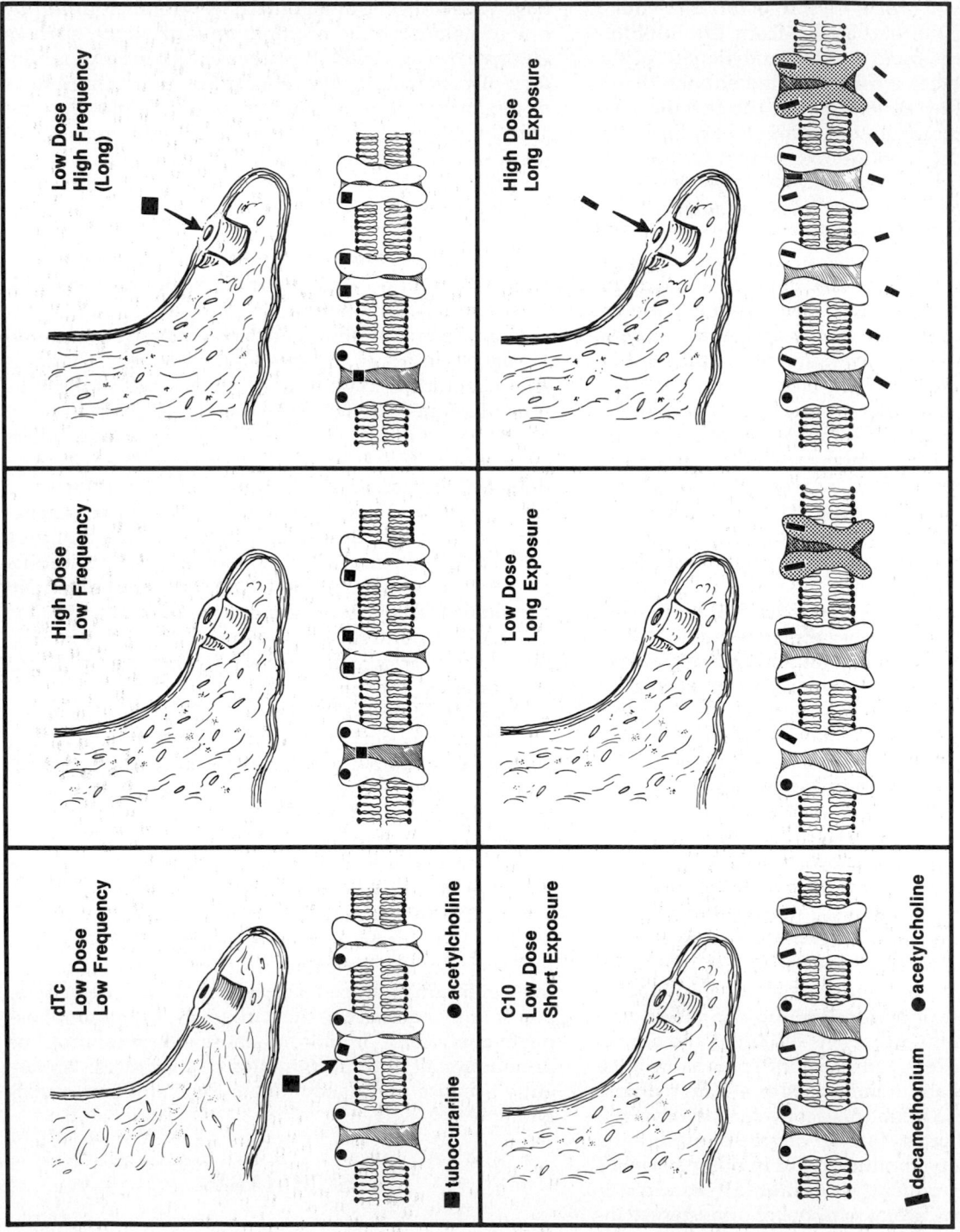

Fig. 20-17. Summary of effects of drug concentration and exposure time on neuromuscular transmission. Top row: tubocurarine. Left to right: when junction is exposed to low concentrations of drug and stimulated slowly (e.g., 1 Hz or less), blockade is primarily classical antagonism of acetylcholine at the recognition site of receptor. Higher concentrations of drug also cause channel blockade. In nerves stimulated at high frequency, drug interferes with mobilization of transmitter. Bottom row: decamethonium. Left to right: initial exposure causes channels to open and depolarize endplate. Longer exposures promote formation of desensitized receptors, channel blockade, and penetration of drug into cytoplasm. In nerves stimulated at high frequency, drug may interfere with mobilization of transmitter.

actions seem to occur by the mechanisms and at the sites described for decades: agonistic and antagonistic actions at postjunctional receptors for depolarizing and nondepolarizing muscle relaxants, and inhibition of postjunctional acetylcholinesterase for reversing agents. An approximate description of neuromuscular drug action may be derived from these actions alone, but it gives a simplistic picture. A more accurately version recognizes that the neuromuscular junction is a complex system and a dynamic one in which the phenomena produced by drugs are composites of action that vary with drugs, dose, activity in the junction, time after administration of the drug, the presence of other anesthetic agents or drugs, and the age and condition of the patient. Figure 20-17 illustrates some of these complexities.

The drawings in the top row of Figure 20-17 depict some of the variations in the actions of tubocurarine as a function of dose and rate of stimulation. The sketch at the left depicts the classical situation in which a junction is exposed to a low concentration of drug and stimulated slowly. Neuromuscular transmission is impeded because tubocurarine prevents access of acetylcholine to its recognition site on the postjunctional receptor. If the concentration of tubocurarine is increased (center), another, noncompetitive action, blockade of the ion channel, is added. If the preparation also is stimulated rapidly (right), prejunctional actions become apparent and add with those occurring at the other side of the junction.

The drawings in the bottom row depict some of the variations in the actions of decamethonium that occur with time after exposure. Initially (left), depolarizing compounds react with the acetylcholine recognition site and, like the transmitter, open ion channels and depolarize the endplate membrane. Unlike the transmitter, they are not subject to hydrolysis by acetylcholinesterase and so remain in the junction. Soon after administration of the drug (center), some receptors are desensitized and, although occupied by an agonist, do not open to allow current to flow and depolarize the area. If the depolarizing relaxant is applied in high concentration and allowed to remain at the junction for a long time (right), then other events occur, including entry of the drug into the channel to obstruct it and to pass through it into cytoplasm. Although not sketched, similar actions occur on prejunctional structures, and the combination of prejunctional and postjunctional effects, plus secondary ones on muscle and nerve homeostasis, result in the complicated phenomenon known as phase II blockade.

The new knowledge of neuromuscular transmission and of muscle relaxants seems to complicate affairs; certainly it was easier to remember things when the mechanism was considered to be only a reaction of cholinergic agonists or antagonists with receptors in the endplate. However, the newer observations on receptors, ion channels, membranes, and prejunctional functions reveal a much broader range of sites and mechanisms of action for both agonists and antagonists, and in doing so they allow a more complete understanding. In recognizing them, we begin to bring our theoretical knowledge closer to explaining the phenomena observed when these drugs are administered to living human beings.

ACKNOWLEDGMENT

I am deeply indebted to my long-time collaborator Kitt Booher for her expert help with the literature on neuromuscular transmission. She is truly a coauthor of this chapter and would be so designated, if she would permit it.

REFERENCES

1. Massoulie J, Bon S: Molecular forms of cholinesterase and acetylcholinesterase in vertebrates. Annu Rev Neurosci 5:57, 1982
2. Dowall MJ, Hawthorne JN (eds): Cellular and Molecular Basis of Cholinergic Function. VCH Publishers/Ellis Horwood, Deerfield Beach, Fla., 1987
3. Ronundo RL: Biogenesis and regulation of acetylcholinesterase. p. 247. In Salpeter MM (ed): The Vertebrate Neuromuscular Junction. Alan R Liss, New York, 1987
4. Taylor P, Schumacher M, MacPhee-Quingley K, et al: The structure of acetylcholinesterase: Relationship to its function and cellular disposition. Trends Neurosci 10:93, 1987
5. Kelly RB: The cell biology of the nerve terminal. Neuron 1:431, 1988
6. Miles K, Huganir RL: Regulation of nicotinic acetylcholine receptors by protein phosphorylation. Mol Neurobiol 2:91, 1988
7. Whittaker VP: The organization of the cholinergic synapse. Keio J Med 37:234, 1988
8. Van der Kloot W: Acetylcholine quanta are released from vesicles by exocytosis (and why some think not). Neuroscience 24:1, 1988
9. Zimmermann H (ed): Cellular and Molecular Basis of Synaptic Transmission. NATO Advanced Science Institute Series H: Cell Biology. Vol. 21. Springer-Verlag, Berlin, 1988
10. Durant NW, Katz RI: Suxamethonium. Br J Anesth 54:195, 1982
11. Betz WJ, Caldwel JH, Kinnamon SC: Increased sodium conductance in the synaptic region of rat skeletal muscle fibres. J Physiol (Lond) 352:189, 1984
12. Rash JE, Walrond JP, Morita M: Structural and functional correlates of synaptic transmission in the vertebrate neuromuscular junction. J Electron Microsc Tech 10:153, 1988
13. Heuser JE, Reese TS: Structural changes after transmitter release at the frog neuromuscular junction. J Cell Biol 88:564, 1981
14. Katz B, Miledi R: Estimates of quantal content during "chemical potentiation" of transmitter release. Proc R Soc Lond [Biol] 215:369, 1979
15. Parnas J, Parnas H: The "Ca-voltage" hypothesis for neurotransmitter release. Biophys Chem 29:85, 1988
16. Valtorta F, Jahn R, Fesce R, et al: Synaptophysin (p38) at the frog neuromuscular junction: Its incorporation into the axo-

lemma and recycling after intense quantal secretion. J Cell Biol 107:2717, 1988

17. Standaert FG: Release of transmitter at the neuromuscular junction. Br J Anaesth 54:131, 1982

18. Lindstrom J, Schoepfer R, Whiting P: Molecular studies of the neuronal nicotinic acetylcholine receptor family. Mol Neurobiol 1:281, 1987

19. Changeux J-P, Revah F: The acetylcholine receptor molecule: Allosteric sites and the ion channel. Trends Neurosci 10:245, 1987

20. Sine SM: Functional properties of human skeletal muscle acetylcholine receptors expressed by the TE671 cell line. J Biol Chem 263:18052, 1988

21. Oswald RE, Papke RL, Lukas RJ: Characterization of nicotinic acetylcholine receptor channels of the TE671 human medulloblastoma clonal line. Neurosci Lett 96:207, 1989

22. Steinbach JH, Ifane C: How many kinds of nicotinic acetylcholine receptors are there? Trends Neurosci 12:2, 1989

23. Maelicke A (ed): Nicotinic Acetylcholine Receptor, Structure and Function. NATO Advanced Research Workshop. Springer-Verlag, New York, 1986

24. Barrantes FJ: Muscle endplate cholinoreceptors. Pharmacol Ther 38:331, 1988

25. McCarthy MP, Stroud RM: Conformational states of the nicotinic acetylcholine receptor from Torpedo californica induced by the binding of agonist, antagonists, and local anesthetics. Equilibrium measurements using tritium-hydrogen exchange. Biochemistry 28:40, 1989

26. Karlin A, DiPaola M, Kao PN, Lobel P: Functional sites and transient states of the nicotinic acetylcholine receptor. p. 43. In Hille B, Fambrough DM (eds): Proteins of Excitable Membranes. Society of General Physiologists and Wiley Interscience, New York, 1987

27. Katz AM, Messinso FC, Herbette L: Ion channels in membranes. Circulation, 65: suppl. 1, 1–2, 1982

28. Dionne VE: Two types of nicotinic acetylcholine receptors at slow fibre end-plates of the garter snake. J Physiol 409:313, 1989

29. Gage PW, Hammill OP: Effects of anesthetics on ion channels in synapses. Int Rev Neurophysiol 25:3, 1981

30. Standaert FG: Donuts and holes: Molecules and muscle relaxants. Semin Anesthesiol 3:251, 1984

31. Hopfield JF, Tank DW, Greengard P, et al: Functional modulation of the nicotinic acetylcholine receptor by tyrosine phosphorylation. Nature 336:477, 1988

32. Spivak CE, Albuquerque EX: Dynamic properties of the nicotinic acetylcholine receptors ion channel complex: Activation and blockade. p. 323. In Hanin I, Goldberg AM (eds): Progress in Cholinergic Biology: Model Cholinergic Synapses. Raven Press, New York, 1982

33. Albuquerque EX, Akaike A, Shaw KP, et al: The interaction of anticholinesterase agents with the acetylcholine receptor-ionic channel complex. Fund Appl Toxicol 4:S27, 1984

34. Creese R, Head SD, Jenkinson DF: The role of the sodium pump during prolonged end-plate currents in guinea-pig diaphragm. J Physiol 384:377, 1987

35. Gu Y, Hall ZW: Characterization of acetylcholine receptor subunits in developing and denervated mammalian muscle. J Biol Chem 363:12878, 1988

36. Witzemann V, Sakmann B: Mechanisms regulating the expression and function of acetylcholine receptor. p. 453. In Zimmermann H (ed): Cellular and Molecular Basis of Synaptic Transmission. NATO Advanced Science Institute Series H: Cell Biology. Vol. 21. Springer-Verlag, Berlin, 1988

37. Merlie JP, Bunonanno A, Carlin B, et al: Coordinate regulation of expression of synaptic proteins in skeletal muscle: Studies with acetylcholine receptor. p. 77. In Hille B, Fambrough DM (eds): Proteins of Excitable Membranes. Society of General Physiologists and Wiley Interscience, New York, 1987

38. Schuetze SM, Role LW: Developmental regulation of nicotinic acetylcholine receptors. Annu Rev Neurosci 10:403, 1987

39. Goudsouzian NG, Standaert FG: The infant and the myoneural junction. Anesth Analg 65:1208, 1986

40. Bowman WC, Marshall IG, Gibb AJ, Harborne AJ: Feedback control of transmitter release at the neuromuscular junction. Trends in Pharmacological Sciences 9:16, 1988

41. Heuser JE: Morphology of synaptic vesicle discharge and reformation at the frog neuromuscular junction. p. 51. In Thesleff S (ed): Motor Innervation of Muscle. Academic Press, Orlando, FL, 1976

42. Matsuda Y, Oki S, Kitaoka K, et al: Scanning electron microscopic study of denervated and reinnervated neuromuscular junction. Muscle Nerve 11:1266, 1988

43. Neher B, Sakmann E, Steinbach JH: The extracellular patch-clamp: A method of resolving currents through individual open channels in biological membranes. Pfluegers Arch 375:219, 1978

44. Sine SM, Steinbach JH: Agonists block currents through acetylcholine receptor channels. Biophys 7 46:277, 1984

21
STATISTICS IN ANESTHESIA

Dennis M. Fisher

Mention of the word *statistics* evokes in many members of the medical community two responses, first, a recognition of its necessity for research, and second, a distaste. This distaste results from a number of sources —the limited (and often incomprehensible) teaching provided in many courses, the inconsistent terminology used by different investigators, the frequency with which statistics is used to mislead rather than clarify, and finally, a distrust of mathematics.

Clinicians who are not knowledgeable about the language and techniques of statistics may believe that journal editors will ensure the appropriateness and accuracy of statistical techniques used in their publications. Unfortunately, this may not be true: several reviews have demonstrated a high incidence of statistical errors in reputable journals.[1,2] In response to these criticisms, one journal, *Circulation Research*, adopted the policy that articles accepted for publication must undergo review by a statistician.[3] This policy has not been widely accepted, probably because of potential delays in the editorial process and the additional costs of using a statistical advisor.

The investigator who completes a research project must organize and analyze the data, draw conclusions, and then communicate the results. To embark on this task, the researcher should first select the variables to be analyzed. Next, data are summarized so that relationships and contrasts can be examined. After the investigator notes the magnitude and direction of these contrasts, scientific judgment must be applied to determine their importance. Only then should the investigator use statistical tools to establish "significance."

In recent decades, emphasis on statistical analysis in research studies has increased. Readers tend to believe that any conclusion accompanied by the statement "$P < 0.05$" is true; conversely, all observations not supported by that statement are believed to be untrue. This emphasis on statistical significance has encouraged investigators to focus their analyses on statistical testing rather than actually examining individual data points.

685

When data have been collected, the investigator might call upon one of several resources such as a hand-held calculator, a computer, or even a statistician (many of whom lack expertise in the statistical concerns relating to medicine). The raw data are entered, along with instructions as to which test is desired, and the investigator is rewarded with a number of statistical results. For example, when data are analyzed by linear regression, the output from a computer program might state "$P <$ 0.001." If the investigator does not understand terms such as *within-groups variance, residual mean square,* or *standard error of the estimate,* the statement "$P <$ 0.001" suggests that the data show a strong statistical association. As we will examine later, for linear regression, the validity of the association is better supported by other statistical statements. However, the uninitiated researcher is usually pleased with the probability associated with this low value and may not devote additional time to interpreting or understanding the results. Of greater importance, the investigator may not realize that these results do not ensure that a statistical difference exists, that the correct statistical test was employed, or even that the study was performed in a manner that permits any conclusions to be drawn.[4]

Gaining a thorough knowledge of statistical techniques requires much time and energy. However, most statistical techniques used in medical research are simple. Emerson and Colditz[5] reviewed the statistical tests employed in original articles published in the *New England Journal of Medicine* from 1978 to 1979. They found that seven statistical techniques (descriptive tests, *t* tests, contingency tables, nonparametric tests, epidemiologic statistics, Pearson correlation, and simple linear regression) composed 82 percent of all the tests used in these studies. A compilation of the statistical tests reported in *Pediatrics*[6] articles demonstrates similar findings, as does a review[7] of the two major American anesthesia journals, *Anesthesiology* and *Anesthesia and Analgesia.*

This chapter introduces the reader to the principles governing these simple statistical tests. First, descriptive statistics (how to examine and describe data) and the concept of probability are discussed. These concepts are then used to examine the principles of inferential statistics (that is, using statistics to draw conclusions). For each statistical test, the mathematical derivation of that test and examples will be provided. The chapter concludes with a guide to the selection of the appropriate statistical test for a variety of research designs as well as a review of some resources for statistical analysis. This chapter is not a definitive treatise on statistics but rather an introduction to basic principles.

DESCRIPTIVE STATISTICS

The initial step in statistical analyses is to categorize and summarize the data, that is, apply the techniques of descriptive statistics.

Types of Data

The most familiar type of data, *data on a ratio scale,* has two characteristics (Table 21-1). First, the size interval between successive units on the measurement scale is constant. For example, the difference between cardiac outputs of 4 and 5 L/min is the same as the difference between cardiac outputs of 7 and 8 L/min. Second, the measurement scale must have a zero point, and this zero value must have physiologic significance. These characteristics permit statements about the ratio of different values on the measurement scale. For example, a drug effect lasting 30 minutes is twice as long as a drug effect lasting 15 minutes.

Data on an interval scale also have constant intervals but lack a true zero point. For example, most measurements of pressure are referenced to atmospheric pressure (approximately 760 mmHg) rather than to a true zero point. The pressure represented by 20 cmH_2O (14.7 mmHg) is not twice as great as the pressure represented by 10 cmH_2O (7.4 mmHg). To caclulate the true ratio, we would have to convert the pressures to absolute measurements by adding the reference zero value, in this case 760 mmHg. Similarly, the temperature represented by 36°C is not twice the temperature represented by 18°C.

For many physiologic variables, there are known numerical differences between subjects. However, the data may indicate only a relative, rather than a measurable, difference between subjects. For example, a patient whose ASA physical status is III is at greater risk of harm from undergoing anesthesia than is the patient having a physical status of I. However, the difference in terms of degree of illness between patients having a physical status of II and those having a status of III is not necessarily the same as the difference between patients having a status of I and those having a status of II. Similarly, an Apgar score of 8 is better than one of 5; how-

TABLE 21-1. Types of Data

Type of Data	Characteristic	Examples
Data on a ratio scale	Measurement scale has constant intervals and a true zero point.	Duration of drug effect, cardiac output
Data on an interval scale	Measurement scale has a constant interval, but no true zero point.	Airway pressure, body temperature
Data on an ordinal scale	Data are ordered or ranked, not measured.	ASA physical status, Apgar scores
Data on a nominal scale	Data are classified not by a numerical measurement but by some quality or attribute.	EEG patterns, survival, genotypes of pseudocholinesterase

ever, the difference between these two scores, in terms of neurobehavioral well-being, is not necessarily the same as the difference between Apgar scores of 5 and 2. These scoring systems are examples of *data on an ordinal scale*. Ordinal scales have arbitrary intervals that describe relative, rather than absolute, relationships between the ranks. They convey less information than data on a ratio or interval scale, because only relative comparisons can be made (e.g., that an Apgar score of 10 is better than a score of 5). In medical literature it is common to see data on an ordinal scale treated as if they were on a ratio or an interval scale. For example, the extent of sensory blockade produced by spinal or epidural anesthesia is often reported in units of dermatomes, although a segment in the sacral region may not be identical, in terms of the amount of anesthetic required to produce loss of sensation, to a segment in the thoracic region. The treatment of ordinal data with statistical techniques more appropriately applied to interval or ratio data is so common as to be widely accepted.[8] Nevertheless, special techniques are available that are more appropriate for the analysis of these types of data.

On occasion, we choose to describe, that is, name, a variable in terms of a quality rather than a quantity. Variables described in this fashion are called *data on a nominal scale*. For example, electroencephalographic waveforms can be identified as α, β, θ, or δ. Similarly, genotypes of pseudocholinesterase are identified by names rather than by numerical measurements.[9] To permit mathematical comparisons, we can obtain ratio-scale measurements of pseudocholinesterase activity for each of the genotypes. Using these ratio-scale measurements rather than the nominal-scale measurements, we can make comparisons of the various groups. Finally, some variables have only two possible attributes. For example, after surgery, a patient is either alive or dead.

The investigator must correctly identify the type of data collected. Only then can the appropriate statistical analysis be applied.

Significant Digits

For all measurements, there are limits to precision. For example, blood pressure is usually measured to the nearest millimeter of mercury; and arterial oxygen (PaO_2) and carbon dioxide ($PaCO_2$) partial pressures are measured to the nearest millimeter or, at best, the nearest tenth of a millimeter of mercury. In neuromuscular studies, because the ulnar nerve is usually stimulated less frequently than once every 5 seconds, onset times cannot be measured with a precision of greater than 5 seconds. Whenever data are reported, a greater degree of precision should not be suggested than really exists.

Populations and Samples

Inherent in statistical analysis of a measured variable is the desire to draw conclusions about that variable. To accomplish this goal, the investigator could measure the variable for the entire population. For example, if we were interested in knowing $PaCO_2$ for all adult patients anesthetized with an end-tidal concentration of isoflurane of 1.0 percent at the University of California, San Francisco, in 1989, we could measure that variable in all eligible subjects. The values for $PaCO_2$ might then be presented in a histogram displaying the number of subjects having each value of $PaCO_2$; the histogram might also display the percentage of subjects having each value of $PaCO_2$ (Fig. 21-1).

Obtaining measurements for all eligible subjects would be cumbersome and expensive. To simplify the task, we might select a smaller sample of the original population and assume that this sample represents the entire population. Values for $PaCO_2$ for a hypothetical sample are shown in Figure 21-2. Note that extreme values (greater than 58 mmHg and less than 36 mmHg) are not represented, nor are certain intermediate values (e.g., 42, 44, 45 mmHg). Using these data, we cannot conclude that $PaCO_2$ is always somewhere be-

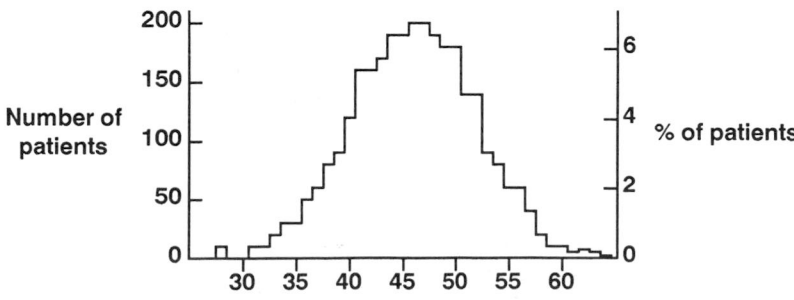

Fig. 21-1. Histogram showing hypothetical values for $PaCO_2$ (mmHg) for all patients undergoing light isoflurane anesthesia at the University of California, San Francisco, during 1989. The x axis represents values for $PaCO_2$. There are two y axes. The left-hand axis represents the actual number of patients with each value of $PaCO_2$; the right-hand axis shows these values as a percentage of the total population.

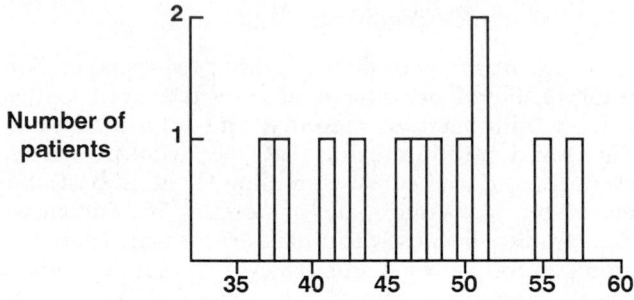

Fig. 21-2. Histogram showing hypothetical values for $PaCO_2$ obtained from 12 subjects undergoing light isoflurane anesthesia. These 12 values represent a sample taken from the values in Figure 21-1.

tween 36 and 58 mmHg during light isoflurane anesthesia, only that extreme values did not occur in this sample. The values obtained from this sample of 12 subjects suggest that during light isoflurane anesthesia, $PaCO_2$ is frequently between 40 and 52 mmHg.

Although measurements have been made on 12 subjects, the purpose of our study was to make predictions about a larger group, the entire population of adults undergoing light isoflurane anesthesia. For this prediction to be valid, we must assume that the sample represents the entire population. If this assumption is not true, the results may not apply to the entire population. For example, Stanley and Webster[10] found that fentanyl, in doses of 50 μg/kg, provided sufficient anesthesia for cardiac surgery; however, subsequent studies suggested that larger doses are necessary for most patients. The studies by Stanley and Webster were conducted in Salt Lake City, a community that is predominantly Mormon. Because Mormons abstain from alcohol and other drugs, the low dose requirement observed by Stanley and Webster may have resulted from the personal habits of the subjects; therefore, this sample may represent the population of Salt Lake City, Utah, but not the population of the United States. Recognizing these types of biases is important. If possible, these biases should be avoided. If they cannot be avoided, they must be stated.

Central Tendency

After the investigator selects the sample population and obtains measurements, the results must then be described. All the measured values could be displayed as in Figure 21-2, or in other formats such as a table. Although these methods of data presentation permit the reader to make judgments about the individual data points, they limit communication about the general nature of the sample. To describe a variable for the entire population, the investigator would like to be able to select the single value from the sample that would represent the center of the entire population, a value known as the *index of central tendency*.[11] If all the values in the sample were identical, the investigator would report that single value. However, for most variables, the sample will contain many different values for individual members.

Mean

The value most widely used to represent the population is the *arithmetic mean*, usually referred to as the mean. The mean is determined by adding all the values of the population and dividing by the number of values in the population. This is described mathematically as population mean = sum of observations/number of observations. When a large number of terms is being summed, a shorthand way of expressing the process, called *summation notation*, is used:

$$\mu = \frac{\sum_{i=1}^{N} X_i}{N} \tag{1}$$

where μ is the population mean, X_i are the individual values, and capital sigma (Σ) means to sum these values. Therefore, this expression is read as follows: μ is equal to the sum of all individual values of X_i from X_I to X_N, divided by N. Since we usually sum all the values of the population, it is conventional to omit several of these symbols and write

$$\mu = \frac{\Sigma X_i}{N} \tag{2}$$

When the investigator is studying a sample rather than the entire population, another term, $\overline{X}$, is used to represent the sample mean. $\overline{X}$ is equal to the sum of all measurements in the sample divided by the number of measurements in the sample. The mean is expressed with the same units as the individual observations.

Median

Alternatively, central tendency might be expressed with the median or the mode. To determine the median, the individual values are ranked from smallest to largest (or from largest to smallest). The *median* is the middle measurement, that is, the value below which half of the values lie and above which the other half lie. Because the median is based on the rankings of the values rather than the magnitude of the individual values, the median is used infrequently in statistics.

Mode

The *mode* is the value that occurs most frequently. With the small number of observations in many medical studies, there will be no mode if each observed value occurs only once.

The arithmetic mean is a valid description of the location of the population only when ratio or interval data are used; for ordinal data, the arithmetic mean has no meaning. For example, the arithmetic mean of 5 is not the appropriate value to describe a sample consisting of subjects having Apgar scores of 0 and 10.[12] Instead, the location of the sample is more accurately described with values such as the median or the mode or, in this case, with individual values.

For many sets of measurements, the arithmetic mean will represent the population accurately. For the measurements of P_ACO_2 during isoflurane anesthesia, the arithmetic mean is $(37 + 38 + \cdots + 57)/12$ or 47 mmHg. Individual values range from 37 to 57 mmHg and most are between 40 and 52 mmHg. Thus, the arithmetic mean of 47 mmHg is "close" to each of the members of the sample and can be considered a fair representative of all the members of the sample.

In contrast, two patients in this small sample had values of 51 mmHg, making this value the mode. Although the mode is theoretically a measure of central tendency, in this instance it lies near one extreme of the sample and therefore does not represent the population. Since the number of members of this sample is even, no value lies exactly in the middle. In such circumstances, the median is taken to be the average of the two values ranked nearest the middle of the population (47 and 48 mmHg, respectively), that is, 47.5 mmHg. Therefore, of the three values describing the location of this population, the mean and median represent the population well, whereas the mode does not. In all statistical analyses, the investigator must examine the values in the sample to determine how the central tendency of the sample can best be described.

Finally, just because we have selected a value to represent the sample does not necessarily imply that this value represents the larger population from which the sample was drawn. For example, our sample might have been biased toward, or away from, certain members of the population; or by chance we might have selected highly unusual members of the population. We must always remember that the mean represents the sample, rather than the population. If we extrapolate conclusions to the population, we must also consider our sampling process and the ability of this sampling process to identify the mean of the population.

Data Transformation

Most samples can be well represented by one of these three indicators of central tendency, particularly the arithmetic mean. However, some samples are not well represented by the arithmetic mean. Feinstein[13] determined that the arithmetic mean for four concentrations of hydrogen ion $(0.3162 \times 10^{-1}, 0.2512 \times 10^{-3}, 0.1995 \times 10^{-6}, 0.1259 \times 10^{-8})$ was 0.0797×10^{-1}. This value is close to the first member of the sample and far from the other three. Rather than use the arithmetic mean to locate the central tendency of the population, he suggested using another indicator, the geometric mean, which is equal to the nth root of the product of each of the observations. Therefore, the geometric mean of these four concentrations would be $[(0.3162 \times 10^{-1}) \times (0.2512 \times 10^{-3}) \times (0.1995 \times 10^{-6}) \times (0.1259 \times 10^{-8})]^{1/4}$ or 0.6683×10^{-5}. In this instance, the geometric mean, being larger than two of the observations and smaller than the other two, is more representative than the arithmetic mean. Alternatively, the hydrogen ion concentrations could be converted to pH values of 1.5, 3.6, 6.7, and 8.9, respectively. The arithmetic mean of these pH values is 5.2, which corresponds to a hydrogen ion concentration of 0.6683×10^{-5}. Thus, the central tendency of hydrogen ion concentration is best expressed using the geometric mean, whereas the central tendency for pH is best expressed using the arithmetic mean.

The above example demonstrates how data might be converted to an easier-to-use form (transformed) by applying simple algebraic processes such as taking the logarithm or square root of each value. Data transformation permits easier manipulation of the data or changes the distribution. Before using a calculator or computer to determine the arithmetic mean, the investigator should examine the data to determine whether the arithmetic mean is representative of the sample and whether transformation may be necessary to improve statistical analysis.

The Normal Distribution

The ability of the arithmetic mean to express the central tendency of the population is a function of the distribution of the values within the population. For many variables, such as P_ACO_2 (shown above), values tend to cluster around a central value, with fewer values being located toward the extremes. If one obtains a sufficiently large sample, for many biologic variables the histogram would assume the shape of a bell (Fig. 21-3A). This distribution, known as the *normal distribution*, was first described by de Moivre[14] but is credited to Karl Gauss, being called the Gaussian distribution. Many statistical tests described in this chapter assume that the population under examination is distributed normally. Because medical studies often use a small sample size, the assumption that resulting data have a Gaussian distribution frequently is not tested.

Populations that do not have a Gaussian distribution may assume a number of different shapes (e.g., Fig. 21-3B & C). For example, administration of an imaginary drug, histodrenaline, might result in the release of histamine in some individuals and in the release of catecholamines in others. Therefore, if we measured the change in blood pressure after administration of this drug, half the subjects might have an increase in blood pressure, while the other half had an equal decrease (Fig. 21-3B). If the mean value were zero, we might be led to believe that histodrenaline had no cardiovascular effects. A more appropriate conclusion would be that the arithmetic mean did not represent the population. The importance of examining the distribution of the data points should now be readily apparent: on occasion, the investigator will find that the arithmetic mean

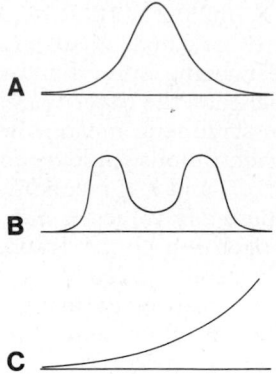

Fig. 21-3. The distribution of values for a population may assume many shapes. One shape frequently encountered in biologic experiments is the normal distribution (**A**). On occasion, distribution may be bimodal (humped) (**B**) or J-shaped (**C**).

should not be used to describe the population. In that case, alternate methods of describing the results of the study, such as a histogram or table, become essential.

Variability

Identifying the central location of the sample is not sufficient to describe the population entirely. For example, had all P_ACO_2 values during isoflurane anesthesia ranged from 44 to 49 mmHg, the mean might have been 47 mmHg. Although the mean for this sample would have been the same as that for the sample described earlier, these two samples probably describe different populations, one having a broad range of P_ACO_2 values during isoflurane anesthesia and the other having a narrow range. Thus, in addition to describing the central location of the sample, we need to describe how dispersed the data are, that is, the variability of the sample.

Mean Deviation

One technique used for this purpose might be to find the average deviation from the mean. However, because some deviations are positive and others negative, their sum is always zero; hence, the average deviation has no value as an indicator of dispersion of the data. Alternatively, the investigator could sum the absolute values of these differences from the mean and divide by *n*, thus producing the *mean absolute deviation*. This technique is mathematically cumbersome and has not become popular.

Sum of Squares

Another approach to the problem of describing how dispersed the data are is to sum the square of the deviations from the mean, a method that eliminates the negative signs and produces positive values. Squaring the

deviations has a second effect: it increases ("weights") the contribution of the values according to their distance from the mean. For example, if the deviations from the mean were −1, −5, +1, and +5, the sum of squared deviations would be 52. A sample containing deviations of −3, −3, +3, and +3 would produce a smaller sum of squared deviations, 36. Although the mean absolute deviation (3) is the same for both samples [(1 + 5 + 5 + 1)/4 or (3 + 3 + 3 + 3)/4], the sample containing values more distant from the mean has the larger sum of squares. This sum of the squared deviations from the mean, known as the *sum of squares* (SS), is a fundamental tool used repeatedly in statistics. It is expressed mathematically as

$$\text{Sample SS} = \Sigma(X_i - \overline{X})^2 \tag{3}$$

Calculating the value of this equation requires two passes through the data: the first pass to sum the individual values to determine the mean value; and the second pass to determine the difference between individual values and the mean. Calculators and computers reduce this to a single step, known as a *machine formula*, which is derived as follows:

$$\text{Sample SS} = \Sigma(X_i^2 - 2X_i\overline{X} + \overline{X}^2) \tag{4}$$

This can be expanded to

$$\text{Sample SS} = \Sigma X_i^2 - \Sigma 2X_i\overline{X} + \Sigma\overline{X}^2 \tag{5}$$

The second part of this equation can be simplified to: $2 \times \overline{X} \times \Sigma X_i$ which is equal to $2 \times (\Sigma X_i/n) \times \Sigma X_i$, or $[2 \times (\Sigma X_i^2/n)]$. Similarly, the third part of the equation can be simplified to $n \times \overline{X}^2$, or $[n \times (\Sigma X_i/n)^2]$. Since $(\Sigma X_i/n)^2$ is equal to $(\Sigma X_i)^2/n^2$ the equation can be simplified to

$$\text{Sample SS} = \Sigma X_i^2 - \frac{(\Sigma X_i)^2}{n} \tag{6}$$

Using this machine formula, we can determine the sum of squares in a single pass through the data; this technique greatly simplifies data manipulation.

Variance

Dividing the sum of squares by the sample size yields the average squared deviation from the mean, also known as the *mean squared deviation* or *population variance, σ^2*:

$$\sigma^2 = \frac{\Sigma(X_i - \mu)^2}{N} \tag{7}$$

This equation is read as follows: population variance is equal to the sum of the squared differences between individual values and the population mean, divided by the sample size. Usually we are dealing with samples rather than populations, and when we calculate the *sample variance*, we must use the sample mean as an estimate of the population mean. If we represent the difference between the sample mean and the population mean as ϵ, equation (7) could be written as

$$\text{Sample variance} = \frac{\Sigma[X_i - (\overline{X} + \epsilon)]^2}{n} \quad (8)$$

As with equation (3), this can be expanded to

$$\text{Sample variance} = \frac{\Sigma(X_i - \overline{X})^2 - 2\Sigma\epsilon(X_i - \overline{X}) + \Sigma\epsilon^2}{n} \quad (9)$$

The first term is what we would obtain had we used the sample mean instead of the population mean to estimate the sample variance. The second term always equals zero, because it is equivalent to the sum of the average deviations from the mean. The third term is equal to $n \times \epsilon^2/n$, or ϵ^2. Thus, the estimates for sample variance differ when it is determined by using sample mean rather than population mean, sample variance being underestimated by the amount ϵ^2. Since we usually do not know the population mean, we typically use the sample mean to calculate sample variance. This, however, produces a biased estimate. We correct for this bias by decreasing the denominator by 1. This process produces a better estimate for sample variance (s^2):

$$s^2 = \frac{\Sigma(X_i - \overline{X})^2}{n - 1} \quad (10)$$

The corrected denominator is known as the *degrees of freedom* (*df*). If there are n values that are squared and summed to determine the sample variance [equation (10)], after one determines the $n - 1$th value, the remaining difference has been predetermined [the sum of the average deviations from the mean $\Sigma(X_i - \overline{X})$ must equal zero]. Thus, the number of independent values used to calculate sample variance differs from the sample size and is known as the degrees of freedom. A more elaborate proof that using $n - 1$ as the denominator yields a less biased estimate is available elsewhere.[15]

Standard Deviation

Although it is possible to express variability of the sample or the population by using the respective variances, this is impractical because the units for variance for a sample are different from those for the population. (Because variance is determined by squaring the differences between individual values and the mean, the units for variance consist of the square of the original units. For example, for $PaCO_2$ values, the units for variance would be [mmHg]^2.) A more common approach is to obtain the square root of the variance, known as the *standard deviation*. As before, the standard deviation for the population (σ) and the standard deviation for the sample (s) differ depending on whether n or $n - 1$ is used in the denominator. In most situations, the standard deviation of the sample, rather than of the population, should be used, even though it is a larger number.

Now we have estimated the central tendency and the variability of the sample, two values that describe the location and dispersion of the entire sample. If the population has a Gaussian distribution, most values lie near the mean and only a few values lie far from the mean. That is, approximately 68 percent of the values lie within the range from one standard deviation above to one standard deviation below the mean. Approximately 95 percent lie within two standard deviations above or below the mean, and more than 99 percent of all values lie within three standard deviations of the mean.*

Returning to the values for $PaCO_2$ during isoflurane anesthesia, we find that the standard deviation is 6.3 mmHg. If we examine values ranging from one standard deviation below the mean (approximately $47 - 6 = 41$ mmHg) to one standard deviation above the mean (approximately $47 + 6 = 53$ mmHg), we find that two-thirds of the values in the sample lie in this range and that one-third lies outside this range. The range from two standard deviations below the mean to two standard deviations above the mean (approximately 34 to 60 mmHg) includes all the values in this sample. If $PaCO_2$ for any subject had been higher than 65 mmHg or lower than 29 mmHg, three or more standard deviations below or above the mean would have been necessary to include those values.

Coefficient of Variation

If the sole information communicated about a sample is that the standard deviation is 6 mmHg, we cannot assess whether variability is large or small. For a mean arterial pressure of 100 mmHg, a standard deviation of 6 mmHg is small; however, for a pulmonary artery pressure of 12 mmHg, a standard deviation of 6 mmHg suggests greater variability. The ratio of standard deviation to the sample mean is known as the *coefficient of variation* and is often expressed as a pecentage. The coefficient of variation is valuable in describing the variability of the sample. Since the units of the numerator and denominator are the same, the coefficient of variation has no units.

Standard Error of the Mean

If we were to repeat our measurements of $PaCO_2$ during isoflurane anesthesia in another 12 subjects, we would probably obtain slightly different results. For example, $PaCO_2$ values might be 34, 36, 40, 41, 44, 44, 47, 48, 48, 49, 54, and 55 mmHg. The mean of this sample would be 45 mmHg and the standard deviation would be 6.5 mmHg. A third sample of 12 subjects might yield a mean of 44 mmHg; additional samples might have

---

* In a Gaussian distribution, 95 percent of all values are actually found within 1.96 (rather than 2.0) standard deviations of the mean and the range of two standard deviations from the mean actually includes 95.44 percent of all values. However, it is common practice to use 2.0, rather than 1.96, standard deviations to describe the 95 pecent variability of populations.

mean values of 43, 44, 48, and 49 mmHg. Which of these mean values best represents the population? Had we not divided these patients into six groups, we would have had a single sample containing 72 members. The mean value for such a sample would have been 46 mmHg. This could be calculated by summing the values for all 72 subjects or by determining the weighted average of the means for the individual groups: $[(12 \times 43) + (12 \times 44) + (12 \times 45) \cdots + (12 \times 49)]/(12 + 12 + \cdots + 12)$ or 3,312/72 or 46 mmHg. These different techniques yield identical results. Since this new mean value, the mean of mean values (also known as the grand mean), was obtained from a larger sample, it better represents the population than each of the other values. As sample size increases, so does the ability of the sample to represent the population from which it came.

Since the sample mean is only an estimate of the mean of the population, we would also like to describe how closely this value approximates the population mean. This is accomplished with the *standard error of the mean* (SEM), more commonly called the standard error (SE). The SE is obtained by dividing the standard deviation of the sample (or population, if appropriate) by the square root of the size of the sample. The term *standard error of the mean* is curious, because this value is neither standard nor an error. This phrase originated during the Industrial Revolution, at which time reproducibility of measurements was important. If one measured the length of an object repeatedly, successive measurements would differ slightly, and an individual measurement would be unlikely to represent the true lenght of the object. Repeating the measurement and determining the average of these measurements provides a better estimate. If we then calculate the SEM value, we determine the "error" with which our measurement was made or how far from the true length the measured values are.

Using our initial set of values for $PaCO_2$ during isoflurane anesthesia, we find that the standard error is $6.3/12^{1/2}$, or 1.8 mmHg. Just as approximately 68 percent of the sample lies within one standard deviation of the mean, approximately 68 percent of all sample means lies within 1 SE of the population mean. As before, increasing the range to 2 SE above and below the population mean increases to approximately 95 percent the likelihood that the sample mean is included. Expanding the range to 3 SE increases the likelihood to more than 99 percent. Note that doubling the population does not decrease the SE by a factor of 2; to decrease the SE by one-half, one would have to increase the population by a factor of 4.

Confidence Limits

These ranges, when used to describe the mean, are called *confidence limits*. The 68 percent confidence limits include all values from 1 SE below the mean to 1 SE above the mean (written as "mean ± SEM" or "mean ± SE"). More commonly reported are the 95 percent confidence limits, which include all values within 2 SE of the mean (mean ± 2 SEM). Since the likelihood is 95 percent that the mean is included in these confidence limits, they are a valuable way to describe both the location and the variability of the mean.

What to Report: Standard Deviation or Standard Error?

When reporting data, investigators must decide whether to report the standard deviation or standard error of the mean. This decision should follow from the purpose of the study, which is, usually, to describe the sample to predict values for the population. Because the standard deviation describes the variability of the sample and, hence, is used to estimate values for the population, it seems that standard deviation should always be reported.

Why, then, are standard errors reported with such frequency? The answer to this question lies in the mathematical relationship between the two values, standard error being standard deviation divided by the square root of the sample size. This relationship means that the standard error is always smaller than the standard deviation; the difference between the two increases as the sample size increases. When describing a sample, it is a too frequent practice to provide the mean ± a value describing variability without identifying whether that value is the standard deviation or the standard error.[16] Since the standard error is the smaller of the two values, it suggests less variability than would the standard deviation.

Two solutions might lessen the ambiguity. First, since it is usually more important to describe the variability of the population rather than the variability of the mean (and the standard error can be calculated by the reader if sample size is reported), perhaps investigators should be required to report only standard deviation rather than standard error. A simpler solution would be to require that all values describing the sample be identified as standard deviation or standard error, a practice occurring with increasing frequency. Whenever standard error is reported, the investigator should ensure that the reader can determine the sample size for that value and thus be able to calculate standard deviation.

z Transformations

If we select a single value from the population, it would be of value to know the location of that value within the population. For example, if we found that 30 minutes after administration of pancuronium, subject A had a serum drug concentration of 150 ng/ml, we might inquire how that subject compared in that regard with other subjects given the same dose. If we knew that the average serum drug concentration for a number of subjects was 200 ng/ml 30 minutes after drug administration, we could conclude that the value for subject A was lower than the mean. However, without knowing the distribution of data for the other subjects, we would not be able to conclude whether this subject had an unusual response. If we also knew the standard deviation for the other subjects, we would be able to better estimate whether this subject differed from others. If the standard deviation for the sample was 40 ng/ml, the value for subject A would be less than two standard deviations from the mean. In contrast, if the standard deviation were 5 ng/ml, the value for subject A would be 10 standard deviations below the mean; such an occurrence would represent an unusual response.

The distance that a value lies from the mean can be expressed mathematically as the difference between that value and the mean divided by the standard deviation (σ). This statistic, known as the *z transformation*, is calculated as

$$z = \frac{X_i - \overline{X}}{\sigma} \qquad (11)$$

If z is large, the new value is far from the mean; if z is small, the value is near to the mean.

Probability

If we measured $P_{A}CO_2$ in a single subject undergoing light isoflurane anesthesia, we might obtain a value of 61 mmHg, a value that occurred infrequently in our other subjects (Fig. 21-1). If the population mean were 46 mmHg and the standard deviation 6 mmHg, the z score would be $(61 - 46)/6$ or 2.5, a value that indicates this subject had an unusual response to light isoflurane anesthesia. If we established that this subject was healthy and that no other obvious reason existed for the greater degree of respiratory depression, we would be able to say that this response is unlikely. However, statistics does not permit us to conclude that the response is abnormal.

The concept of probability attaches a numerical likelihood to the occurrence of an event. Regarding the occurrence of a $P_{A}CO_2$ of 61 mmHg during light isoflurane anesthesia, we can conclude from our other measurements that this event occurs in fewer than 2 percent of all anesthetics; this degree of likelihood is expressed as $P < 0.02$. Is this a "significant" event? Instinct tells us that an event occurring less frequently than once in 50 times is unusual and therefore worthy of notice. Is an event occurring once in 10 times ($P = 0.10$) worthy of notice? By convention, statisticians accept as significant any event that occurs less frequently than once in 20 times ($P < 0.05$). However, no biologic or mathematical rationale exists for choosing 5 percent as the level of statistical significance. R.A. Fisher, a noted statistician, observed that "The value for which $P = 0.05$, or 1 in 20, is 1.96 or nearly 2 [standard deviations]; it is convenient to take this point as a limit in judging whether a deviation is to be considered significant or not. Deviations exceeding twice the standard deviation are thus formally regarded as significant."[17] Later he wrote, "It is usual and convenient . . . to take

5 percent as a standard level of significance . . . [and] to ignore all results which fail to reach this standard. . . ."[18] Although a probability of 5 percent is the usual standard for statistical significance, one publication, the *Journal of Experimental Psychology*, has encouraged a significance level of 1 percent (i.e., $P < 0.01$).[19]

Type I and Type II Errors

The level of probability we select as representing significance, known as α, is also the frequency with which we erroneously conclude that a difference exists when there is no real difference. This is known as a *type I error*, or an α error. Alternatively, we could ask how often we can afford to be wrong. An investigator who repeats an experiment frequently, will eventually select a sample whose mean differs significantly from the population mean. If we select a probability level of 5 percent ($\alpha = 0.05$), we accept a 5 percent chance of being wrong. If the price for being wrong is very great, we might select a stricter criterion for statistical significance, for example, $\alpha = 0.01$.

Thus far, we have focused on the issue of erroneously concluding that a difference exists when none exists in reality. A second issue involves whether we can truly state than no difference exists between two populations. For example, if we were to measure recovery of twitch tension 60 minutes after administration of a dose of pancuronium in one group of subjects and 90 minutes after administration of the same dose in another group, instinct would tell us that more recovery would have occurred in the group studied at 90 minutes. If the samples consisted of two patients each, the variability within each of the groups might be great enough to prevent us from detecting a difference. Within samples of 20 subjects or more, we are more likely to detect a difference. The ability of a statistical test to detect a difference, known as its *power*, depends on the expected difference between groups, the variability within the groups, and the size of the samples. If the sample size is not sufficiently large, we will not be able to detect real differences between groups. This is known as a *type II or β error*.

One-Tailed versus Two-Tailed Comparisons

Thus far, we have considered the idea that a value located toward either extreme of the probability distribution is unlikely to occur. If α equals 0.05 and the distribution is symmetrical, then the 5 percent of values considered unlikely to occur (and therefore worthy of note) would be found equally at both ends of the distribution. That is, the left-hand tail of the curve would contain 2.5 percent of the values, and the right-hand tail of the curve would contain 2.5 percent of the values. This is known as *two-tailed comparison*, because we assume that extreme values are located within both tails of the distribution.

An investigator is often interested in testing a priori assumptions. For example, in assessing the relationship between volume status and blood pressure, we would only be interested in assessing whether blood pressure was lower in hypovolemic patients, because we assume that hypovolemia would decrease, rather than increase, blood pressure. If we performed the two-tailed test, we would be able to answer two questions. First, does blood pressure differ between normovolemic and hypovolemic subjects? If so, is blood pressure higher or lower in hypovolemic patients? If we are interested in only one extreme, we can examine the 5 percent located at one end of the distribution, rather than the 2.5 percent located at each end of the distribution. This is known as a *one-tailed comparison*. If the investigator is able to make an a priori assessment as to the direction of the relationship between groups and is willing to limit statistical evaluation to that issue, a one-tailed test may be appropriate. The investigator must decide to perform a one-tailed comparison before the data are collected. It is inappropriate to examine the data, observe a difference between groups, and then test the significance of the difference using a one-tailed comparison.

Hypothesis Testing and Statistics

Statistics does not permit us to conclude whether or not an association is valid, only whether it is likely or unlikely to occur. For example, if we studied three adults with chronic lung disease whose $PaCO_2$ values were 54, 57, and 59 mmHg, respectively, during isoflurane anesthesia, we might ask whether these patients differed from the adults whose $PaCO_2$ values were measured during isoflurane anesthesia. A statistician would convert this question into a *null hypothesis*, meaning that there is no difference between this sample and the population. The likelihood of this hypothesis would then be tested. If the α were low, for example, less than 5 percent, the statistician would reject the null hypothesis, stating that there is little probability that the sample was selected from the original population. In turn, we can conclude that there is likely to be a difference between these subjects and the original sample.

Before continuing to inferential statistics, we should define certain terms more specifically. The word *statistics* describes not only the name of the discipline that is the subject of this chapter, but also certain numerical entities calculated as part of that discipline. For example, the mean, standard deviation, and variance are all statistics. A statistic is an estimate, based on random sampling of the population, of parameters of the population. In addition, t, F, and a multitude of other symbols represent statistics. Tests employing these statistics are known as *parametric tests;* such tests are based on the actual magnitude of the values. In contrast, tests based on ranking of the values are known as *nonparametric tests*.

INFERENTIAL STATISTICS

After determining the descriptive statistics and noting differences between groups, the investigator would typically like to draw statistical conclusions regarding these differences. To draw these conclusions, the investigator employs a second area of statistics known as *inferential statistics*.

One- and Two-Sample *t* Tests

The most widely used, and misused, statistical test is Student's *t* test, a group of statistical tests designed for analysis of a single group or comparison of two groups. The name of this test refers to a pseudonym used by W.L. Gosset. Gosset's employer, the Guinness Brewing Company, did not permit its employees to publish their research under their own names; however, because of the importance of this work, Gosset was permitted to publish under the name "Student."[20] Gosset's contribution was to develop the *t* distribution. The *z* distribution described earlier is based on an infinite sample size. Gosset recognized that with smaller sample sizes (e.g., less than 30), the distributions differed from the exact bell shape of the Gaussian distribution. In particular, the presence of an extreme value (i.e., one far from the mean) was more likely to occur in a small sample. Gosset examined a variety of distributions of small samples and determined the frequency with which the more extreme values occurred.

Earlier we observed that in an infinitely large, normally distributed sample, 95 percent of all observations fell within 1.96 standard deviations of the mean. Gosset found that with a sample size of 20, a slightly larger range, 2.09 standard deviations, was necessary to include the same 95 percent of the observations. As the sample size decreased to 10, 2.26 standard deviations were necessary; with a sample size of 5, an even larger range, 2.78 standard deviations, was necessary to include 95 percent of all observations. These values (e.g., $t = 2.09$ for $\alpha = 0.05$ and $N = 20$) make up the *t* distribution. Every value in the *t* distribution is associated with a sample size and a value for α. As the sample size becomes large (e.g., greater than 30), the values for the *t* distribution are nearly identical for those for the *z* distribution; with an infinite sample size, they are identical.

These observations were then used to define three statistical tests: the one-sample, the two-sample, and paired-sample *t* tests.

Parametric *t* Tests

One-Sample t *Tests*

An investigator who measures a variable in a single group of subjects may be interested in determining whether the mean for this sample differs from zero (or alternatively, from some other specific value). This analysis can be performed by using the one-sample t test.

To examine the association between diuretic drugs and acid-base status, we might identify a group of patients taking diuretic drugs, obtain arterial blood samples, and determine base excess. A hypothetical set of values is shown in Table 21-2. The mean of these values is 3.0, a fact that might suggest and association between diuretic drugs and alkalosis. However, two of the subjects have negative values and two have zero values. Because a quick and informal appraisal of the data cannot determine whether 3.0 differs significantly from zero, we must use statistical analysis — in this case, the one-sample t test. If we assume that this sample represents the population and that the distribution of these values is normal, we can state with 95 percent confidence that the population mean lies between mean − ($t \times$ SE) and mean + ($t \times$ SE). This statement is similar to an earlier one that the population mean lies between mean − ($1.96 \times$ SE) and mean + ($1.96 \times$ SE). However, the value 1.96 (the z value to include 95 percent of the population) must now be replaced by the value of t appropriate for the sample size (i.e., 2.20). This value can be found on a table of t distribution by locating the row corresponding to the appropriate degrees of freedom (in this case, the value for degrees of freedom is one less than the sample size) and the desired value of α (typically 0.05). Sample values for t distribution are shown in Table 21-3; a more complete listing can be found in any statistical textbook. In this case, the 95 percent confidence limits for the mean are 0.47 and 5.53; these limits do not include the value zero. To de-

TABLE 21-3. Critical Values of the t Distribution (Two-Tailed)

	α		
df	0.05	0.01	0.001
3	3.18	5.84	12.92
4	2.78	4.60	8.61
5	2.57	4.03	6.87
10	2.23	3.17	4.59
20	2.09	2.84	3.85
50	2.01	2.69	3.50
100	1.98	2.63	3.39
1,000	1.96	2.58	3.30
∞	1.96	2.58	3.29

termine the 99 percent confidence limits, we use the t value for $\alpha = 0.01$ and 11 df, 3.11. This results in 99 percent confidence limits of −0.57 and 6.57, a range that does include zero. We can conclude with 95 percent, but not 99 percent, confidence that the use of diuretic drugs is associated with alkalosis.

An alternate approach, more familiar to some readers, is shown in Table 21-4. The division of the mean value by the standard error produces a value for t. This value is compared with a value for t appropriate for the desired level of significance (usually $\alpha = 0.05$ or 5 percent) for the appropriate degrees of freedom. If the value for t exceeds the value from the table (known as the *critical value*), the null hypothesis is rejected, and we would conclude that a difference exists (at the α level) between zero and the mean value for this population. In this instance, the value for t is 2.6. The critical value for t for $\alpha = 0.05$ and 11 df is 2.20; the value for t for α 0.01 and 11 df is 3.11. The value for t exceeds the critical value for α of 0.05 but not for α of 0.01. This fact also leads us to conclude that the mean for this sample differs from zero and that the likelihood is between 95 and 99 percent.

The one-sample t test can also be applied to populations for which mean values are expected to be other than zero. For example, if we were interested in whether 90 mmHg was the mean $PaCO_2$ of smokers, we would determine the difference between 90 mmHg and

TABLE 21-2. Hypothetical Set of Values for Base Excess for Subjects Given Diuretic Drugs

Subject	Base excess (meq/L)
1	0
2	8
3	1
4	6
5	−3
6	7
7	9
8	2
9	1
10	0
11	−1
12	6

$$N = 12$$

$$\text{Mean} = 3.0$$

$$\text{SD} = 3.98$$

$$\text{SE} = 1.15$$

$$df = 11$$

TABLE 21-4. One-Sample Student's t Test Applied to Hypothetical Data from Table 21-2

$$t = \frac{\text{Mean}}{\text{SE}} = 3.0/1.15 = 2.6$$

$$t_{0.05(2),11}{}^a = 2.20$$

$$t_{0.01(2),11}{}^b = 3.11$$

Therefore, $0.01 < P < 0.05$

[a] Read, "the two-tailed t value when $\alpha = 0.05$ and $df = 11$." Notation taken from Zar.[14]
[b] Read, "the two-tailed t value when $\alpha = 0.01$ and $df = 11$."

the mean value for the sample population, divide this value by the standard error of the sample to determine the *t* statistic, and then compare the resulting value with the critical value for *t*.

Two-Sample t Tests

More commonly, we make measurements on two groups of subjects and compare the responses. Such a comparison requires use of the two-sample *t* test. In this form of *t* testing, two independent samples are being compared, that is, an individual datum in one sample is not associated with another datum in the second sample. For example, we might want to compare blood pressure in normovolemic and hypovolemic individuals. Hypothetical values are provided in Table 21-5. In this instance, an informal appraisal of the data would establish that a significant difference exists between the mean values. This difference can be confirmed by using the two-sample *t* test to evaluate the null hypothesis that there is no difference between these two samples, that is, that they come from the same population.

Computation of the *t* statistic for the two-sample test is slightly more complicated than for the one-sample test. In the one sample test, we divided the mean by its

TABLE 21-5. Application of the One-Tailed Two-Sample Student's *t* Test to Hypothetical Sets of Mean Blood Pressure Values for Normovolemic and Hypovolemic Subjects

	Normovolemic Subjects	Hypovolemic Subjects
	77	72
	91	62
	101	51
	81	81
	76	47
	68	74
	72	52
	82	65
N	8	8
Mean	81.0	63.0
SD	10.6	12.3
SE	3.76	4.33

$$SE_{(\bar{X}_1 - \bar{X}_2)} = \left[\frac{10.6^2}{8} + \frac{12.3^2}{8}\right]^{1/2} = 5.74$$

$$t = \frac{\bar{X}_1 - \bar{X}_2}{SE_{(\bar{X}_1 - \bar{X}_2)}} = \frac{(81.0 - 63.0)}{5.74} = 3.1$$

$$t_{0.05(1),14}{}^a = 1.76$$

$$t_{0.01(1),14}{}^b = 2.62$$

Therefore, $P < 0.01$

[a] Read, "the one-tailed *t* value when $\alpha = 0.05$ and $df = 14$."
[b] Read, "the one-tailed *t* value when $\alpha = 0.01$ and $df = 14$."

standard error. With two samples, each sample has its own standard error; we then determine the standard error of the difference between the means. Although the derivation of the standard error between the means is beyond the scope of this chapter (see Feinstein[21]), the equation is similar to that for the one-sample test:

$$SE_{\bar{X}_1 - \bar{X}_2} = (SE_{\bar{X}_1}{}^2 + SE_{\bar{X}_2}{}^2)^{1/2} \qquad (12)$$

Alternate methods are available to calculate the standard error of the difference between means, one of which uses a pooled variance instead of the separate variances of equation (12).[21] Despite the different methods for calculation, the standard errors are similar.

Next, the difference between groups is divided by this standard error; this process produces the now familiar *t* statistic, which is then compared with the critical value from the tables. If the value for *t* exceeds the critical value, the null hypothesis is rejected; if *t* is less than the critical value, the null hypothesis cannot be rejected. An instinctive approach to the comparison between the calculated value for *t* and the critical value is as follows. The numerator is the difference between the mean values, an estimate of the distance between the location of the two samples. The denominator, shown in equation (12), is the standard error of the difference between means, an estimate of the variability within the samples. The ratio of these values estimates how much of the difference between means can be explained by the variability existing in the samples. If the variability within each of the samples is small, only a small difference between mean values should be sufficient to suggest that a difference exists between the samples. In contrast, if the variability within one or both of the samples is great, the difference between the means of the samples must be larger if the investigator is to have confidence that a difference exists between groups.

Before using a table of *t* values to determine the critical value for this example, we should consider one special aspect. In our hypothetical situation, we have been comparing blood pressure in normovolemic and hypovolemic individuals. Our a priori assumption is that blood pressure will be lower, rather than higher, in the hypovolemic group. Therefore, rather than perform a two-tailed comparison that would permit us to assess all possible relationships between the data, it would be appropriate to perform a one-tailed test. Because the critical value for *t* ($\alpha = 0.05$, $df = 14$) is lower for a one-tailed comparison (1.76) than for a two-tailed comparison (2.14), we have increased our chances of detecting a statistically significant difference by using the former.

In this example, the *t* statistic is markedly greater than the critical value; we conclude that it is unlikely ($P < 0.05$) that these two samples were selected from the same population. Therefore, the mean value for blood pressure is lower for these hypovolemic individuals than for normovolemic individuals. Since the *t* statistic is markedly greater than the critical value for $\alpha = 0.05$, we can refer to the table to determine the critical

TABLE 21-6. Application of the Paired *t* Test to Hypothetical Values for Cardiac Output (L/min) Before and After Administration of Pancuronium

Subject	Cardiac Output before Pancuronium (L/min)	Cardiac Output after Pancuronium (L/min)	Change in Cardiac Output (L/min)
1	4.3	5.7	+1.4
2	5.6	5.4	−0.2
3	3.9	4.6	+0.7
4	5.7	7.3	+1.6
5	4.8	6.0	+1.2
6	5.2	5.3	+0.1
Mean	4.92	5.72	0.80
SD	0.72	0.91	0.73
SE	0.29	0.37	0.30

$t = 0.80/0.30 = 2.69$

$t_{0.05(1),5}{}^{a} = 2.01$

Therefore, $P < 0.05$

[a] Read, "the one-tailed *t* value when $\alpha = 0.05$ and $df = 5$."

values for higher levels of significance. With 14 *df*, the one-tailed *t* is 2.62 when $\alpha = 0.01$ and 2.98 when $\alpha = 0.005$. Since the *t* statistic exceeds both these values, we can conclude that the likelihood of these samples being from the same population is extremely small, less than 0.005 or 1 in 200.

Paired-Sample t Tests

On occasion, an investigator obtains measurements before and after an intervention and then studies whether this intervention produced a significant effect. Under these circumstances, when the two samples being compared are in some way related to each other (paired), a *paired-sample* t test, more commonly called a *paired* t *test*, is used. For example, measuring cardiac output before and after the administration of pancuronium might produce the values shown in Table 21-6. In this instance, an informal appraisal of the data suggests a strong difference between the before and after values, since five of six subjects had an increase in cardiac output. The paired *t* test is used to confirm this observation. A new sample is created whose members are equal to the difference between before and after values for each subject. This new sample is then analyzed by the one-sample *t* test. The mean value for this sample is 0.80 L/min, and the standard error is 0.30 L/min. Therefore, the *t* statistic is 2.69, a value that exceeds the critical value of 2.01 (again, we can use a one-tailed test because we assume that pancuronium will increase, not decrease, cardiac output). We would conclude that the before and after measurements are unlikely to be from the same population. This conclusion suggests that pancuronium increases cardiac output.

An alternate statistical approach to this hypothetical situation would be to use the two-sample *t* test (Table 21-7). This test produces a value for *t* of 1.69, which is less than the critical value of 1.81. Despite the greater degrees of freedom for the two-sample test (10) than for the one-sample test (5), the unpaired test does not support our belief that a difference exists between the before and after values and the choice of an incorrect statistical test. This lack of confirmation results because of the variability of the before and after values.

Had the investigator obtained the before measurements in one group of subjects and the after measurements in another group, the paired test would not be applicable. For example, a change in cardiac output from 4 to 6 L/min in one subject means something entirely different than would the measurement of 4 L/min in one subject before pancuronium and the measurement of 6 L/min in a different subject after pancuronium.

Nonparametric *t* Tests: the Mann-Whitney *U* Test

Data on an ordinal scale require special treatment, since determining means and variances for this type of data is usually inappropriate. To make statistical com-

TABLE 21-7. Inappropriate Application of the Two-Sample *t* Test to the Hypothetical Analysis of Data of Table 21-6

$$SE_{(\overline{X}_1 - \overline{X}_2)} = \left[\frac{0.72^2}{6} + \frac{0.91^2}{6} \right] = 0.47$$

$$t = \frac{\overline{X}_1 - \overline{X}_2}{SE_{(\overline{X}_1 - \overline{X}_2)}} = (5.72 - 4.92)/0.47 = 1.69$$

$t_{0.05(1),10}{}^{a} = 1.81$

Therefore, $P > 0.05$

[a] Read, "the one-tailed *t* value when $\alpha = 0.05$ and $df = 10$."

parisons on ordinal data, nonparametric tests, which assess the relative ranks rather than the magnitude of the data, are applied. Most parametric tests have a corresponding nonparametric test.

Nonparametric tests are also valuable for analyzing samples that deviate strongly from the normal distribution. Although parametric tests are based on the assumption that distribution is normal, they are sufficiently powerful (statisticians use the term *robust*) to detect differences even when samples are not distributed normally. However, as the samples stray significantly from a normal distribution, parametric tests lose their ability to detect differences. In contrast, because nonparametric tests analyze only the ranks rather than the individual values, they may detect differences not detected by parametric tests.

The nonparametric test corresponding to the two-sample *t* test is the Mann-Whitney *U* test. With this test, the values in each of the two groups are assigned ranks. The smallest (or largest) value is assigned the rank 1; the next smallest (or next largest), the rank 2. This process continues until the largest (or smallest) value has been assigned the rank equal to the sum of the two sample sizes. If values are tied in rank, they are assigned a value equal to the average of the corresponding ranks. For example, if two samples are tied for ranks 4 and 5, both are assigned rank 4.5. The statistics r_1 and r_2 are equal to the sum of the ranks for groups 1 and 2, respectively. The test statistic, U, is determined by the following equation:

$$U = n_1 n_2 + \frac{n_1(n_1 + 1)}{2} - R_1 \quad (13)$$

The value for U is then compared with critical values for U obtained from a table. The data comparing the blood pressures of normovolemic and hypovolemic subjects (Table 21-5) can be analyzed by using the Mann-Whitney *U* test (Table 21-8). As with the two-sample *t* test, the results of the Mann-Whitney *U* test suggest a difference between the two groups ($P < 0.05$). Nonparametric tests such as the Mann-Whitney *U* test have not been used frequently in the anesthesia literature; however, because they are valuable for data sets that are not normally distributed, they should probably be used more frequently. The nonparametric version of the paired *t* test is the Wilcoxon paired-sample test.

Appropriate Use of the *t* Test

The critical values for *t* are calculated with the assumption that comparisons are being made between only two groups. If the investigator collected data on three groups of subjects, three comparisons would be possible: A versus B, A versus C, and B versus C. If each of these comparisons was made using the two-sample *t* test and $\alpha = 0.05$, we would be accepting a 5 percent risk of committing a type I error for each comparison. For three comparisons, the chance of committing a type I error increases to approximately 3×5 percent,

TABLE 21-8. Nonparametric Comparison of Hypothetical Data from Table 21-5 Using the Mann-Whitney *U* Test

Blood Pressure		Ranks	
Normovolemic	Hypovolemic	Normovolemic	Hypovolemic
77	72	11	7.5
91	62	15	4
101	51	16	2
81	81	12.5	12.5
76	47	10	1
68	74	6	9
72	52	7.5	3
82	65	14	5

$N_1 = 8$

$N_2 = 8$

$R_1 = (11 + 15 + \cdots + 14) = 92$

$R_2 = (7.5 + 4 + \cdots + 5) = 44$

$U = n_1 \times n_2 + n_1 \times (n_1 + 1)/2 - R_1 = 8 \times 8 + 8 \times 9/2 - 92 = 8$

or

$U' = n_1 \times n_2 + n_2 \times (n_2 + 1)/2 - R_2 = 8 \times 8 + 8 \times 9/2 - 44 = 56$

$U_{0.05(2),8,8}{}^a = 51$

$U_{0.01(2),8,8}{}^b = 57$

Therefore, $0.01 < P < 0.05$

[a] Read, "the two-tailed *U* value when $\alpha = 0.05$, $N_1 = 8$, and $N_2 = 8$."
[b] Read, "the two-tailed *U* value when $\alpha = 0.01$, $N_1 = 8$, and $N_2 = 8$."

or 15 percent (actually closer to 14 percent), a level that is usually considered unacceptable. As the number of groups increases, the number of possible comparisons increases such that, with enough groups, the investigator will eventually uncover a nonexistent difference.

Thus, the *t* test is properly used for comparing only two groups. When more than two groups are being compared, other tests, particularly analysis of variance, are more appropriate. If the investigator chooses to use the *t* test to compare more than two groups, a correction must be made to prevent type I errors. When one such correction, the *Bonferroni inequality* (or *correction*), is applied, the α level for each comparison is divided by the number of comparisons to be performed. For example, if the investigator chooses a value of 0.05 for α and three comparisons are possible, a value of 0.0167 for α should be used for each of the comparisons. Then, the investigator is able to state that, overall, the chance of committing a type I error is less than 5 percent.

If the Bonferroni inequality is used, the investigator must decide in advance which of the comparisons will be made. For example, if there are four groups, the investigator may choose to compare group 1 with each of the other groups (for example, if subjects in group 1 were given the placebo and subjects in groups 2 through 4 were given one of three different drugs). In this case, only three of the six possible comparisons will be made. However, it is inappropriate to examine the data and then decide which comparisons to make.

Multisample Tests: Analysis of Variance

Parametric Analysis of Variance

One-Way Analysis of Variance

The *t* test enabled examination of a single group or comparison of two groups. For comparison of three or more groups, another test, *analysis of variance* (also known as *single-factor analysis of variance* or *one-way analysis of variance*) is necessary. Analysis of variance is similar in principle to the two-sample *t* test. Using analysis of variance, we determine two values, one value describing the variability between groups, and the other describing the variability within the groups. For the two-sample *t* test, these values consisted of the difference between mean values and the standard error of the difference between the means. For analysis of variance, the square of corresponding values is used. The variability between groups is called the *between-groups* variance (also the *group variance*); variabilty within groups is called the *within-groups variance* (also the *error variance*). For the two-sample *t* test we divided the difference between the mean of each of the groups by the appropriate standard error; similarly, for analysis of variance, we divide the between-groups variance by the within-groups variance. This process produces the statistic *F*. As with the *t* test, this *F* value is compared with critical values from a table of *F* values: if *F* exceeds the critical value for the desired probability, we conclude that it is unlikely that the difference between the mean values occurred by chance and we reject the null hypothesis.

To determine the between-groups variance, we create a sample consisting of the mean values of the individual groups, determine its sum of squares, and divide by the apropriate degrees of freedom. However, the resulting value estimates the variance of the mean rather than of the population. Since we know that the variance of the mean is equal to the variance of the population divided by sample size (this is equivalent to saying that standard error of the mean is equal to standard deviation divided by the square root of the sample size), we can estimate the between-groups sum of squares by using the following:

$$\text{Between-groups SS} = \sum_{i=1}^{k} n_i (\overline{X}_i - \overline{X})^2 \qquad (14)$$

where *k* is the number of groups and n_i is the number of subjects in each group. the between-group variance (also known as the *between-groups mean square*) is then estimated using this equation:

$$\text{Between-groups MS} = \frac{\sum_{i=1}^{k} n_i (\overline{X}_i - \overline{X})^2}{k - 1} \qquad (15)$$

The within-groups sum of squares is obtained by calculating the sum of squares for each individual group and adding these values. This sum of squares is then divided by the appropriate degrees of freedom (the sum of degrees of freedom of the individual groups, i.e., one less than the size of each group), resulting in the within-groups mean square:

$$\text{Within-groups MS} = \frac{\sum_{i=1}^{k} \left[\sum_{j=1}^{n} (X_{ij} - \overline{X}_i)^2 \right]}{N - k} \qquad (16)$$

where *N* is the total number of subjects in all groups.

The Σ in brackets represents the sum of squares for each of the groups; the outer Σ means to sum these values. Having estimated the between-groups variance the between-groups mean square) and the within-groups variance (the within-groups mean square), we calculate their ratio, *F*:

$$F = \frac{\text{between-groups MS}}{\text{within-groups MS}} \qquad (17)$$

We then refer to a table of *F* values to learn whether this value exceeds the critical value. If *F* exceeds this value, we conclude that the difference between the mean values of the groups was not likely to occur as a result of the variability within groups. Thus, we can reject the null hypothesis and conclude that a difference exists between the groups.

In Table 21-9, analysis of variance is used to compare volumes of distribution for histodrenaline (the imaginary drug causing release of either histamine or epinephrine) in infants, children, and adults. The between-groups variance is 35,060 and the within-groups variance is 2,732.83; the resulting value for *F* is 12.83. Since this value exceeds the critical value for *F* for $\alpha = 0.05$ and the appropriate degrees of freedom (note that we must now consider the number of degrees of freedom in both the numerator and the denominator), we can conclude that it is unlikely that the three samples were selected from the same population.

One-Way Analysis of Variance: Intragroup Comparisons

Using analysis of variance, we tested the null hypothesis that there is no difference between the mean value of any of the multiple groups. If we reject the null hypothesis, we can conclude that at least one of the mean values differs from at least one of the other mean values, not that each of the groups is different from each of the other groups. For example, in Table 21-9, analysis of variance suggests that at least one group differs from the other groups. Examination of the data shows that the mean value for infants differs from the other mean values and that no difference appears to exist between children and adults. To verify this observation, we need to apply multiple comparison tests. These tests fall into one of several categories, depending on whether the

TABLE 21-9. Use of Single-Factor Analysis of Variance to Compare Hypothetical Values for Volume of Distribution (ml/kg) of Histodrenaline[a] in Three Age Groups

	Infants	Children	Adults
	465	291	192
	293	225	212
	371	287	270
	405	302	251
	451	210	290
N	5	5	5
Mean	397	263	243

Grand mean = (397 + 263 + 243)/3 = 301

Between-group
$$SS = 5(397 - 301)^2 + 5(263 - 301)^2 + 5(243 - 301)^2 = 70,120$$

Between-group $df = 3 - 1 = 2$

Between-group MS = 35,060

Infant SS = $(465 - 397)^2 + (293 - 397)^2 + \cdots = 19,096$

Child SS = $(291 - 263)^2 + (225 - 263)^2 + \cdots = 7,134$

Adult SS = $(192 - 243)^2 + (212 - 243)^2 + \cdots = 6,564$

Within-group SS = Infant SS + Child SS + Adult SS = 32,794

Within-group $df = 3(5 - 1) = 12$

Within-group MS = 2,732.83

$$F = \frac{\text{Between-group MS}}{\text{Within-group MS}} = 35060/2732.83 = 12.83$$

$F_{0.05(1),2,12}{}^b = 3.89$

$F_{0.0025(1),2,12}{}^c = 10.3$

Therefore, $P < 0.0025$ that at least one group mean differs from the others.

[a] An imaginary drug causing release of either histamine or epinephrine.
[b] Read, "the one-tailed F value when $\alpha = 0.05$, the between-groups $df = 2$, and the within-groups $df = 12$."
[c] Read, "the one-tailed F value when $\alpha = 0.0025$, the between-groups $df = 2$, and the within groups $df = 12$."

investigator is interested in all possible comparisons between pairs (the number of possible comparisons is equal to one-half the product of the number of groups and the number of groups minus one) or only specific comparisons.

All possible comparisons. A number of tests permit multiple comparisons, for example, the Newman-Keuls test (also known as the Student-Newman-Keuls test or SNK), Duncan's test, the least significant difference test (LSD), Tukey's test, and Scheffe's method. Although there is no consensus regarding the best multiple comparison test, the Student-Newman-Keuls test exemplifies the general procedure and will be described here.

To perform the Student-Newman-Keuls test, the investigator calculates the difference between the means of the largest and the smallest groups, followed by the next largest to the smallest, and so on, until all possible differences have been calculated. The standard error is determined in a manner similar to that for the t test, as the square root of the within-groups mean square (obtained from the analysis of variance) divided by the square root of the size of each of the samples.* The between-groups differences are then divided by the appropriate standard error, much as with the two-sample t test. This process produces the Student-Newman-Keuls statistic, q; critical values for q are also obtainable from a table. In evaluating differences between the extreme means and differences between the less extreme means, the Student-Newman-Keuls test considers the number of ranks (p) between the means being compared.[22] As a result, the critical values for q are based on the number of groups being spanned in the comparison. In Table 21-10, the Student-Newman-Keuls test is applied to the hypothetical data of Table 21-9.

For instructions regarding the use of other multiple comparison tests, the reader is referred to any standard textbook on statistics.

Comparison with the control value. The Student-Newman-Keuls test and other multiple comparison tests are valuable when all possible comparisons must be made. However, the investigator pays a penalty for the opportunity to perform all possible comparisons between pairs, a penalty that may not be acceptable when the investigator is interested in a limited number of comparisons. For example, if subjects were given either placebo or one of four drugs, the investigator may be interested only in the comparison of each of the four drugs with the control state, rather than any comparisons between the four drugs. Although there are 10 (i.e., 5 × 4/2) possible comparisons between the five groups, the investigator is interested in only four of these comparisons.

When an investigator is interested in only the comparisons between the control group and each of the test groups, Dunnett's test is most appropriate. First, the difference between the control mean and the mean of each of the other groups is determined. Then, the standard error is determined: SE = $(2s^2/n)^{0.5}$ where s^2 is the within-groups mean square determined by analysis of variance, and n is the size of each of the groups.† The differences between the control value and each of the

---

* With the Student-Newman-Keuls test, if sample sizes are unequal, the standard error is calculated as

$$\text{SE} = \left[\frac{s^2}{2}\left(\frac{1}{n_a} + \frac{1}{n_b} \right) \right]^{1/2} \tag{18}$$

where s^2 is the within-groups mean square, and n_a and n_b are the sizes of the two samples. Thus, standard error may differ for each of the comparisons if sample sizes differ.

† With Dunnett's test, if group sizes are unequal, standard error is calculated as

$$\text{SE} = \left[s^2 \left(\frac{1}{n_a} + \frac{1}{n_b} \right) \right]^{1/2} \tag{19}$$

where n_a and n_b are sizes of each of the samples.

TABLE 21-10. Application of the Student-Newman-Keuls Test for Multiple Comparisons with the Hypothetical Data from Table 21-9.

	Infants	Children	Adults
Mean	397	263	243
N	5	5	5

Error mean square = 2,732.83

$$SE = \left(\frac{2,732.83}{5}\right)^{1/2} = 23.4$$

Comparison	Difference	SE	q	p^a	$q_{0.05(2),12}{}^b$	Conclusion
Infants vs adults	154	23.4	6.58	3	3.77	$P < 0.05$
Infants vs children	134	23.4	5.73	2	3.08	$P < 0.05$
Children vs adults	20	23.4	0.85	2	3.08	$P < 0.05$

Therefore, the mean value for infants differs from that for children and adults. No difference exists between the mean values for childen and adults.

[a] The number of mean values (groups) across which the comparison is made.
[b] Read, "the q value when $\alpha = 0.05$ and $df = 12$."

other means are then divided by the appropriate standard error; the result is the test statistic, q'. As before, these values are compared with the appropriate critical value. Table 21-11 provides an example of how to apply Dunnett's test to compare systolic blood pressure for four hypothetical groups of subjects.

Specific comparisons. In certain instances, the investigator may desire to make only specific comparisons between groups. For example, in comparing the values for halothane minimum alveolar concentration (MAC) for six ethnic groups (e.g., Chinese, Japanese, German, French, Argentinian, and Peruvian), the investigator may be interested in only three (Chinese versus Japanese, German versus French, and Argentinian versus Peruvian) of the 15 ($6 \times 5/2$) possible comparisons. The multiple comparison tests described above would be inappropriate for this use. If the investigator is interested in only a small number of comparisons, it is occasionally appropriate to perform multiple t tests with the Bonferroni correction (Bonferroni inequality). As mentioned earlier, α values are adjusted to the number

TABLE 21-11. Application of Dunnett's Test to Systolic Blood Pressure for Hypothetical Subjects Given a Placebo or Premedications A, B, or C

	Group 1 (Placebo)	Group 2 (Premed. A)	Group 3 (Premed. B)	Group 4 (Premed. C)
	131	120	97	134
	127	117	105	147
	110	131	112	122
	125	110	121	138
	147	122	100	129
Mean	128	120	107	134
N	5	5	5	5

Error mean square (determined from analysis of variance) = 104.13

Standard errors = $[2(104.13)/5]^{0.5} = 6.45$

Comparison	Difference	SE	q'	p	$q'_{0.05(2),12}{}^a$	Conclusion
1 vs 3	21	6.45	3.25	3	2.42	$P < 0.05$
1 vs 2	8	6.45	1.24	2	2.12	$P > 0.05$
1 vs 4	6	6.45	0.93	2	2.12	$P > 0.05$

Therefore, compared with placebo, premedication B (but not premedication A or C) decreases systolic blood pressure.

[a] Read, "the q' value when $\alpha = 0.05$ and $df = 16$."

of comparisons to be performed. If the investigator is interested in performing three comparisons with an overall significance level of 0.05, the significance level is adjusted to 0.05/3 or 0.0167. For each of the comparisons, a level of 0.0167 must be achieved to permit the investigator to claim a difference between any of the groups. As the number of comparisons increases, the level of significance required by each (0.05 divided by the number of comparisons) is difficult to achieve, and the test becomes overly conservative (i.e., the investigator is unlikely to detect a difference even if one exists). To use Bonferroni's *t* test (the application of the Bonferroni inequality to the two-sample *t* test), the investigator must make an a priori decision as to which comparisons will be made. In the example described above, the choice of comparisons was based on geographic considerations. It is not considered acceptable to perform multiple *t* tests, make an a posteriori decision as to which are the most significant, and then use the Bonferroni inequality based on the number of comparisons that are likely to be significant.

Repeated-Measures (Two-Way) Analysis of Variance

Just as the paired *t* test may detect differences not found with the two-sample *t* test (when the study design has resulted in paired measurements), a paired test corresponding to analysis of variance *(repeated-measures analysis of variance)* may detect differences not found with single-factor analysis of variance. If the investigator obtains more than two measurements on each subject (each measurement on a subject will be called a *treatment*), repeated-measures analysis of variance should be employed. Just as the standard error for the paired *t* test was calculated in a manner different from that for the two-sample *t* test, the denominator for repeated-measures analysis of variance is calculated differently from that for single-factor analysis of variance. The within-subject variability results from two factors, namely, variability inherent to the subject (equivalent to the error variability for single-factor analysis of variance) and the variability resulting from the treatments. This can be stated as:

Within-subject SS = error SS + between-treatments SS

(20)

The within-subject sum of squares is determined by calculating the sum of squares for each subject and determining the sum of these values. The between-treatments (treatment) sum of squares (identical to the between-groups sum of squares for analysis of variance) is calculated from the sample of means for the treatments. The difference between the within-subject sum of squares and the treatment sum of squares is the error sum of squares [equation (20)]. The variances are determined by dividing the sums of squares by the appropriate degrees of freedom; *F* is the ratio of the treatment variance to the error variance.

Repeated-measures analysis of variance, rather than single-factor analysis of variance, should be used when-

TABLE 21-12. Application of Repeated-Measures Analysis of Variance to Hypothetical Data for Heart Rate (beats/minute) Before and After the Simultaneous Administration of Neostigmine and Atropine

	Drug Administration:			
	Before (beats/min)	1 min After (beats/min)	5 min After (beats/min)	15 min After (beats/min)
	67	92	87	68
	92	112	94	90
	58	71	69	62
	61	90	83	66
	72	85	72	69
Mean	70	90	81	71
N	5	5	5	5

Mean of individual subjects
  Subject 1 = 78.5
  Subject 2 = 97.0
  Subject 3 = 65.0
  Subject 4 = 75.0
  Subject 5 = 74.5

Within-subject
$$SS = [(67 - 78.5)^2 + (92 - 78.5)^2 + (87 - 78.5)^2 + (68 - 78.5)^2]$$
$$+ [(92 - 97)^2 + (112 - 97)^2 + \cdots] + [(58 - 65)^2 + \cdots]$$
$$+ [(61 - 75)^2 + \cdots] + [(72 - 74.5)^2 + \cdots] = 1,634$$

Grand mean = $(70 + 90 + 81 + 71)/4 = 78$

Treatment SS = $5(70 - 78)^2 + 5(90 - 78)^2 + 5(81 - 78)^2 + 5(71 - 78)^2 = 1,330$

Treatment $df = 4 - 1 = 3$

Treatment MS = 433.33

Error SS = Within-subject SS − treatment SS = $1,634 - 1,330 = 334$

Error $df = 3(5 - 1) = 12$

Error MS = 25.33

$$F = \frac{\text{Treatment MS}}{\text{Error MS}} = (433.33/25.33) = 17.50$$

$F_{0.05(1),3,12}{}^a = 3.49$

$F_{0.0005(1),3,12}{}^b = 12.7$

Therefore, heart rate at one time interval differs from heart rate at another time interval. A multiple comparison test (such as the Student-Newman-Keuls test or Dunnett's test) is necessary to determine which of these groups differs from the remainder.

[a] Read, "the one-tailed *F* value when α = 0.05, the treatment *df* = 3, and the error *df* = 12."
[b] Read, "the one-tailed *F* value when α = 0.05, the treatment *df* = 3, and the error *df* = 12."

ever two or more measurements are obtained on the same subject.* For example, to assess the effects of neostigmine and atropine on heart rate, we might measure heart rate before drug administration and 1, 5, and 15 minutes after drug administration (Table 21-12).

---

* If repeated-measures analysis of variance is used to compare two measurements, the results will be identical to those of the paired *t* test.

When repeated-measures analysis of variance is performed, F is 17.50, a value that exceeds the critical value. In Table 21-13, these same hypothetical data are analyzed inappropriately by using analysis of variance. When this technique is applied, F is 2.83, a value less than the critical value, despite the greater degrees of freedom. This situation is analogous to that shown in Tables 21-5 and 21-6, in which the paired t test suggested differences not supported by the two-sample t test.

As with analysis of variance, repeated-measures analysis of variance permits the conclusion that at least one group differs from the others regarding heart rate and the administration of neostigmine and atropine. In the example shown in Table 21-12, we were able to conclude that at least one of the groups differs from the others. To determine which of the group means differs, we must apply the multiple comparison tests described earlier.

Nonparametric Analysis of Variance: the Kruskal-Wallis Test and Friedman's Test

A nonparametric version of analysis of variance, the Kruskal-Wallis test, can be used for ordinal data, or for ratio or interval data, particularly those data that are not distributed normally. The test is performed by ranking the values in much the same manner as for the Mann-Whitney U test. The sums of ranks are determined, and a test statistic, H, is calculated:

$$H = \frac{12}{N(N+1)} \sum_{i=1}^{k} \frac{R_i^2}{n_i} - 3(N+1) \qquad (21)$$

where n_i is the number of observations in the kth group,

TABLE 21-13. Inappropriate Application of One-Way Analysis of Variance to the Hypothetical Data from Table 21-12

Grand mean = 78
Between-group SS = $5(70 - 78)^2 + 5(90 - 78)^2 \cdots = 1{,}330$

Between-group $df = 4 - 1 = 3$

Between-group MS = 433.33

Within-group SS = $[(67 - 70) + (92 - 70) + (58 - 70) \cdots]$
$+ [(92 - 90) + (112 - 90) + \cdots]$
$+ [(87 - 81) + (94 - 81)] + \cdots]$
$+ [(68 - 71) + (90 - 71)] + \cdots]$
$= 2{,}510$

Within-group $df = 4(5 - 1) = 16$

Within-group MS = 156.88

$F = \dfrac{\text{Between-group MS}}{\text{Within-group MS}} = 433.33/156.88 = 2.83$

$F_{0.05(1),3,16}{}^a = 3.24$

Therefore, when this inappropriate statistical test is used, $P > 0.05$.

[a] Read, "the one-tailed F value when $\alpha = 0.05$, the between-group $df = 3$, and the within-group $df = 16$."

k is the number of groups, N is the total number of observations, and R_i is the sum of ranks in each group.

The H value is then compared with the critical value obtained from a table. Although a nonparametric version of the Student-Newman-Keuls test exists, it unfortunately requires equal sample sizes for each of the groups.

Friedman's test is a nonparametric version of repeated-measures analysis of variance. As with the Kruskal-Wallis test, ranks, rather than the individual values, are used in the analysis. The test is extremely powerful for the analysis of data in which repeated measures are obtained on the same subject. Nonparametric versions of tests to perform intragroup comparisons (e.g., the Student-Newman-Keuls test) also exist.

Contingency Tables and Chi-Square Analysis

For data on an ordinal or nominal scale, different techniques are available for the presentation and analysis of results. Histograms, which are valuable for presentation of ratio or interval data, are of limited value, since ordinal and nominal data can assume only a limited number of values. To present ordinal or nominal data collected for two or more variables simultaneously, the investigator might use a *contingency table*, that is, a table displaying the frequency of occurrence of events or characteristics. Contingency tables are described by the number of rows and columns they contain, for example, a 2 × 4 contingency table has two rows and four columns. Table 21-14 is an example of a 2 × 2 contingency table depicting the hypothetical incidences of succinylcholine-induced myalgias with "Antisore" (an imaginary defasciculating drug) or placebo. Examination of these data suggests that the incidence of myalgias is markedly lower after administration of Antisore than after administration of a placebo. Statistical confirmation of this observation requires varying the techniques described previously. This section describes analysis of ordinal data using a variation of the z test, followed by an introduction to another variant of the z test, χ^2 analysis.

For the data presented in Table 21-14, the incidence of myalgias in each group can be described as the number of patients having myalgias divided by the total number in that group (N). This ratio, the proportion (p), is analogous to the central location for ratio or

TABLE 21-14. A 2 × 2 Contingency Table Depicting Hypothetical Incidence of Succinylcholine-Induced Myalgias in Subjects Given "Antisore"[a] vs Placebo

	No. of Subjects		
	Myalgias	No Myalgias	Total
Antisore	8	22	30
Placebo	16	9	25
Total	24	31	55

[a] An imaginary defasciculating drug.

interval data. To perform a statistical analysis, we need to determine the standard deviation for these samples. If we assign the value 1 to subjects having the attribute (in this instance, myalgias), the value zero to subjects not having the attribute, and the mean equal to p, we can use equation (7) to determine the sample standard deviation:

$$s = \left[\frac{(1-p)^2 + (1-p)^2 + \cdots + (0-p)^2 + (0-p)^2}{n} \right]^{1/2} \tag{22}$$

This equation can be simplified to

$$s = [p(1-p)]^{1/2} \tag{23}$$

Since standard error of the mean is equal to standard deviation divided by the square root of the sample size, the standard error is equal to

$$SE = \frac{[p(1-p)]^{1/2}}{n^{1/2}} \tag{24}$$

Table 21-15 shows the computation of standard error for each of the hypothetical samples from Table 21-14. Then, to compute the test statistic, we must determine the standard error of the difference between the two proportions:

$$SE_{(p_2 - p_1)} = [\hat{p}(1-\hat{p})/n_1 + \hat{p}(1-\hat{p})/n_2]^{1/2} \tag{25}$$

where $\hat{p}$ is the proportion determined by combining the groups (e.g., 24/55 for the values reported in Table

21-14). This method of calculating the standard error of the difference between two proportions is similar to that used to determine the standard error of the difference between two means in the two-sample t test. The test statistic z is then calculated as

$$z = \frac{p_2 - p_1}{SE_{(p_2 - p_1)}} \tag{26}$$

This value for z is then compared with the critical value obtained from a table. As before, if the value for z exceeds the critical value, the null hypothesis (that the two samples were drawn from the same population) is rejected, and we conclude that a difference probably exists between the two samples.

This approach to determining statistical difference between proportions is mathematically cumbersome, since the investigator must determine several standard deviations and standard errors. An alternate approach, χ^2 analysis, arrives at identical conclusions using many fewer mathematical calculations. To use χ^2 analysis, the investigator creates a second contingency table (Table 21-16), the values of which correspond to the values expected to occur if no difference existed between the two treatments. For example, of the 55 subjects in Table 21-14, 24 had myalgias, the overall incidence being 43.6 percent. Had there been no difference between treatments, we would expect 13 (actually 13.1) of the 30 subjects given Antisore and 11 (actually 10.9) of the subjects given a placebo to experience myalgias. The χ^2 statistic is determined as follows:

$$\chi^2 = \Sigma \frac{(O - E)^2}{E} \tag{27}$$

where O is the observed frequency and E is the expected frequency. If the observed frequencies are similar to the expected frequencies, the squared differences will be small relative to the expected values, and the value for χ^2 will be small. Conversely, large differences between expected and observed values will result in a large value for χ^2. This value for χ^2 is then compared with the critical value. To determine the critical value, we must first determine the degrees of freedom. Unlike the previously discussed statistical techniques, in which the degrees of freedom were a function of the size of the samples, degrees of freedom for χ^2 analysis

TABLE 21-15. Calculation of the Standard Error of a Proportion, the Standard Error of the Difference between Proportions, and the z Statistic for the Hypothetical Data from Table 21-14

For Antisore[a]: $P_1 = 8/30$, $N = 30$

$$SE_{P_1} = \frac{\left[\frac{8}{30}\left(1 - \frac{8}{30}\right) \right]^{1/2}}{30^{1/2}} = 0.081$$

For placebo: $P_2 = 16/25$, $N = 25$

$$SE_{P_2} = \frac{\left[\frac{16}{25}\left(1 - \frac{16}{25}\right) \right]^{1/2}}{25^{1/2}} = 0.096$$

For the difference between Antisore and placebo

$$SE_{(P_2 - P_1)} = \left[\frac{\frac{24}{55}\left(1 - \frac{24}{55}\right)}{30} + \frac{\frac{24}{55}\left(1 - \frac{24}{55}\right)}{25} \right] = 0.134$$

Calculation of the z statistic

$$z = \frac{P_2 - P_1}{SE_{(P_2 - P_1)}}$$

$$z = \frac{0.64 - 0.27}{0.134} = 2.78$$

$z_{0.05}{}^b = 1.96$

[a] An imaginary defasciculating drug.
[b] Read, "the two-tailed z value when $\alpha = 0.05$."

TABLE 21-16. A 2 × 2 Contingency Table of Hypothetical Expected Values for Succinylcholine-Induced Myalgias if No Difference Existed Between "Antisore"[a] and Placebo

	No. of Subjects		
	Myalgias	No Myalgias	Total
Antisore	13.1	16.9	30
Placebo	10.9	14.1	25
Total	24	31	55

[a] An imaginary defasciculating drug.

TABLE 21-17. Calculation of the χ^2 Statistic Using the Hypothetical Data from Table 21-15

$$\chi^2 = \frac{(8-13.1)^2}{13.1} + \frac{(16-10.9)^2}{10.9} + \frac{(22-16.9)^2}{16.9} + \frac{(9-14.1)^2}{14.1}$$
$$= 7.75$$

$\chi^2_{0.05(2),1}{}^a = 3.84$

Therefore, $P < 0.05$

---
^{a} Read, "the two-tailed χ^2 value when $\alpha = 0.05$ and $df = 1$."

TABLE 21-18. Use of the Yate's Correction to Determine χ^2 Statistic for the Hypothetical Data from Table 21-15

$$\chi^2 = \frac{(|8-13.1|-0.5)^2}{13.1} + \frac{(|16-10.9|-0.5)^2}{10.9}$$
$$+ \frac{(|22-16.9|-0.5)^2}{16.9}$$
$$+ \frac{(|9-14.1|-0.5)^2}{14.1} = 6.28$$

$\chi^2_{0.05(2),1}{}^a = 3.84$

Therefore, using the Yate's correction, $P < 0.05$.

---
^{a} Read, "the two-tailed χ^2 value when $\alpha = 0.05$ and $df = 1$."

are a function of the dimension of the contingency table, the product of the number of rows minus one and the number of columns minus one. This contingency table includes two rows and two columns, resulting in $(2-1) \times (2-1)$, or 1 df. The critical value for χ^2 is determined from the χ^2 table using the appropriate degrees of freedom. χ^2 analysis of the data from Table 21-14 is performed in Table 21-17. Note that the value for χ^2, 7.75, approximates the square of the value for z obtained in Table 21-15 (differences are due to rounding errors). This occurrence is due to the fact that χ^2 analysis is mathematically equivalent to z analysis.

Yate's Correction

As mentioned earlier, the population sum of squares underestimates the sample sum of squares; therefore, a correction factor, a smaller denominator (usually $n-1$, instead of n) must be applied to ensure reliable estimates for various statistics such as t and F. A similar problem exists with χ^2 analysis of 2×2 tables. This problem is usually resolved by using the Yate's (continuity) correction. Instead of using equation (27) to calculate χ^2, the following equation is preferable:

$$\chi^2 = \Sigma \frac{(|O-E|-0.5)^2}{E} \tag{28}$$

where $|O-E|$ means the absolute value of $O-E$.

Yate's correction reduces the numerator for each value and produces values for χ^2 that are smaller than those obtained with equation (27). These values are less likely to result in a type I error and should always be used to analyze 2×2 tables. The data from Table 21-14 are reanalyzed by using χ^2 analysis and the Yate's correction in Table 21-18. There is no comparable correction procedure for larger contingency tables.

Larger Contingency Tables

An investigator will frequently obtain data involving more than two groups or possible outcomes. These data can also be presented in contingency tables and analyzed by χ^2 analysis. Table 21-19 provides a larger contingency table (2×4) for hypothetical incidences of vomiting associated with four doses of an imaginary antiemetic drug, "Calm". Determination of the χ^2 statistic is performed in a similar manner, by summing the squared differences between the observed and expected values and then dividing this value by the expected values. The resulting value is then compared with the critical value for χ^2 for 3 df [$(4 < 1) \times (2-1)$].

Limits of Chi-Square Analysis

The assumptions of χ^2 analysis are valid only when certain conditions are met. For 2×2 tables, the expected value for each of the cells must be at least 5 or the resulting value for χ^2 will be biased (i.e., may suggest that a difference exists when, in fact, it does not); if the expected value for one or more cells is less than 5, the Fisher exact test[14] (a test involving binomial distributions) is recommended. For larger tables, the expected value for each cell should be at least 1.0, and no more than 20 percent of the cells should have expected values of less than 5.0. Violating this condition results in biased estimates for χ^2 and should be avoided either by combining columns or rows to form a smaller contingency table or by collecting additional data.

TABLE 21-19. Calculation of the χ^2 Statistic for a 4×2 Contingency Table Representing Hypothetical Incidences of Vomiting with "Calm"^{a}

	Observed Frequency		Expected Frequency	
	Vomiting	No Vomiting	Vomiting	No Vomiting
Placebo	9	11	8.5	11.5
Calm, 1 mg	10	10	8.5	11.5
Calm, 2 mg	8	12	8.5	11.5
Calm, 4 mg	7	13	8.5	11.5
Total	34	46	34	46

$$\chi^2 = \frac{(9-8.5)^2}{8.5} + \frac{(10-8.5)^2}{8.5} + \frac{(8-8.5)^2}{8.5} + \frac{(7-8.5)^2}{8.5}$$
$$+ \frac{(11-11.5)^2}{11.5} + \frac{(10-11.5)^2}{11.5} + \frac{(12-11.5)^2}{11.5} + \frac{(13-11.5)^2}{11.5}$$
$$= 1.02$$

$\chi^2_{0.05(2),3}{}^b = 7.82$.

Therefore, $P > 0.05$.

---
^{a} An imaginary antiemetic drug.
^{b} Read, "the two-tailed χ^2 value when $\alpha = 0.05$ and $df = 3$."

Analysis of Linear Regression and Correlation Coefficient

Earlier in this chapter, statistics was used to compare values for different variables, for example, blood pressure in hypovolemic versus normovolemic patients, blood pressure before and after the administration of pancuronium, and the effects of placebo versus those of premedications. In these analyses, the independent variable was divided into discrete groups. In certain instances, dividing the independent variable into discrete groups may be undesirable or impossible. For example, the subjects in Table 21-5 were categorized as either normovolemic or hypovolemic, despite the fact that there are various degrees of hypovolemia, each of which might be associated with differing amounts of hypotension. To investigate the association between the degree of hypovolemia and the extent of hypotension, the investigator might measure systolic blood pressure while inducing various degrees of hypovolemia by removing blood. These values might then be plotted on a scattergram (Fig. 21-4), which is similar to a two-dimensional histogram.* The scattergram permits the investigator to examine the relationship between the independent variable (in this case, the amount of blood loss) and the dependent variable (blood pressure). Figure 21-4 shows that larger amounts of volume loss are associated with lower blood pressures.

This relationship also could be analyzed with Student's *t* test by dividing the independent variable into two groups, mild hypovolemia (less than 10 ml/kg) and severe hypovolemia (10 to 25 ml/kg). The investigator would find that blood pressure was lower during severe blood loss than during mild blood loss. Moreover, several smaller groups could be formed, depending on the amount of blood loss, thus permitting the use of analysis of variance.

The limitation of these analyses, however, is that they do not describe the apparently linear relationship existing between blood loss and blood pressure observed in Figure 21-4. There is no discrete difference in blood pressure with blood loss of more than or less than 10 ml/kg; instead, the relationship between the two variables appears to be continuous. The slope and the *Y* intercept of the line that best describes that relationship are determined by using *analysis of linear regression*. The equation for this line is

$$\hat{Y} = \alpha X + \beta$$

---

* In a scattergram, the independent variable is plotted on the x axis, the dependent variable on the y axis. When one variable is used to "predict" another (e.g., when one assesses the accuracy of end-tidal PCO_2 to predict $PaCO_2$, end-tidal values should be plotted on the x axis and arterial values on the y axis. When there is no causal relationship between two variables (e.g., if one were to examine the relationship between heart rate and blood pressure in subjects who were hypovolemic), either variable can be plotted on the x axis.

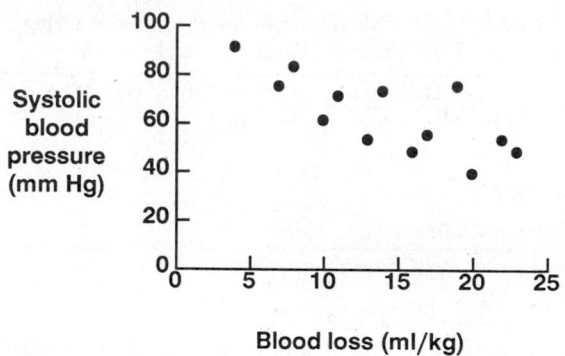

Fig. 21-4. This scattergram results from the plotting of a hypothetical set of values for two variables (in this instance, blood loss and systolic blood pressure) having a linear relationship.

where α is the slope, and β the *Y* intercept, of the line ($\hat{Y}$ is read Y-hat). The line that fits best is one that minimizes the sum of squared differences between the values of *Y* and $\hat{Y}$. This accounts for the other name for linear regression analysis, *least-squares regression*. The distance between each point and the line is equal to $Y - \hat{Y}$, or $Y - (\alpha X + \beta)$; the sum of squared distances can be written as

$$\text{Sum of squared distances} = \Sigma[Y - (\alpha X + \beta)]^2 \quad (29)$$

The reader knowledgeable in calculus will realize that when the partial derivatives of the equation with respect to α and β are equal to zero, the sum of squared distance is minimized. These simultaneous equations can be solved to yield the following equations for slope and intercept of the least-squares regression line:

$$\alpha = \frac{\Sigma(X_i - \overline{X})(Y_i - \overline{Y})}{\Sigma(X_i - \overline{X})^2} \quad (30)$$

$$\beta = \overline{Y} - \alpha\overline{X} \quad (31)$$

Table 21-20 demonstrates analysis of linear regression for the hypothetical data in Figure 21-4. The line produced by this technique (Fig. 21-5) lies close to all the data points. Just as the index of central tendency was a value near the center of the population, the least-squares regression line lies near the center of the values: seven of the data points are above the line and six are below.

Using analysis of linear regression, we were able to minimize the sum of squared distances between this sample of points and the regression line. With a second sample, analysis of linear regression would identify a different (although possibly similar) *best-fit* line. Each different sample would result in a different line, resulting eventually in a family of best-fit lines.

Just as the standard error of the mean describes the variability with which the sample mean located the population mean, so do some statistical techniques assess the variability (*goodness of fit*) of this family of regression lines. The first test, an analysis of variance, evalu-

TABLE 21-20. Analysis of Linear Regression for Data shown in Figure 21-4

$\overline{X} = 14.2$
$\overline{Y} = 62.5$
Slope $= -1.964$
Intercept $= 90.26$
Total sum of squares $= 2,927.3$
Regression sum of squares $= 1,657.5$
Residual sum of squares $= 1,269.8$
Regression mean square $= 1,657.5$
Residual mean square $= 115.4$
$F = 1,657.5/115.4 = 14.4$
$r^2 = 1,657.5/2,927.3 = 0.57$
$r = -0.75$
Standard error of the estimate $= 115.4^{1/2} = 10.7$

ates whether the regression analysis suggests a trend between the independent and dependent variables. The investigator first determines the regression sum of squares, which is equal to the variability resulting from the linear regression:

$$\text{Regression sum of squares} = \Sigma(\hat{Y} - \overline{Y})^2 \qquad (32)$$

This can be simplified to

$$\text{Regression sum of squares} = (\Sigma xy)^2/\Sigma x^2 \qquad (33)$$

where Σxy is another notation for $\Sigma(X_i - \overline{X})(Y_i - \overline{Y})$, and Σx^2 is equivalent to $\Sigma(X_i - \overline{X})^2$, or

$$\text{Regression sum of squares} = \text{slope} \times \Sigma xy \qquad (34)$$

which has 1 *df*.

As with analysis of variance, the total sum of squares can be partitioned into two components, the regression sum of squares and the residual sum of squares, which

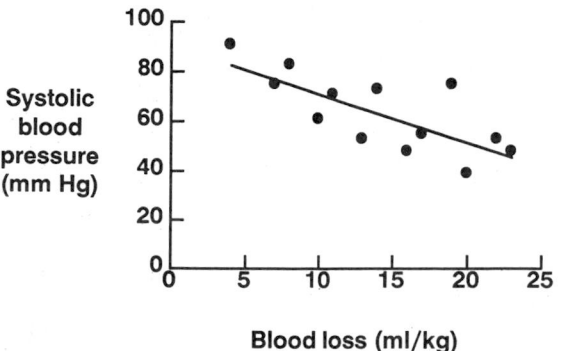

Fig. 21-5. The best-fit line for hypothetical data in Figure 21-4 using analysis of linear regression.

is the variability not accounted for by the regression, that is, the sum of squared distance between Y_i and $\hat{Y}$:

$$\text{Residual sum of squares} = \Sigma(Y_i - \hat{Y})^2 \qquad (35)$$

The residual sum of squares has $N - 2$ *df*. The ratio between the regression mean square and the residual mean square,

$$F = \frac{\text{Regression mean square}}{\text{Residual mean square}} \qquad (36)$$

is then compared with the critical value for F obtained from a table. If F exceeds the critical value, the regression is significant, that is, a relationship exists between the independent and dependent variables. If F is less than the critical value, the slope does not differ from zero, and the analysis does not support the hypothesis that an association exists between the independent and dependent variables.

The residual mean square (often noted as $s^2_{y\cdot x}$) has a second important role. Its square root, $s_{y\cdot x}$, called the *standard error of the estimate* (or occasionally, the *standard error of the regression*) represents the average deviation of y values from the regression line. The standard error of the estimate provides an estimate for regression analysis in a way similar to the way standard deviation describes variability of the sample (i.e., the standard error of the estimate is actually the standard deviation, not the standard error, of the distance between the y values and the regression line). For the sample described in Figure 21-4, the standard error of the estimate is 12.3, a value that represents the average distance of the points from the regression line.

The third method of describing fit to the regression line is by determining the correlation coefficient. The variability of the dependent variable, Y, has already been partitioned into two components, the component that is accounted for by the regression line (the regression sum of squares) and the component that is not accounted for by the regression line (the residual sum of squares). The sum of these sums of squares, the total sum of squares, can also be expressed as

$$\text{Total sum of squares} = (Y_i - \overline{Y})^2 \qquad (37)$$

The ratio of the regression sum of squares to the total sum of squares is equal to the percentage of the variability of one variable explained by the variability of the other variable. This ratio, r^2, is known as the *coefficient of determination*. If the regression line fits the sample exactly, the error sum of squares is equal to zero and the regression sum of squares is equal to the total sum of squares. This results in a coefficient of determination equal to 1. The greater the distance between the values in the sample and the regression line, the larger the value of the error sum of squares and the smaller the value of r^2. The value for r^2 always lies between zero and 1, with larger values implying a better fit between the regression line and the sample. More commonly reported than r^2 is its square root, r, known as the *correlation coefficient* or the *product-moment correlation coefficient.* Since r^2 is always between zero and 1, its square root will always lie between -1 and $+1$, and its sign is identical to that of the slope. The advantage of using the coefficient of determination and the correlation coefficient is that they lack units, whereas the slope of the regression line depends on the magnitude of the units used to express the independent and dependent variables.

In addition to these techniques to evaluate the significance and goodness of fit of a regression line, a number of techniques compare the slopes and positions of two or more regression lines. These techniques can also be applied to two or more dose–response curves or to

The investigator who uses analysis of linear regression must decide which results to report to the reader. It is often tempting to search a computer output for a statement of probability such as $P = 0.02$. Reporting only this value limits the information provided to the reader, since it provides no information as to the goodness of fit of the regression line. This is particularly important with large samples in which it is possible to obtain significant probabilities for the regression line (e.g., $P = 0.05$), despite large standard errors of the estimate and poor coefficients of determination. The variability of the regression analysis is better described by two statistics, the standard error of the estimate and the coefficient of determination (or the correlation coefficient). The standard error of the estimate describes the average distance of the points from the regression line, whereas the coefficient of determination describes the proportion of the variance that can be accounted for by the regression.

Logistic Regression

Certain types of data, for example the relationship between dose and effect, seem appropriate for analysis by using regression techniques. On occasion, effect is recorded in terms of a quantal response (e.g., yes or no) rather than as discrete values; in this instance, analysis of linear regression may not be the appropriate statistical technique. For example, the relationship between the dose of thiopental and loss of the lid reflex is probably sigmoidal, rather than linear, in shape. Forcing a linear analysis onto nonlinear data may produce spurious results, particularly regarding nonlinear portions of the sigmoid curve. For example, because the middle portion of a sigmoid curve is linear, estimations of the ED_{50} (the dose producing 50 percent effect) may be accurate using analysis of linear regression; however, analysis of linear regression is likely to produce flawed estimates for ED_{95} (the dose producing 95 percent effect).

Special techniques are available for the analysis of these types of data. One simple technique that could be accomplished readily without a computer was the probit analysis technique popularized by Litchfield and Wilcoxon.[23] Recently, a technique called logistic regression has become popular. Although the mathemat-

ics of this technique are beyond the scope of this chapter, logistic regression permits the investigator to determine the best sigmoid curve that fits the data. As with linear regression, for each data set, one can determine such values as the ED_{50} and its 95 percent confidence limits; in addition, one can compare two or more curves. Logistic regression is a powerful tool for the analysis of epidemiologic data (e.g., data involving the effects of anesthetic techniques on outcome) and will be seen with increasing frequency in the medical literature.

Sequential Analysis

To compare the results of two treatments, the investigator first estimates the difference in outcomes for each treatment and uses this difference to estimate how many subjects will be required to demonstrate a statistical difference between treatments. Once the study has commenced, the investigator should not analyze the results until the predetermined number of studies has been performed.[24] In addition, should this number of subjects not yield statistically significant results, the investigator should not increase the number of subjects studied until statistical significance is achieved. These requirements are based on the same rationale as support the prohibition against multiple t tests: the test statistic is based on the assumption that only one comparison is to be made between the two treatments.

In certain instances it is vital to determine rapidly which treatment is more efficacious. For example, if the cost of conducting trials is excessive, or if knowledge of an improved therapy might greatly influence morbidity, the investigator might desire to learn very quickly the difference between treatments. Sequential analysis is particularly suited for this purpose.[25] The investigator uses a chart similar to that shown in Figure 21-6. Paired subjects are given treatments (e.g., one subject is given an antiemetic drug; another subject is given a placebo), and their scores regarding some predetermined response (e.g., vomiting) are compared. If scores are the same, or tied (e.g., vomiting occurred in both trials), the results are ignored. If a difference exists that favors the antiemetic drug, a mark is made one unit upward and to the right; if a difference exists that favors the placebo, a mark is made one unit downward and to the right. Once the mark leaves the hatched area, the trial is complete. If the resulting line is above the enclosed area, the trial favors the antiemetic drug; if the resulting line is below the enclosed area, the trial favors the placebo. Completion of the trial beyond the right-hand border indicates that no statistical difference exists between the two treatments. Using sequential analysis, Abramowitz et al.[26] demonstrated the antiemetic effect of droperidol using only 11 untied treatment pairs and a total of 42 subjects. In contrast, Cohen et al.[27] found that the incidence of vomiting was lower in subjects given droperidol than in those given a placebo, but were unable to demonstrate a statistical difference using χ^2 analysis.

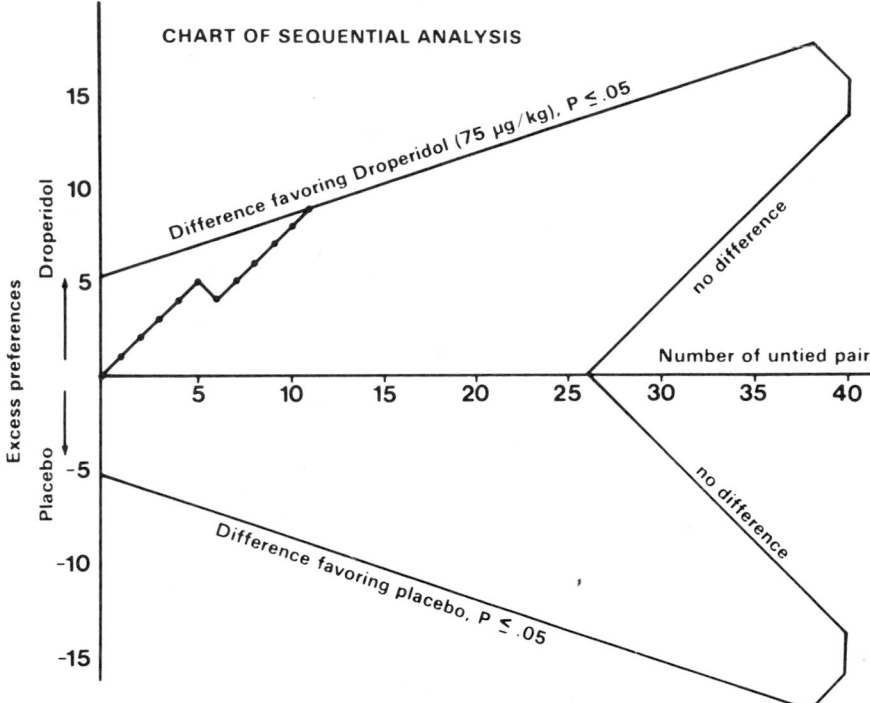

Fig. 21-6. Using sequential analysis, Abramowitz et al.[26] demonstrated that droperidol decreased the incidence of postoperative vomiting. (From Abramowitz et al.,[26] with permission.)

RESEARCH METHODOLOGY AND STUDY DESIGN

Too often, an investigation begins without a well-designed plan regarding the design of the study and the statistical analysis. After the study is under way or completed and the investigators have accumulated a large mass of data, they begin to contemplate its analysis. Unfortunately, in many instances, data are collected in an inappropriate manner or the study was not designed to permit the question of interest to be answered. This chapter is not designed to address the many issues related to study design; instead the reader is referred to other sources such as a recent monograph, "Medical Uses of Statistics,"[28] published by the *New England Journal of Medicine*. Unfortunately, much research effort has been wasted by not considering issues of study design or the type of statistical analysis prior to beginning the study.

STATISTICAL ERRORS

Many clinicians and investigators distrust statistical analysis. Sometimes this distrust is based, in part, on lack of knowledge of the terms used by the investigator or on the inability of the investigator to communicate thoughts clearly. However, distrust also occurs when the data presented in a manuscript appear to contradict the statistical conclusions. For example, one study reported that the elimination half-life of theophyllines was 216 minutes in one group and 72 minutes in a second group, a threefold difference the authors claimed was not statistically significant.[29] In contrast, distribution half-lives for the same groups were 2.7 minutes and 3.0 minutes, a 10 percent difference for which the authors claimed statistical significance ($P < 0.05$). Because neither individual data points nor standard deviations were reported, the reader was unable to examine the data and draw conclusions; thus, the reader can only be suspicious regarding the conclusion.

Perhaps the most common error is presentation of descriptive data without indicating whether the values for variability represent the standard deviation or the standard error. Since there is no consensus or conventional practice regarding which of these should be reported, investigators may be tempted to report the smaller value (suggesting less variability in the data), the standard error, without identifying it as such. The reader may have insufficient information to determine which value is being reported. This problem occurs less frequently than in past years, probably because of the heightened interest in statistics in recent years.[30,31]

Another error is to use sample sizes that are too small to detect expected differences. The denominator used in *t* tests and analysis of variance is the variability within the groups, a value determined by using sample size [see equation (16)]. If sample size is small, the denominator will be large, and the *t* or *F* value will be smaller than it would be with a large sample size. Thus, the investigator may be unable to detect differences between groups.

An additional reason for obtaining the wrong statistical conclusion is the use of the wrong statistical test. This error occurs most frequently when multiple *t* tests are performed without applying the appropriate correction. The resulting type I errors can be avoided by using the appropriate statistical test, such as analysis of variance. Alternately, the investigator might select a test that is inappropriately strict. For example, if three or more measurements were obtained on the same subject, the investigator would be correct in avoiding multiple paired *t* tests. Unless the investigator is knowledgeable of statistical techniques such as repeated-measures analysis of variance, one-way analysis of variance might erroneously be used, a test that ignores the information gained by obtaining repeated measurements on the same subject. Just as the two-sample *t* test may be unable to find differences that can be detected with a paired *t* test (assuming that paired measurements were obtained), a one-way analysis of variance may be unable to find differences that can be detected with the repeated-measures test. Frequently, investigators recognize the value of statistical tests that consider that paired measurements were obtained, but they are unaware that appropriate tests such as repeated-measures analysis of variance exist. In response, they analyze their data first with a one-way analysis of variance (a test that is inappropriately strict), then with paired *t* tests with or without the Bonferroni correction. If the Bonferroni correction is applied, the analysis may be too strict; if it is not applied, the analysis is too lenient. Regardless, the analysis could have been performed more appropriately with a repeated-measures analysis of variance and one of the multiple comparison tests described earlier. Use of one-way analysis of variance instead of the more appropriate repeated-measures analysis of variance occurs frequently in the anesthesia literature. Using a statistical test with inadequate sensitivity often prevents investigators from determining the correct result.

SELECTING THE APPROPRIATE STATISTICAL TEST

Most statistics courses focus attention on the techniques necessary to perform statistical analysis and give the student examples of each statistical test. In contrast, when performing research, the investigator must decide which statistical test is appropriate for the data collected. Because statistics courses emphasize performance of the tests rather than study design and how to select the appropriate test, the investigator may have difficulty selecting the appropriate test. Ironically, with the great availability of hand-held calculators, micro-

computers, and even user-friendly mainframe computers, performing complicated statistical tests is now possible for almost all medical investigators. The greatest difficulty therefore lies in selecting the appropriate test.

The first question the investigator should ask is, "What type of data have I obtained?" If the data are on a nominal scale, the choice of analytic techniques is generally limited to χ^2 analysis. For data on an ordinal scale, the investigator is generally restricted to nonparametric analyses. For data on a ratio or interval scale, a large variety of tests, both parametric and nonparametric, are appropriate. To choose between parametric and nonparametric tests, the investigator should consider the sample size and whether the data are distributed normally. If the data are not distributed normally, a parametric test may not demonstrate statistical significance, because the distribution of critical values is based on the assumption of normality. Because of the small sample size frequently used in many medical studies, nonparametric techniques should probably be used more frequently. The major argument against their use is that, if the data are distributed normally, nonparametric tests are slightly less powerful and may not detect real differences. Typically, the advantage they yield with abnormal distributions significantly outweighs the minor lack of power compared with parametric analyses.

Once the investigator determines the type of data obtained, the data should be displayed in a readily understandable form, such as a histogram or scattergram. Appropriate visual presentation permits the investigator to learn whether the data are distributed normally and also to perform a quick and informal visual analysis. Many analyses can be terminated at this point — if no obvious difference exists between groups, statistical analysis will be fruitless, although an investigator might be able to find an obscure statistical test that produces significance.

The next step is to determine the descriptive statistics (including the mean, standard deviation, and standard error). These statistics describe the location and variability of the sample; in addition, they are prerequisites for subsequent analyses. Only after completing these preliminary steps should the investigator embark on inferential statistics. The choice of which inferential test to use depends on the nature of the data. If the independent variable consists of only a single or paired measurement on one group, the one-sample *t* test should be used. For two groups, the two-sample *t* test should be used. For more than two groups, analysis of variance is the appropriate statistical test, although an investigator may choose the two-sample *t* test with the Bonferroni correction. If measurements have been repeated on the same subject, repeated-measures analysis of variance should be used rather than the paired *t* test. For each of these tests, the investigator may select the parametric or nonparametric version. Finally, if the independent variable is continuous and cannot be divided readily into discrete groups, analysis of linear regression is the appropriate test to apply.

For most of the research reported in the anesthesia literature, these statistical techniques are sufficient. As study design becomes more complicated, more sophisticated techniques may become necessary. Because a more detailed discussion of these tests is beyond the scope of this chapter, the investigator should turn to the resources described below. These resources permit the investigator to design a study for optimal data collection and analysis.

When these guidelines are used, the choice of statistical tests is simple. The most common errors involve the use of multiple *t* tests when analysis of variance is appropriate, or the use of analysis of variance when repeated-measures analysis of variance is appropriate. Once the investigator understands the importance of type I and type II errors, the importance of selecting the appropriate statistical test will become apparent.

STATISTICAL RESOURCES

The techniques described in this chapter should permit the reader to examine a data set, to determine descriptive statistics, and to perform simple tests such as the one-sample or two-sample *t* test. More complicated tests such as analysis of variance or linear regression analysis, if done manually, are tedious and require mathematical precision beyond the ability and scope of many investigators. In addition, mathematical errors occur, which, as the number of calculations increases, may be compounded. To avoid these problems, most investigators turn to a variety of resources. The simplest of these, a scientific calculator (such as those produced by Hewlett-Packard, Texas Instruments, or Casio), permits accurate calculation of means, standard deviations, and standard errors. More sophisticated calculators, particularly those that are programmable, can perform analysis of variance and linear regression analysis.

Microcomputers (e.g., Macintosh, IBM PC) have become commonplace in offices, laboratories, and homes. A variety of statistical packages having various degrees of sophistication are available for these computers. These statistical packages perform complicated analyses with minimal effort.

Users of minicomputers (such as the Digital Equipment Corporation Microvax series) and mainframe computers have additional options for statistical services. Several comprehensive statistical software packages are widely available. The most popular packages are BMDP (Biomedical Statistical Software, University of California Press), SPSS (Statistical Package for the Social Sciences), and SAS (Statistical Analysis Systems).

Regardless of the statistical package, the results must be examined by the investigator. I have found errors in several statistical software packages, one produced lo-

cally and others widely available. On occasion, errors are subtle and may escape notice; in some instances, the errors are obvious to even the casual user. Several steps are available to confirm the accuracy of the statistical package. First, the investigator can use a data set analyzed in a standard textbook; differences between the results offered in the textbook and those from the statistical package should alert the investigator to errors. Second, the investigator should always examine the entire output from the statistical package, not just the statistical results. If the mean values, standard deviations, or other results differ from those predicted from the data, the investigator should be suspicious of the results.

Materials are readily available to guide the investigator toward more sophisticated statistical techniques. Glantz[32] has written an excellent monograph, *Primer of Biostatistics*. Textbooks by Zar,[14] Dixon and Massey,[33] and Colton[34] are also valuable resources, particularly if the investigator has selected a particular test and needs guidance through the individual steps.

In addition, the number of statisticians who have biomedical expertise is increasing. These statisticians have knowledge of the particular problems associated with medical research, including small sample sizes and abnormal distributions. Biostatisticians can be valuable in directing the medical investigator toward the appropriate statistical test, in performing the analyses, and in interpreting the results.

Finally, a word of caution regarding study design. Inexperienced investigators may accumulate a large amount of data before identifying the most appropriate statistical techniques to be used. When an attempt is made to select the appropriate statistical test, the investigator may learn that the data have been collected in a way that prohibits appropriate statistical analysis. This problem can usually be avoided if the investigator considers the issue of statistical analysis before data are collected, particularly if outside advice is necessary. With increasing awareness among anesthesia researchers, these problems should occur less frequently.

SUMMARY

The aim of this chapter has been to provide an introduction to the techniques used in many statistical analyses. Emphasis has been placed on descriptive statistics, particularly on identifying the location and distribution of data. This focus was chosen because of the increasing tendency of investigators to perform complicated analyses using sophisticated statistical techniques without spending sufficient time examining the data. The chapter also emphasized the more common abuses of statistics: reporting variability of the data without identifying whether standard deviation or standard error is being used, and the inappropriate use of multiple *t* tests. Repeated-measures analysis of variance, a statistical technique that is appropriate for many of the studies performed in anesthesia, has been described, with the hope that it will be used with greater frequency.

Undoubtedly, many investigators will continue to view statistical analysis as a necessary evil in research. Despite increased awareness of the abuses of statistics, errors continue to appear in the anesthesia literature (as in all medical literature). However, with time, with improved editorial vigilance, with the availability of newer statistical resources for investigators, and with education for investigators, we are likely to see improvements in the future.

REFERENCES

1. Gore SM, Jones IG, Rytter EC: Misuse of statistical methods: Critical assessment of articles in BMJ from January to March 1976. Br Med J 1:85, 1977
2. Glantz SA: Biostatistics: How to detect, correct and prevent errors in the medical literature. Circulation 61:1, 1980
3. Rosen MR, Hoffman BF: Statistics, biomedical scientists, and circulation research (editorial). Circ Rec 42:739, 1978
4. Feinstein AR: Clinical biostatistics. XXXVII. Demeaned errors, confidence games, nonplussed minuses, inefficient coefficients, and other statistical disruptions of scientific communication. Clin Pharmacol Ther 20:617, 1973
5. Emerson JD, Colditz GA: Use of statistical analysis in *The New England Journal of Medicine*. N Engl J Med 309:709, 1983
6. Hayden GF: Biostatistical trends in *Pediatrics:* Implications for the future. Pediatrics 72:84, 1983
7. Avram MJ, Shanks CA, Dykes MHM, et al: Statistical methods in anesthesia articles: An evaluation of two American journals during two six-month periods. Anesth Analg 64:607, 1985
8. Feinstein AR: Clinical biostatistics. XLIX. The basic data structures used in quantitative indexes. Clin Pharmacol Ther 26:525, 1979
9. Viby-Mogensen J: Succinylcholine neuromuscular blockade in subjects heterozygous for abnormal plasma cholinesterase. Anesthesiology 55:231, 1981
10. Stanley TH, Webster LR: Anesthetic requirements and cardiovascular effects of fentanyl-oxygen and fentanyl-diazepam-oxygen anesthesia in man. Anesth Analg 57:411, 1978
11. Feinstein AR: Clinical biostatistics. L. On choosing a mean and other quantitative indexes to describe the location and dispersion of univariate data. Clin Pharmacol Ther 27:120, 1980
12. Student: Illegal number crunching (letter). Pediatrics 71:864, 1983
13. Feinstein AR: On central tendency and the meaning of mean for pH values (editorial). Anesth Analg 58:1, 1979
14. Zar JH: Biostatistical Analysis. Prentice-Hall, Englewood Cliffs, NJ, 1974
15. Feinstein AR: Clinical biostatistics. LV. The t test and the basic ethos of parametric statistical inference (Part 1). Clin Pharmacol Ther 29:548, 1981
16. Brown GW: Standard deviation, standard error. Which 'standard' should we use? Am J Dis Child 136:937, 1982
17. Fisher RA: Statistical Methods for Research Workers. p. 44. Hafner Press, Macmillan, New York, 1970
18. Fisher RA: The Design of Experiments. 2nd ed. p. 150. Oliver and Boyd, Edinburgh, 1937
19. Melton AW: Editorial. J Exp Psychol 64:553, 1962
20. Student: The probable error of a mean. Biometrika 6:1, 1908
21. Feinstein AR: Clinical biostatistics. LVI. The t test and the basic ethos of parametric statistical inference (Conclusion). Clin Pharmacol Ther 30:133, 1981
22. Schefler WC: Statistics for the Biological Sciences. 2nd ed. p. 136. Addison-Wesley, Reading, MA, 1979
23. Litchfield JT, Wilcoxon F: A simplified method of evaluating dose-effect experiments. J Pharmacol Exp Ther 96:99, 1949
24. McPherson K: Statistics: The problem of examining accumulating data more than once. N Engl J Med 290: 501, 1974
25. Armitage P: Sequential Medical Trials. 2nd ed. Blackwell Scientific Publications, Oxford, 1975
26. Abramowitz MD, Oh TH, Epstein BS, et al: The antiemetic effect of droperidol following outpatient strabismus surgery in children. Anesthesiology 59:579, 1983
27. Cohen SE, Woods WA, Wyner J: Antiemetic efficacy of droperidol and metoclopramide. Anesthesiology 60:67, 1984
28. Mosteller, F, Bailar JC III (eds): Medical Uses of Statistics. NEJM Books, Waltham, MA, 1986
29. Berger JM, Stirt JA, Sullivan SF: Enflurane, halothane, and aminophylline—uptake and pharmacokinetics. Anesth Analg 62:733, 1983
30. Longnecker DE: Support versus illumination: Trends in medical statistics (editorial). Anesthesiology 57:73, 1982
31. Ford I: Can statistics cause brain damage (editorial)? J Cereb Blood Flow Metab 3:259, 1983
32. Glantz SA: Primer of Biostatistics. 2nd ed. McGraw-Hill, New York, 1987
33. Dixon WJ, Massey FJ, Jr: Introduction to Statistical Analysis. 4th ed. McGraw-Hill, New York, 1983
34. Colton T: Statistics in Medicine. Little, Brown, Boston, 1974

Section III

ANESTHESIA MANAGEMENT

22
ANESTHESIA RISK

Alan F. Ross
John H. Tinker

INTRODUCTION

Perhaps the most important epidemiologic work of this century is that of Hammond and Horn,[1] who demonstrated increased mortality in cigarette smokers. Their data were collected over many years, from thousands of people, and despite constant criticism and impediments from the tobacco industry. Persons who smoked were (are) at increased risks of death from a variety of diseases, particularly lung cancer and coronary atherosclerosis.[1,2] Although this is not by any measure a complete success story, nonetheless, thousands of deaths are undoubtedly now prevented. Smoking is at least

initially volitional. In contrast, there are about 24 million surgical operations performed in the United States alone.[3] These patients cannot voluntarily reduce their personal risk from anesthesia, as Hammond, Horn, and many others convinced the public to do with respect to cessation of smoking. In fact, numerous health risks can be reduced, either by personal action (obesity, hypertension, etc.) or by societal pressure (air and water pollution). In contrast, anesthesia risk reduction rests squarely on the shoulders of those who practice our specialty. We cannot ever use the excuse sometimes used by the general physician, "Well, I told him to lose weight, stop smoking . . . ," etc.

The magnitude of the problem of anesthesia risk is major. If overall risk of death due to anesthesia is about 1 : 10,000 anesthetics,[4] then there may be 2,400 deaths primarily due to anesthesia in the United States alone every year. Death from anesthesia is by no means the only risk. Morbidity due to anesthesia ranges from temporary pressure injuries to the comatose vegetating patient.

For several years now, the American Society of Anesthesiologists (ASA) and its Anesthesia Patient Safety Foundation have undertaken major efforts at education and standard setting in an effort to reduce the risks of anesthesia.[5] Large and small groups of anesthesia providers have adopted numerous risk management strategies. Standards of acceptable anesthesia practice are being set by national organizations of anesthesiologists, not by the government.[5,6] Review and accreditation organizations such as the Joint Commission on Accreditation of Healthcare Organizations (JCAHO) have demanded now that "quality assurance" activities have real teeth, that is, that various objective monitors of quality of care in anesthesia be instituted, analyzed, and acted upon. Specific anesthesia providers who do not meet these previously agreed-upon criteria are to be advised and, if necessary, given meaningful sanctions.

To put this in perspective:

> . . . we must evaluate this situation in light of the changing practice of anesthesiology and surgery in the past 20 years. The more obvious of these changes include the broadening of the criteria of operability and patient selection, the development of longer and more stressful procedures, the exposure of the patient to a multiplicity of pharmacologic agents, both before surgery and during anesthesia, and the more accurate reporting of operative mortality. It is obvious that by rarely refusing any patient the benefits of surgery we may expose ourselves to a higher mortality rate.[7]

This statement was made *three decades ago*. Previous writings about anesthesia risk have often cited these explanations. It is time now to look beyond such relatively defensive precepts and face the issue of anesthetic risk with renewed vigor. To quote an individual whose studies of errors and lapses during anesthesia were pioneering in the sense that they convinced leaders in anesthesia that it was time to do something about reducing anesthesia risk: *"Perhaps the most insidious hazard of anesthesia is its relative safety."*[8]

The first so-called anesthetic deaths were described in a remarkable 1858 treatise by John Snow, entitled *On Chloroform and Other Anesthetics*.[9] As A. S. Keats[10] has pointed out, few if any subsequent investigators have gone into such detail or performed specific experiments in an effort to ascertain whether particular deaths were actually due to anesthesia. Using the words of Keats[10]:

> No control study of the hazards of operation without anesthesia or, conversely, anesthesia without operation will ever be performed. The hazards of anesthesia can therefore never be considered independent of a second procedure.

Nonetheless, mortality and morbidity can be directly attributed to anesthesia. Early investigators did their best to raise consciousness to the risks of anesthesia. Sir Robert MacIntosh[11] in a 1948 treatise entitled *Deaths under Anaesthetics* attempted to reduce errors by stating that anesthetic drugs and practices were (are, should be) safe if managed correctly. Ruth,[12] MacIntosh,[11] and Edwards et al.[13] advocated anesthesia study commissions to identify and describe circumstances that resulted in adverse outcomes. They strongly recommended that cases of anesthetic morbidity and mortality be frankly and openly discussed in every hospital. No reasonable anesthetist can argue that deaths and morbidity are not occasionally due to errors, lapses, and preventable failures. Unfortunately, the purported benefit of study commissions in preventing future recurrences is open to question. Many currently accepted techniques might have been judged to constitute malpractice just 20 years ago. To use Keats's[10] example, if a critically ill cardiac patient was given 2 mg/kg morphine and then a vasodilator such as sodium nitroprusside and later died in the operating room, the Beecher and Todd[14] study commission would likely have considered it an anesthetic death in the early 1950s. By 1977, this was daily practice.[15] In 1989, this might be considered uncommon.[16,17] Adoption of innovations in management of critically ill, inherently high-risk patients could be hindered if death should always be judged due to technical error or flaw associated with the innovation. Today in the United States, legitimate quality assurance and mortality and morbidity conference activities conducted by hospital medical staff for the purposes of education and improvement in patient care are reasonably well protected against "discovery" in legal proceedings. The courts can break down this protection, but, we believe, only at the peril of our patients.

Currently, terms such as *risk–benefit ratio* and *outcome studies* have useful roles in assessing anesthetic management, as long as sweeping generalizations from limited data are avoided. Another curious idea that lies behind some demands for zero anesthetic risk is the notion that anesthetic risk can and must be reduced to zero because there is little or no therapeutic benefit of anesthesia per se. No one educated in the myriad complexities and possible disasters inherent in such separate categories as muscle relaxants, inhaled anesthetics, local anesthetics, hypnotics, all the above plus pre-existent patient disease, surgical stress and trespass, plus electromechanical transducers with quasi-computerized monitors and drug delivery systems could rationally conclude that the sum total risk of an anesthetic could or should be zero. Anesthesia performed completely in accordance with current accepted standards can still be associated with major morbidity and mortality.

Some educators hold that browbeating anesthetists-in-training with the concept that all untoward outcomes are due to preventable errors will somehow result in optimal vigilance. We believe that truth, including admission of ignorance of causation when such exists, is a better educational tool. For the beginning anesthetist reading this chapter, our message is that whereas lack of vigilance, ignorance of recent medical advances, errors of omission and commission, and poor medical judgment do contribute greatly to anesthetic morbidity and mortality, nonetheless patients can and do die despite state-of-the-art anesthetic and perioperative care.

DEFINING AND QUANTIFYING ANESTHETIC RISK

The occurrence of perioperative death and morbidity have been used to define anesthetic risk. Yet these indicators are influenced by a variety of factors. For example, among 15 institutions performing coronary artery bypass grafts (CABG), Kennedy et al.[18] reported that perioperative mortality ranged from 0.3 to more than 6 percent for the same operation in groups of patients that could not be told apart by standard disease-severity criteria. In this report, mortality rates were near linearly distributed between these extremes.

Another example of disparate outcomes can be seen by comparing the results published for carotid endarterectomy. Sundt et al.[19] reported an overall stroke/mortality outcome of 3.6 percent (when minor new deficits were included) and 2.5 percent for major deficits plus mortalities following 1,145 operations. In sharp contrast, Easton and Sherman,[20] examining 228 of the same operations in a different institution, reported a stroke-plus-death rate nearly 10 times greater, namely, 21.1 percent.

When overall surgical mortality rates vary so widely, how can the true anesthetic component of the risk be measured? Past investigations have considered that an adverse outcome may be due to anesthesia, surgery, or patient disease. Variations in the definitions of perioperative death (i.e., within 24 hours of surgery to 3 months postoperatively) and differences in anesthetic practice among countries will affect reported incidence of risk. With these considerations in mind, we will review the findings of several major anesthetic risk studies published after 1980, in an effort to establish a modern overall statistic for anesthetic risk. The reader is also referred to reviews by Davies et al.,[21] Derrington and Smith,[22] and Strunin et al.[23]

United Kingdom Studies

Lunn and Mushin[4] and their colleagues at Cardiff, Wales, under a grant from the Nuffield Provincial Hospital Trust, examined deaths occurring within 6 days of anesthesia in five regions of England, Wales, and Scotland. An anonymous and confidential reporting system (which was also voluntary) provided detailed reports from which a committee (including anesthetists, surgeons, and epidemiologists) judged the contributions of anesthesia to the deaths. By 1987, this ongoing study had included well over 1 million anesthetics.[24] The findings first published in 1982 included an overall 6-day perioperative mortality of 0.6 percent.[4] Anesthesia was deemed totally causative for 1 death per 10,000 operations but contributed at least partially to 5 deaths per 10,000 operations.[4,25] *Anesthesia thus contributed to approximately 1 of 12 of the perioperative deaths.* The figure of 1:10,000 deaths totally due to anesthesia is in reasonable agreement with several recent studies of anesthesia mortality.[25–28]

From the data collected, Lunn and Mushin[4] attempted in 1982 to characterize the practice of anesthesia in these regions and came to some rather startling projections. If their study population represented the practice of anesthesia in the whole country (Great Britain), then 300,000 patients per year were not seen by their anesthetist preoperatively; 468,000 per year did not have their arterial blood pressures recorded during their operations; 534,000 per year had operations prior to which their anesthetists had not tested the anesthetic machine; finally, in 1,290,000 cases per year, the electrocardiogram (ECG) was not monitored.[4,25] The most recent update of this remarkable survey was published in 1987, and the above projections from 1982 are not necessarily outdated.[4,24,29,30] In addition to this landmark risk survey, Lunn also contributed to real improvements in epidemiologic techniques for these studies. For example, the importance of several independent opinions about the contribution of anesthesia to a perioperative death was quantitated by Lunn, Hunter, and Scott in 1983.[29] Reports concerning 197 deaths that were received from both the anesthetist and the surgeon were reviewed by two independent assessors. Irreconcilable differences in the assessors' opinions were then settled by an arbitrator. Table 22-1 illustrates the degree with which the assessors agreed with either anesthetist or surgeon concerning the role of anesthesia in the patient's death. This table presents objective evidence of the bias inherent in such voluntary reports.[29]

The most recent major anesthetic risk study is the Confidential Enquiry into Perioperative Deaths (CEPOD) by Buck et al.[24] from the same group of investigators. Three regions of the United Kingdom were studied over 12 months. By this time, the credibility of the ongoing investigations and investigators was such that voluntary cooperation of 95 percent of both anesthetists and surgeons was achieved by use of methods including confidentiality. This confidentiality protec-

TABLE 22-1. Percent of Agreement[a] Between Assessors and Anesthetist and Surgeons

Assessor Agreed with:	Percent Agreement
Anesthetist	33
Surgeon	29
Both	18
Neither	19

[a] Arbitration was required in 16.2% of the cases.
(Adapted from Lunn et al.,[29] with permission.)

tion included "crown privilege," meaning that data sent to the CEPOD were protected from subpoena, since disclosure of any identifying material about individual cases would "be against the public interest and undermine the whole basis for a confidential enquiry."[24] Similar to their earlier studies, determination of causal factors in each death (anesthesia, surgery, or patient disease) was made by assessors. Importantly, the definition of perioperative death was extended to include all deaths occurring within 30 days after surgery to discern whether anesthetic deaths had been missed if only the first 6 days were examined. For approximately 500,000 operations, the overall death rate was 0.7 percent. Of the reports analyzed, anesthesia contributed (partially or totally) to death in 410 cases *but was judged completely responsible for death in only 3 cases.* The incidence of primary anesthetic mortality of this study was therefore 1 per 185,056 operations but 1 per 1,351 for anesthetic-associated deaths.[24,31] Factors believed contributory to the anesthesia-associated deaths are listed in Table 22-2. Anesthesia caused only 1 death in 185,000 operations but contributed in a major way to 7 deaths in 10,000 operations. We believe that the above two statistics could be used *together* in obtaining informed consent. We recognize that anesthetists who have, for some years now, been quoting 1 : 10,000 as the risk of anesthesia death (from the 1982 British survey), may now be tempted to quote 1 : 185,000.[31] This risk statement would be incomplete, in our opinion.

The striking finding from the CEPOD study of 1987[24] was the frequency of preventable human factors and the infrequency of equipment problems. Fatigue was *not* listed as causative or contributory to any of these deaths. Perhaps the United Kingdom has managed this problem well, or perhaps fatigue as a factor is unmentionable in that society. The CEPOD study indicated that improvements in anesthetic care may have occurred compared with the same group's earlier findings.[4,24] By 1987, more patients were seen preoperatively (but still about 18 percent were not).[24] Intraoperative monitoring of blood pressure was now done in over 90 percent and ECG monitoring in over 97 percent of cases.[24] Nonetheless, an inspired oxygen analyzer was in use in only 16 percent of cases in the 1987

CEPOD report from England.[24] We doubt that pulse oximetry and capnometry were commonly employed. The 161-page CEPOD report included 236 data tables.[24] The authors came to the specific conclusions summarized below:

Most overall mortality occurred in elderly patients.

Many surgeons, anesthetists, and hospital staff did not hold regular morbidity and mortality meetings.

There were important differences in supervision of trainees and important regional differences in clinical practice.

A worrisome number of deaths involved junior surgeons and anesthetists who did not seek advice from senior colleagues.

Preoperative assessment and optional resuscitation of patients were sometimes compromised by medically unnecessary haste to operate.

Some patients who were moribund or terminally ill had operations that would not have improved their condition.

There were examples of surgeons operating for conditions for which they were not trained.

There were difficulties in retrieval of patients' records and in transferring patients between hospitals.

French Survey

Beginning in 1977, the French Health Ministry carried out a nationwide survey of major complications that occurred during anesthesia.[25,27,32] The results reflected 198,103 anesthetics surveyed in 460 public and private institutions between 1978 and 1982.[27] During or within 24 hours of anesthesia, 268 major anesthesia-related complications occurred, for an incidence of *1 major complication per 739 anesthetics.* These complications resulted in 67 deaths within 24 hours and 16 comas persisting after 24 hours. When death and coma (expected death) were considered to be due partially or totally to anesthesia, the incidence was 1 : 2,387.[27] Death due totally to anesthesia had an incidence of 1 : 13,207.[27] Although numerically slightly better than the 1 : 10,000 figure reported about the same time from England,[4] it is not possible to say with certainty that it represents a favorable trend. When death *and coma* due totally to anesthesia were considered, the incidence was 1 : 7,924.[27]

It is not unreasonable that an anesthesiologist will perform or be responsible for 750 to 1,000 anesthetics per year. If the above statistics are valid, it is possible that each of us will be responsible for one death every 10 to 15 years; that is, two or three deaths totally attributable to improper anesthesia practice for each anesthesiologist during a career in the specialty. On the other hand, if the most recent British findings are confirmed, perhaps this outlook is better.

The French study analyzed the data with respect to time of complication (induction, maintenance, postanesthetic), location of complication (ward, operating

TABLE 22-2. Factors Responsible for Anesthesia-Related Mortality in CEPOD Study (1987)

Factor	Percent Cases Involved
Failure to apply knowledge	75
Poor standard of practice	30
Failure of organization	25
Lack of experience	24
Failure of equipment	1.7
Fatigue	0.002 (1 case)
Impairment	0

(Adapted from Buck et al.,[24] with permission.)

room, intensive care unit [ICU]), patient age, duration of surgery and ASA physical status.[27,32] These data confirmed other studies in finding that complications occurred more frequently at extremes of age; during and after longer surgical procedures; when there were more preoperative diseases; and in emergency cases. ASA physical status rating was relatively closely related to the anesthesia-related complication rate. A provocative finding was that complications that resulted in death or coma occurred more frequently in the postanesthetic period (50 of 82 cases) than in the operating room. In fact, *postanesthetic respiratory depression accounted for nearly half of the cases (12 of 25) in which death or coma was totally attributed to anesthesia.* The authors stated that most episodes of postoperative respiratory depression occurred in patients who had received narcotic analgesics and/or muscle relaxants "for which antagonists had not been used."[27] The postoperative respiratory depression was compounded by the fact that recovery rooms were not routinely present in France ("about 50 percent of the patients returned directly to the ward after anesthesia").[27] When an accident involving respiratory depression occurred in the operating room, recovery room, or ICU, it was lethal for 29 percent of such patients. If such an accident occurred on the ward, 70 percent of such patients died.[27] The authors should be commended for their report, which identified problems in France in the 1970s similar to those which MacIntosh described in Britain in 1948. Our belief is that such reports do facilitate changes in practice when findings emerge that are disconcerting. It is likely that the ongoing, carefully documented, elegantly understated reports of Lunn, Mushin, and their colleagues in England have had a significant impact on practice and have also contributed materially to reduction in anesthetic mortality.

Australia (New South Wales)

Since 1960, a committee that has included anesthesiologists, surgeons, and obstetricians in New South Wales has conducted an ongoing investigation of deaths and other complications related to anesthesia.[28,33] The committee is notified of deaths because mortality associated with anesthesia is required by law to be reported. Information is gathered by voluntary completion of a questionnaire. Owing to an unbroken record of confidentiality, participation is now over 90 percent.[28] Deaths are classified by anesthesia, surgery, patient disease, or "fortuitous causes" (based on the classification system of Edwards et al.[13]). The extensive period analyzed by this study may facilitate understanding of changes in anesthetic risk over time. The most recent findings were reported by Holland in 1987.[28] There was a significant decrease in the magnitude of anesthesia-related deaths over time. Of the cases that were judged to warrant review, that is, were not clearly due to patient disease, the fraction attributed to anesthesia (partially or totally) decreased from 35 percent to 12.2 percent over

the 35-year period.[28] The New South Wales data base does not include total numbers of anesthetics administered over any time period. This precludes calculation of true rates of anesthetic risk. By estimating these denominators, the authors made a calculation that suggested that it was five times safer to undergo anesthesia in 1987 than in 1960[28,33] (Table 22-3). Holland speculated about several changes that have occurred that may explain the apparent improvement, especially changes in the anesthesia work force. More anesthetics are now administered by trained anesthesiologists, that is, a smaller percentage are administered by nonspecialists. The nonanesthesia medical house officer had been associated with considerable anesthetic mortality in low-risk patients in the early years of 1960 to 1969.[33] This led to a phasing out of the medical house officer as a member of the anesthetic work force.[28] Despite a sixfold increase in the number of anesthesia trainees, their contribution to anesthetic mortality did not increase. Holland[28] speculated that this may be due to better supervision. Does this reflect Professor Holland's bias, since the recommendations followed were in part his own? Could safer anesthetic drugs, better equipment, better preoperative evaluation, etc. all have played roles? The data from New South Wales lead to several questions. When patients were classified according to preoperative condition, the absolute number of deaths decreased over time but the percentages did not. Low-risk patients made up 19.4 percent of the total anesthesia mortality for 1960 to 1969. The percentage of the total anesthesia deaths for 1983 to 1985 was about the same at 18 percent for this group. In other words, *approximately one of five anesthetic deaths continued to occur in the low-risk patients.*[28] Perhaps this argues that improvement in knowledge and skill (and more equipment, safer drugs, etc.) does not necessarily result in increased vigilance. A second concern illustrated by the New South Wales data is the frequency of certain defined errors that contribute to anesthetic mortality. Table 22-4 shows that the top four errors of 1960 to 1969 remain in the top four slots for 1983 to 1985 (although their order in the top four has changed).[28]

Holland's report, therefore, is objective evidence that there have been important advances in anesthesia safety, but it also has identified areas that continue as problems. The efforts of Professor Holland are, by far, the most longstanding of the ongoing contributions to this field. We have immense respect for the difficulties of such an undertaking.

TABLE 22-3. Estimated Risk of Death from Anesthesia in New South Wales, Australia

Year	No. of Deaths	Estimated Anesthetics	Deaths per No. of Anesthetics
1960	55	300,000	1 per 5,500
1970	39	400,000	1 per 10,250
1984	24	550,000	1 per 26,000

(Adapted from Holland,[28] with permission.)

TABLE 22-4. Frequency of Common Errors in Anesthetic Management

Error	1960–1969 Ranking	1983–1985 Ranking
Overdose	1	4
Wrong choice	2	2
Inadequate preparation	3	1
Inadequate crisis management	4	3

(Adapted from Holland,[28] with permission.)

United States

With the adversarial legal situation in the United States, by which is meant that nearly every untoward outcome is scrutinized for possible legal action, plus the curious but well-rooted idea that pain, suffering, and loss of "consortium" can and should somehow be worth money, it is easy to see why the climate in this country is not conducive to valid regional or national assessment of anesthetic risk. Several important contributions have instead been made in specific areas of anesthetic risk.

The counting of postoperative deaths suffers from incomplete reporting, varied definitions of postoperative period, and blurred distinctions between anesthesia and other causes of death. Keenan and Boyan[34] chose instead to study incidence of intraoperative cardiac arrest. Such specific events are usually fairly well documented and may represent a sort of final common pathway for many anesthetic complications (overdose, esophageal intubation, intravascular local anesthetic, etc.).

The data reported by Keenan and Boyan[34] were obtained from 163,240 anesthetics administered over a 15-year period at the Medical College of Virginia Hospital. A total of 449 intraoperative cardiac arrests occurred, most of which were judged related to patient condition and/or surgery. Cardiac arrest solely due to anesthesia occurred in 27 cases (an incidence of 1.7 arrests per 10,000 anesthetics). In 14 of these cases, the patients died, an incidence of death due to anesthesia-related cardiac arrest of 0.9 : 10,000 cases, almost exactly equal to the overall anesthetic death rate reported from England in 1982.[4,34]

The incidence of cardiac arrest during anesthesia was six times more likely during emergency versus elective surgery and three times more likely in children under the age of 12 years. The greatest proportion of the arrests occurred in ASA class III and IV patients, each accounting for 10 of 27 arrests, but 7 arrests occurred in ASA class I or II patients. Failure to ventilate accounted for 45 percent of such arrests, but anesthetic overdose (absolute and relative) caused 55 percent. Three-fourths of the cardiac arrests (20 of 27) were judged avoidable. Death followed arrest more often in ASA class III and IV patients than in ASA class I and II patients. Death followed approximately one-half of the overdose arrests (8 of 15); about one-half of the patients

in whom failure to ventilate caused the arrest (7 of 12); and in one-half of the pediatric patients. In other words, *death followed a witnessed operating room cardiac arrest roughly 50 percent of the time, despite the presence of trained personnel and other support measures.* This result is not encouraging about the efficiency of accepted resuscitative procedures. An important finding in this study was the fact that *more than 50 percent of these cardiac arrests resulted from absolute or relative volatile anesthetic overdoses* (halothane or enflurane-isoflurane was not yet in use). These data seem to confirm the low toxic/therapeutic ratios of these agents reported from animal studies.[35,36] Should these data sound a note of caution? Another important finding was that *progressive bradycardia preceded cardiac arrest in 26 of 27 cases.*[34] Not obvious is whether bradycardia was a sufficiently early sign to be potentially preventative. A previous report[37] on cardiac arrest during anesthesia and surgery had concluded that

> **"if the precipitating cause of cardiac arrest is hypoxemia of respiratory origin (for which there are no commonly used monitors) then diagnosis may be made too late to permit brain survival."**

In the report of Keenan and Boyan,[34] despite a warning (bradycardia) in 96 percent of cases, cardiac arrests resulting from anesthesia occurred. The authors contended that appearance of bradycardia was often treated with atropine, which did "little but waste time,"[34] instead of 100 percent oxygen. The data of Keenan and Boyan[34] were obtained before the widespread use of pulse oximetry and capnography.

The study of Keenan and Boyan[34] was of cardiac arrest resulting from anesthesia and therefore underestimates the incidence of anesthetic death, because complications such as aspiration, hepatic necrosis, or hypoxic cerebral damage may eventually result in death without intraoperative arrest. Despite this, incidence of cardiac arrest may prove a valid statistic to allow comparisons among institutions.

Another important contribution from the United States is the 1988 report from the ASA Professional Liability Committee Closed Claims Study, by Caplan et al.,[38] of unexpected cardiac arrests in healthy patients undergoing spinal anesthesia. During a review of over 900 cases of major anesthetic complications from insurance carrier closed claims, 14 cases of unexplained cardiac arrest were noted in patients who underwent spinal anesthetics judged competently administered. In cases in which sedative agents had been administered to the point where patients were sleeping, cyanosis frequently preceded the arrest. The authors postulated that unappreciated respiratory insufficiency may have been present, despite ventilation that appeared adequate to the anesthetist.[38] The second finding was a possible prior inadequate appreciation of the influence of spinal anesthesia on distribution of blood flow during cardiopulmonary resuscitation. When cardiac arrest occurred, Caplan et al.[38] speculated that perhaps potent inotrope–vasoconstrictors were administered relatively late and/or in insufficient dosage to adequately counteract spinal anesthetic-induced peripheral vasodilation, resulting in too much diversion of cardiopulmonary resuscitation (CPR)-induced blood flow away from the brain (and heart). Despite apparently successful cardiac resuscitation, *only 4 of the 14 patients regained consciousness (3 of these with neurologic deficits)*. These results were much worse than results of out-of-hospital CPRs, which have been reported to result in as many as 41 percent of patients recovering without neurologic deficits.[38]

The report of Caplan et al.[38] is a landmark contribution to the study of anesthetic risk. By careful investigation of a few rare events, a mechanism has been postulated that can now undergo laboratory and/or human investigation. New research should characterize the nature of spinal anesthetic-related respiratory insufficiency and mechanisms preventing effective CPR and neurologic resuscitation.

Summary of Recent Surveys of Anesthesia Risk

Review of the major anesthetic risk surveys of the 1980s finds considerable variation in incidence of anesthesia-related mortality (Table 22-5). Most statistics are still close to the generally accepted modern risk of one death due to anesthesia per 10,000 anesthetics, although a trend toward improvement seems to exist.

USING PAST STUDIES TO BETTER UNDERSTAND MODERN ANESTHETIC RISK

Early Reports (Before 1960)

Anesthetic risk has been studied for decades. As early as 1944, Gillespie[39] noted the problems of distinguishing anesthetic death from other causes and reported an incidence of anesthetic death of 1:1,000. In his personal experience, seven such deaths had occurred over 10 years. Respiratory problems were the most frequent contributing factor. Sir Robert MacIntosh[11] contended in 1948 that anesthetic complications were being repeated owing to lack of communication and that deaths from anesthetics were attributed to quasidiagnoses such as "status lymphaticus." MacIntosh was a pioneer in stressing that real causes such as airway obstruction, inhalation of gastric contents, and narcotic respiratory depression were prominent factors of anesthetic mortality.[11]

In 1951, Ehrenhaft et al.[40] reported 25 cases of cardiac arrest during 71,000 anesthetics at the University of Iowa over 10 years for an incidence of 3.5:10,000. Early therapy for cardiac arrest had consisted of intracardiac injections without survivors. Later in the series, open chest cardiac massage was utilized, with a 28 percent survival rate. By 1985, Keenan and Boyan[34] reported 48 percent survival after intraoperative cardiac arrest. The observation that cyanosis may occur prior to cardiac arrest was reported in 1954 by West[41] in his review of intraoperative cardiac arrests.

Beecher and Todd's[14] landmark multi-institutional survey of 599,548 anesthetics determined a primary anesthesia death rate of 1:2,680. They observed that anesthetic deaths were more frequent at the extremes of age and if curare had been administered, but did not connect the curare deaths to the idea that ventilation should be better supported. Instead, they indicted the drug.[14]

Edwards et al.[13] reported in 1956 on 1,000 cases of anesthetic-related deaths voluntarily and anonymously reported to the Council of the Association of Anaesthetists (United Kingdom). The development of a classification system to separate anesthetic mortality from other causes was a major contribution of this report.[13] In 1956, Dornette and Orth[42] reported 26 cases in which operative death was judged to be primarily caused by anesthesia in a series of 63,105 anesthetics (incidence, 1:2,427). Reevaluation of the case descriptions provided suggests that today we would judge more of their cases to be anesthetic deaths. Moyer and Key[43] addressed the Section on Surgery at the 104th Annual Meeting of the American Medical Association in 1956 and placed anesthetic risk in perspective:

> **Anesthesia has long been incriminated as an important factor in operative risk. . . . Obviously although anesthesia deaths constitute a significant number they are comparatively few when compared to those attributed to surgical error.**

More Recent Reports (1960–1980)

In 1960, Schapira et al.[44] reported an incidence of 1:232 for primary anesthetic deaths; Collins[45] recommended midday breaks to minimize "operating room hypnosis"; and Phillips et al.[46] reported on 1,024 postoperative deaths analyzed by the Baltimore Anesthesia Study Committee. The incidence of primary anesthesia deaths was estimated at 1:7,692 operations. Over 50 percent of the anesthesia-related deaths occurred in the patients' rooms, indicating a need for routine recovery room utilization. In 1961, Jude et al.[47] reported the use

TABLE 22-5. Summary of Anesthesia-Related Mortality in Major Studies of the 1980s

Study	Incidence of Primary Anesthetic Death
United Kingdom Nuffield Hospital Trust, 1982[4]	1:10,000
United Kingdom Confidential Enquiry (CEPOD), 1987[31]	1:185,056
French Survey, 1986[27]	1:13,207[a]
New South Wales, Australia, 1987[28]	1:26,000
United States, 1985[34]	1:10,000[b]

[a] When death and coma were considered, the incidence was 1:7,924.
[b] Deaths after anesthetic cardiac arrest.

of external cardiac massage for cardiac arrests occurring in the operating and recovery rooms. With this technique, they had 24 percent survival.[47] Boba and Landmesser[48] contended that errors of omission were more problematic than those of commission; that is, that it may not be safer to do nothing.

Dripps et al.[49] reported the incidence of primary anesthetic death at 1:852 in 1961. Their incidence differed between general anesthesia at 1:536 and spinal anesthesia at 1:1,560.[49] No deaths occurred in 16,000 ASA class I patients, including those who had received curare.[49] From Australia, Clifton and Hotten[50] reported in 1963 primary anesthetic deaths at an incidence of 1:6,048. The leading causes were inhalation of gastric contents, respiratory obstruction, and circulatory collapse after thiopentone administration.[50] Memery[51] in 1965 reported the incidence of primary anesthetic death in private practice in Massachusetts to be 1:3,145 for surgical anesthetics. No deaths occurred during 45,575 anesthetics administered for obstetric and gynecologic procedures.[51] In 1964, Dinnick[52] implicated hypovolemia, hypoventilation, and gastric aspiration as the most frequent factors associated with anesthetic deaths in new cases reviewed by the Association of Anesthetists (United Kingdom). Other studies included those of Gebbie[53] in 1966 and Minuck[54] in 1967.

In 1968, Harrison[55] reported that anesthesia significantly contributed to death in 1:3,068 operations in Cape Town, South Africa. A later report in 1978[56] demonstrated a decreased incidence, namely, 1:4,537, which was attributed to better monitoring, trainee supervision, decreased case load, and the introduction of recovery rooms.[56] Bodlander[57] in 1975 determined that anesthesia was solely responsible for death in 1:14,075 anesthetics administered in Australia but contributed to 1 death per 1,702 anesthetics. In 1976, Taylor et al.[37] described circumstances associated with 41 cases of cardiac arrest in healthy patients undergoing routine elective surgery. Hypoxia from hypoventilation appeared to be the most frequent contributing factor. Only three of the patients survived and returned to normal activities. Hovi-Viander[58] reported in 1980 primary anesthetic deaths from 100 hospitals of Finland for an incidence of 1:5,059. Factors most frequently involved were problems in fluid management and respiratory insufficiency. In 1980, Turnbull et al.[59] reviewed 195,232 anesthetics administered at Vancouver General Hospital for deaths occurring within 48 hours. Most of these deaths were classified as being due to patient disease. There were 38 "possibly preventable" deaths, giving an incidence of 1:5,138. Goldstein and Keats[60] reviewed earlier risk studies in 1970. Variations in the classification of cause of death, definition of the perioperative period, patient population, and clinical practice certainly influenced the incidences of reported anesthesia-related deaths. A trend toward decreased risk is suggested, nonetheless (Table 22-6).

RISK CLASSIFICATIONS

Risk Indices

A well-known risk index study is the Cardiac Risk Index (CRI), published by Goldman et al.[61] in 1977. It was created as a result of retrospective analysis of 1,001 patients who underwent anesthesia and surgery after undergoing cardiologic evaluation. Several previously identified cardiac risk factors (e.g., recent myocardial infarction, severe congestive failure, etc.) were reidentified. Goldman et al.[61,62] contended that the CRI could be used as a predictor of cardiac risk. Subsequent prospective analyses of the CRI by Jeffrey et al.,[63] Carliner et al.,[64] and Gerson et al.[65] failed to demonstrate that the CRI could predict outcome. The Goldman CRI represents an attempt to correlate preoperative risk factors to outcome. Probably, the reason the CRI did not succeed is that *preoperative risk factors are by no means the only determinants of outcome.*

Similar approaches have been utilized in the anesthesia literature. Some investigators have focused on a single preoperative risk factor such as hypertension.[66]

TABLE 22-6. Estimates of Anesthetic Risk Prior to 1980

Investigator	Year	No. of Anesthetics	Primary Cause	Primary and Associated Cause
Beecher and Todd[14]	1954	599,548	1:2,680	1:1,560
Dornette and Orth[42]	1956	63,105	1:2,427	1:1,343
Schapira et al.[44]	1960	22,177	1:1,232	1:821
Phillips et al.[46]	1960		1:7,692	1:2,500
Dripps et al.[49]	1961	33,224	1:852	1:415
Clifton & Hotten[50]	1963	205,640	1:6,048	1:3,955
Memery[51]	1965	114,866	1:3,145	1:1,082
Gebbie[53]	1966	129,336		1:6,158
Minuck[54]	1967	121,786	1:6,766	1:3,291
Harrison[55]	1968	177,928		1:3,068
Marx et al.[76]	1973	34,145		1:1,265
Bodlander[57]	1975	211,130	1:14,075	1:1,703
Harrison[56]	1978	240,483		1:4,537
Hovi-Viander[58]	1980	338,934	1:5,059	1:1,412

Despite the established medical correlation of hypertension to mortality resulting from stroke and myocardial infarction, Goldman and Caldera[66] did not find a correlation between preoperative hypertension and adverse surgical outcome. Another approach is to analyze all possible risk factors for possible correlation to adverse outcome. Lunn et al.,[67] Farrow et al.,[68] and Fowkes et al.[69] have used an extensive data collection system to assess the impact of various preoperative conditions. Cohen et al.[70] utilized a logistic regression analysis to conclude that age, emergency surgery, complexity of operation, and preoperative disease were partial determinants of mortality. Cohen et al.[70] concluded as follows:

> **Those factors under control of the anesthetist played a relatively minor role in predicting mortality. In fact, patient and surgical factors provided so much information for predicting mortality that a meaningful increase was not shown by the addition of "other" and anesthesia-related factors.**

Tiret et al.[71] generated a multifactorial risk index for prediction of outcome of anesthesia in patients over 40 years of age, using four preoperative factors: ASA physical status, age, complexity of surgical procedure, and urgency of operation. Prospective evaluation will be needed to verify the accuracy of this model.

ASA Physical Status

Anesthesiologists have worked for many years to devise a means to classify preoperative condition.[72] Total operative risk also depends on the proposed surgery and skill of the surgeon, but the classification index was strictly limited to a definition of preoperative physical status. The original ASA-sponsored scheme included six categories[72] and was revised by Dripps et al.[49] in 1961 to its present form of five categories (Table 22-7). Classification can vary according to individual anesthesiologists. Owens[73] found that a group of 255 anesthesiologists, asked by questionnaire to classify 10 hypothetical patients, was unanimous in only six cases. This result can be interpreted as remarkable inconsistency, or the converse. Keats,[74] however, pointed out that physical status was never intended to be a multifactor-

ial index or predictor of outcome. The classification system has facilitated communication and has remained essentially unchanged for almost 50 years. Since physical status is assigned preoperatively, its correlation to outcome and/or its predictive ability were obvious questions and have been addressed by many investigators.

In the 1970 review by Goldstein and Keats[60] of deaths attributable in whole or in part to anesthesia, a total of 41 percent of all such deaths occurred in ASA class I or II patients. These data represented the combined findings of six large anesthesia risk studies.[13,14,48-51] Since these patients were either healthy or had mild systemic disease, Goldstein and Keats' conclusion was that ASA physical status was not a sensitive predictor of anesthetic mortality.[60] An alternative explanation would be that risks of anesthesia and surgery were greater than risks of the patient's coexisting disease. Also, if most or even some "anesthetic deaths" are due to errors, lapses, or technical difficulties, then ASA physical status might not accurately predict risk. Indeed, the smaller but definite proportion of patients in ASA class I or II status who have suffered cardiac arrest or other complications from anesthesia may well be that proportion in whom errors and lapses played the most "pure" roles in outcome.[34]

When the ASA physical status classification has been applied to total operative mortality (deaths resulting from anesthesia, surgery, or patient disease), it *has* been correlated to outcome. Vacanti et al.[75] in 1970 collected 68,388 cases from 11 U.S. Navy hospitals and reported that ASA physical status was somewhat predictive at least of overall outcome. Marx et al.[76] studied 34,145 patients and found ASA physical status to be a reasonable predictor of outcome. Table 22-8 summarizes and compares these two studies.[75,76]

Both studies show trends toward higher mortality for worsening preoperative physical status, but several differences between the studies may be instructive. Although Vacanti et al.[75] found an incidence of perioperative mortality of 7.7 and 9.4 percent in physical status classes III and IV, respectively, Marx et al.[76] reported 23.4 percent and 50.7 percent mortality, respectively, in the same classes. A number of explanations can be advanced, such as a different interpretation of the ASA physical status categories, differences in patient population, and surgical risk. The Vacanti et al.[75] study does not specify the operations performed, whereas Marx et al.[76] specifically included cardiovascular and neurosurgery but not obstetrics. The overall mortality of the Marx et al.[76] study is over four times that of the Vacanti et al.[75] study. The definition of *perioperative period* probably influenced the results, since Vacanti et al.[75] counted only the deaths that occurred in the first 48 postoperative hours, whereas Marx et al.[76] surveyed deaths occurring within 7 days postoperatively (approximately 35 percent of the deaths in Marx's study occurred after 48 hours). Also, neither institution seems to have seriously accepted the ASA physical

TABLE 22-7. ASA Physical Status

Category	Description
I	Healthy patient
II	Mild systemic disease — no functional limitations
III	Severe systemic disease[a] — definite functional limitation
IV	Severe systemic disease[a] that is a constant threat to life
V	Moribund patient not expected to survive 24 hours with or without operation

[a] Whether or not the systemic disease is the disease for which the patient is undergoing surgery.

TABLE 22-8. ASA Physical Status versus Overall Death Rates[a]

Physical Status	Vacanti et al.[75] Death Rates (1970)		Marx et al.[76] Death Rates (1973)	
	Incidence	Percent	Incidence	Percent
I	43:50,703	0.08	11:18,320	0.06
II	34:12,601	0.27	50:10,609	0.40
III	66:3,626	1.82	168:3,820	4.30
IV	66:850	7.76	252:1,073	23.40
V	57:608	9.38	164:323	50.70
Totals	266:68,388	0.39	645:34,145	1.80

[a] Death rates represent overall perioperative mortality, not deaths from anesthesia.

status classification description of class V, since supposedly it is reserved for moribund patients. Both groups had amazing success if their patients listed as class V really fit the accepted definition. When the data of Marx et al.[76] are computed into rate form for the 27 deaths due to anesthesia (Table 22-9), anesthetic-related deaths were much more likely to occur in sicker patients. A similar finding was that of Keenan and Boyan,[34] who examined 27 cases of anesthetic-related cardiac arrest. The majority of these arrests occurred in class III and IV patients and were more likely to result in death (Table 22-10).

In summary, the ASA physical status classification appears to have some predictive ability when applied to overall operative mortality and to anesthetic-related mortality. Whether or not the likelihood of error increases with degree of patient illness is unknown. It may be that the sicker patient who has little physiologic reserve simply cannot tolerate any degree of error.

ANESTHESIA RISK OTHER THAN DEATH

We have thus far focused mostly on anesthetic deaths. Published risks of anesthetic death versus cardiac arrest, hepatic necrosis, and malignant hyperthermia might be useful as comparisons. These risks have in common with death due to anesthesia the fact that they are rare yet dramatic. Table 22-11 indicates that halothane-associated hepatic injury and malignant hyperthermia are considerably less common than anesthetic death. Despite this, the literature contains hundreds of papers devoted to each. The overall concept of anes-

thetic death is much more difficult to study, especially with respect to mechanism.

In assessing anesthesia complications, a distinction between morbidity and mortality must be made. Cohen et al.[79] reported on the incidence of nonfatal complications in a survey of 112,000 anesthetics administered over a 9-year period in a major teaching hospital. The authors concluded *that 17.8 percent of all patients experienced one or more anesthetic complications.* Most of these were considered minor. Nausea and vomiting constituted 50 percent of the total postoperative complications. Sore throat was the second most frequent postoperative complication and is generally considered a minor complication.[79] Despite this general perception, the postoperative sore throat may represent injury to the trachea and may progress to sequela such as laryngeal granuloma.[80-82] Future studies should evaluate the *impact* of these complications, as well as documenting their frequencies.

MORBIDITY AND MORTALITY OF ANESTHETIC MISADVENTURE

Errors or Toxicity?

Keats[10] challenged the assumption that anesthetic death was always due to error or poor judgment. He considered that toxicity of anesthetic agents, variability in patient responses, and adverse drug reactions must also be considered. In his review of early anesthetic risk studies, Keats found that a bias existed toward finding errors rather than looking for toxicity. A good example was that written by Sir Robert MacIntosh[11]:

TABLE 22-9. ASA Physical Status and Anesthetic Deaths

ASA	No. of Cases	No. of Anesthetic Deaths (n = 27)	Incidence
I	18,320	2	1:10,000
II	10,609	1	1:10,000
III	3,820	11	28:10,000
IV	1,073	8	74:10,000
V	323	5	155:10,000

(Data from Marx et al.[76])

TABLE 22-10. ASA Physical Status and Anesthetic-Related Cardiac Arrest

ASA Classes	No. of Anesthetic-Related Arrests (n = 27)	No. of Survivors	Percent Survived
I and II	7	5	70
III and IV	20	8	40

(From Keenan and Boyan,[34] with permission.)

As I hold that there should be no deaths due to anesthetics, I am very uneasy as to how far we are justified in testing new drugs when the correct administration of those already available to us will give excellent operating conditions to the surgeon at negligible risk to the patient.

Keats warned that preoccupation with classification of errors may prevent recognition of drug toxicity. The discoveries of malignant hyperthermia and succinylcholine-induced hyperkalemia did not occur because of a search for errors by an anesthesia review commission. The cyanosis and hypercarbia of malignant hyperthermia might have been attributed to error in airway management by such a commission. Cardiac arrest from succinylcholine might have been attributed to error in resuscitation. The classification of the error might have ended the search for cause.

In response, Hamilton[83] presented an opposing view. While acknowledging that deaths may occur from drug toxicity, he believed that such cases were rare. Errors in management, however, were contended to be common and predictable sources of anesthetic mortality. Concerning the relative contributions of drug toxicity versus error to anesthetic deaths, Hamilton wrote, "In my view error is near the 90 per cent end."[83]

The recent report by Caplan et al.[38] of 14 cases of unexpected cardiac arrest in healthy patients during spinal anesthesia has renewed the "toxicity versus errors" controversy (see above). Caplan et al.[38] can be interpreted on either side of the controversy. A previously unrecognized spinal anesthesia toxicity has perhaps been uncovered. Yet it was an exhaustive investigation for errors that brought these cases to light. They were grouped because no error could be determined.[84]

Misadventures or Errors?

Misadventure is defined as misfortune or bad luck. What might constitute an anesthetic misadventure? Bad luck certainly cannot be held responsible for an esophageal intubation. The Utting et al.[85] report on "human misadventure in anesthesia" analyzed 602 cases that were reported between 1970 and 1977 to the British Medical Defense Union in anticipation of legal action. Included were 277 deaths and 71 cases of cerebral damage. Although drug sensitivity, hepatic failure,

and hyperthermia were considered misadventures, the large majority of these misadventures were attributed to error and were thus not really misadventures at all. Most involved problems with the respiratory system, namely, esophageal intubation, ventilator disconnection, and aspiration.[85] A similar finding was reported by Craig and Wilson[86] in their 1981 survey of anesthetic misadventures. Of the 81 misadventures reported, human error was concluded to be the cause in 65 percent. Failure to perform a preanesthetic check was the most common factor.[86]

A common characteristic of an error is that its occurrence has been previously described. For example, cases of incorrect gas administration were reported by Utting and co-workers[85] because a carbon dioxide or nitrous oxide cylinder had somehow been put in place of an oxygen cylinder. Mushin had described that problem in 1948[87]:

The patient's color fails and the more the nitrous oxide cylinder is turned on, under the impression that it contains the appropriate antidote—lifesaving oxygen—the worse the patient gets. The patient quickly dies unless the mistake is recognized by the anesthetist and rectified. These deaths have been reported for over twenty years with tiresome and lately alarming frequency.

The Mushin reference was itself preceded by wartime fatalities when American green cylinders containing oxygen were confused with English green cylinders containing carbon dioxide.[87] Lest we think it cannot happen again, consider the fact that there is no government standard for cylinder color in the United States. Worse, the international color for oxygen is white, not green.[88] When ASA presidents Dr. Jess Weiss and Dr. Ellison Pierce and others began an earnest and official push toward establishment of standards of anesthesia care in the early 1980s, there was much initial resistance. Physicians proclaimed themselves resentful of attempts to "tell us how to practice," and worried about government or insurance company interference. Nonetheless, when one carefully reads the CEPOD study,[24] the need for standards of care become obvious. We believe that this push, initiated and promulgated by clinical anesthesiologists, not government, *is by far the most important advance in the field of anesthesia risk in the 1980s.*

Critical Incidents

A significant problem in studying risk of anesthesia is that events are infrequent, requiring extensive and tedious data collection. A pioneering alternative approach was that of Cooper and his colleagues,[8,89-92] who used a technique of *critical incident* analysis adopted from the work of Flanagan in 1954.[93] Cooper et al.[8] defined the critical incident in anesthesia:

A critical incident is a human error or equipment failure that could have led (if not discovered or corrected in

TABLE 22-11. Incidence of Several Major Anesthetic Risks

Risk	Incidence	Source
Death	1 : 10,000	Lunn et al.[4]
Cardiac arrest	1.7 : 10,000	Keenan and Boyan[34]
Halothane hepatonecrosis	1 : 35,000[a]	National Halothane Study[77,106]
Malignant hyperthermia	1 : 50,000	International Symposium on Malignant Hyperthermia[78]

[a] 1 : 35,000 *halothane* anesthetics.

time) or did lead to an undesirable outcome, ranging from increased length of hospital stay to death.

In the 1978 report,[91] 47 staff and resident anesthesiologists of one teaching hospital were interviewed by non-physician professionals and asked to report any preventable anesthetic-related errors they had observed or in which they had participated. A total of 359 such incidents were described and their characteristics analyzed. The most frequent incidents included breathing circuit disconnection, syringe swap, and gas supply problems. *Human error was a much more frequent contributor than was equipment failure*, but equipment design contributed to human errors in a significant number of cases (copper kettle controls, oxygen flow knob, etc.). The most frequent factors cited included inadequate total experience and inadequate familiarity with equipment or device, suggesting to the authors that better teaching could have prevented many of the reported errors. Haste, inattention, carelessness, and fatigue were also frequently cited factors.[91]

Two important findings of the studies of Cooper et al. were that critical incidents occurred most frequently *during the maintenance period of anesthesia* and that a number of incidents were detected during "breaks" by the relief anesthetist. The authors suggested that work-rest cycles may be important. This thesis was confirmed in a subsequent report.[89,90]

In the 1984 report, Cooper et al.[8] expanded the study to include 139 anesthesiologists, residents, and nurse anesthetists at four hospitals and obtained descriptions of 1,089 preventable critical incidents. The most frequent critical incidents were similar to those of the earlier report (Table 22-12).[91] Inexperience and lack of vigilance were still cited most frequently (Table 22-13). Fatigue was an infrequent factor. The 1984 report also added a focus on incidents that were associated with substantial negative outcomes, defined as mortality, cardiac arrest, cancelled surgery, or extended postoperative stay. Various respiratory problems, including esophageal intubation and breathing circuit disconnection, plus inhalation and intravenous drug overdoses accounted for many substantial negative outcomes. Significantly, equipment failure accounted for only 4.3 percent of the incidents that resulted in substantial negative outcomes.[8] Critical incidents resulting in substantial negative outcome were more frequent in

TABLE 22-13. Top Five Factors Cited in Critical Incidents

Factor	No. of Incidents
Failure to check	223
First experience with situation	208
Inadequate total experience	201
Inattention or carelessness	166
Haste encouraged by situation	131

(Adapted from Cooper et al.,[8] with permission.)

seriously ill patients (ASA class III or greater), while critical incidents that fortunately did not cause serious harm were more likely in healthy patients (ASA class I). The authors offered several strategies for reducing incidents associated with substantial negative outcomes. These included (1) improved supervision and continued education; (2) specific protocols for preoperative assessment, machine inspection, and personnel changes; (3) additional monitoring of ventilation and oxygenation; (4) better assignment of personnel to cases commensurate with their experience. Although lack of experience was a major factor in Cooper's studies in teaching hospitals, failure to apply already acquired knowledge was the major factor cited in CEPOD.[24] Perhaps if the definitions of these "knowledge and/or experience" categories were standardized, one would find greater similarity between these studies since the CEPOD survey included mostly fully trained practitioners. Presently, we can only conclude that human factors are emphasized in both reports. Recently Cooper et al.[92] developed a system to assess recovery room incidents. Gaba et al.[94] reviewed the error process and suggested that a "chain of accident evolution" causes incidents to become accidents.

DOES ANESTHESIA RISK DEPEND ON WHO ADMINISTERS THE ANESTHESIA?

This question of whether anesthetic risk depends on the anesthesia provider is charged with emotional and political energy and therefore is often avoided in textbooks. Yet, there is much to suggest that major differences in both practice and outcome do exist between

TABLE 22-12. Five Most Frequently Described Critical Incidents

Incident	No. Described
Breathing circuit disconnection during mechanical ventilation	57
Syringe swap	50
Gas flow control technical errors	41
Loss of gas supply	32
Intravenous line disconnection	24

(Adapted from Cooper et al.,[8] with permission.)

individuals and institutions. Such information can be used constructively to direct resources to problem arcas.

A courageous example from another specialty was set by Hotchkiss[95] in 1960 in his report on "Patent Ductus Arteriosus and the Occasional Cardiac Surgeon." Hotchkiss evaluated operative mortality over a 10-year period in 68 nonuniversity hospitals for repair of patent ductus arteriosus, a presumed low-risk procedure. These data were compared with those for university centers. Mortality in nonteaching centers was two to three times that of teaching centers. Explanations included inexperience and lack of support facilities. The average number of cases per nonuniversity hospital was less than one per year. Cardiac catheterization was performed in less than one-half of the hospitals performing the operation. Hotchkiss[95] suggested that if proper facilities and/or experience were not present, a hospital might refer such cases. The current controversy over where organ transplants are done and who performs them is reminiscent of this early admonition by Hotchkiss.

Another example of mortality variation was uncovered by the National Halothane Study.[77,96] Examination of postoperative death rates after general anesthesia in 34 hospitals revealed marked differences. After correction for age, sex, prior surgery, physical status, and year of surgery, mortality rates for six selected operations were evaluated. Despite standardization, overall mortality ranged from 0.7 to about 5 percent. Today, the U.S. government Health Care Finance Agency (HCFA) is releasing raw individual hospital mortality data related to diagnosis only, by hospital name. It is widely understood that accurate "severity of illness" scoring is needed, but no agreed-on method has been established, although several are being tested and advocated.

Differences in outcome may be related to individual anesthesiologists. Slogoff and Keats[97] contended that perioperative myocardial ischemia led to postoperative myocardial infarction. They had the temerity to publish data by individual (numbered) anesthesiologists. One, namely, number 7, appeared to have significantly more patients who developed postoperative myocardial infarctions. Of note is that anesthesiologist number 7's caseload was about one-half the average caseload of the other anesthesiologists and was the smallest of the group. The implication that experience played a role is refuted by the fact that anesthesiologist number 9 had the second smallest caseload, yet had the fewest perioperative myocardial infarctions. The authors' contention that perioperative ischemia might cause infarcts is not satisfying. Anesthesiologist number 4 had almost the same incidence of ischemic episodes as did number 7 but less than one-half the incidence of postoperative infarctions (Table 22-14).[97]

Perhaps the most courageous such individualized report ever published was that of Easton and Sherman,[20] who reported on 228 consecutive carotid endarterectomies, with an overall stroke and/or death rate of ap-

TABLE 22-14. Comparison of Cardiac Anesthesiologists 4, 7, and 9

Anesthesiologist no.	No. of Patients	Arrival Ischemia (%)	Anesthesia Ischemia (%)	Postoperative Infarction (%)
4	118	22	38	5.1
7	64	20	45	12.5
9	95	17	26	1.1
Group average	113	17.8	27.6	4.1

(Adapted from Slogoff and Keats,[97] with permission.)

proximately 20 percent. They knew, of course, that this was nearly 10 times worse than "standard" published rates, and attempted, without success, to find the cause by breaking down their data to individual surgeons (unnamed), also year by year, and several other approaches. They did not find the answer. Interestingly, the influence of anesthesia, either who did it, or which technique, was not examined as a potential contributor to such variations.[20]

It is also disturbing when a particular group of anesthesia providers is identified as having a higher incidence of anesthetic mortality. Holland[28] reported on anesthetic mortality over 25 years in New South Wales, Australia. The contribution of nonspecialist physicians to anesthetic mortality declined over this period. Holland[28] stated that this reflects a "reduction in the general practitioner involvement in anesthesia—a process common to all developed countries as specialization takes hold." Resident medical officers who were not anesthesia trainees contributed significantly to mortality in low-risk patients in the early years, which led to a phasing out of these persons as service members of the anesthetic work force.[28]

The recent CEPOD[24] also noted a nonrandom distribution of mortality among anesthetist personnel. In the three regions studied, consultants (fully trained physician anesthetists) undertook 34 to 49 percent of the cases and were responsible for 12 to 13 percent of the associated anesthetic mortality. Several nonconsultant groups had proportionally more anesthetic-associated deaths. For example, in one region, "other" physician anesthetists undertook 0.6 percent of the cases but were responsible for 33.3 percent of the anesthetic-associated deaths.[24]

In the United States, the issue of relative safety of anesthesia when administered by certified nurse anesthetists (CRNAs) versus physicians is complex and emotional. There are numerous categories that must be taken into account in any valid analysis: CRNAs in independent unsupervised practice; CRNAs supervised by physician anesthesiologists (and in what supervisory ratio, i.e., 1:1 through 1:4 or more); resident physician trainees supervised by faculty physician anesthesiologists (and, again, in what ratio); student nurse anesthetists supervised by either CRNAs or physicians; and physician anesthesiologists doing their own anesthetics.

There are also master's degree physician assistants (PAs) performing anesthesia in the United States. Physician anesthesiologists are either M.D.'s or D.O.'s; are either certified by a specialty board or not (from the United States or elsewhere); are recently trained, long out of training, or never had any (or much) formal training in anesthesia at all. Worse, the better-trained individuals (of any of the above stripes), at a given hospital, either do or do not more often encounter the sickest, highest-risk patients. We hope the student will use the above to read any report of this problem with great care (and skepticism), including that which follows.

The above should also be kept in mind when considering a report by Bechtoldt[98] from the Anesthesia Study Committee of North Carolina. They evaluated 90 anesthetic-related deaths over an 8-year period (1969 to 1976), during which time they estimated that a total of more than 2 million anesthetics were administered. CRNAs working alone administered about one-half of the total. The fewest anesthetics were administered by surgeons and dentists. Anesthesiologists made up the middle group. When mortality was compared among the groups, the surgeon and dentist administrations had the highest mortality. The CRNAs and anesthesiologists had better mortality rates when they worked together (Table 22-15) than when either worked independently. The mortality rates for all groups in this report were less than the modern large-study, generally quoted anesthetic mortality of 1 : 10,000. Perhaps this result relates to the fact that the number of anesthetics administered was only estimated; no risk categorization or adjustment was made to compare outcome results with the different categories of providers. The North Carolina study included cardiac cases, which are often excluded from mortality studies of anesthetic risk. We are concerned that the study was not published in a major peer-reviewed anesthesiology journal.[98]

In 1988, the American Society of Anesthesiologists, collaborating with the Communicable Disease Center of the United States Public Health Service, began a large-scale pilot survey of anesthesia-related morbidity and mortality, with extensive categorization of providers. The pilot study has indicated the feasibility of such an undertaking.[99] If errors, lapses, and/or lack of vigilance do account for significant numbers of anesthetic deaths, then lower levels of training may not necessarily have greater associated anesthetic morbidity and mortality, especially if preoperative physical status is being appropriately matched to skill and experience level. The greatest problem with this type of survey is to obtain valid assessment of patient severity of illness, specifically as it relates to performance of anesthesia. A patient terminally ill with cancer might constitute a relatively low anesthetic difficulty, that is, easy intubation, reasonable cardiovascular health, etc., whereas a patient who has a bull neck, poor but extensive dentition, etc., might not be classified as seriously ill by any of the currently available severity of illness indices, yet pose a major anesthetic challenge. Raw mortality and mortality statistics for the groups of anesthesia providers mentioned above, unless corrected for anesthesia-specific severity of illness (or magnitude of anesthetic challenge), may be dangerously misleading, in the sense that legislators and other payors may become convinced that anesthesia services can be safely "bought" from less well trained groups of people, regardless of patient condition, complexity of required surgery, abnormal position, new techniques, etc.

CHOICE OF ANESTHETIC OR TECHNIQUE AS A FACTOR OF SAFETY

Ether, cyclopropane, fluroxene, and ethylene, owing to their flammability, have been essentially abandoned in the United States. Questions of toxicity and/or safety of today's agents and techniques are not so clear-cut. Such questions are raised when an untoward clinical response is reported in one or a few patients. Multiple such reports stimulate research to prove or disprove toxicity and to understand mechanisms. Over time, the agent is vindicated, abandoned, or used with certain guidelines.

Methoxyflurane, for example, was first noted by Crandell et al.[100] to be associated with high-output renal failure. Other case reports followed. Numerous mechanistic studies followed these early case reports. A control study by Mazze et al.[101] showed that patients anesthetized with methoxyflurane developed a tendency toward antidiuretic hormone-resistant polyuria, while patients similarly anesthetized with halothane did not. Methoxyflurane subsequently has been supplanted by less toxic agents, but when enflurane was introduced, the fact that fluoride can be released stimulated a series of studies about the latter's possible nephrotoxicity. Enflurane was not shown to be nephrotoxic.[102]

Some anesthetic agents can be toxic in certain patients or diseases. Succinylcholine is contraindicated after certain time periods in patients with extensive burns,[103] trauma,[104] spinal cord injuries, and neuromuscular disease[105] because of the risk of hyperkalemia and subsequent cardiac arrest. Although this proscription is part of our knowledge base now, consider the dismay of the clinician previously:

> **Burn dressing. Extensive third degree burns of lower body. . . . Pentothal, succinylcholine intubation. Bradycardia to *arrest*. No response to massage.**
>
> **—A case report by Ament[7]**

TABLE 22-15. Comparative Anesthetic Mortality Rates Among Anesthesia Providers in North Carolina

Anesthesiologist and CRNA	1 : 28,166
Anesthesiologist alone	1 : 24,500
CRNA alone	1 : 20,723
Surgeon or dentist	1 : 11,432

(Adapted from Bechtoldt,[98] with permission.)

Some anesthetic-risk surveys have implicated a particular anesthetic agent as a cause of mortality. Beecher and Todd[14] examined perioperative deaths in a massive multihospital study of 599,548 patients. A particular association was that patients who had received curare had higher mortality. The authors contended that this was an "inherent toxicity" of curare. It is obvious now that this "toxicity" was due to failure to provide respiratory assistance. Edwards et al.[13] illustrated this early lack of appreciation of this problem by this description:

A fit patient was subjected to a long abdominal operation for which he was given thiopentone 1 g, *d*-tubocurarine chloride 15 mg and deep ether anesthesia. Respiration was assisted at first, but later allowed to continue spontaneously. He was flaccid postoperatively and his respiration shallow. On this account he was given a 5% carbon dioxide and oxygen mixture to breathe. Over a period of half an hour his respiration gradually failed.

Although it seems obvious now that failure of reversal of neuromuscular blockade was the culprit in these cases, the controversy went on for several years, until Dripps et al.[49] clarified the issue when they reported that 6,000 physically fit patients had received a muscle relaxant and that none had died. This illustrates the need to understand mechanisms behind the epidemiologic results seen in large-scale studies.

The largest analysis of an anesthetic's potential specific toxicity was the National Halothane Study.[77,96,106] Halothane was similar enough chemically to chloroform to have engendered concern about its hepatic effects at the time of its introduction. Prompted by several case reports of massive hepatic narcosis after halothane anesthesia, the manufacturer warned against the use of halothane in patients with known liver or biliary tract disease. A collaborative retrospective study of 34 institutions and 856,500 cases of general anesthesia was performed to determine whether halothane was in fact a hepatotoxin.

There were 10,171 complete necropsies done, which disclosed 82 cases of massive hepatic necrosis representing approximately 1 case per 10,000 administrations of general anesthesia. The incidence of massive hepatic necrosis following halothane was the same as that with nitrous oxide-barbiturate anesthesia, somewhat more than with ether, and considerably less than with cyclopropane. The hepatic necrosis could be adequately explained by circulatory shock, infection, or vasopressor use *in all but nine patients, seven of which had received halothane.* Thus, the report appeared to show that halothane could be a cause of hepatic necrosis but that the incidence was extremely rare.[106] The report also showed, interestingly enough, that halothane was the *safest* anesthetic then in use, from an overall standpoint.[106]

Occasionally, preoperative medications have been reported to interact adversely with anesthetic agents. A 1972 report[107] described several cardiac surgical patients who were taking oral propranolol preoperatively and who subsequently had poor cardiac function intra-operatively. The authors contended that propranolol was the only temporally associated therapeutic change and therefore blamed its use. Based on a tissue study, it was advocated to stop the drug 2 weeks before elective surgery. Without corroborating research, many physicians discontinued propranolol in patients with coronary artery disease prior to surgery. Eventually it became obvious that discontinuation caused some patients to have exacerbation of anginal symptoms, arrhythmias, and myocardial infarctions.[108,109] The original case report was not entirely to blame, but *there are dangers in making sweeping generalizations from initial reports.* All too often, authors of such reports cannot resist the admonition that a drug or a technique should be used "with caution" in a patient who is taking a drug or has a certain disease. Equally to blame are physicians (and lawyers) who adopt such speculations as fact, without demanding controlled research.

The most recent anesthetic agent to be accused of specific toxicity is isoflurane. In some ways, the story of isoflurane and coronary steal resembles that of propranolol. In 1983, a study of 21 patients undergoing coronary bypass surgery under protocol isoflurane anesthesia was published.[110] Ten of the patients developed signs of myocardial ischemia. The authors concluded that isoflurane was a "powerful" coronary vasodilator, based on coronary sinus flow measurements, and speculated that the ischemia was therefore due to coronary steal. Another explanation, however, was that hypotension (40 percent decrease in mean arterial pressure) had caused the ischemia. After 4 years of controversy, an editorial by Becker[111] concluded that isoflurane was a small vessel coronary vasodilator capable of causing coronary steal and that it was "dangerous" in patients with known coronary artery disease. Professor Becker did not use the term "dangerous" in any comparative sense, that is, addressing the question as to which anesthetic would be specifically safer, not only from the coronary steal standpoint but from the overall patient safety point of view.[111] Since isoflurane has been administered many millions of times in the United States (where coronary artery disease is prevalent), is there really an increased incidence of ischemia and/or infarction with it? If administering 1 percent isoflurane can cause myocardial ischemia in coronary patients, why wasn't this a widespread clinical observation, since Reiz et al.[110] described ischemia in 50 percent of patients studied? Further, like the propranolol study, will there be consequences of a change in practice? Will the incidence of renal toxicity or hepatotoxicity or some other problem increase because isoflurane is avoided? Will narcotic respiratory depression and naloxone pulmonary edema become more common? Probably Dr. Becker's[111] best advice in that unfortunate editorial was, "Clearly these recommendations await further support from carefully controlled randomized studies in humans. . . ." The point of the above example is not to castigate authors who point out that they have had problems with particular anesthetics or techniques. We need these reports, especially after a new drug or technique goes into widespread use. We are not sufficiently sophisticated in our ability to take these reports in stride and to rapidly clarify such issues with carefully designed and controlled studies.

Reports of isoflurane versus other inhalational anesthetics are now appearing. A retrospective analysis by Cucchiara et al.[112] of patients who underwent carotid endarterectomy with halothane, enflurane, or isoflurane demonstrated no significant difference in the number of postoperative myocardial infarctions among the different techniques. The number of fatal myocardial infarctions was lowest in the isoflurane group.

In the mid-1980s, a United States-Canadian multi-institutional prospective study of anesthesia-related outcomes was carried out. The results are not yet published, but a preliminary report (B. R. Brown, personal communication) indicated that no statistically significant differences in outcome could be attributed to a specific anesthetic agent or technique. Isoflurane constituted about one-fourth of the anesthetics.

The controversy of regional versus general anesthesia with respect to patient safety is longstanding. Dripps et al.[49] reported that primary anesthetic deaths were less frequent with regional than with general anesthesia. Yeager et al.[113] randomized 53 high-risk patients to either general anesthesia or epidural anesthesia with light general anesthesia plus postoperative epidural analgesia. The epidural plus light general anesthesia group had fewer total complications and lower hospital costs. A recent review by Scott and Kehlet[114] found morbidity to be less for regional rather than general anesthesia if the surgical procedure was below the umbilicus. Unfortunately, recent studies on the subject are of small numbers of cases. No recent large-scale survey of anesthetic mortality has indicated either regional or general anesthesia to be advantageous.

ANESTHETIC RISKS IN SPECIFIC PATIENT GROUPS

Obstetrics
(Also See Ch. 57)

Several recent reports have characterized maternal mortality in the United States. In a nationwide (50-state) analysis, Kaunitz et al.[115] reported on 2,475 maternal deaths that occurred during 1974 through 1978; an overall U.S. maternal mortality of 15.3 deaths per 100,000 live births. Causes of death are listed in Table 22-16. In 1988, Rochat et al.[116] reported the findings of the Maternal Mortality Collaborative, which was established in 1983 by the American College of Obstetricians and Gynecologists. This survey received voluntary reports of maternal deaths occurring between 1980 and 1985 from all regions of the United States. This study found a maternal mortality ratio of 14.1 deaths per 100,000 live births. The causes of death are also listed in

Table 22-16. If this is a real (circa 0.8 percent) decrease in overall maternal mortality rate (15.3 to 14.1 deaths), these studies appear to indicate that fewer deaths are occurring as a result of embolism, hypertensive disease, hemorrhage, and ectopic pregnancy. In fact, Rochat et al.[116] found that maternal mortality ratios were lower *for all direct causes except anesthesia and cerebrovascular accident.*

Similar data exist from the United Kingdom.[117] The Confidential Enquiry into Maternal Deaths in England and Wales has been acquiring data for 3-year periods over the last 30 years.[118] The most recent report for the years 1979 to 1981 lists similar causes for maternal deaths. Anesthesia is the third most common direct cause of maternal death after hypertensive disease and pulmonary embolism.[119] As in the United States, the overall number of direct maternal deaths has decreased, but anesthesia still contributes significantly to the total.

Endler et al.[120] studied specific causes of anesthesia-related maternal mortality for the years 1972 through 1984 in Michigan. Anesthesia was the primary cause of death in 15 cases, accounting for 6.9 percent of direct maternal deaths. This amounted to 0.82 deaths from anesthesia per 100,000 live births. It is difficult to extrapolate this number to deaths per number of anesthetics, because many mothers giving birth do not receive anesthesia. Also, anesthetics are provided for conditions such as tubal ligation and ectopic pregnancy in patients considered obstetric, when no live birth occurred.

The causes of anesthesia-related maternal mortality are similar to those of other anesthetic deaths, namely, cardiac arrest, intubation problems, and aspiration of gastric contents; cerebral anoxia and complications of regional anesthesia accounted for most of the deaths in the U.S. and U.K. studies. Other risk factors commonly noted were patient age over 30 years, nonwhite race, and obesity. Risk of death from obstetric hemorrhage has been contended to be higher in small hospitals. The issue of cardiac arrest during anesthesia in pregnant patients was addressed by Keenan and Boyan,[34] who found 2 of 27 anesthesia-related cardiac arrests in pregnant patients. One arrest was due to esophageal intuba-

TABLE 22-16. Causes of Maternal Deaths (Percentage of Totals) for Two Periods[a] in the United States

Cause	% Maternal Deaths 1974–1978 (Kaunitz)[115]	% Maternal Deaths 1980–1985 (Rochat)[116]
Embolism	19.8	17.0
Hypertensive disease	17.0	12.3
Ectopic pregnancy	10.2	10.0
Hemorrhage	13.4	9.0
Cerebral vascular accident	4.3	8.4
Anesthesia complications	4.0	7.0

[a] The overall maternal mortality ratio was 15.3 deaths per 100,000 live births for 1974–1978 and 14.2 deaths per 100,000 live births for 1980–1985.

tion and the other to overdose of inhalational anesthetic. Marx[121] pointed out that both of these occurred with general anesthesia, as did most (26 of 27) of the arrests in the Keenan and Boyan[34] report.

A portion of anesthesia-related maternal mortality can be attributed to nonanesthesiologist physicians who administer anesthetics. Grimes and Cates[122] reported three cases of death occurring during first-trimester pregnancy termination, when paracervical block was administered by "the physician." The descriptions of convulsions followed by cardiac arrest suggest that deaths were due to systemic effects of local anesthetics. The authors[122] wrote as follows:

> If tremor, twitching or convulsions occur, the patient should be treated with intravenous diazepam or a rapid acting barbiturate. . . . If convulsions persist, intubation should be instituted with the aid of succinylcholine . . .

Although administration of such drugs is routine for the anesthesiologist, the *expected* consequences, namely, unconsciousness and paralysis, may be difficult to manage for the obstetrician or family physician. While paracervical block raises these concerns most, they apply to any circumstances in which local anesthetics are utilized.

Numerous authors have addressed the question of how to reduce the risks of anesthesia in the obstetric patient.[123-128] Critical to improvement in these risks are factors noted by Gibbs et al.[129] in a national survey of obstetric anesthesia. Questionnaires were sent to chiefs of obstetrics and anesthesiology in almost 1,200 hospitals in the United States, who were divided into groups based on delivery volume. The findings were disquieting. Anesthesiologists (defined to include anesthesia residents) were available full time in only 21 percent of the hospitals and available on nights and weekends in only 15 percent of the hospitals. This was true despite the fact that "anesthesiologists" included resident coverage with on-call faculty at home. The lack of anesthesia coverage was most marked in hospitals that performed less than 500 deliveries per year. For example, personnel performing newborn resuscitation in smaller hospitals were often described as "other." By this category was meant that the individual was not an anesthesiologist, obstetrician, pediatrician, or CRNA. This was the case for 24 percent of the cesarean deliveries and 43 percent of the vaginal deliveries in these hospitals.[129]

Questionnaire responses as to reasons for lack of anesthesiologic involvement included the following[129]:

1. Unpredictability of labor and delivery making coverage difficult, especially in small-volume hospitals
2. High risk of malpractice actions
3. Obstetricians dictation of type and timing of anesthesia provided
4. Insufficient remuneration

Whether the presence of a trained anesthesiologist can

improve maternal or fetal morbidity or mortality cannot be addressed by such a questionnaire study. Clearly, hospital administrations are becoming increasingly aware of their responsibility to ensure first-class anesthetic coverage if they are to continue to have viable obstetric services.

Pediatrics
(Also See Ch. 59)

Specialists in pediatric anesthesia often admonish against the practice of treating pediatric patients as "little adults." Data regarding anesthetic complications in pediatric patients firmly support this warning.[130-136] In the Keenan and Boyan[34] study of cardiac arrests from anesthesia, the incidence in patients less than 12 years old was three times that in patients over 12 years (Table 22-17). Within the pediatric age group, the contrast is more striking. The fact that infants less than 1 year of age are at considerably greater risk than older children has been demonstrated repeatedly in risk studies. Rackow et al.[137] reviewed pediatric cardiac arrests occurring during anesthesia over a 10-year period (1947 to 1956) at Columbia Hospital in New York. Infants (less than 1 year old) composed 12.5 percent of the pediatric population, underwent 4,308 anesthetics, and suffered 28 percent of the arrests (Table 22-18). Rackow et al.[137] noted in children that cardiac arrests were associated with complete recovery in only 16 percent of cases and that death occurred in 68 percent. Intraoperative cardiac arrest in adults has been associated with 50 percent complete recovery, but the Rackow et al.[137] report is from an earlier period.

The most recent data on pediatric anesthesia risk are those of Tiret et al.,[138] who studied major anesthetic complications that occurred in children less than 15 years old during a prospective study of 440 French hospitals between 1978 and 1982. A total of 40,240 anesthetics were included in the survey. Major complications were defined as life-threatening incidents and/or those that resulted in severe sequelae. Twenty-seven such major complications occurred for an incidence of 7:10,000. Twelve of these were cardiac arrests (3:10,000). The group of infants aged less than 1 year comprised only *5 percent* of the anesthetized population of children but suffered *one-half* of all the complications, including one-half of the cardiac arrests (Table 22-19). These data indicate an incidence of cardiac arrest due to anesthesia in infants that was 10 times that in older children. Also, the incidence of all complications

TABLE 22-17. Incidence of Anesthesia-Associated Cardiac Arrest in Pediatric versus Adult Patients

Age Group	No. of Anesthetics	No. of Arrests	Incidence
Less than 12 yrs	12,712	6	4.7:10,000
Over 12 yrs	150,528	21	1.4:10,000

(From Keenan and Boyan,[34] with permission.)

TABLE 22-18. Incidence of Cardiac Arrest in Infants and Children 1947–1956[a]

Patient Group	No. of Anesthetics	No. and Incidence of Cardiac Arrest due to Anesthesia	Cardiac Arrest from All Causes
Infants (<1 yr)	4,308	6 (14:10,000)	7 (16:10,000)
Children (1–12 yrs)	30,191	13 (4.3:10,000)	18 (6:10,000)

[a] Children over age 13 had an incidence of cardiac arrest of 3.9:10,000 from all causes. (Adapted from Rackow et al.,[137] with permission.)

was eight times higher in infants than in older children. Conversely, older children had fewer complications and cardiac arrests than the generally reported adult rates during the same year. Complications in pediatric patients were more frequent for emergency operations, patients with full stomachs, and patients classified higher in ASA physical status (Table 22-20). Complications in infants mainly involved respiratory problems and were most frequent during maintenance rather than during induction of anesthesia. In contrast, children experienced equal amounts of respiratory and circulatory complications, and they were distributed throughout the time period of the anesthetic. The only death that occurred in a child occurred from respiratory depression in the recovery room.[138] One might imagine that congenital airway anomalies and neonatal emergencies accounted for the high incidence of infant complications during anesthesia. Yet the majority of all pediatric complications reported by Tiret et al.[138] were due to typical problems such as aspiration, laryngospasm, bronchospasm, endobronchial intubation, ventilator malfunction, halothane overdose, fluid overload, etc.

Salem et al.[139] described 73 episodes of cardiac arrest in infants and children resulting from anesthesia. Respiratory factors contributed to 37 of these arrests; 12 of the latter progressed to death. Congenital airway problems such as Pierre Robin syndrome, neck contractures, and gargoylism accounted for only 3 of 37 cases and only 1 of the 12 deaths.

Recognizing the special considerations for the pediatric age group, some have implied or suggested that hospitals devoted to children have better anesthetic results. Data provided by Smith[140] are supportive. When data from the Boston Children's Hospital are pooled for the period between 1954 through 1978, 15 anesthetic deaths occurred in 116,784 anesthetized pediatric patients (0 to 10 years old) for an incidence of anesthetic mortality of 1.3:10,000. This is a remarkable record for this protracted period (and no small tribute to Dr. Robert M. Smith), but of course there is no denominator, that is, no way to compare it with risk data for pediatric patients anesthetized in all hospitals.[140]

The importance of the specialist in pediatric anesthesia is also illustrated by Hickey et al.,[141] who reported on 500 consecutive surgeries for congenital heart disease during a 9-month period from 1981 to 1982. Despite the fact that 47 percent of the patients were less than 1 year old, there were no anesthetic deaths. Major complications occurred in four cases, namely, tension pneumothorax in two cases and severe hypotension in two cases.[141] Again, reports of outstanding success from individual hospitals do not constitute standards or population risk, although they certainly do constitute a target to which to aspire.[142–144]

Geriatrics
(Also See Ch. 62)

The landmark 1951 study by Beecher and Todd[14] noted that perioperative deaths were more frequent in the elderly. This finding has been supported by numerous subsequent studies. Goldman et al.[61] reported that age over 70 years was a statistically significant risk factor for development of perioperative cardiac complication and a greater risk factor than symptomatic aortic stenosis, poor general medical condition, site of operation (intraperitoneal, intrathoracic or aortic), or emergency

TABLE 22-19. Incidence of Major Anesthesia Complications in Infants, Children, and Adults

Group	No. of Anesthetics	No. and Incidence of Cardiac Arrests due to Anesthesia	No. and Incidence of All Major Anesthetic Complications
Infants (<1 yr)	2,103	4 (19:10,000)	9 (43:10,000)
Children (1–14 yrs)	38,137	8 (2:10,000)	18 (5:10,000)
Adults[a] (>15 yrs)		7:10,000	15:10,000

[a] Data on adults were simultaneously collected and reported by Tiret et al.[27]
(Adapted from Tiret et al.,[138] with permission.)

TABLE 22-20. Frequency of Major Complications Compared with ASA Class in Pediatric Patients

ASA Physical Status Category	No. of Anesthetics	No. of Complications	Incidence of Complications
I	36,903	14	4 : 10,000
II	1,461	5	34 : 10,000
III	518	6	116 : 10,000
IV and V	122	2	164 : 10,000

(Adapted from Tiret et al.,[138] with permission.)

TABLE 22-21. Risk Groups in Elderly Determined by Preoperative Hemodynamic Assessment

Group	Recommendation
I No functional deficit	Proceed to Surgery
II Mild functional deficit	Proceed to surgery with hemodynamic monitors
III Moderate deficit (could be corrected)	Delay surgery for preoperative therapy
IV Advanced deficit (could not be corrected)	Alternative mode of treatment

(Data from Del Guercio and Cohn.[153])

surgery. Age over 70 increased risk of perioperative cardiac death 10-fold. In a recent study, Cohen et al.[70] again demonstrated increased mortality with advanced age and showed that it was markedly increased for patients greater than 80 years old. Operative mortality rates for patients with specific preoperative conditions (respiratory disease, ischemic heart disease, renal disease) also increased with advancing age.[69] The recent British Confidential Enquiry into Perioperative Deaths (1987) reported a 0.7 percent operative mortality rate for about 0.5 million surgeries but noted that most of the deaths occurred in the elderly, specifically, that 79 percent of the deaths occurred in patients over 65, despite the fact that this age group comprised only 22 percent of all the operations in England for 1986.[24]

Physiologic changes coupled with disease have been proposed to account for these findings, including cardiovascular disease and hypertension, decreased ventilatory reserves, and various renal and hepatic changes.[145-152] Cardiac β-adrenergic receptors may be less responsive or numerous in the elderly.[147] An autopsy study of patients over 90 years of age revealed complete atherosclerotic occlusion of at least one coronary vessel in 70 percent of the patients despite the fact that only 25 percent of the patients had died of myocardial infarction.[148]

A revealing study about the limited physiologic reserve of the elderly was that of Del Guercio and Cohn.[153] These authors studied 148 patients over age 65 who had been evaluated and cleared for surgery by an internist. They then measured hemodynamics preoperatively with pulmonary artery catheters. On the basis of cardiac output, arterial and mixed venous oxygen saturations, filling pressure, and vascular resistance, patients were classified into four groups (Table 22-21) that were then related to the outcome (Table 22-22). The study illustrated the importance of valid preoperative evaluation and the insensitivity of internists providing clinical impressions in this group of elderly.[153] The satisfactory appearance of the patient at rest may mask markedly diminished physiologic reserves. The characterization of an elderly patient as "spry" may be an error if it produces optimism instead of objective preoperative evaluation.[153-164]

A thought-provoking question is raised by the Keenan and Boyan[34] study of cardiac arrests resulting from an-

esthesia, which found no significant predilection for these events in the elderly. Only 2 of 27 such arrests occurred in patients over age 65. Perhaps elderly patients compose too small a percentage of the total surgical population to draw conclusions from these data. Also possible is the notion that very elderly patients might be more carefully watched, or better monitored, or anesthetized by more competent or more experienced personnel. It does highlight the difficulty in discussing anesthesia risk. The oldest, youngest, and sickest patients are not the only ones at risk.

Coronary Artery Disease (Also See Ch. 51)

Postoperative myocardial infarction has long been recognized as a factor contributing to perioperative mortality. It seems to us that a curious evolution has occurred in the literature. Numerous reports defined the now well-known association between previous myocardial infarction and perioperative reinfarction, especially if the prior infarct was recent.[165-186] Recently, the burden of postoperative infarction seems to have been increasingly placed on anesthesia (Table 22-23).[97,177,178] Is this change justified? Are there other factors that may contribute to postoperative infarction? Consider, for example, the physiology of the postoperative state. An intense catabolic state occurs as the body attempts to repair its tissue. The coagulation system is hyperactive. Anemia may decrease oxygen-carrying capacity and re-

TABLE 22-22. Outcome of Elderly Risk Groups

Group[a]	No. of Patients	Outcomes
I	20	All survived surgery
II and III	94	8.5% operative mortality
IV	34	56% cancelled surgery 21% lesser operations—all survived 23% underwent originally proposed surgery—all died

[a] See Table 22-21.
(Data from Del Guercio and Cohn.[153])

TABLE 22-23. Evolution of Literature Concerning Perioperative Infarction

Title	Date
"Myocardial Infarction and Surgery"[165]	1964
"Myocardial Reinfarction after Anesthesia and Surgery"[168]	1978
"Perianesthetic Ischemic Episodes Cause Myocardial Infarctions in Humans—A Hypothesis Confirmed"[178]	1985

quire the heart to do more flow work to compensate. Pain and discomfort add to the abnormal catecholamine milieu. The arachidonic acid cascade may be producing excessive quantities of the vasoconstrictor thromboxane, which also increases platelet adhesiveness. Intense surgical efforts at hemostasis, including massive tissue cauterization, fresh frozen plasma, platelet concentrates, even ε-aminocaproic acid may result in thrombosis and resultant complications.[179,180] The period of anesthesia accounts for only a limited portion of the perioperative period, and it is well known that many postoperative infarctions do not occur until the *third* postoperative day.[171] Nonetheless, it is reasonable to ask whether type of anesthesia or permittance of intraoperative ischemic episodes could be correlated with the occurrence of postoperative myocardial infarction. The most recent surveys of this issue are those of Slogoff and Keats[181] and Tuman et al.,[182] with editorial comment by Mangano.[184]

Slogoff and Keats[181] prospectively studied 1,012 coronary bypass patients who were randomized to receive enflurane, halothane, isoflurane, or sufentanil. New intraoperative myocardial ischemia, indicated by ST-segment depression, was noted in 30.4 percent of all patients. Postoperative myocardial infarction occurred in 4 percent. Mortality in the hospital was the result in 1.6 percent of the patients. In this recent prospective study, after careful statistical analysis, the authors could find no significant differences among the four anesthetic techniques with respect to any of these events (Table 22-24).[23,181,184]

Tuman et al.[182] recently completed a similar but nonrandomized study comparing five commonly employed anesthetic techniques for coronary bypass surgery in patients with coronary artery disease. Again, no differ-

ences in any outcome measure specifically associated with anesthetic technique could be detected (Table 22-25). The authors acknowledged that lack of randomization of techniques may have introduced bias. For example, pulmonary artery pressure monitoring was utilized in over 50 percent of the narcotic-based techniques but in only 25.5 percent of the halothane cases.[181-184]

Another problem exists when studies of anesthesia techniques are undertaken in the coronary bypass patient population. As Mangano[184] points out, other factors such as adequacy of myocardial revascularization and cardioplegia are likely to markedly influence the outcome, especially with respect to postoperative myocardial infarction. How difficult is this problem? If past experience with attempts at separating surgical from anesthetic risk is any indication, the problem of trying to understand the anesthetic contribution to perioperative morbidity after coronary bypass surgery, especially with respect to perioperative myocardial infarction, is indeed difficult.

With respect to perioperative myocardial infarction after *noncardiac surgery*, investigators have pursued this question for over 40 years in surveys and studies involving hundreds of thousands of patients. What do we think we know about this problem? Patients who undergo noncardiac surgery after suffering a prior myocardial infarction are still disturbingly likely to suffer a perioperative infarct. These risks are probably still as follows: circa 5 percent overall reinfarction risk if patient has had a prior myocardial infarction; 15 to 30 percent reinfarction risk if the prior myocardial infarction is less than 3 months old; 10 to 15 percent reinfarction risk if the prior myocardial infarction is 3 to 6 months old.[165-176] Although Rao and El-Etr[177] reported considerably better results in all the above categories in 1983, no corroborating study has emerged. We also believe that operations on the great vessels, thoracic structures, and the upper abdomen are associated with greater risk of perioperative reinfarction in patients with prior myocardial infarction than are other operations.[168] Patients who have successfully undergone CABG surgery are probably at much less risk of undergoing a perioperative myocardial infarction after noncardiac surgery, although this protection probably diminishes in the years after the CABG.[172-174]

TABLE 22-24. Comparison of Four Randomized Anesthetic Techniques with the Incidence of New Myocardial Ischemia Postoperative Infarction, and Death

	Enflurane	Halothane	Isoflurane	Sufentanil
No. of patients	257	253	248	254
New ischemia (%)	28.0	32.8	33.5	28.4
Postoperative Infarction (%)	4.7	3.6	4.0	3.9
Deaths (%)	1.2	2.0	1.2	2.4

(Adapted from Slogoff and Keats,[181] with permission.)

TABLE 22-25. Comparison of Five Anesthetic Techniques with Respect to Incidence of Postoperative Myocardial Infarction and Death

	Fentanyl High Dose	Fentanyl Moderate Dose	Sufentanil	Diazapam-Ketamine	Halothane
No. of patients	240	345	212	250	47
Postoperative infarction (%)	4.7	4.4	4.3	2.8	4.3
Death (%)	4.6	3.2	2.8	1.6	4.3

(Adapted from Tuman et al.,[182] with permission.)

How could the perplexing problem of perioperative myocardial infarction be better addressed? Commissions of surgeons and anesthetists to review each perioperative infarction may not be more fruitful than our past survey-type studies. The results of such surveys may indicate that surgery is a greater factor for infarction in coronary bypass cases than is anesthesia. In the British CEPOD study, surgery was 66 times more frequently a cause of perioperative mortality than was anesthesia.[31,183] If this held true for CABG-perioperative myocardial infarction the number of coronary bypass patients surveyed would need to be greatly expanded to find any differences in anesthetic technique that might affect outcome.

Maybe studying postoperative myocardial infarction in coronary bypass patients is not, after all, a particularly useful marker.[184] Perhaps only the pre-bypass period, before the surgeon touches the heart, should be studied. Perhaps coronary bypass patients should not be studied at all. It appears that the problem of perioperative cardiovascular morbidity, especially perioperative myocardial infarction, is *not* solved and, in fact, may not even have been greatly ameliorated. Slogoff and Keats[97] asked "Does perioperative myocardial ischemia cause postoperative infarction?" They answered "yes," despite the fact that postoperative infarction occurred in only 7 percent of (CABG) patients who had shown perioperative ischemic signs. Why did the other 93 percent of the patients who were ischemic *not* develop infarctions? Could it be, as we have seen before, that we are blaming (or taking credit) ourselves (as anesthesiologists), when in fact the *mechanism* of these perioperative infarcts may lie elsewhere? In the future, we need to carefully study these patients with coronary artery disease perioperatively, with respect to their coagulation dynamics, the arachidonic cascade, and numerous other aspects of their disturbed perioperative physiology. Knight et al.[185] have observed that intraoperative ischemia is not a specific predictor of infarction.

ANESTHETIC RISK REDUCTION

Specific High-Risk Areas

Strategies for reduction of anesthetic risk must include programs directed at specific high-risk areas, for example, unfamiliarity with patient or situation and cardiac arrest, and large-scale efforts to reduce anesthetic risk from all causes. When specific risk issues are identified, energy can be focused. The anesthesia literature is replete with examples of risk management solutions to problems such as the pin index system for gas cylinders, the intraoperative electrocardiogram,[186] cricoid pressure,[187] and development of postanesthetic recovery rooms.

Cardiac arrest is a specific area deserving attention. Such events are infrequent and may still be unrecognized until dangerously late when precious time remaining for salvage is limited. One risk reduction strategy is development of early warning technology. Recognition that failure to provide adequate oxygenation to the patient has been a factor in many such cardiac arrests suggests that widespread application of pulse oximetry and capnography may permit discovery of episodes of ventilator disconnection or esophageal intubation before they progress to cardiac arrest.[188-191] Indeed, the ASA Closed Claims Study has revealed that in the judgment of physician anesthesiologist reviewers, about 30 percent of the claims that were judged preventable at all could have been prevented by use of pulse oximetry and capnometry.[192] Worse, these preventable accidents were by far the most damaging to the patient and the most costly.

Another specific strategy is establishment of protocols to facilitate efficient use of limited time in an emergency. Protocols such as the "difficult intubation drill" or the "peripartum hemorrhage drill" have been useful in obstetric emergencies.[128,193] In reported cases of cardiac arrest, Keenan and Boyan[34] observed that correct measures were often not taken rapidly. For example, nearly all the cardiac arrests (26 of 27) were preceded by progressive bradycardia. They noted the following[34]:

Prompt and appropriate action when bradycardia was first observed would have prevented many of the "avoidable" cardiac arrests. Instead, atropine was administered in many cases, an action that did little but waste time. We feel that the prudent anesthetist should learn to respond *reflexively* to progressive bradycardia by promptly replacing all inhalational anesthetics with 100% oxygen and directing all attention to adequate ventilation.

A similar finding was observed by Caplan et al.[38] in the ASA Closed Claims Study of cases of cardiac arrest occurring during spinal anesthesia. In these cases, the initiation of CPR and ventilation with 100 percent oxygen was appropriate, but pharmacologic support was judged suboptimal.

Large-Scale Anesthetic Risk Reduction Strategies

In 1984, the inaugural meeting of the International Committee on Preventable Anesthesia Morbidity and Mortality (ICPAMM) took place in Boston. Since then, two further meetings have occurred in 1986 in Vienna and in 1988 in Washington, DC, at the World Congress of Anesthesiology. Keats and Siker[194] reviewed the first meeting, which concentrated on establishment of uniform terminology with which to compare results from different countries. Differences in practice were particularly noted in the discussions about monitoring. In the United States since then, minimal acceptable standards for anesthesia have been established by the ASA, the legal implications notwithstanding (see below).

The second meeting in 1986 has also been reviewed.[195] Nineteen countries were represented. Highlights included discussion of international differences in anesthetic morbidity and mortality. Anesthesia was described to be a causal factor in 6 to 17 percent of the perioperative deaths in various countries. Anesthetic mortality was reported as 1:10,000 to 1:25,000 in several large studies. Patient safety activities under way in Canada, France, the United Kingdom, Australia, the Netherlands, and the United States were described. Areas of controversy included the impact of the American legal system on patient safety; advantages and disadvantages of increased monitoring technology; and selection criteria for anesthesia training programs.[195]

In 1986, the ASA adopted Standards for Basic Intraoperative Monitoring (Table 22-26).[196] This followed the example previously set by Harvard Medical School in adopting standards for its hospitals.[6]

It is no surprise that the adoption of any standards was met with criticism. Potential disadvantages were said to include a false sense of security, incorrect information owing to monitoring dysfunction, and legal ramifications. In contrast, others criticized the standards for not being sufficiently stringent. In fact, the only monitors specifically mandated were an inspiratory oxygen analyzer, a ventilator disconnect alarm, an electrocardiogram, and a blood pressure device.[196] Pulse oximetry and capnometry were encouraged, but

were not listed as standards. It should be noted that standards do not *require* the physician to *do* anything (though the physician's insurance carrier may). They are standards for care, set by our professional society. Time and experience will demonstrate the utility of their adoption, although it may be difficult to determine whether mortality and/or morbidity improvements, if they occur at all, are actually results of compliance. Should we be able to agree on basic principles of safe anesthesia practice, and enforce implementation?

THE COST OF PATIENT SAFETY IN ANESTHESIA

The magnitude of the cost of anesthesia risk has been estimated by studies of insurance company payments for anesthesia-related morbidity and mortality. The ASA Committee on Professional Liability has collected data from closed claims (settled or adjudicated) in an effort to identify problem areas. Data from 624 of these cases, each of which resulted in legal action, is published in *Safety and Cost Containment in Anesthesiology*.[5,197] The most common cause of death and brain damage involved the respiratory system. The three most common problems were inadequate ventilation, esophageal intubation, and difficult intubation. The median cost of these settlements was approximately 0.25 million dollars per case, despite the fact that many of these occurred before 1980 (Table 22-27).[5,197]

Table 22-28 compares the incidences of these top three respiratory complications with incidences other respiratory complications in this closed claims study. It should be noted that inadequate FIO_2 was infrequent. A possible explanation is the widespread application of oxygen analyzers in the United States, but if this is so, why did not other monitors, specifically ventilator disconnect alarms and breath sound auscultations, protect as well against inadequate ventilation or esophageal intubation? The answer may be that such monitors may not be sufficiently sensitive or specific and/or may not be optimally located in the system, or that the problem was recognized, but attempts to improve ventilation failed. Pulse oximetry may reduce the incidence of these accidents considerably. Indeed, several U.S. insurance carriers have seen fit recently to offer substantial premium reductions to anesthesiologists who will use the monitor on every case.

The ASA Committee on Professional Liability addressed the question of whether improved monitoring would have prevented patient injury in over 1,000 closed claims cases.[192] In one-third of the cases judged preventable at all, use of a pulse oximeter and capnometer (together) were judged by the anesthesiologist reviewers to potentially prevent the negative outcome. Further, the median cost of the cases judged preventable with pulse oximetry and capnometry was *10 times* that of the cases not judged preventable.[192]

In today's climate of limited resources, the expense

TABLE 22-26. ASA Standards for Basic Intraoperative Monitoring[196]

Standard I	Qualified anesthesia personnel shall be present in the room throughout the conduct of all general anesthetics, regional anesthetics, and monitored anesthesia care.
Standard II	During all anesthetics, the patient's oxygenation, ventilation, circulation, and temperature shall be continually evaluated.

(Data from Pierce.[196])

TABLE 22-27. High Incidence of Respiratory-Related Critical Care Incidents from ASA Closed Claims Preliminary Data

Incident	No. of Cases[a]	Resultant Deaths	Resultant Brain Damage	Range of Settlement Cost
Inadequate ventilation	80 (13%)	61	18	$ 1,500–$6 million
Esophageal intubation	41 (7%)	31	8	$40,000–$3.4 million
Difficult intubation	22 (4%)	9	4	$ 4,500–$4.7 million

[a] Gathered from 624 total cases studied.
(Adapted from Cheney,[197] with permission.)

to improve safety is often raised. Hamilton,[198] instead, challenged,

> Do we believe increasing cost must result in increased patient safety, or that increased patient safety cannot be achieved without increasing costs? I cannot accept that cost and safety are inseparably united — or necessarily functionally related.

Hamilton[198] emphasized that better teaching will improve patient safety at little added cost and that cost containment is best served by eliminating wasteful practice. It is possible that no increased expenditures are needed but rather a shift in the present distribution of funds. Two estimates taken from the literature put the question in perspective. McKay and Noble,[188] in their analysis of critical incidents detected by pulse oximetry, calculated a cost of $2,400 per year to equip a single operating room with pulse oximetry. If that operating room was utilized for 20 cases per week for 50 weeks in the year, the cost of pulse oximetry would be $2.40 per case. The argument is often made that "just one lawsuit saved might justify the cost of the new monitor." We reject that argument, as does Hamilton.[198] If detection of decreased oxygen delivery to vital organs can be achieved earlier with pulse oximetry, and if this prevents mortality and/or morbidity — two separate questions — then patient care is improved. *That* should always be our motive, not "saving lawsuits."[199] This latter statement may sound evangelical or trite, but real patient advocacy must remain our objective.

TABLE 22-28. Comparison of Frequent versus Infrequent Respiratory Complications from the ASA Closed Claims Study

Incident	No. of Cases
Inadequate ventilation	80 (13%)
Esophageal intubation	41 (7%)
Difficult intubation	22 (4%)
Bronchospasm	12 (2%)
Airway obstruction	7 (1%)
Inadvertent extubation	6 (1%)
Inadequate FIO_2	4 (<1%)
Premature extubation	3 (<1%)

(Adapted from Cheney,[197] with permission.)

SUMMARY

Because anesthesia is not directly therapeutic, many have said that there should be no associated mortality or morbidity. We believe this is patent nonsense. The above statement fails to appreciate the true nature of modern surgical anesthesia, a state achieved not by "falling asleep," but rather by artificially overpowering the body's most tenacious defenses with some of the most dangerous drugs known. Anesthesia is an integral part of many therapies. The vast majority of today's operations would be impossible, in fact unknown, without anesthesia. Clearly, there *is* a risk to anesthesia. Unfortunately, a major finding of risk surveys is that many of the complications were avoidable. Faulty technique, poor judgment, failure to apply existing knowledge, coupled with lack of vigilance, all do contribute significantly to anesthetic morbidity and mortality.[8,24,27,28,34,83,91,200–204]

As yet, limited research beyond surveys of the magnitude of the problem has been performed. We have developed dozens of exciting new drugs, monitors, and techniques.[205,206] We understand numerous mechanisms of drug effects, interactions, and toxicities. These developments should continue, but we believe we must also make concerted efforts in two general areas if we are to reduce risk. First, we must bring the trailing edge of anesthesia practice forward, by setting standards that really benefit patients and using quality assurance monitors that have valid clinical importance to highlight problems.[207,208] At the same time, we must try to understand the *mechanisms that underlie the risks of anesthesia*, whether they be complex drug-drug interactions, perioperative cardiovascular morbidity, the psychologic aspects of vigilance, or any other relevant subject.[209–211]

Unfortunately, it is likely that new problems will accompany new technology. There may be a tendency toward undue reliance on gadgets. For example, will tomorrow's residents listen for breath sounds over the chest and stomach or simply glance at the capnograph after tracheal intubation? Do we and will they understand what the squiggles mean?

To us, the best strategy is to restructure our educational priorities toward safety. Perhaps, for example, there are too many lectures devoted to coronary steal and not enough on the significance of bradycardia. Hamilton[198] doubts that any patient ever died "because the anesthesiologist lacked information concerning Hoffman elimination." It is our task and responsibility to establish real priority for patient safety, at least in part through a renaissance in the basic principles of respiratory and circulatory management. Over 30 years ago, Beecher and Todd[14] pointed out that poliomyelitis, which was receiving millions of research dollars, caused fewer deaths per year than did anesthesia. Today, polio is almost unheard of, but anesthetic risks persist. It should be our goal to achieve that kind of progress.

REFERENCES

1. Hammond EC, Horn D: Smoking and death rates: Report on 44 months of follow-up of 187,783 men. Part I. Total mortality. JAMA 166:1159, 1958. Part II. Death rates by cause. JAMA 166:1294, 1958

2. Doll R: Smoking and death rates. JAMA 251:2854, 1984

3. U.S. Bureau of Census: Vital and Health Statistics of the United States. 1988 Ed. Government Printing Office, Washington, DC, 1987

4. Lunn JN, Mushin WW: Mortality associated with anaesthesia. Nuffield Provincial Hospitals Trust, London, 1982

5. Gravenstein JS, Holzer JF (eds): Safety and Cost Containment in Anesthesia. Butterworth Publishers, Stoneham, MA, 1988

6. Eichhorn JH, Cooper JB, Cullen DJ, et al: Standards for patient monitoring during anesthesia at Harvard Medical School. JAMA 256:1017, 1986

7. Ament R: Classification of operating room mortality; review of cases in a pediatric medical center during the 10-year period, 1949–1958. Anesth Analg 39:158, 1960

8. Cooper JB, Newbower RS, Kitz RJ: An analysis of major errors and equipment failures in anesthesia management: Considerations for prevention and detection. Anesthesiology 60:34, 1984

9. Snow J: On chloroform and other anesthetics. p. 107. John Churchill, London, 1858

10. Keats AS: What do we know about anesthetic mortality? Anesthesiology 50:387, 1979

11. MacIntosh RR: Deaths under anaesthetics. Br J Anaesth 21:107, 1948

12. Ruth HS: Anesthesia study commissions. JAMA 127:514, 1945

13. Edwards G, Morton HJV, Pask EA, Wylie WD: Deaths associated with anaesthesia: A report on 1,000 cases. Anaesthesia 11:194, 1956

14. Beecher HK, Todd DP: A study of the deaths associated with anesthesia and surgery. Ann Surg 140:2, 1954

15. Lowenstein E, Hallowell P, Levine FH, et al: Cardiovascular response to large doses of intravenous morphine in man. N Engl J Med 281:1389, 1969

16. Stanley TH, Webster LR: Anesthetic requirements and cardiovascular effects of fentanyl-oxygen and fentanyl-diazepam-oxygen anesthesia in man. Anesth Analg 57:411, 1978

17. Keats AS: The Rovenstine Lecture, 1983: Cardiovascular anesthesia: Perceptions and perspectives. Anesthesiology 60:467, 1984

18. Kennedy JW, Kaiser GC, Fisher LD, et al: Clinical and angio-graphic predictors of operative mortality from the Collaborative Study in Coronary Artery Surgery (CASS). Circulation 63:793, 1981

19. Sundt TM, Sharbrough FW, Piepgras DG, et al: Correlation of cerebral blood flow and electro-encephalographic changes during carotid endarterectomy. Mayo Clin Proc 56:533, 1981

20. Easton JD, Sherman DG: Stroke and mortality rate in carotid endarterectomy: 228 consecutive operations. Stroke 8:565, 1977

21. Davies JM, Strunin L: Anaesthesia in 1984: How safe is it? Can Med Assoc J 131:437, 1984

22. Derrington MC, Smith G: A review of studies of anaesthetic risk, morbidity and mortality. Br J Anaesth 59:815, 1987

23. Strunin L, Forrest JB, Lunn JN, et al: Towards excellence in anaesthesia. Can J Anaesthesia 35:278, 1988

24. Buck N, Devlin HB, Lunn JL: Report on the confidential enquiry into perioperative deaths. Nuffield Provincial Hospitals Trust, London. The Kings Fund Publishing House, London, 1987

25. Lunn JN. Anaesthetic mortality in Britain and France — methods and results of the British study. p. 19. In Vickers MD, Lunn JN (eds): Mortality in Anaesthesia. Springer-Verlag, New York, 1983

26. Smith G, Norman J: Editorial: Complications and medicolegal aspects of anaesthesia. Br J Anaesthesia 59:813, 1987

27. Tiret L, Desmonts JM, Hatton F, Vourc'h G: Complications associated with anaesthesia — a prospective survey in France. Can Anaesth Soc J 33:336, 1986

28. Holland R: Anaesthetic mortality in New South Wales. Br J Anaesth 59:834, 1987

29. Lunn JN, Hunter AR, Scott DB: Anaesthesia related surgical mortality. Anaesthesia 38:1090, 1983

30. Schneider AJL: Assessment of risk factors and surgical outcome. Surg Clin North Am 63:1113, 1983

31. Lunn JN, Devlin HB: Lessons from the confidential enquiry into peri-operative deaths in three NHS regions. Lancet 2:1384, Dec 1987

32. Hatton F, Tiret L, Vourc'h G, et al: Morbidity and mortality associated with anesthesia — French survey: Preliminary results. p. 25. In Vickers MD, Lunn JN (eds): Mortality in Anaesthesia. Springer-Verlag, New York, 1983

33. Holland R: Special committee investigating deaths under anaesthesia: Report on 745 classified cases. Med J Aust 1:573, 1970

34. Keenan RL, Boyan CP: Cardiac arrest due to anesthesia: A study of incidence and causes. JAMA 253:2373, 1985

35. Wolfson B, Kielar CM, Lake C, et al: Anesthetic index — a new approach. Anesthesiology 38:583, 1973

36. Roberts SL, Gilbert M, Tinker JH: Isoflurane has a greater margin of safety than halothane in swine with and without major surgery or critical coronary stenosis. Anesth Analg 66:485, 1987

37. Taylor G, Larson P, Prestrich R: Unexpected cardiac arrest during anesthesia and surgery. JAMA 236:2758, 1976

38. Caplan RA, Ward RJ, Posner K, Cheney FW: Unexpected cardiac arrest during spinal anesthesia. A closed claims analysis of predisposing factors. Anesthesiology 68:5, 1988

39. Gillespie DM: Death during anesthesia. Br J Anaesth 19:1, 1944

40. Ehrenhaft JL, Eastwood DW, Morris LE: Analysis of twenty-seven cases of acute cardiac arrest. J Thorac Surg 22:592, 1951

41. West JP: Cardiac arrest during anesthesia and surgery. Ann Surg 140:623, 1954

42. Dornette WHL, Orth OS: Death in the operating room. Anesth Analg 35:545, 1956

43. Moyer CA, Key AJ: Estimation of operative risk in 1955. JAMA 160:853, 1956

44. Schapira M, Kepes ER, Hurwitt ES: An analysis of deaths in the operating room and within 24 hours of surgery. Anesth Analg 39:149, 1960

45. Collins VJ: Fatalities in anesthesia and surgery: Fundamental considerations. JAMA 172:549, 1960

46. Phillips OC, Frazier TM, Graff TD, DeKornfeld TJ: The Baltimore Anesthesia Study Committee. A review of 1,024 postoperative deaths. JAMA 174:2015, 1960

47. Jude JR, Kouwenhoven WB, Knickerbocker GG: Cardiac arrest: Report of application of external cardiac massage on 118 patients. JAMA 178:85, 1961

48. Boba A, Landmesser CM: Total cardiorespiratory collapse (cardiac arrest): Contributory and causative errors of omission and commission for which anesthesiologists must assume responsibility. NY State J Med 61:2928, 1961

49. Dripps RD, Lamont A, Eckenhoff JE: The role of anesthesia in surgical mortality. JAMA 178:261, 1961

50. Clifton BS, Hotten WIT: Deaths associated with anaesthesia. Br J Anaesthesia 35:250, 1963

51. Memery HN: Anesthesia mortality in private practice. JAMA 194:127, 1965

52. Dinnick OP: Deaths associated with anesthesia. Anaesthesia 19:536, 1964

53. Gebbie D: Anaesthesia and death. Can Anaesth Soc J 13:390, 1966

54. Minuck M: Death in the operating room. Can Anaesth Soc J 14:197, 1967

55. Harrison GG: Anaesthetic contributory death — its incidence and causes. S Afr Med J, Part I, 25 May 1968, p. 514; Part II, 8 June 1968, p. 544.

56. Harrison GG: Death attributable to anaesthesia: A 10 year survey (1967–1976). Br J Anaesth 50:1041, 1978

57. Bodlander FMS: Deaths associated with anaesthesia. Br J Anaesth 47:36, 1975

58. Hovi-Viander M: Death associated with anaesthesia in Finland. Br J Anaesth 52:483, 1980

59. Turnbull KW, Fancourt-Smith PF, Banting GC: Death within 48 hours of anaesthesia at the Vancouver General Hospital. Can Anaesth Soc J 27:159, 1980

60. Goldstein A, Keats AS: The risk of anesthesia. Anesthesiology 33:130, 1970

61. Goldman L, Caldera DL, Nussbaum SR, et al: Multifactorial index on cardiac risk in noncardiac surgical procedures. N Engl J Med 297:845, 1977

62. Goldman L: Cardiac risks and complications of noncardiac surgery. Ann Intern Med 98:504, 1983

63. Jeffrey CC, Kunsman J, Cullen DJ, et al: A prospective evaluation of cardiac risk index. Anesthesiology 58:462, 1983

64. Carliner NH, Fischer ML, Plotnick GD, et al: Routine preoperative exercise testing in patients undergoing major noncardiac surgery. Am J Cardiol 56:51, 1985

65. Gerson MC, Hurst JM, Hertzberg VS, et al: Cardiac prognosis in noncardiac geriatric surgery. Ann Intern Med 103:832, 1985

66. Goldman L, Caldera DL: Risks of general anesthesia and elective operation in the hypertensive patients. Anesthesiology 50:285, 1979

67. Lunn JN, Farrow SC, Fowkes FGR, et al: Epidemiology in anaesthesia. I. Anaesthetic practice over 20 years. Br J Anaesth 54:803, 1982

68. Farrow SC, Fowkes FGR, Lunn JN, et al: Epidemiology in anaesthesia. II. Factors affecting mortality in hospital. Br J Anaesth 54:811, 1982

69. Fowkes FGR, Lunn JN, Farrow SC, et al: Epidemiology in anaesthesia. III. Mortality risk in patients with coexisting physical disease. Br J Anaesth 54:819, 1982

70. Cohen MM, Duncan PG, Tate RB: Does anaesthesia contribute to operative mortality? JAMA 260:2859, 1988

71. Tiret L, Hatton F, Desmonts JM, Vourc'h G: Prediction of outcome of anaesthesia in patients over 40 years: A multifactorial risk index. Stat Med 7:947, 1988

72. Saklad M: Grading of patients for surgical procedures. Anesthesia 2:281, 1941

73. Owens WD: ASA physical status classifications: A study of consistency of ratings. Anesthesiology 49:239, 1978

74. Keats AS: The ASA classification of physical status — a recapitulation. Anesthesiology 49:233, 1978

75. Vacanti CJ, VanHouten RJ, Hill RC: A statistical analysis of relationship of physical status to postoperative mortality in 68,388 cases. Anesth Analg 49:564, 1970

76. Marx GH, Matteo CV, Orkin LR: Computer analysis of post anesthetic deaths. Anesthesiology 39:54, 1973

77. Editorial: The National Halothane Study. JAMA 197:811, 1966

78. Gordon RA, Britt BA, Kalow W (eds): International Symposium on Malignant Hyperthermia. Charles C Thomas, Springfield, IL, 1973

79. Cohen MM, Duncan PG, Pope WDP, Wolkenstein C: A survey of 112,000 anaesthetics at one teaching hospital (1975–83). Can Anaesth Soc J 33:22, 1986

80. Campkin V: Post intubation ulcer of the larynx: Report of a case. Br J Anaesth 31:561, 1959

81. Snow JC, Harano M, Balogh K: Post intubation granuloma of the larynx. Anesth Analg 45:425, 1966

82. Riding JE: Minor complications of general anaesthesia. Br J Anaesth 49:91, 1975

83. Hamilton WK: Unexpected deaths during anesthesia: Wherein lies the cause? Anesthesiology 50:381, 1979

84. Keats AS: Anesthesia mortality — a new mechanism. Anesthesiology 68:2, 1988

85. Utting JE, Gray TC, Shelley FC: Human misadventure in anesthesia. Can Anaesth Soc J 26:472, 1979

86. Craig J, Wilson ME: A survey of anaesthetic misadventures. Anaesthesia 36:933, 1981

87. Mushin WW: Anaesthesia for the Poor Risk, and Other Essays. Charles C Thomas, Springfield, IL, 1948

88. Dorsch JA, Dorsch SE: Understanding Anesthesia Equipment, Construction, Care and Complications. 2nd Ed. Williams & Wilkens, Baltimore, 1984

89. Cooper JB, Newbower RS, Long CD: Human error in anesthesia management. p. 114. In Grundy BL, Gravenstein JS (eds): The Quality of Care in Anesthesia. Charles C. Thomas, Springfield, IL, 1982

90. Cooper JB, Long CD, Newbower RS, Philip JH: Critical incidents associated with intraoperative exchanges of anesthesia personnel. Anesthesiology 56:456, 1982

91. Cooper JB, Newbower RS, Long CD, McPeek B: Preventable anesthesia mishaps: A study of human factors. Anesthesiology 49:399, 1978

92. Cooper JB, Cullen DJ, Nemeskal R, et al: Effects of information feedback and pulse oximetry on the incidence of anesthesia complications. Anesthesiology 67:686, 1987

93. Flanagan JC: The critical incident technique. Psychol Bull 51:327, 1954

94. Gaba DM, Maxwell M, DeAnda A: Anesthetic mishaps: Breaking the chain of accident evolution. Anesthesiology 66:670, 1987

95. Hotchkiss WS: Patent ductus arteriosus and the occasional cardiac surgeon. JAMA 173:244, 1960

96. Moses LE, Mosteller F: Institutional differences in postoper-

ative death rates; commentary on some findings of the National Halothane Study. JAMA 203:150, 1968

97. Slogoff S, Keats AS: Does perioperative myocardial ischemia lead to postoperative myocardial infarction? Anesthesiology 62:107, 1985

98. Bechtoldt AA: Committee on anesthesia study of anesthesia-related deaths: 1969–1976. NC Med J 42:253, 1981

99. Klaucke DN, Rericki DA, Brown RA: Investigation of Mortality and Severe Morbidity Associated with Anesthesia: Pilot Study Final Report. American Association of Anesthesiologists and Centers for Disease Control, Atlanta, GA, 1988

100. Crandell WB, Pappas SG, Macdonald A: Nephrotoxicity associated with methoxyflurane anesthesia. Anesthesiology 27:591, 1966

101. Mazze RI, Shue GL, Jackson SH: Renal dysfunction associated with methoxyflurane anesthesia: A randomized, prospective clinical evaluation. JAMA 216:278, 1971

102. Cousins MJ, Greenstein LR, Hitt BA, et al: Metabolism and renal effects of enflurane in man. Anesthesiology 44:44, 1976

103. Tolmie JD, Joyce TH, Mitchell GD: Succinylcholine danger in the burned patient. Anesthesiology 28:467, 1967

104. Birch AA, Mitchell GD, Playford GA, et al: Changes in serum potassium response in succinylcholine following trauma. JAMA 210:490, 1969

105. Cooperman LH: Succinylcholine-induced hyperkalemia in neuromuscular disease. JAMA 213:1867, 1970

106. Subcommittee on the National Halothane Study of the Committee on Anesthesia, National Academy of Sciences-National Research Council: Summary of the National Halothane Study: Possible association between halothane anesthesia and postoperative hepatic necrosis. JAMA 197:775, 1966

107. Viljoen JF, Estafanous G, Kellner GA: Propranolol and cardiac surgery. J Thorac Cardiovasc Surg 64:826, 1972

108. Alderman EL, Coltart DJ, Wettach GE, Harrison DC: Coronary artery syndromes after sudden propranolol withdrawal. Ann Intern Med 81:625, 1974

109. Miller RR, Olson HG, Amsterdam EA, Mason DT: Propranolol withdrawal rebound phenomenon. N Engl J Med 293:416, 1975

110. Reiz S, Balfors E, Sorensen MB, et al.: Isoflurane—a powerful coronary vasodilator in patients with coronary artery disease. Anesthesiology 59:91, 1983

111. Becker LC: Is isoflurane dangerous for the patient with coronary artery disease? Anesthesiology 66:259, 1987

112. Cucchiara RF, Sundt TM, Michenfelder JD: Myocardial infarction in carotid endarterectomy patients anesthetized with halothane, enflurane or isoflurane. Anesthesiology 69:783, 1988

113. Yeager MP, Glass DD, Neff RK, Brinck-Johnsen T: Epidural anesthesia and analgesia in high risk surgical patients. Anesthesiology 66:729, 1987

114. Scott NB, Kehlet H: Regional anesthesia and surgical morbidity. Br J Surg 75:299, 1988

115. Kaunitz AM, Hughes JM, Grimes DA, et al.: Causes of maternal mortality in the United States. Obstet Gynecol 65:605, 1985

116. Rochat RW, Koonin LM, Atrash HK, Jewett JF, and The Maternal Mortality Collaborative: Maternal Mortality in the United States: Report from the Maternal Mortality Collaborative. Obstet Gynecol 72:91, 1988

117. Moir DD: Maternal mortality and anaesthesia. Br J Anaesth 52:1, 1980

118. Report on Confidential Enquiries into Maternal Deaths in England and Wales, 1979–1981. Department of Health and Social Security, Her Majesty's Stationary Office, London, England, 1986

119. Morgan M: Anaesthetic contribution to maternal mortality. Br J Anaesth 59:842, 1987

120. Endler GC, Marion FG, Sokol RJ, Stevenson LB: Anesthesia-related maternal mortality in Michigan, 1972–1984. Am J Obstet Gynecol 159:187, 1988

121. Marx GF: Comment. Obstet Anesth Digest, p. 110, 1985

122. Grimes DA, Cates W: Deaths from paracervical anesthesia used for first trimester abortion 1972–1975. N Engl J Med 295:1397, 1976

123. Rosen M: Deaths associated with anesthesia for obstetrics (editorial). Anaesthesia 36:145, 1981

124. Roberts RB, Shirley MA: Reducing the risk of acid aspiration during cesarean section. Anesth Analg 53:859, 1974

125. Marx GF: Maternal complications of regional analgesia. Reg Anaesth 6:104, 1981

126. Marx GF: Cardiopulmonary resuscitation of late-pregnant women. Anesthesiology 56:156, 1982

127. Crawford JS: Some maternal complications of epidural analgesia for labour. Anaesthesia 40:1219, 1985

128. Cormack RS, Lehane J: Difficult tracheal intubation in obstetrics. Anaesthesia 39:1105, 1984

129. Gibbs CP, Krischer J, Peckham BM, et al: Obstetric anesthesia: A national survey. Anesthesiology 65:298, 1986

130. Dierdorf SF, Krishna G: Anesthetic management of neonatal surgical emergencies. Anesth Analg 60:204, 1981

131. Richardson MA, Colton RT: Anatomic abnormalities of the pediatric airway. Pediatr Clin North Am 31:821, 1984

132. Badgwell JM, McLeod ME, Friedberg J: Airway obstruction in infants and children. Can Anaesth Soc J 34:90, 1987

133. Diaz JH: Croup and epiglottis in children: The anesthesiologist as diagnostician. Anesth Analg 64:621, 1985

134. Kurth CD, Spitzer AR, Broennle AM, Downes JJ: Postoperative apnea in preterm infants. Anesthesiology 66:483, 1987

135. Roy WL, Lerman J: Laryngospasm in paediatric anaesthesia. Can J Anaesth 35:93, 1988

136. Montoyama EK, Glazener CH: Hypoxemia after general anesthesia in children. Anesth Analg 65:267, 1986

137. Rackow H, Salanitre E, Green LT: Frequency of cardiac arrest associated with anesthesia in infants and children. Pediatrics, p. 697, November, 1961

138. Tiret L, Nivoche Y, Hatton F, et al: Complications related to anaesthesia in infants and children. Br J Anaesth 61:263, 1988

139. Salem MR, Bennett EJ, Schweiss JF, et al.: Cardiac arrest related to anesthesia; contributing factors in infants and children. JAMA 233:238, 1975

140. Smith RM: Anesthesia for Infants and Children. 4th Ed. p. 653. CV Mosby, St. Louis, 1980

141. Hickey PR, Hansen DD, Norwood WI, Castaneda AR: Anesthetic complications in surgery for congenital heart disease. Anesth Analg 63:657, 1984

142. Graff TD, Phillips OC, Benson DW, Kelley G: Baltimore Anesthesia Study Committee: Factors in pediatric anesthesia mortality. Anesth Analg 43:407, 1964

143. Hatch DJ: Anaesthesia for children. Anaesthesia 39:405, 1984

144. Editorial: Complications of anaesthesia in infants and children. Lancet 2:1466, 1988

145. Scott DL: Anaesthetic experiences in 1,300 major geriatric operations. Br J Anaesth 33:354, 1961

146. Cogbill CL: Operation in the aged. Arch Surg 94:202, 1967

147. Lakatta EG: Alterations in the cardiovascular system that occur in advanced age. Fed Proc 38:163, 1979

148. Waller BF, Roberts WC: Cardiovascular disease in the very elderly: Analysis of 40 necropsy patients aged 90 years and over. Am J Cardiol 51:403, 1983

149. Cole WH: Medical differences between the young and the aged. J Am Geriatr Soc 18:589, 1970

150. Editorial: Accounting for perioperative deaths. Lancet 2:1369, 1987

151. Desmeules H, Fourneir L, Tremblay PR: Systematic changes in the elderly patient and their anaesthetic implications. Can Anaesth Soc J 32:184, 1985

152. Kannel WB, McGee D, Gordon T: A general cardiovascular risk profile: The Framingham study. Am J Cardiol 38:46, 1976

153. Del Guercio LRM, Cohn JD: Monitoring operative risk in the elderly. JAMA 243:1350, 1980

154. Roberts AJ, Woodhall DD, Conti R, et al: Mortality, morbidity and cost accounting related to coronary artery bypass graft surgery in the elderly. Ann Thorac Surg 39:426, 1985

155. Palmberg S, Hirsjärvi E: Mortality in geriatric surgery. Gerontology 25:103, 1979

156. Weisfeldt ML: Aging of the cardiovascular system (editorial). N Engl J Med 303:1172, 1980

157. Port S, Cobb FR, Coleman E, Jones RH: Effect of age on the response of the left ventricular ejection fraction to exercise. N Engl J Med 303:1133, 1980

158. Greenburg AG, Saik RP, Pridham D: Influence of age on mortality of colon surgery. Am J Surg 150:65, 1985

159. Mohr DN: Estimation of surgical risk in the elderly: A correlative view. Am Geriatr Soc 31:99, 1983

160. Djokovic JL, Hedley-Whyte J: Prediction of outcome of surgery and anesthesia in patients over 80. JAMA 242:2301, 1979

161. Morley JE, Reese SS: Clinical implications of the aging heart. Am J Med 86:77, 1989

162. Wahba WM: Influence of aging on lung function — clinical significance of changes from age twenty. Anesth Analg 62:764, 1983

163. Morrison JN, Richardson J, Dunn L, Pardy RL: Respiratory muscle performance in normal elderly subjects and patients with COPD. Chest 95:90, 1989

164. Kronenberg RS, Drage GW: Attenuation of the ventilatory and heart rate responses to hypoxia and hypocapnia with aging in normal man. J Clin Invest 52:1812, 1973

165. Topkins MJ, Artusio JF: Myocardial infarction and surgery. Anesth Analg 43:716, 1964

166. Tarhan S, Moffitt EA, Taylor WF, Giuliani ER: Myocardial infarction after general anesthesia. JAMA 220:1451, 1972

167. Arkins R, Smessaert AA, Hicks RG: Mortality and morbidity in surgical patients with coronary artery disease. JAMA 190:485, 1964

168. Steen PA, Tinker JH, Tarhan S: Myocardial reinfarction after anesthesia and surgery. JAMA 239:2566, 1978

169. Fraser JG, Ramachandran PR, Davis HS: Anesthesia and recent myocardial infarction. JAMA 199:318, 1967

170. Eerola M, Eerola R, Kaukinen S, Kaukinen L: Risk factors in surgical patients with verified preoperative myocardial infarction. Acta Anaesthesiol Scand 24:219, 1980

171. Tinker JH: Perioperative myocardial infarction. Semin Anesth 1:253, 1982

172. Scher KS, Tice DA: Operative risk in patients with previous coronary artery bypass. Arch Surg 111:807, 1976

173. Mahar LJ, Steen PA, Tinker JH, et al: Perioperative myocardial infarction in patients with coronary artery disease with and without aorto-coronary artery bypass grafts. J Thorac Cardiovasc Surg 76:533, 1978

174. Crawford ES, Morris GC, Howell JF: Operative risk in pa-tients with previous coronary artery bypass. Ann Thorac Surg 26:215, 1978

175. Foster ED, Davis KB, Carpenter JA, et al: Risk of noncardiac operation in patients with defined coronary disease: The Coronary Artery Surgery Study (CASS) Registry experience. Ann Thorac Surg 41:42, 1986

176. Sapala JA, Ponka JL, Duverrow WSC: Operative and nonoperative risks in the cardiac patient. J Am Geriatr Soc 23:529, 1978

177. Rao TL, Jacobs KH, El-Etr AA: Reinfarction following anesthesia in patients with myocardial infarction. Anesthesiology 59:499, 1983

178. Lowenstein E: Perianesthetic ischemic episodes cause myocardial infarction in humans — a hypothesis confirmed. Anesthesiology 62:103, 1985

179. Clowes GHA, Del Guercio LRM: Circulatory response to trauma of surgical operations. Metabolism 9:67, 1960

180. Seyfer AE, Seaber AV, Dombrose FA, Urbaniak JR: Coagulation changes in elective surgery and trauma. Ann Surg 210, 1980

181. Slogoff S, Keats AS: Randomized trial of primary anesthetic agents on outcome of coronary artery bypass operation. Anesthesiology 70:179, 1989

182. Tuman KJ, McCarthy RJ, Spiess BD: Does choice of anesthetic agent significantly affect outcome after coronary artery surgery? Anesthesiology 70:189, 1989

183. Spence AA: The lessons of CEPOD. Br J Anaesth 60:753, 1988

184. Mangano DT: Anesthetics, coronary artery disease, and outcome: Unresolved controversies. Anesthesiology 70:175, 1989

185. Knight AA, Hollenberg M, London MJ, et al: Perioperative myocardial ischemia: Importance of the preoperative ischemic pattern. Anesthesiology 68:681, 1988

186. Cannard TH, Dripps RD, Helwig J, Jr, et al: Electrocardiogram during anesthesia and surgery. Anesthesiology 21:194, 1960

187. Sellick BA: Cricoid pressure to control regurgitation of stomach contents during induction of anesthesia. Lancet 2:404, 1961

188. McKay WPS, Noble WH: Critical incidents detected by pulse oximetry during anesthesia. Can J Anaesth 35:265, 1988

189. Coté CJ, Goldstein EA, Cote MA, et al: A single-blind study of pulse oximetry in children. Anesthesiology 68:184, 1988

190. An ECRI Technology Assessment: Deaths during general anesthesia. J Health Care Technol 1:155, 1985

191. Archer GW, Marx GF: Arterial oxygen tension during apnea in parturient women. Br J Anaesth 46:358, 1974

192. Tinker JH: Submitted for publication, 1989

193. Tunstal ME: Failed intubation drill. Anaesthesia 31:856, 1976

194. Keats AS, Siker ES: International Symposium on Preventable Anesthetic Morbidity and Mortality, Boston, MA, October, 8–19, 1984. Anesthesiology 63:349, 1985

195. Strunin L, Forrest JB, Lunn JN, et al: Panel summary: Toward excellence in anesthesia. Can J Anaesth 35:278, 1988

196. Pierce EC: Improving anesthesia safety today and in the future: Steps taken by the profession to reduce risks. p. 114. In Gravenstein JS, Holzer JF (eds): Safety and Cost Containment in Anesthesia. Butterworth Publishers, Stoneham, MA, 1988

197. Cheney FW: Anesthesia: Potential risks and causes of incidents. p. 11. In Gravenstein JS, Holzer JF (eds): Safety and Cost Containment in Anesthesia. Butterworth Publishers, Stoneham, MA, 1988

198. Hamilton WK: Patient safety and cost containment. p. 3. In Gravenstein JS, Holzer JF (eds): Safety and Cost Contain-

ment in Anesthesia. Butterworth Publishers, Stoneham, MA, 1988

199. Lunn JN: Anaesthetist, lawyers and the public. Anaesthesia 44:1, 1989

200. Greiss FC, Anderson SG: Elimination of maternal deaths from anesthesia. Obstet Gynecol 29:677, 1967

201. Crawford JS: The anesthetist's contribution to maternal mortality. Br J Anaesth 42:70, 1970

202. Wylie WD: "There but for the grace of God. . . ." Ann R Coll Surg Engl 56:171, 1975

203. Epstein RM: Morbidity and mortality from anesthesia: A continuing problem. Anesthesiology 49:388, 1978

204. Utting JE: Pitfalls in anaesthetic practice. Br J Anaesth 59:877, 1987

205. Mazze RI: Therapeutic misadventures with oxygen delivery systems: The need for continuous in-line oxygen monitors. Anesth Analg 51:787, 1972

206. Cohen DE, Downes JJ, Raphaely RC: What difference does pulse oximetry make? Anesthesiology 68:181, 1988

207. Editorial: NCEPOD (National Confidential Enquiry into Perioperative Deaths). Lancet 2:1320, 1988

208. Hornbein TF: The setting of standards of care. JAMA 256:1040, 1986

209. Allnut MF: Human factors in accidents. Br J Anaesth 59:856, 1987

210. Gaba DM, DeAnda A: A comprehensive anesthesia simulation environment: Recreating the operating room for research and training. Anesthesiology 69:387, 1988

211. Gravenstein JS: Training devices and simulators. Anesthesiology 69:295, 1988

23

PREOPERATIVE EVALUATION

Michael F. Roizen

INTRODUCTION

The ultimate goal of preoperative medical assessment of patients is to reduce the morbidity of surgery. This goal is achieved by optimizing the health of the patient before surgery and by planning the most appropriate perioperative management. Such management relies on uncovering hidden conditions that could cause problems during and after surgery. In this way, the anesthesiologist is able to anticipate problems and plan therapies for their occurrence. The other goals of preoperative assessment—to reduce anxiety and obtain informed consent—are discussed in Chapters 26 and

75, respectively. Although these two subjects will not be discussed in this chapter, most data support the concept that recovery occurs more quickly when the anesthesiologist allays the patient's concerns and informs the patient about what is to come (Ch. 26).[1-4]

In the beginning, preoperative medical assessment relied on only accurate history-taking and physical examination. Then, in the 1960s, multiphasic screening laboratory tests were added to the process. This chapter will evaluate the goals of preoperative medical assessment and the *relative* importance of history-taking, physical examination, and laboratory testing regarding improvement of perioperative outcome.

Since the first edition of *Anesthesia* in 1979, I have attempted not only to describe current practice but also to suggest the need for innovative change. In the first edition (1979) I discussed the lack of benefit from laboratory testing. In the second edition (1986), the chapter described how cost-benefit and benefit-risk analyses again pointed to the need to reduce the amount of laboratory testing. Not surprisingly, the third edition of the chapter also comes to a nontraditional conclusion: that we need to change the way we usually perform preoperative evaluation. This author believes that just as the practice of anesthesia has changed in the last decade, the practice of preoperative evaluation also needs to change.

THE CHANGING NATURE OF PREOPERATIVE EVALUATION

Preoperative evaluation strives to answer three questions: Is the patient in optimal health? Can, or should, the patient's physical or mental condition be improved before surgery? Does the patient have any health problem or use any medications that could unexpectedly influence perioperative events? Of course, such evaluation must include the long-accepted standard practices: review of hospital chart(s) and prior anesthesia records, consultation with the primary care physician, history taking, physical examination, evaluation of laboratory tests obtained, ordering of additional laboratory tests, and discussion of perioperative anesthesia plans (including alternatives for intraoperative and postoperative analgesia) with the patient in a way that provides accurate information and reduces patient anxiety. However, the practice of medicine has changed. The cost-conscious environment of the 1980s has made it difficult for anesthesiologists to achieve these goals using the style of the 1970s and earlier.

For example, the increased need to minimize costs means fewer or no preoperative hospital days for the patient. Over 50 percent of all operations are performed on an outpatient basis, and another 20 to 30 percent are performed as morning admissions. Unfortunately, however, the increasing age of patients often means a greater likelihood of concurrent disease. Unlike in the old days, when the whole night could be spent learning about a medically complex patient, anesthesiologists are now being asked to perform preoperative evaluation as they "run" from case to case. We are being asked to deliver more for less, and to do a more complete job, while administrators and surgeons continue to demand shorter turnover times. In such situations, the anesthesiologist may be justifiably uncomfortable about the adequacy and comprehensiveness of his or her preoperative evaluation. Did I ask the patient whether or not he or she had a drink in the last 12 hours, or whether he or she ever had a problem with drinking? (These are currently the two most sensitive and specific questions to ask a patient when trying to determine the

likelihood of alcoholism.[5]) Did I forget to ask other questions, for example, whether any family members had hepatitis? *It is very difficult to make an adequate preoperative evaluation in 5 to 15 minutes.*

Do we need to change our system? Let us first consider why one performs a preoperative evaluation. These medical assessments provide an important opportunity for physicians to gain the patient's confidence and to reduce perioperative morbidity by confirming the presence of optimal preoperative status and planning perioperative management.[6-17] Because the mortality and morbidity of surgery increase with the severity of pre-existing disease, careful evaluation and treatment should reduce their occurrence.

Clearly, a change is needed if an adequate preoperative assessment is to be accomplished. The anesthesiologist needs to know about the patient to perform these assessments efficiently. I also believe that preoperative evaluation is intrinsically valuable and that interacting with human beings in this way is an enjoyable and productive part of our practice. Also, for the practical-minded, the absence of preoperative assessment is now one of the top three causes of lawsuits against anesthesiologists. Nevertheless, in our current atmosphere there is not enough time to assess the patient preoperatively by using the traditional method. Before solutions to the problem of lack of time for comprehensive assessment are suggested, the importance of preoperative assessment will be evaluated, as well as the conditions that might be sought and determined from such assessment.

UNCOVERING THE PATIENT FACTORS THAT INCREASE THE PERIOPERATIVE RISK OF ANESTHESIA

The chapter provides information the anesthesiologist needs to ensure that his or her patient is asymptomatic from the standpoint of anesthetic risk. The management of patients found to be symptomatic is discussed in Chapter 25. Ensuring that the patient is asymptomatic requires a knowledge of what patient factors increase the perioperative risk of anesthesia, because it is those factors that one must eliminate.

Major surgery usually represents a tremendous assault on the human organism. The body has developed an elaborate defense mechanism to warn it about trauma and to help it escape from trauma. The job of the anesthesiologist is not simply to put the patient to sleep and to wake him or her when surgery is over. It is to maintain homeostasis during the assault or surgery. To do this, the anesthesiologist must interfere with the stress response induced by pain, anticipate periods when the stress response will not be present, plan for treating rare situations that the patient's medical problems may present, and, at the same time, manage the patient's chronic medical conditions.

Even when the stress of surgery is not felt consciously, it evokes a complex physiologic response. Much of this response aims to allow the body to escape trauma. For example, blood flow is diverted from the kidney and liver and is supplied to the heart and head. Also, blood pressure rises. Thus, the system most needed to be in a "good" state of health, the cardiovascular system, has first priority.[8,13–16]

The Search for Potential Problems

Unfortunately, however, illness in other systems affects perioperative risk. The following is a list of relatively common conditions I ensure are not present before assuming the patient is asymptomatic. The increased risk posed by the problems discovered is discussed in Chapters 22 and 25, and optimization of their physical condition or anticipation of potential problems and possible therapies for the problems are the goals of Chapter 25. The evaluation process that follows represents my initial screening procedure for disease. Although the process attempts to be relatively inclusive, it cannot cover all possible conditions that might be encountered when dealing with surgical patients.

Cardiovascular Disease

For the cardiovascular system, I try to ensure that the patient does not have congestive heart failure, cardiomyopathies, unstable (or even stable) ischemic heart disease, valvular or subvalvular heart disease, hypertension, disturbances in cardiac rhythm, pericarditis, arteritis, or other manifestations of atherosclerosis. These are conditions requiring further evaluation to be sure optimal treatment has been achieved prior to surgery (see Ch. 25). Questions cannot be limited to the cardiovascular system. For example, to search for alcoholic cardiomyopathy, the following inquiries are made: Have you had a drink in the last 24 hours and Have you ever had a problem with drinking? As mentioned earlier, these two questions are the most sensitive and specific questions to ask when trying to determine the possibility of alcoholism in a patient.[5] Exercise tolerance is also checked—for example, the patient's ability to walk up stairs, play sports, and perform chores (mowing lawns, making beds, vacuuming) —without getting short of breath. Typical questions regarding the cardiovascular system include the following:

What is the most vigorous activity you've done in the last 3 weeks?
Have you ever had a heart attack, or have you been treated for a possible heart attack?
Do you have heart problems such as skipped heart beats, angina, or chest pain?
Have you been told you have a heart murmur or rheumatic fever?
Have you ever been told you have mitral valve prolapse?

Have you ever had heart or lung surgery?
Have you ever awakened and felt short of breath?
Do you become short of breath after climbing one flight of stairs or after walking a short distance?
Are you able to walk up stairs at the same rate you were able to 5 years ago?
Do your ankles ever swell?
Are you ever short of breath?
Do you ever have chest pains, angina, chest heaviness, or chest tightness?
Do you ever have indigestion *not* associated with overeating?
Have you ever been told by your doctor to exercise or diet to control high blood pressure?
Have you ever been a patient in a critical care unit (cardiac care unit, intensive coronary care unit)?
Do you sleep with more than one pillow at night?
Do you currently take heart medication?
Do you currently take any medication for high blood pressure?
Do you currently take water pills or diuretics?
Do you currently take potassium pills or powder?
Do you currently take anticoagulants or blood thinning medicine?
Have you ever been told to take, or been given, antibiotics before routine dental work?

Some of these questions are asked in a different order, so that the patient is not startled or confused by them, as if they were a "pop quiz." To avoid surprising or confusing the patient, questions are asked in a "set." For instance, all questions related to medication are asked at the same time.

Respiratory and Airway Problems

For the system responsible for gas exchange, the most important consideration is securing of the airway as airway problems cause substantial risk. Therefore, evidence of airway obstruction and restriction of neck and jaw movement is sought. The end result of exposure to toxins (whether environmental or related to smoking) is also sought: emphysema, bronchitis, and chronic infections. My practice is to try to ensure that asthma is not present and that other diseases such as obesity have not progressed to the point of limiting respiratory function. The in-person interview (no matter when performed) is usually quite efficient in revealing the condition of the airway, respiratory reserve, and the possible need for laboratory evaluation such as pulmonary function testing with bronchodilators and/or blood gas analysis. The in-person interview is also the best time for educating the patient about the time needed for cessation of smoking to be beneficial (see Ch. 25). Questions that usually elicit information about the general condition of the mouth and airway and about possible reactions to anesthesia include the following:

Do you wear dentures, a crown, a partial, or a bridge?
Are any of your teeth capped?

Are any of your teeth loose, cracked, or chipped?

Have you ever had anesthesia?

Have you or any blood relative ever had any problems with anesthesia? (This question not only helps reveal possible airway problems but can elicit information about some rarer diseases such as malignant hyperthermia, glucose-6-phosphate dehydrogenase [G6PD] deficiency, acute porphyria, allergies, sickle cell disease, neurologic disorders, and hiatus hernia. It usually also elicits concerns about postoperative nausea and vomiting and thus provides an opportunity to reassure the patient and to use preanesthetic suggestion, for those physicians believing in the value of this practice.)

Can you open your mouth fully?

Do your joints ever click, pop, or hurt?

Have you ever been treated for a problem of the jaw joint (that is, a temporomandibular jaw [TMJ] joint problem)?

Have you ever been hoarse for over a month?

Have you ever had cancer?

Have you ever had, or been treated for, arthritis?

Do you have neck stiffness or problems moving your head?

Have you ever been told that you had diphtheria? (Diphtheria can cause narrowing of the airway.)

The following questions search for lung disease:

Have you ever had pneumonia?

Have you ever undergone lung surgery?

Do you have shortness of breath, wheezing, chest pain, bronchitis, asthma, or emphysema?

Do you cough regularly or frequently?

Do you cough up mucus (sputum or phlegm)?

In the last 4 weeks, have you had a fever, chills, cold, or flu?

Have you ever smoked?

Have you ever smoked half a pack or more of cigarettes a day on a regular basis?

Have you ever smoked a pipe or cigars on a regular basis?

Hepatic and Gastrointestinal Disease

Past or present hepatic disease increases the risk of certain surgical procedures (see Ch. 25), sometimes contributes to abnormal clotting and abnormal pharmacokinetics of drugs, and may present medicolegal concerns (e.g., as in the instance of postanesthetic jaundice). Hepatic disease also increases the risk of surgery for nonhepatic problems (see Ch. 25). Gastrointestinal diseases may increase the potential for aspiration of gastric contents. For example, the gastroparesis of ulcer disease often is accompanied by solid food in the stomach, and inflammatory bowel disease may be accompanied by arthritis of the neck. Gastrointestinal disease also increases the potential for dehydration, electrolyte disturbances, and anemia. The presence of gastrointestinal or hepatic disease can give clues about

possible endocrine, pulmonary, or cardiac disease (e.g., the occurrence of gastritis in the alcoholic patient could indicate a need to search for alcoholic cardiomyopathy). Questions that screen for gastrointestinal or hepatic disease include the following:

Have you ever been diagnosed as having a hiatus hernia?

Have you ever had hepatitis, yellow jaundice, liver disease, or malaria?

Have you ever had gallstones or gallbladder disease?

Are your stools ever bloody or black and tarry?

Have your bowel habits changed this year?

Do you often have diarrhea?

Have you vomited blood or material that looks like coffee grounds in the last 6 months?

Have you lost weight this year without trying?

Has your appetite for food changed in the last year?

Are you eating the same foods you ate a year ago?

Have you had heartburn within the last month?

Are you currently taking antacids, or Tagamet (cimetidine), Zantac (ranitidine), Pepcid (famotidine), or Axid (nizatidine)?

Bleeding Problems

Bleeding can also occur because of a hereditary deficiency of clotting factors or because of an abnormal platelet function or vascular function caused by disease or drugs. The following questions search for such abnormalities:

Have you ever had a blood problem such as anemia or leukemia?

Do your gums bleed when you brush your teeth?

Have you ever had a problem with blood clotting?

Have you ever had a serious bleeding problem?

Have you received a blood transfusion since 1979?

These questions are often asked in two ways, as patients seem to need time to recall such events. For example:

Has a family member or blood relative ever had a serious bleeding problem?

Have you ever had prolonged or unusual bleeding from cuts, nosebleeds, minor bruises, tooth extractions, or surgery?

Have you ever had excessive bleeding that required blood transfusion?

Renal Disease

Renal disease can also contribute to bleeding because of a functional platelet deficit associated with renal impairment (see Ch. 25). In addition, renal insufficiency can increase risk because it produces anemia (prior to, or in the absence of, erythropoietin therapy), electrolyte disturbances, peripheral neuropathy, and abnormalities in drug metabolism and excretion. Renal disease is searched for with the following questions:

Have you ever had any kidney problem?

Have you ever had kidney failure, dialysis, or more than two kidney infections?

Have you ever had kidney stones?

Are you undergoing dialysis for kidney problems?

Have your bowel or bladder functions changed in the last year?

Has your appetite for food changed in the last year? (Voluntary avoidance of foods having a high protein content is a subtle sign of renal disease.)

Endocrine Disturbances

Endocrine disturbances and the end-organ effects of diabetes or thyroid, parathyroid, adrenal (and carcinoid) diseases can increase perioperative risk substantially. For instance, morbidity and mortality increase five- to tenfold because of the nephropathy and autonomic insufficiency of diabetes (see Ch. 25). The following questions help ensure the patient does not have endocrine-related diseases:

Do you wake up at night to urinate? How often?

Have you ever been told you have diabetes or sugar diabetes?

Do you take, or have you taken, steroids, cortisone, or adrenocorticotropic hormone (ACTH) in the last year?

Do you perspire (sweat) much more than others or a great deal every now and then?

Does your face flush or get red every now and then, even when not exercising?

These last two questions attempt to rule out the very hazardous perioperative situations of undiscovered pheochromocytoma and carcinoid syndromes. Both conditions can now be well managed if known (see Ch. 25). Both, however, have a mortality rate of as high as 10 percent if undiscovered prior to operation. The following questions search for symptoms of thyroid and parathyroid disease:

Are you taking, or did you ever take, medicine for thyroid disease, for example, Synthroid (levothyroxine) or I-131?

Do you like the room consistently warmer or colder than your spouse?

Do you have muscle cramps or spasms in your legs more than three times a year?

Neurologic Disease

Physical examination can add significantly to one's impressions and reduce the necessity for some questions, particularly regarding neurologic disease. Nevertheless, to exclude nervous system disease, the following questions are usually asked:

Have you ever had a seizure, convulsion, fit, stroke, or paralysis?

Have you ever been diagnosed as having a tremor?

Do you have, or have you ever had, migraine headaches?

Have you ever had nerve injury, multiple sclerosis, or any disorder of the nervous system?

Have you ever had numbness, tingling, or the feeling of "pins and needles" in your arm or leg that lasted more than 2 hours?

Have you taken antidepressant, sedative tranquilizing, or antiseizure medications in the last year?

Musculoskeletal Disease

My usual practice is to ask about potential musculoskeletal system disease during my search for airway and lung disease, as arthritis affects the ease of securing the airway. Nevertheless, a brief review can include the following questions:

Do you have, or have you ever had, low back pain?

Have you been working your usual job or doing your normal activities in the last week?

Have you taken pain pills or had pain shots in the last 6 months?

Other Areas of Concern

Also included are general items such as whether or not the patient has received recent medical care, has taken medication, or has allergies. Once again, questions are asked about prior exposure to anesthetics and subsequent problems:

When did you last have anesthesia?

Do you have any allergies?

What are you allergic to?

Have you had blood tests in the last 6 months?

Have you had a chest radiograph in the last 2 months?

Have you had an electrocardiogram (ECG) in the last 2 months?

Has your stool been checked for blood in the last year?

Have you been a patient in a hospital, an emergency room, or an outpatient surgery center in the last 2 years? If so, why?

Do you take any medications?

What medicines do you take?

Do you take any medications not prescribed by your doctor, or that you just purchase off the shelf of a drugstore or grocery store?

Also included in this category of questions are items about artificial devices (e.g., hearing aids, false eyes):

Have you ever had a drinking problem?

Do you wear contact lenses?

Do you currently use eye drops prescribed by a doctor?

One area not yet discussed relates to more difficult-to-manage subjects such as establishing the possibility of pregnancy in a minor, asymptomatic hemoglobinopathies when an intense counseling and consultation service is not available, illicit drug use, or the potential for acquired immunodeficiency syndrome (AIDS).

Much like Epstein,[18] I believe such matters should be handled in concert with hospital policy. However, because this kind of information can affect perioperative risk and plans, my usual procedure is to search for clues in the history. If one has taken the time to gain the patient's confidence so that the patient understands one is asking these questions in order to provide better care, success is possible. If one tries to approach these sensitive areas in the 5- to 15-minutes usually allotted, the process ends up being awkward at best and usually not successful. Assuming optimal conditions, the questions that can be asked include the following:

Within the last 2 years, have you taken nonprescription drugs such as cocaine, crack, heroin, or LSD?

Have you been exposed to the body fluids (blood, semen, urine, or saliva) of anyone likely to have the AIDS virus?

Are you in one of the groups at high risk of AIDS (gays, bisexuals, hemophiliacs, or those who have had sex with a prostitute within the last 8 years)?

Would you like to undergo a test to find out whether you have been exposed to the AIDS virus?

It is my belief that AIDS testing will be an especially important consideration from an institutional point of view. In most states, testing requires patient consent. However, the decision not to test may also soon require patient consent. This latter concern may arise because azidothymidine (AZT) has been found to delay the onset of disease in asymptomatic patients infected with HIV.[19]

The Physical Examination

The physical examination again looks for the same conditions sought by history. It consists of the following processes:

Determination of arterial blood pressure in both arms, and in at least one arm 2 minutes after the patient assumes the upright position after lying down. Examination of the pulses, and of the chest, for heaves, thrusts, pulsations, murmurs, and gallops (S_3 and S_4). Examination of the carotid and jugular pulses.

Examination of the chest and auscultation of the bases for subtle rales suggestive of congestive heart failure or for rhonchi, wheezes, and other sounds indicative of lung disease.

Observation of the patient's walk to look for signs of neurologic disease and to assess back mobility and general health. A check of the eyes for abnormal movement and, along with the skin, signs of jaundice, cyanosis, nutritional abnormalities, and dehydration. The skin is checked for clubbing. A functional evaluation of cardiovascular risk can be made from observation of vigor and stamina in walking.

Examination of the airway and mouth for neck mobility, tongue size, oral lesions, and ease of intubation.

Examination of the legs for edema, clubbing, mobility, sensation, and adequacy of hair growth (or skin texture) as signs of circulatory competence. Examination of the legs for bruising.

DETECTING DISEASE: HISTORY, PHYSICAL EXAMINATION AND CHART REVIEW VERSUS LABORATORY TESTS

Because 50 percent of the patients now receiving anesthesia are either outpatients or "come-and-stay" patients (i.e., patients admitted to the hospital after surgery), patients cannot be evaluated preoperatively as they were in the 1970s. A new system had to be developed. Gradually I began using that system for inpatients as well (this process is described later in the chapter). Most anesthesiologists have developed ways of putting the classic pattern (chart review, history, physical exam, and discussion of risk) together so that all of these questions are part of a compassionate flow of thought that helps the patient recall information. A rigid, specific order for questioning is not usually necessary.

The anesthesiologist must remember that male patients tend to deny symptoms, often seeing disease as a sign of frailty. Others believe symptoms represent a disease signaling the end of life. They therefore put off seeking medical help or answering questions until help is imperative. Despite these types of obstacles to the efficient discovery of pertinent information, seeing a patient preoperatively does give the anesthesiologist an advantage in obtaining an accurate history, as no patient views even minor surgery as "minor." All surgery is a major life event for both men and women. Although the anesthesiologist may participate in 1,000 operations a year, few patients undergo more than 5 in their lifetime. Therefore, because patients are usually willing and eager to share all information, the preoperative interview can elicit vital information.

The set of questions asked is extensive, consisting of over 100 items. I believe that use of either a written or automated questionnaire to ask the screening questions, coupled with an in-person interview to pursue positive answers, does not decrease the accuracy or perceived personalized care given (see below).[20]

Other authors have suggested that anesthesiologists forget the history and just use laboratory screening for disease. Review of the literature forces me to disagree strongly: the history — whether obtained personally, by questionnaire (see below), or by automated device (see below), and the investigation of positive answers by an in-person interview — is many times better than laboratory tests in screening for disease. Also, it can be much less expensive and avoids the medicolegal problems and inefficiency associated with testing.

In fact, the data presented below led me to believe that the combination of history (from personal interview or questionnaire supplemented by personal interview) and physical examination is the best tool for optimal evaluation of patients and optimal selection of laboratory tests (i.e., selection of only those tests that have a greater chance of benefiting rather than harming the patient).

The primary problem with ordering batteries of laboratory tests for all patients is that laboratory tests are not very good screening devices for disease. In addition, the "extra" tests that physicians order as a follow-up to supposedly abnormal results on these batteries of tests are costly. More important, however, is the fact that nonindicated tests often represent additional risk to the patient, increase medicolegal risk to the physician, and render operating rooms in outpatient centers and hospitals inefficient.

Laboratory Tests as Effective Screening Devices

The value of routine laboratory testing for preoperative evaluation is dubious. Leonard and co-workers[21] reported that biochemical screening tests had no significant value in the preoperative screening of pediatric patients expected to be hospitalized for less than one week. In another study, Korvin and associates[22] reviewed biochemical tests given routinely to 1,000 patients on hospital admission. None of the tests produced a new diagnosis that was unequivocally beneficial to the patient. In an ambitious, controlled trial of multiphasic screening of 1,500 patients, Olsen and co-workers[23] found no difference in morbidity between control groups and groups subjected to screening tests. Durbridge and colleagues[24] compared 1,500 patients randomly assigned to undergo or not undergo screening tests on admission. No benefit resulted from the 8,363 extra tests performed for the group undergoing screening tests, with respect to length of hospital stay or patient outcome.

Although laboratory tests can aid in assuring that a patient's preoperative condition is optimal once a disease is suspected or diagnosed, as screening devices for the discovery of unknown disease, they have several shortcomings. They frequently fail to uncover pathologic conditions. Second, they detect abnormalities, the discovery of which does not necessarily improve patient care or outcome. Also, they are inefficient in screening for asymptomatic diseases. Finally, most abnormalities discovered on preoperative screening, or even on admission screening for nonsurgical purposes, are not recorded (other than in the laboratory report) or pursued appropriately.

Even for the very elderly, a patient group at higher risk of morbidity and mortality during surgery, the ulti-

mate benefit of routine laboratory screening is doubtful. Domoto et al[25] examined the yield and benefit of a battery of 19 screening laboratory tests performed routinely in 70 functionally intact elderly patients (average age, 82.6 years) who resided at a chronic care facility. The 70 patients underwent 3,903 screening tests. "New abnormal" results occurred in 5 of the 19 screening tests. Most of these "new abnormalities" were only minimally outside the normal range. Only four discoveries (0.1 percent of all tests ordered) led to change in patient management, none of which, Domoto and co-workers concluded, benefited any patient in an important way.

Wolf-Klein et al.[26] retrospectively studied the results of annual laboratory screening on a population of 500 institutionalized and ambulatory elderly patients (average age, 80 years). From the 15,000 tests performed, 756 new abnormalities were discovered, 690 of which were ignored. Sixty-six of the new abnormalities were evaluated; 20 new diagnoses resulted, 12 of which were treated. Two patients of the 500 ultimately may have benefited from eradication of asymptomatic bacteriuria (although eradication of this condition has not been shown to improve the quality of life or to extend life[27-30]).

Studies show that the history and physical examination are the best ways to screen for disease. Delahunt and Turnbull[31] evaluated 803 patients who were assessed preoperatively for varicose vein stripping or inguinal herniorrhaphy. A total of 1,972 tests produced only 63 abnormalities not indicated by history or physical findings. Furthermore, in no instance did the discovery of these abnormalities influence patient management. Another study retrospectively evaluated 690 admissions for elective pediatric surgical procedures.[32] The history and physical examination indicated the probability of abnormalities in all 12 patients for whom an abnormality was found through laboratory testing. Clinical diagnosis, and not laboratory testing, was the apparent basis for any change in operative plans.

Several studies have compared groups of hospitalized patients undergoing routine laboratory screening tests (to supplement the history and physical examination) with groups not undergoing routine screening tests. Would outcome differ? Wood and Hoekelman[33] found that abnormal results from history, physical examination, or laboratory examination changed the preoperative clinical course (for all, surgery was postponed) for 28 of 1,924 children. For 3 of those 28 patients, laboratory tests indicated an abnormality not suggested by history or physical examination. Thus, the history and physical examination dictated the appropriate laboratory testing for all but 3 of 1,924 patients.

A more specific conclusion is also possible. The abnormalities discovered for these three patients were found on chest radiographs. (These children were part of a study comparing perioperative outcome at two hospitals, one that required chest radiographs as a screening test for elective surgery in children and one that did not.) There were no differences noted in anesthetic or perioperative complications between the two groups. Therefore, Wood and Hoekelman recommended that chest radiographs not be obtained routinely for apparently healthy children.

Even in a referral population history and physical examination determine more than 90 percent of the clinical course when a patient is referred for consultation about cardiovascular, neurologic, or respiratory disease.[34] Other studies also have demonstrated that the history and physical examination accurately indicate all areas in which subsequent laboratory testing proves beneficial to patients. For example, Rabkin and Horne[35,36] examined the records of 165 patients having a "new" abnormality on ECG that was "surgically significant" (i.e., a change from a previous tracing that represents a condition possibly affecting perioperative management or outcome). In only two instances were anesthetic or surgical plans altered by the discovery of "new abnormalities" found on ECG but not indicated by history. Thus, even for these 165 patients, for whom the benefits of a laboratory test should have been maximal because abnormalities were detected before surgery, the history or physical examination determined case management most of the time. Furthermore, for one of the two instances of altered case management — a patient who had atrial fibrillation — physical examination should have indicated the need for an ECG. A history or physical examination was not available for the other patient.

In summary, the studies cited point to the lack of benefit from routine laboratory tests as a method of assessing patients preoperatively. Many of these laboratory tests have been shown to be superfluous to patient care management. History and physical examination are considered the most effective ways to screen for disease. Laboratory tests can be used to screen for disease when such tests have proved effective, but are better used to confirm clinical diagnoses or to optimize a patient's condition prior to surgery.

Patient Risk

Unnecessary testing may lead physicians to pursue and treat borderline and false-positive laboratory abnormalities. This observation does not imply that all standard screening tests should be discontinued; some are beneficial, such as the mammogram for all women over 40 years of age,[37] the test for occult blood in stool for all people over 40 years of age,[38] and the Papanicolaou (Pap) smear.[38] However, few studies have examined whether increased testing and the follow-up on false-positive test results adversely affect patients. In one study addressing this issue, Roizen et al.[39] retrospectively examined the adverse effects of chest radiographs on patients. For 606 patients, 386 extra chest radiographs were ordered without indication of need. Among those 386 patients, the discovery of only one

abnormality (an elevated hemidiaphragm probably caused by phrenic nerve palsy) may have resulted in improved care for that patient. On the other hand, the existence of three lung shadows on chest radiographs led to three sets of invasive tests, including one thoracotomy, but no discovery of disease. These procedures caused considerable morbidity, including one pneumothorax and 4 months of disability, for those three patients.

Tape and Mushlin[40] found a similar result when examining the benefits and risks of chest radiographs obtained preoperatively in Rochester, New York. Of 341 patients admitted for vascular surgery, 9 had radiograph findings that led to clinical action. Specifically, *3 patients* (2 with congestive heart failure and 1 with pulmonary fibrosis) *may have benefited* from the findings. However, all 3 patients were known by history to have the disease shown on chest radiographs. In addition, *6 patients were subjected to a potentially detrimental clinical response.* Two had false diagnosis of tuberculosis, with subsequent therapy in 1; 2 others had false diagnosis of nodules; and the last 2 had falsely normal chest radiograph readings. All the beneficial effects attributed to preoperative chest radiographs accrued to patients who had obvious clinical history of pulmonary or cardiac disease. Orkin[41] has further explained the basis of the risk from testing asymptomatic individuals.

In another study, Turnbull and Buck[42] examined the charts of 2,570 patients undergoing cholecystectomy to determine the value of preoperative test. With four possible exceptions, history and physical examination successfully indicated the need for all tests that ultimately benefited the patients. Again, for those 4 patients, it is doubtful if any benefit actually occurred as a result of preoperative tests. Among them was one patient who had emphysema detected only by chest radiograph. This patient had preoperative physiotherapy without subsequent postoperative complication. Two patients had unsuspected hypokalemia (potassium levels of 3.2 and 3.4 mEq/L in blood, respectively) and received treatment prior to operation. Data now in the literature indicate that no harm occurs to patients undergoing surgery with this degree of hypokalemia, and that severe harm may be caused by treating such patients with oral or intravenous administration of potassium (Table 23-1).[43–47] The fourth patient possibly benefiting from preoperative testing had an asymptomatic hemoglobin concentration of 9.9 g/dl and was given a blood transfusion prior to cholycystectomy. Because cholycystectomy is not normally associated with major blood loss, one might conclude that this patient also received no benefit from preoperative laboratory testing and its pursuit, but was exposed to the risk of transfusion. Thus, it is not clear that any patient in this study benefited from preoperative screening tests given without indication for need by history or physical examination.

In another study, only two patients at most (who had eradication of asymptomatic bacteriuria) benefited from the 9,720 screening tests that were obtained.[48] At

TABLE 23-1. Risk of Potassium Supplementation[a]

| | Route of Administration | | | |
	Oral	Intravenous	Oral and IV	All Routes
Number of patients	1,910	2,192	819	921
Death	3 (0.2%)	3 (0.15%)	1 (0.1%)	7 (0.14%)
Life-threatening reaction or death	6 (0.3%)	7 (0.35%)	14 (1.7%)	28 (0.57%)
Hyperkalemia	74 (3.9%)	34 (1.6%)	71 (8.7%)	179 (3.6%)
Other side effects	53 (2.8%)	18 (0.8%)	33 (4.0%)	283 (5.7%)

[a]One in 200 patients given potassium supplementation dies or has a life-threatening reaction.
(Data from Lawson et al.[46,47])

least one patient was seriously harmed from pursuit and treatment of abnormalities on screening tests. For this patient, atrial fibrillation and congestive heart failure developed after institution of thyroid therapy for borderline low thyroxine and free thyroxine index tests. It is unclear whether these investigators examined other patients for potential harm arising from pursuit and treatment of abnormalities on screening tests.

Medicolegal Liability

"Extra testing"—testing that is not warranted by findings on a medical history—does not provide medicolegal protection against liability. A series of studies shows that 30 to 95 percent of all unexpected abnormalities found on preoperative laboratory tests are not noted on the chart before surgery (Table 23-2). This lack of nota-

tion occurs not only at university medical centers but at community hospitals as well. Moreover, failure to pursue an abnormality appropriately poses a greater risk to medicolegal liability than does failure to detect that abnormality.[61] In this way, extra testing increases the medicolegal risk to physicians. In addition, the Health Care Financing Administration is attempting to make failure to pursue abnormalities grounds for charging physicians with inadequate practice.

Effect on Operating Room Schedules

According to hospital administrators in the United States, surgeons say they order preoperative tests to satisfy anesthesiologists: they find it easier just to order all the tests and let the anesthesiologist sort them out. Surgeons also believe it is much more efficient to order

TABLE 23-2. Potential Medicolegal Liability of Unrecorded Abnormalities

Series	Type Test	Unexpected Abnormalities (N)	Unexpected Abnormalities Noted Preoperatively[a] (%)
Lorenzi and Cohen[b]	PT/PTT	20	5
Rabkin and Horne[35,36]	ECG	157	31
Kaplan et al.[49]	CBC/PTT Glucose/SMA 6 }	12[c]	17
Robbins and Rose[50]	PT	23	39
Wood and Hoekelman[33]	Hematocrit	15[c]	27
Parkerson[51,52d]	Multiple	343	38
	Multiple; >10% abnormal	63?	60
Williamson et al.[53d]	Urinalysis	164	17
	FBS	63	32
	Hemoglobin	32	16
Huntley et al.[54d]	Multiple	343	67
Daughaday et al.[55]	Multiple	167	60
Epstein et al.[56d]	T_4	111	60
Wheeler et al.[57]	Hemoglobin	258	71
Kelley and Mamlin[58d]	Multiple	852	64–85
Wolf-Klein et al.[26d]	Multiple	756	7–73 (avg. 50)
Lawrence and Kroenke[59]	Urinalysis	180	29
Umbach et al.[60]	Chest roentgenograms	116	59

[a]Refers to recording of an unexpected abnormality on the patient's chart either preoperatively or anytime other than on the laboratory test report printout.
[b]Personal communication.
[c]Abnormalities potentially significant to perioperative management.
[d]Test not obtained preoperatively.
Abbreviations: PT, prothrombin time; PTT, partial thromboplastin time; ECG, electrocardiogram; CBC, complete blood count; SMA 6, simultaneous multichannel analyses of sodium, potassium, chloride, bicarbonate, urea nitrogen, and creatinine levels in blood; FBS, fasting blood sugar; T_4, thyroxine.

batteries of tests than to have the anesthesiologist, who sees the patient the night before or the morning of surgery, obtain the tests on an emergency basis. This reasoning process overlooks the fact that abnormalities arising from tests done in the battery fashion usually are not discovered until the night before, or the morning of, surgery, if at all. Then, the discovery of abnormal results delays or postpones schedules, as effort and time are wasted to obtain consultant reviews of false-positive or slightly abnormal results.

PREOPERATIVE TESTING

Most hospitals, many anesthesia departments, and now many outpatient surgical centers have rather arbitrary rules and recommendations regarding tests that should be performed before elective surgery. When, with good intentions, anesthesiologists tried to follow those rules, our problems began. The inexpensive multiphasic screening batteries of tests subsequently developed by the Kaiser Hospitals and Health Plan seemed to be the answer to this confusing and arbitrary process.[62] Physicians believed they could now order inexpensive batteries of tests and thus efficiently screen for disease. However, physicians were still trying to figure out which tests to order before surgery, and what to do with the unexpectedly abnormal result on the morning of surgery; Kaiser found that this system of preoperative multiphasic screening was not practical.[63] The system produced so many false-positive and false-negative results that the subsequent harm vastly outweighed any possible benefit. Nevertheless, the notion of "the more testing, the better" is still with us.

The Low Predictive Value of an "Abnormal" Laboratory Test Result

Understanding what constitutes an "abnormal" laboratory test result requires an appreciation of the way "normal" values are determined. A normal range is based on the typical distribution of the Gaussian curve.[64,65] For example, assuming a Gaussian distribution and hemoglobin values of 13.5 to 16.7 g/dl for healthy men, one can expect 5 percent of "normal" healthy men to have a test result outside that range.

Of prime importance in preoperative evaluation is knowing the percentage of abnormal laboratory test values that truly indicates disease. If the anesthetic management of a patient is altered because of test abnormality, that abnormality should indicate a condition that (1) poses a significant risk of perioperative morbidity that can be lessened by preoperative treatment, (2) cannot be discovered through history-taking and physical examination, and (3) is sufficiently prevalent in the population to justify the risk of performing the follow-up test. To be cost-efficient, the test should be sufficiently "sensitive" (have "positivity in disease") and sufficiently "specific" (have "negativity in health").

That is, test results should be positive if the patient has disease and negative if the patient is healthy.[64-67]

We should now consider the significance of false-positive and false-negative results and the prevalence of disease in the test population in relation to abnormal laboratory test results. For example, let us assume that the sensitivity (positivity in disease) of a test is 75 percent: 75 of 100 people who actually have, for example, pneumonia would have the notation "pneumonia" (or some significant abnormality) written as the diagnosis on their chest roentgenogram reports. Let us also assume that the specificity of a test (its negativity in health) is 98.3 percent. That is, 983 of 1,000 people who actually do not have pneumonia will have "without evidence of pneumonia," "normal," or a similar comment on their chest roentgenogram reports. Third, let us assume that 0.5 percent of the asymptomatic population about to undergo routine elective surgery has pneumonia. Given the preceding assumptions, what is the likelihood that a person whose chest roentgenogram report reads "pneumonia" will actually have pneumonia?

If we test 100,000 asymptomatic individuals and 0.5 percent are assumed to be diseased, this would mean that 500 people would have undetected pneumonia. If the sensitivity of chest roentgenograms to pneumonia is assumed to be 75 percent, 375 of these individuals would have abnormal roentgenograms. Then, if specificity is assumed to be 98.3 percent, 97,809 of the 99,500 healthy individuals would have normal chest roentgenogram results. This means that 1,691 (1.7 percent) would have abnormal roentgenogram results. Thus, of 2,066 patients having a diagnosis of pneumonia based on chest roentgenogram, 1,691 (82 percent) of the results would be false-positive. Therefore, it is entirely possible that 82 percent of the chest roentgenograms indicating "infiltrate compatible with pneumonia" in otherwise asymptomatic individuals would actually be describing totally healthy people. Expressed in another way, when the assumptions discussed are applied, the likelihood of an asymptomatic person's actually having pneumonia when the chest roentgenogram report contains that notation is only 18 percent.

Only patients with abnormal test results who actually have disease ("true positives") benefit from laboratory testing. Let us assume that 1.5 percent of the chest radiographs in the under-40 population are positive, and that for each true positive, perioperative mortality is decreased by 50 percent. If we use the 82 percent false-positive rate derived previously, then the number of patients benefiting per 1,000 roentgenograms is 2.7 (true positives per 1,000 = all positives − false-positives, i.e., [1.5 percent × 1,000] − [82 percent × 1.5 percent × 1,000] × 1,000 = 2.7 patients). Therefore, a reduction in operative mortality of 50 percent, or 1 per 10,000 (i.e., 2.7 × 0.5 × 0.0002) gives 0.00027 fewer deaths per 1,000 operations when preoperative chest roentgenograms are obtained.

Translating this figure into the present value for years of life saved per 1,000 roentgenograms yields the following: 0.00027 fewer deaths per 1,000 operations × 22.62 years saved per life saved = 0.0061 years of life. (The figure 22.62 is the present value of 60 more years of life for a 20-year-old, per Neuhauser.[65]) At the University of Chicago, this 0.0061 years of life saved would cost $70,000 (an anterior-posterior and lateral chest roentgenogram costs $70, not including fees for consultations, repeated roentgenograms, or other laboratory tests or procedures). Therefore, each year of life saved by obtaining chest roentgenograms costs about $11,475,000 ($70,000 ÷ 0.0061).

However, just as there are other costs (e.g., pursuing some false-positive chest shadows will result in computed tomographic needle biopsies and lobectomies in totally healthy patients[39–42]), there are other benefits (e.g., treatment of some patients having solitary nodules or mediastinal masses may prolong life). Let us arbitrarily assume that these costs and benefits are equal. One is forced to conclude that screening for an asymptomatic disease having a low prevalence rate is a very expensive and possibly risky procedure.

Laboratory Test Abnormalities in Asymptomatic Populations

Chest Roentgenograms

First, what abnormalities on chest roentgenograms would influence management of anesthesia? Certainly, it may be important to know about the existence of tracheal deviation; mediastinal masses; pulmonary nodules; a solitary lung mass; aortic aneurysm; pulmonary edema; pneumonia; atelectasis; new fractures of the vertebrae, ribs, or clavicles; dextrocardia; or cardiomegaly before proceeding to anesthesia and surgery. However, a chest roentgenogram probably would not detect the degree of chronic lung disease requiring a change in anesthetic technique any better than would the history and physical examination. Table 23-3[25,26,31,33,40,42,48,60,62,68–89] shows the prevalence of conditions that a chest roentgenogram might detect. These data show that abnormalities are rare in the asymptomatic individual. In fact, the risks of chest roentgenogram probably exceed its possible benefits if the patient is asymptomatic and younger than 60 years of age. This analysis is, of course, predicated on maximizing benefit to society in general, as one cannot predict in advance which patients will benefit or which will be harmed.

Electrocardiograms

The incidence of electrocardiographic abnormalities has been determined by studies of patients[62,63] and epidemiologic surveys of healthy people.[69,90,91] The abnormalities on ECG that have the potential to alter management of anesthesia are as follows: atrial flutter or fibrillation; first-, second-, or third-degree atrioventricular block; changes in ST segment suggesting myocar-

dial ischemia or recent pulmonary embolism; premature ventricular and atrial contractions; left or right ventricular hypertrophy; short PR interval; Wolf-Parkinson-White syndrome; myocardial infarction; prolonged QT segment; and tall peaked T waves. What is the incidence of finding these abnormalities on a 12-lead preoperative screening ECG but not on a standard monitor lead 1 or an MCL5 lead applied immediately before induction of anesthesia in the operating room?

Before answering that question, some qualifiers should be mentioned. First, none of the studies on the incidence of electrocardiographic abnormalities excluded patients having histories or physical examinations indicating cardiac problems. Second, the studies do not distinguish those findings evident on monitoring leads from findings evident on only 6- or 12-lead ECGs (Table 23-4).[26,35,36,48,62,75,77,87,90–94]

The data in Table 23-4 and elsewhere[95] show that abnormalities on ECG are relatively common and increase exponentially with age. Averaging all those data indicates that the incidence of abnormal preoperative electrocardiographic results would exceed 10 percent at 40 years of age and would be 25 percent by 60 years of age. These estimates pool abnormalities for both sexes. Clearly, those studies that looked for abnormalities on ECG after first ensuring the patient was asymptomatic (McKee and Scott,[77] Moorman et al.,[94] and Blery et al.[87]) found a much lower incidence of significant abnormalities. McKee and Scott found no abnormalities significant to perioperative care in 160 individuals who had no cardiac symptoms and were under 60 years of age and only two abnormalities in 163 patients over 60 years of age. Moorman and colleagues found only 1 of 275 asymptomatic patients under the age of 46 years, and 7 of 500 asymptomatic patients over the age of 45 years, who had abnormalities on preoperative ECGs. In the study by Blery and co-workers, only 0.6 percent of 2,256 patients under age 40 years who had no cardiac or pulmonary symptoms had an abnormality on preoperative ECG. Our group, Apfelbaum et al.,[93] found no abnormalities on ECG that were significant to perioperative care or that altered perioperative care among patients judged asymptomatic on the basis of results from a video questionnaire. This study will be discussed later in the chapter.

How useful is it to repeat ECGs if the patient has had an ECG within the past 2 years? Rabkin and Horne[35,36] address this question. "New abnormalities" on a subsequent ECG occur with significant frequency—approximately 25 to 50 percent as frequently as all abnormalities occurring on the previous ECG (Table 23-5). Thus, one would be justified in obtaining screening ECGs prior to elective surgery on all patients over 40 years of age, even in those who recently have had an ECG.

Some physicians have questioned even that conclusion. Goldberger and O'Konski[95] believe that the most important potential benefit of the preoperative ECG is detection of previously unrecognized myocardial in-

TABLE 23-3. Screening Chest Roentgenograms: Incidence of Abnormal Test Results, the Discovery of Which Might Change Management of Anesthesia

Age (years)	Series	Patients Examined (N)	Abnormalities[a] (%)	New Abnormalities[b] (%)
0–14	Farnsworth et al.[68]	350	8.9	0.3
0–18	Brill et al.[69]	1,000	1.9	0.7
0–19	Sagel et al.[70]	521	0	0
0–19	Sane et al.[71]	1,500	5.4	2.2
0–19	Wood and Hoekelman[33]	749	4.7	1.2
1–20	Rees et al.[72]	46	0	0
20–29	Sagel et al.[70]	894	1	
21–30	Rees et al.[72]	62	3	
≤30	Loder[73]	437	10.1	0.2
≤30	Hubbell et al.[74]	12	0	0
≥30	Maigaard et al.[75]	1,256	≤4.5	0
0–39	Umbach et al.[60]	305	3.0	
30–39	Sagel et al.[70]	942	2.3	
≤40	Catchlove et al.[76]	29	0	0
≤40	Collen et al.[62]	15,978	2.1	
≤40	Sagel et al.[70]	2,357	1.3	1.3
≤40	McKee and Scott[77c]	26	7.7	3.9
≤40	Combined[60,68–71,73–77d]	6,787	4.0	0.8
40–49	Sagel et al.[70]	928	7.1	
40–49	Umbach et al.[60]	290	6.2	
40–59	Collen et al.[62]	21,489	7.4	
41–50	Hubbell et al.[74]	28	17.9	0
41–50	Rees et al.[72]	119	19	
41–50	McKee & Scott[77c]	53	17	0
30–69	Loder[73]	515	≤6.0	
31–40	Rees et al.[72]	93	13	
31–40	Hubbell et al.[74]	22	22.5	4.5
≥40	Sagel et al.[70]	3,689	23.9	6.0
≥40	Catchlove et al.[76]	50	0	0
≥40	Thomsen et al.[78]	1,823	2.3	0.2
50–59	Umbach et al.[60]	247	10.9	
50–59	Sagel et al.[70]	833	20.3	
51–60	Hubbell et al.[74]	87	36.8	4.4
51–60	Rees et al.[72]	121	40.0	
51–60	McKee and Scott[77c]	85	40.0	0
60–69	Umbach et al.[60]	202	13.3	
60–69	Sagel et al.[70]	977	29.7	
61–70	Boghosian and Mooradian[79]	78	≤49	
>60	Boghosian and Mooradian[79]			
	Without risk factors[c]	44	34.0	
	With risk factors	92	62.0	
>60	Collen et al.[62]	7,196	19.2	
>60	Hubbell et al.[74]	145	44.1	4.8[e]
>60	McKee and Scott[77c]	163	44.2	1.9
61–70	Rees et al.[72]	134	43.3	
61–70	Hubbell et al.[74]	94	36.2	5.4
>65	Sewell et al.[80]	28	21	
≥69	Loder[73]	48	≤72.9	

continued

farction. This risk increases with increasing age. However, even in the highest risk group, men 75 years of age or older, the estimated incidence of unrecognized Q-wave infarction within the preceding 6 months is relatively small (less than 0.5 percent). Goldberger and O'Konski concluded that the risk of obtaining a preoperative ECG and subsequent reactions probably exceeds its benefit if patients are asymptomatic, do not have important risk factors for coronary disease, and are under 45 (men) or 55 (women) years of age.

Hemoglobin, Hematocrit, and White Blood Cell Counts

Wasserman and Gilbert[96] found that of 28 patients having uncontrolled polycythemia (hemoglobin greater than 16 g/dl) who underwent major surgery, 22 (79 percent) had complications and 10 (36 percent) died. That group was compared with a group of 53 patients who had controlled polycythemia (hemoglobin ≤ 16 g/dl) and major surgery; 15 (28 percent) had complications and 3 (5 percent) died. For both groups, most of the

TABLE 23-3. *(continued)* **Screening Chest Roentgenograms: Incidence of Abnormal Test Results, the Discovery of Which Might Change Management of Anesthesia**

Age (years)	Series	Patients Examined (N)	Abnormalities[a] (%)	New Abnormalities[b] (%)
≥?70	Wolf-Klein et al.[26]	500	1.9	
≥70	Sagel et al.[70]	832	41.7	
≥70	Törnebrandt and Fletcher[81]	100	37	8.1?
≥70	Boghosian and Mooradian[79]			
	Without risk factors[c]	58	≤59	
	With risk factors	45	≤64	
≥71	Levinstein et al.[48]	121	84.4	0.9
70–79	Umbach et al.[60]	110	27.2	
71–80	Rees et al.[72]	76	61.8	
71–80	Hubbell et al.[74]	28	57.1	0
>80	Umbach et al.[60]	21	33.3	
>80	Hubbell et al.[74]	23	60.9	8.7
20–89	Fink et al.[82]	127	46	
74–97	Domoto et al.[25]	69	72.5	33
>81	Rees et al.[72]	16	68.8	
?0–?90	Wiencek et al.[83]	403	≤25.1	≤2.4
0–90	Delahunt and Turnbull[31]	860		0
24–90	Tape and Mushlin[40]'	318	33	0
0–?90	Petterson and Janower[84]	1,530	9.8	1.3
0–?90	Turnbull and Buck[42]'	691	5.5	
0–?90	Royal College[85]	3,052	3.8	
0–?90	Rucker et al.[86c]	371	0.3	
0–?90	Blery et al.[87]	2,765	0.7	0.1
0–90+	Weibman et al.[88]'	734	5.0	
0–90+	Muskett and McGreevy[89]	119	29.4	5.0

[a]These data constitute an edited summary of the data presented in various articles, edited to select abnormalities that might change management of anesthesia.
[b]Abnormalities not already known or suspected by history or physical examination.
[c]Patients were asymptomatic.
[d]Combined studies in under-40 population excluding two studies, Rees et al.[72] and Collen et al.[62]
[e]0 percent changed treatment.
['Tape and Mushlin[40] studied vascular surgery patients; Turnbull and Buck,[42] cholecystectomy patients; and Weibman and colleagues,[88] cancer patients.

complications were related to polycythemia (e.g., hemorrhage or thrombosis). Admittedly, this study had deficiencies. It was a retrospective study and no time frame was given. "Minor" surgery was excluded. Also, the study did not explain why polycythemia was controlled preoperatively in some patients but not in others. Nevertheless, results indicated that knowledge and pretreatment of polycythemia decreased perioperative morbidity and mortality.

No such evidence exists for normovolemic anemia. Rothstein[97] concluded that in patients under 3 months of age, hemoglobin should be over 10 g/dl, whereas in children over 3 months of age, hemoglobin of 9 g/dl is adequate. Slogoff[98] concluded that in adults, a hematocrit of 20 percent (hemoglobin of approximately 7 g/dl) is adequate (also see Ch. 48). However, no data confirm the hypothesis that preoperative treatment of moderate or mild normovolemic anemia in asymptomatic patients undergoing surgery involving no major blood loss decreases perioperative morbidity or mortality. Similarly, no data exist regarding the possible harm from abnormal white blood cell counts found preoper-

atively. Therefore, the following ranges of "surgically acceptable values" are arbitrary: for hematocrit, 29 to 57 percent for men and 27 to 54 percent for women; for white blood cell count, 2,400 to $16,000/mm^3$ for both men and women. When values fall outside these ranges, this author recommends seeking an alternative diagnosis before institution of anesthesia or surgery.[99]

How many healthy patients have this degree of abnormality in hematocrit or white blood cell count? No such patient was found among the 223 of 2,010 patients judged healthy by history (i.e., history indicated no need for tests)[49,92] The other limited available data are provided in Table 23-6. If we assume that 10 percent of all abnormalities are outside the "surgically acceptable" range[101] (Table 23-6), and if we apply the benefit-risk analysis described in the section on chest roentgenograms, we would conclude that either preoperative hematocrit or hemoglobin levels should be determined for all female surgical patients and for all male surgical patients over 60 years of age. Red cell antigen screening would be warranted for all patients undergoing procedures involving possible blood loss of

TABLE 23-4. Percentage of Patients Having Abnormalities Determined by Screening Electrocardiograms[a]

Age (yr)	Sex	Series	Patients Examined (N)	Total Abnormalities (%)[b]	Specific Abnormalities (%)			
					LVH	MI	ST Changes	AV Block
16–19	M	Ostrander et al.[91]	216	20.3	17.8	0	0.9	1.4
16–19	F	Ostrander et al.[91]	24	5.9	1.3	0	4.2	0.4
20–29	M	Ostrander et al.[91]	452	14.0	7.1	0.2	6.0	0.7
20–29	F	Ostrander et al.[91]	577	11.3	0.2	0.2	9.9	1.0
20–29	M	Collen et al.[62]	3,000	9.6				
20–29	F	Collen et al.[62]	4,000[c]	9.3				
>30	Either	Maigaard et al.[75]	1,256	<4.5		0.1		
30–39	M	Ostrander et al.[91]	676		3.0	0	6.9	1.3
30–39	F	Ostrander et al.[91]	699		0.4	0.1	11.6	1.6
30–39	M	Collen et al.[62]	4,000[c]	12.1				
30–39	F	Collen et al.[62]	5,000[c]	11.7				
35–44	M	Kannel et al.[90,92]			2.9			
35–44	F	Kannel et al.[90,92]			0.9			
<40	Either	Blery et al.[87d]	2,256	0.6				
<40	Either	Apfelbaum et al.[93d]	510	0				
<40	Either	McKee and Scott[77d]	23	13(0)				
40–49	M	Ostrander et al.[91]	468	24[a]	4.1	1.7	16.1	1.5
40–49	F	Ostrander et al.[91]	474	21[c]	0.6	0.8	17.2	0.6
40–49	M	Collen et al.[62]	4,000[c]	17.6				
40–49	F	Collen et al.[62]	5,000[c]	15.6				
41–50	Either	McKee and Scott[77d]	53	1.9(0)				
<45	?	Moorman et al.[94d]	275	0.4				
45–54	M	Kannel et al.[90,92]			4.8			
45–54	F	Kannel et al.[90,92]			3.6			
>45	?	Moorman et al.[94d]	500	1.4				
50–59	M	Ostrander et al.[91]	330	30[c]	3.3	5.1	20.8	1.2
50–59	F	Ostrander et al.[91]	327	40[c]	3.4	0.9	32.4	2.1
50–59	M	Collen et al.[62]	5,000[c]	24.9				
50–59	F	Collen et al.[62]	6,000[c]	20.7				
51–60	Either	McKee and Scott[77d]	84	23.8(0)				
55–64	M	Kannel et al.[90,92]			10.1			
55–64	F	Kannel et al.[90,92]			4.1			
<60	Either	Rabkin and Horne[35,36]	309	13.5	2.5	1.6	11.0	1.0
>60	Either	Rabkin and Horne[35,36]	503	24.4	2.2	1.9	13.0	0.6
>60	Either	McKee and Scott[77d]	163	42.3(1.3)				
60–69	M	Ostrander et al.[91]	177		8.4	9.0	37.1	4.5
60–69	F	Ostrander et al.[91]	196		10.2	6.1	42.4	4.1
60–69	M	Collen et al.[62]	2,000[c]	35.1				
60–69	F	Collen et al.[62]	3,000[c]	29.7				
64–74	M	Kannel et al.[90,92]			7.1			
65–74	F	Kannel et al.[90,92]			9.6			
>?70	Either	Wolf-Klein et al.[26]	500	11.9				
>70	M	Collen et al.[62]	1,000[c]	52.2				
>70	F	Collen et al.[62]	1,000[c]	41.2				
≥71	Either	Levinstein et al.[48]	121	24.4	0.7	13.8	6.3	3.6
70–79	M	Ostrander et al.[91]	100		7.9	9.9	46.5	7.9
70–79	F	Ostrander et al.[91]	119		11.8	2.5	43.8	6.7
74–97	Either	Domoto et al.[25]	69	27.5				
>80	M	Ostrander et al.[91]	26		11.5	7.7	46.2	19.2
>80	F	Ostrander et al.[91]	43		16.3	4.7	58.2	9.3
0–?90	Either	Blery et al.[87]	2,256	0.6(0.3)				
0–?90	Either	Turnbull and Buck[42]	632	14.6				
0–?90	Either	Muskett and McGreevy[89d]	145	1.3				

[a]All studies are 12-lead studies, except for that of Collen et al.,[62] which is a 6-lead study.
[b]These data constitute an edited summary of data given in several series, edited to select abnormalities that might change management of anesthesia. *Numbers in parentheses indicate abnormalities judged retrospectively by the authors of the paper to be significant to perioperative management.*
[c]Values are approximations that represent "best-guess" numbers from data not explicitly stated in the reports.
[d]Patients were asymptomatic.
Abbreviations: LVH, left ventricular hypertrophy; MI, myocardial infarction; ST changes, changes in the ST segment on electrocardiogram; AV, atrioventricular.

TABLE 23-5. Number and Percentages of Patients Having a New Abnormality on ECG and a Previous ECG[a]

	New Abnormality with a Previously			
	Normal ECG		Abnormal ECG	
Age (yr)	<60	≥60	<60	≥60
No. of pts./total no.	18/180	42/192	24/129	81/310
% new abnormalities	(10%)	(21.9%)	(18.6%)	(26%)
Abnormality:				
T wave	11(6.1%)	18(9.4%)	10(7.8%)	19(6.1%)
ST segment	7(3.9%)	9(4.7%)	6(4.7%)	20(6.4%)
Arrhythmias				
SVT or PVCs	3(1.7%)	7(3.6%)		8(2.6%)
Others, including PACs	3(1.7%)	6(3.1%)	1(0.8%)	1(0.3%)
QRS duration		8(4.2%)	2(1.6%)	14(4.5%)
LVH	3(1.7%)	4(2.1%)	5(3.9%)	7(2.3%)
Q wave	4(2.2%)	3(1.6%)	1(0.8%)	7(2.3%)
Ventricular conduction defects	5(2.6%)	1(0.8%)	7(2.3%)	
AV block	2(1.0%)	3(2.3%)	1(0.3%)	

[a]Numbers in parentheses are percentages of patients. Two-thirds of patients had a previous ECG within 2 years of their new ECG.
Abbreviations: ECG, electrocardiogram; SVT, supraventricular tachycardia; PVCs, premature ventricular contractions; PACs, premature atrial contractions; LVH, left ventricular hypertrophy; AV, atrioventricular.
(Data from Rabkin and Horne[36] and Rabkin and Horne.[37])

TABLE 23-6. Abnormalities Discovered by Screening Hemoglobin Tests and White Blood Cell Counts

Age (years)	Sex	Series	Patients Examined (N)	Hemoglobin Abnormalities (%)	WBC Count Abnormalities (%)
<19	Either	Wood and Hoekelman[33]	1,924	0.8	
<40	M	Collen et al.[62]	6,941	1.9	2.6
<40	F	Collen et al.[62]	9,037	12.6	2.6
≥18	Either	Parkerson[52]	392	18.8	10.7
<40	Either	McKee and Scott[77a]	96[a]	0	0
40–59	M	Collen et al.[62]	11,832	3.1	2.2
40–59	F	Collen et al.[62]	9,657	10.1	2.2
41–50	Either	McKee and Scott[77a]	53[a]	5.7	?
51–60	Either	McKee and Scott[77a]	85[a]	0	0
≥60	M	Collen et al.[62]	4,062	5.6	1.7
≥60	F	Collen et al.[62]	3,134	5.5	1.7
>60	Either	McKee and Scott[77a]	163[a]	6.1	?
>?70	Either	Wolf-Klein et al.[26]	551	33.2	17.4
>71	Either	Levinstein et al.[48]	12.1	27.8	4.0
74–97	Either	Domoto et al.[25]	70	11.4	4.3
Unspecified	Either	Turnbull and Buck[42]	1,005[a]	0.7	0.1
Unspecified	Either	Muskett and McGreevy[89]	199	60.8 / 9.0[b]	34.8 / 5.1[b]
Unspecified	Either	Kaplan et al.[49a]	293	0[b]	0[b]
Unspecified	Either	Gold and Wolfersberger[100a]	3,375	0.33	
Unspecified	Either	Carmalt et al.[101]	278	30.4[c]	
Unspecified	Either	Huntley et al.[54]	119	23	
Unspecified	Either	Williamson et al.[53]	982	3.2	
Unspecified	Either	Blery et al.[87a]	1,728	1.1	

[a]Patients were asymptomatic.
[b]Abnormalities significant to perioperative management.
[c]Carmalt and coworkers found that 24.5 percent were new abnormalities; 2 patients had hemoglobin values less than 8 g/dl, 17 had values of 8 to 10 g/dl, and 21 had values of 10 to 12 g/dl.

more than 2 units/70 kg body weight.[102] White blood cell counts appear to be rarely, if ever, justified for asymptomatic individuals.

Blood Chemistries, Urinalysis, and Clotting Studies

What blood chemistries would have to be abnormal, and how abnormal would they have to be, to justify changing one's perioperative management? Abnormal hepatic or renal function might change the choice and dose of anesthetic or adjuvant drugs. About 1 in 700 supposedly healthy patients is actually harboring hepatitis, and 1 in 3 of those will become jaundiced.[103,104] However, our group found no asymptomatic patient who denied exposure to hepatitis who then became jaundiced after uneventful surgery (MF Roizen, unpublished data from 3,500 patients in a prospective study of the "HealthQuiz," discussed later).[93] These data imply that either the screening history suffices or the incidence of asymptomatic hepatitis is decreasing.

Table 23-7 presents the available data regarding the abnormalities found on screening blood chemistries. Unexpected abnormalities are reported for 2 to 10 percent of patients screened, and these abnormalities lead to many additional tests that usually (approximately 80 percent of cases) have no significance for the patient. Unexpected abnormalities that are significant arise in 2 to 5 percent of patients studied. Of these abnormalities, approximately 70 percent are related to blood glucose[113] and blood urea nitrogen (BUN) levels. The 9 to 20 additional tests on the screening SMAs 12–20 panels lead to very few important discoveries affecting anesthesia. In fact, the false-positive rate is so high (i.e., 96.5 percent for the test for calcium) that the value representing cost versus benefit for most of these tests (even when the tests are free) is negative, as is the value representing benefit versus risk.

If a screening test for hepatitis is desired (because the incidence of hepatitis is 0.14 percent and/or because one wishes to avoid the potential legal problems of postanesthetic jaundice), only three tests seem justified: serum glutamic-oxaloacetic transaminase (SGOT), blood glucose, and BUN. Even then, the last two are indicated only for patients over 60 years of age. In fact, if the data from our group on asymptomatic liver disease can be generalized, no blood chemistry tests are warranted for patients under 60 years of age. Furthermore, if the antibody test that detects "non-A, non-B hepatitis" (now called hepatitis C) proves as useful after infection has occurred, the medicolegal risk posed by postanesthetic jaundice will be even less.[114]

Abnormalities are commonly found on urinalysis (Table 23-8).[25,26,33,42,48,53,54,59,89,100,115] The quality of urinalysis results obtained by dipstick technique has been variable at best.[116] In addition, these abnormal results usually do not lead to beneficial changes in management. Most of the results that do lead to beneficial changes could have been obtained by history or determination of BUN and glucose levels, tests that are already recommended for all patients over 60 years of age. Thus, urinalysis, although initially inexpensive, becomes an expensive test to justify on a cost-benefit basis.

Although measurement of the partial thromboplastin time (PTT) and the prothrombin time (PT) are useful tests to screen patients having a history of bleeding, their values as screening tests for asymptomatic patients has never been shown (Table 23-9).[119,121,122] I believe that Table 23-10 shows the maximum testing one could recommend for asymptomatic individuals. Even then, history-taking would be an even better way to screen for conditions warranting testing.

Other Tests

As mentioned earlier, tests for AIDS and pregnancy and screening for hemoglobinopathy and malignant hyperthermia raise ethical issues that may require close attention to institutional policy and the immediate availability of counseling services. Moreover, all of these tests have associated risks. The physician may therefore decide to limit testing to only "at-risk" populations (e.g., for pregnancy testing, only female patients who believe they may possibly be pregnant).

Testing of the asymptomatic population for AIDS is not likely to be the most effective way of uncovering the disease. Of the more than 100,000 people in the United States who have had AIDS, only 1 person has not been gay, had sex with a prostitute, used intravenously administered drugs and shared needles, been stuck with a needle, cared for a family member with AIDS, or received a blood transfusion after 1979. One program screening for human immunodeficiency virus in asymptomatic individuals was able to produce an "acceptably low false-positive rate" by diagnosing HIV infection only after one sample of blood produced positive results on four different tests, and after a second sample of blood had been used for verification.[123] Thus, for pregnancy, hemoglobinopathies, and AIDS, the history is still best at identifying those at risk for the condition.

In the past, no screening test has existed for malignant hyperthermia other than a personal or family history of the condition. However, one new test may be appearing—the fluidization of a susceptible patient's red cell membrane on exposure to halothane.[124] It is still too early to predict the usefulness of this test as a screening procedure; other screening tests for this disease have not been reliable enough to use for any but "at-risk" individuals (e.g., children with a history of myopathies who are undergoing squint surgery, patients having a family history of problems with anesthesia, or patients with a history of abnormal red appearance, thermoregulation, and reactions to minor stresses) (see Ch. 28).

Even sophisticated laboratory tests have not proved in controlled trials to be better than the history and physical examination in estimating the risk from a diagnosis. This lack of benefit from laboratory testing has

TABLE 23-7. Screening Blood Chemistries: Percentages of Patients Having Abnormalities

Age (years)	Series	Patients Examined (N)	BUN	Cr	Glucose	SGOT	Uric Acid	Cholesterol	Albumin	Total Protein	Ca++	VDRL	Alkaline PTAse	Bilirubin	K+	Phosphate
10–54	Schemel[104]	7,620				0.144										
15–85	Carmalt et al.[101a]	296	1.4	1.0	2.0	0		0.3	0		0.3		0	0	0	0.3
>18	Parkerson[52]	397		1.2	15.8	2.8	7.9	6.1			2.0			1.2	6.6	
>18	Schneiderman et al.[105]	547		9.3		1.3							9.7	3.7		
>18	[Bryan data][106,107]	623	1.1		5.0		4.5		1.4	2.4	1.0				4.0	
>25	Peery[108a]	1,771	18		21	3.1	36	30	0.5	0.5			1.3	3.6	0	
<40	McKee and Scott[77b]	96	0												0	
40–59	Collen et al.[62]	21,489		1.4	5.6	4.6	4.8	2.7	0.3	4.4	1.3	1.9				
41–50	McKee and Scott[77b]	53	0												0	
>40	Collen et al.[62]	15,978		0.8	4.6	3.6	3.4	1.7	0.4	3.5	1.4	0.8				
51–60	McKee and Scott[77b]	85	0												0	
>60	Collen et al.[62]	7,196		2.7	8.3	4.5	6.0	3.0	0.4	3.9	1.5	2.3				
>60	McKee and Scott[77b]	163	2.5												0	
>70	Wolf-Klein et al.[26]	500	24.6	14.5	24.6	9.4	7.7	13.8	20.4	9.9	7.2		23.2	1.7	5.4	
≥71	Levinstein et al.[48]	121	36	10.8	29.0	0.8	7.2	6.9	27.8	19.2	5.6		19.0	0.7	3.0	
74–97	Domoto et al.[25]	70	30		26.5	9.2	8.6	17.2	0	2.1	1.0		9.2	2.1		1.0
All	Wataneeyawech and Kelly[103]	6,540				0.234										
All	Bryan et al.[106]	2,846	1.4		5.6				1.4	0.7	0.3				0.3	
All	Friedman et al.[109]	8,446	3.4	3.3	5.9	2.7	2.7	3.8	1.5	2.5	5.4		3.9	2.4	1.4	
All	Delahunt and Turnbull[31b]	332	0	0											0.3	
All	Young and Drake[110a]	390	6.4	3.7	7.5						2.0				0	
All	Boonstra and Jackson[111a]	12,000									5.0					
All	Whitehead[112]	2,871	3.4		10.0	1.8	9.2	9.3	2.9		9.2		8.3	6.0	4.7	
All	Turnbull and Buck[42b]	995	0.1	0.2	0.7										1.4	
All	Blery et al.[87b]	~2,800	0.1	0.1	0.1											0.5

[a] A high percentage of these findings were analyzed in more depth and found to be clinically unimportant.

[b] Patients were asymptomatic.

Abbreviations: BUN, blood urea nitrogen; Cr, creatinine; SGOT, serum glutamic-oxaloacetic transaminase; CA++, calcium; VDRL, serologic test for syphilis, developed by the Venereal Disease Research Laboratory; PTAse, phosphatase; K+, potassium.

TABLE 23-8. Abnormalities Discovered by Screening Urinalysis

Age (years)	Sex	Series	Patients Examined (N)	Abnormalities (%)	Significant Abnormalities (%)
<19	Either	Wood and Hoekelman[33]	1,859	11.7	0.5
Unspecified	Either	Huntley et al.[54]	119	25	
5-12	F	Cardiff-Oxford[115]	16,800	1.8	
15-?	Either	Lawrence and Kroenke[59]	180	15	
Unspecified	Either	Gold and Wolfersberger[100]	3,375	2.7	
Unspecified	Either	Williamson et al.[53]	982	16.7	
Unspecified	Either	Collen et al.[62]	44,663	14.6	
Unspecified	Either	Muskett and McGreevy[89]	144	22.4	2.6
Unspecified	Either	Turnbull and Buck[42a]	995	4.3	0.1
>?70	Either	Wolf-Klein et al.[26]	550	12.9	
≥71	Either	Levinstein et al.[48]	121	25.8[b]	
74-97	Either	Domoto et al.[25]	70	9.2	

[a]Patients were asymptomatic.
[b]*Note:* Was only 1.4 percent when a dipstick technique was used.

been shown for diagnoses as relatively amenable to laboratory diagnosis as the differential diagnosis of systolic murmurs[125] or assessment of nutritional status.[126]

IMPLEMENTING CHANGE

Any possible benefit of routinely ordering an unselected battery of screening tests is negated by the factors discussed above. Screening laboratory tests appear to be both an extra cost to society and an extra risk to the individual patient. Several studies in addition to that of our group show that testing based on indications of disease found in a patient's history is capable of detecting all of the significant abnormalities revealed by screening tests. (Here, "significant" abnormalities are those whose discovery ultimately benefits the patient.) This practice also avoids some of the risk of nonselective testing.

Recently, many professional societies and national organizations have endorsed the concept of reducing preoperative screening tests by selectively ordering tests based on a patient's history. Professional societies include the American College of Surgeons, the American Society of Anesthesiologists, the American College of Physicians (the Clinical Efficacy Project), the American College of Pediatricians, and the American Society of Radiologists. National organizations include the Food and Drug Administration's panel on preoperative chest roentgenograms, the National Institutes of Health Consensus Panel on Dental Anesthesia, and the Blue Cross/Blue Shield Medical Necessity Panel.

Thus, our desire to increase efficiency, the weight of scientific evidence, and organizational endorsements, combined with changes occurring in health care reimbursement (payment of fixed fees, called "capitated care") and medicolegal liability (higher risk from not pursuing abnormalities than from failure to diagnose), make this an ideal time to change the current pattern of preoperative assessment. I believe that anesthesiologists should forego ordering batteries of tests and, instead order tests selectively, on the basis of medical history. How can this be accomplished efficiently and without greatly increasing physician time and costs? Several strategies are possible.

Possible Methods of Preoperative Evaluation

At least three methods of determining the laboratory tests to be ordered for a patient are possible. The surgeon or anesthesiologist who sees the patient prior to the scheduled procedure can obtain the history and perform the physical. Second, a clinic could be set up in the outpatient facility to perform these two tasks sufficiently early to ensure that the appropriate laboratory tests or consultations can be obtained without a delay in the schedule. Third, a questionnaire answered by the patient could be used to indicate which laboratory tests, if any, would be appropriate.

Regarding the first method, one might ask, Can the appropriate testing be easily generated from the surgeon's preoperative visit? One study found that it could. At the University of California, San Francisco, Kaplan et al.[49] found that even a partial history conveyed enough information to indicate correctly all but 22 abnormalities (none of which affected patient outcome) for over 2,785 preoperative blood tests obtained. (This study counted the complete blood count and simultaneous multichannel analysis of six variables [SMA 6] as one test.) Knowing only the admission diagnosis, previous discharge diagnoses, and scheduled operation, and using previously determined indications for laboratory testing, enabled detection of virtually all abnormalities that would have been detected by routine screening.

The second possibility involves setting up an office clinic where an anesthesiologist would see patients preparatory to surgery. Later sections describe how to make this type of clinic efficient.

The third suggestion for implementing preoperative evaluation involves the use of a patient questionnaire. Several groups have tested the effects and sensitivity of orally administered or written questionnaires as a way

TABLE 23-9. Percentage of Patients Having Coagulation Abnormalities, as Determined by Screening PT, PTT, Platelet Count, or Bleeding Time Tests

Age (years)	Series	Patients Examined (N)	Percentage with Abnormalities of				Percentage with Surgically Significant Abnormalities of			
			PT	PTT	PLT CNT	BT	PT	PTT	PLT CNT	BT
?0–90	Robbins and Rose[50]	1,025		14 (143/1,025)			0 (0/1,025)			
Unspecified	Baranetsky and Weinstein[117]	2,600	0.2 (5/2,600)				0 (0/2,600)			
Unspecified	Barber et al.[118]	1,941 (including 141 with risk factors) 1,800				6(110/1941)[a] 1.5(27/1800)[a]		0.19(2/1800)[a]	?2.2(43/1941)[a]	
?0–90	Blery et al.[87]	~2,900	0.1 (4/2,931)	0.1 (4/2,914)	0.3 (10/3,546)	0.4 (17/3,845)	0 (0/2,931)	0 (0/2,914)	?0.03 (1/3,576)	0 (0/3,845)
0–93	Lorenzi and Cohen (personal communication)	578		3.5 (20/578)			0 (0/578)			
>18	Kaplan et al.[49]	154					0 (0/154)			
>18	Rohrer et al.[119] With risk factors	282	0.6 (1/159)	6.3 (10/159)	8.2 (20/117)	7.4 (14/170)	0.6 (1/154)	?1.4 (?3/159)	?2.6 (?3/117)	?
	Asymptomatic		0.8 (1/123)	2.4 (3/123)	8.0 (13/103)	3.8 (4/105)	0 (0/123)	0 (0/123) (0/154)	0 (0/103)	0 (0/105)
≥71	Levinstein et al.[48]	121			4.0					
Unspecified	Turnbull and Buck[42]	1,005	0 (0/213)	1.5 (3/210)	0 (0/1,005)		0 (0/213)	0 (0/210)	0 (0/1,005)	
Unspecified	Eisenberg et al.[120]	750					0 (0/750)			
Unspecified	Muskett and McGreevy[89]	200	3.9 (5/128)	3.9 (5/126)			0 (0/128)	0 (0/126)		

[a]Number in parentheses = number of patients.
Abbreviations: PT, prothrombin time; PTT, partial thromboplastin time; PLT CNT, platelet count; BT, bleeding time.

TABLE 23-10. Screening Studies That Should Be Performed on Asymptomatic Healthy Patients Scheduled to Undergo "Peripheral" Surgical Procedures Involving No Major Blood Loss

Age (years)	Tests Indicated	
	For Men	For Women
Under 40	None	Hemoglobin or hematocrit
40–59	Electrocardiogram BUN/glucose	Hemoglobin or hematocrit Electrocardiogram BUN/glucose
Over 60	Hemoglobin or hematocrit Electrocardiogram Chest roentgenogram BUN/glucose	Hemoglobin or hematocrit Electrocardiogram Chest roentgenogram BUN/glucose

Abbreviation: BUN, blood urea nitrogen

of linking the patient's medical history to the selection of laboratory tests (Table 23-11; Figs. 23-1 and 23-2).[39,127,128] In 1987, McKee and Scott[77] used patient demographics and 17 orally administered questions to select preoperative tests for 400 patients. Age was found to be the best predictor of abnormalities on preoperative tests. Complications occurred most commonly in older patients who reported positive symptoms on the questionnaire.

A study at our institution determined that the response of patients to written questions could predict all laboratory tests that would produce abnormal results for those patients.[127] After the patient answered the questionnaire, a plastic overlay revealed what tests were indicated. If the patient could not answer the questions, a standard group of tests was ordered. Using such a method, even a tertiary care hospital admitting very sick patients could eliminate over 60 percent of laboratory tests now routinely obtained. The elimination of such tests could reduce patient charges and hospital costs 93 to 97 percent[129] (also, SN Cohen, personal communication).

Blery et al.[87] confirmed these results. Using suspected disease to order preoperative tests selectively for 3,866 consecutive surgical patients, these investigators subsequently questioned anesthetists to assess whether management of the patient suffered from omission of one or more preoperative tests. Only 0.2 percent of omitted tests would have possibly been useful. Table 23-11 provides a protocol similar to that used by Blery and colleagues and our group to indicate which preoperative conditions warrant follow-up laboratory tests (i.e., which suspected abnormalities are most likely to be confirmed by tests).

The protocol outlined in Table 23-11 is a minimum guideline for clinical judgment regarding ordering of laboratory tests. This method requires careful history-taking and physical examination of the patient, with special attention to testing whenever indicators of disease entities are discovered. With the goal of optimizing the patient's preoperative condition, this protocol clearly places the burden of accuracy on the person taking the history.

Errors by Physicians When Ordering Tests

This system has one major problem. *Even when physicians agree to reduce testing by using specific, agreed-upon criteria for selectively ordering tests based on history and physical examination, they still make a surprising number of mistakes when ordering tests.* Approximately 30 to 40 percent of patients who *should* have certain tests (based on agreed-upon criteria such as those in Table 23-11) do not get them, and 20 to 40 percent of patients who should *not* have tests are subjected to them. For instance, Blery and co-workers[87] examined 3,866 surgical patients in France. Even after medical personnel had been educated regarding which criteria indicated a need for which tests, 30 percent of the tests were ordered without need; another 22 percent of tests should have been ordered but were not. Thus, surgeons and anesthesiologists both increased costs and failed to obtain possibly valuable information.

These mistakes occur because integrating the history, physical examination, and indications for laboratory tests is not an easy process. Even when criteria for testing have been previously agreed upon by surgeons and anesthesiologists, the number of variables one must remember makes arriving at the correct conclusions a complex task. As an example, let us now consider how many mistakes are made regarding one commonly used preoperative test.

Charpak et al.[130] examined the value of preoperative screening chest roentgenograms for 3,849 patients. Surgeons and anesthesiologists agreed that any of the following findings on history or physical examination would warrant ordering of a chest roentgenogram: any lung or cardiovascular disease, malignant disease; a current history of smoking in patients older than 50 years of age; major surgical emergencies; immunodepression; or, for immigrants, absence of prior health

TABLE 23-11. Simplified Strategy for Selecting Preoperative Tests

Tests to be Obtained

Suspected Preoperative Conditions	HGB M	HGB F	WBC	PT/PTT	PLT, BT	Elect.	Creat./BUN	Blood Glucose	SGOT/Alk. PTAse	Roentgenogram	ECG	Pregnancy	T/S
Surgical procedure													
With blood loss	X	X											X
Without blood loss													
Neonates	X	X											
Age													
<40 yr		X											
40–59 yr										±	±		
≥60 yr	X	X								X	X		
Cardiovascular disease							X			X	X		
Pulmonary disease										X	X		
Malignancy	X	X	*	*						X			
Radiation therapy			X	X						X	X		
Hepatic disease									X				
Exposure to hepatitis									X				
Renal disease	X	X				X	X						
Bleeding disorder				X	X								
Diabetes						X	X	X			X		
Smoking ≥ 20 pack/yr	X	X								X			
Possible pregnancy												X	
Use of diuretics						X	X				X		
Use of digoxin						X	X				X		
Use of steroids						X		X					
Use of anticoagulants	X	X		X									

Note: Not all diseases are included in this table. Therefore, the physician should use his or her own judgment regarding patients having diseases that are not listed. *Abbreviations:* ±, Perhaps obtain; *, obtain for leukemias only; HGB, hemoglobin (obtain for male [M] or female [F] patients); WBC, white blood cell count; PT prothrombin time; PTT, partial thromboplastin time; PLT, platelet count; BT, bleeding time; Elect., electrolytes (i.e., sodium, potassium, chloride, carbon dioxide, and proteins); Creat./BUN, creatinine or blood urea nitrogen; SGOT/Alk. PTAse, serum glutamic-oxaloacetic transaminase and alkaline phosphatase; T/S, blood typing and screening for unexpected antibodies. (Data from Refs. 39, 49, 87, 127, and 128.)

SKR #2 M.D. Checklist for Ordering Preoperative Laboratory Tests

(Check indication if positive: Only one positive indication is needed per item.)

Patient's Name: _____

Scheduled Operation: _____

Test to Be Obtained   **Indication for Ordering Test**

Hb/Hct

_____ Potentially bloody operation (blood to be crossmatched
        preoperatively)
_____ Known anemia
_____ Bleeding disorder
_____ Hematologic malignancy
_____ Radiation or chemotherapy
_____ Chronic renal failure
_____ Severe chronic disease
_____ Other (specify): _____

_____

WBCs (differential will be
automatic   if   abnormal
WBC (or Hb)

_____ Infection
_____ Disease of WBCs
_____ Radiation or chemotherapy
_____ Immunosuppressive therapy or steroid therapy
_____ Hypersplenism
_____ Aplastic anemia

_____ Check here if you   _____ Collagen vascular disease
wish   differential   in   any   _____ Other (specify): _____
case.
                                 _____

                                 _____

PT/PTT

_____ Known or suspected coagulation abnormality
_____ Anticoagulant therapy or anticipated therapy
_____ Hemorrhage or anemia
_____ Thrombosis
_____ Liver disease
_____ Malabsorption or poor nutrition
_____ Other (specify): _____

_____

Fig. 23–1. Sample checklist for determining which preoperative laboratory tests should be obtained. Hb, hemoglobin; Hct, hematocrit; WBC, white blood cells; PT, prothrombin time; PTT, partial thromboplastin time; SMA 6 and SMA 12, simultaneous multichannel analysis of 6 and 12 blood components, respectively; SIADH, syndrome of inappropriate antidiuretic hormone secretion; ECG, electrocardiogram; CPK, creatinine phosphokinase. (Figure Continues.)

examination. Surgeons made their decision regarding ordering of chest roentgenograms after seeing the patient. Even with this agreement on criteria, of a total of 1,426 chest roentgenograms that should have been ordered for this group of 3,849 patients, 271 chest roentgenograms were ordered but not warranted, and 596 chest roentgenograms were not ordered although warranted. Although clinical judgment may account for some of these discrepancies, most of the chest roentgenograms that were inappropriately ordered or not ordered simply appear to be errors. If so many errors occurred for a single test, even more errors would be likely if patients were subjected to multiple testing.

Preliminary data from studies performed by our group confirm this rate of error.[131] We tested the hypothesis that over the last decade (1979 through 1988),

PLATELETS

_____ Known platelet abnormality
_____ Hemorrhage or purpura
_____ Leukemia
_____ Radiation or chemotherapy
_____ Hypersplenism
_____ Some anemias (aplastic, autoimmune, myelophthisic, pernicious)
_____ Transplant rejection
_____ Other

SMA 6

_____ Age 60 years or older
_____ Use of diuretics
_____ Renal disease
_____ Other fluid or electrolyte abnormality (diarrhea, SIADH, diabetes insipidus, severe liver disease, malabsorption, fever)
_____ Other (specify): _____

SMA 12

_____ Age 60 years or older
_____ Diabetes mellitus
_____ Hypoglycemia
_____ Pancreatic disease
_____ Pituitary disease
_____ Adrenal disease, steroid therapy
_____ Liver disease or exposure to hepatitis
_____ Radiation or chemotherapy
_____ Parathyroid disease

ECG

_____ Age 40 years or older
_____ Known or suspected cardiac abnormality
_____ Other (specify): _____

OTHER TESTS DESIRED
(specify indication):

_____ Urinalysis
_____ Rapid plasma reagin [syphilis screening test]
_____ CPK isoenzymes

OTHERS

_____   (Test name and indication):
_____   _____
_____   _____
                     _____

Fig. 23–1. *Continued*

physicians voluntarily and substantially reduced the ordering of preoperative tests unwarranted by history or physical examination. Reviewing 2,093 medical records from every other year in that period, including one of four operations at one of three study cities, we investigated the indications for, and the performance of, preoperative tests. During this period, the incidence of unwarranted laboratory tests obtained preoperatively decreased from 32.2 to 25.8 percent. This decrease was irregular and varied from operation to operation, from test to test, and from city to city. Furthermore, an unexpected 12 percent decrease (from 92.9 to 80.9 percent) in the ordering of *indicated* preoperative tests also occurred. Overall, 66.9 percent of tests obtained preoperatively in 1979 were not warranted, decreasing to 60.1 percent in 1987. If the possible benefit of ordering only appropriate tests outweighed the possible harm of not ordering a needed test, the net result would still be a benefit to society. Unfortunately, however, the possible benefit for performing a needed test is probably more than twice the possible harm of performing an unnecessary test.

SKR Preoperative Patient Questionnaire

Patient's Name: _____

Age: _____

	Yes	No	Don't Know
1. Do you currently take any of the following medications?			
a. Aspirin (Excedrin, Anacin, Bufferin, Alka-Seltzer)	___	___	___
b. Anticoagulants (blood-thinning medicine)	___	___	___
c. Quinidine or diltiazem, verapamil, nifedipine, propranolol or Inderal (heart rhythm medicines)	___	___	___
d. Diuretics (water pills)	___	___	___
e. Antihypertensive drugs (blood pressure pills)	___	___	___
f. Digitalis (heart pills)	___	___	___
g. Immunosuppressive drugs (e.g., cyclosporin, cyclophosphamide, azathioprine, 6-mercaptopurine)	___	___	___
h. Steroids (e.g., prednisone, prednisolone)	___	___	___
2. Have you ever been treated for cancer with chemotherapy or radiation (x-ray) therapy?	___	___	___
3. Do you currently have any problems with your:			
a. Liver (e.g., cirrhosis, hepatitis, yellow jaundice, malaria)	___	___	___
b. Kidneys (e.g., stones, infection, failure, dialysis)	___	___	___
c. Spleen	___	___	___
d. Blood (e.g., anemia, leukemia, sickle cell disease)	___	___	___
4. Have you or anyone in your family ever had a serious bleeding problem?	___	___	___
5. Have you ever had prolonged or unusual bleeding from nosebleeds, tooth extractions, cuts, or surgery (e.g., tonsilectomy, hernia, hysterectomy)?	___	___	___
6. Do you bleed from your teeth or gums when you brush your teeth?	___	___	___
7. Are your stools sometimes bloody or black and tarry?	___	___	___
8. Have you vomited blood or material that looks like coffee grounds?	___	___	___
9. Have you received a blood tranfusion within the last 6 months?	___	___	___

Fig. 23–2. Sample patient questionnaire for determining which preoperative laboratory tests should be obtained. (Figure Continues.)

I conclude that the pressures to order tests more optimally have not been accompanied by changes in practice patterns that ultimately benefit the patient. In order for a net benefit to accrue to the patient, a better system is needed for obtaining the truly necessary tests and for not ordering the unwarranted ones. On the other hand, punitive measures to reduce testing may save money from testing but impair health.

Thus, just as the need for a more effective system of preoperative evaluation became evident, the preceding study reinforced our belief that the actual methods of ordering tests also needed to change in order to improve the efficiency of the process.

Automating the System for Better Preoperative Evaluations

Can physicians do better at preoperative evaluation than the 5- to 15-minute history prior to induction for outpatients or "come-and-stay" patients (those to be

10. Have you recently had fever or chills, cold, or flu? ___ ___ ___

11. Have you ever been told you have sugar diabetes? ___ ___ ___

12. Do you wake up to urinate more than once a night? ___ ___ ___

13. Do you have muscle cramps or spasms? ___ ___ ___

14. Do you have problems with your lungs or chest (e.g., chest pain, skipped heart beats, high blood pressure)? ___ ___ ___

15. Do you have problems with your lungs or chest (e.g., smoke one pack or more per day, shortness of breath, chest pain, emphysema, asthma, bronchitis? ___ ___ ___

16. Have you recently been exosed to anyone with hepatitis (yellow jaundice)? ___ ___ ___

17. Are you pregnant? ___ ___ ___

18. Is there any possibility that you are pregnant? ___ ___ ___

19. Do you have a cough, or do you cough frequently? ___ ___ ___

20. Do you cough up sputum? ___ ___ ___

21. When you cough up sputum, have you noticed a change in the color or consistency or type of the sputum? ___ ___ ___

22. Do you have epilepsy or suffer from fits or seizures? ___ ___ ___

23. Do you have neck or back problems? ___ ___ ___

24. Have you or any blood relative had problems related to an operation? ___ ___ ___

25. Have you lost weight recently? ___ ___ ___

26. Are you scheduled to have an operation? ___ ___ ___

    If so, which one?_____

27. What medicines do you take?
    1. _____   4. _____
    2. _____   5. _____
    3. _____   6. _____
    Others: _____
    _____

Fig. 23–2. *Continued*

admitted after surgery)? They can, and should, for their patients' sake and their own sake. The British have reached the same conclusion.[132,133] A change in the system of obtaining patient histories and ordering tests has been advocated for even internists.[134–143]

The University of Chicago and at least six other institutions have initiated such a change. At these institutions, computer memory has helped simplify the complex task of integrating history, physical examination, and indications for laboratory tests. Specifically, patients answer a health-related questionnaire that is programmed into a four-button, battery-powered com-

```
HEALTHQUAL  PATIENT SUMMARY          PREOP-1.1            Page 1
COPYRIGHT 1988                                        JAN 14, 1989
IDENTIFICATION NUMBER:  120362880

PATIENT NAME: _____

PHYSICIAN: _____

PRESENT COMPLAINT: _____


The patient's answers to the HealthQuiz may suggest disease in the following systems as
indicated by the following symptoms:

SYSTEM             SYMPTOMS

PULM               RECENT URI _____




SOME ITEMS PERTINENT TO ANESTHESIA CARE ARE:

Patient wears dentures.
Patient has capped teeth.
Patient wears contact lenses.
Patient has allergies. **
Patient  has previously had Anesthesia.


             SUGGESTED LABORATORY TESTS

HCT                                      DIFF
EKG

Consider stool for occult blood

If operation involves insertion of a prosthesis or foreign material, you might obtain a
URINALYSIS to rule out a urinary tract infection.


THE PATIENT REPORTS THAT HE/SHE HAS HAD THE FOLLOWING TESTS
RECENTLY:

Patient's stool has been checked for blood in the last year.
Patient has had a pap smear in the last year.
Patient has had a mammogram in the last year.
```

Fig. 23–3. Actual printout from "HealthQuiz" questionnaire. (© University of Chicago.)

puter device (the "HealthQuiz"*). This device is similar to that used in "Donkey Kong, Jr.," a computer game for children. The box displays questions on its video screen, and the patient answers either yes or no. The device then generates a summary of the patient's health

history (Fig. 23-3) and, on the basis of the patient's answers and previously established criteria, suggests which laboratory tests, if any, would be appropriate. The "HealthQuiz" also gives reminders about items in history that are important to anesthesia care, such as allergies and the existence of capped teeth. Although the anesthesiologist still needs to see the patient, the productivity of the time spent is much greater.

As one preliminary study now under way indicates, laboratory testing generated in this way produces substantial savings. The study involves the University of Manitoba, Duke University, Washington University in

---

* I developed the preoperative video health questionnaire at the University of Chicago to help ameliorate the problem of inefficient preoperative assessments and to evaluate methods of selecting tests. Consequently, the University owns the right to commercialize this product and has indicated an intention to do so.

St. Louis, Tulane University, Archbishop Bergan Hospital in Nebraska, the University of California at Davis, and the University of Chicago. Preliminary data show that $68.70 could be saved per patient. For the 27 million patients receiving anesthesia care nationwide, this savings would amount to $1.85 billion annually. These figures take into consideration only the savings associated with the initial tests. Savings no doubt would be considerably greater if the analysis included the cost of repeated tests and of consultations for false or borderline positive tests, and the costs saved by preventing iatrogenic disease.

The assumptions used to perform the benefit-risk analysis were skewed to overestimate the predictive value of laboratory testing. Thus, for asymptomatic patients, physicians should probably do less laboratory testing rather than more. All physicians have a responsibility to provide optimum care within the bounds of finite resources. If laboratory work for asymptomatic individuals is limited to only that warranted by proven methods, perhaps government would allow the practice of optimum medicine (which tends to be more expensive) for the sick, who need more laboratory work.

Does the system of preoperative evaluation need to change? I believe it does. Physicians need to be available in a "preoperative" office (even if only in the late afternoon) to perform a thorough history, to select tests in a cost-efficient fashion, and to reassure patients. They also need to transmit that preoperative information in a concise fashion to the anesthesiologist providing care for the patient. In the past, anesthesiologists have taken a leading role in adopting system changes and thus making operating rooms safer and anesthesia care less expensive. One of these innovations, pulse oximetry, provides a moment-by-moment measure of the patient's oxygen level and thus reduces the need for extra blood tests. Similarly, physicians can demonstrate to their constituency, the patients, and to their watchdog, the government, that they can change the system of preoperative evaluation to increase efficiency, reduce costs substantially, and improve the quality of care. At the same time, anesthesiologists will reduce their own anxiety about performing the very best evaluation possible.

REFERENCES

1. Egbert LD, Battit GE, Turndorf H, Beecher HK: The value of the preoperative visit by an anesthetist. A study of doctor-patient rapport. JAMA 185:553, 1963
2. Egbert LD, Battit GE, Welch CE, Bartlett MK: Reduction of postoperative pain by encouragement and instruction of patients: A study of doctor-patient rapport. N Engl J Med 270:825, 1964
3. Wolfer JA, Davis CE: Assessment of surgical patients' preoperative emotional condition and postoperative welfare. Nurs Res 19:402, 1970
4. Anderson EA: Preoperative preparation for cardiac surgery facilitates recovery, reduces psychological distress, and re-duces the incidence of acute postoperative hypertension. J Consult Clin Psychol 55:513, 1987
5. Cyr MG, Wartman SA: The effectiveness of routine screening questions in the detection of alcoholism. JAMA 259:51, 1988
6. Vacanti CJ, Van Houten RJ, Hill RC: A statistical analysis of the relationship of physical status to postoperative mortality in 68,388 cases. Anesth Analg 49:564, 1970
7. Lewin I, Lerner AG, Green SH, et al: Physical class and physiologic status in the prediction of operative mortality in the aged sick. Ann Surg 174:217, 1971
8. Goldman L, Caldera DL, Nussbaum SR, et al: Multifactorial index of cardiac risk in noncardiac surgical procedures. N Engl J Med 297:845, 1977
9. Keats AS: The ASA classification of physical status—a recapitulation (editorial). Anesthesiology 49:233, 1978
10. Rehder K: Clinical evaluation of isoflurane. Complications during and after anaesthesia. Can Anaesth Soc J, suppl., 29: S44, 1982
11. Cohen MM, Duncan PG: Physical status score and trends in anesthetic complications. J Clin Epidemiol 41:83, 1988
12. Ziffren SE, Hardford CE: Comparative mortality for various surgical operations in older versus younger age groups. J Am Geriatr Soc 20:485, 1972
13. Hosking MP, Warner MA Lobdell CM, et al: Outcomes of surgery in patients 90 years of age and older. JAMA 261:1909, 1989
14. Tiret L, Hatton F, Desmonts JM, Vourc'h G: Prediction of outcome of anaesthesia in patients over 40 years: A multifactorial risk index. Stat Med 7:947, 1988
15. Marx GF, Mateo CV, Orkin LR: Computer analysis of postanesthetic deaths. Anesthesiology 39:54, 1973
16. Olsson GL, Hallén B: Cardiac arrest during anaesthesia. A computer-aided study in 250,543 anaesthetics. Acta Anaesthesiol Scand 32:653, 1988
17. Bechtoldt AA, Jr: Committee on Anaesthesia Study. Anesthetic-related deaths: 1969–1976. NC Med J 42:253, 1981
18. Epstein B: Controversies in outpatient anesthesia. p. 473. In White PF (ed): Outpatient Anesthesia. Churchill Livingstone, New York (in press)
19. Marwick C: Expanding AIDS drug availability. JAMA 262:1289, 1989
20. Roizen MF, Hendren M, Stocking C, et al: The personal vs. the automated interview: Do patient responses to health questions differ? (abstract). Anesthesiology 71:A334, 1989
21. Leonard JV, Clayton BE, Colley JRT: Use of biochemical profile in Children's Hospital: Results of two controlled trials. Br Med J 2:662, 1975
22. Korvin CC, Pearce RH, Stanley J: Admissions screening: Clinical benefits. Ann Intern Med 83:197, 1975
23. Olsen DM, Kane RL, Proctor PH: A controlled trial of multiphasic screening. N Engl J Med 294:925, 1976
24. Durbridge TC, Edwards F, Edwards RG, Atkinson M: Evaluation of benefits of screening tests done immediately on admission to hospital. Clin Chem 22:968, 1976
25. Domoto K, Ben R, Wei JY, et al: Yield of routine annual laboratory screening in the institutionalized elderly. Am J Public Health 75:243, 1985
26. Wolf-Klein GP, Holt T, Silverstone FA, et al: Efficacy of routine annual studies in the care of elderly patients. J Am Geriatr Soc 33:325, 1985
27. Dontas AS, Kasviki-Charvarti P, Chem L, et al: Bacteriuria and survival in old age. N Engl J Med 304:939, 1981
28. Boscia JA, Kobasa WD, Knight RA, et al: Epidemiology of bacteriuria in an elderly ambulatory population. Am J Med 80:208, 1986

29. Boscia JA, Kobasa WD, Knight RA, et al: Therapy vs no therapy for bacteriuria in elderly ambulatory nonhospitalized women. JAMA 257:1067, 1987

30. Nordenstam GR, Brandberg CÅ, Odén AS, et al: Bacteriuria and mortality in an elderly population. N Engl J Med 314:1152, 1986

31. Delahunt B, Turnbull PRG: How cost effective are routine preoperative investigations? NZ Med J 92:431, 1980

32. Rossello PJ, Cruz AR, Mayol PM: Routine laboratory tests for elective surgery in pediatric patients. Bull Assoc Med Puerto Rico 72:614, 1980

33. Wood RA, Hoekelman RA: Value of the chest x-ray as a screening test for elective surgery in children. Pediatrics 67:477, 1981

34. Sandler G: Costs of unnecessary tests. Br J Med 2:21, 1979

35. Rabkin SW, Horne JM: Preoperative electrocardiography: Its cost-effectiveness in detecting abnormalities when a previous tracing exists. Can Med Assoc J 121:301, 1979

36. Rabkin SW, Horne JM: Preoperative electrocardiography: Effect of new abnormalities on clinical decisions. Can Med Assoc J 128:146, 1983

37. Eddy DM, Hasselblad V, McGivney W, Hendee W: The value of mammography screening in women under age 50 years. JAMA 259:1512, 1988

38. U.S. Preventive Services Task Force [RS Lawrence, chairman]: Guide to Clinical Preventive Services. Report of the U.S. Preventive Services Task Force. Washington, D.C., 1989 (prepublication copy)

39. Roizen MF, Kaplan EB, Schreider BD, et al: The relative roles of the history and physical examination, and laboratory testing in preoperative evaluation for outpatient surgery: The "Starling" curve of preoperative laboratory testing. Anesthesiol Clin North Am 5:15, 1987

40. Tape TG, Mushlin AI: How useful are routine chest x-rays of preoperative patients at risk for postoperative chest disease? J Gen Intern Med 3:15, 1988

41. Orkin FK: Practice standards: The Midas touch or the emperor's new clothes? (editorial). Anesthesiology 70:567, 1989

42. Turnbull JM, Buck C: The value of preoperative screening investigations in otherwise healthy individuals. Arch Intern Med 147:1101, 1987

43. Hirsch IA, Tomlinson DL, Slogoff S, Keats AS: The overstated risk of preoperative hypokalemia. Anesth Analg 67:131, 1988

44. Vitez TS, Soper LE, Wong KC, Soper P: Chronic hypokalemia and intraoperative dysrhythmias. Anesthesiology 63:130, 1985

45. Harrington JT, Isner JM, Kassirerr JP: Our national obsession with potassium. Am J Med 73:155, 1982

46. Lawson DH: Adverse reactions to potassium chloride. Q J Med 43:433, 1974

47. Lawson DH, Hutcheon AW, Jick H: Life threatening drug reactions amongst medical in-patients. Scott Med J 24:127, 1979

48. Levinstein MR, Ouslander JG, Rubenstein LZ, Forsythe SB: Yield of routine annual laboratory tests in a skilled nursing home population. JAMA 258:1909, 1987

49. Kaplan EB, Sheiner LB, Boeckmann AJ, et al: The usefulness of preoperative laboratory screening. JAMA 253:3576, 1985

50. Robbins JA, Rose SD: Partial thromboplastin time as a screening test. Ann Intern Med 90:796, 1979

51. Parkerson GR, Jr: Cost analysis of laboratory tests in ambulatory primary care. J Fam Pract 7:1001, 1978

52. Parkerson GR, Jr: Determinants of physician recognition and follow-up of abnormal laboratory values. J Fam Pract 7:341, 1978

53. Williamson JW, Alexander M, Miller GE: Continuing education and patient care research. Physician response to screening test results. JAMA 201:938, 1967

54. Huntley RR, Steinhauser R, White KL, et al: The quality of medical care: Techniques and investigation in the outpatient clinic. J Chronic Dis 14:630, 1961

55. Daughaday WH, Erickson MM, White W, et al: Evaluation of routine 12-channel chemical profiles on patients admitted to a university general hospital. p. 181. In Benson ES, Strandjord PE (eds): Multiple Laboratory Screening. Academic Press, New York, 1969

56. Epstein KA, Schneiderman LJ, Bush JW, Zettner A: The "abnormal" screening serum thyroxine (T4): Analysis of physician response, outcome, cost and health effectiveness. J Chronic Dis 34:175, 1981

57. Wheeler LA, Brecher G, Sheiner LB: Clinical laboratory use in the evaluation of anemia. JAMA 238:2709, 1977

58. Kelley CR, Mamlin JJ: Ambulatory medical care quality. Determination by diagnostic outcome. JAMA 227:1155, 1974

59. Lawrence VA, Kroenke K: The unproven utility of preoperative urinalysis. Clinical use. Arch Intern Med 148:1370, 1988

60. Umbach GE, Zubek S, Deck H-J, et al: The value of preoperative chest x-rays in gynecological patients. Arch Gynecol Obstet 243:179, 1988

61. Robertson WM: Medical Malpractice: A Preventive Approach. University of Washington Press, Seattle, 1985

62. Collen MF, Feldman R, Siegelaub AB, Crawford D: Dollar cost per positive test for automated multiphasic screening. N Engl J Med 283:459, 1970

63. Collen MF (ed): Multiphasic Health Testing Services. John Wiley & Sons, New York, 1978

64. Kreig AF, Gambino R, Galen RS: Why are clinical laboratory tests performed? When are they valid? JAMA 233:76, 1975

65. Neuhauser D: Cost-effective clinical decision making (commentary). Pediatrics 60:756, 1977

66. Robbins JA, Mushlin AI: Preoperative evaluation of the healthy patient. Med Clin North Am 63:1145, 1979

67. Rembold CM, Watson D: Posttest probability calculation by weights. A simple form of Bayes' theorem. Ann Intern Med 108:115, 1988

68. Farnsworth PB, Steiner E, Klein RM, SanFilippo JA: The value of routine preoperative chest roentgenograms in infants and children. JAMA 244:582, 1980

69. Brill PW, Ewing ML, Dunn AA: The value (?) of routine chest radiography in children and adolescents. Pediatrics 52:125, 1973

70. Sagel SS, Evens RG, Forrest JV, Bramson RT: Efficacy of routine screening and lateral chest radiographs in a hospital-based population. N Engl J Med 291:1001, 1974

71. Sane SM, Worsing RA, Jr, Wiens CW, Sharma RK: Value of preoperative chest x-ray examinations in children. Pediatrics 60:669, 1977

72. Rees AM, Roberts CJ, Bligh AS, Evans KT: Routine preoperative chest radiography in non-cardiopulmonary surgery. Br Med J 1:1333, 1976

73. Loder RE: Routine pre-operative chest radiography: 1977 compared with 1955 at Peterborough District General Hospital. Anaesthesia 33:972, 1978

74. Hubbell FA, Greenfield S, Tyler JL, et al: The impact of routine admission chest x-ray films on patient care. N Engl J Med 312:209, 1985

75. Maigaard S, Elkjaer P, Stefansson T: Vaerdien af praeoperativ rutinerøntgenundersøgelse af thorax og ekg. (English ab-

stract: Value of routine preoperative radiographic examination of the thorax and ECG). Ugeskr Laeger 140:769, 1978

76. Catcholve BR, Wilson RM, Spring S, Hall J: Routine investigations in elective surgical patients. Their use and cost effectiveness in a teaching hospital. Med J Aust 2:107, 1979

77. McKee RF, Scott EM: The value of routine preoperative investigations. Ann R Coll Surg Engl 69:160, 1987

78. Thomsen HS, Gottlieb J, Madsen JK, et al: Rutinemaessig røntgen-undersøgelse af thorax inden kirurgiske indgreg i universel anaestesi. (English abstract: Routine radiographic examination of the thorax prior to surgical intervention under general anesthesia.) Ugeskr Laeger 140:765, 1978

79. Boghosian SG, Mooradian AD: Usefulness of routine preoperative chest roentgenograms in elderly patients. J Am Geriatr Soc 35:142, 1987

80. Sewell JMA, Spooner LLR, Dixon AK, Rubenstein D: Preoperative chest x-rays in elderly patients. Age Ageing 10:165, 1981

81. Törnebrandt K, Fletcher R: Pre-operative chest x-rays in elderly patients. Anaesthesia 37:901, 1982

82. Fink DJ, Fang M, Wyle FA: Routine chest x-ray films in a Veterans Hospital. JAMA 245:1056, 1981

83. Wiencek RG, Weaver DW, Bouwman DL, Sachs RJ: Usefulness of selective preoperative chest x-ray films. A prospective study. Am Surg 53:396, 1987

84. Petterson SR, Janower ML: Is the routine preoperative chest film of value? Appl Radiol, Jan-Feb 70, 1977

85. Royal College of Radiologists Working Party on the Effective Use of Diagnostic Radiology: Preoperative chest radiology. National study by the Royal College of Radiologists. Lancet 2:83, 1979

86. Rucker L, Frye EB, Staten MA: Usefulness of screening chest roentgenograms in preoperative patients. JAMA 250:3209, 1983

87. Blery C, Szatan M, Fourgeaux B, et al: Evaluation of a protocol for selective ordering of preoperative tests. Lancet 1:139, 1986

88. Weibman MD, Shah NK, Bedford RF: Influence of preoperative chest x-rays on the perioperative management of cancer patients (abstract). Anesthesiology 67:A332, 1987

89. Muskett AD, McGreevy JM: Rational preoperative evaluation. Postgrad Med J 62:925, 1986

90. Gordon T, Kannel WB: The Framingham Massachusetts study twenty years later. p. 123. In Kessler II, Levin ML (eds): The Community as an Epidemiologic Laboratory: A Casebook of Community Studies. Johns Hopkins University Press, Baltimore, 1970

91. Ostrander LD, Jr, Brandt RL, Kjelsberg MO, Epstein FH: Electrocardiographic findings among the adult population of a total natural community, Tecumseh, Michigan. Circulation 31:888, 1965

92. Kannel WB, McGee D, Gordon T: A general cardiovascular risk profile: The Framingham study. Am J Cardiol 38:46, 1976

93. Apfelbaum J, Robinson D, Murray WJ, et al: An automated method to validate preoperative test selection: First results of a multicenter study (abstract). Anesthesiology 71:A928, 1989

94. Moorman JR, Hlatky MA, Eddy DM, et al: The yield of the routine admission electrocardiogram. A study in a general medical service. Ann Intern Med 103:590, 1985

95. Goldberger AL, O'Konski M: Utility of the routine electrocardiogram before surgery and on general hospital admission. Critical review and new guidelines. Ann Intern Med 105:552, 1986

96. Wasserman LR, Gilbert HS: Surgical bleeding in polycythemia vera. Ann NY Acad Sci 115:122, 1964

97. Rothstein P: What hemoglobin level is adequate in pediatric anesthesia? Anesthesiol Update 1:2, 1978

98. Slogoff S: Anesthesia considerations in the anemic patient. Anesthesiol Update 2:7, 1979

99. Kowalyshyn TJ, Prager D, Young J: A review of the present status of preoperative hemoglobin requirements. Anesth Analg 51:75, 1972

100. Gold BD, Wolfersberger WH: Findings from routine urinalysis and hematocrit on ambulatory oral and maxillofacial surgery patients. J Oral Surg 38:677, 1980

101. Carmalt MHB, Freeman P, Stephens AJH, Whitehead TP: Value of routine multiple blood tests in patients attending the general practitioner. Br Med J 1:620, 1970

102. Moore SB, Reisner RK, Offord KP: Morning admission for a same-day surgical procedure: Resolution of a blood bank problem. Mayo Clin Proc 64:406, 1989

103. Wataneeyawech M, Kelly KA, Jr: Hepatic diseases unsuspected before surgery. NY State J Med 75:1278, 1975

104. Schemel WH: Unexpected hepatic dysfunction found by multiple laboratory screening. Anesth Analg 55:810, 1976

105. Schneiderman LJ, DeSalvo L, Baylor S, Wolf PL: The "abnormal" screening laboratory results. Its effect on physician and patient. Arch Intern Med 129:88, 1972

106. Bryan DJ, Wearne JL, Viau A, et al: Profile of admission chemical data by multichannel automation: An evaluative experiment. Clin Chem 12:137, 1966

107. Schoen I: Clinical chemistry. A retrospective look at routine screening. Calif Med 108:430, 1968

108. Peery TM: The role of the laboratory in health evaluation, Interim Report No. 77, from the 1964 Technicon International Symposium, New York, in Schoen I: Clinical chemistry, a retrospective look at routine screening. Calif Med 108:430, 1968

109. Friedman GD, Goldberg M, Ahuja JN, et al: Biochemical screening tests. Effect of panel size on medical care. Arch Intern Med 129:91, 1972

110. Young DM, Drake TGH: Unsolicited laboratory information, presented to the College of American Pathologists, Chicago, 18 Oct 1965, in Schoen I: Clinical chemistry, a retrospective look at routine screening. Calif Med 108:430, 1968

111. Boonstra CE, Jackson CE: The clinical value of routine serum calcium analysis. Ann Intern Med 57:963, 1962

112. Whitehead TP: Multiple analyses and their use in the investigation of patients. Adv Clin Chem 14:389, 1971

113. Singer DE, Samet JH, Coley CM, Nathan DM: Screening for diabetes mellitus. Ann Intern Med 109:639, 1988

114. Alter MJ: Non-A, non-B hepatitis: Sorting through a diagnosis of exclusion. Ann Intern Med 110:583, 1989

115. Cardiff-Oxford Bacteriuria Study Group: Sequelae of covert bacteriuria in schoolgirls. A four-year follow-up study. Lancet 1:889, 1978

116. Challand GS: Is ward biochemical testing cheap and easy? Intensive Care World 4:9, 1987

117. Baranetsky NG, Weinstein P: Partial thromboplastin time for screening (correspondence). Ann Intern Med 91:498, 1979

118. Barber A, Green D, Galluzzo T, Ts'ao C-H: The bleeding time as a preoperative screening test. Am J Med 78:761, 1985

119. Rohrer MJ, Michelotti MC, Nahrwold DL: A prospective evaluation of the efficacy of preoperative coagulation testing. Ann Surg 208:554, 1988

120. Eisenberg JM, Clarke JR, Sussman SA: Prothrombin and partial thromboplastin times as preoperative screening tests. Arch Surg 117:48, 1982

121. Ramsey G, Arvan DA, Steward S, Blumberg N: Do preoperative laboratory tests predict blood transfusion needs in cardiac operations? J Thorac Cardiovasc Surg 85:564, 1983

122. Koutts J: Clinching the diagnosis: Assessment of hemostatic function. Pathology 17:643, 1985

123. Burke DS, Brundage JF, Redfield RR, et al: Measurement of the false positive rate in a screening program for human immunodeficiency virus infections. N Engl J Med 319:961, 1988

124. Ohnishi ST, Katagi H, Ohnishi T, Brownell AKW: Detection of malignant hyperthermia susceptibility using a spin label technique on red blood cells. Br J Anaesth 61:565, 1988

125. Lembo NJ, Dell'Italia LJ, Crawford MH, O'Rourke RA: Bedside diagnosis of systolic murmurs. N Engl J Med 318:1572, 1988

126. Baker JP, Detsky AS, Wesson DE, et al: Nutritional assessment: A comparison of clinical judgment and objective measurements. N Engl J Med 306:969, 1982

127. Roizen MF, Kaplan EB, Sheiner LB, et al: Elimination of unnecessary laboratory tests by preoperative questionnaire (abstract). Anesthesiology 61:A455, 1984

128. Kaplan EB, Boeckmann AS, Roizen MF, Sheiner LB: Elimination of unnecessary preoperative laboratory tests (abstract). Anesthesiology 57:A445, 1982

129. Finkler SA: The distinction between cost and charges. Ann Intern Med 96:102, 1982

130. Charpak Y, Blery C, Chastang C, et al: Usefulness of selectively ordered preoperative tests. Med Care 26:95, 1988

131. Roizen MF, Macario A, Thisted R, et al: A tale of three cities—has reassessment of preoperative test value changed physician test-ordering patterns? (abstract). Anesthesiology 71:A1188, 1989

132. Curran J, Chmielewski AT, White JB, Jennings AM: Practice of preoperative assessment by anaesthetists. Br Med J 291:391, 1985

133. Leigh JM, Walker J, Janaganathan P: Effect of preoperative anaesthetic visit on anxiety. Br Med J 285:987, 1977

134. Canadian Task Force on the Periodic Health Examination: The periodic health examination. Can Med Assoc J 121:1193, 1979

135. Finn AF, Jr, Valenstein PN, Burke MD: Alteration of physicians' orders by nonphysicians. JAMA 259:2549, 1988

136. Grady D: Going overboard on medical tests. p 80. Time Apr 25, 1988

137. Fischer AF, Stevenson DK: The consequences of uncertainty. An empirical approach to medical decision making in neonatal intensive care. JAMA 258:1929, 1987

138. Wong ET, Nelson JM: Quality assurance and the clinical laboratory (editorial). JAMA 259:2584, 1988

139. Tierney WM, McDonald CJ, Hui SL, Martin DK: Computer predictions of abnormal test results. Effects on outpatient testing. JAMA 259:1194, 1988

140. Tierney WM, McDonald CJ, Martin DK, et al: Computerized display of past test results. Effect on outpatient testing. Ann Intern Med 107:569, 1987

141. Goldman L, Cook EF, Brand DA, et al: A computer protocol to predict myocardial infarction in emergency department patients with chest pain. N Engl J Med 318:797, 1988

142. Romm FJ, Fletcher SW, Hulka BS: The periodic health examination: Comparison of recommendations and internists' performance. South Med J 74:265, 1981

143. Gluck R, Muñoz E, Wise L: Preoperative and postoperative medical evaluation of surgical patients. Am J Surg 155:730, 1988

24
PULMONARY FUNCTION TESTING

Thomas J. Gal

INTRODUCTION

Pulmonary function testing has assumed an increasing role in the preoperative preparation of many surgical patients. Such preoperative screening is aimed at identifying individuals with abnormal lung function in hopes of altering their outcome by reducing the risk of postoperative ventilation abnormalities and respiratory complications. The subjective information provided by the medical history and the findings on physical examination seldom identify actual abnormalities of respiratory function and are poor predictors of the severity of disease (see Chs. 23 and 25). In contrast, pulmonary function testing provides objective standardized measurements for quantitating the degree of respiratory dysfunction. These tests fall into two major groups. Those that detect abnormalities of gas exchange and those that relate to the mechanical ventilatory function of the lungs and chest wall. This discussion will deal principally with the latter group.

The cornerstone of all pulmonary function testing is clinical spirometry. There are numerous other tests, including some that purport to be useful in identifying mild abnormalities or lung function. This presentation will attempt to review the actual measurement techniques and interpret the physiologic basis and significance of many of these tests. The aim is to provide a better understanding of the defects that each testing scheme identifies. Such information will serve to enhance the anesthesiologist's consultant role and will facilitate the rational perioperative management of the patients who undergo the preoperative screening.

CLINICAL SPIROMETRY

Vital Capacity

The most common measurement of lung function is the vital capacity (VC). This is the largest volume measured after an individual inspires deeply and maximally to total lung capacity (TLC) and then exhales completely to residual volume (RV) into a spirometer. The maneuver is performed without concern for rapidity of effort. Normal values for VC are lower in supine subjects than sitting subjects and vary directly with height and inversely with age. A given VC is generally considered abnormal if it falls below 80 percent of the predicted value. Patients with abnormally low values for VC often have restrictive disease. The decreased VC associated with restrictive disease may result from lung pathology such as pneumonia, atelectasis, and pulmonary fibrosis. It may also occur with a loss of distensible lung tissue such as that following surgical excision. Decreased VC also occurs in the absence of lung disease. In this case, muscle weakness, abdominal swelling, or pain may prevent the patient from obtaining either a full inspiration or a maximum expiratory effort.

Timed Expiratory Spirogram

If after a maximal inspiratory effort a subject exhales as forcefully and rapidly as possible, the exhaled volume is recorded with respect to time and termed the *forced vital capacity* (FVC). The rate of airflow during this rapid forceful exhalation indirectly reflects the flow resistance properties of the airways. In the presence of airway obstruction, FVC tends to be less than the standard slow VC because of air trapping. In healthy subjects, the two maneuvers result in nearly equal measured volumes. Since the FVC maneuver is an artificial one, patients must be instructed carefully and often require practice attempts before performing the test adequately. Generally, three acceptable tracings are required for analysis. These FVC maneuvers must be characterized by a full inspiration to TLC, followed by an abrupt onset of exhalation, and continued maximum effort throughout exhalation to RV. The exhalation should take at least 4 seconds and not be interrupted by coughing, glottic closure, or any mechanical obstruction.[1]

The FVC is reduced by the same conditions that reduce VC. Therefore, in order to identify airway obstruction, flow rates are determined by calculating the volume exhaled during certain time intervals. Most commonly measured is the volume exhaled in the first second, or the forced expiratory volume in 1 second (FEV_1). The FEV_1 is expressed as absolute volume in liters or as a percentage of the forced vital capacity (FEV_1/FVC percent). For the purposes of reporting and calculating values, the largest observed FVC and FEV_1 from any of the three acceptable spirograms are used even if they are not obtained from the same curve.[1] Normal healthy subjects can exhale 75 to 80 percent of their FVC in the first second; the remaining volume is exhaled in an additional 2 or 3 seconds (Fig. 24-1). Diseases such as asthma and bronchitis, which produce airway obstruction, reduce expiratory flow rates and, thus, reduce FEV_1 and FEV_1/FVC percent. Restrictive diseases are not usually associated with airway obstruc-

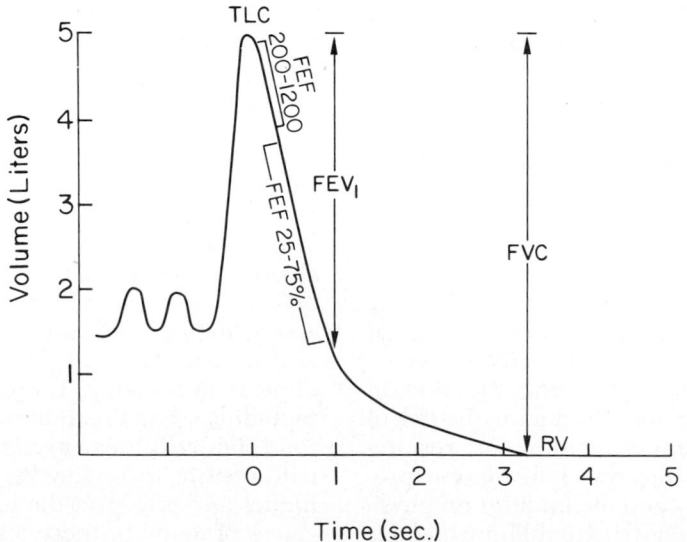

Fig. 24-1. Forced vital capacity (FVC) maneuver in a normal subject. Exhaled volume is plotted against time as the subject expires forcefully, rapidly, and completely to residual volume (RV) after a maximal deep inspiration to total lung capacity (TLC). FEV_1, forced expired volume in 1 second; $FEF_{200-1200}$, forced expiratory flow between 200 and 1,200 ml of expired volume; $FEF_{25-75\%}$, forced expiratory flow over the midportion of vital capacity (i.e., from 25 to 75 percent of expired volume).

TABLE 24-1. Forced Vital Capacity and 1-Second Forced Expiratory Volumes in Disease States

	FVC (L)	FEV$_1$ (L)	FEV$_1$/FVC Percent
Airway obstruction (asthma, bronchitis)	Normal	Decreased	Decreased
Stiff lungs (pneumonia, pulmonary edema, pulmonary fibrosis)	Decreased	Decreased	Normal
Respiratory muscle weakness (myasthenia gravis, myopathies)	Decreased	Decreased	Normal

tion but do cause decreases in FVC. Although the absolute volume of FEV$_1$ may be reduced on a similar basis, the FEV$_1$ expressed as a percentage of FVC is usually normal (i.e., FEV$_1$/FVC $\geqq$ 70 percent). The impact of various mechanical abnormalities on vital capacity and these dynamic lung volumes is summarized in Table 24-1.

The maximal flow rate obtainable at any time during FVC maneuver is termed the *peak flow*, which is measured in liters per second or liters per minute. Peak flow can be measured by drawing a tangent to the steepest part of the FVC spirogram, but this is subject to large errors. More commonly, maximal flow is measured as the average flow during the liter of gas expired after the initial 200 ml during an FVC maneuver (Fig. 24-1). This

is usually designated as *forced expiratory flow* (FEF$_{200-1200}$); however, the term *maximal expiratory flow rate* (MEFR) has also been used. This flow is slightly lower than the true peak flow, which can be measured conveniently with hand-held flowmeters (Fig. 24-2) or more accurately with a pneumotachygraph. Peak flow is markedly affected by obstruction of large airways and is particularly responsive to bronchodilator therapy. Since obtaining repeat measurements is convenient, peak flow rates can be utilized to monitor therapeutic responses in acute asthma. Normal values in healthy males under 40 years of age are typically 500 L/min or more. Values less than 200 L/min in the surgical candidate suggest impaired cough efficiency and strong likelihood of postoperative complications.[2] The test is

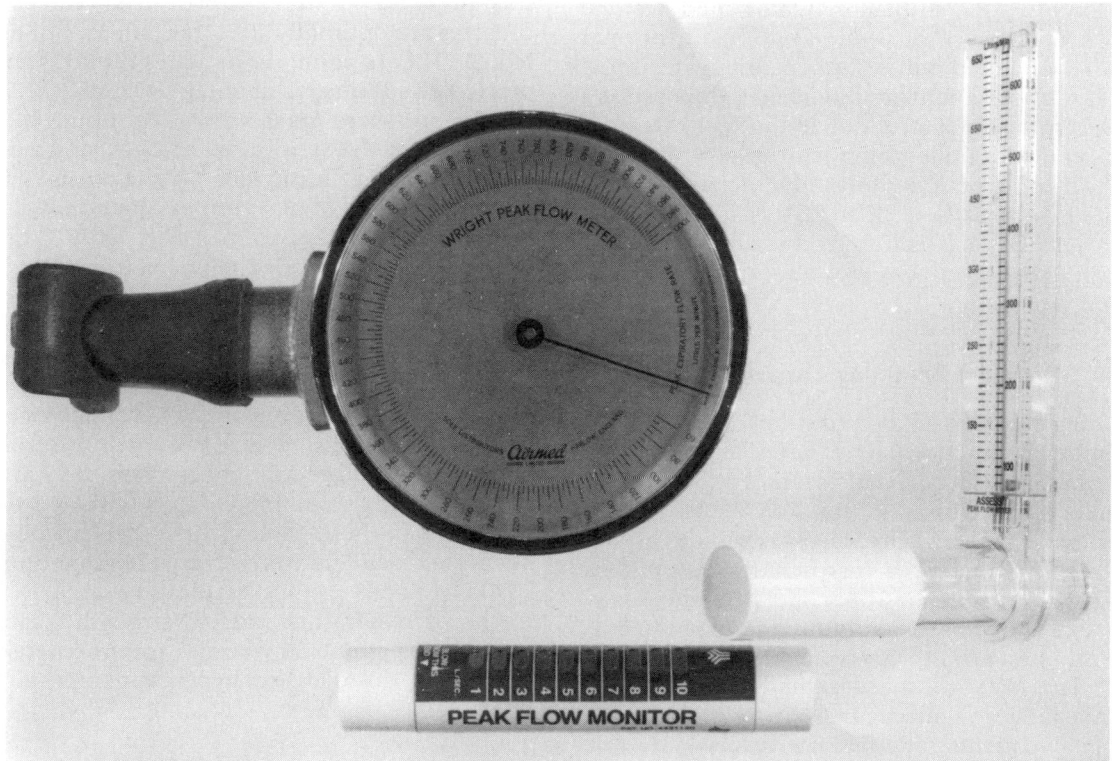

Fig. 24-2. Three hand-held peak flow meters. The classic Wright meter (Air Med Limited, Harlow, England) and the Assess peak flowmeter (Health Scan Products, Cedar Grove, N.J.) provide actual quantitation of peak flow rate; the smaller Peak Flow Monitor (Biotrine Corp., Woburn, Mass.) allows the patient to tape over the holes before blowing. If the flow rate indicated by the first uncovered hole is reached, a hornlike sound is produced by a metal reedlike device within the tube.

much less unpleasant and exhausting for patients than the FVC maneuver and thus provides a valuable tool to identify gross pulmonary disability at the bedside.

Because peak flow is highly dependent on patient effort, the measurement can be quite variable and changes may not solely reflect airway function. In contrast, high degrees of effort are not required to achieve maximal expiratory flow at intermediate and low lung volumes during forced expiration. Therefore, to identify airway obstruction, flow is often measured over the middle half of the FVC (i.e., between 25 and 75 percent of expired volume). This parameter, formerly called the maximal midexpiratory flow, is now referred to as the forced midexpiratory flow ($FEF_{25-75\%}$). Since the flow does not include the initial highly effort-dependent portion of forced expiration, $FEF_{25-75\%}$ is often referred to as "effort-independent." This designation is not entirely appropriate since $FEF_{25-75\%}$ can be decreased by marked reductions in expiratory effort and by a submaximal inspiration preceding the FVC maneuver. The same flow rates may also decrease with truly maximal effort compared to slightly suboptimal effort.[3] This phenomenon, termed *negative effort dependence*, appears to be in part an artifact of measuring volume changes at the mouth rather than actual changes in thoracic gas volume but probably also reflects the dynamic airway compression associated with truly maximal effort.

Values for $FEF_{25-75\%}$ in healthy young men average 4.5 to 5.0 L/s. Because of wide variations in normal subjects, the predicted limits of normal may be as low as 2 L/s. The measurement has often been proposed as a sensitive test for early obstruction in the small airways. However, patients undergoing spirometry for suspected airway obstruction almost always have normal values for $FEF_{25-75\%}$ when FEV_1/FEV is 75 percent or greater.[4] Thus $FEF_{25-75\%}$ is not necessarily more sensitive than FEV_1 in detecting minor abnormalities of the spirogram.

Maximum Breathing Capacity

Dynamic lung function is also routinely evaluated in many pulmonary function laboratories by measuring the maximum breathing capacity or, more specifically, the maximal voluntary ventilation (MVV). This is the largest volume that can be breathed per minute by voluntary effort. The patient is instructed to breathe as hard and fast as possible for 12 seconds. The measured volume is extrapolated to 1 minute and expressed as liters per minute (L/min). Since high rates of airflow are required for MVV, the measurement is significantly affected by changes in airway resistance. MVV is usually reduced in patients with obstructive airway disease and correlates well with FEV_1 measured in liters ($FEV_1 \times 35$ approximates MVV). Discrepancies between the measured MVV and that predicted by FEV_1 often indicate inconsistent patient effort. The MVV as a comprehensive test of ventilatory function is altered by factors other than airway obstruction. These include the elastic properties of the lung and chest wall, respira-

tory muscle strength, learning, coordination, and motivation. In healthy male adults MVV averages 150 to 175 L/min. This extremely high level of ventilatory effort cannot be maintained for much longer than 1 minute. However, approximately 80 percent of the MVV can be maintained by healthy subjects for as long as 15 minutes and up to 60 percent of MVV can be sustained for even longer periods. Abnormally low values (less than 80 percent of predicted) do not identify specific defects but do indicate gross impairment in respiratory function. The unique value of the test in the surgical candidate may lie in its dependence on intangible variables such as cooperation, motivation, and stamina.

Respiratory Muscle Strength

All measurements of pulmonary function that require patient effort (e.g., FVC, FEV_1, peak flow, and MVV) are influenced by the strength of the respiratory muscles. The latter can be specifically evaluated by measurement of maximal static respiratory pressures. The pressures are generated against an occluded airway during a maximal forced inspiratory or expiratory effort and usually measured with simple aneroid gauges.[5] Maximal static inspiratory pressure (PImax) is measured when inspiratory muscles are at their optimal length near RV (Fig. 24-3). Similarly, maximal static expiratory pressure (PEmax) is measured when expiratory muscles are optimally stretched after a full inspiration to near TLC. In young adult males PImax is about -125 cmH_2O and PEmax is about $+200$ cmH_2O.

Thus pressures measured at the mouth include that generated by the respiratory muscles and a portion resulting from the elastic recoil of the respiratory system. The latter is essentially zero at functional residual capacity (FRC). Pressures measured at FRC are slightly less than at the extremes of lung volume (Fig. 24-3) but, unlike the other values, reflect solely the pressure developed by the respiratory muscles.

A PImax of -25 cmH_2O or less indicates severe inability to take a deep breath; a PEmax of less than $+40$ cmH_2O suggests severely impaired coughing ability. Although these pressures are not measured routinely in all pulmonary function laboratories, they are particularly useful in evaluating patients with neuromuscular disorders. In these patients, the vital capacity has long been used to indicate the severity of respiratory muscle weakness and predict respiratory failure. Measurements of respiratory muscle strength identify more readily the patients in whom respiratory muscle weakness is the prime cause of hypercapneic respiratory failure.[6]

PHYSIOLOGIC DETERMINANTS OF MAXIMUM FLOW RATES

The maximal flow rates that can be achieved during pulmonary function testing depend on three factors, each of which is highly dependent on the volume of the

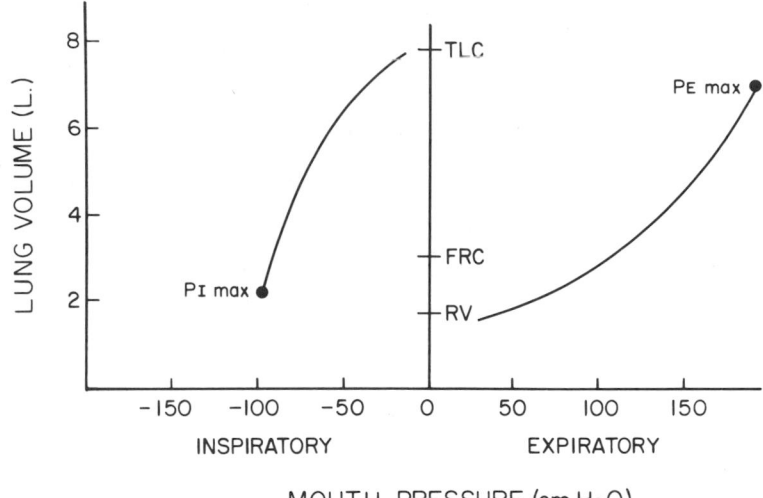

Fig. 24-3. Normal values for maximum static inspiratory (PImax) and expiratory (PEmax) pressures measured at the mouth are plotted as a function of lung volume from residual volume (RV) to total lung capacity (TLC). FRC, functional residual capacity.

lung at the time. One of these factors is the degree of effort, or the driving pressure generated by muscle contraction. The expiratory effort reflected by PEmax is maximal at high lung volumes near TLC and decreases as lung volume decreases (Fig. 24-3). On the other hand, PImax is achieved at low lung volumes near RV and diminishes at higher lung volumes.

Another important determinant of flow is the elastic recoil pressure of the lung (Pl). At all lung volumes from RV to TLC, the lung has a tendency to recoil inward (Fig. 24-4). The Pl, therefore, is greatest at TLC (25 to 30 cmH_2O) and lowest at RV (2 to 3 cmH_2O). This Pl tends to augment flows during expiration and acts to

oppose flow during inspiration. The Pl is opposed by the outward recoil of the chest wall (Pcw), except at very high lung volumes. The recoil pressure of the respiratory system (Prs) is the algebraic sum of Pl + Pcw. Note that Pl and Pcw are equal and opposite at a certain point (i.e., Prs = zero). This volume is the functional residual capacity (FRC), which is the respiratory system's resting volume.

The third factor, which opposes these two driving pressures, is the resistance to flow provided by the airways. This airway resistance (Raw) is determined by the size of the airways. Since airways are largest at high lung volumes and smallest at RV, Raw is greatest at RV

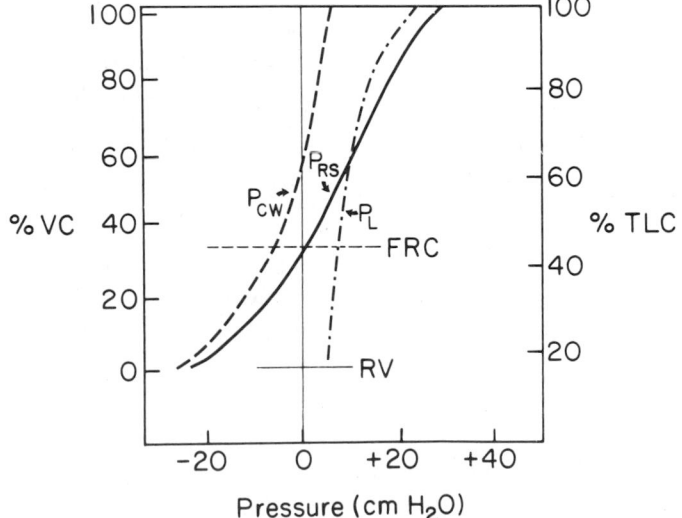

Fig. 24-4. Elastic recoil pressures for the lung (Pl), chest wall (Pcw), and total respiratory system (Prs) are plotted as a function of lung volume. VC, vital capacity; TLC, total lung capacity; RV, residual volume; FRC, functional residual capacity.

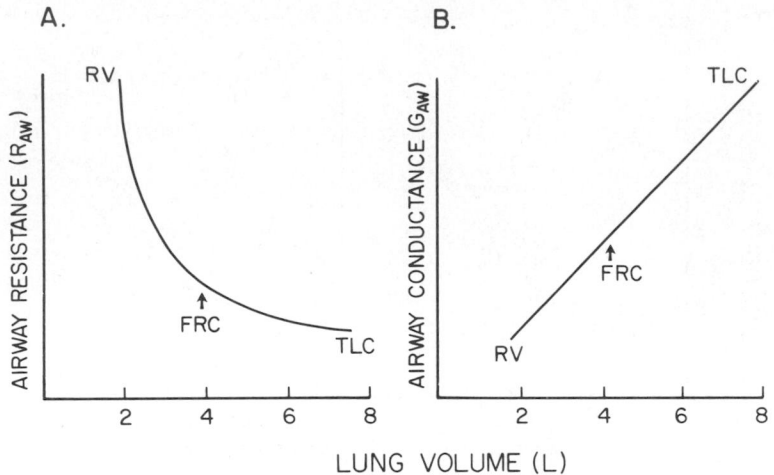

Fig. 24-5. The hyperbolic relationship of airway resistance (Raw) to lung volume (A) is contrasted with the linear relationship (B) of its reciprocal airway conductance (Gaw). RV, residual volume; TLC, total lung capacity; FRC, functional residual capacity.

and least at TLC (Fig. 24-5A). The inverse relationship between Raw and lung volume is not linear. Therefore, the reciprocal of Raw, conductance (Gaw), which is related to lung volume linearly (Fig. 24-5B), is often utilized to identify bronchoconstriction or bronchodilation.

When measuring Raw, another factor that must be considered besides lung volume is the partitioning of the total resistance to airflow. The total respiratory system resistance is composed of an elastic component (chest wall) and a nonelastic component (pulmonary resistance). The chest wall component, which includes diaphragm and abdominal contents as well, contributes about 40 percent of the total respiratory resistance.[7] The remaining 60 percent is pulmonary resistance, which for practical purposes is the same as airway assistance since pulmonary tissue contributes only about 1 percent to pulmonary resistance. Macklem and Mead have further partitioned Raw and shown that approximately 80 percent of the measurable resistance is in the large central airways.[8] The smaller, more peripheral bronchioles account for the remaining 20 percent. Large reductions in the diameter of these small airways may occur without appreciably affecting total Raw. Thus, these airways have been referred to as the "silent zone" of the lungs since early disease in this area often goes undetected.

Flow Volume Relationships

Since all of the determinants of maximal flow are dependent on lung volume, a useful format to assess the flow resistive properties of the airways is to plot flow as a function of volume during the forced vital capacity maneuver. At the beginning of the forced expiration, the rate of flow quickly rises to a maximal or peak value

at a lung volume very near to TLC. As expiration continues, lung volume decreases, airways narrow, resistance increases, and the flow rates progressively decrease. The impact of obstructive airway disease on such flow rates is emphasized in Figure 24-6. In the patients with airway obstruction, flows are reduced over the full range of lung volume from TLC to RV.

The influence of expiratory effort on the flow-volume curves is very important. An individual can actually inscribe different flow-volume curves with differing efforts, although each may have the same FVC (Fig. 24-7). At large lung volumes close to TLC, airflow rises with increasing effort (Curve A). Curves B and C with decreasing effort exhibit decreased flows in this high range of lung volume, but all three curves merge at a point and continue together to RV. At these intermediate and low lung volumes, only moderate effort is needed to produce maximal flow. Since increased expiratory effort has little effect on increasing these flows, there is little difference between the three curves and this portion of the curve is referred to as effort-independent. At this point, flow is largely a function of the other two variables (Pl and Raw). Once again it is important to point out that exaggerated effort may decrease these same flows as with FEV_1 and $FEF_{25-75\%}$.[9]

The rate of airflow during forced expiration is influenced not only by the effort expended but also by the lung volume at which the expiratory maneuver is begun. True maximum flows occur only when expiration is begun at or near TLC. When forced expirations are begun with maximal effort from volumes below TLC (Fig. 24-8), peak flow is lower but flows quickly and conforms to the same performance envelope as if the maneuvers were begun at TLC. Even healthy subjects can exhibit a decreased FEV_1/FVC ratio when the forced expirations are started from such submaximal volumes. Therein lies some of the advantage of a flow-

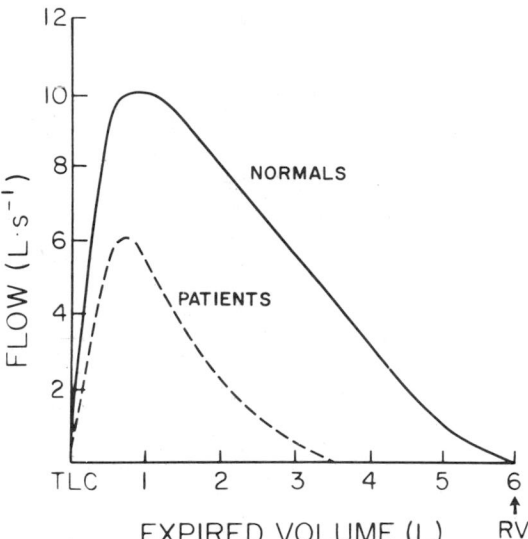

Fig. 24-6. Idealized maximum expiratory flow-volume curves in normal subjects are contrasted with those typically seen in patients with obstructive airway disease. Expiratory flow is plotted as a function of lung volume during maximal expiration from total lung capacity (TLC) to residual volume (RV).

volume plot as opposed to the volume-time tracing with conventional spirometry.

Airway Compression and Flow Limitation

The failure of increasing effort to augment flow over the lower two-thirds of the vital capacity further results from dynamic compression of the airways. This has

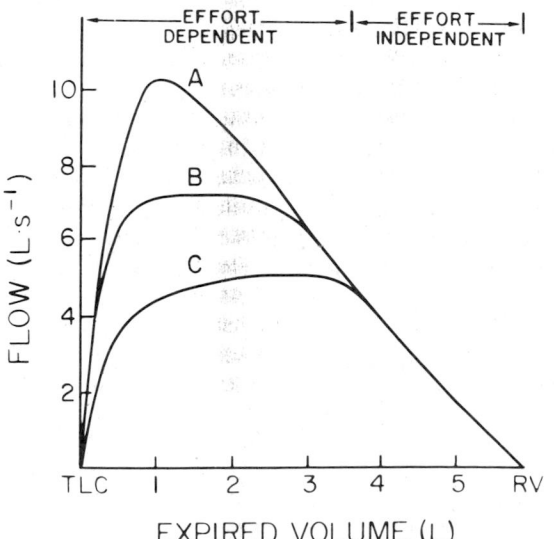

Fig. 24-7. Forced expiratory flow-volume curves in a normal subject. The exhalation from total lung capacity (TLC) to residual volume (RV) was performed at three levels of effort ranging from maximal *(A)* to minimal *(C)*.

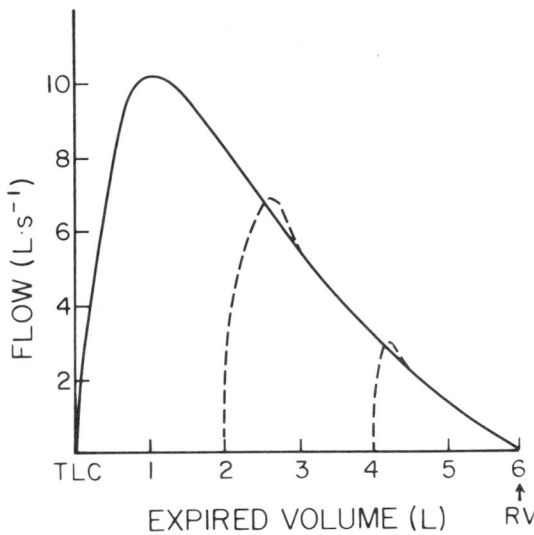

Fig. 24-8. Forced expiratory flow volume curves inscribed during maximal maneuvers performed by beginning at total lung capacity (TLC) and at 2 L and 4 L below TLC.

been described in a model of flow limitation termed the *equal pressure point* (EPP) concept. The pressure head that serves to move air from the alveoli to the mouth is provided by the alveolar pressure (Palv). At any given lung volume, Palv is the sum of lung elastic recoil pressure (Pl) and pleural pressure (Ppl). At any lung volume when there is no flow, such as end inspiration (Fig. 24-9A), Ppl is subatmospheric and counterbalances Pl. Thus, this sum, Palv, is zero, as are pressures at the mouth and through the remaining airways. During forced expiration (Fig. 24-9B), Ppl rises above atmospheric (becomes positive). The increased Palv again is the sum of Pl + Ppl. Pressure is dissipated along the airway in overcoming resistance to flow and finally reaches zero at the mouth. At some point along the airway, the intraluminal pressure falls to a level that equals the surrounding pleural pressure. This site is the EPP. Toward the mouth (downstream) the lateral pressure within the airway lumen is less than the compressing Ppl and the airways tend to collapse. Once maximal flow is reached, further increases in Ppl from increasing effort do not affect airflow in the upstream segment (from EPP toward the alveoli) since the driving pressure along this portion of the airway essentially is equal to Pl. Therein lies the origin of the term *effort-independent*. The increased Ppl simply produces more compression of the downstream airways (from EPP to mouth). Thus increasing effort augments airway compression but fails to increase flow.

The principal value of this dynamic airway compression is in the production of an effective cough. Even though maximum flows may not be reached, the compressed downstream airway develops an increased linear velocity of airflow, which maximizes the removal of secretions along airway walls. At intermediate lung vol-

A

NO FLOW

B

MAXIMUM FLOW

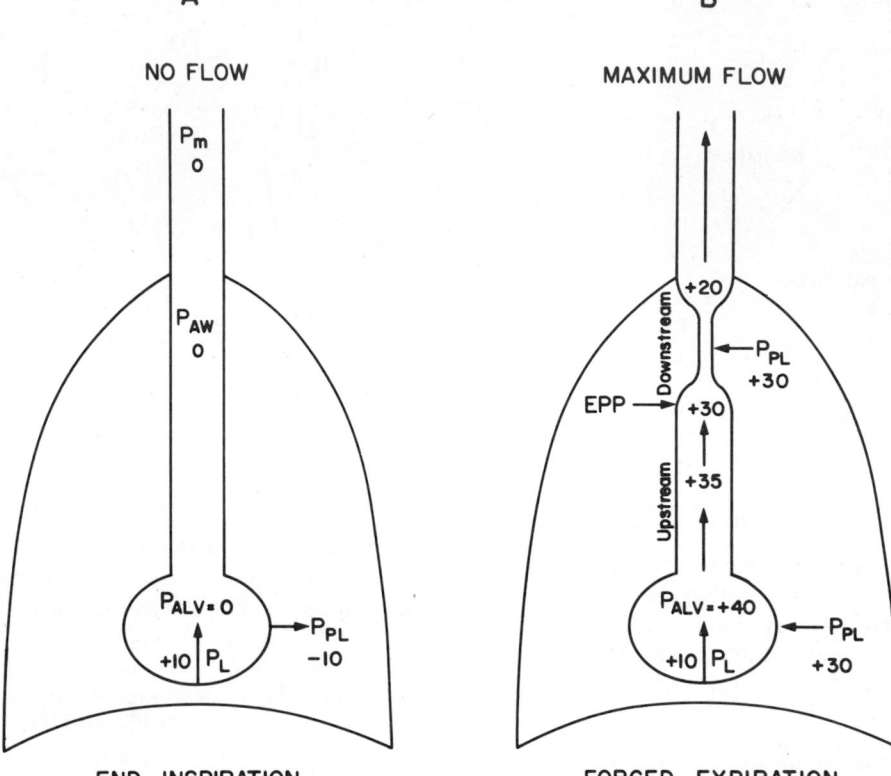

END-INSPIRATION

FORCED EXPIRATION

Fig. 24-9. A model depicting the equal pressure point (EPP) concept of expiratory flow limitation (see text for explanation). Pm, mouth pressure; Paw, intraluminal airway pressure; Pl, lung elastic recoil pressure; Ppl, pleural pressure; Palv, alveolar pressure.

umes EPPs lie in segmental bronchi, but they may move farther upstream toward the alveoli at lower lung volumes. The dynamic compression involves primarily lobar and mainstem bronchi and the intrathoracic trachea. Coughing is, therefore, most effective in removing material from these relatively large airways.

Sites and Mechanisms of Decreased Airflow in Disease

Abnormal expiratory flow rates may be seen in many disease states and may result from alterations in any of the three major determinants of flow (PEmax, Pl, and Raw), as seen in Table 24-2. For example, the patients with neuromuscular disease who may exhibit decreased expiratory flows include those with myasthenia gravis, muscular dystrophy, Guillain-Barré syndrome, and spinal cord transection. Decreased ability to generate expiratory effort is the principal cause of low expiratory flows in these patients, who seldom exhibit increases in Raw or decreased Pl. Other categories of restrictive disease, such as musculoskeletal deformities (kyphoscoliosis, ankylosing spondylitis, and interstitial lung disease), are often associated with near-normal muscle strength. In these situations, expiratory flows may actually be slightly increased because of an in-

creased Pl associated with reductions in lung volume. Reduced lung volumes associated with long-term neuromuscular disease may likewise be associated with increases in Pl that may result in more normal expiratory flow rates.

The classic example of decreased expiratory flow associated with decreased lung recoil (Pl) is emphysema. Here, expiratory muscle strength is usually adequate and lung distension tends to increase airway size, such that Raw is also usually normal. In patients with bronchitis and asthma, on the other hand, airway narrowing is prominent. In these two variants of obstructive lung

TABLE 24-2. Mechanisms for Decreased Expiratory Flow Rates

		Physiologic Variables	
Disease	PEmax	Raw	Pl
Neuromuscular weakness	↓	N	N
Emphysema	N	N	↓
Asthma, bronchitis	N	↑	N
Peripheral airway disease	N	N	N

Abbreviations and Symbols: N, normal; ↑, increased; ↓, decreased; PEmax, maximum statis expiratory pressure; Raw, airway resistance; Pl, lung elastic recoil pressure.

disease the major factor reducing flow is an increased Raw. Early changes in these obstructive lung diseases are often confined to the peripheral airways. Narrowing in these airways does produce reduced expiratory flows at middle and low lung volumes but does not appreciably affect measurements in Raw or the other determinants of airflow.

MEASUREMENT OF AIRWAY OBSTRUCTION

Airway Resistance

Of the standard techniques used to evaluate airway obstruction, airway resistance Raw measurements appear to be the most direct. The technique is rapid and noninvasive and merely requires that a subject pant once or twice per second through a mouthpiece and with a nose clip in place. During normal breathing a major fraction of the resistance to airflow resides in the nose, pharynx, and larynx and can mask changes taking place in the lungs. The use of a mouthpiece bypasses the nose in order to minimize the effects of the upper airway on the measurement. The panting maneuver is likewise uti-

lized to keep the larynx dilated and reduce its influence on the total resistance to airflow. The measurement of Raw requires the subject to sit in a constant volume body plethysmograph ("body box"), which also permits the recording of thoracic gas volume and thereby provides an accurate appraisal of the effects of lung volume on Raw. Lung volume is estimated by utilizing Boyle's law to relate changes in box pressure and mouth pressure; Raw is calculated from changes in box pressure and flow.[10] The subjects initially pant against a closed mouthpiece, usually at end expiration. Thus, thoracic gas volume (FRC) is calculated from relationship of box pressure to mouth pressure (Fig. 24-10). The shutter in the mouthpiece is then opened and continued panting inscribes the relationship between box pressure and flow at the mouth to derive Raw. The upper limit of normal Raw is usually considered to be 2 $cmH_2O \cdot s$. In order to eliminate passive changes in Raw as a result of difference in lung volume, the reciprocal of Raw, airway conductance (Gaw), is calculated. This Gaw is usually divided by the lung volume at which the measurement (usually FRC) is made to obtain specific airway conductance (sGaw). The coefficient of variation (standard deviation/mean $\times$ 100) in normal baseline values for the same subject is usually

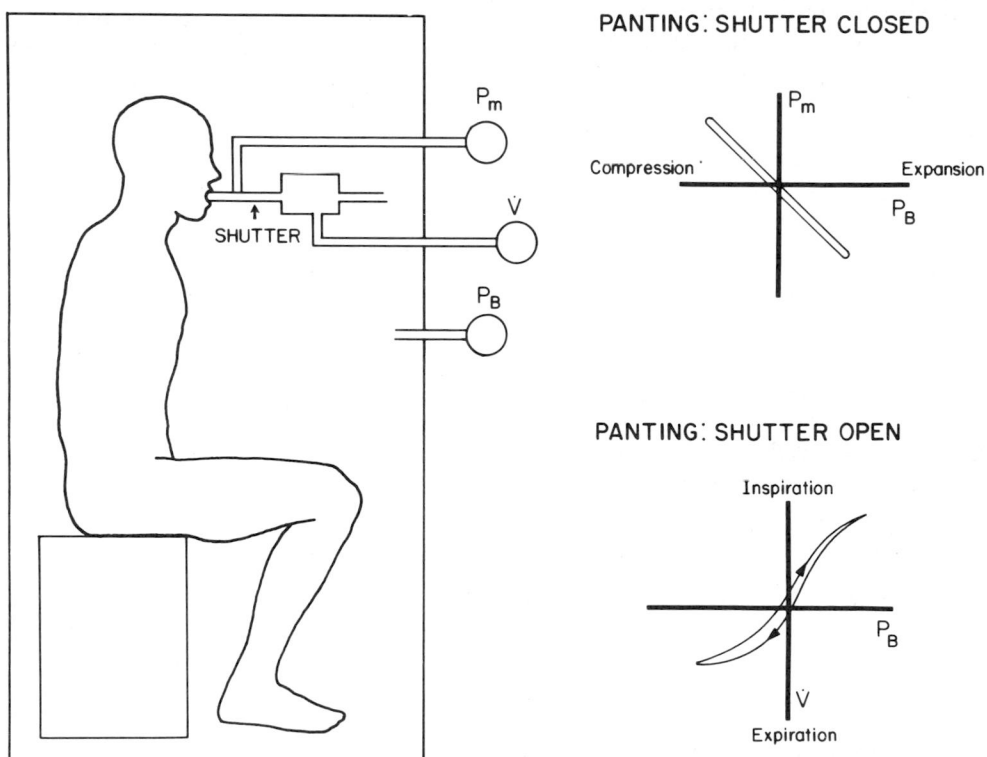

Fig. 24-10. Diagram of the constant volume body plethysmograph to measure airway resistance and lung volume. When subject pants against an obstructed mouthpiece (shutter closed) box pressure (Pb) is plotted against mouth pressure (Pm). Changes in Pb are converted in changes in lung volume by calibrating the box with known volumes of added gas and observing Pb changes. As subject pants through the open mouthpiece, flow (V) replaces Pm on the plot and airway resistance is computed from the relationship between Pb and V.

small (less than 10 percent). Therefore, sGaw is a highly reproducible measurement that can identify changes in the caliber of the intrapulmonary airways. However, a significant portion of normal airway resistance resides in the upper airways. Since the latter can be significantly increased with head flexion,[11] it is important that patients position themselves as erect as possible when attached to the mouthpiece in the body box.

Forced Expiratory Maneuvers

Despite the specificity and sensitivity of Raw measurements, airway obstruction is more commonly evaluated by measurements of maximal forced expiration. The indices obtained from forced expiration, unlike Raw, are determined by a complex interrelationship of flow resistive properties of intrathoracic airways and elastic recoil of the lung. The simplest of such measurements is the peak expiratory flow, which is conveniently measured with a variable orifice flow meter. Since the peak flow occurs early in a forced expiration, flow limitation has not occurred in the airways and, thus, flow is highly dependent on effort and subject cooperation. However, since the variation for the measurement in the same subject is surprisingly low, peak expiratory flow is a fairly reproducible test of airway function.

Another extensively used indirect measure of airway dimensions is the FEV_1. Again, during the first 25 percent of a forced vital capacity maneuver, flow reflects dimensions of the airways between the alveoli and the mouth and is effort-dependent. Although the physiologic parameters governing the remaining flow are complex, FEV_1, like peak flow, is simple and reproducible and, thus, a useful index of airway function. The measurement is subject to day-to-day variability, which is greater in patients with obstructive airway disease than in normal individuals.[12] Thus changes in FEV_1 must exceed 15 percent in order to signify bronchodilation or constriction in patients. The same variability applies to $FEF_{25-75\%}$ measurements. In addition, one must account for the possibilities of negative effort dependence[3] and, more importantly, the changes in FVC that may occur. For example, in the case of bronchodilation, FVC may increase but actually produce a misleading decrease in FEF 25 to 75.[13] Thus the measurement should be adjusted to the same absolute lung volume (i.e., the same segment of FVC below total lung capacity).

Additional assessment of the flow resistive properties of the airways can be obtained from maximal expiratory flow volume (MEFV) curves, which illustrate the relationship between airflow and lung volume during a forced vital capacity maneuver (Fig. 24-6). A typical response when bronchoconstriction is induced consists of diminished flows throughout the whole MEFV curve envelope (Fig. 24-11). Usually ventilatory flows and FVC decrease and RV increases. Therefore, expiratory flows must be measured at the same reference lung

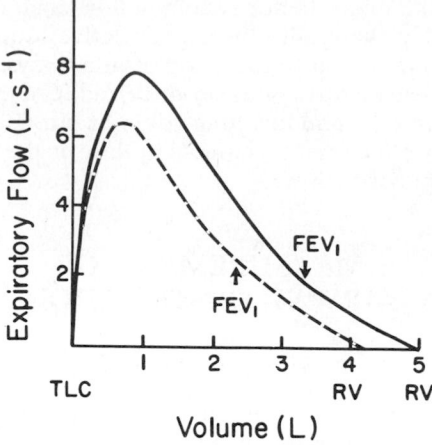

Fig. 24-11. Maximum expiratory flow volume curves before (solid line) and after (broken line) induced bronchoconstriction. Flow is plotted against expired volume expressed in liters from total lung capacity (TLC) to residual volume (RV). Forced 1-second expiratory volumes (FEV_1) are indicated with arrows on each curve.

volume. This is usually at a fixed percentage of the baseline or normal FVC and requires that all curves be superimposed at TLC.

In normal subjects, full inhalation to TLC may remove the bronchoconstriction induced by mechanical stimuli or drugs; in asthmatic subjects, an increase in bronchomotor tone may accompany the same deep inspiration. To overcome these variable effects of a full inspiration on bronchial tone, Bouhuys and co-workers proposed that flows be measured with partial expiratory flow volume (PEFV) curves.[14] In this case, the maximal forced expiration is started at or slightly above the

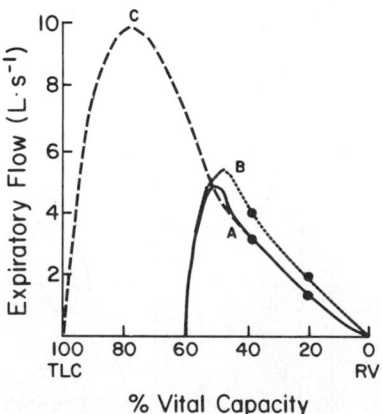

Fig. 24-12. Partial expiratory flow volume curves before *(A)* and after *(B)* bronchodilator treatment. Forced expiration is begun just above midpoint of vital capacity (VC). Flows are quantitated at 20 and 40 percent of VC above residual volume (RV). A reference maximum expiratory curve *(C)* is also inscribed by beginning exhalation from total lung capacity.

middle of FVC (Fig. 24-12). In all cases, the PEFV curve is followed by a full inhalation to TLC and a maximal forced exhalation to RV to obtain a reference MEFV curve. Flows are usually measured between 20 and 40 percent of VC above RV. Since PEFV curves are unaffected by changes in upper airway resistance, they are sensitive to the changes in the intrapulmonary airways and have been suggested as a useful alternative to Raw for detecting bronchoconstrictor and bronchodilator responses and are particularly useful in normal subjects.

Flow-Volume Loops

The finding of reduced peak flow, MVV, and FEV_1 without additional clinical evidence of chronic obstructive lung disease may indicate the presence of an obstructing lesion of the upper airway, larynx, or trachea. In some cases, this obstruction may be suspected by a careful history and physical examination, but in many instances it may simulate diffuse airway obstruction and suggest a marked degree of lung dysfunction. This is most likely to occur in patients for head and neck surgery who may present for operative procedures related to these lesions. Flow-volume (F-V) loops provide a graphic analysis of flow at various lung volumes and have been utilized to discriminate between patients with upper airway obstructive lung lesions. Both flow and volume are plotted simultaneously on an X-Y recorder as subjects inhale fully to total lung capacity (TLC) and then perform an FVC maneuver. This is followed immediately by a maximal inspiration as quickly as possible back to TLC (Fig. 24-13). Expiratory flow decreases over the latter half of the exhaled volume despite the sustained expiratory effort indicated by the high positive pleural pressure. During maximal inspiration, airways do not undergo compression. Rather, with increasing inspiratory effort, airways become distended by the subatmospheric (negative) pleural pressure and flow is increased. Thus, the entire inspiratory portion of the loop, as well as the expiratory curve near TLC, is highly dependent on effort. The ratio of expiratory flow to inspiratory flow at 50 percent of vital capacity (mid-VC ratio) normally is about 1.0. This ratio is particularly useful in identifying the presence of upper airway obstruction, in which case inspiratory flow tends to be reduced more than expiratory flow, and the mid-VC ratio is increased (i.e., >1.0).

Flow-volume loops not only aid in suspecting upper airway obstruction but may help to localize the site and nature of the obstruction. Several characteristic patterns have been described. Perhaps the most common lesion is a fixed obstruction such as a benign stricture resulting from tracheostomy or tracheal intubation. A tumor or mass such as a goiter may also produce a similar picture, as may breathing through a fixed external resistance. No significant change in airway diameter occurs during inspiration or expiration. As a result, expiratory flows show a plateau of constant flow over

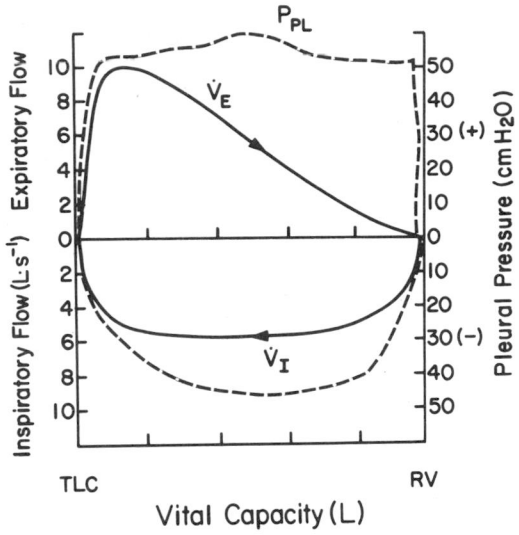

Fig. 24-13. Schematic representation of a maximum inspiratory ($\dot{V}_I$) and expiratory ($\dot{V}_E$) flow volume loop in a normal subject. The pleural pressures (Ppl) associated with the maximal efforts are plotted as a function of lung volume from total lung capacity (TLC) to residual volume (RV). $\dot{V}_I$ and $\dot{V}_E$ at the midpoint (50 percent) of vital capacity are indicated by arrows.

the effort-dependent portion of vital capacity. Inspiratory flows show a similar plateau (Fig. 24-14A). Since both are reduced to nearly the same extent, the mid-VC ratio remains approximately 1.0.

A lesion whose influence varies with the phase of respiration is termed a variable obstruction. Variable extrathoracic obstructions (Fig. 24-14B) are most commonly associated with vocal cord paralysis, which is usually accompanied by inspiratory stridor. A similar pattern occurs with marked pharyngeal muscle weakness in paralyzed volunteers[15] and in those with chronic neuromuscular disorders.[16] The flow pattern occurs occasionally in patients with severe obstructive sleep apnea. During forced inspiration, the negative transmural pressure inside the airway tends to collapse the airway with increasing effort and, thus, reduces inspiratory flow. During expiration the positive pressure within the upper airway tends to decrease the obstruction so that expiratory flow is reduced far less and may even be normal. The mid-VC ratio of expiratory to inspiratory flow is often greater than 2.0.

The other form of variable obstruction occurs intrathoracically and is usually due to tumors of the trachea or major bronchi. During forced expiration, the high pleural pressures decrease airway diameter and may increase obstruction. A plateau flow usually occurs during expiration when the compressed airway lumen assumes its minimal size at the area of the lesion (Fig. 24-14C). During inspiration the lowered pleural pressure surrounding the airway tends to decrease the obstruction, such that the inspiratory portion of the flow-

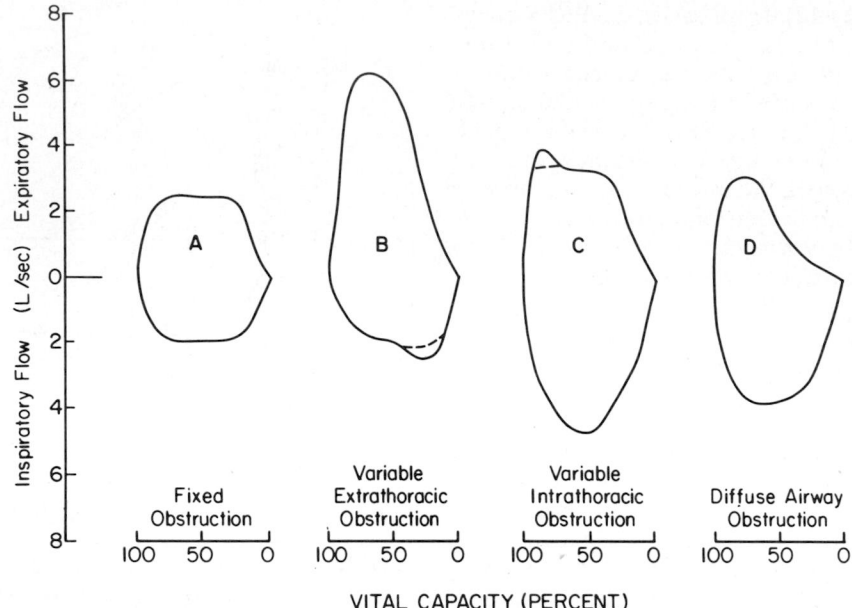

Fig. 24-14. Maximum inspiratory and expiratory flow-volume curves (flow-volume loops) in four types of airway obstruction (**A–D**).

volume loop may be quite normal. The mid-VC ratio of expiratory to inspiratory flow is low, as in the case of diffuse airway obstruction (Fig. 24-14D). However, the shapes of the curves differ. Curve D, an example of diffuse airway obstruction, exhibits abnormal decreased flow in the segment near residual volume. Curve C, on the other hand, demonstrates normal flow in this area.

The physiologic diagnosis of upper airway obstruction is sometimes difficult in the patients with diffuse airway obstruction such as chronic bronchitis or asthma. These conditions themselves produce significant abnormalities of the flow-volume loop (Fig. 24-14D). Therefore, flow-volume loops most clearly identify upper airway obstruction in the absence of significant generalized airway disease.

TESTS OF EARLY LUNG DYSFUNCTION

During the past two decades, interest in disease in the peripheral airways has increased. Several terms, such as *small airway disease, early obstructive lung disease,* and *minimal airway dysfunction,* have been used to describe abnormalities of the small peripheral airways. There has evolved the basic concept that peripheral airway obstruction is a forerunner of chronic bronchitis and emphysema. These processes are thought to be moderately advanced and irreversible by the time routine indices of pulmonary function such as FVC and FEV_1 become abnormal. Numerous tests are used to detect such early lung dysfunction, including measurements of mild abnormal gas exchange, distribution of

ventilation, airway instability, and variables derived from maximum expiratory flow-volume curves.

The initial enthusiasm with which these tests were greeted has been tempered by the complexity of the equipment and the intersubject variability, as compared to the spirometric "gold standard", the FEV_1. Furthermore, such tests probably offer little advantage over spirometry in identifying susceptible smokers who are likely to develop chronic obstructive airway disease.[17] These tests, however, are sensitive indicators of abnormal airway function despite this relative lack of specificity. They have an important place in pulmonary research, and an understanding of their methodology and physiologic principles provides an important perspective for dealing with abnormalities of pulmonary function.

Alveolar-Arterial Oxygen Tension Difference

Abnormally high alveolar-arterial oxygen tension gradients ($AaDO_2$) during room air breathing are quite common in asymptomatic smokers and in patients with minimal signs of chronic bronchitis. Although the $AaDO_2$ is a sensitive means of detecting regional ventilation-perfusion inequalities, the test is not widely used for screening purposes because of the difficulty in measuring alveolar O_2 tension (PAO_2). Unlike arterial O_2 tension (PaO_2), which can be measured, PAO_2 is usually estimated from the alveolar air equation. In this calculation arterial CO_2 tension ($PaCO_2$) is also substituted for alveolar CO_2 ($PACO_2$). The oxygen tension of the warmed and humidified inspired gas in the trachea is represented as PIO_2. As a rule, less CO_2 is produced than

O_2 consumed. This ratio of CO_2 production to O_2 consumption is the respiratory exchange ratio (R), which is usually assumed to be 0.8. A simple calculation for bedside use may be derived by dividing $PaCO_2$ by R or simply multiplying the CO_2 value by 1.25.[18] Therefore, the alveolar gas equation may be written simply as

$$PAO_2 = PIO_2 - \frac{PaCO_2}{R}$$

The normal $AaDO_2$ with subjects breathing room air averages 8 mmHg in normal young persons and increases linearly with age. By the eighth decade the normal values may reach 25 mmHg. This widening of the $AaDO_2$ with age and in disease states results solely from decreases of PaO_2 not PAO_2.

Frequency Dependence of Compliance

Decreases in dynamic compliance with increased rates of breathing occur in asymptomatic smokers and are attributed to small airway dysfunction. This was one of the first tests to be proposed as an indicator of small airway dysfunction and can still be regarded as the standard. Compliance is considered frequency-dependent if the dynamic compliance (C_{DYN}) at any of the increased breathing rates falls to less than 80 percent of the static compliance (C_{STAT}). Most workers have measured C_{DYN} as the change in lung volume during a tidal breath divided by the change in transpulmonary pressure. The C_{STAT} is derived from the slope of an inspiratory static pressure-volume curve over the usual range of tidal volume. Both compliance measurements require the insertion of an esophageal balloon to estimate transpulmonary pressure (difference between esophageal pressure and mouth pressure). Because of the rather sophisticated equipment required and the discomfort associated with balloon insertion, the test is not technically suited for screening purposes. Nevertheless, frequency dependence of compliance is commonly used as a reference for other tests in identifying peripheral airway dysfunction.

In normal lungs, alveoli fill and empty synchronously at all physiologic respiratory rates. Therefore, compliance is not normally dependent on respiratory frequency. Frequency dependence of compliance, on the other hand, implies asynchronous behavior wherein some regions of the lung are moving out of phase with others. The rate at which alveoli respond to a given pressure change by a change in volume is determined by their time constant, the product of their resistance and compliance (R $\times$ C). The more restricted or compliant a unit of lung is, the longer it takes for air to enter or leave.

When various areas of the lung have different time constants, they fill and empty at different rates. During slow breathing, air can still be so equally distributed that C_{DYN} is not altered appreciably. However, during rapid breathing, air moves less rapidly into areas with long time constants, especially those with a high resist-

ance. There is insufficient time to expand these areas. As a result, greater transpulmonary pressure is required to move the same volume of air and C_{DYN} falls.

This asynchronous behavior of lung units is ascribed to obstruction in the small airways. However, other factors may cause time-constant discrepancies throughout the lung and must be eliminated before attributing changes in C_{DYN} solely to small airway disease. These may include abnormal lung elasticity and obstruction in the large central airways such as might occur with a bronchial tumor. In the case of the former, C_{STAT} is abnormal, whereas abnormally increased airway resistance is likely in the latter.

Multiple-Breath Nitrogen Washout

Measurements of the uneven distribution of ventilation are also sensitive to mild airway obstruction. If the resident nitrogen in the lung is washed out by breathing 100 percent oxygen, the concentration of nitrogen decreases as cumulative expired volume decreases. When the distribution of ventilation is normal and uniform, the lung appears to behave as a single compartment, which produces a single exponential washout curve for nitrogen (Fig. 24-15). In the abnormal patient with lung disease and nonuniform ventilation, the curve deviates from the single exponential and appears to contain more than one ventilatory compartment. Different lung units have their nitrogen diluted at different rates. The fast, well-ventilated alveoli cause a rapid decrease in expired nitrogen, whereas slow, poorly ventilated areas produce a prolonged tail on the washout curve. Ingram and Schilder[19] have reported a direct relationship between nitrogen clearance and frequency dependence of compliance. Unequal time constants throughout the

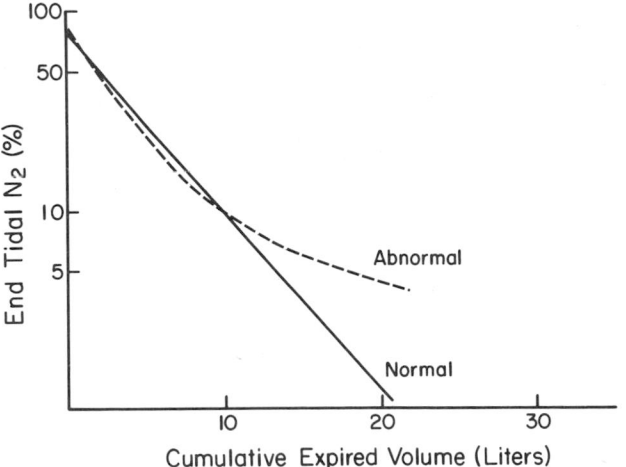

Fig. 24-15. Schematic representation of multiple-breath nitrogen washout curves in a young healthy nonsmoker (normal) and an asymptomatic smoker (abnormal). Expired nitrogen concentration is plotted on a logarithmic scale against cumulative expired volume during pure oxygen breathing.

lung may possibly explain both phenomena. Although multiple breath nitrogen washout appears to be a very sensitive test, appropriate analysis of curves is tedious and requires computerization in order to be practical as a screening test.

Single-Breath Nitrogen Washout

Inequality of ventilation can also be measured by the single breath nitrogen test, which has been used extensively since its original description by Fowler in 1949.[20] The expired nitrogen concentration is measured after inspiration of 1 L of oxygen from FRC. The change in nitrogen concentration between 750 ml and 1,250 ml of expired volume was originally used as an index of uneven ventilation. More recently it was shown that this change in nitrogen concentration can also be measured from the plot of nitrogen versus lung volume in the resident gas technique as used to measure closing volume. Instead of inspiring only 1 L, the patient makes a full inspiration from RV to TLC with pure oxygen. A line of best fit is drawn through the alveolar plateau (phase III, Fig. 24-16) and the increase in nitrogen concentration per liter quantitated. The alveolar nitrogen slope with this technique is less steep than in the original standardized procedure. This results from the fact that oxygen is preferentially distributed to the lung bases when only 1 L is inspired from FRC. The nitrogen in lung apices is less diluted with oxygen than when oxygen is inspired over the whole range of vital capacity. This higher apex to base nitrogen gradient (original standard technique) will produce a steeper rise in exhaled nitrogen than the newer technique, in which less of an apex to base nitrogen gradient is established.

The slope of the alveolar nitrogen plateau (ΔN_2 per-cent/L) is larger in old than in young subjects, reflecting the increasing uneven ventilation with age. Buist and Ross found that ΔN_2 percent/L was less than 2 percent in male nonsmokers regardless of age and as high as 10 percent in smokers.[21] They also noted that nearly half of the asymptomatic smokers they tested had an abnormal alveolar nitrogen slope when compared to their own predicted values. Therefore, quantitative analysis of the alveolar plateau (phase III) appears to be a sensitive test of early changes in the lungs of cigarette smokers. When it is found to be abnormal, there is a reasonable likelihood of structural abnormalities. However, its predictive usefulness is diminished by the large numbers of smokers with mild dysfunction who do not progress to chronic airflow obstruction.[17]

Closing Volume

One of the tests most frequently associated with the concept of small airway obstruction is the measurement of closing volume (CV). The term describes the lung volume at which airways in dependent areas in the lung begin to close or, more precisely, cease contributing to the expired gas. This phenomenon presumably occurs because of gravity-dependent gradients in pleural pressure. At or near residual volume the lower portions of the lungs are subjected to pleural pressures in excess of airway pressures. Hence, airway closure is promoted.

The CV test is designed to detect the lung volume at which these airways begin to close. The basic technique is to tag these "closed" units of lung by giving them a different concentration of a tracer gas than the ones that remain open. As a subject inspires from RV to TLC, a concentration difference for the tracer gas is created between the top and bottom of the lung as a result of differences in distribution of ventilation. During the subsequent slow exhalation, the changing concentration of tracer gas is plotted against lung volume on an X-Y recorder. Two methods utilize this principle to estimate CV: the bolus technique and the resident-gas technique.

The bolus technique employs a bolus of tracer gas. Although xenon and argon were originally used, the easier availability of helium has made it most popular. The technique depends on the principle that a bolus of gas inspired at residual volume will be distributed preferentially to the apical lung areas, because small airways in dependent lung zones are far less patent at these low lung volumes. Therefore, the pre-expiratory concentration gradient created for the tracer gas causes the apical areas to contain most of the marker gas while lower basilar areas contain very little.

The resident gas technique also depends on the creation of a pre-expiratory concentration gradient of marker gas from top to bottom of the lung. However, it differs from bolus technique in two ways. First, the tracer gas is the nitrogen already present or resident in

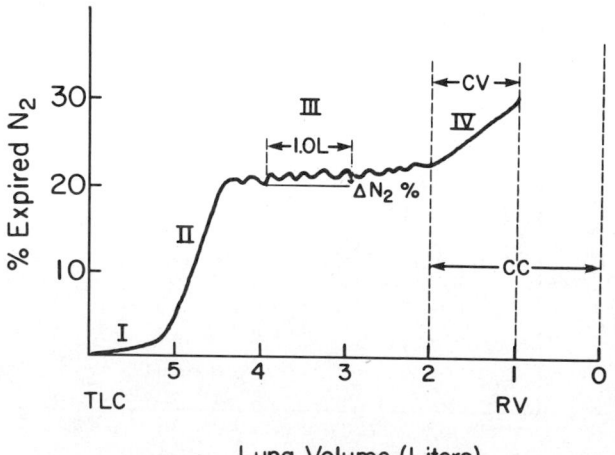

Fig. 24-16. Schematic representation of the plot of nitrogen (N_2) concentration versus expired volume during the closing volume (CV) measurement with resident gas technique. Closing capacity (CC) is the sum of residual volume (RV) and CV. TLC, total lung capacity.

the lungs. Second, there is normally little difference in nitrogen concentration at TLC between the top and bottom of the lung when breathing air. Therefore, a pre-expiratory concentration gradient is artificially created by using oxygen to dilute the nitrogen normally present in the lungs. The nitrogen in all alveoli is not diluted equally. At residual volume the alveoli at the bottom of the lung are smaller than those at the top. At TLC all alveoli reach essentially equal volumes. Thus, during inspiration from residual volume to total lung capacity, the lower basal alveoli undergo almost one and one half times the volume change undergone by the upper or apical alveoli. As a result, the nitrogen in the lower zones is diluted more by the inspired oxygen than is the nitrogen in the upper zones. There is approximately a $2:1$ concentration gradient for nitrogen between top and bottom of the lungs.

Despite fundamental differences in these methods, they yield surprisingly similar information; the plots of marker gas versus lung volume are similar qualitatively and quantitatively. In disease states such as asthma or in normal subjects, after histamine-induced bronchoconstriction, the size of the closing volume measured by the nitrogen method can be significantly smaller than with the bolus technique. Most likely the nitrogen method fails to establish the normal apex-to-base concentration gradient because of "air trapping."

In normal subjects the nitrogen concentration appearing at the mouth after inspiration of 100 percent oxygen changes gradually throughout the expiration. A typical trace displays four basic phases (Fig. 24-16). The first three are familiar from Fowler's original single-breath nitrogen test. Phase I contains expired gas essentially free of marker, representing emptying from the dead space of the apparatus, as well as of the conducting airways (anatomic dead space). Phase II consists of a rapid rise in the concentration of marker gas as alveolar emptying begins. Phase III, or the alveolar plateau, is produced by the mixing of expired air and marker gas from all lung regions, each with different concentrations. The "ripples" appearing during Phase III are termed *cardiogenic oscillations* since they correspond to cardiac systole and are believed to arise as a result of interruptions in gas flow from the dependent lung zones during cardiac systole. The alveolar plateau exhibits a small positive slope even in normal lungs; the extent of this rise has been used as an index of abnormality as discussed previously.

Near the end of expiration, another abrupt increase in tracer gas concentration occurs (phase IV). The point at which Phase IV begins has been designated the closing volume because the dependent airways have presumably closed or, more correctly, have essentially ceased contributing to the expired gas. Now, the exhaled gas arises almost entirely from the upper lung zones, whose concentration of marker gas (in this case, nitrogen) was high. The CV is the difference in volume between the onset of phase IV and RV. Since it represents a portion of the VC maneuver, it is usually expressed as a percentage of VC (CV/VC percent). Most published values for CV in normal healthy subjects in the sitting position fall between 15 and 20 percent of VC.

The terminology is confused by another term, *closing capacity* (CC). This term is used to designate the volume between the onset of Phase IV and zero lung volume; it thus includes CV and RV. Since it is the absolute lung volume at which Phase IV occurs, it is usually expressed as a percentage of total lung capacity (CC/TLC percent).

Although the onset of Phase IV is usually taken to represent a unique volume at which actual closure of the small airways occurs, Hyatt and Rodarte[22] have suggested that rather than closing off, they may merely be emptying more slowly because of dynamic compression and the resultant increased resistance to flow. This impression is based on the evidence that Phase IV occurs at the time the lungs reach flow limitation and continue to empty at a decreased rate despite increasing transpulmonary pressures. This same phenomenon occurs during the later portions of the MEFV curve. In fact, high expiratory flow rates, such as characterize the MEFV curve, can actually increase the lung volume at which Phase IV occurs, presumably because of some dynamic airway compression. Thus, in order to produce a satisfactory trace when measuring CV, one must assure that expiration be performed slowly (about 0.5 L/s). This can be assured by introducing mechanical resistance into the breathing circuit.

Whether the mechanism is closure or compression, most observers have noted significantly increased values for CC in cigarette smokers when compared to nonsmokers of the same age. These findings have been cited as evidence of small airway disease. However, Hoeppner et al.[23] suggest that these changes in CC in smokers reflect a loss of elastic recoil and not necessarily intrinsic small airway pathology. This same relationship between CC and lung elastic recoil is clearly demonstrated by the changes that occur with age. The progressive reduction in lung recoil and its associated tethering action on the bronchioles produce an increase in CC with advancing age, until at age 65, CC exceeds the FRC (CC > FRC) even in the seated individual.[24] Young children who exhibit reduced values for lung elastic recoil likewise have increased closing capacities.[25] The smallest CC values occur in subjects during the late teens, when maximal values for static elastic recoil are observed.

Regardless of whether an increased CV represents intrinsic airway disease or parenchymal disease with loss of elastic recoil, the sensitivity of the measurement renders it a likely indicator of early functional abnormality that may represent early obstructive lung disease. The relative simplicity of equipment and the lack of discomfort to the patient further enhance the acceptance of CV as a screening tool. Perhaps the major obstacle to its wider application has been the difficulty of establishing well-defined limits of normality because of variability between measurements even under ideal conditions.[26]

Maximum Expiratory Flow Rates

The frictional resistance of the small airways affects flows at low lung volumes (i.e., after more than 50 percent of FVC has been expired). Reduced values for flow at the "foot" of the MEFV curve (Fig. 24-6) have often been observed in smokers compared to nonsmokers, when no differentiations were possible on the basis of FEV_1 measurements. Unfortunately, normal variations make quantitation and interpretation of these flows at low lung volumes sometimes difficult. Thus, although they may specifically reflect the state of the peripheral airways and afford a useful comparison of populations or groups, they are less able to establish with certainty whether a given individual is normal or slightly abnormal.

Because of this difficulty in defining abnormal flows at low lung volumes, a modification of the maneuver has been devised for better detecting of mild airway obstruction. MEFV curves inscribed after inspiring a gas mixture of low density (80 percent helium and 20 percent oxygen) are compared with those obtained while breathing air. Maximum flow ($\dot{V}$max) in normal individuals is dependent on the density of the gases breathed and increases with gases of low density. However, this is true during the FVC maneuver only as long as the equal pressure points (EPPs) remain predominantly in the larger, more central airways. In these airways most of the resistance to airflow is due to convective acceleration and turbulence, both of which are density-dependent. At lung volumes in the last 25 percent of the VC, the EPPs move upstream toward the alveoli and lie in the smaller peripheral airways, where resistance to laminar flow predominates. Gases of low density, such as helium, do not significantly lower resistance to laminar flow since the latter is independent of gas density. Therefore, the increased flows that result from the helium-oxygen mixture no longer occur and flows are identical to those with air breathing. The lung volume at which this occurs is the volume of isoflow (Viso$\dot{V}$),[27] usually measured from residual volume (RV) and expressed as percentage of VC (Fig. 24-17). Another means of analyzing the helium response compares the flow at 50 percent of VC with He/O_2 to that breathing air. The increase in flow with the helium mixture is expressed as a fraction or percentage of the flow in air and is designated as Δ $\dot{V}$max.[50]

In patients with obstructive lung disease, because of diminished elastic recoil and increased resistance of small upstream airways, the EPPs lie in the small airways even at higher lung volumes. As a result of this peripheral airway obstruction, flow is less density-dependent. Therefore, Δ $\dot{V}$max[50] should decrease and Viso$\dot{V}$ increase compared to those in normal individuals. The Viso$\dot{V}$ in normal subjects usually occurs at 10 to 15 percent of VC. A value greater than 25 percent would be considered abnormal.

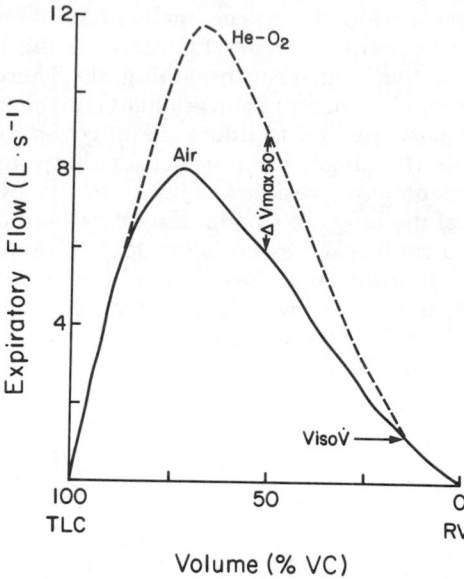

Fig. 24-17. Maximum expiratory flow volume curves with air and with a helium-oxygen mixture. Viso$\dot{V}$, volume of isoflow, the point at which flows with both gases become equal; Δ $\dot{V}$max[50], increase in flow at midpoint of vital capacity with helium-oxygen compared to air; TLC, total lung capacity; RV, residual volume.

The reduced values for Δ $\dot{V}$max[50] and elevated Viso$\dot{V}$ in smokers have been thought to be a result of the airflow resistance in the small peripheral airways where the flow regime is independent of density. Unfortunately the response to breathing helium is highly variable even among subjects with normal airways. This rather nonuniform response to helium has led to questioning previous interpretations of Δ $\dot{V}$max[50] as an index of peripheral airway obstruction. Interindividual variations in lung recoil and central airway geometry also appear to contribute significantly to the density dependence of maximal flow.[28]

PULMONARY FUNCTION TESTING IN SURGICAL PATIENTS
(Also See Chs. 25 and 50)

Significant postoperative changes in pulmonary function occur in many surgical patients and include such phenomena as reduced lung volumes, rapid shallow breathing, and impaired gas exchange. These alterations in pulmonary function may be induced by the anesthetic, the surgical procedure, the associated body position, or the medications administered immediately postoperatively. These changes, which occur in normal patients, may be more severe in patients who undergo surgery with compromised pulmonary function and thus lead to postoperative pulmonary complications. Such complications usually include bronchospasm, bronchitis with purulent sputum, disabling cough, pneumonia, and respiratory failure as indicated by altered blood gases. However, other pulmonary problems, such as aspiration, pulmonary embolus, congestive heart failure, and bleeding disorders in the lung, may also be aggravated by pre-existing abnormalities of lung function.

Although there is no general agreement concerning which particular patients should be studied preoperatively, the following types of patients are usually considered candidates for screening of preoperative pulmonary function:

1. Patients with any evidence of chronic pulmonary disease
2. Heavy smokers with history of persistent cough
3. Patients with chest wall and spinal deformities
4. Morbidly obese patients
5. Elderly patients (>70 years of age)
6. Patients for thoracic surgery
7. Patients for upper abdominal surgery

Initial identification of most of these patients is accomplished by history, physical exam, and chest radiographs. The question of which pulmonary function studies are appropriate for preoperative evaluation then arises. The more sophisticated lung function tests, such as phase III of the CV test, frequency dependence of compliance, and volume of isoflow, can detect the early phases of early mild lung dysfunction. The objective of testing in the preoperative setting, however, is not to detect early lung disease but rather to predict the likelihood of pulmonary complications. No single test appears to be the best predictor of risk. The optimal scheme for evaluating patients preoperatively is by means of arterial blood gas analysis and clinical spirometry. The FEV_1, FVC, FEV_1/FVC, percent, peak flow, and forced midexpiratory flow can be and usually are obtained from a single spirometric study.

The decision about whether the observed values in a given patient are normal or abnormal requires comparing the measured values with predicted standard reference values. The most widely used normal standards are values reported by Morris et al.[29] These were determined from measurements in 1,000 healthy nonsmokers residing in a relatively pollution-free environment. Normal limits are set by regression equations derived from studies such as that in large groups of normal subjects. An acceptable method to establish normal limits for general use is to define the lower limit of normal as a point $1.64 \times SEE$ (the SD of regression line) below the mean value for the same age and height on the regression line. With this approach 95 percent of the normal population should fall within the normal range. The widely used convention setting lower limits of normal at 80 percent of the predicted value should be avoided.[30]

Abnormalities on spirometric tests have been shown to correlate with the incidence of postoperative pulmonary complications.[2] However, it must be emphasized that the incidence and severity of postoperative pulmonary complications are not directly related to the severity of preoperative lung dysfunction. The site of the surgical incision is probably far more important, since upper abdominal and thoracic surgical procedures are associated with far more frequent problems. Obesity, patient age, and extent of smoking history are of considerable importance also.

The emphasis in evaluating preoperative pulmonary function is largely based on predicting the risk of postoperative complications. The identification of abnormal lung function, in particular, obstructive airway disease, is also important to reduce intraoperative and anesthetic morbidity. A reduced FEV_1/FVC, for example, not only documents the presence of airway obstruction but also suggests the likelihood of increased airway reactivity. The site and nature of many surgical procedures often provide very little latitude for choosing between regional and general anesthesia. In patients with airway obstruction and irritable airways, instrumentation such as laryngoscopy and endotracheal intubation is fraught with the hazard of provoking reflex bronchoconstriction, particularly under light anesthesia. In many patients with obstructive airway disease achieving the deep levels of inhalation anesthesia required to blunt airway reflexes[31] is difficult because of poor ventilation perfusion matching, and, if they are achieved, they are poorly tolerated by the cardiovascular system. Thus it is important to utilize prophylactic measures to minimize airway responses. These may include anticholinergics and β-adrenergic agonists inhaled as aerosols preoperatively and intravenous opioids and lidocaine prior to airway instrumentation.

Patients with an abnormal low FEV_1 preoperatively are likely to develop severe hypercapnia when allowed to breathe spontaneously under general anesthesia.[32] The magnitude of the carbon dioxide rise is directly related to the reduction in FEV_1. It, therefore, appears prudent to control ventilation in such patients. With controlled ventilation low respiratory rates (<10/min) are desirable to minimize ventilation perfusion mismatch, which largely arises because of the prolonged time constants of the obstructed airways. Low inspiratory flow rates were also thought to be desirable because of this obstruction to minimize excessive peak airway pressures and hence pulmonary barotrauma and circulatory disturbances. Recent studies,[33,34] however, have shown that a high inspiratory flow rate in such patients produced improved gas exchange that was not complicated by barotrauma or circulatory depression. Important consequences of the increased inspiratory flow rate were reduced inspiratory time and consequently increased time allowed for exhalation. This increased expiratory time allows more complete emptying of alveoli that must do so through high-resistance airways. Conversely, with a shorter expiratory time and a lower inspiratory flow these alveoli neither empty completely nor receive as much air at the same distending pressures. In addition to all of these considerations, the anesthetic technique should ideally be tailored to allow prompt awakening at the end of the operation with as few sequelae as possible and minimal residual anesthesia.

EVALUATION OF THE PATIENT FOR LUNG RESECTION
(Also See Ch. 50)

Resection of lung tissue results in a greater impairment in postoperative lung function than most other types of surgery. These patients require a more extensive pulmonary evaluation, particularly if removal of an entire lung is anticipated. A major aim of the evaluation is to decide whether the resectional surgery can be tolerated without compromising pulmonary function to a degree that the patient dies of pulmonary insufficiency or is severely disabled. The long-term ability to withstand such lung resection relates to the amount and functional status of the lung parenchyma removed and more importantly to the function of the remaining lung tissue. Removal of lung from an already compromised patient may be followed by inadequate gas exchange, pulmonary hypertension, and incapacitating degree of dyspnea.

Although much of the emphasis in this area is on long-term disability in the pneumonectomy patient, it is important to note that in patients undergoing lobectomy the immediate impact on pulmonary function may be as great because of surgical trauma to the remaining tissue of the same lung. The pulmonary function studies must be viewed in light of the patient's age, status of the cardiovascular system, and cooperation and motivation. Data in pneumonectomy patients indicate that whole lung removal will be tolerated if the preoperative pulmonary function meets the following criteria[35]: (1) FEV_1 greater than 2 L and FEV_1/FVC ratio of at least 50 percent, (2) MVV greater than 50 percent of predicted, (3) ratio of residual volume to total lung capacity less than 50 percent.

If any of these criteria is not met, more sophisticated tests of split lung function are indicated. Usually, these consist of xenon radiospirometry to assess ventilation and use of macroaggregates of iodine or technetium to scan perfusion. The relative contribution of each lung to either total ventilation or perfusion can then be used to predict postoperative pulmonary function. A predicted postoperative FEV_1 of at least 800 ml is required before allowing pneumonectomy. The risk of significant resting carbon dioxide retention appears to be high with lower FEV_1 values. If surgery is still contemplated in the face of this low predicted FEV_1, an invasive study is recommended. The pulmonary artery of the lung to be removed is subjected to occlusion by a balloon. If pulmonary hypertension (mean pulmonary arterial pressure > 35 mmHg) and arterial hypoxemia (PaO_2 < 45 mmHg) do not occur, it is concluded that the remaining lung may be able to accommodate the entire cardiac output. Such a patient may be allowed to undergo surgery in spite of failure to fulfill the mechanical ventilatory criteria. The indications for performing this invasive procedure are not agreed on universally, but Olsen et al.[35] believe that balloon occlusion, if feasible, should be performed when the less invasive studies are inconclusive.

Predicting post pneumonectomy FEV_1 with split lung function testing has been at times disappointing and inaccurate, and it may not provide the best way of predicting postoperative cardiopulmonary function.[36] The primary advantage of such testing is the low level of invasiveness compared to those of pulmonary artery occlusion and bronchospirometry, which radiospirometry essentially supplanted. The latter may in turn be supplanted by preoperative studies of exercise capacity. Recent observations suggest that a patient's maximal oxygen uptake during exercise ($\dot{V}O_2$ max) was an accurate means of preoperatively identifying patients likely to develop post-thoracotomy morbidity.[37] Thus many patients who otherwise might have been considered inoperable on the basis of FEV_1 values might be considered to be operative candidates because of their performance and high $\dot{V}O_2$ max during exercise.

PREOPERATIVE MEASURES TO IMPROVE LUNG FUNCTION

The basic goal of preoperative pulmonary function testing is to alter outcome by reducing the morbidity and mortality associated with postoperative pulmonary complications. The assumption is that the patients identified as abnormal may benefit from therapeutic measures to improve lung function and thus have reduced likelihood of postoperative complications. Several groups have applied such therapy to their poor-risk patients and demonstrated a decrease in the postoperative complications to levels approaching those in patients with normal lung function.[38–40]

Usually the therapy is carried out for 48 to 72 hours prior to surgery. However, it is equally important that the measures be continued postoperatively as well. Although a detailed discussion of such prophylaxis and therapy is beyond the scope of this presentation, the regimen is aimed largely at removing secretions, eliminating infection, and reversing bronchospasm. Therapy typically consists of the items listed in Table 24-3. It appears unreasonable to expect more than a slight reversibility in airflow obstruction and arterial blood gases in stable patients with such a 48- to 72-hour regi-

TABLE 24-3. Preoperative Measures to Improve Lung Function

Cessation of smoking	
Chest physiotherapy	(Percussion, vibration, postural drainage)
Bronchodilators	(Oral theophyllines, inhaled β-agonists, anticholinergics)
Expectorants	(Glycerol guaiacolate)
Forced fluids	(3 L orally per day)
Sustained deep inspiration	(Incentive spirometer)

men.[41] Gracey et al.[42] attempted to improve pulmonary function preoperatively in patients with chronic obstructive pulmonary disease with such a standardized regimen. Although this therapy produced changes in several tests of pulmonary function that were statistically significant, the functional significance of the changes was doubtful. Nevertheless the incidence of complications was dramatically reduced as in other studies. There are no definitive data that can identify whether this reduced complication rate results specifically from the preparation regimen, use of specific agents or techniques, or added attention paid to patients with identified airway obstruction.

Clearly patients whose clinical history and physical examination suggest the presence of pulmonary disease are at increased risk if spirometric testing produces abnormal results. It is far from clear exactly what should be done for such patients with abnormal test results short of an abbreviated regimen of preoperative preparation and intraoperative concern for controlling airway reactivity. Equally uncertain is which test best predicts risk and what further testing is appropriate for patients with abnormal spirometry, particularly those about to undergo pulmonary resection.

REFERENCES

1. American Thoracic Society: Standardization of spirometry—1987 update. Am Rev Respir Dis 136:1285, 1987
2. Stein M, Koota GM, Simon M, et al: Pulmonary evaluation of surgical patients. JAMA 181:765, 1962
3. Suratt PM, Hooe DM, Owens DA, Antharvedi A: Effect of maximal versus submaximal expiratory effort on spirometric values. Respiration 42:233, 1981
4. Gelb AF, Williams AJ, Zamel N: Spirometry: FEV_1 vs FEF 25–75 percent. Chest 84:473, 1983
5. Black LF, Hyatt RE: Maximal respiratory pressures: Normal values and relationship to age and sex. Am Rev Resp Dis 103:641, 1971
6. Braun NMT, Arora NS, Rochester DF: Respiratory muscle and pulmonary function in polymyositis and other proximal myopathies. Thorax 38:616, 1983
7. Ferris BG, Mead J, Opie LH: Partitioning of respiratory flow resistance in man. J Appl Physiol 19:653, 1964
8. Macklem PT, Mead J: Resistance of central and peripheral airways measured by a retrograde catheter. J Appl Physiol 22:395, 1967
9. Krowka MJ, Enright PL, Rodarte JR, Hyatt RE: Effect of effort on measurement of forced expiratory volume in one second. Am Rev Respir Dis 136:829, 1987
10. Dubois AB, Botelho SY, Comroe JH: A new method for measuring airway resistance in man using a body plethysmograph: Values in normal subject and in patients with respiratory disease. J Clin Invest 35:327, 1956
11. Suratt PM, Gal TJ, Hooe DM: Effect of head flexion on airway resistance measured in a body plethysmograph. Br J Dis Chest 75:204, 1981
12. Rozas, CJ, Goldman AL: Daily spirometric variability: Normal subjects and subjects with chronic bronchitis with and without airflow obstruction. Arch Intern Med 142:1287, 1982
13. Cockroft DW, Berscheid BA: Volume adjustment of maximum mid expiratory flow: Importance of changes in total lung capacity. Chest 78:595, 1980
14. Bouhuys A, Hunt VR, Kim BM, Zapletal A: Maximum expiratory flow rates in induced bronchoconstriction in man. J Clin Invest 48:1159, 1969
15. Gal TJ, Arora NS: Respiratory mechanics in supine subjects during progressive partial curarization. J Appl Physiol 52:57, 1982
16. Vincken WG, Elleker MG, Cusio MG: Flow-volume loop changes reflecting respiratory muscle weakness in chronic neuromuscular disorders. Am J Med 83:673, 1987
17. Buist AS, Vollmer WM, Johnson LR, McCamant LE: Does the single breath N_2 test identify the smoker who will develop chronic airflow limitation. Am Rev Respir Dis 137:293, 1988
18. Snider GL: Interpretation of the arterial oxygen and carbon dioxide partial pressures. Chest 63:801, 1973
19. Ingram RH, Schilder DP: Association of decrease in dynamic compliance with a change in gas distribution. J Appl Physiol 23:911, 1967
20. Fowler WS: Lung function studies. III: Uneven pulmonary ventilation in normal subjects and in patients with pulmonary disease. J Appl Physiol 2:283, 1949
21. Buist AS, Ross BB: Quantitative analysis of the alveolar plateau in the diagnosis of early airway obstruction. Am Rev Respir Dis 108:1078, 1973
22. Hyatt RE, Rodarte JR: "Closing volume," one man's noise—other men's experiment. Mayo Clin Proc 50:17, 1975
23. Hoeppner VH, Cooper DM, Zamel N, et al: Relationship between elastic recoil and closing volume in smokers and nonsmokers. Am Rev Respir Dis 109:81, 1974
24. LeBlanc P, Ruff F, Milic-Emili J: Effects of age and body position on airway closure in man. J Appl Physiol 28:448, 1970
25. Mansell A, Bryan C, Levision H: Airway closure in children. J Appl Physiol 33:711, 1972
26. McFadden ER, Holmes B, Kiker R: Variability of closing volume measurements in normal man. Am Rev Respir Dis 111:135, 1975
27. Hutcheon M, Griffin P, Levison H, et al: Volume of isoflow, a new test in detection of mild abnormalities of lung mechanics. Am Rev Respir Dis 110:458, 1974
28. Castille RG, Hyatt RE, Rodarte JR: Determinants of maximal expiratory flow and density dependence in normal humans. J Appl Physiol 49:897, 1980
29. Morris JF, Koski A, Johnson LC: Spirometric standards for healthy nonsmoking adults. Am Rev Respir Dis 102:57, 1971
30. Clausen JL: Prediction of normal values. pp 49–59. In Clausen JE (ed): Pulmonary Function Testing Guidelines and Controversies. Orlando, Fla., Grune & Stratton, 1984
31. Yakaitis RW, Blitt CD, Angiullo JP: End tidal halothane concentration for endotracheal intubation. Anesthesiology 47:386, 1977
32. Pietak S, Weenig CS, Hickey RF, et al: Anesthetic effects on ventilation in patients with chronic obstructive pulmonary disease. Anesthesiology 42:160, 1975
33. Connors AF, McAferee D, Gray BA: Effect of inspiratory flow rate on gas exchange during mechanical ventilation. Am Rev Respir Dis 124:537, 1981
34. Tuxen DV, Lane S: The effects of ventilatory pattern on hyperinflation, airway pressures, and circulation in mechanical ventilation of patients with severe airflow obstruction. Am Rev Respir Dis 136:872, 1987
35. Olsen GN, Block AJ, Swenson EW, et al: Pulmonary function evaluation of the lung resection candidate: A prospective study. Am Rev Respir Dis 111:379, 1975
36. Ladurie ML, Ranson, Bitker B: Uncertainties in the expected value for forced expiratory volume in one second after surgery. Chest 90:222, 1986
37. Smith TP, Kinasewitz GT, Tucker WY, et al: Exercise capacity

as a predictor of post-thoracotomy morbidity. Am Rev Respir Dis 129:730, 1984

38. Stein M, Cassara EL: Preoperative pulmonary evaluation and therapy for surgery patients. JAMA 211:787, 1970
39. Milledge JS, Nunn JF: Criteria of fitness for anaesthesia in patients with chronic obstructive lung disease. Br Med J 3:670, 1975
40. Williams CD, Brenowitz JB: "Prohibitive" lung function and major surgical procedures. Am J Surg 132:703, 1976
41. Petty TL, Brink GA, Miller NW, Corsello PR: Objective functional improvement in chronic airway obstruction. Chest 57:216, 1970
42. Gracey DR, Divertie MB, Didier EP: Preoperative pulmonary preparation of patients with chronic obstructive pulmonary disease: A prospective study. Chest 76:123, 1979

25

ANESTHETIC IMPLICATIONS OF CONCURRENT DISEASES

Michael F. Roizen

Continued

INTRODUCTION

This chapter discusses patients who have conditions requiring special preoperative evaluation and intraoperative management. As with "healthy" patients (also see Ch. 23), it is the history and physical examination of these patients that most accurately predict not only the associated risks but also the likelihood that a monitoring technique or change in therapy will be beneficial or necessary for survival. Those instances in which specific information should be sought in the history-taking, physical examination, or laboratory evaluations are emphasized. Although controlled studies to confirm that optimizing a patient's preoperative physical condition will result in lower morbidity have not been performed for most diseases, it is logical to assume that such is the case. Studies showing the benefits of optimizing specific preoperative conditions are highlighted. The fact that such preventive measures would cost less than treating the morbidity that would otherwise occur is an important consideration in a cost-conscious environment. Examples of determining the costs of such benefits can be found in Chapter 23 in the section on preoperative preparation of the patient with cardiovascular disease. Conditions discussed in this chapter are (1) diseases involving the endocrine system and disorders of nutrition; (2) diseases involving the cardiovascular system; (3) disorders of the respiratory and immune systems; (4) diseases of the CNS, neuromuscular diseases, and mental disorders; (5) diseases involving the kidney, infectious diseases, and disorders of electrolytes; (6) diseases involving the gastrointestinal (GI) tract or the liver; (7) diseases involving hematopoiesis and various forms of cancer; and (8) diseases of aging or that occur more commonly in the aged, as well as chronic and acute medical conditions requiring drug therapy (also see Chs. 57–59 and 62).

THE ROLE OF THE PRIMARY CARE PHYSICIAN OR CONSULTANT

The role of the primary care physician or consultant is not to select or suggest anesthetic or surgical methods but, rather, to optimize the patient's preoperative status regarding those conditions that increase the morbidity and mortality associated with surgery.

Optimizing a patient's preoperative condition is a cooperative venture between the anesthesiologist and the internist, pediatrician, surgeon, or family physician. If the primary care physician cannot affirm that the patient is in the very best physical state attainable (for that patient) by that physician and his or her consultants, the anesthesiologist and the physician should do what is necessary to optimize that condition. Failing to consult with the primary care physician preoperatively is as risky as not checking the oxygen in the spare tanks. In fact, statements that describe the preoperative physical condition of the patient (e.g., "This patient is in optimum shape," and "I believe the mitral stenosis is more severe than the slight degree of mitral insufficiency") are much more useful to the anesthesiologist than are statements that suggest perioperative procedures ("Prevent hypoxia and hypotension").[1] Internists, pediatricians, and family practitioners usually have little knowledge of the problems, physiologic processes, and drug properties and reactions related to anesthesia.

Although information about the perioperative period is being introduced to physician consultants, such material is currently descriptive, elementary, and incomplete and rarely describes how anesthetic considerations should modify the primary care physician's management of pathophysiologic conditions.[2] Without understanding the physiologic changes that occur perioperatively, it is difficult to prescribe the appropriate therapy. It is therefore part of the anesthesiologist's job to educate the patient's consultants as to what information is needed from the preoperative consultation.

DISEASES INVOLVING THE ENDOCRINE SYSTEM AND DISORDERS OF NUTRITION

Pancreatic Disorders

Preoperative Diabetes Mellitus

This section makes five major points regarding diabetes:

1. Although the presence of diabetes has long been as-

sumed to increase perioperative risk, results from epidemiologic studies segregating the effects of diabetes per se from those of the organ system and complications of diabetes (e.g., cardiac and vascular disease), and of old age may not support this assumption. Surgical mortality rates for the diabetic population are on average five times higher than those for the nondiabetic population.[3-5] However, in epidemiologic studies in which diabetes itself was segregated from the complications of diabetes (including cardiac and vascular disease) and old age, this finding was questioned.[5-8] Similarly, if diabetics undergoing major vascular surgery are compared with nondiabetics who are matched for type of surgery, age, sex, weight, and complicating diseases, there is no difference in the mortality rate or the number of postoperative complications.[7]

2. Because diabetes represents at least two disease processes, perioperative management may differ between them.

3. A current debate exists as to how closely the blood glucose levels of diabetic patients should be controlled. Chronic "tight" control of type I diabetes probably prevents, retards, or even ameliorates, to some degree, some of the chronic complications of diabetes. However, the debate centers on how great the benefit of tight control is, and what the benefit-risk ratio is. Evidence indicates tight control of blood glucose might be a benefit for the pregnant diabetic (and her future offspring)[9] (also see Ch. 57), for the diabetic undergoing cardiopulmonary bypass[10] (also see Ch. 51), and for those undergoing (global) CNS ischemia[11-12] (also see Chs. 54 and 74). Little evidence indicates that tight control is of substantial benefit to any other group; the benefit-risk ratio of tight control has not been examined in any other group of patients.

4. Different regimens permit almost any degree of perioperative control of blood glucose levels, but the tighter the control desired, the more frequently blood glucose levels must be monitored. Three treatment regimens are outlined.

5. The major risk factors for diabetics undergoing surgery are the end-organ diseases associated with diabetes: cardiovascular dysfunction, renal insufficiency, and neuropathies;[3-4,7-8,13] thus, a major focus of the anesthesiologist should be preoperative evaluation and treatment of these diseases to ensure optimal preoperative conditions of the patient.

Pancreatic islets are composed of at least three cells: alpha cells that secrete glucagon, beta cells that secrete insulin, and delta cells that contain secretory granules. Insulin is first synthesized as proinsulin, converted to insulin by proteolytic cleavage, and then packaged into granules within the beta cells. A large quantity of insulin, normally about 200 units, is stored in the pancreas, and continued synthesis is stimulated by glucose. There is a basal, steady-state release of insulin from the beta granules and additional release that is controlled by stimuli external to the beta cell. Basal insulin secretion continues in the fasted state and is of key importance in the inhibition of catabolism and ketoacidosis. Glucose and fructose are the primary and most important regulators of insulin release. Other stimulators of insulin release include amino acids, glucagon, gastrointestinal hormones (gastrin, secretin, cholecystokinin-pancreozymin, and enteroglucagon), and acetylcholine. Epinephrine and norepinephrine inhibit insulin release by stimulating α-adrenergic receptors, and they stimulate its release at β-adrenergic receptors.

Diabetes mellitus is a heterogeneous group of disorders that have the common feature of a relative or absolute lack of insulin. It is characterized by a multitude of hormone-induced metabolic abnormalities, by a diffuse microvascular lesion, and by long-term end-organ complications. Diabetes can be divided into two very different diseases which share these end-organ abnormalities. Type I diabetes is associated with autoimmune diseases and has a concordance rate of 40 to 50 percent (that is, if one of a pair of monozygotic twins had diabetes, the likelihood that the other twin would have diabetes is 40 to 50 percent). In type I, the patient is insulin-deficient and is prone to ketoacidosis if insulin is withheld. For type II diabetes, the concordance rate is 100 percent (that is, the genetic material is both necessary and sufficient for the development of type II diabetes). The patients are not prone to develop ketoacidosis in the absence of insulin, and they have peripheral insulin resistance.

Type I and type II diabetes differ in other ways as well. Contrary to a long-standing belief, patient age does not allow a firm distinction between type I and type II diabetes; an older person can develop type I diabetes.[14] A diabetes-producing variant of coxsackie B4 virus has been isolated from the pancreas of a patient who died of diabetic ketoacidosis (type I diabetes). This virus also was recovered from mice bred to be diabetes-prone after inoculation of the virus had produced hyperglycemia and pancreatic beta-cell necrosis coincident with rising antibody titers.[15] Thus, the intrinsic genetic "vulnerability" in insulin-dependent type I diabetes mellitus may consist of diminished capacity of beta cells to survive exposure to potentially damaging extrinsic agents.

Non-insulin-dependent (type II) diabetics compose 90 percent of the 10 million diabetics in America; they tend to be elderly, overweight, relatively resistant to ketoacidosis, and prone to the development of a hyperglycemic, hyperosmolar, nonketotic state. Plasma insulin levels are normal or elevated but are relatively low for the level of blood glucose.

Currently, therapy for type II diabetes usually begins with dietary management alone but may progress to the use of oral hypoglycemic medications that act by stimulating release of insulin by pancreatic beta cells and by improving the tissue responsiveness to insulin by reversing the post-binding abnormality. The common orally administered drugs are tolazamide (Tolinase) and tolbutamide (Orinase). The newer sulfonylureas include glyburide (Micronase) and glipizide (Glucotrol); these have a longer blood glucose-lowering effect, which persists for 24 hours or more, and fewer drug-drug interactions. Oral hypoglycemic drugs may produce hypoglycemia for as long as 50 hours after intake (chlorpropamide [Diabinese] has the longest half-life). Occasionally, physicians advocating tight control of blood sugar levels give insulin to "maturity-onset" insulin-dependent diabetic patients twice a day, or even more frequently.

Insulin-dependent diabetics tend to be young, nonobese, and prone to the development of ketoacidosis. Plasma insulin levels are low or nonmeasurable, and therapy requires insulin replacement. Patients with insulin-dependent diabetes experience an increase in their insulin requirements in the postmidnight hours, and this may result in early-morning hyperglycemia (dawn phenomenon). This accelerated glucose production and impaired glucose utilization are due to nocturnal surges in growth hormone secretion.[16]

Acute complications for the diabetic patient include hypoglycemia, diabetic ketoacidosis, and hyperglycemic, hyperosmolar, nonketotic coma. Diabetic patients also are subject to a series of long-term complications, including cataracts, neuropathies, retinopathy, and angiopathy involving peripheral and myocardial vessels, that lead to considerable morbidity and premature mortality. Many of these complications will bring the diabetic patient to surgery. The evidence that hyperglycemia itself accelerates these complications or that tight control of blood sugar levels decreases the rapidity of the progression of microangiopathic disease is very suggestive but not definitive.[17-20] A controversy now exists as to how tightly blood sugar levels should be controlled chronically in diabetic patients. The controversy centers on whether attempts to attain normal blood sugar levels are a greater benefit than risk to diabetic patients.[21]

The perioperative management of the diabetic patient may affect surgical outcome. Physicians advocating tight control of blood glucose levels point to the evidence of increased wound-healing tensile strength and decreased wound infections in animal models of diabetes (type I) under tight control.[22,23]

It has been known for many years that neuropathy, atherosclerosis, and small-vessel disease may contribute to wound failure. Experimental studies suggest that hyperglycemia itself may cause deficient wound healing. Several investigators have shown that diabetic animals have delayed healing with poor collagen formation and poor tensile strength of deep surgical wounds.[15] These abnormalities can be corrected by administration of insulin. Goodson and Hunt reported that obesity, insulin resistance, hyperglycemia, and depressed leukocyte function interfere with collagen synthesis and lead to impaired wound healing.[22] They demonstrated slowing of granulocyte influx and retardation of early capillary ingrowth. Synthesis of protocollagen and collagen was decreased in the wounds of diabetic animals. In insulin-deficient animals, administration of insulin is crucial for early development of granulation tissue and for subsequent fibroblast growth and collagen synthesis.[24] Insulin is necessary in the early stages of the inflammatory response but seems to have no effect on collagen formation after the first 10 days.

In studies of corneal wounds, identical healing rates were observed in diabetic and nondiabetic animals and human subjects. Healing epithelial wounds have minimal leukocyte infiltration and, unlike deep wounds, are not dependent on collagen synthesis for the integrity of the tissue. Thus, simple epithelial repair is not inhibited in the diabetic patient, whereas the repair of deeper wounds is impaired with respect to collagen formation and defense against bacterial growth.

Infections account for two-thirds of postoperative complications and about 20 percent of perioperative deaths in diabetic patients. Experimental data suggest many factors that may make diabetics vulnerable to infection. Many alterations in leukocyte function have been demonstrated in hyperglycemic diabetics, including decreased chemotaxis and impaired phagocytic activity of granulocytes, as well as reduced intracellular killing of pneumococci and staphylococci.[25,26] When diabetic patients are treated aggressively and blood glucose levels are maintained below 250 mg/dl, the phagocytic function of granulocytes is improved and intracellular killing of bacteria is restored to near-normal levels.[27]

It has been thought that diabetic patients experience more infections in clean wounds than do nondiabetics. In a review of 23,649 surgical patients, the rate of wound infection in clean incisions was found to be 10.7 percent in diabetics, as compared to 1.8 percent in nondiabetics.[28] However, when age is accounted for, the difference in the incidence of wound infection in diabetic surgical patients compared to that in nondiabetic patients is not statistically significant. In addition, hyperglycemia may worsen neurologic outcome after intraoperative cerebral ischemia.

Recent information regarding the relationship between blood glucose and neurologic recovery after a global ischemic event may have important implications for perioperative diabetic management. In a study of 430 consecutive patients resuscitated after out-of-hospital cardiac arrest, mean blood glucose levels were found to be higher in patients who never awakened (341 ± 13 mg/dl) than in those who did (262 ± 7 mg/dl).[28a] Among patients who awakened, those with persistent neurologic deficits had higher mean glucose levels (286 ± 15 mg/dl) than did those without deficits (251 ± 7 mg/dl). These results are consistent with the finding that hyperglycemia during a stroke is associated with poorer short- and long-term neurologic outcomes. The question remains what is cause and what is effect; does the high glucose level predispose to a bad outcome, or does a bad outcome predispose to high glucose levels? If high glucose levels predispose to bad outcomes, the mechanism for the association of hyperglycemia with ischemic brain damage is not known. However, the possibility that blood glucose is a determinant of brain damage following global ischemia is supported by some animal studies after global CNS ischemia,[11] but not by others after focal CNS ischemia.[12] The preponderance of data after CNS ischemia seems to favor an effect of glucose on CNS recovery. Until better data are available, there will be those who argue that the diabetic patient about to undergo surgery in which hypotension or reduced cerebral flow may occur should have a blood glucose level below 250 mg/dl during a period of cerebral ischemia. There are some special situations that may also influence how tightly one should manage the patient's glucose level: surgery requiring cardiopulmonary bypass, and emergency surgery in patients already suffering from diabetic ketoacidosis or hyperosmolar nonketotic coma.

Twelve years ago, diabetics undergoing coronary artery bypass (CABG) surgery had a perioperative mortality rate of 5 percent, compared to 1.5 percent for nondiabetics.[29] In this study, and in most other studies of diabetic patients undergoing CABG surgery, important additional risk factors or confounding variables were not considered, including the incidence and extent of hypertension, ventricular dysfunction, congestive heart failure, or severity of coronary artery disease.

In 1980, a study of 340 diabetics and 2,522 nondiabetics undergoing CABG surgery demonstrated only a moderate increase in the operative mortality for diabetics (1.8 percent versus 0.6 percent).[29] In the postbypass phase, patients with diabetes have required inotropic therapy and intra-aortic balloon pump support five times more frequently than nondiabetics.[10] There are several possible reasons. Diabetics with angina have more extensive coronary artery disease than do nondiabetic patients. They are also more likely to have hypertension, cardiomegaly, diffuse hypokinesis, and prior myocardial infarction. Insulin-dependent diabetics with coronary artery disease appear to have stiffer ventricles with greater elevation to left ventricular end-diastolic pressure than do matched nondiabetic controls.[10] During cardiopulmonary bypass, hypothermia and stress reactions decrease the response to insulin and result in marked hyperglycemia (even when the perfusate and IV solutions do not contain glucose). These changes are exaggerated in the diabetic patient, and insulin administration may have little effect until rewarming is achieved. In a number of recently reported cases, inotropic agents were ineffective in maintaining cardiac contractility, although filling pressures, sinus rhythm, serum electrolytes, and blood gases were adequate. The blood sugar was high in each case. After IV infusion of insulin, effective myocardial contractions returned, allowing easy and rapid bypass weaning.[10] A cautious prognosis needs to be given to the diabetic coronary-bypass patient with poor ventricular function, since the surgical mortality may be 10 to 15 percent.[29]

Many diabetics requiring emergency surgery for trauma or infection have significant metabolic decompensation, including ketoacidosis. Often little time is available for stabilization of the patient, but even a few hours may be sufficient for correction of fluid and electrolyte disturbances that are potentially life-threatening. It is futile to delay surgery in an attempt to eliminate ketoacidosis completely if the underlying surgical condition will lead to further metabolic deterioration. The likelihood of intraoperative cardiac arrhythmias and hypotension resulting from ketoacidosis will be reduced if volume depletion and hypokalemia are at least partially treated.

Insulin therapy is initiated with a 10-unit IV bolus of regular insulin, which is followed by continuous insulin infusion. The rate of infusion is determined most easily if one divides the last serum glucose value by 150 (or 100 if the patient is receiving steroids, has an infection, or is overweight). The actual amount of insulin administered is less important than regular monitoring of glucose, potassium, and pH. Because the number of insulin-binding sites is limited, the maximum rate of glucose decline is fairly constant, averaging 75 to 100 mg/dl/h regardless of the insulin dose.[30] During the first 1 to 2 hours of fluid resuscitation, the glucose level may fall more precipitously. When the serum glucose reaches 250 mg/dl, the IV fluid should include 5 percent dextrose.

The volume of fluid required for therapy varies with overall deficits; it ranges from 3 to 5 liters, but it can be as high as 10 liters. Despite losses of water in excess of losses of solute, sodium levels are generally normal or reduced. Factitious hyponatremia caused by hyperglycemia or hypertriglyceridemia may result in this seeming contradiction. The plasma sodium concentration decreases by about 1.6 mEq/L for every 100-mg/dl increase in plasma glucose above normal. Initially, normal saline is infused at the rate of 250 to 1,000 ml/h, depending on the degree of volume depletion and on the cardiac status. Some measure of left ventricular volume should be monitored in diabetics who have a history of myocardial dysfunction. About one-third of the estimated fluid deficit is corrected in the first 6 to 8 hours, and the remaining two-thirds over the next 24 hours.

The degree of acidosis present is determined by measurement of arterial blood gases and an increased anion gap $[Na^+ - (Cl^- + HCO_3^-)]$. Acidosis with an increased anion gap (≥ 16 mEq/L) in the acutely ill diabetic may be caused by ketones in ketoacidosis, lactic acid in lactic acidosis, increased organic acids from renal insufficiency, or all three. In ketoacidosis, the plasma levels of acetoacetate, β-hydroxybutarate, and acetone are increased. Plasma and urinary ketones are measured semiquantitatively with the Ketostix and Acetest tablets. The role of bicarbonate therapy in diabetic ketoacidosis is controversial. Myocardial function and respiration are known to be depressed at a blood pH below 7.0 to 7.10; yet rapid correction of acidosis with bicarbonate therapy may result in alterations in central nervous system function and structure. This may be caused by (1) paradoxical development of CSF and CNS acidosis resulting from rapid conversion of bicarbonate to carbon dioxide and diffusion of the acid across the blood-brain barrier, (2) altered CNS oxygenation with decreased cerebral blood flow, and (3) development of unfavorable osmotic gradients. After treatment with fluids and insulin, β-hydroxybutarate levels decrease rapidly, whereas acetoacetate levels may remain stable or even increase before declining. Plasma acetone levels remain elevated for 24 to 42 hours, long after blood glucose, β-hydroxybutarate, and acetoacetate levels have returned to normal; the result is continuing ketonuria.[30] Persistent ketosis, with a serum bicarbonate level of less than 20 mEq/L in the presence of a normal glucose level, represents a continued need for intracellular glucose and insulin for reversal of lipolysis.

The most important electrolyte disturbance in diabetic ketoacidosis is depletion of total body potassium. The deficits range from 3 mEq/kg body weight up to 10 mEq/kg body weight. Rapid declines in serum potassium level occur, reaching a nadir within 2 to 4 hours after the start of IV insulin administration. Aggressive replacement therapy is required. The potassium administered moves into the intracellular space with insulin as the acidosis is corrected. Potassium is also excreted in the urine with the increased delivery of sodium to the distal renal tubules that accompanies volume expansion. Phosphorus deficiency in ketoacidosis caused by tissue catabolism, impaired cellular uptake, and increased urinary losses may result in significant muscular weakness and organ dysfunction. The average phosphorus deficit is approximately 1 mmol/kg body weight. Replacement is needed if the plasma concentration falls below 1.0 mg/dl.[30]

Thus management of intraoperative glucose might be influenced by specific situations, such as type of operation, pregnancy, expected global CNS insult, bias of the patient's primary care physician, or type of diabetic. Type I diabetic patients definitely need insulin and might be considered candidates for tight control of blood glucose levels. Type II diabetic patients have insulin and may not benefit from tight perioperative control.

The key to managing blood glucose levels in diabetic patients perioperatively is to set clear goals and then to monitor blood glucose levels frequently enough to adjust therapy to achieve those goals. Three regimens that afford various degrees of perioperative control of blood glucose levels are listed below.

Classic "Nontight Control" Regimen

Aim: To prevent hypoglycemia. To prevent ketoacidosis and hyperosmolar states.

Protocol:

1. Day before surgery: Patient should be given nothing by mouth after midnight; glass of orange juice should be at the bedside for emergency use.
2. At 6 A.M. on day of surgery, institute intravenous fluids using plastic cannulae and a solution containing 5 percent dextrose, infusion at the rate of 125 ml/h/70-kg body weight.
3. After intravenous infusion is instituted, give one-half the usual morning insulin dose subcutaneously.
4. Continue 5 percent dextrose solutions through operative period, giving at least 125 ml/h/70-kg body weight.
5. In recovery room monitor blood glucose concentrations and treat with a sliding scale.

Such a regimen has been found to meet its goals.[31]

"Tight Control" Regimen 1

Aim: To keep plasma glucose levels between 79 and 200 mg/dl; this practice may improve wound healing and prevent wound infections.

Protocol:

1. Evening before operation, determine preprandial blood glucose level.
2. Through a plastic cannula, begin intravenous infusion of 5 percent dextrose in water at the rate of 50 ml/h/70-kg body weight.
3. Next, "piggyback" (Fig. 25-1) to the dextrose infusion an infusion of regular insulin (50 units in 250 ml or 0.9 percent sodium chloride) and an infusion pump. Before attaching this piggyback line to the dextrose infusion, flush the line with 60 ml of infusion mixture and discard the flushing solution. This approach saturates insulin-binding sites of the tubing.[32]
4. Set the infusion rate, using the following equation: Insulin (units/h) = plasma glucose (mg/dl)/150 (Note: This denominator should be 100 if patient is taking corticosteroids, e.g., 100 mg of prednisone a day).
5. Repeat measurements of blood glucose levels every 4 hours as needed and adjust insulin appropriately to obtain blood glucose levels of 100 to 200 mg/dl.
6. Day of surgery: Intraoperative fluids and electrolytes are managed by continuing to administer non-dextrose containing solutions, as described in steps 3 and 4.
7. Determine plasma glucose level at the start of operation and every 2 hours for the rest of the 24-hour period. Adjust insulin dosage appropriately.

Although I have not needed to treat hypoglycemia (i.e., blood glucose levels of less than 50 mg/dl), I have been prepared to do so with 15 ml of 50 percent dextrose in water. Under such circumstances, the insulin

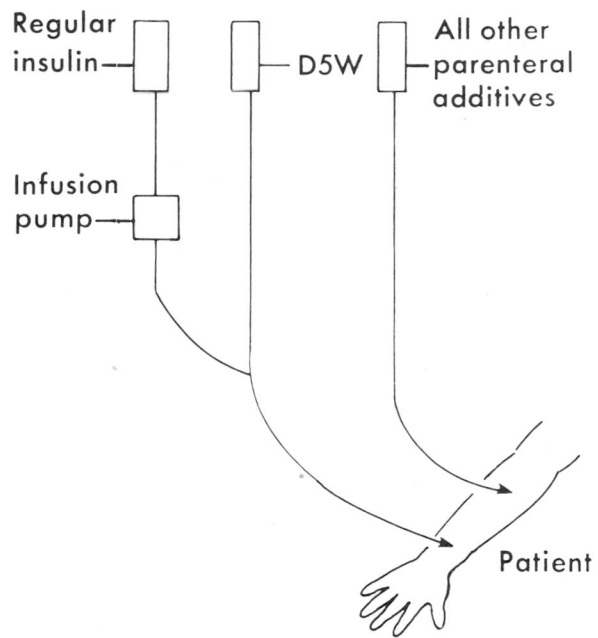

Fig. 25-1. Arrangement of intravenous lines for infusion of regular insulin in a regimen tightly controlling blood glucose levels in diabetic patients undergoing surgery.

infusion would be terminated. Such a regimen has been found to accomplish its goals, even in very "brittle" diabetics (i.e., those extremely resistant to treatment) given high doses of steroids.[33]

"Tight Control" Regimen 2

Aim: Same as for Tight Control Regimen 1

Protocol:

1. Obtain a "feedback mechanical pancreas" and set the controls for the desired plasma glucose regimen.
2. Institute appropriate two intravenous lines.

This last regimen may well supersede all others if the cost of a mechanical pancreas can be reduced and if control of hyperglycemia is shown to make a meaningful difference perioperatively.

Despite the fact that hyperglycemic type I diabetic patients have a higher incidence of wound infections, a lower wound-healing tensile strength, and a higher incidence of renal transplant rejections than do normal patients,[25,28] it does not necessarily follow that short-term tight control of blood glucose levels perioperatively would reduce morbidity and mortality. For example, in one study, the incidence of perioperative mortality was 11 times greater for diabetic patients than for asymptomatic healthy patients.[34] However, in several other studies[4-8,35] no increase in wound or systemic infections or in any measure of perioperative morbidity or mortality could be attributable to diabetes

itself. Also, when corrections were made for age and end-organ disease (cardiovascular) in those five studies, the increases in morbidity for diabetic patients seemed to disappear.[4-8,35]

Perhaps only wound healing and rate of infection are important factors during the perioperative period. However, the debate concerns whether control of hyperglycemia itself lowers the incidence of any of the complications associated with diabetes. One editorial implied that tight perioperative control of blood sugar levels would decrease the incidence of infections and increase the quality of wound healing.[36] While many would welcome such a study, no data to support those implications yet exist.

Other Conditions Associated with Diabetes

Diabetes is associated with microangiopathy (in retinal and renal vessels), peripheral neuropathies, autonomic dysfunction, and infection.

Before surgery, assessment and optimization of treatment of the potential and potent end-organ effects of diabetes are at least as important as an assessment of the diabetic's current overall metabolic status. Information about a diabetic patient that might merit special attention before surgery includes the therapeutic (including dietary) and exercise regimens, adequacy of glucose control, prior surgical and anesthetic responses, and presence of end-organ effects of diabetes. Basic laboratory examinations might include fasting blood sugar, electrolytes, BUN or creatinine levels, and an electrocardiogram. Scheduling the operative procedure early in the day avoids prolonging the catabolic state and minimizes the risk of preoperative hypoglycemia.

Patients with severe diabetic autonomic neuropathy are at an increased risk for gastroparesis and consequent aspiration and for intraoperative and postoperative cardiorespiratory arrest. Recent data indicate that diabetics who exhibit signs of autonomic neuropathy, such as early satiety, lack of sweating, lack of pulse rate change with inspiration or orthostatic maneuvers, and impotence, have a very high incidence both of painless myocardial ischemia[37,38] and of gastroparesis. Some authors have successfully used 10 mg of metoclopramide preoperatively to facilitate gastric emptying of solids. Interference with respiration by pneumonia or by anesthetics, pain medications, or sedative drugs appears to be the precipitating cause in most cases of sudden cardiorespiratory arrest. Measuring the degree of sinus arrhythmia or beat-to-beat variability provides a simple, accurate test for significant autonomic neuropathy. The difference between maximum and minimum heart rate on deep inspiration is normally 15 beats/min, but was found to be 5 beats/min or less in all patients who sustained cardiorespiratory arrest.[38]

Other characteristics of patients with autonomic neuropathy include postural hypotension with a decrease in blood pressure of more than 30 mmHg, resting tachycardia, nocturnal diarrhea, and dense peripheral neuropathy. Diabetics with significant autonomic neuropathy may have impaired respiratory responses to hypoxia and are particularly susceptible to the action of drugs that have depressant effects. Such patients may warrant very close, continuous cardiac and respiratory monitoring for 12 to 24 hours postoperatively, although such logical treatment has not, as yet, been tested in a rigorous, controlled trial. Thus, in the absence of these conditions, I would favor outpatient surgery for the diabetic (Table 25-1).

Perhaps most important, diabetic patients have an increased incidence of atherosclerosis and all its complications. Such patients are particularly susceptible to episodes of painless myocardial ischemia and cardiovascular instability.[37-39] As with other endocrinopathies, the cardiovascular system should be a focus of the anesthetist's attention for the diabetic patient.

Insulinoma and Other Causes of Hypoglycemia

Hypoglycemia can be caused by such diverse entities as a pancreatic islet cell adenoma or carcinoma, large hepatoma, large sarcoma, alcohol ingestion, hypopituitarism, adrenal insufficiency, altered physiology after gastric surgery, hereditary fructose intolerance, or galactosemia and the recently discovered autoimmune hypoglycemia. The last three entities cause postprandial reactive hypoglycemia. Since restriction of oral intake prevents severe hypoglycemia, the practice of giving the patient nothing by mouth and infusing small amounts of a solution containing 5 percent dextrose greatly lessens the possibility of postprandial reactive hypoglycemia. The other causes of hypoglycemia can cause serious problems during the perioperative period.[41]

The symptoms of hypoglycemia fall into two groups: adrenergic excess (tachycardia, palpitations, tremulousness, or diaphoresis) and neuroglycopenia (headache, confusion, mental sluggishness, seizures, or coma). Since all these symptoms may be masked by anesthesia, blood glucose levels should be determined frequently to ensure that hypoglycemia is not present. Because manipulation of an insulinoma can result in massive insulin release, this tumor probably should be operated on only at centers having a mechanical pancreas: such machines have on-line blood glucose analysis and a glucose infusion setup.

A different point of view was expressed by Muir and colleagues,[42] who managed 38 patients undergoing insulinoma resection. Every 15 minutes they noted the plasma glucose concentration in these patients, in whom a mechanical pancreas produced no increase in plasma glucose. Although 9 of the 38 patients became significantly hypoglycemic (i.e., plasma glucose concentrations < 50 mg/dl), in only 4 of 253 measurements before resection did glucose concentration decrease more than 20 mg/dl in any 15-minute period. Muir et al.[42] believe that intermittent sampling of plasma glucose (every 15 minutes) may be satisfactory as long as the plasma glucose concentration is kept at ≥ 60 mg/dl. In this series, the absence or presence of a hyperglycemic rebound after tumor resection was not of predictive value in determining completeness of insulinoma resection(s). The other causes of hypoglycemia do not involve release of insulin in such vast quantities (or at all), and therefore less frequent (every 1 to 2 hours) intraoperative blood glucose determinations and continuous dextrose infusion appear to be sufficient.

Disorders of Nutrition

Hyperlipidemias and Hypolipidemias

Hyperlipidemia may result from obesity, estrogen or corticoid therapy, uremia, diabetes, hypothyroidism, acromegaly, alcohol ingestion, liver disease, inborn errors of metabolism, or pregnancy. Hyperlipidemia may cause premature coronary or peripheral vascular disease or pancreatitis.[43] Hypercholesterolemia, a form of hyperlipidemia, appears to be associated with premature atherosclerosis. Most cholesterol is carried in serum by low-density lipoprotein (LDL), whereas approximately 30 percent of total serum cholesterol is carried by high-density lipoprotein (HDL). High density-lipoprotein cholesterol is carried in roughly equivalent amounts on two types of HDL: on a less dense HDL_2 subfraction that is negatively associated with coronary artery disease, and on a more dense HDL_3 subfraction that is unrelated to coronary artery disease.[44] In atherosclerosis, LDL, and not HDL, is probably the risk factor. Levels of HDL are 25 percent higher in women than in men; low levels of HDL in women are associated with premature atherosclerosis. Cigarette smoking lowers HDL levels, whereas regular strenuous exercise and small daily intake of alcohol raise HDL levels. However, alcohol increases HDL_3, the HDL subfraction thought to be inert with respect to coronary artery disease;[44] octogenarians have high levels of HDL.

Although controlling diet remains the major treat-

TABLE 25-1. Should a Diabetic Be an Outpatient or a Morning Admittance Patient?

Outpatient If	Morning Admittance Patient If
Can evaluate history in advance	Cannot evaluate history
End-organ disease does not require invasive monitoring	End-organ disease requires invasive monitoring
Prehydration is available or is not necessary	Needs careful prehydration
No CNS ischemia or cardiopulmonary bypass is planned	CNS ischemia is present or cardiopulmonary bypass is planned
Not pregnant	Pregnant
Patients can determine blood glucose level	Patients cannot determine blood glucose level
Vested home "mate"	No vested individual
Can take temperature or look for "red" wound	Cannot take temperature or look for "red" wound
Plan higher admit rate (no data)	Financially unsuitable

ment modality for all types of hyperlipidemia, clofibrate (Atromid-S) and gemfibrozil, used to treat hypertriglyceridemia, can cause myopathy, especially in patients with hepatic or renal disease; clofibrate is also associated with an increased incidence of gallstones. Cholestyramine binds bile acids, as well as oral anticoagulants, digitalis drugs, and thyroid hormones. Nicotinic acid causes peripheral vasodilation and probably should not be continued through the morning of surgery. Probucol (Lorelco) decreases the synthesis of apoprotein A1; its use is rarely associated with fetid perspiration and/or prolongation of the QT interval, and sudden death in animals. Lovastatin is a drug that blocks HMG CoA reductase, the rate-limiting enzyme of cholesterol synthesis.

Hypolipidemic conditions are rare diseases often associated with neuropathies, anemia, and renal failure. Although anesthetic experience with hypolipidemic conditions has been limited, some specific recommendations can be made: continuation of caloric intake and intravenous administration of protein hydralysates and glucose throughout the perioperative period.

Obesity

Twenty to 50 percent of adults in the United States weigh more than 20 percent above what is considered the optimum body weight for their height. The pathophysiologic consequences of obesity involve every major organ system. Many of the metabolic, hormonal, and physiologic changes associated with obesity (e.g., insulin resistance, decreased number of insulin receptors, and subsequent diabetes mellitus) can be induced by overfeeding normal subjects and can be reversed by weight reduction. Obesity itself, its complications, and its treatment have significance for the anesthesiologist. Being 30 percent overweight is associated with a 40 percent increase in the chance of dying from heart disease and with a 50 percent increase in the chance of dying from a stroke. Obesity is also associated with higher perioperative morbidity and mortality.[45]

Massively obese individuals with carbon dioxide retention are called pickwickian, alveolar hypoventilation being the hallmark of this condition. Other components of the pickwickian syndrome are somnolence, hypoxemia, failure of the right side of the heart, and secondary polycythemia. These patients often have right ventricular failure (also see Ch. 31 for monitoring considerations).

Although many conditions associated with obesity (diabetes, cholelithiasis, cirrhosis) contribute to morbidity, the main concerns for the anesthesiologist are derangements of the cardiopulmonary system.[46,47] Cardiac output must increase approximately 0.1 L/min to perfuse each kilogram of adipose tissue. As a result, obese patients often have hypertension, which can cause cardiomegaly and left ventricular failure. Care should be taken to use a blood pressure cuff of correct size when quantitating the degree of hypertension present.

The obese may have limited cardiac reserve and a poor tolerance for stress induced by hypotension, hypertension, tachycardia, or fluid overload associated with the preoperative period. Airway obstruction frequently occurs because of the abundant soft tissue in the upper airway. Functional residual capacity is reduced, as the weight of the torso and abdomen makes diaphragmatic excursions more difficult and more position-dependent. Thus, preoperative assessment should include not only history-taking and physical examination accentuating cardiopulmonary problems but also an electrocardiographic (ECG) examination (looking specifically for left or right ventricular hypertrophy, ischemia, and conduction defects). If obesity is severe, arterial blood gases should also be analyzed to quantitate the degree of hypoventilation and to aid in assessing the most appropriate time to extubate the trachea. More extensive pulmonary function tests and preoperative treatment of any treatable abnormality (such as infectious and bronchospastic components of pulmonary disease) may be indicated for the obese patient who smokes or has pulmonary symptoms (e.g., a chronic cough, sputum production, wheezing, shortness of breath at rest or on minor exertion).

Other features of obesity are of interest to the anesthesiologist as well. Obese patients have an increased volume and acidity of gastric juices preoperatively, perhaps indicating the wisdom of premedicating such patients with cimetidine, ranitidine, Bicitra, glycopyrrolate, and metoclopramide.[48,49] In addition, obese individuals may metabolize lipophilic drugs to a greater degree (and for longer periods) than their thin counterparts. More fluorine is produced from enflurane given to obese patients than to thin ones.[50] One would assume that responses to drugs stored in fat (e.g., narcotics, barbiturates, volatile anesthetics) would be prolonged in the obese. However, there is no evidence that use of the more soluble anesthetics delays recovery time in obese subjects.[51] Further, an increased incidence of wound infections, deep vein thromboses, and pulmonary emboli occurs; the last two probably should be guarded against with subcutaneous heparin and early ambulation.[52]

The anesthesiologist also needs to be aware of conditions caused by remedies to obesity. Drastic dieting can produce acidosis, hypokalemia, and hyperuricemia; protein hydrolysate liquid diets are associated with intractable ventricular arrhythmias.[53] These problems seem to have disappeared as the diets have changed from hydrolyzed collagen fasts to the presently used very low calorie diet.[54] Metabolic complications of jejunoileal bypass include hypokalemia, hypocalcemia, hypomagnesemia, anemia, renal stones, gout, and liver abnormalities. An attempt to reverse these abnormal conditions should be made prior to anesthesia and may consist of infusing solutions containing amino acids. Because of the high morbidity associated with jejunoileal bypass, this procedure has been supplanted by gastric plication or bypass surgery. However, long-term data about the chronic morbidity of these two procedures are not available.

Drug treatment for obesity also has implications for the anesthesiologist. Amphetamines (and probably mazindol) given acutely increase anesthetic requirements; by contrast, chronically administered amphetamines decrease anesthetic requirements (see the section on chronic drug therapy). Amphetamines may interfere with the action of vasoactive drugs given to treat hypotension or hypertension. Fenfluramine (a drug that inhibits the serotonergic system) may decrease both anesthetic requirement and blood pressure.

Anorexia Nervosa, Bulimarexia, and Starvation

Many endocrine and metabolic abnormalities occur in the patient with anorexia nervosa, a condition of starvation to the point of 40 percent loss of normal weight, hyperactivity, and a psychiatrically distorted body image. Many patients resort to impulsive behavior, including suicide attempts; intravenous drug usage is present to a much larger degree than in the general population. Acidosis, hypokalemia, hypocalcemia, hypomagnesemia, hypothermia, diabetes insipidus, and severe endocrine abnormalities mimicking panhypopituitarism need attention prior to anesthesia and surgery. Similar problems occur in bulimarexia, also termed bulimia, a condition that may be present in 50 percent of female college students.[55] As in severe protein deficiency (kwashiorkor), anorexia nervosa and bulimarexia may be accompanied by ECG alterations, including prolonged QT interval, AV block and other arrhythmias, sensitivity to epinephrine,[56] and cardiomyopathy.[55,57] Total depletion of body potassium makes addition of potassium to glucose solutions useful; however, fluid administration can precipitate pulmonary edema in these patients. Thus, invasive monitoring (radial artery and pulmonary artery catheterization) may be indicated for anorectic, bulimarexic, and malnurtured patients requiring emergency surgery. Elective surgery probably should be delayed until abnormalities are treated.

Hyperalimentation (Total Parenteral Nutrition) (Also See Ch. 73)

For patients receiving hyperalimentation (i.e., TPN) hypertonic glucose calories are concentrated in the normal daily fluid requirements in solutions containing protein hydrolysates, soybean emulsions (i.e., Intralipid), or synthetic amino acids. Major benefits of total parenteral nutrition (TPN) or enteral nutrition have been reported in fewer complications postoperatively and shorter hospital stays per patients scheduled to have no oral feeding for 7 days or who were malnourished preoperatively.[59,60] Starker and colleagues found that response to TPN, as monitored by serum albumin levels predicted postoperative outcome.[61] The group

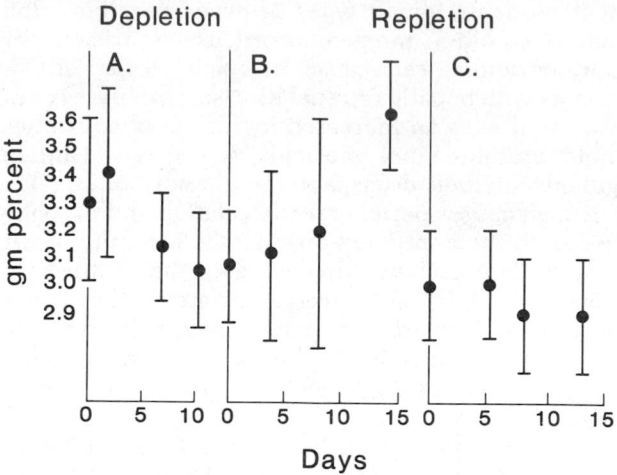

Fig. 25-2. (A–C) Variations in serum albumin levels during administration of hyperalimentation (repletion), predicted response, and outcome of surgery. Those patients who responded (Fig. B) to nutritional support with increased albumin levels had significantly better outcome than those whose albumin level did not increase (Fig. C). (See text for a more complete explanation.) (Redrawn from Starker et al.,[766] with permission.)

with a rise in serum albumin with TPN exhibited diuresis, weight loss, and fewer complications (1 of 15 patients) than the group that gained weight and had a fall in serum albumin (8 of 16 patients had 15 complications (Fig. 25–2). The major complications of hyperalimentation are sepsis and metabolic abnormalities. The central lines used for TPN require application of an absolutely aseptic technique and should not be used as an intravenous route for drug administration.

Major metabolic complications of TPN relate to deficiencies and to development of hyperosmolar states. Complications of hypertonic dextrose can develop if the patient has insufficient insulin (diabetes mellitus) to metabolize the sugar or if insulin resistance occurs (e.g., because of uremia, burns, or sepsis).[58]

Gradual decrease in the infusion rate of TPN prevents the hypoglycemia that can occur on abrupt discontinuance. Thus, the infusion rate of TPN should be decreased the night before anesthesia and surgery. The main reason for slowing or discontinuing TPN before anesthesia is to avoid intraoperative hyperosmolarity secondary to accidental rapid infusion of the solution or hypoglycemia if the infusion is discontinued because of the high levels of endogenous insulin and lower levels of glucose present in usual crystalloid solutions.[58] Hypophosphatemia is a particularly serious complication that results from the administration of phosphate-free or phosphate-depleted solutions for hyperalimentation. The low serum phosphate level causes shifts of the oxygen dissociation curve to the left. Thus, the resulting low 2,3-diphosphoglycerate and ATP levels mean that cardiac output must increase for oxygen delivery to remain the same. Hypophosphatemia of < 1.0 mg/dl blood may cause hemolytic anemia, cardiac failure, tachypnea, neurologic symptoms, seizures, and death. In addition, long-term TPN is associated with deficiencies in trace metals such as copper (refractory anemia), zinc (impaired wound healing), and magnesium. For these reason, I have adopted the following practices.[58] The infusion of TPN or enteral nutrition is reduced beginning the night before surgery, substituting 5 or 10 percent dextrose solution preoperatively. If serum glucose phosphate and potassium concentrations (measured preoperatively) are abnormal, they are restored to within normal limits. Strict asepsis is maintained. Conversely, one could continue infusing the TPN solution by using a pump system or enteral nutrition, strictly maintaining its normal rate and asepsis, administering all fluids through a different intravenous site, and performing a rapid sequence induction of anesthesia (for those who received enteral nutrition).

Adrenocortical Malfunction*

Three major classes of hormones—androgens, glucocorticoids, and mineralocorticoids—are secreted by the adrenal cortex.[62-65] A characteristic clinical syndrome is associated with excess or deficiency of each class. In addition, the widespread use of steroids may result in inability of the adrenal cortex to respond normally to the demands placed on it by surgical trauma and subsequent healing.[66-78] An anesthetic, etomidate, profoundly limits adrenal reserves. Thus, anesthesiologists frequently come into contact with abnormalities of adrenocortical function.

Controlled comparisons of perioperative management for individuals who have disorders of adrenal function are lacking.[64] However, a review of the possible pathophysiologic changes in the adrenal cortex and techniques for their management should enable us to improve the perioperative care of patients with adrenal abnormalities.

Physiologic Properties of Adrenocortical Hormones

Androgens

Androstenedione and dehydroepiandrosterone, weak androgens arising from the adrenal cortex,[79] constitute major sources of androgens in women. Excess secretion of androgen causes masculinization, pseudopuberty, or female pseudohemaphroditism. With some tumors, androgen is converted to an estrogenic substance, in which case feminization results.[79] No special anesthetic evaluation is needed for such patients. Some congenital enzyme defects that cause androgen abnormalities also result in glucocorticoid and mineralocorticoid abnormalities that should be evaluated prior to

surgery.[79] Most of these patients are treated with exogenous gluco- and mineralocorticoids and consequently need supplementation of these hormones perioperatively (see below).

Glucocorticoids

The principal glucocorticoid, cortisol, is an essential regulator of carbohydrate, protein, lipid, and nucleic acid metabolism.[80] Cortisol is believed to exert its biologic effects through a sequence of steps initiated by hormone binding to stereospecific, intracellular cytoplasmic receptors. This bound complex stimulates nuclear transcription of specific messenger RNAs (mRNAs). These mRNAs are then translated to give rise to proteins that mediate the ultimate effects of hormones.[80]

Most cortisol is bound to corticosterone-binding globulin (CBG, transcortin). It is the relatively small amounts of unbound cortisol that enter cells to induce actions or to be metabolized. Conditions that induce changes in the amount of CBG include liver disease and nephrotic syndrome, both of which result in decreased circulating levels of CBG, and estrogen administration and pregnancy, which result in increased CBG production. Total serum cortisol levels may become elevated or depressed under these conditions that alter the amount of bound cortisol, and yet the unbound, active form of cortisol is present in normal amounts. The most accurate measure of cortisol activity is the level of urinary cortisol, that is, the amount of unbound, active cortisol filtered by the kidney.

The serum half-life of cortisol is 80 to 110 minutes.[71] However, since cortisol acts through intracellular receptors, pharmacokinetics based on serum levels is not a good indicator of cortisol activity. After a single dose of glucocorticoid, serum glucose is elevated for 12 to 24 hours; improvements in pulmonary function in patients with bronchial asthma can still be measured 24 hours after glucocorticoid administration.[71,81] Treatment schedules for glucocorticoid replacement are based, therefore, not on the measured serum half-life but on the well-documented, prolonged end-organ effect of these steroids. Hospitalized patients requiring chronic glucocorticoid replacement therapy are usually treated twice daily, with a slightly higher dose given in the morning than in the evening to stimulate the normal diurnal variations in cortisol levels.[75] For patients who require parenteral "steroid coverage" during and after surgery (see later paragraphs), administration of glucocorticoid every 8 to 12 hours is appropriate.[62,70] Relative potencies of glucocorticoids are listed in Table 25 – 2. Cortisol is inactivated primarily in the liver and is excreted as 17-hydroxycorticosteroid. Cortisol is also filtered and excreted unchanged into the urine.

The synthetic glucocorticoids vary in their binding specificity in a dose-related manner. When given in supraphysiologic doses (more than 30 mg/day), cortisol and cortisone bind to mineralocorticoid receptor sites and cause salt and water retention and loss of potassium and hydrogen ions.[71,82] When these steroids are administered in maintenance doses of 30 mg/day or less, patients require a specific mineralocorticoid for electrolyte and volume homeostasis.[71] Many other steroids do not bind to mineralocorticoid receptors, even at high doses, and have no mineralocorticoid effect (see Table 25-2).[71]

Secretion of glucocorticoids is regulated by pituitary ACTH. ACTH is synthesized from a precursor molecule (preopiomelanocortin) that breaks down to form an endorphin (β-lipotropin) and ACTH.[83] Episodic secretion of ACTH has a diurnal rhythm normally greatest during the early morning hours and is regulated at least in part by light-dark cycles. Its secretion is stimulated by release of corticortropin-releasing hormone (CRF) from the hypothalamus.[62,63,82,83] (An abnormality in the diurnal rhythm of corticoid secretion has been implicated as a cause of "jet lag.") Cortisol and other glucocorticoids exert negative feedback at both pituitary and hypothalamic levels to inhibit secretion of ACTH and CRF.[62,63,82,83]

Mineralocorticoids

Aldosterone, the major mineralocorticoid secreted in humans, comes from the zona glomerulosa of the adrenal cortex and causes reabsorption of sodium and secretion of potassium and hydrogen ions, thereby contributing to electrolyte and volume homeostasis.[62,63,84] This action is most prominent in the distal renal tubule but also occurs in salivary and sweat glands. The major regulator of aldosterone secretion is the renin-angiotensin system. Juxtaglomerular cells in the cuff of the renal arterioles are sensitive to decreased renal perfusion pressure or volume and, consequently, secrete renin.[84] Renin splits the precursor angiotensinogen (from the liver) into angiotensin I, which is further converted by a converting enzyme, primarily in lung, to angiotensin II. Mineralocorticoid secretion is increased by increased angiotensin II, increased potas-

sium concentration, and, to a lesser degree, ACTH.[62,63,84]

Adrenocortical Hormone Excess

Glucocorticoid Excess

Glucocorticoid excess (Cushing syndrome) resulting from either endogenous oversecretion or chronic treatment with high-dose glucocorticoids produces a moon-faced, plethoric individual having a centripetal distribution of fat (truncal obesity and skinny extremities), thin skin, easy bruising, and striae. Muscle wasting is common, but the heart and diaphragm are usually spared. These patients often have osteopenia due to decreased formation of bone matrix and impaired absorption of calcium. Fluid retention and hypertension are common; hypertension (because of increases in renin substrate and vascular reactivity caused by glucocorticoid) is present. Such patients may also have hyperglycemia and even diabetes mellitus resulting from inhibition of peripheral use of glucose, as well as anti-insulin action and concomitant stimulation of gluconeogenesis.[62,63,85]

The most common cause of Cushing syndrome is administration of glucocorticoids for such conditions as arthritis, asthma, and allergies.[62,64] In such conditions, the adrenal glands atrophy and cannot respond to stressful situations (e.g., the perioperative period) by secreting more steroid. Thus, additional glucocorticoids may be required perioperatively (see the section, *The Patient Taking Steroids for Other Reasons*). Spontaneous Cushing syndrome may be caused by pituitary production of ACTH (60 to 70 percent of all spontaneous cases), which is usually associated with pituitary microadenoma, or nonendocrine ectopic ACTH production (principally by tumors of the lung, pancreas, or thymus).[62,63,85] Ten to 20 percent of cases of spontaneous Cushing syndrome are caused by an ACTH-independent process, either an adrenal adenoma or carcinoma.

Special preoperative considerations for patients having Cushing syndrome include regulating diabetes and hypertension and ensuring that intravascular fluid volume and electrolyte concentrations are normal. Ectopic ACTH production may cause marked hypokalemic alkalosis.[62-64]. Treatment with the aldosterone antagonist spironolactone will stop the potassium loss and help mobilize excess fluid. Because of the high incidence of severe osteopenia and the risk of fractures, meticulous attention to patient positioning is necessary.[64] In addition, glucocorticoids are lympholytic and immunosuppressive, increasing the patient's susceptibility to infection.[86-88] The tensile strength of healing wounds decreases in the presence of glucocorticoids,[86] an effect at least partially reversed by topical administration of vitamin A.[86]

Specific considerations pertain to the surgical approach for each cause of Cushing syndrome. For example, nearly three-fourths of the cases of spontaneous

TABLE 25-2. The Relative Potency and Equivalent Doses for Commonly Used Glucocorticoids

Steroids	Relative Glucocorticoid Potency[a]	Equivalent Glucocorticoid Dose (mg)
Short-acting		
Cortisol (hydrocortisone)	1	20
Cortisone	0.8	25
Prednisone	4	5
Prednisolone	4	5
Methylprednisolone	5	4
Intermediate-acting		
Triamcinolone	5	4
Long-acting		
Betamethasone	25	0.60
Dexamethasone	30	0.75

[a] Data from Axelrod.[71]

Cushing disease result from a pituitary adenoma that secretes ACTH.[85] Our perioperative treatment for patients who have Cushing disease and a pituitary microadenoma differs from that for patients who have a pituitary adenoma associated with amenorrhea and galactorrhea.[85] The Cushing patient tends to bleed more easily and (on the basis of anecdotal evidence) tends to have a higher central venous pressure (CVP). Thus, during trans-sphenoidal tumor resection in such patients, I routinely monitor CVP and maintain it in the low end of the normal range. Such monitoring is needed only infrequently in other cases of trans-sphenoidal resection of microadenoma.

Ten to 15 percent of patients with Cushing syndrome have adrenal overproduction of glucocorticoids from an adrenal adenoma or carcinoma.[64] If either unilateral or bilateral adrenal resection is planned, I normally begin administering glucocorticoids at the start of tumor resectioning. Although no definitive studies exist, I normally give 100 mg of hydrocortisone hemisuccinate or hydrocortisone phosphate every 8 to 12 hours intravenously. I reduce this amount over 3 to 6 days until a maintenance dose is reached. Beginning on day 3, I also give 9α-fluorocortisol (a mineralocorticoid), 0.05 to 0.1 mg/day. In certain patients, both steroids may require several adjustments.[62-63] This therapy is continued in the patient who has undergone bilateral resection. In the patient who has undergone unilateral adrenal resection, therapy is individualized according to the status of the remaining adrenal gland. At the University of California, San Francisco (UCSF), the incidence of pneumothorax in adrenal resection approaches 20 percent; its diagnosis is sought and treatment begun before the wound is closed.

Bilateral adrenalectomy with Cushing syndrome has a high incidence of postoperative complications and a perioperative mortality rate of 5 to 10 percent; it often results in permanent mineralocorticoid and glucocorticoid deficiency.[89] Ten percent of patients with Cushing syndrome who undergo adrenalectomy have an undiagnosed pituitary tumor. After reduction of high levels of cortisol by adrenalectomy, the pituitary tumor enlarges.[85] These pituitary tumors are potentially invasive and may produce large amounts of ACTH and melanocyte-stimulating hormone (MSH), thereby increasing pigmentation.[62,63,85]

Adrenal adenomas are usually treated surgically, and often the contralateral gland resumes functioning after several months. Frequently, however, the effects of carcinomas are not cured by surgery. In such cases, administration of inhibitors of steroid synthesis such as metyrapone or o,p'-DDD[2,2 bis (2-chlorophenyl-4-chlorophenyl)-1,1-dichloroethane] may ameliorate some symptoms but may not improve survival. These drugs and the aldosterone antagonist spironolactone may aid in reducing symptoms in the case of ectopic ACTH secretion if the primary tumor proves unresectable. Patients given these adrenal suppressants are also placed on chronic glucocorticoid replacement therapy (that is, the goal of therapy is complete adrenal suppression). These patients should be considered to have suppressed adrenal function, and glucocorticoid replacement should be increased perioperatively.

Mineralocorticoid Excess

Excess mineralocorticoid activity (common with glucocorticoid excess, since most glucocorticoids have some mineralocorticoid properties) leads to potassium depletion, sodium retention, muscle weakness, hypertension, tetany, polyuria, inability to concentrate urine, and hypokalemic alkalosis.[62,90] These symptoms constitute primary hyperaldosteronism, or Conn syndrome (a cause of low-renin hypertension, as renin secretion is inhibited by the effects of the high levels of aldosterone).

Primary hyperaldosteronism is present in 0.5 to 1 percent of hypertensive patients who have no other known cause of hypertension.[90] Primary hyperaldosteronism most often results from unilateral adenoma, although 25 to 40 percent of patients have been found to have bilateral adrenal hyperplasia. Intravascular fluid volume, electrolyte concentrations, and renal function should be restored to within normal limits preoperatively by administering the aldosterone antagonist spironolactone. The effects of spironolactone are slow in onset and increase for 1 to 2 weeks.[90] A patient having a serum potassium level of 2.9 mEq/L may have a deficit of body potassium of as little as 40 mEq or as much as 400 mEq.[91-94] Frequently, at least 24 hours is required to restore potassium equilibrium.[91-94] A normal serum potassium level does not necessarily imply correction of a total body deficit of potassium. In addition, patients with Conn syndrome have a high incidence of hypertension and ischemic heart disease; hemodynamic monitoring should be appropriate for the degree of cardiovascular impairment.[95] A retrospective anecdotal study indicated that intraoperative hemodynamic status was more stable when blood pressure and electrolytes were controlled preoperatively with spironolactone than when other antihypertensive drugs were used.[65] However, the efficacy of optimizing the perioperative status of patients with disorders of glucocorticoid or mineralocorticoid secretion has not been clearly established. I have assumed that gradual restoration of a normal condition is good medicine and therefore decreases perioperative morbidity and mortality.

Adrenocortical Hormone Deficiency

Glucocorticoid Deficiency

Withdrawal of steroids or suppression of synthesis by steroid therapy is the leading cause of underproduction of corticosteroids.[64] The management of this type of glucocorticoid deficiency is discussed in the section, *The Patient Taking Steroids for Other Reasons.* Other causes of adrenocortical insufficiency include defects in ACTH secretion and destruction of the adrenal gland by cancer, tuberculosis, hemorrhage, or an autoimmune mechanism; some forms of congenital adrenal hyperplasia (see previous discussion); and administration of cytotoxic drugs.

Primary adrenal insufficiency (Addison's disease) is caused by a local process within the adrenal gland that leads to destruction of all zones of the cortex and causes both glucocorticoid and mineralocorticoid deficiency if the insufficiency is bilateral. Autoimmune disease is the most common cause of primary (nonexogenous) bilateral ACTH deficiency.

Autoimmune destruction of the adrenals may be associated with other autoimmune disorders, such as Hashimoto's thyroiditis. Enzymatic defects in cortisol synthesis also cause glucocorticoid insufficiency, compensatory elevations of ACTH, and congenital adrenal hyperplasia.[79] Because adrenal insufficiency usually develops slowly, such patients develop marked pigmentation (from excess ACTH trying to stimulate an unproductive adrenal gland) and cardiopenia (apparently secondary to chronic hypotension).[63,64]

Secondary adrenal insufficiency occurs when ACTH secretion is deficient, often because of a pituitary or hypothalamic tumor. Treatment of pituitary tumors by surgery or radiation may result in hypopituitarism and consequent adrenal failure.[62-64]

If glucocorticoid-deficient patients are not stressed, they usually have no perioperative problems. However, acute adrenal crisis (Addisonian crisis) can occur when even a minor stress (for example, upper respiratory infection) is present.[63,95,96] In the preparation of such a patient for anesthesia and surgery, hypovolemia, hyperkalemia, and hyponatremia should be treated.[74] Since these patients cannot respond to stressful situations, we traditionally recommended that they be given a maximum stress dose of glucocorticoids (about 300 mg hydrocortisone/70 kg body weight/day) perioperatively. Symreng and colleagues[69] gave 25 mg of hydrocortisone phosphate IV to adults at the start of the operative procedure, followed by 100 mg IV over the next 24 hours. Since using the minimum drug dose that will cause an appropriate effect is desirable, this latter regimen seems attractive. Such a regimen has not been used widely enough to show whether it will be as successful as the regimen with maximum doses (see the section, *The Patient Taking Steroids for Other Reasons*). However, evidence is accumulating that less steroid supplementation does not cause problems (see later discussion), and we now recommend giving 100 mg of hydrocortisone phosphate intravenously every 12 hours.[64,70]

Mineralocorticoid Deficiency

Hypoaldosteronism, a less common condition,[97] can be congenital or can occur after unilateral adrenalectomy or prolonged administration of heparin. It can also be a consequence of long-standing diabetes and renal failure. Nonsteroidal inhibitors of prostaglandin synthesis may also inhibit renin release and exacerbate this condition in patients who have renal insufficiency.[97,98] Plasma renin activity levels are below normal and fail to increase appropriately in response to sodium restriction or diuretic drugs. Most symptoms are caused by hyperkalemic acidosis rather than hypovolemia; in fact, some patients are hypertensive. These patients can have severe hyperkalemia, hyponatremia, and myocardial conduction defects.[97] These defects can be treated successfully by administering mineralocorticoids (9α-fluorocortisol, 0.05 to 0.1 mg/day) preoperatively.[97] Doses must be carefully titrated and monitored to avoid an increase in hypertension.

The Patient Taking Steroids for Other Reasons

Perioperative Stress and the Need for Corticoid Supplementation

Many experimental studies and other (mostly anecdotal) reports concerning the adrenal responses of normal patients to the perioperative period and responses of patients taking steroids for other diseases indicate the following:

1. Perioperative stress relates to the degree of trauma and the depth of anesthesia. Deep general or regional anesthesia causes the usual intraoperative glucocorticoid surge to be postponed to the postoperative period.[99-101]
2. Few patients who have suppressed adrenal function have perioperative cardiovascular problems if they do not receive supplemental steroids perioperatively.[62,67-78]
3. Occasionally, a patient who chronically takes steroids becomes hypotensive perioperatively, but this event has only rarely been documented sufficiently to implicate glucocorticoid or mineralocorticoid deficiency as the cause.[62,67-78]
4. Although it occurs rarely, acute adrenal insufficiency can be a life-threatening event.[62,67-78]
5. There is little risk in giving these patients high-dose steroid coverage perioperatively.[69,70,96]

In a recent well-controlled study of glucocorticoid replacement in primates, the investigators clearly defined the life-threatening events that can be associated with inadequate perioperative corticosteroid replacement.[70] This study further defined the physiologic and hemodynamic consequences of inadequate cortisol replacement, and the authors suggest an alternative dose regimen that if substantiated, will alter current management methods and possibly improve patient safety. In this study, adrenalectomized primates and sham-operated controls were maintained on physiologic doses of steroids for 4 months. The animals were then randomized to receive subphysiologic (one-tenth the normal cortisol production), physiologic, and supraphysiologic (10 times the normal cortisol production) doses of cortisol for 4 days preceding abdominal surgery (cholecystectomy). Hemodynamic variables were measured with arterial and pulmonary-artery catheters. The animals were maintained on their randomized dosage schedules during and after surgery. The group receiving subphysiologic doses of steroid perioperatively had a significant increase in postoperative mortality. The death rates in the physiologic and supraphysiologic replacement groups were the same and did not differ from that for sham-operated controls. Death in the subphysiologic replacement group was related to severe hypotension associated with a significant decrease in systemic vascular resistance (SVR) and a reduced left ventricular stroke work index (LVSWI). The filling pressures of the heart were unchanged compared to those in control animals. There was, therefore, no evidence of hypovolemia or severe congestive heart failure. Despite the low SVR, the animals did not become tachycardic. All of these responses are compatible with the previously documented interaction of glucocorticoids and catecholamines, suggesting that glucocorticoids mediate catecholamine-induced increases in cardiac contractility and maintenance of vascular tone.[80]

The investigators used a sensitive measure of wound healing by studying hydroxyproline accumulation. All treatment groups, including that which received supraphysiologic doses of glucocorticoids, had the same capacity for wound healing. Furthermore, there were no adverse metabolic consequences of supraphysiologic corticosteroid doses given perioperatively.

This well-conducted study confirms several "old wives' tales" concerning patients who have inadequate adrenal function, either resulting from underlying disease or secondary to administration of exogenous steroids. Inadequate replacement of corticosteroids perioperatively can lead to Addisonian crisis and death. Administration of supraphysiologic doses of steroids for a short time perioperatively caused no discernible complications. However, as will be discussed later, there are at least theoretical negative consequences when large doses of steroids are given. It is clear that inadequate corticosteroid coverage can cause death. What is not so clear is what dose of steroid for replacement therapy should be recommended. The authors of the previously discussed study on monkeys were reluctant to recommend simple physiologic steroid replacement doses for human patients perioperatively. We

agree that a prospective, randomized double-blind trial in patients receiving physiologic doses of steroids is needed before current recommendations are modified.[69,70] In any case, we never supplement perioperatively with a dose lower than that which the patient has already been receiving.[71]

Which patients definitely need supplementation? If in doubt, how can one determine a patient's need for supplementation with glucocorticoids? Since the risk is low, I normally provide supplementation for any patient who has received steroids within a year.[66-87] Data indicate that topical application of steroids (even without use of occlusive dressings) can suppress normal adrenal responses for as long as 9 months to 1 year (Table 25-3).[66,71]

How can one determine when adrenal responsiveness has returned to normal? The morning plasma cortisol level does not reveal whether the adrenal cortex has recovered sufficiently to ensure that cortisol secretion will increase adequately to meet the demands of stress.[102] Inducing hypoglycemia with insulin has been advocated as a sensitive test of pituitary-adrenal competence but is impractical and probably a more dangerous practice than simply administering glucocorticoids.[102] If the plasma cortisol concentration is measured during acute stress, a value of $>25 \mu g/dl$ assuredly (and a value of $>15 \mu g/dl$ probably) indicates normal pituitary-adrenal responsiveness. In another test of pituitary-adrenal sufficiency, the baseline plasma cortisol level is determined. Then, 250 μg of synthetic ACTH (cosyntropin) is given, and plasma cortisol is measured 30 to 60 minutes later.[73] An increase in plasma cortisol of 6 to 20 $\mu g/dl$ or more is normal.[103] A normal response indicates recovery of pituitary-adrenal axis function. A lesser response usually indicates pituitary-adrenal insufficiency, possibly requiring perioperative supplementation with steroids.

Usually laboratory data defining pituitary-adrenal adequacy are not available before surgery. However, rather than delay surgery or test most patients, I assume that any patient who has taken steroids at any time in the preceding year has suppressed pituitary-adrenal functioning and will require perioperative supplementation.

Under perioperative conditions, the adrenal glands secrete 116 to 185 mg of cortisol daily.[101] Under maximum stress, they may secrete 200 to 500 mg/day.[101] A

TABLE 25-3. Recovery of Hypothalamic-Pituitary Adrenal Function after Withdrawal of Steroids

Recovery Time (months)	Plasma 17-Hydroxycorticoid Values	Plasma ACTH Values	Adrenal Response to Exogenous ACTH	Response to Metyrapone
1	Low[a]	Low	Low	Low
2–5	Low	High[b]	Low	Low
6–9	Normal	Normal	Low	Low
>9	Normal	Normal	Normal	Normal

[a] Various subjective manifestations of mild adrenal insufficiency occur during this stage.
[b] The diurnal rhythm of the plasma concentrations is qualitatively normal during this stage.
(Data from Graber et al.[73])

good correlation exists between the severity and duration of the operation and the response of adrenal gland.[101] Major surgery would be represented by procedures such as colectomy and minor surgery by procedures such as herniorrhaphy. In one study of 20 patients during major surgery, the mean maximal concentration of cortisol in plasma was 47 μg/dl (range 22 to 75 μg/dl). Values remained above 26 μg/dl for a maximum of 72 hours after surgery. During minor surgery, the mean maximal concentration of cortisol in plasma was 28 μg/dl (range 10 to 44 μg/dl).

Although the precise amount required has not been established, I usually administer intravenously the maximum amount of glucocorticoid that the body manufactures in response to a maximal stress (i.e., approximately 200 mg/day of hydrocortisone phosphate/ 70 kg of body weight.[69,70,99,100] For minor surgical procedures, I usually give hydrocortisone phosphate intravenously, 100 mg/day/70 kg body weight. Unless infection or some other perioperative complication develops, I decrease this dose by approximately 25 percent a day until oral intake can be resumed. At this point, the usual maintenance dose of glucocorticoids can be employed.

Risks of Supplementation

Rare potential risks of perioperative supplementation with steroids include aggravation of hypertension, fluid retention, inducement of stress ulcers, and psychiatric disturbance. Although data are not available to assess the incidences of these risks, two common complications of short-term perioperative supplementation with glucocorticoids are described in the literature: abnormal wound healing and increased rate of infections.[67–78,83–88,104–105] This evidence is inconclusive, however, as it relates to acute glucocorticoid administration and not to chronic administration of glucocorticoids with increased doses at times of stress. Ehrlich and Hunt[86] found that moderate to large doses of steroids exerted their morphologic effects best within 3 days of injury. These workers postulated that the inhibition of the early inflammatory process by steroids after wounding was responsible for delayed healing. Vitamin A was found to protect somewhat against delayed healing, presumably because of its effect on stabilizing lysosomes.[86] In contrast to these studies that suggest a deleterious effect of perioperative glucocorticoid administration on wound healing in rats, a recent study of primates suggests that high doses of glucocorticoid, administered perioperatively, did not impair sensitive measures of wound healing.[70] Other data give us no better insight into these problems.[67–78,83–87] Such data are not conclusive regarding a short-term increase in supplementation. However, an overall assessment of these results suggests that short-term perioperative supplementation with steroids has a small but definite deleterious effect on wound healing that is perhaps partially reversed by topical administration of vitamin A.

Information regarding the risk of infection from peri-operative supplementation with glucocorticoids is also unclear. Winstone and Brook[106] reported four cases of septicemia among 18 surgical patients given perioperative supplementation with glucocorticoids. No similar complications occurred in 17 others who were also taking glucocorticoids but who were not given perioperative supplementation. In a controlled study of 100 patients given perioperative supplementation with glucocorticoids, 11 wound infections occurred in the group treated with steroids, and only 1 occurred in the control group.[104] Test subjects and controls were not matched for underlying disease. By contrast, Jensen and Elb[105] found no change in the incidence of wound infections or of other infections in an uncontrolled series of 419 patients subjected to surgery and perioperative supplementation with glucocorticoids. Oh and Patterson[96] found only one minor suture abscess in 17 steroid-dependent asthmatic patients undergoing 21 surgical procedures. Thus, although data indicate that the risk of infection to the patient chronically taking steroids is real, such data are inadequate to conclude that perioperative supplementation with steroids increases that risk.

Adrenal Cortex Function in the Elderly (Also See Ch. 62)

The adrenal gland shows a marked decline in androgen production with age. There is a progressive reduction in adrenal androgen production in individuals more than 40 years old.[107] This lack of androgen activity has no known implications for anesthesia.

Plasma levels of cortisol are unaffected by increasing age. Levels of corticosterone-binding globulin are also unaffected by age; this suggests that a normal fraction of free cortisol (1 to 5 percent) is present in elderly patients. Several investigators have noted a progressively impaired ability of the aged patient to metabolize and excrete glucocorticoids. In normal elderly individuals, the quantity of 17-hydroxycorticosteroids excreted is reduced by one-half by the seventh decade. This undoubtedly reflects reduced renal function that occurs with aging. When excretion of cortisol metabolites is expressed as a function of creatinine clearance, the age difference disappears. Further reductions in cortisol clearance may be due to impaired hepatic metabolism of circulating cortisol.

The rate of secretion of cortisol is decreased by 30 percent in the elderly. This is an appropriate compensatory mechanism for maintaining a normal level of cortisol in the face of its decreased hepatic and renal clearance. It is important to the anesthesiologist that the reduced cortisol production can be overcome during periods of stress and that the elderly display an entirely normal adrenal response to administration of ACTH and to stresses such as hypoglycemia.

Both under- and overproduction of glucocorticoids are generally considered diseases of younger individuals. The highest incidence of Cushing disease, of either pituitary or adrenal origin, occurs during the third decade of life. The most common cause of spontaneous Cushing disease is benign pituitary adenoma.[85] However, in patients more than 60 years old who develop Cushing disease, the most likely cause is adrenal carcinoma or ectopic ACTH production from tumors usually located in the lung, pancreas, or thymus.

Effect of Etomidate on Adrenal Function (Also See Ch. 9)

It has been demonstrated repeatedly that even a single dose of etomidate, used for induction of anesthesia, causes suppression of adrenal function.[108] The clinical significance of adrenal suppression by etomidate is unknown, but there is justifiable concern over its continued use without steroid supplementation.

Etomidate is an imidazole sedative-hypnotic that induces rapid loss of consciousness with minimal cardiovascular depression even in compromised patients. Etomidate has been administered in two clinical settings — as a bolus for induction of anesthesia and as a continuous infusion for prolonged sedation in an ICU setting. The pattern of adrenal suppression appears to be dose- and time-related, and it differs with the duration of administration.[107]

Etomidate inhibits two essential adrenocortical enzymes, 11 β-hydroxylase and cholesterol side-chain cleavage enzyme, in rats and in humans.[109] We believe that it is important to clarify the difference between the adrenal suppression by etomidate and the stated goal of several anesthesiologists to provide stress-free anesthesia. It would appear that providing a level of anesthesia that prevents grimacing, sweating, extreme elevations of blood pressure and heart rate, and an outpouring of the neurohumoral mediators of stress is evidence that we have adequately depressed CNS function and protected our patients from some of the unwanted side effects of surgery. This goal is different from the inhibition of peripheral adrenocortical enzymes of etomidate that occurs as an unwanted and possibly harmful side effect of the drug.

Thus, it has been documented that adrenal reserve is compromised for at least 24 hours after a single induction dose of etomidate in most patients.[110] Should hypotension or electrolyte abnormalities associated with adrenal insufficiency (hyponatremia and hyperkalemia) occur in a patient who has recently received etomidate, we agree with previous suggestions[108,109] that corticosteroids should be administered in stress doses (for example, cortisol, 100 mg every 12 hours) and be tapered as noted in the section, *The Patient Taking Steroids for Other Reasons.*

Adrenal Medullary Sympathetic Hormone Excess: Pheochromocytoma

Fewer than 0.1 percent of all cases of hypertension are caused by pheochromocytomas, catecholamine-producing tumors derived from chromaffin tissue. Nevertheless, these tumors are clearly important to the anesthetist, since 25 to 50 percent of hospital deaths in patients with pheochromocytomas occur during induction of anesthesia or during operative procedures for other causes.[111] Although usually found in the adrenal medulla, these vascular tumors can occur anywhere, such as in the right atrium, the spleen, the broad ligament of the ovary, or the organs of Zucherkandl at the bifurcation of the aorta. Malignant spread, which occurs in fewer than 15 percent of pheochromocytomas, usually proceeds to venous and lymphatic channels with a predisposition for the liver. Occasionally the occurrence of this tumor is familial and/or part of the pluriglandular-neoplastic syndrome known as multiple endocrine adenoma-type IIa (consisting of medullary carcinoma of the thyroid, and parathyroid adenoma or hyperplasia and pheochromocytomas) or type IIb (consisting of medullary carcinoma of the thyroid, marfanoid appearance, mucosal neuromas, and pheochromocytomas) as an autosomal dominant trait. Often bilateral tumors are found in the familial form. Localization of tumors can be done with MRI or CT scans, MIBG nuclear scanning, ultrasonography, or IVP studies (in decreasing order of combined sensitivity and specificity).

Symptoms and signs that may be solicited preoperatively and that are suggestive of pheochromocytoma are excessive sweating; headache; hypertension; orthostatic hypotension; previous hypertensive or dysrhythmic response to induction of anesthesia or to abdominal examination; paroxysmal attacks of sweating, headache, tachycardia, and hypertension; glucose intolerance; polycythemia; weight loss; and psychological abnormalities. Despite more than 2,000 articles in the literature about pheochromocytomas, little is known about what factors in care affect perioperative morbidity.[112-115]

Although no controlled, randomized, prospective clinical studies have studied the value of preoperative use of adrenergic receptor-blocking drugs, the use of such drugs is generally recommended before surgery. These drugs probably reduce the complications of hypertensive crisis, the wide blood pressure fluctuations during manipulation of the tumor (especially until venous drainage is obliterated), and the myocardial dysfunction that occur perioperatively. The reduction in mortality associated with resection of pheochromocytoma from 40 to 60 percent to the current 0 to 6 percent occurred when α-adrenergic receptor blockade was introduced as preoperative preparatory therapy for such patients (Table 25–4).[114]

α-Adrenergic receptor blockade with prazosin or phenoxybenzamine restores plasma volume by counteracting the vasoconstrictive effects of high levels of catecholamines. This reexpansion of fluid volume is often followed by a decrease in hematocrit. Because some patients may be very sensitive to the effects of phenoxybenzamine, it should initially be given in doses of 20 to 30 mg/70 kg orally once or twice a day. Most patients usually require 60 to 250 mg/day. Efficacy of therapy should be judged by a reduction in symptoms (especially sweating) and a stabilization of blood pres-

TABLE 25-4. Preoperative Mortality Associated with Resectioning of Pheochromocytoma

Year of Series	Study	Mortality (%)	No. Patients In Series
1951	Apgar (review)	45	91
1951	Apgar	33	12
1963	Stackpole	13	100
Earlier than 1960	Mayo Clinic	0–26	101 (?)
Later than 1960	Mayo Clinic	2.9 (?)	44 (?)
Earlier than 1960	Modlin (without α blockade)	18	17
Later than 1967	Modlin (with α blockade)	2	41
1976	Scott	3	33
1976–1983	Roizen	0	36

(Data abstracted from studies discussed in Roizen et al.[114])

sure. In patients who have carbohydrate intolerance because of inhibition of insulin release mediated by α-adrenergic receptor stimulation, α-adrenergic receptor blockade may reduce fasting blood sugar levels. In patients who exhibit ST-T changes on ECG, long-term preoperative α-adrenergic receptor blockade (1 to 6 months) has been shown to result in ECG and clinical resolution of catecholamine-induced myocarditis.[113-115]

β-Adrenergic receptor blockade with propranolol is suggested for patients who have persistent dysrhythmias or tachycardia,[112-116] because these conditions can be precipitated or aggravated by α-adrenergic receptor blockade. β-adrenergic receptor blockade should not be used without concomitant α-adrenergic receptor blockade, lest the vasoconstrictive effects of the latter go unopposed, thereby increasing the risk of dangerous hypertension.

The optimal duration of preoperative therapy with phenoxybenzamine has not been studied. Most patients require 10 to 14 days, as judged by the time needed to stabilize blood pressure and to ameliorate symptoms. On the basis of my experience, this is a minimal period of time.[113,114,116] Since the tumor spreads slowly, little is lost by waiting until medical therapy has optimized the patient's preoperative condition. Accordingly, the following criteria are recommended:

1. No in-hospital blood pressure reading higher than 165/90 mmHg should be evident for 48 hours before surgery. We often measure arterial blood pressure for 1 hour in a stressful environment (our postanesthesia care unit) every minute. If no blood pressure reading is greater than 165/90, then this criterion is considered satisfied.
2. Orthostatic hypotension should be present, but blood pressure on standing should not be lower than 80/45 mmHg.
3. The ECG should be free of ST-T changes.
4. No more than one premature ventricular contraction should be present every 5 minutes.

Other drugs, including prazocin and calcium chan-

nel blocking drugs, have also been used to achieve suitable degrees of α-adrenergic blockade prior to surgery.

Although specific anesthetic drugs have been recommended, I believe that optimal preoperative preparation, a gentle induction of anesthesia, and good communication between surgeon and anesthesiologist are most important. Virtually all anesthetic agents and techniques (including isoflurane, sufentanil, fentanyl, and regional anesthesia) have been used with success. In fact, all agents studied are associated with a high rate of transient intraoperative arrhythmias (Table 25-5).[113] Because of ease of use, I prefer to give phenylephrine hydrochloride (Neo-Synephrine) or dopamine for hypotension and nitroprusside for hypertension. Phentolamine (Regitine) has too long an onset and duration of action. Once the venous supply is secured, and if intravascular volume is normal (as measured by pulmonary wedge pressure), normal blood pressure usually results. However, some patients become hypotensive, occasionally requiring massive infusions of catecholamines. On rare occasions, patients remain hypertensive intraoperatively. Postoperatively, about 50 percent remain hypertensive for 1 to 3 days—and initially have markedly elevated but declining plasma catecholamine levels—at which time all but 25 percent become normotensive. It is important to interview other family members and perhaps advise them to inform their future anesthetist about the potential for such familial disease.

Hypofunction or Aberration in Function of the Sympathetic Nervous System (Dysautonomia)

Disorders of the sympathetic nervous system include Shy-Drager syndrome, Riley-Day syndrome, Lesch-Nyhan syndrome, Gill familia dysautonomia, diabetic dysautonomia, and the dysautonomia of spinal cord transection.

Although individuals can function well without an adrenal medulla,[117] a deficient peripheral sympathetic nervous system occurring late in life poses major problems for many facets of life[118-130]; nevertheless, a perioperative sympathectomy or its equivalent has been recommended by some.[131-142] One of the main functions of the sympathetic nervous system appears to be the regulation of blood pressure and of intravascular fluid volume during changing of body position. Common features of all the syndromes of hypofunctioning of the sympathetic nervous system are orthostatic hypotension and decreased beat-to-beat variability in heart rate. These conditions can be caused by deficient intravascular volume, deficient baroreceptor function (as also occurs in carotid artery disease[143a]), abnormalities in CNS function (as in Wernicke or Shy-Drager syndrome[119]), deficient neuronal stores of norepinephrine (as in idiopathic orthostatic hypotension[120] and diabetes[13]), or deficient release of norepinephrine (as in traumatic spinal cord injury[117,118]). These patients may have an increased number of available adrenergic re-

TABLE 25-5. Incidence of Perioperative Complications in a Randomized Study of Patients Undergoing Resectioning of Pheochromocytoma Under One of Four Anesthetic Techniques

	Anesthetic[a]			
	Enflurane (6)	Halothane (6)	Droperiodol and Fentanyl (7)	Regional (5)
Ventricular tachycardia				
Needing no treatment	5	5	6	5
Needing treatment	0	1	1	0
Vasodilator needed				
Intraoperatively	6	6	7	5
Postoperatively	0	1[b]	1[b]	0
Vasopressor needed				
Intraoperatively	0	1	1	0
Postoperatively	0	0	0	0
Myocardial infarction[c]	0	0	0	0
Renal failure[c]	0	0	0	0
Congestive heart failure[c]	0	1	1	1
Stroke[c]	0	0	0	0
Death[c]	0	0	0	0

[a] Number of patients shown in parentheses.
[b] Not all the abnormally secreting tumor tissue was removed from the patient.
[c] Occurring postoperatively.
(Data from Roizen et al.[113])

ceptors (a compensatory response) and an exaggerated response to sympathomimetic drugs.[144] In addition to other abnormalities, such as retention of urine or feces and deficient heat exchange, hypofunctioning of the sympathetic nervous system is often accompanied by renal amyloidosis. Thus, electrolyte and intravascular fluid volume status should be evaluated preoperatively. Because many of these patients have cardiac abnormalities, intravascular fluid volume might be assessed preoperatively using a Swan-Ganz catheter rather than by CVP measurement (also see Ch. 31).

Since functioning of the sympathetic nervous system is not predictable in these patients, I usually employ slow gentle induction of anesthesia and treat sympathetic excess or deficiency by infusing, with careful titration, drugs that directly constrict (phenylephrine) or dilate (nitroprusside) blood vessels or that stimulate (isoproterenol) or depress (esmolol) heart rate. I prefer these drugs to agonists or antagonists, which may indirectly release catecholamines. A 20 percent perioperative mortality rate for 2,600 patients with spinal cord transection has been reported,[128] indicating that such patients are difficult to manage and deserve particularly close attention.

After reviewing 300 patients with spinal cord injury, Kendrick et al.[145] concluded that autonomic hyperreflexia syndrome does not develop if the lesion is below spinal dermatome T7. If the lesion is above spinal dermatome T7 (the splanchnic outflow), 60 to 70 percent of the patients experience extreme vascular instability. The trigger to this instability, or mass reflex involving noradrenergic and motor hypertonus,[121] can be a cuta-

neous, proprioceptive, or visceral stimulus (full bladder is a common initiator). The sensation enters the spinal cord and causes a spinal reflex, which in normal individuals is inhibited from above. Sudden increases in blood pressure are sensed in the pressure receptors of the aorta and carotid sinus. The resulting vagal hyperactivity produces bradycardia, ventricular ectopia, or various degrees of heart block. Reflex vasodilation may occur above the level of the lesion, resulting in flushing of the head and neck.

Depending on the length of time since spinal cord transection, other abnormalities may occur. Acutely (i.e., less than 3 weeks from the time of spinal injury), retention of urine and feces is common and, by elevating the diaphragm, may impair respiration. Disimpaction of the intestine alleviates this respiratory problem. Hyperesthesia is present above the lesion; reflexes and flaccid paralysis are present below the lesion. The intermediate time period (3 days to 6 months) is marked by a hyperkalemic response to depolarizing drugs.[127] The chronic phase is characterized by a return of muscle tone, positive Babinski's sign, and frequently, the occurrence of hyperreflexia syndromes (e.g., mass reflex; see above).

Thus, in addition to meticulous attention to perioperative intravascular volume and electrolyte status, the anesthesiologist should know — by history taking, physical examination, and laboratory data — the status of the patient's myocardial conduction (as revealed by ECG), the status of renal functioning (by noting the ratio of creatinine to blood urea nitrogen), and the condition of respiratory muscle (by determining the ratio of forced expiratory volume in 1 second to forced vital capacity (i.e., FEV_1/FVC) (also see Ch. 24). The anesthesiologist could also have obtained a chest roentgenogram if atelectasis or pneumonia was suspected on history-taking or physical examination. Temperature control, presence of bone fractures or decubitus ulcers, and normal functioning of urination and defecation systems must be assessed. Confirmation of the last prevents postoperative pneumonia or atelectasis caused by high positioning of the diaphragm.

Thyroid Dysfunction

The major thyroid hormones are thyroxine (T_4), a product of the thyroid gland, and the more potent 3,5,3-triiodothyronine (T_3), a product of both the thyroid and the extrathyroidal enzymatic deiodination of thyroxine. Approximately 80 percent of T_3 is produced outside the thyroid gland. Production of thyroid secretions is maintained by secretion of thyroid-stimulating hormone (TSH) in the pituitary, which in turn is regulated by secretion of thyrotropin-releasing hormone (TRH) in the hypothalamus. Secretion of TSH and TRH appears to be negatively regulated by T_4 and T_3. Whether all effects of thyroid hormones are mediated by T_3, or if T_4 has intrinsic biologic activity, remains unclear.

Thyroid hormones create their effects through several mechanisms. Binding of T_3 to high-affinity nuclear receptors and the subsequent activation of DNA-directed mRNA synthesis may account for the anabolic growth and developmental effects, plus some calorigenic effect, of thyroid hormones. Thyroid hormone also causes an increased concentration of adrenergic receptors,[143] which may account for many of its cardiovascular effects.

Since T_3 has a greater biologic effect than does T_4, one would expect the diagnosis of thyroid disorders to be based on levels of T_3. However, this is not usually the case. The diagnosis of thyroid disease is confirmed by one of several biochemical measurements: levels of free T_4 or of total serum concentrations of T_4, and by the "free T_4 index." This index is determined by multiplying total T_4 (free and bound) by the T_3 resin uptake. The T_3 resin uptake measures the extra quantity of serum protein binding sites. This measurement is necessary because thyroxine-binding globulin (TBG) is abnormally high during pregnancy, hepatic disease, and estrogen therapy (all of which would elevate total T_4 levels). For measurements of the total hormone concentration in serum to be interpreted reliably, it is necessary to have data on the percentage of bound hormone. The T_3 resin uptake test provides this information. In this test, ^{131}I-labeled T_3 is added to a patient's serum and allowed to reach an equilibrium binding stage. Then a resin is added which binds the remaining radioactive T_3. The resin uptake is greater if the patient has fewer TBG binding sites. In normal patients, the resin T_3 uptake (RT_3U) is 25 to 35 percent. When the serum TBG is elevated, the RT_3U is diminished. When the serum TBG is diminished, as in the

nephrotic syndrome, in conditions in which glucocorticoids are increased, or in chronic liver disease, the RT_3U is increased.

The free T_4 index and the free T_3 index are frequently used as measures of a patient's serum T_4 and T_3 hormone concentration. To obtain these indices, one multiplies the concentration of total serum T_4 or total serum T_3 by the measured RT_3U. The values of these two indices are normal if a primary alteration in binding, but not in secretion, of thyroid hormone occurs.

Hyperthyroidism can be diagnosed by measurement of the levels of TSH after administration of TRH. Although administering TRH normally increases TSH levels in blood, even a small increase in the T_4 or T_3 level in blood abolishes this response. Thus, a subnormal or absent serum TSH response to TRH is a very sensitive indicator of hyperthyroidism. In one group of disorders involving hyperthyroidism, serum TSH levels are elevated in the presence of elevated levels of free thyroid hormone.

Measurement of the alpha subunit of TSH has been helpful in identifying the rare patients who have a pituitary neoplasm and who usually have increased alpha-subunit concentrations. Some patients are clinically euthyroid in the presence of elevated levels of total T_4 in serum. Certain drugs, notably gallbladder dyes, propranolol, glucocorticoids, and amiodarone, block the conversion to T_3 of T_4, thus elevating T_4 levels. Severe illness also slows this conversion. Levels of TSH are often high in situations where the rate of this conversion is decreased. In hyperthyroidism, cardiac function and responses to stress are abnormal; return of normal cardiac function parallels the return of TSH levels to normal values.

Hyperthyroidism

Although hyperthyroidism is usually caused by the multinodular diffuse enlargement in Grave's disease (also associated with disorders of the skin and/or eyes), it can also be associated with pregnancy,[146] thyroiditis (with or without neck pain), thyroid adenoma, choriocarcinoma, or TSH-secreting pituitary adenoma. Five percent of women have been reported to suffer thyrotoxic effects 3 to 6 months post partum, and they tend to have recurrences with subsequent pregnancies. Major manifestations of hyperthyroidism are weight loss, diarrhea, warm moist skin, weakness of large muscle groups, menstrual abnormalities, nervousness, jitteriness, intolerance to heat, tachycardia, cardiac arrhythmias, mitral valve prolapse,[147] and heart failure. When the thyroid is functioning abnormally, the system most threatened is the cardiovascular system. When diarrhea is severe, dehydration should be corrected preoperatively. Mild anemia, thrombocytopenia, increased serum alkaline phosphatase, hypercalcemia, muscle wasting, and bone loss frequently occur in hyperthyroidism. Muscle disease usually involves proximal muscle groups; it has not been reported to cause respiratory muscle paralysis. In the apathetic form of hyperthyroidism (seen most commonly in persons over 60 years of age), cardiac effects dominate the clinical picture.[148,149] These signs and symptoms include tachycardia, irregular heart beat, atrial fibrillation, heart failure, and occasionally papillary muscle dysfunction.[147-149]

Although β-adrenergic receptor blockade can control heart rate, its use is fraught with hazard in the patient already experiencing congestive heart failure (CHF). However, decreasing heart rate may improve heart pumping function. Thus, hyperthyroid patients who have fast ventricular rates, who are in congestive heart failure, and who require emergency surgery are given propranolol or esmolol guided by changes in pulmonary artery wedge pressure and their condition. If slowing the heart rate with a small dose of propranolol (i.e., 0.05 mg) or esmolol 50 μg/kg does not aggravate heart failure, I administer more propranolol or esmolol. I believe that we should aim to avoid imposing surgery on any patient whose thyroid function is clinically abnormal. Therefore, I believe only "life-or-death" emergency surgery should preclude making the patient pharmacologically euthyroid, a process that can take 2 to 6 weeks. Antithyroid medications include propylthiouracil or methimazole, both of which decrease synthesis of thyroxine. Propylthiouracil also decreases conversion of thyroxine into the more potent T_3. However, the literature indicates a trend toward preoperative preparation with propranolol and iodides alone.[150,151] This approach is quicker (i.e., 7 to 14 days versus 2 to 6 weeks); it shrinks the thyroid gland, as does the more traditional approach; and it treats symptoms but may not correct abnormalities in left ventricular function.[152] Regardless of approach, antithyroid drugs should be administered chronically and on the morning of surgery. When emergency surgery is necessary before the euthyroid state is achieved, or if hyperthyroidism gets out of control during surgery, intravenous administration of 0.2 to 10 mg of propranolol or 50 to 500 μg/kg of esmolol should be titrated to restore normal heart rate (assuming the absence of CHF) (see above). Also, intravascular fluid volume and electrolyte balance should be restored. However, administering propranolol or esmolol does not invariably prevent "thyroid storm."[153]

No controlled study has demonstrated clinical advantages of any anesthetic drug over another for surgical patients who are hyperthyroid. Review of cases done at the University of California, San Francisco, from 1968 to 1982 reveals that virtually all techniques and anesthetic agents have been employed without adverse effects being even remotely attributable to agent or technique. Furthermore, although some authors have recommended that anticholinergic drugs (especially atropine) be avoided because they interfere with the sweating mechanism and cause tachycardia, atropine has been given as a test for adequacy of antithyroid treatment. Because patients are now subject to operative procedures only when euthyroid, the traditional "steal" of the heavily premedicated hyperthyroid patient to the operating room has vanished.

The patient having a large goiter and an obstructed airway can be handled in the same way as any other patient having problematic airway management. Preoperative medication should avoid excessive sedation, and an airway should be established, often with the patient awake. A firm armored endotracheal tube is preferable and should be passed beyond the point of extrinsic compression. It is most useful to examine computed tomographic (CT) scans of the neck preoperatively to determine the extent of compression. Maintenance of anesthesia usually presents little difficulty. Postoperatively, extubation should be performed under optimal circumstances for reintubation, in case the tracheal rings have been weakened and the trachea collapses.

Of the many possible postoperative complications (nerve injuries, bleeding, and metabolic abnormalities), "thyroid storm" (discussed below), bilateral recurrent nerve trauma, and hypocalcemic tetany are the most feared. Bilateral recurrent laryngeal nerve injury (by trauma or edema) causes stridor and laryngeal obstruction due to unopposed adduction of the vocal cords and closure of the glottic aperture. Immediate endotracheal intubation is required, usually followed by tracheostomy to ensure an adequate airway. This rare complication occurred only once in over 30,000 thyroid operations at the Lahey Clinic. Unilateral recurrent nerve injury often goes unnoticed because of compensatory overadduction of the uninvolved cord. However, we often test vocal cord function before and after this surgery by asking the patient to say "e" or "moon." Unilateral nerve injury is characterized by hoarseness and bilateral nerve injury by aphonia. Selective injury of adductor fibers of both recurrent laryngeal nerves leaves the abductor muscles relatively unopposed, and pulmonary aspiration is a risk. Selective injury of abductor fibers leaves the adductor muscles relatively unopposed, and airway obstruction can occur. Bullous glottic edema, an additional cause of postoperative respiratory compromise, has no specific cause or known preventive measure.

The intimate involvement of the parathyroid gland with the thyroid gland can result in inadvertent hypocalcemia during surgery for thyroid disease. Complications relating to hypocalcemia are discussed in the section, *Hypocalcemia*, below.

Because postoperative hematoma can compromise the airway, neck and wound dressings should be examined for evidence of bleeding before a patient is discharged from the recovery room.

Thyroid Storm

"Thyroid storm" is the name for the clinical diagnosis of a life-threatening illness in a patient whose hyperthyroidism has been severely exacerbated by illness or operation. Thyroid storm is manifested by hyperpyrexia, tachycardia, and striking alterations in consciousness.[154,155] No laboratory tests are diagnostic of thyroid storm, and the precipitating (nonthyroidal) cause is the major determinant of survival. Therapy can include blocking the synthesis of thyroid hormones by administering antithyroid drugs, blocking the release of preformed hormone with iodine, meticulous attention to hydration and supportive therapy, and correcting the precipitating cause. Blocking the sympathetic nervous system with reserpine, guanethidine, or α- and β-receptor antagonists may be exceedingly hazardous and requires skillful management and constant monitoring of the critically ill patient.

Hypothyroidism

Hypothyroidism is a common disease, occurring in 5 percent of a large adult population in Great Britain, in 3 to 6 percent of a healthy older population in Massachusetts, and in 4.5 percent of a medical clinic population in Switzerland. Usually hypothyroidism is subclinical, serum concentrations of thyroid hormones are in the normal range, and only serum TSH levels are elevated.[156,157] In such patients, hypothyroidism may have little or no perioperative significance. However, a recent retrospective study of 59 mildly hypothyroid patients found that more hypothyroid patients than control subjects required prolonged postoperative intubation (9/59 versus 4/59) and had significant electrolyte imbalances (3/59 versus 1/59) and bleeding complications (4/59 versus 0/59).[158] Because only a small number of charts were examined, these differences did not reach statistical significance.

In the less frequent occurrences of overt hypothyroidism, relative lack of thyroid hormone results in slow mental functioning, slow movement, dry skin, intolerance to cold, depression of the ventilatory responses to hypoxia and hypercarbia,[159] impaired clearance of free water, slow gastric emptying, and bradycardia. In extreme cases, cardiomegaly, heart failure, and pericardial and pleural effusions manifest as fatigue, dyspnea, and orthopnea.[160] Hypothyroidism is often associated with amyloidosis, which may produce an enlarged tongue, abnormalities of the cardiac conduction system, and renal disease. Hypothyroidism decreases anesthetic requirement slightly.[161] The tongue may be enlarged in the hypothyroid patient even in the absence of amyloidosis, and this may hamper endotracheal intubation.

Ideal preoperative management of hypothyroidism consists of restoring normal thyroid status: I routinely administer the normal dose of T_3 or T_4 the morning of surgery even though these drugs have long half-lives (1.4 to 10 days). For patients with myxedema coma requiring emergency surgery, T_3 can be given intravenously (with fear of precipitating myocardial ischemia, however) while supportive therapy is undertaken to restore normal intravascular fluid volume, body temperature, cardiac function, respiratory function, and electrolyte balance.

Treating hypothyroid patients having symptomatic coronary artery disease poses special problems and may require compromises in the general practice of preoperatively restoring euthyroidism with drugs.[162] Although both T_4 and propranolol may be given, adequate amelioration of both ischemic heart disease and hypothyroidism may be difficult to achieve. The need for thyroid therapy must be balanced against the risk of aggravating anginal symptoms. One review suggested early consideration for coronary artery revascularization.[162] It advocated initiating thyroid replacement therapy in the ICU soon after the patient's arrival from the operating room and myocardial revascularization surgery. However, several deaths due to arrhythmia and CHF as well as cardiogenic shock with infarction have occurred while patients who were not given thyroid therapy were awaiting surgery. Thus, there is need for consideration of true emergency coronary artery revascularization in patients having both severe coronary artery disease and significant hypothyroidism.

In hypothyroidism, respiratory control mechanisms do not function normally.[159] However, the response to hypoxia and hypercarbia and the clearance of free water become normal with thyroid replacement therapy.[159,160] Drug metabolism is anecdotally reported to be slowed, and awakening times from sedatives are reported to be prolonged during hypothyroidism. However, no formal study of the pharmacokinetics and pharmacodynamics of sedatives or anesthetic agents has been published. These concerns disappear when thyroid function is normalized preoperatively. Addison's disease (with its relative steroid deficiency) is more common in hypothyroidism, and some endocrinologists routinely treat noniatrogenic hypothyroid patients with stress doses of steroids perioperatively. The possibility that this steroid deficiency exists should be considered if the patient becomes hypotensive perioperatively. Body heat mechanisms are inadequate in hypothyroid patients, and temperature should be monitored and maintained, especially in patients requiring emergency surgery. Because there is an increased incidence of myasthenia gravis in hypothyroid patients, it may be advisable to use a twitch monitor to guide muscle relaxant administration (see Ch. 12).

Thyroid Nodules and Carcinoma

Identifying malignancy in a solitary thyroid nodule is a difficult and important procedure. Males and patients with previous radiation to the head and neck have an increased likelihood of malignant disease in their nodules. Often, needle biopsy and scanning are sufficient for the diagnosis, but occasionally an excisional biopsy is needed. Papillary carcinoma accounts for more than 60 percent of all thyroid carcinomas. Simple excision of lymph node metastases appears to be as efficacious for patient survival as are radical neck procedures.

Medullary carcinoma is the most aggressive form of thyroid carcinoma. It is associated with familial incidence of pheochromocytoma, as are parathyroid adenomas. For this reason, a history should be obtained for patients who have a surgical scar in the thyroid region, so that the possibility of occult pheochromocytoma can be ruled out.

Disorders of Calcium Metabolism

The three substances that regulate the serum concentrations of calcium, phosphorus, and magnesium—parathyroid hormone, calcitonin, and vitamin D—act on bone, kidney, and gut. Parathyroid hormone stimulates bone resorption and inhibits renal excretion of calcium, two conditions that lead to hypercalcemia. Calcitonin can be considered an antagonist to parathyroid hormone. Through its metabolites, vitamin D aids in absorption of calcium, phosphate, and magnesium from the gut and facilitates the bone resorptive effects of parathyroid hormone.[163]

Hyperparathyroidism and Hypercalcemia

Primary hyperparathyroidism most commonly begins in the third to fifth decades of life. Its incidence is two to three times higher in women than in men. Primary hyperparathyroidism is usually the result of enlargement of a single gland, commonly an adenoma and very rarely a carcinoma. Hypercalcemia almost always occurs. The normal total serum calcium level is 8.6 to 10.4 m/dl as measured in most laboratories. The value is dependent on the albumin level, declining 0.8 mg/dl for each 1 gm/dl drop in albumin. Calcium binding to albumin is pH-dependent; binding decreases with acidic pH and increases with alkaline pH. It should be noted that serum calcium and not ionized calcium decreases with decreases in albumin levels. Although ionized calcium is the clinically significant fraction, the cost and technical difficulties of stabilizing the electrodes used for measurement have limited the available assays.

Many of the prominent symptoms of hyperparathyroidism are a result of the hypercalcemia that accompanies it. Regardless of the cause, hypercalcemia can cause any of a number of symptoms, the most prominent of which appear in the renal, skeletal, neuromuscular, and gastrointestinal systems, including: anorexia, vomiting, constipation, polyuria, polydipsia, lethargy, confusion, formation of renal calculi, pancreatitis, bone pain, and psychiatric abnormalities. Free intracellular calcium initiates and/or regulates muscle contraction, release of neurotransmitters, secretion of hormones, enzyme action, and energy metabolism.

Nephrolithiasis occurs in 60 to 70 percent of patients with hyperparathyroidism. Sustained hypercalcemia can result in tubular and glomerular disorders, including proximal (type II) renal tubular acidosis. Polyuria and polydipsia are common complaints.

Skeletal disorders related to hyperparathyroidism are osteitis fibrosa cystica and simple diffuse osteopenia. There is a fivefold increase in the rate of bone turnover in patients with hyperparathyroidism compared to that in normal controls. Patients may have a history of frequent fractures or complain of bone pain.

Since free intracellular calcium initiates or regulates muscle contraction, neutrotransmitter release, hormone secretion, enzyme action, and energy metabolism, abnormalities in these end organs are often symptoms of hyperparathyroidism. Patients may experience profound muscle weakness, especially in proximal muscle groups, as well as muscle atrophy. Depression, psychomotor retardation, and memory impairment may occur. Lethargy and confusion are frequent complaints.

Peptic ulcer disease is more common in these patients than in the rest of the population. Production of gastrin and gastric acid is increased. Anorexia, vomiting, and constipation may also be present.

Approximately one-third of all hypercalcemic patients are hypertensive; the hypertension usually resolves with successful treatment of the primary disease.[164] Long-standing hypercalcemia can lead to calcifications in the myocardium, blood vessels, brain, and kidney. Cerebral calcifications may cause seizures, whereas renal calcifications lead to polyuria that is unresponsive to vasopressin.

The most useful confirmatory test for hyperparathyroidism is a radioimmunoassay for parathyroid hormone. In hyperparathyroid patients, the hormone levels are abnormal for a given level of calcium. The level of inorganic phosphorus in serum is usually low but may be within normal limits. Alkaline phosphatase is elevated if considerable skeletal involvement is present.

Glucocorticoid administration reduces the level of calcium in the blood in many other conditions that cause hypercalcemia but usually not in primary hyperparathyroidism. In sarcoidosis, multiple myeloma, vitamin D intoxication, and some malignant diseases, all of which can cause hypercalcemia, administration of glucocorticoids may lower the serum calcium through an effect on gastrointestinal absorption. This effect occurs to a lesser degree in primary hyperparathyroidism.

Hypercalcemia may also occur as a consequence of secondary hyperparathyroidism in patients who have chronic renal disease. When phosphate excretion decreases as a result of a lower nephron mass, serum calcium levels fall because of deposition of calcium and phosphate in bone. Parathyroid hormone secretion subsequently increases, whereas the fraction of phosphate excreted by each nephron increases. Eventually, the chronic intermittent hypocalcemia of chronic renal failure leads to chronically high levels of serum parathyroid hormone and hyperplasia of the parathyroid glands.

What should be done for asymptomatic patients with primary hyperparathyroidism has become the subject of a major controversy. Symptomatic primary hyperparathyroidism is usually treated surgically. If the patient refuses surgery, or if other illnesses make surgery inadvisable, using medical management instead is often difficult. This difficulty occurs when hyperfunctioning parathyroid glands secrete more hormone as the serum calcium is lowered, as if the calcium setpoint for feedback regulation of parathyroid hormone secretion had been raised.

Preoperative Considerations for Patients with Hyperparathyroidism

Patients with moderate hypercalcemia who have normal renal and cardiovascular function present no special preoperative problems. The electrocardiogram should be examined preoperatively and intraoperatively for shortened PR or QT intervals (Fig. 25–3). Because severe hypercalcemia can result in hypovolemia, normal intravascular volume and electrolyte status should be restored before anesthesia and surgery are begun.

Management of hypercalcemia can include increasing the urinary calcium excretion by means of hydration and diuresis. Restoration of intravascular volume, augmentation of urinary sodium excretion, and administration of diuretics (furosemide is commonly employed) usually increase urinary calcium excretion substantially. Complications of these interventions include hypomagnesemia and hypokalemia.

In emergency situations, vigorous expansion of intravascular volume usually reduces serum calcium to a safe level (less than 14 mg/dl); administration of furosemide also is often helpful in such situations. Phosphate should be given to correct hypophosphatemia, because hypophosphatemia decreases calcium uptake into bone, increases calcium absorption from the intestine,

and stimulates breakdown of bone. Hydration and diuresis, accompanied by phosphate repletion, suffice as management of most hypercalcemic patients. If additional intervention is needed, glucocorticoids, mithramycin, or calcitonin may be given. Corticosteroids inhibit further gastrointestinal calcium absorption. Mithramycin lowers calcium levels by approximately 2 mg/dl in 36 to 48 hours through its effect on osteoclasts. Its toxic effects include thrombocytopenia, decreased levels of clotting factors, hepatotoxicity, azotemia, proteinuria, hypocalcemia, hypophosphatemia, and hypokalemia. Most of these can be reversed simply by discontinuation of the drug. Consultation with an endocrinologist or oncologist is advisable before mithramycin is given, because it has a narrow therapeutic-to-toxic ratio.

Calcitonin lowers serum calcium levels through direct inhibition of bone resorption. It can decrease serum calcium levels within minutes after its intravenous administration. Calcitonin is less effective than phosphate or mithramycin, however, for patients with hypercalcemia caused by hyperparathyroidism. Side effects include urticaria and nausea.

It is especially important to know whether hypercalcemia has been chronic, because serious cardiac, renal, or CNS abnormalities may have resulted.

Hypocalcemia

Hypocalcemia (caused by hypoalbuminemia, hypoparathyroidism, hypomagnesemia, or chronic renal disease) is not usually accompanied by a clinically evident cardiovascular disorder. However, myocardial contractility does vary directly with levels of blood ionized calcium, although contractility decreased only 20 percent when ionized calcium levels changed from 1.68 to 1.34 mmol/L.[166] The clinical signs of hypocalcemia are clumsiness; convulsions; laryngeal stridor; depression; muscle stiffness; paresthesia (oral and perioral); parkinsonism; tetany; Chvostek's sign; dry, scaly skin, brittle nails, and coarse hair; low serum concentrations of calcium; prolonged QT intervals; soft tissue calcifications; and Trousseau's sign.

Hypocalcemia delays ventricular repolarization, hence increasing the QT_c interval (normal, 0.35 to 0.44 seconds). With electrical systole thus prolonged, the ventricles may fail to respond to the next electrical impulse from the SA node, causing 2:1 heart block. Prolongation of the QT interval is a moderately reliable electrocardiographic sign of hypocalcemia, not for the population as a whole, but for the individual patient.[167] Thus, following the QT interval as corrected for heart rate (Fig. 25–3) is a useful but not always accurate means of monitoring hypocalcemia. Congestive heart failure may also occur with hypocalcemia, but this is rare. Since congestive heart failure in patients with coexisting heart disease is reduced in severity when calcium and magnesium ion levels are restored to normal, these levels should be normal before surgery.[165,166] Sud-

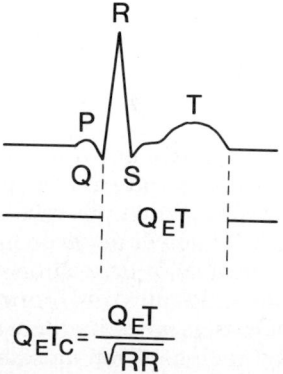

Fig. 25-3. The QT_c interval (termed Q_ET_c, properly to indicate that it begins with the start of the Q wave, lasts for the entire QT interval, ends with the end of the T wave, and is corrected for heart rate) is measured as illustrated. RR is RR interval in seconds.[165]

den decreases in blood levels of ionized calcium (as with chelation therapy) can result in severe hypotension.

Patients with hypocalcemia may have seizures. These may be focal, Jacksonian, petit mal, or grand mal in appearance, indistinguishable from such seizures in the absence of hypocalcemia. Patients may also have a type of seizure called cerebral tetany, which consists of generalized tetany followed by tonic spasms. Therapy with standard anticonvulsants is ineffective and may even exacerbate these seizures (by an anti-vitamin D effect). In long-standing hypoparathyroidism, calcifications may appear above the sella, representing deposits of calcium in and around small blood vessels of the basal ganglia. These may be associated with a variety of extrapyramidal syndromes.

The most common cause of *acquired* hypoparathyroidism is surgery of the thyroid or parathyroid glands. Other causes include therapy with iodine 131, hemosiderosis, neoplasia, and granulomatous disease. *Idiopathic* hypoparathyroidism has been divided into three categories: an isolated persistent neonatal form, branchial dysembryogenesis, and multiple endocrine deficiency autoimmune candidiasis (MEDAC).

Pseudohypoparathyroidism and pseudopseudohypoparathyroidism are rare hereditary disorders characterized by short stature, obesity, rounded face, and shortened metacarpals. Patients with pseudohypoparathyroidism have hypocalcemia and hyperphosphatemia despite high serum levels of parathyroid hormone. These patients have a deficient end-organ response to parathyroid hormone.

Since treatment of hypoparathyroidism is not surgical, hypoparathyroid patients who come to the operating room are those who require surgery for an unrelated condition. Their calcium, phosphate, and magnesium levels should be measured both pre- and postoperatively. Patients with symptomatic hypocalcemia should be treated with intravenous calcium gluconate before surgery. Initially, 10 to 20 ml of 10 percent calcium gluconate may be given at a rate of 10 ml/min. The effect on serum calcium levels is of short duration, but a continuous infusion with 10 ml of 10 percent calcium gluconate in 500 ml of solution over 6 hours helps to maintain adequate serum calcium levels.

The objective of therapy is to have symptoms under control prior to surgery and anesthesia. In patients with chronic hypoparathyroidism, the objective is to maintain the serum calcium level in the lower half of the normal range. A preoperative ECG should be obtained and the QT_c interval calculated. The QT_c value may be used as a guide to the serum calcium level if a rapid laboratory assessment is not possible.

The intimate involvement of the parathyroid gland with the thyroid gland can result in unintentional hypocalcemia during surgery for diseases of either organ. Because of the affinity of their bones for calcium, this relationship is especially important for patients having advanced osteitis. Internal redistribution of magnesium and/or calcium ions may occur (into "hungry bones") after parathyroidectomy, causing hypomagnesemia and/or hypocalcemia. The most prominent manifestations of acute hypocalcemia are distal paresthesias and muscle spasm (tetany). Potentially fatal complications of severe hypocalcemia include laryngeal spasm and hypocalcemic seizures. Clinical sequelae of magnesium deficiency include cardiac arrhythmias (principally ventricular tachyarrhythmias), hyocalcemic tetany, and neuromuscular irritability that is independent of hypocalcemia (tremors, twitching, asterixis, and seizures).

In addition to monitoring total serum calcium or ionized calcium postoperatively, one can test for Chvostek's sign and Trousseau's sign. (Note that serum calcium and not ionized calcium is dependent on albumin level, declining about 0.8 mg/dl for each 1 g/dl drop in serum albumin level.) Because Chvostek's sign can be elicited in 10 to 15 percent of individuals who are not hypocalcemic, an attempt should be made to elicit it preoperatively to ensure its appearance is meaningful. Chvostek's sign is a contracture of the facial muscles produced by tapping the ipsilateral facial nerves at the angle of the jaw. Trousseau's sign is elicited by applying a blood pressure cuff at a level slightly above the systolic level for a few minutes. The resulting carpopedal spasm, with contractions of the fingers and inability to open the hand, stems from the increased muscle irritability in hypocalcemic states, which is aggravated by ischemia produced by the blood pressure cuff.

Pituitary Abnormalities

Anterior Pituitary Hypersecretion

The anterior pituitary gland consists of five identified secretory cell types: somatotrophs (growth hormone [GH]), corticotrophs (adrenocorticotropin [ACTH]), lactotrophs (prolactin), gonadotrophs (luteinizing hormone [LH] and follicle-stimulating hormone [FSH]), and thyrotrophs (thyrotropin [TSH]). The secretion of these pituitary hormones is regulated largely by a negative feedback loop by hypothalamic regulatory hormones and by signals that originate from the target site of pituitary action. Six hypothalamic hormones have been characterized: dopamine, the prolactin-inhibiting hormone; somatostatin, the growth hormone release-inhibiting hormone; growth hormone-releasing hormone (GHRH); corticotropin-releasing hormone (CRH); gonadotropin-releasing hormone (GnRH or LHRH); and thyrotropin-releasing hormone (TRH). Most pituitary tumors (more than 60 percent) are hypersecretory and are classified according to the excess production of a specific anterior pituitary hormone.

The three most common disorders of pituitary hypersecretion are those related to excesses of prolactin (amenorrhea, galactorrhea, and infertility), ACTH (Cushing syndrome), or growth hormone (acromegaly). In addition to knowing the pathophysiologic processes of the disease involved, the anesthesiologist must determine whether the patient recently underwent air pneumoencephalography. If so, nitrous oxide should not be used; this practice lessens the risk of intracranial hypertension from gas collection. CT scanning of the sella has largely replaced neuroencephalography.

Acromegaly is a syndrome that presents with characteristic facies, weakness, enlargement of the hands (often to the point of rendering the usual oximeter probes difficult to use) and feet, thickening of the tongue (often to the point of making endotracheal intubation difficult), and enlargement of the nose and mandible with spreading of the teeth (often to the point of requiring larger than normal laryngoscope blades).[168] The patient may even appear myxedematous. Other findings include abnormal glucose tolerance and osteoporosis. The most specific test for acromegaly is measurement of growth hormone before and after glucose. The typical acromegalic has very elevated fasting levels of GH (usually above 10 mg/ml), and the levels do not change appreciably after oral glucose. In the normal state, glucose markedly suppresses the GH level. A few patients with active acromegaly have normal levels of fasting GH but do not suppress with glucose. The drug L-dopa, which normally causes an elevation of GH in normal subjects, in the acromegalic either has no effect or lowers GH levels. More than 99 percent of cases of acromegaly are a result of pituitary adenoma. Thus, the primary treatment of acromegaly is trans-sphenoidal surgery. If the pituitary tumor is not totally removed, patients are often offered external pituitary irradiation. If suprasellar extension exists, conventional transfrontal hypophysectomy is often employed. The dopaminergic agonist bromocriptine can lower GH levels, but long-term follow-up with this drug is still lacking.

The effects of excessive growth hormone stem from both direct actions of the hormone on tissue and stimulation of the production of somatomedins. Excessive growth hormone often results in retention of sodium and potassium, inhibition of the peripheral action of insulin (which can result in diabetes mellitus), and occurrence of premature atherosclerosis (often associated with cardiomegaly). Exertional dyspnea may be related to either heart failure or respiratory insufficiency due to kyphoscoliosis. Cardiac arrhythmias are common.[169] Preoperative evaluation of the patient with acromegaly might begin by determining whether significant cardiac, hypertensive, pulmonary, or diabetic problems exist. If so, preoperative evaluation should proceed along the lines described in sections discussing those topics. In addition, difficulty with endotracheal intubation should be anticipated in the acromegalic patient; lateral neck films or CT scans of the neck and direct or indirect visualization can identify the patient who has subglottic stenosis or an enlarged tongue, mandibles, epiglottis, or vocal cords.[168,170] If placement of an arterial line is necessary, a brachial or femoral site may be preferable to a radial site.[171]

Prolactin has been one of the most interesting markers to identify patients with pituitary tumors. Elevated prolactin levels are often but not invariably associated with galactorrhea. Females commonly present with amenorrhea, and males present with impotence. Optimal therapy for prolactin-secreting tumors is still being evaluated: the dopamine agonist bromocriptine can be extremely effective in controlling the prolactin level and restoring gonadotropin function.[172] However, in females who wish to become pregnant, the concern that pregnancy will cause rapid growth of these tumors may make a surgical procedure more desirable. In medical centers with the most extensive experience, 80 percent of patients with prolactin levels less than 200 ng/ml are initially cured by surgery. However, the relapse rate is as high as 50 percent within 5 years. But pituitary irradiation has not been uniformly successful. Over the last 10 years it has become apparent that most prolactin-secreting pituitary tumors can be treated medically with the dopamine-receptor antagonist bromocriptine. Bromocriptine can also be used to shrink tumor size prior to surgery. Its side effects include orthostatic hypotension, gastroparesis (possible increased risk of aspiration), constipation, and nasal congestion (possible need for oral intubation).[172] Thus, the treatment of microadenomas is currently being reevaluated. However, with large prolactin-secreting tumors (macroadenomas), loss of other pituitary function is common and evaluation of thyroid and adrenocortical status is indicated. Preoperative preparation of patients with Cushing syndrome is discussed in the section on adrenocortical hormone excess.

Anterior Pituitary Hypofunction

Anterior pituitary hypofunction results in deficiency of one or more of the following hormones: GH, TSH, ACTH, prolactin, or gonadotropin. Preoperative preparation of those individuals chronically deficient in ACTH and TSH is discussed above. No special preoperative preparation is required for the patient deficient in prolactin or gonadotropin; deficiency in growth hormone can result in atrophy of cardiac muscle, a condition that may necessitate preoperative cardiac evaluation. However, anesthetic problems have not been documented in patients with isolated growth hormone deficiency. Acute deficiencies are another matter.

Acute pituitary deficiency is often caused by bleeding into a pituitary tumor. In surgical specimens of resected adenomas, as many as 25 percent show evidence of hemorrhage. Such patients often present with acute headache, visual loss, nausea or vomiting, ocular palsies, disturbances of consciousness, fever, vertigo, or hemiparesis. In such patients, rapid trans-sphenoidal decompression should be accompanied by consideration of replacement therapy including glucocorticoids.

Posterior Pituitary Hormone Excess and Deficiency

The secretion of vasopressin, or antidiuretic hormone (ADH), is increased by increased serum osmolality or the presence of hypotension. Inappropriate secretion of vasopressin, without relation to serum osmolality, results in hyponatremia and fluid retention. This inappropriate secretion can result from a variety of CNS lesions; from drugs such as nicotine, narcotics, chlorpropamide, clofibrate, vincristine, vinblastine, and cyclophosphamide; and from pulmonary infections, hypothyroidism, adrenal insufficiency, and ectopic production from tumors. Preoperative management of the surgical patient with inappropriate secretion of vasopressin includes appropriate treatment of the causative disorders and restriction of water. Occasionally, drugs that inhibit the renal response to ADH (e.g., lithium or demeclocycline) should be administered preoperatively to restore normal intravascular volume and electrolyte status.

Most of the clinical features associated with syndrome of inappropriate antidiuretic hormone (SIADH) are related to hyponatremia and the resulting brain edema; these features include weight gain, weakness, lethargy, mental confusion, obtundation, and disordered reflexes and may progress, finally, to convulsions and coma. This form of edema rarely leads to hypertension.

SIADH should be suspected in any patient with hyponatremia who excretes urine that is hypertonic relative to plasma. The following laboratory findings further support the diagnosis[173]:

1. Urinary sodium >20 mEq/L
2. Low serum levels of BUN, creatinine, uric acid, and albumin
3. Serum sodium <130 mEq/L
4. Plasma osmolality <270 mOsm/L
5. Urine hypertonic relative to plasma

The response to water loading is a useful means of evaluating the patient with hyponatremia. Patients with SIADH are unable to excrete dilute urine even after water loading. Assay of ADH in blood can confirm the diagnosis.[173]

Patients with mild to moderate symptoms of water intoxication can be treated with restriction of fluid intake to about 500 to 1,000 ml/day. Patients with severe water intoxication and CNS symptoms may need vigorous treatment, with intravenous (IV) administration of 200 to 300 ml of 5 percent saline solution over several hours, followed by fluid restriction.

Treatment should be directed at the underlying problem. If SIADH is drug-induced, the drug should be withdrawn. Inflammation should be treated with appropriate measures, and neoplasms should be managed with surgical resection, irradiation, or chemotherapy, whichever is indicated.

At present, no drugs that can suppress release of ADH from the neurohypophysis or from a tumor are available. Dilantin and narcotic antagonists such as naloxone and butorphanol have some inhibiting effect on physiologic ADH release but are clinically ineffective in patients with SIADH. Drugs blocking the effect of ADH on renal tubules include lithium, which is rarely used because its toxicity often outweighs its benefits, and

demethylchlortetracycline in doses of 900 to 1,200 mg/day. The latter drug interferes with the ability of the renal tubules to concentrate urine, causing excretion of isotonic or hypotonic urine and thereby lessening hyponatremia. Demethylchlortetracycline can be used for ambulatory patients with SIADH in whom it is difficult to accomplish fluid restriction.

When a patient with SIADH comes to the operating room for any surgical procedure, fluids are managed by measuring the central volume status by CVP or PA lines and by frequent assays of urine osmolarity, plasma osmolarity, and serum sodium, often into the immediate postoperative period. Despite the common impression that SIADH is frequently seen in elderly patients in the postoperative period, studies have shown that the patient's age and the type of anesthetic used have no bearing on the postoperative development of SIADH. It is not unusual to see many patients in the neurosurgical intensive care unit suffering from this syndrome. The diagnosis is usually one of exclusion. Patients with SIADH usually require only fluid restriction; very rarely is hypertonic saline needed.

Lack of ADH, which results in diabetes insipidus (DI), is caused by pituitary disease, brain tumors, infiltrative diseases such as sarcoidosis, head trauma, or lack of renal response to ADH. The last can occur with such diverse causes as hypokalemia, hypercalcemia, sickle cell anemia, obstructive uropathy, or renal insufficiency. Preoperative treatment of diabetes insipidus consists of restoring normal intravascular volume by replacing urinary losses and by giving daily fluid requirements intravenously.

Perioperative management of patients with DI is based upon the extent of the ADH deficiency. Management of a patient with complete DI and a total lack of ADH usually does not present any major problems as long as side effects of the drug are avoided and as long as that status is known prior to surgery. Just before surgery, such a patient is given the usual dose of DDAVP intranasally or an intravenous bolus of 100 milliunits of aqueous vasopressin, followed by constant infusion of 100 to 200 milliunits/h. All of the intravenous fluids given intraoperatively should be isotonic, so that the risk of water depletion and hypernatremia is reduced. Plasma osmolality should be measured every hour both intraoperatively and in the immediate postoperative period. If the plasma osmolality goes well above 290 mOsm/L, hypotonic fluids should be administered; the rate of the intraoperative vasopressin infusion should be increased to more than 200 milliunits/h.

In patients who have a partial deficiency of ADH, it is not necessary to use aqueous vasopressin perioperatively unless the plasma osmolality rises above 290 mOsm/L. Nonosmotic stimuli, for example, volume depletion and stress of surgery, usually cause the release of large quantities of ADH in the perioperative period. Consequently, these patients require only frequent monitoring of plasma osmolality during this period.

Because of the side effects, the dose of vasopressin should be limited to that necessary for control of diuresis.[174,175] This limit is applicable especially to patients who are pregnant or who have coronary artery disease, because of the oxytoxic and coronary-artery-constricting properties of vasopressin.[175]

Another problem for anesthesiologists is the care of patients who come to the operating room with a vasopressin drip for treatment of bleeding from esophageal varices. In these situations, the vasoconstrictive effect of vasopressin on the splanchnic vasculature is being used to decrease bleeding. Such patients are often volume-depleted and may have concomitant coronary artery disease. Since vasopressin has been shown to decrease oxygen availability markedly, primarily because of a decreased stroke volume and heart rate,[174] monitoring of tissue oxygen delivery may be useful. In 1982 Nikolic and Singh[176] reported on a patient with a history of angina pectoris who received a combination of cimetidine and vasopressin for esophageal varices and who developed bradyarrhythmias and AV block, requiring a pacemaker. Cessation of either of these drugs alleviated the symptoms on two occasions. This indicates that the combination of cimetidine and vasopressin could be deleterious to patients because of the combined negative inotropic and arrhythmogenic effects of the two drugs.

DISEASES INVOLVING THE CARDIOVASCULAR SYSTEM

Hypertension (Also See Ch. 22)

Because of the controversy regarding the appropriateness of preoperative treatment of hypertension, the original articles that stimulated this controversy will be evaluated. Smithwick and Thompson[177] and Brown[178] reported overall mortality rates of 2.5 to 3.6 percent, respectively, in hypertensive patients undergoing sympathectomy between 1935 and 1947. These values were five or six times higher than values for normotensive patients undergoing similar operations. Obviously, these patients were not randomly assigned to treatment or nontreatment groups, and no attempt was made to ensure that end-organ disease was equivalent in the two groups. In 1929, Sprague[179] analyzed the records of 75 patients with hypertensive cardiac disease and found that 24 (32 percent) died during or shortly after operations employing general anesthesia.

In the early part of this century, severely ill patients did not do well perioperatively; however, whether preoperative treatment would have improved surgical outcome is still not known. The evolution of drug therapy for hypertension was hampered in the late 1950s and early 1960s by the publication of case reports of severe hypotension and bradycardia in patients receiving antihypertensive drugs before surgery. The tailoring of anesthetic dose to patient condition and the realization that sympatholytic antihypertensive drugs decreased anesthetic requirement[180] caused such case reports to disappear from the literature. A more recent prospec-

tive controlled double-blind study by the Veterans Administration (VA) provided a rationale for lifelong treatment of hypertension: such treatment decreased the incidence of stroke, CHF, and progression to renal insufficiency and to accelerated (malignant) hypertension (Table 25-6).[181,182] Berglund et al.[183] found a decrease in deaths due to myocardial infarction when patients were treated for mild-to-moderate hypertension. Other studies have confirmed the beneficial effect of treating hypertension, even for patients with diastolic pressures of 90 to 104 mmHg.[184] One study has indicated caution in adding diuretics to therapeutic limits in therapy for the patient with an abnormal ECG whose blood pressure does not decrease after administration of the usual doses of diuretic drugs (see the section, *Hypokalemia,* below).[185] Other studies in experimental models of hypertension indicate that treatment results in a regression of cardiac hypertrophy and in autonomic nerve alterations of hypertension.[186] United States government statistics reveal significant decreases (greater than 50 percent) in the death rate from stroke from 1969 to 1986. Deaths related to hypertensive cardiovascular disease and to myocardial infarction have decreased dramatically since 1974, accounting for most of the decrease in cardiovascular death in this time period, and this decrease (at least in localized communities) correlates with successful control of hypertension. This strong evidence from the VA studies and the epidemiologic data have led to the belief that all patients with a diastolic blood pressure above 90 mmHg should be treated, regardless of age. However, the question is, Should elective surgery be postponed and patient and physician schedules disrupted, so that treatment can be instituted and stabilized? Several schools of thought exist, the two oldest represented by the study conducted by Prys-Roberts et al.[187] in 1971 and by Goldman and Caldera[188] in 1979. Five other studies (Bedford and Feinstein,[189] Asiddao et al.,[190] Stone et al.,[132] Flacke et al,[133] and Ghignone et al.[134]) have also been cited. Unfortunately, all seven studies have deficiencies that prevent the establishment of a definitive answer to this question.

Critical Analysis of the Data of Prys-Roberts et al.

The followers of Prys-Roberts et al.[187] believe that preoperative treatment of hypertension lowers the inci-

TABLE 25-6. Effect of Treatment on Morbidity in Hypertension (Average Diastolic BP 90 to 114 mmHg)

	Control Group	Treatment Group
5-yr morbidity	55%	18%
Death	19/194	8/186
Terminating CHF	5	0
Terminating stroke	6	0
All CHF	11	0
All strokes	20	5

Abbreviations: BP, blood pressure; CHF, congestive heart failure.
(Data from Veterans Administration Cooperative Study Group on Antihypertensive Agents.[182])

dence of perioperative morbidity and mortality. In this study, three groups were compared: a control group consisting of 7 elderly normotensive patients having an average mean arterial blood pressure of 89.5 mmHg; a group of 7 hypertensive patients whose high blood pressure was not treated preoperatively (4 were being treated not for high blood pressure but for its complications) who had an average mean arterial blood pressure (MABP) of 129.5 mmHg; and a group of 15 hypertensive patients whose high blood pressure was treated preoperatively and who had an average MABP of 129.9 mmHg. The same doses of thiopental and halothane were given to all groups of patients, and measurements of absolute change in MABP, cardiac arrhythmias, and ECG evidence of ischemia were made. Patients with untreated hypertension had the greatest absolute fall in blood pressure and the highest percentage of arrhythmias and ischemia.

Several flaws in study design create serious doubt as to whether the relationship between preoperative treatment of hypertension and perioperative morbidity has been evaluated objectively in this investigation. First, the wisdom of administering the same dose of anesthetic to both groups of patients should be questioned. If the anesthetic dose had been titrated to the anesthetic needs of the patient, would the results have been different? Second, blood pressure did not differ between the treated and untreated groups. In addition, at least four of the seven hypertensive patients who were not treated for high blood pressure were "sicker" than any of the hypertensive patients who were treated. Why some patients were treated for hypertension and others were not was not explained; selection definitely did not occur on a random basis. Finally, it was not stated whether surgery was similar for all groups.

This study does indicate that patients who are sick preoperatively have more problems perioperatively than do healthy patients. This has been shown many times (see Ref. 191 for recent evidence of this, and review). However, from these data, the efficacy of preoperative treatment of hypertension cannot be established. This study and others by the same group provide useful data regarding the hemodynamic consequences of anesthesia when a standard technique is used on patients who have untreated hypertension.

Critical Analysis of the Data of Goldman and Caldera

The school of thought represented by Goldman and Caldera[188] advocates that preoperative treatment of hypertension does not affect outcome. Goldman and Caldera state that their study is a prospective one. However, the only prospective aspect of their study appears to be that patients were examined preoperatively. These investigators compared surgical outcome for three groups: sick hypertensive patients whose high blood pressure was treated preoperatively; less sick hypertensive patients whose high blood pressure was "undertreated" preoperatively; and less sick, only mod-

erately hypertensive patients who received no treatment preoperatively. No differences in outcome between groups was found.

This study has several flaws in design. Patients were not randomly assigned regarding preoperative treatment, undertreatment, or nontreatment of hypertension. Also, sicker patients were allocated to the treated hypertensive group (Table 25-7), thus biasing study results toward favoring nontreatment of hypertension.

Other flaws concern statistical methods. Only 34 of the 117 patients who were hypertensive at the time of surgery had diastolic blood pressure of at least 100 mmHg (Table 25-7). If morbid complications were assumed to be 20 percent in the untreated group, and if treatment was assumed to reduce morbidity 50 percent, then by power analysis,[192] Goldman and Caldera[188] would have had to compare approximately 237 patients to have an 80 percent chance of finding a difference at a confidence level of 0.05 percent. If a lower rate of morbidity in the untreated group (e.g., 15 percent) and a lesser reduction in the rate of morbidity (e.g., 33 percent) were assumed, then even more patients would have to be studied to be 80 percent sure no difference occurred, even at the 0.05 confidence level. For example, if morbid complications were assumed to be 15 percent in the untreated group, and if treatment were assumed to reduce morbidity 33 percent, 764 patients would have had to be studied in each group to be 80 percent certain no difference occurred, the confidence level being 0.05. These major flaws in study design make it impossible to ascertain whether preoperative treatment of hypertension decreased perioperative morbidity.

Critical Analysis of the Data of Bedford and Feinstein

Bedford and Feinstein[189] and their supporters believe that instability of blood pressure is the condition most frequently predicting morbid perioperative complications. In their study, the responses of three groups to rapid-sequence induction were compared prospectively. Patients were allocated to groups based on the initial admitting room blood pressures (BP) and the average presurgical in-hospital blood pressure: Group I (30 patients) had BP less than 140/90 mmHg during and after admission (normal BP group); group II (12 patients) had BP greater than 140/90 mmHg on admission but less than 140/90 mmHg during hospitalization (labile BP group); group III (8 patients) had BP greater than 140/90 mmHg during and after admission (hypertensive BP group). Whether any of the patients in the labile or hypertensive BP groups were under treatment for hypertension, had end-organ complications of hypertension (such as ischemic heart disease), or were told they were hypertensive was not stated. Patients were given standard (i.e., not tailored to the patient's condition) premedication (morphine, diazepam, and atropine) and a standard rapid-sequence induction (thiopental, 3 to 4 mg/kg IV, succinylcholine, 1.5

TABLE 25-7. Analysis of Treatment Groups Used by Goldman and Caldera[188] to Evaluate Effectiveness of Preoperative Treatment of Hypertension in Surgical Patients

Preoperatively Hypertensive Patients	(n)	Preoperatively			
		Diastolic BP > 100 mmHg (n)	BUN > 30 mg% (n)	Angina or CHF (%)	TIAs (%)
Treated successfully[a]	79	0	8	47	13
Treated unsuccessfully	40	34	13	40	18
Not treated	77		1	26	4

[a] These data demonstrate that the patients who were the sickest before surgery were allocated to this group, thereby biasing results toward nontreatment.

Abbreviations: BP, blood pressure; CHF, congestive heart failure; TIA, transient ischemic attacks.

mg/kg, IV). After intubation, heart rate and blood pressure increased significantly in all three groups. The increase was greatest in the labile BP group, rising from a mean BP of 102 ± 5 to 152 ± 4 mmHg. Eight of 12 patients in that group required additional thiopental and/or vasodilating drugs to normalize blood pressure, and 2 of 12 developed transient ST segment depression in lead II. No patient in either of the other two groups required similar treatment or had ST segment changes on ECG.

Thus, this study does indicate that patients with labile blood pressure may require more careful titration of anesthetic drugs than those whose blood pressure is either normal or high but stable. However, we do not know whether the results would have been different if the anesthetic had been titrated to the anesthetic needs of the individual patient. Nor do we know whether the groups had equivalent baseline end-organ disease. We do not even know how many patients were being treated for hypertension. Therefore, these data do not shed light on the efficacy of preoperative treatment of hypertension.

Critical Analysis of the Data of Asiddao et al.

The study of Asiddao et al.[190] is cited by those advocating preoperative treatment of hypertension. In this study, records of 166 cases of unilateral carotid endarterectomy were reviewed to investigate the association of preoperative and intraoperative factors with perioperative complications. The authors found that postoperative hypertension (i.e., systolic blood pressure > 200 mmHg or diastolic blood pressure > 110 mmHg) and transient postoperative neurologic deficits occurred more commonly in the 21 patients with poor preoperative control of blood pressure (BP > 170/95 mmHg) (52 and 23.8 percent, respectively) than in the 79 patients with adequate blood pressure control (BP < 170/95 mmHg) (35 and 2.5 percent, respectively) or in the 66 normotensive patients (17 and 1.5 percent, respectively). No statistically significant difference was found between the groups regarding permanent neurologic sequelae of surgery or the rate of myocardial ischemia.

The study by Asiddao et al. does not tell us whether postoperative hypertension caused the transient neurologic deficits or whether these deficits resulted in a compensation of postoperative hypertension. We also do not know whether the three groups were equivalent in end-organ manifestations of preoperative disease. Nor does the study tell us why blood pressure was not controlled preoperatively in some patients or whether preoperative normalization of high blood pressure would have reduced the rate of postoperative complications. This study does tell us that patients with high blood pressure before surgery are likely to have high blood pressure after surgery.

Critical Analysis of the Data of Stone et al.

Stone et al.[132] gave one of a variety of β-adrenergic blocking drugs or a placebo as preoperative medication to a group of mildly hypertensive patients and, knowing to which group the patients were assigned, the investigators then looked for ischemic episodes. They observed a significantly greater incidence of brief ischemic episodes during induction and emergence in the untreated patients compared with patients receiving a β-adrenergic blocking drug as premedication (Table 25-8). Although, on the surface, the results seem to clearly establish the efficacy of β-blocking drugs in reducing perioperative ischemic episodes in patients who are mildly hypertensive preoperatively, there are two limitations to this study which might cause us to temper our enthusiasm. First, there seems to be a problem with

TABLE 25-8. Myocardial Ischemia and Sympathectomy in "Mildly" Hypertensive Patients

	Control Group	Mildly Hypertensive Patients Receiving β-Adrenergic Receptor Blocking Drug Immediately Preoperatively
Developed myocardial ischemia	11	2
No evidence of myocardial ischemia	28	87

(Data from Stone et al.[132])

the randomization; although characteristics of the groups are not statistically different, they are numerically different. One wonders, therefore, whether bias was introduced by the fact that the control group underwent more vascular operations and had more preexisting coronary artery disease than did the treatment groups. Second, the observers' awareness of which patients belonged to which treatment group could introduce insidious and subtle differences in management, such as provision of inadequate anesthesia, a closer search for myocardial ischemia, or a more lengthy sampling of ECG strips in the control group. Although one wishes one could perform a double-blind study in such a situation, and maybe it is possible to do so, the effect upon heart rate induced by β-adrenergic blockade may make this difficult. The authors clearly note the limitations of their study and should be congratulated for not extrapolating or expanding their conclusions beyond that allowed by the data.

Some may comment that the tachycardia that was allowed to occur was severe, indicating inadequate anesthesia, and that the authors have merely demonstrated that β-adrenergic blockade takes the place of a skillful anesthesiologist. I hesitate to come to that conclusion, as I believe these investigators really tried to provide the best anesthesia care possible. I doubt whether even the subtle bias of an unblinded study could have caused this degree of inadequate anesthesia, but one must consider that possibility. Nevertheless, this study, and two recently published papers,[133,134] demonstrating that clonidine depressed sympathetic nervous system responses during anesthesia, all imply that modifying the response of the sympathetic nervous system, whether on the α-adrenergic side with clonidine, or the β-adrenergic side with one of the β-adrenergic blocking drugs used by Stone et al.,[132] may be all that is needed preoperatively in the mildly hypertensive patient. Although such may prove to be true, I believe the significant limitations of the cited studies make this currently unclear.

Recommendations

Although preoperative systolic blood pressure has been found to be a significant predictor of postoperative morbidity,[132,190,193–195] no data definitively establish whether preoperative treatment of hypertension reduces perioperative risk. Until a definitive study (which is, unfortunately, extremely difficult to conduct) is performed, I recommend that preoperative treatment of the patient with hypertension be based on the following beliefs: (1) the patient should be educated as to the importance of the life-long treatment of hypertension[196,197] even isolated systolic hypertension, and (2) perioperative hemodynamic fluctuations are less frequent in treated than in untreated hypertensive patients (as demonstrated by Prys-Roberts et al.[187] and confirmed by Goldman and Caldera[188]) and that hemody-

namic fluctuations have some relationship to morbidity. The data of Stone et al.[132] imply that rapid correction of blood pressure may be all that is needed. Data from animals that reveal declining renal function with acute reductions in arterial blood pressure accentuate the risks of acute blood pressure reduction,[198] yet the hazards of blood pressure fluctuations and acute hypertension may be serious in the untreated hypertensive.[199] Modern drug therapy for hypertension appears to reduce these risks but does so with a decrement in quality of life that causes many patients to wish to forego such medications.[200]

In addition to deciding whether a hypertensive patient needs treatment and ensuring that none of the complications of antihypertensive drugs is present, preoperative management should include a search for end-organ damage secondary to hypertension, that is, changes in the CNS and coronary arteries, myocardium, aorta, carotid arteries, kidneys, and peripheral blood vessels. Such injury may affect perioperative management. For example, the presence of renal disease may alter the choice and dosage of anesthetic drugs. Similarly, the recent occurrence of myocardial ischemia may warrant a delay in elective surgery. Knowing the location of myocardial ischemia would indicate which ECG lead should be monitored intraoperatively (also see Ch. 32). Also, to guide intraoperative regulation of blood pressure and to judge the effects of therapy, I obtain multiple blood pressure readings in both arms while the patient is in various positions.

I use such preoperative data to determine the individualized range of values I consider tolerable by a particular patient during and after surgery. That is, if blood pressure is 180/100 mmHg and heart rate 96 beats/min on admission with no signs or symptoms of myocardial ischemia, I feel confident that the patient can tolerate these levels during surgery. If during the night blood pressure decreases to 80/50 mmHg and heart rate to 48 beats/min and the patient does not wake with signs of a new cerebral deficit, I believe he or she can tolerate safely such levels during anesthesia. Therefore, from preoperative data, I derive an individualized set of values for each patient. I then try to keep cardiovascular variables within that range and, in fact, plan prior to induction what therapies to use to accomplish that goal (e.g., administration of more/less anesthesia, nitroglycerin or nitroprusside/dopamine, dobutamine, phenylephrine, or propranolol/isoproterenol, atropine) (Fig. 25–4). I believe this sort of planning is especially important in the patient with suspected cardiovascular disease and relatively unimportant in the totally healthy patient. I do not know for certain that keeping cardiovascular variables within an individualized range of acceptable values improves surgical outcome, but I do believe that such a plan reduces morbidity. For example, in several studies, major intraoperative deviations in blood pressure and/or heart rate from the preoperative level have been correlated with the occurrence of myocardial ischemia.[187–190,193–195,201,202]

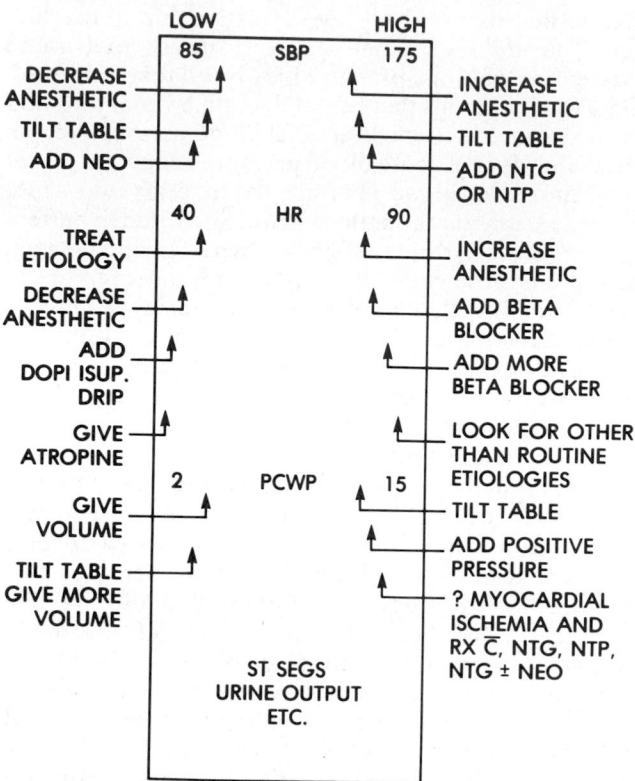

Fig. 25-4. Window of acceptable values. This hypothetical range of "safe" cardiovascular values for one patient illustrates possible therapies that might be employed if actual perioperative values approached the high or low end of that range. The range of safe values, variables treated, and therapies are tailored to the patient and surgical situation. SBP, systemic blood pressure; NTG, nitroglycerin; NTP, nitroprusside; HR, heart rate; PCWP, pulmonary capillary wedge pressure; NEO, Neo-Synephrine; DOPI ISUP, dopamine or Isuprel.

Ischemic Heart Disease

Identifying Ischemic Heart Disease

Any of the following conditions may indicate the presence of ischemic heart disease: a history of viselike chest pain, with or without radiation to the inner arm or neck; dyspnea on exertion, on exposure to cold, with defecation, or after eating; orthopnea; paroxysmal nocturnal dyspnea; nocturnal coughing; nocturia; previous or current peripheral or pulmonary edema; history of myocardial infarction (MI); family history of coronary artery disease; diagnosis of MI by ECG or elevated levels of enzymes; and cardiomegaly. Other patients who should be suspected of having ischemic heart disease include those who have diabetes, hypertension (especially if they are cigarette smokers or hyperlipemic[18–20,203,204]), left ventricular hypertrophy on ECG or echocardiogram,[204–206] peripheral vascular disease,[204–210] carotid bruits,[209–212] asymptomatic ca-

rotid artery occlusion,[209,210] or unexplained tachycardia or fatigue.

The more difficult question to answer is, How common is ischemic heart disease in asymptomatic patients or in patients having a normal ECG but predisposing conditions? The history appears to be the best indicator of coronary artery disease. Tomatis et al.[207] recorded coronary angiograms for "nearly all patients" who presented for aortoiliac reconstruction or resection of an abdominal aortic aneurysm. Of those having normal ECG results and histories not suggestive of coronary artery disease, 38 percent had stenosis of at least 50 percent in one or more coronary arteries, and 14 percent had stenosis of at least 75 percent in one or more coronary arteries. The percentages of patients with stenosis were the same for asymptomatic patients having abnormal ECG findings. However, a normal ECG result was not sensitive in ruling out significant stenosis when vascular disease was present: 44 percent of patients having normal ECGs and peripheral vascular disease had stenosis of at least 50 percent in one or more coronary arteries; and 30 percent had stenosis of at least 75 percent.

Hertzer et al.[208] found that angina and a history of myocardial disease reliably indicated coronary artery disease. These investigators studied 1,000 patients having peripheral vascular disease. Of the 500 patients having normal ECG results and no history of myocardial disease, 37 percent had narrowing of at least 70 percent in one or more coronary arteries. In contrast, of those suspected of coronary artery disease because of history and/or ECG results, 78 percent had narrowing of at least 70 percent in one or more coronary arteries. Also, patients who currently had angina had a 66 percent incidence of either severe correctable or severe inoperable coronary artery disease, whereas those who had peripheral vascular disease but no angina had an incidence of only 22.5 percent.

Although there is a great deal written about asymptomatic myocardial ischemia, patients with myocardial ischemia are not silent: that is, although the episodes of myocardial ischemia may be silent, the patient's history gave an indication of risk for coronary artery disease (CAD) in all 165 patients studied by Rabkin and Horne,[213,214] who had ECG evidence of CAD. Such has also been the finding of our own studies[215] and several others when age ≥ 70 years has been added to the clinical history indicating myocardial ischemia (chest pain, typical or atypical; dyspnea on exertion or exposure to cold, with defecation, or after eating; nocturnal coughing; nocturia; previous or current peripheral or pulmonary edema; history of myocardial infarction; family history of CAD; cardiomegaly; abnormal ECG results; diabetes; hypertension; hyperlipemia; left ventricular hypertrophy; peripheral vascular disease; cigarette smoking; carotid artery bruits; peripheral vascular surgery; unexplained tachycardia).

Several studies of asymptomatic carotid artery disease have shown very high perioperative mortality rates and life risk from associated ischemic heart disease.[209,210,212] Barnes and Marszalek[210] found perioperative mortality rates of 18.2 and 15 percent, respectively, for patients having an asymptomatic carotid bruit or occlusive disease but a rate of only 2.1 percent for patients undergoing similar peripheral vascular procedures who did not have a carotid bruit. Whereas the existence of asymptomatic carotid bruits did not predict the site of stroke or greatly influence the incidence of perioperative stroke,[209-212] it did predict mortality from ischemic heart disease (Table 25-9). Another point of view is found in the retrospective case-controlled review of strokes after CABG surgery.[213] In that review, strokes after CABG surgery were 3.9 times more likely to occur if carotid bruit was present preoperatively than if such was not present. The group was too small to determine whether site of bruit predicted site of stroke. Benchimol et al.[205] showed that 15 percent of patients with triple-vessel coronary artery disease have a normal resting ECG.

The important point to remember is that the history is the best indicator of coronary artery disease; in most series, the sensitivity and specificity of the history in indicating such disease range from 80 to 91 percent[203-208,213-219] and has higher sensitivity and specificity than most tests in indicating such disease (also see Ch. 23 for the definition of sensitivity and specificity).

Perioperative Morbidity

The presence of coronary artery disease, its severity, the time of most recent myocardial tissue death, the arteries affected, and complications and treatment of the disease are important information to the anesthesiologist. These variables influence the manner in which anesthesia is given and, in fact, may determine whether anesthesia and surgery should be postponed.

Previous Myocardial Infarction

Numerous epidemiologic studies[95,194,195,220-229] (Table 25-10) have shown that if previous myocardial infarction precedes surgery by less than 6 months, the periop-

erative reinfarction rate is 5 to 86 percent and mortality rate 23 to 86 percent. (This 5 to 86 percent value is 1.5 to 10 times higher than the value when previous myocardial infarction and subsequent surgery are separated by more than 6 months.) After 6 months, the perioperative reinfarction rate seems to stabilize at 2 to 6 percent. An investigation by Schoeppel et al.[227] studying a small number of patients produced a 0 percent mortality rate in the first year after infarction but a perioperative reinfarction rate of 16.7 percent and a mortality rate of 67 percent for patients experiencing perioperative reinfarction. Since the incidence and timing of perioperative reinfarction in the Schoeppel et al. study differ so much from those variables in the other studies listed in Table 25-10, I have put little emphasis on that study. However, for all 11 of the studies listed in Table 25-10, the overall reinfarction rates are similar.[95,194,195,220-229]

The study of Rao et al.[95] deserves special comment because it proposes to show a vast decrease in perioperative reinfarction rate attributable to the use of modern monitoring techniques. These investigators compared the rates of perioperative reinfarction and mortality at their institution for 364 patients having previous MIs operated on between 1973 and 1976 with the rates for 733 patients having prior MIs operated on between 1976 and 1982. The authors attribute the reduction in overall perioperative reinfarction rate (from 7.7 to 1.9 percent) and in each time period (i.e., from 36 to 5.8 percent when surgery occurs within 3 months of a previous MI) to invasive monitoring and rapid treatment of cardiovascular variables when values deviated from normal values. These two practices apply to both the intraoperative period and the first 72 postoperative hours. (The 72-hour period may be especially important, as virtually all of the 11 studies and others showed that reinfarction was most likely to occur 24 to 96 hours after surgery (Table 25-11).[95,194,195,220-234] Most of the reduction in perioperative reinfarction rate was found in patients over 65 years of age.

The editorial evaluating the Rao et al. study stated that the use of historical controls may have biased the conclusions.[235] Also, a different patient mix, improved skills of the surgeon and anesthetist, and other unidentified or unmeasured changes over time may have contributed to the reduction in reinfarction rate. Other workers have pointed out that certain surgical procedures (such as ophthalmic operations) have low perioperative reinfarction rates,[225-227, 236,237] whereas others (such as vascular operations[226,232-234,238-242]) have high reinfarction rates. The study by Rao et al. does confirm the fact that the perioperative reinfarction rate is higher in the first 6 months after a previous MI. Postponement of surgery for patients who have had an MI less than 6 months earlier should reduce mortality associated with anesthesia. The less severe the coronary artery disease, the more similar the patient's anticipated survival curve to that of patients who do not have coronary artery disease[244] and, probably, the less the perioperative risk.[245-247]

TABLE 25-9. Carotid Artery Bruits and the Risk of Stroke in Elective Surgery

Study	Incidence of Stroke in Patients	
	With Bruits	Without Bruits
Ropper et al.[211]	1/104	4/631
Of those having vascular surgery	1/37	4/130
Barnes et al.[209]	5/85[a]	0/364
Perioperative deaths	10.6%	0.3%
Reed et al.[213]		
CABG surgery; 54 strokes	13/54[b]	4/54[b]

[a] All patients included in this study were undergoing vascular surgery. These 85 patients also had either a bruit or significant carotid artery obstruction or both.
[b] Case-control study. Authors examined incidence of carotid bruit in patients who developed strokes after CABG surgery.
Abbreviation: CABG, coronary artery bypass graft.

TABLE 25-10. Incidence of Perioperative Myocardial Infarction or

Time from MI Operation (months)	Arkins et al.[220] 1963 (Mort.)	Topkins and Artusio[221] 1959–1963 (Reinf.)	(Mort.)	Fraser et al.[222] 1960–1964 (Mort.)	Tarhan et al.[223] 1975–1976 (Reinf.)	(Mort.)	Sapala et al.[224] 1970–1974 (Reinf.)	(Mort.)	Steen et al.[225] 1980 (Reinf.)	(Mort.)
0–3	40% 11/27	54.5% 12/22	*	38% 19/38	37% 3/8	*	86% 6/7	86% 6/7	27% 2/18	
4–6	*		*	*	16% 3/19	*			11% 2/18	
7–12	*	25.0% 9/36	*	*	5% 2/42	*				
13–18	*	22.4% 11/49	*	*	4% 1/27	*				
19–24	*		*	*	4% 1/21	*	5.7% 9/159	1.9% 3/159	5.4% 30/544	
25–36	*	5.9% 3/51	*	*	5% 11/232	*				
>36	*	1.0% 5/493	*	*						
Unknown	*	42.8% 3/7	*	*	5.6% 7/73	*				
Total patients with MI	*	6.5% 43/658	4.7% 31/658	*	6.6% 28/422	3% 15/422	9% 15/166	5.4% 9/166	6.1% 36/587	4.2% 25/587

* Mortality not stated.
Abbreviations: MI, myocardial infarction; Mort., mortality; Reinf., reinfarction.

Other Predictive Preoperative Information

Treadmill exercise testing, bicycle ergometer, dipyridamole-thallium imaging, preoperative Holter monitoring, noninvasive imaging, and cardiac catheterization also add information to the history, increasing our knowledge about the likelihood of cardiac disease and perioperative cardiac function.[218,232–234,239–243,248–251] The electrocardiographic criteria for myocardial ischemia during or after exercise consist of at least 1 mm of J-point depression with downsloping or horizontal ST segments; slowly upsloping ST segment depression, defined as being 2 mm of ST depression, measured at 80 ms from the J point; and ST segment elevation (Fig. 25-5).[218] Other responses to treadmill testing predictive of severe multivessel or of left main stem coronary artery disease include ST segment depression exceeding 2.5 mm; serious ventricular arrhythmias at low heart rates, or early (first 3 minutes) onset of ischemic ST segment depression; and/or prolonged duration of the ischemic ST segment depression in the posttest recovery period (> 8 minutes).[218]

Nonelectrocardiographic responses to treadmill testing that predict severe coronary artery disease include low achieved heart rates (≤ 120 beats/min), systolic hypotension (decrease of > 10 mmHg) in the absence of hypovolemia or antihypertensive medications, rise in diastolic blood pressure to > 110 mmHg, and inability to exercise beyond 3 minutes. The treadmill test responses predictive of severe multivessel and/or left main coronary artery disease are listed in Table 25-12.

Clearly, however, the response to the test must be interpreted in light of the patient's history and with knowledge that it is more predictive for men than for women (Table 25-13).[218]

Inability to increase heart rate (CRI) above 90 beats/min after supine bicycle exercise for 2 minutes at 50 rev/min has been shown to predict perioperative myocardial infarction with 80 percent sensitivity. This test is claimed by its investigators to have better sensitivity (80 percent) with a small sacrifice in specificity (53 percent) than the Goldman cardiac risk index (CRI) (sensitivity 60 percent, specificity 64 percent). This same group recommended this test for the group of geriatric patients with low risk (according to Goldman CRI) to identify the "false negatives" of the Goldman CRI or geriatric patients at risk for perioperative myocardial infarction. Limitations to this test, however, are recognized in patients with impaired joint mobility, dementia, muscle weakness, claudication, or exertional angina.[234] Ejection fractions of over 50 percent (and normal left ventricular size on plain chest roentgeno-

TABLE 25-11. When Do Myocardial Infarctions Occur after Vascular Surgery?

Authors	Year Published	Examined Prospectively	Postoperative Day 0	Day 1	Day 2	Day 3	Day 4
Plumlee et al.[230]	1972	No	11/24	3/24	1/24	2/24	
Tarhan et al.[223]	1972	No		14/71	8/71	22/71	13/71
Rao et al.[95]	1983	No		8/28	7/28	10/28	3/28
		No		3/14	4/14	7/14	
Becker and Underwood[231]	1987	?	11/28	6/28	9/28	0/28	1/28
Total (4 studies)			22	34	29	41	17

Mortality in Patients with Previous Myocardial Infarction

von Knorring[229] 1981 (Reinf.)	(Mort.)	Goldman et al.[226] 1975-1976 (Reinf.)	(Mort.)	Eerola et al.[194] 1970-1974 (Reinf.)	(Mort.)	Schoeppel et al.[227] 1980 (Reinf.)	(Mort.)	Rao et al.[95] 1973-1976 (Reinf.)	(Mort.)	Rao et al.[95] 1976-1982 (Reinf.)	(Mort.)
25% 4/16	*	4.5% 1/22	23% 5/22	8% 1/12	8% 1/12	0% 0/1	0% 0/1	30% 4/11	*	5.8% 3/52	*
			5.9% 1/12	5.9% 1/17	0% 0/1	0% 0/8	0% 0/8	26% 8/31	*	2.3% 2/36	*
18% 2/11	*	0% 0/13						5% 6/127	*	1.0% 1/104	*
			8% 1/13					5% 6/114	*	1.6% 4/258	*
11% 10/89	*			4.9% 4/82	12% 1/82	0% 0/10	0% 0/10	5% 4/81	*	1.7% 4/235	*
		3.3% 2/66	3.3% 2/66			0% 0/26	0% 0/26				
22% 9/41	*										
15.9% 25/157	4% 7/157		8.9% 9/109			5.7% 3/53	3.8% 2/53	7.7% 28/364	4.1% 15/364	1.9% 14/733	0.7% 5/733

gram) predict good perioperative cardiac function and survival.[247-250]

For dipyridamole thallium scanning, patients received dipyridamole (0.56 mg/kg) intravenously over 4 minutes while their heart rate, blood pressure, and ECG were monitored. After an additional 2 minutes, when dipyridamole's effect was considered maximal, 2 mCi of thallium 201 was administered intravenously. Five minutes after administration of thallium, initial images were taken for 8 consecutive minutes. Delayed images were obtained 3 hours later. The anterior, 45 degree, and 70 degree LAO projections were taken each time. Dipyridamole causes vasodilation and increase in coronary blood flow. Since stenotic vessels cannot dilate normally, areas of myocardium supplied by them will take up less thallium during scanning than areas sup-

ECG Patterns indicative of Myocardial Ischemia

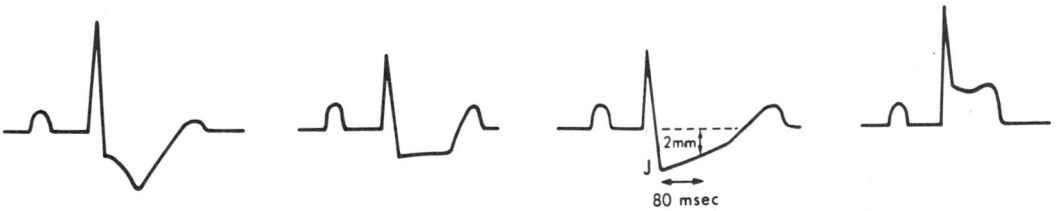

ECG Patterns not indicative of Myocardial Ischemia

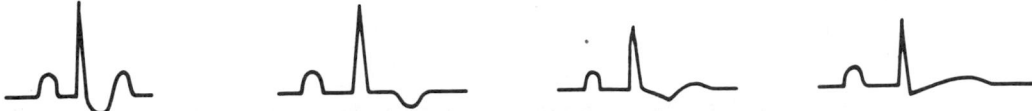

Fig. 25-5. Electrocardiographic criteria for myocardial ischemia consist of at least 1 mm of J-point depression with downsloping or horizontal ST segments; slowly upsloping ST-segment depression, defined as 2 mm of ST depression measured 80 ms from the J point; and ST-segment elevation. Whereas ST-segment depression indicates nontransmural ischemia, ST-segment elevation often connotes more severe degrees of ischemia reflecting transmural injury. The structure of the ST-segment slope is predictive for the severity of coronary disease shown angiographically, with downsloping ST depression indicating severe two- and three-vessel coronary artery disease more often than does either horizontal and slowly upsloping ST depression, and ST-segment elevation indicating high-grade, usually proximal, arterial obstruction in patients without previous myocardial infarction. (From Goldschlager,[218] with permission.)

TABLE 25-12. Treadmill Test Responses Predictive of Severe Multivessel and/or Left Main Coronary Artery Disease

Electrocardiographic responses
  ST-segment response
    Downsloping
    Elevation
  ST-segment depression exceeding 2.5 mm
  Serious ventricular arrhythmias occurring at low heart rates (120 to 130 beats/min)
  Early onset (first 3 minutes) of ischemic ST-segment depression or elevation
  Prolonged duration in the post-test recovery period ($\geq$ 8 minutes) of ischemic ST-segment depression

Nonelectrocardiographic criteria
  Low achieved heart rate ($\leq$ 120 beats/min)
  Hypotension[a] ($\geq$ 10 mmHg fall in systolic pressure)
  Rise in diastolic blood pressure ($\geq$ 110 to 120 mmHg)
  Low achieved rate-pressure product ($\leq$ 15,000)
  Inability to exercise beyond 3 minutes

[a] In the absence of antihypertensive medications or hypovolemia of any cause.
(Modified from Goldschlager,[218] with permission.)

plied by normal vessels and will show up as filling defects on immediate image. On the late images, after the vasodilation has resolved, thallium redistributes to these previously underperfused areas.

Dipyridamole infusion resulted in an increase of heart rate of 17 beats/min, decrease in systolic blood pressure of 17 mmHg, and chest pain in 30 percent of patients, which is reversible with 125 mg of aminophylline intravenously. ECGs are examined for ischemic changes defined as $\geq$ 1 mm horizontal or downsloping ST-segment depression. Myocardial regions on initial and delayed images were graded as being normal, as showing fixed deficits (without redistribution), or as showing one or more segments with thallium redistribution (with or without evidence of fixed deficits). Initial studies[239,240,243] have shown this test to be valuable in further stratifying high risk as assessed by five clinical factors (congestive heart failure [CHF], diabetes mellitus, history of ventricular ectopy, angina, and history of MI). Of patients with thallium redistribution 45 percent suffered PMI, whereas 7 percent of patients without redistribution had PMI (p = 0.001). This test has been suggested to be valuable in stratifying patients

with intermediate risk as assessed by five clinical factors (Q waves on resting ECG, history of ventricular ectopy, diabetes, age > 70 years, and angina) that were identified by logistic regression on several clinical findings and Goldman Indices and Dripp classes. Fletcher[243] found the test superior to clinical assessment in identification of high-risk patients for further angiographic study or prophylactic CABG or intensive intra- and postoperative management. This test may reveal redistribution in instances where coronary narrowing is only 40 to 60 percent and may aid in the management of higher-risk patients with invasive monitoring and prompt medicating of hemodynamic changes and artificially decrease the incidence of PMI in the studies of thallium scan cited. Since in all these studies the results of thallium scans were made known to the caretakers, those patients with positive scans may have received more invasive monitoring, as well as coronary angiography, angioplasty, medications, and CABG. The discriminating capacities of this test may improve with further classification of redistribution segment by size and number and by additional projections.

Twenty-four to 48-hour Holter monitoring of intermediate risk patients has recently been shown to be effective in detecting asymptomatic ischemia with an excellent negative predictive value and a fair positive predictive value for postoperative cardiac complications. Preoperative ischemia increases risk of intraoperative ischemia three- to fourfold. Goldman and colleagues[241] studied 176 vascular surgery patients who were asymptomatic for ischemic cardiac disease and found preoperative ischemia on Holter monitoring to be an independent factor with high correlation for significant postoperative cardiac complications (such as infarction, unstable angina, and ischemic pulmonary edema). In this series, 24- to 48-hour Holter monitoring detected two of three patients with positive stress test results and four patients with postoperative cardiac complications who did not have a history suggestive of ischemic heart disease. With an overall sensitivity of 92 percent, specificity of 88 percent, positive predictive value of 38 percent, and negative predictive value of 99 percent, this test may be a test of choice for evaluating intermediate-risk patients who have no suggestive history or for those patients unable to undergo an exercise

TABLE 25-13. Electrocardiographic Response to Treadmill Exercise of Angiographically Demonstrated Coronary Disease

Clinical Characteristics	Prevalence of Coronary Artery Disease (%)	Predictive Accuracy of a Positive Test (%)	Predictive Accuracy of a Negative Test (%)
Asymptomatic	5	10–20	95–100
Noncardiac chest pain	10–25	45–50	80–85
Cardiac chest pain			
Atypical, or probable, angina	50–70	80–85	65–70
Typical, or definite, angina	85–95	95–100	50–55

(Modified from Goldschlager,[218] with permission.)

stress test. Limitations of this method are seen in patients with left bundle branch block (LBBB), left ventricular hypertrophy, with strain, and ST-T changes with digoxin because of the difficulties in analyzing ST-segment changes.

Studies of visual interpretation of the coronary angiogram suggest that the physiologic effects of most coronary artery obstruction cannot be determined accurately by conventional angiographic approaches.[251]

Recent studies have concentrated on the identification and stratification of risks in the intermediate-risk group of patients who will benefit most from a preoperative cardiac work-up and risk assessment. Goldman[226] prospectively studied 1,001 patients over 40 years of age undergoing a broad variety of emergency and elective surgery. He found by multiple regression analysis that nine factors correlated independently with development of life-threatening or fatal cardiac complications: (1) presence of an S_3 gallop, JVD, or CHF; (2) history of MI in the preceding 6 months; (3) rhythm other than sinus; (4) >5 PVC/min; (5) intraperitoneal, intrathoracic, or aortic surgery; (6) age >70 years; (7) significant valvular aortic stenosis; (8) emergency surgery; (9) poor general medical condition. On the basis of this study he developed a method of computing CRI (Table 25-14). This study suggests that history and physical examination account for 29 of 53 points in assessing cardiac risk of the general surgical population and that initial history and physical examination permit selection of intermediate-risk patients for further evaluation. Eagle[239] studied 200 vascular surgery patients, a population with a high incidence of cardiovascular disease, and found independent risk factors by logistic regression to be as follows: Q waves on resting ECG, history of ventricular ectopy, diabetes, age >70 years, angina, and CHF. Again multiple regression studies suggest that initial clinical evaluation suffices for selecting patients for further evaluation.

Thus, the major signposts of perioperative myocardial function we can obtain before surgery are history of ischemic pain and its relationship to exercise, and history of CHF. The usefulness of this information is enhanced slightly by ECG and non-ECG responses to bicycle or treadmill exercise, determination of ejection fraction, and use of an echocardiogram, nuclear imaging, nuclear imaging after dipyridamole, or angiogram.[218,232–234,239–243,249–251]

Relationship to Previous Coronary Artery Bypass Grafting

Much of the information upon which altered perioperative anesthetic management of ischemic heart disease is based derives from studies of patients undergoing aortic to coronary artery bypass grafting (CABG) procedures. Although CABG relieves angina and increases exercise tolerance (as did many placebo operations and medications before it),[253] improved survival occurs only for patients having significant left main coronary artery disease[242,254,255] and for those with mild to moder-

TABLE 25-14. Computation of the Cardiac Risk Index

Criteria	Points
1. History	
(a) Age >70 yr	5
(b) MI in previous 6 mon	10
2. Physical examination	
(a) S_3 gallop or JVD	11
(b) Important VAS	3
3. Electrocardiogram	
(a) Rhythm other than sinus or PACs on last preoperative ECG	7
(b) >5 PVCs/min documented at any time before operation	7
4. General status	
$PO_2 < 60$ or $PCO_2 > 50$ mmHg, $K < 3.0$ or $HCO_3 < 20$ mEq/L, $BUN > 50$ or $Cr > 3.0$ mg/dl, abnormal SGOT, signs of chronic liver disease, or patient bedridden from noncardiac causes	3
5. Operation	
(a) Intraperitoneal, intrathoracic, or aortic operation	3
(b) Emergency operation	4
Total possible	53 points

To calculate a patient's score, the number of points from all factors he or she possesses are summed.
Patients are further segregated into class I (0–5 points), with a risk of 1–7 percent of major complications; class II (6–12 points), risk 7–11 percent; class III (13–25 points), risk 14–38 percent; and class IV (≥26 points), risk 30–100 percent.
Abbreviations: MI, myocardial infarction; JVD, jugular vein distention; VAS, valvular aortic stenosis; PACs, premature atrial contractions; ECG, electrocardiogram; PVCs, premature ventricular contractions; PO_2, partial pressure of oxygen; PCO_2, partial pressure of carbon dioxide; K, potassium; HCO_3, bicarbonate; BUN, blood urea nitrogen; Cr, creatinine; and SGOT, serum glutamic-oxaloacetic transaminase.
(Modified from Goldman et al.,[768] with permission. Risk calculations from Goldman et al.,[226] Detsky et al.,[233] and Jeffrey et al.[252])

ate impairment of left ventricular function.[251,256,257] However, a potential additional benefit of CABG surgery has been suggested. Reduced perioperative morbidity during subsequent noncardiac surgical procedures may be an additional benefit of surviving CABG surgery.[208,246,257,258] To provide definitive data for this hypothesis, a randomized controlled study would be necessary: CABG surgery may constitute a "survival test"; that is, it may cause reinfarction and/or death in those patients who would have had an MI or who would have died after the noncardiac surgery.[246] This appears to be a likely conclusion, since those patients who do poorly during and after CABG surgery are those with poor left ventricular function and increased left ventricular end-diastolic pressure.[259] Patients with these same cardiovascular conditions also have increased perioperative risk after noncardiac surgery.[208,226,232–234,239–243,247,249,251] Therefore, one proposal to decrease perioperative risk in patients severely disabled with angina (or ischemic heart disease) is to study the coronary arteries and to perform percutaneous transluminal coronary angioplasty or CABG surgery, if indicated, prior to their noncardiac surgery. Hertzer et al.[208] did just this. Knowing that survival after vascular surgery depends mainly on preserving myocardial function,

Hertzer et al. obtained coronary angiograms from, and proposed CABG surgery, when appropriate, for 1,001 consecutive patients needing peripheral vascular surgery (regardless of degree of suspicion of coronary artery disease prior to angiogram). CABG was believed to be indicated in 251 patients, of whom 226 underwent CABG with 12 (5.13 percent) operative deaths and 130 of whom subsequently underwent peripheral vascular procedures with only one death. Do these figures imply that mortality was decreased or increased by the CABG procedure? Did some patients not undergo their initially indicated vascular procedure because of morbidity associated with CABG? (Why 26 patients who initially were scheduled for peripheral vascular procedures did not have them after their CABG procedure is not revealed in the report.) Thus, the hypothesis that CABG surgery decreases the morbidity and mortality rates in patients undergoing subsequent noncardiac surgery remains a hypothesis. As stated earlier, this hypothesis deserves to be studied in a randomized clinical trial.

Summary of Preoperative and Intraoperative Factors That Correlate with Perioperative Morbidity

To summarize a large number of studies, preoperative findings that correlate with perioperative morbidity and that can be corrected prior to operation are as follows: (1) recent MI (within 6 months),[95,194,220-229] (2) severe CHF (i.e., severe enough to produce rales, an S_3 gallop, or distention of the jugular vein),[95,224,226,232-243,247,259] (3) severe angina (see Table 25-15 for classifications of severity of angina),[226,232-243,247,261] (4) heart rhythm other than sinus,[224,226,232-234] (5) premature atrial contractions,[226] (6) more than five premature ventricular contractions per minute,[224,226] and (7) blood urea nitrogen levels higher than 50 mg percent, or potassium levels lower than 3.0 mEq/L.[226]

Preoperative factors that correlate with perioperative risk but that cannot be altered include (1) old age (perioperative risk increases with age),[191,226,232-243,262,263] (2) significant aortic stenosis,[226,264] (3) emergency operation,[95,191,220,226,232-234,247] (4) cardiomegaly,[226,232-234,247,265] (5) history of CHF,[95,224,226,232-243,247] (6) angina (or history of angina or ischemia) on ECG,[95,218,224,226,232-243,247,266] (7) abnormal, ST-segment or inverted or flat T waves on ECG,[226,232,234,266] abnormal QRS complex on ECG,[226] and (8) significant mitral regurgitant murmur.[226]

Significant intraoperative factors that may be avoided or altered that correlate with perioperative risk are as follows: (1) unnecessary use of vasopressors,[267,268] (2) unintentional hypotension[95,195,225,226] (this point is controversial, however, as some investigators have found that unintentional hypotension does not correlate with perioperative morbidity[263,268]), (3) high rate-pressure product (i.e., if the product of heart rate times systolic blood pressure exceeds 11,000),[269] and (4) long operations.[95,220,225,226]

TABLE 25-15. New York Heart Association's and the Canadian Cardiovascular Society's Classifications of Angina

NYHA's	CCS's
I. Ordinary physical activity, such as walking or climbing stairs, does not cause angina. Angina with strenuous or rapid prolonged exertion at work or recreation or with sexual relations.	I. Ordinary physical activity, such as walking and climbing stairs, does not cause angina. Angina with strenuous or rapid or prolonged exertion at work or recreation.
II. Slight limitation of ordinary activity. Walking or climbing stairs rapidly, walking uphill, walking or stair climbing after meals, or in cold, or in wind, or under emotional stress, or only during a few hours after awakening. Walking more than two blocks on the level or more than one flight of stairs at a normal pace and in normal conditions.	II. Slight limitation of ordinary activity. Walking or climbing stairs rapidly, walking uphill, walking or stair climbing after meals, in cold, in wind, or when under emotional stress, or only during the few hours after awakening. Walking more than two blocks on the level and climbing more than one flight of ordinary stairs at a normal pace and in normal conditions.
III. Marked limitation of ordinary physical activity. Walking one or two blocks on the level and climbing one flight of stairs in normal conditions and at a normal pace. "Comfortable at rest."	III. Marked limitation of ordinary physical activity. Walking one to two blocks on the level and climbing more than one flight in normal conditions.
IV. Inability to carry on any physical activity without discomfort—anginal syndrome may be present at rest.	IV. Inability to carry on any physical activity without discomfort—anginal syndrome *may be* present at rest.

Significant intraoperative factors that correlate with perioperative morbidity and probably cannot be avoided are (1) emergency surgery and (2) thoracic or intraperitoneal surgery or above-the-knee amputations.[224-226,232-247,262]

Although the evidence for the factors provided above is fairly substantial, virtually none of the data derive from prospective randomized studies indicating that treatment of the above conditions reduces the perioperative risk to patients with ischemic heart disease. Nevertheless, all logic dictates that such treatment does reduce risk. Thus, the goal in giving anesthesia to patients with ischemic heart disease is to have the patient in the best preoperative condition obtainable, by treating those conditions that correlate with perioperative risk. Then one monitors intraoperatively for conditions that correlate with perioperative risk and, by that monitoring and attentiveness to detail, avoids those circumstances that lead to perioperative risk. Although local anesthesia may reduce perioperative risk,[224,236] epidemiologic studies do not reveal significant differences in perioperative morbidity for patients with ischemic heart disease who are given local anesthesia as opposed to general anesthesia.

Preoperative Evaluation

Preoperative evaluation of the patient with ischemic heart disease should include a review of the clinical course of any previous myocardial infarctions and a review of studies made subsequent to those events. Since the patients most likely to benefit are those who have severe coronary artery disease (i.e., multivessel left mainstem coronary artery disease) and ejection fractions of 21 to 50 percent,[270,271] some strategies have been devised to limit routine exercise testing, dipyrida-

mole-thallium scanning, Holter monitoring, and angiographic testing to only such patients (Figs. 25-6 to 25-8).[270,271] Thus, the fact that these studies have been, or are being, performed implies something about the patient's cardiac function.

The preoperative evaluation should also include a review of exercise studies, Holter monitoring results, dipyridamole-thallium scans, and coronary angiogram, in order to determine which ECG lead to monitor for ischemia. Although, in theory, the ECG lead that first reveals ischemia or best represents the stenosed artery on exercise should be the first to reveal ischemia in the operating room, no study has confirmed this assumption. If no exercise or coronary angiographic study has been performed, precordial lead V_5 is preferred.[272,273]

Currently, the only known way to increase oxygen

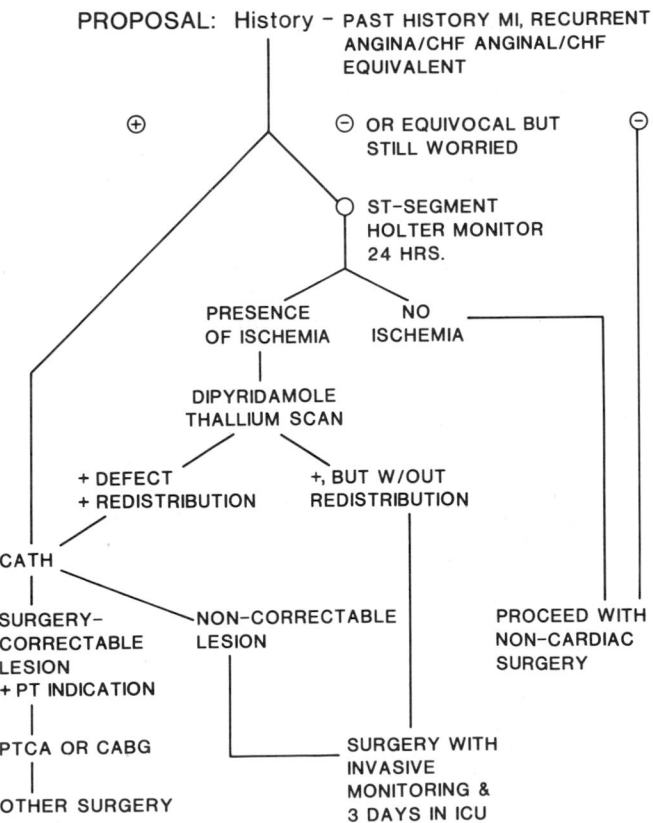

Fig. 25-6. Assessment of cardiac risk in a patient about to undergo vascular surgery. If clinical index is high, coronary arteriography (CATH) is recommended with subsequent coronary artery bypass grafting (CABG) or percutaneous transluminal coronary angioplasty (PTCA) for those with correctable lesions and patient (PT) consent. Equivocal history is followed by Holter monitoring and dipyridamole thallium scanning if positive. (See text.)

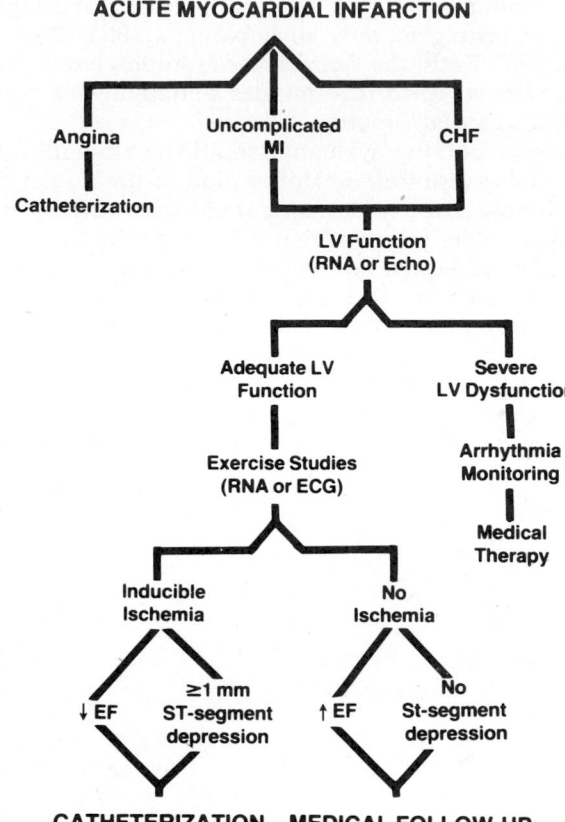

Fig. 25-7. Strategy for identifying patients who should undergo cardiac catheterization after acute myocardial infarction. This strategy is based on clinical assessment, evaluation of left ventricular (LV) function by radionuclide angiography (RNA) or echocardiography, analysis of arrhythmias, and stress testing. MI, acute myocardial infarction; CHF, overt congestive heart failure; EF, ejection fraction. (From Epstein et al.,[271] with permission.)

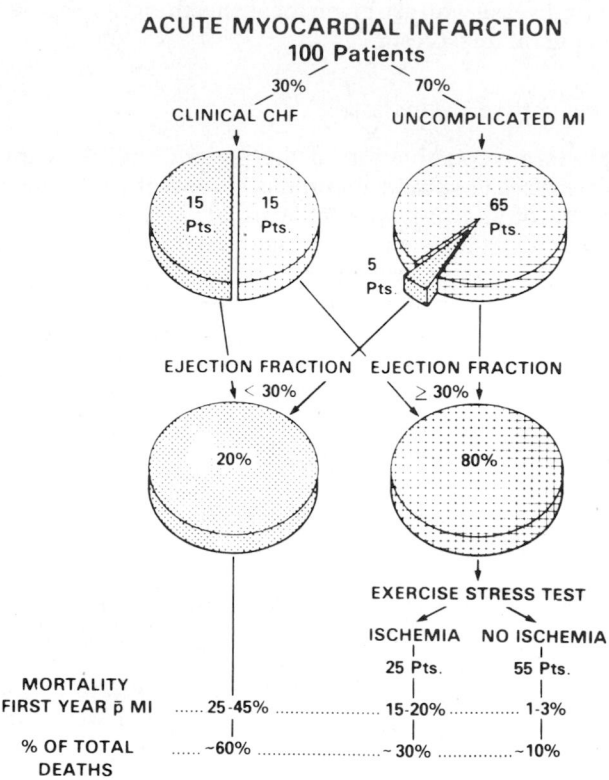

Fig. 25-8. First-year mortality rates for patients with acute myocardial infarction, according to subgroup. Hatched areas represent patients with ejection fractions of more than 30 percent; stippled areas represent patients with ejection fractions of less than 30 percent. (The percentages are, by necessity, rough approximations.) MI, acute myocardial infarction; CHF, overt congestive heart failure. (From Epstein et al.,[271] with permission.)

supply to the myocardium of patients with coronary artery stenosis is to maintain diastolic blood pressure, hemoglobin concentration, and oxygen saturation. Therefore, the main goal of anesthesia practice for such patients has been to decrease the determinants of myocardial oxygen demand[1]: heart rate, ventricular wall tension, and contractile performance.[238,274,275] Thus, medical management to accomplish the goal of preserving all viable myocardial tissue may include (1) administration of β-adrenergic receptor blocking drugs (propranolol, esmolol, or metoprolol) to decrease contractility and heart rate, and (2) vasodilation [with nitroglycerin (or its "long-acting" analogues), nitroprusside, hydralazine, or prazosin] to decrease ventricular wall tension.[132-134,275] The goal of anesthesia management should be the same, although no prospective controlled studies have documented a decrease in perioperative morbidity by reducing preload or afterload or by decreasing heart rate. However, the goal of keeping cardiovascular variables within an acceptable range and the rate–pressure product below the threshold for

angina appears appropriate.[95,201,202,260,274–276] The use of Swan-Ganz catheters for this type of patient is described in Chapter 31, and the intraoperative management of ischemic heart disease patients is discussed in further detail in Chapter 51.

Briefly, I believe drugs given chronically (e.g., antihypertensive medications) should be continued through the morning of surgery. The topic of chronic drug therapy is discussed in more detail in the last section of this chapter. Finally, a patient with a subendocardial MI has been assumed to be at less perioperative risk than a patient with a transmural MI. This assumption is now being questioned in medical circles.[277] Thus, patients with a subendocardial MI should be treated no differently than those with a transmural MI.

Valvular Heart Disease

Major alterations in the preoperative management of patients with valvular heart disease have been made regarding the use of anticoagulant therapy and are now based on the causes of disease. Although preoperative and intraoperative management of patients with valvular heart disease are discussed in Chapter 51, a few important points concerning preoperative care are emphasized here. Of prime importance is realizing that stenotic lesions are managed in a fashion exactly opposite that for regurgitant lesions. Therefore, the type of lesion that exists should be determined preoperatively. Although the causes of various forms of valvular heart disease have not changed, the relative frequency has. Rheumatic valvulitis is much less common today than in the 1970s, and syphilitic aortitis has all but disappeared. Now common are congenital bicuspid aortic stenosis, mitral valve prolapse, hypertrophic cardiomyopathy (also called asymmetric septal hypertrophy or subvalvular aortic stenosis), and mitral valve insufficiency due to calcification.

The prognosis and, presumably, the perioperative risk for patients with valvular heart disease depend on the stage of the disease.[264] Although stenotic lesions progress faster than regurgitant lesions, regurgitant lesions secondary to infective endocarditis, rupture of chordae tendineae, or ischemic heart disease can be rapidly fatal. Left ventricular dysfunction is common in the late stage of valvular heart disease. Once again history and physical examination appear to be the most sensitive and specific indicators of disease and disease stage (Table 25-16).[278]

Preoperative maintenance of drug therapy can be crucial: the patient with aortic stenosis can deteriorate rapidly with the onset of atrial fibrillation or flutter, as the atrial component to left ventricular filling can be critical in maintaining cardiac output. One of the most serious complications of valvular heart surgery and of valvular heart disease prior to surgery are cardiac arrhythmias. Conduction disorders and chronic therapy with antiarrhythmic and inotropic drugs are discussed elsewhere in this chapter. The reader is referred elsewhere in this book (Ch. 52) or to other references[279,280] for discussion of the management of the child with congenital heart disease for noncardiac surgery.

Mitral Valve Prolapse

Mitral valve prolapse, perhaps the most frequent valvular abnormality, occurs in 5 to 17 percent of otherwise healthy people. It is associated with atrioseptal secundum defects,[281-283] thoracic skeletal abnormality (due to time of development of these structures), and, for unknown reasons, migraine anxiety neurosis, and autonomic dysfunction. Hereditary transmission has been proposed as occurring through autosomal dominance with reduced expressivity in humans. Mitral valve prolapse is also associated with von Willebrand's syndrome and polycystic kidney disease, and the presence of one condition requires a search (by at least history and physical examination) for the other. This valvular lesion presents either asymptomatically or with palpitations, dyspnea, atypical chest pain, dizziness, syncope, or sudden death. Supraventricular arrhythmias (associated with atrioventricular bypass tracts and the pre-excitation syndrome) occur in over 50 percent of patients with mitral valve prolapse. Ventricular arrhythmias (usually in surgery) occur in 45 percent of such patients, bradyarrhythmias in 25 percent, and sudden death in 1.4 percent.[281-284] The frequent occur-

TABLE 25-16. Bedside Diagnosis of Systolic Murmurs: Sensitivity, Specificity, and Predictive Value of Diagnostic Maneuvers

Maneuver	Response	Murmur	Sensitivity (%)	Specificity (%)	Predictive Value Positive (%)	Predictive Value Negative (%)
Inspiration	Increase	Right-sided	100	88	67	100
Expiration	Decrease	Right-sided	100	88	67	100
Müller maneuver	Increase	Right-sided	15	92	33	81
Valsalva maneuver	Increase	Hypertrophic cardiomyopathy	65	96	81	92
Squatting to standing	Increase	Hypertrophic cardiomyopathy	95	84	59	98
Standing to squatting	Decrease	Hypertrophic cardiomyopathy	95	85	61	99
Leg elevation	Decrease	Hypertrophic cardiomyopathy	85	91	71	96
Handgrip	Decrease	Hypertrophic cardiomyopathy	85	75	46	95
Handgrip	Increase	Mitral regurgitation and ventricular septal defect	68	92	84	81
Transient arterial occlusion	Increase	Mitral regurgitation and ventricular septal defect	78	100	100	87
Amyl nitrite inhalation	Decrease	Mitral regurgitation and ventricular septal defect	80	90	84	87

(Adapted from Lembo et al.,[278] with permission.)

rence of transient cerebral ischemia has resulted in the chronic use of aspirin or anticoagulants in patients with mitral valve prolapse, and the potential for endocarditis has led to the recommendation for prophylaxis with antibiotics prior to known bacteremic events,[281-285] and the avoidance of head-up positions and decreased afterload in such patients.

Preoperative Antibiotic Prophylaxis for Endocarditis

Patients who have any form of valvular heart disease, as well as those with intracardiac (ventricular septal or atrial septal defects) or intravascular shunt, should be protected against endocarditis at the time of known bacteremic event. Endocarditis has occurred in a sufficiently significant number of patients with hypertrophic cardiomyopathy (subvalvular aortic stenosis, asymmetric septal hypertrophy) and mitral valve prolapse to warrant including such patients in the prophylaxis regimen.

Is endotracheal intubation a bacteremic event? Bacteremia occurs after the following events at these rates: dental extraction, 30 to 80 percent; brushing of teeth, 20 to 24 percent; use of oral irrigation devices, 20 to 24 percent; barium enema, 11 percent; transurethral prostate resection, 10 to 57 percent; upper gastrointestinal endoscopy, 8 percent; nasotracheal intubation, 16 percent (4 of 25 patients); and orotracheal intubation, 0 percent (0 of 25 patients).[286,287] Thus, although bacteremia from orotracheal intubation is rare, I believe that, for patients with valvular heart disease, prophylaxis should be given before instrumentation of the gallbladder, GI tract, oropharynx, or genitourinary tract. The choice of antibiotic for prophylaxis should be aimed at the most commonly occurring (i.e., most numerous) pathogen (Table 25-17A).[288] Note these prophylactic regimens should be altered to prevent sepsis after specific surgical procedures (Table 25-17B).[289] Guidelines of the American Heart Association state that all antimicrobial prophylaxis should be started 30 minutes to 1 hour, rather than 24 hours, before a known bacteremic event, so as to reach therapeutic levels without superinfecting the patient with unusual pathogens.[288,289]

Cardiac Valve Prostheses and Anticoagulant Therapy, and Prophylaxis for Deep Venous Thrombosis

Prothrombin time should be within 20 percent of control at the time of operation, or an appreciable risk is incurred.[290] Therefore, to produce a normal prothrombin time on the day of surgery, chronic anticoagulant therapy should be suspended in surgical patients having cardiac valve prostheses. This can be done with safety several days before surgery if the prosthesis is an aortic valve. However, because the risk of thromboem-

---

TABLE 25-17A. Endocarditis Prophylaxis: Recommended Antibiotic Regimens

	Dosage for Adults	Dosage for Children
Dental and upper respiratory procedures (i.e., tonsilloadenoidectomy, bronchoscopy, nasal intubation, nasogastric tube placement)		
Oral		
Penicillin V	2 g 1 hour before procedure and 1 g 6 hours later	>60 lb: adult dosage <60 lb: half adult dosage
Penicillin allergy: erythromycin	1 g 1 hour before procedure and 500 mg 6 hours later	20 mg/kg 1 hour before procedure and 10 mg/kg 6 hours later
Parenteral		
Ampicillin	2 g IM or IV 30 minutes before procedure	50 mg/kg IM or IV 30 minutes before procedure
plus gentamicin	1.5 mg/kg IM or IV 30 minutes before procedure	2.0 mg/kg IM or IV 30 minutes before procedure
Penicillin allergy: vancomycin	1 g IV infused slowly over 1 hour beginning 1 hour before procedure	20 mg/kg IV infused slowly over 1 hour beginning 1 hour before procedure
Gastrointestinal and genitourinary procedures (i.e., GI or GU surgery, or instrumentation or surgery involving a tissue possibly contaminated with GI or GU organisms)		
Parenteral		
Ampicillin	2 g IM or IV 30 minutes before procedure	50 mg/kg IM or IV 30 minutes before procedure
plus gentamicin	1.5 mg/kg IM or IV 30 minutes before procedure	2.0 mg/kg IM or IV 30 minutes before procedure
Penicillin allergy: vancomycin	1 g IV infused slowly over 1 hour beginning 1 hour before procedure	20 mg/kg IV infused slowly over 1 hour beginning 1 hour before procedure
plus gentamicin	1.5 mg/kg IM or IV 30 minutes before procedure	2.0 mg/kg IM or IV 30 minutes before procedure
Oral		
Amoxicillin	3 g 1 hour before procedure and 1.5 g 6 hours later	50 mg/kg 1 hour before procedure and 25 mg/kg 6 hours later

The frequently used cephalosporins are not recommended. A single dose of the parental drugs is probably adequate, because bacteremias after most oral cavity and diagnostic procedures are of short duration. However, one or two follow-up doses may be given at 8- to 12-hour intervals in selected patients, such as hospitalized patients judged to be at higher risk.
(Adapted from Committee on Prevention of Rheumatic Fever and Bacterial Endocarditis,[288] with permission.)

TABLE 25-17B. Prevention of Wound Infection and Sepsis in Surgical Patients

Nature of Operation	Likely Pathogens	Recommended Drugs	Adult Dosage Before Surgery[a]
Clean			
Cardiovascular			
Prosthetic valve and other open-heart surgery, pacemaker implantation[b]	*Staphylococcus epidermidis, S. aureus, Corynebacterium* sp., enteric gram-negative bacilli, fungi	Cefazolin or vancomycin[c]	1 g IV
Arterial reconstructive surgery involving the abdominal aorta, a prosthesis, or a groin incision	*S. aureus, S. epidermidis*, enteric gram-negative bacilli	Cefazolin or vancomycin[c]	1 g IM/IV 1 g IV
Orthopaedic			
Total joint replacement, internal fixation of proximal femoral fracture	*S. aureus, S. epidermidis*	Cefazolin or vancomycin[c]	1 g IM/IV 1 g IV
Clean-contaminated			
Head and neck			
Entering oral cavity or pharynx	*S. aureus*, streptococci, oral anaerobes	Cefazolin	1 g IM/IV
Gastroduodenal	Enteric gram-negative bacilli, gram-positive cocci	High risk or gastric bypass only: cefazolin	1 g IM/IV
Biliary tract	Enteric gram-negative bacilli, group D streptococci, *Clostridia*	High risk only: cefazolin	1 g IM/IV
Colorectal	Enteric gram-negative bacilli, anaerobic bacteria, group D streptococci	Oral: neomycin plus erythromycin base	1 g of each at 1 PM, 2 PM, and 11 PM the day before the operation[d]
		Parenteral: cefoxitin or clindamycin plus gentamicin or tobramycin	1 g IV 600 mg IV 1.5 mg/kg IM/IV
Appendectomy	Enteric gram-negative bacilli, anaerobic bacteria	Cefoxitin	1 g IV
Vaginal or abdominal hysterectomy	Enteric gram-negative bacilli, anaerobes, group B and D streptococci	Cefazolin	1 g IM/IV
Cesarean section	Same as for hysterectomy	High risk only: cefazolin	1 g IV after cord clamping
Abortion	Same as for hysterectomy	First trimester in patients with previous pelvic inflammatory disease: aqueous penicillin G Second trimester: cefazolin	1 million units IV 1 g IM/IV
Dirty			
Ruptured viscus	Enteric gram-negative bacilli, anaerobes, group D streptococci	Clindamycin plus gentamicin or tobramycin or cefoxitin with or without gentamicin or tobramycin	600 mg IV q6h 1.5 mg/kg q8h IM/IV 1g q4-8h IV 1.5 mg/kg q8h IM/IV
Traumatic wound	*S. aureus*, group A strep, *Clostridia, Pasteurella multocida*[e]	Cefazolin	1 g q8h IM/IV

[a] Parenteral prophylactic antimicrobials for clean and clean-contaminated surgery can be given as a single dose just before the operation. For prolonged operations, additional intraoperative doses should be given q4-8h for the duration of the procedure. For dirty surgery, therapy should usually be continued for 5 to 10 days.
[b] Prophylaxis not needed for pacemaker implantation in centers with low incidence of infection.
[c] For hospitals in which methicillin-resistant *S. aureus* and *S. epidermidis* frequently cause wound infections after these procedures.
[d] After appropriate diet and catharsis (RL Nichols in GL Mandell et al, eds., Principles and Practice of Infectious Diseases, 2nd Ed., Churchchill Livingstone, New York, 1985, p. 1641).
(From Abramowicz,[289] with permission.)

bolism is greater with mitral valve prostheses (5 percent) than with aortic valve prostheses (1 to 3 percent), patients having mitral valve prostheses should have rapid reversal of oral anticoagulation with vitamin K the day before surgery or fresh frozen plasma on the day of surgery. For resumption of anticoagulant therapy after surgery, rapid anticoagulation with heparin 12 hours postoperatively has proved successful in patients with mitral valve prostheses.[291,292] In patients with new aortic valve prostheses, resumption of anticoagulant therapy should start 2 days after surgery. Regional anesthetic techniques might be avoided, although controversy exists on this issue.[293-301] Many practitioners do not hesitate to use regional anesthesia in the face of prophylaxis for deep venous thrombosis.[297,298,301]

Deep venous thromboses are so common in postoperative patients that almost 1 percent of postsurgical patients die of fatal pulmonary embolism (Table 25-18).[302] Because of this high mortality risk, prophylaxis against DVT is gaining widespread acceptance; and thus, prophylaxis often begins with 5,000 units of heparin given subcutaneously 2 hours prior to surgery.[302-304] Other trials have shown equal effect with low-molecular-weight heparin (which is associated with less theoretical risk of bleeding) and external pneumatic compression.[303,305] Persuading surgeons to use the latter technique may allow more assurance in using regional anesthesia. Such an option, however, is not available for the patient with a prosthetic valve.

Another problem that can arise is managing the preg-

TABLE 25-18. Incidence of Deep Venous Thrombosis, Fatal Pulmonary Embolism, and Recommended Prophylaxis

| Type of Surgery | Incidence of | | | Recommended Prophylaxis |
	Deep Vein Thrombosis (%)	Proximal Deep Vein Thrombosis (%)	Fatal Pulmonary Embolism (%)	
General				
Age > 40 yr	30	3–15	0.8	
Age > 60 yr	50			
Malignancy	50–60			
Thoracic	30			
Vascular				
Aortic repair	26			Low-dose heparin with or without compression stockings or external pneumatic compression
Peripheral	12			
Urologic				
Open prostatectomy	40			
TURP	10			
Other urologic	30–40			
Major gynecologic				
With malignancy	40			
Without malignancy	10–20			
Neurosurgery				
Craniotomy	20–40			External pneumatic compression
Laminectomy	4–25		1.5–3	
Orthopaedic				
Total hip replacement	40–78	30	1.8–3.4	Low-dose heparin and DHE or warfarin or adjusted-dose heparin or low-molecular-weight heparin
Hip fracture	48–75		3–10	
Tibial fracture	45			
Total knee	57			External pneumatic compression or warfarin or low-dose heparin
Head, neck, chest wall	11			
Medical				
Acute MI	30	6		
Stroke	60–75			
Acute spinal injury	60–100			
Other bed-bound	26			

nant patient with a prosthetic valve during delivery. It is recommended that warfarin be replaced by subcutaneous heparin during the peripartum period. During labor and delivery, elective induction is advocated with discontinuance of all anticoagulant therapy, as indicated for the particular valve prosthesis (discussed above).[306]

Auscultation of the prosthetic valve should be performed preoperatively to verify normal functioning (Fig. 25-9).[307] Abnormalities in such sounds warrant preoperative consultation and verification of functioning.

Cardiac Conduction Disturbances

Cardiac Arrhythmias (Also See Chs. 31 and 32)

Bradyarrhythmias, especially if profound or associated with dizziness or syncope, are generally managed with pacemakers. However, on rare occasion, chronic bifascicular block (right bundle branch block with left anterior or posterior hemiblock, or left bundle branch block with combined left anterior and posterior hemiblocks) even when only first-degree heart block is present, progresses to complete heart block and sudden perioperative death. But this is a rare occurrence. In five studies, fewer than 2 percent of the approximately 160 patients with bifascicular block progressed to complete heart block perioperatively.[308-312] On the other hand, such patients have a high 5-year mortality rate (160 of 554 patients, or 35 percent).[313] Most of the deaths were related to tachyarrhythmias or MI—events usually not preventable by pacemakers. Thus, the presence of bifascicular block on ECG should make the anesthesiologist more worried about associated coronary artery disease or left ventricular dysfunction. Nevertheless, these patients rarely have complete heart block perioperatively. Therefore, prophylactic preoperative insertion of temporary pacing wires for bifascicular block does not seem warranted. However, a central route should be established in advance in the event a temporary pacemaker needs to be inserted. The actual pacemaker equipment and appropriate personnel should be immediately available and tested regularly since symptomatic heart block does occur perioperatively in more than 1 percent of patients.[308-312]

Premature ventricular contractions (PVCs) of more than 5 per minute on preoperative examination correlate with perioperative cardiac morbidity.[226,233,234,247] To the classic criteria for treating PVCs (the presence of R-on-T couplets, the occurrence of more than three PVCs per minute, multifocality of PVCs) must be added frequent (> 10/h over a 24-hour period) and repetitive ventricular beats. Electrophysiologic and programmed ventricular stimulation studies are being used to indicate and guide treatment for patients with ischemic heart disease or recurrent arrhythmias and for survivors of out-of-hospital sudden death.[314,315] Although such patients are often treated with antiarrhythmic therapy, attention to their underlying condition should be a focus of our preoperative management. Chronic antiarrhythmic therapy is discussed in the last section of this chapter.

Premature atrial contractions and cardiac rhythm other than sinus also correlate with perioperative cardiac morbidity.[226,233] These arrhythmias may be more a marker of poor cardiovascular reserve than a specific cause of perioperative cardiac complications.

Prosthesis type	Mitral Prosthesis	Acoustic Characteristics	Aortic Prosthesis	Acoustic Characteristics
Ball Valves	*(diagram: SEM, MC, S₂, MO)*	1) A_2-MO interval 0.07-0.11 sec. 2) MO > MC 3) II-III/VI Systolic ejection murmur (SEM) 4) No diastolic murmur	*(diagram: S₁, S₂, AO, AC)*	1) S_1-AO interval 0.07 sec. 2) AO > AC 3) II/VI harsh SEM 4) No diastolic murmur
Disc Valves	*(diagram: SEM, DM, MC, S₂)*	1) A_2-MO interval 0.05-0.09 sec. 2) MO is rarely heard 3) II/VI SEM is usually heard 4) I-II/VI diastolic rumble is usually heard	*(diagram: SEM, S₁, P₂, AC)*	1) S_1-AO interval 0.04 sec. 2) AO is uncommonly heard, AC is usually heard 3) II/VI SEM is usually heard 4) Occasional diastolic murmur
Porcine Valves	*(diagram: SEM, DM, MC, S₂, MO)*	1) A_2-MO interval 0.1 sec. 2) MO is audible 50% 3) I-II/VI apical SEM 50% 4) Diastolic rumble ½-⅔	*(diagram: SEM, S₁, P₂, AC)*	1) S_1-AO interval 0.03-0.08 sec. 2) AO is uncommonly heard, AC is usually heard 3) II/VI SEM in most 4) No diastolic murmur
Bileaflet Valve (St. Jude)			*(diagram: SEM, S₁, P₂, AO, AC)*	1) AO and AC commonly heard 2) A soft SEM is common

Fig. 25-9. Summary of the normal acoustic characteristics of valve prostheses according to type and location. SEM, systolic ejection murmur; DM, diastolic murmur; S_1, first heart sound; S_2, second heart sound; P_2, pulmonary second sound; A_2, aortic second sound; AO, aortic valve opening sound; AC, aortic valve closure sound; MO, mitral valve opening sound; MC, mitral valve closure sound. (From Smith et al.,[307] with permission.)

Preexcitation syndrome is the name for supraventricular tachycardias associated with atrioventricular bypass tracts.[316] Successful treatment, which is predicated on an understanding of the clinical and electrophysiologic manifestations of the syndrome, consists of preoperative and intraoperative techniques that avoid release of sympathetic substances and other vasoactive substances, and hence tachyarrhythmias.[316-318]

Pacemakers

The types of pacemakers and indications for their use have changed significantly since 1980. More than 90 percent of pacemakers are inserted for bradyarrhythmias, either after tachycardia (brady–tachy syndrome) or by themselves, that is, sick sinus syndrome or atrioventricular conduction disorders. The rate of pacemaker insertion has also declined by over 40 percent since 1980; in 1984 a publication by the American College of Cardiology and American Heart Association of indications for pacemaker insertion codified these changes in practice patterns. The most common pacemaker for such dysfunction is the ventricular R-wave inhibited (demand) type (VVI) (letter codes are described later and in Table 25-19). More complex pacemakers are now being employed to provide better cardiac output in stressful situations and to decrease myocardial wall stress[319] or to treat ventricular tachyarrhythmias. Lithium batteries now allow a pacemaker to have a 5- to 10-year life span. Programmable pacemakers are adjustable for sensitivity and rate. Atrial pacemakers fired by an outside radiofrequency source now allow termination of reentrant or pre-excitation atrial arrhythmias; similarly, ventricular pacemakers can be used to terminate supraventricular tachycardia and recurrent ventricular tachycardia.[320] Thus, in addition to learning about the patient's underlying disease, current condition, and drug therapy, the anesthesiologist must learn, preoperatively, the following information about any implanted pacemaker[320]:

1. The indication for placement of the pacemaker and the default rhythm (i.e., what rhythm occurs if the pacemaker does not capture).
2. The type of pacemaker (demand, fixed, or radiofrequency), the chamber paced, and the chamber sensed. Pacemakers have traditionally been given a five-letter code (Table 25-19). (However, most pacemakers implanted since 1980 have codes consisting of only the first three letters. The *first letter* indicates the chamber paced (i.e., V = ventricle, A = atrium, D = double or both). The *second letter* indicates the chamber sensed (i.e., V = ventricle, A = atrium, O = none). The *third letter* indicates the sensing pattern (i.e., O = no sensing, fixed mode; I = inhibited, demand pacer; T = triggered, meaning that the sensing of an electrical impulse triggers a pacemaker spike). For example, a VOO pacemaker paces the ventricle, does not sense and is in a fixed mode. In other words, it is a fixed-rate ventricular pacemaker. A VVI pacemaker paces the ventricle, senses the ventricle, and is inhibited. It is a ventricular-inhibited demand pacemaker. A DVI pacemaker paces both atrium and ventricle, senses only the ventricle, and is inhibited. Thus, it is a sequential atrioventricular demand pacemaker that fires when it does not sense intrinsic ventricular activity.
3. How to detect deterioration in battery function (increased rate or decreased rate).
4. How to change the mode or to fire the pacemaker if it is of the radiofrequency type. (These procedures should not only be learned by the anesthesiologist but also demonstrated to him or her. Also, the magnet and/or programming device should be in or near the operating room at the time of surgery.)
5. The current rate and sensitivity settings of the pacemaker.
6. Whether the pacemaker is currently functioning and how well.

Because demand pacemakers can sense electrocautery, which sometimes inhibits pacemaker firing, asystole can occur in the pacemaker-dependent patient. Most pacemakers can be converted to a fixed rate, and the anesthesiologist should do the following: (1) have the cardiologist demonstrate how this is done, and (2) have the necessary magnet and/or programming device available in the operating room. In addition, the ground plate should be as far from the pulse generator and lead as possible, a bipolar form of electrocautery should be used, and, if possible, some measure of blood flow should be monitored, that is, Doppler detector, pulse oximetry that is unaffected by electrocautery, or intra-arterial line. The rationale for the latter measure is that electrocautery temporarily affects the accuracy of electrocardiographic results; since asystole could occur during this period, a measure of blood flow is necessary. Currently, at least 12 manufacturers pro-

TABLE 25-19. Traditional Five-Letter Code for Pacemaker Systems

1st Letter Chamber Paced	2nd Letter Chamber Sensed	3rd Letter Mode of Response	4th Letter (if Used) Programmable Features	5th Letter (if Used) Arrhythmia Treatment
A = atrium	A = atrium	T = triggered	P = programmable	B = burst
V = ventricle	V = ventricle	I = inhibited	M = multiprogrammable	N = normal
D = double	D = double	D = double	O = not programmable	S = scanning
	O = none	O = not applicable		E = external

duce a total of more than 50 types of pacemakers, each having a different default program. A default program is the secondary program (i.e., the generator circuit) to which the primary program will revert if it senses problems in the initial circuit. Since default programs differ, pacemaker malfunction will present differently depending on the brand and model. Thus, it is necessary to learn before surgery how problems will manifest with each pacemaker during surgery.[320]

The most common cause of temporary pacemaker malfunction is lack of contact between the electrode wire and the endocardium. Pacemaker spikes continue to exist on the ECG oscilloscope even when no myocardial contractions propel blood. This situation has occurred with muscular exertion, blunt trauma, cardioversion, and positive-pressure ventilation.[321] Treatment consists of advancing the electrode until it captures, administering isoproterenol (if that worked in the past), external pacing, or, failing that, cardiopulmonary resuscitation.

During the preoperative examination, the anesthesiologist must also assess the progression of underlying disease (e.g., CHF, electrolyte disorders, and the condition of all systems related to the underlying disease).[319] Antiarrhythmic therapy and its implications are discussed in the last section of this chapter.

DISORDERS OF THE RESPIRATORY AND IMMUNE SYSTEMS

General Preoperative Considerations

The main purpose of preoperative testing is to identify patients at risk of perioperative complications and to institute appropriate perioperative therapy. Also, preoperative assessment can establish baseline function and the feasibility of surgical intervention. Whereas numerous investigators have used pulmonary function tests that define inoperability or high- versus low-risk groups for pulmonary complications, few have been able to demonstrate that the performance of any specific preoperative or intraoperative measure reliably decreases perioperative pulmonary morbidity or mortality. Since routine preoperative pulmonary testing and care are discussed extensively in Chapters 24 and 71, the current discussion limits itself to assessing the effectiveness of such care.

In fact, only four randomized prospective studies indicate a benefit of preoperative preparation. Stein and Cassara[322] randomly allocated 48 patients to undergo preoperative therapy (cessation of smoking, use of antibiotic treatment for purulent sputum, and use of bronchodilating drugs, postural drainage, chest physiotherapy, and ultrasonic nebulizer) or no preoperative therapy. The no-treatment group had mortality of 16 percent and morbidity of 60 percent, as opposed to the

0 to 20 percent rates, respectively, for the treatment group. In addition, the treatment group spent an average of 12 postoperative days in the hospital, compared with 24 days for the 21 survivors in the no-treatment group.

Collins et al.[323] prospectively examined the benefits of preoperative antibiotics, perioperative chest physiotherapy and therapy with bronchodilating drugs, and routing postoperative analgesia (morphine) on postoperative respiratory complications in patients with chronic obstructive pulmonary disease (COPD). Of those therapies, only preoperative treatment with antibiotics had a beneficial effect.

Warner and colleagues[324] collected data retrospectively about smoking history and prospectively (concurrently) about pulmonary complications for 200 patients undergoing CABG surgery. They documented that 8 weeks or more of smoking cessation was associated with a 66 percent reduction in postoperative pulmonary complications. Smokers who stopped for less than 8 weeks actually had an increase (from 33 percent for current smokers to 57.1 percent for recent quitters) in the rate of one or more of the six complications surveyed: purulent sputum with pyrexia; need for respiratory therapy care; bronchospasm requiring therapy; pleural effusion and/or pneumothorax necessitating drainage; segmental pulmonary collapse, as confirmed by radiograph; or pneumonia necessitating antibiotic therapy. Although others have found both shorter and longer periods of cessation of smoking prior to cardiovascular benefits[325-328] and hematologic benefits,[329,330] this is one of the few studies that show both harmful and beneficial outcomes for pulmonary status from the same maneuver—smoking cessation. Since anesthesiologists rarely see their patients 8 weeks or more prior to surgery, this presents a dilemma: if you are unable to advise a smoker to stop 8 weeks or more before surgery, is continued smoking preferable? Perhaps these data will give further impetus to institution of preoperative assessment clinics where anesthesiologists will be able to advise and counsel patients about risk reduction.

Celli and co-workers[331] performed a randomized prospective controlled trial of intermittent positive-pressure breathing (IPPB), versus incentive spirometry, versus deep breathing exercises in 81 patients undergoing abnormal surgery. The groups exposed to a respiratory therapist (regardless of treatment given) had more than a 50 percent lower incidence of clinical complications (30 to 33 percent versus 88 percent) and shorter hospital stays than the control group. Thus, this third prospective study indicates that any concern about lung function on the part of someone knowledgeable in maneuvers designed to clear lung secretions improves outcome.

Bartlett et al.[332] randomly assigned 150 patients undergoing extensive laparotomy to one of two groups. One group received preoperative instruction in, and postoperative use (10 times/h) of, incentive spirometry. The other group received similar medical care but no incentive spirometry. Only 7 of 75 patients using incentive spirometry had postoperative pulmonary complications, as opposed to 19 of 75 in the control group. However, other studies have not shown a benefit for specific treatments or have been too contaminated with bias to have a clear result emerge. Lyager et al.[333] randomly assigned 103 patients undergoing biliary or gastric surgery to receive either incentive spirometry with preoperative and postoperative chest physiotherapy, or only preoperative and postoperative chest physiotherapy. No difference in postoperative course or pulmonary complications was found between the two groups. Other studies have shown a specific benefit (i.e., above that provided by routine care) for chest physiotherapy and IPPB. These studies are usually poorly controlled, not randomized, and/or retrospective in design; these deficiencies probably substantially bias the results.[334-336] Although randomized prospective studies showed no benefit or actual harm from chest physiotherapy and IPPB on the resolution of pneumonia[337,338] or postoperative pulmonary complications,[323,331,336,338-340] the four studies cited above[322,323,331,332] and numerous retrospective studies[324,334-336] strongly suggest that preoperative evaluation and treatment of patients with pulmonary disease actually decrease perioperative respiratory complications.

The evaluation of dyspnea is especially useful and so warrants discussion here (for a review of the specific pulmonary function tests that identify high-risk groups, see Ch. 24). Boushy et al.[341] found that grades of preoperative dyspnea correlated with postoperative survival. (The grades of respiratory dyspnea are provided in Table 25-20). Mittman[342] demonstrated an increased risk of death after thoracic surgery from 8 percent in patients without dyspnea to 56 percent in patients who were dyspneic. Similarly, Reichel[343] found that no patients died after pneumonectomy if they were able to complete a preoperative treadmill test for 4 minutes at the rate of 2 mph on level ground. Other studies have found that history and physical examination of the asthmatic subject can also predict the need for hospitalization.[344] Other than dyspnea, what preoperative conditions make postoperative respiratory complications more likely? (see Refs. 345, 346, and also Ch. 71). The important information and conditions to search for during the history-taking and physical examination are as follows:

1. Dyspnea.
2. Coughing and production of sputum. Sputum, if present, should be Gram-stained and cultured, and appropriate antibiotic treatment should be instituted.
3. Recent respiratory infection. Viral respiratory infections affect respiratory function, giving rise to increased airflow obstruction that may persist for as long as 5 weeks.[347,348] These infections also adversely affect respiratory mechanisms responding to bacteria. However, whether the incidence of complications in normal children is lessened by waiting 5 weeks until the symptoms of respiratory infections have disappeared is open to question.[349-351]
4. Hemoptysis.
5. Wheezing and prior use of bronchodilating drugs and corticosteroids. Wheezing often suggests potentially reversible airway obstruction but is a notoriously poor indicator of the degree of obstruction. In addition, all wheezing is not bronchospasm. Cardiac and other pulmonary causes must be differentiated from asthma.[352,353] Drug therapy for asthma should be ascertained and optimized if possible. Asthmatics have a fourfold increase in perioperative respiratory complications.
6. Pulmonary complications from previous surgery. Prolonged endotracheal intubation after surgery can be required by many conditions, most probably respiratory and neuromuscular disorders.
7. A history of smoking. The incidence of respiratory complications is higher among tobacco smokers than among nonsmokers.[324,334,335,354]
8. Age, general history of the patient, and any other significant physical findings. Although other disease conditions probably increase respiratory risk, this hypothesis has not been adequately documented. Old age definitely increases respiratory and cardiac risk.[324,333,354,355] Cardiovascular history and examinations are obviously important for risk by themselves and especially for signs of pulmonary hypertension, such as right ventricular lift (i.e., lift over the lower sternum), fixed and widely split second heart sound, and S_4 gallop at the left sternal border.
9. Breathing frequency and form. Pursed lips, cyanosis, and use of accessory muscles should be noted.
10. Body habitus:
    a. Abnormalities of the chest wall, trauma, kyphoscoliosis with restrictive lung disease. Development of a barrel chest is a late manifestation of obstructive lung disease.
    b. Obesity. A weight 30 percent over ideal weight

TABLE 25-20. Grade of Dyspnea Caused by Respiratory Problems (Assessed in Terms of Walking on the Level at a Normal Pace)

Category	Description
0	No dyspnea while walking on the level at a normal pace
I	"I am able to walk as far as I like provided I take my time"
II	Specific (street) block limitation ("I have to stop for a while after one or two blocks")
III	Dyspnea on mild exertion ("I have to stop and rest while going from the kitchen to the bathroom")
IV	Dyspnea at rest

(Modified from Boushy et al.,[341] with permission.)

doubles the incidence of respiratory complications.[337,354,356]

11. Adequacy of upper airway, presence of tracheal deviation, ease of face mask application, ease of endotracheal intubation.

12. Presence of rales, rhonchi, wheezing, diaphragmatic excursion, air movement, and ratio of expiratory to inspiratory times.

13. Site of proposed surgery. Upper abdominal surgery increases the incidence of perioperative pulmonary complications.[322,335,345,357]

Chapters 24 and 71 review the value of the chest roentgenograms and pulmonary function tests in identifying patients with preoperative pulmonary disease as well as which tests should be ordered and for whom. Any patient who will require postoperative ventilatory support should undergo preoperative testing. Although the ideal pulmonary function test guaranteeing success or predicting poor outcome that can be improved by therapy has yet to be found, a maximum breathing capacity less than 40 or 50 L/min/70 kg, a FVC_1/FVC less than 40 percent of predicted, or a maximum midexpiratory flow rate of less than 50 L/min is a relatively good predictor of complications for surgery involving resection of lung.[334,335,342-345,358-360] To these now is added the diffusing capacity of the lung for carbon monoxide (DLCO).[359,360] DLCO decreases with fixed obstructive lung disease (i.e., emphysema) but remains normal in bronchospastic disease. In one study, when preoperative DLCO was less than 60 percent of predicted, the mortality rate was 25 percent and pulmonary morbidity rate was 45 percent, whereas a DLCO of 100 percent or greater of predicted was associated with a 0 percent mortality rate and a 11 percent pulmonary morbidity rate. A subsequent study confirmed these findings.[360] Although I've always tried to reduce laboratory studies, these may prove useful in the patient with COPD needing pulmonary surgery. Further analysis is necessary to determine whether the finding of a normal DLCO may allow expansion of the usual spirometric criteria to permit successful pulmonary resection in patients who are currently excluded as candidates for such operations. I conduct such tests on any patient with dyspnea of grade II or higher or on any patient who shows significant abnormalities or risk on the 13 factors listed.

Despite the lack of definitive data establishing the efficacy of preoperative pulmonary testing and therapy, I recommend the following approach:

1. Eradicate acute infections and suppress chronic infections by using appropriate diagnostic measures and antibiotic treatment.

2. Relieve bronchospasm by using bronchodilating drugs and document such relief with measurements of forced expiratory volume at one second (also see Chs. 24 and 71).

3. Institute measures to improve sputum clearance and to familiarize the patient with respiratory therapy equipment (incentive spirometry) and postural drainage maneuvers. Initiate practice coughing and deep-breathing exercises (also see Chs. 24 and 71).

4. Treat uncompensated right ventricular heart failure with digoxin, diuretics, oxygen, and drugs that decrease pulmonary vascular resistance (e.g., hydralazine).[361]

5. Use low-dose heparin prophylactically to decrease the incidence of venous thrombosis (and pulmonary emboli).[302-304]

6. Encourage reduction or cessation of smoking 8 weeks or more prior to surgery.[324] Although the debate about smoking cessation includes more than pulmonary risk, cardiovascular, hematologic, and aspiration risks also have not been shown to be responsive to short-term cessation.[324-330] Perhaps the benefit of using a major life event, an operation, to motivate smoking cessation is worth the increased short-term risk that encouraging cessation within a day or two of surgery would entail; the latter hypothesis remains to be tested. Even young people who smoke only one-half to one pack of cigarettes per day exhibit abnormalities in respiratory function.[362]

Specific Diseases

Pulmonary Vascular Diseases

Pulmonary vascular diseases include pulmonary hypertension secondary to heart disease (postcapillary disorders), parenchymal lung disease (pulmonary precapillary disorders), pulmonary embolism, and cor pulmonale from chronic obstructive pulmonary disease (COLD).[363] Optimal preoperative management of these conditions requires treatment of the underlying disease.[363-366] Because pulmonary embolism can be especially difficult to diagnose, it is crucial to be especially alert to the possibility of this disease. The clinical findings of pulmonary emboli are not always present or specific for the diagnosis. The history may include tachypnea, dyspnea, palpitations, syncope, chest pain, or hemoptysis. Physical examination can reveal a pleural rub, wheezing, rales, a fixed and split second heart sound, right ventricular lift, or evidence of venous thromboses, none of which is present in most patients. If the ECG shows a S_1-Q_3 pattern, lung perfusion scans can be obtained to rule out the diagnosis of pulmonary emboli. A high degree of suspicion is necessary to warrant angiography and anticoagulation or fibrinolytic therapy. If possible, the reactivity of the pulmonary vasculature should be determined, for it may be enhanced or decreased by such agents as nifedipine, hydralazine, nitroglycerin, prazosin, tolazoline, and phentolamine. Monitoring of pulmonary artery pressure is often required; preoperative measures should be undertaken to ensure that the patient is not exposed to conditions that elevate pulmonary vascular resistance (i.e., hypoxia, hypercarbia, acidosis, lung hyperinflation, hypothermia)[367] or that decrease blood volume (prolonged restriction of fluid intake) or systemic vascular resistance.

Infectious Diseases of the Lung

Preoperative evaluation and treatment should follow the basic guidelines outlined in the introduction to this section; treatment of the underlying disease should be completed before all but emergency surgery is performed. To repeat, viral respiratory infections do affect respiratory function, giving rise to increased airflow obstruction (especially in the small airways) that may persist for at least 5 weeks.[347] Viral respiratory infections also adversely affect respiratory defense mechanisms against bacteria.[348] Within 5 weeks of an upper respiratory tract infection, children may have an increased incidence of perioperative respiratory tract complications.[349-351]

Chronic Obstructive Pulmonary Diseases

Treatment of COPD (reactive airways) may include the use of β-adrenergic drugs, parasympatholytic agents (especially for exercise-induced asthma), and corticosteroids.[368] An estimated 5 percent of the population has bronchospasm. There is now a trend toward the use of topically applied steroids, such as beclomethasone dipropionate, which are inactivated after absorption. However, in large doses, these "topical" steroids can suppress adrenal function, and supplemental systemic corticosteroids may be needed at times of stress (see the earlier discussion under the section on adrenocortical malfunction). Preoperative assessment must include knowledge of drug regimens and effects, as these drugs can have dangerous interactions with anesthetic agents (see last section of this chapter). No known interaction between the inhaled anticholinergic ipratropium bromide and muscle relaxants has been reported. It is important to note that patients can feel fine at rest but must be tested with exercise or spirometry to document the degree of current bronchospasm. Furthermore, symptomatic response to bronchodilators in the asymptomatic patient may not predict whether or not the patient responds to bronchodilator therapy. An estimated 10 percent of asthmatic patients exhibit sensitivity to aspirin and may react not only to compounds containing aspirin but also to tartrazine, yellow dye no. 5, indomethacin, and aminopyrine.[369] Chronic obstructive pulmonary disease takes several forms. Bronchial asthma, which occurs in 3 to 5 percent of the population, is characterized by reversible airway obstruction. When airway obstruction is partially reversible (by steroids or adrenergic mediators), it is often accompanied by chronic bronchitis.[370] Some of these drugs may improve aspects of lung function other than bronchial muscle tone.[370] Chronic bronchitis almost always exists if there is a history of chronic cough and production of sputum on most days for 3 months a year for at least 2 years. These patients are (or almost always have been)

smokers, although environmental and occupational or genetic predisposition may contribute to hypertrophy of mucous glands in major airways, to hyperplasia of goblet cells, and to edema and inflammation of the airways. They will have a decreased DLCO; patients with pure bronchospasm will have a normal DLCO. Hyperinflation of airspaces, abnormal dilatation, and destruction of acinar units distal to the terminal bronchiole define emphysema. Cystic fibrosis is characterized by dilatation and hypertrophy of bronchial glands, mucous plugging of peripheral airways, and often bronchitis, bronchiectasis, and bronchiolectasis. For all these conditions, the measures recommended earlier in this section, as well as appropriate hydration to allow for mobilization of secretions, should be followed.

Interstitial and Immune Lung Diseases

Included in this heterogeneous group of diseases are the hypersensitivity lung diseases, environmental exposure diseases, the inorganic dust diseases, radiation-induced lung disease, sarcoidosis, the collagen-vascular disorders (systemic lupus erythematosus, polymyositis, dermatomyositis, Sjögren syndrome, rheumatoid arthritis, systemic sclerosis), Goodpasture syndrome, idiopathic pulmonary hemosiderosis, Wegener's granulomatosis, and the autoimmune diseases.[371] The gallium 67 scan localizes pulmonary inflammation and has proved an accurate method of assessing autoimmune pulmonary function disturbance as well as the response to steroid therapy.[372] Many of these disorders affect not only the lungs but the blood vessels, the conduction system of the heart, the myocardium, the joints (including those of the upper airway and larynx), and the renal, hepatic, and/or CNS as well. The reader is referred to a textbook of internal medicine to aid in understanding the pathophysiologic processes and full preoperative assessment of these conditions. Therapy for these conditions includes use of anti-inflammatory drugs, corticosteroids, and immunosuppressive drugs.

Neoplasms

Solitary nodules consist of tumors that are less than 6 cm in diameter, are surrounded by lung parenchyma, and are not associated with adenopathy or pleural effusion. The cure rate for bronchogenic carcinoma presenting as a solitary nodule is 70 percent — much better than the "cure" rate for other presentations.[373] (It should be remembered that tuberculosis can mimic cancer so closely that surgery has even been performed.[374]) Blood studies including calcium and alkaline phosphatase levels and liver function studies help confirm that the neoplasm has not disseminated. If these studies and history and physical examination show no abnormal findings, it is unlikely that bone, brain, or hepatic NMR or CT imaging techniques will indicate metastasis. Surgery need not await the results of these tests, as few patients not found to have metastatic disease by simple blood tests, history, and physical examination will prove to have such disease detected by these scans. Survival is dependent upon tissue staging and age of patients.[374a,375] Oat cell (small cell) carcinoma of the lung and bronchial adenomas are known for their secretion of endocrinologically active substances, such as ACTH-like hormones. Squamous cell cancers in the superior pulmonary sulcus produce Horner syndrome as well as a characteristic pain in the areas served by the eighth cervical nerves and first and second thoracic nerves. These tumors are now treated with preoperative radiation; surgical resection leads to an almost 30 percent "cure" rate.

Anaphylaxis, Anaphylactoid Responses, and Allergic Disorders Other Than Those Related to Lung Diseases and Asthma

Anaphylactic and Anaphylactoid Reactions

Anaphylaxis is a severe life-threatening allergic reaction. The term *allergic* applies to immunologically mediated reactions, as opposed to those caused by pharmacologic idiosyncrasy, by direct toxicity or drug overdosage, or by drug interaction.[376] Anaphylaxis is the typical immediate hypersensitivity reaction (type 1). Such reactions are produced by the immunoglobulin E (IgE)-mediated release of pharmacologically active substances. These mediators in turn produce specific end-organ responses in the skin (urticaria), the respiratory system (bronchospasm and upper airway edema), and the cardiovascular system (vasodilation, changes in inotropy, and increased capillary permeability). Vasodilation occurs at the level of the capillary and post-capillary venule, leading to erythema, edema, and smooth muscle contraction. This clinical syndrome is called *anaphylaxis*. By contrast, the term *anaphylactoid reaction* denotes an identical or very similar clinical response that is not mediated by IgE or (usually) an antigen–antibody process.[377]

In anaphylactic reactions, an injected substance can serve as the allergen itself. Low-molecular-weight agents are believed to act as haptens that form immunologic conjugates with host proteins. The offending substance, whether hapten or not, may be the parent compound, a nonenzymatically generated product, or a metabolic product formed in the patient. When an allergen binds immunospecific IgE antibodies on the surface of mast cells and basophils, histamine[378] and eosinophilic chemotactic factors of anaphylaxis (ECF-A) are released from the storage granules in a calcium- and energy-dependent process.[379] Other chemical mediators, including slow-reacting substance of anaphylaxis (SRS-A), which is a combination of three leukotrienes, other leukotrienes,[380] kinins, platelet activating factors, adenosine, chemotactic factors, heparin, tryptase, chymase, and prostaglandins, including the potent bronchoconstrictor prostaglandin D_2, are rapidly synthesized and subsequently released in response to cellular activation.

The end-organ effects of the mediators produce the clinical syndrome of anaphylaxis. Usually a first wave of symptoms, including vasodilation and a feeling of impending doom, is followed quickly by the second wave as the cascade of mediators amplifies the reactions. In a sensitized individual, the onset of the signs and symptoms caused by these mediators is usually immediate but may be delayed 2 to 15 minutes or, in rare instances, as long a $2\frac{1}{2}$ hours after the parenteral injection of antigen.[381,382] After oral administration, manifestations may occur at unpredictable times.[379]

In addition, there are multiple effector processes by which biologically active mediators can be generated to produce an anaphylactoid reaction. Activation of the blood coagulation and fibrinolytic systems, of the kinin-generating sequence, or of the complement cascade can produce the same inflammatory substances that result in an anaphylactic reaction. The two mechanisms known to activate the complement system are called classical and alternate. The classical pathway can be initiated through IgG or IgM (transfusion reactions) or plasmin.[383] The alternate pathway can be activated by lipopolysaccharides (endotoxin), drugs (Althesin,[377] radiographic contrast media[384]), membranes (nylon tricot membranes for bubble oxygenators,[385] cellophane membranes of dialyzers,[386] vascular graft material[387]), and perfluorocarbon artificial blood.[388] In addition, histamine can be liberated independently of immunologic reactions.[377] Mast cells and basophils release histamine in response to chemicals or drugs. Most narcotics can release histamine,[389,390] producing an anaphylactoid reaction, as can radiographic contrast media,[384] *d*-tubocurarine[391] and thiopental.[392] What makes some patients susceptible to histamine release in response to drugs is unknown, but hereditary and environmental factors may play a role.

Chymopapain, an agent used to treat herniated nucleus pulposus enzymatically, is associated with a 0.35 to 2 percent incidence of anaphylactic and anaphylactoid reactions. This agent is now used much less frequently than before but still has its advocates, who point to a better risk/benefit ratio than that of more invasive therapies.[393] Sensitization of some of the general population occurs because chymopapain or close structural relatives are present in papaya, meat tenderizer, some beers, toothpastes, and cosmetics. However, it is not clearly known whether all vasoactive reactions to chymopapain are anaphylactic: chymopapain may have a direct (nonimmunologic) action on mast cells and thus initiate an anaphylactoid reaction. Women are 3 to 10 times more likely to have anaphylactic or anaphylactoid reactions to chymopapain than are men, the incidence being 0.1 to 0.5 percent for men and 0.7 to 1.5 percent for women. Two of the 1,049 men and 11 of the 536 women in the phase III clinical trials of Chymodiactin (chymopapain) experienced serious anaphylactic reactions after administration of chymopapain.[394]

These reactions were manifested by bronchospasm in 2 subjects, severe hypotension in 13, laryngeal edema in 2, and rash or pilomotor changes in 9. Eleven of the 13 survived.

Since release of Chymodiactin by the Food and Drug Administration (FDA) in November 1982, the incidence of anaphylactic reactions has dropped slightly from that in the phase III trials, the incidence now being approximately 0.3 percent in men and 0.8 percent in women for the first 80,000 patients treated (R. McDermott, personal communication). Two of the anaphylactic reactions were fatal. We believe that the successful outcome for most such reactions has come about through vigilance when administering the drug and pretreatment of the patient with antihistamines and hydration.

Intravenous contrast material is probably the most frequently used agent causing anaphylactoid reactions. Since diagnostic (skin and other) tests are helpful only in IgE-mediated reactions, pretesting is not useful in contrast reactions. Pretreatment with diphenhydramine, cimetidine (or ranitidine), and corticosteroids has been reported useful in preventing or ameliorating anaphylactoid reactions due to intravenous contrast material,[395,396] and perhaps to narcotics and chymopapain.[397] Unfortunately, very large doses of steroids (1 g of methylprednisolone intravenously) may be necessary to obtain a beneficial effect.[398,399] The efficacy of large-dose steroid therapy has not been confirmed. Other common substances associated with anaphylactic or anaphylactoid reactions that might merit preoperative therapy include antibiotics, volume expanders, and blood products (Table 25-21).[376,400–403] The anesthesiologist should be prepared preoperatively to treat an anaphylactic or anaphylactoid response.

Sometimes a patient with a history of anaphylactic or anaphylactoid reaction must receive a substance suspected of producing such a reaction (e.g., iodinated contrast material). Also, some patients have a higher than average likelihood of having a reaction. In such instances, pretreatment and therapy for possible anaphylactic and anaphylactoid reactions should be well planned.[376] Although virtually all evidence on these subjects is merely anecdotal, enough consistent thought recurs through the literature to justify proposing an optimal approach to these problems. First, predisposing factors should be sought; the patient with a history of atopy or allergic rhinitis should be suspected as being at risk. Because anaphylactic and anaphylactoid reactions to contrast media occur 5 to 10 times more frequently in patients with a previously suspected reaction, one might consider giving such patients both H_1- and H_2-receptor antagonists for 16 to 24 hours before exposing them to a suspected allergen.[394,396,397] The H_1-receptor antagonist appears to require this much time to act on the receptor.[396] Volume status should be optimized,[376] and perhaps large doses of steroids (2 g of hydrocortisone) should also be administered before exposing patients to agents associated with a high incidence of anaphylactic or anaphylactoid reactions.[398,399,404,405] Older patients present a special problem: they are at more risk of having complications from both pretreatment (especially vigorous hydration) and therapy for anaphylactic reactions. Perhaps drugs likely to trigger anaphylactic or anaphylactoid reactions should be avoided, or the treatment protocol altered, for this group.

Primary Immunodeficiency Diseases

The primary immunodeficiency diseases usually present early in life with recurrent infections. Along with survival due to antibiotic and antibody treatment have come new prominent features: cancer, and allergic and autoimmune disorders. Heredity angioneurotic edema is an autosomal dominant genetic disease characterized by episodes of angioneurotic edema involving the subcutaneous tissues and submucosa of the GI tract and the airway and often presenting as abdominal pain. These patients have a functionally impotent inhibitor or a deficiency of an inhibitor to the complement component C1. Treatment of an acute attack is supportive because epinephrine, antihistamines, and corticosteroids often fail to work. Plasma transfusions have been reported to resolve attacks or to make them worse (theoretically by supplying either Cl esterase inhibitor or previously depleted complement components). The severity of attacks can be prevented or decreased by drugs that are either plasmin inhibitors (such as ϵ-aminocaproic acid and tranexamic acid) or androgens (such as danazol). Because trauma can precipitate acute attacks, prophylactic therapy with danazol, intravenous ϵ-aminocaproic acid, plasma, or all three, is recommended prior to elective surgery. Reports have also described the successful use of a partially purified C1-esterase inhibitor in two patients.[406,407]

Most of the 1 in 700 persons who have selective IgA deficiency (i.e., <5 mg/dl) have repeated serious infections or connective tissue disorders.[408] The infections commonly involve the respiratory tract (e.g., sinusitis, otitis) or GI tract (presenting as diarrhea and/or malab-

TABLE 25-21. Incidence of Anaphylactic or Anaphylactoid Reactions to Some Common Agents

Agent	Incidence
Plasma protein	
Plasma protein derivative	0.019
Human serum albumin	0.011
Dextran 60/75	0.069
Dextran 40	0.007
Starch	
Hydroxyethyl starch	0.085
Penicillin	0.002[a]
Chymopapain	0.3–1.5

[a]Fatal reactions.
(Data from Ring and Messmer,[400] Levy et al.,[376] and Moss et al.[394])

sorption). If the patient has rheumatoid arthritis, Sjögren syndrome, or systemic lupus erythematosus, the anesthetist should consider the possibility of isolated IgA deficiency. However, patients with this disorder can be otherwise healthy. Since patients may develop antibodies to IgA if previously exposed to IgA (as might occur from a previous blood transfusion), subsequent blood transfusions can cause anaphylaxis even when they contain washed erythrocytes. Transfusion should therefore consist of blood donated by another IgA-deficient patient.

Many immunomodulators are now being tried to augment cancer treatments;[409] no interactions between these modulators, or effects on the incidence of immune reactions during anesthesia, or interactions with anesthetic effects have been reported except for with immune-suppressing agents (see last section of this chapter).

DISEASES OF THE CNS, NEUROMUSCULAR DISEASES, AND PSYCHIATRIC DISORDERS

Taking the history and performing the physical examination suggested in Chapter 23 should help identify almost all patients with significant neurologic or mental disease. Historical information warranting further investigation includes the previous need for postoperative ventilation in a patient without inordinate lung disease (indicating the possibility of metabolic neurologic disorders such as porphyria, alcoholic myopathy, other myopathies, neuropathies, and neuromuscular disorders such as myasthenia gravis) and the use of drug therapy (steroids; guanidine; anticonvulsant, anticoagulant, and antiplatelet drugs; lithium; tricyclic antidepressent drugs; phenothiazines; butyrophenones). Although preoperative treatment of most neurologic disorders has not been reported to lessen perioperative morbidity, knowledge of the pathophysiologic characteristics of these disorders is important in planning intraoperative and postoperative management. Thus, preoperative knowledge about these disorders and their associated conditions (such as cardiac dysrhythmias with Duchenne muscular dystrophy or respiratory and cardiac muscle weakness in dermatomyositis) may reduce perioperative morbidity. A major goal of neurologic evaluation is to determine the site of the lesion in the nervous system. Such localization is essential for accurate diagnosis and appropriate management. (Disorders accompanied by increased intracranial pressure and cerebrovascular disorders are discussed in Ch. 54.)

Coma

Little is known about anesthesia for the comatose patient, but, as for all other conditions, it is imperative to know the cause of the coma, so that drugs that might worsen the condition or that might not be metabolized because of organ dysfunction can be avoided. First the patient should be observed. Yawning, swallowing, or licking of the lips implies a "light" coma with major brain stem function intact. If consciousness is depressed but respiration, pupillary reactivity to light, and eye movements are normal and no focal motor signs are present, metabolic depression is likely. Abnormal pupillary responses may indicate hypoxia, hypothermia, local eye disease, or drug intoxication with belladonna alkaloids, narcotics, or glutethimide; pupillary responses may also be abnormal, however, after use of eye drops. Other metabolic causes of coma include uremia, hypoglycemia, hepatic coma, alcohol ingestion, hypophosphatemia, myxedema, and hyperosmolar nonketotic coma. Except in extreme emergencies, such as uncontrolled bleeding or perforated viscus, care should be taken to render the patient as metabolically normal as possible before surgery. This practice lessens any confusion regarding the cause of intraoperative and postoperative problems. However, too rapid correction of uremia or hyperosmolar nonketotic coma can lead to cerebral edema, a shift of water into the brain due to a reverse osmotic effect caused by the dysequilibrium of urea concentration. The physical examination can be extremely helpful preoperatively in assessing the prognosis.[410–414] Arms flexed at the elbow (decorticate posture) imply bilateral hemisphere dysfunction but intact brain stem, whereas extension of legs and arms (bilateral decerebrate posture) implies bilateral damage to structures at the upper brain stem or deep hemisphere level. Seizures are often seen in uremia and in other metabolic encephalopathies. Hyper-reflexia and upward-pointing toes suggest a structural CNS lesion or uremia, hypoglycemia, or hepatic coma; hyporeflexia and downward-pointing toes with no hemiplegia generally indicate no structural CNS lesion.

Epileptic Seizures

Epileptic seizures result from paroxysmal neuronal discharges of abnormally excitable neurons. Seizures can be generalized (arising from deep midline structures in the brain stem or thalamus, usually without aura or focal features during the seizure), partial focal motor, or sensory seizures (the initial discharge comes from a focal unilateral area of brain, often preceded by an aura). As with cerebrovascular accidents (CVAs) and coma, knowing the origin may be crucial to understanding the pathophysiologic processes of the disease and to managing the intraoperative and postoperative course. Epileptic seizures can arise from discontinuation of sedative hypnotic drugs or alcohol, use of narcotics, uremia, traumatic injury, neoplasms, infection, congenital malformation, birth injury, drug usage (amphetamines, cocaine), hypercalcemia or hypocalcemia, and vascular disease and vascular accidents.[412] Thirty percent of epileptic seizures have no known cause. Most partial seizures are caused by structural brain abnormalities (secondary to tumor, trauma, stroke, infection, and other causes). The epileptic patient requires no special anesthetic management other than that for the underlying disease. Anticonvulsant medications should be given in the therapeutic range[415-417] and continued through the morning of surgery; they should also be given postoperatively. Appropriate treatment of status epilepticus may include general anesthesia.[417] High concentrations of enflurane (especially with hyperventilation) can be associated with EEG evidence of epileptic activity and tonic-clonic movements.[418,419] These seizures, however, do not appear to have serious sequelae.[420] Enflurane anesthesia does not appear to increase seizure activity in patients with a history of convulsive disorders; it even suppresses seizures induced by electroshock, pentylene-tetrazole, strychnine, picrotoxin, or bemegride.[419-421] Thus, other than the use of current drug therapy and heeding precautions taken for the underlying disease, no known changes in perioperative management seem indicated.

Infectious Diseases of the CNS, Degenerative Disorders of the CNS, and Headache

Many of the degenerative CNS disorders have been traced to slowly developing viral diseases. No special perioperative anesthetic considerations appear to apply for infectious disorders of the CNS other than those for increased intracranial pressure and avoiding occupational exposures (also see Ch. 54). What prophylactic measures to take if one comes into contact with meningococcal disease or other infectious CNS disease is not well established.[422]

Parkinson's disease is a degenerative disorder of the CNS that may or may not be caused by a virus. Clinically, Parkinson's disease, chronic manganese intoxication, phenothiazine or butyrophenone toxicity, Wilson's disease, Huntington's chorea, traumatic boxing injury, and carbon monoxide encephalopathy all present with similar features: bradykinesia, muscular rigidity, and tremor. The substantia nigra degenerates, and the clinical signs presumably result from decreased production of dopamine in the neurons of the basal ganglia leading to the putamen and caudate nucleus. The effects of this dopaminergic deficiency may be compounded by the unopposed effects of cholinergic neurons bordering the basal ganglia. Therapy is thus directed either at increasing the neuronal release of dopamine, or the receptor's response to dopamine; or the direct stimulation of the receptor by bromocriptine and lergotrile; or implanting dopaminergic tissue; or decreasing cholinergic activity. New therapies with the monamine oxidase inhibitor, deprenyl, to slow the progression of disease appear promising.[423] There is not enough experience with this drug in the perioperative milieu to make proscriptions about its use. Anticholinergic agents have been the initial drugs of choice; they

decrease tremor more than muscle rigidity. Since dopamine does not pass the blood–brain barrier (BBB), its precursor, L-dopa (levodopa), is used. Unfortunately, L-dopa is decarboxylated to dopamine in the periphery and can cause nausea, vomiting, and arrhythmia. These side effects are diminished by administration of α-methylhydrazine (Carbidopa), a decarboxylase inhibitor that does not pass the BBB. Refractoriness to L-dopa develops, and the drug is now used only when symptoms cannot be controlled with other anticholinergic medications. "Drug holidays" have been suggested as one way of restoring the effectiveness of these compounds, but cessation of such therapy may result in a marked deterioration of function and the need for hospitalization.[424] Therapy for Parkinson's disease should be continued through the morning of surgery; such treatment seems to decrease drooling, the potential for aspiration, and ventilatory weakness.[424-426] Reinstituting therapy promptly after surgery is important,[424-426] as is avoiding such drugs as phenothiazines and butyrophenones (droperidol) that compete with dopamine at the receptor.[427]

Dementia, a progressive decline in intellectual function, can be caused by treatable infections (e.g., syphilis, cryptococcosis, coccidioidomycosis, tuberculosis), myxedema, vitamin B_{12} deficiency, chronic drug or alcohol intoxication, metabolic causes (liver and renal failure), neoplasms, untreatable infections (Creutzfeldt-Jakob syndrome), or decrease of acetylcholine in the cerebral cortex (Alzheimer's disease). This last condition occurs in over 0.5 percent of Americans.[413,428] Although such patients are often given cholinergic agonists, controlled trials of these drugs have not shown benefit as yet.[428] Creutzfeldt-Jakob disease has been transmitted inadvertently by surgical instruments and corneal transplants; the causative virus is not inactivated by heat, disinfectants, or formaldehyde.

More than 90 percent of patients with chronic recurring headaches are diagnosed as having migraine, tension, or cluster headaches. The mechanism of tension or cluster headaches may not differ qualitatively from that for migraine headaches; all may be manifestations of labile vasomotor regulation.[429] The treatment for cluster and migraine headaches centers around ergotamine and its derivatives. Other drugs and therapies that may be effective are propranolol, calcium channel inhibitors, cyproheptadine, prednisone, antihistamines, tricyclic antidepressant drugs, phenytoin, diuretic drugs, and biofeedback.[430a] Giant cell arteritis and glaucoma are other causes of headache that might benefit from treatment before surgery. No other special treatment is indicated preoperatively for the patient who has a well-delineated cause for headaches. Acute migraine attacks can sometimes be terminated by ergotamine tartrate aerosol or by injection of dihydroergotamine mesylate intravenously; general anesthesia has also been used. I normally continue all prophylactic headache medicines, except aspirin (because of the potential for bleeding), through the morning of surgery.

Back Pain, Neck Pain, and Spinal Canal Syndromes

Acute spinal cord injury is discussed earlier in the section on autonomic dysfunction. Little is written about the anesthetic management of syndromes related to herniated disk, spondylosis (usually of advancing age), and the congenital narrowing of the cervical and lumbar canal that gives rise to symptoms of nerve-root compression.[430,431] Recent reports stress the importance of the vascular component in the mechanism of damage to the spinal cord and hence the theoretical desirability of slight hypertension perioperatively.[432] One report suggests the use of awake intubation, a fiberoptic bronchoscope, and evoked potential monitoring.[430] The preoperative management of the patient about to undergo chemonucleolysis is discussed earlier in the section on anaphylaxis. Other than the common-sense approach of seeking neurological consultation or, if necessary, using awake positioning of patients in a comfortable position prior to emergency root-decompression procedures, no special procedures appear to be necessary.

Demyelinating Diseases

Demyelinating diseases constitute a diffuse group of diseases ranging from those with no known causes (such as multiple sclerosis) to those that follow infection, vaccination (such as Guillain-Barré syndrome), or antimetabolite treatment of cancer. Therefore, demyelinating disease can present with very diverse symptoms. Apparently, there is a risk of relapse of these diseases immediately after surgery.[433] The risk of relapse may occur because of rapid electrolyte changes in the perioperative period. Such might be avoided, and perioperative steroid use has been advocated.[434] Thus far, no mode of treatment has been shown to alter these disease processes, although ACTH, steroids, and plasmapheresis may ameliorate or abbreviate a relapse, especially of multiple sclerosis. Such an effect is consonant with the hypothesis of an immunologic disorder as the cause of these diseases.

Metabolic Diseases

Included in the category of metabolic diseases is nervous system dysfunction secondary to porphyrias, alcoholism, uremia, hepatic failure, and vitamin B_{12} deficiency. The periodic paralysis that can accompany thyroid disease is discussed under neuromuscular disorders, following this section.

Alcoholism or heavy alcohol intake is associated with acute alcoholic hepatitis (also see Ch. 56) (the activity of which declines as alcohol is withdrawn), myopathy and cardiomyopathy that can be severe, and withdrawal syndromes. The best questions to ask in seeking a history of alcohol intake are, "Have you ever had a drinking problem?" and "Have you had a drink in the last 24 hours?" These questions have a higher sensitivity and specificity than many other longer series of questions about alcoholism (see Ch. 23).[435] Within 6 to 8 hours of withdrawal, the patient may become tremulous, a state that usually subsides within days or weeks. Alcoholic hallucinosis and withdrawal seizures generally occur within 24 to 36 hours. These seizures are generalized grand mal attacks; when focal seizures are manifest, other causes should be sought. Delirium tremens usually appears within 72 hours of withdrawal and is often preceded by tremulousness, hallucinations, or seizures. These three occurrences combined with perceptual distortions, insomnia, psychomotor disturbances, autonomic hyperactivity, and, in a large percentage of cases, another potentially fatal illness (such as bowel infarction or subdural hematoma) comprise delirium tremens. This syndrome is now treated with benzodiazepines. Nutritional disorders of alcoholism include alcoholic hypoglycemia and hypothermia, alcoholic polyneuropathy, Wernicke-Korsakoff syndrome, and cerebellar degeneration. In alcoholic patients (i.e., those who drink at least 2 six-packs of beer or 1 pint of whiskey per day, or the equivalent), emergency surgery and anesthesia (despite alcoholic hepatitis) are not associated with worsening abnormalities of liver enzymes.[436] In addition, about 20 percent of alcoholic patients also have COPD. Thus, the patient who gives a history of alcohol abuse warrants careful examination of many systems to quantify his or her preoperative physical status.

Although hepatic failure can lead to coma with high-output cardiac failure, unlike uremia, it does not lead to chronic polyneuropathy. Uremic polyneuropathy is a distal symmetric sensorimotor polyneuropathy that may be improved by dialysis. The use of depolarizing muscle relaxants has been questioned in polyneuropathies (also see Ch. 12). I believe that patients who have a neuropathy associated with uremia should not be given succinylcholine because of a possible exaggerated hyperkalemic response.

Pernicious anemia caused by vitamin B_{12} deficiency may result in subacute combined degeneration of the spinal cord, its signs being similar to those of chronic nitrous oxide toxicity. Both pernicious anemia and N_2O toxicity are associated with peripheral neuropathy and disorders of the pyramidal tract and posterior column (which governs fine motor skills and the sense of body position). Combined system disease can also occur without anemia, as can N_2O toxicity in dentists and N_2O abusers. Patients with B_{12} deficiency and anemia, if treated with folate, improve hematologically but progress to dementia and severe neuropathy. Thus, intramuscular administration of 100 μg of vitamin B_{12} before giving folate to the patient who has signs of combined system degeneration may be prudent.

The porphyrias are a constellation of metabolic diseases resulting from an autosomally inherited lack of functional enzymes active in the synthesis of hemoglobin. Figure 25-10 schematically depicts the abnormalities resulting from these enzyme deficits. It is important to note that types 1, 3, and 4 can cause life-threatening neurologic abnormalities. These types of porphyrias are characterized by the presence of aminolevulinic acid (ALA) and/or porphobilinogen (PBG) in urine, whereas porphyria cutanea tarda, which is not associated with neurologic sequelae, is not.[437,438] In acute intermittent porphyria, the typical pattern consists of acute attacks of colicky pain, nausea, vomiting, severe constipation, psychiatric disorders, and lesions of the lower motor neuron, which can progress to bulbar paralysis. Certain drugs can induce the enzyme ALA synthetase, exacerbating the disease process.[437-440] These sensitizing drugs include barbiturates, meprobamate, chlordiazepoxide, glutethimide, diazepam, hydroxydione, phenytoin, imipramine, pentazocine, birth control pills, ethyl alcohol, sulfonamides, griseofulvin, and ergot preparations. Patients often have attacks at times of infection, fasting, or menstruation. Administration of glucose suppresses ALA synthetase activity and prevents or ablates acute attacks. Drugs used in anesthetic management that are reported to be safe for patients with porphyria include neostigmine (Prostigmin), atropine, gallamine, succinylcholine, *d*-tubocurarine, pancuronium, nitrous oxide, procaine, propanidid, etomidate, meperidine, fentanyl, morphine, droperidol, promazine, promethazine, and chlorpromazine.[437-440] Although ketamine has been used,[439] postoperative psychoses attributable to the disease may be difficult to distinguish from those possibly caused by ketamine. In addition, although ketamine and etomidate are reported to be safe in humans, they have been reported to be porphyrinogenic in a rat model.[439]

Neuromuscular Disorders

The category of neuromuscular disorders includes those affecting all major components of the motor unit: motor neuron, peripheral nerve, neuromuscular junction, and muscle. Neuropathies may involve all components of the nerve, producing sensory, motor, and autonomic dysfunction, or may preferentially involve one or the other component. Myopathies may involve proximal or distal muscles, or both.

Myasthenia gravis (also see Ch. 12) is a disorder of the muscular system caused by partial blockade or destruction of nicotinic acetylcholine receptors by IgG antibodies. This syndrome is characterized by fluctuating ophthalmoplegia, ptosis, and bulbar, respiratory, or limb weakness and confirmed by a beneficial response to cholinergic drugs.[440a,441] These patients often have other autoimmune diseases, including rheumatoid arthritis and hypothyroidism. Thirty-three percent of patients with myasthenia gravis have bulbar symptoms (and hence are subject to problems with disposing of secretions) at presentation, and over 60 percent at some time during life. This symptom should not be confused with respiratory muscle weakness, which occurs much less commonly.

The severity of the disease correlates with the ability of the antibodies to decrease the number of available acetylcholine receptors.[440a] Treatment of myasthenia is usually begun with anticholinesterase agents but, in moderate and severe disease, progresses to steroids and thymectomy.[440a,441] Immunosuppressive drugs and plasmapheresis are begun if these more conservative measures fail.[440a,441] One major problem for the anesthesiologist involves the use of muscle relaxants and their reversal.[442,443] Since much of the care of myasthenia gravis patients involves tailoring the amount of anticholinesterase medication to the maximal muscle strength of the patient, derangement of the course of the disease during surgery could necessitate reassessment of the drug dosage. For that reason, several researchers recommend withholding all anticholinergic drugs for 6 hours before surgery and reinstituting medicine postoperatively with extreme caution, because the sensitivity of these patients to such drugs may have changed. In addition, there has been some concern that anticholinergic drugs may facilitate a high incidence of bowel anastomotic leaks in those patients who have undergone bowel anastomoses. Small doses of succinylcholine can be used to facilitate endotracheal intubation, and tiny doses of nondepolarizing drugs can be used for intraoperative relaxation not obtained by regional anesthesia or volatile agents. Controlled ventilation is usually required for 24 to 48 or more hours postoperatively.[441-444] This practice is especially important for patients who have had myasthenia gravis for more than 6 years, for those who have COLD, for those having a daily pyridostigmine requirement of 750 mg or more who have significant bulbar weakness, and for those whose vital capacity is less than 40 ml/kg.[443-446]

The Eaton-Lambert syndrome (myasthenic syndrome) is characterized by proximal limb muscle weakness. Strength or reflexes may increase with repetitive effort. These patients have a decreased release of acetylcholine at the neuromuscular junction. Guanidine therapy enhances the release of acetylcholine from nerve terminals and improves strength. Most men who have this syndrome also have small cell carcinoma of the lung or other malignancy, whereas women often have malignancy, sarcoidosis, thyroiditis, or a collagen-related vascular disease. In addition, these patients have increased sensitivity to both depolarizing and nondepolarizing muscle relaxants.[447] There is also an autonomic nervous system defect in this syndrome with gastroparesis, orthostatic hypotension, and urinary retention.[447]

Dermatomyositis and polymyositis are characterized by proximal limb muscle weakness with dysphagia. These conditions are associated with malignancy or collagen-related vascular disease, often involving respiratory and cardiac muscle.

Periodic paralysis is another disease in which sensitivity to muscle relaxants increases. Periodic weakness

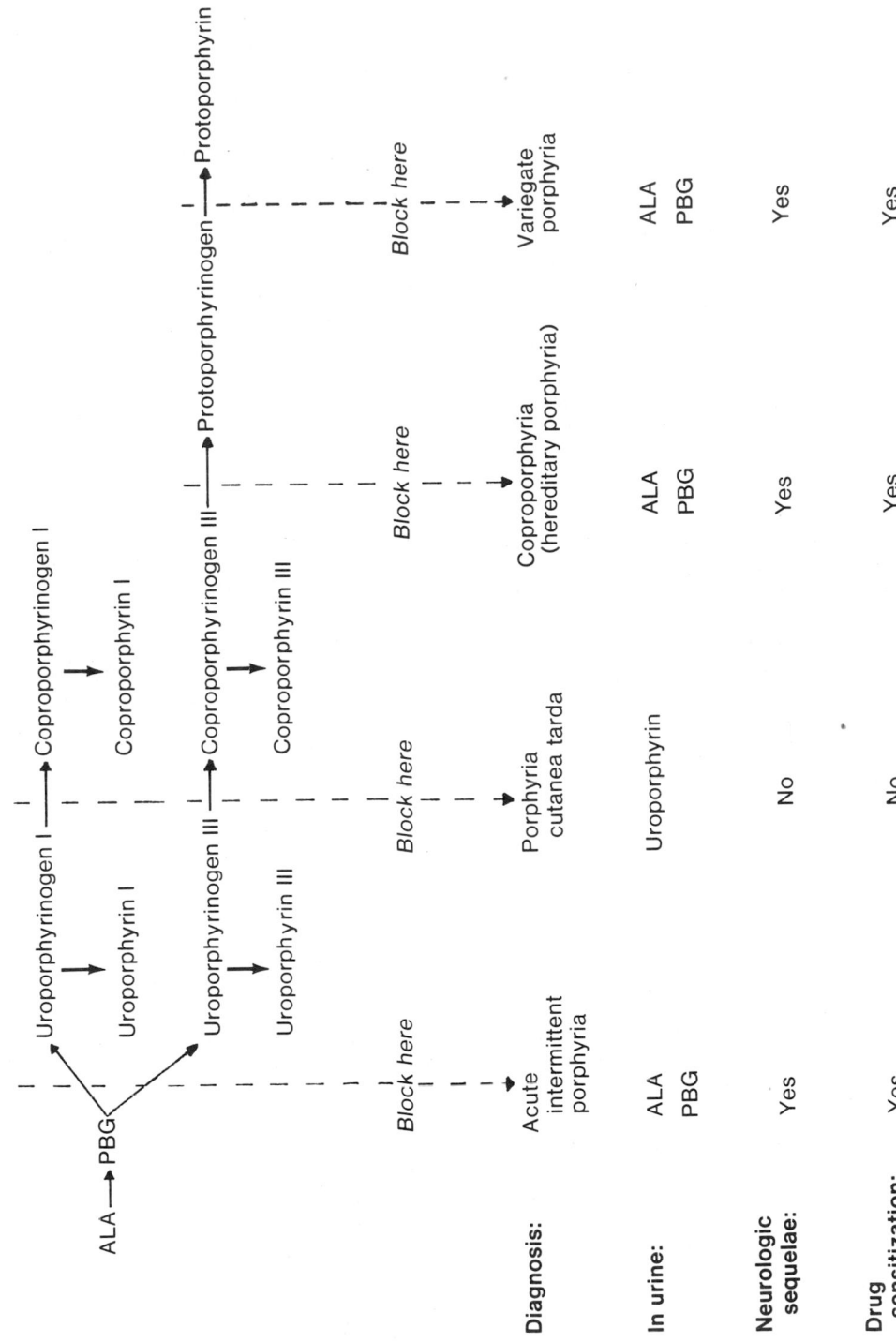

Fig. 25-10. Scheme depicting functional enzyme deficits for some of the porphyrias. ALA, aminolevulinic acid; PBG, porphobilinogen.

starts in childhood or adolescence and is precipitated by rest after exercise, sleep, cold, surgery, or pregnancy. Hypokalemic and hyperkalemic forms exist and are associated with cardiac arrhythmias. Like thyrotoxic periodic paralysis, these hypokalemic and hyperkalemic forms usually spare the respiratory muscles. Anesthetic management consists of minimizing stress and maintaining normal fluid and electrolyte states and body temperature.[447]

Muscular dystrophy patients now survive into their late twenties. Complicating their disease are respiratory infections, kyphoscoliosis, muscle contractions, and cardiac abnormalities. Duchenne muscular dystrophy is a sex-linked recessive disease, the most common of the muscular dystrophies. It occurs after 5 years of age, at which time patients experience a rapid progression of muscle disease that leads to incapacity in their teens. Cardiac involvement is common when the disease affects proximal and pelvic muscles, and respiratory failure is a common cause of death. Limb-girdle muscular dystrophy is not as severe as Duchenne muscular dystrophy; it occurs later in life, has cardiac involvement, and is transmitted as an autosomal recessive trait. Facioscapulohumeral muscular dystrophy (FSHMD) is a disease of autosomal dominant inheritance that has a mild clinical form in adolescence. Patients with FSHMD have a normal lifespan without an increased risk of cardiac complications; however, postoperative respiratory deaths have been recorded. Myotonic dystrophy is a disease in which continued active contraction of the muscles persists after voluntary effort or stimulation has ceased. This autosomal dominant inherited disease begins at 20 to 40 years of age and is associated with cardiomyopathy, baldness, testicular atrophy, cataracts, intellectual and emotional abnormalities, and premature death in the 50- to 60-year age range. The facial, sternocleidomastoidal, distal, and pharyngeal muscles become weak and atrophy. Since the disease involves the muscles themselves, and not their innervation, conduction anesthesia cannot produce adequate relaxation of tonic muscles. Gastric dilatation has also been reported to be a problem, as has malignant hyperthermia. As with the other forms of muscular dystrophies, most problems in myotonic dystrophy arise from cardiac arrhythmias and inadequacies of the respiratory muscles. With all the forms of muscular dystrophy, as with all the neuropathies (discussed earlier), problems related to exaggerated serum potassium release following administration of depolarizing muscle relaxants have been reported (also see Ch. 12).

Malignant hyperthermia (MH) (also see Ch. 28) in the patient or in a relative of the patient merits careful history-taking and at least consideration of performing a test for susceptibility to MH. Prophylaxis with intravenous dantrolene sodium (Dantrium) may also be warranted (also see Ch. 28). In a minority of cases, MH has been associated with recognizable musculoskeletal abnormalities such as strabismus, ptosis, myotonic dys-

trophy, hernias, kyphoscoliosis, muscular dystrophy, central core disease, and marfanoid syndrome. What to do for the patient with previous masseter spasm, or trismus, is a matter of considerable debate. We prepare for MH (clean machine, nontriggering agents, MH cart in room) but do not routinely perform muscle biopsy or prescribe dantrolene prophylaxis.[449,450] Malignant hyperthermia occurs most frequently among children and adolescents, the incidence being 1 in 14,000 anesthetic administrations. The incidence increases to 1 in 2,500 among patients requiring squint surgery.[451] Questions to ask the parents during preoperative evaluation include the following: Does your child get rigid when upset? Does your child sweat profusely when upset? However, the sensitivity and specificity of such questions in predicting malignant hyperthermia are not confirmed. The reader is referred to Chapter 28 for a complete discussion of the screening procedure to use.

Down Syndrome (Trisomy 21)

Down syndrome (trisomy 21) occurs 1.5 times in 1,000 live births. It is associated with congenital cardiac lesions, such as endocardial cushion defects (40 percent), ventricular septal defects (27 percent), patent ductus arteriosus (12 percent), and tetralogy of Fallot (8 percent), necessitating prophylactic antibiotics prior to predictable bactemic events; with upper respiratory infections; with atlanto-occipital instability (in about 15 percent of patients,[452] in which it is asymptomatic in the majority of patients) and laxity of other joints; with thyroid hypofunction (50 percent); with an increased incidence of subglottic stenosis; and with enlargement of the tongue.[453] No abnormal responses to anesthetics or anesthetic adjuvants have been substantiated. A reported sensitivity to atropine has been disproved, although administration of atropine to any patient given digoxin for atrial fibrillation should be done with extreme care.[453] Examination for these conditions should precede surgery.

Predicting Preoperatively Which Neurologic Patients Will Have Increased Intracranial Pressure During Surgery

Symptoms and signs of increased intracranial pressure include morning headache or headache made worse by coughing, nausea, vomiting, disturbances of consciousness, history of large tumors, tumors involving the brain stem, neck rigidity, and papilledema. Patients having these signs, large ventricles as seen on roentgenograms or images of the brain, or edema surrounding supratentorial tumors should be considered at risk of intraoperative intracranial hypertension. Such patients may benefit from preoperative treatment or anesthetic management that assumes this possibility (also see Ch. 54).[454]

Other preoperative considerations in patients with neurologic disease that can cause intracranial hypertension are the associated hypoventilation and hypoxia in patients who have severe hemiplegia and the presence of subarachnoid bleeding or other forms of intracranial hemorrhage (especially likely in women given heparin who have two or more cerebral infarcts on CT scan).[454a] A large percentage (59 of 184 patients) with strokes or transient ischemic attacks (TIAs) have a possible cardiac cause of their stroke.[456] The drugs used to prevent cerebral arterial spasm,[455] calcium-channel blockers, are discussed in the last section of this chapter.

Mental Disorders

Perhaps the most important preoperative consideration for patients with mental disorders, in addition to developing rapport with them, is understanding their drug therapy and its effects and side effects. Lithium, tricyclic antidepressants, phenothiazines, butyrophenones, and monoamine oxidase (MAO) inhibitors are used in these patients.[456a] These drugs have potent effects and side effects that are discussed in the last section of this chapter.

RENAL DISEASE, INFECTIOUS DISEASES, AND ELECTROLYTE DISORDERS

One may ask why preoperative preparation of the patient with renal disease is discussed in the same section as preoperative preparation of the patient with an infectious disease. Although it is commonly recommended that no surgery except emergency or curative (e.g., drainage of an abscess) be performed in patients with infectious disease, it has become evident that renal insufficiency can be caused by antimicrobial agents[457] and that sepsis, not shock, is probably the leading cause of acute postoperative renal failure.[458] The linking of renal failure to electrolyte disorders is more obvious: the kidney is the primary organ for regulating body osmolality and fluid volume and has a major role in the excretion of the end products of metabolism. In performing these functions, the kidney becomes intimately involved in the excretion of electrolytes.

The patient with renal insufficiency whose own kidneys are still functioning is distinct not only from the patient with end-stage renal disease whose renal functions are provided by a dialysis machine, but also from the patient who has a transplanted kidney. These three groups of patients require quite different preoperative preparation. In addition, acute changes in renal function present quite a different problem than do chronic alterations in function. Certain renal diseases require different preoperative preparation than others, but generally renal disease of any origin presents the same preoperative problems (also see Chs. 18, 34, and 55).

Renal Disease

Causes and Systemic Effects of Renal Disorders

The nephrotic syndrome may develop in patients with glomerular diseases without disturbing tubular function. The soundness of tubular function is an important consideration, as tubular dysfunction with attendant uremia presents quite different problems than does glomerular disease with only the nephrotic syndrome. This is not to minimize the adverse effects of glomerular disease; the nephrotic syndrome consists of massive proteinuria and consequent hypoalbuminemia. The resulting reduction in plasma oncotic pressure diminishes plasma volume; this calls forth compensatory mechanisms that result in retention of sodium and water. As a result, a common clinical finding in nephrotic syndrome is edema. Thus, patients with the nephrotic syndrome may have excess total body water and decreased intravascular volume. In addition, diuretic drugs are often given in attempts to decrease edema. Thus, the estimation of intravascular volume status is an essential preoperative consideration in patients with the nephrotic syndrome and diminished tubular renal function who do not yet require hemodialysis.

However, in patients with the nephrotic syndrome in whom renal tubular function has been preserved, hypovolemia appears to be a significant cause of deteriorating tubular renal function.[459-462] Consequently, I advocate the same intense preoperative, intraoperative, and postoperative fluid management for patients with the nephrotic syndrome as I do for patients with diminished tubular function. Admittedly, no randomized study shows that close control of intravascular volume status in these groups of patients preserves renal tubular function (or any other measure of perioperative morbidity) to a greater degree than does less rigid control.

Uremia, the end result of renal tubular failure (i.e., failure of the concentrating, diluting, acidifying, and filtering functions) presents in many ways. Changes occur in the cardiovascular, immunologic, hematologic, neuromuscular, pulmonary, and endocrine systems, as well as in bone. These alterations are ascribed either to the toxic end products of protein metabolism or to an imbalance in the functioning of the kidney. As the number of functioning nephrons diminishes, the still-functioning nephrons attempt to increase some solute and body composition preservation functions at the expense of other functions, such as the excretion of phosphate. The accumulation of phosphate increases parathormone levels, which in turn produces osteodystrophy. Osteodystrophy can be managed by restricting dietary phosphate, by administering gels (such as aluminum hydroxide or carbonate) that bind with intestinal phosphate, by giving supplemental calcium, or by performing parathyroidectomy.[463,464]

Certain alterations in uremia, such as neuropathy, are most logically attributed to an accumulation of toxic metabolites.[465] Peripheral neuropathy is most often sensory and of the lower extremities but may also be motor; peripheral neuropathies are often improved with hemodialysis and can be dramatically reversed with transplantation.[465] The use of depolarizing muscle relaxants in patients with peripheral neuropathy is controversial; it is discussed in the section on neuropathies (also see Ch. 12). Along with the altered volume states and cardiac complications in uremic patients, autonomic neuropathy may contribute to hypotension during anesthesia. Atherosclerosis is often accelerated in uremic patients; hypertension, with its attendant consequences, is very common.

Cardiac failure (especially episodic) occurs frequently in uremic patients because of the presence of many adverse conditions: anemia with increasing myocardial work, hypertension, atherosclerosis, and altered volume states. Pericarditis can present with pericardial rub alone or with pain (with or without hemorrhage). Cardiac tamponade should be ruled out on the basis of clinical features and by echocardiography if this diagnosis is seriously suspected preoperatively. Also, cardiac tamponade should be treated or planned for preoperatively.

If anemia exists, its severity generally parallels the degree of uremia; chronically uremic patients seem to adapt well to anemia. No hard data substantiate the need to give a preoperative blood transfusion to a chronically uremic patient, even when preoperative hematocrit is as low as 16 or 18 vol %. One of the major reasons not to transfuse blood in patients having end-stage renal disease has recently been disproved: data show that the more blood transfusions a transplant recipient receives before transplant, the greater the chance that the transplant will function successfully.[466,467] This immunosuppressive effect of transfusions is now routinely used in transplantation. However, the recent development of recombinant human erythropoietin may obviate the need for transfusions in chronically uremic patients in the future. Administration of recombinant human erythropoietin to patients in chronic and progressive renal failure showed an average increase in hematocrit of 10 percent above baseline within 3 weeks with no serious side effects.[468,469] The balancing of the immunosuppressive uses of blood transfusions versus the benefits of erythropoietin and risks of transfusion remains to be determined. In uremic patients, coagulation and platelet adhesiveness may be abnormal and factor III activity decreased. Even those uremic patients not given corticosteroids or immunosuppressive drugs may demonstrate abnormal immunity, perhaps meriting increased attention regarding the procedures that lessen patient cross-contamination.

Uremic patients exhibit a wide variety of metabolic and endocrinologic disorders,[463,470] including impaired carbohydrate tolerance, insulin resistance, type IV hyperlipoproteinemia, hyperparathyroidism, autonomic insufficiency, hyperkalemia, and anion gap acidosis (caused by the inability of the kidneys to reabsorb filtered bicarbonate and to excrete sufficient ammonium into the urine[470]). Also, the excretion and pharmacokinetics of drugs is different in uremic patients than in normal patients. In addition, the complications of hemodialysis include hepatitis B (and persistent hepatitis B antigenemia), nutritional deficiencies, electrolyte and fluid imbalances, and mental disorders. Because these conditions can lead to serious perioperative morbidity, they should be evaluated before surgery. No data, however, substantiate the hypothesis that preoperative optimization of these metabolic and endocrinologic disorders reduces perioperative risk in the uremic patient.

As with uremic patients, preoperative optimization of volume status is paramount in patients with kidney stones. Seventy-five percent of all kidney stones are composed of calcium oxylate. Patients with these stones often take diuretic drugs, avoid calcium-rich foods, or restrict their intake of salt. Prevention of dehydration by institution of intravenous fluid therapy at the same time that oral intake is restricted may be as important for these patients as it is for patients with struvate or uric acid stones. Struvate stones often result from urinary infection. Uric acid stones can be prevented by treatment with allopurinol, by preoperative hydration, or by alkalization of the urine. Acidosis may contribute to stone formation. Thus, again, optimal intravascular volume status is important in preventing stones and preserving renal function. More thorough discussion of renal function and physiology is discussed in Chapter 18. Chapter 55 deals with the complexities of managing patients for renal surgery and other urologic procedures.

Creatinine clearance in conjunction with free water clearance appears to be the most accurate means of quantifying, for pharmacokinetic purposes, the degree of decreased renal function[471-474] (also see Ch. 34). In the patient with stable renal function, creatinine clearance, which is a rough estimate of glomerular filtration rate (GFR), can be approximated by noting the serum creatinine levels: a doubling of creatinine level represents a halving of glomerular filtration rate. Thus, a patient with a stable serum creatinine level of 2 mg/dl would have a GFR of approximately 60 ml/min. A stable serum creatinine level of 4 mg/dl would accompany a GFR of approximately 30 ml/min, and a stable serum creatinine of 8 mg/dl would accompany a GFR of 15 ml/min or less. When pregnancy and considerable edema are not present and the serum creatinine level is stable, the following formulas can be used to estimate creatinine clearance and free water clearance[470-472,475]:

$$\text{Creatinine clearance} = \frac{[140 - \text{age (yr)}] \times [\text{body weight (kg)}]}{72 \times \text{serum creatinine (mg/dl)}}$$

$$\text{Free water clearance} = \text{urine flow (ml/h)} - \left[\frac{\text{urine osmolality (mOsm/L)} \times \text{urine flow (ml/h)}}{\text{plasma osmolality (mOsm/L)}}\right]$$

Note that renal function must be stable. Unstable renal

function often is associated with changes in serum creatinine levels that lag by several days. Although knowing the serum creatinine level is more useful than knowing the blood urea nitrogen level, the latter provides some information, as discussed in the next section.

Free water clearance is a measure of renal concentrating ability and is normally −25 to −100 ml/h, becoming more positive in renal insufficiency states. It, however, may also become more positive in patients with head injury or high blood alcohol levels, or after aggressive fluid infusion, and administration of diuretics.[474]

The Patient with Insufficient but Functioning Kidneys

I believe that one of the greatest challenges for the anesthesiologist is presented by those patients whose insufficient renal function must be preserved during surgery. The many uremic symptoms and great perioperative morbidity associated with uremia can probably be avoided by attention to detail in the preoperative and perioperative management of patients with insufficient but still functioning kidneys.[458-462,475,476] First, studies demonstrate that acute postoperative renal failure is associated with an extremely high mortality rate. Moreover, acute perioperative renal failure is most likely to occur in patients who have renal insufficiency before surgery, are more than 70 years of age and have preoperative left ventricular dysfunction.[477,478] Proper hydration before surgery probably decreases mortality following acute renal failure due to radiocontrast agents.[460-462] Clues as to the presence of hypovolemia or hypervolemia should be sought from the history and physical examination (e.g., weight loss or gain, thirst, edema, orthostatic hypotension and tachycardia, flat neck veins, dry mucous membranes, decreased skin turgor). In seriously ill patients, insertion of a pulmonary arterial catheter will permit more precise monitoring of intravascular fluid volume. To preserve normal renal function, infusion of saline, mannitol, furosemide, or low dose dopamine has been recommended.[479-485] This should be done cautiously, however, because saline infusions and mannitol can lead to fluid overload and myocardial damage; also, diuretic drugs given intraoperatively can produce postoperative hypovolemia, which worsens renal function. Maintaining normal intravascular fluid volume can be guided by pulmonary capillary wedge pressure. At UCSF maintaining normal intravascular fluid volume prevented impairment of renal function after abdominal aortic reconstruction, even when urinary volumes were low.[486] Other causes of deterioration in function in chronic renal insufficiency are low cardiac output or low renal blood flow (in prerenal azotemia, whether because of cardiac failure or because of fluid depletion from diuretic drugs, BUN often increases disproportionately to increases in creatinine), urinary tract infection, use of nephrotoxic drugs, hypercalcemia, and hyperuricemia. These conditions and drugs should be avoided; if any of these conditions exists, it should be treated preoperatively.

The Patient Undergoing Dialysis

Because the patient undergoing dialysis has already lost natural renal functioning, the emphasis in preoperative assessment shifts toward protecting other organ systems and toward optimally maintaining vascular access sites for cannulation. Usually this does not require invasive monitoring. Emphasis is placed on intravascular fluid volume and electrolyte status, which can be ascertained by knowing when the patient last underwent dialysis, how much weight was normally gained or lost with dialysis and whether fluid loss was peritoneal or intravascular, and what electrolyte composition the blood was dialyzed against. Although preoperative dialysis may benefit patients who have hyperkalemia, hypercalcemia, acidosis, neuropathy, and fluid overload, the resulting dysequilibrium between fluid and electrolytes can cause problems. Because hypovolemia induced by dialysis can lead to intraoperative hypotension, we try to avoid weight and fluid reduction when giving preoperative dialysis. Also, hypopnea has been found to occur during and after dialysis when the dialysate contained acetate.[487] Avoiding an acetate bathing solution may prevent this cause of hypoventilation.

The Patient Who Has Had a Renal Transplant

More than 70,000 patients have received renal transplants (compared with 50,000 currently undergoing dialysis in the United States). Approximately 55 percent are still alive, although one-third must undergo dialysis.[467] When such patients have subsequent surgery, the state of their renal function must be determined (i.e., whether they have normal renal function, insufficient but still functioning kidneys, or end-stage renal disease requiring hemodialysis). Descriptions of side effects from immunosuppressive drugs should also be sought. Drugs used pre- and intraoperatively to prevent acute rejection themselves have serious side effects that encourage close monitoring of blood glucose[33] and cardiovascular function.[488] Because renal transplant places patients at much higher risk of infection, all effort at avoiding invasive monitoring and at preventing patient cross-contamination should be taken.

Drugs in Renal Failure

Patients with renal azotemia have a threefold or greater risk of an adverse drug reaction than do those with normal renal function.[489-492] Risk is increased by either excessive pharmacologic effects (secondary to high blood levels of a drug or its metabolite, such as the metabolite of meperidine), to physiologic changes in target tissues induced by the uremic state (such as excessive sedation in the uremic patient having standard blood levels of sedative hypnotic drugs), or to excessive administration of electrolytes with drugs (e.g., penicillin standardly has 1.7 mEq of potassium/1 million units).[489-492] Administration of standard doses of drugs dependent on renal excretion for their elimination can result in drug accumulation and enhanced pharmacologic effect. Dosing guidelines about many drugs used by anesthesiologists for patients with and without renal failure were provided by Bennett et al.[489] and Gibson.[492]

Infectious Disease

Since it is commonly recommended that no surgery except emergency or essential (e.g., drainage of an abscess) be done in patients with infectious disease, and since renal insufficiency is known possibly to be caused by antimicrobial agents,[457,460,462] renal function and organ damage due to renal insufficiency should be assessed preoperatively in the patient with infectious disease. Guidelines for prophylactic antibiotics, summarized in Tables 25-17A and B, help prevent sepsis from bacteremic interventions.[289,493,494] Sepsis has become a leading cause of postoperative morbidity,[458,461,462] probably through a decrease in systemic vascular resistance related to activation of the complement system. Thus, attention to the effects of antibiotic drugs must be supplemented by attention to intravascular volume status.[460-462,494,495] The degree of impairment of the infected organ and its effect on anesthesia should be assessed. For instance, endocarditis merits examination of volume status, antibiotic and other drug therapy and side effects,[496] myocardial function, and renal, pulmonary, neurologic, and hepatic function: those organ systems that endocarditis can affect.

At least two other considerations merit preoperative consideration: patient isolation to prevent contamination and patient infectivity to the physician. Both concerns are real. Nosocomial infection is a major source of postsurgical morbidity.[497-503] Acquired immunodeficiency syndrome (AIDS)[504] and many forms of hepatitis (A, B, and non-A, non-B [hepatitis C]) appear to be due to viral infections but require direct contact with blood or body fluids. Screening for specific viruses or for the chronic end-organ effects of these viruses[505] is now being done to reduce the risk of infection to both recipients and health care personnel during blood transfusions. Usual precautions appear to be effective.[506] These two considerations are the focus of at least two published volumes.[507,508]

Electrolyte Disorders
(Also See Chs. 32, 38, and 47)

Disorders of calcium, magnesium, and phosphate balance were discussed in the section on diseases involving the endocrine system and disorders of nutrition.

Hyponatremia and Hypernatremia

Electrolyte disorders are usually detected by determining the levels of electrolytes in serum. These concentrations reflect the balance between water and electrolytes. The osmolality of all body fluids is normally maintained within the narrow physiologic range of 285 to 290 mOsm/kg H_2O. Because of the permeability of biologic membranes, intra- and extra-cellular osmolality are almost always equal and can be estimated by the following formula:

$$2[Na^+](mEq/L) + \frac{[glucose]\ (mg/dl)}{18} + \frac{BUN\ (mg/dl)}{2.8} = mOsm/kg$$

Therefore, disturbances in serum sodium reflect alterations in glucose metabolism, renal function, or accumulation of body water. The last can be affected by disturbances in thirst, antidiuretic hormone release, and renal function. Thus, hyponatremia reflects a relative excess of free water and can occur when total body sodium increases (as in edematous disorders), when total body sodium is normal (as in excesses of free water because of inappropriate secretion of antidiuretic hormone), or when total body sodium decreases (as occurs with too-aggressive use of diuretic drugs). Definition of the cause defines treatment. The anesthesiologist is faced with the question, What levels of electrolytes require treatment prior to anesthesia? Although slowly developing hyponatremia usually produces few symptoms, the patient may be lethargic and apathetic. Chronic hyponatremia is better tolerated than acute hyponatremia because of mechanisms regulating intracellular fluid volume that alleviate brain edema; the loss of other solutes from the cell decreases the osmotic movement of water into cells. Despite this, severe chronic hyponatremia (i.e., serum sodium levels < 123 mEq/L) can cause brain edema.[509] By contrast, acute hyponatremia may manifest with severe symptoms requiring emergency treatment: profound cerebral edema with obtundation, coma, convulsions, and disordered reflexes and thermoregulatory control.[509] Depending on the cause and relative total sodium and water content, treatment can range from administering hypertonic saline or mannitol (with or without diuretic drugs) to restricting fluids or administering other drugs.[509-512] Because neurologic damage may develop if the serum sodium concentration is increased too rapidly, the rate of rise should not exceed 1 mEq/L/h.[434,512] After the serum sodium concentration has reached 125 mEq/L, therapy may consist of water restriction; more rapid correction may result in CNS demyelination.[434,512] In hyponatremic patients who have excess total body water secondary to inappropriate secretion of antidiuretic hormone (SIADH), serum levels can be corrected by giving furosemide, 1 mg/kg, and hypertonic saline to replace loss of electrolytes in urine.[510-512] The diagnosis of SIADH is discussed earlier in this chapter.

In neither acute nor chronic hyponatremia is it necessary to restore serum sodium levels to their normal levels; brain swelling usually disappears at a serum sodium level of 130 mEq/L. This leaves us with the question, What levels of serum sodium make anesthesia more risky? Since no data exist to answer this question, to allow for some error in caring for patients, I have arbitrarily chosen a flexible 131 mEq/L concentration as the lower sodium limit for elective surgery. A discussion of intraoperative hyponatremia in patients undergoing transurethral prostatectomy can be found in Chapter 55.

Hypernatremia occurs much less commonly than hyponatremia. It is often iatrogenic in origin (e.g., can be caused by failure to provide sufficient free water to the patient who is unconscious or who has had a recent stroke-induced deficit of the thirst mechanism) and can occur in the presence of low, normal, or excess total body sodium. The primary symptoms of hypernatremia relate to brain cell shrinking. Because too rapid correction of hypernatremia can lead to cerebral edema and convulsions, correction should be made gradually. Again, with no data to support this stance, I believe that all patients undergoing surgery should have serum sodium concentrations of less than 150 mEq/L prior to anesthesia.

Hypokalemia and Hyperkalemia

Hypokalemia and hyperkalemia are also discussed in Chapters 32, 38, and 47. The relationship between the measured potassium concentration in serum and the total body potassium stores can best be described using a scattergram.[92,513] Only 2 percent of total body potassium is stored in plasma (4,200 mEq in cells and 60 mEq in extracellular fluid). In normal individuals, 75 percent of the 50 to 60 mEq/L of total body potassium is stored in skeletal muscle, 6 percent in red blood cells, and 5 percent in the liver. Thus, a 20 to 25 percent change in potassium levels in plasma could represent a change in total body potassium of 1,000 mEq or more, if the change were chronic, or as little as 10 to 20 mEq if the change were acute.

As with serum sodium levels,[509] acute changes in serum potassium levels appear to be less well tolerated than chronic changes. Chronic changes are relatively well tolerated because of the equilibration of serum and intracellular stores that takes place over time to return the resting membrane potential of excitable cells to near normal.

Hyperkalemia can result from factitious elevation of potassium (as in red blood cell hemolysis); excessive exogenous potassium from sources such as salt substitutes, or in large amounts, bananas; cellular shifts in potassium (owing to metabolic acidosis, tissue and muscle damage after burns, use of depolarizing muscle relaxants or intense catabolism of protein), and decreased renal excretion (as occurs in renal failure, renal insufficiency with trauma, therapy with potassium-sparing diuretic drugs[511] or mineralocorticoid deficiency). The major danger in anesthetizing patients who have disorders of potassium balance appears to be abnormal cardiac function, that is, both electrical disturbances[514–517] and poor cardiac contractility.[515,516] Hyperkalemia lowers the resting membrane potential of excitable cardiac cells and decreases the duration of the myocardial action potential and upstroke velocity.

This decreased rate of ventricular depolarization, plus the beginning of repolarization in some areas of the myocardium while other areas are still being depolarized, produces a progressively widening QRS complex that merges with the T wave into a sine wave on ECG. Above a potassium level of 6.7 mEq/L,[514] the degree of hyperkalemia and the duration of the QRS complex correlate well. This correlation is even better than the correlation between the serum potassium level and changes in the T wave. Nevertheless, the earliest manifestations of hyperkalemia are narrowing and peaking of the T wave. Although not diagnostic of hyperkalemia, T waves are almost invariably peaked and narrow when serum potassium levels are 7 to 9 mEq/L. When serum potassium levels exceed 7 mEq/L, atrial conduction disturbances appear as manifested by a decrease in P-wave amplitude and by an increase in the PR interval. Supraventricular tachycardia, atrial fibrillation, premature ventricular contractions, ventricular tachycardia, ventricular fibrillation, or sinus arrest may all occur. The ECG and cardiac alterations of hyperkalemia are potentiated by low serum levels of calcium and sodium. Intravenous administration of saline, bicarbonate, glucose with insulin (1 unit/2 g glucose), and calcium can reverse these changes by shifting some extracellular potassium into the cell. Kayexalate (sodium polystyrene sulfonate) enemas can be given to bind potassium in the gut in exchange for sodium. Dialysis against a hypokalemic solution will also decrease serum potassium levels. However, in the hyperkalemic patient, hypoventilation can be dangerous during anesthesia,[514–517] because each 0.1 pH unit change can produce a 0.4 to 1.5 mEq/L change in serum potassium levels in the opposite direction. For example, if pH decreases from 7.4 to 7.3, serum potassium levels could increase from 5.5 to 6.5 mEq/L.[517,518]

Hypokalemia can be caused by inadequate intake of potassium, excessive GI losses (through diarrhea, vomiting, nasopharyngeal suctioning; chronic use of laxatives, or ingestion of cation-exchange resins, as occur in certain wines), excessive renal losses (because of use of diuretic drugs, renal tubular acidosis, chronic chloride deficiency, metabolic alkalosis, mineralocorticoid excess, excessive ingestion of licorice, use of antibiotics, ureterosigmoidoscomy and diabetic ketoacidosis), and shifts of potassium from extracellular to intracellular compartments (as occur in alkalosis, insulin administration, β-adrenergic agonist administration or stress, barium poisoning, and periodic paralysis). As with hyperkalemia, knowledge of the cause of potassium deficiency and its appropriate preoperative evaluation and treatment may be as important as treatment of the deficiency itself. Also like hyperkalemia, hypokalemia may reflect small or vast changes in total body potassium. Acute hypokalemia may be much less well tolerated than chronic hypokalemia. The major worrisome manifestations of hypokalemia pertain to the circulatory system, both the cardiac and peripheral components. In addition, however, chronic hypokalemia results in muscle weakness, hypoperistalsis, and nephropathy.

The cardiovascular manifestations of hypokalemia include autonomic neuropathy (which results in orthostatic hypotension and decreased sympathetic reserve), impaired myocardial contractility, and electrical conduction abnormalities that can result in sinus tachycardia, atrial and ventricular arrhythmias, and disturbances of intraventricular conduction that can progress to ventricular fibrillation. That these are real concerns for the hypokalemic patient has been attested to too many times.[514-516,518-520] In addition to arrhythmias, the ECG reveals widening of the QRS complex, ST-segment abnormalities, progressive diminution of the T-wave amplitude, and progressive increase in the U-wave amplitude.[521] Surawicz[514] found these changes to be present invariably when serum potassium levels decreased to below 2.3 mEq/L. Although U waves are not specific to hypokalemia, they are sensitive indicators of the condition. Replenishing the total body potassium deficit for a depletion reflected by a serum deficit of 1 mEq/L (e.g., from 3.3 to 4.3 mEq/L) may require 1,000 mEq of potassium. Even if this amount could be given instantaneously (and it should not be replenished at a rate exceeding 250 mEq/day), it would take 24 to 48 hours to equilibrate in all tissues.[93,94] The potassium-depleted myocardium is unusually sensitive to digoxin, calcium, and, most important, potassium. Rapid potassium infusion can produce as severe arrhythmias in the hypokalemic patient as does hypokalemia itself.[94,522-524]

Thus, the decision about proceeding with surgery and anesthesia in the face of acute or chronic depletions or excesses of potassium depends on many factors.[525-529] One must know the cause and treatment of the underlying condition creating the electrolyte imbalance and the effect of that imbalance on perioperative risk and physiologic processes. The urgency of the operation, the degree of electrolyte abnormality, the medications given, the acid-base balance, and the suddenness or persistence of the electrolyte disturbance are all considerations.

Retrospective epidemiologic studies attribute significant risk to administration of potassium (even chronic oral administration).[526,527] In one study, 1,910 of 16,048 consecutive hospitalized patients were given oral potassium supplements. Of these, hyperkalemia contributed to death in seven, making the incidence of complications of potassium therapy one in 250 patients. Armed with such data, many internists do not prescribe oral potassium therapy for patients given diuretic drugs. Yet such patients frequently become moderately hypokalemic.[511,530,531] Modest hypokalemia occurs in 10 to 50 percent of patients given diuretic drugs. Should surgery be delayed to subject such patients to the risks of potassium therapy?

Two studies investigated whether modest hypokalemia was a problem by prospectively seeking arrhythmias on ECG in patients with various preoperative potassium levels.[528,529] No difference in the incidence of arrhythmias was found among 25 normokalemic (K > 3.4 mEq/L) patients, 25 moderately hypokalemic (K = 3 to 3.4 mEq/L) patients, and 10 severely hypokalemic (K < 2.9 mEq/L) patients.[528] The insensitivity of the eye or of even Holter recordings for short periods[532] (which seem not to have been obtained in this study) indicates that confirming studies are needed.

Other studies indicate that modest hypokalemia can have severe consequences.[531,533,534] Holland and co-workers[534] treated 21 patients with 50 mg hydrochlorothiazide twice a day for 4 weeks. These patients had a history of becoming hypokalemic during diuretic therapy; none of them had cardiac disease or was taking other medication. Before and after diuretic therapy, 24-hour ambulatory ECGs were recorded. This study is also subject to the limitations of Holter monitoring.[532] Seven of the 21 patients (33 percent) developed ventricular ectopy, including complex ventricular ectopy (multifocal PVCs, ventricular couplets, ventricular tachycardia). Potassium repletion decreased the number of ectopic ventricular beats per patient from 71.2 to 5.4/h. Apparently, some patients are sensitive to even minor potassium depletion. In the Multiple Risk Factor Intervention Trial involving 361,662 patients, of whom over 2,000 were treated for hypertension with diuretics, the reduction in serum potassium after diuretic therapy was greater for those with PVCs.[531] Therefore, although I recommend that hypokalemic patients be given potassium supplements, this issue is not clear.[535]

My personal criteria for preoperative potassium therapy are as follows. As a rule, I believe all patients undergoing elective surgery should have normal serum potassium levels. However, I do not recommend delaying surgery if the serum potassium level is above 2.9 mEq/L or below 5.9 mEq/L, if the cause of potassium imbalance is known, and if the patient is in otherwise optimal condition. This range of safe potassium levels is arbitrary and has changed from 3.3 in 1979, to 3.1 in 1986, to 2.9 in 1990 on the lower side and from 5.6 in 1979, to 5.7 in 1986, and to 5.9 in 1990 on the upper side as more data have become available on the safety of preoperative hypokalemia and the dangers of replacing potassium in a hospital environment[526-529] (see Table 23-1). I subject all patients with end-stage renal failure to dialysis (using the same arbitrary safe range) before all surgical procedures except truly emergency ones (as in the instance of imminent exsanguination). In 1978, Tanifuji and Eger[536] determined the relationships between electrolyte status and anesthetic requirement in dogs that may represent intraoperative considerations: hyponatremia and hypoosmolality decreased MAC, hypernatremia increased MAC, and hyperkalemia did not affect anesthetic requirement.

GASTROINTESTINAL AND LIVER DISEASES

The reader should also see the discussion of porphyrias in the section on neurologic disease; the discussion of nutritional deficiencies in the section on disorders of nutrition; and pediatric disorders, such as transesophageal fistula, in Chapters 59 and 73.

Gastrointestinal Disease

The Preoperative Search for Diverse Associated Disorders in Gastrointestinal Disease

Although preoperative preparation of the GI tract is usually the responsibility of the surgeon, and although the GI tract frequently does not need to be extensively evaluated by the anesthesiologist, GI disease can, and often does, cause derangements in many or all other systems. Such disturbances can affect the safety of anesthesia for the patient. Thus, the anesthesiologist may need not only to optimize the patient's condition through extensive preoperative preparation but also to have knowledge of disease processes and their effects in order to guide the patient smoothly through the perioperative period. The major advances of correcting fluid and electrolyte disorders and of optimizing nutritional status before surgery now allow surgery to be performed in patients with GI disease previously deemed to be at too great a risk and may have lessened the risk for others.[57-61,537,538] Still, in patients with GI disease, a thorough evaluation of intravascular fluid volume and electrolyte concentrations and nutrition is essential, including an evaluation of the supervening side effects of these therapies (e.g., hypophosphatemia from parenteral nutrition, hyperkalemia or cardiac arrhythmias from too vigorous a treatment of hypokalemia, and congestive heart failure from too rapid or too vigorous treatment for hypovolemia).

In addition to vast alterations in fluids, electrolytes, and nutrition that can occur with such diverse GI diseases as neoplasms and pancreatitis, patients with GI disorders can have bowel obstruction, vomiting, or hypersecretion of acid. These effects may merit rapid induction of anesthesia with application of cricoid pressure or awake endotracheal intubation, preoperative nasogastric suctioning, or preoperative use of histamine-receptor blocking agents (also see Ch. 40).[537,538] Clotting abnormalities may need to be corrected, since the fat-soluble vitamin K (often malabsorbed) is necessary for synthesis of factors V, VII, IX, and X in the liver (also see Ch. 56). Liver disease is often associated with GI disease and, if severe enough, can also result in deficiency of clotting factors synthesized by the liver.

Other factors should be remembered in any preoperative evaluation of the patient with GI disease. First, closed spaces containing gas expand by absorbing nitrous oxide. This expansion can lead to ischemic injury and/or GI viscus rupture.[539] Second, GI surgery predisposes the patient to sepsis; sepsis and decreased peripheral vascular resistance can lead to massive fluid requirements, cardiac failure, and renal insufficiency. Recently the wound infection rate has been declining; this decrease may be attributable to the use of better technique or to more appropriate prophylactic use of

antibiotics.[289,540] Third, patients with GI disease may have many other associated disorders not directly related to the GI tract. For example, they may be anemic from deficiencies in iron, intrinsic factor, folate, or vitamin B_{12}. They may also manifest neurologic changes from combined-system disease. Respiration may be impaired because of heavy cigarette smoking, peritonitis, abscess, pulmonary obstruction, previous incisions, aspirations, or pulmonary embolism (as occurs with ulcerative colitis or with thrombophlebitis in the bedridden).[541] They may also have hepatitis, cholangitis, or side effects from antibiotic drugs or other medications, massive bleeding with anemia and shock, or psychological derangements. Since GI disease can be accompanied by so many diverse associated disorders, the clinician clearly must search for other system involvement and preoperatively assess and treat such disorders appropriately. Discussion of two specific diseases, ulcerative colitis and carcinoid tumors, will highlight the importance of other-system involvement in GI disease.

Ulcerative Colitis and Carcinoid Tumors as Examples of Gastrointestinal Disease Affecting Other Systems

Patients with ulcerative colitis often have psychological problems. They may also have phlebitis; deficiencies in iron, folate, or vitamin B_{12}; anemia; or clotting disorders caused by malabsorption. They may be malnourished, dehydrated, or have electrolyte abnormalities. In addition, ulcerative collitis can be accompanied by massive bleeding; bowel obstruction or perforation or toxic megacolon, causing respiratory compromise; hepatitis; arthritis; iritis; spondylitis; or diabetes secondary to pancreatitis.

The site of origin of carcinoid tumors in more than 75 percent of patients is the gastrointestinal tract.[542] Within the gastrointestinal tract, carcinoid tumors have been documented to occur from the esophagus to the rectum. The most frequent site is the appendix, but carcinoids in this location rarely, if ever, metastasize or produce the carcinoid syndrome. Tumors arising in the ileocecal region have the highest incidence of metastases. Carcinoid tumors originating from other than the gastrointestinal tract have been reported in such other sites as the head and neck, lung, gonads, thymus, breast and urinary tract. Cardiac involvement, although frequently reported, is usually limited to right-sided valvular and myocardial plaque formation.

Not all patients with carcinoid tumors have symptoms attributable to hormone secretion by the tumor. The most comprehensive series in the literature indicates that only 7 percent of patients have the carcinoid syndrome: flushing, diarrhea and valvular heart disease. Of those with the syndrome, approximately 74 percent manifest cutaneous flushing, 68 percent have intestinal hypermotility, 41 percent exhibit cardiac symptoms, and wheezing occurs in 18 percent. Factors influencing symptoms include the location of the tumor as well as the particular hormones produced and secreted. Although it is generally believed that if patients do not exhibit the carcinoid syndrome the tumors are not producing serotonin (5-hydroxytryptamine), this may not be the case. Approximately 50 percent of patients with carcinoid tumors of the gastrointestinal tract demonstrate evidence of serotonin (5-HT) production, as manifested by elevated levels of urinary 5-hydroxyindoleacetic acid (5-HIAA) excretion. The carcinoid syndrome is usually associated with ileal carcinoid tumors that have metastasized to the liver. Presumably the liver clears mediators released from the tumor. Impairment of this clearing ability by the metastatic tumor results in the carcinoid syndrome.

The majority of patients with carcinoid tumors and increased urinary 5-HIAA have typical carcinoid tumors originating from the midgut (ileum or jejunum). Such patients excrete only small amounts of 5-hydroxytryptophan (5-HPT). Patients with atypical carcinoid tumors which originate from the foregut (bronchus, stomach, and pancreas) excrete large amounts of 5-HT and 5-HTP as well as moderately increased levels of 5-HIAA.

Although there is general agreement that serotonin is responsible for the diarrhea experienced by patients with carcinoids, other neurohumoral agents may contribute to the flushing and hypotension.[542-544] These include dopamine, histamine, and some of the neuropeptides such as substance P, neurotensin, vasoactive intestinal peptides, and somatostatin.

The net physiologic effect of circulating serotonin represents a composite of both direct action (mediated by serotonin receptors) and indirect action (mediated through modulation of adrenergic neurotransmission). The existence of several subtypes of serotonin receptors may account for the different effects of serotonin on various serotonin-sensitive tissue beds. Indirect actions are effected through alterations in catecholamine release and depend on the level of circulating serotonin.

Serotonin has little, if any, direct effect on the heart. With elevated levels, however, positive chronotropic and inotropic myocardial effects may occur, mediated through release of noradrenaline (norepinephrine). Effects of serotonin on the vasculature include both vasoconstriction and vasodilatation.

Alterations in gastrointestinal function attributed to serotonin include increased motility and net secretion of water, sodium chloride, and potassium by intestine. Serotonin reportedly causes bronchoconstriction in many animals but rarely in humans. Asthmatics are a possible exception.

Carcinoid tumors frequently present as diarrhea with fluid and electrolyte abnormalities. Because these tumors secrete vasoactive substances, patients can exhibit hypotension or hypertension with the flush of vasoactive substance release. Vasoactive substances can be released from the tumor by any number of substances including catecholamines. Thus, the anesthesiologist must tread a line between avoiding substances that release histamine (such as a *d*-tubocurarine and morphine) and creating anesthesia so light that painful stimuli activate a sympathetic stress response.[545-548] The anesthesiologist must also be ready and able to treat hypotension, decreased peripheral vascular resistance, bronchospasm, and hypertension. α-Adrenergic receptor blockade with the phenothiazines, butyrophenones, or phenoxybenzamine and β-adrenergic receptor blockade with propranolol have been advocated to prevent catecholamine-mediated release of vasoactive substances; these practices, however, can lead to hypotension.

If severe hypotension occurs, the drug of choice is either angiotensin (now commercially unavailable in the United States but an approved drug that is available by contacting CIBA-GIGY) or vasopressin. However, the vasoactive substances released by carcinoid tumors cause fibrosis of heart valves, often resulting in pulmonic stenosis or tricuspid insufficiency. To increase cardiac output in the patient with tricuspid insufficiency, the anesthesiologist should avoid drugs or situations that increase pulmonary vascular resistance (e.g., angiotensin, vasopressin, acidosis, hypercarbia, hypothermia) (also see Chs. 51 and 52). In addition, if large amounts of serotonin are produced (equal to 200 mg/day of 5-hydroxyindoleacetic acid, a metabolic product of serotonin), then niacin deficiency with pellagra (as occurs with diarrhea, dermatitis, and dementia) can develop.

Medical therapy is employed to treat the manifestations of serotonin production by carcinoid tumors. The serotonin antagonists cyproheptadine and methysergide block the effects of serotonin, especially on the gastrointestinal tract. Fenclonine (parachlorophenylalanine), which inhibits tryptophan hydroxylase, the rate-limiting step in serotonin synthesis, is also used to treat diarrhea.

Ketanserin is a prototypical selective $5HT_2$ receptor antagonist that blocks the actions mediated through the $5HT_2$ receptor, including serotonin-induced vasoconstriction, bronchoconstriction, and platelet aggregation. It does, however, also possess α-adrenergic antagonist activity. Ketanserin may be used to treat hypertension in patients with the carcinoid syndrome. Prophylactic use of this agent has been reported in one carcinoid patient undergoing surgery; hemodynamic stability was maintained despite elevated levels of serotonin throughout the procedure.

Acute elevation of plasma kinin activity in carcinoid patients has been postulated for many years as the explanation for the symptoms of the carcinoid syndrome. Physiological effects of kinins are known to include vasodilation of smaller, resistance vessels and stimulation of release of histamine from mast cells. The latter action potentiates their own vasodilating properties and further reduces systolic and diastolic blood pressure. In addition, increases in vascular permeability may lead to edema formation. Kinins are not known to affect the myocardium directly.

Steroids have been reported to be effective for treatment of symptoms associated with bronchial carcinoid tumors. Prophylactic preoperative administration as well as intraoperative therapeutic use have been reported, but controlled studies of beneficial effects are lacking.

Aprotinin, like steroids, inhibits the kallikrein cascade. This agent is believed to be capable of blocking the proteinase activity of kallikrein. A dramatic clinical response has been reported in some cases.

A subset of patients with symptoms of the carcinoid syndrome excrete histamine at increased levels in their urine. Histamine causes vasodilation of small blood vessels, leading to flushing and lowered total peripheral resistance. The rate of force of myocardial contraction are increased as is cardiac output. Histamine is known to cause bronchoconstriction, particularly in patients with bronchial asthma and other pulmonary diseases. Its role in carcinoid bronchospasm, if any, is uncertain. Histamine receptor-blocking drugs have been used with some success in alleviating the flushing associated with the carcinoid syndrome. H_2 antagonism alone was just as effective as combination therapy in preventing symptoms; pure H_1 antagonism, however, was ineffective.

Phenothiazines have been used preoperatively and perioperatively in patients with the carcinoid syndrome. Leukocyte interferon has also been reported to decrease symptoms in patients with the carcinoid syndrome.

Catecholamines aggravate symptoms of the carcinoid syndrome, presumably by stimulating hormone release by the tumor. The mechanism by which this occurs remains obscure. Adrenergic receptors have not been demonstrated in carcinoid tumors, nor do these tumors usually have neural innervation. Perhaps adrenergic stimuli work through their mechanical effects on the gut and vessels to stimulate release of tumor products. Treatment of patients with carcinoid tumors by means of α- and β-adrenergic antagonists has been beneficial in ameliorating flushing in some instances but ineffective for other patients.

Clonidine has been demonstrated to reduce flushing in a patient with a carcinoid tumor. The mechanism of action was presumed to be presynaptic inhibition of noradrenaline release.

Results of prospective studies on somatostatin used to ameliorate symptoms of the carcinoid syndrome have been encouraging. In several case reports involving a total of 38 patients, all but 2 patients had rapid, dramatic improvement in flushing.[542-544] Similar results have been obtained in patients with diarrhea. It would appear that somatostatin holds promise as a major treatment advance for patients with the carcinoid syndrome.

It might logically be concluded that preoperative preparation of the patient with carcinoid syndrome might proceed similarly to that of the patient with pheochromocytoma: titrating adrenergic, histaminic, and serotonergic receptor-blocking drugs to maximum effect while monitoring intravascular volume status and adding somatostatin prior to surgery. Although this approach is logical, preoperative symptoms do not correlate with perioperative ones, and only the last two therapeutic options (intravascular fluid status optimization and administration of somatostatin) seem likely to be effective.

Many patients also develop bronchospasm with or without flushing when vasoactive substances are released. Thus, a patient with a carcinoid tumor may be well, or may be severely incapacitated by pulmonary, neurologic, nutritional, fluid, electrolytic or cardiovascular disturbances.[542-544] Thus, the GI system by itself may not need extensive preoperative preparation, but GI disease can cause disturbances in any or all other systems that require both extensive preoperative preparation to optimize patient condition and preoperative knowledge of disease physiology and effects by anesthesiologists in order to guide patients through the perioperative period smoothly. In addition, the anesthesiologist's understanding of the nature of the surgery probably aids in determining the system involvement caused by GI disorder.

Liver Disease

What are the risks of giving anesthesia to patients with acute liver disease who require emergency surgery? What are the risks of giving anesthesia to patients with chronic impairment of liver function? What can be done to minimize these risks? Since hepatic function and physiology are discussed in Chapter 56, I will mention only that the liver performs many functions: it synthesizes (e.g., proteins, clotting factors), detoxifies the body of both drugs and the products of normal human metabolism, excretes waste products, and stores and supplies energy. Thus, tests of liver function assess synthesis (cholesterol levels, prothrombin time, albumin levels), cellular integrity (SGOT, alanine transaminase, LDH, alkaline phosphatase), the liver's ability to detoxify the body (e.g., ammonia, direct bilirubin, or lidocaine levels), and the liver's ability to excrete certain substances (BSP retention, total bilirubin levels).

In examining the effects of anesthesia (with or without surgery) on liver function, and in examining ways to reduce risk in patients with pre-existing liver disease, investigators have often looked at one or more of these tests, or, more commonly, at major end points of morbidity (jaundice) or mortality. The evidence can be summarized as follows: without anesthesia or surgery, approximately 1 in 7 to 800 patients who are otherwise healthy and scheduled for surgery will have abnormal preoperative results for liver function tests; of these patients, 1 in 3 will develop jaundice (also see Ch. 23 for these studies).[549,550] In our preliminary study, *every* patient with abnormal liver function tests has been symptomatic preoperatively.[215] Thus perhaps the risk is less than described (see Ch. 23).

All anesthetics tested (general, narcotic-nitrous oxide, and regional) have caused transient abnormalities in liver function tests. These abnormalities were magnified by upper intra-abdominal surgery and occurred regardless of pre-existing liver disease.[436,551-564] Patients with abnormal preoperative liver function tests obviously will have a higher incidence of abnormal results on postoperative liver function tests.[436,551,556-558,560,561] Lacking in the literature are investigations that studied patients with compromised hepatic function, to determine how to decrease the risk of surgery and anesthesia. In addition to pre-existing hepatic disease and the operative site, hypokalemia, hypotension, sepsis, and the need for blood transfusion all contribute to postoperative hepatic dysfunction. Thus, anesthesia and surgery probably exacerbate hepatic disease and this obviously increases morbidity and mortality.[436,553,554,556,560,561] Only one study, and that in alcoholic liver disease, has implied otherwise.[436]

The main goal of the anesthesiologist is to avoid making the hepatic disease (with perhaps its metabolic and CNS toxicity) worse and thereby increasing the chance of renal failure, coma, and death.[565] Studies of portal hypertension have shown that mortality can be 50 percent when preoperative serum albumin concentrations are lower than 3 g/dl, preoperative serum bilirubin levels are greater than 3 mg/dl, and ascites and encephalopathy are present and even higher with a grossly abnormal prothrombin time. By contrast, mortality decreases to 10 percent when preoperative serum albumin levels are 3 to 3.5 g/dl, preoperative serum bilirubin levels are 2 to 3 mg/dl, prothrombin time is normal and encephalopathy is absent. The risks of anesthetizing a patient with chronic liver disease not requiring portacaval shunt are detailed only sporadically but appear to be greater than those associated with anesthetizing a healthy patient.[549-572]

Should halothane be given to patients with hepatitis or biliary tract disease? The National Halothane Study did not find that halothane caused massive hepatic necrosis, or any other hepatic abnormality, more frequently than did any other anesthetic agent[561] and in fact demonstrated its safety in biliary tract surgery. Prospective studies have been contradictory at best as to whether repeat exposures to halothane within a short time elevate liver enzyme levels to a greater degree than do other anesthetic agents.[571-574] Because the incidence of hepatitis attributable only to halothane would be very low, very large groups would have to be studied. The incidence of postoperative jaundice and hepatitis not attributable to halothane is much greater than the incidence of hepatitis attributable only to halothane, and the absence of differentiating pathologic features makes halothane hepatitis difficult to exclude as a possibility. Newer tests imply an immunologic basis to either the hepatitis or liver dysfunction continuing after the initial mechanism (e.g., if hypoxia begets the injury, the immune mechanism continues it), and are supported by resolution of the prolonged case of halothane hepatitis after treatment.[593] Although other cases that have resolved after steroid therapy have been presented, those cases did not, in fact, have a long enough period of time prior to the beginning of their resolution when the disease was stable to conclude that the steroids made a difference and that this was not the natural course of the disease. One case is not conclusive but certainly implies that a controlled trial should be instituted.

More sensitive tests of hepatocellular dysfunction after anesthesia and surgery, such as glutathione-S-transferase, reveal impairment more frequently.[592] One is left to conclude that both metabolic and immunologic mechanisms can contribute to hepatocellular dysfunction after anesthesia and surgery. Are these related to anesthesia or surgery? Internists almost always point to anesthesia and must be educated to shed light on their bias.

Thus, the strong bias of internists makes halothane hepatitis a popular diagnosis, despite the higher incidence of viral and drug hepatitides.[436,574-591] Another factor producing possible bias is the fact that animal models of halothane hepatitis incorporate liver hypoxia or pretreatment with polyvinylchlorides, conditions that can themselves adversely affect liver function. Thus, no irrefutable evidence implicating halothane as being better or worse than any other anesthetic for the patient with pre-existing liver disease exists. However, should liver disease worsen postoperatively, the tendency is to blame halothane. Anesthesia is certainly less likely than hypoxia, trauma, viral hepatitis, drug-induced hepatitis or sepsis to cause serious hepatic injury.[215,549,594] No one has yet determined whether a time limit exists within which repeat exposure to an anesthetic is more dangerous than exposure to various anesthetics or after which repeat anesthesia is as safe as a first exposure to anesthetic.

What should physicians do to prevent contracting hepatitis from, or giving it to, patients? If the hepatitis B vaccine proves as safe as its initial trials suggest, and if the risk of anesthesia personnel acquiring the disease and perhaps its chronic sequelae is as great as studies suggest, it would be cost-effective for anesthesia personnel to be given the vaccine.[595-597] What should the physician with hepatitis B do to prevent infecting patients? That subject is discussed in detail elsewhere.[598]

Liver disease severe enough to affect hepatic synthesis can impair the detoxification of many drugs,[491-494,599-601] including muscle relaxants[599-601] (also see Ch. 12), and can disturb coagulation (also see Ch. 48). Administration of fresh-frozen plasma may be needed to correct coagulation disorders.

HEMATOLOGIC DISORDERS AND ONCOLOGIC DISEASE

Hematologic Disorders

Anemia and Polycythemia: General Considerations

Chapter 23 discussed the evidence that normovolemic anemia or polycythemia increases perioperative morbidity. Wasserman and Gilbert[602] evaluated two groups of patients undergoing major surgery. Of 28 patients with uncontrolled polycythemia (hemoglobin >16 g/dl), 22 (79 percent) had complications and 10 (36 percent) died. Of 53 patients having controlled polycythemia (hemoglobin <16 g/dl), 15 (28 percent) had complications and 3 (5 percent) died. In both groups, most of the complications were related to polycythemia (for example, hemorrhage or thrombosis). Although this study has deficiencies (e.g., the study was retrospective in design, no time frame of study was given, "minor" surgery was excluded, and no statement was provided as to why polycythemia was controlled preoperatively in some patients and not in others), its results indicate that knowledge and pretreatment of polycythemia might decrease perioperative morbidity and mortality.

No such evidence exists for normovolemic anemia. Rothstein[603] concluded that in children under 3 months of age, hemoglobin should be over 10 g/dl, whereas in older children, hemoglobin of 9 g/dl is adequate. Slogoff[604] concluded that in adults, a hematocrit of 20 percent (hemoglobin of ~7 g/dl) is adequate. However, no data confirm the hypothesis that treatment of moderate or mild normovolemic anemia in asymptomatic patients undergoing surgery involving no major blood loss decreases perioperative morbidity or mortality. Perhaps the duration of anemia is important also, because, with time, the cardiovascular system adjusts to anemia by increasing cardiac output.[604] Thus, there are no specific preoperative routines for anemia itself.

However, because anemia can be a hallmark of many other diseases possibly affecting perioperative anesthetic management, the preoperative presence of anemia requires a search for, and treatment of, the underlying cause. For instance, anemia could indicate renal insufficiency or a drug reaction, both of which could alter anesthetic management. For this reason, the cause of anemia should be known preoperatively. Similarly, polycythemia can be a primary disease (such as polycythemia vera) or secondary to smoking, use of diuretic drugs, chronic use of androgens, hypoxia, or other forms of chronic lung/heart disease. Phlebotomies are quite effective for patients whose polycythemia is mild. Cerebral blood flow improves when hematocrit is kept below 45 percent.[605–607] No prospective controlled study has been performed on humans regarding a possible decrease in perioperative morbidity or wound healing[607–609] from perioperative treatment of anemia or polycythemia. The time of most danger to the patient may be the early recovery room period, during which time oxygen delivery to the lungs is perhaps at its worst (also see Ch. 68). When religious convictions prohibit blood transfusion and the patient is anemic or may become anemic, therapeutic options include autotransfusion[610] and use of blood substitutes.[611] Although the latter has fallen into disrepute because of effects on reticuloendothelial function, other substitutes probably will become available,[612] and synthetic erythropoietin will find greater use in preoperative prophylaxis and preoperative predeposit pro-

grams.[468,469,613] This subject is discussed in more detail in Chapter 49.

Several forms of anemia present special situations, such as sickle cell anemia, hereditary spherocytosis, and the autoimmune hemolytic anemias.

Sickle Cell Anemia and Related Hemoglobinopathies

The sickle cell syndromes comprise a family of hemoglobinopathies caused by abnormal genetic transformation of amino acids in the heme portion of the hemoglobin molecule.[614] The sickle cell syndromes arise from a mutation in the beta-globin gene that changes the sixth amino acid from valine to glutamic acid. A major pathologic feature of sickle cell disease is the aggregation of irreversibly sickled cells in blood vessels. The molecular basis of sickling is aggregation of deoxygenated hemoglobin molecules along their longitudinal axis.[614] This abnormal aggregation distorts the cell membrane and produces a sickle shape. Irreversibly sickled cells become dehydrated and rigid and can cause tissue infarcts by impeding blood flow and oxygen to tissues.[615,616] Some other abnormal hemoglobins interact with hemoglobin S to various degrees, giving rise to symptomatic disease in patients heterozygous for hemoglobin S and one of the other hemoglobins such as the hemoglobin of thalassemia (hemoglobin C).

Two-tenths of 1 percent of the black population in America has sickle cell-thalassemia disease (hemoglobin SC); these patients also have end-organ disease and symptoms suggestive of organ infarction. For such patients, perioperative considerations should be similar to those for patients with sickle cell disease (hemoglobin SS), discussed later.

Whereas 8 to 10 percent of American blacks have the sickle cell trait (hemoglobin AS), 0.2 percent are homozygous for the sickle cell hemoglobin and have sickle cell anemia. The sickle cell trait should not be considered a disease, because hemoglobin AS cells begin to sickle only when oxygen saturation of hemoglobin is below 20 percent. No difference has been found between normal persons (those with hemoglobin AA) and those with hemoglobin AS regarding survival rates or incidence of severe disease, with one exception: patients with hemoglobin AS have a 50 percent increase in pulmonary infarctions. However, single case reports of a perioperative death and a perioperative brain infarct in two patients with hemoglobin AS disease do exist,[616,617] and a report of death believed due to aortocaval compression during general anesthesia that resulted in a sickling crisis does exist.[618] Those authors recommend frequent measurement of oxygen saturation (pulse oximetry) in multiple areas of the body, including ear and toe in pregnant patients.

The pathologic end-organ damage that occurs in sickle cell states is attributable to three processes: the sickling of cells in blood vessels, an occurrence that causes infarcts and consequent tissue destruction secondary to tissue ischemia; hemolytic crisis secondary to hemolysis; and aplastic crises that occur with bone marrow exhaustion and can rapidly result in severe anemia. Logic dictates that patients currently in a crisis should not be operated upon except for extreme emergencies, and then only after exchange transfusion.[615-619]

Since sickling is increased with lowered oxygen tensions, acidosis, hypothermia, and the presence of more desaturated hemoglobin S, current therapy includes keeping the patient warm and well hydrated, giving supplemental oxygen, maintaining high cardiac output, and not creating areas of stasis with pressure or with tourniquets. Meticulous attention to these practices in those periods when we usually do not pay most careful attention (i.e., waiting in the preinduction area) or when gas exchange may be most unmatched to cardiovascular-metabolic demands (early postoperative period) may be important in lessening morbidity. Even following these measures routinely with no special emphasis placed on the periods described reduced mortality to 1 percent in several series of patients with sickle cell syndromes.[617-620] Retrospective review of patient charts led the authors of those studies to conclude that, at most, a 0.5 percent mortality rate could be attributed to the interaction between sickle cell anemia and anesthetic agent.

Can this rate be decreased?[620-622] Several authors have advocated using partial exchange transfusions perioperatively. In children with sickle cell anemia and acute lung syndromes, partial exchange transfusion improved clinical symptoms and blood oxygenation. Also, serum bilirubin levels decreased in patients with acute liver injury. Clinical improvement of pneumococcal meningitis and cessation of hematuria in papillary necrosis also accompanied exchange transfusion.[623] The goal of exchange transfusion is to increase the concentration of hemoglobin A to 40 percent and the hematocrit to 35 percent. The 40 percent figure is an arbitrary one, as no controlled studies have established the threshold ratio of hemoglobin A to S that would render blood not able to sickle in vivo. To achieve the 40 percent ratio in a 70-kg adult, about 4 units of washed erythrocytes would have to be exchanged; the system is inexpensive but efficient. The possible decrease in preoperative morbidity after partial exchange transfusion has not been compared with the risks of exchange, except in one study,[620] which found the risks of exchange to exceed the benefits. In that retrospective review of 82 surgical procedures performed between 1978 and 1986 in 60 patients, no advantage was noted in preoperative exchange transfusion as measured by a decrease in postoperative complication. (However, only the sickest may have received exchange as patients were not randomly allocated to exchange or nonexchange groups.) A slight increase in postoperative atelectasis requiring treatment was seen in those patients who received preoperative transfusions. Over 50 percent of patients receiving transfusions had a postoperative complication.

Patients who began with a hematocrit over 36 percent had a lower complication rate.[620] Therefore, my recommendation is to pay meticulous attention to preventing conditions that increase sickling or cause infection and to limit exchange transfusion to crisis situations. Induction of hyponatremia has recently been shown to abort acute sickle cell crisis; however, this treatment is still experimental.[625] Other conditions are common in sickle cell syndromes: pulmonary dysfunction with increased shunt, renal insufficiency, gallstones, small myocardial infarcts, priapism, stroke, aseptic necrosis of bones and joints, ischemic ulcers, retinal detachments from neovascularization, and complications of repeated transfusions.

In thalassemia, globin structures are normal but, because of gene deletion, the rate of synthesis of either the α or β chains of hemoglobin (α- and β-thalassemia, respectively) is reduced.[626] Bone marrow transplantation and pharmacologic manipulation of hemoglobin F synthesis are being tried in these hemoglobinopathies, as is direct gene replacement therapy. These syndromes are common in Southeast Asia, India, and the Middle East and in individuals of African descent. In thalassemia, facial deformity from erythropoietin stimulated ineffective erythropoiesis (ineffective secondary to genetic inability to produce useful hemoglobin) has been reported to make endotracheal intubation difficult.[626] This one case report has not been amplified upon, and there are no reports of this complication for patients with sickle cell anemia. However, the anemia associated with these syndromes often produces a compensatory hyperplasia of the erythroid marrow, which in turn is associated with severe skeletal abnormalities.[627]

Glucose 6-phosphate dehydrogenase (G6PD) deficiency (a sex-linked recessive trait) is also reported to occur in approximately 8 percent of African-American men. Young cells have normal activity, but older cells are grossly deficient compared with normal cells. A deficiency in this enzyme results in hemolysis of the erythrocyte and formation of Heinz bodies. Red cell hemolysis can also occur after administration of drugs that produce substances requiring G6PD for detoxification (e.g., methemoglobin, glutathione, and hydrogen peroxide). Drugs to be avoided are sulfa drugs, quinidine, prilocaine, lidocaine, antimalarial drugs, antipyretic drugs, non-narcotic analgesics, vitamin K analogues, and perhaps sodium nitroprusside.

Hereditary Spherocytosis, Elliptocytosis, and Autoimmune Hemolytic Anemias

Congenital abnormalities of the erythrocyte membrane are becoming better understood. In elliptocytosis and hereditary spherocytosis, the membrane is more permeable to cations and more susceptible to lipid loss when cell energy is depleted than is the membrane of the normal red blood cell. Both hereditary spherocytosis (present in 1 in 5,000 people) and hereditary elliptocytosis are inherited as autosomal dominant traits. In both, defects in the membrane are thought to result from mutation of spectrin, a structural protein of the membrane cytoskeleton.[628] Although the therapeutic role of splenectomy in these diseases is not fully defined, in severe disease, splenectomy is known to improve the shortened lifespan of the red blood cell 100 percent (from 20 to 30 days to 40 to 70 days). Because splenectomy does predispose the patient to gram-positive septicemia (particularly pneumococcal), perhaps patients should be given pneumococcal vaccine preoperatively prior to predictable bacteremic events. No specific problems relating to anesthesia have been reported for these disorders.

The autoimmune hemolytic anemias include cold antibody anemia, warm antibody anemia (idiopathic), and drug-induced anemias.[629,630] The cold antibody hemolytic anemias are mediated by immunoglobulin M or G antibodies, which, at room temperature and below cause red blood cells to clump. When these patients are given blood transfusions, the cells and all fluid infusions must be warm, and body temperature must be maintained meticulously at 37°C if hemolysis is to be prevented. Warm antibody (or "idiopathic" hemolytic anemia) is a difficult management problem characterized by chronic anemia, the presence of antibodies active against red blood cells, positive Coombs' test, and difficulty in cross-matching blood. For patients undergoing elective surgery, autologous transfusions, predeposit with or without erythropoietin stimulation,[613] and blood from rare Rh-negative red blood cell donors and/ or the patient's first-degree relatives can be used. In emergency situations, the possibility of autotransfusions, splenectomy, or corticosteroid treatment should be discussed with a hematologist knowledgeable in this area. Drug-induced anemias have three mechanisms: receptor-type hemolysis, in which a drug (e.g., penicillin) binds to the membrane of the red blood cell, and the complex stimulates formation of an antibody against the complex; "innocent bystander" hemolysis, in which a drug (e.g., quinidine, sulfuramide) binds to a plasma protein, thereby stimulating an antibody (IgM) that cross-reacts with an erythrocyte; and autoimmune hemolysis, in which the drug stimulates production of an antibody (IgG) that cross-reacts with the erythrocyte. Drug-induced hemolytic anemias generally cease when drug therapy ends. In emergency situations, the least incompatible cells available should be used for blood transfusion.

Granulocytopenia

In patients who have fewer than 500 granulocytes/ml blood and established sepsis, granulocyte transfusion has been shown to prolong life.[631] One study has questioned this finding.[632] Although logic might appear to dictate giving granulocyte transfusions prophylactically to patients with fewer than 500 granulocytes/ml blood who will undergo bacteremic events, the effectiveness of this practice has not been studied extensively and is controversial.[633,634]

Platelet Disorders

Although inherited platelet disorders are rare, acquired disorders are quite common. Both conditions cause skin and mucosal bleeding, whereas defects in plasma coagulation produce deep tissue bleeding or delayed bleeding.[635] Perioperative treatment of inherited platelet disorders (Glanzmann's thrombasthenia, Bernard-Souliep syndrome, Hermansky-Pudlak syndrome) consists of platelet transfusions. ε-Aminocaproic acid (EACA) has recently been used successfully (experimentally, 1 g/70 kg/4 h) to decrease perioperative bleeding in thrombocytopenic patients. The much more common acquired disorders may respond to one of several therapies. Immune thrombocytopenias, such as those associated with lupus erythematosus, idiopathic thrombocytopenic purpura, uremia, hemolytic-uremic syndrome, platelet transfusions, heparin, and thrombocytosis may respond to steroids, splenectomy, platelet pheresis, or alkylating agents or may require platelet transfusions, plasma exchange, whole blood exchange transfusion, or may not respond to anything.[633-637] By far the largest number of platelet abnormalities consist of drug-related defects in the aggregation and release of platelets. Aspirin irreversibly acetylates platelet cyclo-oxygenase, the enzyme that converts arachidonic acid to prostaglandin endoperoxidases. Because cyclo-oxygenase is not regenerated in the circulation within the lifespan of the platelet, and because this enzyme is essential for the aggregation of platelets, one aspirin may affect platelet function for a week. All other drugs that inhibit platelet function (vitamin E, indomethacin, sulfinpyrazone, dipyridamole, tricyclic antidepressant drugs, phenothiazines, furosemide, steroids) do not irreversibly inhibit cyclo-oxygenase function; thus, these drugs disturb platelet function for only 24 to 48 hours. If emergency surgery is needed before the customary 8-day period for platelet regeneration after aspirin, or if the 2-day period for other drugs has not elapsed, administration of 2 to 5 units of platelet concentrates will return platelet function in a 70-kg adult to an adequate level and platelet-induced clotting dysfunction to normal.[635,638-640] Only 30,000 to 50,000 normally functioning platelets/mm³ are needed for normal clotting. One platelet transfusion will increase the platelet count from 4,000 to 20,000/ml blood; platelet half-life is about 8 hours.[635,638-640]

Hemophilia and Related Clotting Disorders

Abnormalities in blood coagulation owing to defects in plasma coagulation factor are either inherited or acquired. Inherited disorders include X-linked hemophilia A (a defect in factor VIII activity), von Willebrand's diseases (defect in von Willebrand's component of factor VIII), hemophilia B (a sex-linked deficiency of factor IX activity), and other less common disorders. The sex-linked origin of some of these disorders means that hemophilia occurs almost exclusively in male offspring of female carriers; men do not transmit the disease to their male offspring. In elective surgery, levels of the deficient coagulation factor should be assayed 48 hours before surgery and the level restored to 40 percent of normal before surgery. One unit of factor concentrate per kilogram of body weight normally increases factor concentration by 2 percent. Thus, in the individual essentially devoid of activity, administration of 20 units/kg body weight would be required as an initial dose. Since half-life is 6 to 10 hours for factor VIII and 8 to 16 hours for factor IX, one should give approximately 1.5 units/h/kg of factor VIII or 1.5 units/2 h/kg of factor IX. Additional administration of factors VIII and IX should be guided by the activity of the clotting factors for about 6 to 10 days postoperatively.[641–643]

These factors are available in various preparations: cryoprecipitate, which contains 20 units/ml, is obtained from regular donors (the risk of hepatitis being 1 : 200 for 5-ml lots) or from fresh-frozen plasma (which contains 1 unit/ml). Some risk of transmitting hepatitis and AIDS accompanies these transfusions.[644–646] Current screening of blood for AST or ALT levels is believed to result in a much lower risk of non-A, non-B hepatitis and even AIDS from transfusion. Antigenic testing for the HIV viruses should theoretically further decrease the risk of their transmission by blood products. Heat treatment is reported to reduce these risks substantially. Factor IX, but not factor VIII, is contained in prothrombin complex concentrates; however, these concentrates may contain activated clotting factors, leading to disseminated intravascular clotting and a high risk of hepatitis. In addition, although EACA or tranexamic acid (0.5 mg/kg) is sometimes administered as a fibrinolytic inhibitor, these substances carry with them a significant risk of disseminated intravascular coagulation. Additional hazards of modern therapy include acute and chronic hepatitis, AIDS, hypersensitivity reactions, psychic trauma, chronic pain with narcotic addiction, and inhibition of factors, especially VIII.

Approximately 10 percent of patients with either hemophilia A or B develop an antibody that inactivates factor VIII or IX (fresh-frozen plasma fails to increase clotting factor activity after incubation with the patient's plasma). These acquired anticoagulants are usually composed of immunoglobulin G, are poorly removed by plasmapheresis, and are variably responsive to immunosuppressive drugs. Use of prothrombin complex concentrates can be lifesaving but carries the risk of disseminated intravascular coagulation and hepatitis.

Vitamin K deficiency is discussed in the section on liver disease. To review, vitamin K-dependent clotting factors (II, VII, IX, and X) require vitamin K for the postsynthetic addition of γ-carboxyl groups to glutamate residues; administration of vitamin K or fresh-frozen plasma can correct these deficiencies.

Patients who come to the operating room having received many units of blood (as in massive GI bleeding) may have deficient clotting. This impaired clotting is caused initially by depletion of platelets (which occurs after approximately 10 to 15 units of blood has been given and later, by depletion of coagulation factors (see Ch. 48).[647,648] Treatment of these deficiencies can be corrected with platelet concentrates (each concentrate is normally suspended in 50 ml of fresh plasma; thus, coagulation factors are also replaced).

Urokinase, streptokinase, and tissue plasminogen activator have been used to treat pulmonary embolism, deep-vein thrombosis, and arterial occlusive disease. These drugs accelerate the lysis of thrombi and emboli, in contrast to heparin, which may prevent but not dissolve a thrombus. Bleeding complications associated with these fibrinolytic agents result from dissolution of hemostatic plugs and can be quickly reversed by discontinuing the medication and replenishing plasma fibrinogen with cryoprecipitate or plasma. However, cryoprecipitate and plasma are seldom needed preoperatively because the fibrinolytic activity of urokinase and streptokinase usually dissipates within an hour of discontinuing their administration. However, insufficient data have accumulated to prescribe ideal preoperative preparation and intraoperative management of hemostasis in patients recently treated with urokinase, streptokinase, or tissue plasminogen activator. Postponing surgery for three half-lives of the drug (increases in plasmin activity in blood can be assayed for at least 4 to 8 hours) may not be possible, and observing the operative field for meticulous attention to hemostasis may not suffice.[649] The process may be even more complex in the vascular or cardiac patient who requires heparin administration intraoperatively. To correct fibrinogen deficiency in such patients, some clinicians administer fibrinogen before surgery and EACA at the time of heparin administration. I usually delay or avoid giving EACA until heparin is administered to minimize the risk of thrombosis.

Desmopressin is now being tried in high blood loss operations as a routine measure to decrease bleeding and transfusion requirements. Such therapy began as a treatment for platelet dysfunction in von Willebrand's disease but has since expanded to routine use in patients undergoing cardiovascular surgery and frequent use in other high blood loss operations. This increased use occurred because desmopressin was found to decrease bleeding and transfusion requirements.[650] Whether the side effects of desmopressin exceed the benefits remains to be determined and will probably influence how routine its administration becomes.

The problem of patients on oral anticoagulants is discussed in the cardiovascular section of this chapter.[290–305] Regional anesthetic techniques might be avoided in patients given anticoagulant drugs.[290–305] Whether these regional techniques should also be avoided in patients treated prophylactically with low-dose subcutaneous heparin has not been studied. The effects of heparin sulfate can be reversed by titrating protamine, using activated clotting time as a guide. Our group usually gives approximately 1 mg of protamine per 3 to 4 mg of heparin administered within the last 8 hours. Pharmacologic research is searching for specific molecular subtypes of heparin that have different anticoagulant potency, binding affinities for antithrombin III, antithrombotic effects, and platelet aggregating effects. The search is for a "new" heparin preparation that will block thrombosis without causing clinical bleeding. Such a development might change our ways of monitoring clotting function. Determining bleeding time, platelet count, partial thromboplastin time (PTT) and prothrombin time will identify almost all problems in the patient with a suspected clotting or bleeding disorder (also see Ch. 48). As explained in Chapter 23, these screening tests probably should not be obtained in asymptomatic patients.

Oncologic Disease

Patients with malignant tumors may be otherwise healthy or desperately ill with nutritional, neurologic, metabolic, endocrinologic, electrolyte, cardiac, pulmonary, renal, hepatic, hematologic, or pharmacologic disabilities. Thus, determining the other disabilities accompanying malignant tumors requires evaluating all systems. Abnormalities frequently accompanying such tumors include hypercalcemia either by direct bone invasion or by ectopic elaboration of parathyroid hormone or other bone-dissolving substance, uric acid nephropathy, hyponatremia (especially with small cell, or oat cell, carcinoma of the lung), nausea, vomiting, anorexia and cachexia, fever, tumor-induced hypoglycemia, intracranial metastases (10 to 20 percent of all cancers), peripheral nerve or spinal cord disorders, meningeal carcinomatosis, toxic neuropathies secondary to anticancer therapy, and paraneoplastic neurologic syndromes (dermatomyositis, Eaton-Lambert syndrome, myopathies, and distal neuropathies). Many patients with malignant tumors are given large doses of analgesics and should be kept comfortable during the perioperative period; avoiding drug dependence is of no practical importance in terminally ill patients.[651-653] Marijuana (tetrahydrocannabinol) depresses the CNS vomiting center and may be more effective than the phenothiazines or butyrophenones in suppressing nausea associated with cancer and its therapy; it decreases anesthetic requirements 15 to 30 percent.[654]

The toxicity of cancer chemotherapy relates to the agents used and to the dose. For radiation therapy, damage occurs when the following doses are exceeded: lungs, 1,500 rad; kidneys, 2,400 rad; heart, 3,000 rad; spinal cord, 4,000 rad; intestine, 5,500 rad; brain, 6,000

rad; and bone, 7,500 rad. The toxicities of biologic therapy and immunomodulating therapies relate to the change in immune function they cause.[409] Alkylating agents cause bone marrow depression, including thrombocytopenia, alopecia, hemorrhagic cystitis, nausea, and vomiting. The alkylating agents including cyclophosphamide and mechlorethamine can act as anticholinesterase and prolong neuromuscular blockade.[655] The antineoplastic alkaloids vincristine and vinblastine produce, respectively, peripheral neuropathies and SIADH, and myelotoxicity. Cisplatin also produces peripheral neuropathies and severe nausea. Nitrosoureas can cause severe hepatic and renal damage, as well as bone marrow toxicity, myalgias, and paresthesia. Folic acid analogues such as methotrexate (MTX) produce bone marrow depression, ulcerative stomatitis, pulmonary interstitial infiltrates, GI toxicity, and occasionally severe liver dysfunction. Fluorouracil (5-FU) and floxuridine (FUDR), both pyrimidine analogues, cause bone marrow toxicity, megaloblastic anemia, nervous system dysfunction, and hepatic and GI alterations. Purine analogues (mercaptopurine, thioguanine) have bone marrow depression as their primary toxic effect. Anthracycline antibiotics (doxorubicin, daunorubicin, mithramycin, mitomycin C, bleomycin) can all cause pulmonary infiltrates, cardiomyopathies (especially doxorubicin and daunorubicin), myelotoxicity, and GI, hepatic, and renal disturbances.

The wisdom of anesthetizing patients given bleomycin has been questioned. A retrospective study by Goldiner et al.[656] reported postoperative deaths in five consecutive patients given bleomycin. All five patients died of postoperative respiratory failure. Using the same anesthetic technique, Goldiner et al.[656] then anesthetized 12 patients, limited the inspired oxygen concentration to 22 to 25 percent perioperatively, and replaced much of the blood loss with colloids rather than crystalloids. None of the 12 patients died. These investigators postulated that bleomycin caused epithelial cell edema that progressed to necrosis of type I alveolar cells, fluid leakage into the alveolar space, and formation of "hyaline membranes" similar to that occurring in oxygen toxicity.[658] Goldiner et al. believe that this pathophysiologic similarity indicates a possible synergistic relationship between oxygen and bleomycin. However, LaMantia and coworkers[657] retrospectively analyzed charts of 16 patients undergoing surgery after bleomycin therapy. Thirteen patients were given oxygen at inspired concentrations of 37 to 45 percent. No instances of postoperative respiratory failure occurred. Thus, data are currently available to support all practices regarding oxygen administration to patients given bleomycin. My preference is to keep inspired oxygen concentrations at the lowest level providing adequate tissue oxygenation. When in doubt about side effects in patients undergoing cancer chemotherapy, my practice is to seek advice from two experts.

PATIENTS GIVEN DRUG THERAPY FOR CHRONIC AND ACUTE MEDICAL CONDITIONS

A steadily increasing number of potent drugs are being used to treat disease; the average hospitalized patient receives over 10 drugs. Many drugs have side effects that might make anesthesia more risky or patient management more difficult. Knowing the pharmacologic properties and potential side effects of commonly used drugs helps the anesthesiologist avoid pitfalls during anesthesia and surgery. The first step in avoiding such pitfalls is to obtain a drug history from the patient. Then, for every drug, medicine, and over-the-counter preparation the patient is using, the anesthesiologist should know the name, classification of drug, diseases and conditions for which it is prescribed, and common side effects. Having such knowledge before surgery helps one to avoid making mistakes that can turn minor side effects into life-threatening situations. If necessary, the anesthesiologist should return to the patient's bedside to search for signs or symptoms of these effects. Unnecessary drugs should be discontinued for at least three, and preferably five, half-lives of the drugs. This period should be longer if metabolites of the drug have activity and longer half-lives. For needed or beneficial drugs, the optimal dose should be determined in consultation with the treating physician; the optimal dose is that which maximizes the ratio of therapeutic value to risk of drug toxicity. Drug side effects should be sought and either corrected preoperatively or at least planned for in anesthetic management. For instance, if a patient is made hypokalemic with diuretic drugs, hypokalemia might be corrected before surgery or, perhaps even better, hyperventilation could be avoided during surgery (see earlier section on hypokalemia). This type of reasoning and planning is best done at least 1 week before surgery. Ideally, the surgeon, internist, and anesthesiologist should communicate regarding these topics well in advance of surgery. Understanding the side effects of chronic drug therapy that affect the sympathetic nervous system requires some knowledge of basic pharmacologic characteristics of the sympathetic nervous system.[659,660]

Pharmacologic Processes in the Sympathetic Nervous System

The autonomic nervous system is discussed in detail in Chapter 14. A sympathetic neuron consists of a cell body and its nucleus, a long axon, and many nerve terminals. Enzymes responsible for synthesizing dopamine, norepinephrine, and epinephrine are made in the cell body, transported by a tube system (rapid axoplasmic transport) down the axon to the terminal where the neurotransmitters are made, and then stored in granules (Fig. 25-11). The sympathetic neuron makes neurotransmitters from either phenylalanine or tyrosine. Tyrosine hydroxylase, the rate-limiting enzyme, aids in converting tyrosine to dopa, which is decarboxylated by 1-aromatic acid decarboxylase to dopamine. Dopamine is taken up into granules, where it remains in that form or is converted by dopamine-α-hydroxylase to norepinephrine. The granules are little packets of neurotransmitters whose contents are released when an action potential reaches the nerve endings. In some nerve endings (and in the adrenal medulla), norepinephrine leaves the granules, is methylated in the cytoplasm to epinephrine, and then reenters a different group of intracellular granules.

Norepinephrine, dopamine, and epinephrine exert their physiologic effect by interacting with an appropriate receptor at the target tissue. The primary receptor acts through intermediary messenger systems (includ-

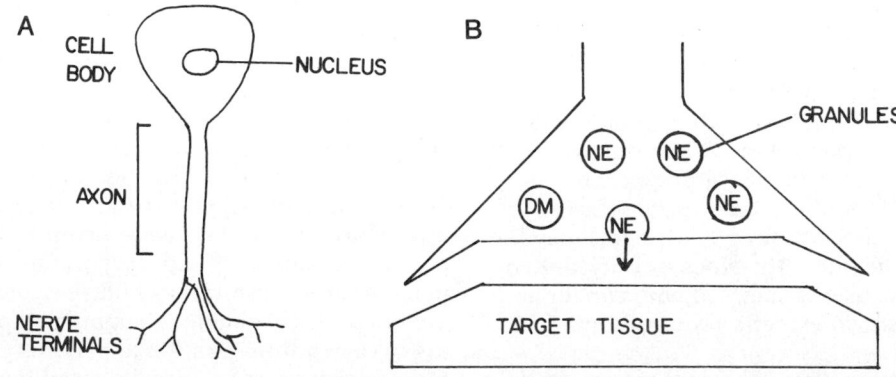

Fig. 25-11. A sympathetic neuron consists of **(A)** a cell body and its nucleus, a long axon, and **(B)** multiple nerve terminals (shown enlarged). Enzymes responsible for the synthesis of dopamine (DM), norepinephrine (NE), and epinephrine are made in the cell body, transported by a tube system (rapid axoplasmic transport) down the axes to the terminal where the transmitters are made, and stored in granules. (Modified from Axelrod,[767] with permission.)

ing cyclic-AMP and/or G-stimulatory or G-inhibitory proteins) and/or can change conformation (and thus affinity for ligands) of bordering or neighboring receptors. These bordering or neighboring receptor effects may account for many of the multitude of effects associated with catecholamines. The three major kinds of catecholamine receptors are α-adrenergic, β-adrenergic, and dopaminergic. These receptors are subdivided as follows:

α_1: stimulation constricts vascular smooth muscle and thus increases peripheral vascular resistance.

α_2: stimulation inhibits the release of norepinephrine itself (constituting negative feedback to the sympathetic neuron). These are largely presynaptic, although postsynaptic vasoconstricting α_2 receptors exist on blood vessels.

β_1: stimulation increases heart rate and the strength of cardiac contractions.

β_2: stimulation causes dilation of smooth muscles of the blood vessels and airway, relaxation of uterine smooth muscle, and a variety of endocrine effects, including secretion of renin.

β_3: stimulation results in a greater release of norepinephrine from the sympathetic neuron (constituting positive feedback to the sympathetic neuron).

Dopamine-1: stimulation causes dilation of vascular smooth muscle, notably of renal and mesenteric blood vessels.

Dopamine-2: stimulation inhibits release of norepinephrine (presynaptic) and may also inhibit, via its ganglionic actions, the ·release of acetylcholine. The class of dopamine receptors involved in locomotion, inhibiting intestinal motility (the antagonism of which

accounts for the increase in gastric emptying by metoclopramide), and vomiting is not yet clear. These different effects may be caused by slight differences in receptor conformations.

The action of sympathomimetic substances is terminated through an unusual process: the nerve ending recaptures most norepinephrine from the target tissue using an active reuptake system (Fig. 25-12). Obviously, blockage of this system permits more norepinephrine to remain free to cause physiologic effects. In addition to this reuptake system, two enzymes transform catecholamines metabolically: monoamine oxidase (MAO) and catechol-*o*-methyltransferase (COMT) (Fig. 25-12).

Antihypertensive Drugs

Many antihypertensive agents and almost all mind-altering drugs affect sympathetic neuronal storage, uptake, metabolism, or release of neurotransmitters. For instance, the antihypertensive drug reserpine depletes the granules of norepinephrine, epinephrine, and dopamine in both the brain stem and the periphery. The depletion of transmitters in sympathetic nerve endings renders drugs such as ephedrine and metaraminol ineffective, since such drugs act primarily by releasing catecholamines (Fig. 25-13). Guanethidine depletes granular norepinephrine and affects only the peripheral sympathetic system. In amounts used clinically, reserpine decreases MAC 20 to 30 percent, whereas guanethidine has no effect on anesthetic requirements.[180] In addition to causing a lack of response to indirectly acting vasopressors, reserpine may cause a denervation

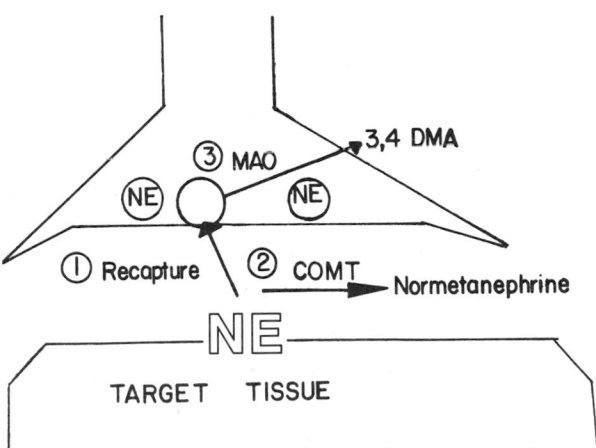

Fig. 25-12. The action of norepinephrine (NE) is terminated primarily through recapture of norepinephrine from the target tissue (i.e., recycling of NE back into the granules of the nerve terminal). The action of NE can also be terminated by metabolism of NE by catechol-*o*-methyltransferase (COMT) and/or monoamine oxidase (MAO).

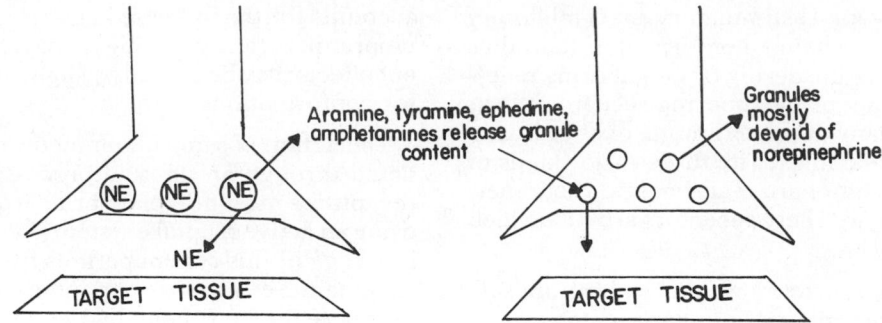

Fig. 25-13. Antihypotensive drugs such as metaraminol (Aramine), tyramine, and ephedrine release catecholamines from the granules of the nerve terminal. Therefore, if little norepinephrine (NE) is left within the granules (as after treatment with methyldopa, reserpine, or guanethidine), little norepinephrine is released.

supersensitivity and hyperresponsiveness (with hypertension and/or tachycardia) to the usual doses of direct-acting sympathetic amines, such as phenylephrine (Neo-Synephrine), isoproterenol, norepinephrine, epinephrine, and dopamine.[659-662] Thus, in patients who have been treated with drugs that alter sympathetic neurotransmitter release, uptake, metabolism, or receptor function, some problems may occur: hypotension, hypertension, and/or bradycardia should be treated by titrating doses of direct-acting vasoconstrictors, such as phenylephrine (Neo-Synephrine); vasodilators, such as nitroprusside; or chronotropic drugs, such as atropine, isoproterenol, or dopamine.

Another group of antihypertensive agents are the "false neurotransmitters." False neurotransmitters replace norepinephrine in the granules at the nerve ending. α-Methyldopa (Aldomet) becomes α-methyldopamine, which is further metabolized to α-methyl-norepinephrine (Fig. 25-14). In some nerve endings and for some receptors, α-methyldopamine or α-methylnorepinephrine is more potent than dopamine or norepinephrine as dopaminergic or α-adrenergic receptor stimulants. However, at most nerve endings, the false neurotransmitters are less potent stimulants, and this lesser degree of stimulation is one means by which their antihypertensive action is produced. Alternately, α-methyldopa may act by stimulating the brain stem sympathetic nervous system. When this system antagonizes the peripheral sympathetic nervous system, the activity of the latter decreases and blood pressure is reduced. Through its central effect, α-methyldopa decreases anesthetic requirements 20 to 40 percent.[180]

In addition to altering the response to exogenously administered vasopressors, these neurotransmitter-depleting drugs can also produce side effects: psychic depression, nightmares, drowsiness, nasal stuffiness, diar-

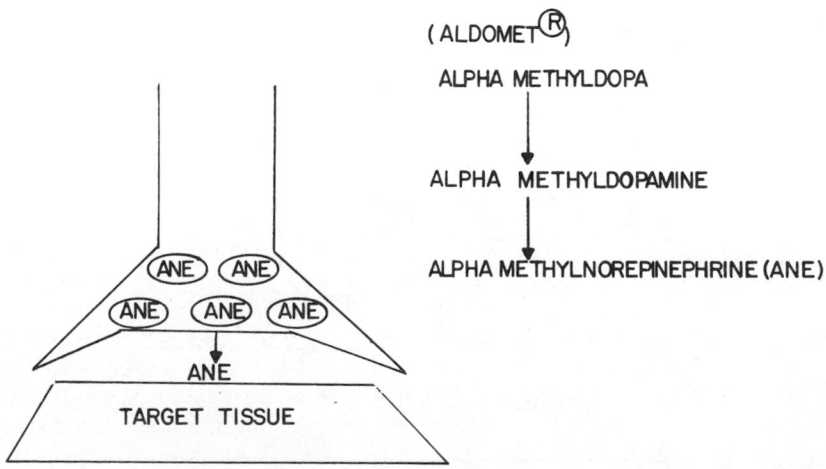

Fig. 25-14. In the granules of the nerve terminal, α-methyldopa (Aldomet) is converted enzymatically to α-methyldopamine by the same enzyme that converts dopa to dopamine. α-Methyldopamine is converted to α-methylnorepinephrine by the same enzyme that converts dopamine to norepinephrine.

rhea, bradycardia, and orthostatic hypotension with impotence (reserpine). Guanethidine can cause orthostatic hypotension, bradycardia, asthma, diarrhea, and inhibition of ejaculation. α-Methyldopa is associated with drowsiness, orthostatic hypotension, bradycardia, diarrhea, acute or chronic hepatitis, cirrhosis, and autoimmune hemolytic anemia (i.e., positive Coombs' test result).[662] Because of these side effects, angiotensin-converting enzyme inhibitors (captopril, enalapril, lisinopril, enalaprilat) are being used more and more as first line drugs and appear to improve the antihypertensive patient's quality of life.[200] They may be associated with more peripheral vasodilation and hypotension on induction of anesthesia than are sympatholytics, however.[663]

Catecholamine or sympathetic receptor blocking drugs affect the three major types of catecholamine receptors: α-adrenergic, β-adrenergic, and dopaminergic. The existence of subdivisions (e.g., β_1, β_2) suggested the possibility that some drugs would be found to affect only one set of receptors. For example, terbutaline is used more frequently than isoproterenol because terbutaline is said to exert a preferential effect on β_2-receptors (i.e., to dilate bronchial smooth muscle), thereby avoiding the cardiac stimulation produced by drugs that stimulate β_1-receptors. In fact, selectivity is dose related. At a certain dose, a direct β_2-receptor stimulating drug will affect only those receptors, but at a higher dose will stimulate both β_1- and β_2-receptors. The effect of a given dose varies with each patient. A certain dose may stimulate β_1- and β_2-receptors in one patient but neither receptor in another patient. More and more selective blocking drugs are being developed in hopes of widening the margin between β_1- and β_2- and α-adrenergic effects. However, ultimately, more selectivity is desired than even this. It would be advantageous to be able to decrease heart rate without changing myocardial contractility, or to increase contractility without changing heart rate. Such is the goal of much drug research and of the development of dobutamine (see Chs. 14 and 16). However, to date, all such selectivity appears to be dose related, even for dobutamine.[664]

Metoprolol (Lopressor) and atenolol (Tenormin) (both β_1-adrenergic receptor blocking drugs) and propranolol, timolol, esmolol, pindolol, oxprenolol, acebutolol, carteolol, penbutolol, and nadolol are the only widely available β-adrenergic receptor blocking drugs used for chronic therapy in the United States. Because nadolol has poor lipid solubility, it has a long elimination half-life (17 to 24 hours) and does not cross the blood-brain barrier readily. Although nadolol should be associated with fewer CNS side effects such as fatigue, nightmares, and depression, we do not know that definitely yet. The ability to use it on a once daily basis should increase patient compliance. Although selective β-adrenergic receptor blocking drugs should be more appropriate in patients with increased airway resistance or diabetes, this advantage is apparent only when low doses are used. The use of β-adrenergic receptor blocking drugs has become widespread, as these drugs treat everything from angina and hypertension to priapism and stage fright. They appear to decrease morbidity and mortality in patients who have initially survived myocardial infarction,[139,140,665-667] and may be useful in decreasing the incidence of myocardial ischemia preoperatively,[132,140,665-667] especially when anesthesia is delivered in such a way as to foster tachycardia were the β-adrenergic receptor blocking drug not present.[132]

At present, propranolol is the standard for β-adrenergic receptor blocking drugs. Smulyan et al.[668] studied the problems of adult patients on long-term propranolol hydrochloride therapy who must undergo abdominal surgery. Because such patients cannot take oral medications postoperatively for many days, they must be protected against perioperative sympathetic stimulation and the propranolol withdrawal syndrome. A continuous intravenous infusion of propranolol (3 mg/h, regardless of the patient's weight) given postoperatively accomplished these goals: postoperative serum propranolol levels and β-adrenergic receptor blockade returned to their "usual" preoperative levels. The hypotensive and bradycardic effects of propranolol and general anesthesia appear to be additive.[669] Esmolol, because of its shorter half-life (3 to 10 minutes) is quickly replacing propranolol in critical care (including anesthesia) settings, as errors in therapy or side effects, such as increased airway resistance, vanish much more quickly than were propranolol administered.[670] Propranolol does not affect anesthetic requirements,[671] and one would expect the same lack of effect from other "pure" β-adrenergic receptor blocking drugs.

α-Adrenergic-receptor blocking drugs include phentolamine, prazosin, phenoxybenzamine, the phenothiazines, and the butyrophenones (such as droperidol). Dopaminergic receptor antagonists include the antischizophrenic medicines (phenothiazines and butyrophenones) and metoclopramide. The receptor-blocking drugs inhibit the action of sympathomimetic drugs at the receptor in a dose-related fashion. Thus, propranolol lowers blood pressure by blocking the tendency of norepinephrine and epinephrine to increase the rate and force of the contractions of the heart (and perhaps also their tendency to increase the secretion of renin). To overcome this blockade, one need only provide more β-receptor stimulating drug. Thus, high doses of vasopressors may be needed to increase blood pressure in a patient given large doses of propranolol.

When administration of β-adrenergic receptor blocking drugs is terminated, sympathetic stimulation often increases, as if the body had responded to the presence of these drugs by increasing sympathetic neuron activity. Thus, propranolol withdrawal can be accompanied by a hyper-β-adrenergic condition that increases myocardial oxygen demands. Administering propranolol or metoprolol can cause bradycardia, CHF, fatigue, dizziness, depression, psychoses, bronchospasm, and Peyronie's disease.[662] Side effects of the dopaminergic receptor blocking drugs are discussed later in this chapter.

Prazosin (Minipress) is an α_1-adrenergic receptor blocking drug used to treat both hypertension and ischemic cardiomyopathy because it dilates both veins and arteries. It is associated with vertigo, palpitations, depression, dizziness, weakness, and anticholinergic effects.

Brain stem sympathomimetic drugs stimulate α-adrenergic receptors in the brain stem. Clonidine (Catapres), a drug with a half-life of 12 to 24 hours, is an α_2-adrenergic receptor stimulant. Presumably, α_2-adrenergic agonists including clonidine, guanabenz, and guanfacine (Tenex) lower blood pressure through the central brain stem adrenergic stimulation referred to previously. They may also be used to treat opiate, cocaine, food, and tobacco withdrawal. Occasionally, withdrawal from clonidine can precipitate a sudden hypertensive crisis, analogous to that occurring on withdrawal from propranolol, causing a hyper-β-adrenergic condition. The degree of hypertensive crisis following clonidine withdrawal is now being debated. (Although intravenous clonidine is not available in the United States, a skin patch of clonidine is approved.) Tricyclic antidepressant drugs, and presumably phenothiazines and the butyrophenones, interfere with the action of clonidine. Although administering a butyrophenone (e.g., droperidol) to a patient given clonidine chronically could theoretically precipitate a hypertensive crisis, none has been reported. Clonidine administration can be accompanied by drowsiness, dry mouth, orthostatic hypotension, bradycardia, and impotence. In dogs, acute clonidine administration decreases anesthetic requirements by 40 to 60 percent; chronic administration decreases requirements by 10 to 20 percent.[133,134,672,673] Because of the relative safety of these drugs, and their ability to decrease anesthetic requirements, block narcotic-induced muscle rigidity, and provide pain relief, their popularity preoperatively is increasing.[133,134,672-674]

Three other classes of antihypertensive drugs affect the sympathetic nervous system indirectly: diuretic drugs, arteriolar dilators, and slow (calcium) channel-blocking agents. Thiazide diuretic drugs are associated with hypochloremic alkalosis, hypokalemia, hyperglycemia, hyperuricemia, and hypercalcemia. The potassium-sparing diuretic drug spironolactone is associated with hyperkalemia, hyponatremia, gynecomastia, and impotence. All diuretic drugs can cause dehydration. The thiazide diuretics and furosemide appear to prolong neuromuscular blockade.[675] The arteriolar dilator hydralazine can cause a lupuslike condition (usually with renal involvement), nasal congestion, headache, dizziness, congestive heart failure, angina, and GI disturbances.

The slow-channel calcium ion antagonists (also called calcium channel-blocking drugs) inhibit the transmembrane influx of calcium ions into cardiac and vascular smooth muscle. Such inhibition reduces heart rate (negative chronotropy), depresses contractility (negative inotropy), decreases conduction velocity (negative dromotropy), and dilates coronary, cerebral, and systemic arterioles (Fig. 25-15).[676] Verapamil, diltiazem, and nifedipine all produce such effects, but to varying degrees, and apparently by similar but different mechanisms.[677] Nifedipine is the most potent of the three as a smooth muscle dilator, while verapamil and diltiazem have negative dromotropic and inotropic effects, and vasodilating properties. Diltiazem has weak vasodilating properties as compared with nifedipine and has less atrioventricular conduction effect than does verapamil. Thus, verapamil and diltiazem can increase the PR interval and produce atrioventricular block. In fact, reflex activation of the sympathetic nervous system may be necessary during administration of diltiazem, and especially during verapamil therapy, to maintain normal conduction. Clearly, verapamil and diltiazem must be titrated very carefully when a patient is already taking a β-adrenergic receptor blocking drug,[678] or when adding β-blocking drugs to the patient already taking verapamil or diltiazem.

The use of calcium channel blocking drugs has several important implications for anesthetic management.[676,679-695] First, the effects of inhalational and narcotic anesthetic agents and of nifedipine in decreasing systemic vascular resistance, blood pressure, and contractility may be additive.[676,680-684] Similarly, verapamil and anesthetics (inhalational anesthetics, nitrous oxide, and narcotics) increase atrioventricular conduction times and additively decrease blood pressure, systemic vascular resistance, and contractility.[682-684,692,695] Second, verapamil, and presumably the other calcium channel blocking drugs, have been found to decrease anesthetic requirements by 25 percent.[679] These agents can produce neuromuscular blockade; potentiate both depolarizing and nondepolarizing neuromuscular blocking drugs; and, in at least one type of myopathy (Duchenne's muscular dystrophy), can even precipitate respiratory failure.[687,688,693] Finally, since slow-channel activation of calcium is necessary to cause spasms of cerebral and coronary vessels, bronchoconstriction, and normal platelet aggregation, these drugs may have a role in treating ischemia of the nervous system, bronchoconstriction, and unwanted clotting disorders perioperatively.[685,687,689,690] All three drugs are highly protein bound and may displace or be displaced by other drugs that are also highly protein bound (e.g., lidocaine, bupivacaine, diazepam, disopyramide, and propranolol).[690] Adverse consequences can be minimized by titrating inhalational or narcotic agent to hemodynamic and anesthetic effects. By monitoring for side effects, the anesthetist can prevent side effects from becoming serious (S. Slogoff and co-workers, personal communication). Hemodynamic, but not electrophysiologic, changes usually can be reversed by ad-

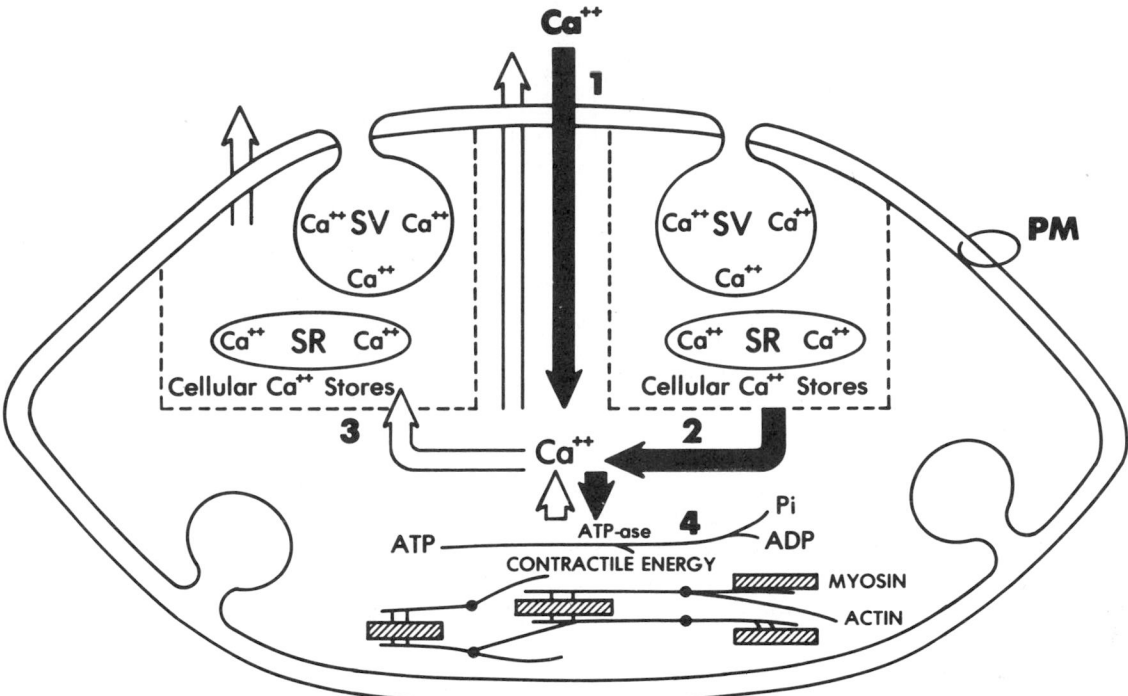

Fig. 25-15. Schematic drawing of smooth muscle cell showing calcium flux and possible sites of interference by halothane and nifedipine. The concentration of calcium (Ca^{++}) in the cytoplasm increases (black arrows) because of entry through the plasma membrane (PM) and release from surface vesicles (SV) or the sarcoplasmic reticulum (SR). When the concentration of cytoplasmic Ca^{++} is sufficiently high, ATP is activated. The splitting of ATP by ATPase provides the interaction and contraction of actin filaments and myosin particles constituting muscle fibers. The concentration of cytoplasmic Ca^{++} decreases (white arrows) with the return of Ca^{++} to cellular stores and the extracellular transport of Ca^{++}. Both halothane and nifedipine probably (1) inhibit the entry of Ca^{++} and (2) may also interfere with cytoplasmic Ca^{++} flux by reducing the release of Ca^{++} by the SR, by (3) reducing storage and reuptake, or by (4) blocking ATPase and/or the contractile mechanism. (From Tosone et al.,[676] with permission.)

ministering calcium.[694] Reversal of electrophysiologic effects may occur if industrial doses of β-adrenergic agonists are given.

Mood-Altering Drugs

Mood-altering drugs are the most frequently prescribed medications in the United States. They include MAO inhibitors (Fig. 25-12), phenothiazines, tricyclic antidepressant drugs, and drugs of abuse such as cocaine.

Monoamine oxidase inhibitors (MAOIs)— isocarboxazid (Marplan), phenelzine (Nardil), pargyline (Eutonyl), tranylcypromine (Parnate), and deprenyl—irreversibly bind to the enzyme MAO and thereby increase intraneuronal levels of amine neurotransmitters (serotonin, norepinephrine, dopamine, epinephrine, octopamine). This increase is associated with an antidepressant effect, an antihypertensive effect, an antinarcoleptic effect, liver enzyme elevation, and in delaying the onset of Parkinson's disease (deprenyl).[623] Since there are two forms of the enzyme

(MAO-A and MAO-B) that are selective in vitro for substrate (MAO-A is selective for serotonin, dopamine, and norepinephrine; MAO-B for tyramine and phenylethylamine), presumably MAOIs that are selective for MAO-A or MAO-B would have different effects.[696] Such is not known for sure, as deprenyl (selegiline, Eldepryl), an MAOI-B selective drug, improves a dopamine deficiency state, parkinsonism.[423] Interactions between MAO inhibitors and a variety of foods and drugs containing indirectly acting sympathomimetic substances such as ephedrine or tyramine (found especially in the aged cheeses) can occur for as long as 2 weeks after the last dose of MAO inhibitor is given. The most serious effects of this interaction are convulsions, and hyperpyrexic coma (especially after narcotics). Anesthetic management for a patient given an MAO inhibitor can be chaotic: for this reason it is widely accepted practice to discontinue MAO inhibitors at least 2 to 3 weeks before any planned operation.[697-702] An alternate point of view has recently been expressed regarding severely psychotic patients or emergency surgery.[696,703] Clearly, the risk of discontinuing MAOIs must be weighed against the risk of suicidal tendencies in some patients deprived of MAOIs. There are no reported experiences of interactions between narcotics and deprenyl, so judgments about possible worsening of Parkinson's disease and continuing MAOIs have no basis in data. It should be noted that severe reactions have occurred when too short an interval existed between administration of MAOIs and tricyclic antidepressants.[702] Emergency surgery on patients given MAO inhibitors can be punctuated by hemodynamic instability. Regional block can be attempted as treatment for postoperative pain to avoid having to give narcotics. Case reports of hyperpyrexic coma following administration of most narcotics exist in humans, and animal studies document a 10 to 50 percent incidence of hyperpyrexic coma in animals that were pretreated with MAO inhibitors and then given a variety of narcotics.[425,697-702] These reactions appear to be treated best using therapy supporting vital functions.

Alternate drugs for the treatment of severe depression include the tricyclic antidepressant drugs: amitriptyline (Elavil, Endep), imipramine (Imavate, Tofranil, Presamine), despiramine (Norpramine), doxepin (Adapin, Sinequan), and nortriptyline (Aventyl).[702] Tricyclic antidepressant drugs block the reuptake of neurotransmitters and cause their acute release. If given chronically, these drugs decrease noradrenergic catecholamine stores. Tricyclic antidepressant drugs also produce side effects similar to those produced by atropine (dry mouth, tachycardia, delirium, urinary retention) and can cause ECG changes (changes in T wave, prolongation of the QRS complex, bundle branch block or other conduction abnormalities, or premature ventricular contractions). Although arrhythmias induced by tricyclic antidepressants have been treated successfully with physostigmine, bradycardia has sometimes occurred.[702] Drug interactions with tricyclic antidepressants include those related to the blockade of the reuptake of norepinephrine (such as interference with the action of guanethidine) and fatal dysrhythmias after halothane and pancuronium.[704-707] Such interactions, although predictable for a population of patients, may not alter an individual's threshold for arrhythmias.

The effectiveness of phenothiazines and butyrophenones in schizophrenia suggests a dopamine-receptor blocking action. In addition, these drugs possess varying degrees of parasympathetic stimulation and ability to block α-adrenergic receptors. The phenothiazines include chlorpromazine (Thorazine, Chlor-PZ), promazine (Sparine), trifluompromazine (Vesprin), fluphenazine (Prolixin), trifluoperazine, prochlorperazine (Compazine), and many others. The butyrophenones include droperidol and haloperidol (Haldol). Both phenothiazines and butyrophenones produce sedation, depression, and antihistaminic, antiemetic, and hypothermic responses. They are also associated with cholestatic jaundice, impotence, dystonia, and photo-

sensitivity. Other side effects associated with phenothiazines include orthostatic hypotension (partly due to α-adrenergic blockade) and ECG abnormalities, such as prolongation of the QT or PR intervals, blunting of T waves, depression of the ST segment, and on rare occasion, premature ventricular contractions and torsades du pointes.[702,706,707]

Several important drug interactions are noteworthy for the phenothiazine derivatives. The effects of CNS depressants (especially narcotics and barbiturates) are enhanced by concomitant administration of phenothiazines. Also, CNS seizure threshold is lowered by administration of phenothiazines which should be avoided in patients who are epileptic or withdrawing from any drug that depresses the CNS. The antihypertensive effects of guanethidine are blocked by tricyclic antidepressant drugs and phenothiazines.[662] Lithium carbonate is used to treat manic depression; it is more effective in preventing mania than in relieving depression. In excitable cells, lithium mimics sodium, decreasing the release of neurotransmitters both centrally and peripherally. Lithium prolongs neuromuscular blockade[708,709] and may decrease anesthetic requirements because it blocks brain stem release of norepinephrine, epinephrine, and dopamine.

Psychoactive drugs such as amphetamines (including methamphetamines and their smokable derivative in crystal form, known as "ice"), and cocaine acutely release norepinephrine, epinephrine, and dopamine and block their reuptake. When taken chronically, they deplete the nerve endings of these neurotransmitters.

Drugs that appear to increase central α-adrenergic release increase anesthetic requirement, whereas drugs that appear to decrease central α-adrenergic release decrease anesthetic requirements. (This may not be the mechanism by which they alter anesthetic requirement, but it is a convenient way of remembering the alteration.) Drugs that affect only the β-adrenergic receptors do not alter anesthetic requirements.[133,134,180,671-673,710,711]

Sympathomimetic Drugs
(Also See Ch. 14)

Many antiasthmatic drugs (bronchodilators) such as terbutaline, aminophylline, and theophylline are sympathomimetic drugs that can interact with the volatile anesthetics to cause cardiac arrhythmias. Halothane (and to some degree most other volatile anesthetics) sensitizes the myocardium to exogenous catecholamines.[712-715] Sensitization means that the minimum dose of exogenous epinephrine administered intravenously needed to produce premature ventricular contractions would be lower in individuals anesthetized with halothane than in awake individuals.

How much epinephrine is safe to give when halothane is the anesthetic? Katz and Bigger[712] reported that administering 0.15 ml/kg of a 1/100,000 epinephrine solution per 10-minute period (not to exceed 0.45

ml/kg of a 1/100,000 solution/h) was safe. Several studies have shown that lidocaine given with epinephrine affords extra protection, and that enflurane and isoflurane are less sensitizing than halothane.[713-715] Since halothane is a potent bronchodilator,[716] it may be the best choice for anesthetizing patients with asthma.[717] However, this may not be the case; many asthmatic patients are already taking exogenous catecholamines such as xanthines as chronic bronchodilator therapy.

Xanthines are effective bronchodilators because they produce β-adrenergic stimulation in two ways: they cause release of norepinephrine[718,719] and also inhibit the breakdown of adenosine 3',5'-cyclic monophosphate (cyclic AMP),[720] the mediator of many of the actions of β-adrenergic receptor agonists.[345] Phosphodiesterase catalyzes the breakdown of cyclic AMP. Thus, inhibition of phosphodiesterase by theophylline increases the concentration of cyclic AMP. Marcus et al.[718] and Westfall and Fleming[719] showed that at least 40 percent of the inotropic effects of aminophylline are due to its ability to release norepinephrine directly. Infusion of aminophylline also increases excretion of catecholamines in urine.[721] Experimentally, aminophylline decreases the threshold for ventricular fibrillation.[722]

Plasma theophylline levels of 5 mg/L are needed to reduce abnormally high airway resistance. No further beneficial effects are obtained when levels exceed 20 mg/L, and, instead, toxic effects appear.[723,724] Theophylline (aminophylline is a combination of 85 percent theophylline and 15 percent ethylenediamine) is metabolized largely by the liver, less than 10 percent being excreted unchanged in the urine. The average half-life is 4.4 ± 1.15 hours in adults, and clearance is 1.2 ml/min/kg.[723,724] Significant liver disease or pulmonary edema can decrease clearance of the drug by one-half and by one-third, respectively.[725] Cigarette smokers clear aminophylline more rapidly than nonsmokers.[726]

An interaction between aminophylline and halothane appears to be a predictable, frequent occurrence: of 16 dogs anesthetized with 1 percent halothane and given high-dose bolus injections of aminophylline, 12 had ventricular arrhythmias and 8 had ventricular tachycardia or fibrillation.[727-729] Thus, it is advisable to wait three drug half-lives after the last dose of aminophylline is given (i.e., approximately 13 hours in normal individuals) before using halothane to anesthetize an asthmatic patient. Using another anesthetic that is a bronchodilator[716] but less likely to predispose the patient to catecholamine-induced arrhythmias[713-715] (such as enflurane or isoflurane) might be an alternative in patients who must be given aminophylline or other exogenous sympathomimetic drugs before or during surgery.[730]

Other Drugs

Drugs other than those discussed earlier in this chapter have implications for anesthetic management. These discussed therapies include anticoagulants and fibrinolytics (in hematologic section), endocrinologic preparations excluding birth control pills but including corticosteroids (in the section on endocrinologic disease), antihypertensives (earlier in this section and in cardiovascular diseases), anticonvulsants (in the section on neurologic disorders), and cancer chemotherapeutic agents (in the section on oncology).

Antiarrhythmic Drugs

Antiarrhythmic drugs include local anesthetics (lidocaine, procaine), anticonvulsant (phenytoin) or antihypertensive (propranolol) drugs, calcium channel blocking agents, or primary antiarrhythmic drugs. These drugs are classified into five major categories: local anesthetics that alter phase 0 and phase 4 depolarization (quinidine, procainamide, and flecainide); local anesthetics that affect only phase 4 depolarization (lidocaine, tocainide, phenytoin, encainide); β-adrenergic receptor antagonists; antiadrenergic drugs (bretylium, disopyramide, amiodarone); and calcium entry blockers. These drugs are discussed elsewhere in this chapter or in Chapter 14. A useful reference with suggestions about drug therapy for cardiac arrhythmias and monitoring of side effects was published by the *Medical Letter on Drugs and Therapeutics*.[731] Lack of adverse reports does not indicate that all these drugs should be continued through the time of surgery; pharmacokinetic studies have not yet determined whether anesthesia (or anesthesia with specific agents) alters the volume of distribution or clearance of these drugs to an extent sufficient to warrant changing the dosage or dosage schedule in the perioperative period. The dearth of reports on this subject may be due to a lack of significant drug interaction or to a lack of awareness that untoward events could be due to such an interaction.

The pharmacologic characteristics of the various antiarrhythmic drugs can affect anesthetic management. Disopyramide is similar to quinidine and procainamide in its antiarrhythmic effectiveness. Disopyramide is mainly excreted by the kidneys, but hepatic disease increases its half-life. This drug often produces anticholinergic effects including tachycardia, urinary retention, and psychosis. Hepatitis has also been reported to have occurred after its use.[731] Little is known of the interaction of bretylium with anesthetic agents. Because bretylium blocks the release of catecholamines, chronic therapy with this drug has been associated with hypersensitivity to vasopressors.[731] Quinidine is dependent on the kidneys for excretion, can have vagolytic effects that can decrease atrioventricular block, and is associated with blood dyscrasias and GI disturbances.[731] Most of the antiarrhythmic agents enhance a nondepolarizing neuromuscular blockade. Reports confirm this enhancement for quinidine, phenytoin, lidocaine, procainamide, and propranolol.[732-741] Amiodarone, an antiadrenergic drug used to treat recurrent supraventricular and ventricular tachycardias, causes a peripheral neuropathy and has been associated with hypertension, bradyarrhythmias, and a lower cardiac output during anesthesia.[742] It has a half-life of 29 days, and pharmacologic effects persist for over 45 days after its discontinuance.[743] No data document such an effect for depolarizing muscle relaxants.

Antibiotics

Many antibacterial agents are nephrotoxic and/or neurotoxic and many prolong neuromuscular blockade (also see Ch. 12).[735-741] The only antibiotics devoid of neuromuscular effects appear to be penicillin G and the cephalosporins.[740] Most enzyme-inducing drugs do not increase the metabolism of enflurane or isoflurane. However, isoniazid appears to induce the microsomal enzymes responsible for the metabolism of at least enflurane, increasing the possibility of fluorine-associated renal damage after enflurane.[744] Appropriate antibiotic prophylaxis for surgery (see Table 25-17A, B) requires knowledge of the probability of infection for that type of surgical procedure, and, if the incidence of infection warrants it, a drug regimen directed against the most likely infecting organisms.[289]

Digitalis

Digitalis preparations have a limited margin of safety, the risk of toxicity increasing with hypokalemia.[745] Although there is good rationale for administering digoxin prophylactically prior to surgery,[371] I generally avoid doing so because potassium concentrations can fluctuate widely during anesthesia due to fluid shifts, ventilatory acid-base derangements, and adjuvant treatments,[746,747] and because intraoperative arrhythmias caused by digitalis toxicity may be difficult to differentiate from those having other sources. Digitalis intoxication can present with such diverse cardiac arrhythmias as junctional escape rhythm, premature ventricular contractions, ventricular bigeminy or trigeminy, junctional tachycardia, paroxysmal atrial tachycardia with or without block, sinus arrest, sinus exit block, Mobitz type I or II blocks, or ventricular tachycardia.[745] However, anesthetic agents appear to protect against digitalis toxicity, at least in animal studies.[747-750] A titrated cardioversion technique using at first 10, then 20, 30, 40, 50, 75, 100, 150, and 200 joule doses resulted in safe cardioversion in the presence of digitalis and diazepam or midazolam hypnosis.[751] For patients in atrial fibrillation, the ventricular response should guide the choice of dose of digitalis.

Medications for Glaucoma (Also See Ch. 64)

Medications for glaucoma include two organophosphates, echothiophate and isoflurophate. These drugs inhibit serum cholinesterase, which is responsible for hydrolysis and inactivation of succinylcholine and the ester-type local anesthetics such as procaine, chloroprocaine, and tetracaine.[752,753] These ester-type local anesthetics should be avoided in patients treated with eye drops containing organophosphate. Other medications and their side effects related to anesthesia (from the National Registry for Drug-Induced Ocular Side Effects, Oregon Health Sciences University, 3181 SW Sam Jackson Park Road, Portland, Oregon 97201 [503-279-8456]) are listed in Table 25-22.

Magnesium, Cimetidine, and Oral Contraceptives

Magnesium is given to treat eclampsia; it can cause neuromuscular blockade by itself and potentiates neuromuscular blockade by both nondepolarizing and depolarizing muscle relaxants.[754,755] Cimetidine reduces hepatic blood flow and inhibits enzymatic degradation of drugs by the liver. Thus, higher blood levels and prolonged elimination half-lives may result when drugs that are metabolized by the liver (e.g., lidocaine, procaine, some narcotics and propranolol) are given to patients chronically or acutely taking cimetidine.[756,757] The risk of postoperative venous thrombosis increases when oral contraceptives are used preoperatively.[758,759] Whereas some authorities recommend changing from oral contraceptives to topical methods of birth control 2 to 4 weeks before surgery,[760] no controlled study has established whether birth control pills should be stopped before surgery or what the resulting incidence of pregnancy would be. Other authorities recommend preventing venous thromboembolism by using low-dose heparin, guided by a determination of efficacy and cost-effectiveness.[302-304]

Interrupting a Drug Regimen before Surgery

As stated earlier, if a drug is needed for treatment preoperatively, it should be continued through surgery. It often must be specifically requested, as many patients and nurses perceive the NPO status to include a proscription on drugs.[761] The only exceptions to this general rule of not altering preoperative drug therapy might pertain to (1) MAO inhibitors; (2) anticoagulants and fibrinolytics if surgical hemostasis is needed; (3) nicotinic acid; and (4) dosage adjustments for insulin and corticosteroids. These recommendations require that the anesthesiologist be aware of the pharmacologic characteristics, interactions, and anesthetic implications of drugs described earlier in this chapter.[425,760-765]

When in doubt about a disease or a drug, I consult the following textbooks: *Harrison's Principles of Internal Medicine; Anesthesia and Uncommon Diseases: Pathophysiologic and Clinical Correlations; Anesthesia and Co-Existing Disease; To Make the Patient Ready for Anesthesia: Medical Care of the Surgical Patient; Anesthetic Implications of Congenital Anomalies in Children; Pharmacology and Physiology in Anesthetic Practice; Medical Care of the Surgical Patient: A Problem-Oriented Approach to Management;* and *Goodman and Gilman's The Pharmacologic Basis of Therapeutics.* Following this, it is wise to consult two people who are experts

TABLE 25-22. Common Ophthalmologic Agents and Their Anesthetically Important Interactions

Glaucoma: Primary goal is to reduce IOP by—	
Miotics and epinephrine: increase outflow of aqueous humor	
β-Blockade and carbonic anhydrase inhibitors: reduce production of aqueous humor	
Osmotic agents: transiently decrease volume	

Agent (Trade Name)	Toxicities and Specific Treatments
Miotics	
Parasympathomimetics	
Pilocarpine (Adsorbocarpine, Isopto Carpine, Pilocar, Pilocel)	
Carbachol	
Acetylcholinesterase inhibitors	*Tox:* hypersalivation, sweating, N/V, bradycardia, hypotension,
Physostigmine	bronchospasm, CNS effects, coma, respiratory arrest, death
Demecarium	
Isoflurophate (Floropryl)	*Rx:* atropine, pralidoxime (Protopam)
Echothiophate (Echodide, Phospholine)	*Ix:* succinylcholine—prolonged apnea (agents must be D/C'd 4 wks prior)
Epinephrine (Epitrate, Murocoll, Mytrate, Epifrin, Glaucon, Epinal, Eppy)	*Tox:* (rare) tachycardia, PVCs, hypertension, headache, tremors
	Ix: avoid agents that sensitize to catecholamines, e.g., halothane
β-Blockers	
Timolol (Timoptic)	*Tox:* J-blockade with bradycardia, exacerbation of asthma, CNS
Betaxolol (Betopic (?β-1 selective))	depression, lethargy, confusion
Levobunolol (Betagan)	Synergy noted with systemic agents
Carbonic anhydrase inhibitors	
Acetazolamide (Diamox)	*Tox:* Anorexia, GI disturbances, "general miserable feeling," and
Dichlorphenamide (Daranide, Oratrol)	malaise, paresthesias, diuresis, hypokalemia (transient), renal
Ethoxzolamide (Cardrase, Ethamide)	colic and calculi, hyperuricemia, thrombocytopenia, aplastic
Methazolamide (Neptazane)	anemia, acute respiratory failure in patients with COPD
Osmotic agents	
Glycerin (Glyrol, Osmoglyn)	*Tox:* Dehydration, hyperglycemia, nonketotic hyperosmolar coma
Isosorbide (Ismotic)	(rare). Fatalities with mannitol secondary to CHF or intracranial
Urea (Urevert, Ureaphil)	bleed.
Mannitol (Osmitrol)	Urea may cause thrombosis
Intraocular acetylcholine (Miochol)	*Tox:* hypotension, bradycardia
	Rx: atropine

Mydriatics and cycloplegics: Provide pupillary dilatation and paralysis of accommodation—	
Anticholinergics block muscarinic receptors; paralyzing in iris	
α-Adrenergics contract the dilator of the iris	

Agent (Trade Name)	Toxicities and Specific Treatments
Anticholinergics	
Atropine (Atropisol, Bufopto, Isopto Atropine)	*Tox:* dry mouth, flushing, thirst, tachycardia seizure, hyperactivity,
Cyclopentolate, alone (Cyclogyl) or with phenylephrine-homatropine (Cyclomydril)	transient psychosis, rare coma and death
Scopolamine tropicamide (Homatrocel, Isopto Homatropine, Isopto Hyoscine, Murocoll #19, Mydriacyl)	*Rx:* physostigmine
α-Adrenergics	
Phenylephrine (Efricel, Mydfrin, Neo-Synephrine)	*Tox:* tachycardia, HTN, PVCs, MI, agitation
Hydroxyamphetamine (Paredrine)	

Abbreviations: IOP, intraocular pressure; Tox, toxicity; Rx, treatment; Ix, interaction; N/V, nausea and vomiting; D/C'd, discontinued; GI, gastrointestinal; PVCs, premature ventricular contractions; COPD, chronic obstructive pulmonary disease; CHF, congestive heart failure; HTN, hypertension; MI, myocardial ischemia.

about the drug or disease and then to determine who is best able to care for the patient. Should one of these be best qualified, one should then watch that person care for the patient. Remember, few prospective controlled studies have been done to show that any preoperative technique, treatment, or management decreases perioperative risk. However, common sense and foreknowledge of potential pitfalls as well as diligence in avoiding those pitfalls should reduce avoidable perioperative complications.

REFERENCES

1. Hamilton WK: Do let the blood pressure drop and do use myocardial depressants! Anesthesiology 45:273, 1976
2. Medical consultation. p. 22. In Medical Knowledge Self-Assessment Program VIII, Part A, Book 1. American College of Physicians, Philadelphia, 1988.
3. Mundth ED: Cholecystitis and diabetes mellitus. N Engl J Med 267:642, 1962
4. Walsh DB, Eckhauser FE, Ramsburgh SR, et al: Risk asso-

ciated with diabetes mellitus in patients undergoing gallbladder surgery. Surgery 91:254, 1982

5. Fowkes, FGR, Lunn JN, Farrow SC, et al: Epidemiology in anesthesia. III: Mortality risk in patients with coexisting physical disease. Br J Anaesth 54:819, 1982

6. Douglas JS, King SB, Craver JM, et al: Factors influencing risk and benefit of coronary bypass surgery in patients with diabetes mellitus. Chest 80:369, 1981

7. Hjortrup A, Rasmussen BF, and Kehlet H: Morbidity in diabetic and nondiabetic patients after major vascular surgery. Br Med J 287:1107, 1983

8. Ransohoff DF, Miller GL, Forsythe SB, Hermann RE: Outcome of acute cholecystitis in patients with diabetes mellitus. Ann Intern Med 106:829, 1987

9. Kenepp NB, Shelley WC, Gabbe SG, et al: Fetal and neonatal hazards of maternal hydration with 5% dextrose before cesarean section. Lancet 1:1150, 1982

10. Frater RWM, Oka Y, Kadish A, et al: Diabetes and coronary artery surgery. Mt Sinai J Med 49:237, 1982

11. Lanier WL, Stangland KJ, Scheithauer BW, et al: The effects of dextrose infusion and head position on neurologic outcome after complete cerebral ischemia in primates: examination of a model. Anesthesiology 66:39, 1987

12. Zasslow MA, Pearl RG, Shuer LM, et al: Hyperglycemia decreases acute neuronal ischemic changes after middle cerebral artery occlusion in cats. Stroke 20:519, 1989

13. Burgos LG, Ebert TJ, Asiddao C, et al: Increased intraoperative cardiovascular morbidity in diabetes with autonomic neuropathy. Anesthesiology 70:591, 1989

14. Cahill GF, Jr, McDevitt HO: Insulin-dependent diabetes mellitus: the initial lesion. N Engl J Med 304:1454, 1981

15. Yoon J-W, Austin M, Onodera T, et al: Virus-induced diabetes mellitus. N Engl J Med 300:1173, 1979

16. Campbell PJ, Bolli GB, Cryer PE, et al: Pathogenesis of the dawn phenomenon in patients with insulin-dependent diabetes mellitus. N Engl J Med 312:1473, 1985

17. White NH, Waltman SR, Krupin T, et al: Reversal of neuropathic and gastrointestinal complications related to diabetes mellitus in adolescents with improved metabolic control. J Pediatr 99:41, 1981

18. Stern MP, Rosenthal M, Haffner SM: A new concept of impaired glucose tolerance: relation to cardiovascular risk. Atherosclerosis 5:311, 1985

19. Brenner BM: Hemodynamically mediated glomerular injury and the progressive nature of kidney disease. Kidney Int 23:647, 1983

20. Christlieb AR, Warram JH, Królewski AS, et al: Hypertension: the major risk factor in juvenile-onset insulin-dependent diabetics. Diabetes 30: suppl 2, 90, 1981

21. Olson RL, Leichter S, Warram J, et al: Deaths among patients using continuous subcutaneous insulin infusion pumps—United States. MMWR 31:80, 1982

22. Goodson WH, III, Hunt TK: Studies of wound healing in experimental diabetes mellitus. J Surg Res 22:221, 1977

23. Rosen RG, Enquist IF: The healing wound in experimental diabetes. Surgery 50:525, 1961

24. Gottrup F, Andreassen TT: Healing of incisional wounds in stomach and duodenum: the influence of experimental diabetes. J Surg Res 31:61, 1981

25. Bagdade JD: Phagocytic and microbiological function in diabetes mellitus. Acta Endocrinol 83: suppl 205, 27, 1976

26. Nolan CM, Beaty HN, Bagdade JD: Further characterization of the impaired bactericidal function of granulocytes in patients with poorly controlled diabetes. Diabetes 27:889, 1978

27. McMurry JF: Wound healing with diabetes mellitus. Better glucose control for better wound healing in diabetics. Surg Clin North Am 64:769, 1984

28. Cruse PJ, Foord R: A 5-year prospective study of 23,649 surgical wounds. Arch Surg 107:206, 1973

28a. Longstreth WT, Inui TS: High blood glucose level on hospital admission and poor neurological recovery after cardiac arrest. Ann Neurol 15:59, 1984

29. Johnson WD, Pedraza PM, Kayser KL: Coronary artery surgery in diabetics: 261 consecutive patients followed four to seven years. Am Heart J 104:823, 1982

30. Kreisberg RA: Diabetic ketoacidosis: new concepts and trends in pathogenesis and treatment. Ann Intern Med 88:681, 1978

31. Walts LF, Miller J, Davidson MB, et al: Perioperative management of diabetes mellitus. Anesthesiology 55:104, 1981

32. Peterson L, Caldwell J, Hoffman J: Insulin adsorbance to polyvinyl chloride surfaces with implications for constant-infusion therapy. Diabetes 25:72, 1976

33. Meyer EJ, Lorenzi M, Bohannon NV, et al: Diabetic management by insulin infusion during major surgery. Am J Surg 137:323, 1979

34. Farrow SC, Fowkes FGR, Lunn JN, et al: Epidemiology in anaesthesia. II: Factors affecting mortality in hospital. Br J Anaesth 54:811, 1982

35. Galloway JA, Shuman CR: Diabetes and surgery. A study of 667 cases. Am J Med 34:177, 1963

36. Palumbo PJ: Blood glucose control during surgery (editorial). Anesthesiology 55:94, 1981

37. Kannel WB, McGee DL: Diabetes and cardiovascular disease. JAMA 241:2035, 1979

38. Page MM, Watkins PJ: Cardiorespiratory arrest and diabetic autonomic neuropathy. Lancet 1:14, 1978

39. Garcia MJ, McNamara PM, Gordon T, et al: Morbidity and mortality in diabetics in the Framingham population: sixteen year follow-up study. Diabetes 23:105, 1974

40. Heino A: Operative and postoperative nonsurgical complications in diabetic patients undergoing renal transplantation. Scand J Urol Nephrol 22:53, 1988

41. Schreider BD, Uitvlugt A, Roizen MF: Anesthesia for patients with insulinoma and other causes of hypoglycemia. Anesthesiol Clin North Am 5:357, 1987

42. Muir JJ, Endres SM, Offord K, et al: Glucose management in patients undergoing operation for insulinoma removal. Anesthesiology 59:371, 1983

43. Schaefer EJ, Levy RI: Pathogenesis and management of lipoprotein disorders. N Engl J Med 312:1300, 1985

44. Haskell WL, Camargo C, Jr, Williams PT, et al: The effect of cessation and resumption of moderate alcohol intake on serum high-density-lipoprotein subfractions. N Engl J Med 310:805, 1984

45. Andres R: Effect of obesity on total mortality. Int J Obesity 4:381, 1980

46. Fox GS, Whalley DG, Bevan DR: Anaesthesia for the morbidly obese. Experience with 110 patients. Br J Anaesth 53:811, 1983

47. Taylor RR, Kelly TM, Elliott CG, et al: Hypoxemia after gastric bypass surgery for morbid obesity. Arch Surg 120:1298, 1985

48. Vaughan RW, Bauer S, Wise L: Volume and pH of gastric juice in obese patients. Anesthesiology 43:686, 1975

49. Wilson SL, Mantena NR, Halverson JD: Effects of atropine, glycopyrrolate, and cimetidine on gastric secretions in morbidly obese patients. Anesth Analg 60:37, 1981

50. Bentley JB, Vaughan RW, Miller MS, et al: Serum inorganic

fluoride levels in obese patients during and after enflurane anesthesia. Anesth Analg 58:409, 1979

51. Cork RC, Vaughan RW, Bentley JB: General anesthesia for morbidly obese patients—an examination of postoperative outcomes. Anesthesiology 54:310, 1981

52. Pasulka PS, Bistman BR, Benotti PN, Blackburn GL: The risk of surgery in obese patients. Ann Intern Med 104:540, 1986

53. Sours HE, Frattali VP, Brand CD, et al: Sudden death associated with very low calorie weight reduction regimens. Am J Clin Nutr 34:453, 1981

54. Wadden TA, Stunkard AJ, Brownell KD: Very low calorie diets: their efficacy, safety and future. Ann Intern Med 99:675, 1983

55. Balaa MA, Drossman DA: Anorexia nervosa and bulimia: the eating disorders. Dis Month 31:1, 1985

56. Miletich DJ, Albrecht RF, Seals C: Responses to fasting and lipid infusion of epinephrine-induced dysrhythmia during halothane anesthesia. Anesthesiology 48:245, 1987

57. Wharton BA, Howells GR, McCann RA: Cardiac failure in kwashiorkor. Lancet 2:384, 1967

58. Schneider AJL, Biebyck JF: Intraoperative management of patients receiving total parenteral nutrition. Clin Anaesthesiol 1:647, 1983

59. Rombeau JL, Barot LR, Williamson CE, et al: Preoperative total parenteral nutrition and surgical outcome in patients with inflammatory bowel disease. Am J Surg 143:139, 1982

60. Askanazi J, Hensle TW, Starker PM, et al: Effect of immediate postoperative nutritional support on length of hospitalization. Ann Surg 203:236, 1986

61. Starker PM, La Sala PA, Askanazi J, et al: The responses to TPN, a form of nutritional assessment. Ann Surg 198:720, 1983

62. Goldmann DR: The surgical patient on steroids. p. 113. In Goldmann DR, Brown FH, Levy WK, et al (eds): Medical Care of the Surgical Patient: A Problem-Oriented Approach to Management. JB Lippincott, Philadelphia, 1982

63. Smith RJ, Dluhy RG, Williams GH: Endocrinology. p. 115. In Vandam LD (ed): To Make the Patient Ready for Anesthesia: Medical Care of the Surgical Patient. Addison-Wesley, Menlo Park, Calif., 1984

64. Lampe GH, Roizen MF: Anesthesia for patients with abnormal function at the adrenal cortex. Anesthesiol Clin North Am 5:245, 1987

65. Hanowell ST, Hittner KC, Kim YD, et al: Anesthetic management of primary aldosteronism. Anesthesiol Rev 9:36, 1982

66. Rabinowitz IN, Watson W, Farber EM: Topical steroid depression of the hypothalamic-pituitary-adrenal axis in psoriasis vulgaris. Dermatologica 154:321, 1977

67. Knudsen L, Christiansen LA, Lorentzen JE: Hypotension during and after operation in glucocorticoid-treated patients. Br J Anaesth 53:295, 1981

68. Oyama T: Hazards of steroids in association with anaesthesia. Can Anaesth Soc J 16:361, 1969

69. Symreng T, Karlberg BE, Kågedal B, et al: Physiological cortisol substitution of long-term steroid-treated patients undergoing major surgery. Br J Anaesth 53:949, 1981

70. Udelsman R, Ramp J, Gallucci WT, et al: Adaptation during surgical stress: a reevaluation of the role of glucocorticoids. J Clin Invest 77:1377, 1986

71. Axelrod L: Glucocorticoid therapy. Medicine (Baltimore) 55:39, 1976

72. Danowski TS, Bonessi JV, Sabeh G, et al: Probabilities of pituitary-adrenal responsiveness after steroid therapy. Ann Intern Med 61:11, 1964

73. Graber AL, Ney RI, Nicholson WE, et al: Natural history of pituitary-adrenal recovery following long-term suppression with corticosteroids. J Clin Endocrinol Metab 25:11, 1965

74. Ackerman GL, Nolan GM: Adrenocortical responsiveness after alternate-day corticosteroid therapy. N Engl J Med 278:405, 1968

75. Nichols T, Nugent CA, Tyler FH: Diurnal variation in suppression of adrenal function by glucocorticoids. J Clin Endocrinol Metab 25:343, 1965

76. Sampson PA, Brooke BN, Winstone NE: Biochemical confirmation of collapse due to adrenal failure. Lancet 1:1377, 1961

77. Sampson PA, Winstone NE, Brooke BN: Adrenal function in surgical patients after steroid therapy. Lancet 2:322, 1962

78. Streck WF, Lockwood DH: Pituitary adrenal recovery following short-term suppression with corticosteroids. Am J Med 66:910, 1979

79. White PC, New MI, Dupont B: Congenital adrenal hyperplasia. N Engl J Med 316:1519, 1987

80. McPartland RP: Metabolic and pharmacologic actions of glucocorticoids. p. 85. In Mulrow PJ (ed): The Adrenal Gland. Elsevier, New York, 1986

81. Ellul-Micallef R, Borthwick RC, McHardy GJR: The time-course of response to prednisolone in chronic bronchial asthma. Clin Sci 47:105, 1974

82. Fauci AS, Dale DC, Balow JE: Glucocorticoid therapy: mechanisms of action and clinical considerations. Ann Intern Med 84:304, 1976

83. Krieger DT, Liotta AS, Brownstein MJ, et al: ACTH, β-lipoprotein, and related peptides in brain, pituitary, and blood. Recent Prog Horm Res 36:277, 1980

84. Hollenberg NK, Williams GH: Hypertension, the adrenal and the kidney: lessons from pharmacologic interruption of the renin-angiotensin system. Adv Intern Med 25:327, 1980

85. Tyrrell JB, Brooks RM, Fitzgerald PA, et al: Cushing's disease. Selective trans-sphenoidal resection of pituitary microadenomas. N Engl J Med 298:753, 1978

86. Ehrlich HP, Hunt TK: Effects of cortisone and vitamin A on wound healing. Ann Surg 167:324, 1968

87. Myerowitz RL, Medeiros AA, O'Brien TF: Bacterial infection in renal homotransplant recipients: a study of fifty-three bacteremic episodes. Am J Med 53:308, 1972

88. Dale DC, Fauci AS, Wolff SM: Alternate-day prednisone. Leukocyte kinetics and susceptibility to infections. N Engl J Med 291:1154, 1974

89. Ernest I, Ekman H: Adrenalectomy in Cushing's disease: a long-term follow-up. Acta Endocrinol, suppl, 160:3, 1972

90. Weinberger MH, Grim CE, Hollifield JW, et al: Primary aldosteronism: diagnosis, localization, and treatment. Ann Intern Med 90:386, 1979

91. Moore FD, Edelman IS, Olney JM, et al: Body sodium and potassium. III:Inter-related trends in alimentary, renal and cardiovascular disease; lack of correlation between body stores and plasma concentration. Metabolism 3:334, 1954

92. Jasani BM, Edmonds CJ: Kinetics of potassium distribution in man using isotope dilution and whole-body counting. Metabolism 20:1099, 1971

93. Johnson JE, Hartsuck JM, Zollinger RM, Jr, et al: Radiopotassium equilibrium in total body potassium: studies using ^{43}K and ^{42}K. Metabolism 18:663, 1969

94. Surawicz B, Chlebus H, Mazzoleni A: Hemodynamic and electrocardiographic effects of hyperpotassemia: differences in response to slow and rapid increases in concentration of plasma K. Am Heart J 73:647, 1967

95. Rao TLK, Jacobs KH, El-Etr AA: Reinfarction following anesthesia in patients with myocardial infarction. Anesthesiology 59:499, 1983

96. Oh SH, Patterson R: Surgery in corticosteroid-dependent asthmatics. J Allergy Clin Immunol 53:345, 1974

97. Schambelan M, Sebastian A: Hyporeninemic hypoaldosteronism. Adv Intern Med 24:385, 1979

98. Zusman RM: Prostaglandins and water excretion. Annu Rev Med 32:359, 1981

99. Oyama T, Taniguchi K, Jin T, et al: Effects of anaesthesia and surgery on plasma aldosterone concentration and renin activity in man. Br J Anaesth 51:747, 1979

100. Namba Y, Smith JB, Fox GS, et al: Plasma cortisol concentrations during caesarean section. Br J Anaesth 52:1027, 1980

101. Knowlton AI: Addison's disease: A review of its clinical course and management. p. 329. In Christy NR (ed): The Human Adrenal Cortex. Harper & Row, New York, New York, 1971

102. Landon J, Greenwood FC, Stamp TCB, et al: The plasma sugar, free fatty acid, cortisol, and growth hormone response to insulin, and the comparison of this procedure with other tests of pituitary and adrenal function. II. In patients with hypothalamic or pituitary dysfunction or anorexia nervosa. J Clin Invest 45:437, 1966

103. Wood JB, Frankland AW, James VHT, et al: A rapid test of adrenocortical function. Lancet 1:243, 1965

104. Engquist A, Backer OG, Jarnum S: Incidence of postoperative complications in patients subjected to surgery under steroid cover. Acta Chir Scand 140:343, 1974

105. Jensen JK, Elb S: Per- og postoperative komplikationer hos tidligere kortikosteroidbehandlede patienter. Nord Med 76:975, 1966

106. Winstone NE, Brooke BN: Effects of steroid treatment on patients undergoing operation. Lancet 1:973, 1961

107. Migeon C, Keller A, Lawrence B, Shepard T: DHA and androsterone levels in human plasma. Effect of age and sex: day-to-day and diurnal variations. J Clin Endocrinol Metab 17:1051, 1957

108. Wagner RL, White PF: Etomidate inhibits adrenocortical function in surgical patients. Anesthesiology 61:647, 1984

109. Wagner RL, White PF, Kan PB, et al: Inhibition of adrenal steroidogenesis by the anesthetic etomidate. N Engl J Med 310:1415, 1984

110. Zurick AM, Sigurdsson H, Koehler LS, et al: Magnitude and time course of perioperative adrenal suppression with single dose etomidate in male adult cardiac surgical patients. Anesthesiology 65:A248, 1986

111. St John Sutton MG, Sheps SG, Lie JT: Prevalence of clinically unsuspected pheochromocytoma: Review of a 50-year autopsy series. Mayo Clin Proc 56:354, 1981

112. Desmonts JM, le Houelleur J, Remond P, et al: Anaesthetic management of patients with pheochromocytoma: a review of 102 cases. Br J Anaesth 49:991, 1977

113. Roizen MF, Horrigan RW, Koike M, et al: A prospective randomized trial of four anesthetic techniques for resection of pheochromocytoma. Anesthesiology 57:A43, 1982

114. Roizen MF, Hunt TK, Beaupre PN, et al: The effect of alpha-adrenergic blockade on cardiac performance and tissue oxygen delivery during excision of pheochromocytoma. Surgery 94:941, 1983

115. Schaffer MS, Zuberbuhler P, Wilson G, et al: Catecholamine cardiomyopathy: an unusual presentation of pheochromocytoma in children. J Pediatr 99:276, 1981

116. Roizen MF, Schreider BD, Hassan SZ: Anesthetic for patients with pheochromocytoma. Anesthesiol Clin North Am 5:269, 1987

117. Kopin IJ, Lake CR, Ziegler M: Plasma levels of norepinephrine. Ann Intern Med 88:671, 1978

118. Riley CM, Day RL, Greeley DM, et al: Central autonomic dysfunction with defective lacrimation. I: Report of five cases. Pediatrics 3:468, 1949

119. Shy GM, Drager GA: A neurologic syndrome associated with orthostatic hypotension: a clinico-pathologic study. Arch Neurol 2:511, 1960

120. Ziegler MG, Lake CR, Kopin IJ: The sympathetic nervous system defect in primary orthostatic hypotension. N Engl J Med 296:293, 1977

121. Naftchi NE, Wooten GF, Lowman EW, et al: Relationship between serum dopamine-β-hydroxylase activity, catecholamine metabolism, and hemodynamic changes during paroxysmal hypertension in quadraplegia. Circ Res 35:850, 1974

122. Cohen CA: Anesthetic management of a patient with the Shy-Drager syndrome. Anesthesiology 35:95, 1971

123. Kirtchman MM, Schwartz H, Papper EM: Experiences with general anesthesia in patients with familial dysautonomia. JAMA 170:529, 1959

124. McCaughey TJ: Familial dysautonomia as an anaesthetic hazard. Can Anaesth Soc J 12:558, 1965

125. Meridy HW, Creighton RE: General anaesthesia in eight patients with familial dysautonomia. Can Anaesth Soc J 18:563, 1971

126. Desmond J: Paraplegia: problems confronting the anaesthesiologist. Can Anaesth Soc J 17:435, 1970

127. Gronert GA, Theye RA: Pathophysiology of hyperkalemia induced by succinylcholine. Anesthesiology 43:89, 1975

128. Jousse AT, Wynne-Jones M, Breithaupt DJ: A follow-up study of life expectancy and mortality in traumatic transverse myelitis. Can Med Assoc J 98:770, 1968

129. Bevan DR: Shy-Drager syndrome. A review and a description of the anaesthetic management. Anaesthesia 34:866, 1979

130. Malan MD, Crago RR: Anaesthetic considerations in idiopathic orthostatic hypotension and the Shy-Drager syndrome. Can Anaesth Soc J 26:322, 1979

131. Roizen MF: Should we all have a sympathectomy at birth? Or at least preoperatively? Anesthesiology 68:482, 1988

132. Stone JG, Foëx P, Sear JW, et al: Myocardial ischemia in untreated hypertensive patients. Effect of a single small oral dose of a beta-adrenergic blocking agent. Anesthesiology 68:495, 1988

133. Flacke JW, Bloor BC, Flacke WE, et al: Reduced narcotic requirement by clonidine with improved hemodynamic and adrenergic stability in patients undergoing coronary bypass surgery. Anesthesiology 67:11, 1987

134. Ghignone M, Calvillo O, Quintin L: Anesthesia and hypertension: the effect of clonidine on perioperative hemodynamics and isoflurane requirements. Anesthesiology 67:3, 1987

135. Yeager MP, Glass DD, Neff RK, Brinck-Johnsen T: Epidural anesthesia and analgesia in high-risk surgical patients. Anesthesiology 66:729, 1987

136. Roizen MF, Lampe GH, Benefiel DJ, et al: Is increased operative stress associated with worse outcome? (abstract) Anesthesiology 67:A1, 1987

137. Bland JHL, Lowenstein E: Halothane-induced decrease in experimental myocardial ischemia in the non-failing canine heart. Anesthesiology 45:287, 1976

138. Klassen GA, Bramwell RS, Bromage PR, Zborowska-Sluis DT: Effect of acute sympathectomy by epidural anesthesia on the canine coronary circulation. Anesthesiology 52:8, 1980

139. Maroko DR, Braunwald E: Modification of myocardial infarction size after coronary occlusion. Ann Intern Med 79:720, 1973

140. Norris RM, Clarke ED, Sammel NL, et al: Protective effect of propranolol in threatened myocardial infarction. Lancet 2:907, 1978

141. Levine JD, Dardick SJ, Roizen MF, et al: The contribution of sensory afferents and sympathetic efferents to joint injury in experimental arthritis. J Neurosci 6:3423, 1986

142. Feigl EO: The paradox of adrenergic coronary vasoconstriction. Circulation 76:737, 1987

143. Williams LT, Lefkowitz RJ, Watanabe AM, et al: Thyroid hormone regulation of β-adrenergic receptor number. J Biol Chem 252:2787, 1977

143a. Wade JG, Larson CP, Hickey RF, et al: Carotid endarterectomy and carotid chemoreceptor and baroreceptor function in man. N Engl J Med 282:823, 1970

144. Hui KKP, Conolly ME: Increased numbers of beta receptors in orthostatic hypotension due to autonomic dysfunction. N Engl J Med 304:1473, 1981

145. Kendrick WW, Scott JW, Jousse AT, et al: Reflex sweating and hypertension in traumatic transverse myelitis. Treatm Serv Bull (Ottawa) 8:437, 1953

146. Amino N, Mori H, Iwatani Y, et al: High prevalence of transient postpartum thyrotoxicosis and hypothyroidism. N Engl J Med 306:849, 1982

147. Channick BJ, Adlin EV, Marks AD, et al: Hyperthyroidism and mitral-valve prolapse. N Engl J Med 305:497, 1981

148. Forfar JC, Miller HC, Toft AD: Occult thyrotoxicosis: a correctable cause of "idiopathic" atrial fibrillation. Am J Cardiol 44:9, 1979

149. Davis PJ, Davis FB: Hyperthyroidism in patients over the age of 60 years. Clinical features in 85 patients. Medicine (Baltimore) 53:161, 1974

150. Toft AD, Irvine WJ, Sinclair I, et al: Thyroid function after surgical treatment of thyrotoxicosis: a report of 100 cases treated with propranolol before operation. N Engl J Med 298:643, 1978

151. Feek CM, Sawers JSA, Irvine WJ, et al: Combination of potassium iodide and propranolol in preparation of patients with Graves' disease for thyroid surgery. N Engl J Med 302:883, 1980

152. Forfar JC, Muir AL, Sawers SA, Toft AD: Abnormal left ventricular function in hyperthyroidism: evidence for a possible reversible cardiomyopathy. N Engl J Med 307:1165, 1982

153. Eriksson M, Rubenfeld S, Garber AJ, et al: Propranolol does not prevent thyroid storm. N Engl J Med 296:263, 1977

154. Roizen MF, Becker CE: Thyroid storm: a review of cases at University of California, San Francisco. Calif Med 115(4):5, 1971

155. Mackin JF, Canary JJ, Pittman CS: Thyroid storm and its management. N Engl J Med 291:1396, 1974

156. Murkin JM: Anesthesia and hypothyroidism: a review of thyroxine physiology, pharmacology, and anesthetic implications. Anesth Analg 61:371, 1982

157. Sawin CT, Castelli WP, Hershman JM, et al: The aging thyroid: thyroid deficiency in the Framingham Study. Arch Intern Med 145:1386, 1985

158. Weinberg AD, Brennan MD, Gorman CA, et al: Outcome of anesthesia and surgery in hypothyroid patients. Arch Intern Med 143:893, 1983

159. Zwillich CW, Pierson DJ, Hofeldt FD, et al: Ventilatory control in myxedema and hypothyroidism. N Engl J Med 292:662, 1975

160. Bough EW, Crowley WF, Ridgway EC, et al: Myocardial function in hypothyroidism. Relation to disease severity and response to treatment. Arch Intern Med 138:1476, 1978

161. Babad AA, Eger EI, II: The effects of hyperthyroidism and hypothyroidism on halothane and oxygen requirements in dogs. Anesthesiology 29:1087, 1968

162. Levine HD: Compromise therapy in the patient with angina pectoris and hypothyroidism: a clinical assessment. Am J Med 69:411, 1980

163. Bone HG, III, Snyder WH, III, Pak CYC: Diagnosis of hyperparathyroidism. Annu Rev Med 28:111, 1977

164. Weidmann P, Massry SG, Coburn WJ, et al: Blood pressure effects of acute hypercalcemia. Ann Intern Med 76:741, 1972

165. Hensel P, Roizen MF: Patients with disorders of parathyroid function. Anesthesiol Clin North Am 5:287, 1987

166. Lang RM, Fellner SK, Neumann A, et al: Left ventricular contractility varies directly with blood ionized calcium. Ann Intern Med 108:524, 1988

167. Rumancik WM, Denlinger JK, Nahrwold ML, et al: The QT interval and serum ionized calcium. JAMA 240:366, 1978

168. Southwick JP, Katz J: Unusual airway difficulty in the acromegalic patient: indications for tracheostomy. Anesthesiology 51:72, 1979

169. McGuffin WL, Sherman BM, Roth J, et al: Acromegaly and cardiovascular disorders: a prospective study. Ann Intern Med 81:11, 1974

170. Hassan SZ, Matz G, Lawrence AM, et al: Laryngeal stenosis in acromegaly: a possible cause of airway difficulties associated with anesthesia. Anesth Analg 55:57, 1976

171. Campkin TV: Radial artery cannulation: potential hazard in patients with acromegaly. Anaesthesia 35:1008, 1980

172. Molitch ME, Elton RL, Blackwell RE, et al: Bromocriptine as primary therapy for prolactin-secreting macroadenomas: results of a prospective multicenter study. J Clin Endocrinol Metab 60:698, 1985

173. Weiss NM, Robertson GL: Water metabolism in endocrine disorders. Semin Nephrol 4:303, 1984

174. Berk JL, Hagen JF, Fried VJ: The effect of vasopressin on oxygen availability. Ann Surg 189:439, 1979

175. Corliss RJ, McKenna DH, Sialers S, et al: Systemic and coronary hemodynamic effects of vasopressin. Am J Med Sci 256:293, 1968

176. Nikolic G, Singh JB: Cimetidine, vasopressin and chronotropic incompetence. Med J Aust 2:435, 1982

177. Smithwick RH, Thompson JE: Splanchnicectomy for essential hypertension. JAMA 152:1501, 1953

178. Brown BR: Anesthesia and essential hypertension. p. 41. In Hershey SG (ed): ASA Refresher Courses in Anesthesiology. Vol. 7. JB Lippincott, Philadelphia, 1979

179. Sprague HB: The heart in surgery. An analysis of results of surgery on cardiac patients during the past ten years at the Massachusetts General Hospital. Surg Gynecol Obstet 49:54, 1929

180. Miller RD, Way WL, Eger EI, II: The effects of alpha-methyldopa, reserpine, and guanethidine on minimum alveolar

anesthetic requirement (MAC). Anesthesiology 29:1153, 1968

181. Veterans Administration Study on Antihypertensive Agents: Effects of treatment on morbidity in hypertension. JAMA 202:1028, 1967

182. Veterans Administration Cooperative Study Group on Antihypertensive Agents: Effects of treatment on morbidity in hypertension: results in patients with diastolic blood pressure averaging 90 through 114 mm Hg. JAMA 213:1143, 1970

183. Berglund G, Wilhelmen L, Sannerstedt R, et al: Coronary heart-disease after treatment of hypertension. Lancet 1:1, 1978

184. Hypertension Detection and Follow-up Program Cooperative Group: The effect of treatment on mortality in "mild" hypertension. N Engl J Med 307:976, 1982

185. Multiple Risk Factor Intervention Trial Research Group: Multiple risk factor intervention trial. Risk factor changes and mortality results. JAMA 248:1465, 1982

186. Ayobe MH, Tarazi RC: Reversal of changes in myocardial β-receptors and inotropic responsiveness with regression of cardiac hypertrophy in renal hypertensive rats (RHR). Circ Res 54:125, 1984

187. Prys-Roberts C, Meloche R, Foëx P: Studies of anesthesia in relation to hypertension. I: Cardiovascular responses of treated and untreated patients. Br J Anaesth 43:122, 1971

188. Goldman L, Caldera DL: Risks of general anesthesia and elective operation in the hypertensive patient. Anesthesiology 50:285, 1979

189. Bedford RF, Feinstein B: Hospital admission blood pressure: a predictor for hypertension following endotracheal intubation. Anesth Analg 59:367, 1980

190. Asiddao CB, Donegan JH, Whitesell RC, et al: Factors associated with perioperative complications during carotid endarterectomy. Anesth Analg 61:631, 1982

191. Cohen MM, Duncan PG: Physical Status Score and trends in anesthetic complications. J Clin Epidemiol 41:83, 1988

192. Fleiss JL: Statistical Methods for Rates and Proportions. Wiley, New York, 1973, p 178

193. Schneider AJL, Knoke JD, Zollinger RM, Jr, et al: Morbidity prediction using pre- and intraoperative data. Anesthesiology 51:4, 1979

194. Eerola M, Eerola R, Kaukinen S, et al: Risk factors in surgical patients with verified preoperative myocardial infarction. Acta Anaesthesiol Scand 24:219, 1980

195. Mauney FM, Ebert PA, Sabiston DC: Postoperative myocardial infarction: a study of predisposing factors, diagnosis and mortality in a high risk group of surgical patients. Ann Surg 172:497, 1970

196. Garraway WM, Whisnant JP: The changing pattern of hypertension and the declining incidence of stroke. JAMA 258:214, 1987

197. Rutan GH, Kuller LH, Neaton JD, et al: Mortality associated with diastolic hypertension and isolated systolic hypertension among men screened for the Multiple Risk Intervention Trial. Circulation 77:504, 1988

198. Okuda S, Onoyama K, Motomura K, et al: Effect of acute reduction in blood pressure on renal function of rats with diseased kidneys. Nephron 45:311, 1987

199. Mayhan WG, Faraci FM, Heistad DD: Disruption of the blood-brain barrier in cerebrum and brain stem during acute hypertension. Am J Physiol 251:H1171, 1986

200. Croog SH, Levine S, Testa MA, et al: The effects of antihypertensive therapy on the quality of life. N Engl J Med 314:1657, 1986

201. Slogoff S, Keats AS: Does perioperative myocardial ische-

mia lead to postoperative myocardial infarction? Anesthesiology 62:107, 1985

202. Slogoff S, Keats AS: Further observations on perioperative myocardial ischemia. Anesthesiology 65:539, 1986

203. Garber AM, Sox HC, Littenberg B: Screening asymptomatic adults for cardiac risk factors: the serum cholesterol level. Ann Intern Med 110:622, 1989

204. Gordon T, Kannel WB: The Framingham, Massachusetts, study twenty years later. p. 123. In Kessler II, Levin ML (eds): Community as an Epidemiologic Laboratory: A Casebook of Community Studies. Johns Hopkins University Press, Baltimore, 1970

205. Benchimol A, Harris CL, Desser KB, et al: Resting electrocardiogram in major coronary artery disease. JAMA 224:1489, 1973

206. Levy D, Garrison RJ, Savage DD, et al: Left ventricular mass and the incidence of coronary heart disease in an elderly cohort: the Framingham heart study. Ann Intern Med 110:101, 1989

207. Tomatis LA, Fierens EE, Verbrugge GP: Evaluation of surgical risk in peripheral vascular disease by coronary angiography: a series of 100 cases. Surgery 71:429, 1972

208. Hertzer NR, Beven EG, Young JR, et al: Coronary artery disease in peripheral vascular patients. A classification of 1000 angiograms and results of surgical management. Ann Surg 199:223, 1984

209. Barnes RW, Liebman PR, Marszalek PB, et al: The natural history of asymptomatic carotid disease in patients undergoing cardiovascular surgery. Surgery 90:1075, 1981

210. Barnes RW, Marszalek PB: Asymptomatic carotid disease in the cardiovascular surgical patient: is prophylactic endarterectomy necessary? Stroke 12:497, 1981

211. Ropper AH, Wechsler LR, Wilson LS: Carotid bruit and the risk of stroke in elective surgery. N Engl J Med 307:1388, 1982

212. Heyman A, Wilkinson WE, Heyden S, et al: Risk of stroke in asymptomatic persons with cervical arterial bruits. A population study in Evans County, Georgia. N Engl J Med 302:838, 1980

213. Reed GL, Singer DE, Picard EH, DeSanctis RW: Stroke following coronary-artery bypass surgery: a case-control estimate of the risk from carotid bruits. N Engl J Med 319:1246, 1988

214. Rabkin SE, Horne JM: Preoperative electrocardiography: effect of new abnormalities on clinical decisions. Can Med Assoc J 128:146, 1983

215. Apfelbaum J, Robinson D, Murray WJ, et al: An automated method to validate preoperative test selection: first results of a multicenter study (abstract). Anesthesiology 71:A928, 1989

216. Borer JS, Brensike JF, Redwood DR, et al: Limitations of the electrocardiograhic response to exercise in predicting coronary artery disease. N Engl J Med 293:367, 1975

217. Proudfit WL, Shirey EK, Sones FM: Selective CINE coronary angiography: correlation with clinical finding in 1000 patients. Circulation 33:901, 1966

218. Goldschlager N: Use of the treadmill test in the diagnosis of coronary artery disease in patients with chest pain. Ann Intern Med 97:383, 1982

219. Weiner DA, Ryan TJ, McCabe CH, et al: Exercise stress testing. Correlations among history of angina, ST-segment response and prevalence of coronary-artery disease in the Coronary Artery Surgery Study (CASS). N Engl J Med 301:230, 1979

220. Arkins R, Smessaert AA, Hicks RG: Mortality and morbidity

in surgical patients with coronary artery disease. JAMA 190:485, 1964

221. Topkins MJ, Artusio JF: Myocardial infarction and surgery: a five year study. Anesth Analg 43:715, 1964

222. Fraser JG, Ramachandran PR, Davis HS: Anesthesia and recent myocardial infarction. JAMA 199:318, 1972

223. Tarhan S, Moffitt EA, Taylor WF, et al: Myocardial infarction after general anesthesia. JAMA 199:318, 1972

224. Sapala JA, Ponka JL, Duvernow WFC: Operative and non-operative risks in the cardiac patient. J Am Geriatr Soc 23:529, 1975

225. Steen PA, Tinker JH, Tarhan S: Myocardial reinfarction after anesthesia and surgery. JAMA 239:2566, 1976

226. Goldman L, Caldera DL, Southwick FS, et al: Cardiac risk factors and complications in noncardiac surgery. Medicine (Baltimore) 57:357, 1978

227. Schoeppel SL, Wilkinson C, Waters J, et al: Effects of myocardial infarction on perioperative cardiac complications. Anesth Analg 62:493, 1983.

228. Knapp RB, Topkins MJ, Artusio JF, Jr: The cerebrovascular accident and coronary occlusion in anesthesia. JAMA 182:332, 1962

229. von Knorring J: Postoperative myocardial infarction: a prospective study in a risk group of surgical patients. Surgery 90:55, 1981

230. Plumlee JE, Boettner RB: Myocardial infarction during and following anesthesia and operation. South Med J 65:886, 1972

231. Becker RC, Underwood DA: Myocardial infarction in patients undergoing noncardiac surgery. Cleve Clin J Med 54:25, 1987

232. Eagle KA, Boucher CA: Cardiac risk of noncardiac surgery. N Engl J Med 321:1330, 1989

233. Detsky AS, Abrams HB, McLaughlin JR, et al: Predicting cardiac complications in patients undergoing non-cardiac surgery. J Gen Intern Med 1:211, 1986

234. Gerson MC, Hurst JM, Hertzberg VS, et al: Cardiac prognosis in noncardiac surgery. Ann Intern Med 103:832, 1985

235. Lowenstein E, Yusuf S, Teplick RS: Perioperative myocardial reinfarction: A glimmer of hope—a note of caution (editorial). Anesthesiology 59:493, 1983

236. Backer CL, Tinker JH, Robertson DM, et al: Myocardial reinfarction following local anesthesia for ophthalmic surgery. Anesth Analg 59:257, 1980

237. Wolf GL, Lynch S, Berlin I: Intra-ocular surgery with general anesthesia. Arch Ophthalmol 93:323, 1975

238. Roizen MF: Anesthesia goals for surgery to relieve or prevent visceral ischemia. p. 171. In Roizen MF (ed): Anesthesia for Vascular Surgery. Churchill Livingstone, New York, 1990.

239. Eagle KA, Coley CM, Newell JB, et al: Combining clinical and thallium data optimizes preoperative assessment of cardiac risk before major vascular surgery. Ann Intern Med 110:859, 1989

240. Boucher CA, Brewster DC, Darling RC, et al: Determination of cardiac risk by dipyridamole-thallium imaging before peripheral vascular surgery. N Engl J Med 312:389, 1985

241. Raby KE, Goldman L, Creager MA, et al: Correlation between preoperative ischemia and major cardiac events after peripheral vascular surgery. N Engl J Med 321:1296, 1989

242. Lette J, Waters D, Lapointe J, et al: Usefulness of the severity and extent of reversible perfusion defects during thallium-dipyridamole imaging for cardiac risk assessment before noncardiac surgery. Am J Cardiol 64:276, 1989

243. Fletcher JP, Antico VF, Gruenwald S, Kershaw LZ: Dipyridamole-thallium scan for screening of coronary artery disease prior to vascular surgery. J Cardiovasc Surg 29:666, 1988

244. Bruschke AVG, Proudfit WL, Sones FM: Progress study of 590 consecutive nonsurgical cases of coronary disease followed 5–9 years. Circulation 47:1147, 1973

245. Diamond GA, Forrester JS: Analysis probability as an aid in the clinical diagnosis of coronary-artery disease. N Engl J Med 300:1350, 1979

246. Mahar LJ, Steen PA, Tinker JH, et al: Perioperative myocardial infarction in patients with coronary artery disease with and without aorta-coronary bypass grafts. J Thorac Cardiovasc Surg 76:533, 1978

247. Kennedy JW, Kaiser GC, Fisher LD, et al: Clinical and angiographic predictors of operative mortality from the Collaborative Study in Coronary Artery Surgery (CASS). Circulation 63:793, 1981

248. Podrid PJ, Graboys TB, Lown B: Prognosis of medically treated patients with coronary-artery disease with profound ST-segment depression during exercise testing. N Engl J Med 305:1111, 1981

249. Rozanski A, Berman D, Gray R, et al: Preoperative prediction of reversible myocardial asynergy by postexercise radionuclide ventriculography. N Engl J Med 307:212, 1982

250. Mangano DT, Hedgcock MW, Wisneski JA: Noninvasive prediction of ventricular dysfunction: coronary artery disease. Anesthesiology 57:A21, 1982

251. White CW, Wright CB, Doty DB, et al: Does visual interpretation of the coronary arteriogram predict the physiologic importance of a coronary stenosis? N Engl J Med 310:819, 1984

252. Jeffrey CC, Kunsman J, Cullen DJ, Brewster DC: A prospective evaluation of cardiac risk index. Anesthesiology 58:462, 1984

253. Benson H, McCallie DP: Angina pectoris and the placebo effect. N Engl J Med 300:1424, 1979

254. Oberman A, Kouchoukos NT, Harrell RR, et al: Surgical versus medical treatment in disease of the left main coronary artery. Lancet 2:591, 1976

255. Takaro T, Hultgren HN, Lipton MJ, et al: The VA cooperative randomized study of surgery for coronary arterial occlusive disease. II:Subgroup with significant left main lesions. Circulation 54:suppl. 3, III107, 1976

256. Vliestra RE, Assad-Morell JL, Frye RL, et al: Survival predictors in coronary artery disease: medical and surgical comparisons. Mayo Clin Proc 42:85, 1977

257. Reed RC, Murphy ML, Hultgren HN, et al: Survival of men treated for chronic stable angina pectoris. A cooperative randomized study. J Thorac Cardiovasc Surg 75:1, 1978

258. Crawford ES, Morris GC, Howell JF, et al: Operative risk in patients with previous coronary artery bypass. Ann Thorac Surg 26:215, 1978

259. Hultgren HN, Pfeifer JF, Angell WW, et al: Unstable angina: comparison of medical and surgical management. Am J Cardiol 39:734, 1977

260. Roizen MF, Beaupre PN, Alpert RA, et al: Monitoring with two-dimensional transesophageal echocardiography. J Vasc Surg 1:300, 1984

261. The Criteria Committee of the New York Heart Association, Kossman CE (chairman): Diseases of the heart and blood vessels. In Nomenclature and Criteria for Diagnosis. 6th Ed. Little, Brown, Boston, 1964

262. Santos AL, Gelperin A: Surgical mortality in the elderly. J Am Geriatr Soc 23:42, 1975

263. Driscoll AC, Hobika JH, Etsten BE, et al: Clinically unrec-

ognized myocardial infarction following surgery. N Engl J Med 264:633, 1961

264. O'Keefe JH, Shub C, Rettke SR: Risk of noncardiac surgical procedures in patients with aortic stenosis. Mayo Clin Proc 64:400, 1989

265. Cohn PF, Gorlin R, Cohn LH, et al: Left ventricular ejection fraction as a prognostic guide in surgical treatment of coronary and valvular heart disease. Am J Cardiol 34:136, 1974

266. Charlson ME, Mackenzie CR, Ales K, et al: Surveillance for postoperative myocardial infarction after noncardiac operations. Surgery Gynecol Obstet 167:407, 1988

267. Smith JS, Roizen MF, Cahalan MK, Benefiel DJ: Does anesthetic technique make a difference? Augmentation of systolic blood pressure during carotid endarterectomy: effects of phenylephrine versus light anesthesia and of isoflurane versus halothane on the incidence of myocardial ischemia. Anesthesiology 69:846, 1988

268. Riles TS, Kopelman I, Imparato AM: Myocardial infarction following carotid endarterectomy: a review of 683 operations. Surgery 85:249, 1979

269. Nachlas MM, Abrams SJ, Goldberg MM: The influence of arteriosclerotic heart disease on surgical risk. Am J Surg 101:447, 1961

270. Sanz G, Castañer A, Bertriu A, et al: Determinants of prognosis in survivors of myocardial infarction: a prospective clinical angiographic study. N Engl J Med 306:1065, 1982

271. Epstein SE, Palmeri ST, Patterson RE: Evaluation of patients after acute myocardial infarction. Indications for cardiac catheterization and surgical intervention. N Engl J Med 307:1487, 1982

272. Roy WL, Edelist G, Gilbert B: Myocardial ischemia during non-cardiac surgical procedures in patients with coronary-artery disease. Anesthesiology 51:393, 1979

273. Kaplan JA, King SB: The precordial electrocardiographic lead (V_5) in patients who have coronary-artery disease. Anesthesiology 45:570, 1976

274. Braunwald E: Thirteenth Bowditch Lecture: the determinants of myocardial oxygen consumption. Physiologist 12:65, 1969

275. Pasternack PF, Grossi EA, Baumann FG, Riles TS: Beta blockade to decrease silent myocardial ischemia during peripheral vascular surgery. Am J Surg 158:113, 1989

276. Robinson BF: Relation of heart rate and systolic blood pressure to the onset of pain and angina pectoris. Circulation 25:1073, 1967

277. Cannon DS, Levy W, Cohen LS: The short- and long-term prognosis of patients with transmural and nontransmural myocardial infarction. Am J Med 61:452, 1976

278. Lembo NJ, Dell'Italia LJ, Crawford MH, O'Rourke RA: Bedside diagnosis of systolic murmurs. N Engl J Med 318:1572, 1988

279. Hollinger I: Diseases of the cardiovascular system. p. 93. In Katz R, Steward D (eds): Anesthesia and Uncommon Pediatric Diseases. WB Saunders, Philadelphia, 1987

280. Noonan JA: Association of congenital heart disease with syndromes or other defects. Pediatr Clin North Am 25:797, 1978

281. Nishimura RA, McGoon MD, Shub C, et al: Echocardiographically documented mitral-valve prolapse: long term follow-up of 237 patients. N Engl J Med 313:1305, 1985

282. Schlant RC, Felner JM, Miklozek C, et al: Mitral valve prolapse. DM 26(10):1, 1980

283. Bor DH, Himmelstein DU: Endocarditis prophylaxis for patients with mitral valve prolapse: a quantitative analysis. Am J Med 76:711, 1984

284. Swartz MH, Teicholz LE, Donoso F: Mitral valve prolapse: A review of associated arrhythmias. Am J Med 62:377, 1977

285. Clemens JD, Horwitz RI, Jaffe CC, et al: A controlled evaluation of the risk of bacterial endocarditis in persons with mitral-valve prolapse. N Engl J Med 307:776, 1982

286. Berry FA, Blanketbaker WL, Ball CG: A comparison of bacteremia occurring with nasotracheal and orotracheal intubation. Anesth Analg 52:873, 1973

287. Shull HJ, Greene BM, Allen SD, et al: Bacteremia with upper gastrointestinal endoscopy. Ann Intern Med 83:212, 1975

288. Committee on Prevention of Rheumatic Fever and Bacterial Endocarditis of the American Heart Association: Prevention of bacterial endocarditis. Circulation 70:1123A, 1984

289. Abramowicz M (ed): Antimicrobial prophylaxis for surgery. Med Lett 27:105, 1985

290. Tinker JH, Tarhan S: Discontinuing anticoagulant therapy in surgical patients with cardiac valve prostheses: observations in 180 operations. JAMA 239:738, 1978

291. Cade JF, Hunt D, Stubbs KP, et al: Guidelines for the management of oral anticoagulant therapy in patients undergoing surgery. Med J Aust 2:292, 1979

292. Katholi RE, Nolan SP, McGuire LB: The management of anticoagulant during noncardiac operations in patients with prosthetic heart valves: a prospective study. Am Heart J 96:163, 1978

293. De Angelis J: Hazards of subdural and epidural anesthesia during anticoagulant therapy: a case report and review. Anesth Analg 51:676, 1972

294. Edelson RN, Chernik NL, Posner JB: Spinal subdural hematomas complicating lumbar puncture. Arch Neurol 31:134, 1974

295. Brem SS, Hafler DA, Van Uitert RL, et al: Spinal subarachnoid hematoma: a hazard of lumbar puncture resulting in reversible paraplegia. N Engl J Med 303:1020, 1981

296. Owens EL, Kasten GW, Hessel EA II: Spinal subarachnoid hematoma after lumbar puncture and heparinization: a case report, review of the literature, and discussion of anesthetic implications. Anesth Analg 65:1201, 1986

297. Rao TLK, El-Etr AA: Anticoagulation following placement of epidural and subarachnoid catheters: an evaluation of neurologic sequelae. Anesthesiology 55:618, 1981

298. Odoom JA, Sih IL: Epidural analgesia and anticoagulant therapy: experience with one thousand cases of continuous epidurals. Anaesthesia 38:254, 1983

299. Kane RE: Neurologic deficits following epidural or spinal anesthesia. Anesth Analg 60:150, 1981

300. Locke GE, Giorgio AJ, Biggers SL, Jr, et al: Acute spinal epidural hematoma secondary to aspirin-induced prolonged bleeding. Surg Neurol 5:293, 1976

301. Reddy NB, Rao TLK: Regional anesthesia for vascular surgery of the lower extremities: considerations regarding anticoagulation. p. 367. In Roizen MF (ed): Anesthesia for Vascular Surgery. Churchill Livingstone, New York, 1990

302. International Multicentre Trial: Prevention of fatal postoperative pulmonary embolism by low doses of heparin. Lancet 2:45, 1975

303. Consensus Conference: Prevention of venous thrombosis and pulmonary embolism. JAMA 256:744, 1988

304. Collins R, Scrimgeour A, Yusuf S, Peto R: Reduction in fatal pulmonary embolism and venous thrombosis by perioperative administration of subcutaneous heparin. N Engl J Med 318:1162, 1988

305. Gallus A, Raman K, Darby T: Venous thrombosis after elec-

tive hip replacement—the influence of preventive intermittent calf compression and or surgical technique. Br J Surg 70:17, 1983

306. Lutz DJ, Noller KL, Spittell JA, Jr, et al: Pregnancy and its complications following cardiac valve prostheses. Am J Obstet Gynecol 131:460, 1978

307. Smith ND, Raizada V, Abrams J: Auscultation of the normally functioning prosthetic valve. Ann Intern Med 95:594, 1981

308. Pastore JO, Yurchak PM, Janis KM, et al: The risk of advanced heart block in surgical patients with right bundle branch block and left axis deviation. Circulation 57:677, 1978

309. Berg GR, Kotler MN: The significance of bilateral bundle branch block in the preoperative patient. A retrospective electrocardiographic and clinical study in 30 patients. Chest 59:62, 1971

310. Rooney S-M, Goldiner PL, Muss E: Relationship of right bundle-branch block and marked left axis deviation to complete heart block during general anesthesia. Anesthesiology 44:64, 1976

311. Kunstadt D, Punja M, Cagin N, et al: Bifascicular block: a clinical and electrophysiologic study. Am Heart J 86:173, 1973

312. Venkataraman K, Madias JE, Hood WB, Jr: Indications for prophylactic preoperative insertion of pacemakers in patients with right bundle branch block and left anterior hemiblock. Chest 68:501, 1975

313. McAnulty JH, Rahimtoola SH, Murphy E, et al: Natural history of "high-risk" bundle-branch block. Final report of a prospective study. N Engl J Med 307:137, 1982

314. Ruskin JN, DiMarco JP, Garan H: Out-of-hospital cardiac arrest. Electrophysiologic observations and selection of long-term antiarrhythmic therapy. N Engl J Med 303:607, 1980

315. Ruberman W, Weinblatt E, Frank CW, et al: Repeated 1 hour electrocardiographic monitoring of survivors of myocardial infarction at 6 month intervals: arrhythmia detection and relation to prognosis. Am J Cardiol 47:1197, 1981

316. Prystowsky EN: Diagnosis and management of the pre-excitation syndromes. Curr Probl Cardiol 13:225, 1988

317. Sadowski AR, Moyers JR: Anesthetic management of the Wolff-Parkinson-White syndrome. Anesthesiology 51:553, 1979

318. Rose MR, Koski G: Anesthesia in patients with Wolff-Parkinson-White syndrome (abstract). Anesthesiology 69:A146, 1988

319. Kruse I, Arnman K, Conradson T-B, et al: A comparison of the acute and long-term hemodynamic effects of ventricular inhibited and atrial synchronous ventricular inhibited pacing. Circulation 65:846, 1982

320. Shapiro WA, Roizen MF, Singleton MA, et al: Intraoperative pacemaker complications. Anesthesiology 63:319, 1985

321. Thiagarajah S, Azar I, Agres M, et al: Pacemaker malfunction associated with positive-pressure ventilation. Anesthesiology 58:565, 1983

322. Stein M, Cassara EL: Preoperative pulmonary evaluation and therapy for surgery patients. JAMA 211:787, 1970

323. Collins CD, Darke CS, Knowelden J: Chest complications after upper abdominal surgery: their anticipation and prevention. Br Med J 1:401, 1968

324. Warner MA, Offerd KP, Warner ME, et al: Role of preoperative cessation of smoking and other factors in postoperative pulmonary complications: a blinded prospective study of coronary artery bypass patients. Mayo Clin Proc 64:609, 1989

325. Robinson K, Conroy RM, Mulcahy R: When does the risk of acute coronary heart disease in ex-smokers fall to that in non-smokers? A retrospective study of patients admitted to hospital with a first episode of myocardial infarction or unstable angina. Br Heart J 62:16, 1989

326. Rosenberg L, Kaufman D, Helmrich S, Shapiro S: The risk of myocardial infarction after quitting smoking in men under 55 years of age. N Engl J Med 313:1511, 1985

327. Gordon T, Kannell WB, McGee D: Death and coronary attacks in men after giving up smoking: a report from the Framingham Study. Lancet 2:1345, 1974

328. Jajich CL, Ostfeld AM, Freeman DH, Jr: Smoking and coronary heart disease mortality in the elderly. JAMA 252:2831, 1984

329. Ernst E, Matrai A: Abstention from chronic cigarette smoking normalizes blood rheology. Atherosclerosis 64:75, 1987

330. Galae G, Davidson RJL: Haematological and haemorheological changes associated with cigarette smoking. J Clin Pathol 38:978, 1985

331. Celli BR, Rodriguez KS, Snider GL: A controlled trial of intermittent positive pressure breathing, incentive spirometry, and deep breathing exercises in preventing pulmonary complications after abdominal surgery. Am Rev Respir Dis 130:12, 1984

332. Bartlett RH, Brennan ML, Gazzaniga AB, et al: Studies on the pathogenesis and prevention of postoperative pulmonary complications. Surg Gynecol Obstet 137:925, 1973

333. Lyager S, Wernberg M, Rajani N, et al: Can postoperative pulmonary conditions be improved by treatment with the Bartlett-Edwards incentive spirometer after upper abdominal surgery? Acta Anaesthesiol Scand 23:312, 1979

334. Tisi GM: Preoperative evaluation of pulmonary function: validity, indications, benefits. Am Rev Respir Dis 119:293, 1979

335. Hedley-Whyte J, Burgess GE, Feeley TW, et al: Critical analysis of preventive measures. p. 119. In Applied Physiology of Respiratory Care. Little, Brown, Boston, 1976

336. Pontoppidan H: Mechanical aids to lung expansion in non-intubated surgical patients. Am Rev Respir Dis 122:109, 1980

337. Graham WGB, Bradley DA: Efficacy of chest physiotherapy in the resolution of pneumonia. N Engl J Med 299:624, 1978

338. Connors AF, Jr, Hammon WE, Martin RJ, et al: Chest physical therapy. The immediate effect on oxygenation in acutely ill patients. Chest 78:559, 1980

339. Cottrell JE, Siker ES: Preoperative intermittent positive pressure breathing therapy in patients with chronic obstructive lung disease: effect on postoperative pulmonary complications. Anesth Analg 52:258, 1973

340. Forthman HJ, Shepard A: Postoperative pulmonary complications. South Med J 62:1198, 1969

341. Boushy SF, Billing DM, North LB, et al: Clinical course related to preoperative pulmonary function in patients with bronchogenic carcinoma. Chest 59:383, 1971

342. Mittman C: Assessment of operative risk in thoracic surgery. Am Rev Respir Dis 84:197, 1961

343. Reichel J: Assessment of operative risk of pneumonectomy. Chest 62:570, 1972

344. Fischl MA, Pitchenik A, Gardner LB: An index predicting relapse and need for hospitalization in patients with acute bronchial asthma. N Engl J Med 305:783, 1981

345. Wiener-Kronish JP, Matthay MA: Preoperative evaluation.

p. 683. In Murray J, Nadel J (eds): Textbook of Respiratory Medicine. WB Saunders, Philadelphia, 1988

346. Roukema JA, Carol EJ, Prins JG: The prevention of pulmonary complications after upper abdominal surgery in patients with non-compromised pulmonary status. Arch Surg 123:30, 1988

347. Hall WJ, Douglas RG, Hyde RW, et al: Pulmonary mechanics after uncomplicated influenza A infection. Am Rev Respir Dis 113:141, 1976

348. Green GM, Jakab GJ, Low RB, et al: Defense mechanisms of the respiratory membrane. Am Rev Respir Dis 115:479, 1977

349. Tait AR, Ketcham TR, Klein MJ, et al: Perioperative respiratory complications in patients with upper respiratory tract infections. Anesthesiology 59:A433, 1983

350. Tait AR, Knight PR: The effects of general anesthesia on upper respiratory tract infections in children. Anesthesiology 67:930, 1987

351. DeSoto H, Patel RI, Soliman IE, Hannallah RS: Changes in oxygen saturation following general anesthesia in children with upper respiratory infection signs and symptoms undergoing otolaryngological procedures. Anesthesiology 68:276, 1988

352. Fishman AP: Cardiac asthma—a fresh look at an old wheeze. N Engl J Med 320:1346, 1989

353. Baughman RP, Loudon RC: Stridor: Differentiation from wheezing or upper airway noise. Am Rev Respir Dis 139:1407, 1989

354. Latimer RG, Dickman M, Day WC, et al: Ventilatory patterns and pulmonary complications after upper abdominal surgery determined by preoperative and postoperative computerized spirometry and blood gas analysis. Am J Surg 122:622, 1971

355. Tarhan S, Moffitt EA, Sessler AD, et al: Risk of anesthesia and surgery in patients with chronic bronchitis and chronic obstructive pulmonary disease. Surgery 74:720, 1973

356. Gould AB: Effect of obesity on respiratory complications following general anesthesia. Anesth Analg 41:448, 1962

357. Knudson J: Duration of hypoxemia after uncomplicated upper abdominal and thoraco-abdominal operations. Anaesthesia 25:372, 1970

358. Boysen PG, Block AJ, Moulder PV: Relationship between preoperative pulmonary function tests and complications after thoracotomy. Surg Gynecol Obstet 152:813, 1981

359. Furguson MK, Little L, Rizzo L, et al: Diffusing capacity predicts morbidity and mortality after pulmonary resection. J Thorac Cardiovasc Surg 96:894, 1988

360. Markos J, Mullan BP, Hillman DR, et al: Preoperative assessment as a predictor of mortality and morbidity after lung resection. Am Rev Respir Dis 139:902, 1989

361. Selzer A, Walter RM: Adequacy of preoperative digitalis therapy in controlling ventricular rate in postoperative atrial fibrillation. Circulation 34:119, 1966

362. Neiwoehner DE, Kleinerman J, Rice DB: Pathologic changes in the peripheral airways of young cigarette smokers. N Engl J Med 291:755, 1974

363. Enson Y: Pulmonary heart disease: relation of pulmonary hypertension to abnormal lung structure and function. Bull NY Acad Med 53:551, 1977

364. Edwards WD, Edwards JE: Clinical primary pulmonary hypertension: three pathologic types. Circulation 56:884, 1977

365. Reves JT, Groves BM, Turkevich D: The case for treatment of selected patients with primary pulmonary hypertension. Am Rev Respir Dis 134:342, 1986

366. Stein PD, Willis PW, III, DeMets DL: History and physical examination in acute pulmonary embolism in patients without preexisting cardiac or pulmonary disease. Am J Cardiol 47:218, 1981

367. Domino KB, Wetstein L, Glasser SA, et al: Influence of mixed venous oxygen tension ($P\bar{v}O_2$) on blood flow to atelectatic lung. Anesthesiology 59:428, 1983

368. Mendella LA, Manfreda J, Warren CPW, et al: Steroid response in stable chronic obstructive pulmonary disease. Ann Intern Med 96:17, 1982

369. Settipane GA, Dudupakkam RK: Aspirin intolerance. III: Subtypes, familial occurrence and cross reactivity with tartrazine. J Allergy Clin Immunol 56:215, 1975

370. Aubier M, De Troyer A, Sampson M, et al: Aminophylline improves diaphragmatic contractility. N Engl J Med 305:249, 1981

371. Crystal RG, Bitterman PB, Rennard SI, et al: Interstitial lung disease of unknown cause: disorders characterized by chronic inflammation of the lower respiratory tract. N Engl J Med 310:154, 1984

372. Baughman RP, Fernandez M, Bosken CH, et al: Comparison of gallium-67 scanning, bronchoalveolar lavage, and serum angiotensin-converting enzyme levels in pulmonary sarcoidosis: predicting response to therapy. Am Rev Respir Dis 129:676, 1984

373. Williams DE, Pairolero PC, Davis CS, et al: Survival of patients surgically treated for stage I lung cancer. J Thorac Cardiovasc Surg 82:70, 1981

374. Pitlik SD, Fainstein V, Bodey GP: Tuberculosis mimicking cancer—a reminder. Am J Med 76:822, 1984

374a. Ginsberg RJ, Hill LD, Eagan RT, et al: Modern thirty-day operative mortality for surgical resections in lung cancer. J Thorac Cardiovasc Surg 86:654, 1983

375. Sherman S, Guidot CE: The feasibility of thoracotomy for lung cancer in the elderly. JAMA 258:927, 1987

376. Levy JH, Roizen MF, Morris JM: Anaphylactic and anaphylactoid reactions: a review. Spine 11:282, 1986

377. Watkins J: Anaphylactoid reactions to I.V. substances. Br J Anaesth 51:51, 1979

378. Bristow MR, Ginsburg R, Harrison DC: Histamine and the human heart: the other receptor system. Am J Cardiol 49:249, 1982

379. Austen KF: Systemic anaphylaxis in the human being. N Engl J Med 291:661, 1974

380. Michelassi F, Landa L, Hill RD, et al: Leukotriene D$_4$: a potent coronary artery vasoconstrictor associated with impaired ventricular contraction. Science 217:841, 1982

381. Smith PL, Kagey-Sobotka A, Bleecker ER, et al: Physiologic manifestations of human anaphylaxis. J Clin Invest 66:1072, 1980

382. Delage C, Irey NS: Anaphylactic deaths: a clinicopathologic study of 43 cases. J Forensic Sci 17:525, 1972

383. Murano G: The "Hageman" connection: interrelationships of blood coagulation, fibrino(geno)lysis, kinin generation, and complement activation. Am J Hematol 4:409, 1978

384. Lasser EC, Lang JH, Hamblin AE, et al: Activation systems in contrast idiosyncrasy. Invest Radiol 15:suppl. 6, S2, 1980

385. Chenoweth DE, Cooper SW, Hugli TE, et al: Complement activation during cardiopulmonary bypass. N Engl J Med 304:497, 1981

386. Craddock PR, Fehr J, Brigham KL, et al: Complement and leukocyte-mediated pulmonary dysfunction in hemodialysis. N Engl J Med 296:769, 1977

387. Roizen MF, Rodgers GM, Valone FH, et al: Anaphylactoid reactions to vascular graft material presenting with vasodi-

lation and subsequent disseminated intravascular coagulation. Anesthesiology 71:331, 1989

388. Vercellotti GM, Hammerschmidt DE, Craddock PR, et al: Activation of plasma complement by perfluorocarbon artificial blood: probable mechanism of adverse pulmonary reactions in treated patients and rationale for corticosteroid prophylaxis. Blood 59:1299, 1982

389. Lorenz W, Doenicke A, Schöning B, et al: The role of histamine in adverse reactions to intravenous agents. p. 169. In Thornton JA (ed): Adverse Reactions of Anaesthetic Drugs. Elsevier/North Holland Biomedical Press, Amsterdam, 1981

390. Rosow CE, Moss J, Philbin DM, et al: Histamine release during morphine and fentanyl anesthesia. Anesthesiology 56:93, 1982

391. Moss J, Rosow CE, Savarese JJ, et al: Role of histamine in the hypotensive action of *d*-tubocurarine in humans. Anesthesiology 55:19, 1981

392. Hirshman CA, Peters J, Cartwright-Lee I: Leukocyte histamine release to thiopental. Anesthesiology 56:64, 1982

393. McCulloch JA: Chemonucleolysis: experience with 2000 cases. Clin Orthop 146:128, 1980

394. Moss J, McDermott DJ, Thisted RA, et al: Anaphylactic/anaphylactoid reactions in response to Chymodiactin (chymopapain). Anesth Analg 63:253, 1984

395. Millbern SM, Bell SD: Prevention of anaphylaxis to contrast media. Anesthesiology 50:56, 1979

396. Kaliner M, Sigler R, Summers R, et al: Effects of infused histamine: analysis of the effects of H-1 and H-2 histamine receptor antagonists on cardiovascular and pulmonary responses. J Allergy Clin Immunol 68:365, 1981

397. Philbin DM, Moss J, Akins CW, et al: The use of H_1 and H_2 histamine antagonists with morphine anesthesia: a double-blind study. Anesthesiology 55:292, 1981

398. Hammerschmidt DE, White JG, Craddock PR, et al: Corticosteroids inhibit complement-induced granulocyte aggregation: a possible mechanism for their efficacy in shock states. J Clin Invest 63:798, 1979

399. Halevy S, Altura BT, Altura BM: Pathophysiological basis for the use of steroids in the treatment of shock and trauma. Klin Wochenschr 60:1021, 1982

400. Ring J, Messmer K: Incidence and severity of anaphylactoid reactions to colloid volume substitutes. Lancet 1:466, 1977

401. Ring J, Stephan W, Brendel W: Anaphylactoid reactions to infusions of plasma protein and human serum albumin. Clin Allergy 9:89, 1979

402. Ellison N, Behar M, MacVaugh H, et al: Bradykinin, plasma protein fraction, and hypotension. Ann Thorac Surg 29:15, 1978

403. Milner LV, Butcher K: Transfusion reactions reported after transfusion of red blood cells and of whole blood. Transfusion 18:493, 1978

404. Barach EM, Nowak RM, Lee TG, et al: Epinephrine for treatment of anaphylactic shock. JAMA 251:2118, 1984

405. Schleimer RP, MacGlashan DW, Gillespie E, et al: Inhibition of basophil release by anti-inflammatory steroids. J Immunol 129:1632, 1982

406. Del Pizzo A: Hereditary angioneurotic edema. Anesthesiol Rev 5:41, 1978

407. Hosea SW, Santaella ML, Brown EJ, et al: Long-term therapy of hereditary angioedema with danazol. Ann Intern Med 93:809, 1982

408. Oxelius V-A, Laurell A-B, Lindquist B, et al: IgG subclasses in selective IgA deficiency. Importance of IgG2-IgA deficiency. N Engl J Med 304:1476, 1981

409. Fauci AS, Rosenberg SA, Sherwin SA, et al: Immunomodulators in clinical medicine. Ann Intern Med 106:421, 1987

410. Levy DE, Caronna JJ, Singer BH, et al: Predicting outcome from hypoxic-ischemic coma. JAMA 253:1420, 1985

411. Plum F, Posner JB: The Diagnosis of Stupor and Coma. 2nd Ed. FA Davis, Philadelphia, 1972

412. Lowenstein DH, Massa SM, Rowbotham MC, et al: Acute neurologic and psychiatric complications associated with cocaine abuse. Am J Med 83:841, 1987

413. Barry PP, Moskowitz MA: The diagnosis of reversible dementia in the elderly, a critical review. Arch Intern Med 148:1914, 1988

414. Boguosslavsky J, Meineberg O: Eye-movement disorders in brain-stem and cerebellar stoke. Arch Neurol 44:141, 1987

415. Drugs for epilepsy. Med Lett Drugs Ther 31:1, 1989

416. Montouris GD, Fenichel GM, McLain LW, Jr: The pregnant epileptic: a review and recommendations. Arch Neurol 36:601, 1979

417. Delgado-Escueta AV, Wasterlain C, Treiman DM, et al: Management of status epilepticus. N Engl J Med 306:1337, 1982

418. Joas TA, Stevens WC, Eger EI, II: Electroencephalographic seizure activity in dogs during anesthesia. Br J Anaesth 43:739, 1971

419. Buzello W, Jantzen K, Scholler KL: The influence of Ethrane on the electro- and pentylene-tetrazol-convulsions in mice. Anaesthesist 24:118, 1975

420. Wollman H, Smith AL, Neigh JL, et al: Cerebral blood flow and oxygen consumption in man during electroencephalographic seizure patterns associated with Ethrane anesthesia. p. 246. In Brock M, Fieschi C, et al (eds): Cerebral Blood Flow. Springer-Verlag, Berlin, 1969

421. Opitz A, Brechts B, Stenzel E: Enflurane anaesthesia for epileptic patients. Anaesthesist 26:329, 1977

422. Preventing spread of meningococcal disease. Med Lett Drugs Ther 23:37, 1981

423. The Parkinson Study Group: Effect of deprenyl on the progression of disability in early Parkinson's disease. N Engl J Med 321:1364, 1989

424. Diamond SG, Markham CH, Hoehn MM, et al: Multi-center study of Parkinson mortality with early versus later dopa treatment. Ann Neurol 22:8, 1987

425. Schwartz AJ, Wollman H: Anesthetic considerations for patients on chronic drug therapy: L-dopa, monamine oxidase inhibitors, tricyclic antidepressants and propranolol. p. 99. In Hershey SG (ed): ASA Refresher Courses in Anesthesiology. Vol. 4. JB Lippincott, Philadelphia, 1976

426. Ngai SH: Parkinsonism, levodopa, and anesthesia. Anesthesiology 37:344, 1972

427. Wiklund RA, Ngai SH: Rigidity, and pulmonary edema after Innovar in a patient on levodopa therapy: report of a case. Anesthesiology 35:545, 1971

428. Terry RD, Katzman R: Senile dementia of the Alzheimer type. Ann Neurol 14:497, 1983

429. Raskin NH, Appenzeller O: Major Problems in Internal Medicine. Vol. 19: Headache. WB Saunders, Philadelphia, 1980

430. Ovassapian A, Land P, Schafer MF, et al: Anesthetic management for surgical corrections of severe flexion deformity of the cervical spine. Anesthesiology 58:370, 1983

430a. Saper JR: Drug treatment of headache: changing concepts and treatment strategies. Semin Neurol 7:178, 1987

431. Dahm LS, Dickson JH, Harrison GH: Perioperative and anesthetic management in the patient with scoliosis. Anesthesiol Rev 9:13, 1982

432. Ferguson RJ, Caplan LR: Cervical spondylitic myelopathy. Neurol Clin 3:373, 1985

433. Baskett PJF, Armstrong R: Anaesthetic problems in multiple sclerosis: are certain agents contraindicated? Anaesthesia 25:397, 1970

434. Rojiani AM, Prineas JW, Cho ES: Protective effect of steroids on electrolyte-induced demyelination. J Neuropathol Exp Neurol 46:495, 1987

435. Cyr MG, Wartman SA: The effectiveness of routine screening questions in the detection of alcoholism. JAMA 259:51, 1988

436. Zinn SE, Fairley HB, Glenn JD: Liver function in patients with mild alcoholic hepatitis, after enflurane, nitrous oxide-narcotic, and spinal anesthesia. Anesth Analg 64:487, 1985

437. Tschudy DP, Valsamis M, Magnussen CR: Acute intermittent porphyria: clinical and selected research aspects. Ann Intern Med 83:851, 1975

438. Ellefson RD: Porphyrinogens, porphyrins, and the porphyrias. Mayo Clin Proc 57:454, 1982

439. Harrison GG, Moore MR, Meissner PN: Porphyrinogenicity of etomidate and ketamine as continuous infusions: screening in the DDC-primed rat model. Br J Anaesth 57:420, 1985

440. Blekkenhorst GH, Harrison GG, Cook ES, et al: Screening of certain anaesthetic agents for their ability to elicit acute porphyric phases in susceptible patients. Br J Anaesth 52:759, 1980

440a. Drachman DB, Adams RN, Josifek LF, et al: Functional activities of autoantibodies to acetylcholine receptors and the clinical severity of myasthenia gravis. N Engl J Med 307:769, 1982

441. d'Empaire G, Hoaglin DC, Perlo VP, et al: Effect of prethymectomy plasma exchange on postoperative respiratory function in myasthenia gravis. J Thorac Cardiovasc Surg 89:592, 1985

442. Eisenkraft JB, Book WJ, Mann SM et al: Resistance to succinylcholine in myasthenia gravis: a dose response study. Anesthesiology 69:760, 1988

443. Miller RD: Myasthenia gravis. p. 148. In Wilkinson PL, Ham J, Miller RD (eds): Clinical Anesthesia. Case Selections from the University of California, San Francisco. CV Mosby, St Louis, 1980

444. Eisenkraft JB, Papatestas AE, Kahn CH, et al: Predicting the need for postoperative mechanical ventilation in myasthenia gravis. Anesthesiology 65:79, 1986

445. Rolbin SH, Levinson G, Shnider SM, et al: Anesthetic considerations for myasthenia gravis and pregnancy. Anesth Analg 57:441, 1978

446. Leventhal SR, Orkin FK, Hirsh RA: Prediction of the need for postoperative mechanical ventilation in myasthenia gravis. Anesthesiology 53:26, 1980

447. Miller J, Lee C: Muscle diseases. p. 621. In Katz J, Benumof J, Kadis LB (eds): Anesthesia and Uncommon Diseases: Pathophysiologic and Clinical Correlations. 3rd Ed. WB Saunders, Philadelphia, 1989

448. Smith CL, Bush GH: Anesthesia and progressive muscular dystrophy. Br J Anaesth 57:1113, 1985

449. Schwartz L, Rockoff MA, Koka BV: Masseter spasm with anesthesia: incidence and implications. Anesthesiology 61:772, 1984

450. Rosenberg H: Trismus is not trivial (editorial). Anesthesiology 67:453, 1987

451. Britt BA (ed): Malignant hyperthermia. Int Anesthesiol Clin 17:1, 1979

452. Pueschel SM, Scola FH: Atlantoaxial instability in individuals with Down syndrome: epidemiologic, radiographic, and clinical studies. Pediatrics 80:55, 1987

453. Kobel M, Creighton RE, Steward DJ: Anaesthetic considerations in Down's syndrome: experience with 100 patients and a review of the literature. Can Anaesth Soc J 29:593, 1982

454. Bedford RF, Morris L, Jane JA: Intracranial hypertension during surgery for supratentorial tumor: correlation with preoperative computed tomography scans. Anesth Analg 61:430, 1982

454a. Allen GS, Ahn HS, Preziosi TJ, et al: Cerebral arterial spasm—a controlled trial of nimodipine in patients with subarachnoid hemorrhage. N Engl J Med 308:619, 1983

455. Ramirez-Lassepas M, Quinones MR: Heparin therapy for stroke: hemorrhagic complications and risk factors for intracerebral hemorrhage. Neurology (NY) 34:114, 1984

456. Rem JA, Hachinski VC, Boughner DR, Barnett HJ: Value of cardiac monitoring and echocardiography in TIA and stroke patients. Stroke 16:950, 1985

456a. Drugs for psychiatric disorders. Med Lett Drugs Ther 31:13, 1989

457. Appel GB, Neu HC: The nephrotoxicity of antimicrobial agents. N Engl J Med 296:663, 722, 784, 1977

458. Fischer RP, Polk HC, Jr: Changing etiologic patterns of renal insufficiency in surgical patients (editorial). Surg Gynecol Obstet 140:85, 1975

459. Brenowitz JB, Williams CD, Edwards WS: Major surgery in patients with chronic renal failure. Am J Surg 134:765, 1977

460. Bennett WM, Luft F, Porter GA: Pathogenesis of renal failure due to aminoglycosides and contrast media used in roentgenography. Am J Med 69:767, 1980

461. Myers BD, Moran SM: Hemodynamically medicated acute renal failure. N Engl J Med 314:97, 1986

462. Shusterman N, Strom BL, Murray TG, et al: Risk factors and outcome of hospital-acquired acute renal failure: a clinical epidemiologic study. Am J Med 83:65, 1987

463. Feldman HA, Singer I: Endocrinology and metabolism in uremia and dialysis: a clinical review. Medicine (Baltimore) 54:345, 1975

464. Walser M: Nutritional management of chronic renal failure. Am J Kidney Dis 1:261, 1982

465. Raskin NH, Fishman RA: Neurologic disorders in renal failure. N Engl J Med 294:143, 204, 1976

466. Vincenti F, Duca RM, Amend W, et al: Immunologic factors determining survival of cadaver-kidney transplants: the effect of HLA serotyping, cytotoxic antibodies and blood transfusions on graft survival. N Engl J Med 299:793, 1978

467. Rao KV, Anderson RC, O'Brien TJ: Factors contributing for improved graft survival in recipients of kidney transplants. Kidney Int 24:210, 1983

468. Eschbach JW, Egrie JC, Downing MR, et al: Correction of the anemia of end-stage renal disease with recombinant human erythropoietin: results of a combined phase I and II clinical trial. N Engl J Med 316:73, 1987

469. Eschbach JW, Kelly MR, Haley NR, et al: Treatment of the anemia of progressive renal failure with recombinant human erythropoietin. N Engl J Med 321:158, 1989

470. Burke GR, Gulyassy PF: Surgery in the patient with renal disease and related electrolyte disorders. Med Clin North Am 63:1191, 1979

471. Baek SM, Brown RS, Shoemaker WC: Early prediction of acute renal failure and recovery. Ann Surg 177:253, 1973

472. Landes RG, Lillehei RC, Lindsay WG, et al: Free water clearance and the early recognition of acute renal insuffi-

ciency after cardiopulmonary bypass. Ann Thorac Surg 22:41, 1976

473. Shin B, Isenhower NN, McAslan TC, et al: Early recognition of renal insufficiency in post-anesthetized trauma victims. Anesthesiology 50:262, 1979

474. Shin B, Mackenzie CF, Helrich M: Creatinine clearance for early detection of posttraumatic renal dysfunction. Anesthesiology 64:605, 1986

475. Rowe JW, Andres R, Tobin JD, et al: The effect of age on creatinine clearance in men: A cross-sectional and longitudinal study. J Gerontol 31:155, 1976

476. Abel RM, Buckley MJ, Austen WL: Etiology, incidence and prognosis of renal failure following cardiac operations. J Thorac Cardiovasc Surg 71:323, 1976

477. Hilberman M, Myers BD, Carrie BJ, et al: Acute renal failure following cardiac surgery. J Thorac Cardiovasc Surg 77:880, 1979

478. Koning HM, Koning AJ, Leusink JA: Serious acute renal failure following open heart surgery. Thorac Cardiovasc Surg 33:283, 1985

479. Kleinknecht D, Ganeval D, Gonzalez-Duque LA, et al: Furosemide in acute oliguric renal failure: a controlled trial. Nephron 17:51, 1976

480. Anderson RJ, Linas SL, Berns AS, et al: Nonoliguric acute renal failure. N Engl J Med 296:1134, 1977

481. Siegel DC, Cochin A, Geocaris T, et al: Effects of saline and colloid resuscitation on renal function. Ann Surgery 177:51, 1971

482. Miller TR, Anderson RJ, Linas SL, et al: Urinary diagnostic indices in acute renal failure. Ann Intern Med 89:47, 1978

483. Hanley MJ, Davidson K: Prior mannitol and furosemide infusion in a model of ischemic acute renal failure. Am J Physiol 241:F556, 1981

484. Davis RF, Lappas DG, Kirklin JK, et al: Acute oliguria after cardiopulmonary bypass: renal functional improvement with low-dose dopamine infusion. Crit Care Med 10:852, 1982

485. Polson RJ, Park GR, Lindop MJ, et al: The prevention of renal impairment in patients undergoing orthotopic liver grafting by infusion of low dose dopamine. Anaesthesia 42:15, 1987

486. Alpert RA, Roizen MF, Hamilton WK, et al: Intraoperative urinary output does not predict postoperative renal function in patients undergoing abdominal aortic revascularization. Surgery 95:707, 1984

487. Dolan MJ, Whipp BJ, Davidson WD, et al: Hypopnea associated with acetate hemodialysis: carbon dioxide-flow-dependent ventilation. N Engl J Med 305:72, 1981

488. Roth S, O'Connor M: Adverse cardiopulmonary sequelae after OKT3 administration (abstract). Anesthesiology 71:A944, 1989

489. Bennett WM, Aronoff GR, Morrison G, et al: Drug prescribing in renal failure: dosing guidelines for adults. Am J Kidney Dis 3:155, 1983

490. Rubin AL, Stenzel KH, Reidenberg MM: Symposium on drug action and metabolism in renal failure. Am J Med 62:459, 1977

491. Benet L (ed): The Effect of Disease States on Drug Pharmacokinetics. Am Pharmaceutical Assoc/Am Pharmaceutical Sci, Washington, DC, 1976

492. Gibson TP: Renal disease and drug metabolism: an overview. Am J Kidney Dis 8:7, 1986

493. Keighley MRB: Antibiotics in biliary disease: the relative importance of antibiotic concentrations in the bile and serum. Gut 17:495, 1976

494. Root RK, Hierholzer WJ, Jr: Infectious disease. p. 709. In Melmon KL, Morelli HF (eds): Clinical Pharmacology: Basic Principles in Therapeutics. 2nd Ed. Macmillan, New York, 1978

495. Robinson JA, Klodnycky ML, Loeb HS, et al: Endotoxin, prekallikrein, complement and systemic vascular resistance: sequential measurements in man. Am J Med 59:61, 1975

496. The Medical Letter on Drugs and Therapeutics Handbook of Antimicrobial Therapy. The Medical Letter, New Rochelle, N.Y., 1988

497. Platt R, Polk BF, Murdock B, et al: Mortality associated with nosocomial urinary-tract infection. N Engl J Med 307:637, 1982

498. Albert RK, Condie F: Hand-washing patterns in medical intensive-care units. N Engl J Med 304:1465, 1981

499. Farber BF, Kaiser DL, Wenzel RP: Relation between surgical volume and incidence of postoperative wound infection. N Engl J Med 305:200, 1981

500. Gross PA, Neu HC, Aswapokee P, et al: Deaths from nosocomial infections: experience in a university hospital and a community hospital. Am J Med 68:219, 1980

501. Bryan CS, Reynolds KL: Bacteremic nosocomial pneumonia: analysis of 172 epidoses from a single metropolitan area. Am Rev Respir Dis 129:668, 1984

502. Maki DG, Botticelli JT, Le Roy ML, Thielke TS: Prospective study of replacing administration sets for intravenous therapy at 48- vs 72-hour intervals: 72 hours is safe and cost-effective. JAMA 258:1771, 1987

503. Maki DG, Ringer M: Evaluation of dressing regimens for prevention of infection with peripheral intravenous catheters: gauze, a transparent polyurethane dressing, and an iodophor-transparent dressing. JAMA 258:2396, 1987

504. Popovic M, Sarngadharan MG, Read E, et al: Detection, isolation, and continuous production of cytopathic retroviruses (HTLV-III) from patients with AIDS and pre-AIDS. Science 224:497, 1984

505. Aach RD, Szmuness W, Mosley JW, et al: Serum alanine aminotransferase of donors in relation to the risk of non-A, non-B hepatitis in recipients: the transfusion-transmitted viruses study. N Engl J Med 304:989, 1981

506. Dworsky ME, Welch K, Cassady G, et al: Occupational risk for primary cytomegalovirus infection among pediatric health-care workers. N Engl J Med 309:950, 1983

507. Committee on Infections Within Hospitals, American Hospital Association: Infection Control in the Hospital. American Hospital Association, Chicago, 1979

508. Committee on Control of Surgical Infections, Altemeier WA (ed): Manual of Control of Infection in Surgical Patients. JB Lippincott, Philadelphia, 1976

509. Arieff AI, Llacki F, Massry SG: Neurologic manifestations and morbidity of hyponatremia: correlation with brain water and electrolytes. Medicine (Baltimore) 55:121, 1976

510. Rose BD: New approach to disturbances in the plasma sodium concentration. Am J Med 81:1033, 1986

511. Laski ME: Diuretics: mechanism of action and therapy. Semin Nephrol 6:210, 1986

512. Ayus JC, Krothapalli RK, Arieff AI: Changing concepts in the treatment of severe symptomatic hyponatremia: rapid correction and possible relation to central pontine myelinolysis. Am J Med 78:897, 1985

513. Muldowney FP, Williams RT: Clinical disturbances in serum sodium and potassium in relation to alteration in total exchangeable sodium, exchangeable potassium and total body water. Am J Med 35:768, 1963

514. Surawicz B: Relationship between electrocardiogram and electrolytes. Am Heart J 73:814, 1967

515. Sack D, Kim ND, Harrison CE, Jr: Contractility and subcel-

lular calcium metabolism in chronic potassium deficiency. Am J Physiol 226:756, 1974

516. Wong KC, Vitez TS: Electrolyte imbalance. Semin Anesth 2:161, 1983

517. Goggin MJ, Joekes AM: Gas exchange in renal failure. I: Dangers of hyperkalaemia during anaesthesia. Br Med J 2:244, 1971

518. Wright BD, Di Giovanni AJ: Respiratory alkalosis, hypokalemia and repeated ventricular fibrillation associated with mechanical ventilation. Anesth Analg 48:467, 1969

519. Edwards R, Winnie AP, Ramamurthy S: Acute hypocapneic hypokalemia: an iatrogenic anesthetic complication. Anesth Analg 56:786, 1977

520. Lawson NW, Butler GH, Rat CT: Alkalosis and cardiac arrhythmias. Anesth Analg 52:951, 1973

521. Aldinger KA, Samaan NA: Hypokalemia with hypercalcemia. Prevalence and significance in treatment. Ann Intern Med 87:571, 1977

522. Wong KC, Kawamura R, Hodges MR, et al: Acute intravenous administration of potassium chloride to furosemide pretreated dogs. Can Anaesth Soc J 24:203, 1977

523. Kawamura R, Wong KC, Hodges MR: Intravenous potassium chloride in hypokalemic dogs pretreated with digoxin. Anesth Analg 57:108, 1978

524. Kunin AS, Surawicz B, Sims EAH: Decrease in serum potassium concentrations and appearance of cardiac arrhythmias during infusion of potassium with glucose in potassium-depleted patients. N Engl J Med 266:228, 1962

525. Wilkinson PL, Ham J, Miller RD: Preoperative hyperkalemia and elective surgery. p. 54. In Wilkinson PL, Ham J, Miller RD (eds): Clinical Anesthesia. Case Selections from the University of California, San Francisco. CV Mosby, St Louis, 1980.

526. Lawson DH: Adverse reactions to potassium chloride. Q J Med 43:433, 1974

527. Lawson DH, Hutcheon AW, Jick H: Life threatening drug reactions amongst medical in-patients. Scott Med J 24:127, 1979

528. Vitez TS, Soper LE, Wong KC, Soper P: Chronic hypokalemia and intraoperative dysrhythmias. Anesthesiology 63:130, 1985

529. Hirsch IA, Tomlinson DL, Slogoff S, Keats AS: The overstated risk of preoperative hypokalemia. Anesth Analg 67:131, 1988

530. Dyckner T, Wester PO: Ventricular extrasystoles and intracellular electrolytes before and after potassium and magnesium infusions in patients on diuretic treatment. Am Heart J 97:12, 1979

531. Cohen JD, Neaton JD, Prineas RJ, Daniels KA: Diuretics, serum potassium and ventricular arrhythmias in the multiple risk factor intervention. Am J Cardiol 60:548, 1987

532. Morganroth J, Michelson EL, Horowitz LN, et al: Limitations of routine long-term electrocardiographic monitoring to assess ventricular ectopic frequency. Circulation 58:408, 1978

533. Duke M: Thiazide-induced hypokalemia: association with acute myocardial infarction and ventricular fibrillation. JAMA 239:43, 1978

534. Holland OB, Nixon JV, Kuhnert L: Diuretic-induced ventricular ectopic activity. Am J Med 70:762, 1981

535. Harrington JT, Isner JM, Kassirerr JP: Our national obsession with potassium. Am J Med 73:155, 1982

536. Tanifuji Y, Eger EI, II: Brain sodium, potassium and osmolality: Effect on anesthetic requirement. Anesth Analg 57:404, 1978

537. Lennard-Jones JE: Medical treatment of ulcerative colitis. Postgrad Med J 60:797, 1984

538. May RJ, Long BW, Gardner JD: H_2-histamine receptor blocking agents in the Zollinger-Ellison syndrome. Ann Intern Med 87:668, 1977

539. Eger EI, II, Saidman LJ: Hazards of nitrous oxide anesthesia in bowel obstruction and pneumothorax. Anesthesiology 26:61, 1965

540. Hospital Infections Branch, Bacterial Diseases Bureau of Epidemiology, CDC: Trends in surgical wound infection rates. MMWR 29:27, 33, 1980

541. Ross AHM, Smith MA, Anderson JR, et al: Late mortality after surgery for peptic ulcer. N Engl J Med 307:519, 1982

542. Longnecker M, Roizen MF: Patients with carcinoid syndrome. Anesthesiol Clin North Am 5:313, 1987

543. Kvols LK, Moertel CG, O'Connell MJ, et al: Treatment of the malignant carcinoid syndrome: evaluation of a long-acting somatostatin analogue. N Engl J Med 315:663, 1986

544. Quantrini M, Basilisco G, Conte D, et al: Effects of somatostatin infusion in four patients with malignant carcinoid syndrome. Am J Gastroenterol 78:149, 1983

545. Roizen MF, Moss J, Henry DP, et al: Effect of general anesthetics on handling- and decapitation-induced increases in sympathoadrenal discharge. J Pharmacol Exp Ther 204:11, 1978

546. Shnider SM, Wright RG, Levinson G, et al: Uterine blood flow and plasma norepinephrine changes during maternal stress in the pregnant ewe. Anesthesiology 50:524, 1979

547. Philbin DM, Coggins CH: Plasma antidiuretic hormone levels in cardiac surgical patients during morphine and halothane anesthesia. Anesthesiology 49:95, 1978

548. Muldoon SM, Moss J, Freas W, et al: The effects of anaesthetics on the sympathoadrenal system. Clin Anaesthesiol 2:289, 1984

549. Wataneeyawech M, Kelly KA, Jr: Hepatic diseases, unsuspected before surgery. NY State J Med 75:1278, 1975

550. Schemel WH: Unexpected hepatic dysfunction found by multiple laboratory screening. Anesth Analg 55:810, 1976

551. Clark R, Doggart J, Tavery T: Changes in liver function after different types of surgery. Br J Anaesth 48:119, 1976

552. Stevens WC, Eger EI II, Joas TA, et al: Comparative toxicity of isoflurane, halothane, fluroxene, and diethyl ether in human volunteers. Can Anaesth Soc J 20:357, 1973

553. Gelman SI, Fowler KC, Smith LR: Liver circulation and function during isoflurane and halothane anesthesia. Anesthesiology 61:726, 1984

554. Akdikem S, Flanagan TV, Landmesser CM: A comparative study of serum glutamic pyruvic transaminase changes following anesthesia with halothane, methoxyflurane, and other inhalation agents. Anesth Analg 45:819, 1966

555. Strunin L: Preoperative assessment of the patient with liver dysfunction. Br J Anaesth 50:25, 1978

556. Harville DD, Summerskill WH: Surgery in acute hepatitis—cause and effects. JAMA 184:257, 1963

557. Farman JV: Anaesthesia in the presence of liver disease and for hepatic transplantation. Br J Anaesth 44:946, 1972

558. Viegas O, Stoelting RK: LDH_5 changes after cholecystectomy and hysterectomy in patients receiving halothane, enflurane or fentanyl. Anesthesiology 51:556, 1979

559. Smith AA, Volpitto PP, Gramling ZW, et al: Chloroform, halothane and regional anesthesia: a comparative study. Anesth Analg 52:1, 1973

560. Ronk W: Liver function chemistries after enflurane and narcotic-N_2O anesthesia. AANA J 46:507, 1978

561. The National Halothane Study, Bunker JP, Forrest WH,

Mosteller F, et al (eds): A Study of the Possible Association Between Halothane Anesthesia and Postoperative Hepatic Necrosis. US Government Printing Office, Washington, D.C., 1969

562. Evans C, Evans M, Pollock AV: The incidence and causes of postoperative jaundice. Br J Anaesth 46:520, 1974

563. Shingu K, Eger EI, II, Johnson BH, et al: Effect of oxygen concentration, hyperthermia, and choice of vendor on anesthetic-induced hepatic injury in rats. Anesth Analg 62:146, 1983

564. La Mont JT: Postoperative jaundice. Surg Clin North Am 54:637, 1974

565. Black PM: Predicting the outcome from hypoxic-ischemic coma: medical and ethical implications. JAMA 254:1215, 1985

566. Dawson JL: The incidence of postoperative renal failure in obstructive jaundice. Br J Surg 52:663, 1965

567. Green J, Beyar R, Sideman S, et al: The "jaundiced heart": a possible explanation for postoperative shock in obstructive jaundice. Surgery 100:14, 1986

568. Aranha GV, Sontag SJ, Greenlee HB: Cholecystectomy in cirrhotic patients: a formidable operation. Am J Surg 143:55, 1982

569. Metcalf AMT, Dozois RR, Wolff BG, Beart RW, Jr: The surgical risk of colectomy in patients with cirrhosis. Dis Colon Rectum 30:529, 1987

570. Resnick RH, Iber FL, Ishihara AM, et al: A controlled study of the therapeutic portacaval shunt. Gastroenterology 67:843, 1974

571. Wright R, Eade OE, Chisholm M, et al: Controlled prospective study of the effect on liver function of multiple exposures to halothane. Lancet 6:817, 1975

572. Trowell J, Peto R, Smith AC: Controlled trial of repeated halothane anaesthetics in patients with carcinoma of the uterine cervix treated with radium. Lancet 1:821, 1975

573. Allen PJ, Downing JW: A prospective study of hepatocellular function after repeated exposures to halothane or enflurane in women undergoing radium therapy for cervical cancer. Br J Anaesth 49:1035, 1977

574. Fee JPH, Black GW, Dundee JW, et al: A prospective study of liver enzyme and other changes following repeat administration of halothane and enflurane. Br J Anaesth 51:1133, 1979

575. Dykes MHM: Is halothane hepatitis chronic active hepatitis? (editorial). Anesthesiology 46:233, 1977

576. Vergani D, Tsantoulas D, Eddleston ALWF, et al: Sensitization to halothane—altered liver components in severe hepatic necrosis after halothane anesthesia. Lancet 2:801, 1978

577. Bréchot C, Nalpas B, Couroucé A-M, et al: Evidence that hepatitis B virus has a role in liver-cell carcinoma in alcoholic liver disease. N Engl J Med 306:1384, 1982

578. Thomas FB: Chronic aggressive hepatitis induced by halothane. Ann Intern Med 81:487, 1974

579. Berman M, Alter JH, Ishak KG, et al: The chronic sequelae of non-A, non-B hepatitis. Ann Intern Med 91:1, 1979

580. Sipes I, Brown B: An animal model of hepatotoxicity associated with halothane anesthesia. Anesthesiology 45:622, 1976

581. Klatskin G, Kimberg DV: Recurrent hepatitis attributable to halothane sensitization in an anesthetist. N Engl J Med 280:515, 1969

582. Douglas HJ, Eger EI, II, Biava CG, et al: Hepatic necrosis associated with viral infection after enflurane anesthesia. N Engl J Med 296:553, 1977

583. Gall EA: Report of the pathology panel: National Halothane Study. Anesthesiology 29:233, 1968

584. Wright EC, Seeff LB, Berk PD, et al: Treatment of chronic active hepatitis. An analysis of three controlled trials. Gastroenterology 73:1422, 1977

585. Reynolds TB: Chronic hepatitis: current dilemmas. Am J Med 69:485, 1980

586. Alter MJ: Non-A, Non-B hepatitis: sorting through a diagnosis of exclusion. Ann Intern Med 110:583, 1989

587. Stoelting RK, Blitt CD, Cohen PJ, Merin RG: Hepatic dysfunction after isoflurane anesthesia. Anesth Analg 66:147, 1987

588. Plummer JL, Hall PM, Jenner M, et al: Effect of treatment with phenobarbitone or isoniazid on hepatotoxicity due to prolonged subanesthetic halothane inhalation. Pharmacol Toxicol 62:74, 1988

589. Hubbard AK, Roth TP, Gandolfi AJ, et al: Halothane hepatitis patients generate an antibody response toward a covalently bound metabolite of halothane. Anesthesiology 68:791, 1988

590. Farrell G, Prendergast D, Murray M: Halothane hepatitis: detection of constitutional susceptibility factor. N Engl J Med 313:1310, 1985

591. Nomura F, Hatano H, Iida S, Onishi K: Halothane hepatotoxicity and reductive metabolism of halothane in acute experimental liver injury in rats. Anesth Analg 67:448, 1988

592. Hussey AJ, Howie J, Allan LG, et al: Impaired hepatocellular integrity during general anaesthesia, as assessed by measurement of plasma glutathione S-transferase. Clin Chim Acta 161:19, 1986

593. Moore DH, Benson GD: Prolonged halothane hepatitis: prompt resolution of severe lesion with corticosteroid therapy. Dig Dis Sci 31:1269, 1986

594. Lewis JH, Zimmerman HJ, Ishak KG, Mullick FG: Enflurane hepatotoxicity: a clinicopathologic study of 24 cases. Ann Intern Med 98:984, 1983

595. Stevens CE, Taylor PE, Rubinstein P, et al: Safety of the hepatitis B vaccine. N Engl J Med 312:375, 1985

595a. Richter JM, Silverstein MD, Schapiro R: Suspected obstructive jaundice: a decision analysis of diagnostic strategies. Ann Intern Med 99:46, 1983

596. Berry AJ, Isaacson IJ, Hunt D, et al: The prevalence of hepatitis B viral markers in anesthesia personnel. Anesthesiology 60:6, 1984

597. Mulley AG, Silverstein MD, Dienstag JL: Indications for use of hepatitis B vaccine, based on cost-effectiveness analysis. N Engl J Med 307:644, 1982

598. Naulty JS, Reves JG, Tobey RR, et al: Hepatitis and operating room personnel: an approach to diagnosis and management. Anesth Analg 56:360, 1977

599. Duvaldestin P, Agoston S, Henzel D, et al: Pancuronium pharmacokinetics in patients with liver cirrhosis. Br J Anaesth 50:1131, 1978

600. Orko R, Ailia A, Rosenberg PH: Effect of biliary obstruction on muscle relaxation with vecuronium. Eur J Anaesthesiol 5:9, 1988

601. Arden JR, Lynam DP, Castagnoli KP, et al: Vecuronium in alcoholic liver disease: a pharmacokinetic and pharmacodynamic analysis. Anesthesiology 68:771, 1988

602. Wasserman LR, Gilbert HS: Surgical bleeding in polycythemia vera. Ann NY Acad Sci 115:122, 1964

603. Rothstein P: What hemoglobin level is adequate in pediatric anesthesia? Anesthesiol Update 1(24):2, 1978

604. Slogoff S: Anesthesia considerations in the anemic patient. Anesthesiol Update 2(7):1, 1979

605. Thomas DJ, Du Boulay GH, Marshall J, et al: Effect of hematocrit on cerebral blood flow in man. Lancet 2:941, 1977

606. York EL, Jones RL, Menon D, et al: Effects of secondary polycythemia on cerebral blood flow in chronic obstructive pulmonary disease. Am Rev Respir Dis 121:813, 1980

607. Thomas DJ: Whole blood viscosity and cerebral blood flow (editorial). Stroke 13:285, 1982

608. Crystal GJ, Rooney MW, Salem MR: Myocardial blood flow and oxygen consumption during isovolemic hemodilution alone and in combination with adenosine-induced controlled hypotension. Anesth Analg 67:539, 1988

609. Heughan C, Grislis G, Hunt TK: The effect of anemia on wound healing. Ann Surg 179:163, 1974

610. Lichtiger B, Dupuis JF, Seski J: Hemotherapy during surgery for Jehovah's Witnesses: a new method. Anesth Analg 61:618, 1982

611. Tremper KK, Friedman AE, Levine EM, et al: The preoperative treatment of severely anemic patients with a perfluorochemical oxygen-transport fluid, Fluosol-DA. N Engl J Med 307:277, 1982

612. Greenburg AG: Blood substitutes: where are we? Surg Annu 15:13, 1983

613. Goodnough LT, Rudnick S, Price TH, et al: Increased preoperative collection of autologous blood with recombinant human erythropoietin therapy. N Engl J Med 321:1163, 1989

614. Embury SH: The clinical pathophysiology of sickle cell disease. Annu Rev Med 37:361, 1986

615. Heller P, Best WR, Nelson RB, et al: Clinical implication of sickle cell trait and glucose-6-phosphate dehydrogenase deficiency in hospitalized black male patients. N Engl J Med 300:1001, 1979

616. Dalal FY, Schmidt GB, Bennett EJ, et al: Sickle-cell trait, a report of a postoperative neurological complication. Br J Anaesth 46:387, 1974

617. Oduro KA, Searle JF: Anaesthesia in sickle-cell states: a plea for simplicity. Br Med J 4:596, 1972

618. Dunn A, Davies A, Eckert G, et al: Intraoperative death during caesarean section in a patient with sickle-cell trait. Can J Anaesth 34:67, 1987

619. Homi J, Reynolds J, Skinner A, et al: General anesthesia in sickle-cell disease. Br Med J 1:1599, 1979

620. Bischoff RJ, Williamson A, III, Dalali MJ, et al: Assessment of the use of transfusion therapy perioperatively in patients with sickle cell hemoglobinopathies. Ann Surg 435, 1988

621. Morrison JC, Wiser WL: The use of prophylactic partial exchange transfusion in pregnancies associated with sickle cell hemoglobinopathy. Obstet Gynecol 48:516, 1976

622. Morrison JC, Whybrew WD, Bucovaz ET: Use of partial exchange transfusion preoperatively in patients with sickle cell hemoglobinopathies. Am J Obstet Gynecol 132:59, 1978

623. Lanzkowsky P, Shende A, Karayalcin G, et al: Partial exchange transfusion in sickle cell anemia: use in children with serious complications. Am J Dis Child 132:1206, 1978

624. Tuck SM, James CE, Brewster EM, et al: Prophylactic blood transfusion in maternal sickle cell syndromes. Br J Obstet Gynecol 94:121, 1987

625. Rosa RM, Bierer BE, Thomas R, et al: A study of induced hyponatremia in the prevention and treatment of sickle-cell crisis. N Engl J Med 303:1138, 1980

626. Orr D: Difficult intubation: a hazard in thalassemia. A case report. Br J Anaesth 39:585, 1967

627. Pootrakul P, Hungsprenges S, Fucharoen S, et al: Relation between erythropoiesis and bone metabolism in thalassemia. N Engl J Med 304:1470, 1981

628. Lux SE, Wolfe LC: Inherited disorders of the red cell membrane skeleton. Pediatr Clin North Am 27:463, 1980

629. Frank MM, Schreiber AD, Atkinson JP, et al: Pathophysiology of immune hemolytic anemia. Ann Intern Med 87:210, 1979

630. Loque G, Rosse W: Immunologic mechanisms in autoimmune hemolytic disease. Semin Hematol 13:277, 1976

631. Alavi JB, Root RK, Djerassi I, et al: A randomized clinical trial of granulocyte transfusion for infection in acute leukemia. N Engl J Med 296:706, 1977

632. Winston DJ, Ho WG, Gale RP: Therapeutic granulocyte transfusions for documented infections: a controlled trial in ninety-five infectious granulocytopenic episodes. Ann Intern Med 97:509, 1982

633. Strauss RG, Connett JE, Gale RP, et al: A controlled trial of prophylactic granulocyte transfusions during initial induction chemotherapy for acute myelogenous leukemia. N Engl J Med 305:597, 1981

634. Quie PG: The white cells: use of granulocyte transfusions. Rev Infect Dis 9:189, 1987

635. Petrovitch CT: The bleeding patient. p. 465. In Roizen MF (ed): Anesthesia for Vascular Surgery. Churchill Livingstone, New York, 1990

635a. Lacey JV, Penner JA: Management of idiopathic thrombocytopenic purpura in the adult. Semin Thromb Hemost 3:160, 1977

636. Kelton JG: Management of the pregnant patient with idiopathic thrombocytopenic purpura. Ann Intern Med 99:796, 1983

637. Tyler DC: Anesthetic management of hemolytic-uremic syndrome. Anesthesiol Rev 9:23, 1982

638. Simpson MB: Platelet function and transfusion therapy in the surgical patient. p. 51. In Schiffer CJ (ed): Platelet Physiology and Transfusion. American Association of Blood Banks, Washington, D.C., 1978

639. Davis DW, Steward DT: Unexplained excessive bleeding during operation: role of acetylsalicylic acid. Can Anaesth Soc J 24:452, 1977

640. Majerus PW, Miletich JP: Relationships between platelets and coagulation factors in hemostasis. Annu Rev Med 29:41, 1978

641. Evans BE: Dental treatment for hemophiliacs: evaluation of dental program (1975–1976) at the Mount Sinai Hospital International Hemophilia Training Center. Mt Sinai J Med 44:409, 1977

642. Zauber NP, Levin J: Factor IX levels in patients with hemophilia B (Christmas disease) following transfusion with concentrates of factor IX or fresh frozen plasma (FFP). Medicine (Baltimore) 56:213, 1977

643. Gralnick HR, Coller BS, Schulman NR, et al: Factor VIII. Ann Intern Med 86:598, 1977

644. Curran JW, Lawrence DN, Jaffe H, et al: Acquired immunodeficiency syndrome (AIDS) associated with transfusions. N Engl J Med 310:69, 1984

644a. Safety of therapeutic products used for hemophilia patients. MMWR 37:441, 1988

645. Briere RO: Serum ALT levels: effect of sex, race, and obesity on unit rejection rate. Transfusion 28:392, 1988

646. Bove JR: Transfusion-transmitted diseases: current problems and challenges. Prog Hematol 14:123, 1986

647. Miller RD: Complications of massive blood transfusions. Anesthesiology 39:82, 1973

648. Sherman LA: Alterations in hemostasis during massive transfusion. p. 51. In Nusbacher J (ed): Massive Transfusion. American Association of Blood Banks, Washington, D.C., 1978

649. Lee KF, Manchell J, Rankin JS, et al: Immediate versus delayed coronary grafting after streptokinase treatment: postoperative blood loss and clinical results. J Thorac Cardiovasc Surg 95:216, 1988

650. Czer LS, Bateman TM, Gary RJ, et al: Treatment of severe platelet dysfunction and hemorrhage after cardiopulmonary bypass: reduction in blood product usage with desmopressin. J Am Coll Cardiol 9:1139, 1987

651. Marks RM, Sachar EJ: Undertreatment of medical inpatients with narcotic analgesics. Ann Intern Med 78:173, 1973

652. Brigden ML, Barnett JB: A practical approach to improving pain control in cancer patients. West J Med 146:580, 1987

653. Vitez TS, Way WL, Miller RD, et al: Effect of delta-9-tetrahydrocannabinol on cyclopropane MAC in the rat. Anesthesiology 38:525, 1973

654. Cancer chemotherapy. Med Lett Drugs Ther 29:29, 1987

655. Chung F: Cancer, chemotherapy, and anesthesia. Can Anaesth Soc J 29:364, 1982

656. Goldiner P, Carlon GC, Cvitkovic E, et al: Factors influencing postoperative morbidity and mortality in patients treated with bleomycin. Br Med J 1:1664, 1978

657. LaMantia KR, Glick JH, Marshall BE: Supplemental oxygen does not cause respiratory failure in bleomycin-treated surgical patients. Anesthesiology 60:65, 1984

658. Singer MM, Wright F, Stanley LK, et al: Oxygen toxicity in man: a prospective study in patients after open-heart surgery. N Engl J Med 283:1473, 1970

659. Weiner N, Taylor P: Neurohumoral transmission and the autonomic nervous system. p. 66. In Gilman AG, Goodman LS, Rall TW, et al (eds): Goodman and Gilman's The Pharmacological Basis of Therapeutics. 7th Ed. Macmillan, New York, 1985

660. Lake CR, Chernow B, Feuerstein G, et al: The sympathetic nervous system in man: its evaluation and the measurement of plasma NE. p. 1. In Ziegler MG, Lake CR (eds): Norepinephrine. Williams & Wilkins, Baltimore, 1984.

661. Burn JH, Rand MJ: Actions of sympathomimetic amines on animals treated with reserpine. J Physiol (Lond) 144:314, 1958

662. Drugs for hypertension. Med Lett Drugs Ther 31:25, 1989

663. Woodside J, Jr, Garner L, Bedford RF, et al: Captopril reduces the dose requirement for sodium nitroprusside induced hypotension. Anesthesiology 60:413, 1984

664. Sethna DH, Gray RJ, Moffitt EA, et al: Dobutamine and cardiac oxygen balance in patients following myocardial revascularization. Anesth Analg 61:917, 1982

665. The Norwegian Multicenter Study Group: Timolol-induced reduction in mortality and reinfarction in patients surviving acute myocardial infarction. N Engl J Med 304:801, 1981

666. Sleight P: Beta-adrenergic blockade after myocardial infarction (editorial). N Engl J Med 304:837, 1981

667. Frishman WH, Furberg CD, Friedewald WT: β-Adrenergic blockade for survivors of acute myocardial infarction. N Engl J Med 310:830, 1984

668. Smulyan H, Weinberg SE, Howanitz PJ: Continuous propranolol infusion following abdominal surgery. JAMA 247:2539, 1982

669. Slogoff S, Keats AS, Hibbs CW, et al: Failure of general anesthesia to potentiate propranolol activity. Anesthesiology 47:504, 1977

670. Girard D, Shulman BJ, Thys DM, et al: The safety and efficacy of esmolol during myocardial revascularization. Anesthesiology 65:157, 1986

671. Tanifuji Y, Eger EI, II: Effect of isoproterenol and propranolol on halothane MAC in dogs. Anesth Analg 55:383, 1976

672. Kaukinen S, Pyykkö K: The potentiation of halothane anaesthesia by clonidine. Acta Anaesthesiol Scand 23:107, 1979

673. Bloor BC, Flacke WE: Reduction in halothane anesthetic requirement by clonidine, an alpha-adrenergic agonist. Anesth Analg 61:741, 1982

674. Weinger MB, Segal IS, Maze M: Dexmedetomidine, acting through central alpha-2 adrenoceptors, prevents opiate-induced muscle rigidity in the rat. Anesthesiology 71:242, 1989

675. Miller RD, Sohn YJ, Matteo RS: Enhancement of *d*-tubocurarine neuromuscular blockade by diuretics in man. Anesthesiology 45:442, 1976

676. Tosone SR, Reves JG, Kissin I, et al: Hemodynamic responses to nifedipine in dogs anesthetized with halothane. Anesth Analg 62:903, 1983

677. Millard RW, Grupp G, Grupp IL, et al: Chronotropic, inotropic, and vasodilator actions of diltiazem, nifedipine, and verapamil. Circ Res 52:suppl. I, I29, 1983

678. Braunwald E: Mechanism of action of calcium-channel-blocking agents. N Engl J Med 307:1618, 1982

679. Maze M, Mason DM: Verapamil decreases the MAC for halothane in dogs. Anesth Analg 62:274, 1983

680. Reves JG, Kissin I, Lell WA, et al: Calcium entry blockers: uses and implications for anesthesiologists. Anesthesiology 57:504, 1982

681. Springman SR, Redon D, Rusy BF: The effect of nifedipine on the circulation during morphine-N_2O and halothane anesthesia in dogs. Anesth Analg 62:284, 1983

682. Hysing ES, Chelly JE, Doursout M-F: Cardiovascular effects of and interaction between calcium blocking drugs and anesthetics in chronically instrumented dogs. III: Nicardipine and isoflurane. Anesthesiology 65:385, 1986

683. Merin RG, Chelly JE, Hysing ES, et al: Cardiovascular effects of and interaction between calcium blocking drugs and anesthetics in chronically instrumented dogs. IV: Chronically administered oral verapamil and halothane, enflurane, and isoflurane. Anesthesiology 66:140, 1987

684. Kapur PA, Matarazzo DA, Fung DM, Sullivan KB: The cardiovascular and adrenergic actions of verapamil or diltiazem in combination with propranolol during halothane anesthesia in the dog. Anesthesiology 66:122, 1987

685. Fanta CH, Drazen JM: Calcium blockers and bronchoconstriction (editorial). Am Rev Respir Dis 127:673, 1983

686. Epstein SE, Rosing DR: Verapamil: Its potential for causing serious complications in patients with hypertrophic cardiomyopathy. Circulation 64:437, 1981

687. Dale J, Landmark KH, Myhre E: The effects of nifedipine, a calcium antagonist, on platelet function. Am Heart J 105:103, 1983

688. Zalman F, Perloff JK, Durant NN, et al: Acute respiratory failure following intravenous verapamil in Duchenne's muscular dystrophy. Am Heart J 105:510, 1983

689. White BC, Gadzinski DS, Hoehner PJ, et al: Effect of flunarizine on canine cerebral cortical blood flow and vascular resistance post cardiac arrest. Ann Emerg Med 11:119, 1982

690. McAllister RG, Jr: Clinical pharmacokinetics of calcium channel antagonists. J Cardiovasc Pharmacol 4:suppl. 3, S340, 1982

691. Kapur PA, Flacke WE: Epinephrine-induced arrhythmias and cardiovascular function after verapamil during halothane anesthesia in the dog. Anesthesiology 55:218, 1981

692. Zimpfer M, Fitzal S, Tonzcar L: Verapamil as a hypotensive agent during neuroleptanaesthesia. Br J Anaesth 53:885, 1981

693. Durant NN, Nguyen N, Katz RL: Potentiation of neuromuscular blockade by verapamil. Anesthesiology 60:298, 1984

694. Nugent M, Tinker JH, Moyer TP: Verapamil worsens rate of development and hemodynamic effects of acute hyperkalemia in halothane anesthetized dogs: effects of calcium therapy. Anesthesiology 60:435, 1984

695. Lalka SG, Rhodes RS, Lina AA, et al: Effect of calcium entry and β blockade during infrarenal aortic clamping. J Surg Res 46:246, 1989

696. Michaels I, Serrins M, Shier NQ, Barash PG: Anesthesia for cardiac surgery in patients receiving monoamine oxidase inhibitors. Anesth Analg 63:1014, 1984

697. Evans-Prosser CDG: The use of pethidine and morphine in the presence of monamine oxidase inhibitors. Br J Anaesth 40:279, 1968

698. Campbell GD: Dangers of monamine oxidase inhibitors. Br Med J 1:750, 1963

699. Rogers KJ, Thornton JA: The interaction between monamine oxidase inhibitors and narcotic analgesics in mice. Br J Pharmacol 36:470, 1969

700. Sjoqvist F: Psychotropic drugs. 2: Interaction between monoamine oxidase (MAO) inhibitors and other substances. Proc R Soc Med 58:967, 1965

701. Monamine oxidase inhibitors for depression. Med Lett Drugs Ther 31:11, 1989

702. Drugs for psychiatric disorders. Med Lett Drugs Ther 31:13, 1989

703. El-Ganzouri AR, Ivankovich AD, Braverman B, McCarthy R: Monoamine oxidase inhibitors: should they be discontinued preoperatively? Anesth Analg 64:592, 1985

704. Edwards RE, Miller RD, Roizen MF, et al: Cardiac effects of imipramine and pancuronium during halothane and enflurane anesthesia. Anesthesiology 50:421, 1979

705. Kosanin R: Anesthetic considerations in patients on chronic tricyclic antidepressant therapy. Anesthesiol Rev 8:38, 1981

706. Veith RC, Raskind MA, Caldwell JH, et al: Cardiovascular effects of tricyclic antidepressants in depressed patients with chronic heart disease. N Engl J Med 306:954, 1982

707. Richelson E, El-Fakahany E: Changes in the sensitivity of receptors for neurotransmitters and the actions of some psychotherapeutic drugs. Mayo Clin Proc 57:576, 1982

708. Hill GE, Wong KC: Lithium carbonate and neuromuscular blocking agents. Anesthesiology 46:122, 1977

709. Martin BA, Kramer PM: Clinical significance of the interaction between lithium and a neuromuscular blocker. Am J Psychiatry 139:1326, 1982

710. Johnston RR, Way WL, Miller RD: Alteration of anesthetic requirements by amphetamine. Anesthesiology 36:357, 1972

711. Stoelting RK, Creasser CW, Martz RC: Effect of cocaine administration on halothane MAC in dogs. Anesth Analg 54:422, 1975

712. Katz RL, Bigger JT: Cardiac arrhythmias during anesthesia and operation. Anesthesiology 33:193, 1970

713. Joas TA, Stevens WC: Comparison of the arrhythmic doses of epinephrine during Forane, halothane and enflurane anesthesia in dogs. Anesthesiology 35:48, 1971

714. Johnston RR, Eger EI, II, Wilson C: A comparative interaction of epinephrine with enflurane, isoflurane and halothane in man. Anesth Analg 55:709, 1976

715. Horrigan RW, Eger EI, II, Wilson CB: Epinephrine-induced arrhythmias during enflurane anesthesia in man: a nonlinear dose–response relationship and dose-dependent protection from lidocaine. Anesth Analg 57:547, 1978

716. Hirshman CA, Bergman NA: Halothane and enflurane protect against bronchospasm in an asthma dog model. Anesth Analg 57:629, 1978

717. Shnider SM, Papper EM: Anesthesia for the asthmatic patient. Anesthesiology 22:886, 1961

718. Marcus ML, Skelton CL, Graver LE, et al: Effects of theophylline on myocardial mechanics. Am J Physiol 222:1361, 1972

719. Westfall DP, Flemming WW: Sensitivity changes in the dog heart to norepinephrine, calcium and aminophylline resulting from pretreatment with reserpine. J Pharmacol Exp Ther 159:98, 1968

720. Rall TW, West TC: The potentiation of cardiac inotropic responses to norepinephrine by theophylline. J Pharmacol Exp Ther 139:269, 1963

721. Atuk NO, Blaydes C, Westervelt FB, et al: Effect of aminophylline on urinary excretion of epinephrine and norepinephrine in man. Circulation 35:745, 1967

722. Horwitz LN, Spear JF, Moore EN, et al: Effect of aminophylline on the threshold for initiating ventricular fibrillation during respiratory failure. Am J Cardiol 35:376, 1975

723. Mitenko PA, Ogilvie RI: Pharmacokinetics of intravenous theophylline. Clin Pharmacol Ther 14:509, 1973

724. Patterson JW, Shenfield GM: Bronchodilators. Parts I and II. Br Thorac Tuberc Assoc Rev 4:25, 61, 1974

725. Piafsky KM, Ogilvie RI: Dosage of theophylline in bronchial asthma. N Engl J Med 292:1218, 1975

726. Hunt SN, Jusko WJ, Yurchak AM: Effect of smoking on theophylline disposition. Clin Pharmacol Ther 19:546, 1975

727. Takaori M, Loehning RW: Ventricular arrhythmias induced by aminophylline during halothane anaesthesia in dogs. Can Anaesth Soc J 14:79, 1967

728. Takaori M, Loehning RW: Ventricular arrhythmias during halothane anaesthesia: effect of isoproterenol, aminophylline, and ephedrine. Can Anaesth Soc J 12:275, 1965

729. Roizen MF, Stevens WC: Multiform ventricular tachycardia due to the interaction of aminophylline and halothane. Anesth Analg 57:738, 1978

730. Stirt JA, Berger JM, Sullivan SF: Lack of arrhythmogenicity of isoflurane following administration of aminophylline in dogs. Anesth Analg 62:568, 1983

731. Treatment of cardiac arrhythmias. Med Lett Drugs Ther 31:35, 1989

732. Harrah MD, Way WL, Katzung BG: The interaction of d-tubocurarine with antiarrhythmic drugs. Anesthesiology 33:406, 1970

733. Telivuo L, Katz RL: The effects of modern intravenous local anesthetics on respiration during partial neuromuscular block in man. Anaesthesia 25:30, 1970

734. Miller RD, Way WL, Katzung BG: The potentiation of neuromuscular blocking agents by quinidine. Anesthesiology 28:1036, 1967

735. Pittinger CB, Eryasa Y, Adamson R: Antibiotic-induced paralysis. Anesth Analg 49:487, 1970

736. Singh YN, Harvey AL, Marshall IG: Antibiotic induced-paralysis of the mouse phrenic nerve-hemidiaphragm preparation, and reversibility by calcium and by neostigmine. Anesthesiology 48:418, 1978

737. Pittinger CB, Adamson R: Antibiotic blockade of neuromuscular function. Annu Rev Pharmacol 12:169, 1972

738. Becker LD, Miller RD: Clindamycin enhances a non-depo-

larizing neuromuscular blockade. Anesthesiology 45:84, 1976

739. Sampson IH, Miller R: Antibiotics: Their relevance to the anesthesiologist, a review. Anesthesiol Rev 5:43, 1978

740. Snavely SR, Hodges GR: The neurotoxicity of antibacterial agents. Ann Intern Med 101:92, 1984

741. McIndewar IC, Marshall RJ: Interactions between the neuromuscular blocking drug Org NC45 and some anaesthetic, analgesic and antimicrobial agents. Br J Anaesth 53:785, 1981

742. Navalgund AA, Alifimoff JK, Jakymec AJ, Bleyaert AL: Amiodarone-induced sinus arrest successfully treated with ephedrine and isoproterenol. Anesth Analg 65:414, 1986

743. Kannan R, Nademane K, Hendrickson JA, et al: Amiodarone kinetics after oral doses. Clin Pharmacol Ther 31:438, 1982

744. Rice SA, Sbordone L, Mazze RI: Metabolism by rat hepatic microsomes of fluorinated ether anesthetics following isoniazid administration. Anesthesiology 53:489, 1980

745. Beller GA, Smith TW, Abelmann WH, et al: Digitalis intoxication. N Engl J Med 284:989, 1971

746. Hurlbert BJ, Edelman JD, David K: Serum potassium levels during and after terbutaline. Anesth Analg 60:723, 1981

747. Morrow DH: Anesthesia and digitalis toxicity. VI: Effect of barbiturates and halothane on digoxin toxicity. Anesth Analg 49:305, 1970

748. Pratila MG, Pratilas V: Anesthetic agents and cardiac electromechanical activity. Anesthesiology 49:338, 1978

749. Logic JR, Morrow DH: The effect of halothane on ventricular automaticity. Anesthesiology 36:107, 1972

750. Ivankovich AD, Miletich DJ, Grossman RK, et al: The effect of enflurane, isoflurane, fluroxene, methoxyflurane and diethyl ether on ouabain tolerance in the dog. Anesth Analg 55:360, 1976

751. Ali N, Dais K, Banks T, Sheikh M: Titrated electrical cardioversion in patients on digoxin. Clin Cardiol 5:417, 1982

752. Adverse systemic effects from ophthalmic drugs. Med Lett Drugs Ther 24:53, 1982

753. Pantuck EJ, Pantuck CB: Cholinesterases and anticholinesterases. p. 143. In Katz RL (ed): Muscle Relaxants. Excerpta Medica, Amsterdam, 1975

754. Ghoneim MM, Long JP: The interaction between magnesium and other neuromuscular blocking agents. Anesthesiology 32:23, 1970

755. Del Castillo J, Engback L: The nature of neuromuscular block produced by magnesium. J Physiol (Lond) 124:370, 1954

756. Feely J, Wilkinson GR, McAllister CB, et al: Increased toxicity and reduced clearance of lidocaine by cimetidine. Ann Intern Med 96:592, 1982

757. Lam AM, Parkin JA: Cimetidine and prolonged post-operative somnolence. Can Anaesth Soc J 28:450, 1981

758. Vessey MD, Doll R, Fairbairn AS, et al: Postoperative thromboembolism and the use of oral contraceptives. Br Med J 3:123, 1970

759. Greene GR, Sartwell PE: Oral contraceptive use in patients with thromboembolism following surgery, trauma, or infection. Am J Public Health 62:680, 1972

760. Interruption of a drug regimen before anesthesia. Med Lett Drugs Ther 16:19, 1974

761. Wyld R, Nimmo WS: Do patients fasting before and after surgery receive their prescribed drug treatment? Br Med J 296:744, 1988

762. Cullen BF, Miller MG: Drug interactions and anesthesia: a review. Anesth Analg 58:413, 1979

763. Smith NT, Miller RD, Corbascio AN: Drug Interactions in Anesthesia. Lea & Febiger, Philadelphia, 1981

764. Update: Drugs in breast milk. Med Lett Drugs Ther 21:21, 1979

765. Halsey MJ: Drug interactions in anaesthesia. Br J Anaesth 59:112, 1987

766. Starker PM, Group FE, Askanazi J, et al: Serum albumin levels as an index of nutritional support. Surgery 91:194, 1982

767. Axelrod J: Neurotransmitters. Sci Am 230:58, 1974

768. Goldman L, Caldera DL, Nussbaum SR, et al: Multifactorial index of cardiac risk in noncardiac surgical procedures. N Engl J Med 297:845, 1977

26
PSYCHOLOGICAL PREPARATION AND PREOPERATIVE MEDICATION

J. Lance Lichtor

INTRODUCTION

The primary reasons for medicating patients before surgery are to relieve anxiety, induce sedation, promote hemodynamic stability, minimize the chances of aspiration of acid gastric contents, provide analgesia (especially with regional anesthesia), prevent postoperative nausea and vomiting, and control infection. Other considerations include production of amnesia and control of oral secretions.

Patients about to undergo surgery can be quite frightened. What seems like a minor procedure to the anesthesiologist and surgeon may represent a major ordeal to the patient. A visit with the anesthesiologist before surgery is often very effective in allaying anxiety. Alternatively, the patient may be given drugs that calm him or her before anesthesia, and that lessen or prevent certain side effects of the anesthetics.

The existence of specific situations affects the decision regarding premedication. For example, the use of premedication in outpatient surgery may hinder early ambulation and discharge from the hospital on the day of surgery (also see Ch. 65). In other instances, however, premedication may actually facilitate early ambulation and discharge. For the patient undergoing major surgery, especially one who has pre-existing hypertension or coronary artery disease, certain drugs given preoperatively may prevent dangerous increases in arterial blood pressure and heart rate that could cause myocardial ischemia.

Special considerations regarding premedication are also given to patients at risk of aspiration of gastric contents during surgery (see Ch. 40). Various drugs or anesthetic techniques that precipitate postoperative nausea and possibly vomiting might be avoided because they can prolong the time spent in the recovery room or, in the case of ambulatory surgery patients, the hospital. On the other hand, some drugs given preoperatively may help to reduce nausea after anesthesia and surgery.

Although some patients request amnesia, this may not always be a desirable goal, especially for the outpatient (also see Ch. 65), as drug effect can extend beyond surgery and delay discharge from the hospital. Although narcotics are useful for analgesia, they can also precipitate nausea. For intraoral or bronchoscopic examination, administration of anticholinergics (which also reduce nausea) may be worthwhile. However, the resulting dry mouth can be quite uncomfortable. Transdermal administration of anticholinergics has been successful in reducing nausea without causing sedation or excessive dryness of the mouth. Finally, surgeons may request preoperative administration of antibiotics to safeguard against wound infection.

ANXIETY, SEDATION, AND PREMEDICATION

The Incidence of Anxiety

Patients who undergo surgery tend to be anxious. Although anxiety usually exists long before the patient is brought to the preoperative holding area, in some instances, it does not peak until after surgery. In one study, 52 consecutive patients completed a questionnaire used for assessment of anxiety (the Profile of Mood States[1]) at two times: the afternoon before surgery and approximately 1 hour before surgery (in the preoperative holding area, before any anesthetic had been given).[2] Levels of anxiety in the preoperative holding area, although relatively high, were predicted by, and not significantly different from, those measured the previous afternoon. In another study, the level of anxiety was measured daily from 4 days before hospital admission to several days after surgery.[3] Anxiety was high

before admission, between admission and surgery, and 2 days after surgery (Fig. 26-1). In a third study, psychological variables were measured for 8 patients admitted for total hip replacement.[4] Measurements were made for 2 days before surgery and then daily after surgery until discharge of the patient from the hospital. Tension and anxiety were moderate before surgery but increased considerably during the first 2 days after surgery and subsequently decreased until the day of discharge. Similarly, fatigue peaked on the second postoperative day and then returned to its preoperative level on the ninth day after surgery. The lowest level of vigor also occurred on the second day after surgery.

The Uncertain Relationship between Anxiety and Functional Outcome

One assumes that the amount of anxiety reported by a patient would affect his or her recovery. The evidence for this conclusion, however, is not strong. The relationship between preoperative anxiety and objective measures of functional outcome—the most commonly used being postoperative pain—varies. In one study, 80 patients undergoing laparoscopy for sterilization or investigation of infertility were given one of three treatments: routine care, routine care plus a minimally informative preparatory booklet, or routine care plus a maximally informative booklet.[5] Patients given the most information fared the best. Measure of preoperative anxiety were lower. After surgery, pain and "state anxiety" were lower. ("State anxiety" is a transitory emotional state, as opposed to "trait anxiety," a personality disposition to anxiety.) Recovery (both in the hospital and over the first 6 days after going home) was quicker. In addition, these patients had higher scores for vigor after discharge from the hospital and returned to normal activities more quickly. In another study, similarly favorable results occurred with preoperative dissemination of information to patients.[6] Patients given audiovisual instructions before surgery needed significantly less narcotic analgesia in the first 24 hours after surgery than did a control group.

Results from other studies, however, seem to preclude any broad conclusions about anxiety and outcome. In one study, 111 patients were given one of the following kinds of information: a tape-recorded description of what occurs perioperatively ("procedure information"); procedure information, with elaboration on some of the sensations accompanying the procedure ("sensation information"); or procedure and sensation information, with instruction on selected coping strategies, such as diaphragmatic breathing, effective coughing, and other techniques.[7] Subsequent evaluation of outcome in terms of intensity of pain, distress, or certain physical complications revealed no differences among groups. Therefore, the type of information provided appears irrelevant to outcome. Another study evaluated the significance of trait anxiety to state anxiety and outcome.[8] Among 118 women undergoing

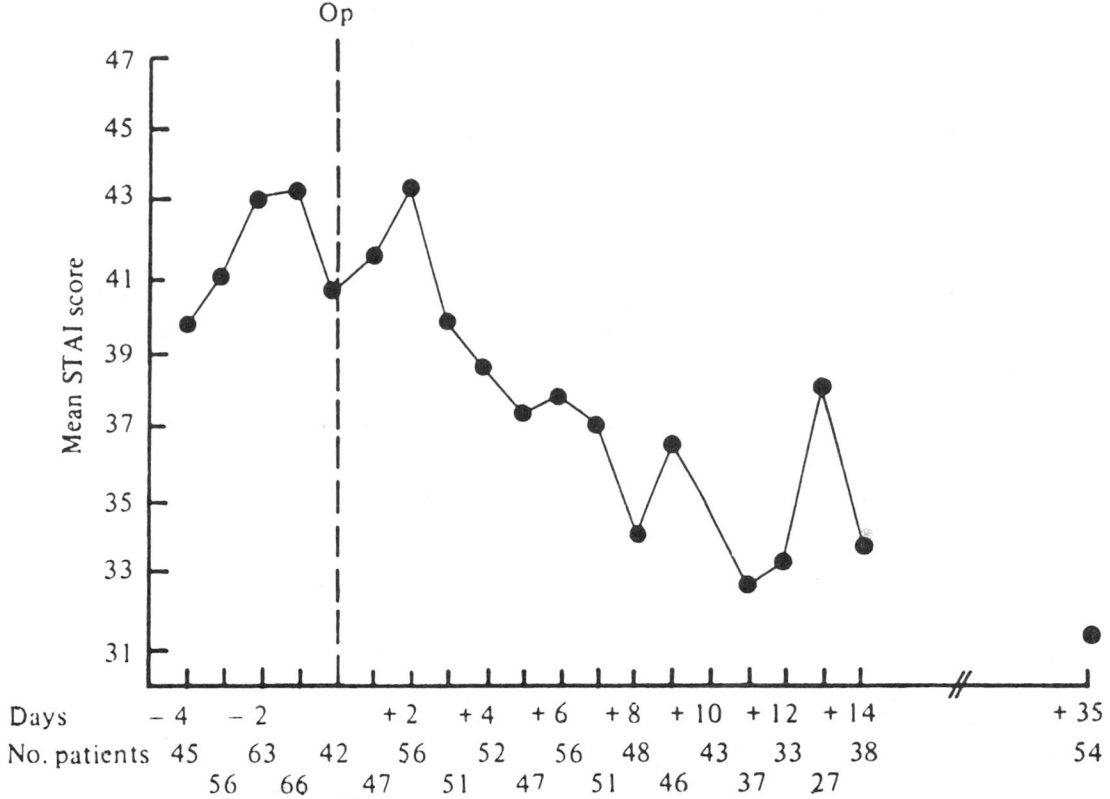

Fig. 26-1. Mean scores for the State-Trait Anxiety Inventory (STAI), which were obtained daily beginning 4 days before surgery, at home, at the time of admission to the hospital, and up to 35 days after surgery (at this time, most patients had been discharged). "Op" indicates day of surgery. The level of anxiety was high not only before surgery but also at 2 days after surgery. (From Johnston,[3] with permission of Cambridge University Press.)

laparoscopic surgery for sterility or investigation of infertility, the existence of trait anxiety was predictive of increases in state anxiety 6 to 8 weeks before hospitalization, as well as on the morning of surgery. However, trait anxiety had little effect on measures of outcome such as pain, arterial blood pressure, heart rate, and the need for pain medication, not only on return of the patient to the ward from the operating room but also 2 hours later. In a third study, results depended on the type of method used to measure pain. High levels of preoperative state anxiety and a high degree of preoperative information were predictive of the amount of pain a patient felt postoperatively when pain was assessed on a five-point scale.[9] This was not true, however, when pain was assessed using an adjective checklist. Furthermore, the amount of postoperative analgesic required by the patient was related to the amount of information the patient possessed before surgery, but not by the level of presurgical anxiety.

Results also vary when investigators use measures other than pain to determine the relationship between preoperative anxiety and postoperative outcome. One study used postoperative complications as the measure of outcome.[10] Eighty-one patients about to undergo minor surgery were given either routine or detailed information about the anesthetic and surgical procedure. The amount of information given preoperatively did not affect the level of anxiety but did influence the incidence of postoperative complications. Patients given detailed preoperative information had fewer postoperative complaints (i.e., slow cerebral functioning, shivering, and vomiting). Another study added the possible effects of age in its investigation of preoperative anxiety and postoperative outcome.[11] Subjects consisted of healthy old and young men undergoing elective hernia repair. The two age groups did not differ significantly in the degree of anxiety experienced before surgery. However, the older patients who were anxious had more days of disability and more complications than did either the older patients who were not anxious or the young patients (both anxious and not anxious).

When preoperative anxiety and postoperative cognitive function were examined in 45 older patients (60 to 82 years old, average age 70.9 years) undergoing total hip replacement, no relationship between the two was found, although the more anxious patients did tend to have fewer cognitive changes.[12]

A small study of 15 patients undergoing prostatectomy used postoperative impotence as the measure of outcome in its investigation of psychologic state.[13] By using the mini Minnesota Multiphasic Personality Inventory and a structured interview, researchers found that impotence after surgery was related to anxiety before surgery.

However, another study of 76 female patients undergoing major gynecologic surgery and 70 male patients undergoing major abdominal surgery found no significant relationship between preoperative fear and anxiety and any aspect of postoperative recovery.[14] In fact, some data suggest that patients who are anxious or worried before surgery may be better able to deal with postsurgical stress than those who are free of anxiety and do not worry. For example, among 73 patients undergoing major elective gynecologic surgery, those who scored moderately high on a "worries scale" (an evaluative tool assessing anxiety associated with hospitalization and surgery) had better and earlier recovery than those who scored low.[15]

Relief of preoperative anxiety may improve postoperative outcome in patients with cardiac disease.[16] Patients given extensive preparation for cardiac surgery seem to have less anxiety, better physical recovery (as perceived by nurses), and lower incidence of postoperative hypertension. An earlier study of patients who had myocardial infarctions showed that emotional changes during transfer from a coronary care unit resulted in higher urinary levels of catecholamines at the time of transfer, and that cardiovascular complications occurred less frequently in patients who were prepared for transfer.[17]

Thus, the evidence for a relationship between preoperative anxiety and postoperative recovery varies. Why some studies found a benefit to outcome from relief of anxiety and others did not is not clear. Many factors influence postoperative recovery. At the very least, the control of anxiety is a humane goal and should be attempted for every patient.

Relieving Anxiety

Nonpharmacologic Methods

The purpose of the anesthesiologist's preoperative visit is not only to assess fitness and preparation for surgery but also to calm the patient. Certain nonpharmacologic techniques are very effective in reducing anxiety. The classic study of Egbert et al.[18] found that a preoperative visit by an anesthesiologist was more effective in decreasing anxiety than administration of a barbiturate. Other authors have also confirmed the value of a preoperative visit. Patients given maximally informative preparatory booklets before surgery have less anxiety than those given minimally informative booklets or only routine care.[5] Preoperative assurance from nonanesthesia staff and the use of booklets also reduce preoperative anxiety. However, use of such booklets is less effective than a preoperative visit by the anes-

thesiologist.[19] Audiovisual instructions also reduce preoperative anxiety.[6]

Elicitation of the relaxation response is an anxiety-reducing technique in which the subject focuses attention on a positive or neutral theme and passively ignores distracting thoughts.[20] This practice decreases oxygen consumption and lowers arterial blood pressure in both unmedicated and medicated hypertensive patients (Table 26-1).[21] Patients with ischemic heart disease and premature ventricular contractions (PVCs) who practiced relaxation had a lower incidence of PVCs, especially during sleep.[22]

Although the relaxation technique has also been used to help hospitalized patients who have difficulty with sleep,[23] it has had only limited use in patients about to undergo surgery. Patients undergoing cholecystectomy who practiced relaxation had significantly less state anxiety and lower cortisol levels 1 day after surgery than did a control group.[24] Patients who had spinal surgery and practiced relaxation needed fewer days of hospitalization and less pain medication and complained less (as noted by nurses) than did an equivalent control group (Table 26-2).[25] In another study, relaxation training was given to ambulatory patients scheduled for excision of a skin cancer without general anesthesia.[26] The relaxation response was elicited for 20 min/day until the day of surgery; the control group spent 20 min/day reading. Patients who were taught the relaxation response said their anxiety was highest before entering the study; control patients said their anxiety was greatest during surgery and when facing the results of biopsy. However, anxiety levels (as assessed by the State-Trait Anxiety Inventory[27]) were the same immediately before and after surgery for both the control and study groups.

Unlike drugs, which can exert their effect relatively quickly, these nonpharmacologic methods of relieving anxiety are best started at least 24 hours before surgery. Increasingly, hospitals and anesthesia departments are arranging preoperative visits with an anesthesiologist at least 24 hours before surgery, so that these nonpharmacologic methods can be applied.

Relaxation techniques are clearly effective in reducing anxiety, even to the extent of reducing preoperative arterial blood pressure and other biochemical indices of stress. Unfortunately, these techniques are time-consuming for both the patient and medical personnel. However, in a time of cost containment, one hopes that methods will be found to use these nondrug techniques.

Drugs That Relieve Anxiety and Induce Sedation

Although historically many classes of drugs (e.g., barbiturates and antihistamines) have been used to reduce anxiety and induce sedation, benzodiazepines are at present the drugs most commonly used. As a result, prime emphasis will be placed on the use of this type of drug for premedication.

TABLE 26-1. Elicitation of the Relaxation Response Decreases Oxygen Consumption and Arterial Blood Pressure in Both Medicated and Unmedicated Hypertensive Patients

Variable	Reference	Subject (No.; BP; Medication)	Effect of Eliciting the Relaxation Response
Oxygen consumption	Beary & Benson[255]	17; normal	O_2 consumption ↓ 13%; CO_2 elimination ↓ 12%; respirations ↓ 4/min.[a]
BP	Benson et al.[256]	22; hypertensive, unmedicated	Mean systolic BP ↓ from 146 to 139 mmHg[b]; diastolic BP ↓ from 95 to 91 mmHg[c]
	Benson et al.[257]	14; hypertensive, medicated	Mean systolic BP ↓ from 146 to 135 mmHg[a]; diastolic BP ↓ from 92 to 87 mmHg[d]
	Datey et al.[258]	10; hypertensive, unmedicated	Mean BP ↓ from 134 to 102 mmHg[d]
		22; hypertension well controlled	Drug requirement ↓ to 32% of original in 59% of patients[d]
		15; hypertension inadequately controlled	Drug requirement ↓ to 29% of original in 40% of patients
	Little et al.[259]	60 hypertensive parturients given: (1) relaxation training; (2) biofeedback and relaxation training; or (3) no training.	Treatment ↓ systolic and diastolic BPs; need for admission to hospital: <1/3 of treatment groups, 2/3 of control group
	Patel[260,261]	20; hypertensive, medicated	Treatment ↓ mean BP from 121 to 101 mmHg and ↓ drug requirement by 41%
		20 age- and sex-matched hypertensive controls	No change in either variable
	Peters et al.[262]	126 normotensive office workers	Systolic BP ↓ 6.7 mmHg[b]; diastolic BP ↓ 5.2 mmHg[b] (The higher the initial BP, the greater the decrease)

[a] $P < 0.01$.
[b] $P < 0.001$.
[c] $P < 0.002$.
[d] $P < 0.05$.
Abbreviations: ↓, decreased; BP, blood pressure; "medicated" and "unmedicated" refer to antihypertensive drugs.

Comparative Effects of Benzodiazepines

Midazolam. Midazolam is a water-soluble benzodiazepine having an initial distribution half-life of 7.2 minutes and an elimination half-life of 2.5 hours (range, 2.1 to 3.4 hours).[28] The metabolites of midazolam have negligible soporific effects,[29] and midazolam does not produce thrombosis or thrombophlebitis in humans or in animals 48 hours after injection.

The ability of midazolam to reduce anxiety has been demonstrated reliably over a range of doses administered by various routes (e.g., 15 mg orally [PO], 7.5 to 10.0 mg or 0.115 mg/kg intravenously [IV], 0.07 to 0.10 mg/kg intramuscularly [IM]) (Table 26-3).[30-38] Although orally administered midazolam is effective against anxiety, in the United States this drug can only be given intravenously or intramuscularly.

Midazolam can also provide amnesia. A double-blind crossover study evaluated amnesia in patients 20 to 48 years of age who underwent two endoscopies over 30 days.[39] Patients were randomly assigned to receive either midazolam (0.07 mg/kg IV) or diazepam (0.15 mg/kg IV) and then 20 mg of hyoscine butylbromide. Seventy-four percent of the patients given midazolam, but only 17 percent of those given diazepam, could not remember insertion of the endoscope 24 hours later.

TABLE 26-2. Effect of Relaxation Training on Different Aspects of Pain after Spinal Surgery

	Patients Given Relaxation Training	Control Group
Days in hospital	5.6	7.6[a]
Complaints (% of patients)	10.1	17.2[b]
Administration of drugs		
Meperidine (mg)	426.5	1,019.4[a]
Acetaminophen (tablets)	4.9	10.2[b]
Morphine (mg)	30 (1 patient)	60 (5 patients)

[a] $P < 0.05$.
[b] $P < 0.01$.
(Adapted from Lawlis et al.,[25] with permission.)

TABLE 26-3. Midazolam Effectively Reduces Anxiety over a Range of Dosages Administered by Various Routes

Reference	Procedure	Dose of Midazolam	Sedation Assessed by:	Sedation Assessment:	Reduction in Anxiety Assessed by:	Reduction in Anxiety Assessment:
Barclay et al.[112]	Oral surgery	0.115 mg/kg IV	Observer Patient	6/15, excellent or good 15/15, excellent or good		
Barker et al.[33]	Oral surgery	0.14 mg/kg IV vs. 0.29 mg/kg IV of D	Observer	Onset time shorter with M (3.1 min) than with D (3.4 min)[a]	Observer	Patients less anxious with M than D[b]
Clark et al.[111]	Oral surgery	7.5 to 10 mg IV	Observer	M: 5% good, 90% excellent P: 35% good, 29% excellent		
Driessen et al.[35]	Bronchoscopy	15 mg PO	Patient	53% good, 40% excellent	Observer	82% good, 18% fair
Forrest et al.[36]	Ambulatory urologic surgery	15 mg PO	Linear scale	Greater with M than P[c]	Linear scale Observer	No overall difference between groups Greatest reduction with M
O'Boyle et al.[38]	Oral surgery	15 mg PO			Adjectives Linear scale	No difference from control Moderate[d]
Raybould and Bradshaw[30]	Ambulatory surgery	7.5 and 15 mg PO	Linear scale Observer	Greater with 7.5 mg M than P but NS; greater with 15 mg M at 30 and 60 min[e] Greater with 7.5 mg M at 60 min[f]; greater with 15 mg M at 30[d] and 60 min[c]	Linear scale	M 7.5 mg not different from P; 15 mg significant[e]
Reinhart et al.[31]	Urologic surgery	0.1 mg/kg IM	Observer	13/27 asleep 30 min after injection; 20/27 asleep after 60 min; and 16/27 lightly asleep after 90 min	Observer	No patient anxious 60 min after injection
van der Bijl et al.[37]	Oral surgery	0.1 mg/kg IV	Observer		Observer	M: all patients slightly anxious P: 50% moderately anxious, 50% severely anxious
van Wijhe et al.[32]	Orthopedic surgery	0.07 mg/kg IM	Observer Linear scale	Greater than control[c] Greater than control[c]	Observer Linear scale	Decrease in anxiety[c] Decrease in anxiety[c]
Vinik et al.[34]	Elective surgery	0.07 mg/kg IM	Observer	Significant sedation up to 60 min after injection[e]	Linear scale	Significantly less anxiety[e]

Modes of assessment: "Observer": assessment by an individual who was not the patient, and who was unaware of the study design (i.e., "blinded"); "patient": the patient reported his or her feelings directly; "linear scale": the patient used a linear scale to assess his or her feelings; "adjectives": a score obtained by rating a series of adjectives to measure a feeling.

[a]$P = 0.001$.
[b]$P < 0.02$.
[c]$P < 0.001$.
[d]$P < 0.05$.
[e]$P < 0.01$.
[f]$P < 0.025$.

Abbreviations: M, midazolam; P, placebo; D, diazepam. NS, not statistically significant.

Nine percent of those given midazolam and 61 percent of those given diazepam could remember that the endoscope was inserted.

Nausea occasionally occurs after administration of benzodiazepines such as midazolam.[40] Whether premedication with midazolam itself actually causes nausea is difficult to ascertain, as this practice has not been well studied. However, when midazolam is used for induction of anesthesia, the incidence of nausea is very low.[41,42] It is interesting to note that the antagonism of midazolam sometimes increases nausea. In one double-blind study of 100 patients having induced abortion under midazolam anesthesia, patients given the benzodiazepine antagonist flumazenil (RO 15-1788) had a higher incidence of nausea and/or vomiting in the recovery room (16 percent) than did patients given placebo (4 percent).[43] In another study, the use of physostigmine and glycopyrrolate for reversal of midazolam-induced sedation was associated with nausea in five of eight volunteers and/or with vomiting in three.[44]

Administration of midazolam for premedication should be undertaken very cautiously in the elderly, who are more sensitive to the sedative effects than younger individuals (also see Ch. 62). For example, the dose of intravenously administered midazolam necessary to produce adequate sedation in 800 consecutive patients about to undergo upper gastrointentinal endoscopy was markedly lower with age (Fig. 26-2).[45] Because the rate of reduction was approximately 15 percent per decade, a dose of midazolam of 0.1 mg/kg IV in a 60-year-old patient would be equivalent to a dose of 0.03 mg/kg IV in a 90-year-old patient and a dose of 0.15 mg/kg in a 20-year-old patient. In a similar study of elderly patients, midazolam (0.07 mg/kg IV) was given to 40 patients for sedation prior to endoscopy of the esophagus, stomach, and duodenum.[46] Although less effective in the young, this dose was very effective as a sedative in the elderly, as based on time to sedation, adequacy of sedation, and absence of gagging during the procedure.

The effectiveness of midazolam (0.3 mg/kg) for induction of anesthesia in unpremedicated young (<50 years) and older (>50 years) patients has also been studied.[47] An inverse relationship existed between the age of the patients and the time to loss of consciousness. Effectiveness was more reliable, and anesthetic induction times were significantly shorter, in patients over 50 years of age than in younger patients.

To summarize, midazolam is an effective sedative and anxiolytic. Although the dose must be tailored to each patient, midazolam usually provides effective sedation at 0.07 to 0.15 mg/kg in a 20-year-old, with a

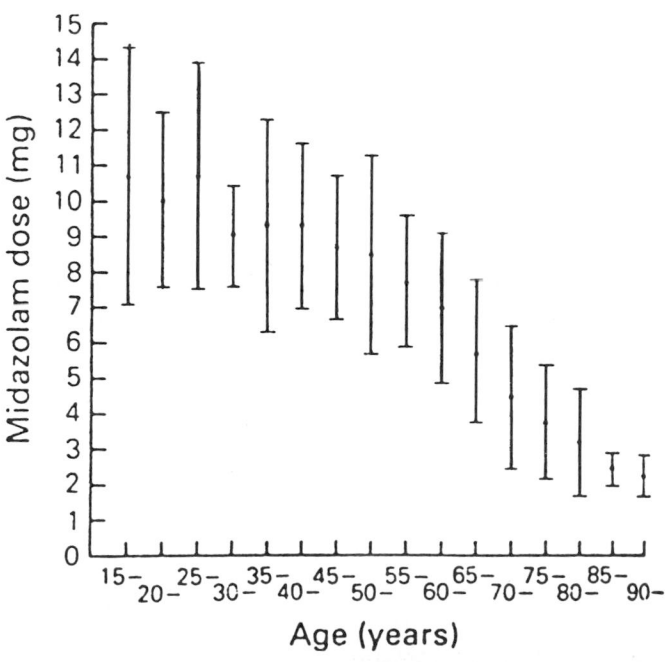

Fig. 26-2. The mean dose (±SD) of intravenous midazolam that is required to produce adequate sedation before upper gastrointestinal endoscopy decreases with age. (From Bell et al.,[45] with permission.)

decrease in dose of approximately 15 percent per decade. Sedation is effective for 20 to 40 minutes. These same doses of midazolam effectively relieve anxiety, although this area has not been studied as thoroughly as has sedation. Midazolam does not increase, and may even decrease, incidence of nausea and vomiting after surgery. Cardiovascular, respiratory, and psychomotor depression are side effects one needs to consider when using midazolam; these issues will be discussed in greater detail below. Reves et al.[48] provide a comprehensive summary of the pharmacologic characteristics and use of this drug (see also Ch. 9).

Diazepam. Unlike midazolam, diazepam is available in tablet form in the United States. This eliminates the need for injection and makes it a popular drug for reducing preoperative anxiety. Furthermore, diazepam is very effective in relieving anxiety before surgery.[49,50] However, as explained below, the current trend regarding use of benzodiazepines is to limit diazepam to oral administration and to give midazolam when intravenous or intramuscular administration is desired. When diazepam is given orally, at least 1 hour must elapse before its anxiolytic effects are measurable. This time lag makes it difficult to use diazepam to premedicate patients "on call." However, the drug is effective for several hours.

The potency of diazepam for sedation seems to be about one-half to one-fourth that of midazolam. In one study, a dose of midazolam of 0.05 to 0.15 mg/kg IV produced sedation similar to that produced by a dose of diazepam of 0.1 to 0.3 mg/kg IV.[51] Sedation was measured at three times: 2 to 3 minutes after injection, during injection of local anesthetic, and during surgery.

In the past, diazepam has been used extensively. Unfortunately, the injectable form uses propylene glycol for solubility, which produces not only pain on injection but also a high incidence of thrombophlebitis. The availability of other, shorter-acting water-soluble anxiolytics such as midazolam that do not produce pain on administration has decreased the popularity of diazepam, especially as a parenteral anxiolytic agent. When 10 mg of diazepam was injected into the largest available vein, thrombosis or thrombophlebitis developed in 23 percent of patients 2 to 3 days after injection, and in 39 percent at 7 to 10 days.[52] The incidence of thrombosis was significantly lower after injection into large antecubital veins than after injection into smaller vessels. Also, venous thrombosis occurred more frequently in older patients (Fig. 26-3).

When diazepam is injected intravenously, plasma levels decrease in a smooth biexponential fashion, the distribution half-life being 1 hour and the excretion half-life being 32.9 ± 8.8 hours (mean $\pm$ SD) (Fig. 26-4).[53] Concentrations of the major metabolite in plasma, desmethyldiazepam, can be detected after 2 hours and decreases only after 36 hours. This metabolite has pharmacologic properties similar to those of the parent drug; the long half-life of the metabolite,

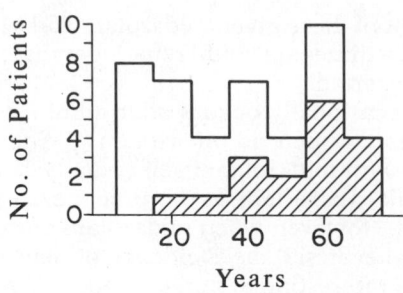

Fig. 26-3. The incidence of venous thrombosis at 7 to 10 days after intravenous injection of 10 mg of diazepam increases with age. The clear area represents the total number of patients given diazepam. The crosshatched area represents the number of patients having venous thrombosis. (From Hegarty and Dundee,[52] with permission.)

coupled with the long excretion half-life of the parent drug, may account for the long action of diazepam.[54] Orally administered diazepam is well absorbed from the intestine, with plasma levels reaching a peak 60 minutes after ingestion.[55] If atropine or narcotics are given at approximately the same time as oral administration of diazepam, the plasma concentrations of diazepam are lower than if diazepam were given by itself. In contrast, if metoclopramide is administered at the time of ingestion of diazepam, plasma concentrations of diazepam are higher. These effects are attributed to decreased or increased gastric emptying. Injection of diazepam into the gluteal region, particularly into fat instead of muscle, results in low plasma levels of the drug.[56]

Ingestion of food also affects the pharmacokinetics of diazepam. In one study, subjects were given diazepam intravenously and, 5 hours later, one of the following: mineral water, a predominantly carbohydrate meal, or a meal heavy in fat. Serum levels of diazepam were significantly higher in both groups given food (Fig. 26-5).[57] Although the actual mechanism is not clear, ingestion of food may increase serum levels of diazepam because the drug is excreted in the bile and reabsorbed from the intestine. These high serum levels of diazepam were associated with the recurrence of fatigue.

Diazepam has amnesic properties but is less effective than midazolam. Five percent of patients given 10 mg of diazepam intravenously and 40 percent of patients given 20 mg of diazepam intravenously could not remember being taken to the operating room or experiencing induction of anesthesia.[58] Amnesia is more profound, however, when diazepam is combined with other drugs. After administration of 10 mg of diazepam with 0.4 mg of scopolamine, the incidence of amnesia increased to 63 percent. The incidence of amnesia in-

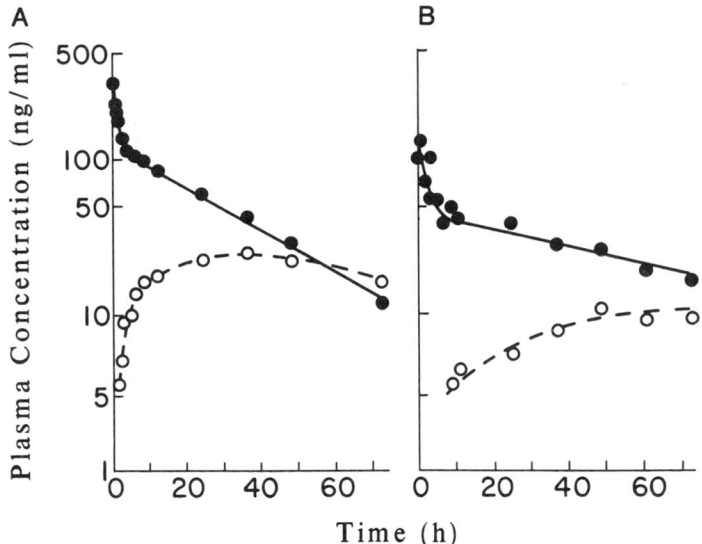

Fig. 26-4. Plasma concentration versus time curves for diazepam (solid line) and desmethyldiazepam (broken line) after intravenous injection of diazepam (0.1 mg/kg) in two asymptomatic adults having no laboratory evidence of disease: a 20-year-old (**A**) and a 67-year-old (**B**). The elimination half-life of diazepam was 21.6 hours for the younger person and 51.9 hours for the older person. (From Klotz et al.,[63] with permission.)

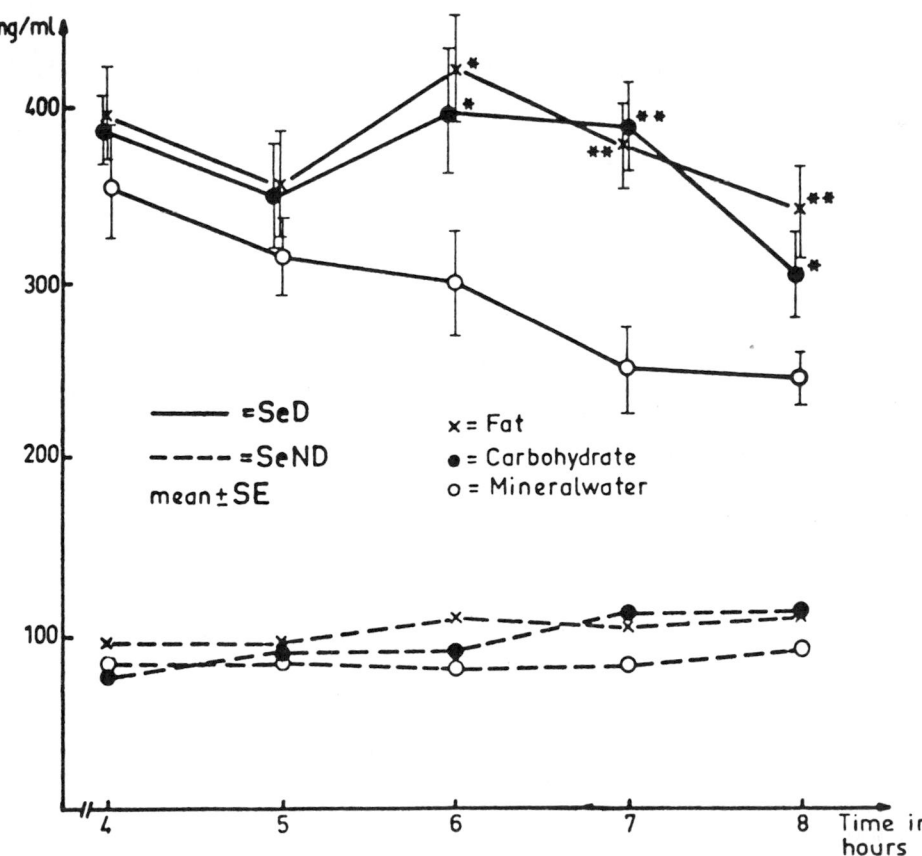

Fig. 26-5. Serum Levels of diazepam (solid lines, "SeD") and *N*-desmethyldiazepam (broken lines, "SeND") after ingestion of mineral water, carbohydrate, or fat. Asterisks indicate significant differences from values obtained with mineral water (*$P < 0.05$ and **$P < 0.01$). (From Linnoila et al.,[57] with permission.)

creased to 35 percent when 10 mg of diazepam was combined with 50 mg of meperidine and to 70 percent when meperidine was increased to 100 mg. The incidence of amnesia was 20 percent after 10 mg of diazepam with 15 mg of morphine. In one study, patients were shown different cards; 6 hours later, after a minor gynecologic operation, they were asked to recall the pictures.[59] The incidence of amnesia was highest (16 percent) when cards were shown 2 to 3 minutes after injection of diazepam (10 mg IV); for 16 percent of patients, amnesia was still in effect 20 to 30 minutes after injection.[59]

A similar study tested the effect orally administered diazepam on recall 6 hours after a minor gynecologic operation.[60] Amnesia was in effect 20 to 30 minutes after administration and persisted for 90 minutes. The incidence of failure to recall was 70 percent 90 minutes after 20 mg of diazepam and 40 percent after 10 mg of diazepam. Diazepam (5 mg IV) was no better than placebo: at 90 minutes, the incidence of failure to recall was 0 percent after 5 mg of diazepam and 7.5 percent after placebo.

Diazepam also raises the seizure threshold and thus protects against seizures caused by local anesthetics (see Ch. 13). For example, the incidence of convulsions in mice after administration of lidocaine, bupivacaine, or etidocaine was lower when mice were pretreated with diazepam, lorazepam, or midazolam.[61] Similar findings have been reported for rhesus monkeys.[62] Diazepam is therefore sometimes given before regional anesthesia to raise the seizure threshold. However, no controlled study on patients undergoing regional anesthesia has demonstrated that the routine use of benzodiazepines effectively reduces the incidence of seizures.

As with all benzodiazepines, the elimination half-life of diazepam is longer in older subjects than in young subjects (Fig. 26-4). After either intravenous or oral administration of diazepam, the elimination half-life increases from 20 hours in 20-year-olds to approximately 90 hours in 80-year-olds, the correlation coefficient for half-life versus age being 0.83.[63] This prolongation of elimination half-life is attributed primarily to an increase in the initial volume of distribution of the drug.

The activity of this drug, however, does not depend on plasma concentration alone. At equal plasma levels, the central nervous system of elderly patients is increasingly sensitive to the depressant effects of diazepam. For example, for patients undergoing cardioversion, the correlation between age and dose, as well as between age and plasma level of the drug required to produce unresponsiveness to vocal stimuli, is a negative one.[64] Dose requirements decrease approximately 10 percent per decade (Fig. 26-6). Another study evaluated age and the infused dose of diazepam just adequate to allow peroral endoscopic intubation.[65] At this state of relaxation, patients respond verbally to verbal stimulation but fall asleep without such stimulation. The dose of diazepam appropriate for endoscopic intubation decreased with age. The rate of metabolism of desmethyl-

diazepam is also affected by age. In the elderly, the initial presence and peak values of the drug were observed later, and the metabolite was present at lower concentrations.[63]

In summary, diazepam, like midazolam, is an effective sedative and anxiolytic. For a 20-year-old person weighing 70 kg, intravenous injection of 10 to 20 mg of diazepam provides effective sedation; this dose should be reduced by 10 percent per decade. Because thrombosis or thrombophlebitis can result after intravenous injection of diazepam, the usual practice is to limit diazepam to only oral administration, given just prior to transfer of the patient from the ward to the operating room. Oral administration requires at least 1 hour before the onset of measurable sedative or anxiolytic effects. The plasma half-life of the drug is much longer than that of midazolam, because the metabolite of diazepam has an effect similar to that of the parent drug. In the clinical setting, residual drowsiness affecting recovery is not much different from that with midazolam, especially because of the effects of anesthesia and surgery. This issue and the effect of diazepam on cardiac and pulmonary function will be considered in greater detail below.

Lorazepam. As a sedative, lorazepam is approximately four times as potent as diazepam. For example, an oral dose of 2.5 mg of lorazepam produces as much drowsiness as does 10 mg of diazepam.[66] However, the onset of action is much slower and the duration of action much longer with lorazepam. Even with intravenous injection, an unexplained delay of 40 minutes occurs before peak drug effect.[67] The duration of action is about three or four times greater than that of equivalent doses of diazepam. After an intravenous dose, the mean elimination half-life is 14 to 15 hours for lorazepam, 2.5 hours for midazolam, and 30 hours for diazepam.[68] Unlike diazepam, lorazepam is not transformed to pharmacologically active metabolites. Lorazepam causes fewer venous sequelae after intravenous injection than does diazepam. Assessed 7 to 10 days after injection, such sequelae have occurred in 15 percent of patients given lorazepam and in 39 percent of patients given diazepam.[52]

Several studies have shown the effectiveness of lorazepam as a preoperative anxiolytic.[69-74] In addition, elimination of recall lasts much longer after lorazepam than after diazepam.[70] Patients given lorazepam did not recall events 1 1/2 to 6 hours after injection; 50 percent of patients did not recall most events of the day. In contrast, after diazepam or placebo, the incidence of recall was high. Patients also remain sleepy for a longer period after lorazepam than after diazepam[72] or triazolam.[74] Nonetheless, in one study, four patients who had been given meperidine and atropine as premedicants for an earlier operation preferred lorazepam, which they said made them feel more relaxed (see the section, *Narcotics*, below).[73]

The long duration of action and the prolonged time to

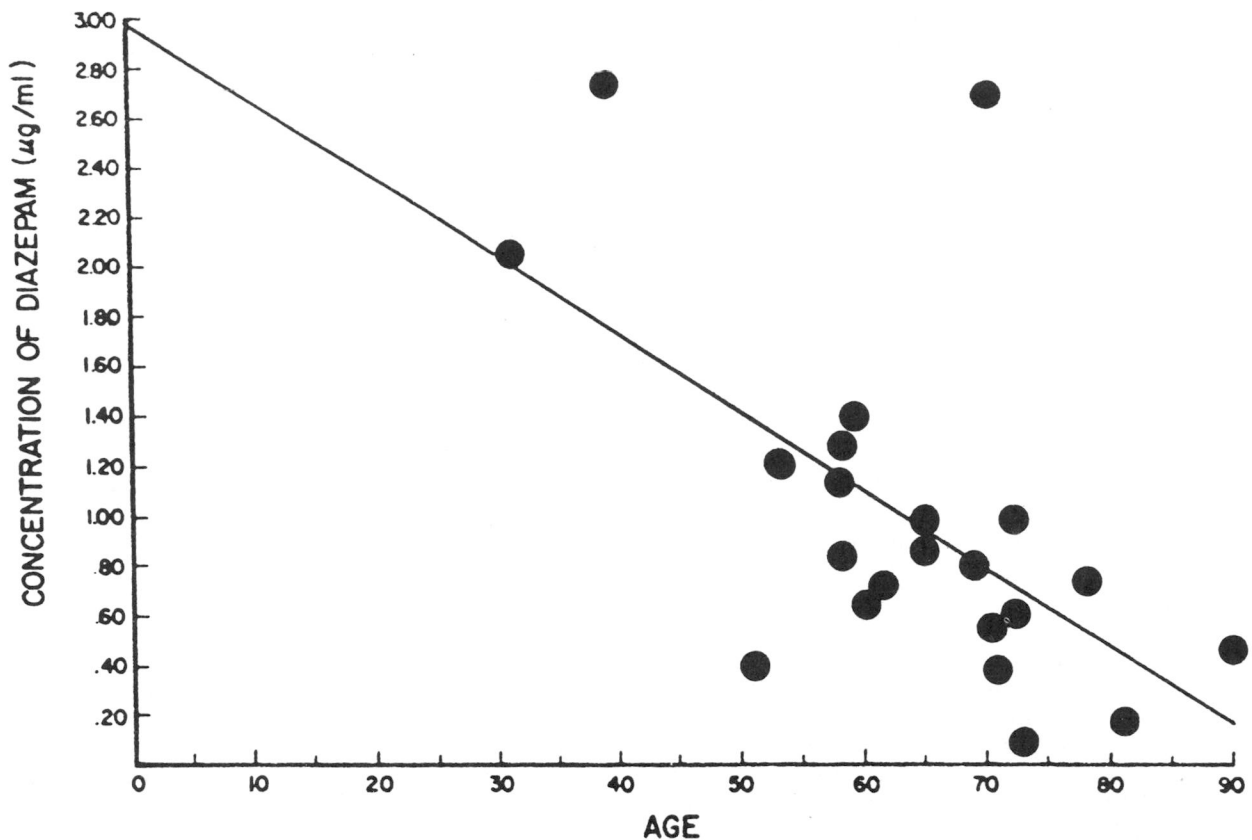

Fig. 26-6. The plasma concentration of diazepam necessary to eliminate responsiveness to vocal stimuli decreases with age. Equation for the regression line: $2.98 - 0.31 \times$ age. (From Reidenberg et al.,[64] with permission.)

effectiveness of lorazepam may make this drug unsuitable for certain situations (for example, as a premedicant for ambulatory patients immediately before surgery). Lorazepam may be useful for anxious patients seen by a surgeon or an anesthesiologist at least 1 day before surgery, in that the drug can be given several hours or even the night before a procedure. Lorazepam is so effective as an amnesic agent, however, that outpatients may not remember why they came to the surgical center. Lorazepam may also be useful when one desires profound amnesia for a longer period of time (e.g., during coronary artery bypass grafting).

One study compared the sedative and anxiolytic effects of lorazepam (0.06 mg/kg), given 90 minutes preoperatively, with those of morphine (0.1 mg/kg IM) and scopolamine (0.006 mg/kg, IM), given 60 minutes preoperatively.[75] The patients did not differ with respect to levels of sedation or anxiety either before or after premedication. Fentanyl, 100 μg/kg, was used as the primary anesthetic. After induction, hypertension (increase in arterial blood pressure of more than 20 percent above control) occurred more frequently among patients given morphine-scopolamine than among those given lorazepam. After induction and after intubation, hypotension (defined as a decrease in arte-

rial blood pressure of more than 20 percent below control) was more frequent in the lorazepam group. However, no patient had new electrocardiographic changes indicative of ischemia.

A comprehensive review by Ameer and Greenblatt[76] provides additional information about lorazepam.

Triazolam. Triazolam, used extensively as a hypnotic agent, has a plasma half-life of 2.3 hours.[77] This relatively short half-life may make triazolam a useful preoperative anxiolytic. However, study results have been mixed. In one study, 90 patients undergoing minor gynecologic surgery received sedation with oral administration of 0.25 mg of triazolam, 10 mg of diazepam, or placebo 2 hours before anesthesia.[78] Although both diazepam and triazolam produced sedation, a linear analog scale showed that only diazepam reduced anxiety. In another study, 58 female patients undergoing laparoscopy were given oral administration of 0.25 mg of triazolam, 2 mg of lorazepam, or placebo.[74] Evaluation of an adjective test list used for assessment of anxiety showed that both triazolam and lorazepam reduced anxiety significantly. The relatively short half-life and ability of triazolam to be administered orally may warrant closer examination of the drug as an anxiolytic.

Problems Associated with Relief of Anxiety and Induction of Sedation with Benzodiazepines

Cardiovascular and Respiratory Function. Over a 2-year period, premedication with midazolam was associated with 40 deaths.[79] As a result, the Public Citizen Health Research Group, a nonprofit consumer organization that guards against unsafe food and drugs, filed a petition with the Food and Drug Administration (FDA) to restrict the use of midazolam. A congressional investigation into the FDA approval of midazolam linked use of the drug with serious side effects and deaths, and accused the FDA of failing to gather all available data before clearing the drug for general use.[80] However, many of the deaths that have occurred after administration of midazolam have involved elderly patients undergoing endoscopy with poor monitoring of vital signs. Many deaths also involved elderly patients who were debilitated and also monitored inadequately. These patients were given midazolam for sedation (with or without narcotics) in lieu of a general anesthetic (B.H. Medd, M.D., Hoffmann-La Roche, Inc., personal communication).

All of this attention has resulted in a lowering of the total doses recommended for administration of midazolam. Originally, the range of total doses approved for intravenous administration of midazolam to sedate adults was 0.1 to 0.15 mg/kg, the maximum dose being on rare occasion 0.2 mg/kg.[81] The recommended range for elderly patients was 0.07 to 0.10 mg/kg. One year later, evaluation of clinical experience resulted in a lowering of the recommended dose for intravenous sedation in adults to 0.1 mg/kg.[82] Most recently, the total recommended dose is no more than 5 mg (Versed product information sheet, issued May 1988). In any regard, a drug such as midazolam should always have been given as a titration rather than as a bolus injection. Although initial estimates judged the potency of the drug to be approximately twice that of diazepam, more recent clinical experience indicates that midazolam is three or four times more potent than diazepam.[83]

The benzodiazepines, used both alone and with other drugs (particularly narcotics), cause hypotension in some patients. In normal volunteers, midazolam (0.15 mg/kg) reduced systolic arterial blood pressure by 5 percent and diastolic pressure by 10 percent; this effect persisted for at least 20 minutes.[84] The decrease in arterial blood pressure after a 0.05 mg/kg IV dose of midazolam is similar to that caused by diazepam at 0.15 mg/kg.[85] Furthermore, if patients have heart disease, hypotension can be more profound. One study gave patients who were undergoing coronary artery bypass grafting either midazolam (0.2 mg/kg IV) or diazepam (0.5 mg/kg IV).[86] Both groups were generally hemodynamically stable. However, at 5 minutes after induction, systolic blood pressure had decreased 34 percent in those given midazolam and 18 percent in those given diazepam. Apnea occurred in 9 of 20 patients given midazolam and in none of the patients given diazepam.

Benzodiazepine-induced hypotension can be much more severe when narcotics are also given, especially if patients have cardiac disease. In one report, four patients scheduled for cardiac surgery or abdominal aortic aneurysm resection had severe hypotension when sufentanil was used as an induction agent at least 30 minutes after intramuscular or intravenous administration of 2 to 4 mg of lorazepam.[87] A similar case of severe hypotension with sufentanil occurred after an intramuscular dose of 5 mg of midazolam.[88]

Giving midazolam in conjunction with fentanyl has approximately the same effect. After induction of anesthesia for coronary artery bypass grafting, mean arterial pressure decreased 17 percent in patients given fentanyl (10 μg/kg IV) and then midazolam (0.25 mg/kg IV).[89] In another study, induction of anesthesia that included fentanyl (75 μg/kg) was followed by a 24 percent decrease in mean arterial blood pressure after a 0.075 mg/kg dose of midazolam, and a 32 percent decrease after a 0.15 mg/kg dose of midazolam.[90] After the higher dose, the lowest mean arterial blood pressure was 45 mmHg and 10 of 12 patients had mean blood pressures below 70 mmHg.

The benzodiazepines blunt baroreflex control of heart rate. One study evaluated the pressor baroreflex slope that results from plotting changes in systolic blood pressure after administration of phenylephrine against the PR interval: the slope decreased after either diazepam (0.4 mg/kg) or midazolam (0.3 mg/kg).[91] Changes were maximal (45 percent with diazepam and 43 percent with midazolam) when the plasma concentrations of the drugs were highest. This loss of baroreflex control, however, is not as great as that occurring with halogenated anesthetic agents.[92]

Three anecdotal cases of ventricular irritability have been reported after preoperative sedation with midazolam.[93] One of the three patients had an abnormal echocardiogram. However, other studies of patients with coronary artery disease who were given midazolam have reported no ventricular irritability.[86,89,90]

The benzodiazepines can also depress respiratory function. For 100 patients undergoing endoscopy, the average initial baseline oxygen saturation of 95 percent decreased to 92 percent after intravenous administration of midazolam and to 89 percent during endoscopy.[94] Oxygen saturation decreased to below 80 percent in 7 percent of these patients (Fig. 26-7). Response to carbon dioxide is also blunted by benzodiazepines. When ventilatory and mouth occlusion pressure responses to carbon dioxide were measured in healthy volunteers after diazepam (0.3 mg/kg) or midazolam (0.15 mg/kg), the ventilatory response curves were flatter than those of control groups.[95] This decrement is not as severe as that associated with narcotics.[96]

Ventilatory depression with midazolam is much more profound in patients with chronic obstructive pulmonary disease (COPD) than in normal individuals. One study described the ventilatory effects of giving a 15-second intravenous injection of 0.2 mg/kg of mida-

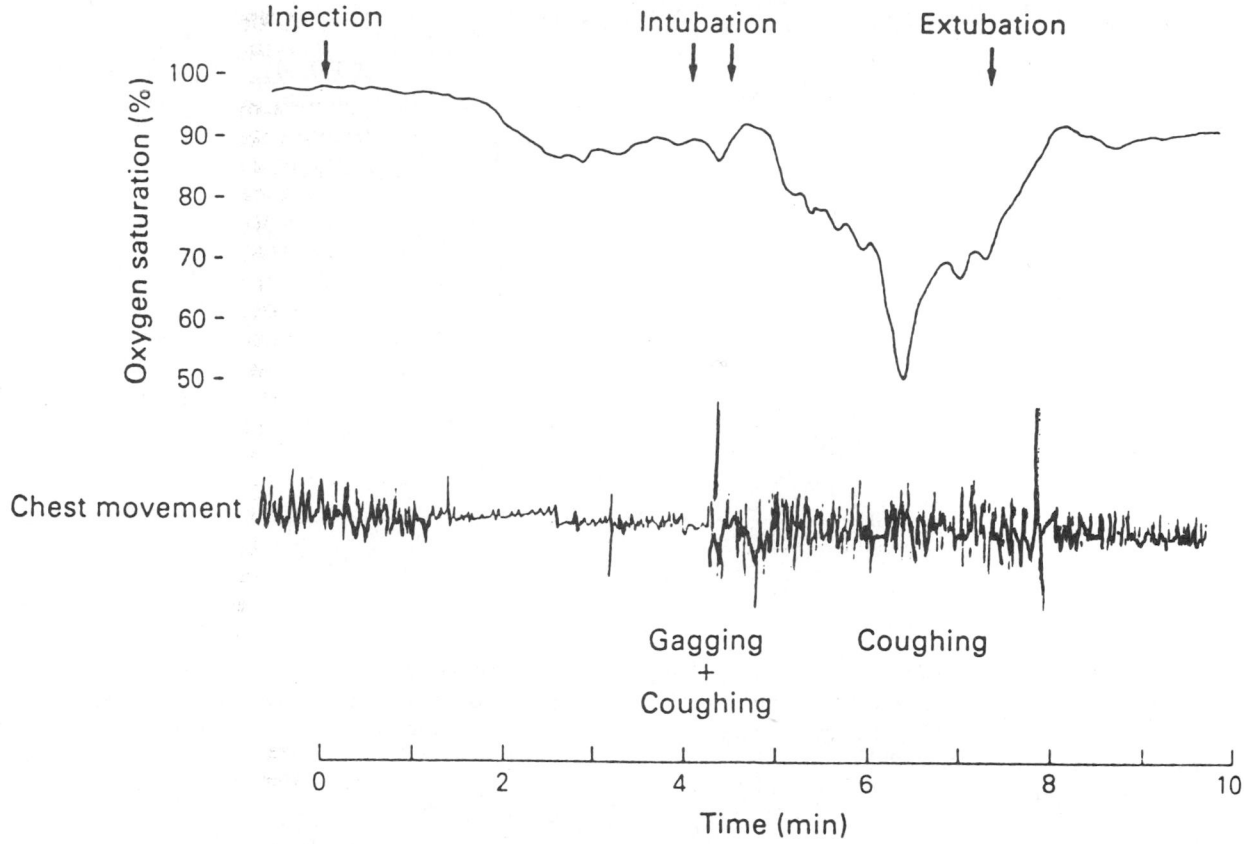

Fig. 26-7. Oxygen saturation and chest wall movements decreased in a patient after injection of midazolam during gastroscopy. After introduction of the gastroscope, the patient coughed and oxygen saturation decreased even more. (From Bell et al.,[94] with permission.)

zolam to patients with COPD.[97] Within 15 minutes, the slope for the carbon dioxide response curve returned to 33 percent of control in patients with COPD and to 75 percent of control in normal patients (Fig. 26-8). The levels of sedation were similar for the two groups.

Psychomotor Function. Another concern is that the fatigue associated with preoperative administration of anxiolytics may prevent the scheduled discharge of patients on the day of surgery (see Ch. 65). Even when no surgery has taken place, fatigue has played an important part in certain widely publicized accidents involving human error.[98–100] No epidemiologic study has yet attempted to show the relationship between the lingering effects of anesthetics and the occurrence of accidents. In general, benzodiazepines do delay recovery from anesthesia.

Recovery from anesthesia is initially slower when anxiolytics have been administered preoperatively. Studies of nonpatient subjects have shown that the longer excretion rates of anxiolytics result in longer depression of psychomotor function. However, with the exception of lorazepam, which has a much longer effect than the other anxiolytics, the times to discharge

from the hospital do not differ for patients who are and are not given premedicant anxiolytics.

Another study of nonpatient volunteers assessed recovery from anesthesia after intravenous administration of sedatives.[101] Subjects given diazepam (0.3 mg/kg) had impaired perceptual speed (the speed with which subjects could find well-known symbols in a mass of material) for 5 hours, and impaired postural stability for as long as 7 hours after drug administration. Control subjects given saline showed no such effects. Elsewhere, subjects given diazepam (0.15 mg/kg) had impaired coordination and reaction times for up to 2 hours after drug administration.[102] Results of various psychomotor tests (letter deletion, visual reaction time, addition, and seven-digit recall) given to volunteers after intravenous injection of either 5 mg of midazolam or 10 mg of diazepam seem to indicate that midazolam is more than twice as potent as diazepam.[103] After 3 hours, this effect showed signs of reversal, the subjects given midazolam improving more rapidly than those given diazepam (Fig. 26-9).

Although such studies clearly demonstrate the prolonged effects of the benzodiazepines, the clinical significance of these findings is less clear. For example,

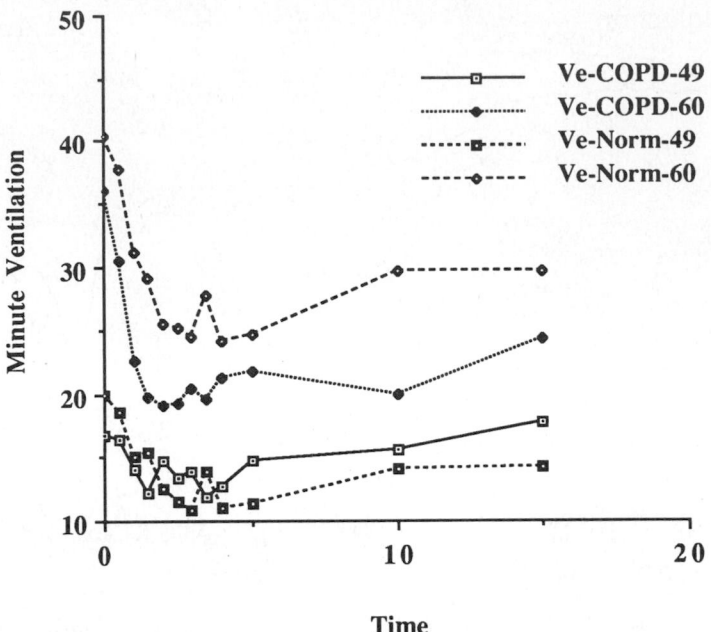

Fig. 26-8. After intravenous injection of midazolam, 0.2 mg/kg, ventilatory depression in response to low levels of carbon dioxide (49 or 60 mmHg) was much greater in subjects with chronic obstructive pulmonary disease ("Ve-COPD-49" and "Ve-COPD-60") than in normal subjects ("Ve-Norm-49" and "Ve-Norm-60"). (From Gross et al.,[97] with permission.)

when 15 mg of midazolam was administered to patients undergoing excisional breast biopsy, their performance on a letter cancellation task was similar to baseline by 4 hours after surgery or 6 hours after drug administration.[104]

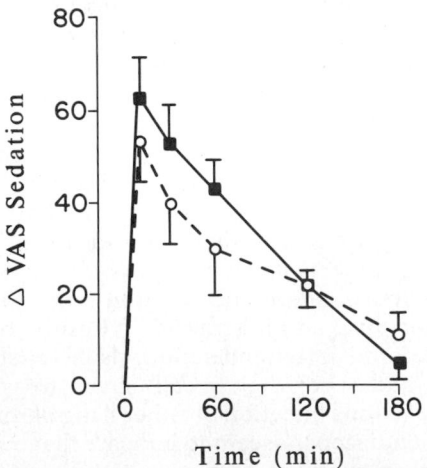

Fig. 26-9. Mean change in the subjective visual analogue scale (VAS) after sedation with diazepam (light circles) or midazolam (dark squares). Initially, sedation was greater after 5 mg of midazolam than after 10 mg of diazepam. By 80 minutes after drug injection, however, sedation with diazepam began to exceed that with midazolam. (From Galletly et al.,[103] with permission.)

Comparison of midazolam with diazepam in terms of the return of psychomotor function has not produced as many differences as one might expect. Outpatients given either local anesthesia and diazepam (0.2 mg/kg IV) or one of two doses of midazolam (0.05 or 0.10 mg/kg IV) for bronchoscopy did not differ in their ability to perform a visualization test, an aiming test, and a perceptual speed test.[105] Two hours after drug administration, performance was similar to that before sedation. However, at this time, 17 percent of patients given the higher dose of midazolam (0.1 mg/kg) were unable to walk a straight line, whereas patients given diazepam or the lower dose of midazolam were able to do so. Another study reported that the level of sedation during recovery, the discharge times, and postoperative Trieger test scores were similar for patients given diazepam at a dose of 0.1 to 0.3 mg/kg and those given midazolam at a dose of 0.05 to 0.15 mg/kg.[51] A third study assessed not only drug-related differences in test scores but also recall.[106] Anesthesia for outpatient gynecologic surgery was induced and maintained with intravenous administration of either midazolam (0.07 mg/kg) or diazepam (0.15 mg/kg), both given with fentanyl (1.5 μg/kg) and then etomidate. When measured at either 30 minutes or 3 hours after surgery, there was no difference in scores on performance tests, recall of operative events, or recall of pain on injection of etomidate.

Because of its very long duration of action, some physicians avoid using lorazepam for outpatient ambulatory surgery. Oral administration of 2 and 4 mg of lorazepam with pentobarbital has impaired hand-eye coordination for 4 and 8 hours, respectively.[107] Using a paper and pencil test, one study assessed possible drug-related differences in psychomotor performance of 58 female patients undergoing laparoscopy.[74] Patients were given 0.25 mg of triazolam, 2 mg of lorazepam, or placebo as oral premedication. When tested 2 hours after laparoscopy, the number of patients who had lower-than-median test results was higher with lorazepam (15/18) than with triazolam (6/17) or placebo (6/18).

The results of psychomotor performance tests after anesthesia must be interpreted carefully. A necessary limitation on the interpretation of any study involves the nature of the tasks and their relationship to actual functioning. For example, does a delay in visual reaction time mean that a patient is indeed more likely to have an automobile accident? Another limitation is that some patients perceive psychomotor testing as trivial and irrelevant. Others view the tests as a contest and therefore spend more effort on them than they would on normal daily activities. In either case, the tests may not provide a true measure of a patient's ability to function once he or she leaves the hospital. Finally, even though certain drug regimens may decrease performance, this side effect usually does not constitute the primary reason for a longer hospital stay. That is, patients normally do not stay in the hospital because they are too sleepy but, rather, because they are perhaps nauseous.

One study of ambulatory patients supports this conclusion. Patients were given either placebo or 5 mg of midazolam intramuscularly, followed by 100 μg of fentanyl, 1 mg of oxymorphone, or placebo immediately before induction.[108] Although various measures of recovery did not differ between groups, more patients given placebo became nauseous. Furthermore, the patients who had nausea or vomiting had longer hospital stays. Thus, despite the theory that benzodiazepines prolong outpatient stay, actual clinical studies do not seem to support that conclusion. In fact, as discussed more fully later, benzodiazepines may shorten overall hospital stay.

Amnesia. The potential for amnesia after premedication is another concern, especially for patients undergoing ambulatory surgery. One anecdotal report of several patients given 2 mg of midazolam intravenously in the preoperative waiting area said that these patients not only did not remember meeting their surgeon or anesthesiologist before the operation, but also wondered whether they had been present for the operation.[109] No controlled studies have shown that retrograde amnesia has occurred in patients given midazolam or diazepam.[38,84,110] Amnesia does occur after administration of benzodiazepines.[38,51,60,111,112] In one study, 42 percent of patients given a placebo, but only 2.8 percent of patients given midazolam (0.1 mg/kg IM), could remember induction of anesthesia for cervical dilation and uterine curettage ($P <$ 0.0001).[113] It is interesting to note, however, that so many patients given placebo could not remember induction.

After administration of lorazepam, amnesia can persist for quite a while. For example, 70 to 80 percent of patients given 4 mg of lorazepam intravenously had amnesia that lasted as long as 4 hours.[114] A 2-mg intrave-

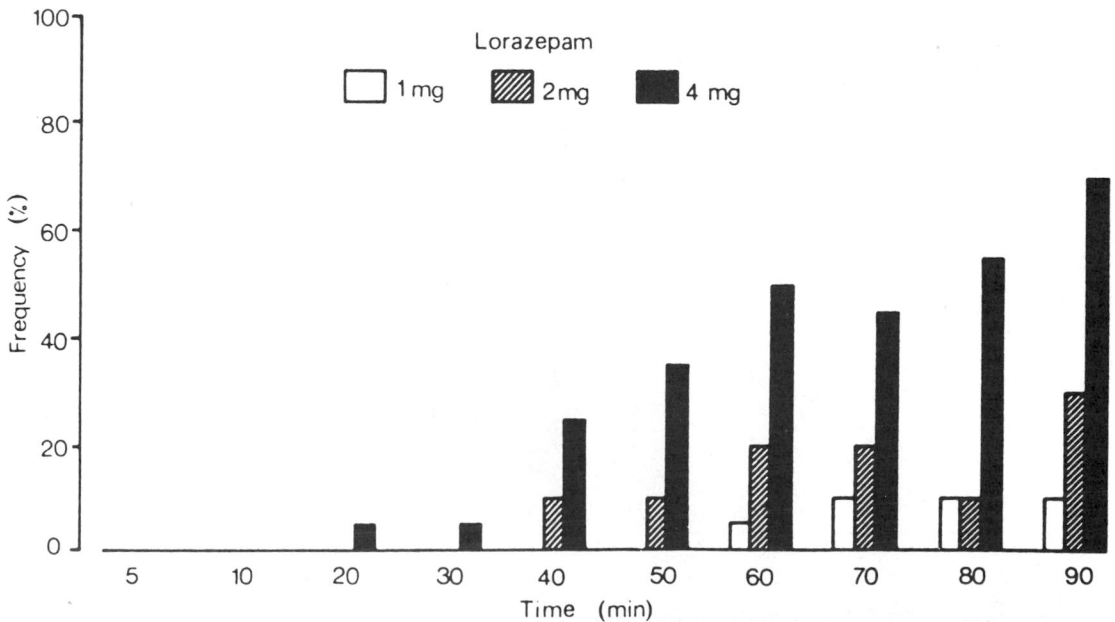

Fig. 26-10. Percent frequency of failure to recognize a previously seen stimulus (picture postcard), shown at the times indicated, after oral administration of 1, 2, or 4 mg of lorazepam. Recall was assessed 6 hours after surgery. (From McKay and Dundee,[60] with permission.)

nous dose produced amnesia in 50 percent of patients; the latency period was 30 minutes, and the duration of action was 30 minutes (Fig. 26-10; compare with diazepam, Fig. 26-11).

Recommendations

This author uses the following criteria regarding use of benzodiazepines. If the patient has been seen at least 24 hours before a scheduled procedure and is judged to need preoperative medication because of an expressed desire or anxiety that cannot be relieved with comforting, oral administration of *diazepam*, 10 mg/70 kg body weight, is prescribed for 6:00 a.m. on the day of surgery. If surgery is scheduled for 1:00 p.m. or later, the drug should be taken at 8:00 a.m. on the day of surgery. When patients are seen for the first time in the preoperative holding area and seem to need medication (again, because of an expressed desire, anxiety that cannot be relieved with assurances, or, on rare occasion, the ineffectiveness of a previously administered dose of diazepam), midazolam is administered intravenously with or without a narcotic. The initial dose of midazolam is 0.03 mg/kg.

PROMOTING HEMODYNAMIC STABILITY WITH PREMEDICATION

Hypertensive patients who have coronary artery disease are particularly likely to have extremes of blood pressure before, during, and after surgery.[115-118] Intra-

operative hypertension is treated by precise adjustment of the level of anesthesia and/or by administration of antihypertensive agents. In spite of these measures, arterial blood pressure can become extremely high, especially when hypertension already exists, during intense stimulation (e.g., laryngoscopy or sternotomy), or during emergence from anesthesia. Individuals who take antihypertensive medication should continue these drugs up to the time of surgery. Patients who have hypertension that is well controlled before surgery usually have relatively stable blood pressure during surgery, whereas those whose hypertension is not well controlled may have extreme hypotension or hypertension during the procedure.[119]

Clonidine, an α_2-Adrenergic Agonist

Recently, preoperative administration of α_2-adrenergic agonists has been shown to reduce intraoperative extremes of blood pressure. Of these agents, clonidine has been studied most extensively. Unlike antihypertensive drugs such as guanethidine, propranolol, and captopril, which act peripherally, clonidine affects the central release of catecholamines. Thus, as with other drugs affecting the central release of adrenergics,[120-122] clonidine not only reduces anesthetic requirement (as represented by the minimum alveolar concentration [MAC] of an anesthetic; also see Ch. 30) but also decreases extremes in arterial blood pressure during anesthesia.[123] Indeed, part of the reason that clonidine decreases extremes in blood pressure during anesthesia may be that it reduces anesthetic requirement.

Halothane anesthesia can be potentiated by the administration of clonidine. A crossover study of eight

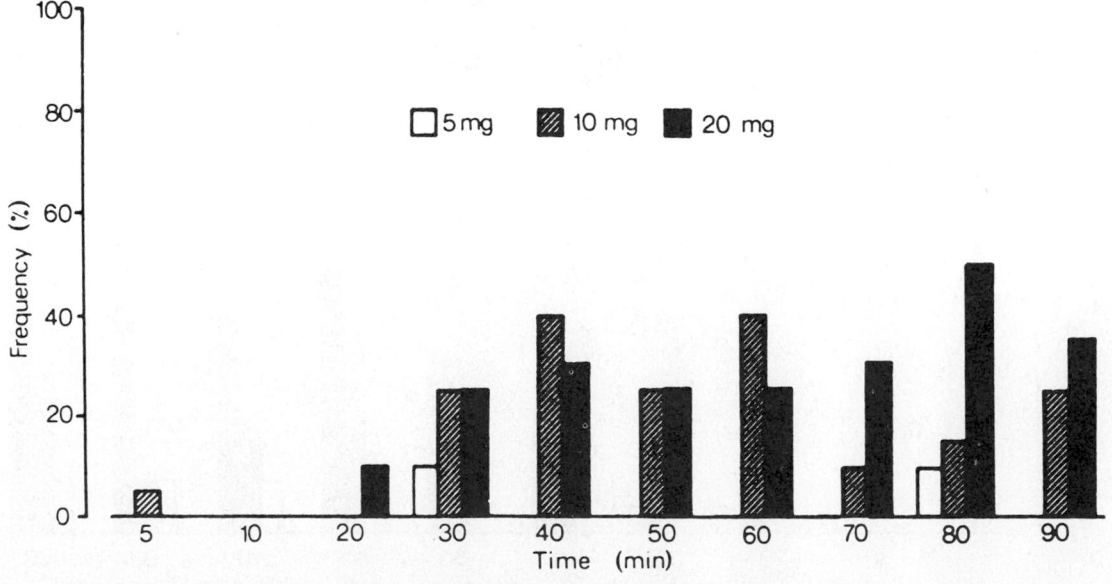

Fig. 26-11. Percent frequency of failure to recognize a previously seen stimulus (picture postcard), shown at the times indicated, after oral administration of 5, 10, or 20 mg of diazepam. Recall was assessed 6 hours after surgery. (From McKay and Dundee,[60] with permission.)

rabbits given either placebo or clonidine subcutaneously for 3 days showed that the MAC for halothane was 1.29 percent in unpremedicated rabbits but 1.09 percent in premedicated animals.[124] A single 5- or 20-μg/kg dose of clonidine in dogs reduced MAC as much as 42 percent at 2.3 hours and 48 percent at 2.6 hours, respectively.[125] In effect, clonidine exhibited a "ceiling": the higher dose did not reduce MAC to a greater extent than did the lower dose. Acute administration of clonidine reduces MAC to a greater extent than chronic administration, possibly because of the development of tolerance to the drug.[126,127] The ceiling effect in the reduction of MAC is not as apparent with azepexole, a more highly selective α_2-adrenergic agonist.[128] Azepexole causes both sedation and analgesia indistinguishable from that produced by general anesthesia.

No formal MAC studies with clonidine have been performed on human beings. However, MAC is lower when clonidine is given. In one study of patients with a history of arterial hypertension who were undergoing cardiopulmonary bypass, the addition of an orally administered 5-μg/kg dose of clonidine to premedication with morphine and lorazepam 90 minutes before induction reduced the requirement for fentanyl by 45 percent, as assessed by electroencephalogram.[129]

A similar study of patients undergoing elective abdominal, head and neck, or orthopedic surgery reported a 40 percent reduction in the requirement for isoflurane and a significant decrease in the need for narcotic supplementation.[130] Another study also noted the effect of clonidine on the requirement for isoflurane, which was used to induce hypotension in patients undergoing middle-ear or nasal surgery and on the need for supplemental doses of labetalol.[131] Patients given a 0.6-mg oral dose of clonidine 2 hours before surgery required less isoflurane for induction (2 versus 3 percent, $P < 0.05$) or maintenance (1.4 versus 2.3 percent, $P < 0.01$) of controlled hypotension than did control patients. Also, fewer patients given clonidine needed supplemental doses of labetalol (1/10 versus 5/10).

Clonidine also reduces the requirement for sufentanil.[132] Patients undergoing cardiopulmonary bypass were given 200 or 300 μg of clonidine orally 90 minutes before transport to the operating room. A second dose of 200 or 300 μg was given via nasogastric tube 5 hours after the first dose, before initiation of cardiopulmonary bypass and hypothermia. Patients given clonidine had a 40 percent lower requirement for sufentanil, significantly shorter times to extubation, and, for reasons that are not entirely clear, a lower incidence of postoperative shivering.

The fact that MAC decreases with clonidine implies that hemodynamic variability also decreases. In most instances, unless blood pressure stays the same, the amount of anesthetic required does not change. Several studies have investigated the issue of hemodynamic variability with clonidine. In one study (discussed earlier), patients undergoing elective abdominal, head and neck, or orthopedic surgery after pretreatment with clonidine had significantly less variability in heart rate ($P < 0.05$) and systolic ($P < 0.01$) and diastolic ($P < 0.05$) blood pressures.[130] In addition, these patients had significantly slower heart rate during recovery (mean $\pm$ SD, 79 $\pm$ 10 beats/min with clonidine versus 101 $\pm$ 23 beats/min for controls; $P < 0.01$). After intubation, heart rate was 10 percent higher in patients pretreated with clonidine but 25 percent higher in controls. Transient ischemic changes occurred on the electrocardiograms of two of the untreated (control) patients whose heart rate exceeded 100 beats/min.

In another study of hemodynamic changes associated with endotracheal intubation of American Society of Anesthesiologists (ASA) I and II patients scheduled for elective surgery, the mean maximal increase in heart rate was lowest in patients pretreated with clonidine.[133] However, the changes in mean arterial blood pressure associated with intubation did not differ significantly between the pretreatment and control groups. In addition, during endotracheal intubation, the incidence of bigeminy on the electrocardiogram was higher for unpretreated patients (7/40) than for pretreated patients (0/23). Twenty-one women undergoing breast surgery after administration of clonidine (4.5 μg/kg) 2 hours earlier had smaller mean ($\pm$SD) increases in postintubation heart rate (14 $\pm$ 11 beats/min versus 25 $\pm$ 11 beats/min) and systolic blood pressure (8 $\pm$ 8 mmHg versus 27 $\pm$ 21 mmHg) than untreated (control) patients.[134]

Hemodynamic stability has also been greater in elderly patients. Elderly patients given clonidine (5 μg/kg) 90 to 120 minutes before arrival at the operating room for elective ophthalmic surgery under general anesthesia had less cardiovascular response to tracheal intubation than did control patients.[135] The increase in intraocular pressure was also less, being 10 percent with pretreatment and 53 percent without pretreatment (Fig. 26-12). Presumably, this difference is attributable to either a reduction in the production of aqueous humor or an increase in the facility for outflow of aqueous humor.

Side effects of clonidine administration, including marked sedation and dryness of the mouth, were common in many of the investigations mentioned. These side effects were related to the plasma concentration of the drug.[136] In addition, severe hypotension or bradycardia occasionally occurred. For example, in one study of hemodynamic changes associated with tracheal intubation, ASA I and II patients undergoing elective surgery were given 225 to 375 μg of clonidine, according to weight.[133] Patients had been excluded from study if marked hypotension and bradycardia occurred during induction: two patients had systolic blood pressure of less than 70 mmHg and heart rate of less than 40 beats/min). Nevertheless, significantly more pretreated patients than control patients had bradycardia (< 45 beats/min) in the recovery room.

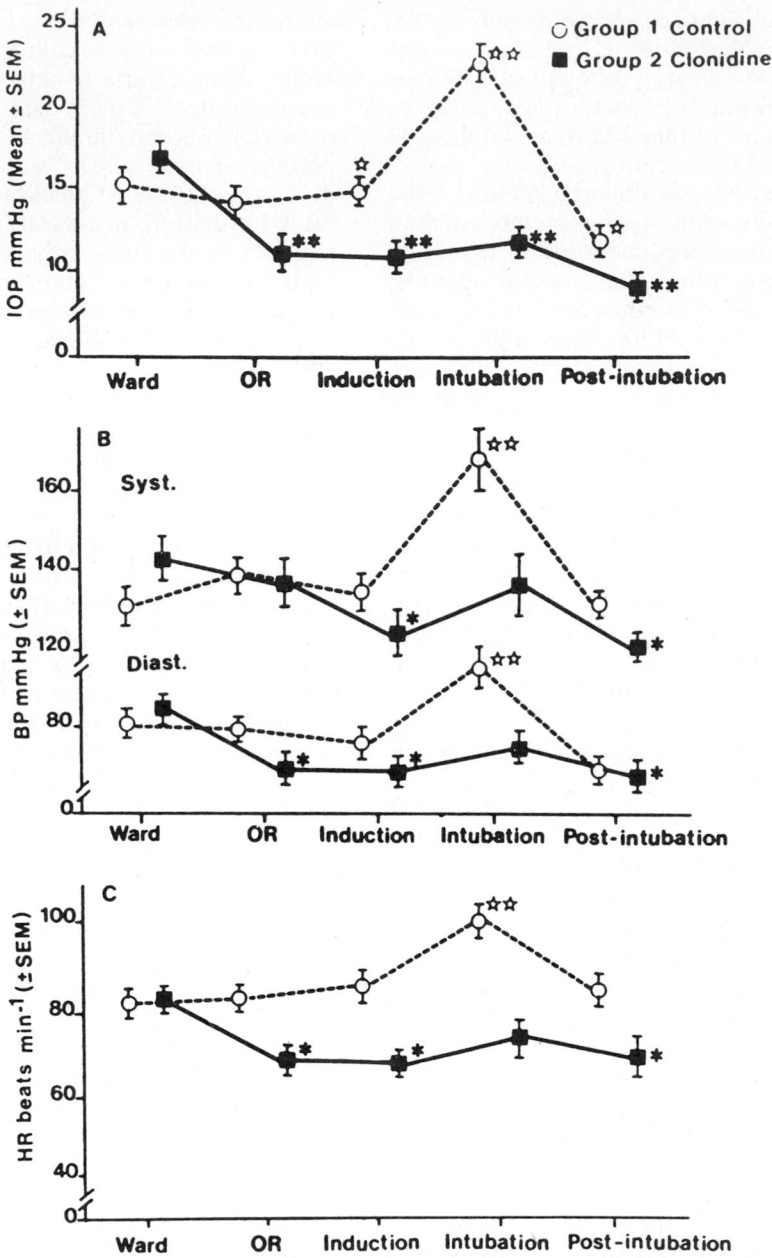

Fig. 26-12. Intraocular pressure (IOP), blood pressure (BP), and heart rate (HR) in patients given clonidine (an α_2-adrenergic agonist) before elective ophthalmic surgery under general anesthesia. Variables were measured before premedication (Ward), on arrival at the operating room ("OR"), after induction ("Induction"), within 3 minutes of endotracheal intubation ("Intubation"), and 8 minutes after endotracheal intubation ("Post-intubation"). *$P < 0.05$ and **$P < 0.01$, when values were compared with values on the ward. ☆$P < 0.05$ and ☆☆$P < 0.001$, when values for a given measurement were compared between groups. (From Ghignone et al.,[135] with permission.)

Recommendations

Although α_2-adrenergic agonists are not specifically anxiolytics, their potential as premedication is an attractive alternative, or perhaps addition to, the use of benzodizepines. This possibility is especially pertinent to individuals who are hypertensive before surgery and to those likely to become hypertensive during surgery. However, these agents have not yet become as popular as the benzodiazepines. Much of the work regarding the use of α_2-adrenergic agonists has been published only recently and focuses on one drug, clonidine.

DECREASING THE RISK OF ASPIRATION OF GASTRIC CONTENTS

The Risk of Aspiration

Patients who undergo surgery are at some risk of aspiration of gastric contents (see also Ch. 40). The volume and pH of the aspirated matter determine the extent of pulmonary damage. Pulmonary damage can occur if the volume is 25 ml and the pH is ≤ 2.5.[137] If pH is only 1.0, aspirated volumes as low as 0.3 mg/kg can incur a very high mortality rate.[138] Various studies of gastric pH and volume have shown that unpremedicated patients are at significant risk of aspiration of acidic gastric contents. Studies on outpatients report that the mean pH of gastric contents varies from 1.86 to 2.34 and that mean volume ranges from 25.6 to 45.48 ml.[139-143] Also, the percentage of outpatients having residual volumes ≥ 25 ml (and pH ≤ 2.5) is estimated to be 36 to 56 percent.

Conflicting evidence in the literature indicates that outpatients may be at greater risk of aspiration than inpatients. For example, one study comparing gastric volume and pH in 21 inpatients and 21 outpatients found that although average pH did not differ, outpatients had greater gastric volumes than inpatients.[144] Four of the outpatients had gastric volumes greater than 75 ml (pH < 2.0), values that were much more extreme than those seen in outpatients in most other studies. On the other hand, a similar study of 25 inpatients and 25 outpatients found no difference in gastric volume, gastric pH, or number of patients at risk of aspiration.[141]

Certain categories of patients (e.g., pregnant or morbidly obese patients or patients with hiatal hernia) may be at greater risk of aspiration. Also, smokers may be particularly prone to morbidity from aspiration. In a study of smokers versus nonsmokers undergoing outpatient surgery, the average gastric volume ($\pm$SD) was 8.6 ± 5.6 ml for nonsmokers but 18.8 ± 10.8 ml for patients who had smoked on the day of surgery.[145] Furthermore, 4 of the 19 smokers had gastric volume of more than 25 ml and gastric pH of 2.0 or less. In contrast, a similar study of outpatients found no difference in the average volume of aspirated material or its pH.[146] However, in this study, unlike the previous one, smokers were told not to smoke after midnight of the night before surgery and all patients were premedicated with diazepam (15 mg PO) 1 hour before surgery.

Although smoking itself may not increase gastric acidity, some association does exist between increased anxiety and smoking.[147] Some association also exists between increased anxiety and increased gastric acidity. A study of gastric pH measured in two patients during psychotherapy indicated that secretion of hydrocholoric acid increased during periods of anxiety.[148] Diazepam reduces gastric secretion and total acid output, presumably because it reduces anxiety.[149] In a review of their own work and that of others, Gray and Ramsey[150] gave examples of the relationship between various stress factors (such as burns, surgery, fractures, and emotions) and increased gastric acidity.

How Long Should a Patient Be "NPO"?

To decrease the risk of aspiration of gastric contents, patients are routinely asked not to eat or drink anything (*non per os* "nothing by mouth") for at least 6 to 8 hours before surgery. However, patients may take medicines with a sip of water if they do so at least 2 hours before the procedure. In fact, taking a small amount of liquid 2 hours before surgery may actually increase gastric pH and promote gastric emptying. One study of patients given diazepam orally with 50 ml of water and a similar group given diazepam intramuscularly found that gastric volume was smaller (median volume, 1.5 versus 20 ml) and pH higher (median pH, 2.4 versus 1.8) for patients given diazepam and water.[151] When 100 cc of water was ingested 2 hours before surgery without a pill but in conjunction with an intramuscular premedicant (meperidine and promethazine), gastric volume and pH, although variable, were the same regardless of ingestion of water.[152]

Ingestion of other fluids and even food seems not to affect gastric volume and pH greatly. In one study, patients either drank orange juice or coffee 2 to 3 hours before surgery or fasted overnight.[153] The incidence of gastric volume exceeding 25 ml and of gastric pH less than 2.5 did not differ for the groups. Similarly, the volume and pH of gastric contents did not differ between patients given tea or coffee with milk and one slice of buttered toast on the morning of surgery and those who had fasted.[154] In this last study, the time between breakfast and surgery in the nonfasting group ranged from 2 to 4 hours, the shortest interval being 105 minutes. In the patient having the shortest interval, 5 ml of gastric contents (pH 4.1) was aspirated. Because an 18-gauge tube was used for aspiration of stomach contents, large fragments of food may not have been aspirated.

One study used Bromsulphathalein (BSP) to measure residual gastric volume and pH in outpatients.[155] Patients were given BSP in 10 ml of water and then either 150 ml of water or no additional fluid. Those given the extra water had a significantly lower residual gastric volume than those given no additional fluid (mean $\pm$ SD, 20.6 ± 14.1 ml versus 29.9 ± 18.2 ml). Gastric pH did not differ between groups. When 150 mg of ranitidine is ingested orally with 150 ml of water, mean ($\pm$SD) gastric volume decreases even further (from 17.6 ± 14.5 ml without ranitidine to 8.3 ± 7.3 ml with ranitidine) and gastric pH increases (from 1.75 ± 0.94 to 5.52 ± 1.79).[156]

One group of authors found that gastric volumes were greater if patients were given 100 cc rather than 50 cc of water with oral diazepam (0.3 mg/kg); 32 ml of gastric contents were aspirated with 100 cc of water and 16 ml was aspirated with 50 cc of water.[157] Values for pH did not differ between groups. This study assessed gastric volumes from 1.5 to 6 hours after premedication. The longer period from premedication to determination of gastric volume is not unlike the standard 6- to 8-hour fast.

The preceding data show the difficulty of making firm conclusions about how long a patient should be NPO. In *Basics of Anesthesia*, Stoelting and Miller[158] draw the following conclusions:

> Fasting before elective surgery . . . after midnight is recommended in the hope of minimizing gastric fluid volume at the time of induction of anesthesia. Nevertheless, complete emptying of the stomach can never be guaranteed. Furthermore, foods pass through the stomach at variable and unpredictable rates, sometimes taking up to 12 hours. In contrast, water and crystalloid-containing solutions have a 50 percent emptying time of only 12 minutes to 20 minutes. Therefore, it may be illogical to have a single guideline for solid and liquid ingestion before induction of anesthesia for elective operations. Indeed, gastric fluid volumes are less in patients receiving 150 ml of water 2 hours to 3 hours before induction of anesthesia compared with patients who are fasted. It is possible that a liquid bolus stimulates gastric peristalsis and thus gastric emptying. For this reason, it does not seem logical to forbid ingestion of small volumes of liquids before elective surgery. Clearly, this recommendation does not apply to solid foods or to patients at known risk for slow gastric emptying (obese, parturients, opioids included in preoperative medication, diabetes mellitus, gastrointestinal disease).

The recommendation that a patient be NPO for 6 to 8 hours prior to anesthesia and surgery probably still applies.

Drugs That Decrease Gastric Volume and Increase Gastric pH (Also See Ch. 40)

H₂ Receptor Antagonists

Cimetidine and ranitidine are reversible, competitive drugs that antagonize the action of histamine on H₂ receptors. In this way, they inhibit gastric secretion in response to acetylcholine, histamine, or gastrin and reduce concentration of hydrogen ions. The effect of cimetidine begins 60 to 90 minutes after administration and lasts for at least 3 hours.[159] In patients with duodenal ulcers, cimetidine reduces acid secretion by 95 percent for at least 5 hours. Ranitidine is four to six times as potent as cimetidine. Therefore, because the elimination half-lives are similar for the two drugs (2 to 3 hours) and ranitidine is often administered at half the dose of cimetidine, the effects of ranitidine usually last longer (8 to 12 hours).[160] Clearly, H₂ receptor antagonists raise gastric pH and decrease gastric volume during surgery.[161-163]

Cimetidine inhibits metabolism of a drug by impairing its biotransformation by cytochrome P-450. Therefore, the action of drugs that are dependent on the cytochrome P-450 microsomal enzyme system (such as diazepam) is potentiated when such drugs are taken with cimetidine.[164] Potentiation occurs after as little as 1 day of therapy with cimetidine and a single injection of diazepam. Cimetidine can also affect the metabolism of midazolam and increase plasma concentrations of the drug.[165] The effect of lorazepam, which is not transformed by the cytochrome P-450 microsomal enzyme system but by glucuronic acid, is not potentiated by cimetidine.[166] Cimetidine also decreases blood flow in the liver by 25 percent after acute administration during fasting and by 33 percent after chronic administration. Thus, drugs such as propranolol, the hepatic elimination of which depends on blood flow in the liver, are eliminated from the body more slowly when given in conjunction with cimetidine.[167] Hence, resting heart rate is markedly lower after administration of propranolol and cimetidine than after administration of propranolol alone.

Other drug interactions with cimetidine (with recommendations for therapy in parentheses) include the following: oral anticoagulants (e.g., warfarin [monitor coagulation variables], theophylline [decrease maintenance dose by 50 percent but do not change loading dose], phenytoin and carbamazepine [reduce maintenance dose by 33 percent], and lidocaine [reduce maintenance dose by 50 percent]).[168] Cimetidine also reduces clearance of bupivacaine.[169]

Unlike cimetidine, ranitidine has a much weaker effect on cytochrome P-450. In most studies, the interaction of ranitidine with other drugs has not produced statistically significant differences.[170]

Famotidine and nizatidine, two new H₂ receptor antagonists, are similar to cimetidine and ranitidine. On an equimolar basis, famotidine is approximately 7.5 times more potent than ranitidine and 20 times more potent than cimetidine. For healing duodenal ulcers, a 20-mg dose of famotidine twice daily or a 40-mg dose at bedtime is as effective as standard doses of cimetidine and ranitidine.[171] Nizatidine is three times more potent than cimetidine.[172] Both nizatidine and famotidine, like ranitidine but unlike cimetidine, do not bind to cytochrome P-450 to any degree and hence do not interfere with the hepatic metabolism of various drugs.[173] For example, cimetidine inhibits the hepatic elimination of diazepam in humans by approximately 45 percent, whereas ranitidine, nizatidine, and famotidine do not. Although a 40-mg oral dose of famotidine is equivalent to a 300-mg oral dose of ranitidine in terms of increasing gastric pH,[174] one study found slightly higher gastric volumes after 150 mg of oral ranitidine than after 40 mg of oral famotidine.[175] To date, no data have been published regarding patients undergoing surgery after administration of nizatidine.

This class of drugs sometimes causes mental confusion, particularly in elderly patients (Fig. 26-13),[176] and usually within 48 hours of the first dose. Deterioration in mental function occasionally follows acute deterioration in renal or hepatic function. Symptoms include restlessness, confusion, disorientation, agitation, hallucinations, focal twitching, seizures, unresponsiveness,

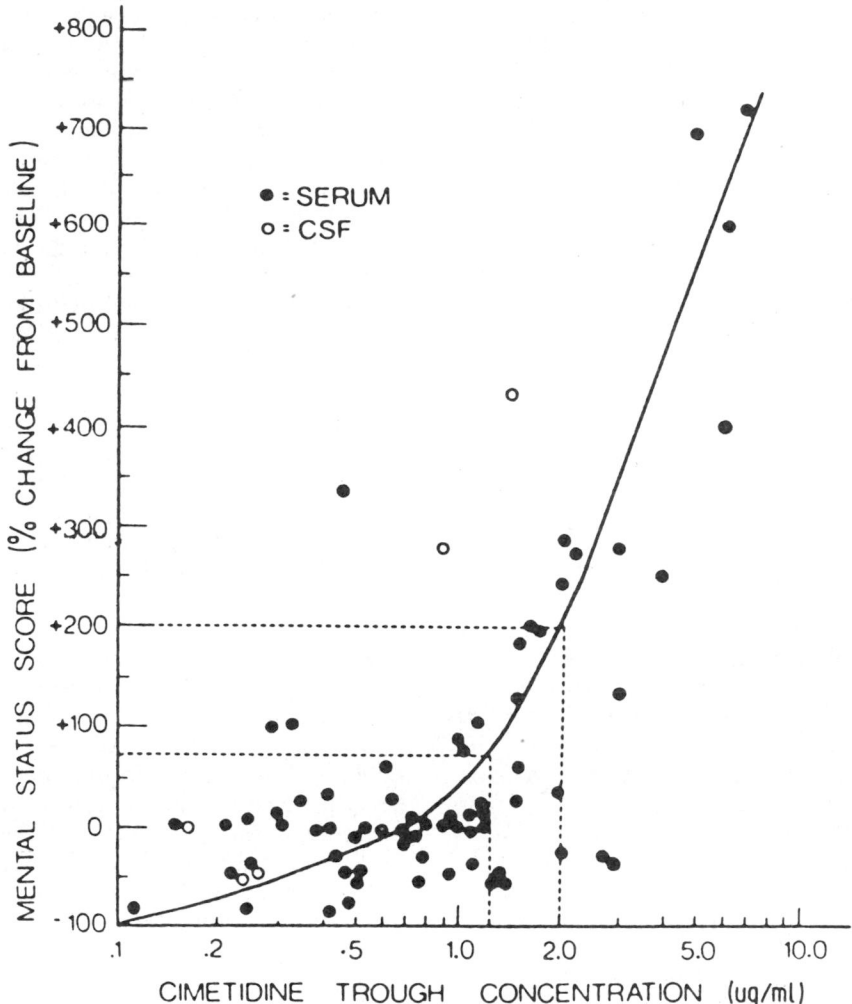

Fig. 26-13. Cimetidine, an H_2 receptor antagonist, sometimes causes mental confusion. This figure shows the relationship between trough concentrations of cimetidine in serum and cerebrospinal fluid (CSF) and scores of mental status. Because almost one-third of patients had impaired mental status before administration of cimetidine, the unit of measurement used for mental status was the percentage change from baseline. A 200 percent increase over baseline was judged to constitute significant mental impairment. A normal trough concentration of cimetidine is less than 1.25 μg/ml. (From Schentag et al.,[176] with permission.)

and apnea. This syndrome is associated with trough concentrations of cimetidine of more than 2.0 μg/ml. Confusion is much less common with ranitidine.[177,178]

Sodium Citrate

Recently, the use of soluble antacids such as sodium citrate or Bicitra has become popular. (Bicitra is a commercial preparation of sodium citrate and citric acid in a sugar-free base). Aspiration of soluble antacids produces less severe hypoxia and lung abnormalities than does aspiration of nonabsorbable antacids such as Mylanta.[179] Alka-Seltzer Effervescent solution (active ingredient, sodium citrate) is also an effective soluble antacid.[180]

Although administration of soluble antacids does raise gastric pH, it can also increase gastric volume. The following study illustrates this point by using the values for gastric pH and volume that are commonly considered critical to pulmonary damage if aspiration occurs, namely $\leq$ 2.5 for pH and $\geq$ 25 ml for volume (if pH $\leq$ 2.5).[140] Specifically, outpatients were given 0 (controls), 15, or 30 ml of Bicitra orally. Both doses of Bicitra decreased the percentage of patients having gastric contents at the critically low pH level (from 88 percent for controls to 32 percent with 15 ml of Bicitra, and to 16 percent with 30 ml of Bicitra). However, both doses of Bicitra increased the percentage of patients having gastric contents at the critically high level for volume (pH being $\leq$ 2.5) (i.e., from 36 percent for controls to 56 percent with 15 ml of Bicitra and to 84 percent with 30 ml of Bicitra).

A study of 16 women undergoing general anesthesia for cesarean section found that 30 ml of sodium citrate increased gastric pH above 3.5 in all patients.[181] The average ($\pm$SD) gastric volume was 26.1 ± 28.6 ml. These researchers had asked their patients to roll 90 degrees to each side to increase mixing of the antacids with stomach contents.

One group of investigators demonstrated that very small volumes of sodium bicarbonate can increase gastric pH without affecting gastric volume.[182] To determine the volume of gastric contents, these researchers removed as much gastric fluid as possible while patients were anesthetized. They then injected a volume of 8.4 percent sodium bicarbonate that was equal to 5 percent of the volume of gastric fluid. For most patients, 1.60 ml (mean value) of sodium bicarbonate increased gastric pH to 7.0, an effect that lasted for 120 minutes.

Metoclopramide

Metoclopromide is a dopamine antagonist that increases pressure of the lower esophageal sphincter, speeds gastric emptying, and prevents or alleviates nausea and vomiting.[183] Administration of metoclopramide in combination with other drugs reduces gastric volume to an even greater extent. For example, when 10 mg of intravenous metoclopramide was included with either 15 or 30 ml of Bicitra, the percentages of patients having gastric volume at the critically high level (≥ 25 ml) decreased from 56 and 84 percent to 28 and 36 percent, respectively.[140] Similarly, mean ($\pm$SE) gastric fluid volume was 51 ± 2.33 ml for patients given cimetidine alone but only 12.05 ± 0.79 ml for patients given both cimetidine and metoclopramide.[184] Gastric pH was treated more effectively with cimetidine than with metoclopramide, although none of the patients given both drugs had gastric pH lower than 2.5. When 300 mg of oral cimetidine was given at bedtime and then repeated the morning of surgery with 10 mg of oral metoclopramide, the risk of pulmonary damage from aspiration of gastric contents was essentially eliminated.[185] That is, gastric pH was ≥ 5 ml and gastric volume was ≤ 25 ml for all patients.

Metoclopramide is also an effective antiemetic.[186] A side benefit of giving metoclopramide before surgery may be less nausea and vomiting, not only during but also after surgery, especially for patients undergoing regional anesthesia. The duration of action of metoclopramide is relatively brief, however, and published reports contain conflicting views about its effectiveness. One study of patients undergoing anesthesia with fentanyl, nitrous oxide, and succinylcholine for therapeutic abortion found that 10 mg of intravenous metoclopramide given 2 to 10 minutes before induction of anesthesia did not decrease postoperative nausea and vomiting.[187] However, patients given this drug were able to sit up, walk, and leave the hospital sooner than

were control patients. The reason for this was not clear. Similarly, intramuscular administration of 10 or 20 mg of metoclopramide before minor gynecologic surgery under methohexital and nitrous oxide anesthesia did not decrease nausea and vomiting after surgery.[188] On the other hand, a 0.15 mg/kg dose of intravenous metoclopramide did reduce the incidence of postdelivery nausea (from 36 percent with placebo to 12 percent) and vomiting (from 15 percent with placebo to 0 percent) in patients undergoing elective cesarean section under epidural anesthesia with fentanyl supplementation.[189] Nausea was assessed at the time of clamping of the umbilical cord.

Two other studies of women undergoing outpatient gynecologic procedures under mask anesthesia produced similar results. In one study, women given metoclopramide had significantly less postoperative nausea and vomiting (4/48) than did control patients (9/53).[190] In the second study, women given either 2.5 mg of droperidol or 10 mg of metoclopramide intravenously before induction of anesthesia (with fentanyl, pentothal, etomidate, and nitrous oxide by face mask) had a significantly lower incidence of nausea or vomiting (21 percent after droperidol, 26 percent after metoclopramide, and 47 percent after placebo).[191]

One reason for the conflicting views concerning the effectiveness of metoclopramide as an antiemetic may be that the doses being used have been too low. For example, oral doses of 0.15 to 0.3 mg/kg have not been effective in preventing emesis induced by cisplatin, an antineoplastic drug given to cancer patients, whereas intravenous doses of 2 mg/kg have been much more effective.[192] These higher doses, however, have not been used perioperatively.

Metoclopramide is a very safe drug; overdoses of up to 100 times the recommended amount have been tolerated without serious consequences.[193] The most common side effects involve the central nervous system and include lassitude, drowsiness, transient agitation, and motor restlessness; dystonia occurs in approximately 1 percent of patients, most frequently the young.[194] The extrapyramidal reactions usually occur within 36 hours of the start of treatment and are rare after a single dose. One patient had extreme agitation 10 minutes after 10 mg of metoclopramide and 0.2 mg of glycopyrrolate given intravenously.

Similar case reports describe a variety of side effects after administration of small doses of metoclopramide in combination with phenothiazines or related drugs.[195] Also, two anecdotal reports describe supraventricular or sinus tachycardia after administration of metoclopramide.[196,197] In both instances, heart rate returned to normal within 1 hour. However, one investigation reported that 11 patients undergoing cardiac catheterization for valvular or ischemic heart disease were given 20 mg of metoclopramide intravenously with no serious cardiac sequelae, including no change in heart rate.[198] In the same study, electrocardiographic recording of His-bundle activity in four patients showed no changes in conduction from before to after administration of metoclopramide.

Recommendations

In my practice, sodium citrate and metoclopramide or an H₂ receptor antagonist is routinely administered to patients at risk of acid aspiration, particularly those with hiatal hernia, the morbidly obese, and parturients. Although the idea of feeding patients clear liquids as little as 2 hours before surgery seems attractive, this practice is currently not recommended on a routine basis.

NARCOTICS AND ANTICHOLINERGICS FOR PREOPERATIVE MEDICATION

Narcotics

Narcotics can be administered preoperatively to decrease pain and anxiety before surgery, to sedate the patient, and to control hypertension on tracheal intubation. In addition, meperidine (but not morphine or fentanyl) is sometimes helpful in controlling shivering in the operating or recovery room.[199,200] However, treatment is usually instituted at the time of shivering and not in anticipation of the event.

The effectiveness of narcotics in relieving anxiety is controversial. Use of fentanyl has been particularly fashionable because it is erroneously believed to have a relatively shorter duration of action than meperidine or morphine. Various assessments of fentanyl for preoperative anxiety have been made: fentanyl is effective in relieving anxiety[201]; it is useful when given with diazepam[202,203]; it is less effective than midazolam[204]; and it is no more effective than administration of no medication at all.[202,205] Most studies examining the relationship between fentanyl and anxiety used either no controls or only a single dose of the drug.

Narcotics, particularly fentanyl, alfentanil, and sufentanil, are useful in controlling hypertension on tracheal intubation (Fig. 26-14). A linear relationship exists between increasing doses of narcotic premedication and preventing increases in systolic pressure.[206-208] However, after tracheal intubation, systolic, diastolic, and mean arterial blood pressures sometimes decrease below baseline values measured in patients not given narcotic premedication.[209,210]

Nausea can also be a problem after narcotics. Although administration of alfentanil (10 μg/kg) 1 minute before induction of anesthesia for cesarean section was successful in preventing hypertension during tracheal intubation, 12 of 21 patients had postoperative nausea.[211] In contrast, control patients had hypertension on tracheal intubation, but only 3 of 16 had postoperative nausea. Elsewhere, a study of 1,020 patients undergoing uterine curettage and cervical dilation compared

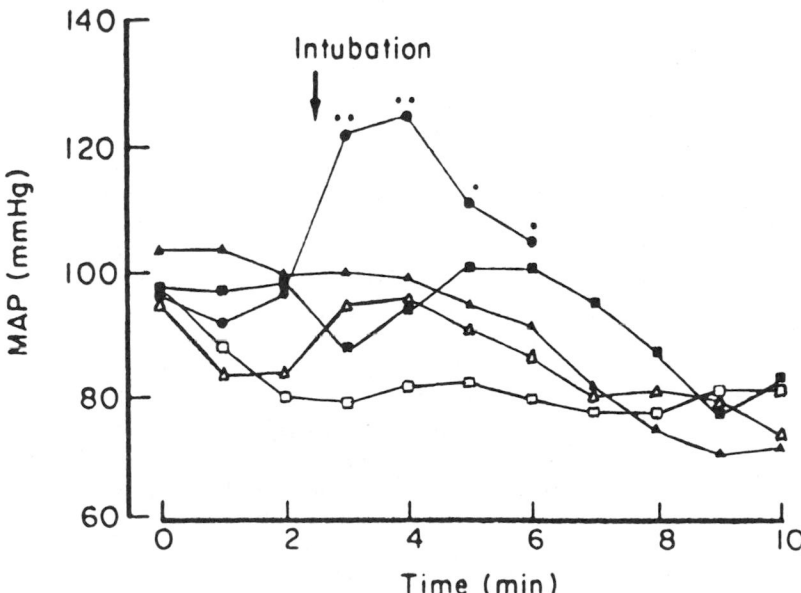

Fig. 26-14. Plotting mean arterial pressure (MAP) against time after laryngoscopy and intubation shows that narcotics control the hypertension associated with tracheal intubation. Five groups were studied: controls, who were given saline (●); those given 15 μg/kg (△) or 30 μg/kg (□) of alfentanil intravenously after administration of thiopental; and those given 5 μg/kg of fentanyl before (■) or after (▲) administration of thiopental. Asterisks indicate significant increases (*$P < 0.05$ and **$P < 0.01$). (From Black et al.,[208] with permission.)

the incidence of nausea and vomiting after administration of one of three drug regimens.[212] The drugs were given 60 to 90 minutes before surgery and consisted of 0.6 mg of atropine by itself or in combination with 10 mg of morphine or 50 mg of meperidine. Vomiting occurred more frequently after morphine (in 49 percent of patients) than after meperidine (36 percent) or atropine alone (29 percent). The incidence of nausea and vomiting was greatest with morphine (67 percent), less with meperidine (51 percent), and least with atropine alone (46 percent).

Other reports have confirmed that premedication with nalbuphine,[213,214] meperidine,[213] morphine,[113,215,216] fentanyl,[214,217–219] butorphanol,[217] or alfentanil[219,220] increases the incidence of nausea or vomiting. Fortunately, administration of atropine with narcotics can decrease nausea or vomiting.[215] Later sections discuss the possibility that postoperative nausea may prolong recovery time in ambulatory patients.

Narcotics slow gastric emptying time and thus sometimes increase gastric volume. One study of patients given either an opioid (meperidine) and an anticholinergic or a benzodizepine found a trend—although not a significant one—toward larger gastric volumes after premedication with narcotics.[154] Decreased respiratory drive and even apnea may also result after administration of narcotics.

This author limits his use of narcotics for premedication to the following situations: for relief or preoperative pain, for regional anesthesia, and for attenuation of the cardiovascular response to endotracheal intubation (e.g., in patients with a history of hypertension).

Anticholinergics

Anticholinergic drugs are becoming less popular as premedicants. Nevertheless, for procedures involving intraoral or bronchoscopic examination, the tendency of anticholinergics to decrease salivation can be useful. If topical intraoral anesthetics are to be used, dilution of the anesthetic by saliva can be prevented by administration of antisialagogues. However, the dry mouth produced by these drugs is very uncomfortable. Patients awaiting anesthesia who are deprived of fluids as well as anxious may have a dry mouth without the use of anticholinergics. One group of investigators found this to be true in 26 to 50 percent of patients 1 hour after administration of a placebo on the day of surgery.[220]

All anticholinergics are rather similar in their ability to decrease salivation. When 0.2 mg of glycopyrrolate was compared with 0.6 mg of atropine or 0.4 mg of scopolamine in a double-blind study of patients anesthetized with diethyl ether, the antisialic actions of all three drugs were similar.[221] However, glycopyrrolate produced less tachycardia, pyrexia, and blurred vision than did atropine, and its sedative effect was less than that of scopolamine. Another study of similar dosages also found the antisialic actions of all three drugs to be approximately the same.[222] In a third study, significant

dryness resulted 60 to 90 minutes after atropine was administered either orally or intramuscularly; glycopyrrolate also produced significant dryness at 60 minutes after intramuscular administration of either 0.2 or 0.4 mg.[223] Two milligrams of atropine given orally was similar in antisialic action to 1.0 mg of atropine given intramuscularly.

Anticholinergics have little ability to prevent conditions critical to acid aspiration. For example, one study reported that administration of glycopyrrolate (4 to 5 μg/kg IM) 45 to 90 minutes before induction of anesthesia in outpatients failed to increase gastric pH or reduce gastric volume.[141] Combining anticholinergics with metoclopramide causes little change in lower esophageal sphincter tone; in contrast, administration of metoclopramide alone increases barrier pressure.[224]

CONTROLLING POSTOPERATIVE NAUSEA WITH PREOPERATIVE MEDICATION

Nausea, with or without vomiting, is probably the most common complication after surgery. An ambulatory surgery center in Phoenix, Arizona, reported that 30 percent of their patients had postoperative nausea and 20 percent had emesis.[225] Also, postoperative nausea and vomiting occur more frequently in women than in men. When 554 patients were given a variety of premedicant drugs and an ether-nitrous oxide anesthetic, nausea occurred in 81 percent of the women and in 43 percent of the men.[226] A similar study of 300 patients reported figures of 55 percent for women and 23 percent for men.[227] Age was not a factor in either of these two studies. Although a third study of 2,528 patients also reported a higher incidence of vomiting for women than men, particularly after age 20, vomiting decreased with age for both sexes (Fig. 26-15).[228]

Pregnant ambulatory patients have a higher incidence of nausea before surgery than nonpregnant patients. For example, preoperative nausea and vomiting occurred in 38 percent of 66 patients scheduled for first trimester abortion but in only 8 percent of 66 nonpregnant patients undergoing minor gynecologic procedures.[229]

Drugs given for premedication should not exacerbate the problem of postoperative nausea and vomiting. The use of narcotics, as already discussed, may increase postoperative nausea. On the other hand, drugs such as metoclopramide may help alleviate this condition. Two other drugs, droperidol and transdermally administered scopolamine, are particularly useful and are discussed below. Others, including prochlorperazine, hydroxyzine, perphenazine, benzquinamide, promazine, and trimethobenzamide, are frequently used in the recovery room and may be given as premedicants. However, they have not been investigated in controlled studies for premedication and will not be discussed here.

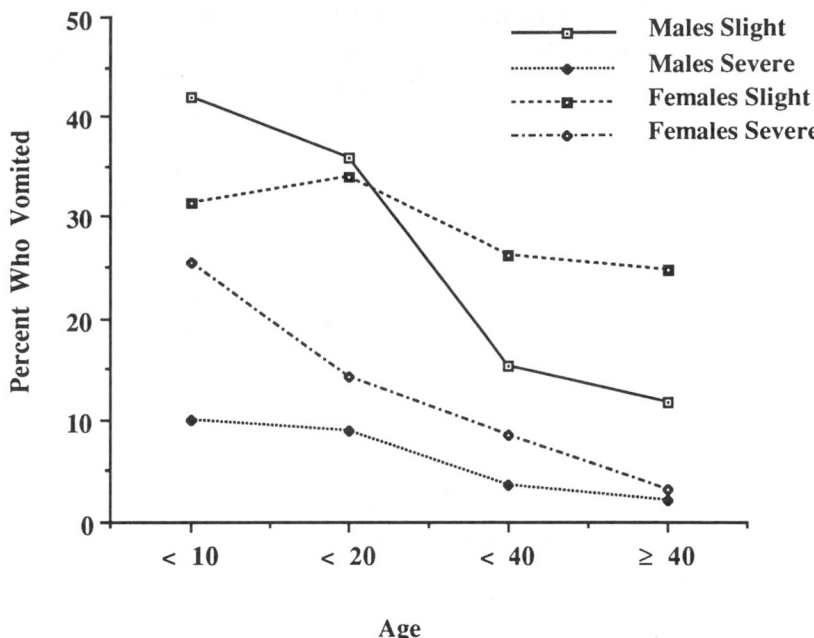

Fig. 26-15. In general, the incidence of postoperative vomiting is higher for female patients than for male patients and decreases with age for both sexes. (From Burtles and Pecket,[228] with permission.)

Droperidol

Droperidol has been variably successful as an antiemetic in patients undergoing surgery. In some studies, low doses seemed to be more effective than high doses. Importantly, the recovery of patients who receive the drug is not a problem. The effects of low doses of droperidol (0.25 and 0.5 mg IV) and placebo, administered immediately after induction of anesthesia, were studied in patients given prostaglandin for termination of pregnancy.[230] All treatment groups had similar incidences of nausea and vomiting before surgery (49 and 29 percent, respectively). There was no significant difference in preoperative and postoperative vomiting in the placebo group. In contrast, both doses of droperidol effectively reduced nausea after surgery (from 48 to 21 percent with the lower dose and from 49 to 19 percent with the higher dose). Unexpectedly, a significant decrease in postoperative vomiting (from 27 to 10 percent) occurred only with the lower dose of droperidol. The fact that the lower dose but not the higher dose was effective makes this author uncomfortable with the study's conclusion that administration of 0.25 mg of droperidol at induction may enhance recovery by reducing nausea and vomiting. Recovery times were similar for all three groups.

A second study compared droperidol (0.25 and 1.25 mg IV) with placebo in patients undergoing ambulatory dental surgery.[231] The lower dose of droperidol reduced the incidence of nausea (35 percent with placebo versus 10 percent with low-dose droperidol) without delaying recovery time, as judged by the time to open-

ing of the eyes on command. The higher dose of droperidol did not reduce nausea and significantly prolonged recovery time by 2 minutes. However, discharge times did not differ. When placebo was compared with droperidol (2.5 mg IV) given during spinal anesthesia, after delivery of the infant by cesarean section, the incidence of nausea was 40 percent with saline and 12 percent with droperidol.[232]

In contrast, a study of 100 patients undergoing ambulatory oral surgery did not find droperidol more effective than saline in relieving nausea.[233] The incidence of nausea and vomiting overall was 18 and 7 percent, respectively, in patients given droperidol (0.014 mg/kg IV) and 27 and 11 percent, respectively, in patients given saline. This change was not statistically significant. At 6 to 12 hours after anesthesia, the number of nauseated patients was slightly higher with droperidol than with saline. The time to orientation was similar for both groups. More patients given saline could walk a straight line at 30 minutes after anesthesia, but this number was not significantly different between groups at 60 minutes. Perceptual speed was better at both 30 and 60 minutes with saline.

The relative effectiveness of droperidol versus metoclopramide in decreasing nausea and vomiting also varies. When intravenous doses of 1.25 mg of droperidol and 10 mg of metoclopramide were compared, neither drug decreased nausea and vomiting.[187] However, patients given metoclopramide were able to sit up and walk and were discharged from the hospital earlier than were control patients. Another study found different results. Both droperidol (2.5 mg IV) and metoclopramide (10 mg IV) decreased the incidence of nausea and vomiting. It is interesting to note that although patients treated with either drug were no more sedated than those given placebo, patients given droperidol complained of significantly less postoperative pain than those given metoclopramide.[191]

Transdermally Administered Scopolamine

Scopolamine is very effective in preventing motion sickness. However, when it is administered orally or parenterally, its duration of action is short and the incidence of side effects is high. The solution to these problems was found by delivering the drug through the skin. A patch applied behind the ear produces very low blood levels of scopolamine and is effective for up to 72 hours. A modified radioreceptor assay was able to detect scopolamine in only 4 of 12 volunteers given the drug in this manner.[234] For these four patients, plasma concentrations of the drug peaked after 8 hours and were thereafter relatively stable. Side effects of scopolamine include dry mouth, drowsiness, blurred vision, and mydriasis. Anisocoria has occurred on occasion because of transfer of scopolamine to the eye by finger after touching the patch.[235,236] Because scopolamine produces a dry mouth, the drug has been given transdermally to treat sialorrhea and drooling, or for patients undergoing surgery for lesions of the mouth, larynx, or pharynx.[237]

Several studies have compared the effectiveness of transdermally administered scopolamine with more traditional methods of relieving motion sickness and nausea. When experimental motion sickness was induced in volunteers, motion-induced symptoms decreased 63 percent with transdermal scopolamine, 75 percent with oral scopolamine, and 86 percent with a combination of promethazine and ephedrine.[238] In a study of 96 female patients undergoing superficial short-stay surgery, patients were randomly selected to receive one of the following: transdermal scopolamine 45 to 60 minutes before induction of anesthesia, droperidol (1.25 mg IV) 5 minutes before the end of surgery, or placebo.[239] Even though sedation was greater after droperidol, both transdermal scopolamine and droperidol were able to reduce nausea over the following 24 hours. The incidence of actual vomiting on the ward, however, did not differ between groups. Visual disturbances were more frequent after transdermal scopolamine. When the effects of transdermal scopolamine and placebo were compared for 40 patients undergoing minor gynecologic surgery, patients given transdermal scopolamine the evening before surgery had significantly less nausea (45 percent) than those given placebo (75 percent) (Fig. 26-16).[240] Perhaps the early application of the patch in this study allowed attainment of effective steady-state plasma concentrations of the drug.

Prophylactic transdermal administration of scopolamine has also been successful in reducing the incidence and severity of nausea associated with epidural morphine in women undergoing major gynecologic surgery.[241]

A review by Clissold and Heel[242] provides additional information about this drug.

Recommendations

I consider drug treatment for nausea only when patients have a history of severe nausea and vomiting after anesthesia or when patients report the tendency to become nauseated easily (e.g., they become carsick easily). If the patient is seen more than 24 hours before the procedure, transdermal scopolamine is given, with instructions to apply the patch the night before the procedure. Otherwise, 0.25 mg of droperidol is administered in the operating room immediately before induction of anesthesia.

PREOPERATIVE ADMINISTRATION OF ANTIBIOTICS

Regarding infection, surgical wounds may be said to be clean, potentially contaminated (e.g., as in procedures entering a bronchus, the gastrointestinal tract, or the oropharyngeal tract), contaminated, or dirty.[243] "Clean" wounds generally involve little contamination by bacteria, the most common sources of infection being the patient's skin, the operating room environment, and the surgical team. Because gross contamination or active infection relates to the inoculum soiling the wound, prophylactic administration of antibiotics is of little use for operations that are clean or that present little risk of sepsis. Antibiotics may be useful, however, in decreasing the incidence of wound infections during certain types of procedures: trauma or burn surgery; surgery in areas having infection, heavy contamination, impoverished blood supply, or considerable tissue destruction; and lengthy operations.[244,245] Antibiotics are also used when active infection exists remote from the operative site. Other candidates for prophylactic administration of antibiotics are patients who are obese, diabetic, old, or malnourished; those whose immune system is suppressed; and those taking steroids.[244,245] However, this practice must not be taken lightly, as some individuals can become hypersensitive, and use of antibiotics can increase the resistance of indigenous hospital flora to these drugs.

Prophylactic administration of antibiotics is most effective when the agent is given at the time of, or immediately before, exposure to possible pathogens. Guinea pigs given antibiotics before bacterial contamination had significantly less severe cutaneous infection than control animals; antibiotics given 3 to 5 hours after bacterial inoculation were ineffective.[246] A similar study used experimentally induced lesions to evaluate the effectiveness of antibiotics over time. As the time be-

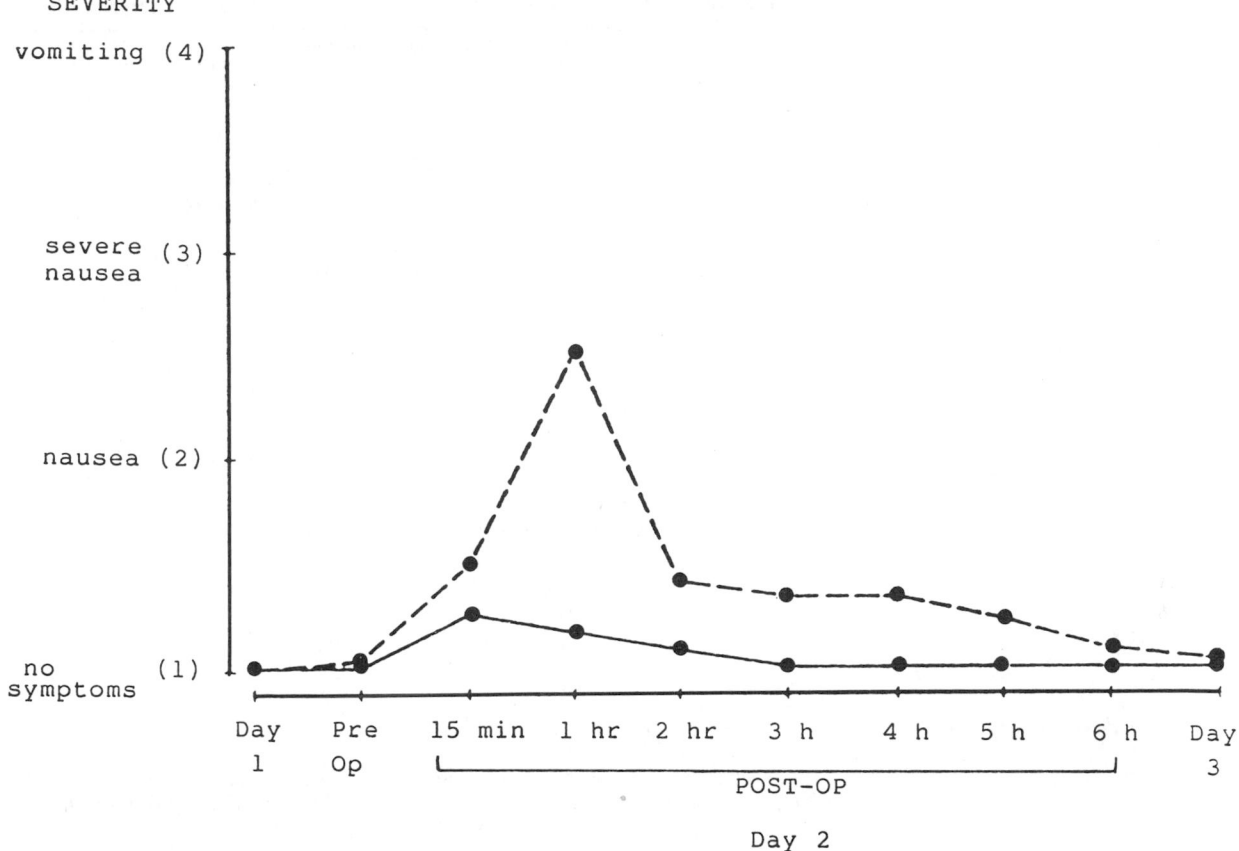

Fig. 26-16. Transdermal administration of scopolamine (solid line) but not placebo (broken line) given the evening before surgery effectively controls postoperative nausea and vomiting (average levels are shown). (From Tolksdorf et al.,[240] with permission.)

tween injection of bacteria and administration of antibiotic increased, the effectiveness of the antibiotic decreased.[247] By 3 hours, the resulting lesion was similar in size to that produced in control animals.

The cephalosporins are particularly suited as prophylactic antibiotics because they are effective for a wide range of bacteria. A retrospective study of 5,288 patients in 1974 cited the cephalosporins as the most popular antibiotics administered prophylactically.[248] No one cephalosporin, however, has been shown to be more effective than another.[249] For one thing, at the $P < 0.05$ level of statistical significance, and using a "clean" operation and an infection rate of 2 percent, the number of patients required to show a 50 percent decrease in the rate of infection would still exceed 2,000. The number of patients enrolled in such studies is usually much lower.

Antimicrobial prophylaxis is also useful in preventing endocarditis when valvular heart disease, prosthetic heart valve, or other cardiac abnormality is present in patients undergoing procedures associated with transient bacteremia.[250] Patients with mitral valve prolapse are also at greater risk of endocarditis, particularly those with thickened, redundant leaflets or a pre-

viously known systolic murmur.[251-253] Streptococci from the mouth, enterococci from the gastrointestinal or genitourinary tract, and staphylococci from the skin can cause endocarditis, and antimicrobials used for prophylaxis of endocarditis are directed toward these organisms. Endotracheal intubation may not be an indication for prophylaxis with antibiotics unless intubation is associated with other procedures warranting prophylaxis.[254] Table 26-4 provides suggestions for antibiotic regimens to prevent endocarditis.

SUMMARY

The preoperative visit is an essential step in preparing the patient for anesthesia and surgery. Although time-consuming for both the patient and medical personnel, nonpharmacologic methods should first be attempted for attenuating anxiety. The use of drugs for relief of persistent anxiety before surgery is desirable and, at the very least, humane. Therapy to reduce anxiety and/or blood pressure preoperatively tends to decrease anesthetic requirements. The practice of providing prophylaxis for acid aspiration of gastric contents for all pa-

TABLE 26-4. Recommended Antibiotic Regimens for Patients Needing Prophylaxis for Bacterial Endocarditis

	Dose and Time of Administration	
	Before Surgery	After First Dose
For dental procedures		
Standard therapy[a]		
(choose one):		
Penicillin V	2.0 g PO, 1 h	1.0 g PO, 6 h
Aqueous penicillin G	2×10^6 units IV or IM, 30–60 min	1×10^6 units IV or IM, 6 h
For those allergic to penicillin		
Erythromycin	1.0 g PO, 1 h	500 mg PO, 6 h
Maximal therapy[b]		
(administer both):		
Ampicillin	1.0–2.0 g IV or IM, 30 min	1.0–2.0 g IV or IM, 8 h
Gentamicin	1.5 mg/kg IV or IM, 30 min	1.5 mg/kg IV or IM, 8 h
or administer the following after		
the first dose of the above regimen:		
Penicillin V		1.0 g PO, 6 h
For those allergic to penicillin		
Vancomycin	1.0 g IV slowly over starting 1 h before	Not necessary
For gastrointestinal/genitourinary procedures		
Standard therapy		
(administer both):		
Ampicillin	2.0 g IV or IM, 30–60 min	2.0 g IV or IM, 8 h
Gentamicin	1.5 mg/kg IV or IM, 30–60 min	1.5 mg/kg IV or IM, 8 h
For those allergic to penicillin		
(administer both):		
Vancomycin	1.0 g IV slowly over 1 h, starting 1 h before	1.0 g IV slowly over 1 h, 8–12 h
Gentamicin	1.5 mg/kg IV or IM, 1 h	1.5 mg/kg IV or IM, 8–12 h
For low-risk procedures[c]		
Amoxicillin	3.0 g PO, 1 h	1.5 g PO, 6 h

[a]"Standard therapy" is warranted for all dental procedures causing gingival bleeding and for surgery of the oral/respiratory tract.
[b]"Maximal therapy" is warranted for patients at particularly high risk (e.g., those with prosthetic heart valves or surgically constructed systemic-pulmonary shunts).
[c]"Low-risk therapy" is appropriate for gastrointestinal/genitourinary procedures such as liver biopsy, upper gastrointestinal endoscopy, or proctosigmoidoscopy without biopsy, barium enema, uncomplicated vaginal delivery, and brief bladder catheterization with sterile urine.
(Adapted from Shulman et al.,[254] with permission.)

tients is controversial. Although some drugs do increase gastric pH and decrease gastric volume, these drugs have side effects and unknown effectiveness in reducing the actual incidence of aspiration and its associated morbidity. Nausea can be a problem, as it prolongs the stay in the recovery room, or, in the case of ambulatory surgery patients, the hospital. For this reason, drugs that contribute to nausea are undesirable, and drug therapy that can help to alleviate this problem may be considered. Table 26-5 summarizes the basic

TABLE 26-5. Suggestions for Preoperative Medication for Adults Undergoing Elective Surgery

Suggestion	Example
1. Patient visit and interview by anesthesiologist the day before surgery.	
2. Benzodiazepine to treat insomnia the night before surgery.	Triazolam, 0.125 to 0.25 mg/70 kg PO
3. Benzodiazepine (preferably orally) 1–2 h before surgery. Water up to 150 ml may stimulate gastric emptying.	Diazepam 10 mg/70 kg PO
4. Substitute opioid (intramuscularly) for #3 if analgesia is desired. Opioids may delay gastric emptying.	Morphine, 10 mg/70 kg IM
5. In rare cases, scopolamine (intramuscularly) 1–2 h before surgery if reliable sedation and amnesia are desired; otherwise, follow recommendation #7 or do not administer an anticholinergic.	0.2 to 0.4 mg/70 kg
6. Consider H_2 antagonist (orally) 1–2 h before surgery. Administration with up to 150 ml of water may be the most predictable method of reducing gastric fluid volume and increasing gastric fluid pH.	Cimetidine, 300 mg PO
7. Glycopyrrolate (intramuscularly) when patient is ready to be transported to the operating room, if an antisialic effect is desired.	0.2 to 0.3 mg/70 kg

(Adapted from Stoelting and Miller,[158] with permission.)

considerations regarding preoperative preparation of the patient.[158] Preoperative administration of antibiotics is useful for some types of surgery, and antibiotics are routinely included for patients at risk of bacterial endocarditis.

REFERENCES

1. McNair DM, Lorr M, Droppleman LF: Profile of Mood States. Educational and Industrial Testing, San Diego, 1971
2. Lichtor JL, Johanson CE, Mhoon D, et al: Preoperative anxiety: Does anxiety level the afternoon before surgery predict anxiety level just before surgery? Anesthesiology 67:595, 1987
3. Johnston M: Anxiety in surgical patients. Psychol Med 10:145, 1980
4. Vögele C, Steptoe A: Physiological and subjective stress responses in surgical patients. J Psychosom Res 30:205, 1986
5. Wallace LM: Psychological preparation as a method of reducing the stress of surgery. J Human Stress 10:62, 1984
6. Weis OF, Sriwatanakul K, Weintraub M, Lasagna L: Reduction of anxiety and postoperative analgesic requirements by audiovisual instruction. Lancet 1:43, 1983
7. Ziemer MM: Effects of information on postsurgical coping. Nurs Res 32:282, 1983
8. Wallace LM: Trait anxiety as a predictor of adjustment to and recovery from surgery. Br J Clin Psychol 26:73, 1987
9. Scott LE, Clum GA, Peoples JB: Preoperative predictors of postoperative pain. Pain 15:283, 1983
10. Elsass P, Eikard B, Junge J, et al: Psychological effect of detailed preanesthetic information. Acta Anaesthesiol Scand 31:579, 1987
11. Linn BS, Linn MW, Jensen J: Surgical stress in the healthy elderly. J Am Geriatr Soc 31:544, 1983
12. Simpson CJ, Kellett JM: The relationship between pre-operative anxiety and post-operative delirium. J Psychosom Res 31:491, 1987
13. Zohar J, Meiraz D, Maoz B, Durst N: Factors influencing sexual activity after prostatectomy: A prospective study. J Urol 116:332, 1976
14. Wolfer JA, Davis CE: Assessment of surgical patients' preoperative emotional condition and postoperative welfare. Nurs Res 19:402, 1970
15. Johnston M, Carpenter L: Relationship between pre-operative anxiety and post-operative state. Psychol Med 10:361, 1980
16. Anderson EA: Preoperative preparation for cardiac surgery facilitates recovery, reduces psychological distress, and reduces the incidence of acute postoperative hypertension. J Consult Clin Psychol 55:513, 1987
17. Klein RF, Kliner VA, Zipes DP, et al: Transfer from a coronary care unit. Arch Intern Med 122:104, 1968
18. Egbert LD, Battit GE, Turndorf H, Beecher HK: The value of the preoperative visit by an anesthetist. JAMA 185:553, 1963
19. Leigh JM, Walker J, Janaganathan P: Effect of preoperative anaesthetic visit on anxiety. Br Med J 2:987, 1977
20. Benson H, Beary JF, Carol MP: The relaxation response. Psychiatry 37:37, 1974
21. Benson H: Systemic hypertension and the relaxation response. N Engl J Med 296:1152, 1977
22. Benson H, Alexander S, Feldman CL: Decreased premature ventricular contractions through use of the relaxation response in patients with stable ischaemic heart-disease. Lancet 2:380, 1975
23. Berlin RM: Management of insomnia in hospitalized patients. Ann Intern Med 100:398, 1984
24. Holden-Lund C: Effects of relaxation with guided imagery on surgical stress and wound healing. Res Nurs Health 11:235, 1988
25. Lawlis GF, Selby D, Hinnant D, McCoy CE: Reduction of postoperative pain parameters by presurgical relaxation instructions for spinal pain patients. Spine 10:649, 1985
26. Domar AD, Noe JM, Benson H: The preoperative use of the relaxation response with ambulatory surgery patients. J Human Stress 13:101, 1987
27. Spielberger CD, Gorsich RL, Lushene RE: Manual for the State-Trait Anxiety Inventory. Consulting Psychologists Press, Palo Alto, Calf., 1970
28. Greenblatt DJ, Locniskar A, Ochs HR, Lauven PM: Automated gas chromatography for studies of midazolam pharmacokinetics. Anesthesiology 55:176, 1981
29. Dundee JW: New I.V. anaesthetics. Br J Anaesth 51:641, 1979
30. Raybould D, Bradshaw EG: Premedication for day case surgery: A study of oral midazolam. Anaesthesia 42:591, 1987
31. Reinhart K, Dallinger-Stiller G, Dennhardt R, et al: Comparison of midazolam, diazepam and placebo I.M. as premedication for regional anaesthesia: A randomized double-blind study. Br J Anaesth 57:294, 1985
32. van Wijhe M, de Voogt-Frenkel E, Stijnen T: Midazolam versus fentanyl/droperidol and placebo as intramuscular premedicant. Acta Anaesthesiol Scand 29:409, 1985
33. Barker I, Butchart DGM, Gibson J, et al: I.V. sedation for conservative dentistry. A comparison of midazolam and diazepam. Br J Anaesth 58:371, 1986
34. Vinik HR, Reves JG, Wright D: Premedication with intramuscular midazolam: A prospective randomized double-blind controlled study. Anesth Analg 61:933, 1982
35. Driessen JJ, Smets MJW, Goey LS, Booij LHDJ: Comparison of diazepam and midazolam as oral premedicants for bronchoscopy under local anesthesia. Acta Anaesthesiol Belg 33:99, 1982
36. Forrest P, Galletly DC, Yee P: Placebo controlled comparison of midazolam triazolam and diazepam as oral premedicants for outpatient anaesthesia. Anaesth Intensive Care 15:296, 1987
37. van der Bijl P, Roelofse JA, de v. Joubert JJ, Breytenbach HS: Intravenous midazolam in oral surgery. Int J Oral Maxillofac Surg 16:325, 1987
38. O'Boyle CA, Harris D, Barry H, et al: Comparison of midazolam by mouth and diazepam I.V. in outpatient oral surgery. Br J Anaesth 59:746, 1987
39. Bianchi Porro G, Baroni S, Parente F, Lazzaroni M: Midazolam versus diazepam as premedication for upper gastrointestinal endoscopy: A randomized, double-blind, crossover study. Gastrointest Endosc 34:252, 1988
40. Feldmeier C, Kapp W: Comparative clinical studies with midazolam, oxazepam and placebo. Br J Clin Pharmacol 16:suppl 1, 151S, 1983
41. Berggren L, Eriksson I: Midazolam for induction of anaesthesia in outpatients: A comparison with thiopentone. Acta Anaesthesiol Scand 25:492, 1981
42. Reves JG, Vinik R, Hirschfield AM, et al: Midazolam compared with thiopentone as a hypnotic component in balanced anaesthesia: A randomized, double-blind study. Can Anaesth Soc J 26:42, 1979
43. Wolff J, Carl P, Clausen TG, Mikkelsen BO: Ro 15-1788 for

postoperative recovery. A randomised clinical trial in patients undergoing minor surgical procedures under midazolam anaesthesia. Anaesthesia 41:1001, 1986

44. Alexander CM, Gross JB: Sedative doses of midazolam depress hypoxic ventilatory responses in humans. Anesth Analg 67:377, 1988

45. Bell GD, Spickett GP, Reeve PA, et al: Intravenous midazolam for upper gastrointestinal endoscopy: A study of 800 consecutive cases relating dose to age and sex of patient. Br J Clin Pharmacol 23:241, 1987

46. Brophy T, Dundee JW, Heazelwood V, et al: Midazolam, a water-soluble benzodiazepine, for gastroscopy. Anaesth Intensive Care 10:344, 1982

47. Dundee JW, Halliday NJ, Loughran PG, Harper KW: The influence of age on the onset of anaesthesia with midazolam. Anaesthesia 40:441, 1985

48. Reves JG, Fragen RJ, Vinik HR, Greenblatt DJ: Midazolam: Pharmacology and uses. Anesthesiology 62:310, 1985

49. Dionne RA, Goldstein DS, Wirdzek PR: Effects of diazepam premedication and epinephrine-containing local anesthetic on cardiovascular and plasma catecholamine responses to oral surgery. Anesth Analg 63:640, 1984

50. Jakobsen H, Hertz JB, Johansen JR, et al: Premedication before day surgery. A double-blind comparison of diazepam and placebo. Br J Anaesth 57:300, 1985

51. White PF, Vasconez LO, Mathes SA, et al: Comparison of midazolam and diazepam for sedation during plastic surgery. Plast Reconstr Surg 81:703, 1988

52. Hegarty JE, Dundee JW: Sequelae after the intravenous injection of three benzodiazepines—diazepam, lorazepam and flunitrazepam. Br Med J 2:1384, 1977

53. Klotz U, Antonin K-H, Bieck PR: Pharmacokinetics and plasma binding of diazepam in man, dog, rabbit, guinea pig and rat. J Pharmacol Exp Ther 199:67, 1976

54. Randall LO, Scheckel CL, Banziger RF: Pharmacology of the metabolites of chlordiazepoxide and diazepam. Curr Ther Res 7:590, 1965

55. Gamble JAS, Gaston JH, Nair SG, Dundee JW: Some pharmacological factors influencing the absorption of diazepam following oral administration. Br J Anaesth 48:1181, 1976

56. Gamble JAS, Dundee JW, Assaf RAE: Plasma diazepam levels after single dose oral and intramuscular administration. Anaesthesia 30:164, 1975

57. Linnoila M, Korttila K, Mattila MJ: Effect of food and repeated injections on serum diazepam levels. Acta Pharmacol Toxicol 36:181, 1975

58. Pandit SK, Dundee JW, Keilty SR: Amnesia studies with intravenous premedication. Anaesthesia 26:421, 1971

59. Dundee JW, Pandit SK: Anterograde amnesic effects of pethidine, hyoscine and diazepam in adults. Br J Pharmacol 44:140, 1972

60. McKay AC, Dundee JW: Effect of oral benzodiazepines on memory. Br J Anaesth 52:1247, 1980

61. de Jong RH, Bonin JD: Benzodiazepines protect mice from local anesthetic convulsions and deaths. Anesth Analg 60:385, 1981

62. Ausinsch B, Malagodi MH, Munson ES: Diazepam in the prophylaxis of lignocaine seizures. Br J Anaesth 48:309, 1976

63. Klotz U, Avant GR, Hoyumpa A, et al: The effects of age and liver disease on the disposition and elimination of diazepam in adult man. J Clin Invest 55:347, 1975

64. Reidenberg MM, Levy M, Warner H, et al: Relationship between diazepam dose, plasma level, age, and central nervous system depression. Clin Pharmacol Ther 23:371, 1978

65. Giles HG, MacLeod SM, Wright JR, Sellers EM: Influence of age and previous use on diazepam dosage required for endoscopy. Can Med Assoc J 118:513, 1978

66. Dundee JW, McGowan WAW, Lilburn JK, et al: Comparison of the actions of diazepam and lorazepam. Br J Anaesth 51:439, 1979

67. Dundee JW, Lilburn JK, Nair SG, George KA: Studies of drugs given before anaesthesia. XXVI: Lorazepam. Br J Anaesth 49:1047, 1977

68. Greenblatt DJ, Shader RI, Franke K, et al: Pharmacokinetics and bioavailability of intravenous, intramuscular, and oral lorazepam in humans. J Pharm Sci 68:57, 1979

69. Conner JT, Katz RL, Bellville JW, et al: Diazepam and lorazepam for intravenous surgical premedication. J Clin Pharmacol 18:285, 1978

70. Fragen RJ, Caldwell N: Lorazepam premedication: Lack of recall and relief of anxiety. Anesth Analg 55:792, 1976

71. Milligan DW, Howard MR, Judd A: Premedication with lorazepam before bone marrow biopsy. J Clin Pathol 40:696, 1987

72. Paymaster NJ: Lorazepam (WY 4036) as a pre-operative medication. Anaesthesia 28:521, 1973

73. Magbagbeola JAO: A comparison of lorazepam and diazepam as oral premedicants for surgery under regional anaesthesia. Br J Anaesth 46:449, 1974

74. Thomas D, Tipping T, Halifax R, et al: Triazolam premedication. A comparison with lorazepam and placebo in gynaecological patients. Anaesthesia 41:692, 1986

75. Thomson IR, Bergstrom RG, Rosenbloom M, Meatherall RC: Premedication and high-dose fentanyl anesthesia for myocardial revascularization: A comparison of lorazepam versus morphine-scopolamine. Anesthesiology 68:194, 1988

76. Ameer B, Greenblatt DJ: Lorazepam: A review of its clinical pharmacological properties and therapeutic uses. Drugs 21:161, 1981

77. Eberts FS, Jr, Philopoulos Y, Reineke LM, Vliek RW: Triazolam disposition. Clin Pharmacol Ther 29:81, 1981

78. Pinnock CA, Fell D, Hunt PCW, et al: A comparison of triazolam and diazepam as premedication agents for minor gynaecological surgery. Anaesthesia 40:324, 1985

79. U.S. is asked to sharply limit use of sedative. Sect. I, p. 37. New York Times, Feb 14, 1988

80. Leary WE: House report faults F.D.A. approval of sedative. Section C, p. 11. New York Times, Oct 18, 1988

81. Physicians' Desk Reference. 41st Ed. Medical Economics Co., Oradell, N.J. 1987, p 1685

82. Physicians' Desk Reference. 42nd Ed. Medical Economics Co., Oradell, N.J., 1988, p 1754

83. Khanderia U, Pandit SK: Use of midazolam hydrochloride in anesthesia. Clin Pharmacol 6:533, 1987

84. Forster A, Gardaz JP, Suter PM, Gemperle M: I.V. midazolam as an induction agent for anaesthesia: A study in volunteers. Br J Anaesth 52:907, 1980

85. Sunzel M, Paalzow L, Berggren L, Eriksson I: Respiratory and cardiovascular effects in relation to plasma levels of midazolam and diazepam. Br J Clin Pharmacol 25:561, 1988

86. Samuelson PN, Reves JG, Kouchoukos NT, et al: Hemodynamic responses to anesthetic induction with midazolam or diazepam in patients with ischemic heart disease. Anesth Analg 60:802, 1981

87. Spiess BD, Sathoff RH, El-Ganzouri ARS, Ivankovich AD: High-dose sufentanil: Four cases of sudden hypotension on induction. Anesth Analg 65:703, 1986

88. West JM, Estrada S, Heerdt M: Sudden hypotension associated with midazolam and sufentanil (letter). Anesth Analg 66:693, 1987

89. Massaut J, d'Hollander A, Barvais L, Dubois-Primo J: Haemodynamic effects of midazolam in the anaesthetized patient with coronary artery disease. Acta Anaesthesiol Scand 27:299, 1983

90. Heikkilä H, Jalonen J, Arola M, et al: Midazolam as adjunct to high-dose fentanyl anaethesia for coronary artery bypass grafting operation. Acta Anaesthesiol Scand 28:683, 1984

91. Marty J, Gauzit R, Lefevre P, et al: Effects of diazepam and midazolam on baroreflex control of heart rate and on sympathetic activity in humans. Anesth Analg 65:113, 1986

92. Kotrly KJ, Ebert TJ, Vucins E, et al: Baroreceptor reflex control of heart rate during isoflurane anesthesia in humans. Anesthesiology 60:173, 1984

93. Arcos GJ: Midazolam-induced ventricular irritability (letter). Anesthesiology 67:612, 1987

94. Bell GD, Reeve PA, Moshiri M, et al: Intravenous midazolam: A study of the degree of oxygen desaturation occurring during upper gastrointestinal endoscopy. Br J Clin Pharmacol 23:703, 1987

95. Forster A, Gardaz J-P, Suter PM, Gemperle M: Respiratory depression by midzolam and diazepam. Anesthesiology 53:494, 1980

96. Knill R, Cosgrove JF, Olley PM, Levison H: Components of respiratory depression after narcotic premedication in adolescents. Can Anaesth Soc J 23:449, 1976

97. Gross JB, Zebrowski ME, Carel WD, et al: Time course of ventilatory depression after thiopental and midazolam in normal subjects and in patients with chronic obstructive pulmonary disease. Anesthesiology 58:540, 1983

98. Asch DA, Parker RM: The Libby Zion case. One step forward or two steps backward? N Engl J Med 318:771, 1988

99. Price WJ, Holley DC: The last minutes of flight 2860: An analysis of crew shift work scheduling. p. 287. In Reinberg A, Vieux N, Andlauer P (eds): Night and Shift Work: Biological and Social Aspects. Pergamon Press, Oxford, 1981

100. Ehret CF: New approaches to chronohygiene for the shift worker in the nuclear power industry. p. 103. In Reinberg A, Vieux N, Andlauer P (eds): Night and Shift Work. Biological and Social Aspects. Pergamon Press, Oxford, 1981

101. Korttila K, Ghoneim MM, Jacobs L, Lakes RS: Evaluation of instrumented force platform as a test to measure residual effects of anesthetics. Anesthesiology 55:625, 1981

102. Korttila K, Linnoila M: Recovery and skills related to driving after intravenous sedation: Dose-response relationship with diazepam. Br J Anaesth 47:457, 1975

103. Galletly D, Forrest P, Purdie G: Comparison of the recovery characteristics of diazepam and midazolam. Br J Anaesth 60:520, 1988

104. Nightingale JJ, Norman J: A comparison of midazolam and temazepam for premedication of day case patients. Anaesthesia 43:111, 1988

105. Korttila K, Tarkkanen J: Comparison of diazepam and midazolam for sedation during local anaesthesia for bronchoscopy. Br J Anaesth 57:581, 1985

106. Clyburn P, Kay NH, McKenzie PJ: Effects of diazepam and midazolam on recovery from anaesthesia in outpatients. Br J Anaesth 58:872, 1986

107. Stoller KP, Belleville JP, Belleville JW: Visual tracking following lorazepam or pentobarbital. Anesthesiology 45:565, 1976

108. Shafer A, White PF, Urquhart ML, Doze VA: Outpatient premedication: Use of midazolam and opioid analgesics. Anesthesiology 71:495, 1989

109. Philip BK: Hazards of amnesia after midazolam in ambulatory surgical patients (letter). Anesth Analg 66:97, 1987

110. Liu S, Miller N, Waye JD: Retrograde amnesia effects of intravenous diazepam in endoscopy patients. Gastrointest Endosc 30:340, 1984

111. Clark MS, Silverstone LM, Coke JM, Hicks J: Midazolam, diazepam, and placebo as intravenous sedatives for dental surgery. Oral Surg Oral Med Oral Pathol 63:127, 1987

112. Barclay JK, Hunter KM, McMillan W: Midazolam and diazepam compared as sedatives for outpatient surgery under local analgesia. Oral Surg Oral Med oral Pathol 59:349, 1985

113. Raeder JC, Breivik H: Premedication with midazolam in outpatient general anaesthesia. A comparison with morphine-scopolamine and placebo. Acta Aanesthesiol Scand 31:509, 1987

114. Pandit SK, Heisterkamp DV, Cohen PJ: Further studies of the antirecall effect of lorazepam: A dose-time-effect relationship. Anesthesiology 45:495, 1976

115. Bassell GM, Lin YT, Oka Y, et al: Circulatory response to tracheal intubation in patients with coronary artery disease and valvular disease. Bull NY Acad Med 54:842, 1978

116. Edde RR: Hemodynamic changes prior to and after sternotomy in patients anesthetized with high-dose fentanyl. Anesthesiology 55:444, 1981

117. Wynands JE, Townsend GE, Wong P, et al: Blood pressure response and plasma fentanyl concentrations during high- and very high-dose fentanyl anesthesia for coronary artery surgery. Anesth Analg 62:661, 1983

118. Hanson EL, Kane PB, Askanazi J, et al: Comparison of patients with coronary artery or valve disease: Intraoperative differences in blood volume and observations of vasomotor response. Ann Thorac Surg 22:343, 1976

119. Prys-Roberts C, Meloche R, Foëx P: Studies of anaesthesia in relation to hypertension. I: Cardiovascular responses of treated and untreated patients. Br J Anaesth 43:122, 1971

120. Johnston RR, Way WL, Miller RD: Alteration of anesthetic requirement by amphetamine. Anesthesiology 36:357, 1972

121. Stoelting RK, Creasser CW, Martz RC: Effect of cocaine administration on halothane MAC in dogs. Anesth Analg 54:422, 1975

122. Miller RD, Way WL, Eger El II: The effects of alpha-methyldopa, reserpine, guanethidine, and iproniazid on minimum alveolar anesthetic requirement (MAC). Anesthesiology 29:1153, 1968

123. Longnecker DE: Alpine anesthesia: Can pretreatment with clonidine decrease the peaks and valleys? (editorial). Anesthesiology 67:1, 1987

124. Kaukinen S, Pyykkö K: The potentiation of halothane anaesthesia by clonidine. Acta Anaesthesiol Scand 23:107, 1979

125. Bloor BC, Flacke WE: Reduction in halothane anesthetic requirement by clonidine, an alpha-adrenergic agonist. Anesth Analg 61:741, 1982

126. Laverty R, Taylor KM: Behavioural and biochemical effects of 2-(2,6-dichlorophenylamino)-2-imidazoline hydrochloride (St 155) on the central nervous system. Br J Pharmacol 35:253, 1969

127. Paalzow G: Development of tolerance to the analgesic effect of clonidine in rats. Cross-tolerance to morphine. Naunyn Schmiedebergs Arch Pharmacol 304:1, 1978

128. Maze M, Vickery RG, Merlone SC, Gaba DM: Anesthetic and hemodynamic effects of the alpha$_2$-adrenergic agonist, azepexole, in isoflurane-anesthetized dogs. Anesthesiology 68:689, 1988

129. Ghignone M, Quintin L, Duke PC, et al: Effects of clonidine on narcotic requirements and hemodynamic response during induction of fentanyl anesthesia and endotracheal intubation. Anesthesiology 64:36, 1986

130. Ghignone M, Calvillo O, Quintin L: Anesthesia and hypertension: The effect of clonidine on perioperative hemodynamics and isoflurane requirements. Anesthesiology 67:3, 1987

131. Woodcock TE, Millard RK, Dixon J, Prys-Roberts C: Clonidine premedication for isoflurane-induced hypotension: Sympathoadrenal responses and a computer-controlled assessment of the vapour requirement. Br J Anaesth 60:388, 1988

132. Flacke JW, Bloor BC, Flacke WE, et al: Reduced narcotic requirement by clonidine with improved hemodynamic and adrenergic stability in patients undergoing coronary bypass surgery. Anesthesiology 67:11, 1987

133. Orko R, Pouttu J, Ghignone M, Rosenberg PH: Effect of clonidine on haemodynamic responses to endotracheal intubation and on gastric acidity. Acta Anaesthesiol Scand 31:325, 1987

134. Pouttu J, Scheinin B, Rosenberg PH, et al: Oral premedication with clonidine: Effects on stress responses during general anaesthesia. Acta Anaesthesiol Scand 31:730, 1987

135. Ghignone M, Noe C, Calvillo O, Quintin L: Anesthesia for ophthalmic surgery in the elderly: The effects of clonidine on intraocular pressure, perioperative hemodynamics, and anesthetic requirement. Anesthesiology 68:707, 1988

136. Keränen A, Nykänen S, Taskinen J: Pharmacokinetics and side-effects of clonidine. Eur J Clin Pharmacol 13:97, 1978

137. Roberts RB, Shirley MA: Reducing the risk of acid aspiration during cesarean section. Anesth Analg 53:859, 1974

138. James CF, Modell JH, Gibbs CP, et al: Pulmonary aspiration —effects of volume and pH in the rat. Anesth Analg 63:665, 1984

139. Manchikanti L, Canella MG, Hohlbein LJ, Colliver JA: Assessment of effect of various modes of premedication on acid aspiration risk factors in outpatient surgery. Anesth Analg 66:81, 1987

140. Manchikanti L, Grow JB, Colliver JA, et al: Bicitra® (sodium citrate) and metoclopramide in outpatient anesthesia for prophylaxis against aspiration pneumonitis. Anesthesiology 63:378, 1985

141. Manchikanti L, Roush JR: Effect of preanesthetic glycopyrrolate and cimetidine on gastric fluid pH and volume in outpatients. Anesth Analg 63:40, 1984

142. Pandit SK, Kothary SP, Pandit UA, Mirakhur RK: Premedication with cimetidine and metoclopramide. Effect on the risk factors of acid aspiration. Anaesthesia 41:486, 1986

143. Manchikanti L, Colliver JA, Roush JR, Canella MG: Evaluation of ranitidine as an oral antacid in outpatient anesthesia. South Med J 78:818, 1985

144. Ong BY, Palahniuk RJ, Cumming M: Gastric volume and pH in outpatients. Can Anaesth Soc J 25:36, 1978

145. Wright DJ, Pandya A: Smoking and gastric juice volume in outpatients. Can Anaesth Soc J 26:328, 1979

146. Adelhøj B, Petring OU, Frøsig F, et al: Influence of cigarette smoking on the risk of acid pulmonary aspiration. Acta Anaesthesiol Scand 31:7, 1987

147. Spielberger CD, Jacobs GA: Personality and smoking behavior. J Pers Assess 46:396, 1982

148. Mahl GF, Karpe R: Emotions and hydrochloric acid secretion during psychoanalytic hours. Psychosom Med 15:312, 1953

149. Birnbaum D, Karmeli F, Tefera M: The effect of diazepam on human gastric secretion. Gut 12:616, 1971

150. Gray SJ, Ramsey CG: Adrenal influences upon the stomach and the gastric responses to stress. Recent Prog Horm Res 13:583, 1957

151. Hjortsø E, Mondorf T: Does oral premedication increase the risk of gastric aspiration? Acta Anaesthesiol Scand 26:505, 1982

152. McGrady EM, Macdonald AG: Effect of the preoperative administration of water on gastric volume and pH. Br J Anaesth 60:803, 1988

153. Hutchinson A, Maltby JR, Reid CRG: Gastric fluid volume and pH in elective inpatients. Part I: Coffee or orange juice versus overnight fast. Can J Anaesth 35:12, 1988

154. Miller M, Wishart HY, Nimmo WS: Gastric contents at induction of anaesthesia. Is a 4-hour fast necessary? Br J Anaesth 55:1185, 1983

155. Sutherland AD, Maltby JR, Sale JP, Reid CRG: The effect of preoperative oral fluid and ranitidine on gastric fluid volume and pH. Can J Anaesth 34:117, 1987

156. Maltby JR, Sutherland AD, Sale JP, Shaffer EA: Preoperative oral fluids: Is a five-hour fast justified prior to elective surgery? Anesth Analg 65:1112, 1986

157. Brocks K, Jensen JS, Schmidt JF, Jørgensen BC: Gastric contents and pH after oral premedication. Acta Anaesthesiol Scand 31:448, 1987

158. Stoelting RK, Miller RD: Basics of Anesthesia. 2nd Ed. Churchill Livingstone, New York, 1989

159. Richardson CT: Effect of H₂-receptor antagonists on gastric acid secretion and serum gastrin concentration. Gastroenterology 74:366, 1978

160. Douglass WW: Histamine and 5-hydroxytryptamine (serotonin) and their antagonists. p. 624. In Gilman AG, Goodman LS, Rall TW, Murad F (eds): Goodman and Gilman's the Pharmacological Basis of Therapeutics. 7th Ed. Macmillan, New York, 1985

161. Stock JGL, Sutherland AD: The role of H₂ receptor antagonist premedication in pregnant day care patients. Can Anaesth Soc J 32:463, 1985

162. Durrant JM, Strunin L: Comparative trial of the effect of ranitidine and cimetidine on gastric secretion in fasting patients at induction of anaesthesia. Can Anaesth Soc J 29:446, 1982

163. Harris PW, Morison DH, Dunn GL, et al: Intramuscular cimetidine and ranitidine as prophylaxis against gastric aspiration syndrome—a randomized double-blind study. Can Anaesth Soc J 31:599, 1984

164. Klotz U, Reimann I: Delayed clearance of diazepam due to cimetidine. N Engl J Med 302:1012, 1980

165. Klotz U, Arvela P, Rosenkranz B: Effect of single doses of cimetidine and ranitidine on the steady-state plasma levels of midazolam. Clin Pharmacol Ther 38:652, 1985

166. Patwardhan RV, Yarborough GW, Desmond PV, et al: Cimetidine spares the glucuronidation of lorazepam and oxazepam. Gastroenterology 79:912, 1980

167. Feely J, Wilkinson GR, Wood AJJ: Reduction of liver blood flow and propranolol metabolism by cimetidine. N Engl J Med 304:692, 1981

168. Sedman AJ: Cimetidine-drug interactions. Am J Med 76:109, 1984

169. Noble DW, Smith KJ, Dundas CR: Effects of H-2 antagonists on the elimination of bupivacaine. Br J Anaesth 59:735, 1987

170. Smith SR, Kendall MJ: Ranitidine versus cimetidine: A comparison of their potential to cause clinically important drug interactions. Clin Pharmacokinet 15:44, 1988

171. Berardi RR, Tankanow RM, Nostrant TT: Comparison of famotidine with cimetidine and ranitidine. Clin Pharmacol 7:271, 1988

172. Callaghan JT, Bergstrom RF, Rubin A, et al: A pharmacokinetic profile of nizatidine in man. Scand J Gastroenterol 136(suppl):9, 1987

173. Pasanen M, Arvela P, Pelkonen O, et al: Effect of five structurally diverse H_2-receptor antagonists on drug metabolism. Biochem Pharmacol 35:4457, 1986

174. Gallagher EG, White M, Ward S, et al: Prophylaxis against acid aspiration syndrome. Single oral dose of H2-antagonist on the evening before elective surgery. Anaesthesia 43:1011, 1988

175. Escolano F, Castaño J, Pares N, et al: Comparison of the effects of famotidine and ranitidine on gastric secretion in patients undergoing elective surgery. Anaesthesia 44:212, 1989

176. Schentag JJ, Cerra FB, Calleri G, et al: Pharmacokinetic and clinical studies in patients with cimetidine-associated mental confusion. Lancet 1:177, 1979

177. Silverstone PH: Ranitidine and confusion (letter). Lancet 1:1071, 1984

178. Epstein CM: Ranitidine and mental confusion (letter). Lancet 1:1071, 1984

179. Eyler SW, Cullen BF, Murphy ME, Welch WD: Antacid aspiration in rabbits: A comparison of Mylanta and Bicitra. Anesth Analg 61:288, 1982

180. Chen CT, Toung TJK, Haupt HM, et al: Evaluation of the efficacy of Alka-Seltzer Effervescent in gastric acid neutralization. Anesth Analg 63:325, 1984

181. Abboud TK, Curtis J, Earl S, et al: Efficacy of clear antacid prophylaxis in obstetrics. Acta Anaesthesiol Scand 28:301, 1984

182. Faure EA, Lim HS, Block BS, et al: Sodium bicarbonate buffers gastric acid during surgery in obstetric and gynecologic patients. Anesthesiology 67:274, 1987

183. Albibi R, McCallum RW: Metoclopramide: Pharmacology and clinical application. Ann Intern Med 98:86, 1983

184. Rao TLK, Madhavareddy S, Chinthagada M, El-Etr AA: Metoclopramide and cimetidine to reduce gastric fluid pH and volume. Anesth Analg 63:1014, 1984

185. Manchikanti L, Marrero TC, Roush JR: Preanesthetic cimetidine and metoclopramide for acid aspiration prophylaxis in elective surgery. Anesthesiology 61:48, 1984

186. Proctor JD, Chremos AN, Evans EF, Wasserman AJ: An apomorphine-induced vomiting model for antiemetic studies in man. J Clin Pharmacol 18:95, 1978

187. Cohen SE, Woods WA, Wyner J: Antiemetic efficacy of droperidol and metoclopramide. Anesthesiology 60:67, 1984

188. Dundee JW, Clarke RSJ, Howard PJ: Studies of drugs given before anaesthesia. XXIII: Metoclopramide. Br J Anaesth 46:509, 1974

189. Chestnut DH, Vandewalker GE, Owen CL, et al: Administration of metoclopramide for prevention of nausea and vomiting during epidural anesthesia for elective cesarean section. Anesthesiology 66:563, 1987

190. Miller CD, Anderson WG: Silent regurgitation in day case gynaecological patients. Anaesthesia 43:321, 1988

191. Madej TH, Simpson KH: Comparison of the use of domperidone, droperidol and metoclopramide in the prevention of nausea and vomiting following gynaecological surgery in day cases. Br J Anaesth 58:879, 1986

192. Gralla RJ: Metoclopramide. A review of antiemetic trials. Drugs 25(suppl 1):63, 1983

193. Schulze-Delrieu K: Metoclopramide. N Engl J Med 305:28, 1981

194. Pinder RM, Brogden RN, Sawyer PR, et al: Metoclopramide: A review of its pharmacological properties and clinical use. Drugs 12:81, 1976

195. Caldwell C, Rains G, McKiterick K: An unusual reaction to preoperative metoclopramide. Anesthesiology 67:854, 1987

196. Bevacqua BK: Supraventricular tachycardia associated with postpartum metoclopramide administration. Anesthesiology 68:124, 1988

197. Shaklai M, Pinkhas J, De Vries A: Metoclopramide and cardiac arrhythmia (letter). Br Med J 2:385, 1974

198. Thorburn CW, Sowton E: The hemodynamic effects of metoclopramide. Postgrad Med J 49(suppl 4):22, 1973

199. Casey WF, Smith CE, Katz JM, et al: Intravenous meperidine for control of shivering during caesarean section under epidural anaesthesia. Can J Anaesth 35:128, 1988

200. Pauca AL, Savage RT, Simpson S, Roy RC: Effect of pethidine, fentanyl and morphine on post-operative shivering in man. Acta Anaesthesiol Scand 28:138, 1984

201. Conner JT, Herr G, Katz RL, et al: Droperidol, fentanyl and morphine for I.V. surgical premedication. Br J Anaesth 50:463, 1978

202. Dionne RA: Differential pharmacology of drugs used for intravenous premedication. J Dent Res 63:842, 1984

203. Scamman FL, Klein SL, Choi WW: Conscious sedation for procedures under local or topical anesthesia. Ann Otol Rhinol Laryngol 94:21, 1985

204. Van de Velde A, Camu F, Claeys MA: Midazolam for intramuscular premedication: Dose-effect relationships compared to diazepam, fentanyl and fentanyl-droperidol in a placebo controlled study. Acta Anaesthesiol Belg 37:127, 1986

205. Morrison JD: Studies of drugs given before anaesthesia. XXII: Phenoperidine and fentanyl, alone and in combination with droperidol. Br J Anaesth 42:1119, 1970

206. Stockham RJ, Stanley TH, Pace NL, et al: Fentanyl pretreatment modifies anaesthetic induction with etomidate. Anaesth Intensive Care 16:171, 1988

207. Kirby IJ, Northwood D, Dodson ME: Modification by alfentanil of the haemodynamic response to tracheal intubation in elderly patients. A dose-response study. Br J Anaesth 60:384, 1988

208. Black TE, Kay B, Healy TEJ: Reducing the haemodynamic responses to laryngoscopy and intubation. A comparison of alfentanil with fentanyl. Anaesthesia 39:883, 1984

209. Van Aken H, Meinshausen E, Prien T, et al: The influence of fentanyl and tracheal intubation on the hemodynamic effects of anesthesia induction with propofol/N_2O in humans. Anesthesiology 68:157, 1988

210. Kay B, Nolan D, Mayall R, Healy TEJ: The effect of sufentanil on the cardiovascular responses to tracheal intubation. Anaesthesia 42:382, 1987

211. Dann WL, Hutchinson A, Cartwright DP: Maternal and neonatal responses to alfentanil administered before induction of general anaesthesia for caesarean section. Br J Anaesth 59:1392, 1987

212. Dundee JW, Kirwan MJ, Clarke RSJ: Anaesthesia and premedication as factors in postoperative vomiting. Acta Anaesthesiol Scand 9:223, 1965

213. Chestnutt WN, Clarke RS, Dundee JW: Comparison of nalbuphine, pethidine and placebo as premedication for minor gynaecological surgery. Br J Anaesth 59:576, 1987

214. Bone ME, Dowson S, Smith G: A comparison of nalbuphine with fentanyl for postoperative pain relief following termination of pregnancy under day care anaesthesia. Anaesthesia 43:194, 1988

215. Riding JE: Post-operative vomiting. Proc R Soc Med 53:671, 1960

216. Lundgren S: Comparison of rectal diazepam and subcutaneous morphine-scopolamine administration for outpatient sedation in minor oral surgery. Acta Anaesthesiol Scand 29:674, 1985

217. Pandit SK, Kothary SP, Pandit UA, Mathai MK: Comparison

of fentanyl and butorphanol for outpatient anaesthesia. Can J Anaesth 34:130, 1987

218. White PF, Coe V, Shafer A, Sung ML: Comparison of alfentanil with fentanyl for outpatient anesthesia. Anesthesiology 64:99, 1986

219. Brown EM, Kunjappan VE, Alexander GD: Fentanyl/alfentanil for pelvic laparoscopy. Can Anaesth Soc J 31:251, 1984

220. Forrest WH, Jr, Brown CR, Brown BW: Subjective responses to six common preoperative medications. Anesthesiology 47:241, 1977

221. Sengupta A, Gupta PK, Pandey K: Investigation of glycopyrrolate as a premedicant drug. Br J Anaesth 52:513, 1980

222. Mirakhur RK, Reid J, Elliott J: Volume and pH of gastric contents following anticholinergic premedication. Anaesthesia 34:453, 1979

223. Mirakhur RK, Dundee JW, Connolly JDR: Studies of drugs given before anaesthesia. XVII: Anticholinergic premedicants. Br J Anaesth 51:339, 1979

224. Fell D, Cotton BR, Smith G: IM atropine and regurgitation (letter). Br J Anaesth 55:256, 1983

225. Dawson B, Reed WA: Anaesthesia for day-care surgery: A symposium (III). Anaesthesia for adult surgical out-patients. Can Anaesth Soc J 27:409, 1980

226. Knapp MR, Beecher HK: Postanesthetic nausea, vomiting, and retching. Evaluation of the antiemetic drugs dimenhydrinate (Dramamine), chlorpromazine, and pentobarital sodium. JAMA 160:376, 1956

227. Howat DDC: Anti-emetic drugs in anaesthesia. A double blind trial of two phenothiazine derivatives. Anaesthesia 15:289, 1960

228. Burtles R, Peckett BW: Postoperative vomiting. Some factors affecting its incidence. Br J Anaesth 29:114, 1957

229. Sutherland AD, Stock JG, Davies JM: Effects of preoperative fasting on morbidity and gastric contents in patients undergoing day-stay surgery. Br J Anaesth 58:876, 1986

230. Millar JM, Hall PJ: Nausea and vomiting after prostaglandins in day case termination of pregnancy. The efficacy of low dose droperidol. Anaesthesia 42:613, 1987

231. O'Donovan N, Shaw J: Nausea and vomiting in day-case dental anaesthesia. The use of low-dose droperidol. Anaesthesia 39:1172, 1984

232. Santos A, Datta S: Prophylactic use of droperidol for control of nausea and vomiting during spinal anesthesia for cesarean section. Anesth Analg 63:85, 1984

233. Valanne J, Korttila K: Effect of a small dose of droperidol on nausea, vomiting and recovery after outpatient enflurane anaesthesia. Acta Anaesthesiol Scand 29:359, 1985

234. Muir C, Metcalfe R: A comparison of plasma levels of hyoscine after oral and transdermal administration. J Pharm Biomed Analysis 1:363, 1983

235. McCrary JA, Webb NR: Anisocoria from scopolamine patches. JAMA 248:353, 1982

236. Price BH: Anisocoria from scopolamine patches (letter). JAMA 253:1561, 1985

237. Talmi YP, Finkelstein Y, Zohar Y, Laurian N: Reduction of salivary flow with Scopoderm TTS. Ann Otol Rhinol Laryngol 97:128, 1988

238. Graybiel A, Knepton J, Shaw J: Prevention of experimental motion sickness by scopolamine absorbed through the skin. Aviat Space Environ Med 47:1096, 1976

239. Tigerstedt I, Salmela L, Aromaa U: Double-blind comparison of transdermal scopolamine, droperidol and placebo against postoperative nausea and vomiting. Acta Anaesthesiol Scand 32:454, 1988

240. Tolksdorf W, Meisel R, Müller P, Bender H-J: Transdermales Scopolamin (TTS-Scopolamin) zur Prophylaxe Postoperativer Übelkeit und Erbrechen. Anaesthesist 34:656, 1985

241. Loper KA, Ready LB, Dorman BH: Prophylactic transdermal scopolamine patches reduce nausea in postoperative patients receiving epidural morphine. Anesth Analg 68:144, 1989

242. Clissold SP, Heel RC: Transdermal hyoscine (scopolamine). A preliminary review of its pharmacodynamic properties and therapeutic efficacy. Drugs 29:189, 1985

243. Postoperative wound infections: The influence of ultraviolet irradiation of the operating room and of various other factors. [Report of an ad hoc committee of the Committee on Trauma, National Academy of Sciences-National Research Council.] Ann Surg 160(suppl 2):1, 1964

244. Nichols RL: Use of prophylactic antibiotics in surgical practice. Am J Med 70:686, 1981

245. Hunt TK: Surgical wound infections: An overview. Am J Med 70:712, 1981

246. Miles AA, Miles EM, Burke J: The value and duration of defence reactions of the skin to the primary lodgement of bacteria. Br J Exp Pathol 38:79, 1957

247. Burke JF: The effective period of preventive antibiotic action in experimental incisions and dermal lesions. Surgery 50:161, 1961

248. Shapiro M, Townsend TR, Rosner B, Kass EH: Use of antimicrobial drugs in general hospitals. N Engl J Med 301:351, 1979

249. Kaiser AB: Overview of cephalosporin prophylaxis. Am J Surg 155(suppl):52, 1988

250. Prevention of bacterial endocarditis. Med Lett 26:3, 1983

251. Clemens JD, Horwitz RI, Jaffe CC, et al: A controlled evaluation of the risk of bacterial endocarditis in persons with mitral-valve prolapse. N Engl J Med 307:776, 1982

252. Danchin N, Voiriot P, Briancon S, et al: Mitral valve prolapse as a risk factor for infective endocarditis. Lancet 1:743, 1989

253. Marks AR, Choong CY, Sanfilippo AJ, et al: Identification of high-risk and low-risk subgroups of patients with mitral-valve prolapse. N Engl J Med 320:1031, 1989

254. Shulman ST, et al: Prevention of bacterial endocarditis. A statement for health professionals by the Committee on Rheumatic Fever and Infective Endocarditis of the Council on Cardiovascular Disease in the Young. Circulation 70:1123A, 1984

255. Beary JF, Benson H: A simple psychophysiologic technique which elicits the hypometabolic changes of the relaxation response. Psychosom Med 36:115, 1974

256. Benson H, Rosner BA, Marzetta BR, Klemchuk HP: Decreased blood pressure in borderline hypertensive subjects who practiced meditation. J Chronic Dis 27:163, 1974

257. Benson H, Rosner BA, Marzetta BR, Klemchuk HP: Decreased blood pressure in pharmacologically treated hypertensive patients who regularly elicited the relaxation response. Lancet 1:289, 1974

258. Datey KK, Deshmukh SN, Dalvi CP, Vinekar SL: "Shavasan": A yogic exercise in the management of hypertension. Angiology 20:325, 1969

259. Little BC, Hayworth J, Benson P, et al: Treatment of hypertension in pregnancy by relaxation and biofeedback. Lancet 1:865, 1984

260. Patel CH: Yoga and bio-feedback in the management of hypertension. Lancet 2:1053, 1973

261. Patel C: 12-month follow-up of yoga and bio-feedback in the management of hypertension. Lancet 1:62, 1975

262. Peters RK, Benson H, Peters JM: Daily relaxation response breaks in a working population. II: Effects on blood pressure. Am J Public Health 67:954, 1977

27
IMMEDIATE PREINDUCTION PERIOD

Robert L. Willenkin

The Patient
The Equipment
The Surgeon

The Positioning of the Patient
The Overall Plan

There are fundamental considerations that must be attended to before anesthesia is induced. The preparation and decisions that are made from the moment the anesthesiologist starts to organize the administration of anesthesia to the moment of its induction are critical links in the total anesthetic care of a patient. During this period, the anesthesiologist reviews the basic management plan, ensures that the environment and use of equipment are consistent with that plan, and assesses the current status of the patient (Table 27-1).

This chapter discusses the essential planning and tasks common to almost all anesthetic procedures. Other chapters describe the requirements for special patients or procedures. As with many other aspects of anesthesia, an organized, logical strategy for thinking about this period helps the anesthesiologist function efficiently and prevent errors. The period immediately before induction of anesthesia can be divided arbitrarily into five sections: the patient, equipment, surgeon, initial positioning of the patient, and overall plan.

THE PATIENT

For most aspects of anesthesia, the preparation immediately before anesthesia is approximately the same for all patients. Nevertheless, it is useful to ask the question, What is special about this patient at this time, and what will I do about it?

In addition to information gained in the earlier preanesthesia assessment (see Chs. 22 through 26 and 28), new information can be obtained by reviewing the patient's chart at this time: (1) the latest progress notes; (2) laboratory results (hemoglobin, electrolyte and blood enzyme levels, electrocardiograms, radiograms); (3) test results (e.g., from pulmonary and cardiac function tests); (4) name, dose, and time of administration of medications; (5) nature, time, and amount of last oral intake; (6) nature, time, and amount of intravenous fluids; (7) patient's temperature; (8) nurses' comments; and (9) the consent form for operation or procedure.

In the period immediately before induction of anesthesia, the anesthesiologist greets the patient and re-establishes the relationship formed at the preanesthesia visit. The identity of the patient and the procedure to be performed are verified. Also assessed are the degree of anxiety, the readiness for surgery, and whether the patient is comfortable. If deemed advisable, more premedication may be given intravenously after the intravenous infusion is started. To confirm the patient's agreement, it is helpful to repeat briefly the previously discussed anesthesia plan.

At this time, the anesthesiologist also reviews any special circumstances, such as the refusal or agreement for

TABLE 27-1. Fundamental Considerations for the Basic Management of Anesthesia in the Period Immediately before Induction of Anesthesia

General Consideration	Specifics
Patient	Medical history, surgical consent form, present health status, patient-physician relationship, special needs, special requests, intravenous catheters, monitoring lines
Equipment	Gas supplies, anesthesia machine, monitors, small equipment, drugs
Surgeon	Surgical plan, operative site, patient position, surgical time and requirements, plans for postoperative care
Positioning of the patient	Supine position, potential injuries, prevention of injuries
Overall plan	Management plan, anticipated problems, alternatives, safety

blood transfusion, use of autologous blood in reserve, notification of relatives, and preferences for body position immediately after surgery. If special aspects of postoperative management have been agreed to (the use of epidural narcotics, patient-controlled analgesia, respiratory exercises), these, too, are discussed again as a reminder for both the anesthesiologist and the patient (also see Chs. 68 and 69). If the patient plans to leave the hospital on the day of surgery, the plan for transportation and assistance is reviewed.

The presence or absence of prostheses (dentures, hearing aids, artificial eyes) is confirmed. It is also useful to recheck the condition of the teeth, noting on the anesthesia record the absence of teeth or the presence of abnormal teeth. One or more catheters are inserted intravenously, taking into consideration the location of the surgical procedure, the intraoperative position of the patient, the anticipated blood and fluid requirements, and the possible use of continuous infusion of drugs. Intravenous catheters are placed by using a sterile technique, local anesthesia, and a sterile bandage over the puncture site, and with concern for the patient's comfort. The size of the catheters should be adequate for the highest rates of fluid administration in a "worst-case" scenario. Needles must be handled with great care and disposed of promptly in appropriate containers to minimize the risk of inadvertent needle punctures into either the patient or health care personnel.

If invasive monitoring is planned, time of catheter placement is determined. Arterial and brachial central venous pressure catheters may be inserted either before or after transport of the patient to the operating room (see Ch. 31). Insertion of catheters into the internal jugular and subclavian veins usually occurs in the operating room either before or after induction of anesthesia. The choice depends on the anesthesiologist's judgment regarding the patient's hemodynamic stability and the need for monitoring of venous pressure during induction of anesthesia.

At this time, certain questions need to be addressed: Is this patient in optimum condition for anesthesia? Is there anything else I need to do? Specific practices help assess the patient's current condition. Blood pressure values obtained with the patient supine and sitting, or in the reverse Trendelenburg position, reveal the status of blood volume. The current state of bronchospasm can be determined by questioning the patient, auscultating the chest for breath sounds, and observing the character of breathing. Patients with a history of angina must undergo evaluation of current symptoms (see Chs. 23 through 25). Finally, results of tests of the patient's current status (arterial blood gas tensions, serum potassium level, hematocrit, blood clotting studies) are the basis for further decision making regarding the anesthesia plan.

THE EQUIPMENT

It is the personal responsibility of the anesthesiologist to verify the proper functioning of all equipment. Although it is appropriate and efficient to use technicians and aides to help with equipment, the ultimate responsibility for the safe use of anesthesia equipment cannot be delegated.

Gas supplies are inspected first. High-pressure hoses are connected to centrally supplied oxygen and nitrous oxide. If the anesthesia machine has suitable pressure gauges, the pressure in the central line is observed and should be at least 50 psi. A simple and quick safety check consists of turning on the oxygen flow and oxygen analyzer to verify delivery of oxygen from what is labeled the central oxygen supply. This verification is critically important whenever any repair work has been done anywhere along the oxygen delivery lines. Next, the valve on at least one oxygen cylinder should be opened and its pressure checked to see that at least a 1-hour supply of oxygen is present. Because the oxygen in E cylinders exists as a compressed gas at room temperature, pressure and volume are proportional. A full E cylinder contains approximately 625 L of oxygen at about 2,200 psi. Thus, a 1-hour supply at 2 L/min, about 120 L, corresponds to a gauge pressure of approximately 500 psi.

Although not as vital as for oxygen, it is important to look at the pressure of the nitrous oxide cylinder. The pressure in a cylinder of nitrous oxide is not as useful a guide to content as is the pressure in a cylinder of oxygen, because the nitrous oxide in full E cylinders exists as a liquid at room temperature. As long as any liquid is present in the cylinder, the pressure will be approximately 750 psi at room temperature. However, just at the point when the liquid is exhausted and pressure starts to decrease, the volume of nitrous oxide in the tank is about 215 L. At 3 L/min, this is approximately a

1-hour supply. As nitrous oxide is further removed, the content of the cylinder can now be calculated from the pressure-volume relationship. For example, when the pressure is 350 psi, approximately 100 L remains.

Flow meters and flow control valves should be observed for proper motion and stability throughout their expected range of use. The oxygen flush valve is checked to see that it releases a high flow of oxygen. A crude check for leaks can be made by turning on oxygen and nitrous oxide, kinking the outflow hose to prevent gas outflow from the machine, and watching the flow meters. They should descend a little and stabilize. No change means that a significant leak exists. A second way of checking for leaks between tanks and flow meters is to disconnect the hoses from central gas supplies, close all flow meters, open and close oxygen and nitrous oxide tanks, and observe the gas pressure gauges. A decrease in pressure over a few minutes signifies a leak.

Vaporizers should be checked for adequate amounts of liquid anesthetic agents, smooth functioning of controls, and closed filling caps.

The circle system can be examined for leaks by closing the exhaust ("pop-off") valve, obstructing the patient end of the Y-piece, filling the system with gas to a pressure of 30 to 40 mmHg, turning off all gas flows, and watching the airway pressure gauge. A decrease in pressure indicates a leak. The amount of leakage can be quantified by turning on a flow of gas just sufficient to maintain a stable system pressure. This amount of flow equals the amount of leakage at that pressure. The pop-off valve and scavenger system are then checked by releasing the system pressure (i.e., by opening the pop-off valve while the Y-piece is still occluded). Controllable release of pressure results from a properly functioning pop-off valve and an open, unoccluded scavenger system. The carbon dioxide absorbent should be observed for appropriate color. Inspiratory and expiratory valves and circle resistance are checked by inspiring into and expiring from each hose of the circle system while oxygen is flowing and vaporizers are turned off. This practice verifies, by smell, that the vaporizers are not releasing volatile agents when the controls are in the "off" position.

The oxygen analyzer is calibrated, preferably at two concentrations, but at least at around 21 percent oxygen, and its alarm is checked. Other meters and alarms for pressure, volume, and respiratory frequency are activated and checked. The ventilator is turned on, observed for appropriate functioning, and adjusted approximately to the anticipated requirements of the patient. All hoses and connections are tested for tightness. Electric power lines are checked. Anesthesia machine drawers, shelves, and wheels are checked for stability and smoothness of functioning.

Small equipment and work space are checked and organized for efficient functioning. This inspection includes laryngoscopes, endotracheal tubes, suctioning tools, suction flow and negative pressure, airways, nerve stimulators, intravenous fluids and equipment, towels, adhesive tape, and gloves. Syringes are labeled with drug name and concentration. Proper disposal facilities for both needles and other materials need to be accessible.

Monitors should be tested and calibrated according to manufacturers' guidelines. Such devices include arterial blood pressure cuff (manual or automatic), electrocardiograph, temperature indicator, pulse oximeter, respirometer, gas analyzers, pressure monitors, and brain function monitors.

Other pieces of equipment are activated and checked: temperature blanket, rapid blood administrator, blood warmer, infusion devices, and humidifiers. Finally, the ground fault detector should be observed while all electrical devices, including electrocautery equipment, are turned on.

These tests should be performed before the first use of the day, and most are repeated quickly before every patient. If done efficiently, these tests can be carried out in less than 15 minutes and provide reasonable assurance of proper functioning of equipment. Equipment testing should be documented on the anesthesia record.

Equipment is discussed in greater detail in Chapters 7, 11, and 29.

THE SURGEON

If the operating room team is to function effectively and efficiently, communication among all members of the team must be good. It is useful to review the surgical plan with the surgeon, including positioning of the patient, operative site, type of incision, expected length of the procedure, anticipated difficulties, and special requirements. Examples of special requirements are the need for the absence of paralysis during use of a surgical nerve stimulator, the need for regulation of blood pressure, and the constraints of monitoring evoked potentials. Management of special problems regarding Jehovah's Witnesses or patients with "do-not-resuscitate" orders must be discussed and agreed upon by all affected persons.

If postoperative pain management might include epidurally or intrathecally administered narcotics, patient-controlled analgesia, or peripheral nerve blocks, these plans also should be discussed and agreed upon (see Ch. 69).

THE POSITIONING OF THE PATIENT

For most procedures, anesthesia is induced with the patient in the supine position (Fig. 27-1). The head is elevated and extended, and the neck is flexed slightly;

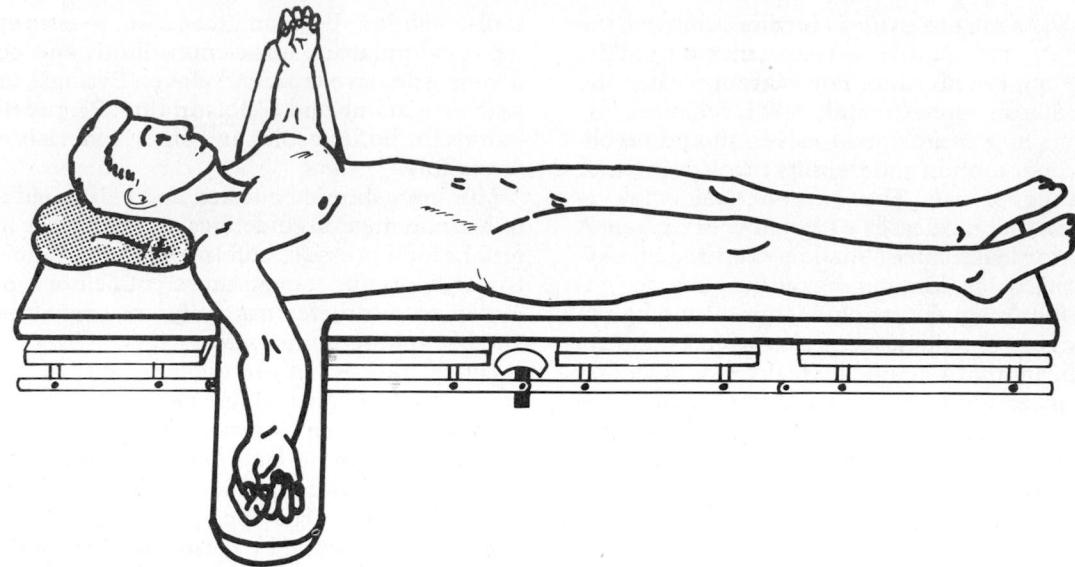

Fig. 27-1. The supine position. The head is elevated. The arms are extended 90 degrees with slight flexion and external rotation of the elbow.

this is called the "sniffing" position. Arms may be placed alongside the trunk or extended and placed on arm boards. Patients are generally more comfortable if their hips, knees, and elbows are flexed slightly. Padding may be used to maintain the normal lumbar vertebral curve, which tends to flatten after anesthesia is established, especially when muscle relaxants or spinal or epidural anesthesia is used. For more detailed description of the supine and "lawn chair" positions, see discussions by Smith[1] and Martin.[2] After the position is established, personnel should ask whether the patient is comfortable.

Anesthetized patients are vulnerable to injury from pressure or stretching of nerves, vessels, joints, or skin. Several critical areas need special attention. Arms placed at the side should be positioned on the operating table pad and restrained by sheets to prevent abduction and consequent pressure from the anesthesia screen or the edge of the operating table. The elbows should be rotated externally to prevent pressure on the ulnar nerves. If arms are abducted, the angle should be 90 degrees or less, with slight elevation of the supporting surface and slight flexion and external rotation of the elbow. Legs should be supported uniformly to minimize pressure on the heels. Support of the head with a pad distributes pressure on the occiput. Elderly, very thin, or cachectic patients need special care of all bony prominences, especially the sacrum.

Injuries from pressure, stretching, or kinking have been reported for almost every major peripheral nerve. The most frequent injuries involve the ulnar, brachial plexus, sciatic, femoral, common peroneal, saphenous, anterior tibia, obturator, and lateral femoral cutaneous nerves.[3,4]

Positioning of the patient *after* induction of anesthesia is described in Chapter 42.

THE OVERALL PLAN

The anesthesiologist reviews the entire management plan during this time (Table 27-2). Patient problems, surgical requirements, and choice of anesthetic agents

TABLE 27-2. ASA Basic Standards for Preanesthesia Care

These standards apply to all patients who receive anesthesia or monitored anesthesia care. Under unusual circumstances (e.g., extreme emergencies), these standards may be modified. When this is the case, the circumstances shall be documented in the patient's record.

Standard I: An anesthesiologist shall be responsible for determining the medical status of the patient, developing a plan of anesthesia care, and acquainting that patient or the responsible adult with the proposed plan.

The development of an appropriate plan of anesthesia care is based upon

1. Reviewing the medical records
2. Interviewing and examining the patient to
   a. Discuss the medical history, previous anesthetic experiences, and drug therapy
   b. Assess those aspects of the physical condition that might affect decisions regarding perioperative risk and management
3. Obtaining and/or reviewing tests and consultations necessary to the conduct of anesthesia
4. Determining the appropriate prescription of preoperative medications as necessary to the conduct of anesthesia

The responsible anesthesiologist shall verify that the above has been performed properly and documented in the patient's record.

(From American Society of Anesthesiologists,[5] with permission.)

and techniques are all part of a detailed plan that includes specific steps for induction and maintenance of anesthesia, awakening from anesthesia, and postoperative care. This is the time to review potential problems, methods of preventing and recognizing those problems, initial therapeutic steps, and alternative solutions. Because the anesthesiologist is required to resolve both common and rare but dangerous problems, the management plan must anticipate both likely and unlikely events. To maximize problem solving, the anesthesiologist must plan for not only the initial techniques of diagnosis and management but also alternative methods if initial approaches fail. He or she must also consider the consequences of positioning of the patient—and of changes in that position—and design preventive measures to avoid complications.

One orderly system of mental preparation consists of the following practices:

1. Read the operating room schedule for name and anatomic site of operation.
2. Read the patient's consent form in the chart to ensure that it agrees with the schedule.
3. Review the patient's verbal comments regarding the procedure to be performed.
4. Review patient data to determine existing and potential problems.
5. Review all steps of the total anesthetic plan from induction to postoperative care and consider alternatives for each step.
6. Anticipate possible problems with both patient and apparatus. Consider what can be done to prevent, diagnose, and manage these problems and what alternative are available or should be made available.
7. Verify availability of blood (homologous or autologous), blood products, or ancillary drugs (such as antibiotics, heparin) if likely to be needed.
8. Prepare anesthesia records and document significant patient data.
9. Document equipment check.
10. Think safety: equipment safety, electrical safety, patient safety, and personal safety against exposure to anesthetic gases and infectious disease.

REFERENCES

1. Smith BL: The traditional supine position. p. 33. In Martin JT (ed): Positioning in Anesthesia and Surgery. 2nd Ed. WB Saunders, Philadelphia, 1987
2. Martin JT: The lawn chair (contoured supine) position. p. 37. In Martin JT (ed): Positioning in Anesthesia and Surgery. 2nd Ed. WB Saunders, Philadelphia, 1987
3. Cheney FW: Anesthesia: Potential risks and causes of incidents. p. 11. In Gravenstein JS, Holzer JF (eds): Safety and Cost Containment in Anesthesia. Butterworths, Boston, 1988
4. Dornette WHL: Compression neuropathies: Medical aspects and legal implications. Int Anesthesiol Clin 24(4):201, 1986
5. American Society of Anesthesiologists: Basic Standards for Preanesthesia Care. American Society of Anesthesiologists, Park Ridge, IL, 1987

28

MALIGNANT HYPERTHERMIA

Gerald A. Gronert
Scott R. Schulman
John Mott

INTRODUCTION

The popular term *malignant hyperthermia* (MH) refers to a clinical syndrome classically observed during general anesthesia—rapidly increasing temperature (as great as 1°C/5 min) and a high mortality rate. This results from acute uncontrolled increases in skeletal muscle metabolism that may proceed to severe rhabdomyolysis. The early mortality rate reached 70 percent; with earlier diagnosis, this decreased to 28 percent, and the advent of dantrolene in 1979 dropped the rate to less than 10 percent.[1] Wilson's group apparently first used the term *malignant hyperthermia* in print in 1966, several months before Gordon independently referred to malignant hyperpyrexia.[2,3] A recent Danish survey indicates an incidence of fulminant MH of 1 in 250,000 anesthetics. However, when only the potent agents and succinylcholine are considered, fulminant MH occurred in 1 in 62,000 anesthetics. Suspected MH occurred in 1 of 16,000 anesthetics overall, and in 1 of 4,200 anesthetics involving potent volatile agents and succinylcholine.[4] A layman's organization has been set up for public education and communication among affected families (Malignant Hyperthermia Association of the United States [MHAUS], Box 3231, Darien, Connecticut 06820), and a 24-hour 7-day telephone service has been created for emergency consultation (MH hotline: 209-634-4917; request index zero, MH consultant). The North American MH Registry collates findings from biopsy centers in Canada and the United States and provides access to specific patient data, either via the hotline or via direct contact with Dr. Marilyn Lar-

935

ach, Department of Anesthesiology, Pennsylvania State University, Hershey Pennsylvania. A recent comprehensive review of MH is the postgraduate educational symposium in the *British Journal of Anaesthesia*, volume 60, February 1988. Eight articles provide an indepth review of MH.

HISTORY

In 1929 Ombrédanne described anesthesia-induced postoperative hyperthermia and pallor in children with significant mortality (Ombrédanne's syndrome) but did not detect familial relationships.[5] In 1960 Denborough and Lovell[6] described a 21-year-old Australian with an open leg fracture who was more anxious about anesthesia than about surgery, since 10 of his relatives had died during or after anesthesia. Further evaluations of affected families came from Locher in Wausau, Wisconsin, in conjunction with Britt et al. in Toronto, Canada.[7] Direct skeletal muscle involvement rather than central loss of temperature control was established by recognition of increased muscle metabolism or muscle rigidity early in the syndrome, of low-threshold contracture responses by Kalow and Britt,[8] and of elevated values for creatine phosphokinase (CK).

The pig, when inbred for muscle development (e.g., the Landrace, Pietrain, or Poland China), provides an excellent animal model. This model evolved from earlier reports describing unsuitable pork[9]; the stresses of the abattoir resulted in accelerated metabolism and rapid deterioration of the muscle, resulting in pale soft exudative (PSE) pork.[10] The incidence of PSE increased with breeding patterns designed to produce rapid growth rate and superior muscling. This increased incidence led to the term porcine stress syndrome (PSS).[11] Any stresses, such as separation, shipping, weaning, fighting, coitus, and slaughter, could lead to increased metabolism, acidosis, rigidity, fever, and death.

In 1966 Hall et al.[12] reported MH induced by halothane and succinylcholine (SCh) in stress-susceptible swine. The human and porcine forms are virtually identical, when the clinical and laboratory changes of anesthesia-induced MH are compared. Harrison[13] in 1975 described the efficacy of dantrolene in preventing and treating porcine MH, which was confirmed by a multihospital evaluation of dantrolene used to treat unanticipated human episodes that occurred during anesthesia.[14]

There is now little doubt that MH in swine is a manifestation of a generalized susceptibility to stress; the role of the sympathetic nervous system is unclear. Williams[15] and Hall and associates[16] proposed a direct involvement of the sympathetic nervous system in initiating MH; Gronert suggested a secondary involvement, whether MH was induced by anesthesia[17] or by factors involved with stress in the absence of anesthetic agents.[18] Stress-induced MH in humans occurs less frequently than in swine.

Malignant hyperthermia presents several paradoxes. In 1979 Halsall et al.[19] noted that anesthetics are inconsistent in their ability to trigger MH and are therefore frequently ineffective in triggering episodes in affected humans; this may be related to delay of the response by various depressants and nondepolarizing muscle relaxants.[20] Conversely, nontriggering anesthetics can be associated with apparent MH episodes, even in humans partially protected by dantrolene.[21,22] Finally, evaluation for susceptibility to MH requires either an anesthetic challenge or an invasive destructive test (e.g., muscle biopsy). The best indicator is an unequivocal clinical episode; next best is the in vitro muscle contracture test.

CLINICAL SYNDROME

The onset of MH can be acute and rapid, particularly during induction of anesthesia with an inhaled anesthetic or with the use of SCh. Frequently, however, the onset is delayed for hours and may not become overt until the patient is in the recovery room. Regardless of the time of onset, once initiated, the course of MH can be extraordinarily rapid. When clinical signs, such as muscle rigidity, tachycardia, or fever, suggest malignant hyperthermia, the association with MH is not strong unless more than one abnormal sign is noted. When there is but a single suggestive adverse sign, the diagnosis is usually not MH.[23]

The volatile anesthetics and SCh cause affected subjects to undergo a striking increase in metabolism, both aerobic and anaerobic, resulting in intense production of heat, carbon dioxide, and lactate and an associated respiratory and metabolic acidosis.[24] These reactions markedly alter whole-body acid-base balance and temperature because of the large proportion of skeletal muscle to body weight (40 to 50 percent) and are magnified as temperature increases. Whole-body rigidity occurs in almost all pigs and in 75 percent of humans. The temperature may exceed 43°C (109.4°F), $PaCO_2$ may exceed 100 mmHg, and pHa may be less than 7.00. Associated with this is increased permeability of muscle with increased serum potassium, ionized calcium, CK, myoglobin, and serum sodium.[24] Later, serum potassium and calcium levels decrease; muscle edema may occur. Sympathetic hyperactivity is frequently the first sign of this increased metabolism (tachycardia, sweating, hypertension). With metabolic exhaustion, cellular permeability may increase with accompanying generalized edema, including acute cerebral edema. As MH progresses, disseminated intravascular coagulopathy and cardiac or renal failure may develop. One must remember that MH is a disorder of increased metabolism—it need not involve increased temperature, for example, if heat loss is greater than production, or if cardiac output plummets early.

The clinical MH syndrome can occur as a "final common path" in certain situations that may not specifically involve susceptibility to MH. This is somewhat analogous to observing Raynaud's phenomenon in the absence of Raynaud syndrome. Examples include instances of exaggerated heat stroke, some cases of the neuroleptic malignant syndrome, and various myopathies involving constantly and precariously altered permeability of cellular membranes and intracellular organelles, such as Duchenne's muscular dystrophy.

TRISMUS-MASSETER SPASM

Trismus-masseter spasm is defined as jaw muscle rigidity in association with limb muscle flaccidity after administration of SCh. Its causes had been considered entirely pathologic and included MH, myotonia, probably some other myopathies, or unknown etiology. There is now compelling evidence that trismus occurs as a unique property of jaw muscle in some normal people. Not all accept this theory; re-evaluation of trismus continues, particularly in regard to the controversy about its management.

Until recently, most believed that trismus signified MH 50 percent of the time, on the basis of contracture testing and incidence of clinical MH in those patients.[24] This incidence mandated that anesthesia be stopped and treatment or evaluation for MH begun. However, two retrospective American studies document a 1 percent incidence of trismus in children given SCh after an inhalation induction with halothane.[25,26] Although this rather high incidence contrasts with the 0.01 percent incidence reported in Denmark,[4] it nonetheless forces a re-examination of trismus. The results suggest that either susceptibility occurs more frequently than previously thought, or that trismus may occur in normal people. Because clinical MH had not occurred in the patients in these reports,[25,26] the latter possibility (i.e., that trismus can occur in normal people) seemed more likely. Several findings support this supposition: masseter muscles have unusual fiber types that respond with slow tonic contractures.[27] In vitro, halothane predisposes normal skeletal muscle to development of a contracture upon exposure to SCh.[28] In vivo, normal children under deep anesthesia with halothane or enflurane have tighter jaw muscles after SCh is given.[29,30]

Therefore, trismus may be a benign response on many occasions and one position (Gronert) is that anesthesia may be continued safely.[31] But, should a volatile agent be continued in this situation? Rosenberg suggests use of nontriggering agents, if anesthesia must be continued.[31] Anesthesiologists must remember that MH will occur in a few of these trismus patients. Thus, there must be the usual careful monitoring that would detect signs of MH (F_ECO_2, pulse, temperature, muscle tone elsewhere in the body, heat loss, venous or arterial blood gases as needed, examination of urine for myoglobin). The other position (Rosenberg) is that anesthesia should always be halted if possible, and the patient observed for signs of MH and treated if these de-

velop.[31,32] Regardless, it is vitally important that patients who develop trismus undergo testing for MH susceptibility. Collection of such data will help further our understanding of MH and provide the means whereby we can determine the relationship of masseter spasm to MH.

THEORY

MH is a myopathy, usually subclinical, that features an acute loss of intracellular control of calcium. Normally, the wave of depolarization from end plate to transverse tubule is somehow transferred to the sarcoplasmic reticulum (SR), resulting in release of calcium (Fig. 28-1). The free ionized unbound intracellular calcium concentration within the muscle cell increases from the relaxed level of 10^{-7} M to about 5×10^{-5} M. This increase in calcium removes the troponin inhibition from the contractile elements, resulting in muscle contraction. The intracellular calcium pumps rapidly transfer calcium ion back into the SR, and relaxation occurs when the concentration is less than the mechanical threshold. Both contraction and relaxation require ATP (i.e., both are energy-related processes that consume ATP). Dantrolene, the therapeutic wonder drug for MH, blocks SR calcium release without altering calcium reuptake.[24,33]

The clinical and laboratory data in swine and humans indicate decreased control of intracellular calcium, resulting in a release of free unbound ionized calcium from storage sites that normally keep a muscle relaxed. Aerobic and anerobic metabolism increase to provide more ATP to drive the calcium pumps that maintain calcium homeostasis across the sarcolemma into extracellular fluid and into the sarcoplasmic reticulum and mitochondria. Rigidity occurs when unbound myofibrillar calcium approaches the contractile threshold. Originally, many believed that clinical episodes reflected two different phases or types of MH, namely rigid and nonrigid. This is no longer a common opinion; it is unlikely that rigid and nonrigid MH are different entities.[24,33]

Many believe that MH may involve a generalized disorder of membrane permeability for calcium in virtually all tissues, because of calcium's role in so many functions.[34] However, direct support of this ubiquitous involvement is lacking. A similar theory of calcium dysfunction in muscular dystrophies proposes a slower process, eventually resulting in an unmanageable calcium accumulation in intracellular organelles, with ultimate dissolution and muscle damage.[35]

ABNORMALITIES

Abnormalities are functional rather than structural, as MH is a disorder of function.[24,33] These abnormalities can be consistently demonstrated by examination of function, particularly during certain stresses or stimulation.

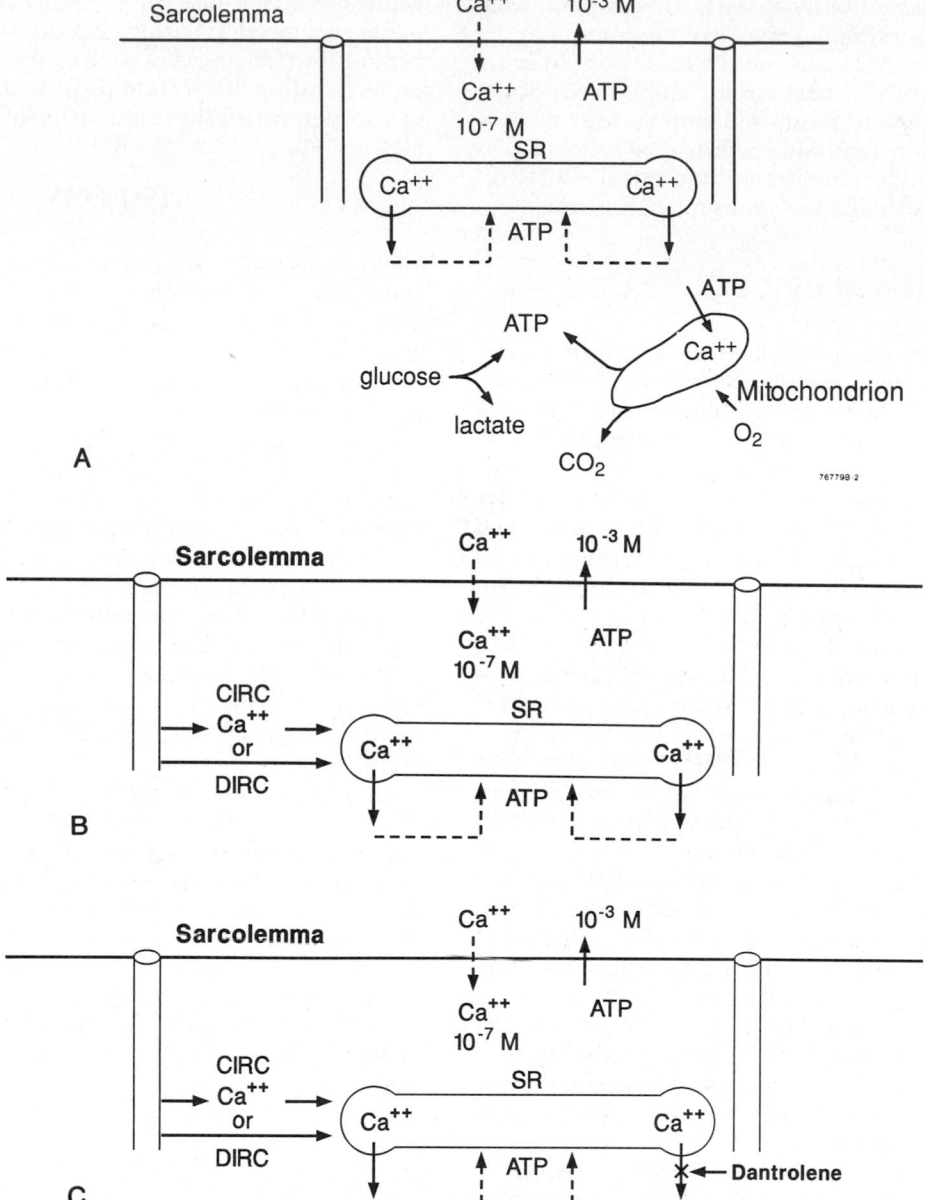

Fig. 28-1. **(A)** Diagram of relaxed skeletal muscle. Calcium fluxes can occur across the sarcolemma, sarcoplasmic reticulum (SR, between the transverse tubules), and mitochondrion. Calcium transport across the sarcolemma or into the intracellular organelles requires energy (ATP). ATP is produced by glycolysis or by aerobic metabolism. **(B)** In the left half of the figure, calcium-induced release of calcium (CIRC) and depolarization-induced release of calcium (DIRC) are shown as possible mechanisms for transfer of the wave of depolarization from transverse tubule to SR. DIRC has been the more accepted explanation for this process in skeletal muscle, and CIRC in cardiac muscle.[103] In DIRC, the changes with depolarization are transferred directly or by a voltage sensibility that results in SR calcium release. In CIRC, the wave of depolarization produces a minuscule release of calcium at the transverse tubule that causes massive SR calcium release. CIRC may occur in susceptible skeletal muscle once MH begins. (See text for details.) **(C)** In the right half of the figure, dantrolene is shown blocking SR calcium release without altering reuptake of calcium back into the SR. (See text for details.) (Modified from Gronert,[207] with permission.)

Skeletal Muscle

Skeletal muscle is the one tissue with proven abnormalities in MH, although pig erythrocyte membranes should probably also be included. Affected human muscle frequently has no histologic defect, or else has protean nonspecific pathology so variable that none can be directly attributed to MH. These include central cores, internal nuclei, target fibers, supercontracted fibrils, and marked variation in fiber diameter.[36]

Metabolism, Enzymatic Considerations, and Heat Production

Affected muscle has greater responses to various stimuli than does normal muscle, whether pig[37,38] or human.[39] Aerobic metabolism (oxygen consumption, $\dot{V}O_2$) and glycolytic metabolism increase dramatically. Anesthetics that trigger MH include the potent volatile anesthetics, classically halothane, and the depolarizing muscle relaxants, such as SCh. There is an approximate 3-fold increase in $\dot{V}O_2$ and a 15- to 20-fold increase in blood lactate, with related acid-base imbalances. The earliest changes appear in the venous effluent from skeletal muscle as decreases in pH or PO_2, or as increases in PCO_2, lactate, potassium, or temperature.[24,37] The increases in lactate occur before there are signs of tissue hypoxia, as shown by venous PO_2 values. These presumed nonhypoxic increases in lactate indicate increased energy demands, for a decrease in ATP alters the balance between NAD and NADH (oxidized and reduced forms, respectively, of nicotinamide adenine dinucleotide), forcing an increase in lactate production. The earliest changes in the venous effluent also occur prior to the increases in heart rate, temperature, and circulating catecholamines.[24,37] The most sensitive early sign during anesthesia is an increase in expired CO_2 (during constant ventilation).[39]

Although different enzyme systems could be abnormal in affected muscle depending on species and genetic influences, the same metabolic changes occur in the extracellular fluid. Studies of proposed abnormal enzymes, including adenylate kinase,[38,40,41] adenylate cyclase,[42,43] and glutathione peroxidase,[44,45] are negative or inconclusive.

Heat production during acute MH derives from aerobic metabolism, glycolysis, neutralization of hydrogen ions, and hydrolysis of high-energy phosphate compounds involved in ion transport and contraction-relaxation.[46] Calculation shows initial heat production to be due to increased aerobic metabolism; subsequent heat production is due to lactate formation. Precise calculations of the expended energy are difficult because of unsteady metabolic and circulatory states, variable and uncontrolled heat loss, and production of heat by neutralization of acid.

Contractures

The muscle rigidity that occurs during MH episodes is a contracture rather than a contraction. A contracture is similar to a muscle cramp; it is nonpropagated and prolonged and can be irreversible. A contraction is the usual form of muscle movement; it is due to a propagated wave of depolarization and is brief and reversible. Contractures are used in tissue baths in the laboratory to study various aspects of MH. Unfortunately, satisfactory samples of tissue are difficult to obtain; an intact muscle fiber undamaged from tendon to tendon is preferred. Human intercostal muscle provides this, but at the expense of a thoracotomy; a unique porcine forelimb dissection provides intact extensor muscle.[47] Most contracture studies use cut muscle, usually excised from quadriceps muscle; these specimens function satisfactorily in a bath but deteriorate quickly as a result of injury currents from the cut ends.[8,48-51] A further modification is the skinned fiber, in which the sarcolemma and portions of the transverse tubules are either stripped away mechanically[52] or "eaten away" chemically.[53] The tissue bath now becomes the intracellular environment, and laboratory manipulations directly affect function of intracellular organelles. Responses of all these preparations are qualitatively similar; the cut muscle preparation develops much less tension.

Although tension can vary as a result of amounts of calcium available to the fibrils,[52,53] in general they are exposed to contracture-producing drugs acting via the sarcoplasmic reticulum (SR), either directly or indirectly. These drugs include caffeine, halothane or other potent volatile anesthetics, and potassium. Succinylcholine 1.1 mM can produce contractures in the tissue bath environment, but this is apparently due to the preservative rather than to SCh itself.[54] Most laboratories report their results in terms of the amount of caffeine required to raise tension by 1 g, for example, the caffeine- or halothane-caffeine-specific concentration proposed by Kalow and associates.[55] This applies to caffeine-specific concentration or halothane-caffeine-specific concentration. However, this approach fails to account for differences in tension due to varying cross-sectional area, or other variations in methodology or interpretation. Gronert attempted to correct for this problem by expressing tension as the fraction of the peak observed tension.[49,50] Whatever the method or drug, abnormal bundles produce low threshold responses.

Older controversies concerning contractures have been discussed elsewhere.[24] Most recent is that concerning the use of halothane and caffeine in combination.[56] Detractors believe that the broad range of responses proves a lack of precision; proponents hold that the broader range indicates a spectrum of susceptibility.[56,57]

Intrafibrillar Proteins

The lack of consistent correlation of fiber type or fiber proteins with abnormal function underscores the difficulties in analyzing this disorder[58-65] — stress is necessary to detect the abnormality.

Calcium Factors

Several studies support the theory that MH is a disorder of calcium control: (1) The SR is the intracellular organelle primarily responsible for control of intracellular calcium transients, and mitochondria serve a secondary reserve function in binding calcium. When intracellular calcium levels increase beyond the capabilities of the SR, the mitochondria begin to bind calcium. Thus, during acute MH, porcine muscle mitochondria begin to store calcium, and this process is reversed after treatment with dantrolene.[62] (2) Intrafibrillar ionized calcium in unstimulated MH-susceptible human intercostal muscle is elevated, as measured with a calcium-selective microelectrode.[66,67] However, it is paradoxical to have an increase in resting intracellular ionized calcium (also observed by the same authors in porcine studies[68]), as such increases in intracellular calcium should be associated with increased resting metabolism. This has not been observed in susceptible humans or pigs.[24,37,38] It may be that the trauma of cellular microelectrode puncture evokes a stress response resulting in the increases in intracellular ionized calcium levels, as normal levels were observed when the intracellular calcium-selective dye Fura-2 was used to measure calcium.[69] (3) Intracellular calcium levels increased with initiation of porcine MH and were reversed by treatment with dantrolene.[62,69,70] The calcium content of skeletal muscle of susceptible humans and pigs is generally but not always less than normal.[24] Calcium antagonists generally affect smooth or cardiac muscle more than skeletal muscle and have contradictory effects in MH: they block contractures in affected human muscle in vitro,[71,72] are associated with hyperkalemia and potentially increased mortality in vivo when used in conjunction with dantrolene,[73–75] and do not prevent or effectively treat MH in susceptible pigs.[76,77] Further, because of the risk of hyperkalemia with calcium antagonists and dantrolene, there is the added hazard that the hyperkalemia could trigger MH in susceptible skeletal muscle.[78]

**Electrophysiologic Measurements —
Surface Membrane**

Recent studies in humans demonstrate a shorter electromechanical delay of contraction with a faster rate of relaxation.[79,80] In regard to rate of relaxation, there was some overlap of data between normal and susceptible, thus precluding its direct use in testing for susceptibility. EMG studies in swine vary, including longer motor unit potential with greater amplitude,[81] increased contraction and half-relaxation times,[82] and prolonged time from stimulus to onset of contraction.[83] However, this latter finding could not be confirmed in other studies.[84] Multiple pulse stimulation of porcine muscle (six pulses with 5-millisecond spacing) demonstrated an increase in tension and an increased rate of rise of tension in susceptible pigs; this difference was accentuated after dantrolene was given, as the susceptible pig muscle recovered much more effectively from the effects of dantrolene than did that of the normal animals.[84] This again suggests abnormally increased calcium transients via intracellular organelles. Susceptible pigs also demonstrate a slower relaxation time after tetanus during exposure to halothane.[85] This was not seen in normal animals. This change in tetanic relaxation may be due to a fatiguelike effect similar to that noted with intracellular acidosis.[85] During slaughter, affected swine are found to have a lower (and rapidly declining) resting membrane potential than that of normal swine.[86,87] This may contribute to the rapid decline of muscle pH and energy stores as this is prevented or attenuated by curarization and ventilation to maintain oxygenation.[86] This implies that muscle membrane depolarization rather than sympathetic stress per se induces the hypermetabolism during slaughter.

A previous report had indicated that halothane depolarized the surface membrane of susceptible swine muscle, a result that reinforced the concept that depolarization was perhaps universally important in triggering MH.[88] However, the findings of depolarization by halothane could not be confirmed upon subsequent reexamination in the same laboratory.[89] The second study differed somewhat — barium depolarization was greater in susceptible muscle, but there was no difference in regard to potassium or halothane. There was a species difference in the two studies, Poland China in the original report, and Pietrain in the follow-up study. Both studies involved limb muscle, but, to the senior author of the present paper, Pietrains appear to develop greater contractures in back and trunk muscles than in hind limbs, and the reverse may hold for the Poland China. Notwithstanding, this slow onset depolarization with halothane[88] could not be confirmed in a second species of susceptible pig.[89] Halothane does lower mechanical threshold in both susceptible and normal muscle, predisposing susceptible muscle toward the development of a contracture.[90] Data suggesting that muscle acetylcholinesterase activity is increased in susceptible animals may reflect a compensatory adaptation to the increased response of skeletal muscles secondary to abnormal intrafibrillar calcium transients.[91]

Intracellular Organelles

Sarcoplasmic Reticulum

Sarcoplasmic reticulum releases and reaccumulates calcium so rapidly that it is difficult to measure these processes accurately. In addition, SR binds calcium at physiologic concentrations more effectively than do mitochondria, suggesting that the latter have a reserve function in this regard. Calcium binding is estimated by the rate and capacity of calcium accumulation by isolated SR in the absence of oxalate; the binding rate is less than that of intact SR; this deficiency is corrected in part by oxalate, which greatly increases the duration and capacity for binding. This is now known as calcium uptake rather than binding; however, the function of these isolated vesicles may not correspond to the mechanism or character of calcium binding or uptake in situ.

Some of the difficulty lies with the inability to load SR vesicles with sufficient labeled calcium.[24]

The key to explaining MH is the link between the transverse tubule of skeletal muscle and the SR (Fig. 28-1A). Muscle physiologists have not yet explained this critical area of excitation-contraction coupling; it appears to be of likely concern in identifying the abnormality of MH. But there have been exciting new developments regarding the structure of this link and the involved receptors.[92] Recent studies identify the ryanodine receptor of skeletal muscle as a factor in the transfer of depolarization from the transverse tubule to SR to produce an intracellular release of calcium.[92] Further, in susceptible swine, the ryanodine receptor has an altered calcium dependence with a markedly lower threshold for ryanodine inhibition of contractile activity.[93] This may bear directly upon the mechanism of MH at a cellular level. Examination of the effects of volatile anesthetics upon skeletal muscle indicates that halothane does not act on the action potential of susceptible muscle via specific effects on sodium channels.[94] The volatile anesthetics alter calcium release from SR at concentrations below their clinical effectiveness; at least in the rabbit, this alteration occurs at concentrations below those that alter calcium uptake.[95] Of the numerous studies of SR function, the findings are variable, dependent in part on variable experimental conditions; in general they demonstrate diminished function in MH muscle.[24,33] However, this decreased function is insufficient in itself to account for MH. One theory is that a mitochondrial phospholipase A2, perhaps in conjunction with changes in calmodulin activity, may indirectly alter SR function via release of fatty acids that then cause SR calcium release.[96] More recent data suggest that a triglyceride lipase may be more important in heat and energy metabolism than phospholipase A2 in the abnormalities of SR.[97]

Several studies demonstrate abnormal calcium-induced release of calcium (CIRC) in susceptible muscle.[98-100] The usual normal transfer of depolarization from the transverse tubule to the SR is believed to occur by a depolarization-induced release of calcium (DIRC).[33] CIRC may represent an abnormal pathway that is activated once MH is triggered (Fig. 28-1B). As mentioned above, ryanodine receptors may participate in this.[92,93] Although room temperature studies had suggested that dantrolene would not block CIRC, this apparent lack of correlation with the physiology of MH is explained by the fact that dantrolene blocks this response at 37° C but not at 22° C.[98-100]

The specific action of dantrolene in halting the hypermetabolism of MH indirectly aids in evaluating SR action in MH. Dantrolene inhibits calcium release from SR without affecting reuptake (Fig. 28-1C). Therefore, abnormal SR function involves calcium release via those factors acting somewhere beyond the end plate and up to and including the SR calcium-release mechanism. The specific defect is likely to remain unidentified until muscle physiologists determine the precise mechanism of excitation-contraction coupling between the transverse tubule and the SR.[24,33]

Mitochondria

The mitochondrion provides the greatest supply of ATP via aerobic metabolism; secondarily, it binds and stores calcium. As with SR, isolated mitochondria have diminished function in MH muscle as compared with normal muscle, but this again is insufficient to account for MH by itself.[24,101] Respiratory and calcium-binding activities are reduced, but there is little evidence for intracellular calcium release by MH triggers. However, there is evidence of muscle mitochondrial binding and accumulation of calcium during acute MH.[62] In these studies, pigs were studied by biopsy before and during MH and after treatment with dantrolene, and mitochondrial functions were analyzed elegantly.[62,101] Halothane enhances calcium release from isolated mitochondria under anerobic conditions, but this is not likely related to the initiation of MH.[24] Increased phospholipase or triglyceride lipase activity may alter SR function because of their effect in releasing long chain fatty acids that uncouple mitochondrial respiration and cause SR calcium release.[96,97] This theory has not been confirmed. Mitochondrial uncoupling had originally been proposed as a cause of MH, but this has been theoretically and empirically discounted.[24,101]

Mitochondrial deficiencies do not explain the diminished aerobic responses in MH. $\dot{V}O_2$ consistently increases about 3-fold during MH, in contrast to the 10-fold increase possible during severe exercise.[24,33] In view of the serious acid-base imbalances and depletion of muscle energy stores, this increase seems paradoxically low. Perhaps $\dot{V}O_2$ and hence ATP production by mitochondria are limited during MH by several factors, including mitochondrial calcium binding (as a reserve function to supplement that by SR), intracellular acid-base, and electrolyte aberrations.[24,62,101]

Implications of Findings in Skeletal Muscle

Volatile anesthetics and SCh apparently represent a stress for skeletal muscle, as they perturb the membranes and disturb calcium homeostasis. In general, normal muscle can withstand and compensate for these stresses. But in susceptible muscle the membrane perturbation induced by halothane or the depolarization induced by succinylcholine may cause an earlier calcium release that itself strikingly stimulates greater calcium release.[24,33,98-100] (For discussion of CIRC, see the section, *Sarcoplasmic Reticulum*, above.) Coupled with the lower mechanical contractile threshold, an early MH response may result. Although MH-susceptible muscle may briefly tolerate these stresses, a cascading cycle of increasing metabolism, temperature, and acidosis eventually results. These findings suggest abnormal excitation-contraction coupling in affected skeletal muscle, a conclusion supported by various studies.[83-85] Normal muscle can respond abnormally with extreme prolonged effort, such as the overstraining disease or capture myopathy of wild animals after prolonged chase.[102]

Heart

Myocardial function is severely altered during human and porcine MH. Initially tachycardia and arrhythmias occur and are followed by hypotension, decreased cardiac output, and eventual cardiac arrest. The controversy is whether the heart is primarily abnormal, as a consequence of dysfunction directly related to MH, as in skeletal muscle, or whether the heart is affected secondarily by the hyperthermia, acidosis, hyperkalemia, and increased membrane permeability.[24,33] Porcine data suggest a secondary involvement. Increased myocardial oxygen consumption during MH is related to the β-agonist stimulation of sympathetic activation without lactate production or potassium efflux that would be suggestive of a primary MH response.[103] Porcine myocardium does not respond abnormally to even high doses of various sympathetic and inotropic stimulants. These include various β- and α-adrenergic agonists, adenosine, carbachol,[104] and carbon dioxide, calcium, digoxin, and potassium.[78] Cardiac symptomatology in MH cannot be explained by altered function of α- and β-receptors, adenosine receptors, or cholinoceptors.[104]

Human myocardial abnormalities were inferred by a higher incidence of sudden death in members of susceptible families[105] and by the occurrence of nonspecific cardiomyopathies and abnormal thallium scans in affected patients.[106] However, right ventricular biopsies have demonstrated only artifactual changes.[107] Although this could reflect the difficulty in identifying a functional abnormality by means of structural analysis, the evidence for myocardial involvement remains indirect and is not strong, despite the claims of enthusiastic proponents.[108] The greater mortality statistically associated with use of some cardiac drugs may not reflect a causal relationship—these drugs may have been used in patients with more fulminant episodes.[33,108] Myocardial stress can result in gradual changes in the protein structure of the myofibrils.[109] One might expect that pigs, with their recognized higher frequency of awake MH episodes, would provide evidence for some myocardial abnormalities, whether acquired or inherited. Again, the evidence suggests myocardial dysfunction only during acute MH.[110] Genetic selection for skeletal muscle need not result in abnormalities in other structures, such as the myocardium.[78,103,104]

Central Nervous System

Central nervous system involvement during fulminant human MH appears to be secondary to increased temperature, acidosis, hyperkalemia, and hypoxia. The extreme picture of coma, areflexia, unresponsiveness, and fixed, dilated pupils suggests acute cerebral edema and intracranial hypertension. Recovery is variable and is related to the duration and severity of the MH episode. Severe fever itself, to 42.5°C, may result in a virtually flat EEG and coma, but recovery is still possible.[111]

Earlier findings had suggested that the central nervous system might be instrumental in initiating and maintaining MH. Kerr et al.[112] suggested that neural activity was important in porcine MH because muscle rigidity induced by halothane could be prevented in limbs paralyzed by an epidural anesthetic but could not be prevented in the unanesthetized limbs of the same animal. This phenomenon was also described during an apparent episode of MH in a patient receiving epidural anesthesia.[113] However, these studies did not include metabolic measurements, and other porcine data contradict these early studies; for example, spinal anesthesia was found not to prevent the metabolic changes induced by halothane in the paralyzed limbs, even when rigidity did not occur.[17] Further support for this concept, namely, that an MH episode need not be related to neural integrity, is provided by clinical episodes in which the application of a limb tourniquet prevented rigidity in the isolated limb at a time when whole-body rigidity existed during acute episodes.[114,115] Early brain involvement during MH is unlikely, for cerebral oxygen consumption and lactate production are not increased in swine during MH.[116]

Sympathetic Nervous System

Whether activation of the sympathetic nervous system by MH is a primary or secondary response is controversial. First, "fight, fright, or flight" can initiate an MH episode in susceptible swine without anesthetic agents.[11] Second, signs of sympathetic overactivity occur in human and in porcine MH.[15-17,24,37,38] Finally, circulating levels of epinephrine and norepinephrine increase markedly during MH (e.g., from less than 1 ng/ml up to 30 ng/ml).[15-17,24,33,117]

Many authors believe that although the sympathetic responses are probably secondary, they do produce many of the changes observed during MH episodes. For example, the increases in circulating catecholamines follow rather than precede the changes in muscle metabolism and acid-base balance.[37] Yet this catecholamine response is not essential for the development of halothane-induced MH in swine; total spinal blockade and the accompanying sympathetic denervation failed to affect the onset, development, or characteristics of halothane-induced MH, while the increases in circulating epinephrine and norepinephrine were completely blocked.[17] Sympathetic hyperactivity likely produces the hyperglycemia and a major portion of the early hyperkalemia, via hepatic efflux.[118] The later hyperkalemia appears to be due more to potassium efflux from muscle, when hepatic blood flow is reduced. β-Agonist effects also result in pronounced myocardial stimulation.[103]

With the dramatic course of acute episodes of MH, particularly in stressed, awake swine, the sympathetic nervous system must be part of this response. However, data to support this conclusion are either weak or indirect. Studies in humans involving measurements of metabolism and responses during exercise demonstrate, at most, subtle abnormal responses.[119,120] Some of these have been interpreted as sympathetic dysfunction.[120] Porcine data fail to show differences in regard to central nervous amines[121] or circulating dopamine β-hydroxylase and platelet monoamine oxidase (MAO).[122] Controlled studies in swine demonstrate apparent triggering of MH by the α-agonist, phenylephrine.[123] However, earlier studies had shown that when MH is provoked by succinylcholine, lactate production increased before the hyperthermia. Thus the increased temperature followed the increase in metabolism. In the study involving phenylephrine, the increase in muscle temperature preceded the increase in lactate. This suggests that the triggering factor was more likely a secondary phenomenon related to vasoconstriction in muscle or skin, resulting in ischemia or decreased heat loss. Hypoxia or hyperthermia are recognized triggers of such hypermetabolism in susceptible muscle.[24] Furthermore, α- and β-agonists do not result in increased metabolism in susceptible porcine muscle when metabolism is measured directly.[18]

Williams believes that sympathetic stimulation causes MH via vasoconstriction by norepinephrine.[15,117] He claims that susceptible pigs produce more heat as a result of constantly greater metabolism. This is counterbalanced by greater heat loss, unless a vasoconstrictive event tips the balance in favor of heat retention. This results in increased temperature and provokes the cascade of events leading to fulminant MH. However, several findings contradict Williams's theory. First, basal oxygen consumption in sedated susceptible pigs is not greater than normal.[37,38] Second, infusion of norepinephrine to blood levels of 140 ng/ml did not result in initiation of MH.[124] Even with the concomitant use of sodium nitroprusside to maintain muscle perfusion during these extreme vasoconstrictive stimuli, there was no evidence of increased aerobic or anaerobic metabolism in the susceptible pigs. In contrast, when halothane and succinylcholine were introduced immediately thereafter, there were obvious signs of increased metabolism compatible with MH.[124] Third, clinical MH is unchanged when the acute catecholamine response is blocked by the sympathetic denervation of total spinal anesthesia.[17]

Sympathetic antagonists may protect from or ameliorate episodes of MH by lowering body temperature and modifying acid-base changes.[125] This protection has been found to be variable and, when demonstrated, has been attributed to an effect on sympathetic-induced MH. It seems more likely that the α-antagonists merely increase heat loss and potentially increase muscle perfusion. β-Antagonists attenuate metabolism and fever during MH, yet do not improve survival.[125] In large doses, they completely block the myocardial stimulation that occurs during porcine MH, but this stimulation of metabolism is secondary to β-agonist effects without evidence of active myocardial MH.[103] Thus, although Wingard's theory[105] resulted in a variety of investigations and counterinvestigations over the ensuing 15 years, there is still no direct evidence that the sympathetic nervous system initiates or plays an important primary role in malignant hyperthermia. As will be discussed later, other factors—certain anesthetic agents that perturb membranes, and certain depolarizing factors, such as succinylcholine during anesthesia or acetylcholine with increased muscle tension or activity[33]—appear more important.

Blood

Abnormalities in human or porcine blood cells have been suggested by variations in ionic permeability, fragility, cholesterol content, leukocyte antigens, or temperature-dependent sensitivity of the erythrocyte membrane.[24,33,126–131] Changes are relatively consistent in swine[126] but not in humans.[129–131] A deficiency of plasma pseudocholinesterase, including the fluoride-resistant gene, has occasionally and inconsistently been associated with MH.[132] Disseminated intravascular coagulation frequently occurs during MH, with varying severity. Although a number of causes have been proposed, the most likely appears to be release of tissue thromboplastin during fever, acidosis, hypoxia, hypoperfusion, and gross alterations in membrane permeability of various body tissues.[33]

Miscellaneous

Although the porcine liver may show structural mitochondrial differences between susceptible and normal animals, functional studies (e.g., studies of metabolism) uniformly fail to demonstrate a direct involvement of hepatic metabolism in MH.[33] Pulmonary changes during MH appear to be secondary to the systemic manifestations. These include tachypnea, hyperventilation, $\dot{V}/\dot{Q}$ abnormalities, increased blood and expired PCO_2, decreased blood PO_2, and ultimately pulmonary edema. The increase in whole-body CO_2 stores during MH is better reflected by measurements of mixed venous blood than of arterial.[37,38] Renal function during active MH is altered indirectly (i.e., oliguria and anuria secondary to shock, ischemia, cardiac failure, myoglobinuria, and myoglobinemia). Pigs may have a decreased insulin response to glucose loads, but insulin responses are not consistently abnormal in affected humans. The hyperglycemia that occurs during active MH is probably partly due to sympathetic overactivity. Smooth muscle does not respond abnormally in susceptible pigs.[133]

TRIGGERING OF MALIGNANT HYPERTHERMIA

An acute MH episode may be the combined result of a series of minor defects in several areas leading to minor increases in metabolism, heat production, and acid loads. It likely involves abnormal calcium gradients, perhaps in several areas of the muscle cell. These may then lead to a cyclical cascade of increased energy demands, increased energy production, and hyperthermia. The control of enzyme systems and energy production is lost with increasing cellular temperature and acidosis.[24] In addition, the threshold for thermal inactivation of cellular function is less in susceptible than in normal muscle.[18] Many of the tissue and organ changes that occur during fulminant MH may be in part secondary and due to insufficient blood flow for metabolic demands, leading to the breakdown of cell membranes with resultant edema and further loss of perfusion.[33]

Acute episodes depend on three variables. These are a genetic (perhaps rarely acquired) predisposition, the absence of inhibiting factors, and the presence of a sufficiently potent anesthetic or nonanesthetic trigger.[33]

Depolarization may be a significant factor in MH reactions whether these are anesthetic-induced or "awake." (1) The mechanical threshold of susceptible muscle is lower than that of normal muscle and therefore predisposes to easier development of a muscle contracture. Further halothane decreases the mechanical threshold of muscle.[90] (2) SCh and carbachol (an equivalent of acetylcholine with prolonged duration) depolarize both normal and susceptible muscle and both trigger susceptible but not normal muscle.[18,24] (3) Electrical stimulation triggers susceptible but not normal muscle.[134] (4) Nondepolarizing muscle relaxants delay MH episodes.[24,135] Evidence against this theory of depolarization is the action of 4-aminopyridine, which increases acetylcholine release at the end plate but does not trigger hypermetabolism in susceptible swine.[136] Thus, extreme muscle activity or tension, either in the awake susceptible subject or in the susceptible individual with increased muscle tension induced during anesthesia, results in exaggerated metabolism in susceptible subjects.[33]

Anesthetic Triggering

Anesthetic drugs that can trigger MH include halothane, enflurane, isoflurane, sevoflurane, methoxyflurane, cyclopropane, and ether, as well as SCh and decamethonium. The onset may be explosive when SCh is used.[24] Inbred susceptible swine are identified predictably during an inhalation induction with a potent volatile anesthetic; they develop pronounced hindlimb rigidity within 5 minutes.[50] Prior exercise even an hour before induction of anesthesia increases the severity and hastens the onset of these attacks in swine.[24,33] The use of depressant drugs such as barbiturates or tranquilizers and the use of nondepolarizing muscle relaxants delay the onset of MH, sometimes for hours.[20, 135]

Susceptible humans respond less predictably than swine to these triggers. Many affected humans have previously tolerated potent triggers without visible difficulty.[19] This unpredictability might be related to the duration of anesthesia, premedication, and/or induction agents that delay or mask early manifestations of MH. Some patients have developed MH episodes during anesthesia that did not involve recognized triggering agents; this has even occurred despite partial protection with dantrolene.[21,22] (However, one of these cases resembled acute interstitial pulmonary edema more than MH.[22]) The intravenous use of prophylactic dantrolene in appropriate doses may eliminate this phenomenon.[137] Obviously, the mechanism of anesthetic triggering in humans is unsolved.

Anesthetic triggering may depend on depolarization or perturbation of the surface membrane, as has been shown for SCh and halothane (in susceptible swine muscle). Succinylcholine probably triggers MH via effects on the end plate, whereas halothane acts on surface membranes or internal membrane systems of the fibril. It is not known how volatile anesthetics act on SR or mitochondria in the intact organism; however, data on isolated preparations imply that these effects are insufficient to trigger MH. If changes in membrane excitability or mechanical threshold are major skeletal muscle factors related to the initiation of MH, then purely environmental or pharmacologic factors could induce susceptibility to MH in the absence of a genetic predisposition (see the section, *Implications of Findings in Skeletal Muscle*). MH episodes in patients with lymphoma suggest such a possibility, but there is no information contradicting a genetic role in these patients.[138]

Succinylcholine has several variant responses that can occur singly or in combination (Table 28-1): (1) a muscle contracture, also noted in muscle that is myotonic or denervated; (2) a change in muscle membrane permeability without contracture, resulting in the release of CK and myoglobin from muscle (even in normal patients, SCh releases CK and myoglobin from muscle in small amounts; this is exaggerated in the presence of halothane and attenuated by curare; myoglobin release can be fairly marked even in the absence of obviously discolored urine[139]); and (3) an increase in metabolism, as in MH, usually associated with both muscle contracture and increased membrane permeability.[24] Although succinylcholine is a valuable and preferred relaxant in certain situations, its use presents a small but significant risk, partly as detailed above, and partly in the patient with occult muscle disease who may develop an abrupt cardiac arrest after its use, in association with hyperkalemia and rhabdomyolysis. Cases such as these occur rarely, but regularly, and occasionally present serious problems in resuscitation.[140]

Nitrous oxide has been proposed as a weak trigger of human MH because it twice produced fever in an 11-year-old girl undergoing dental care.[24] However, nitrous oxide is a most unlikely trigger because it has been used repeatedly as the basic anesthetic in MH-susceptible humans and swine without triggering MH. Hy-

TABLE 28-1. Actions of Succinylcholine

Normal	Pathologic	
1. Profound relaxation[a]	1. Contracture	Myotonia Denervation MH
2. 0.5–1.0 mEq/L increase in K$^+$	2. Hyperkalemia	Denervation MH Disuse atrophy (modest increase)
3. Slight increase in $\dot{V}O_2$ secondary to fasciculations and ion pumping	3. Metabolic mayhem Increased $\dot{V}O_2$	MH Denervation contracture
4. Slight increase in CK and myoglobin[b]	4. Rhabdomyolysis	Duchenne's myopathy Other myopathies MH
5. Bradycardia, especially second dose	5. Cardiac arrest	Duchenne's myopathy Occult myopathies MH Secondary to hyperkalemia

[a] Tonic eye and jaw muscles may develop a contracture.
[b] Attenuated by pretreatment, exaggerated by potent volatile agents.
Abbreviations: K$^+$, serum potassium; MH, malignant hyperthermia; CK, creatine phosphokinase; $\dot{V}O_2$, oxygen consumption.

perbaric nitrous oxide does not produce MH in susceptible swine even in concentrations causing apnea.[141]

Nondepolarizing muscle relaxants block the effects of succinylcholine in triggering MH. They also delay or attenuate the effects of the volatile anesthetics.[20,135] Although pancuronium has been reported to trigger porcine or human MH, this is an unlikely possibility. *d*-Tubocurarine has been incriminated as an MH trigger because it produced fever in two susceptible children.[24] *d*-Tubocurarine has been associated with greater lactate production in susceptible pigs exposed to environmental stress[24] (but it has not been shown to be a trigger of MH in susceptible swine); it does produce a contracture in denervated muscle, suggesting that it may have a mild depolarizing action that is not apparent under usual conditions.[142]

The effects of nondepolarizing muscle relaxants are reversed by cholinergic agonists. Because carbachol, and presumably acetylcholine, can provoke porcine MH,[18] reversal by cholinergic agents of the effects of nondepolarizing relaxants could conceivably trigger MH. However, 4-aminopyridine, which increases acetylcholine release, does not trigger MH in swine[136] and antagonism of a nondepolarizing neuromuscular blockade has been performed without untoward events in affected humans.[143]

Episodes of MH have been reported during various operative procedures, during general or regional anesthesia, and in extremes of ages. Anxiety reactions may precipitate an apparent MH response.[144] Prior fever or SCh-induced trismus should not be ignored even if the patient survived without obvious mishap.[145] The youngest known case involved an episode of muscle rigidity occurring in utero just prior to birth.[146] Presumably the fetus inherited susceptibility from his father that was triggered by anesthetic agents given to his mother.

Delayed onset of MH, up to 25 hours,[147] may be due either to depressed MH responses (by various drugs) in a susceptible person or to prolonged anesthetic stresses in a normal person. Ponies can develop a bizarre form of MH during halothane and SCh anesthesia—despite progression to high fever, acidosis, rigidity, and cardiovascular collapse during 3 hours of anesthesia, all six survived with symptomatic treatment.[148] There may be species differences, as humans, pigs, dogs, cats, and horses have a more virulent form of MH.[24,33]

It was previously believed that amide local anesthetics, such as lidocaine, could trigger MH.[24,33] Further support for this supposition was provided by a report of an MH episode occurring during epidural anesthesia with lidocaine; the report suggested that the amide anesthetics in large doses might trigger MH.[113] However, the evidence for this is weak. Animal data demonstrating calcium release from the SR by amide anesthetics involve mM concentrations, which are difficult to achieve clinically.[24,33] Second, the most susceptible species, inbred swine, is not triggered into MH even when enormous doses of lidocaine are administered intravenously.[149] Third, it is ironic that Britt first commented about the possible efficacy of intravenous local anesthetics in treating MH,[8] when one of the two cases she was referring to involved treatment with intravenous lidocaine.[150] Despite a recurrence, the patient improved. Finally, amide anesthetics are now routinely used for nerve block anesthesia in susceptible patients undergoing muscle biopsy, without untoward events.[151]

Awake Triggering

Swine can be triggered into MH episodes with environmental stress (see the section, *History*). Specific factors include exercise, heat stress, anoxia, apprehension, and excitement.[24] That these responses may be related to muscle movement or to increased temperature is suggested by the following findings: (1) susceptible swine in vitro or in vivo react with abnormally increased oxygen consumption and lactate production to carbachol or heat (41° to 42°C) but not to α- and/or β-sympathetic agonists,[18,152] and (2) the abnormal responses are blocked or delayed by nondepolarizing relaxants.[20,24,86,135]

In the absence of anesthetic drugs, the mechanism of triggering in swine is hypothesized as follows. Progression of MH results from a hypermetabolic response to a neurotransmitter in association with normal or unchanged responses to sympathetic stimulation. Muscle activity occurs during exercise, excitement, and sympathetic stimulation. This contractile activity, resulting from end-plate effects of acetylcholine apparently produces elevated uncontrolled levels of intracellular ionized calcium, the ultimate reasons for which are unknown, but that are related to exaggerated responses of susceptible muscle as compared with those seen in normal muscle. The elevation in intracellular calcium results in greater than normal muscle oxygen consumption and lactate production. The β-sympathetic stimulation accompanying excitement may further increase lactate production. These combined metabolic effects result in respiratory and metabolic acidosis, hyperthermia, and secondary adrenergic stress responses. Accompanying α-sympathetic stimulation produces vasoconstriction with decreased heat loss and perhaps limited muscle perfusion. Increased temperature or relative ischemia can exacerbate the metabolic changes and the combined acidosis, so that these cascade into a vicious circle of fulminant metabolism, acidosis and hyperthermia, further loss of control of calcium, and eventual cardiovascular collapse.[24,33]

Several findings suggest that human MH unrelated to anesthesia may occur: (1) Susceptible families may have an increased incidence of unexplained sudden deaths.[105] (2) These families may develop a nonspecific cardiomyopathy.[106,107] (3) There are now a series of case reports relating heat stroke, sudden and unexpected death, unusual stress and fatigue, and myalgias to possible awake MH episodes.[153-158] Although it is difficult to be certain how many of these represent human MH episodes in the absence of the anesthetic environment, some of these probably reflect that. However, the incidence of possible awake episodes in humans is undoubtedly still rare and, in the absence of any family or personal history of such, the susceptible individual should be advised to live his or her usual everyday life. Precautions need be taken in general only in the anesthetic environment. We must further remember that supposed mechanisms explaining porcine MH in the awake state may not be applicable to human awake MH.

GENETICS

Inheritance of MH is probably via two or three genes or alleles as opposed to solely dominant or recessive factors. The offspring are thus the average of the parents in

this regard, and the pattern of inheritance may vary from dominant to recessive. Data from worldwide testing centers suggest that most human inheritance is autosomal dominant, and that penetrance (i.e., clinical presentation) is variable. Inheritance in pigs is uniformly reported as recessive, but these opinions are based on determinations of susceptibility by halothane challenge. This technique detects only the most susceptible pigs and may miss those with lesser susceptibility.[50,159] These apparently normal pigs, when challenged with a combination of halothane and succinylcholine, can have dramatic MH responses. In a single population study of Ontario boars, the incidences of affected pigs were 1.5 percent, based on a 5-minute halothane challenge (786 pigs), and 18 percent, based on a halothane-succinylcholine challenge (123 pigs).[160] One attempt at testing for susceptibility in pigs with both SCh and halothane suffered from the inadequacies of small doses of SCh, ventilation only by mask in pigs after receiving SCh, and absence of blood gas measurement.[161] In my experience, although halothane detected susceptible pigs, both SCh-halothane and blood gas analysis were necessary to establish that a pig was not susceptible. Some pigs with negative results to the halothane-alone challenge had positive results with the combination of halothane and SCh.[50]

DIAGNOSIS

Diagnosis of acute episodes is more difficult than treatment. MH is a disorder of increased metabolism, the early signs of which may be subtle or masked. Its onset may be delayed until the patient is emerging from the anesthetic. MH must be distinguished from other disorders with similar signs, such as hyperthyroidism, pheochromocytoma, and neuroleptic malignant syndrome (NMS). Some rare families manifest repeated hyperthermia during or after anesthesia, despite pretreatment with dantrolene and other various precautions.[162] These episodes do not feature clinical or laboratory evidence of MH. Thus, part of the differential diagnosis includes familial fever.[162] When the diagnosis is obvious, that is, fulminant MH or SCh-induced rigidity with rapid metabolic changes, there is marked hypermetabolism and heat production and there may be little time left for specific therapy to prevent death or irreversible sequelae. One could make the diagnosis directly with measurements of increased expired carbon dioxide during constant ventilation.[38] However, other causes must first be ruled out, such as increased temperature, a stuck valve with increased inspired carbon dioxide, and hyperthyroidism. In general, MH would not be expected to occur in any patient given barbiturate-nitrous oxide-opiate-tranquilizer-nondepolarizing relaxant anesthesia, although there are rare exceptions.[21,22] When volatile anesthetics or succinylcholine are used, MH should be suspected when there is undue tachycardia, tachypnea, arrhythmias, mottling of the skin, cyanosis, increased temperature, muscle rigidity, sweating, or unstable blood pressure. If any of the preceding abnormalities occurs, signs of increased metabolism, acidosis, or hyperkalemia must be sought. Analysis of arterial blood gases will demonstrate metabolic acidosis and may show respiratory acidosis if the patient is unable to increase ventilation as metabolism increases. Central venous oxygen and carbon dioxide levels change more markedly than do those in arterial blood; therefore, end-expired carbon dioxide or central venous carbon dioxide levels are a more accurate reflection of whole-body carbon dioxide stores.[38] Venous carbon dioxide, unless the blood drains an area of increased metabolic activity, should have PCO_2 levels only about 5 mmHg greater than that of expected or measured $PaCO_2$. Suggested limits for venous blood include 55 mmHg for PCO_2 and 35 mmHg for PO_2, assuming that PaO_2 is greater than 100 mmHg. If $PaCO_2$ is greater than 60 mmHg and base deficit is −5 to −7 mEq/L or more, the diagnosis is established (again assuming that other factors have been ruled out). In small children, particularly those who have had no oral food or fluid for a prolonged period, base excess may be −5 mEq/L because of their smaller energy stores.

ASSOCIATION WITH OTHER DISORDERS

Brownell has written a comprehensive review of MH and its relationship to other diseases.[163] The King-Denborough syndrome, characterized by short stature, musculoskeletal abnormalities, and mental retardation, is definitely associated with susceptibility to MH.[164] Duchenne's muscle dystrophy and central core disease[24] can also be associated with episodes of malignant hyperthermia. Further, Duchenne patients can respond to anesthesia with sudden acute difficult-to-resuscitate cardiac arrest or sudden acute rhabdomyolysis,[165,166] even without the use of SCh.[167] Patients with occult myopathies of any type, and not necessarily related to malignant hyperthermia or to the use of SCh, may develop these potentially and rapidly disastrous anesthetic events.[140]

Other disorders have an inconstant association with MH, wherein susceptibility sometimes may be involved but not always. These include crib death or the sudden infant death syndrome (SIDS), neuroleptic malignant syndrome, and heat stroke.[33] Succinylcholine induces contractures in myotonic muscle, which could be confused with MH. Myotonic goats develop brief rigidity after SCh but, even with the concomitant use of halothane, show no evidence for MH.[168] A recent report suggests an association between myotonia and MH; it demonstrates that positive contracture responses may be observed in patients who have developed rigidity after SCh and/or who have myotonia.[169] Our bias is that an association with clinical episodes of MH has not been demonstrated; in myotonia, there appears to be rigidity in the absence of serious metabolic abnormalities. The association with SIDS is not supported by results from other MH diagnostic centers.[170]

The neuroleptic malignant syndrome is due to central effects of chronic administration of psychoactive drugs (e.g., butyrophenones, phenothiazines, MAO inhibitors, lithium, or a combination of these drugs). These result in a "slow onset MH" with varied symptoms. There are three key elements of pathophysiology: (1) the patient usually develops an impairment of motor function with generalized rigidity, akinesis, and/or extrapyramidal disturbances; (2) deterioration in mental status occurs, with coma, stupor, and/or delirium; (3) hyperpyrexia develops, with deterioration and lability of other "vegetative" functions, resulting in diaphoresis, blood pressure and heart rate fluctuations, and tachypnea. The picture may be quite similar to that of acute MH, but the onset generally requires several days to several weeks. Treatment involves discontinuation of the drugs and symptomatic control of temperature, acid-base balance, intravenous fluid balance, and muscle tone. Recovery is slow because the drug effects dissipate very slowly.

The specific etiology of NMS has been postulated as a spontaneous or iatrogenic derangement of the central nervous system dopaminergic system. Neuroleptic agents often result in antagonism or depression of the actions of dopamine centrally. In addition, withdrawal of L-dopa may precipitate the syndrome. The reaction may not be specifically drug related, however, as a similar neuropsychiatric syndrome called lethal catatonia has also been described. Obviously, this syndrome could occur more easily in MH-susceptible patients,[171] but patients need not be susceptible to develop NMS.[172–174] Evidence obtained during general anesthesia suggests that NMS may not be associated with susceptibility to MH, for these patients have been observed to respond favorably to electroshock therapy and have tolerated the use of SCh without evidence of clinical malignant hyperthermia.[175,176] This lack of MH may be due in part to the fact that only a single trigger (i.e., SCh) was used during a brief anesthetic. Nonetheless, careful metabolic monitoring disclosed no evidence of MH.[176] If the muscle rigidity is due to centrally acting drugs, the usual nondepolarizing relaxants will help to ease this. However, endotracheal intubation and controlled ventilation may be required. With sufficient fever and electrolyte imbalances, the muscle rigidity could be a contracture, and then only dantrolene would be an effective relaxant. Dantrolene may be the relaxant of choice anyway, because it can reduce muscle tone without paralysis so that spontaneous ventilation may continue. These patients can be very ill. Additional therapy includes bromocriptine as a dopamine receptor agonist to counteract the theorized impairment of dopaminergic neurotransmission in the striatum and the frontal limbic system. A major disadvantage of bromocriptine is that it is an oral preparation that must be given by gastric tube in these very sick patients.

TREATMENT

Discontinuation of the trigger may be adequate treatment for acute MH if the onset is slow or if there was a brief administration of the trigger. However, if MH is fulminant (i.e., $PaCO_2$ greater than 60 mmHg and increasing, mixed venous PCO_2 greater than 90 mmHg and increasing, base excess less than -5 mEq/L and falling, and temperature increasing 1°C/15 min), then adequate therapy is urgently needed for survival. In some patients cardiac output falls rapidly, and there are minor metabolic and acid-base changes because of minimal tissue perfusion. This can result in rapid demise.

Dantrolene is the only known specific therapeutic drug, but must be given while adequate muscle perfusion is present.[177] It is also important to use symptomatic therapy to control body temperature, acid-base balance, and renal function. Adjunctive drugs are seldom necessary if proper treatment is begun soon enough. Dantrolene appears to be a virtual miracle drug for MH, whether porcine[13] or human.[14] It rapidly halts the increases in metabolism (Fig. 28-2) and secondarily results in a return to normal levels of catecholamines and potassium. The homeostatic mechanisms

of the body then rapidly restore arterial blood pressure, heart rate, and sympathetic hyperactivity back toward normal.

For clinical use, dantrolene is packaged in 20-mg bottles with sodium hydroxide with a pH value of 9 to 10 (otherwise it will not dissolve) and mannitol (to make the solution isotonic). Dantrolene must be dissolved in sterile water rather than solutions such as 5 percent dextrose in water or bicarbonate because the extra molecules in solution lead to a salting-out effect with greater difficulty in dissolving dantrolene. If it does not dissolve immediately, producing a clear yellow to yellow-orange color, it should be heated under tap water or autoclaved for a few minutes. In a dire emergency, it should be administered through a blood filter without worrying about crystals. In a fulminant episode in a larger adult, as many as 10 bottles may be required to provide the therapeutic dose of 2 mg/kg. This will require the full-time efforts of three or four people. Preoccupation with facets of therapy other than dantrolene can accomplish control of symptomatic factors but lead to the patient's demise as a result of uncontrolled metabolic mayhem within the cells, leading to cell destruction. Dantrolene administration is the key therapy.

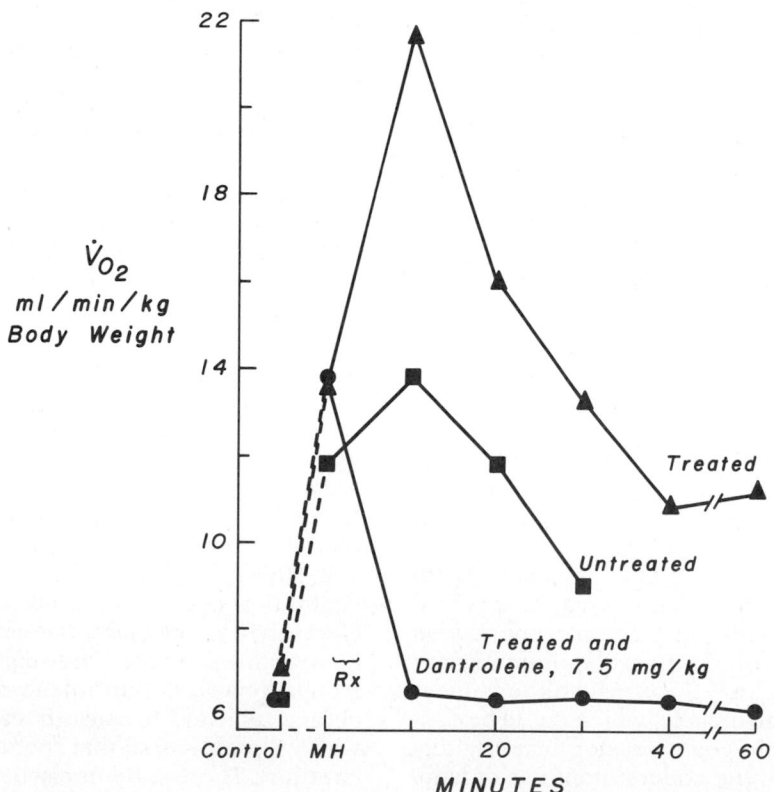

Fig. 28-2. Contrasts among groups of swine (five pigs per group) for three treatment options during acute fulminant MH: none (untreated, ■); treated (symptomatic treatment only, ▲); and treated and dantrolene (symptomatic treatment plus dantrolene, ●). VO$_2$, whole-body oxygen consumption. (From Gronert et al.,[208] with permission.)

Dantrolene acts by inhibiting SR calcium release without affecting reuptake (Fig. 28-1C). Its site of action, then, includes all factors between the neuromuscular junction and the SR (i.e., sarcolemma, transverse tubule, the "bridge" between the tubule and the SR, and the SR itself).[177] Dantrolene in high doses does not paralyze, as the effect plateaus; twitch tension is inhibited more than the response to a tetanic stimulus.[178] Peak effects include moderate muscle weakness with adequate strength for deep breathing and coughing. The therapeutic dose may be repeated every 5 minutes for a total dose of 10 mg/kg. Dantrolene does not have serious side effects unless given for longer than 3 weeks. It may then result in cholestatic hepatic dysfunction. Oral preparations, used for patients with spastic disorders, result eventually in serious hepatic dysfunction similar to that observed with chlorpromazine.

Acute therapy for MH can be summarized as follows:

1. Discontinue all anesthetic agents and hyperventilate the patient with 100 percent oxygen. Normal ventilation is that required to remove metabolic carbon dioxide. Therefore, with increased aerobic metabolism, normal ventilation, by definition, increases anyway. However, carbon dioxide production is also increased because of neutralization of fixed acid by bicarbonate. Therefore, hyperventilation is needed to remove this additional carbon dioxide.
2. Repeat dantrolene, 2 mg/kg, every 5 minutes to a total dose of 10 mg/kg.
3. Administer bicarbonate, approximately 2 to 4 mEq/kg. Continued efflux of lactate from skeletal muscle may result in recurrent acidosis[179] because lactate slowly crosses the muscular cellular membrane to extracellular fluid.
4. Control fever by whatever means are available, including iced fluids, surface cooling, cooling of body cavities with sterile iced fluids, and heat exchanger with a pump oxygenator. One should not become so preoccupied with cooling techniques and other busy work that he or she neglects the prime factor in therapy: IV administration of dantrolene. Cooling should be halted at about 38 to 39°C to prevent inadvertent hypothermia.
5. Monitor urinary output to prevent shock kidneys or acute tubular necrosis,[138] as well as to examine for myoglobinuria.
6. Further therapy is guided by blood gases, temperature, arrhythmia, muscle tone, and urinary output.
7. Some recommend steroids in large doses.[24]
8. Perform blood studies (electrolytes, liver profile, BUN, lactate, glucose), coagulation studies (prothrombin time, fibrinogen, ATPP, fibrinolytic split products, platelet count) and serum hemoglobin and myoglobin and urine hemoglobin and myoglobin studies.

Repetition of the drugs or laboratory studies depends on the clinical course. Dantrolene should probably be repeated every 10 to 15 hours (as this is its half-life) for several doses.[137,180] If there are no signs of recurrence, dantrolene may be discontinued.

Treatment of the hyperkalemia should be done slowly. Plasma K^+ must be serially monitored, as it may be an important factor in treatment (e.g., persistently elevated K^+ may prevent defibrillation).[181] The most effective way to lower serum potassium is reversal of MH by effective doses of dantrolene. The administration of calcium to counteract hyperkalemia is risky. Hypokalemia frequently follows the period of hyperkalemia. The use of calcium to treat hypocalcemia, which frequently occurs during human MH or rhabdomyolysis, is not effective. Calcium administration is indicated only for related arrhythmias or for poor cardiac function.[182] However, when indicated, calcium and cardiac glycosides may be used, as their administration to the susceptible pig does not trigger MH.[78,183,184] They can be life-saving during persistent hyperkalemia.[184] Arrhythmias may be treated with either procainamide or lidocaine.

Permanent neurologic sequelae, coma or paralysis, may occur in advanced cases, probably secondary to inadequate cerebral oxygenation and perfusion for the increased metabolism and, because of the fever, acidosis and potassium release. Even satisfactory care during anesthesia may not prevent neurologic complications. Measurements of intracranial pressure may help in evaluating cerebral edema.

Disseminated intravascular coagulation or consumptive coagulopathy may be caused by hemolysis, increased release of tissue thromboplastins due to increased cellular permeability or overt tissue damage, shock secondary to inadequate capillary perfusion, or some other mechanism in fulminant MH. The best treatment is adequate therapy of MH to prevent stagnation of peripheral blood flow and to lower temperature. Other care is symptomatic and may require heparin.

Among the ineffective therapeutic adjuncts are drugs that are calcium antagonists in cardiac and smooth muscle, drugs such as nimodipine, verapamil, nifedipine, and diltiazem, or sympathetic antagonists such as propranolol. Calcium antagonists do not increase porcine survival.[76,77] Further, they may interact with dantrolene to produce hyperkalemia; this can result in retriggering of MH[78] or in profound myocardial depression.[73-75] The calcium antagonists act primarily on surface membranes of cardiac or smooth muscle, whereas the efficacy of dantrolene is related to inhibition of calcium release from the sarcoplasmic reticulum. β-Sympathetic antagonists do not increase survival in porcine MH,[125] although propranolol prevents the increased myocardial oxygen consumption.[103] This is not a desirable therapeutic goal in treating acute MH, as increased cardiac function is necessary for survival. Ketanserin, a serotonin blocker, is not effective in either prevention or treatment of porcine MH.[185]

Early diagnosis and treatment of MH are obviously essential. The complications that may arise are all difficult to treat and may lead to serious and permanent sequelae.[186] Finally, retriggering may occur even with dantrolene therapy, as the initial dose of the drug is redistributed, metabolized, or excreted.

ANESTHESIA FOR SUSCEPTIBLE PATIENTS

If dantrolene is given in the preoperative period, it should be administered intravenously in a dose of approximately 2 mg/kg just prior to induction of anesthesia.[137] This prevents the uncertainty of predictive blood levels associated with the oral route. Although dantrolene can be given orally and predictably provide therapeutic blood levels, this requires higher doses, preoperative hospitalization, and risk of prolonged weakness or prolongation of the effects of nondepolarizing muscle relaxants.[177,187-189] Data from the maternal-fetal sheep model indicate that there is rapid equilibration between the mother and the fetus but that fetal levels were approximately 10 percent those of the mother.[190] In general, dantrolene is not recommended pre partum or for the small infant because it has an apparent sedative effect. At delivery, if dantrolene is needed for the mother, it is preferable to withhold its administration until after the cord is clamped.

Anesthesia should consist of nitrous oxide, barbiturates, opiates, tranquilizers, and nondepolarizing muscle relaxants. Propofol and etomidate are unlikely triggers, although their use in susceptible subjects has not been reported (Table 28-2). Potent volatile agents such as halothane, enflurane, or isoflurane and the depolarizing muscle relaxants such as SCh and decamethonium must be avoided, even in the presence of dantrolene. Some human patients have developed a hypermetabolic state despite these precautions[21,22]; however, these patients have always responded favorably to intravenous dantrolene. The present consensus is that, in most instances, preoperative dantrolene is not needed in susceptible patients, as the use of nontriggering agents is almost always associated with uneventful anesthesia. Unusual triggering aspects of MH

remain; it is hoped that they will be explained with subsequent research.

Regional anesthesia is safe and may be preferred for certain procedures in susceptible patients. Amide anesthetics had been considered dangerous in susceptible patients because they induce or worsen contractures in vitro as a result of their effect in increasing calcium efflux from the SR.[24,33] However, these effects require millimolar concentrations of these drugs, far greater than the plasma values achieved in clinical usage. But, because of these theoretical considerations, procaine was proposed as a therapeutic drug for MH and lidocaine was condemned as dangerous. Eventually porcine and human studies demonstrated the lack of danger of amide anesthetics,[24,33,150,151] and, at the present time, ester or amide anesthetics may be used safely.[151] Further, intravenous lidocaine was used as long ago as 1970 to treat acute MH without apparent harm and with apparent good results.[33,150]

It no longer appears necessary to provide a noncontaminated anesthetic machine by flushing with oxygen for a number of hours.[191] Removal or sealing of the vaporizers, replacement of the fresh gas outlet hose, and use of a disposable circle with a flush of 6 L/min for 5 minutes suffice.[192] There is an equally satisfactory and economical method—use of a nitrous oxide blender instead of an anesthetic machine.[193]

One should discuss the anesthetic care with the patient with the confidence that all will be done to avoid difficulties with MH and, should any problems occur, the appropriate drugs, knowledge, and skills are immediately at hand. Some physicians are overly cautious in handling MH patients to the point that medical precautions and apprehension are magnified to an exaggerated degree. Many of these patients have undergone certain procedures, such as dental analgesia or obstetric anesthesia, without problems before the diagnosis of susceptibility was made. With a confident approach by the physician, the patient will enter the therapeutic environment in a relaxed and comfortable state of mind. Anxiety and stress are minimal, and the patient is reassured by confidence in the doctor's ability to monitor appropriately and to provide proper treatment for any difficulties.

EVALUATION OF SUSCEPTIBILITY

The subject of evaluating susceptibility has been comprehensively reviewed.[194] The suspect patient has a personal or family history of anesthetic problems, unexpected family deaths, or trismus. Evaluation includes a history and physical examination for detection of subclinical abnormality. A genealogy going back two generations with specific information about anesthetic exposure and agents will estimate the likelihood of adequate exposure to triggering agents. Measurements of blood CK provide a basic screening tool. CK values, when determined in a resting, fasting state without re-

TABLE 28-2. Drugs in MH Susceptible Patients

Unsafe	Safe
Volatile anesthetics[24]	Tranquilizers in general (except chlorpromazine)
Halothane	
Enflurane	Opiates
Isoflurane	Barbiturates
Sevoflurane	Etomidate, propofol[a]
	Ketamine[24]
Relaxants	Nondepolarizing relaxants (except curare, a weak depolarizer)[142]
Succinylcholine[24]	
	Amide anesthetics[151]
	Ester anesthetics
	Epinephrine[18,124]
	Norepinephrine[124]
	Digitalis drugs[78]
	Calcium[78,183]
	Dantrolene[177]

[a] Probably safe; no relevant reports.

cent trauma, reflect muscle membrane stability. The CK is elevated in about 70 percent of affected people and most swine. When CK is elevated in a close relative of a known susceptible person, then this relative may be considered susceptible to MH without further testing. If the CK is normal on several occasions, there is no predictive value, and a muscle biopsy is necessary for contracture studies. Investigations of these specimens, performed at several centers around the world, use exposures to halothane, caffeine, halothane plus caffeine, or potassium. Contracture thresholds are perhaps 95 percent reliable in evaluating susceptibility.[194] Porcine data suggest that cell injury may skew responses toward susceptible.[195] This aspect has not been directly studied in human biopsy specimens. It is known, however, that the pattern of mixed fiber types in human muscle precludes caffeine thresholds directly related to specific fiber types, such as have been seen at times in the pig.[196] Contracture responses are sometimes positive in patients with myopathies that bear no direct relationship to MH; one cannot be certain in these cases that the positive biopsy indicates susceptibility.[197] Patients must not be given dantrolene before the biopsy, as this could mask the response of abnormal muscle to contracture producing drugs.[194]

The predictive value (percentage of positive results that are true positive) or efficiency (percentage of all results that are true, whether positive or negative) of contracture in determining susceptibility cannot be estimated.[198] False-positive results due to cautious interpretation are masked because the patient will never be exposed to triggering agents. No false-negative results have been reported. The tests currently used are sensitive (frequency of positive results in true positives) in that positive results correlate well with MH survivors and with susceptibility in pigs determined by anesthetic challenge in vivo. Specificity (frequency of negative results in true negatives) will become known as patients with normal evaluations are subjected to known MH triggers for routine anesthesia. All these epidemiologic considerations are complicated by the variations in metabolic responses observed in MH-susceptible humans during anesthesia.

For the student of anesthesia, it is only important to remember that susceptible individuals have a lower threshold to the contracture-producing drugs than do normal individuals. However, the muscle specimen must be viable (i.e., twitch when stimulated electrically), as the contracture threshold may vary if the fiber is degenerating or acutely deteriorating.[50,51,195] A major controversy in regard to testing concerns the simultaneous use of caffeine and halothane. Experts agree that the use of each drug alone in the tissue bath is accurate in identifying susceptibility. However, their combined use yields, in a given population, a wide range of thresholds. Some interpret this variation as the broad range inherent in a test that lacks precision.[56] Others interpret this as a spectrum of susceptibility, with those at the lower end being more susceptible and those at the

higher end being less susceptible.[57] The standardization of contracture testing, organized by the Canadian MH Association, MHAUS, and the North American MH Registry, should help to eliminate differences in protocols among the testing laboratories in North America, as well as define more precisely the thresholds in normal people to caffeine alone, to halothane alone, or to the combination of caffeine and halothane. These should then provide greater accuracy in diagnostic biopsies.

What is needed in MH testing is an accurate noninvasive or nondestructive measure of susceptibility. Nuclear magnetic resonance probably has the greatest promise.[199] The difficulty is to standardize a stress, such as forearm ischemia, that will differentiate susceptible tissue from normal. In the absence of stress, susceptible individuals or tissues are not different from normal. As with so many tests, a major problem is to establish conditions whereby there is no overlap between the ranges of normal and susceptible responses. A nondestructive test introduced by Klipp and Britt of Toronto involved the increase in ionized calcium produced by halothane in lymphocytes. Unfortunately, there was overlap between results in pigs[200] and in humans,[201] and the positive test results could not be confirmed by another laboratory.[202] Other newer and as yet unconfirmed tests of susceptibility include halothane-induced disorders of red cell membranes[127,128] and the use of a calcium ionophor that, in susceptible Pietrain pigs, elevated intracellular calcium concentrations in intercostal muscle.[203] In this particular situation there was a clear differentiation of normal versus susceptible muscle. We cannot at present predict the applicability of this test in humans or in muscle other than the intercostal.

Other older tests that could not be confirmed include phosphorylase ratio,[204] platelet ATP depletion,[205] thin strip muscle calcium uptake,[206] and assay of glutathione peroxidase.[44,45] Several years ago the Europeans standardized their protocol for contracture testing among the laboratories in England, Scandinavia, and continental Europe.[194] This protocol resulted in more precise definition of control values and what appeared to be more accurate diagnosis of susceptibility. It is hoped that the major effort now ongoing in the United States and Canada will develop an analogous standardized approach among the various laboratories, with similar better results.

SUMMARY

Malignant hyperthermia is the anesthesiologists' disease. It is a subclinical myopathy that is unmasked upon exposure to the potent agents or succinylcholine; then skeletal muscle acutely and unexpectedly increases its oxygen consumption and lactate production, resulting in greater heat production, respiratory and metabolic acidosis, muscle rigidity, sympathetic stimulation, and increased cellular permeability. The best-accepted theory is that MH is caused by an inability to control calcium concentrations within the muscle fiber and that it may involve a generalized alteration in cellular or subcellular membrane permeability. Diagnosis is made on the basis of extraordinary temperature and acid-base and muscle aberrations. Specific treatment is the action of dantrolene on muscle calcium movements; symptomatic treatment is by reversal of acid-base and temperature changes. Evaluation of affected families is guided by measurements of circulating creatine phosphokinase and by analysis of drug-induced contractures in muscle biopsy specimens. Either general or regional anesthesia is safe for patients susceptible to MH, provided that if a general technique is chosen, care is taken to specially prepare the anesthesia machine and to avoid all anesthetic trigger agents.

Awake stress regularly triggers susceptible swine into typical MH episodes if it excites them. There are a few case reports of this in susceptible humans. Research in MH has yielded new insights into the physiology of metabolism. Challenges for the future include identification of the gene or genes responsible for MH and elucidation of the mechanism that links exposure to the subsequent loss of calcium control.

REFERENCES

1. Ranklev E, Fletcher R: Investigation of malignant hyperthermia in Sweden. Acta Anaesth Scand 30:693, 1986
2. Wilson RD, Nichols RJ, Jr, Dent TE, et al: Disturbances of the oxidative-phosphorylation mechanism as a possible etiological factor in sudden unexplained hyperthermia occurring during anesthesia. Anesthesiology 27:231, 1966
3. Gordon RA: Malignant hyperpyrexia during general anaesthesia. Can Anaesth Soc J 13:415, 1966
4. Ording H: Incidence of malignant hyperthermia in Denmark. Anesth Analg 64:700, 1985
5. Ombrédanne L: De l'influence de l'anesthesique-employé dans la genèse des accidents post-opératoires de paleur-hyperthermie observés chez les nourrissons. Rév Med Fr 10:617, 1929
6. Denborough MA, Lovell RRH: Anaesthetic deaths in a family. Lancet 2:45, 1960
7. Britt BA, Locher WG, Kalow W: Hereditary aspects of malignant hyperthermia. Can Anaesth Soc J 16:89, 1969
8. Kalow W, Britt BA, Terreau ME, et al: Metabolic error of muscle metabolism after recovery from malignant hyperthermia. Lancet 2:89, 1970
9. Herter M, Wilsdorf G: Die Bedeutung des Schweines fur die Fleischversorgung. Berlin, Arbeiten der Deutscher Landwirtschaft-Gesellschaft, Vol. 270, 1914
10. Briskey EJ: Etiological status and associated studies of pale, soft, exudative porcine musculature. Adv Food Res 13:89, 1964
11. Topel DG, Bicknell EJ, Preston KS, et al: Porcine stress syndrome. Mod Vet Pract 49:40, 1968
12. Hall LW, Woolf N, Bradley JWP, et al: Unusual reaction to suxamethonium chloride. Br Med J 2:1305, 1966
13. Harrison GG: Control of the malignant hyperpyrexic syndrome in MHS swine by dantrolene sodium. Br J Anaesth 47:62, 1975
14. Kolb ME, Horne ML, Martz R: Dantrolene in human malignant hyperthermia: A multicenter study. Anesthesiology 56:254, 1982
15. Williams CH: Some observations on the etiology of the fulminant hyperthermia—stress syndrome. Persp Biol Med 20:120, 1976
16. Lucke JN, Hall GM, Lister D: Malignant hyperthermia in the pig and the role of stress. Ann NY Acad Sci 317:326, 1979
17. Gronert GA, Milde JH, Theye RA: Role of sympathetic activity in porcine malignant hyperthermia. Anesthesiology 47:411, 1977
18. Gronert GA, Milde JH, Taylor SR: Porcine muscle responses to carbachol, α and β adrenoceptor agonists, halothane or hyperthermia. J Physiol (Lond) 307:319, 1980
19. Halsall PJ, Cain PA, Ellis FR: Retrospective analysis of anaesthetics received by patients before susceptibility to malignant hyperpyrexia was recognized. Br J Anaesth 51:949, 1979
20. Gronert GA, Milde JH: Variations in onset of porcine malignant hyperthermia. Anesth Analg 60:499, 1981
21. Fitzgibbons DC: Malignant hyperthermia following preoperative oral administration of dantrolene. Anesthesiology 54:73, 1981
22. Ruhland G, Hinkle AF: Malignant hyperthermia after oral and intravenous pretreatment with dantrolene in a patient susceptible to malignant hyperthermia. Anesthesiology 60:159, 1984
23. Larach MG, Rosenberg H, Larach DR, Broennle AM: Prediction of malignant hyperthermia susceptibility by clinical signs. Anesthesiology 66:547, 1987
24. Gronert GA: Malignant hyperthermia. Anesthesiology 53:395, 1980
25. Schwartz L, Rockoff MA, Koka BV: Masseter spasm with anesthesia: Incidence and implications. Anesthesiology 61:772, 1984
26. Carroll JB: Increased incidence of masseter spasm in children with strabismus anesthetized with halothane and succinylcholine. Anesthesiology 67:559, 1987
27. Butler-Browne GS, Eriksson P-O, Laurent C, Thornell L-E: Adult human massceter muscle fibers express myosin isozymes characteristic of development. Muscle Nerve 11:610, 1988
28. Fletcher JE, Rosenberg H: In vitro interaction between halothane and succinylcholine in human skeletal muscle: Implications for malignant hyperthermia and masseter muscle rigidity. Anesthesiology 63:190, 1985
29. van der Spek AFL, Fang WB, Ashton-Miller JA, et al: The effects of succinylcholine on mouth opening. Anesthesiology 67:459, 1987
30. van der Spek AFL, Fang WB, Ashton-Miller JA, et al: Increased masticatory muscle stiffness during limb muscle flaccidity associated with succinylcholine administration. Anesthesiology 69:11, 1988
31. Gronert GA, Rosenberg H: Management of patients in whom trismus occurs following succinylcholine. Anesthesiology 68:653, 1988
32. Rosenberg H: Trismus is not trivial. Anesthesiology 67:453, 1987
33. Gronert GA, Mott J, Lee J: Aetiology of malignant hyperthermia. Br J Anaesth 60:253, 1988
34. Britt BA: Aetiology and pathophysiology of malignant hyperthermia. p. 11. In Britt BA (ed): Malignant Hyperthermia. Martinus Nijhoff, Boston, 1987
35. Duncan CJ: Role of intracellular calcium in promoting muscle damage: A strategy for controlling the dystrophic condition. Experientia 34:1531, 1978
36. Harriman DGF: Malignant hyperthermia myopathy—a critical review. Br J Anaesth 60:309, 1988
37. Gronert GA, Theye RA: Halothane-induced porcine malig-

nant hyperthermia: Metabolic and hemodynamic changes. Anesthesiology 44:36, 1976

38. Verburg MP, Oerlemans FTJ, van Bennekom CA, et al: In vivo induced malignant hyperthermia in pigs. I: Physiological and biochemical changes and the influence of dantrolene sodium. Acta Anaesthesiol Scand 28:1, 1984

39. Rutberg H, Hakanson E: Malignant hyperthermia: Clinical course and metabolic changes in two patients. Acta Anaesth Scand 30:211, 1986

40. Cerri CG, Willner JH, Britt BA, et al: Adenylate kinase deficiency and malignant hyperthermia. Hum Genet 57:325, 1981

41. Marjanen LA, Denborough MA: Effect of halothane on adenylate kinase in porcine malignant hyperpyrexia. Clin Chim Acta 122:225, 1982

42. Sim ATR, White MD, Denborough MA: Effects of adenylate cyclase activators on porcine skeletal muscle in malignant hyperpyrexia. Br J Anaesth 59:1557, 1987

43. Willner JH, Cerri CG, Wood DS: High skeletal muscle adenylate cyclase in malignant hyperthermia. J Clin Invest 68:1119, 1981

44. Schanus EG, Schendel F, Lovrien RE, et al: Malignant hyperthermia (MH): Porcine erythrocyte damage from oxidation and glutathione peroxidase deficiency. Prog Clin Biol Res 55:323, 1981

45. Duthie GG, Arthur JR: Blood antioxidant status and plasma pyruvate kinase activity of halothane-reacting pigs. Am J Vet Res 48:309, 1987

46. Hall GM, Bendall JR, Lucke JN, et al: Porcine malignant hyperthermia. II: Heat production. Br J Anaesth 48:305, 1976

47. Gallant EM: Porcine skeletal muscle for physiological studies. Experientia 35:709, 1979

48. Ellis FR, Harriman DGF, Keaney NP, et al: Halothane-induced muscle contracture as a cause of hyperpyrexia. Br J Anaesth 43:721, 1971

49. Gronert GA: Contracture responses and energy stores in quadriceps muscle from humans age 7–82 years. Hum Biol 52:43, 1980

50. Gronert GA: Muscle contractures and ATP depletion in porcine malignant hyperthermia. Anesth Analg 58:367, 1979

51. Rosenberg H, Reed S: In vitro contracture tests for susceptibility to malignant hyperthermia. Anesth Analg 62:415, 1983

52. Takagi A, Sunohara N, Ishihara T, et al: Malignant hyperthermia and related neuromuscular diseases: Caffeine contracture of the skinned muscle fibers. Muscle Nerve 6:510, 1983

53. Britt BA, Frodis W, Scott E, et al: Comparison of the caffeine skinned fibre tension (CSFT) test with the caffeine-halothane contracture (CHC) test in the diagnosis of malignant hyperthermia. Can Anaesth Soc J 29:550, 1982

54. Galloway GJ, Denborough MA: Suxamethonium chloride and malignant hyperpyrexia. Br J Anaesth 58:447, 1986

55. Kalow W, Britt BA, Richter A: The caffeine test of isolated human muscle in relation to malignant hyperthermia. Can Anaesth Soc J 24:678, 1977

56. Rosenberg H: International workshop on malignant hyperpyrexia. Anesthesiology 54:530, 1981

57. Nelson TE, Flewellen EH, Gloyna DF: Spectrum of susceptibility to malignant hyperthermia—diagnostic dilemma. Anesth Analg 62:545, 1983

58. Nelson TE, Schochet SS Jr: Malignant hyperthermia: A disease of specific myofiber type? Can Anaesth Soc J 29:163, 1982

59. Gallant EM: Histochemical observations on muscle from normal and malignant hyperthermia-susceptible swine. Am J Vet Res 41:1069, 1980

60. Niebroj-Dobosz I, Mayzner-Zawadzka E: Experimental por-

cine malignant hyperthermia: The activity of certain transporting enzymes and myofibrillar calcium-binding protein content in the muscle fiber. Br J Anaesth 54:885, 1982

61. Lorkin PA, Lehmann H: Malignant hyperthermia in pigs: A search for abnormalities in Ca^{2+} binding proteins. FEBS Lett 153:81, 1983

62. Stadhouders AM, Viering WAL, Verburg MP, et al: In vivo induced malignant hyperthermia in pigs. III: Localization of calcium in skeletal muscle mitochondria by means of electronmicroscopy and microprobe analysis. Acta Anaesthesiol Scand 28:14, 1984

63. Walsh MP, Brownell AK, Littman V, et al: Electrophoresis of muscle proteins is not a method for diagnosis of malignant hyperthermia susceptibility. Anesthesiology 64:473, 1986

64. Whistler T, Isaacs H, Badenhorst M: No abnormal low molecular weight proteins identified in human malignant hyperthermic muscle. Anesthesiology 64:795, 1986

65. Marjanen LA, Denborough MA: Electrophoretic analysis of proteins in malignant hyperpyrexia susceptible skeletal muscle. Int J Biochem 16:919, 1984

66. Lopez JR, Alamo L, Caputo C, et al: Intracellular ionized calcium concentration in muscles from humans with malignant hyperthermia. Muscle Nerve 8:355, 1985

67. Lopez JR, Medina P, Alamo L: Dantrolene sodium is able to reduce the resting ionic $[Ca^{2+}]$ in muscle from humans with malignant hyperthermia. Muscle Nerve 10:77, 1987

68. Lopez JR, Allen P, Alamo L, et al: Dantrolene prevents the malignant hyperthermic syndrome by reducing free intracellular calcium concentration in skeletal muscle of susceptible swine. Cell Calcium 8:385, 1987

69. Iaizzo PA, Klein W, Lehmann-Horn F: Fura-2 detected myoplasmic calcium and its correlation with contracture force in skeletal muscle from normal and malignant hyperthermia susceptible pigs. Pflugers Arch 411:648, 1988

70. Lopez JR, Allen PD, Alamo L, et al: Myoplasmic free $[Ca^{2+}]$ during malignant hyperthermia episode in swine. Muscle Nerve 11:82, 1988

71. Iwatsuki N, Koga Y, Imaha K: Calcium channel blocker for treatment of malignant hyperthermia (correspondence). Anesth Analg 62:861, 1983

72. Ilias WK, Williams CH, Fulfer RT, et al: Diltiazem inhibits halothane-induced contractions in malignant hyperthermia-susceptible muscles in vitro. Br J Anaesth 57:994, 1985

73. Saltzman LS, Kates RA, Corke BC, et al: Hyperkalemia and cardiovascular collapse after verapamil and dantrolene administration in swine. Anesth Analg 63:272, 1984

74. Rubin AS, Zablocki AD: Hyperkalemia, verapamil, and dantrolene. Anesthesiology 66:246, 1987

75. Yoganathan T, Casthely PA, Lamprou M: Dantrolene-induced hyperkalemia in a patient treated with diltiazem and metoprolol. J Cardiothor Anesth 2:363, 1988

76. Harrison GG, Wright IG, Morrell DF: The effects of calcium channel blocking drugs on halothane initiation of malignant hyperthermia in MHS swine and on the established syndrome. Anaest Intensive Care 16:197, 1988

77. Gallant EM, Foldes FF, Rempel WE, et al: Verapamil is not a therapeutic adjunct to dantrolene in porcine malignant hyperthermia. Anesth Analg 64:601, 1985

78. Gronert GA, Ahern CP, Milde JH, et al: Effect of CO_2, calcium, digoxin, and potassium on cardiac and skeletal muscle metabolism in malignant hyperthermia susceptible swine. Anesthesiology 64:24, 1986

79. Backman E, Lennmarken C, Rutberg H, et al: Skeletal muscle contraction characteristics *in vivo* in malignant hyperthermia susceptible patients. Acta Neurol Scand 77:278, 1988

80. Lennmarken C, Rutberg H, Henriksson KG: Abnormal relaxation rates in subjects susceptible to malignant hyperthermia. Acta Neurol Scand 75:81, 1987

81. Steiss JE, Bowen JM, Williams CH: Electromyographic evaluation of malignant hyperthermia-susceptible pigs. Am J Vet Res 42:1173, 1982

82. Campion DR, Eikelenboom G, Cassens RG: Isometric contractile properties of skeletal muscle from stress susceptible and stress resistant pigs. J Anim Sci 39:68, 1972

83. Nelson TE, Flewellen EH, Arnett DW: Prolonged electromechanical coupling time intervals in skeletal muscle of pigs susceptible to malignant hyperthermia. Muscle Nerve 6:263, 1983

84. Quinlan JG, Iaizzo PA, Gronert GA, et al: Use of dantrolene plus multiple pulses to detect stress-susceptible porcine muscles. J Appl Physiol 60:1313, 1986

85. Gallant EM, Goettl VM: Porcine malignant hyperthermia: Halothane effects on force generation in skeletal muscles. Muscle Nerve 12:56, 1989

86. Bendall JR: The effect of pre-treatment of pigs with curare on the postmortem rate of pH fall and onset of rigor mortis in the musculature. J Sci Food Agric 17:333, 1966

87. Schmidt GR, Goldspink G, Roberts T, et al: Electromyography and resting membrane potential in longissimus muscle of stress-susceptible and stress-resistant pigs. J Anim Sci 34:379, 1972

88. Gallant EM, Godt RE, Gronert GA: Role of plasma membrane defect of skeletal muscle in malignant hyperthermia. Muscle Nerve 2:491, 1979

89. Gallant EM: Porcine malignant hyperthermia: No role for plasmalemma depolarization. Muscle Nerve 11:785, 1988

90. Gallant EM, Gronert GA, Taylor SR: Cellular membrane potential and contractile threshold in mammalian skeletal muscle susceptible to malignant hyperthermia. Neurosci Lett 28:181, 1982

91. Mickelson JR, Thatte HS, Beaudry TM, et al: Increased skeletal muscle acetylcholinesterase activity in porcine malignant hyperthermia. Muscle Nerve 10:723, 1987

92. Timmerman M, Ashley C: Excitation-contraction coupling. Bridging the gap. J Muscle Cell Motil 9:367, 1988

93. Mickelson JR, Gallant EM, Litterer LA, et al: Abnormal sarcoplasmic reticulum ryanodine receptor in malignant hyperthermia. J Biol Chem 263:9310, 1988

94. Ruppersberg JP, Rudel R: Differential effects of halothane on adult and juvenile sodium channels in human muscle. Pflugers Arch 412:17, 1988

95. Nelson TE, Sweo BA: Ca^{2+} uptake and Ca^{2+} release by skeletal muscle sarcoplasmic reticulum: Differing sensitivity to inhalational anesthetics. Anesthesiology 69:571, 1988

96. Cheah KS, Cheah AM, Waring JC: Phospholipase A2 activity, calmodulin, Ca^{2+} and meat quality in young and adult halothane-sensitive and halothane-insensitive British Landrace pigs. Meat Sci 17:37, 1986

97. Fletcher JE, Rosenberg H, Michaux K, et al: Triglyceride lipase, not phospholipase A2, activity is elevated in skeletal muscle from malignant hyperthermia susceptibles. Anesthesiology 69:A413, 1988

98. Ohta T, Endo M: Inhibition of calcium-induced calcium release by dantrolene at mammalian body temperature. Proc Jpn Acad 62:329, 1986

99. Mickelson JR, Ross JA, Reed BK, et al: Enhanced Ca^{2+}-induced calcium release by isolated sarcoplasmic reticulum vesicles from malignant hyperthermia susceptible pig muscle. Biochim Biophys Acta 862:318, 1986

100. Nelson TE: SR function in malignant hyperthermia. Cell Calcium 9:257, 1988

101. Ruitenbeek W, Verburg MP, Janssen AJM, et al: In vivo induced malignant hyperthermia in pigs. II: Metabolism in skeletal muscle mitochondria. Acta Anaesthesiol Scand 28:9, 1984

102. Harthoorn AM, van der Walt K, Young E: Possible therapy for capture myopathy in captured wild animals. Nature 247:577, 1974

103. Gronert GA, Theye RA, Milde JH, et al: Catecholamine stimulation of myocardial oxygen consumption in porcine malignant hyperthermia. Anesthesiology 49:330, 1978

104. Bohm M, Roewer N, Schmitz W, et al: Effects of beta- and alpha-adrenergic agonists, adenosine, and carbachol in heart muscle isolated from malignant hyperthermia susceptible swine. Anesthesiology 68:38, 1988

105. Wingard DW: Malignant hyperthermia—acute stress syndrome of man? p. 79. In Henschel EO (ed): Malignant Hyperthermia: Current Concepts. Appleton-Century-Crofts, East Norwalk, Conn., 1977

106. Huckell VF, Staniloff HM, Britt BA, et al: Cardiac manifestations of malignant hyperthermia susceptibility. Circulation 58:916, 1978

107. Mambo NC, Silver MD, McLaughlin PR, et al: Malignant hyperthermia susceptibility: A light and electron microscopic study of endomyocardial biopsy specimens from nine patients. Hum Pathol 11:381, 1980

108. Britt BA: Malignant hyperthermia. p. 291. In Orkin FK, Cooperman LH (eds): Complications in Anesthesiology. JB Lippincott, New York, 1982

109. Hammond GL, Lai Y-K, Markert CL: Diverse forms of stress lead to new patterns of gene expression through a common and central metabolic pathway. Proc Natl Acad Sci USA 79:3485, 1982

110. Kawamoto M, Yuge O, Kikuchi H, et al: No myocardial involvement in nonrigid malignant hyperthermia. Anesthesiology 64:93, 1986

111. Cabral R, Prior PF, Scott DF, et al: Reversible profound depression of cerebral electrical activity in hyperthermia. Electroencephalogr Clin Neurophysiol 42:697, 1977

112. Kerr DD, Wingard DW, Gatz EE: Prevention of porcine malignant hyperthermia by epidural block. Anesthesiology 42:307, 1975

113. Klimanek J, Majewski W, Walencik K: A case of malignant hyperthermia during epidural analgesia. Anaesth Resus Int Ther 4:143, 1976

114. Drury PME, Gilbertson AA: Malignant hyperpyrexia and anaesthesia. Br J Anaesth 42:1021, 1970

115. Satnick JH: Hyperthermia under anesthesia with regional muscle flaccidity. Anesthesiology 30:472, 1969

116. Artru AA, Gronert GA: Cerebral metabolism during porcine malignant hyperthermia. Anesthesiology 53:121, 1980

117. Williams CH, Dozier SE, Buzello W, et al: Plasma levels of norepinephrine and epinephrine during malignant hyperthermia in susceptible pigs. J Chromatogr 344:71, 1985

118. Hall GM, Lucke JN, Orchard C, et al: Porcine malignant hyperthermia. VIII: Leg metabolism. Br J Anaesth 54:941, 1982

119. Rutberg H, Hakanson E, Hall GM, et al: Effects of graded exercise on leg exchange of energy substrates in malignant hyperthermia susceptible subjects. Anesthesiology 67:308, 1987

120. Green JH, Ellis FR, Halsall PJ, et al: Thermoregulation, plasma catecholamine and metabolite levels during submaximal work in individuals susceptible to malignant hyperpyrexia. Acta Anaesth Scand 31:122, 1987

121. Bardsley ME, Wheatley AM, Fowler CJ, et al: Metabolism of

monoamines in malignant hyperthermia-susceptible pigs. Br J Anaesth 54:1313, 1982

122. Dantzer R, Hatey F: Plasma dopamine-beta-hydroxylase and platelet monoamine oxidase activities in pigs with different susceptibility to the malignant hyperthermia syndrome induced by halothane. Reprod Nutr Dev 21:103, 1981

123. Hall GM, Lucke JN, Lister D: Porcine malignant hyperthermia. V: Fatal hyperthermia in the Pietrain pig, associated with the infusion of α-adrenergic agonists. Br J Anaesth 49:855, 1977

124. Gronert GA, White DA: Failure of norepinephrine to initiate porcine malignant hyperthermia. Pflugers Arch 411:226, 1988

125. Lister D, Hall GM, Lucke JN: Porcine malignant hyperthermia. III: Adrenergic blockade. Br J Anaesth 48:831, 1976

126. Heffron JJA, Mitchell G: Influence of pH, temperature, halothane and its metabolites on osmotic fragility of erythrocytes of malignant hyperthermia-susceptible and resistant pigs. Br J Anaesth 53:499, 1981

127. Ohnishi ST, Katagi H, Ohnishi T, et al: Detection of malignant hyperthermia susceptibility using a spin label technique on red blood cells. Br J Anaesth 61:565, 1988

128. Thatte HS, Addis PB, Thomas DD, et al: Temperature-dependent abnormalities of the erythrocyte membrane in porcine malignant hyperthermia. Biochem Med Metabol Biol 38:366, 1987

129. Godin DV, Herring FG, MacLeod PJM: Malignant hyperthermia: Characterization of erythrocyte membranes from individuals at risk. J Med 12:35, 1981

130. Rosenberg H, Fischer CA, Reed SB, et al: Platelet aggregation in patients susceptible to malignant hyperthermia. Anesthesiology 5:621, 1981

131. Lutsky I, Witkowski J, Henschel EO: HLA typing in a family prone to malignant hyperthermia. Anesthesiology 56:224, 1982

132. Hall GM: Plasma cholinesterase and malignant hyperthermia. Br J Anaesth 53:199, 1981

133. Mitchell HW, Denborough MA: Smooth muscle contracture in malignant hyperpyrexia. Br J Anaesth 52:637, 1980

134. Ahern CP, Milde JH, Gronert GA: Electrical stimulation triggers porcine malignant hyperthermia. Res Vet Sci 39:257, 1985

135. Hall GM, Lucke JN, Lister D: Porcine malignant hyperthermia. IV: Neuromuscular blockade. Br J Anaesth 48:1135, 1976

136. Hall GM, Cooper GM, Lucke JN, et al: 4-Aminopyridine fails to induce porcine malignant hyperthermia. Br J Anaesth 52:707, 1980

137. Flewellen EH, Nelson TE, Jones WP, et al: Dantrolene dose response in awake man: Implications for management of malignant hyperthermia. Anesthesiology 59:275, 1983

138. Simmons PS, Smithson WA, Gronert GA, et al: Acute myelogenous leukemia and malignant hyperthermia in a patient with type lb glycogen storage disease. J Pediatr 105:428, 1984

139. Brustowicz RM, Moncorge C, Koka BV: Metabolic responses to tourniquet release in children. Anesthesiology 67:792, 1987

140. Delphin E, Jackson D, Rothstein P: Use of succinylcholine during elective pediatric anesthesia should be reevaluated. Anesth Analg 66:1190, 1987

141. Gronert GA: Hyperbaric nitrous oxide and malignant hyperpyrexia. Br J Anaesth 53:1238, 1981

142. McIntyre AR, King RE, Dunn Al: Electrical activity of denervated mammalian skeletal muscle as influenced by D-tubocurarine. J Neurophysiol 8:297, 1945

143. Ording H, Nielsen VG: Atracurium and its antagonism by neostigmine (plus glycopyrrolate) in patients susceptible to malignant hyperthermia. Br J Anaesth 58:1001, 1986

144. Fletcher R, Ranklev E, Olsson AK, et al: Malignant hyperthermia syndrome in an anxious patient. Br J Anesth 53:993, 1981

145. Lips FJ, Newland M, Dutton G: Malignant hyperthermia triggered by cyclopropane during cesarean section. Anesthesiology 56:144, 1982

146. Sewall K, Flowerdew RMM, Bromberger P: Severe muscular rigidity at birth: Malignant hyperthermia syndrome? Can Anaesth Soc J 27:279, 1980

147. Murphy AL, Conlay L, Ryan JF, et al: Malignant hyperthermia during a prolonged anesthetic for reattachment of a limb. Anesthesiology 60:149, 1984

148. Hildebrand SV, Howitt BA: Succinylcholine infusion associated with hyperthermia in ponies anesthetized with halothane. Am J Vet Res 44:2280, 1983

149. Harrison GG, Morrell DF: Response of MHS swine to IV infusion of lignocaine and bupivacaine. Br J Anaesth 52:385, 1980

150. Katz D: Recurrent malignant hyperpyrexia during anesthesia. Anesth Analg 49:225, 1970

151. Berkowitz A, Rosenberg H: Femoral nerve block with mepivacaine for muscle biopsy in malignant hyperthermia patients. Anesthesiology 62:651, 1985

152. Ording H, Hald A, Sjontoft E: Malignant hyperthermia triggered by heating in anaesthetized pigs. Acta Anaesth Scand 29:698, 1985

153. Gronert GA, Thompson RL, Onofrio BM: Human malignant hyperthermia: Awake episodes and correction by dantrolene. Anesth Analg 59:377, 1980

154. Ranklev E, Fletcher R, Krantz P: Malignant hyperpyrexia and sudden death. Am J Forens Med Pathol 6:149, 1985

155. Haverkort-Poels PJE, Joosten EMG, Ruitenbeek W: Prevention of recurrent exertional rhabdomyolysis by dantrolene sodium. Muscle Nerve 10:45, 1987

156. Hunter SL, Rosenberg H, Tuttle GH, et al: Malignant hyperthermia in a college football player. Physician Sportsmed 15:77, 1987

157. Britt BA: Combined anesthetic- and stress-induced malignant hyperthermia in two offspring of malignant hyperthermic-susceptible parents. Anesth Analg 67:393, 1988

158. Feuerman T, Gade GF, Reynolds R: Stress-induced malignant hyperthermia in a head-injured patient case report. J Neurosurg 68:297, 1988

159. Mitchell G, Heffron JJA: The occurrence of pale, soft, exudative musculature in Landrace pigs susceptible and resistant to the malignant hyperthermia syndrome. Br Vet J 136:500, 1980

160. Seeler DC, McDonell WN, Basrur PK: Halothane and halothane/succinylcholine induced hyperthermia (porcine stress syndrome) in a population of Ontario boars. Can J Comp Med 47:284, 1983

161. Webb AJ, Imlah P, Carden AE: Succinylcholine and halothane as a field test for the heterozygote at the halothane locus in pigs. Anim Prod 42:275, 1986

162. Lee DS, Adams JP, Zimmerman JE: Malignant hyperthermia: A possible new variant. Can Anaesth Soc J 32:268, 1985

163. Brownell AKW: Malignant hyperthermia: Relationship to other diseases. Br J Anaesth 60:303, 1988

164. Steenson AJ, Torkelson RD: King's syndrome with malignant hyperthermia potential outpatient risks. Am J Dis Child 141:271, 1987

165. Sethna NF, Rockoff MA, Worthen HM, et al: Anesthesia-related complications in children with Duchenne muscular dystrophy. Anesthesiology 68:462, 1988

166. Wang JM, Stanley TH: Duchenne muscular dystrophy and malignant hyperthermia—two case reports. Can Anaesth Soc J 33:492, 1986

167. Sethna NF, Rockoff MA: Cardiac arrest following inhalation induction of anaesthesia in a child with Duchenne's muscular dystrophy. Can Anaesth Soc J 33:799, 1986

168. Newberg LA, Lambert EH, Gronert GA: Failure to induce malignant hyperthermia in myotonic goats. Br J Anaesth 55:57, 1983

169. Heiman-Patterson T, Martino C, Rosenberg H, et al: Malignant hyperthermia in myotonia congenita. Neurology 38:810, 1988

170. Ellis FR, Halsall PJ, Harriman DGF: Malignant hyperpyrexia and sudden infant death syndrome. Br J Anaesth 60:28, 1988

171. Caroff SN, Rosenberg H, Fletcher JE, et al: Malignant hyperthermia susceptibility in neuroleptic malignant syndrome. Anesthesiology 67:20, 1987

172. Tollefson G: A case of neuroleptic malignant syndrome: In vitro muscle comparison with malignant hyperthermia. J Clin Psychol Pharm 2:266, 1982

173. Krivosic-Horber R, Adnet P, Guevart E, et al: Neuroleptic malignant syndrome and malignant hyperthermia. In vitro comparison with halothane and caffeine contracture tests. Br J Anaesth 59:1554, 1987

174. Araki M, Takagi A, Higuchi I, et al: Neuroleptic malignant syndrome: Caffeine contracture of single muscle fibers and muscle pathology. Neurology 38:297, 1988

175. Addonizio G, Susman VL: ECT as a treatment alternative for patients with symptoms of neuroleptic malignant syndrome. J Clin Psychol 48:102, 1987

176. Geiduschek J, Cohen SA, Khan A, et al: Repeated anesthesia for a patient with neuroleptic malignant syndrome. Anesthesiology 68:134, 1988

177. Harrison GG: Dantrolene—dynamics and kinetics. Br J Anaesth 60:279, 1988

178. Krarup C: The effect of dantrolene on the enhancement and diminution of tension evoked by staircase and by tetanus in rat muscle. J Physiol (Lond) 311:389, 1981

179. Gronert GA, Ahern CP, Milde JH: Treatment of porcine malignant hyperthermia: Lactate gradient from muscle to blood. Can Anaesth Soc J 33:729, 1986

180. Allen GC, Cattran CB, Peterson RG, et al: Plasma levels of dantrolene following oral administration in malignant hyperthermia-susceptible patients. Anesthesiology 69:900, 1988

181. Marchildon MB: Malignant hyperthermia. Arch Surg 117:349, 1982

182. Knochel JP: Serum calcium derangements in rhabdomyolysis. N Engl J Med 305:161, 1981

183. Harrison GG, Morrell DF, Jaros GG: Acute calcium homeostasis in MHS swine. Can Anaesth Soc J 34:377, 1987

184. Murakawa M, Hatano Y, Magaribuchi T, et al: Should calcium administration be avoided in treatment of hyperkalemia in malignant hyperthermia? Anesth Analg 67:604, 1988

185. Ording H, Hald A, Sjontoft E: Ketanserin and malignant hyperthermia in pigs. Acta Anesth Scand 30:7, 1986

186. Jensen AG, Bach V, Werner MU, et al: A fatal case of malignant hyperthermia following isoflurane anesthesia. Acta Anaesth Scand 30:293, 1986

187. Oikkonen M, Rosenberg PH, Bjorkenheim J-M, et al: Spinal block, after dantrolene pretreatment, for resection of a thigh muscle herniation in a young malignant hyperthermia susceptible man. Acta Anaesth Scand 31:309, 1987

188. Watson CB, Reierson N, Norfleet EA: Clinically significant muscle weakness induced by oral dantrolene sodium prophylaxis for malignant hyperthermia. Anesthesiology 65:312, 1986

189. Driessen JJ, Wuis EW, Gielen MJM: Prolonged vecuronium neuromuscular blockade in a patient receiving orally administered dantrolene. Anesthesiology 62:523, 1985

190. Craft JB, Goldberg NH, Lim M, et al: Cardiovascular effects and placental passage of dantrolene in the maternal-fetal sheep model. Anesthesiology 68:68, 1988

191. Ritchie PA, Cheshire MA, Pearce NH: Decontamination of halothane from anaesthetic machines achieved by continuous flushing with oxygen. Br J Anaesth 60:859, 1988

192. Beebe JJ, Sessler DI: Preparation of anesthesia machines for patients susceptible to malignant hyperthermia. Anesthesiology 69:395, 1988

193. Donahue PJ, Schulz J: An alternative to purging an anesthetic machine for patients in whom malignant hyperthermia is a possibility. Anesthesiology 69:1023, 1988

194. Ording H: Diagnosis of susceptibility to malignant hyperthermia in man. Br J Anaesth 60:287, 1988

195. Gallant EM, Fletcher TF, Goettl VM, et al: Porcine malignant hyperthermia: Cell injury enhances halothane sensitivity of biopsies. Muscle Nerve 9:174, 1986

196. Ording H, Hansen U, Skovgaard LT: Age, fiber type composition and in vitro contracture responses in human malignant hyperthermia. Act Anaesth Scand 32:121, 1988

197. Heiman-Patterson TD, Rosenberg H, Fletcher JE, et al: Halothane-caffeine contracture testing in neuromuscular diseases. Muscle Nerve 11:453, 1988

198. Galen RS, Gambino SR: Beyond Normality. New York, John Wiley & Sons, 1975

199. Olgin J, Argov Z, Rosenberg H, et al: Non-invasive evaluation of malignant hyperthermia susceptibility with phosphorus nuclear magnetic resonance spectroscopy. Anesthesiology 68:507, 1988

200. Klip A, Ramlal T, Walker D, et al: Selective increase in cytoplasmic calcium by anesthetic in lymphocytes from malignant hyperthermia-susceptible pigs. Anesth Analg 66:381, 1987

201. Klip A, Britt BA, Elliott ME, et al: Anaesthetic-induced increase in ionized calcium in blood mononuclear cells from malignant hyperthermia patients. Lancet 1:463, 1987

202. Smiley R, Greenberg S, Silverstein SC: Anesthetics increase cytosolic calcium in mononuclear cells from normal and MH-susceptible patients. Anesthesiology 69:A418, 1988

203. Reiss G, Monin G, Lauer C: Comparative effects of the ionophore A23187 on the mechanical responses of muscle in normal Pietrain pigs and pigs with malignant hyperthermia. Can J Physiol Pharmacol 64:248, 1986

204. Traynor CA, Van Dyke RA, Gronert GA: Phosphorylase ratio and susceptibility to malignant hyperthermia. Anesth Analg 62:324, 1983

205. Britt BA, Scott EA: Failure of the platelet-halothane nucleotide depletion test as a diagnostic or screening test for malignant hyperthermia. Anesth Analg 65:171, 1986

206. Nagarajan K, Fishbein WN, Muldoon SM, et al: Calcium uptake in frozen muscle biopsy sections compared with other predictors of malignant hyperthermia susceptibility. Anesthesiology 66:680, 1987

207. Gronert GA: Malignant hyperthermia. Semin Anesth 2:197, 1983

208. Gronert GA, Milde JH, Theye RA: Dantrolene in porcine malignant hyperthermia. Anesthesiology 44:488, 1976

29
FUNDAMENTAL PRINCIPLES OF MONITORING INSTRUMENTATION

Kevin K. Tremper
Steven J. Barker

Mechanical Measurements
  Principles of Mechanics; Energy and Work
  Monitoring of Intravascular Blood Pressure
Measurements of Fluid and Flows
  Fluids at Rest
  Fluids in Motion
  Sound and the Doppler Effect
Measurements of Electricity and Magnetism
  Electricity
  Processing of Small Signals
  Magnetism
  Relationships between Current and
    Magnetic Field

Measurements of Light
  Electromagnetic Radiation
  Absorption, Reflection, Scattering, and
    Transmission of Light
  Engineering Design of Optically Based
    Monitoring Devices
Electrochemical and Thermal Transducers
  Electrochemical Sensors
  Thermal Sensors
Statistical Considerations

Patient monitoring has been a key aspect of anesthesiology since its beginnings as a medical specialty. As the specialty has grown more sophisticated and complex, so have the monitors and the data they present. The stethoscope, sphygmomanometer, and electrocardiogram are now supplemented by the pulse oximeter, expired gas analyzer, processed electroencephalogram, evoked potential monitor, transesophageal echocardiograph, and a host of others. The complexity of some of these devices is intimidating, and we are tempted to regard them as incomprehensible "black boxes" that provide us with clinical data. However, to do so would be to shirk an important part of our clinical responsibility. We must be able not only to understand and interpret the data from our monitors but also to anticipate and recognize errors associated with their use. We cannot accomplish this without understanding how these devices work.

The purpose of this chapter is to provide a comprehensive description and understanding of the scientific foundation for the design and function of our most commonly used monitors. We have divided the chapter into sections based on the method by which a physiologic variable is converted to an electrical or mechanical signal. As shown in Figure 29-1, a physiologic event generates a nonelectric form of energy such as pressure, temperature, or light. A transducer then converts the energy to a signal, which is usually electrical. The transducer signal is processed electrically, and the output is transmitted to a display device for interpretation or to a storage device for later use.

In some forms of monitoring (e.g., transesophageal echocardiography), the processing of signals that occurs between the transducer and the display is very sophisticated. We will discuss the scientific principles governing this type of signal processing only when it is crucial to understanding how a particular monitor works. We will also discuss mechanical and chemical methods of converting physiologic events into useful signals. Therefore, the discussion will involve applications of some basic principles of physics, chemistry, and engineering. Each principle will be derived or explained using a minimum of mathematical complexity and will then be applied to specific monitoring devices. Finally, we will address the problem of assessing the accuracy of monitors, a topic that may help the reader evaluate the steady barrage of published data regarding the performance of new devices.

While the intent of this chapter is to be comprehensive, less detailed descriptions of the monitors and more emphasis on their clinical use can be found in Chapters 30 to 38.

MECHANICAL MEASUREMENTS

Principles of Mechanics; Energy and Work

Many measurements made in the operating room are based on the mechanics of solids and fluids. For example, the mechanics of harmonic oscillators govern the behavior of intravascular pressure transducer systems. This first section on the principles of mechanics will stress basic concepts more than applications. In contrast, subsequent sections will spend more time applying basic concepts to monitoring instrumentation.

At this point, we need to clarify a common source of confusion, the terms units and dimensions. A *dimension* is the measure one uses to describe a physical quantity. For example, length is the dimension used to describe distance, height, and width. In mechanics, the dimensions of all quantities can be expressed as some combination of the three fundamental variables of mass *(M)*, length *(L)*, and time *(T)*. In thermodynamics, a fourth dimension (heat or temperature) must be added. *Units* are specific ways of measuring a given dimension. For example, meters, feet, furlongs, and light-years are all units of the dimension length. We will use Système International d'Unités (SI) units throughout this chapter, supplementing these with "common" units when appropriate. The SI units expressing mass, length, and time are kilograms, meters, and seconds, respectively.

Virtually all classic concepts regarding mechanics are based on Newton's second law of motion,[1] which states that force equals mass times acceleration:

$$F = m\mathbf{a} \tag{1}$$

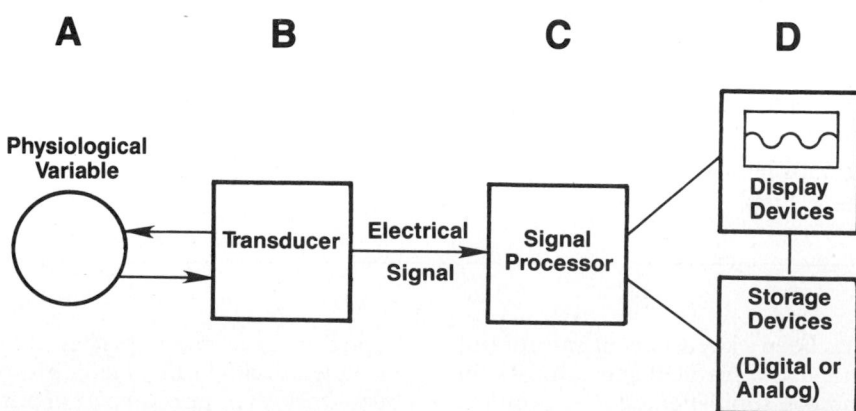

Fig. 29-1. In this schematic representation of the monitoring process, a physiologic event **(A)** produces a form of nonelectric energy. A transducer **(B)** converts this energy to a signal (usually electrical). The signal is processed **(C)** to quantitate the physiologic variable or other related variables (e.g., cardiac output is quantitated from temperature curves obtained using a thermodilution technique). The processed output **(D)** is displayed for interpretation or stored in analog or digital form for later use.

In this equation, force and acceleration are vectors (in this chapter, shown as boldface italics), and mass is a scalar (i.e., it has magnitude but no direction). The SI unit for force is the newton (N), and the units for mass and acceleration are the kilogram (kg) and meter per second squared (m/s²). One newton is the force necessary to give a mass of 1 kg an acceleration of 1 m/s².

Because all monitors convert one form of energy to another, the concept of energy existing in different forms is basic to the subject of monitoring. We will use Newton's second law to discuss kinetic energy, potential energy, and work. Consider a particle of mass m acted on by the force of gravity (Fig. 29-2). Gravitational force F_g is proportional to the mass of the object: $F_g = m \times g$. At the earth's surface, the proportionality constant g is 9.8 N/kg. The gravitational force on an object is often called its "weight." Note that weight is expressed in newtons, whereas mass is expressed in kilograms. (In English units, weight is expressed in pounds and mass in slugs: $g = 32.2$ lb/slug.)

Now, suppose that at time $t = 0$, we release the particle in Figure 29-2 from height $z = 0$ and allow it to fall. According to equation (1), the particle falls with the following acceleration:

$$a = F_g/m, \qquad F_g = mg$$

Therefore,

$$a = mg/m = g \qquad (2)$$

Thus, the constant g is not only the force of gravity per unit mass, it is also the acceleration in m/s² of a free-falling object. We now wish to solve equation (2) for the

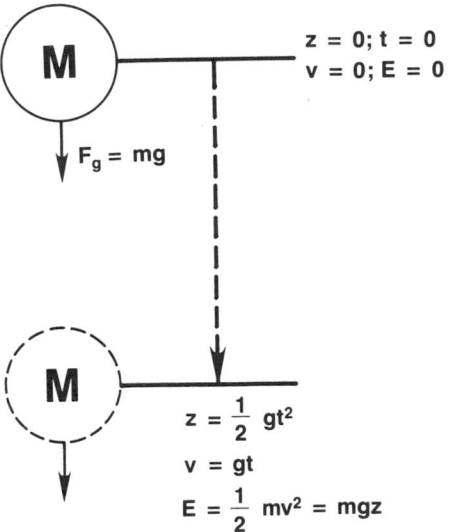

Fig. 29-2. Mass m initially located at height $z = 0$, acted upon by gravitational force mg. At time $t = 0$, the mass is released and accelerates downward according to the equation $F = ma$. As the particle falls, potential energy is converted into kinetic energy (eq. [6] in text).

object's position z as a function of time t. Acceleration a is the time derivative of velocity v, or the second derivative of position z:

$$a = dv/dt = d^2z/dt^2 = g \qquad (3)$$

Integrating twice with respect to time produces:

$$dz/dt = gt \qquad (3a)$$

$$z = (1/2)gt^2 \qquad (3b)$$

After 1 second, the particle has a velocity of 9.8 m/s and has fallen 4.9 m; after 2 seconds, it has a velocity of 19.6 m/s and has fallen 19.6 m (eq. [3]). By integrating equation (1) twice, we find the motion of a particle falling from rest.

Kinetic energy is defined as

$$E_k = (1/2)mv^2 \qquad (4)$$

The dimensions of kinetic energy are ML^2/T^2, and the SI unit is the kilogram-meter²/second² or joule. For the falling particle example, equation (3b) can be solved for t and substituted into equation (3a) to yield

$$v = dz/dt = \sqrt{2gz} \qquad (5)$$

Substituting equation (5) into equation (4) produces

$$E_k = (1/2)mv^2 = mgz \qquad (6)$$

The kinetic energy resulting from the fall is thus proportional to the height of the fall and the mass of the object. The quantity mgz is the decrease in *potential energy* or *gravitational potential* E_p of the object. Equation (6) shows that the kinetic energy acquired in falling distance z equals the decrease in potential energy during the fall. This sequence illustrates a general principle of conservation of energy:

$$E_k + E_p = \text{constant} \qquad (7)$$

This law holds in the absence of friction or other means by which energy is dissipated (i.e., converted into heat or radiation). Kinetic energy is energy in the form of motion, whereas potential energy is stored energy that can be converted into motion. There are many forms of potential energy in anesthesia. For example, a great deal of potential energy is stored in compressed gas cylinders. The magnitude of this energy is realized if one of these cylinders ruptures and potential energy is converted rapidly, and with disastrous consequences, to kinetic energy.

Work is an important concept related to energy. If we move an object by applying a force to it, the work done is defined as the force exerted times the distance moved during the application of force:

$$W = Fd \qquad (8)$$

In our example of a mass m allowed to fall a distance z under a gravitational force mg, the work required to restore the mass to its starting position ($z = 0$) is

$$
\begin{aligned}
W &= \text{force} \times \text{distance} \\
&= mg \times z \\
&= mgz \\
&= E_p
\end{aligned}
\tag{9}
$$

That is, the work required to restore the original configuration is equal to the potential energy that was converted to kinetic energy during the fall. The same dimensions and units are used for both work and energy. In general, work can increase either kinetic or potential energy.

Monitoring of Intravascular Blood Pressure

An excellent example of how this understanding of mechanics helps us optimize monitoring can be seen by examining the workings of a fluid-coupled transducer system that measures intravascular blood pressure. Figure 29-3 shows the common configuration of an intra-arterial cannula connected by means of fluid-filled tubing to a pressure transducer. Through displacement of a diaphragm, the transducer converts pressure into an electrical signal. Most transducers used in measurement have some form of electrical energy as their output.

The transducer system of Figure 29-3 is mechanically analogous to the harmonic oscillator shown in Figure 29-4. The harmonic oscillator consists of a mass m that is free to move only in the x direction. The mass is acted

upon by three forces: an external driving force F_e, a spring force ($F_s = -kx$), and a damping force [$F_d = -c(dx/dt)$]. The spring force is proportional to displacement from equilibrium, and the damping force is proportional to velocity. The minus signs indicate that the last two forces are *restoring forces:* that is, they tend to drive the mass back toward its origin ($x = 0$). In the transducer analogy, the external driving force is the actual arterial pressure, and m is the mass of all the fluid within the transducer, tubing, and cannula. The spring represents the elasticity of the transducer diaphragm and the plastic tubing, and damping results from friction of the fluid moving to and fro within the tubing.

As a first approximation, we model the actual arterial pressure waveform as a sine wave: $F = A \sin(2\pi ft)$, where A is amplitude and f is frequency. We now have mathematical expressions for all three forces, which we can substitute into equation (1) ($F = ma$) to solve for motion of the mass. Solution of the resulting harmonic oscillator equation shows that the mass moves in a sinusoidal fashion with the same frequency f as the driving force:

$$
x(t) = D \sin(2\pi ft + \phi),
\tag{10}
$$

where $x(t)$ is the position of the mass at time t, D is the amplitude of the motion, and ϕ is a phase shift angle. In our pressure transducer analogy, $x(t)$ represents the output of the transducer in response to a sinusoidal arterial pressure wave. The most relevant part of this solution is the response amplitude D, which is plotted

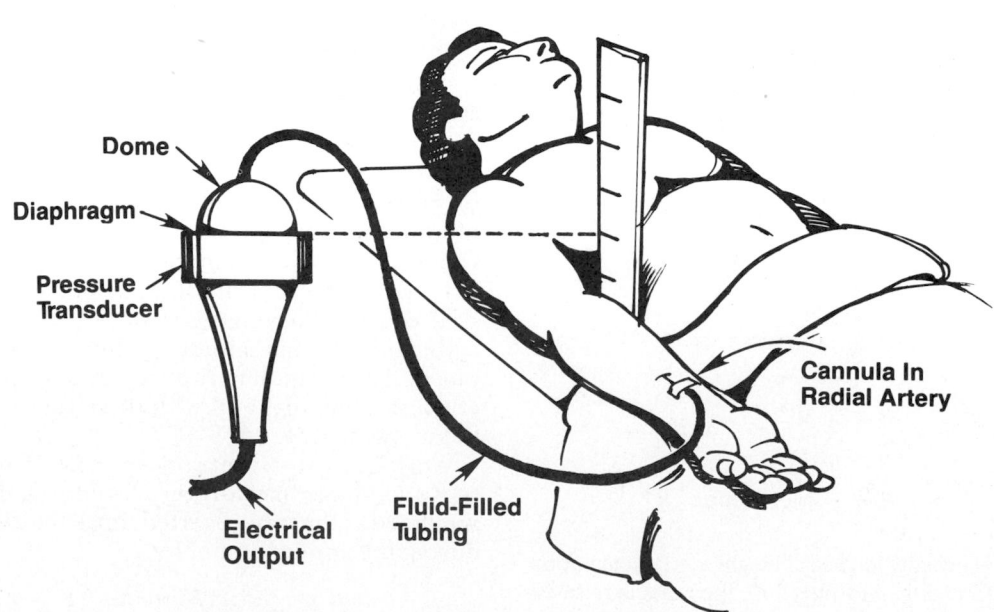

Fig. 29-3. In the most common configuration for intra-arterial monitoring of blood pressure, the arterial cannula is connected to a pressure transducer by means of fluid-filled tubing. This system is analogous to the harmonic oscillator shown in Figure 29-4.

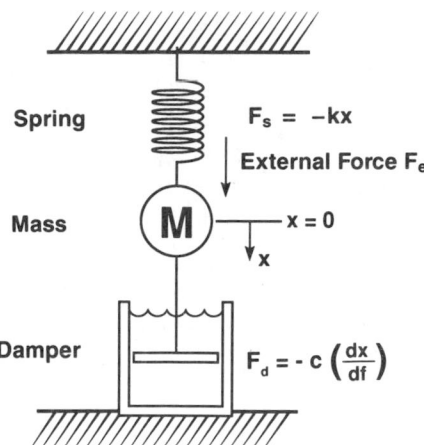

Fig. 29-4. In a forced, damped harmonic oscillator, mass *m* can move in only one direction and has three forces acting on it: spring force F_s, damping force F_d, and external driving force F_e.

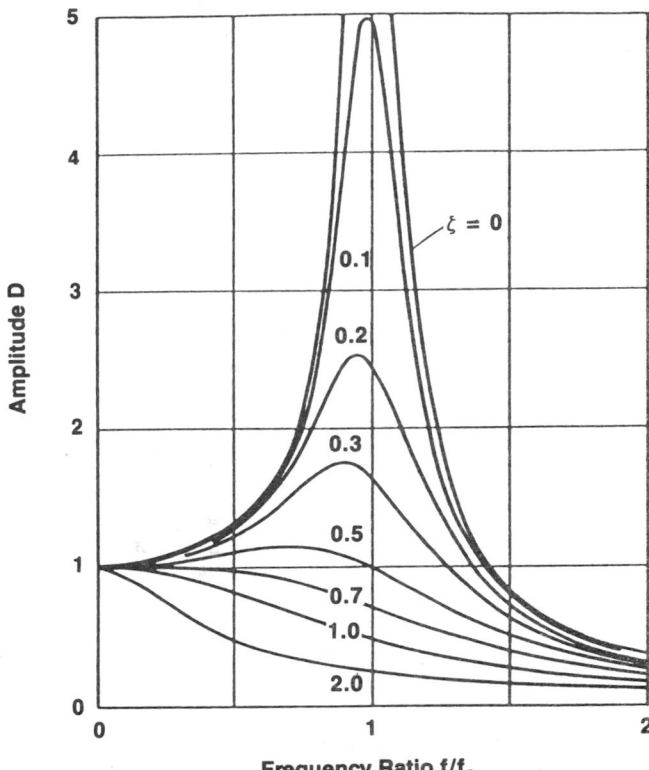

Fig. 29-5. Amplitude *D* of the forced harmonic oscillator is plotted against the ratio of driving frequency *f* to resonant frequency f_0. Curves are shown for various values of the damping coefficient ζ. At $\zeta = 0.2$ (damping coefficient of a typical clinical system), the maximum amplification is approximately 2.5.

against the driving frequency *f* in Figure 29-5.[2] This figure shows some important properties of fluid-coupled transducers and other harmonic oscillators. One of these is the existence of a *resonant frequency, f_0*, which is defined as follows:

$$f_0 = (1/2\pi) \sqrt{k/m} \qquad (11)$$

(Remember, *m* is the mass of the system and *k* is the elasticity, or *spring constant*.) At this frequency, the amplitude of the motion becomes infinite if there is no damping. This is illustrated by the uppermost curve in Figure 29-5, labeled $\zeta = 0$. All real systems possess some damping, making the amplitude at resonance finite. ζ is a *damping coefficient*, defined as follows

$$\zeta = c/\sqrt{2km} \qquad (12)$$

As we increase the amount of damping (i.e., friction), we observe a decrease in the peak amplitude at resonance, and the frequency at which the peak occurs decreases slightly (Fig. 29-5).

Even though the arterial pressure waveform is not actually sinusoidal, Figure 29-5 shows the most important characteristics of the pressure transducer response. Any combination of catheter, tubing, and transducer can be characterized by two quantities: a resonant frequency f_0 and a damping coefficient ζ. Gardner[3] measured these quantities for many transducer and tubing systems; most systems have resonant frequencies of 10 to 20 cycles/s, or hertz (Hz), and damping coefficients of 0.2 to 0.3. Observation of Figure 29-5 reveals that the maximum amplification factor (the ratio of transducer output to input waveform amplitude) at resonance is near 2.0.

If the resonant frequency is 10 Hz (600 cycles/min), one might conclude that amplification plays little role in the clinical range of pulse rates, which are 5 to 10 times smaller. However, the arterial pressure wave-

form is not a sine wave. It can be represented as a summation of sine waves (a *Fourier series*) of frequencies up to many times the pulse rate.[4] It is these higher *harmonic* frequencies that are amplified most and that yield the spiked appearance of the poorly processed arterial waveform. Depending on the shape of the actual arterial pressure wave, this distortion can introduce a 20 to 40 percent "overshoot" error in systolic blood pressure readings. Even worse, this error is dependent on pulse rate, so that an error determined for a particular patient at the beginning of an anesthetic may not remain constant.

From this discussion, we can easily predict how to optimize the performance of a pressure transducer system. First, the resonant frequency (f_0) should be as high as possible. Therefore, the value for *k* in equation (11) should be large (i.e., the spring should be "stiff"), and the value for *m* should be small. That is, the cannula and pressure tubing should be as stiff and inelastic as possible. To minimize the mass of the moving fluid, the tubing should be short in length and small in diameter. Judging from Figure 29-5, the optimal damping coefficient would be 0.4 to 0.5. One should also carefully eliminate air bubbles from the system, as these add elasticity and friction and thereby lower the resonant frequency. In a clinical system, one can determine the approximate f_0 and ζ of a transducer system if graphic output is available. If the high-pressure flush is turned on and then quickly off at a high chart speed (50 mm/s), the tracing oscillates through several cycles at a frequency near f_0. The damping coefficient can be found by determining the ratio of amplitudes of successive peaks on the tracing.

This is a practical example of how fundamental principles of mechanics can be used to predict and optimize the performance of monitoring systems. These concepts of mechanics will recur in later sections of this chapter. Readers interested in further coverage of the subject are directed to several intermediate texts on the mechanics of particles and rigid bodies.[5-9] The historically inclined reader should refer to the original works of Sir Isaac Newton and Lord Kelvin.[1,10]

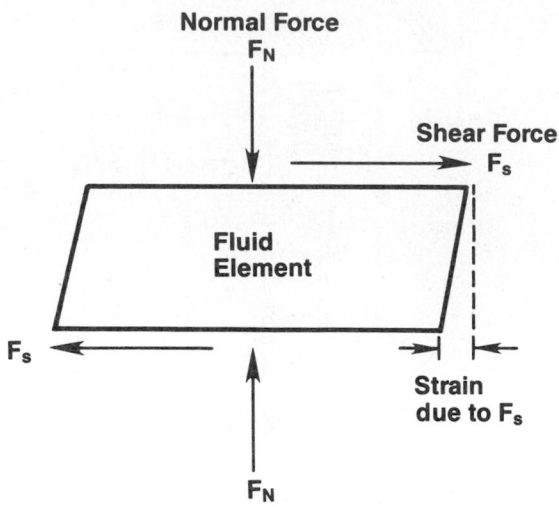

Fig. 29-6. For a fluid element subjected to a shearing or tangential force, shear stress is the tangential force per unit area of surface. The element continuously deforms or "strains" as long as the shear stress is applied. For *Newtonian fluids*, the rate of strain is proportional to stress.

MEASUREMENTS OF FLUIDS AND FLOWS

Fluids at Rest

Measurements of fluids and flows have numerous applications in anesthesiology, particularly in the area of monitoring. An understanding of some of the laws of fluid behavior is essential if one is to use even simple devices such as the flowmeters on an anesthesia machine. In addition, flows of various liquids and gases in the human body are crucial to homeostasis, and one major emphasis in monitoring is continuous measurement of these flows. In this section, we will describe basic principles of fluid mechanics and apply these to the monitoring of gas flows and blood flow.

Basic Principles of Hydrostatics

A fluid is matter that continuously deforms when subjected to a shearing stress. That is, as long as one applies a tangential or shear force to a fluid element (Fig. 29-6), the fluid continues to change shape. By contrast, solid matter subjected to a shearing stress changes its shape to only a fixed extent and then reaches a new, constant shape. For solids, the stress is proportional to the change in shape or *strain*. For fluids stress is proportional to the rate of change or *rate of strain*. If one applies normal (perpendicular) forces to a fluid (Fig. 29-6), the fluid tends to respond in one of two ways. One group of fluids, liquids, is highly resistant to compression and changes its volume very little. The second group of fluids, gases, can be compressed or expanded readily by normal forces. In general, these two phases of matter are very distinct from one another; the few exceptions are not important to our discussion. Often a material can exist as both a liquid and a gas; water, halothane, and carbon dioxide are examples of interest to anesthesiologists. Understanding these distinctions

prevents a common misuse of terms. Physicians sometimes say "fluid" when they really mean "liquid." The question, Do you use air or fluid to test loss of resistance in an epidural? is meaningless, because air is a fluid.

We have already implied that forces on fluids fall into two categories: shear (tangential) forces and normal (perpendicular) forces. If one gradually shrinks the imaginary fluid element in Figure 29-6 to infinitesimal size, the shear force divided by the area of the surface on which it is exerted is called the *shear stress*. In this same limit, the normal force per unit area is called the *pressure* (also called *static pressure*). Pressure is defined at every point within a moving fluid, and its values vary with both positions (x,y,z) and time (t). The dimensions for pressure are force/area, or, in terms of mass-length-time, M/LT^2. The SI unit for pressure is the newton per square meter, which is called the pascal (Pa). Because the pascal is a very small unit of pressure, the kilopascal (kPA) is more commonly used. The English unit for pressure is the pound per square foot (lb/ft²); lb/in² is also often used. The pressure exerted by the earth's atmosphere at sea level (called one *atmosphere*, 1 atm) is 101.3 kPa, or 2,116 lb/ft², or 14.7 lb/in².

The Pressure Manometer

A liquid manometer is a simple and reliable means of monitoring pressure. It simply uses the weight of a measured column of liquid to balance the pressure exerted against the liquid. We have defined weight as being the force exerted by gravity on a mass m ($F_g = mg$). To determine the weight of a column of liquid of known volume (Fig. 29-7), one must first know the mass

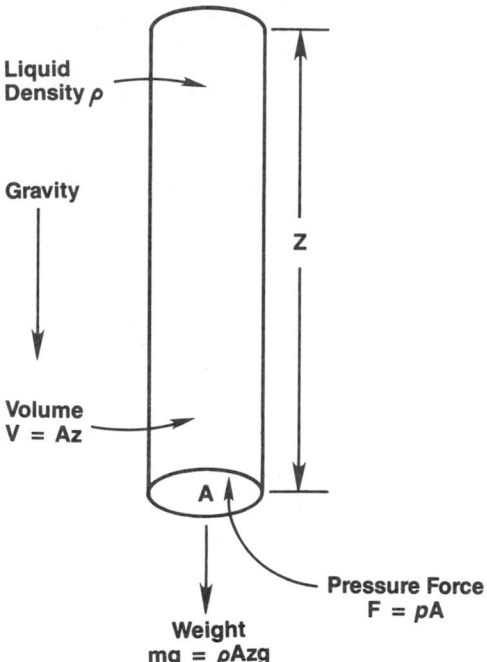

Fig. 29-7. For this cylindrical, vertical column of liquid, the density of the liquid is ρ; the cross-sectional area and height of the cylinder are A and z, respectively; and the volume of liquid is $V = Az$. The weight of the column, ρAzg, is balanced by the pressure on the bottom surface, pA.

per unit volume, or density, of the liquid. Density has dimensions of M/L^3, and the SI units are kilograms per cubic meter (kg/m³). Because liquids are almost incompressible, density is not influenced by pressure (but is influenced by temperature). The density of water at room temperature is 997.8 kg/m³, or 1.0 gram per cubic centimeter (g/cm³).

The pressure p exerted by the bottom of the column of liquid in Figure 29-7 can be determined as follows. If the cross-sectional area of the liquid cylinder is A and the height of the cylinder is z, then its volume is $V = Az$. If the liquid has a density of ρ, the mass of the column is $m = \rho Az$, and its weight is $mg = \rho Azg$. The liquid column exerts this force (i.e., its weight) on its base (area A), thus creating the following pressure on the base:

$$p = \text{force/area} = \rho Azg/A = \rho gz \qquad (13)$$

The pressure of the manometer is therefore independent of its cross-sectional area A; it depends on only the density of the working fluid and the vertical height of the column. For example, the working fluid used by sphygmomanometers to measure arterial blood pressure is mercury, the density of which is 13,600 kg/m³ (13.6 g/cm³, or 13.6 times the density of water). The relationship of pressure to height of the column is thus

$$p \text{ (pascals)} = \rho gz = 13,600 \times 9.8 \ z \text{ (meters)}$$
$$= 1.33 \times 10^5 z \text{ (meters)} \qquad (14)$$

If pressure is expressed in kilopascals and height in millimeters, equation (14) becomes p (kPa) $= 0.133 \ z$ (mm). That is, the pressure exerted by 1 millimeter of mercury (mmHg), also called a *torr*, equals 0.133 kPa. One atmosphere of pressure equals 760 mmHg or 101.3 kPa. Water is also used as the working fluid in manometers, as in the measurement of central venous or intracranial blood pressure. Manometers can accurately measure mean blood pressure but not rapid fluctuations in pressure such as those occurring in an arterial waveform. The mass of the liquid column slows the response to these rapid changes in pressure, as discussed earlier.

Fluids in Motion

Basic Principles of Fluid Dynamics

Understanding the motion of fluids (fluid dynamics) is also important to anesthesiologists. In particular, measuring the volume or velocity of flow is the purpose of a number of monitors, ranging from simple gas flowmeters on the anesthesia machine to complex Doppler cardiac output devices. We will now discuss basic principles of fluid dynamics as they apply to measurement of flow.

The equations governing the motion of fluids are expressions of Newton's second law, $\boldsymbol{F} = \boldsymbol{ma}$ (eq. [1]). Forces associated with fluids fall into three major categories: gravity, pressure, and friction. In the example using manometers, the gravitational force per unit volume of fluid is simply ρg, acting in the vertical direction. Pressure forces are actually the result of *differences* in pressure from one point to another and are expressed mathematically as the negative of the pressure gradient. (The *pressure gradient* is a vector in the direction of maximum rate of pressure increase, having magnitude equal to the pressure derivative in that direction.) Friction is proportional to viscosity, the physical property of a fluid that relates shear stress (tangential force, Fig. 29–6) to rate of strain.

The equations of motion expressing these forces and fluid accelerations in three dimensions are the Navier-Stokes equations.[11] Although these equations can be formidably complex, the level of accuracy needed for most anesthesia-related applications requires use of only a simplified version. For example, for many measurements of flow, frictional or "viscous" forces are neglected and the fluid is assumed to be incompressible. Even anesthetic gases passing through a breathing circuit usually can be regarded as incompressible because the changes in density occurring in the circuit are small. In this situation, the Navier-Stokes equations can be integrated to yield the familiar Bernoulli equation:

$$P_0 = p + (1/2)\rho U^2 + \rho gz \qquad (15)$$

where P_0, the *stagnation pressure*, is constant along streamlines (imaginary lines that are everywhere parallel to the velocity vector), and U is the magnitude of the fluid velocity. The Bernoulli equation can be thought of as a balance of potential and kinetic energy, as expressed earlier in equation (7). The pressure and gravity terms in equation (15) represent forms of potential energy, and $(1/2)\rho U^2$ represents the kinetic energy per unit volume of fluid. As kinetic energy increases, potential energy decreases and vice versa. For example, as an airway narrows, the flow velocity increases and pressure therefore decreases. Such a decrease in pressure in the airway lumen may contribute to further narrowing of a diseased airway that has poor external tethering.

Flowmeters

Equation (15) shows the relationship between velocity and pressure of a fluid in a flow that meets the conditions described. For flows in tubes, the manometer technique provides an easy method of measuring mean pressure. Therefore, the simplest flowmeters apply a combination of these two principles to a tube of changing cross-sectional diameter. For example, the Venturi flowmeter shown in Figure 29-8 consists of a tube of varying cross-sectional area that has two ports for measurement of pressure. The Bernoulli equation for points 1 and 2 in the figure becomes

$$p_1 + (1/2)\rho U_1^2 = p_2 + (1/2)\rho U_2^2 \tag{16}$$

Here the gravity terms have cancelled out because the tube is horizontal, but these terms are usually negligible for gas flows in any direction.

The volume of the fluid flow Q (also called flux) at both locations must be the same, as no fluid is entering or leaving through the tube walls. The dimensions and SI units for the volume of fluid flow are L^3/T and m^3/s, respectively. This volume is determined at each cross-section of the tube by multiplying the average velocity U by the cross-sectional area A:

$$Q = U_1 A_1 = U_2 A_2 \tag{17}$$

Assuming that A_1, A_2, p_1, and p_2 are known, we now have two equations for the two unknowns U_1 and U_2. Solving these for the velocity U_1 produces

$$U_1 = \sqrt{[2(p_2 - p_1)]/[\rho(1 - A_1^2/A_2^2)]} \tag{18}$$

To find the volume of the flow (Q), we merely multiply this result by A_1. Note that velocity is proportional to the square root of the pressure drop, or that the pressure change varies as velocity squared. For a given U_1, magnitude of flow velocity, the pressure drop varies as the square of the ratio of the areas, or the fourth power of the ratio of the diameters. If we choose A_2 greater than A_1 (i.e., if we reverse the flow direction shown in Fig. 29-8), equation (18) implies that p_2 is greater than p_1. In this case, the pressure *increases* in the direction of flow, a change that initially seems contrary to intuition.[12]

The bobbin flowmeters (also called *variable-orifice flowmeters*) in anesthesia machines use a similar principle. These devices consist of a slightly tapered vertical tube and a bobbin or ball that fits inside the tube (Fig. 29-9). The cross-sectional area of the ring-shaped gap between the bobbin and the tube wall is proportional to the height of the bobbin. Because changes in the cross-sectional area of flow are abrupt rather than gradual (as in Fig. 29-8), the Bernoulli equation does not accurately describe this type of flow. The flow above the bobbin (i.e., downstream) is highly turbulent, and turbulence is a condition that dissipates kinetic energy into heat. However, introduction of an empirical constant C_d enables one to use the same formulation as in equation (18):

$$Q = C_d A \sqrt{[2(p_1 - p_2)]/\rho} \tag{19a}$$

and

$$p_1 - p_2 = (1/2\rho Q^2)/(C_d^2 A^2), \tag{19b}$$

where C_d is a dimensionless constant called the *discharge coefficient*. This constant varies with the shape of the orifice and with the value for another dimensionless parameter, the *Reynolds number* (Re).[12] The Reynolds number, the overall ratio of inertial forces to vis-

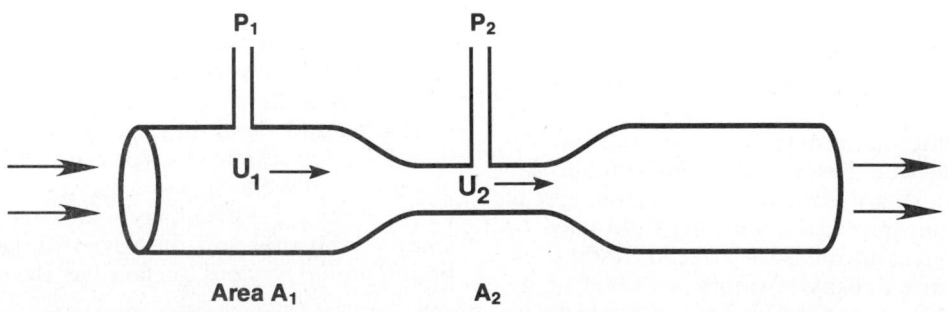

Fig. 29-8. The Venturi flowmeter consists of a straight tube of slowly varying cross-sectional area. It contains two ports for measurement of pressure, the cross-sectional areas of which are A_1 and A_2. As the tube narrows, the velocity of fluid flow increases from U_1 to U_2, and pressure decreases according to the Bernoulli equation. Velocity is proportional to the square root of the change in pressure.

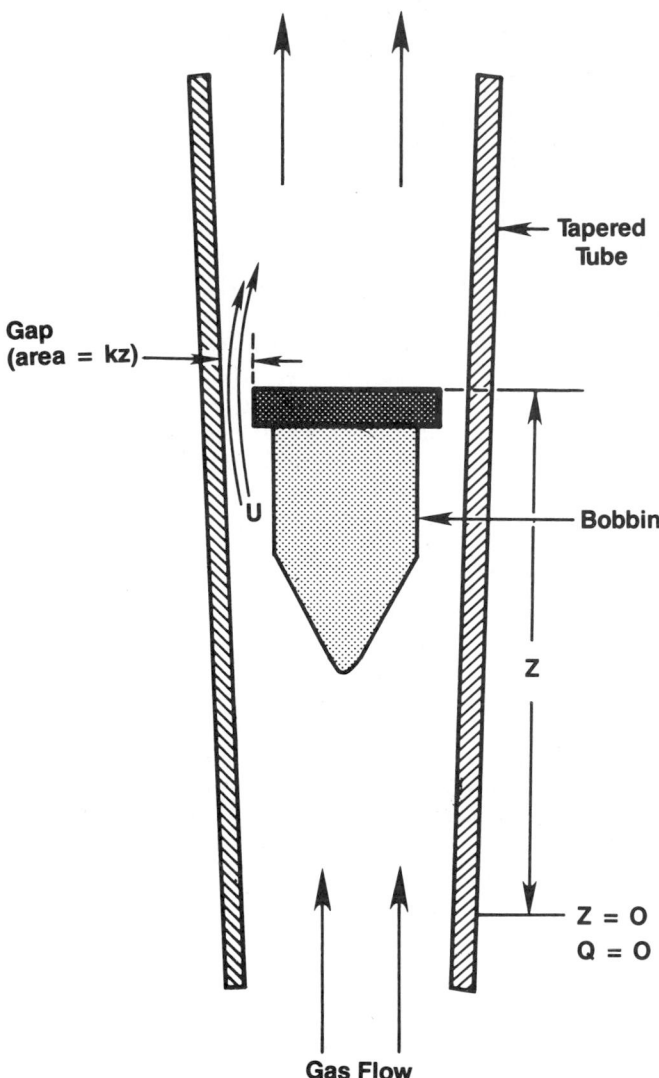

Fig. 29-9. In the variable-orifice or "bobbin" flowmeter, the gap between the bobbin and the wall of the tapered tube is proportional to the height of the bobbin. The pressure force on the bobbin equals its weight when the bobbin is stationary. The volume of flow (Q) is then proportional to the area of the gap and thus to the height (z) of the bobbin. k, constant; U, velocity of the flow.

cous forces in a particular flow, is determined as follows:

$$Re = \rho UL/\mu \qquad (20)$$

where U is mean flow velocity, L is a characteristic length for the flow (in our flowmeter, L is the diameter of the tube), and μ is the viscosity of the fluid. The dimension for viscosity is M/LT. The value for the Reynolds number is important to any fluid flow, as it determines some of the most important characteristics of the flow. For example, the transition from laminar or "smooth" flow to turbulent flow is determined by the shape of the flow and the Reynolds number.[13] Flow in a

long, straight, smooth-walled tube becomes turbulent at an Re value of approximately 2,300.[14] On the other hand, flow through an abrupt orifice such as that of the flowmeter in Figure 29-9 becomes turbulent at a Reynolds number of less than 100.

Returning now to the function of the flowmeter, one can see that as gas flows upward through the tapered tube, the bobbin begins to rise. As the bobbin rises, cross-sectional area of the orifice A increases because of the taper of the tube; therefore, the drop in pressure ($p_1 - p_2$) decreases (eq. [19b]). The bobbin reaches an equilibrium position for a given volume of flow Q when the pressure lifting the bobbin is exactly equal to the weight of the bobbin. In this type of flowmeter, the pressure difference is fixed by the bobbin weight, and the area of the orifice varies with the volume of the flow; hence the name *variable-orifice flowmeter*. Equations (19a) and (19b) show that calibration of these flowmeters depends on both the density and the viscosity of the gas: density ρ appears explicitly, and viscosity μ appears in the dependence of C_d on the Reynolds number. If we use the wrong gas in a particular flowmeter, equations (19a) and (19b) and the viscosity and density of the new gas enable us to predict the change in calibration.[15]

Sound and the Doppler Effect

Basic Principles of Sound Transmission

Several modern monitors use the fundamental principles of sound transmission and reflection and the Doppler effect. These range from the relatively simple precordial Doppler ultrasound probe for detection of air embolism to the sophisticated esophageal echocardiograph.

Sound waves are small fluctuations in pressure, density, and velocity that can propagate through matter of any form: solid, liquid, or gas. Unlike electromagnetic waves, sound cannot propagate through a vacuum. Sound is called a *longitudinal wave* because the motion of the particles occurs in the same direction as wave propagation (Fig. 29-10). In contrast, waves on the surface of the ocean are *transverse waves* because the motion of the particles is mainly perpendicular to the direction of wave propagation.

The simplest sound wave to represent mathematically is a sinusoidal wave propagating in one dimension:

$$p' = p_0 \sin [(2\pi/\lambda)(x - at)] \qquad (21)$$

where p' is the pressure fluctuation, λ is the wavelength (distance between waves), x is the coordinate in the direction of propagation, and a is the speed of propagation, or the speed of sound. Although most sounds we hear are made up of waves far more complex than this simple sine wave, all sounds can be represented as a summation of sine waves of different frequencies; this Fourier series has already been discussed. A note from a musical instrument consists of a sine wave at the *funda-*

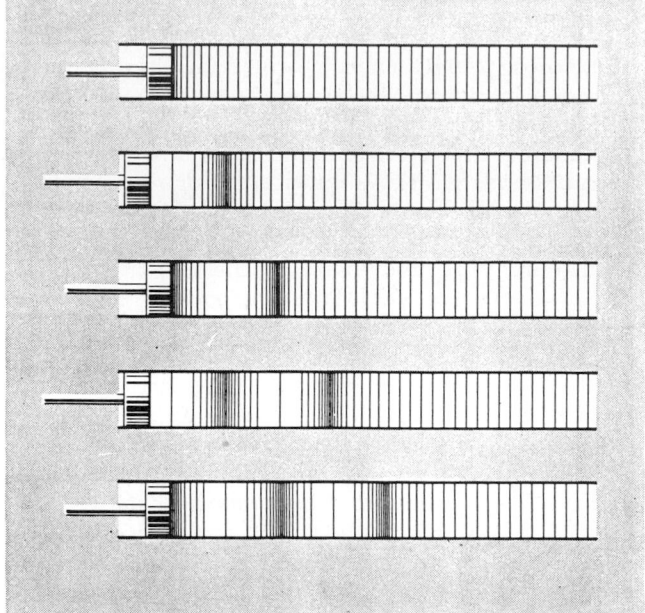

Fig. 29-10. Sound waves generated by a moving piston in a tube. Sound is said to be a "longitudinal" wave because the fluid particles move in the direction of wave propagation.

mental frequency plus many *harmonics*. Harmonics are sine waves at frequencies that are multiples of the fundamental frequency. Fortunately for our ears, all of these many frequencies propagate at the same speed, *a*. That is, the speed of sound is independent of frequency. For ideal gases, the speed of sound is proportional to the square root of temperature.[16] The speed of sound in air at room temperature is 344 m/s, or 1,129 ft/s, or 770 miles per hour (mph). At an altitude of 13,000 m (40,000 ft), where the usual temperature is $-57°C$, the speed of sound is only 295 m/s or 661 mph. The speed of sound is much higher in liquids than in gases. For example, the speed of sound through water at 15°C is 1,450 m/s. In solids, the speed of sound varies greatly, ranging from 54 m/s in rubber to 6,000 m/s in granite.

The amplitude of a sound wave is measured by the root mean square (RMS) value of the pressure fluctuations. This value is called the *sound pressure level* (SPL). Because the range of SPL values is often very wide, a logarithmic scale is used:

$$\text{SPL} = 20 \log (p^*/P_0) \qquad (22)$$

where p^* is the RMS pressure fluctuation and P_0 is a reference pressure, chosen as the lowest sound pressure detectable by the human ear. This pressure representing the threshold of hearing is 2×10^{-8} kPa at a sound frequency of 2 kHz (2,000 cycles/s). The units in this SPL scale are called *decibels*. Thus, a sound pressure of 2×10^{-8} kPa corresponds to an SPL of zero decibels (0 dB), the lowest audible sound level [$(p^*/P_0 = 1$; log (1) = 0)]. Quiet conversation has an SPL of approxi-

mately 40 to 50 dB, or a pressure of 10 to 300 times that of the threshold of hearing. Prolonged exposure to sound levels greater than 90 dB causes permanent hearing impairment. An SPL of 120 dB is at the threshold of pain; this corresponds to the noise level of a jet engine at 30 m or a live rock concert.

When sound waves encounter a sudden change in the properties of the conducting medium, some of the sound is transmitted through the new medium and some of it is reflected or "scattered" in many directions. Although the mathematics of this process is complex, one conclusion is readily apparent: the greater the mismatch in density and compressibility between the two media, the more sound is reflected. In 1896, Lord Rayleigh showed that changes in the compressibility of a medium produce monopole acoustic sources and that changes in density produce dipole sources.[17] The quantity that best determines the degree of reflection at an interface between two media is the ratio *(R)* of the products of density (ρ) and the speed of sound *(a)* through the two media:

$$R = (\rho_1 a_1)/(\rho_2 a_2). \qquad (23)$$

We can easily see that the greatest "acoustic mismatch" in the body occurs between the solid tissues and the lungs. Both the density and speed of sound are much lower in the air-filled lungs than in solid tissues. Therefore, ultrasonography cannot "look" through the lungs to tissues or organs on the other side. The second greatest mismatch occurs between soft tissues and bone, the latter having a much higher ρa than the former.

In 1842, Christian Johann Doppler first described the apparent change in pitch of a sound that occurred when either the source of the sound or the listener was moving.[18] This *Doppler effect* now has several applications in patient monitoring, including precordial and esophageal Doppler ultrasound devices that measure local blood velocities or cardiac output. If a sound source radiating a frequency *f* is stationary and the listener is moving (Fig. 29-11A), the wavelength of the waves can be determined by the equation

$$\lambda = a/f \qquad (24)$$

because the time between wavefronts is $1/f$, and the waves are moving at the speed of sound *a*. If the listener moves toward the source at speed V_0, his velocity relative to the moving wavefronts is $(a + V_0)$. The number of wavefronts the listener encounters per unit time is therefore

$$f' = \text{velocity/distance between waves} = (a + V_0)/\lambda \quad (25)$$

Because the sound frequency for a stationary listener is $f = a/\lambda$ (eq. [24]), the frequency f' heard by the moving listener becomes

$$f' = (a + V_0)/\lambda = f + (V_0/\lambda) = f + (V_0 f/a)$$
$$= f[1 + (V_0/a)] \qquad (26)$$

The apparent frequency of the listener is thus increased

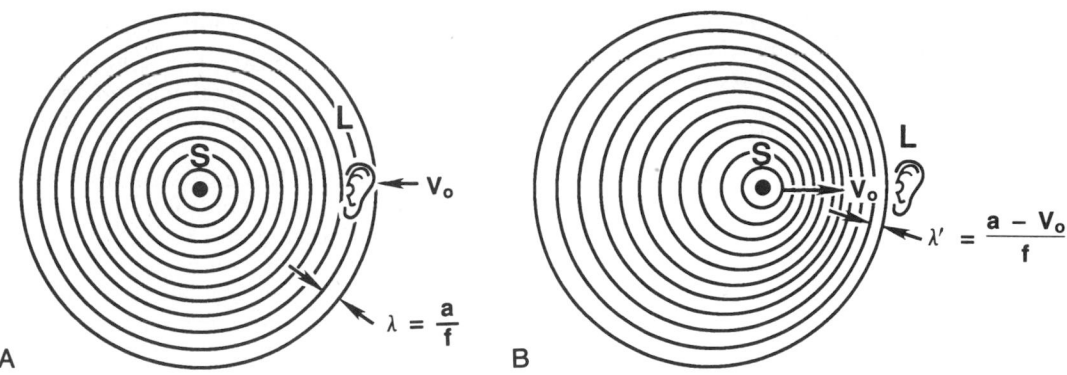

Fig. 29-11. (A) The Doppler effect when the source of sound is stationary and the listener is moving. The waves propagate at speed a, and the listener moves toward the source at speed V_0. Therefore, the number of wavefronts per unit time encountered by the listener is $(a + V_0)/\lambda$, where λ equals the wavelength (distance between waves). (B) The Doppler effect when the source of sound is moving and the listener is stationary. The source moves toward the listener a distance of V_0/f during each vibration, so that the distance between wavefronts in the direction of the listener is $(a - V_0)/f$, where f equals frequency at the source.

by the factor $[1 + (V_0/a)]$. A listener moving toward the source at half the speed of sound hears a frequency 1.5 times that of a stationary listener.

Now consider a stationary listener and a source moving at speed V_0, as shown in Figure 29-11B. The wavefronts are no longer concentric circles; they are more closely spaced in the direction the source is moving. If the frequency of the sound emitted at the source is f, then during each vibration, the source moves a distance V_0/f. The wavelength in the direction of motion is thus shortened by V_0/f, becoming $\lambda' = (a - V_0)/f$. The waves themselves are traveling at speed a, so that the frequency heard by the stationary listener is

$$f' = a/\lambda' = af/(a - V_0) = f[1/(1 - V_0/a)] \qquad (27)$$

Now, if the source is moving at half the speed of sound toward the listener, the apparent frequency doubles. Compare this with the preceding situation in which the listener is moving and the apparent frequency increases by only 50 percent.

Doppler ultrasound systems combine the two situations shown in Figure 29-11. The initial acoustic source is a stationary transducer, and the sound from this device is scattered from a moving target (e.g., red blood cells). The scattered sound then returns to a stationary listener: the receiving transducer. In effect, the target is a moving listener hearing a stationary source; the target then reradiates the sound as a moving source toward a stationary listener. The frequency heard by the receiving transducer is obtained by combining equations (26) and (27):

$$f' = f\left[\frac{1 + V/a}{1 - V/a}\right]. \qquad (28)$$

In this example, we have assumed that the target is moving toward the ultrasound transducers at speed V. If the target is moving at half the speed of sound, the observed frequency is increased by a factor of 3! Because changes in the frequency of sine waves can be measured precisely, the Doppler principle provides a very accurate method of measuring the velocities of moving sound reflectors. At the high frequencies often used (5 megahertz, MHz, or more), objects as small as red corpuscles can scatter enough sound for detection.

Echocardiography

Using recently developed esophageal transducers, echocardiography has become a popular intraoperative monitoring technique.[19,20] Sound waves in the 2- to 10-MHz range are transmitted toward the heart in short bursts or pulses. After each pulse, the transducer passively listens to the reflected echoes from various tissues. The ability to place the transducer in the esophagus is advantageous, as sound does not then have to pass through air spaces or bone on its way to and from the heart. The speed of sound through the heart and surrounding soft tissues is a nearly constant 1,540 m/s. Thus, the elapsed time between transmission of the pulse and receipt of the echo provides the distance to the reflecting structure. The sound beam from the transducer is projected in a narrow "searchlight" pattern, so that the exact direction of reflecting structures is also known.

In early echocardiography, the sound beam was aimed in a fixed direction and the intensity of the echo was plotted against distance from the transducer. The resulting display was called motion-mode (M-mode) or "one-dimensional" echocardiogram. Because it looks in only on direction, M-mode echocardiography provides very limited information. However, it can sample very rapidly in this one direction, being able to change its display up to 1,000 times/s. Therefore, M-mode echocardiography provides excellent time resolution of rapidly moving objects such as mitral valve leaflets. Modern ultrasound imagers vary the direction of the sound beam by sweeping it through an arc of roughly 90 degrees. This sweep produces a two-dimensional (2-D) echocardiogram that shows reflecting structures in a plane. Although 2-D echocardiography shows much more of the heart at a given time, its time resolution is slower than that of M-mode echocardiography: the former can produce only 15 to 100 pictures/s.[21]

Two-dimensional echocardiography has recently incorporated Doppler analysis.[22,23] Moving reflectors shift the frequency of the reflected signal (eq. [28]). This shift is indicated by a change in color of the display, in which red usually indicates motion toward the transducer and blue indicates motion away from the transducer. This seems an unfortunate choice of colors, as a light source (e.g., a star) moving *away* from the observer is shifted toward the red end of the spectrum.

Many aspects of anesthesiology and physiology rely on an understanding of the physics of fluids. Several good introductory and intermediate texts are available.[11-13,16,24-26] In the field of acoustics, the classic text is that of Lord Rayleigh[17]; more modern books are also helpful.[27,28]

MEASUREMENTS OF ELECTRICITY AND MAGNETISM

Most monitors in the operating room and intensive care unit use electrical or magnetic phenomena. As shown in Figure 29-1, nearly all transducers have some form of electrical energy as their output, and the subsequent signal processing and data display are entirely electrical. This section reviews some basic principles of electricity and magnetism; these principles are then applied to specific monitors. Particular emphasis is placed on techniques monitoring physiologic "signals" that are electrical in nature (i.e., electrocardiography and electroencephalography). This section also discusses mass spectrometry as a practical application of the principles of electromagnetism.

Electricity

Basic Principles of Electricity and Circuits

Before discussing specific applications, let us review some fundamental principles governing electricity and circuits. There are only two types of electrical charge: *positive* and *negative*, so named by Benjamin Franklin in the 1700s.[29,30] Franklin knew that in some materials (*conductors*), these charges were free to move, whereas in other materials (*insulators* or *dielectrics*), they were not. Franklin also realized that like charges create a repulsive force and that opposite charges create an attractive force. However, it was Coulomb in 1785 who first showed that the force (F) between two point electric charges follows an inverse-square law[31]:

$$F = (1/4\pi\epsilon_0)(q_1 q_2/r^2) \tag{29}$$

where q_1 and q_2 are the magnitudes of the charges in units of coulombs, r is the distance separating the charges, and ϵ_0 is the *permittivity constant*. The electric force vector is directed along the line between the two charges; a positive force in equation (29) indicates repulsion (q_1 and q_2 are of the same sign). The force vector that would be exerted on a unit charge at a given point in space is called the *electric field* at that location. The electric field E is a vector with a magnitude and direction specified at every point in space.

A battery can be thought of as an electrochemical device that generates positive charges at one conducting terminal and negative charges at another. If the two battery terminals are connected by a conductor, charges flow from one terminal to the other, creating an *electric current* I, defined as the quantity of charge flowing per unit time. Although it is actually the negative charges (electrons) that move in metallic conductors, the direction of the current is defined in terms of the direction in which positive charges would flow were they free to move. The SI unit for electric current is the coulomb per second, or ampere (A).

If the material connecting the two terminals is a less-than-perfect conductor, as all materials are, the battery must provide the electrical field required to move charges through this resistance (Fig. 29-12). If an electrical force F is applied through a distance d to move a unit charge between points A and B, then we know from a previous discussion (eq. [8]) that the work done on the charge is $W = Fd$. We now define the work done in moving a unit charge from point A to point B (Fig. 29-12) as the *potential difference V* between these two points. The dimensions of potential difference are force × distance/charge or work/charge, and the SI unit is the joule per coulomb, or volt (V). The potential difference generated by a battery between its terminals is called the *electromotive force* (EMF) of the battery.

Let us now connect a particular conductor to the

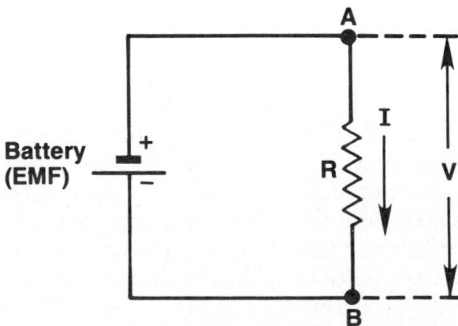

Fig. 29-12. Schematic of battery and resistor. The battery uses chemical energy to generate electromotive force (EMF), which provides the electric field required to move current I through resistance R. The potential difference V across the resistor is proportional to current and resistance (i.e., $V = IR$).

terminals of several batteries having different values for EMF. For most metals at constant temperature, the relationship between the potential difference V and current I is linear (Ohm's law):

$$V = IR \qquad (30)$$

where R is *resistance*, its dimensions being force $\times$ length $\times$ time/charge^2, and its SI unit the volt per ampere, or ohm (Ω). Although many materials do not obey Ohm's law (eq. [30]), most metals do. The resistance of metals generally increases with temperature but for carbon varies inversely with temperature.

The amount of work done per unit time, or rate of work, is called the *power* (P). The dimensions of power are force $\times$ distance/time or ML^2/T^3, and the SI unit is the joule per second, or watt (W). Another common unit of power is the *horsepower*, which equals 746 W. The power required to drive a current I through a resistance R is easy to calculate. For each unit charge moved from point A to B (Fig. 29-12), the amount of work done is the potential difference V. The quantity of charge being moved between the two points per unit time is the current I. The total work done per unit time is thus the product of the two (work/time = work/charge $\times$ charge/time):

$$P = VI \qquad (31)$$

We can use equation (30), Ohm's law, to eliminate either V or I from this expression:

$$P = I^2 R = V^2/R \qquad (32)$$

The power used to drive current through a resistance is dissipated as heat. Current flowing through a fixed resistance thus generates heat in proportion to the square of the current (eq. [32]). If the current is doubled, heat production quadruples. This *Joule heating* causes electrical equipment to become warm. It also produces the local heating around an electrocautery electrode and causes electrical skin burns at sites of high current density. Current density J is simply the current per unit cross-sectional area of the conductor. Common units for heat are related to power units as follows: 1 W = 0.239 cal/s = 0.860 kcal/h.

Multiple resistances to the same battery or power supply can occur in two ways: in series (Fig. 29-13A) or in parallel (Fig. 29-13B). Resistances occurring in series are additive, because the same current I must pass through them all:

$$V = IR_1 + IR_2 + IR_3 = I(R_1 + R_2 + R_3) = IR_s \quad (33)$$

The series resistance R_s is simply the sum of all the individual resistances. For resistances occurring in parallel, the current through the individual resistors varies, but all have the same potential difference V:

$$I_1 = V/R_1, \qquad I_2 = V/R_2, \quad \text{and} \quad I_3 = V/R_3 \quad (34)$$

The total current from the battery is the sum of the three branch currents:

$$I = I_1 + I_2 + I_3 = V(1/R_1 + 1/R_2 + 1/R_3) = V/R_p \quad (35a)$$

where

$$1/R_p = 1/R_1 + 1/R_2 + 1/R_3 \qquad (35b)$$

R_p is the net resistance, which is thus less than the smallest of the parallel resistances.

This discussion of combining resistances is valid

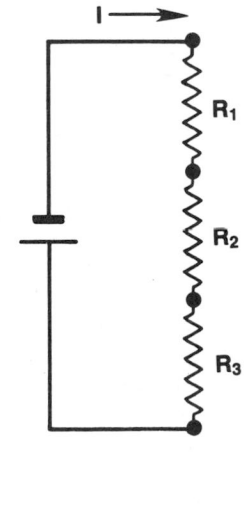

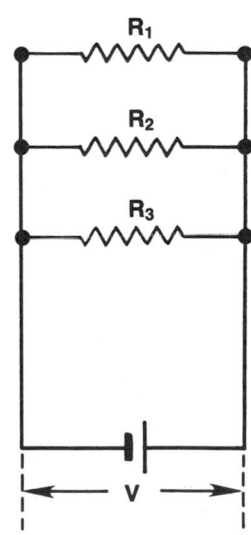

A

B

Fig. 29-13. **(A)** Resistances occurring in series to a battery. Current I is the same in R_1, R_2, and R_3. According to Ohm's law, the net series resistance is the sum of the individual resistances ($R_p = R_1 + R_2 + R_3$). **(B)** Resistances occurring in parallel to a battery. R_1, R_2, and R_3 each have the same potential difference (V) given by the electromotive force of the battery. The total current I is the sum of the three branch currents. The reciprocal of the net parallel resistance is the sum of the reciprocals of the individual resistances ($1/R_p = 1/R_1 + 1/R_2 + 1/R_3$).

whether the source of EMF is a direct current (dc) battery or an alternating current (ac) generator such as that used to deliver commercial electrical power. The EMF or voltage of an ac supply varies sinusoidally with time:

$$V(t) = A \sin (2\pi f t) \qquad (36)$$

where A is the amplitude or peak voltage, and f is the frequency of the power supply (60 Hz in the United States, 50 Hz in Europe). The specified voltage of an ac supply generally refers to the RMS value of $V(t)$, which equals 0.707 times the peak value (A) for a sinusoidal waveform.

The physiologic *signal* for an electrocardiogram (ECG) or electroencephalogram (EEG) is a small fluctuating voltage measured on the surface of the skin. The amplitudes of these voltages are on the order of 1.5 millivolts (mV) for the ECG and 0.1 mV for the EEG. These small signals travel through relatively long wires before reaching the electronic amplifiers that boost their amplitudes, and are therefore subject to interference and attenuation from several sources. One of these sources is *capacitance*, a property that provides an alternative conductive pathway for ac signals. A capacitor is a device that can accumulate charge but does not conduct direct current, as shown by the example of the parallel plate in Figure 29-14. The charge Q accumulated on the two parallel plates is proportional to the applied potential difference V; hence, $Q = CV$. The proportionality constant C is called the capacitance and has dimensions of charge²/(force × distance). The SI unit for capacitance is the coulomb per volt, or *farad* (F), which is such a large unit that use of smaller units —the *microfarad* (10^{-6} F) and *picofarad* (10^{-12} F)— has become common. A capacitor stores charge, and thereby electrical potential energy, in a way analogous to the storage of mechanical potential energy by a spring.

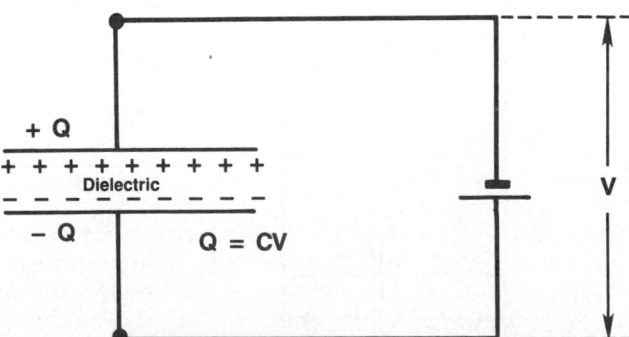

Fig. 29-14. The parallel plate capacitor consists of two conducting parallel plates separated by a dielectric (insulator). When a potential difference V is applied, opposite charges Q accumulate on the two plates. Current ceases to flow, and no further charge accumulates when $Q = CV$, where C is the capacitance of the plates.

If we apply a dc voltage V to a capacitor at time $t = 0$, current flows until the capacitor builds up a charge $Q = CV$, at which time the current reaches zero. (The current falls exponentially from time $t = 0$, as given by $I = (V/R)\exp(-t/RC)$, where R is the internal resistance of the battery.) The effective resistance or *reactance* of a capacitor to a dc voltage is therefore infinite after an initial transient (a temporary current caused by a sudden change in voltage). However, for an ac-applied voltage, the charges stored on the capacitor plates must alternate in sign, and so a current flows to and from the capacitor while the charge is changing. Higher ac frequencies require faster rates of change of charge and hence higher currents. The *capacitive reactance* for an ac voltage (the ratio of the peak voltage to the peak current) is thus given by the following equation:

$$R_c = 1/(2\pi f C) \qquad (37)$$

where f is frequency. Note that at very high frequencies, R_c approaches zero and the capacitor becomes a *short circuit*. One can now see why unwanted or "stray" capacitances between EEG signal wires and electrical ground have some importance.

Capacitances often occur in series or parallel. For capacitors connected in parallel (Fig. 29-15A), the potential difference V is the same across all three capacitors and the total accumulated charge Q is the sum of the individual charges:

$$Q = Q_1 + Q_2 + Q_3 = (C_1 + C_2 + C_3)V = C_p V \qquad (38)$$

where C_p is the net parallel capacitance. Thus, C_p is the sum of the individual capacitances. For capacitances connected in series (Fig. 29-15B), one uses the fact that the charges on each of the three capacitors must be the same. Thus, the potential differences are as follows:

$$V_1 = Q/C_1, \qquad V_2 = Q/C_2, \quad \text{and} \quad V_3 = Q/C_3 \qquad (39)$$

The total potential difference is the sum of these three series potentials:

$$\begin{aligned} V &= V_1 + V_2 + V_3 = Q(1/C_1 + 1/C_2 + 1/C_3) \\ &= Q/C_s \end{aligned} \qquad (40)$$

where C_s is the net series capacitance, derived as follows:

$$1/C_s = 1/C_1 + 1/C_2 + 1/C_3 \qquad (41)$$

Capacitors connected in series combine in the same way as resistors connected in parallel.

Capacitive reactance and resistance are two forms of impedance, the property of materials that describes their resistance to electrical currents. One additional form of impedance, inductance, will be discussed later under the subject of magnetism.

Electrocardiography and Electroencephalography

Electrical potentials on biologic surfaces, including those manifesting on the ECG and EEG, are too small to observe directly and must be amplified and processed

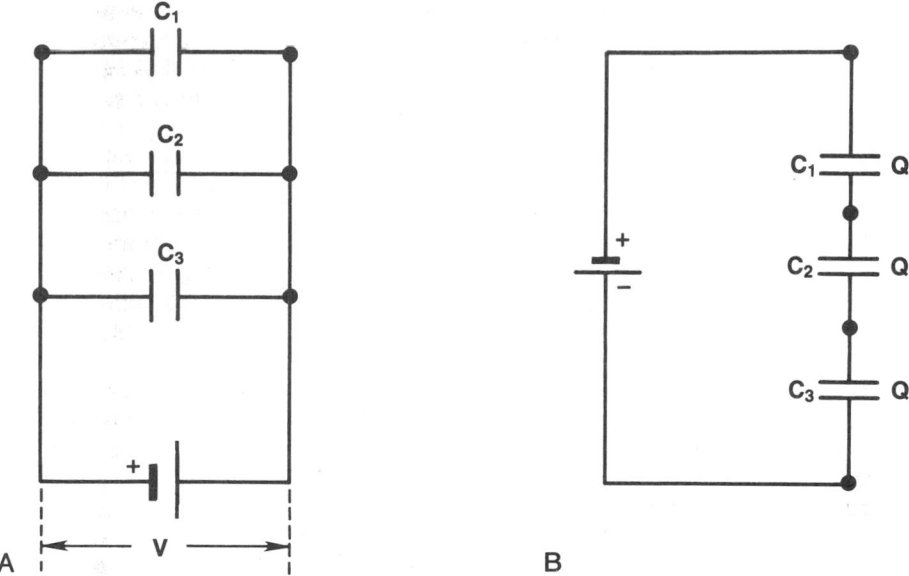

Fig. 29-15. (A) Capacitors connected in parallel to a battery. The potential differences V across individual capacitors C_1, C_2, and C_3 are the same, and the total charge is cumulative. The net parallel capacitance is the sum of the individual values. **(B)** Capacitors connected in series to a battery. The charges Q on C_1, C_2, and C_3 are the same, and the potential differences are additive. The reciprocal of the net series capacitance is the sum of the reciprocals of the individual values.

before display. As noted, ECG potentials on the skin are in the 1-mV range, and EEG potentials are near 0.1 mV. On the other hand, near-field somatosensory evoked potentials (SSEPs) are in the 5-microvolt (μV) range (1 μV = 10^{-6} V) and far-field SSEPs are another order of magnitude smaller.[32-34] Thus, the problems of signal transmission and processing become progressively more difficult.

Figure 29-16 shows why electrical potentials on biologic surfaces are so small.[35] The electrical potentials generated by the heart are measured by two skin electrodes, A and B. The contact of the electrode with the skin effectively forms a capacitor with the dry, keratinized layer forming the dielectric between the two parallel plates. Because the keratinized epidermis is not a perfect insulator, shunt resistance R_s occurs in parallel with skin capacitance C_s. This resistance would be a megaohm (MΩ) (10^6 Ω) or more if the electrode were dry. However, the use of conducting electrolyte jelly reduces resistance to a few hundred ohms. Impedance between electrode and skin is thus highest for a dc voltage and becomes smaller at high frequencies (eq. [37]).

Before reaching the skin, the current from the source of EMF (the heart) passes through a network of resistors representing tissue impedances. The series resistors R_1 and R_2 represent the impedance of tissues located between the heart and the surface of the body. The shunt resistors R_3, R_4, and R_5 represent conduction pathways leading between the two pathways from the heart to the electrodes. Because tissues tend to be arranged in concentric layers below the surface, and because imped-

ance between two points within the same tissue is generally less than that between equally spaced points in different tissues, these shunt resistances tend to have lower values than the series resistances. The network shown in Figure 29-16 forms a *voltage divider*.

Clearly, lower shunt resistances or higher series resistances result in smaller ECG signal voltages at points A and B. Furthermore, capacitance C_s presents a lower impedance to higher-frequency signals than to low-frequency signals (eq. [37]). The actual biologic potential from the heart is not a sine wave but can be represented as a summation of sine waves, as in the case of the pressure waveform discussed earlier. The skin capacitance passes the higher harmonics of this Fourier series in preference for the lower ones, thus distorting the shape of the original waveform.

Processing of Small Signals

The preceding example illustrates how a capacitor can form a *high-pass filter* (i.e., a filter that tends to pass the higher frequencies and attenuate the lower ones). The simplest high-pass filter is shown in Figure 29-17A. The source of fluctuating EMF, V_i, is connected to the filter output through capacitance C. This output is also connected to a ground by means of a *load resistor R*. (*Ground* refers to a conductor that is always held at an electrical potential of 0 V. A ground provides an infinite source of, or "sink" for, electrons for conductors maintained at any nonzero potential.) If the capacitive

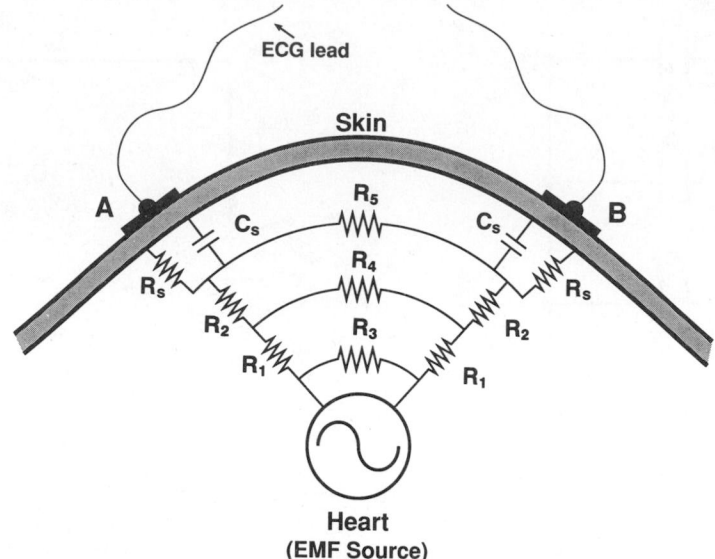

Fig. 29-16. Schematic representation of surface potentials picked up by the electrocardiograph (ECG). The source of electromotive force (EMF), the heart, is connected to the ECG surface electrodes by means of series resistors (R_1, R_2, R_s) and shunt resistors (R_3, R_4, R_5). Skin also possesses a capacitance, C_s.

reactance (eq. [37]) is R_c, the output voltage V_0 of this divider is

$$V_0/V_i = R/(R_c + R)$$
$$= R/(1/2\pi fC + R)$$
$$= 2\pi fRC/(1 + 2\pi fRC) \qquad (42)$$

Note that as frequency f approaches infinity, V_0 approaches V_i. As f approaches zero, V_0 approaches zero. At very low frequencies, a doubling in frequency (raising f by an octave) doubles the output voltage V_0. We use a logarithmic decibel scale to define *gain*, as we did for sound pressure levels (eq. [22]):

$$\text{gain (dB)} = 20 \log (V_0/V_i) \qquad (43)$$

Doubling V_0 thus represents a change in gain of 6 dB ($20 \times \log 2$), so that the low-frequency slope of this single-stage, high-pass filter is described as 6 dB per octave.

The high-pass filter of Figure 29-17A can be converted to a low-pass filter by simply reversing the locations of the resistor and capacitor (Fig. 29-17B). The capacitor would then be shunting the high-frequency components of the signal to ground, while allowing the low frequencies to pass through. The formula for voltage divider for this filter becomes

$$V_0/V_i = R_c/(R_c + R)$$
$$= 1/2\pi fC/(1/2\pi fC + R)$$
$$= 1/(1 + 2\pi fRC) \qquad (44)$$

Now, as f approaches infinity, the output V_0 approaches zero. As f approaches zero, V_0 becomes equal to V_i. Contrast this with the behavior of the high-pass filter (Fig. 29-17A; eq. [42]). If we combine a high-pass filter

with a low-pass filter in series, we obtain a *band-pass filter*, which passes only the signal components whose frequencies lie between the upper and lower band-pass limits. The slope of the "skirts" can be made greater than 6 dB per octave by using more sophisticated filters than those shown in Figure 29-17. The ECG and almost all other analog signal processors incorporate band-pass filters to remove noise at frequencies above and below the range of interest. Low-frequency noise in the ECG originates from respiration or other patient motion, whereas high-frequency noise comes from electrocautery or other electrical equipment. A frequency band from 0.05 to 100 Hz is considered adequate for diagnostic purposes. Modern ECG monitors often allow selection of two band-pass filter modes. The one labeled diagnostic is the wide-band mode, usually 0.05 to 100 Hz. The monitoring mode incorporates a narrower band-pass (e.g., from 0.1 to 50 Hz). Although this mode "cleans up" the signal by reducing motion artifacts and 60-Hz interference, it also distorts the QRS complex; such distortion can lead to erroneous interpretation of ST segments.[36]

Because of their small amplitudes, biologic potentials require considerable amplification as well as filtering before display or interpretation. These small signals, carried by unshielded wires (e.g., ECG leads), are subject to interference from a variety of sources in the operating room: 60-Hz power lines, electrical lights, and electrocautery. These sources of electromagnetic radiation (discussed below) can induce spurious voltages that are superimposed on the desired signal. To minimize this electrical "noise," biologic potentials are processed through a differential amplifier (Fig. 29-18). The output of a differential amplifier is proportional to

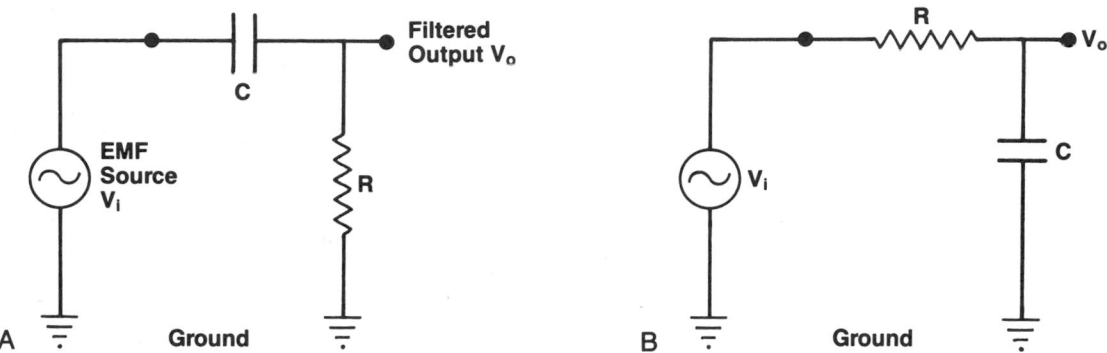

Fig. 29-17. **(A)** The resistance-capacitance high-pass filter. Capacitor *C* presents lower impedance to a source of high-frequency fluctuating electromotive force (EMF), V_i, allowing more current to flow through load resistor *R*. Output voltage V_0 thus increases with frequency. **(B)** The resistance-capacitance low-pass filter. The capacitor tends to shunt high frequencies to ground while leaving low frequencies unattenuated. Combining the two filters in Figs. A and B yields a band-pass filter, which attenuates all signal frequencies outside the designated pass band.

the *difference* between the voltages applied to the two inputs. If the two wires leading to these inputs are kept close together, the interference signals from electromagnetic noise are the same in both. This *common-mode signal* is removed by the subtraction of the two inputs. The common-mode rejection property makes the differential amplifier well suited to the measurement of biologic potentials and other small signals.

The shunt resistances shown in Figure 29-16 (R_3, R_4, R_5) require that ECG and other surface electrodes be placed far apart to maximize the surface potentials. On the other hand, common-mode interference is made worse when electrodes and leads are farther apart. Electrocautery is a particularly difficult source of interference, because the high frequencies used (near 10^6 Hz) make it a more efficient electromagnetic radiator. The electric fields induced in the body by electrocautery lie mainly in the direction between the cautery probe and the grounding pad. Therefore, if ECG electrodes are placed in a line perpendicular to this direc-

tion, the cautery-induced voltages at the two electrodes are nearly the same and are rejected as a common-mode signal. Although this explanation has been over-simplified, electrocautery-induced interference with the ECG can certainly be reduced by judicious selection of an ECG axis.

If a dc voltage is applied between two body-surface electrodes, current flows through the tissues between them. Although the electrical current in metals consists entirely of electron flow, in tissues, both positive and negative ions migrate. Negative ions tend to accumulate at the positive electrode (the *anode*), and positive ions accumulate at the negative electrode (the *cathode*). This collection of *anions* and *cations* near each electrode creates its own EMF, and this force opposes the EMF that set up the original current. The current therefore decreases, so that the effective impedance between the electrodes increases.

This phenomenon, which is called *polarization of electrodes*, has two harmful effects. First, the increased

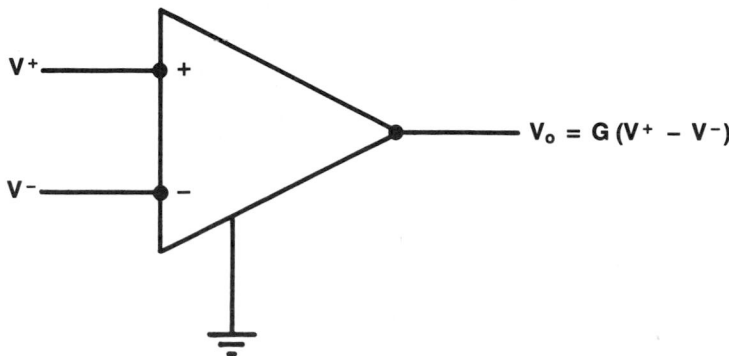

Fig. 29-18. The differential amplifier. Output voltage V_0 is proportional to the difference between the two input voltages V$^+$ and V$^-$. Both inputs are isolated from ground. The differential amplifier is used in many small-signal applications because it removes the "common-mode" signal representing interference with the desired biologic signal. $G = V_0/(V^+ - V^-)$.

impedance from polarization can attenuate the ECG signal for several seconds after defibrillation or dc cardioversion. Such attenuation could be misinterpreted as a lack of electrical activity, resulting in inappropriate administration of a second shock. The second consequence of prolonged application of dc voltage is accumulation of a local concentration of toxic ions near electrode sites, a condition that can cause burns or tissue necrosis. A partial solution to the problem is use of a nonpolarizable electrode, such as a silver and silver chloride combination. This electrode can act as a source of, or "sink" for, both anions and cations, thereby minimizing accumulation of ions. Most disposable ECG electrodes now use such materials. However, even these electrodes are nonpolarizable for only a limited time, and application of prolonged dc voltages between any tissue electrodes must be prevented.

Magnetism

Basic Principles of Magnetism

Although magnetic phenomena have been known for centuries, their relationship to electricity was first reported in 1820 by Oersted, who observed that an electric current in a wire caused movement of a compass needle.[30] An electric current was also found to attract certain metals (iron, nickel, cobalt), which were then called *ferromagnetic*. This discovery led to the concept of magnetic flux density, or *magnetic induction*, a vector that is defined as follows. If a particle having charge q moving at velocity v experiences a force directed perpendicular to the direction of motion, a magnetic field is present. The magnetic force is proportional to the product of the charge q, the velocity vector v, and the induction B of the field, according the following relationship:

$$F = qv \times B \qquad (45)$$

The product of the vectors v and B is the *cross-product*, which is a vector perpendicular to both v and B, having magnitude $vB \sin \theta$, where θ is the angle between v and B. The direction of the force can be determined by applying the "right-hand rule": when the right thumb points in the direction of v and the index finger points in the direction of B, the palm faces the direction of F. The direction of an electrical force is specified by the electric field E. However, to determine the direction of magnetic force, one must know the directions of both induction B and velocity v.

The dimensions of induction B are force/charge/velocity, and the SI unit is the newton/coulomb per meter/second, defined as the *tesla*. An older unit of induction still in use is the *gauss*, which equals 10^{-4} teslas. The earth's magnetic field has an induction of approximately 0.5 gauss in the United States, directed roughly 60 degrees downward from the horizontal. The induction of a magnetic resonance imager is 1 to 2 teslas, or 40,000 times the strength of the earth's field.

Mass Spectrometry

The mass spectrometer, once an esoteric laboratory research tool, is now a common operating room monitor of the concentrations of respiratory gases. This device operates on the principle that a moving ion of each species of gas, when exposed to a magnetic field, has a certain trajectory, based on the ratio of the charge of the ion to its mass (q/m). For a particle of charge q moving at velocity v in an electric field E and a magnetic induction B, the force on the particle is

$$F = qE + qv \times B \qquad (46)$$

As shown in Figure 29-19, the mass spectrometer first ionizes and accelerates the gas molecules by means of an electric field E. The moving ions then pass through a magnetic field oriented perpendicular to their direction of motion (directed off the page in Fig. 29-19). The sideways magnetic force deflects the trajectory of each type of particle through angle α. The deflecting force is proportional to charge q (eq. [46]), and the sideways acceleration from this force is inversely proportional to mass m (eq. [1]). Therefore, the angle of deflection α is a function of q/m. This angle and the ion flux are determined by photodetectors, and the concentration of each species of gas is thereby found.

Relationships between Current and Magnetic Field

The magnetic force on a moving particle given by equation (45) can also be used to derive the force exerted on a wire carrying a current through a magnetic field. If a length L of wire carrying current I is placed in a field of strength B oriented perpendicular to the wire, the force exerted on the wire is

$$F = ILB \qquad (47)$$

The direction of the force can be determined using the right-hand rule, as described. Because a magnetic field exerts a force on any moving charge or current, it is not surprising that an electric current itself generates a magnetic field. For the simplest case of a long, straight wire carrying a current I, the magnetic induction B at a distance r from the wire is proportional to I/r. The direction of B lies in a series of concentric circles in a plane perpendicular to the wire. The relationship between electric current and the induced magnetic field is called *Ampere's law*.[37]

In 1831, Faraday discovered the final link between electricity and magnetism: a loop of wire moved through a stationary magnetic field experiences an "induced" electric current, as shown in Figure 29-20A.[38] If the motion of the wire or the direction of the magnetic field is reversed, the current reverses. In Figure 29-20B, when the switch is closed and current begins to flow through loop B, the magnetic field created by loop B induces a current through loop A. When the current

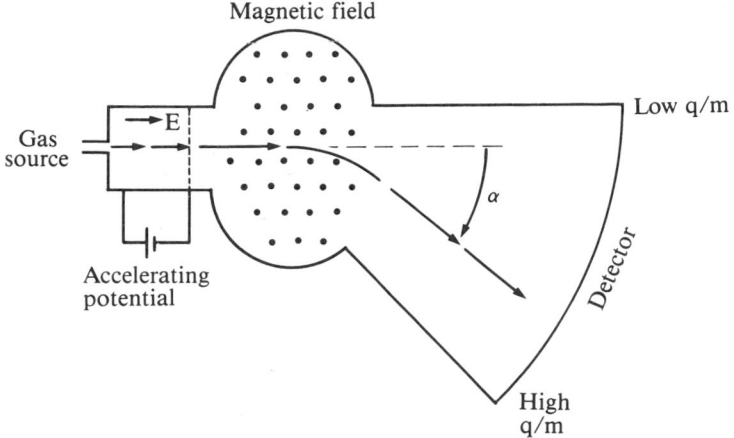

Fig. 29-19. The mass spectrometer. Gas molecules at low pressure are ionized and accelerated by an electric field *E*. The ions then pass through a perpendicular magnetic field *B* that deflects their trajectories through an angle α. This deflection angle, determined by the ratio of charge to mass (q/m) of the ions, is used to identify the species of gas.

through loop B reaches a constant value, the current through A falls to zero. Thus, it is the *rate of change* of the magnetic field that causes the induced current in both cases. The description of the relationship between the two is called the *Faraday law of electromagnetic induction*.

Electric generators and transformers are applications of Faraday's law. A generator is a device that changes mechanical energy into electrical energy by moving loops of wire through a stationary magnetic field, or vice versa: either the field or the wire can be moving. By inducing electric current in these wires, the mechanical power required to turn the generator is converted into electrical power, which can be either ac or dc, depending on the switching connections to the wires.

A transformer is a device that transfers energy from one current circuit to another, usually with a change in voltage. The transformer consists of two sets of wire coils near each other, operating on the principle shown in Figure 29-20B. The changing magnetic field produced by the varying current in the primary coil induces a current in the secondary coil. The ratio of the voltage in the secondary coil to that in the primary coil equals the ratio of the numbers of loops in the secondary and primary coils. Transformers work only for alter-

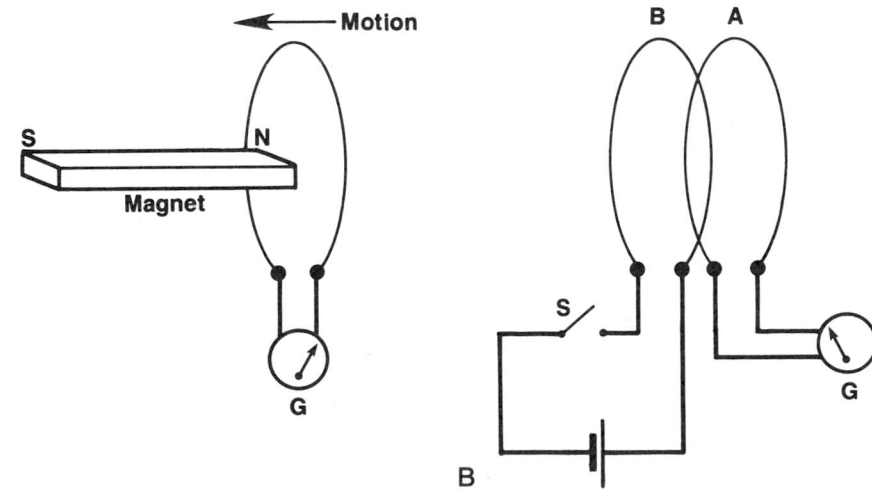

Fig. 29-20. **(A)** A loop of wire moving through a magnetic field induces an electric current. As long as the wire is moving in relation to the magnet, current flows through galvanometer G. **(B)** A changing current in one loop induces a current in a nearby loop by means of its magnetic field. When switch S is closed and current begins to flow in loop B, induced current flows through loop A. When the current through loop B reaches a steady value, the current through loop A ceases.

nating current. They are commonly used in the operating room to isolate power supplies for equipment from electrical ground, thus increasing safety.

Electromagnetic Flowmeters

The electromagnetic flow probe uses the same principle as the electric generator to measure the flow of an electrically conducting fluid (e.g., blood) in a tube. As shown in Figure 29-21, the probe applies a magnetic field B perpendicular to the direction of flow. Because the conducting fluid is moving, ions in the fluid are subject to a magnetic force directed perpendicular to both the field and the direction of motion (eq. [45]). This force drives positive ions to one side and negative ions to the other, thus setting up an EMF across the tube. The flow probe measures the induced EMF with a pair of electrodes in the wall of the tube. If the tube in question is a blood vessel, the measuring electrodes can be placed on the outer wall. In actual practice, a rapidly alternating magnetic field is used and the induced EMF is alternating current. Although these flow probes can measure blood flow through large vessels accurately and instantaneously, they have several limitations. The cross-sectional area of the vessel must be known in order to compute volume flow (flux). Also, the blood vessel must be dissected free to place the transducer around it. Consequently, transducers of different sizes must be available.

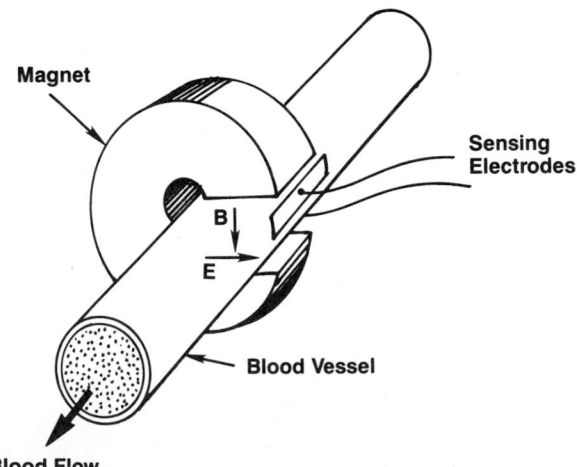

Fig. 29-21. The electromagnetic flow probe measures the flow of an electrically conducting fluid (in this case, blood) in a tube by applying a magnetic field *(B)* perpendicular to the direction of flow. As the conducting fluid flows through the magnetic field, positive ions are deflected to one side and negative ions to the other, setting up an electric field *(E)* perpendicular to both the magnetic field and the direction of flow. This electric field creates an electromotive force (EMF) between the sensing electrodes that is related to the volume of flow.

Inductance

When a current flowing through a coil of wire is changing, the resulting varying magnetic field induces an EMF in that same coil. This induced EMF opposes the original current. This phenomenon is called *self-induction*, the third type of electrical impedance; resistance and capacitance are the first and second. The self-induced EMF is proportional to the time derivative of the current through the coil:

$$V = L(dI/dt) \qquad (48)$$

The constant L is called the *inductance* of the coil; its SI unit is the volt-second per ampere, which is called the *henry* (H). For a sinusoidally varying ac voltage of frequency f, the reactance (ratio of peak voltage to peak current) of an inductor is given by $2\pi fL$. Thus, the inductor has no impedance to a dc voltage ($f = 0$), whereas the capacitor has infinite impedance to a dc voltage. The voltage-current relationships and reactances of the three types of impedance are summarized in Table 29-1.

All electrical cables and leads possess a small amount of inductance as well as resistance, which implies that their impedance will increase at high frequencies. Unwanted inductance can thus limit the high-frequency response of electronic signal processing equipment.

This section has focused on fundamental principles of electromagnetism and their application in monitoring. For the interested reader, there are many good texts describing these principles in more mathematical detail,[39-42] as well as some fascinating historical sources.[29-31,37,38,43] We have also discussed electronic components and circuits superficially, and there are a number of good introductory texts on this subject as well.[44-48]

MEASUREMENTS OF LIGHT

The most complex optical transducer in use today in the operating room was also the first monitor employed—the human eye. Although the eye is invaluable as a patient monitor, it has two basic limitations. First, it can be easily distracted. Second, it does not monitor quantitatively. The past decades have seen several new monitoring systems that use optical sensors to

TABLE 29-1. The Voltage-Current Relationships and Reactances for Three Types of Impedance

Impedance (SI Unit)	Voltage	Reactance for ac Signal
Resistance (ohm)	IR	R
Capacitance (farad)	Q/C	$1/(2\pi fC)$
Inductance (henry)	$L(dI/dt)$	$2\pi fL$

Abbreviations: SI, Système International d'Unités; AC, alternating current; I, electric current; R, resistance; Q, charge; C, capacitance, a proportionality constant; f, frequency; L, inductance of the coil, a constant; d, differential; t, time.

measure physiologic variables quantitatively by absorption or reflection of light. This section describes the basic principles governing these optically based monitors.

Electromagnetic Radiation

Every substance having a temperature above absolute zero ($-273°C$) emits electromagnetic radiation. All electromagnetic radiation travels at the same velocity, the speed of light (c). This velocity varies only with the medium in which the radiation travels. In a vacuum, the speed of light is 2.9979×10^8 m/s, or approximately 186,000 mi/s. The form of radiant energy associated with heat, thermal radiation, is just a portion of the electromagnetic spectrum. As a propagating periodic wave, electromagnetic radiation can be characterized by a frequency f or a wavelength λ, the two being related by the speed of light:

$$f = c/\lambda \tag{49}$$

Wavelength can be expressed in meters, micrometers (μm, 10^{-6} m), nanometers (nm, 10^{-9} m), or angstroms (Å) (10^{-10} m). Figure 29-22A illustrates the breadth of the electromagnetic spectrum, ranging from cosmic rays (wavelength of 10^{-5} nms) to radio and television waves (wavelength of 1 to 10 m). Visible light comprises a very narrow portion of this spectrum, ranging from violet light at 430 nm to red light at 690 nm (Fig. 29-22B). Monitoring devices commonly use light in the visible and infrared range.

As we shall see, the energy of electromagnetic radiation is directly proportional to its frequency. Light in the x-ray and ultraviolet range contains sufficient energy to ionize molecules. Visible and ultraviolet light can stimulate chemical reactions. However, when red or infrared radiation is absorbed, the energy is sufficient only to increase vibrational and rotational energies in the molecules. Because chemical reactions are not induced, exposure of living tissues to red and infrared light is safe. The SI unit for luminous intensity of light is the *candela*. One candela is the luminous intensity emitted by a black surface having an area of 1/600,000 of a square meter at the temperature of melting platinum (2,046°K).[49] A more frequently used measure of the intensity of light is the candle, which is defined as 1/60 of the intensity of light emitted from one square centimeter of a black surface at a temperature of 2,046°K.

Light Sources

Visible and infrared light demonstrates several properties common to all electromagnetic radiation. Light represents a form of energy that, when passing through matter, may be reflected, transmitted, or absorbed. Although light itself cannot be stored, it can be converted into some other form of energy such as electricity, chemical energy, or heat. In addition, light can be generated from other forms of energy, including heat (incandescence), electrical (gas discharge), and chemical (photoluminescence) energies, each of which will be

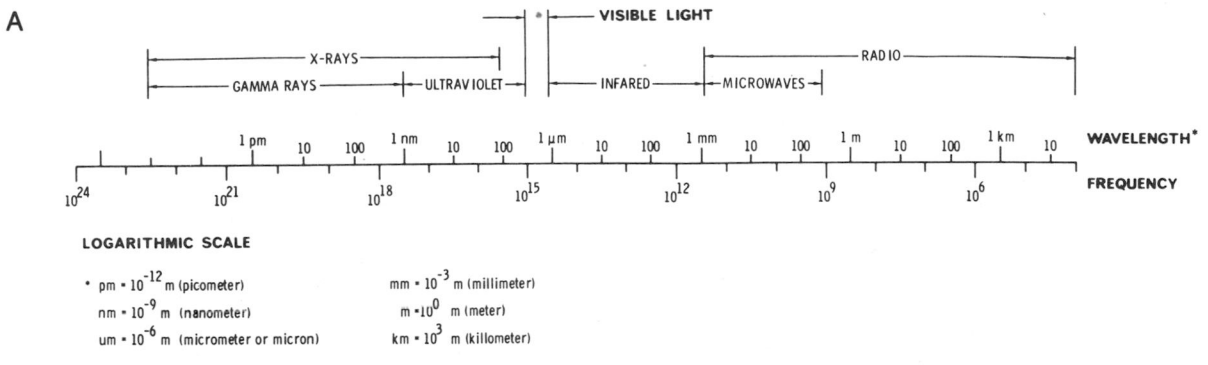

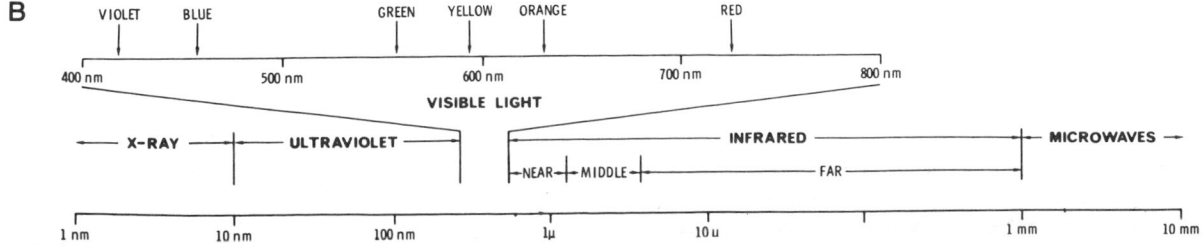

Fig. 29-22. **(A)** The electromagnetic spectrum. **(B)** The optical spectrum. Monitoring devices most frequently use light in the visible and near-infrared range.

discussed. The light produced by these mechanisms can be described in terms of the composition, intensity, and direction of its wavelengths. As noted previously for arterial pressure and acoustic waveforms, any periodic wave can be expressed as a summation of sine waves (Fourier series).

Generating light from heat (thermal emission) produces a spectrum of radiation generally confined to the regions of infrared, visible, and ultraviolet light. The total emissive power of a surface is related to its temperature:

$$Q = KT^4 \qquad (50)$$

where Q = total radiation energy per unit surface area in watts per square centimeter (W/cm²); K = the Stefan-Boltzmann constant (5.67×10^{12} W/cm²/°K⁴; and T = absolute temperature (°K). As the temperature rises, the intensity of radiation increases as the fourth power of T, and the peak wavelength of emission decreases from that of infrared light to that of visible light (Fig. 29-23).[15] When the surface temperature approaches 6,000°K, the emission occupies most of the visible light spectrum and appears white like sunlight. This inverse relationship between peak emission wavelength and temperature is known as Wein's displacement law. The peak emission wavelength is more a

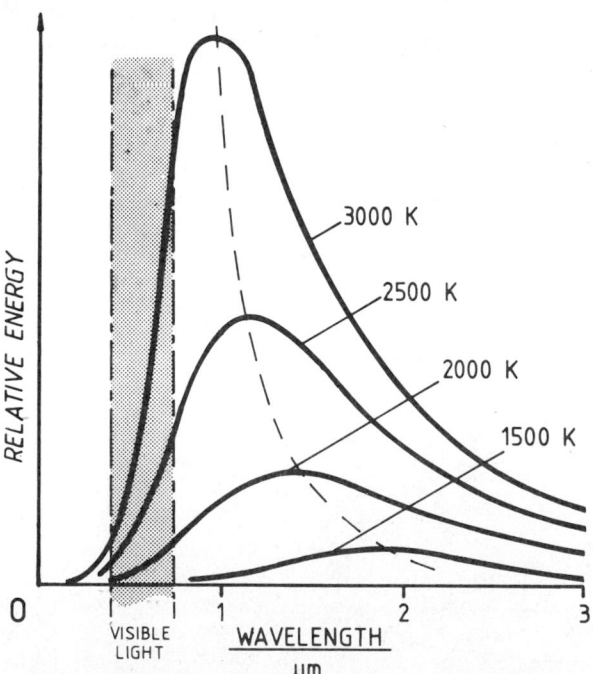

Fig. 29-23. Electromagnetic radiation is emitted from all objects having a temperature higher than absolute zero. The peak wavelength of this emission, which is in the near-infrared range, decreases as the temperature of the emitting source increases. The phenomenon is called Wein's displacement law. (From Mushin and Jones,[15] with permission.)

function of the temperature of the emitter than the material of which the emitter is composed.

In contrast to thermal emission, electrochemical emitters produce a spectrum of single wavelengths or narrow bands that are characteristic of the emitting material. This photochemical emission is not described by classic electromagnetic wave theory but by the quantum theory developed by Planck and Einstein. A detailed description of their theory is beyond the scope of this text but can be summarized briefly as follows.

The quantum theory postulates that when matter emits or absorbs energy, it does so in discrete packets, or *quanta*, of energy. The energy (E) of these electromagnetic radiation quanta is proportional to their frequency. The proportionality constant is called *Planck's constant, h*:

$$E = hf, \qquad (51)$$

where E = the energy of the photon in joules or electron volts (eV; 1 eV = 1.6×10^{-19} J); and h = Planck's constant (6.63×10^{-34} J-s).

When the wavelengths of these energy quanta are in or near the visible range of light, they are referred to as *photons*. Photons of a specific energy are either emitted or absorbed by a material that is changing between two given energy states. Single atoms can increase their energy state by having their electrons change from a lower to a higher energy level (Fig. 29-24).[50] The frequency of light emitted when an electron changes to a lower energy level can easily be calculated. For an electron in a hydrogen atom that drops from an E_3 level to an E_2 level (Fig. 29-24), the frequency of emitted light is

$$
\begin{aligned}
f &= (E_3 - E_2)/h \\
&= (12.09 - 10.20 \text{ eV})/(6.63 \times 10^{-34} \text{ J-s}) \\
&\quad \times 1.6 \times 10^{-19} \text{ J/eV} \\
&= 4.56 \times 10^{21}/\text{s}
\end{aligned} \qquad (51a)
$$

The hydrogen atom, having only one electron and one proton, has fewer possible energy levels than a complex atom having many electrons. Molecular energy can also take the form of translational motion (velocity), and polyatomic molecules can absorb additional energy by increasing their vibrational or rotational energy states. Consequently, a complex molecule having many atoms and electrons can emit and absorb energy at so many levels that the resulting spectrum appears to be a continuum of emitted or absorbed energy, as opposed to discrete quanta. The absorption or emission wavelength spectrum can be used as a "fingerprint" to identify a substance. Because this spectrum is a property of the substance, a specific material absorbs and emits light of the same energy spectrum. This phenomenon is known as *Kirchhoff's law:* "A substance which emits light of a certain wavelength at a given temperature can also absorb light of the same wavelength at that temperature."[15] Therefore, if radiation from a heated source emitting a continuous spec-

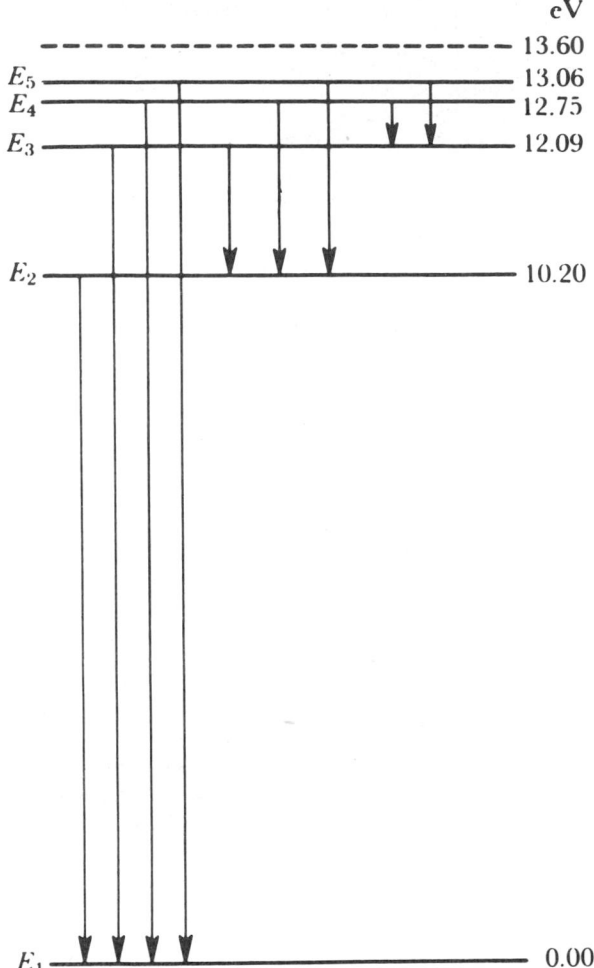

eV

E_5 —————————————————— 13.60
E_4 ——— 13.06
E_3 ——— 12.75
——— 12.09

E_2 ——— 10.20

E_1 ——— 0.00

Fig. 29-24. This figure is a schematic illustration of the energy levels (e.g., E_1, E_2) of the electronic orbitals of the hydrogen atom. The energy of each level listed in electron volts (eV) may be converted to joules (1 eV = 1.6×10^{-19} J). As an electron changes from one energy level to another, it must either absorb or emit energy equal to the difference between the two energy levels. If this energy is in the form of electromagnetic radiation, its frequency (f) can be easily determined by $\Delta E = hf$, where h = Planck's constant (6.63×10^{-34} J-s).

trum is passed through a vapor, the absorption spectrum obtained is deficient in those wavelengths that the vapor itself would emit if it were raised to the same high temperature. This fact provides the basis for all absorption spectrophotometry.

The discussion of light sources thus far has described broad-spectrum polychromatic emitters and narrow-spectrum monochromatic emitters. If a specific wavelength of light is needed in a device, that wavelength can be produced by using either a broad-spectrum emitter and light filters, or a narrow-spectrum emitter, if one is available for that wavelength.

The light-emitting diode (LED) is a remarkable solid-state monochromatic (single-wavelength) emitter.

Diodes, like other solid-state devices, are produced from pure crystals of semiconductive material such as silicon or germanium. A current flows in these semiconductors only when a specific threshold EMF is applied. This minimum energy is required to move electrons into a higher energy state within the crystal so they can move freely and conduct electricity. The electron moves from a *valence band* up to a *conduction band* (Fig. 29-25). The number of electrons in the outer shell and the energy required to boost them into higher levels can be varied by adding "impurity" atoms having more or fewer electrons. This process is called *doping*. If the impurity adds excess electrons (negative charges), it is called an *n-type semiconductor*. Conversely, if the impurity produces a deficiency of electrons, or "holes" (positive charges) as they are called, it is referred to as a *p-type semiconductor*. An LED is produced from the junction of a *p-* and an *n-type* semiconductor.[51] Light is emitted at the *p-n* junction when electrons flowing across the junction drop into a lower energy state and emit photons (Fig. 29-25). LEDs are commercially available in the visible and infrared light ranges. Even though, in theory, a specific LED should emit only one wavelength of light, in fact, there is a narrow emission spectrum having a peak or center wavelength. In addition, as stated for thermal emitters, this peak or center wavelength shifts as a function of the temperature of the diode. LEDs may also have multiple emission peaks because of changes in several levels of electron energy.

When dilute gases of simple molecules or atoms are excited electrically, they emit discrete spectral lines related to the allowable electronic energy states. This process is called *gas discharge* and is used in neon lights and lasers. This method of generating light is not used in clinical monitoring devices, with the exception of lasers, which are used in Raman scattering. Lasers are discussed in more depth in the section, *Raman Scattering*.

Light Detectors

Monitoring devices that use light emission in their transducers require a matched light detection system. The retina of the eye is a complex light detector, sensitive to a wide range of intensities emanating from many polychromatic emitters. Light detection systems are based on the same basic principle of physics governing light sources (i.e., Kirchhoff's law). Detector systems can then be classified into two general categories: thermal and photoelectric detectors.[52]

Thermal detectors can be further subdivided into two types, thermoelectric and thermoexpansion sensors.[52] Two examples of thermoelectric sensors are thermocouples and thermopiles. A *thermocouple* is an electrical circuit used to measure temperature (Fig. 29-26). It is composed of two metals having conduction band electrons at different energy levels. If one of the two metal junctions is kept at a different temperature from

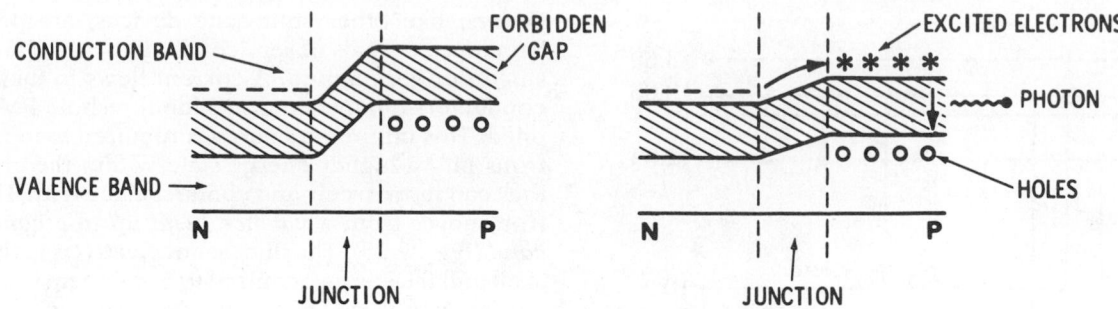

Fig. 29-25. A light-emitting diode (LED) is formed from the junction of a *p-n* semiconductor, as illustrated in the schematic. The frequency of emitted light is determined by the difference in energy levels between the electrons at the junction. See text for fuller explanation of *p-* and *n*-type semiconductors and LEDs. (From Mims,[51] with permission.)

the other, electrons tend to flow from the higher energy level to the lower energy levels, causing a small EMF. One junction is kept at a reference temperature while the other metal junction acts as the sensor. A *thermopile* is a solid-state photodetecting device that employs many microscopic thermocouples in series. The surface of the thermopile absorbs light, causing a small temperature change in the microthermocouples. This change in turn produces a voltage change in the detector circuit. A thermopile is a broad-spectrum light detector, just as a thermal emitter is a broad-spectrum light source.

A normal mercury thermometer is an example of a thermoexpansion device. Light is absorbed by the mercury, thereby increasing its translational energy and expanding and increasing the height of the column of thermometer fluid. Early infrared gas analyzers used sealed chambers of carbon dioxide (CO_2) as a thermopneumatic detecting system. Carbon dioxide is known to absorb infrared light, which heats the CO_2 gas and causes it to expand. As a result, pressure in the CO_2 cell increases. The pressure in the cell causes movement of a diaphragm, which is calibrated to the intensity of light at the specific wavelength absorbed by CO_2.

Photoelectric detectors also fall into two groups, photodiodes and photoconductive devices.[52] The *photodiode* is a solid-state device produced from a *p-n* junction of semiconductor material and is analogous in principle to a light-emitting diode (Fig. 29-27). When light is absorbed, electrons flow across the *p-n* junction and produce a small current. Most photodiodes absorb light from the visible to near-infrared range and are therefore ideal mates to the light-emitting diode.

A *photoconductor* is another solid-state light-detecting device, similar in principle to the photodiode. It is usually made of lead sulfide. When a bias voltage is applied across the device, a small current flows. When light hits the detector, photons are absorbed, boosting more electrons into the conduction band and thus allowing current to flow more easily (i.e., decreasing the

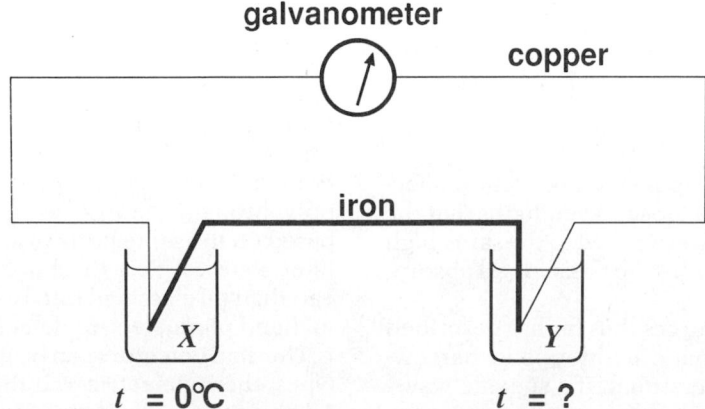

Fig. 29-26. A thermocouple is an electrical circuit used to measure temperature. Two dissimilar metals (usually wires) are joined at the ends. The electrons of these metals have different energy levels. If the two junctions have different temperatures, a voltage results (the Seebeck effect). Absorption of radiation induces a change in temperature in the sensing element, which is called the "hot" junction. The other junction, the "cold" junction, is shielded from radiation and kept at a reference temperature. (From Wilson and Hawkes,[52] with permission.)

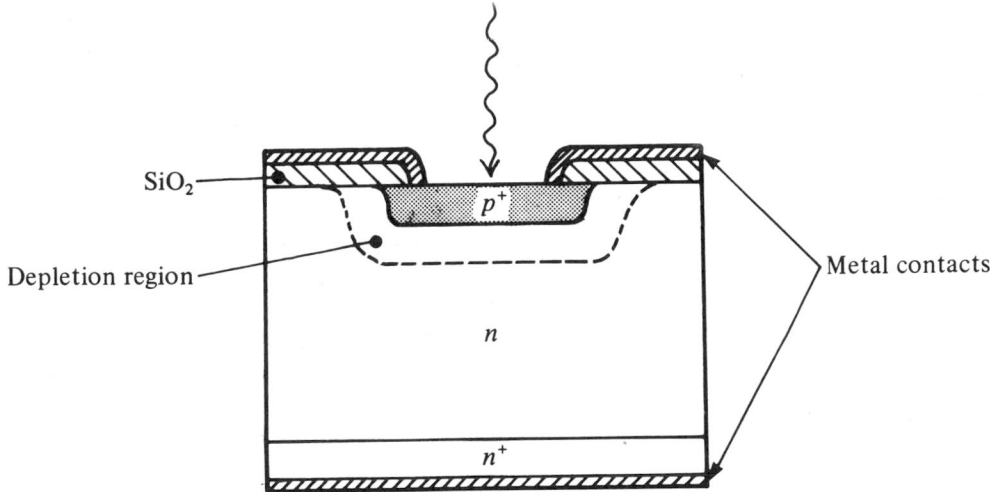

Fig. 29-27. Typical silicon oxide (SiO_2) photodiode structure for photoconductive operation. A junction is formed between a heavily "doped" p-type material ($p+$) and a lightly "doped" n-type material so that the depletion region extends well into the n-type material. "Doping" is the addition of "impurity" atoms having more or fewer electrons than the original substance, the purpose being to create either p- or n-type material. (From Wilson and Hawkes,[52] with permission.)

resistance of the circuit). Photoconductors can be used as light detectors over a wider range of wavelengths than photodiodes.

Absorption, Reflection, Scattering, and Transmission of Light

Light Absorption and the Beer-Lambert Law

When light passes through matter, it is transmitted, absorbed, or reflected. The relative absorption or reflection of light is used in several monitoring devices to estimate the concentrations of dissolved solutes. The field of absorption spectrophotometry is based on the Beer-Lambert law. This optical law is a composite. The first part, Lambert's law, states that when a parallel beam of light falls on a semitransparent, homogeneous substance, the intensity of the transmitted light decreases exponentially as distance through the substance increases:

$$\log I_i / I_t \propto d \tag{52}$$

where I_t = the intensity of the transmitted light; I_i = the intensity of light incident to the substance; and d = the distance the light is transmitted, or the path length of the light. The second part, Beer's law, states that if a parallel beam of light is transmitted a known distance through a clear solution with a dissolved solute, the intensity of the transmitted light decreases exponentially as the concentration of solute increases. Beer's law assumes that the solvent is transparent to the frequency of light used, whereas the solute is at low concentration (C) and absorbs the frequency of light used:

$$\log I_i / I_t \propto C \tag{53}$$

Combining these laws produces

$$\log I_i / I_t = dCE \tag{54}$$

where E is an absorbance coefficient called the *molar extinction coefficient* for the specific solute. The Beer-Lambert law is illustrated in Figure 29-28.[53] The right side of equation (54) represents the absorbance (A) of the system:

$$A = dCE \tag{55}$$

The Beer-Lambert law can then be written in the form

$$I_t = I_i e^{-A} \tag{56}$$

The molar extinction coefficient (E) is a constant for the given molecular species at a specified wavelength. Figure 29-29 is a plot of the molar extinction coefficients for the most common species of hemoglobin as functions of wavelength in the red and infrared range.[53] For multiple solutes, absorbance (eq. [55]) is rewritten as follows:

$$A = d_1 C_1 E_1 + d_2 C_2 E_2 + d_3 C_3 E_3 + d_4 C_4 E_4 \tag{57}$$

Because the distance of light transmission (d) is the same for all four solutes,

$$A = d(C_1 E_1 + C_2 E_2 + C_3 E_3 + C_4 E_4) \tag{57a}$$

If absorbance is measured at a specific wavelength λ and the extinction coefficients at that wavelength are known for the four species, the preceding equation would contain four unknowns: $C_1, C_2, C_3,$ and C_4. Four wavelengths (i.e., four equations) would be needed to solve for these four unknowns.

Laboratory oximeters measure the concentration of the four species of hemoglobin using this system of

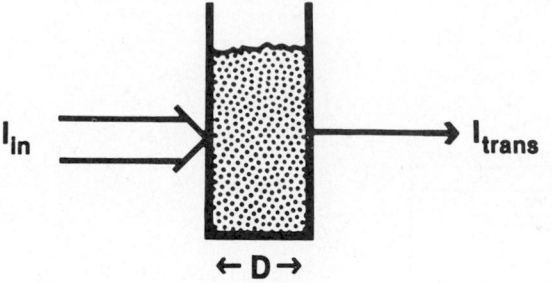

Fig. 29-28. The Beer-Lambert Law. The concentration of a known solute dissolved in a clear solution can be determined by measuring the intensity of the incident light (I_{in}) and the intensity of the transmitted light (I_{trans}) if the path length *(D)*, the wavelength of light, and the extinction coefficient of the solute are known. (From Payne and Severinghaus,[79] with permission.)

Beer-Lambert equations. These devices transmit four or more wavelengths through a cuvette filled with a solution of lysed red blood cells. If methemoglobin and carboxyhemoglobin were not present in the blood sample, then the concentrations of oxyhemoglobin and reduced hemoglobin could be determined by using only two wavelengths of light. Note in Figure 29-29 that at approximately 805 nm, the extinction coefficients for oxyhemoglobin and reduced hemoglobin are the same.

The point at which extinction coefficients are equal is called an *isobestic point.* If an oximeter used this wavelength of light and no methemoglobin or carboxyhemoglobin were present, equation (57a) would reduce to

$$A = dE_{805}(C_1 + C_2) \tag{57b}$$

Thus, the sum of $C_1 + C_2$ (i.e., oxyhemoglobin and reduced hemoglobin) could be determined with one wavelength at the isobestic point.

The Beer-Lambert law can be applied to measuring concentration in mixtures of gases and vapors, as well as dilute liquid solutions. Some of the engineering principles involved in applying this basic Beer-Lambert theory to the development of monitoring devices will be discussed later.

Light Reflection

The preceding discussion illustrates how light absorption can be used to measure the concentration of a solute. Incident light that is reflected or back-scattered from a solute can also be analyzed to determine concentration. The theory pertaining to reflected light from dissolved particles is more complex than the theory of absorption spectrophotometry, because the intensity of reflected light depends on not only the concentration of the solute but also the depth of penetration of the light into the solution. The equations govern-

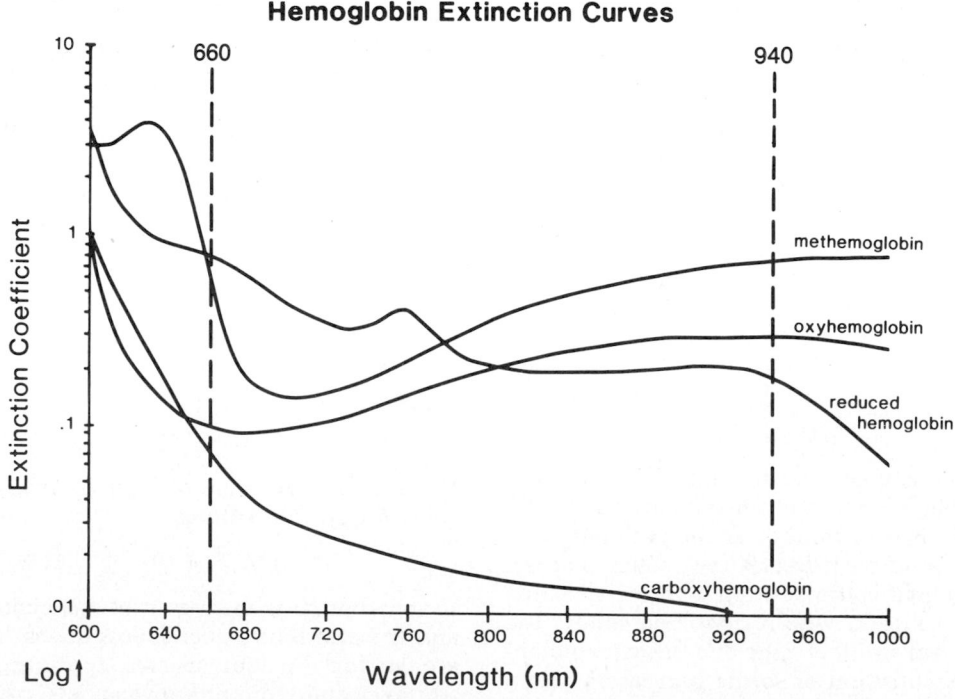

Fig. 29-29. Extinction coefficients are plotted against the transmitted light absorbance spectra in the wavelength range of interest (red and infrared range) for four species of hemoglobin. Any point in which two species have the same extinction coefficient is known as an isobestic point. An isobestic point occurs for oxyhemoglobin and reduced hemoglobin at 805 nm. (Courtesy of Susan Manson, Biox/Ohmeda, Boulder, Colo.)

ing reflectance are therefore semiempirical but similar to those of absorption spectrophotometry.

The primary application of reflectance spectrophotometry in clinical monitoring is that of the Oximetric pulmonary artery catheter.[54] This device continuously monitors the saturation of hemoglobin with oxygen in mixed venous blood ($S\bar{v}O_2$) by means of fiberoptic transmission of reflected light from a catheter placed in the pulmonary artery. The general principle is that oxyhemoglobin reflects more red light than does reduced hemoglobin, whereas in the infrared wavelengths, the two hemoglobins species reflect similarly (Fig. 29-30). Early clinical devices developed in the 1960s use the following linear relationship to calibrate hemoglobin saturation empirically to the ratio of the intensities of reflected light.[54]

$$S\bar{v}O_2 = A + Br \qquad (58)$$

where A and B are calibration constants, and r is the ratio of the intensities of reflected red and infrared light. Unfortunately, this assumption of a linear relationship was not sufficiently accurate. Linearity was affected by pH, hematocrit, and blood flow velocity.[54] Adding a third wavelength of light and a more complex nonlinear empirical relationship resulted in more accurate estimations of saturation.

Technical problems with calibration, vessel wall artifact, and quality of fiberoptics delayed the development of these monitors until the 1980s. Early devices were either calibrated in vitro using milk of magnesia as a uniform reflecting suspension or calibrated in vivo by obtaining a sample of mixed venous blood.[54] Improvements in production of plastic fiberoptics and the development of digital processing for rejection of artifacts

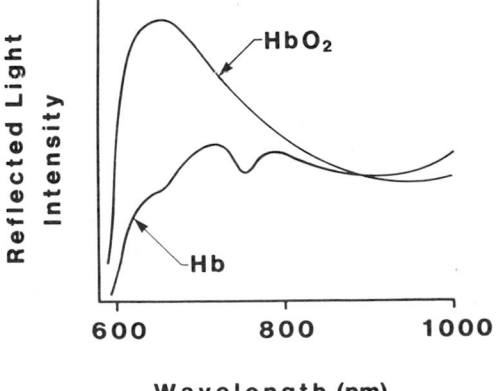

RELATIVE REFLECTION
OF Hb AND HbO$_2$

Fig. 29-30. The relative intensity of reflected light from reduced hemoglobin (Hb) and oxyhemoglobin (HbO$_2$) is plotted as a function of the wavelength of light. (From Sprindy and Senelly,[80] with permission.)

ultimately led to the production of reliable fiberoptic catheters. The algorithms for calculating $S\bar{v}O_2$ assume that no dyshemoglobins (i.e., no carboxyhemoglobin or methemoglobin) are present. The presence of these dyshemoglobins may lead to erroneous results.[55]

Raman Scattering

We stated earlier that light of a specific energy can be absorbed by, or emitted from, a substance depending on its allowable levels of vibrational, rotational, and electronic energy. Another absorption and reemission phenomenon of light scattering occurs in a very small percentage of interactions. In this process, *Raman scattering*, light in the visible and ultraviolet range is absorbed by molecules of a substance, thereby producing unstable vibrational or rotational energy states,[56] schematically illustrated in Figure 29-31.[57] Because these excited states are unstable, some of the absorbed energy is immediately re-emitted, allowing the molecule to relax into a stable state. Raman scattering occurs very infrequently; therefore, most photons pass through the gas sample without taking part in this particular absorption-re-emission phenomenon. If the intensity of the transmitted light is sufficiently great, the Raman-scattered signal can be measured and used to identify the molecules within the gas sample. Because the signal is scattered light, it is emitted in all directions relative to the incident beam.[56,57] The Raman light is of low intensity, so it is best to measure it at right angles to the high-intensity exciting beam (Fig. 29-32).

An advantage of Raman scattering over gas analysis based on absorption of infrared light is that a spectrum of Raman scattering lines can be used to identify all types of molecules in the gas phase. Because it involves only vibrational and rotational energy states, Raman scattering cannot be used to identify single atoms. As discussed below, infrared absorption can be used to analyze molecules having a dipole moment and, therefore, cannot be used to identify oxygen or nitrogen. A disadvantage of Raman scattering as a clinical tool is the requirement for a very high-intensity light source to produce the small Raman-scattered signal. Therefore, the advent of lasers has increased the clinical usefulness of Raman scattering. Currently, argon lasers are used as light sources for gas analyzers based on this technique.[57]

The laser (an acronym of "light amplification by stimulated emission of radiation") is a source of high intensity monochromatic light. It is a gas discharge in which electrons are excited into a metastable energy state. This means that the electrons will linger in this higher energy state longer than usual. Through electrical stimulation within a vacuum tube, a large number of the electrons are excited to this metastable state. As they collide, multiple photons of the same wavelength are emitted. If the laser tube has mirrors on the opposite ends and a length that is a multiple of the wavelength of the emitted light, amplification occurs as photons are

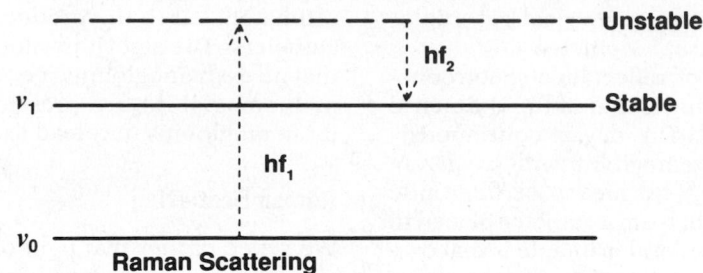

Fig. 29-31. Schematic illustration of the unstable energy states that are the basis of Raman scattering. Note that the energy levels produced are unstable when a particle drops to a stable energy state, emitting the "surplus" energy as a Raman-scattered photon. (From Gravenstein et al.,[56] with permission.)

reflected back and forth. One of the mirrors is designed to allow a portion of the light to be transmitted, producing an "exit beam" of coherent, high-intensity monochromatic light. (*Coherent* means that the wave packets of all emitted photons are in phase with one another, a property that is unique to laser light.) In theory, light-emitting diodes also produce monochromatic light; however, diodes cannot produce light of such high intensity.

Photoluminescence Quenching and the Optode

Photoluminescence is another photon emission process that occurs as an excited electron drops to a lower energy level. The initial excitation of electrons is produced by shining light on a luminescent material. Luminescent dyes emit light of a predictable intensity and frequency, given the intensity and frequency of the incident light. Specific dyes in which the process of lumi-

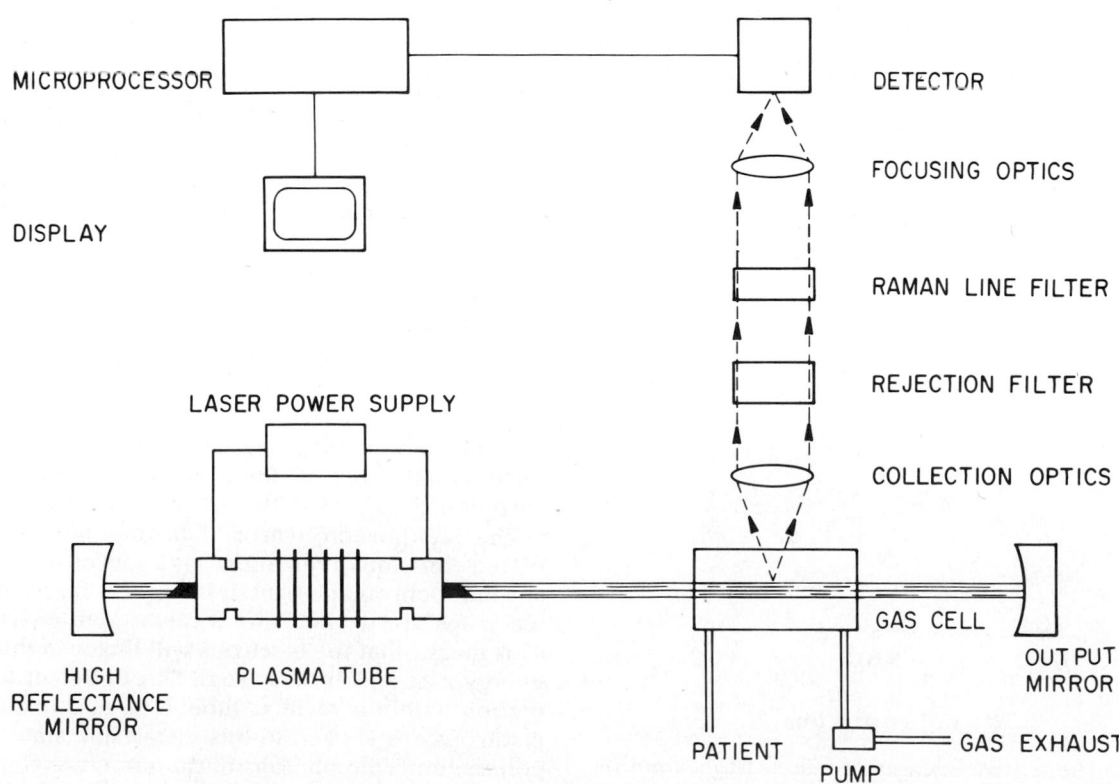

Fig. 29-32. Block diagram of the Raman spectrometer. Note that the Raman signal is collected at right angles to the laser beam. (From Westenskow et al.,[57] with permission.)

nescence is competitively inhibited by oxygen molecules are available.[58] This phenomenon, *luminescence quenching*, can be used to measure the concentration of oxygen. When more oxygen is present, more luminescence is quenched (Fig. 29-33).[59] Here the dye is illuminated with light of a specific frequency, causing electrons to rise to a higher energy level. As these electrons decay to a lower energy level, the excess energy can either be emitted as photons or added to the vibrational or rotational energy states of oxygen molecules.[58] The concentration of oxygen is inversely related to the intensity of the luminescent light (Fig. 29-34). The relationship governing this phenomenon is the Sterm-Volmer equation[59]:

$$I_{PO_2} = I_O/(1 + KPO_2) \qquad (59)$$

where I_{PO_2} = the light intensity of the luminescent signal at the PO_2 being measured; I_0 = the intensity of the luminescent signal in the absence of oxygen; PO_2 = the partial pressure of oxygen; and K = the constant for quenching.

A new fiberoptic device using the phenomenon of photoluminescence quenching for determination of oxygen concentration in the surrounding medium is called an *optode*. This device has the advantages of being small and simple to operate. The optode sensor consists of a small fiberoptic strand having a dye-encapsulated tip. Optodes can also measure pH and carbon dioxide partial pressure by addition of other dyes in the same small fiberoptic probe.[60] Initial studies have demonstrated the clinical potential of a 0.5-mm-diameter optode for continuous intraarterial monitoring of blood gases.[59–61]

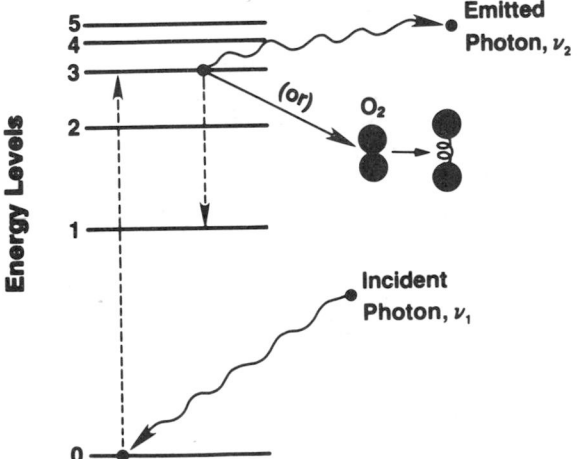

Fig. 29-33. The fluorescence quenching phenomenon. An electron of the fluorescent dye is excited to a higher energy level by an incident photon (ν_1). This excited electron can return to a lower energy level by either emitting a photon (ν_2) or interacting with an oxygen molecule and raising the latter to a higher vibrational energy levels. (From Barker et al.,[59] with permission.)

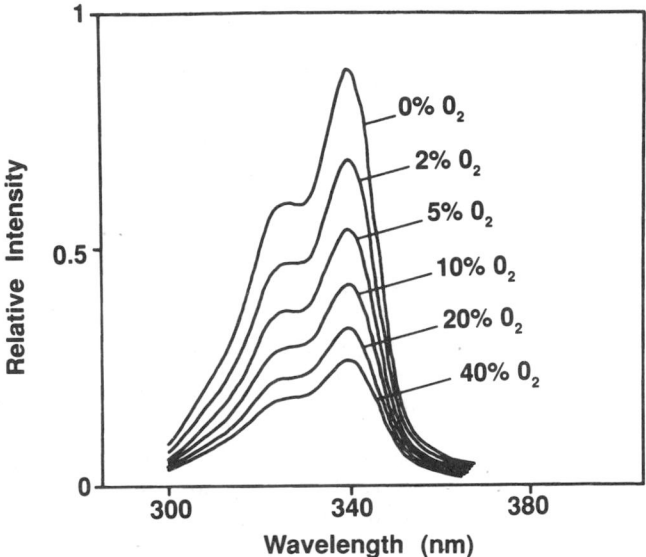

Fig. 29-34. The intensity of luminesced light *(I)* at various concentrations of oxygen. The relative light intensity of luminesced light is plotted against wavelength of light (λ) for oxygen concentrations of zero to 40 percent. The luminescent dye used is pyrene butyric acid. Note the large change in the intensity of luminesced light at oxygen concentrations of 0 to 2 percent oxygen, as compared with the relatively small change at concentrations of 20 to 40 percent. This result suggests that luminescence quenching techniques would be more accurate at lower oxygen tensions. (From Ellis,[81] with permission.)

Fiberoptic Transmission

Light has the ability not only to be reflected, absorbed, or transmitted through a substance but also to be refracted or bent as it travels from one medium to another. The speed of light depends on the medium through which the light is traveling. The refractive index of a substance (μ, which is dimensionless) is defined as the speed of light in a vacuum (c) divided by the speed of light in that substance (v):

$$\mu = c/v \qquad (60)$$

As light traverses one substance to another, its frequency remains constant. Therefore, according to equation (49), the wavelength of light must change.

Some newer monitoring devices transmit and receive optical signals through fiberoptic strands. A fiberoptic fiber ("light pipe") operates on the principle of total internal reflection. Each fiber consists of a central core of glass or plastic surrounded by cladding of another material having a much lower refractive index than the core material. Light incident on the interface of the two materials undergoes almost total internal reflection. Because of this mechanism, light can be transmitted efficiently down the fiber (Fig. 29-35). Individual fibers having very small diameters in the range of 50 to 100 μm can be produced. The use of fiberoptics in

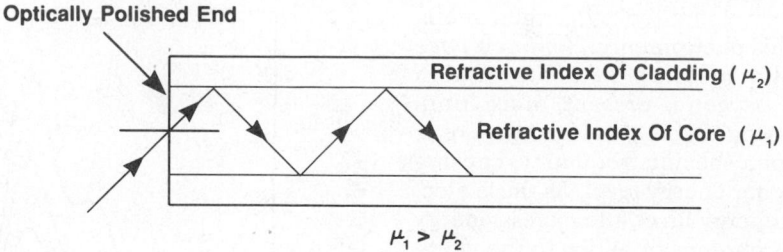

Fig. 29-35. This figure shows how light is transmitted by fiberoptic strands ("light pipes"), which are made of glass or plastic. Almost total internal reflection can be produced if the fiber is coated with a material having a refractive index (μ_2) that is much higher than that of the core fiber (μ_1). These fibers can be produced so that they have very small diameters (less than 1 μm) and they transmit light at high efficiency.

clinical monitoring has made possible the transmission of optical information to and from locations that would otherwise be impossible to monitor directly (e.g., the pulmonary artery).

Engineering Design of Optically Based Monitoring Devices

Thus far we have reviewed some of the basic principles of physics governing optically transduced devices. Production of a reliable, easily used clinical instrument involves many engineering design problems. The following section briefly discusses such problems for two commonly used operating room monitors employing optical transducers, the pulse oximeter and the capnometer.

Pulse Oximeters

Oximeters are devices that use the Beer-Lambert law to determine the concentration of hemoglobin. The first oximeters were not in vitro laboratory devices but noninvasive monitors employed in aviation research during World War II. These devices transilluminated tissue (the earlobe) with light of two wavelengths. One wavelength was sensitive to changes in oxyhemoglobin, and the other was not. In effect, the earlobe acted as a cuvette containing the solute hemoglobin. For a fascinating review of the development of pulse oximetry, the reader is referred to Severinghaus and Astrup.[62]

Before specific engineering problems are discussed, we need to define specifically what is being measured. Adult blood usually contains four species of hemoglobin: oxyhemoglobin (HbO_2), reduced hemoglobin (Hb), methemoglobin (MetHb), and carboxyhemoglobin (COHb) (Fig. 29-29). Except in pathologic conditions, methemoglobin and carboxyhemoglobin occur in only low concentrations. Because the first definitions of the saturation of hemoglobin with oxygen were based on early measurements of arterial oxygen saturation (SaO_2), they include only the two types of hemoglobin that participate in oxygen transport, HbO_2 and Hb[53]:

$$\text{functional } SaO_2 = [Hbo_2/(HbO_2 + Hb)] \times 100\%. \quad (61)$$

Development of in vitro laboratory oximeters capable of measuring many wavelengths made it possible to measure all four forms of hemoglobin. As a result, the ratio of any one species to the total hemoglobin present, the *fractional saturation*, could be determined[53]:

$$\text{fractional } SaO_2 = [HbO_2/(HbO_2 + Hb + COHb + MetHb)] \times 100\%. \quad (62)$$

From the earlier discussion of the Beer-Lambert law, it follows that an oximeter requires four wavelengths of light to measure fractional saturation. What might not be so obvious is that it also requires four wavelengths of light to measure functional saturation if MetHb and COHb are present. Even tough these two species do not appear in the definition of functional saturation, if present, they absorb light. Therefore, their possible effects must be taken into account when calculating the concentration of any species in the solution (Fig. 29-29; eq. [55]).

The pulse oximeter is an example of a device that requires substantial signal processing of the optically transduced physiologic data. The heavy dependence of the pulse oximeter on signal processing is typical of the newer generation of monitors. Although the principle governing pulse oximetry is straightforward, the application of this principle to manufacture of a clinically useful device involves significant engineering problems.[63] This section describes the clinical and physiologic problems involved in designing clinically useful oximeters and the engineering solutions to these problems. The discussion is divided into (1) basic design, (2) variability in center wavelengths of light emitted by LEDs, and (3) management of signal artifacts.

Basic Design of Pulse Oximeters

Noninvasive oximeters measure red and infrared light transmitted through, and reflected by, a tissue bed. Accurate estimation of SaO_2 using this method entails several technical problems. First, there are many light absorbers in the path of transmitted light other than arterial hemoglobin (e.g., skin, soft tissue, and venous and capillary blood). The pulse oximeter takes into account the effect of absorption of light by tissue and

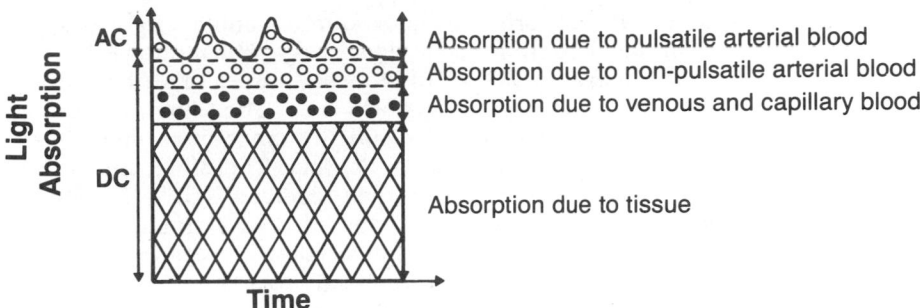

Fig. 29-36. Schematic representation of the absorption of light by living tissues. Note that arterial blood (the ac component) is the only pulsatile component in the series of light absorbers in living tissues. The dc component represents all of the nonpulsatile absorbers. (Adapted from Ohmeda Pulse Oximeter Model 3700 Service Manual,[83] with permission.)

venous blood by assuming that only arterial blood pulsates. Figure 29-36 illustrates schematically the series of absorbers in a typical sample of living tissue. At the top of the figure is the "ac" component, which represents absorption of light by the pulsating arterial blood. The "dc" (baseline) component represents absorption of light by the tissue bed, including venous, capillary, and nonpulsatile arterial blood. The pulsatile expansion of the arteriolar bed increases the path length (eq. [55]), thereby increasing absorbance. Pulse oximeters use only two wavelengths of light: 660 nm (red light) and 940 nm (near-infrared light). The pulse oximeter first determines the ac component of absorbance at each wavelength and then divides this value by the corresponding dc component to obtain a "pulse-added" absorbance that is independent of the intensity of incident light. The oximeter then calculates the ratio R of these pulse-added absorbances, which is empirically related to SaO_2[53]:

$$R = (ac_{660}/dc_{660})/(ac_{940}/dc_{940}). \qquad (63)$$

Figure 29-37 shows a typical pulse oximeter calibration curve. The actual curves used in commercial devices are based on experimental studies in human volun-

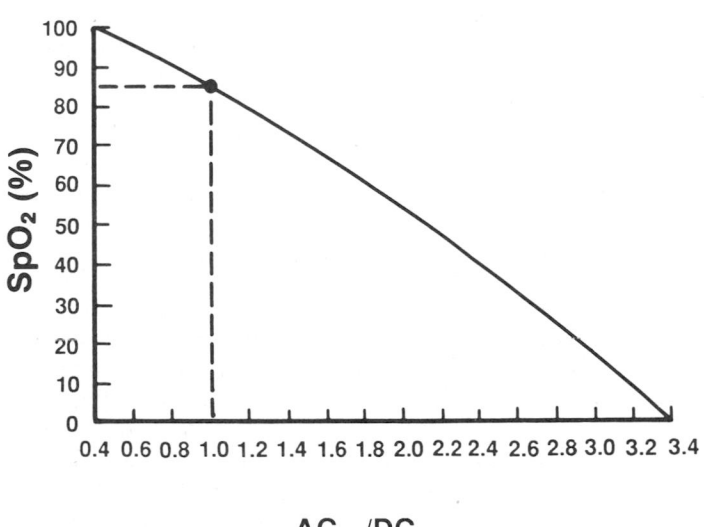

$$R = \frac{AC_{660}/DC_{660}}{AC_{940}/DC_{940}}$$

Fig. 29-37. A typical pulse oximeter calibration curve. Note that arterial oxygen saturation (SaO_2) is estimated from the ratio *(R)* of the pulse-added red absorbance at 660 nm (ac_{660}/dc_{660}) to the pulse-added infrared absorbance at 940 nm (ac_{940}/dc_{940}). The ratios of red to infrared absorbances vary from approximately 0.4 at 100 percent saturation to 3.4 at 0 percent saturation. Note also that the ratio of red to infrared absorbance is 1.0 at a saturation of approximately 85 percent. Although approximate determinations of this curve can be made on a theoretical basis, accurate predictions of saturation by the pulse oximeter (SpO_2) require experimental data. (Adapted from Pologe,[63] with permission.)

teers. Note that when the ratio of red to infrared absorbance is 1.0, saturation is 85 percent. This fact has clinical implications, which will be discussed later.

It was a fortuitous coincidence of technology and physiology that allowed the development of solid-state pulse oximetric sensors.[63] Light-emitting diodes are available over a relatively narrow range of the electromagnetic spectrum. Among the available wavelengths are some that not only pass through skin but also are absorbed by both oxyhemoglobin and reduced hemoglobin. For best sensitivity, the difference between the ratios of the absorbances of HbO_2 and Hb at the two wavelengths should be maximized. As seen in Figure 29-29, at a wavelength of 660 nm, reduced hemoglobin absorbs approximately 10 times as much light as does oxyhemoglobin. At the infrared wavelength of 940 nm, the absorption coefficient of oxyhemoglobin is greater than that of reduced hemoglobin.

Variability in Center Wavelengths

The LEDs used in pulse oximetric sensors are not ideal sources of monochromatic light: there is a narrow spectral range over which they emit light. The center wavelength of the emission spectrum varies even among diodes of the same type produced by the same manufacturer.[63] This variation can be ±15 nm. As seen in Figure 29-29, a shift in LED center wavelength changes the measured extinction coefficient and thus produces an error in the estimate of saturation. This source wavelength effect is greatest for the red wavelength (660 nm), because the extinction curves have a steeper slope at this wavelength.

Manufacturers have found two possible solutions to this problem. Some test all the LEDs and reject those that are outside the specified wavelength tolerances (e.g., 660 ± 5 nm). This process is expensive because of the number of LEDs rejected. That is, a narrower acceptable range increases not only accuracy but also the number of rejected LEDs. Other manufacturers program the pulse oximeter to accept several ranges of LED center wavelengths for both the red and infrared wavelengths, allowing the device to correct internally for different wavelengths.[63] This approach permits the manufacturer to use more of the available LEDs but requires a more sophisticated device that has a mechanism for identifying the sensor LED wavelengths to the pulse oximeter. Incompletely compensated variation in LED wavelength does not change the ability of the pulse oximeter to describe trends in changes in saturation but produces probe-to-probe variability in the absolute measurement of SaO_2.[63]

Signal Artifacts

Probably the most difficult engineering problem in designing pulse oximeters involves the identification of the ripple absorbance pattern of the arterial blood in a sea of electromagnetic artifacts. Artifacts have three major sources: ambient light, low perfusion (low ac-to-dc signal ratio), and motion (high ac-to-dc signal ratio). All of these sources of artifacts produce a poor signal-to-noise ratio. The photodiodes used in the sensor to detect light cannot differentiate one wavelength of light from another. Therefore, the detector does not know whether received light originates from the red-light LED, the infrared-light LED, or the room lights.

This problem is solved by alternating the red and infrared LED sources. The red LED is turned on first, and the photodiode detector produces a current resulting from the red LED plus the room lights. Next, the red LED is turned off, and the infrared LED is turned on. The photodiode signal then represents the infrared LED plus the room lights. Finally, both LEDs are turned off, and the photodiode generates a signal from the room lights alone. This sequence is repeated hundreds of times a second. In this way, the oximeter attempts to eliminate light interference even in a quickly changing background of room light.[63] Some sources of fluctuating light can cause problems in spite of this clever design. Clinically, artifacts from ambient light can be minimized by covering the sensor with an opaque shield.

Another engineering problem is that of low ac-to-dc signal ratio. When a small pulsatile absorbance signal is detected, the pulse oximeter amplifies the signal and estimates saturation from the ratio of the amplified absorbances. In this way, the pulse oximeter can estimate saturation values for a wide range of patients who generate different amplitudes for pulsatile absorbance. Unfortunately, as with a radio receiver, when a weak signal is amplified, the background noise or "static" is also amplified. At the highest amplifications (which can be up to a billion times, or 180 dB), the pulse oximeter may analyze this noise signal and generate a value from it (an SpO_2). Because the noise is usually equal in both the red and infrared signals, the ratio of the two is near unity (1.0), producing a saturation of approximately 85 percent (Fig. 29-37). This problem could be demonstrated in early pulse oximeters by placing a piece of paper in the sensor between the photodiode and the LED. Most early models amplified the background noise in searching for a pulse until they eventually displayed a pulse and saturation value.

To prevent this type of artifact, manufacturers have now incorporated minimum values for signal-to-noise ratio, below which the device displays no value for SpO_2. Some oximeters also display a low-signal-strength error message; yet others display a plethysmographic wave for visual identification of noise.

Patient motion (high ac-to-dc signal ratio) may be the most difficult artifact to eliminate. Engineers have tried several approaches to this problem, beginning with increasing the signal-averaging time. If the device averages its measurements over a longer time period, the effect of an intermittent artifact is less. This longer averaging period also slows the response time to an acute change in SaO_2. Most pulse oximeters allow the user to select one of several time-averaging modes. In addition, the designer can use sophisticated algorithms to identify and reject spurious signals. These algorithms may assess the ac-to-dc signal ratio or may check the validity of the estimate of saturation by calculating its rate of change. For example, if the estimate of saturation changes from 95 to 50 percent in 0.1 s, this sudden change may not be averaged into the displayed SpO_2, or it may be given a lower weighing factor. As stated earlier, these methods of eliminating artifacts may also affect the accuracy and response time of the pulse oximeter.[64]

Capnometers

A *capnometer* is a device that rapidly measures the concentration of carbon dioxide (CO_2) in the airway. Although mass spectrometers and gas analyzers based on Raman scattering have been used for this purpose, the infrared absorption technique is most popular. This method operates on the principle that the concentration of CO_2 can be determined by passing infrared light of a particular wavelength (approximately 4.3 μm) through a very small amount of expired gas. The CO_2 then absorbs the infrared light in proportion to the concentration of CO_2 (Fig. 29-38). As with other absorption spectrophotometers, the infrared CO_2 analyzer is based on the Beer-Lambert law.

Figure 29-39 illustrates schematically the components of a double-beam CO_2 analyzer. The light source is a broad-spectrum emitter that includes the absorption peak of interest for CO_2 (4.3 μm).[56] Next, a filter (the monochromator) allows only the wavelength of interest to be transmitted. The light is then split into parallel beams, one passing through a sample chamber having an unknown concentration of CO_2 and the other passing through a chamber having a known concentration of CO_2 (the *reference chamber*). The two chambers have the same optical characteristics. The windows on these chambers are made of sapphire, because glass would absorb infrared light. the beams from the two chambers pass through a rotating disk or chopper wheel that alternately allows the light from each beam to reach the detector. Early CO_2 analyzers were constructed in this fashion so that a single source of light and a single detector could be used. Consequently, variations in the light source or detector system would affect both beams equally and not change the relative intensity of the transmitted light. The gas sample to be analyzed is circulated through the sample chamber to provide continuous measurement of carbon dioxide.

There are two practical problems to be solved when designing a clinical capnometer. The first is the mechanical problem of using sufficiently small tubing to obtain and analyze the respiratory gas sample as

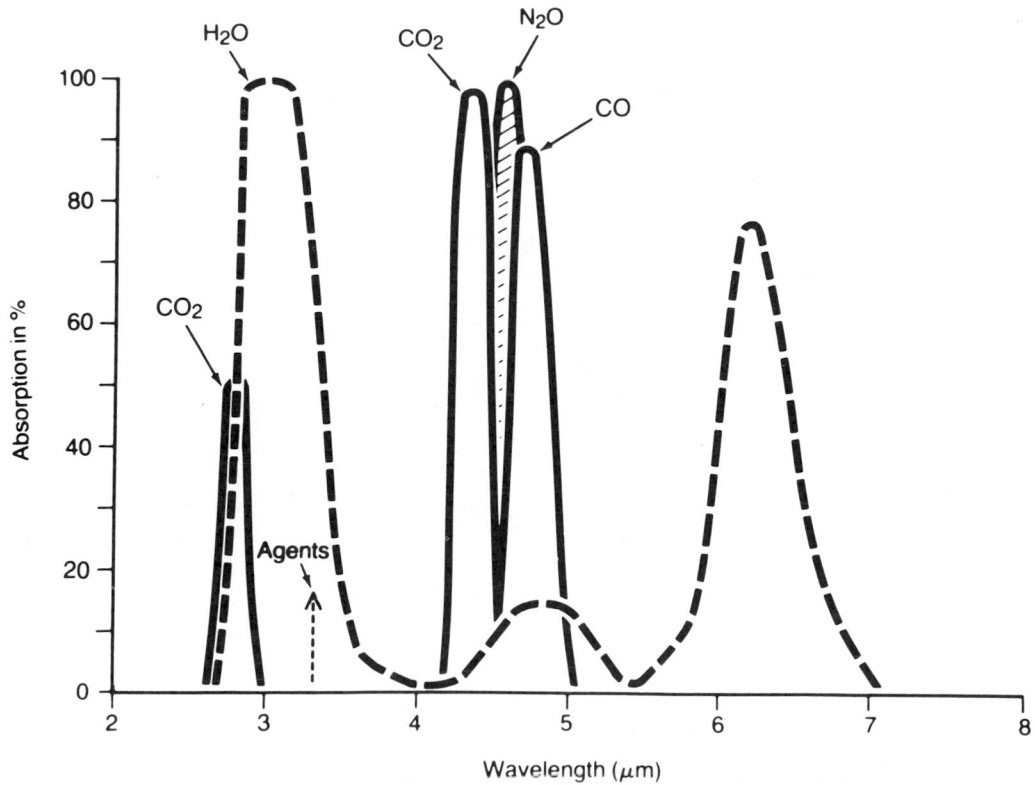

Fig. 29-38. Absorption spectra of anesthetic gases ("agents") and respiratory gases in the red and infrared range. (From Craver,[84] with permission.)

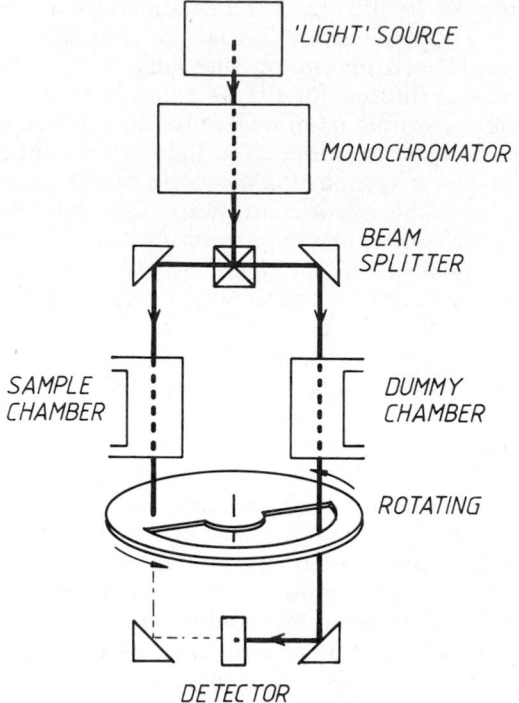

Fig. 29-39. Schematic of the components of a parallel-beam carbon dioxide analyzer. (See text for full description.) (From Mushin and Jones,[15] with permission.)

quickly as possible without clogging the analyzer with humidity. The second problem is minimizing the interference of other gases when measuring CO_2.

Minimizing Response Time of the Capnometer

Most clinical capnometers use a vacuum pump to sample respiratory gases from the patient's airway. That is, gas is aspirated from an adapter in the airway through a capillary tube and into the measuring chamber (Fig. 29-40).[65] For this configuration (sidestream or aspiration-type capnometers), two factors affect response time: the time delay caused by the sampling system and the response time of the infrared analyzer.[56] The time delay involved in sampling depends on the volume of the tubing (i.e., its length and internal diameter) and the flow rate at which gas is sampled. Practical considerations dictate that for dedicated capnometers, the length of the sampling tube be 8 to 10 ft. Consequently, the delay or lag time for the sample to reach the infrared analyzer can be minimized only by using small-caliber tubing. Unfortunately, if the tubing is extremely small, it is easily clogged by droplets of condensed water. For most clinical capnometers, the sampling flow rate is 150 cc/min and the diameter of the sampling tube is near 1 mm, resulting in a time delay of approximately 1 s. Higher sampling flow rates decrease the lag time but may cause errors: during the expiratory cycle, fresh

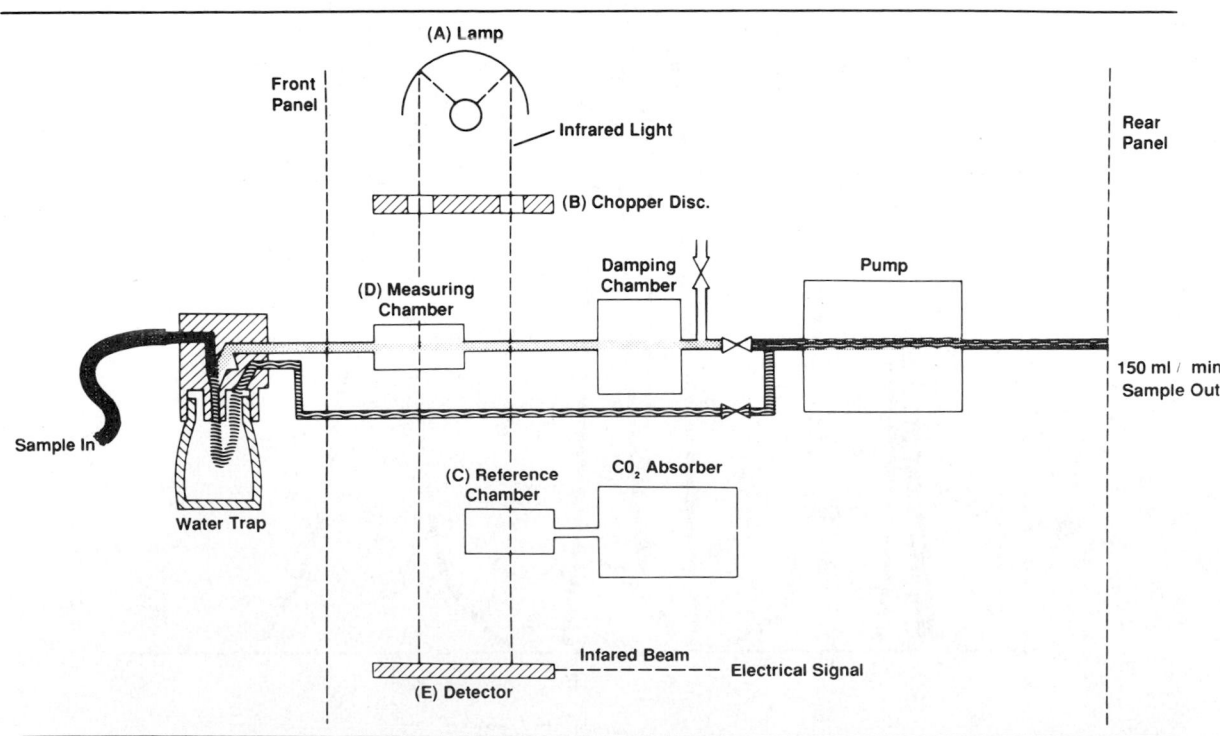

Fig. 29-40. Schematic of a typical "sidestream" or "aspiration-type" capnometer used clinically. (See text for full description.) (From Mogue and Rantala,[65] with permission.)

gas may inadvertently be sampled along with the expired gas. Patient size, respiratory rate, and site of sampling in the ventilatory circuit may all contribute to sampling errors.[56,66-68]

The response time of the infrared analyzer depends on the volume of the sample cell, the flow rate, and the time required to process the data. The response time (or *rise time*) is usually 50 to 150 milliseconds. Light sources for these sidestream capnometers are broad-spectrum incandescent or thermal emitters. The light detectors are usually photoconductors or thermopiles, both of which are sensitive to infrared light in the 4-μm range and have fast response times.

The second method of sampling respiratory gas is to place a very small infrared detector directly in the patient's breathing circuit. This configuration is called a *mainstream capnometer*. Hewlett-Packard developed the first mainstream capnometer in the late 1970s by modifying and miniaturizing the standard infrared detection system (Fig. 29-41).[69] The primary distinction of a mainstream capnometer is that the patient is actually breathing through the measurement chamber. This type of system eliminates the time delay inherent in aspiration-type devices.

Mainstream capnometers do have their own problems, however. First, the entire infrared system must be small and light enough to be placed directly in the airway circuit. To this end, a single-beam detection system was developed by alternating light of two wavelengths. These two alternating light beams are produced by a rotating disk with optical filters. Sealed cells of CO_2 and nitrogen are used as optical filters in the Hewlett-Packard system.

Recently, a solid-state mainstream detection system

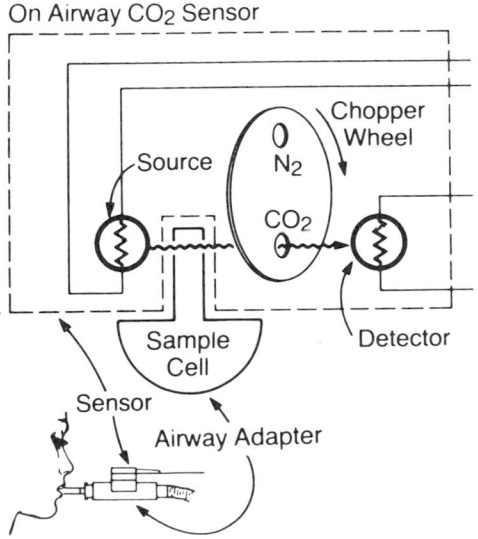

On Airway CO_2 Sensor

Chopper Wheel

Source

N_2

CO_2

Sample Cell

Detector

Sensor

Airway Adapter

Fig. 29-41. Schematic of Hewlett-Packard's "mainstream" capnometer showing the miniaturized infrared detection system placed directly in the patient's breathing circuit. (From Gravenstein et al.,[56] with permission.)

was developed by Novametrix (Wallingford, Connecticut). This device produces the same results as the Hewlett-Packard mainstream system but does not use a rotating disk. The light source is a thermal source that flashes, producing a broad-band emission in pulses. The light passes through the airway sample cell and then impinges on a dual detector. Each detector is coated with a thin filter that allows only the frequencies of interest to be transmitted to the photoconductor beneath. The ratio of these two filtered signals is calibrated to the concentration of CO_2 (personal communication, Mark Tuccillo, project manager, Novametrix Medical Systems, Inc.).

Minimizing Interference from Other Gases

Infrared radiation may be absorbed by any molecule that is both asymmetric and polyatomic. The molecule must not only be asymmetric but also must have allowable vibrational energy levels that will alter the molecule's dipole moment. Therefore, single atoms, such as helium, argon, and hydrogen, and symmetric molecules, such as oxygen and nitrogen, will not absorb infrared radiation. Asymmetric molecules such as carbon dioxide, water vapor, nitrous oxide, and anesthetic agents will absorb infrared radiation. As illustrated in Figure 29-38, the infrared absorption peaks for some of these molecules, especially nitrous oxide, overlap with the absorption peaks for carbon dioxide.

There are two ways of correcting for this interference by nitrous oxide. First, the capnometer can use an additional wavelength of light to measure the concentration of nitrous oxide independently. Corrections for nitrous oxide interference can then be programmed into the capnometer. This type of correction is possible in a sidestream capnometer because the size of the infrared detection system is not limited. However, independent measurement of nitrous oxide is not currently feasible with mainstream capnometers, for which size of the detector is of primary concern. Therefore, mainstream capnometers have manual correction switches that the user must activate when nitrous oxide is present.

A second process can also interfere with absorption of light. In this process (*collision broadening* or *pressure broadening*), the molecules do not themselves absorb infrared light.[56] When a carbon dioxide molecule absorbs light, it must increase its vibrational energy level. These levels depend on factors both internal and external to the molecule. Internal forces relate to the atoms within the molecule—their atomic weights and bond energies. External forces consist of intramolecular forces and collisions with other molecules. In this way, high concentrations of gases that do not absorb infrared light directly (such as nitrogen and oxygen) can affect the absorption bands of carbon dioxide. For clinical purposes, collision-broadening interference is most significant for nitrous oxide, oxygen, and nitrogen. Because of the almost certain presence of nitrous oxide and oxygen in the gas mixture, clinical capnometers incorporate corrections for both gases.

Capnometers are spectrophotometers that have been adapted for clinical use for the specific detection of carbon dioxide. They are calibrated in vitro with known concentrations of carbon dioxide, or, in the case of mainstream capnometers, with calibrated sample cells. Many practical considerations regarding the design of this transducer influence the accuracy of the displayed carbon dioxide waveform. On the other hand, analysis of the absorption data involves relatively little signal processing when compared with pulse oximetry.

ELECTROCHEMICAL AND THERMAL TRANSDUCERS

Electrochemical Sensors

Two electrochemical sensors that have found a place in clinical monitoring are the Clark oxygen electrode and the Severinghaus carbon dioxide electrode. In 1956, Leland Clark presented an electrochemical cell that could measure oxygen partial pressure rapidly.[70] This electrode is an electrical cell consisting of a platinum cathode and a silver anode (Fig. 29-42). As in any resistive circuit, an increase in voltage increases current. However, this electrochemical cell does not obey Ohm's law (eq. [30]) but rather exhibits a plateau. That is, for a certain range of voltages, current does not increase with voltage but does increase with oxygen tension in the cell. The following electrochemical reaction takes place at the cathode:

$$O_2 + 2H_2O + 4e^- \longrightarrow 4OH^-. \qquad (64)$$

The electric current is proportional to the rate of oxygen consumption at the cathode. Clark's polarographic oxygen electrode has been used for more than 30 years to measure oxygen tension in blood gas machines and inspired oxygen meters. Several attempts have been made to manufacture miniaturized Clark electrodes for continuous intravascular monitoring of arterial oxygen tension. These devices met with limited success because of the technical difficulties of producing an electrochemical sensor small enough to fit within an arterial cannula. Intraoperative use involves an additional concern. Halothane is also reduced at the cathode of a Clark electrode, thereby increasing the current; this change is interpreted as an increase in oxygen tension.[71] Because of the development of less expensive optode oxygen sensors (described previously), the Clark electrode, used intravascularly, will probably never find widespread use.

The Clark electrode has found clinical application, however, as a noninvasive monitor of oxygenation in the form of the transcutaneous oxygen sensor. In 1972, Huch et al.[72] found that a heated Clark electrode placed on the skin surface of an infant could measure oxygen tension continuously and noninvasively and that this

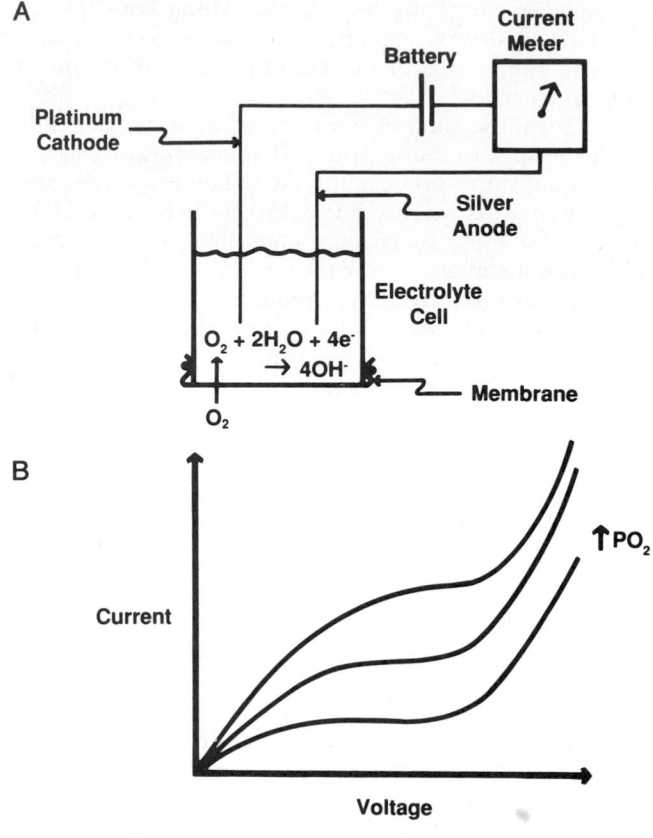

Polarogram

Fig. 29-42. **(A)** A schematic of the Clark polarographic oxygen electrode. The circuit consists of a voltage source (battery) and a current meter connected to a platinum cathode and a silver anode. These electrodes are immersed in an electrolyte cell. A membrane permeable to oxygen but not to the electrolyte covers one surface of the cell. Oxygen diffuses through the membrane and reacts at the platinum cathode with water to produce hydroxyl ions. The current meter measures the current produced by the electrons consumed in this reaction at the cathode. **(B)** Plotting current against the voltage between the two electrodes (i.e., the polarizing voltage) produces a polarogram. In the range of 600 mV, a plateau exists in the polarogram. The plateau occurs at higher currents as the oxygen tension in the cell is increased. (From Tremper and Waxman,[82] with permission.)

value was similar to that of arterial oxygen tension. Application of these sensors to older patients under various clinical conditions revealed that oxygen values obtained transcutaneously represented oxygen tensions for a heated skin surface and that such values are affected by changes in skin thickness, skin perfusion, and other physiologic variables affecting oxygen transport to the skin surface.[73]

When a Clark electrode is modified for use as a transcutaneous sensor, it must be heated and miniaturized.

Both of these modifications shorten the life of the electrolyte. A standard Clark electrode in a blood gas machine contains several milliliters of electrolyte kept at 37°C. A transcutaneous oxygen electrode contains only one drop of electrolyte, and the sensor is heated to a temperature of approximately 44°C. This elevated temperature causes the electrolyte to evaporate more quickly (the vapor pressure of water increases with temperature). The combination of a one-drop reservoir existing in a heated electrode could cause complete evaporation of the electrolyte within a few hours. To lower the vapor pressure of the electrolyte and thus slow evaporation, propylene glycol is usually added to the electrolyte.

Direct application of the transcutaneous sensor to the skin may damage the fragile membrane surface of the electrode. When the Clark electrode is placed in a blood gas machine, its membrane is well protected within the device. When placed in a transcutaneous sensor, however, the membrane is applied directly to the skin surface and is subject to mechanical trauma. In an attempt to increase membrane life, thicker membranes have been used, but these can slow the response of the sensor. None of these modifications is entirely satisfactory, and transcutaneous sensors do require constant maintenance to ensure proper performance.

The Severinghaus electrode used in the blood gas machine to measure carbon dioxide has also been modified to measure carbon dioxide transcutaneously.[74] This carbon dioxide-measuring electrochemical cell is referred to as a secondary sensing device, because it is actually a pH-sensitive glass electrode incorporated within an electrolyte cell (Fig. 29-43). Carbon dioxide diffuses through a membrane into the cell, where it reacts with water, producing carbonic acid. The pH-sensitive glass electrode reacts to the change in the concentration of hydrogen ions by producing a small electromotive force, which can then be calibrated to the partial pressure of carbon dioxide.[75] Since its introduction in 1958, the Severinghaus carbon dioxide electrode has been incorporated into the blood gas analyzer as its carbon dioxide measuring sensor. In the mid-1970s, this electrode was also miniaturized and adapted for transcutaneous measurement of carbon dioxide. Its advantages and disadvantages are similar to those of the transcutaneous oxygen sensor, as it also has a small reservoir of electrolyte that exists in a heated cell having a fragile membrane surface. However, if cared for properly, the device is very effective in monitoring carbon dioxide tension noninvasively.

When a Severinghaus electrode is heated to 44°C and applied to the surface of the skin, the measured CO_2 tension is roughly 60 mmHg when the arterial PCO_2 is 40 mmHg. This CO_2 tension at the heated skin surface has been attributed to metabolic production of CO_2 in tissue, a process that is exaggerated by heating. Although transcutaneous PO_2 values faithfully follow trends of arterial PCO_2, clinical acceptance of the technique was limited because the values were con-

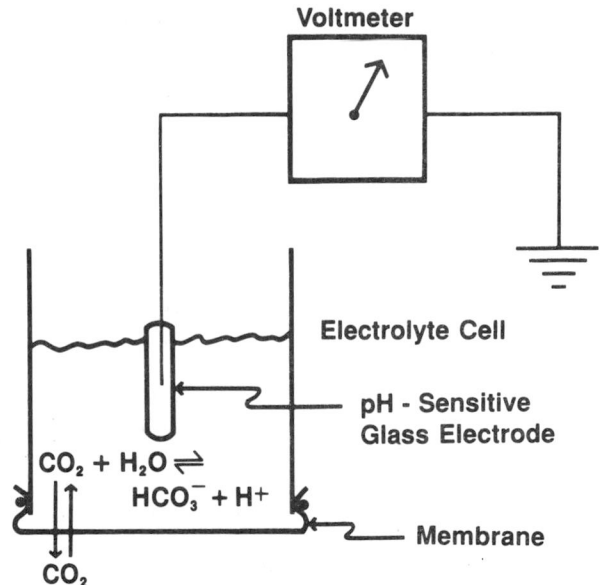

Fig. 29-43. A schematic of a Severinghaus carbon dioxide electrode. This device consists of a pH-sensitive glass electrode referenced to a silver-silver chloride electrode. The glass electrode is immersed in an electrolyte cell having a carbon dioxide-permeable membrane covering on the surface. Carbon dioxide diffuses into the cell, reacts with water in the cell, and produces carbonic acid. The pH electrode then detects the change in pH. (From Tremper and Waxman,[82] with permission.)

siderably higher than arterial PCO_2 values. To improve clinical acceptance, two adjustment methods were proposed to "correct" values for transcutaneous PCO_2.[75] One method is based on the known physiologic effect of temperature on CO_2 tension in normal blood and on the known metabolic rate of CO_2 production in skin. The other "correction" is purely empirical and applies a multiplicative factor derived from clinical data.[76] Both adjustment methods reduce the value for transcutaneous PCO_2 by approximately 30 to 40 percent. Newer transcutaneous monitors automatically incorporate this adjustment into the electronic calibration.

Thermal Sensors

Temperature quantifies the tendency of an object to gain or lose heat when in contact with another object of different temperature. Heat is the energy materials possess because of molecular motion and intermolecular forces (i.e., internal or thermal energy). Heat transfers spontaneously from an object of higher temperature to one of lower temperature if the two are in contact. In gases, temperature is a quantitative measure of the kinetic energy of molecular motion per unit mass. Commonly used temperature scales are arbitrarily defined for convenience. In 1742, Celsius proposed a temperature scale using the freezing point of water as 0°C and the boiling point of water at one atmospheric pressure as 100°C. A temperature of absolute zero can be defined as the point at which the molecules in a substance are in their lowest possible energy state. This condition occurs at −273.15°C or, in SI units, 0°K.

The amount of heat (energy) required to raise the temperature of 1 g of a substance by 1°C is called the *specific heat*. The calorie, a common heat unit, is the amount of heat required to raise the temperature of 1 g of water from 14.5 to 15.5°C. One calorie is equal to 4.184 J. The total amount of heat energy an object contains depends on its composition (specific heat), its temperature, and its mass. For example, although a cup of 60°C coffee is much hotter than a 30°C swimming pool, the coffee contains much less total thermal energy than the water in the pool.

Basic Principles Regarding Measurement of Temperature

There are three general types of techniques for measuring temperature: those based on expansion of a material as the temperature of the material increases, those based on changes in electrical properties with temperature, and those based on optical properties of a material. As heat is added to most substances (gases, liquids, or solids), the motion of the molecules increases, causing the volume of the material to expand at constant pressure. Depending on the material, this expansion can be calibrated linearly to changes in temperature. Liquids are most commonly used, specifically, mercury, because its effective range extends from its freezing point of −39°C to approximately 250°C. Mercury thermometers have two general disadvantages. They require 2 to 3 minutes for complete thermal equilibration (mercury has a high specific heat). Also, they are enclosed in a glass tube, which may break and injure the patient. Thermometers based on the expansion of gas (the Borden tube) or metal (the bimetallic strip) are frequently used as thermostats because they respond slowly to transient changes in temperature.

Electrical techniques for measuring temperature can be subdivided into three categories: resistance thermometers, thermistors, and thermocouples. Resistance thermometers operate on the principle that the electrical resistance of metals increases with temperature. These devices most frequently use a platinum wire as the temperature-sensitive resistor; a battery; and a galvanometer to measure current, which can be calibrated to temperature. The platinum wire is incorporated into a Wheatstone bridge circuit, which accurately measures very small changes in resistance.

Compared with a platinum thermometer, a thermistor is a semiconductor that displays the opposite behavior with regard to electrical resistance. Specifically, as the thermistor is heated, its resistance decreases. This change in resistance is exponential, roughly following the equation

$$R = Ae^{B/T} \qquad (65)$$

where R = the resistance (Ω; T = the absolute temperature (°K), and A and B are constants. As discussed earlier, the semiconductor conducts electricity more easily when energy is added by increasing the number of electrons in the conducting energy band. Thermistors, being solid-state devices, can be manufactured as extremely small devices and therefore have a fast response to change in temperature (i.e., little heat is needed to increase their temperature).

A thermocouple is produced at the junction of two different metal conductors (Fig. 29-26). Many of the electrons in a metal run freely at various energy levels or conduction bands. When two metals having different conduction-band energies are placed in contact, the electrons at the junction tend to move from the higher energy level to the lower energy level, thereby producing a small electromotive force (the *Seebeck effect*). This small voltage is a function of the difference in temperature between the two metal junctions (Fig. 29-26). One of the junctions is kept at a known reference temperature; the other reflects the temperature being measured.

One type of device used to measure temperature does not have to come into direct physical contact with the object being measured. The infrared temperature sensor measures energy radiated from an object and uses that information to determine the temperature of the object. As discussed earlier in the section, *Electromagnetic Radiation*, all exposed surfaces emit electromagnetic radiation in proportion to their absolute temperatures to the fourth power (the Stefan-Boltzmann equation, eq. [50]). When two objects are in optical contact, the net heat transfer is related to the difference between the fourth power of their absolute temperature:

$$Q_{1,2} = K(T_1^4 - T_2^4) \qquad (66)$$

where $Q_{1,2}$ = the net heat transfer (W/cm^2), K = the Stefan-Boltzmann constant, and T_1 and T_2 = absolute temperatures of the two objects (°K).

A simplified version of the way the infrared optical thermometer works is as follows: The front end of the optical thermometer is a telescope focused on an object, the temperature of which is being measured. The telescope collects a sample of infrared radiation from the object and focuses it on an infrared detector. The detector then produces a proportional signal that is the electrical analogue of the incoming infrared radiation and, hence, the temperature of the object. This electrical signal, which is proportional to T_4, is linearized to yield an output voltage proportional to temperature.

In reality, the Stefan-Boltzmann law is valid only for a *black body*, (i.e., a perfect radiating source). A black-body surface is a total radiation absorber and perfect emitter that allows no reflection or transmission of light. Because tissue surfaces do not act as black bodies, corrections about the emissive power of such surfaces must be made.

Thermodilution Cardiac Output

Thermistor probes are most commonly used in clinical monitoring of patient temperature because they are inexpensive, small, and flexible. For these reasons, the thermistor probe is also used to measure cardiac output determined by the thermodilution technique. Computation of cardiac output performed in this manner is, in effect, a heat balance for the right side of the heart. (A heat balance is a method of accounting for all heat in a process or change involving transfer of heat.) The technique consists of quick injection of a known volume of a sterile solution (usually 10 ml of 5 percent dextrose in water) into the right side of the heart while a sensor notes the temperature of the blood in the pulmonary artery. It is assumed that the cold injected solution equilibrates thermally with the blood as it perfuses the pulmonary artery but that the solution does not acquire heat from other tissues. The following equation is the solution of this heat balance[77]:

$$CO = [\rho_i C_i V_i (T_b - T_i)(60 C_r)]/[(\rho_b C_b) \int_0^\infty T_b(t) dt] \quad (67)$$

where CO = cardiac output (liters per minute); ρ_i and ρ_b are the densities of the injectate and blood, respectively; C_i and C_b are the heat capacities of the injectate and the blood, respectively; V_i = the volume of the injectate; T_b and T_i = temperature of the blood and injectate, respectively; C_r = a computational constant that corrects for the rising temperature of the injectate; and $\int_0^\infty T_b(t) dt$ = the area under the thermodilution curve. Because the injectate warms as it is injected through the catheter before mixing with the blood, the correction factor C_r is applied to the equation.

Thermistors are ideal temperature sensors for thermodilution cardiac output because they respond quickly and can be miniaturized to fit in the tip of a 5 French or 7 French pulmonary artery catheter.

STATISTICAL CONSIDERATIONS (Also See Ch. 21)

Over the past decade, invasive and noninvasive monitoring techniques have been developed to produce continuous estimates of physiologic variables that were previously able to be measured only intermittently. Many examples have been described in this chapter. Continuous real-time monitoring has obvious advantages over discrete measurement of vital physiologic variables. In addition, noninvasive techniques add no potential morbidity of their own. As these new methods appear, however, the questions of primary importance are, How accurate are they? Is the new technique sufficiently accurate to replace the old one? and, a question often asked by clinicians, How do these two methods correlate?

Many studies evaluating the accuracy of a new method analyze the data merely by presenting linear regression and correlation coefficients. In linear regression (also called the *method of least squares*), one finds the straight line that best "fits" a given set of data points. This method calculates the slope and intercept of the line minimizing the sum of the squares of the deviations of the data from the line. A linear regression line can be found for any set of paired x and y values, even if they are completely unrelated. The slope and intercept of a linear regression line provide little or no information about how well the results of two methods of measurement agree.

The correlation coefficient (r) is also not a measure of agreement but of association. A high positive correlation coefficient (i.e., an r value approaching 1.0) implies a high degree of linear association but does not provide any information about the absolute value of either of the variables being compared. The r value can also be significantly affected by the range over which the data are collected, although this range may have no bearing on the accuracy of either measurement technique.

Studies comparing two methods of measuring the same variable are called *methods-comparison studies*.[78] Bland and Altman[78] have suggested a simple method of analyzing and presenting these data, in order to answer the question, Is the new method sufficiently accurate to replace the old method? First, one must decide what degree of accuracy is required of the measurement. This requirement should be determined by clinicians who use the measurement to make decisions about patient care. Once the desired accuracy has been established, methods-comparison data can be analyzed to determine whether the new method meets this minimum requirement.

As mentioned, the methods-comparison analysis is appropriate when the two methods measure the same physiologic variable (e.g., oxygen saturation determined by pulse oximeter versus that measured by a cooximeter using an arterial blood sample, or cardiac output determined by thermodilution technique versus that estimated by precordial Doppler probe). Unfortunately, noninvasively monitored variables are often compared with fundamentally different, although related, physiologic variables. For example, end-expired carbon dioxide tension ($ETPCO_2$) is often compared with arterial carbon dioxide tension ($PaCO_2$) measured by analysis of arterial blood gases. Because $ETPCO_2$ and $PaCO_2$ are not the same variable, the two should not be compared to assess the accuracy of measurement techniques. The difference between these two variables is proportional to the amount of alveolar dead space ventilation. Increased alveolar dead space ventilation does not make the capnometer less accurate; it just means that the physiologic variable of $ETPCO_2$ provides different information than $PaCO_2$ would provide. By way of analogy, one would not assess the accuracy of an inspired oxygen meter by comparing its readings with measurements of oxygen tension obtained from arterial blood samples. However, comparing the usefulness of two measuring techniques that help the clinician to make clinical decisions may be a much different process than comparing the two for accuracy. For, if saturation determined by cooximeter were to change in a way that differed from saturation determined by pulse oximeter, the clinician could not substitute changes in one measurement for changes in the other measurement when making clinical decisions.

Nevertheless, the accuracy of measurements is an important factor to consider. Errors in measurement come in two forms: systematic errors and random errors. Systematic errors overestimate or underestimate the measured variable. The systematic error may vary within the range of measurements. Random error relates to the precision and tolerances of each step (or device) in the measurement process, from the transducer to the display. Random error may also vary within the range of the measurements. Average systematic error is obtained by determining the mean difference (d) between the paired values of simultaneous measurements using the two methods. Random error is obtained by determining the standard deviation (SD) of the differences between the paired measurements.

Table 29-2 provides an example. It lists 20 values for oxygen saturation, as estimated by pulse oximeter (SpO_2), and 20 values for oxygen saturation, as determined by simultaneous analysis of arterial blood (SaO_2). The difference between the two measurements is presented in the third column. The mean difference

TABLE 29-2. A Methods-Comparison Analysis for Two Methods of Determining Oxygen Saturation of Blood[a]

SaO_2 (%)	SpO_2 (%)	d
99	99	0
95	97	−2
98	98	0
89	91	−2
82	84	−2
98	99	−1
90	91	−1
89	88	1
97	99	−2
95	93	2
89	87	2
90	89	1
93	94	−1
94	96	−2
98	95	3
97	98	−1
83	84	−1
91	90	1
99	99	0
93	91	2
		−0.2 ± 1.6

[a] Bias (mean d) = −0.2%; precision (SD) = ±1.6%; limits of agreement ([mean d − 2 SD] to [mean d + 2 SD]) = −3.4 to 3.0%.
Abbreviations: SaO_2, oxygen saturation, as determined by oximetric analysis of gases in arterial blood samples; SpO_2, oxygen saturation, as estimated by pulse oximetry; d, the difference between the two measurements.

(d) between the two measures (systematic error) is called the *bias*. The standard deviation of the differences (random error) is often called the *precision*. For roughly 95 percent of the data pairs, the differences fall between (mean d − 2 SD) and (mean d + 2 SD) (more precisely, between [mean d − 1.96 SD] and [mean d + 1.96 SD], assuming a "normal" or Gaussian distribution). This range is referred to as the *limits of agreement*. If these limits of agreement are within an acceptable degree of accuracy, then the new measure may replace the old one with regard to accuracy (but not necessarily with regard to interpretation, as positive changes in one could still be associated with negative changes in the other).

Figure 29-44 is a bias plot, in which difference between the two simultaneously obtained measurements is plotted against their mean. It would be incorrect to plot the difference against the measurement by either one of the methods, because the difference is affected by errors in both methods. The data are plotted in this way to bring out any trends of the bias (or SD) that occur within the range of the measured variable. The calculated bias implicitly assumes a fixed offset throughout the entire range of data, and this may not be correct. The assessment of random error as the standard deviation of the differences also assumes a constant variability throughout the data range; this may also be an incorrect assumption. For example, in Table 29-2, the value for SaO_2 is slightly lower than the value for SpO_2 (a bias of −0.2 percent), and the standard deviation of the difference (SD) is ±1.6 percent. This implies that 95 percent of the data points fall between −3.4 and +3.0 percent. These data yield a correlation coefficient of $r = 0.95$, a high value that should not be surprising. One expects to find a high degree of association between measured oxygen saturation and oxygen saturation provided by a device designed to estimate saturation noninvasively. The question is not how well associated these two variables are but whether the noninvasive method is sufficiently accurate (and changes in the same direction) to justify replacement of the traditional method (i.e., sampling of arterial blood) with the newer method.

In any real situation, it is impossible to determine exactly the "true" value of a measured variable. Error in the form of noise is present in every measurement technique. Much of the electronic processing of data from the transducer attempts to separate this "noise" from the true physiologic signal. Before the advent of sophisticated digital microprocessing, much of this rejection of artifacts was performed by the observer. Even with modern electronic processing, it is still often easier and more accurate for the observer to identify artifacts. Therefore, many monitors provide continuous analog signals representing the variable being measured. The human brain can often identify and interpret abnormal waveforms better than the most sophisticated electronic processor. For example, it is still not possible for a computer to read script handwriting,

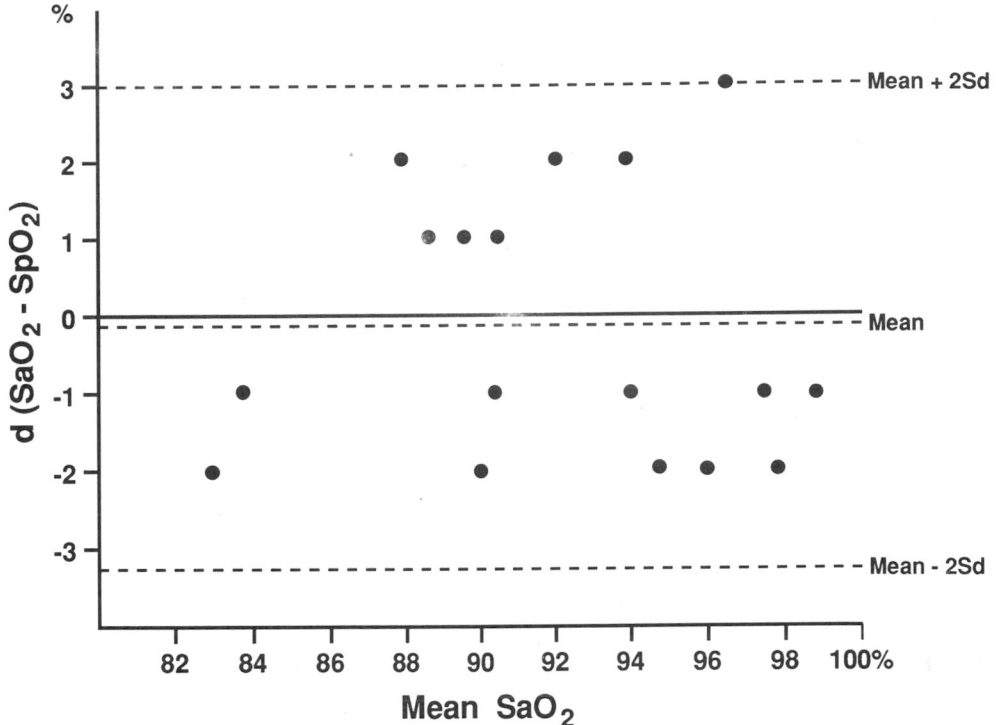

Fig. 29-44. In this bias plot, the difference between paired values for oxygen saturation is plotted against the average of the two paired values. The line for mean difference d (bias) is drawn at -0.2 percent. The standard deviation (SD) of the differences (precision) is ± 1.6 percent. Lines are drawn at the points representing (bias $+$ 2 SD) and (bias $-$ 2 SD) to give the limits of agreement. Ninety-five percent of the data points fall within these limits of agreement. SaO_2, oxygen saturation, as determined by oximetric analysis of arterial blood samples; SpO_2, oxygen saturation, as estimated by pulse oximetry.

whereas most grade-school children can. With this thought in mind, clinicians should interpret all data provided by new and old monitoring techniques in the context of the clinical situation. As the technology becomes more sophisticated, there is always a possibility that "bugs" within the processing algorithms may provide misleading information.

REFERENCES

1. Sir Isaac Newton's Mathematical Principles of Natural Philosophy and His System of the World. University of California Press, Berkeley: 1934
2. Tse FS, Morse IE, Hinkle RT: Mechanical Vibrations: Theory and Applications. 2nd Ed. Allyn and Bacon, Boston, 1978
3. Gardner RM: Direct blood pressure measurement—dynamic response requirements. Anesthesiology 54:227, 1981
4. Mathews J, Walker RL: Mathematical Methods of Physics. WA Benjamin, New York, 1964
5. Meriam JL: Engineering Mechanics: Statics and Dynamics. John Wiley & Sons, New York, 1978
6. Ginsberg JH, Genin J: Statics, Dynamics: Combined Version. John Wilcy & Sons, New York, 1977
7. Goldstein H: Classical Mechanics: Addison-Wesley Publishing, 1950
8. Likins PW: Elements of Engineering Mechanics. McGraw-Hill, New York, 1973
9. Beer FP, Johnston ER, Jr: Vector Mechanics for Engineers: Statics. 3rd Ed. McGraw-Hill, New York, 1977
10. Thompson W (Lord Kelvin): Principles of Mechanics. Dover, New York, 1962
11. Landau LD, Lifshitz EM: Fluid Mechanics. Addison-Wesley Publishing, Reading, Mass., 1959
12. Streeter VL, Wylie EB: Fluid Mechanics. 7th Ed. McGraw-Hill, New York, 1979
13. Schlichting H: Boundary-Layer Theory. McGraw-Hill, New York, 1968
14. Reynolds O: On the experimental investigation of the circumstances which determine whether the motion of water shall be direct or sinuous, and the law of resistance in parallel channels. Philos Trans R Soc Lond 174:935, 1883
15. Mushin WW, Jones PL: Physics for the Anaesthetist. 4th Ed. Blackwell Scientific Publications, Oxford, Boston, 1987
16. Liepmann HW, Roshko A: Elements of Gasdynamics. John Wiley & Sons, New York, 1957
17. Rayleigh JWS: The Theory of Sound. Dover, New York, 1945
18. Resnick R, Halliday D: Physics for Students of Science and Engineering. John Wiley & Sons, New York, 1960
19. Cahalan MK, Litt L, Botvinick EH, Schiller NB: Advances in noninvasive cardiovascular imaging: implications for the anesthesiologist. Anesthesiology 66:356, 1987
20. Clements FM, de Bruijn NP: Perioperative evaluation of re-

gional wall motion by transesophageal two-dimensional echocardiography. Anesth Analg 66:249, 1987

21. Feigenbaum H: Echocardiography. 4th Ed. Lea & Febiger, Philadelphia, 1986

22. Ascah KJ: Doppler echocardiography. In Miller DD et al (eds): Clinical Cardiac Imaging. McGraw-Hill, New York, 1987

23. Kisslo J, Adams D, Mark DB (eds): Basic Doppler Echocardiography. Churchill Livingstone, New York, 1986

24. Sabersky RH, Acosta AJ, Hauptmann EG: Fluid Flow, a First Course in Fluid Mechanics. 2nd Ed. Macmillan, New York, 1971

25. Batchelor GK: Introduction to Fluid Dynamics. Cambridge University Press, London, 1967

26. Kuethe AM, Chow C-Y: Foundations of Aerodynamics: Bases of Aerodynamic Design. John Wiley & Sons, New York, 1976

27. Kinsler LE et al: Fundamentals of Acoustics. 3rd Ed. John Wiley & Sons, New York, 1982

28. Rossing TD: The Science of Sound: Musical, Electronic, Environmental. Addison-Wesley Publishing, Reading, Mass., 1981

29. Meyer HW: A History of Electricity and Magnetism. Cambridge, Mass., MIT Press, 1972

30. Benjamin P: A History of Electricity. Arno Press, New York, 1975

31. Priestley J: The History and Present State of Electricity, with Original Experiments. Johnson Reprint Corp., New York, 1966

32. Grundy BL: Intraoperative monitoring of sensory-evoked potentials. Anesthesiology 58:72, 1983

33. Peterson DO, Drummond JC, Todd MM: Effects of halothane, enflurane, isoflurane, and nitrous oxide on somatosensory evoked potentials in humans. Anesthesiology 65:35, 1986

34. McPherson RW, Sell B, Traystman RJ: Effects of thiopental, fentanyl, and etomidate on upper extremity somatosensory evoked potentials in humans. Anesthesiology 65:584, 1986

35. Pilkington PC, Plonsey R: Engineering Contributions to Biophysical Electrocardiography. Institute of Electrical and Electronics Engineers (IEEE) Press, New York, 1982

36. Reitan JA, Barash PG: Noninvasive monitoring. In Saidman (ed): Monitoring in Anesthesia. 2nd Ed. Butterworth, Boston, 1984

37. Maxwell JC: A Treatise on Electricity and Magnetism. 3rd Ed. Dover, New York, 1954

38. Faraday M: Experimental Researches in Electricity. Dover, New York, 1966

39. Jackson JD: Classical Electrodynamics. John Wiley & Sons, New York, 1962

40. Bleaney BI, Bleaney B: Electricity and Magnetism. 3rd Ed. Oxford University Press, London, 1976

41. Sears FW: Electricity and Magnetism. 2nd Ed. Addison-Wesley Publishing, Reading, Mass., 1958

42. Rojansky V: Electromagnetic Fields and Waves. Prentice-Hall, Englewood Cliffs, N.J., 1971

43. Bordeau S: Voltz to Hertz: The Rise of Electricity. Burgess Publishing, Minneapolis, 1982

44. Simpson RE: Introductory Electronics for Scientists and Engineers. Allyn and Bacon, Boston, 1987

45. Smith RJ: Electronics: Circuits and Devices. 3rd Ed. John Wiley & Sons, New York, 1987

46. Malcolm Dr, Jr: Fundamentals of Electronics. 2nd Ed. Breton Publishers, Boston, 1987

47. Cox JF, Everett SR: Electronic Principles: Integrated and Discrete. Prentice-Hall, Englewood Cliffs, N.J., 1987

48. Horowitz M: Elementary Electricity and Electronics: Component by Component. Tab Books, Blue Ridge Summit, Pa., 1986

49. Weast RC (ed): Handbook of Chemistry and Physics. 49th Ed. Chemical Rubber Company, Cleveland, Ohio, 1968

50. Miller F: College Physics. 4th Ed. Harcourt, Brace, Jovanovich, New York, 1977

51. Mims FM, III: Optoelectronics. HW Sams, Indianapolis, Ind., 1975

52. Wilson J, Hawkes JFB: Optoelectronics: An Introduction. Prentice-Hall, Englewood Cliffs, N.J., 1983

53. Tremper KK, Barker SJ: Pulse oximetry. Anesthesiology 70:98, 1989

54. Fahey PJ: Continuous Measurement of Blood Oxygen Saturation in the High Risk Patient: Theory and Practice in Monitoring Mixed Venous Saturation. Vol. 2. Beach International, San Diego, Calif., 1985

55. Barker SJ, Tremper KK, Hyatt J: Effects of methemoglobinemia on pulse oximetry and mixed venous oximetry. Anesthesiology 70:112, 1989

56. Gravenstein JS, Paulus DA, Hayes TJ: Capnography in Clinical Practice. Butterworths, Boston, 1989

57. Westenskow DR, Smith KW, Coleman DL, et al: Clinical evaluation of a Raman scattering multiple gas analyzer for the operating room. Anesthesiology 70:350, 1989

58. Opitz N, Lübbers DW: Theory and development of fluorescence-based optochemical oxygen sensors: Oxygen optodes. Int Anesthesiol Clin 25(3):177, 1987

59. Barker SJ, Tremper KK, Hyatt J, et al: Continuous fiberoptic arterial oxygen tension measurements in dogs. J Clin Monit 3:48, 1987

60. Shapiro BA, Cane RD, Chomka CM, et al: Evaluation of a new intraarterial blood gas system in dogs (abstract). Crit Care Med 15:361, 1987

61. Barker SJ, Tremper KK, Heitzmann HA, et al: A clinical study of fiberoptic arterial tension (abstract). Crit Care Med 15:403, 1987

62. Severinghaus JW, Astrup PB: History of blood gas analysis. Int Ancsthesiol Clin 25(4), 1987

63. Pologe JA: Pulse oximetry: Technical aspects of machine design. Int Anesthesiol Clin 25(3):137, 1987

64. Wukitsch MW, Petterson MT, Tobler DR, Pologe JA: Pulse oximetry: Analysis of theory, technology, and practice. J Clin Monit 4:290, 1988

65. Mogue LR, Rantala B: Capnometers. J Clin Monit 4:115, 1988

66. Badgwell JM, McLeod ME, Lerman J, Creighton RE: End-tidal PCO_2 measurements sampled at the distal and proximal ends of the endotracheal tube in infants and children. Anesth Analg 66:959, 1987

67. Schieber RA, Namnoum A, Sugden A, et al: Accuracy of expiratory carbon dioxide measurements using the coaxial and circle breathing circuits in small subjects. J Clin Monit 1:149, 1985

68. From RP, Scamman FL: Ventilatory frequency influences accuracy of end-tidal CO_2 measurements. Anesth Analg 67:884, 1988

69. Soloman RJ: A reliable, accurate CO_2 analyzer for medical use. Hewlett-Packard Journal, p. 3, September 1981

70. Clark LC, Jr: Monitor and control of tissue oxygen tensions. Trans Am Soc Artif Intern Organs 2:41, 1956

71. Severinghaus JW, Weiskopf RB, Nishimura M, Bradley AF: Oxygen electrode errors due to polarographic reduction of halothane. J Appl Physiol 31:640, 1971

72. Huch R, Huch A, Lübbers DE: Transcutaneous measurement of blood PO_2 (tcPO_2)—method and application in perinatal medicine. J Perinat Med 1:183, 1973

73. Tremper KK, Barker SJ: Transcutaneous oxygen measure-

ment: Experimental studies and adult applications. Int Anesthesiol Clin 25(3):67, 1987

74. Severinghaus JW: A combined transcutaneous PO_2-PCO_2 electrode with electrochemical HCO_3^- stabilization. J Appl Physiol 51:1027, 1981

75. Severinghaus JW, Stafford M, Bradley AF: tcP_{CO_2} electrode design, calibration and temperature gradient problems. Acta Anaesthesiol Scand [Suppl]68:118, 1978

76. Monaco F, McQuitty JC, Nickerson BG: Calibration of a heated transcutaneous carbon dioxide electrode to reflect arterial carbon dioxide. Am Rev Respir Dis 127:322, 1983

77. Ganz W, Donoso R, Marcus HC, et al: A new technique for measurement of cardiac output by thermodilution in man. Am J Cardiol 27:392, 1971

78. Bland JM, Altman DG: Statistical methods for assessing agreement between two methods of clinical measurement. Lancet 1:307, 1986

79. Payne JP, Severinghaus JW (eds): Pulse Oximetry. Springer-Verlag, Berlin, 1986

80. Sprindy JM, Senelly KM: The Oximetric Opticath Oximetric system: p. 62. In Fahey PJ (ed): Theory and Development, Continuous Measurement of Blood Oxygen Saturation in the High Risk Patient. Oximetric, Mountain View, Calif., 1985

81. Ellis RA: Vascular patterns of the skin. In Montagna W, Ellis RA (eds): Blood Vessels and Circulation. Pergaman Books, Oxford, 1961

82. Tremper KK, Waxman KS: Transcutaneous monitoring of respiratory gases. p. 1. In Nochomovitz ML, Cherniak NS (eds): Noninvasive Respiratory Monitoring. Churchill Livingstone, New York, 1986

83. Ohmeda Pulse Oximeter Model 3700 Service Manual. Ohmeda, Boulder, Colo., 1986

84. Craver CD: A special collection of Infrared Spectra from the Coblentz Society, Inc. The Coblentz Society, Kirkwood, Mo., 1980

30

MONITORING DEPTH OF ANESTHESIA

Donald R. Stanski

INTRODUCTION

The conceptual approaches to defining depth of anesthesia are extremely varied, ranging from in-depth, scientific discussions of the minimum alveolar anesthetic concentration (MAC)[1] to clinical, anecdotal descriptions of "light," "moderate," or "deep" anesthesia.[2] The range of these approaches indicates that no single conceptualization of depth of anesthesia is satisfactory.

The chapter is divided into three general sections. The first discusses two related topics: the evolving definitions of depth of anesthesia and the problem of recall and wakefulness. The many attempts to define "depth of anesthesia" make one realize that our knowledge of the specific attributes of the drugs we use in clinical practice has to be incorporated into our understanding of this phrase. Currently, the diverse nature of these drugs makes it almost impossible to define depth of anesthesia in a unifying manner. Although modern techniques and drugs increase the intraoperative and postoperative safety of anesthesia care, the unfortunate consequence of this otherwise advantageous effect is the occasional occurrence of intraoperative prevent recall and awareness during surgery.

The second section of this chapter involves basic pharmacologic concepts relevant to the scientific investigation of depth of anesthesia. This brief review prepares the reader for the third section, which discusses specific drugs and clinical situations.

The third section of this chapter has two subsections. The first discusses clinical measures of anesthetic depth that derive directly from the patient. Each discussion begins with a review of the scientific approaches available for individual drugs and culminates in the more subjective clinical approaches used in anesthetic practice. The second section discusses three electrophysiologic approaches to assessing depth of anesthesia. This represents the application of technology to the issue of quantitation of anesthetic drug effect and depth of anesthesia.

DEPTH OF ANESTHESIA AND INTRAOPERATIVE RECALL OR WAKEFULNESS

The word *anesthesia* was first used by the Greek philosopher Dioscorides in the first century A.D. to describe the narcotic effect of the plant mandragora. The word reappeared in the 1771 *Encyclopaedia Britannica*, where it was defined as a "privation of the senses."[3] After the introduction of ether anesthesia by Morton in 1846, Oliver Wendell Holmes used the word to describe the new phenomenon that made surgical procedures possible.

Defining Depth of Anesthesia

Plomley was the first, in 1847, to define depth of anesthesia.[4] He described three stages: intoxication, excitement (both conscious and unconscious), and deeper levels of narcosis. In that same year, John Snow described "five degrees of narcotism" for ether anesthesia.[5] The first three stages encompassed induction of anesthesia; the last two, surgical anesthesia. Eleven years later, he turned his attention to chloroform.[6] Snow's excellent characterizations of ether and chloroform anesthesia described the conjunctival reflex; regular, deep, automatic breathing; movement of the eyeballs; and inhibition of the intercostal muscles. Many of these clinical signs were later "rediscovered."[7] Because oxygen was not readily available until the early 1900s, Snow and his successors tried to minimize the use of deep anesthesia to decrease morbidity and mortality.

The early 1900s saw the introduction of premedication with sedatives or opioids. Also, anesthetics with more rapid onset, such as nitrous oxide and ethylene, became available. Therefore, the anesthetic excitement phase could be traversed more rapidly with the use of preanesthetic medication and inhaled anesthetics with a rapid onset of action.

In 1937, Guedel[8] published his classic description of the clinical signs of ether anesthesia. He used clear physical signs involving somatic muscle tone, respiratory patterns, and ocular signs (Fig. 30-1) to define four stages. In the *first stage*, analgesia, characterized by slow, regular breathing with the diaphragm and intercostal muscles and the presence of the lid reflex, the subject experiences complete amnesia, analgesia, and sedation. In the *second stage* (delirium), the subject experiences excitement, unconsciousness, and a dream state with uninhibited activity. Ventilation is irregular and unpredictable. Reflex dilatation of the pupils occurs, the lid reflex is intact, and the risk of clinically important reflex activity (e.g., vomiting, laryngospasm, or arrhythmias) increases. The *third stage* (surgical anesthesia) consists of four progressive planes. Plane 1 is characterized by slight somatic relaxation, regular periodic breathing, and active ocular muscles. During plane 2, breathing changes, inhalation becomes briefer than exhalation, and a slight pause separates inhalation and exhalation. The eyes become immobile. In plane 3, the abdominal muscles are completely relaxed, and diaphragmatic breathing is very prominent. The eyelid reflex is absent. In plane 4, the intercostal muscles are completely paralyzed, and paradoxical rib cage movement occurs. Breathing is irregular and pupils are dilated. In Guedel's *fourth stage* (respiratory paralysis) muscles become flaccid and eyes widely dilated. Car-

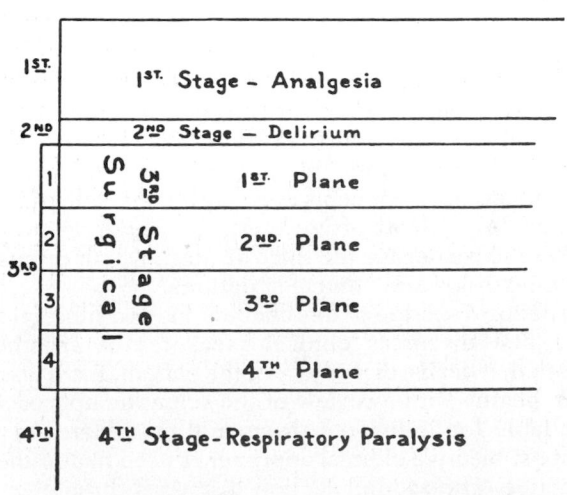

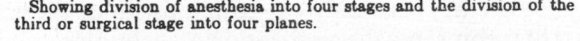

A Showing division of anesthesia into four stages and the division of the third or surgical stage into four planes.

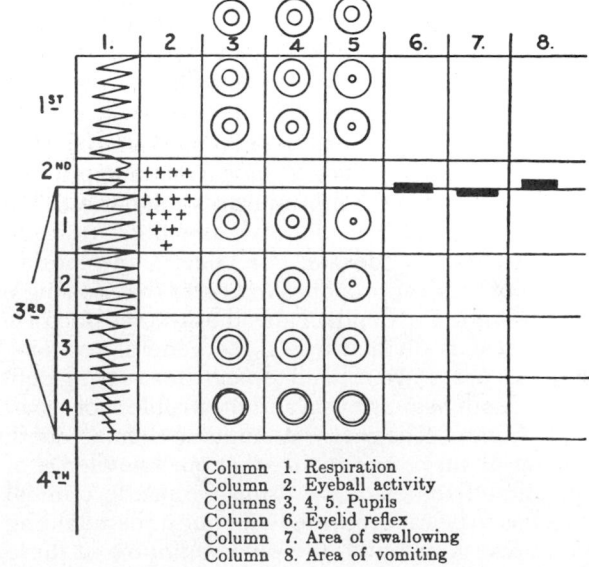

B

Column 1. Respiration
Column 2. Eyeball activity
Columns 3, 4, 5. Pupils
Column 6. Eyelid reflex
Column 7. Area of swallowing
Column 8. Area of vomiting

Fig. 30-1. Guedel's classic text described the stages and planes of ether anesthesia (**A**) and then related them to clinical signs or relevant reflexes (**B**). (From Guedel,[8] with permission.)

diovascular and respiratory arrest occur, as does cardiovascular collapse.

In 1954, Artusio[9] expanded Guedel's description of ether analgesia (stage 1) into three planes. In plane 1, the patient has no amnesia or analgesia. In plane 2, the patient has total amnesia and partial analgesia. In plane 3, the patient has complete analgesia and amnesia, but is comfortable and responsive to verbal stimulation; there is little depression of reflexes. Artusio observed that once patients were anesthetized past stage II (delirium) to the deeper anesthesia of stage III, they could be brought back and forth between stage III and plane 3 of stage II without ever exhibiting stage II. The clinical signs of depth of anesthesia defined by Guedel and others had significant practical utility for the administration of ether, cyclopropane, and chloroform anesthesia.

Beginning in 1942, small doses of the muscle relaxant *d*-tubocurarine were used with the deep levels of ether anesthesia that produced plane 2 or 3 of Guedel's stage III. Respiration was assisted when necessary. Over time, the dose of *d*-tubocurarine began to increase as fully controlled ventilation became commonplace. Anesthesiologists soon realized they could combine controlled ventilation and large doses of muscle relaxants with low concentrations of inhaled anesthetics to reduce the risk of toxicity (cardiovascular and respiratory depression) and increase the speed of emergence from anesthesia. However, the use of muscle relaxants eliminated two valuable types of clinical signs of depth of anesthesia: the rate and volume of respiration and the degree of muscle relaxation induced by the anesthetic.[10] A 1945 editorial in *Lancet* discussed the clinical problems that muscle relaxants would create,[11] and descriptions of patient awareness during surgery later began to appear in the literature.[12]

In 1957, Woodbridge examined the diverse use of anesthetic drugs at that time.[13] He defined anesthesia as having four components: (1) sensory blockade of afferent nerve impulses; (2) motor blockade of efferent impulses; (3) reflex blockade of the respiratory, cardiovascular, or gastrointestinal tract; and (4) mental block, sleep, or unconsciousness. Different drugs could be used to achieve each effect. However, Woodbridge made no effort to define methods of assessing each of these components.

In a 1986 letter to the editor, Pinsker[14] described his conceptualization of *anesthesia* as a broad descriptive term, comparable to the idea of "sickness," in that the source is not one mechanism but rather several components. Anesthesia has three components: paralysis, unconsciousness, and attenuation of the stress response. Any drug or combination of drugs that reversibly provides these three conditions could be used in anesthesia. Paralysis or absence of movement or skeletal muscle tone in the operative field might be achieved by neural blockade or nondepolarizing muscle relaxants. Attenuation of the stress response could be defined only poorly because of limited knowledge of the nature of stress. In contrast, heart rate and blood pressure are clinically measurable components of stress. Unconsciousness, which consists of amnesia and hypnosis, is also a parameter that could not be well defined. No universal end point serves as the basis for the rational administration of drugs to achieve unconsciousness. Presently, an absence of recall is the only objective criterion for unconsciousness (hypnosis or amnesia).

These definitions of anesthesia by Woodbridge and Pinsker produced meaningful concepts that have advanced our understanding of the definition of anesthesia but not necessarily the issue of depth of anesthesia.

In a 1987 editorial, Prys-Roberts[15] made a meaningful contribution to the investigation of depth of anesthesia by redefining which elements are truly relevant to anesthesia. He began by observing that depth of anesthesia is difficult to define because anesthetists have approached the issue in terms of the drugs available to them rather than the patient's needs during surgery. In contrast, Prys-Roberts believes that the noxious stimulation of surgery induces a variety of reflex responses that may be independently modified to the benefit of the patient. One important premise of Prys-Roberts is that pain is the conscious perception of noxious stimuli. Thus, he defines anesthesia as the state in which, as a result of drug-induced unconsciousness, the patient neither perceives nor recalls noxious stimuli. The loss of consciousness is considered a threshold event, an all-or-none (quantal) phenomenon. By this definition, there can be no degrees of anesthesia, nor any variable depths of anesthesia. He then defined anesthesia in terms of the drugs producing unconsciousness and modification of noxious stimuli, classifying them by pharmacologic properties of the drugs and not by their ability to produce components of the state of anesthesia.

Prys-Roberts focused his concepts on the body's response to noxious stimuli, which he defined as factors causing potential or actual cell damage—either mechanical, chemical, thermal, or radiation. Figure 30-2 shows the somatic and autonomic responses to noxious stimuli. In this scheme one reads from left to right and from top to bottom to see the order in which reflex responses are suppressed by anesthetic drugs. For example, somatic responses include both sensory and motor activity. Sensory input obtained through the central nervous system (CNS) can originate from somatic or visceral tissue. The subject must be conscious to perceive pain. Low concentrations of inhaled or intravenously administered anesthetics can eliminate recall of pain but allow a motor response. The motor response to noxious stimuli is typically an all-or-none reflex withdrawal of the stimulated part. Eger et al.[16] used this movement response as a clinical end point in developing the concept of minimal alveolar concentration (MAC) of anesthetic necessary to eliminate such movement in 50 percent of subjects; MAC was used to quantitate the potency of inhaled anesthetics. The concentrations of anesthetics required to eliminate somatic

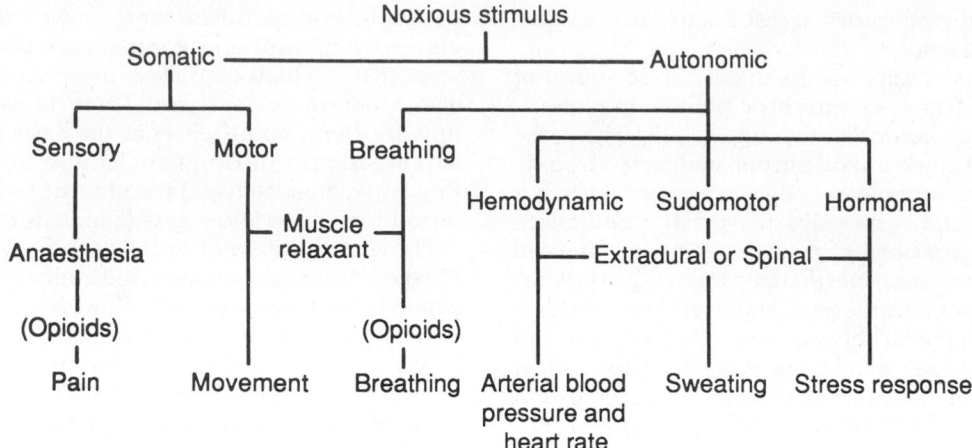

Fig. 30-2. Depth of anesthesia can be defined by the suppression of clinically relevant responses to noxious stimuli, as proposed by Prys-Roberts. (Adapted from Prys-Roberts,[15] with permission.)

motor response are higher than those necessary to induce unconsciousness and to eliminate perception of pain.

The response on the respiratory system is part of the autonomic response described by Prys-Roberts. The motor response to noxious stimuli can involve both an increase in tidal volume and the frequency of breathing. This ventilatory response may occur even if there is no somatic motor response to surgical stimulation. A higher concentration of anesthetic is required to suppress the breathing response than is required to suppress the somatic response to noxious stimuli.

Prys-Roberts divided autonomic responses into three categories. The hemodynamic response consists of autonomic responses to noxious stimuli, namely, increased sympathoadrenal activity that elevates arterial blood pressure and heart rate. The sudomotor response consists of sweating. Release of hormones is an extremely difficult response to eliminate completely.

Prys-Roberts considers pain relief, muscle relaxation, and suppression of autonomic activity as discrete pharmacologic events. These events may be engendered by specific drugs. Some drugs can produce all of these end points; others can achieve only one or two. The only feature common to most anesthetics is the suppression of sensory perception and the production of unconsciousness. Prys-Roberts considered the inclusion of muscle relaxation in the definition of the anesthetic state illogical and confusing. Although muscle relaxation is necessary for laryngoscopy and surgical access, it is neither a component of anesthesia nor an alternative to adequate anesthesia.

The satisfactoriness of the definition of anesthesia has evolved with the drugs used in clinical practice. With ether, the clinical signs described by Guedel were clinically relevant and depth of anesthesia was well defined. The use of potent inhaled anesthetics, opioids, and intravenously administered anesthetics in modern practice has precluded simple, unifying definitions. In my view, the approach of Prys-Roberts to anesthesia, which emphasizes the type of noxious stimuli and the specific class of drug that eliminates that response, is the concept most appropriate for current clinical practice.

Recall and Wakefulness

Before the first induction of anesthesia in 1846, surgical operations were uncommon. Robertson[17] has unearthed two descriptions of the torture suffered by victims of surgical operations performed before the introduction of anesthesia. Despite the introduction of surgical anesthesia, however, the vivid descriptions of pain during surgery have not been eliminated completely. Reports of awareness and recall under anesthesia still occur in the literature.

Vickers[18] has described two degrees of inadequate depth of anesthesia: (1) the recall, or retention in memory, of an event that occurred while under anesthesia: "awareness" is equivalent to "recall"; (2) the responsiveness to auditory input, also called "wakefulness." Wakefulness has been described as a patient's responding to a verbal command during or after surgery without recall of the stimulus. The recall of intraoperative anesthetic events is of greatest relevance to clinical anesthesia and is the main impetus for monitoring depth of anesthesia. The "detection of meaningful auditory input" under anesthesia, a less well-defined area of CNS perception, is of limited clinical significance.

In some clinical situations, the risk of intraoperative recall is high. Bogetz and Katz[19] examined the incidence of recall in 51 patients having surgical procedures after major trauma. Thirty-seven (with a stable hemodynamic status) were able to receive drugs for induction and maintenance of anesthesia. In this group, 4 had intraoperative recall. Of the 4 patients 2 considered this awareness their worst hospital experience. Fourteen of the 51 subjects were so severely injured and hemodynamically unstable that no anesthetic was administered for at least 20 minutes of surgery. Six of 14 of these patients (43 percent) recalled events from their surgery. Two of the latter subjects considered this intraoperative awareness the worst aspect of their hospital experience. Bogetz and Katz could not identify factors predicting which patients would have recall.

Intraoperative recall has been well described in patients given general anesthesia for cesarean section.[20] A prospective study of 150 obstetric patients reported a 2 percent incidence of intraoperative recall, a 17 percent incidence of unpleasant dreams, and a 7 percent incidence of recall of pain.[21] Anesthetic technique was not consistent in this study. Major literature reviews of awareness in anesthesia for the general surgical population have cited a 1 to 2 percent incidence of intraoperative recall.[22,23] Wilson et al.[24] reported a 1 percent incidence of awareness, a 2 percent incidence of dreaming, and an 8 percent incidence of hallucinations in 490 adult patients. No correlation existed between the incidence of mental aberrations and anesthetic agent, sex, or length or type of surgery. Hutchinson's[25] prospective study of 656 patients reported only 6 patients who had recall or intraoperative dreams. All 6 had been given nitrous oxide, oxygen, and muscle relaxants. No recall occurred in patients given potent inhaled anesthetics. However, the use of potent inhaled anesthetics does not guarantee lack of recall.[26,27]

Intraoperative awareness or recall has occurred with high-dose opioid anesthesia. In one case report, the patient had intraoperative awareness and hypertensive crises after fentanyl (96 μg/kg) and diazepam (0.28 mg/kg) following morphine and scopolamine preanesthetic medication.[28] Previous case reports using high-dose opioid anesthesia had not documented a significant hemodynamic response associated with intraoperative awareness.[29,30]

Two clinical signs possibly predicting the occurrence of recall are movement and autonomic response. The use of muscle relaxants can eliminate the movement response, leaving only autonomic activity as a measure of intraoperative awareness. To circumvent the problem of complete muscle paralysis, Tunstall[31,32] used the isolated forearm technique to allow the possibility of movement during and after administration of muscle relaxants. This procedure involves application of a tourniquet to an extremity before the administration of muscle relaxants. Because the muscles do not receive the relaxant, the extremity is not paralyzed and can be monitored for movement.

This technique has been used to study the relationship of muscle movement to intraoperative recall. Schultetus et al.[33] used the isolated arm technique to compare the incidence of movement and recall in patients given ketamine, thiopental, or a combination of the two induction drugs for cesarean section. For 11 of 24 subjects given thiopental (2 mg/kg) or the combination of ketamine (0.5 mg/kg) and thiopental (2 mg/kg) movement occurred in the isolated arm. Four of the 24 patients had dreams, whereas only 3 of 24 had intraop-

erative recall. In 12 subjects given only ketamine (1 mg/kg), one had a movement response and none had recall.

Russell[34,35] has shown that the incidence of movement with the isolated arm technique can vary markedly with the choice of anesthetic. The incidence of intraoperative movement was 44 percent after nitrous oxide and fentanyl anesthesia but only 7 percent after continuous infusion of etomidate with fentanyl. The high incidence of wakefulness (as judged by movement) in the nitrous oxide/fentanyl group caused the investigators to terminate the study. Although the incidence of movement was high, the incidence of intraoperative recall was low (only one subject).

Other investigators have not been able to correlate other clinical signs of light anesthesia to the isolated arm movement response.[36] Also, the effects of ischemia from prolonged inflation of the tourniquet at pressures above arterial blood pressure on this methodology are unknown. Abouleish and Taylor[37] could not correlate movement, size of pupils, or changes in blood pressure with awareness or dreams in patients given morphine (0.2 mg/kg) and diazepam (0.1 mg/kg) after cesarean section. The preceding studies suggest that the occurrence of movement in an isolated extremity is not a good predictor of intraoperative recall.

Detection of Auditory Input

Although the patient may not overtly recall a stimulus or an event, auditory input can register in the brain during apparently adequate surgical anesthesia. Auditory and verbal input must be "meaningful"; however, for input to "register," hypnosis may be needed to elicit recall.

Levinson[38] performed the classic study of detection of meaningful auditory input under anesthesia. Ten volunteers undergoing dental surgery were given thiopental followed by nitrous oxide and diethyl ether. Monitoring the electroencephalogram for an irregular slow-wave, high-voltage pattern allowed the anesthetist to maintain a similar depth of anesthesia in all patients. This electroencephalographic (EEG) pattern was considered equivalent to moderate to deep ether anesthesia. During surgery, the anesthetist provided verbal stimulation for the patient in the form of an intraoperative crisis, saying that cyanosis was present and then treated appropriately. All 10 patients had no spontaneous recall of the intraoperative crisis. Under hypnosis, however, 4 could remember the frightening words in exact detail. An additional 4 remembered someone's speaking to them. All 8 became anxious and either emerged spontaneously from their hypnotic trance or refused to continue exploring the event. One subject had activation of the EEG pattern when the intraoperative crisis occurred, but no recall of the event.

Blacher[39] described his efforts to duplicate Levinson's experiment using noxious, threatening verbal stimuli and hypnosis for subsequent recall. He reported similar findings but did not complete the project, considering it too inhumane. Benign verbal stimuli did not produce significant evidence of auditory recall. He postulates that a noxious or critical event was required.

Bennett et al.[40] randomly assigned 33 subjects to receive either no intraoperative verbal stimuli or a personalized but nonthreatening instruction to pull on their ears during a postoperative interview. Anesthesia was maintained with nitrous oxide, halothane, or enflurane. All subjects given the intraoperative suggestion did not recall the event. The incidence of pulling of the ears during the postoperative interview was significantly higher for patients given the intraoperative message than for those not given it.

These three studies suggest that perception of auditory input can occur during even adequate anesthesia. Other studies, however, have reported negative findings when attempting to study this phenomenon.[41,42]

There is little information regarding the postoperative consequences of intraoperative recall. Blacher[43] described a traumatic post-cardiac-surgery neurosis involving anxiety and irritability, repeated nightmares, preoccupation with death, and reluctance to discuss these symptoms. He attributed this postoperative state to the patient's being awake and paralyzed during open heart surgery. These patients responded favorably to assurances that their postoperative difficulties may have been caused by awareness during surgery. Larson[44] has disputed Blacher's data linking postoperative neurosis with intraoperative awareness.

Although there is much literature regarding intraoperative recall and wakefulness, much of it is anecdotal. As a result, our understanding of the factors relevant to patient recall or wakefulness is limited. There are several reasons for this. The incidence of intraoperative recall is low (1 to 2 percent). Therefore, extremely large numbers of patients would have to be studied to identify the factors that predispose a patient to recall. Most investigators cannot or will not have group sizes of 200 to 1,000 subjects for research on recall. Also, the ethical implications of this research are significant. Ethically, one cannot subject patients to an anesthetic that imposes a moderate or high risk of intraoperative recall. Finally, the measurement tools tend to be subjective. Frequently, one relies on the patient's verbal interpretation of the occurrence of intraoperative recall. The clinical implications of complex psychometric testing such as that performed by Eich et al.[42] are not known. For these reasons, we know very little about how to ensure that intraoperative recall will not occur in every patient. Although certain drugs used in anesthesia have very specific effects in combating recall (e.g., scopolamine, lorazepam), we still do not know whether routine use of these drugs will guarantee lack of intraoperative recall.[45] It is an unproven assumption that careful monitoring of the depth of anesthesia will result in reliable and predictable prevention of intraoperative awareness. Much more research and understanding is needed

in the factors that cause awareness and its prevention in anesthesia.

PHARMACOLOGIC PRINCIPLES OF MEASURING DEPTH OF ANESTHESIA

Before discussing the clinical and electrophysiologic methods of measuring depth of anesthesia, one must understand the pharmacologic concepts governing the relationship of the dose of an anesthetic agent, its concentration in the blood, and the pharmacologic response it produces.[46] Figure 30-3 depicts a situation in which a dose of drug is given to obtain a desired anesthetic response. Pharmacokinetic and pharmacodynamic concepts govern the relationship between drug dose and response. The body's interaction with the drug, through distribution and elimination, governs the concentration that is ultimately available at the site of action. Once the drug reaches the site of action, it interacts with components of the body to create the pharmacologic effect. Figure 30-3 shows that the dose–response relationship is the interaction between its pharmacokinetic and pharmacodynamic components. To quantitate a change in anesthetic dose requirement one must be able to distinguish these components. Depth of anesthesia is a pharmacodynamic measurement.

Measurement of the effect of an anesthetic drug, which is the essence of measurement of depth of anesthesia, depends primarily on three factors: (1) the equilibration of the concentrations of the drug in plasma with the concentration at the drug's site of action and with the measured drug effect; (2) the appropriate characterization of the relationship between drug concentration and drug effect; and (3) the influence of noxious stimuli. To understand these issues, one must address the following questions: (1) When assessing depth of anesthesia, what methods of drug administration are important, and what site does one use to measure the concentration of the drug? (2) How does one model the relationship between concentration of drug and depth of anesthesia? (3) What pharmacokinetic and pharmacodynamic characteristics must be considered when measuring depth of anesthesia?

Equilibration of Drug Concentration and Effect

Figure 30-4 is a theoretical representation of the relationships among time, drug concentration, and drug effect when an anesthetic drug is administered intravenously at two different rates. The curves for time versus effect (Fig. 30-4A) show that rapid administration quickly produces the maximal drug effect, whereas slow administration achieves the same maximal drug effect over a longer period of time.

Curves for the resulting plasma concentration versus time (Fig. 30-4B) show that rapid administration pro-

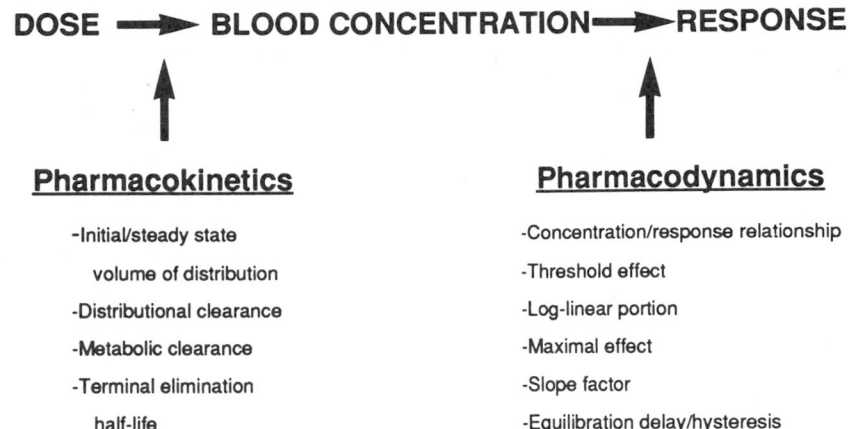

DOSE ➞ BLOOD CONCENTRATION➞RESPONSE

Pharmacokinetics

-Initial/steady state
 volume of distribution
-Distributional clearance
-Metabolic clearance
-Terminal elimination
 half-life

Pharmacodynamics

-Concentration/response relationship
-Threshold effect
-Log-linear portion
-Maximal effect
-Slope factor
-Equilibration delay/hysteresis

Fig. 30-3. The pharmacokinetic and pharmacodynamic components of the dose–response relationship.

duces a peak plasma concentration and peak effect that are separated by time. With slow administration, peak effect and peak plasma concentration occur almost simultaneously. Slow administration of the drug results in relatively stable plasma concentrations near the end of the infusion.

Fig. 30-4C shows the relationship between plasma concentration and drug effect. Rapid administration of the anesthetic drug results in significant hysteresis (or disequilibrium) between concentration and effect. Hysteresis occurs because the relationship between plasma concentration and drug effect during the upstroke of the administration is consistently different than the relationship after termination of the infusion, at which time plasma concentration and drug effect are decreasing. In contrast, slow administration of the drug produces a sigmoid-shaped curve. Once the threshold concentration for detectable drug effect is reached, increasing concentrations result in increasing effect until a maximum or plateau occurs. The disequilibrium or hysteresis seen with rapid administration of the drug occurs because the concentration of the drug in plasma

does not match the actual concentration at the site of action. In contrast, slow administration allows drug concentrations in the plasma and at the site of action to equilibrate.

The ideal body site for measurement of a drug concentration is the biologic fluids immediately surrounding the site of drug action (i.e., the receptor or CNS membrane). Because this is impossible in an intact organism, one must sample at sites that are less than ideal. One is left with the measurement of drug concentration in blood or plasma for intravenously administered drugs, or inspired or end-tidal gas concentrations for potent inhaled anesthetics. The most important principle in sampling for measurement of plasma concentrations of a drug is to obtain a representative sample of blood that is in equilibrium with the biologic fluids at the site of action. Because slow administration of a drug allows equilibration, the direct measurement of drug concentrations in plasma can be related to the drug concentrations at the site of effect.

In the case of rapid intravenous administration of drugs, the disequilibrium between the concentration of

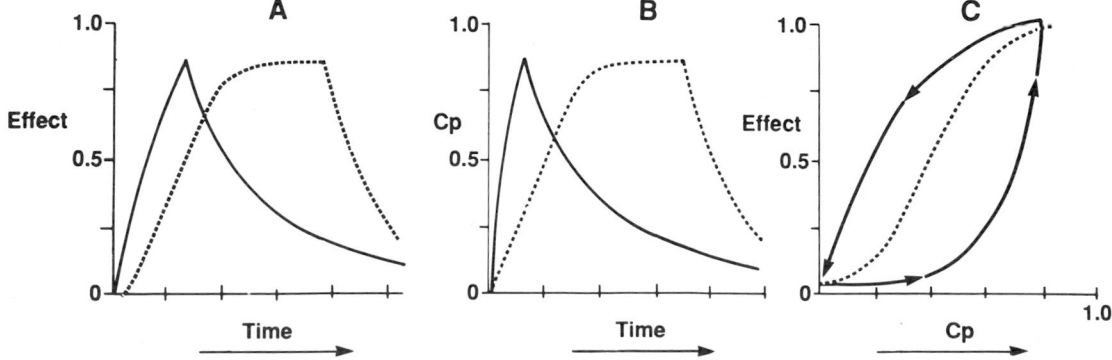

Fig. 30-4. The effect of rapid (solid line) versus slow (broken line) intravenous administration of an anesthetic on the relationships among **(A)** time and drug effect, **(B)** time and plasma concentration of the anesthetic (Cp), and **(C)** plasma concentration of the anesthetic and drug effect. For all panels, 1.0 represents the maximal drug effect that can be achieved or the peak plasma concentration of the anesthetic.

the drug in plasma and the concentration at the effect site means that a plasma sample cannot be used directly to determine the relationship between concentration and response. However, once this lag has been recognized, it is possible to use mathematical modeling concepts to estimate its magnitude.[47,48] Specifically, a first-order rate constant, K_{e0}, can be estimated from plasma concentration and effect data. This rate constant can be used to estimate the half-time of equilibration between drug concentrations in blood and at the site of effect, $T_{1/2}K_{e0}$. $T_{1/2}K_{e0}$ is governed by physiologic and physicochemical properties, such as the perfusion of blood at the site of action, the diffusion of blood at the site of action, the solubility of the drug at the site of action, and the time required to initiate and translate drug receptor interactions into measurable pharmacologic effect.

The choice of arterial versus venous sites for blood sampling also can become a relevant issue when obtaining representative samples of plasma. Venous blood samples can reflect local tissue uptake of drug (i.e., muscle and skin uptake if sampled in an extremity) and therefore are less than ideal. Sampling of biologic fluids from the site of action of anesthetic drugs is not physically possible under most circumstances. Arterial blood sampling reflects the concentration of drug being delivered to all tissues and thus may be the most representative sampling site. Appropriate modeling must be undertaken to eliminate disequilibrium between arterial concentration and effect.

A similar concept also applies to potent inhaled anesthetics. Eger and Bahlman[49] have shown that the concentration and partial pressure of anesthetic in arterial

blood, alveoli, and brain are approximately equal after 15 minutes of administration of an anesthetic inhaled at a constant expired concentration. The easy measurement of the alveolar concentration of anesthetic in expired gas provides a convenient way of assessing the concentrations of potent inhaled anesthetics for subsequent evaluation of depth of anesthesia. The alveolar concentration of anesthetic in expired gas is in equilibration with the concentration in arterial blood, which has equilibrated with the concentration of the drug in the brain.

Characterizing the Relationship between Drug Concentration and Effect

The ideal measurement of drug effect has several basic characteristics. A stable baseline effect that has minimal variability must occur. Also, as the drug concentration increases, the effect should increase in a continuous fashion that is measurable with high resolution. Finally, the effect should reach some maximal plateau, after which an increase in drug concentration does not further increase effect.

Figure 30-5A shows the concentration-effect relationship one expects to see under these ideal conditions. This sigmoid-shaped curve has four characteristics that can be quantitated. The baseline effect and maximal effect are the extremes of drug response. The midpoint between baseline and maximal effect is commonly referred to as the Cp_{50}, or the plasma concentration of drug that results in 50 percent of maximal effect. This parameter indicates the potency of the drug and

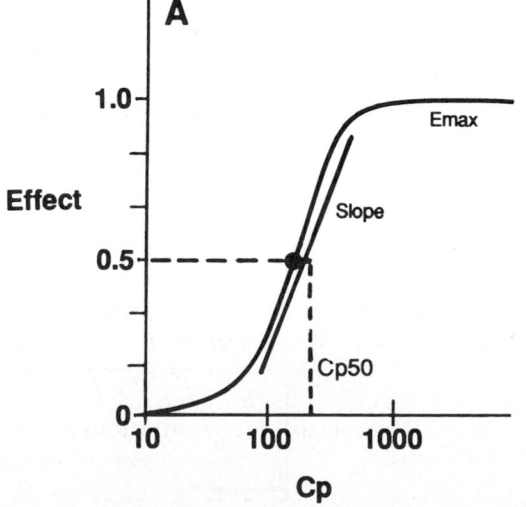
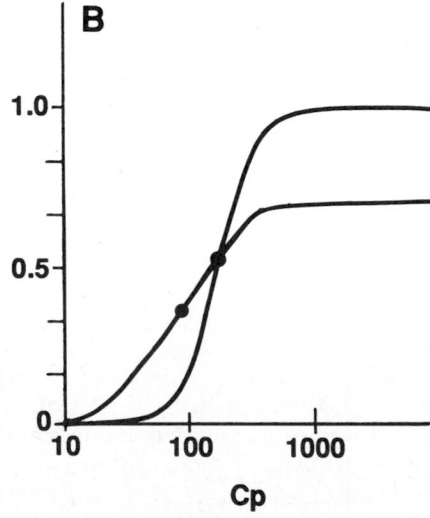

Fig. 30-5. **(A)** A sigmoidal relationship between plasma concentration of a drug (Cp) and drug effect has the following characteristics: Emax, the maximal drug effect; Cp_{50}, the plasma concentration of the drug that produces 50 percent of maximal effect; and the slope of the curve (or rate of change). **(B)** The two concentration–response curves for two anesthetics having different maximal effects. The solid dots indicate the Cp_{50} values. Cp_{50} values are not comparable when values for Emax differ. On the effect axis, 1.0 represents the maximal possible drug effect; on the Cp axis, drug concentration is expressed in arbitrary units.

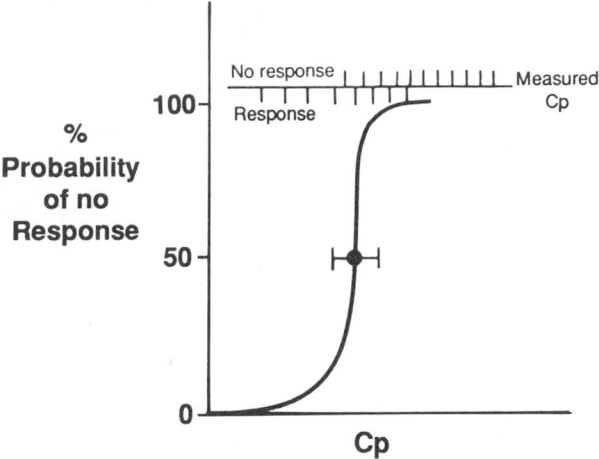

Fig. 30-6. By means of logistic regression, one can use response/no-response data ("quantal" data) to construct the probability of no-response. The solid dot represents the Cp_{50} value (i.e., the plasma concentration of a drug producing a 50 percent probability of no response).

the sensitivity of the individual to that drug. Finally, one can also measure the slope, or rate of change, of the curve. Although generation of the drug concentration versus effect curve is a powerful tool in assessing depth of anesthesia, it is important to understand some of the limitations of this methodology. Figure 30-5B provides such curves for two drugs with different maximal effects. If the maximal effects differ, the Cp_{50}s cannot be used to compare drug potency or individual sensitivity to the drugs.[50]

Many drug effects do not increase in a continuous fashion. Frequently, drug effect is an all-or-none ("quantal") response (that is, the organism responds in some way or not at all). Therefore, when the response is quantal, only the presence or absence of a defined drug effect can be noted. However, one can construct drug concentration versus response curves using quantal data. Although data would include only the two extremes of "response" or "no response," it is possible to use mathematical techniques such as logistic regression or probit or logit analysis to construct the probability of no response.[51] Figure 30-6 provides an example of the curve that results when drug concentration is plotted against the percentage probability of no drug response. The Cp_{50} now represents the midpoint of the probability curve, or the concentration that has a 50 percent probability of producing no response. The drug concentrations that result in both responses and no responses define the Cp_{50}. If the drug concentrations causing both response and no response are large, the variability of the estimated value for Cp_{50} increases. The slope of the curve can also change. When examining drug concentration versus quantal response data, it is important to examine the raw data used to generate the fitted function, as well as the variability associated with the estimated Cp_{50}. Quantal response data are more limiting than continuous data regarding interpretation of data. A quantal response represents only a single point in a theoretical continuous relationship between drug concentration and effect.[50]

Study Design and Choice and Application of Stimuli

To measure depth of anesthesia, one must apply some appropriate form of stimulus to the CNS and then observe the clinical response. This is the essence of Prys-Roberts' definition of depth of anesthesia.[15] The stimulus should have several characteristics: (1) It should be measurable and reproducible. (2) If the stimulus cannot be measured readily, it should be supramaximal, so that variations in the degree of stimulation do not change the nature of the response. (3) The time between initiation of stimulation and the occurrence of peak response must be known reasonably well. The response to stimulation must occur rapidly. Given the usually finite period of time between initiation of the stimulation and the occurrence of the clinical response, it is critically important that the concentration of anesthetic drug be relatively stable during this time. If the concentrations fluctuate markedly, meaningful information cannot be gathered.

Good methodology in the assessment of depth of anesthesia attempts to achieve pharmacokinetic equilibrium in which the drug concentrations in plasma do not change rapidly. This condition is desired because the drug concentrations would then be relatively constant. This state of affairs "freezes" the pharmacokinetic component. The appropriate stimulus can then be applied and a finite period of time allowed to measure other drug responses. This ideal situation would allow the effective separation of pharmacokinetic and pharmacodynamic components of the dose–response relationship.

SPECIFIC DRUGS AND CLINICAL SITUATIONS

This section describes the scientific approaches used for potent inhalational anesthetics, opioids, and intravenously administered hypnotics used to induce anesthesia. After the scientific approaches, a discussion of more subjective approaches relevant to the clinical practice of anesthesia will be presented.

Clinical Measures of Depth of Anesthesia

The following clinical measures of depth of anesthesia are derived directly from the patient. The measures of anesthetic effect represent normal physiologic responses that can be quantitated and are used in clinical practice. Electrophysiologic techniques will be discussed in a later section.

Depth of Anesthesia and Inhaled Anesthetics

The Movement Response and the MAC Concept

The purposeful movement of a body part in response to noxious perioperative stimuli is one of the most useful clinical signs of depth of anesthesia. Using this movement to quantitate depth of anesthesia induced by potent inhaled anesthetics, Eger and colleagues[16,52] defined minimum alveolar concentration (MAC) of inhaled anesthetic as that concentration required to prevent 50 percent of subjects from responding to a painful stimulus with "gross purposeful movement." Readers are referred to the excellent review articles that document the development of the MAC concept and its many applications in anesthesia.[1,53,54] The MAC concept has four basic components: (1) An all-or-none (quantal) movement response must occur after applications of supramaximal noxious stimulus. (2) End-tidal concentrations of anesthetic in the alveoli, considered an equilibrated sample site, are used as an indication of the concentration of anesthetic in the brain. (3) Appropriate mathematical quantitation of the relationship between the alveolar concentration of anesthetic and the quantal response is used to estimate MAC. (4) MAC can be quantitated for altered physiologic and pharmacologic states.

For determination of MAC in humans, the standard noxious stimulus has been the initial surgical skin incision.[16] Skin incision represents a reproducible form of supramaximal surgical stimulation. There has been no systematic examination of other perioperative surgical stimuli (e.g., peritoneal traction) representing more profound surgical manipulation than skin incision or endotracheal intubation. For determination of MAC in animals, the standard stimulus has been application of a surgical clamp to the base of the tail. After examining other noxious stimuli in dogs Eger et al.[16] concluded that tail clamping represented the most noxious stimulation that was clinically reproducible and not exces-

sively traumatic. Response to stimulation must entail a positive, gross, purposeful muscular movement, usually of the head or extremities. Twisting or jerking of the head is considered a movement response, but twitching or grimacing is not. Coughing, rigidity, swallowing, and chewing are not considered positive movement responses, nor is movement of an incised extremity.

The MAC concept has been expanded by evaluating other clinical end points or stimuli. Stoelting et al.[55] determined the minimum alveolar concentration of anesthetic that would allow opening of the eyes on verbal command during emergence from anesthesia ("MAC awake"). This stimulation is less intense than surgical skin incision, and response occurs at lower concentrations of anesthetic than movement to skin incision. Yakaitis et al.[56] determined the minimum alveolar concentration of anesthetic that would inhibit movement and coughing during endotracheal intubation ("MAC intubation"). This event is significantly more stimulating than skin incision; therefore, elimination of the subsequent response requires higher concentrations of anesthetic than does elimination of the movement response. Finally, Roizen et al.[57] investigated the minimum alveolar concentrations of anesthetic necessary to prevent adrenergic response to skin incision ("MAC blockade of autonomic response [BAR]"), as measured by the concentration of catecholamine in venous blood. Figure 30-7 provides the curves representing the relationship between the concentration of halothane and the probability of response for (1) MAC awake, (2) MAC skin incision, (3) MAC intubation, and (4) MAC BAR. One sees a family of concentration–response curves, whose separation depends on the noxious stimuli used to elicit the response.

A second component of the MAC concept involves the use of the alveolar concentration of an anesthetic as an indication of drug concentration. Because the concentration of gas is defined as a percentage of one atmosphere, it is independent of barometric pressure and elevation. Additionally, partial pressures of inhaled anesthetics at equilibrium should be similar in all body parts (e.g., alveolus, blood, and brain). Thus, the measured end-tidal concentration of anesthetic (representative of the alveolar concentration) is in direct proportion to the underlying concentration in the brain. Because cerebral blood perfusion is large, it is possible to achieve an equilibration of end-tidal, alveolar, arterial, and brain anesthetic partial pressures within 15 minutes of exposure to a constant end-tidal anesthetic concentration.

Eger and Bahlman[49] quantitated the difference between arterial concentrations of halothane and the end-tidal expired concentrations of halothane. If the difference between the inspired and end-tidal anesthetic concentrations were less than 10 percent, the difference between the end-tidal and arterial concentrations would be minimal. In the early literature on MAC, the end-tidal concentration of anesthetic was frequently called the "anesthetic dose," and the MAC relationship was referred to as a "dose–response curve."

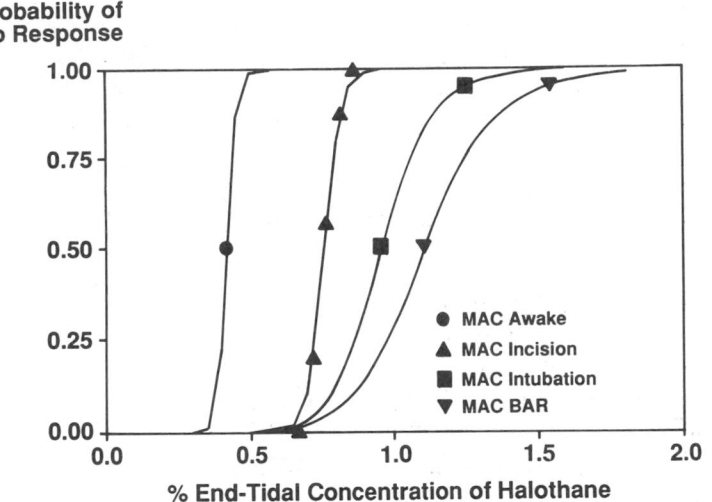

Fig. 30-7. The end-tidal concentration of halothane is plotted against the probability of no response for three different stimuli: a verbal command, skin incision, and endotracheal intubation. For MAC awake, only the concentration producing 50 percent probability of response/no response was available. For movement, multiple concentration–response data points were available. For MAC intubation and MAC BAR, the 50 percent and 95 percent probability points were used. This figure shows that, during halothane anesthesia, the concentration–response curves differ, depending on the stimuli used. (Data from Refs. 55–57 and 59.)

However, Waud and Waud[50] pointed out that this terminology was incorrect, as the MAC concept really describes a concentration versus response relationship. They also believed that a major contribution of the MAC concept was to turn attention from the inspired concentration of an anesthetic to the equilibrated alveolar concentration of the anesthetic, a more accurate and precise reflection of the concentration of the drug in the brain.

A third component of the MAC concept involves using appropriate mathematical approaches to quantitate the relationship between concentration and response. The original MAC concept of Eger and colleagues used a "bracketing approach" in humans and animals. In an individual patient, a fixed end-tidal concentration of anesthetic was achieved, and the response to a single skin incision was observed. Depending on the patient's response or lack of response, the next patient received a higher or lower concentration. A single measurement was obtained per patient. Patients were studied over a range of end-tidal concentrations. They were placed in groups of four; the subject having the lowest end-tidal (alveolar) concentration of anesthetic was the first to be studied. For each group, the percentage of patients moving in response to stimulation was plotted against the average end-tidal concentration for that group. A visual line of "best fit" through these points yielded the concentration at which 50 percent of patients would respond (i.e., the MAC). Figure 30-8 is an example of this analysis, using the concentration versus response data gathered for halothane alone, halothane with morphine premedication, and halothane with 70 percent nitrous oxide. Both morphine premedication

and 70 percent nitrous oxide decreased the MAC value for halothane.[58]

In animal studies, it was possible to manipulate the end-tidal concentration of anesthetic and to apply the tail clamp stimuli on multiple occasions. A MAC value can be obtained for each animal by sequentially increasing or decreasing the end-tidal concentrations to bracket the value between movement and no movement. de Jong and Eger[59] extended the analysis of MAC data by using more appropriate mathematical and statistical techniques to quantitate the relationship between alveolar anesthetic concentration and response-no response data. A nonlinear logistic regression analysis was used to estimate the probability of no movement at any given end-tidal concentration.[51] The logistic regression analysis produced values for MAC to those produced by the bracketing technique. Logistic regression allowed estimation of the variance associated with the estimate of MAC. It was also possible to extrapolate the probability of movement from 50 percent to any given probability within the curve. Thus evolved the concept of an end-tidal concentration of anesthetic that inhibited response in 95 percent of patients.

Waud and Waud[50] have argued that MAC defines only one point on a hypothetical curve that plots the concentration of anesthetic against one index of depth of anesthesia.[50] Because there are no other experimentally defined points on this curve, one cannot be certain that such curves are indeed parallel for different anesthetics. This lack of certainty theoretically limits one's ability to infer that multiples or fractions of MAC represent equal levels of CNS depression for different anes-

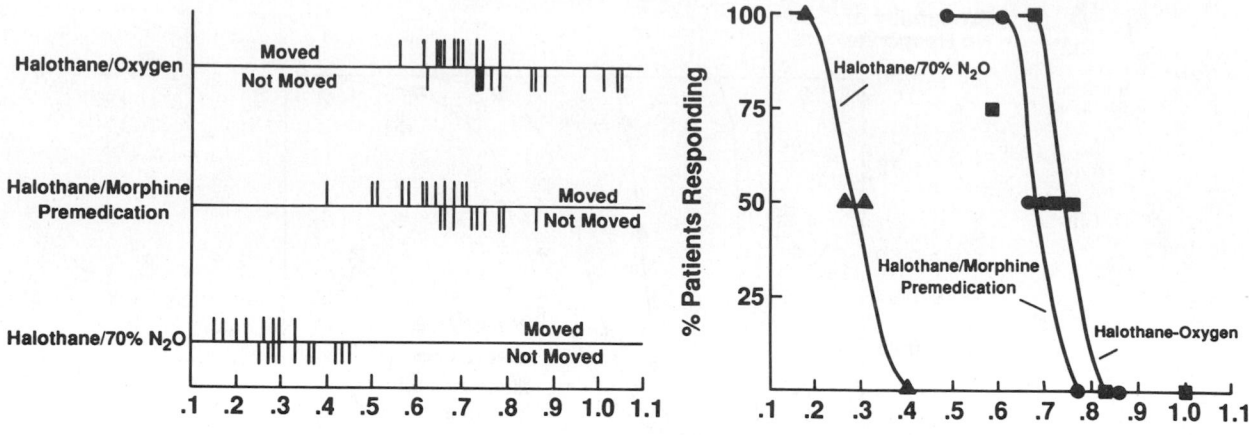

Alveolar Concentration of Halothane

Fig. 30-8. The minimal alveolar concentration necessary to prevent movement in 50 percent of subjects subjected to a noxious stimulus (MAC) was determined for three combinations of halothane: (1) with oxygen only; (2) with oxygen and a morphine premedication (0.15 mg/kg IM), and (3) with 70 percent nitrous oxide. The anesthetic requirement for halothane is greatly decreased by nitrous oxide, and less so by premedication with nitrous oxide. (Adapted from Saidman and Eger,[58] with permission.)

thetics. To address this issue properly and to define the complete curve for anesthetic concentration versus response adequately, one would need a continuous measure of anesthetic effect. As no such clinical measure is currently available, indirect reasoning must be applied to the question of the soundness of adding MAC multiples or of combining MAC values for different anesthetics. Investigators have examined the relationship between MAC skin incision and MAC intubation,[56] which are more noxious and less noxious stimuli, respectively, than MAC awake.[55] When different inhaled anesthetics are compared, the ratio of MAC skin incision to MAC intubation or MAC awake is relatively constant. When the possible relationship between synergism and antagonism of four different potent inhaled anesthetics was examined relative to nitrous oxide, no evidence of a relationship could be demonstrated.[60] Thus, there is only indirect evidence that MAC values can be added.

A fourth feature of MAC is that it has served as a sensitive tool to determine the interaction of other anesthetics and CNS drugs with the inhaled anesthetics. Other drugs used in anesthesia decrease anesthetic requirement, as measured by a reduction in MAC. In addition, numerous altered physiologic states (e.g., aging) change the requirements for inhaled anesthetics. Several review articles have described the many studies applying the MAC concept to the clinical practice and science of anesthesia.[1,53,54] Table 30-1 summarizes the results of these studies regarding the factors that affect MAC.

Other Clinical Responses

The movement response to noxious stimuli is not commonly used in clinical practice. The extensive use of

muscle relaxants makes interpretation of movement both difficult and imprecise in most clinical circumstances. Therefore, other signs have been investigated as possible clinical measures of depth of anesthesia: the rate and volume of ventilation in spontaneously breathing subjects, eye movement, the diameter and reactivity of pupils to light, heart rate, arterial blood pressure, and autonomic signs such as sweating.

TABLE 30-1. Factors That Affect MAC

Effect on MAC	Factors (Study Subjects)
Decrease	Hypothermia (animals)
	Severe hypotension (animals)
	Age (humans)
	Narcotics, ketamine (humans, animals)
	Benzodiazepines, barbiturates (humans, animals)
	Chronic administration of amphetamine (animals)
	Reserpine, α-methyldopa (animals)
	Cholinesterase inhibitors (animals)
	Intravenous local anesthetics (humans, animals)
	Pregnancy (animals)
	Hypoxemia ($PaO_2 < 40$ mmHg) (animals)
	Anemia (< 4.3 ml O_2/100 ml blood) (animals)
	α_2-Agonists (animals)
Increase	Hyperthermia (animals)
	Hyperthyroidism (animals)
	Alcoholism (humans)
	Acute administration of dextroamphetamine (animals)
No effect	Duration of anesthesia (humans, animals)
	Sex (humans, animals)
	Metabolic acid-base status (animals)
	Hypercarbia and hypocarbia (humans, animals)
	Isovolemic anemia (animals)
	Hypertension (animals)

Abbreviation: MAC, minimum alveolar concentration of an anesthetic required to abolish movement in 50 percent of patients, in response to a noxious stimulus. (Data from Cullen,[1] Quasha et al.,[53] and Cullen.[54])

It has not been possible to use these clinical signs to generate uniform measures of depth of anesthesia for inhaled anesthetics. Although some clinical signs do correlate with depth of anesthesia for certain inhaled anesthetics, the same cannot be said for other inhaled anesthetics. In the most complete systematic study of clinical signs and inhaled anesthetics, Cullen et al.[61] examined the relationship between alveolar concentration of inhaled anesthetics and clinical signs of depth of anesthesia in both volunteers and surgical patients. Clinical signs were found to change in usefulness over time. For example, during the first hour of halothane anesthesia, decreasing mean arterial blood pressure was the only useful clinical sign of depth of anesthesia. That is, increasing concentrations of halothane caused a progressive decrease in arterial blood pressure, whereas heart rate remained constant. Also pupils were constricted and nonreactive, and there was no eye movement or tearing. However, after 5 hours of halothane anesthesia, further increases in concentration no longer caused a decrease in arterial blood pressure. This previously useful sign of depth of anesthesia had been eliminated. For cyclopropane, diethyl ether, and fluroxene, only pupillary dilation and reduced pupillary activity correlated with changes in the concentration of anesthetic. Mean arterial blood pressure did not change as the concentration of anesthetic increased.

Cullen and co-workers also found that skin incision modified most clinical signs of drug effect. For example, during anesthesia with halothane and oxygen, heart rate, respiratory tidal volume, and pupil diameter increased after skin incision. Systolic and diastolic blood pressures and respiratory rate did not change. After 12 minutes of surgical incision and manipulation (and unchanged concentrations of halothane), heart rate, tidal volume, and pupil diameter decreased to preincision levels. The clinical response during isoflurane/oxygen anesthesia was different. After skin incision, systolic and diastolic blood pressures and heart rate increased. The pupils dilated in some subjects. No patient moved in response to incision. In general, the increases in blood pressure and heart rate persisted throughout the first hour of surgery, even though higher concentrations of isoflurane were being given. In summary, it has not been possible to make generalizations about clinical responses other than movement for objective research on depth of anesthesia induced by inhaled agents. Although anesthesiologists use these signs extensively to monitor depth of anesthesia clinically, they do so on a qualitative rather than quantitative basis.

Eger's[62] recent review of the subjective interpretation of clinical signs of depth of anesthesia found increasing pupil diameter to be of slight value during halothane, enflurane, isoflurane, or methoxyflurane anesthesia. Premedication with opioids eliminates the usefulness of this clinical end point. Pupillary response to light is rapid and brisk with small amounts of the inhaled anesthetic; however, the response soon becomes sluggish, increasing as depth of anesthesia in-

creases, and pupils do not respond at deeper levels. Eye movements may suggest a low level of anesthesia. Eyelash and corneal reflexes disappear once a surgical level of anesthesia has been achieved and normally do not return at useful surgical depths of anesthesia.

Decreasing arterial blood pressure is the most commonly used sign of increasing depth of anesthesia for halothane or enflurane anesthesia. However, many factors modify the balance between the increase in autonomic cardiovascular activity caused by surgical stimulation and the depression in cardiovascular function caused by potent inhaled anesthetics. These factors include blood volume, cardiac contractility, sympathetic tone, age, and acid-base status. Surgical stimulation also increases blood pressure to a variable degree. Change in blood pressure is also not a useful clinical sign for inhaled anesthetics that cause sympathetic stimulation, such as cyclopropane, diethyl ether, and fluroxene. Pulse rate is a relatively poor sign, as it can be influenced by many factors. Pulse rate is modulated by baroreceptor function, which is sensitive to arterial pressure and its changes. Some anesthetics, such as enflurane and isoflurane, can actually increase pulse rate independent of the surgical stimulation or changes in blood pressure. Such an increase might lead to incorrect decisions regarding dosage.

All inhaled anesthetics depress ventilation and can ultimately cause apnea. This clinical sign is only useful during spontaneous ventilation. Inhaled anesthetics decrease tidal volume in a dose-related fashion, whereas respiratory rate increases in an amount that may sustain minute ventilation (but not necessarily alveolar minute ventilation) at normal levels. Surgical stimulation modifies respiratory depression, frequently returning alveolar minute ventilation to normal values. At light levels of anesthesia with inhaled anesthetics, adverse respiratory events such as breathholding, coughing, and laryngospasm may occur. These respiratory events are very sensitive to the nature and degree of noxious stimulation. Normally, deeper levels of anesthesia eliminate these reflex responses.

For potent inhaled anesthetics, the MAC concept has provided clinical anesthesia with an abundant body of knowledge regarding factors that affect depth of anesthesia and the requirement for anesthetic agents. It is unfortunate, however, that the movement response is not used extensively in clinical practice. The many clinical measures that have poor or unpredictable utility when evaluated scientifically (blood pressure or pulse) have become the mainstay of clinical assessment of depth of anesthesia.[61]

Depth of Anesthesia and Opioids

Opioid analgesics are used extensively for premedication, as a supplement to regional and general anesthesia, as the primary anesthetic agent, and as an analgesic for postoperative pain. The narcosis produced by these agents through specific receptor systems within the CNS decreases autonomic, endocrine, and somatic responses to noxious stimulation. However, efficient use of opioids that maximizes benefit and limits toxicity can be challenging. The difficulty arises when one attempts to monitor opioid drug effects rapidly and carefully during their intraoperative application.

Narcotics as Anesthetics

In 1947, Neff et al.[63] used meperidine as an intravenous supplement to nitrous oxide/oxygen anesthesia in what is now known as a "balanced anesthesia" technique. The later use of opioids as complete anesthetics coincided with the development of cardiac surgery and intensive care in the early 1960s. Providing anesthesia for patients with severe valvular or congenital heart disease without causing cardiovascular collapse was problematic. These early cardiac surgery patients were extremely ill and had little or no circulatory reserve. In the late 1960s, however, Lowenstein et al.[64] noticed the hemodynamic stability of patients undergoing mechanical ventilation who were frequently given large doses of intravenous morphine to suppress respiration. This observation encouraged Lowenstein and co-workers to become the first to administer morphine (0.5 to 3.0 mg/kg) as a complete anesthetic. The resulting cardiovascular stability in acutely ill patients with acquired valvular heart disease was impressive. As cardiac surgery advanced in methodology, patients with ischemic heart disease began to undergo surgical anesthesia. Unfortunately, morphine anesthesia was less satisfactory for these patients (who had hypertension, tachycardia, and awareness during surgery) than for those with valvular heart disease.[65]

In 1978, Stanley and Webster[66] introduced the concept of high-dose fentanyl for cardiac anesthesia. This technique minimized the undesirable effects of morphine on induction and provided better hemodynamic stability in patients with ischemic heart disease. As clinical experience with fentanyl increased, however, investigators found that even increasingly large doses of fentanyl could not always produce a complete anesthetic state in all subjects.[67] This discovery raised the important issue of whether opioids were complete anesthetics.

Human and animal studies show that opioids are not complete anesthetics. For example, Wynands et al.[68] used moderate to large doses of fentanyl and measured plasma concentrations at defined surgical stimuli (intubation, skin incision, sternotomy, aortic root dissection) in patients with good ventricular function undergoing coronary surgery. Figure 30-9 shows the relationships among drug concentrations, stimulation, and hemodynamic response. In approximately 20 percent of patients, even high plasma concentrations of fentanyl (greater than 15 ng/ml) did not eliminate hemodynamic responses, defined as being a 20 percent increase in systolic blood pressure. These results were confirmed by Hynynen and colleagues.[69]

The innovative methods of Murphy and Hug[70] in mea-

suring depth of opioid anesthesia also address the issue of whether opioids are complete anesthetics. These investigators examined the ability of fentanyl to decrease enflurane MAC. They first anesthetized the animal with enflurane and determined MAC. Several infusions of fentanyl at progressively higher rates were used to obtain a constant steady-state plasma concentration of fentanyl in each animal. After each increase in infusion rate, enflurane MAC was determined again. Measurement of opioid concentrations in blood samples ensured that several different steady-state plasma concentrations of fentanyl were obtained in each animal. Murphy and Hug found that even high plasma concentrations of fentanyl (> 20 ng/ml) did not decrease enflurane MAC beyond 60 to 70 percent of its initial value (Fig. 30-10). That is, there was a ceiling to the enflurane-sparing effect. Morphine, sufentanil, and alfentanil also decrease enflurane MAC and have a similar ceiling effect.[71-73]

Stimulation by tail clamping in dogs anesthetized with sufentanil and enflurane produces nearly equivalent increases in heart rate and blood pressure, whether the animals move or not.[71] This observation suggests that hemodynamic and somatic signs are not equally good indicators of depth of anesthesia. When the agonist-antagonist analgesics butorphanol and nalbuphine were examined by using this model, enflurane MAC could only be decreased 11 and 8 percent, respectively.[73] Therefore, the agonist-antagonist analgesics have markedly lower maximal anesthetic effects (Fig. 30-4) than the pure opioid agonists. Even massive doses of fentanyl (3,000 μg/kg with no use of supplemental analgesics) produce a very temporary and transient anesthetic state, as judged by absence of response to tail clamping.[74]

Ardnt et al.[75,76] attempted to develop a trained, unanesthetized, spontaneously breathing dog model to examine the relationship between plasma concentration of fentanyl or alfentanil and clinical signs of depth of anesthesia. They measured hemodynamic and movement responses at low opioid doses that produced moderate ventilatory depression. Interpretation of their data is confounded by their use of increasingly large intravenously administered bolus doses of each opioid. Thus, all plasma concentrations of opioids were measured in a non-steady-state environment, and an unknown degree of disequilibrium existed between drug concentration and clinical responses. However, their data appear to confirm the observation of Hug and colleagues that the plasma concentration of fentanyl and alfentanil at which maximal anesthetic effects occur in dogs are very similar to those for humans.

As mentioned earlier, different investigations show that high-dose opioid anesthesia does not induce complete anesthesia. It has not been possible to identify why or which 30 to 40 percent of patients undergoing coronary artery bypass will have a hemodynamic response to noxious stimuli during even high plasma concentrations of fentanyl. Therefore, it has not been possible to

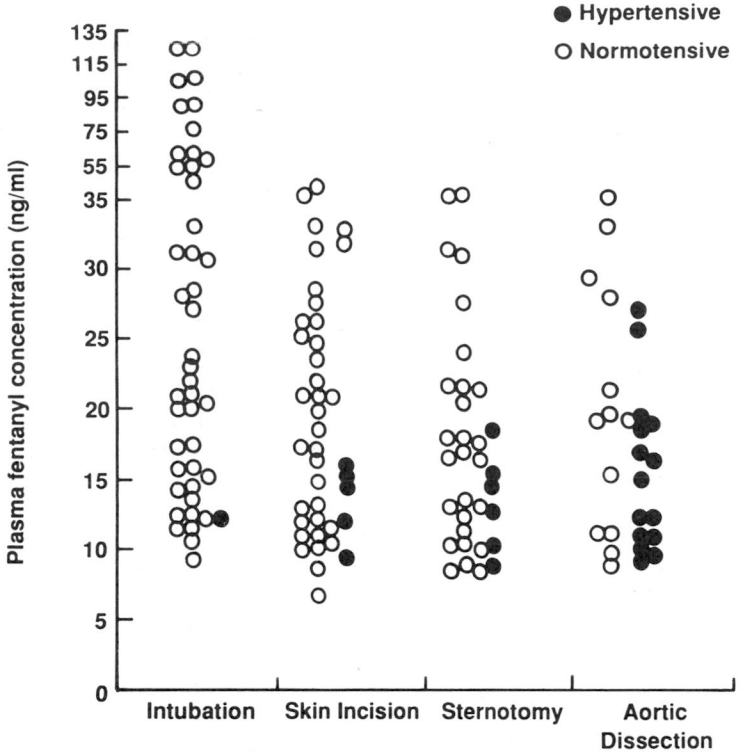

Fig. 30-9. The plasma concentration of fentanyl at the time of certain clinical stimuli, along with the presence or absence of hypertension. During sternotomy and aortic dissection, even high plasma concentrations of fentanyl (> 15 ng/ml) do not always prevent hypertension. (Adapted from Wynands et al.,[68] with permission.)

use autonomic responses to noxious stimuli as reliable and predictable measures of depth of anesthesia. If a patient shows clinical signs of responsiveness, the administration of additional opioid *may or may not* result in hemodynamic control. If it does not, the extra opioid will certainly prolong postoperative respiratory depression and may delay emergence from anesthesia. Thus, there exist no consistent and reliable clinical signs that can be used to quantitate depth of anesthesia induced by opioids. Current clinical practice supplements high-dose opioids with amnestic drugs (benzodiazepines) or low concentrations of potent inhaled anesthetics. Profound hypertensive or tachycardic responses are treated with vasodilating and cardiovascular depressant drugs. Empirically, additional opioid may be given, and, if no response occurs, vasodilating drugs are administered.

Whereas opioids are used alone for cardiovascular procedures, these drugs are usually accompanied by nitrous oxide for surgical procedures involving no postoperative mechanical ventilation. By itself, 70 percent nitrous oxide provides approximately 0.7 MAC anesthesia. Nitrous oxide also interacts profoundly with opioids, markedly decreasing the amount of opioid necessary to provide surgical anesthesia. When alfentanil is

used with oxygen, plasma concentrations of approximately 1,500 to 2,000 ng/ml are needed to suppress hemodynamic response in most patients.[77] The addition of 70 percent nitrous oxide decreases this plasma concentration to approximately 300 ng/ml.[78] A similar degree of potentiation occurs with fentanyl.

Clinical Signs of Inadequate Anesthesia and Plasma Concentration of Opioids

Ausems and colleagues[78] have used pharmacodynamic modeling concepts to relate clinical signs of inadequate opioid anesthesia to plasma concentrations of the drug. In their study, patients were premedicated with a benzodiazepine, anesthesia was induced with alfentanil (150 µg/kg) and the trachea was intubated with the aid of succinylcholine. Anesthesia was maintained with 70 percent nitrous oxide and a variable-rate infusion of alfentanil. The infusion was titrated to the following clinical end points: (1) an increase in systemic arterial blood pressure greater than 15 mmHg above the patient's normal value; (2) heart rate exceeding 90 beats/min in the absence of hypovolemia; (3) somatic responses, such as body movements (minimal muscle paralysis allowed physical movement), swallowing,

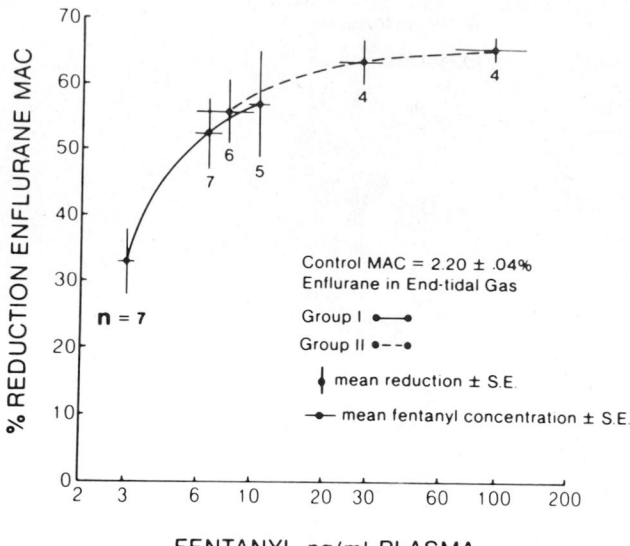

Fig. 30-10. The percentage reduction in enflurane MAC as a function of the logarithm of the plasma concentrations of fentanyl. Each point represents the mean concentration (± SEM) for fentanyl in plasma and the average percentage (± SEM) reduction in enflurane MAC. The numbers of dogs below the vertical standard-error bars indicate the number per data point. (From Murphy and Hug,[70] with permission.)

coughing, grimacing, or opening of the eyes; and (4) autonomic signs of inadequate anesthesia (lacrimation, flushing, or sweating). If any clinical signs occurred, the infusion rate was increased 25 to 50 $\mu g/kg/hr$ and a small bolus dose (7 $\mu g/kg$) was given. Good hemodynamic control was possible in all subjects. If, however, no clinical signs occurred, the infusion rate was decreased at regular 15-minute intervals.

Table 30-2 shows the incidence of response to intraoperative noxious stimuli in 37 patients; three different types of surgical procedures are represented. Although hypertension was the most common clinical response, the other three clinical measures occurred a significant number of times. The authors could not predict which patients would have somatic responses, tachycardia, or hypertension. Measurement of plasma concentrations made it possible to describe the concentration versus response relationship for different perioperative stimuli. Figure 30-11A shows the relationship between the plasma concentration of alfentanil and response/no response for three clinical end points: intubation, skin incision, and skin closure. Regarding elimination of response to noxious stimulation, intubation required significantly higher plasma concentrations of alfentanil than skin incision; and skin closure, significantly lower concentrations than skin incision.

Use of logistic regression made it possible to define Cp_{50} values for these clinical events (Table 30-3). The plasma concentrations of alfentanil were varied in the individual subject during surgery to obtain multiple response/no response data points after which a curve plotting plasma concentration against response was constructed for each subject (Fig. 30-11B).[79] Especially noteworthy are the steep slope of the individual curves and the moderate pharmacodynamic variability among individuals. Table 30-3 demonstrates that upper abdominal surgery required significantly higher plasma concentrations of alfentanil than lower abdominal or breast surgery.

The rapid blood-brain equilibration of alfentanil means that a given plasma concentration has a close relationship to CNS concentration and therefore to drug effect.[80] Drugs having a slower rate of blood-brain equilibration (e.g., fentanyl, sufentanil, morphine) would be less amenable to the kind of pharmacodynamic analysis of the plasma concentration versus clinical effect relationship used by Ausems and co-workers.

The approach to opioid administration presented by

TABLE 30-2. Response of 37 Patients to Noxious Intraoperative Stimulation during Anesthesia with Alfentanil and Nitrous Oxide[a]

	Surgical Procedure		
	Breast	Lower Abdominal	Upper Abdominal
No. of patients	12	14	11
Hemodynamic responses	4	4	5
Hypertension	(1–7)	(1–7)	(1–7)
Tachycardia	0	1	3
	(0–1)	(0–4)	(1–7)
Somatic responses	2	5	2
(Body movement, swallowing, coughing, grimacing, eye opening)	(0–4)	(0–9)	(0–6)
Other autonomic signs of inadequate anesthesia	0	0	1
(Lacrimation, flushing, sweating)	(0–1)	(0–3)	(0–2)

[a] Data are presented as the median number of response episodes per patient. The numbers in parentheses represent the range of number of episodes among the patients in each group. Hypertension, increase in systemic arterial systolic blood pressure of more than 15 mmHg above the patient's normal value; tachycardia, heart rate above 90 beats/min in the absence of hypovolemia. (Data from Ausems et al.[79])

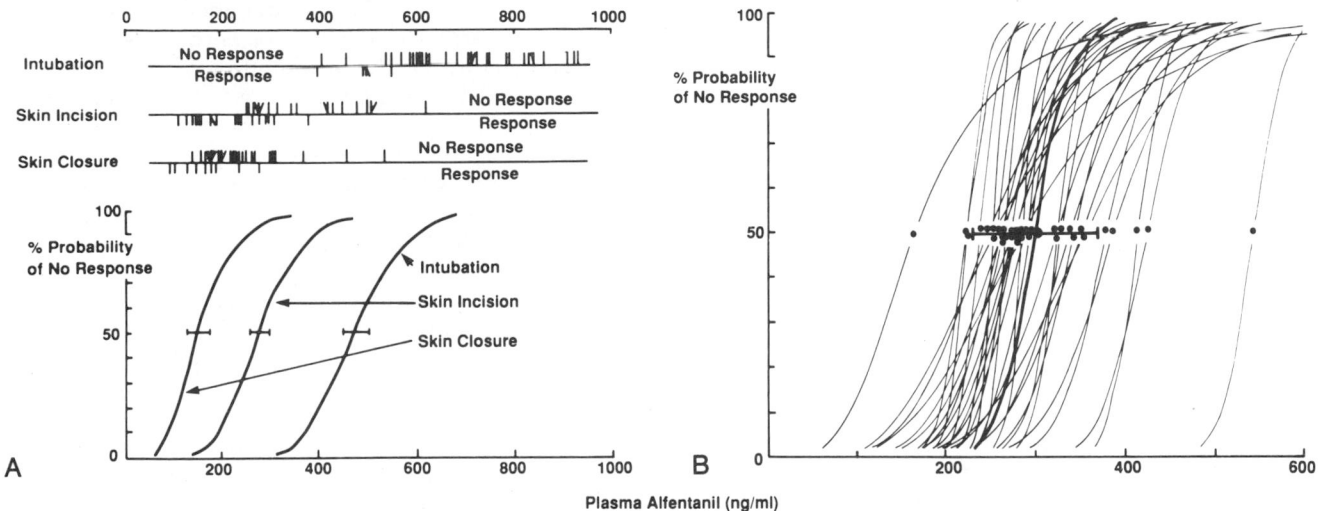

Fig. 30-11. (A) The relationship between the plasma concentration of alfentanil and response/no response at three specific events of short duration. The quantal data are characterized with logistic regression in the lower panel. _____ indicates the ± SE for the Cp_{50} (the plasma concentration of alfentanil producing a 50 percent probability of no response). (B) The plasma concentration of alfentanil versus the probability of no response for each of 34 patients during the intra-abdominal phase of lower abdominal surgery. Dots represent the Cp_{50} values, and the heavy dark line represents the average response of the 34 patients. (Fig. A from Ausems et al.,[78] with permission; Fig. B from Ausems et al.,[79] with permission.)

Ausems and colleagues provided useful insight into the clinical assessment of depth of anesthesia. Overdosage with opioids cannot be judged intraoperatively. Only at the end of anesthesia, when spontaneous ventilation should occur, does one know whether administration of opioids has been excessive. To prevent overdosage, Ausems and co-workers proposed using a variable rate of infusion in which one titrates plasma concentrations to clinical effect to find the lowest possible effective rate of opioid administration. To achieve this end point, one must look for clinical signs of inadequate anesthesia. Once the infusion rate causing inadequate anesthe-sia has been determined, one increases the rate slightly, thus providing adequate anesthesia. The steep slope of the concentration versus response curve for alfentanil (Fig. 30-11) demonstrates that a small increase in the plasma concentration of the drug rapidly converts inadequate anesthesia (100 percent probability of response to stimuli) to adequate anesthesia. Because of the moderate variability in the pharmacokinetics of alfentanil, in the process of titrating dose against clinical effect and pharmacodynamics, this individual titration is necessary for each patient. This concept is most applicable to alfentanil, which has rapid blood to brain equilibration.[80] It has not been shown to be clearly applicable for the other opioids. Intermittent intravenous bolus administration of opioids is not as efficient as variable-rate infusion when titrating plasma concentrations of opioids to clinical effects.[79]

Depth of Anesthesia and Intravenously Administered (Nonopioid) Anesthetics

Few scientifically sound and clinically relevant approaches exist for defining depth of anesthesia induced by intravenously administered hypnotics used to induce anesthesia. Traditionally, these intravenous anesthetics have been used only for induction of anesthesia. Only recently have they been infused for maintenance of anesthesia where assessment of depth of anesthesia becomes more relevant and complex.

Assessing Depth During Induction of Anesthesia

Induction of anesthesia consists of a rapid intravenous bolus injection of a hypnotic anesthetic (i.e., thiopental, etomidate). Plasma concentrations peak within 1/2 to 1

TABLE 30-3. Cp_{50} Values for Perioperative Events and Intraoperative Manipulation Associated with Three Kinds of Surgical Procedures during Alfentanil Anesthesia

Event	Cp_{50} (ng/ml)
Single events[a]	
Intubation	475 ± 28
Skin incision	279 ± 20
Skin closure	150 ± 23
Spontaneous ventilation	233 ± 13
Intraoperative manipulation[b]	
Breast surgery (*n* = 12)	270 ± 63
Lower abdominal (*n* = 14)	309 ± 44
Upper abdominal (*n* = 11)	412 ± 135

[a] Standard error of estimated value for parameter.
[b] Values are presented as mean ± SD.
Abbreviation: Cp_{50}, the plasma concentration of a drug producing a 50 percent chance of suppressing response to a certain stimulus.
(Data from Ausems et al.[79])

minute and decline rapidly on redistribution of the drug. The rapidly changing plasma concentrations cause a corresponding fluctuation in the degree of CNS depression. Depth of anesthesia increases rapidly (causing loss of consciousness), peaks, and then decreases as plasma concentrations decline. The CNS depression lags behind the plasma concentrations, manifesting as hysteresis on curves plotting effect against plasma concentration. All of the concepts discussed earlier regarding non-steady-state conditions produced by rapid administration of a drug make assessment of the relationship of plasma concentration and depth of anesthesia difficult, if not impossible.

Clinical end points that are useful in assessing depth of anesthesia during induction include loss of verbal responsiveness, loss of eyelid reflex, and loss of corneal reflex. Typical stimulation occurring during induction of anesthesia includes laryngoscopy and intubation, which constitute profoundly noxious stimuli. Frequently, response to these two procedures cannot be eliminated completely with only the intravenously administered anesthetic. In one study, administration of thiopental (6 mg/kg) was followed by an average increase in systolic blood pressure of 53 mmHg on laryngoscopy and intubation.[81] In another study, administration of thiamylal (4 mg/kg) was followed by an increase in mean arterial blood pressure from 92 mmHg (control) to 136 mmHg on laryngoscopy.[82] Because most intravenous anesthetics do not provide significant analgesia, the hemodynamic response to major noxious stimuli is great, even when large doses are given. Thus, assessment of depth of anesthesia using clinically relevant noxious stimuli such as laryngoscopy and intubation requires the concurrent administration of other analgesic drugs (opioids or nitrous oxide) to provide reasonable and clinically acceptable hemodynamic control.

Most research on estimating depth of anesthesia induced by intravenous anesthetics has focused on the relationship between dose and response. For example, Brett and Fisher[83] reported that the dose of thiopental associated with a 50 percent probability of no movement in response to a firm squeeze of the trapezius muscle was 3 to 7 mg/kg for adults and more than 7 mg/kg for infants 1 to 11 months of age. It is possible that a larger initial volume of distribution or a more rapid redistribution (both pharmacokinetic mechanisms) in infants accounts for the difference in dose requirement (Fig. 30-3). It is also possible that brain sensitivity to thiopental differs for infants and adults. Dose–response studies cannot differentiate between these two very different mechanisms.

Assessing Depth During Maintenance of Anesthesia

Sear et al.[84,85] proposed the concept of minimum infusion rate (MIR) to compare anesthetic requirements for intravenous anesthetics. After opioid premedication, these investigators induced anesthesia with a bolus injection and then started a maintenance infusion of an anesthetic. Nitrous oxide (67 percent) was administered concurrently. The stimulation of laryngoscopy and intubation was prevented by use of a mask for ventilation. After approximately 25 minutes of the maintenance infusion, the authors recorded movement or no movement in response to the initial surgical incision. Appropriate mathematical techniques related the rate of infusion to the percentage of subjects who moved. The authors could then estimate the 50 percent effective dose (ED_{50}) and 95 percent effective dose (ED_{95}) infusion rates from their patient population. This methodology then was used to examine the effect of age on the requirements for Althesin (a combination of the steroids alphadolone and alphaxolone) and methohexital. Increasing age decreases the ED_{50} infusion rate for both intravenous anesthetics. No blood concentrations of the drugs were measured using this methodology.

The minimum infusion rate concept, as presented by Sear and co-workers, addresses some of the limitations of studies investigating the relationship between bolus dose of intravenous anesthetic and subsequent response. The method uses the movement response to skin incision, which is analogous to the MAC concept. An intravenous bolus injection of an anesthetic combined with a maintenance infusion can produce a steady-state plasma concentration of the drug. Unfortunately, the minimum infusion rate is also affected by the pharmacokinetic properties of the drug—specifically, clearance—in addition to the anesthetic requirement or responsiveness of the CNS. Again, this approach is incapable of effectively separating the pharmacokinetic and pharmacodynamic components of the dose–response relationship.

Becker[86] presents one of the few studies that quantitate the relationship between plasma concentrations of an intravenous anesthetic (in this case, thiopental) and clinical measures of depth of anesthesia. First, studying patients anesthetized with 67 percent nitrous oxide and thiopental (group I), Becker found that the corneal reflex and movement response to a firm squeeze of the trapezius muscle correlated highly with the movement response to surgical stimulation (cervical dilation or skin incision). He then related the plasma concentration of thiopental to three clinical signs (loss of the eyelid reflex, loss of the corneal reflex, and absence of movement in response to squeezing of the trapezius muscle) in another group of patients given thiopental-oxygen anesthesia (group II). Anesthesia was induced with thiopental 2 to 2.5 mg/kg, followed by an intravenous infusion of 1 to 1.5 mg/kg/min. Patients were observed for the three clinical signs. Arterial blood samples drawn at these clinical end points were analyzed for both total plasma concentration and free (or unbound) plasma concentrations of thiopental. Plasma levels of thiopental gathered under these pseudo-steady-state conditions, especially free or unbound plasma levels, are believed to be accurate predictors of brain levels of the drug and, thus, good indicators of depth of anesthesia. The eyelid reflex was lost at significantly lower levels of thiopental than corneal reflex or movement response. Similar plasma concentrations of thiopental were needed for loss of corneal reflex and loss of movement response to squeeze of the trapezius muscle, both of which had been found to correlate highly with loss of movement in response to skin incision. Becker did not report hemodynamic responses to the corneal or trapezius stimulus.

For the patients given 67 percent nitrous oxide (group I) the plasma concentrations of thiopental necessary to achieve the same surgical end points were decreased as much as 71 percent lower than those of patients given only thiopental. As yet, the methodology demonstrated by Becker has not been applied to other clinical situations in which estimation of depth of anesthesia induced by thiopental would be appropriate.

In clinical practice, intravenously administered anesthetic drugs are frequently combined with other drugs that provide additional analgesia (narcotics, nitrous oxide, potent inhaled anesthetics). As indicated earlier, large intravenously administered doses of thiopental are less than effective in eliminating hemodynamic response to relevant clinical stimuli such as laryngoscopy and intubation.[81,82] Fentanyl decreases the anesthetic requirement for thiopental by providing antinociceptive effects that thiopental does not provide.[87] Clinically, the hemodynamic response to laryngoscopy and intubation is most commonly used to assess depth of anesthesia. The use of muscle relaxants to ease endotracheal intubation precludes use of the movement response. Because laryngoscopy and intubation are single events, if clinical depth is inadequate (e.g., in the event of profound hemodynamic response), additional intravenous anesthetics, opioids, or maintenance anesthetic agents are rapidly administered. When precise hemodynamic control becomes important (as in coronary artery disease), larger doses of opioids are used instead of intravenously administered anesthetics. Unfortunately, the scientific basis for the clinical use of intravenously administered anesthetics is less well developed than our knowledge of potent inhaled anesthetics or opioids. Also, the assessment of anesthetic depth when intravenous anesthetics are used as maintenance anesthetics has not been developed.

Electrophysiologic Approaches to Measuring Depth of Anesthesia

The Spontaneous Electroencephalogram

The realization that anesthetic drugs affect the electroencephalogram and alter the EEG dates back to the discovery that the brain produces electrical activity.[88] In 1875, Caton[89] used chloroform to convince himself that the electrical oscillations from the brain were indeed biologic in origin. In the 1920s and 1930s, when electronic amplifiers allowed the recording of these small voltages through the skull, Berger[90] measured the influence of chloroform on the electroencephalogram. In 1937, Gibbs et al.[91] reported that anesthetics changed EEG activity from low-voltage fast waves to high-voltage slow waves and postulated that the electroencephalogram might be used to measure the effects of anesthesia. In 1952, Faulconer[92] demonstrated with ether that the depth of anesthesia, based on recognition of EEG patterns, correlated with the arterial concentration of ether. He also demonstrated that the presence of nitrous oxide lowered the arterial concentration of ether necessary to produce a given EEG effect.

The electroencephalogram can be considered a measure of depth of anesthesia for several reasons. It represents cortical electrical activity derived from summated excitatory and inhibitory postsynaptic activity, which are controlled and paced by subcortical thalamic nuclei. This electrical activity has direct physiologic correlates that are relevant to depth of anesthesia. Cerebral blood flow and cerebral metabolism are related to the degree of EEG activity.[93] Anesthetic drugs affect both cerebral physiology and EEG patterns. The electroencephalogram is a noninvasive indicator of cerebral function when the patient is unconscious and unresponsive. Although recording of the raw electroencephalograph involves accumulating a large amount of information and EEG paper, new computer analysis techniques can summarize and distill the EEG into a condensed, descriptive format (the "processed" electroencephalogram).[94,95]

All anesthetics change the underlying raw EEG signal.[96] Figure 30-12 indicates the raw EEG changes that occur with administration of thiopental or fentanyl, including changes in the voltage and frequency of the signals. Techniques such as use of fast Fourier transform and aperiodic waveform analysis are being used to extract univariate (single-value) parameters that can be related to drug concentration and clinical depth of anesthesia.[94,95] In Figure 30-13, aperiodic waveform analysis was used to process the signal and extract the number of waves per second for thiopental; for fentanyl the fast Fourier transform was used to derive the spectral edge (the frequency below which 95 percent of the EEG power is located). Using the processed electroencephalogram requires that one choose EEG parameters that can be appropriately used as measures of drug effect or depth of anesthesia.

The electroencephalogram is a valuable tool because it reflects cerebral physiology, is a continuous and noninvasive measure, and changes markedly on administration of anesthetic drugs. However, numerous studies have concluded that the electroencephalogram is not a meaningful measure of depth of anesthesia. Galla et al.[97] examined raw electroencephalogram signals for 43 patients and correlated EEG patterns with clinical signs of anesthesia. A discrepancy seemed to exist between the clinical signs and EEG patterns, especially during emergence from, and induction of, anesthesia. During induction, clinical signs indicated that the patients were more lightly anesthetized than EEG patterns

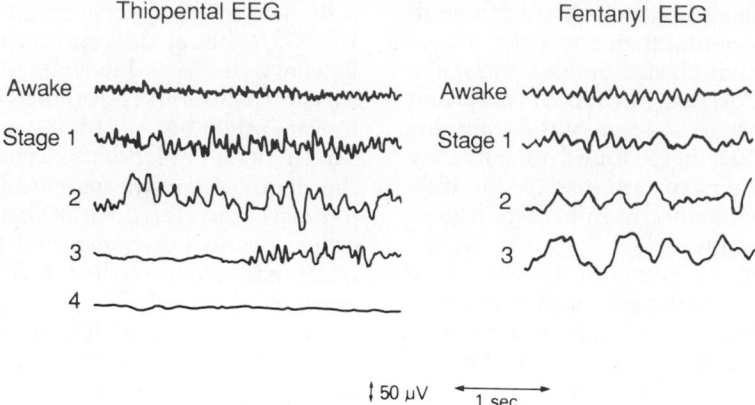

Fig. 30-12. Increasing plasma concentrations of thiopental or fentanyl produce a characteristic progression of changes on the electroencephalogram (EEG). In stage 1, the frequency and amplitude of waveforms increase (thiopental). In stage 2, both drugs produce a decrease in frequency and an increase in amplitude. In stage 3, thiopental produces a burst-suppression pattern and finally, an isoelectric EEG. Fentanyl has its maximal fentanyl effect in stage 3—large, slow delta waves.

suggested, whereas on emergence, clinical signs indicated greater depth. Levy[98] examined processed electroencephalogram signals during induction and before bypass in cardiac surgery patients given potent inhaled anesthetics and opioids. He examined a series of univariate descriptors, including median frequency (the frequency below which 50 percent of the electroencephalogram power is located) and spectral edge (the frequency below which 95 percent of the electroencephalogram power is located). He concluded that the multimodal electroencephalogram activity observed in 64 percent of the cases precluded the use of single univariate parameters to describe the anesthetic state. Ber-

ezowskyj et al.[99] had similar findings using power spectral analysis of patients given nitrous oxide, opioid, and halothane for anesthesia. Clinical assessment of depth of anesthesia did not correlate well with EEG patterns.

Why have these clinical studies indicated that the electroencephalogram is not useful for determining depth of anesthesia? These studies involved the use of numerous types of anesthetic drugs given concurrently in an uncontrolled manner. Different anesthetics are known to cause different EEG effects.[96] Winter has described EEG patterns as representing a multidirection continuum (rather than merely a progressive depression) of CNS modulation ranging from excitation (sei-

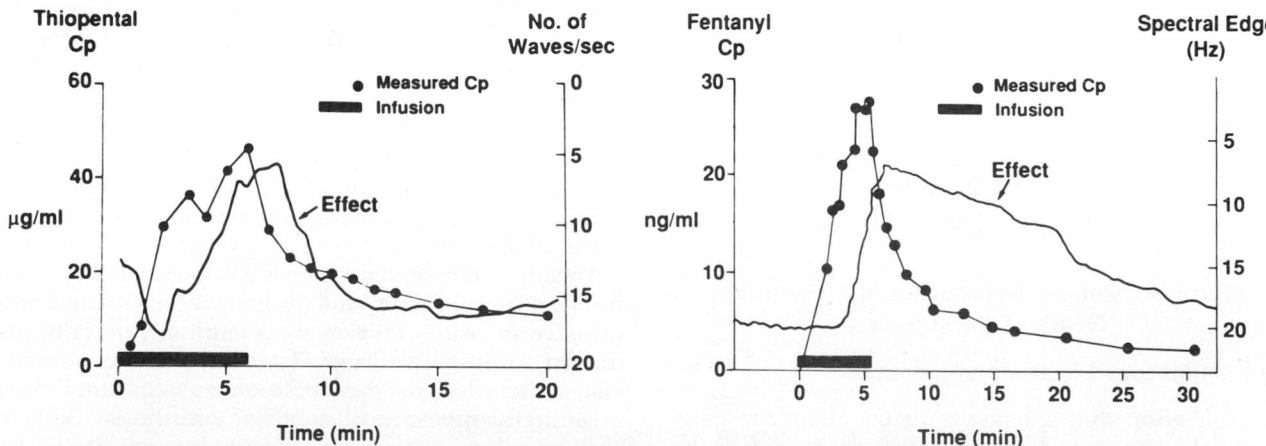

Fig. 30-13. The relationships between (1) the plasma concentration (Cp) of thiopental or fentanyl and time and (2) the response on the processed electroencephalogram and time. The two drugs were characterized in different ways. Aperiodic waveform analysis provided the number of waves per second produced by thiopental. The fast Fourier transform was used to estimate the spectral edge produced by fentanyl. Note the biphasic effect of thiopental on the EEG: the number of waves first increases and then decreases as the plasma concentration of thiopental increases. Note also the lag or hysteresis between plasma concentration and electroencephalographic effect for each drug.

zures) to depression (anesthesia).[100] Because of the diverse nature of drug-induced EEG effects, there is very little understanding or predictability regarding the combined action of several drugs on the raw or processed electroencephalogram. The complexity of the presence of numerous drugs makes it unrealistic to expect simple relationships to emerge between the electroencephalogram and clinical depth of anesthesia. One must first understand how drug concentration relates to EEG effects and clinical depth of anesthesia for individual anesthetic drugs before one can expect to make progress regarding the combined effects of several anesthetic drugs.

Using the Electroencephalogram to Measure the Effects of Anesthetics

Concentrations of anesthetics can be related to derived parameters on the processed electroencephalogram for most anesthetic drugs (Table 30-4). The successful correlation of drug concentration to processed electroencephalogram response is due to the ability to monitor both variables in an intensive manner. Measuring multiple plasma concentrations in any one individual produces a pharmacokinetic profile. Having a recording of the processed electroencephalogram available makes it possible to examine several parameters that might be useful measures of drug effect.[112] Pharmacodynamic modeling can then link the two.

To date, choosing the most appropriate EEG parameter has been an empirical decision based on the following pharmacologic criteria: The baseline value for the parameter should be stable and vary only minimally. The parameter should be able to characterize the maximal EEG changes created by the drug. As drug concentration increases, the parameter should change in a consistent and predictable fashion. During rapid administration, there should be a lag (hysteresis) between change in plasma concentration and change in the parameter. On discontinuation of the drug, as plasma concentrations decrease, the parameter should recover to its baseline (awake state) value.

TABLE 30-4. Derived Parameters of Processed EEG Signals That Have Been Used to Describe the Effects of Anesthetics

	Anesthetic Drug
Parameters of fast Fourier transform analysis	
Spectral edge[80,101,107,113]	Thiopental, halothane, fentanyl, enflurane, alfentanil, sufentanil
Median frequency[102,108,109–111]	Etomidate, isoflurane, methohexital, ketamine
Parameters for aperiodic analysis[114–116]	
Total number of waves/sec	Thiopental, fentanyl, sufentanil, alfentanil, morphine
Total power at 1 Hz	
Cumulative power at 3 Hz	
Cumulative power at 4 Hz	
Frequency at 90% cumulative power	

Examination of raw electroencephalograms obtained during administration of thiopental or fentanyl shows distinct differences between these two drugs. Low concentrations of thiopental first produce EEG activation (that is, increase in the frequency and voltage of EEG signals) and then EEG slowing. Ultimately a burst suppression pattern and an isoelectric electroencephalogram occur. In contrast, fentanyl does not cause activation but progressive slowing and finally, slow delta waves (3 to 4 Hz). Increasing the concentration of fentanyl does not cause further EEG slowing.

To characterize the electroencephalogram produced by thiopental, investigators have used aperiodic waveform analysis, a method that estimates the number of EEG waves per second (Fig. 30-13). This parameter is attractive because it allows one to estimate when zero waves per second (i.e., an isoelectric electroencephalogram) would occur from thiopental. In contrast, the fast Fourier transform is unable to characterize an isoelectric electroencephalogram. Parameters that measure frequency (including spectral edge and median frequency) become unstable when the electroencephalogram is isoelectric. The fast Fourier transform is able to provide effective and practical waveform analysis for fentanyl (Fig. 30-13) because isoelectric electroencephalograms do not occur with opioids.

Figure 30-14 shows the relationship between plasma concentration and two EEG parameters when fentanyl and thiopental are administered as a rapid infusion. For both drugs, the lag between change in plasma concentration and its EEG effect is noticeable. The use of pharmacodynamic modeling can remove this disequilibrium.

The electroencephalogram has been used to determine whether disease states or differing physiologic conditions affect anesthetic requirements. Homer and Stanski[101] found that the dose requirement for thiopental decreased with age. The electroencephalogram showed that this decrease was not caused by a change in brain sensitivity to the drug. The plasma concentration necessary to achieve one-half of the maximal electroencephalogram slowing (the EC_{50}) was not related to age. Rather, a change in distribution pharmacokinetics appears to account for the decrease in thiopental dose requirement. Results have been similar for the intravenous anesthetic etomidate.[102] However, for fentanyl and alfentanil, the decrease in dose requirement with age was found to be caused by an age-related change in brain sensitivity, as measured by the EC_{50}, and not by a change in distribution-phase pharmacokinetics.[103]

Correlating EEG Effect with Clinical Measures of Depth of Anesthesia

One approach to examining the relationship of EEG effect to clinical depth of anesthesia asks the following question: Do EEG changes occur at the same anesthetic drug concentrations that produce certain clinical end points? In Figure 30-15 therapeutic plasma concentrations of fentanyl have been plotted against spectral

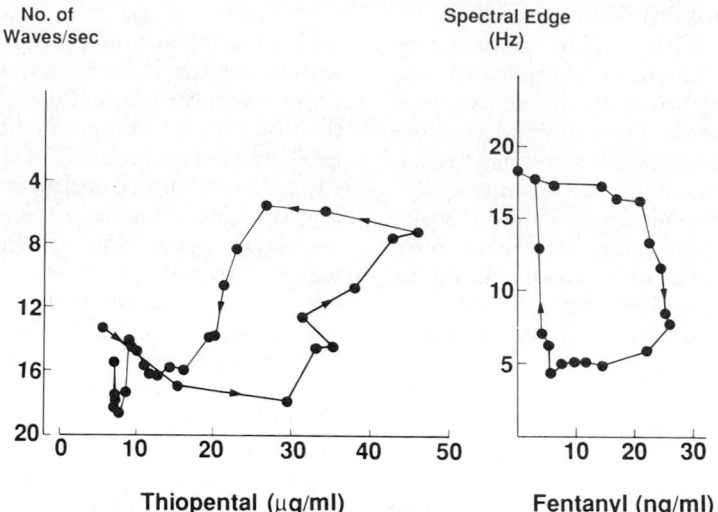

Fig. 30-14. The relationship between the plasma concentrations of thiopental or fentanyl and the electroencephalographic (EEG) parameter representing drug effect for each. These data are the same as indicated in Figure 30-13, except that the time factor has been removed. The disequilibrium or hysteresis between plasma concentration and EEG drug effect is obvious. This lag indicates that for both drugs, the site of action in the central nervous system differs kinetically from that of plasma. Pharmacodynamic modeling can be used to estimate the degree of hysteresis and to predict the steady-state EEG response.

edge. Data in the literature were used to define the therapeutic plasma concentrations for fentanyl at different clinical end points (e.g., analgesia and respiratory depression). The relationship between spectral edge and plasma concentration of opioid was derived from the data of Scott et al.[80] This figure demonstrates that the electroencephalogram would not be useful in assessing postoperative pain relief, as EEG changes have not begun to occur. Also, EEG changes reach a plateau at

plasma concentrations of fentanyl necessary for anesthesia with only oxygen and fentanyl. Therefore, the electroencephalogram would not be useful in monitoring depth of anesthesia induced by high doses of fentanyl. The EEG change with fentanyl is maximal in the therapeutic range associated with nitrous oxide/oxygen anesthesia. It should be noted that the curve for plasma concentration of fentanyl versus EEG effect was derived for nonsurgical subjects. It is not known

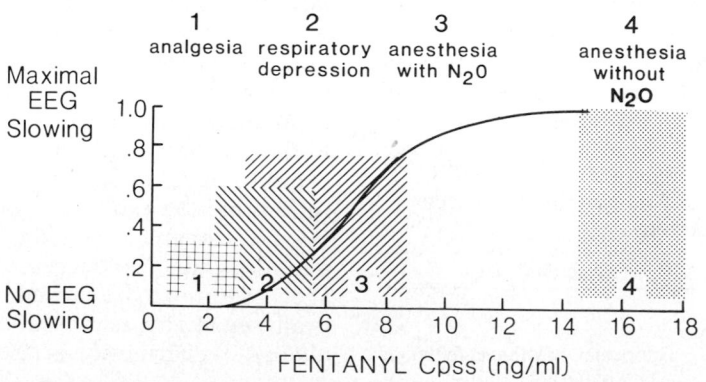

Fig. 30-15. The steady-state plasma concentration of fentanyl (Cpss) (with hysteresis removed) is plotted against the degree of electroencephalographic (EEG) effect as a solid line. The EEG effect of fentanyl manifests as the degree of slowing of the spectral edge. In the background is the steady-state therapeutic plasma concentration of fentanyl needed for four clinical end points: *(1)* postoperative analgesia, *(2)* respiratory depression, *(3)* intraoperative anesthesia with nitrous oxide, and *(4)* intraoperative anesthesia with only oxygen. Note that the change in spectral edge induced by fentanyl occurs at plasma concentrations similar to those needed for anesthesia with nitrous oxide. Therefore, the electroencephalogram may be useful in monitoring depth of anesthesia for this type of anesthetic. (From Ebling et al.,[131] with permission.)

whether noxious surgical stimuli can change the EEG response to fentanyl and possibly shift the curve to the right.

Inadequate anesthesia generally causes EEG activation. Peripheral noxious stimuli reach the brain via afferent systems that pass through the ascending reticular activating systems of the brain stem. These systems regulate corticocerebral function and thus affect the underlying electroencephalogram pattern. Noxious stimuli can cause three kinds of changes on the electroencephalogram: (1) desynchronization with the appearance of 20- to 60-Hz fast rhythms (electroencephalogram activation); (2) the appearance of 6- to 10-Hz spindles; and (3) bursts of 1- to 3-Hz slow waves.[104] These patterns vary with individual anesthetics and with the nature of stimulation.[105] For example, during light levels of thiopental anesthesia in dogs (steady-state plasma concentrations of 15 to 27 μg/ml), supramaximal stimulation of the sciatic nerve caused EEG activation and increased cerebral metabolic oxygen requirement and blood flow 15 percent.[106] During deep levels of thiopental anesthesia (37 to 49 μg/ml), stimulation produces no change in these variables. There seems to be a distinct threshold concentration of thiopental that blocks the response to noxious stimuli during anesthesia in animals.

Rampil and Matteo[107] examined the changes in hemodynamic variables and the EEG spectral edge frequency during laryngoscopy and intubation. Thiopental (3 to 5 mg/kg) was given as a rapid intravenous bolus, with 75 to 100 mg of lidocaine and fentanyl (1 to 1.5 μg/kg). Laryngoscopy was performed and hemodynamic responses recorded. A spectral edge frequency greater than 14 Hz was associated with a 40 percent increase in systolic blood pressure, whereas a spectral edge frequency of less than 14 Hz was associated with only a 12 percent increase.

For the intravenous anesthetics etomidate and ketamine, an orderly progression of clinical CNS depression occurs as the EEG median frequency slows.[108,109] For etomidate, the awake median frequency is 9.5 Hz, loss of consciousness occurs at 4.8 Hz, the corneal reflex is absent at 2 Hz, and a burst-suppression pattern occurs at 1.6 Hz. As the concentration of etomidate decreases, the electroencephalogram and clinical measures recover in parallel. The burst-suppression pattern disappears at a median frequency of 1.8 Hz, the corneal reflex returns at 2.0 Hz, responsiveness occurs at 4.7 Hz, and orientation occurs at 6.6 Hz. Ketamine exhibits a similar orderly progression in terms of clinical depth of anesthesia and EEG median frequency.

In one study, concentrations of isoflurane and nitrous oxide 1.3 and 1.5 MAC, respectively, were associated with an EEG median frequency of less than 5 Hz and an adequate intraoperative anesthesia.[110] For all 14 patients, the median frequency was greater than 5 Hz when the subjects were conscious and responsive.

Schwilden et al.[111] have used the electroencephalogram to provide closed-loop feedback control of methohexital anesthesia in humans. The median frequency parameter was used to monitor the electroencephalogram, and a combined pharmacokinetic and pharmacodynamic model was used to establish the feedback control. A median frequency of 2 to 3 Hz was chosen as the desired EEG level. During the experiment, 75 percent of all measured median frequencies were in the preset range of 2 to 3 Hz. To achieve this, however, the investigators had to stimulate their subjects at 1.5-minute intervals with six different acoustic and tactile stimuli. If the noxious stimulus was not applied, the electroencephalogram feedback was not adequate. This study is intriguing in that the electroencephalogram was used with a closed feedback system to determine the dose of anesthetic administered: the ultimate application of control theory to the practice of anesthesia. The need of the system for constant delivery of noxious stimuli reveals our limited understanding of how afferent CNS input alters the electroencephalogram and EEG drug effects.

An appropriate processed electroencephalogram parameter that will distill the raw electroencephalogram into a measure that reflects anesthetic drug effect and depth of anesthesia must be chosen. Although many different EEG parameters and processing techniques can be used, at present no clear criteria or statistical approaches exist for choosing the ideal parameter.[112] A second important issue involves the absence of a "gold standard" for measurement of clinical depth of anesthesia. As discussed earlier, clinical measures of depth of anesthesia are limited, and their scientific quantitation is complex. Thus, if one does not have a clinical "gold standard" against which to compare changes on the electroencephalogram, how can one accurately determine the usefulness of this recording in assessing depth of anesthesia? Finally, there has been little systematic investigation of how the effects of relevant perioperative noxious stimuli affect the electroencephalogram.

Can the electroencephalogram be used to measure depth of anesthesia? To date, given the typical clinical environment in which multiple drugs are given and clinical end points are not clearly defined, the success in determining depth of anesthesia with EEG parameters has been limited.[113-116] Much of this limitation reflects our lack of understanding of the effects of interactions of anesthetic drugs on the electroencephalogram, our inability to choose the most appropriate EEG parameters, and our lack of a gold standard of clinical drug effect as a reference for EEG effects. All is not lost, though! Considerable success has been attained in examining individual anesthetic agents and relating certain EEG parameters to measured concentrations of drugs. The ultimate application of the electroencephalogram—measurement of depth of anesthesia—will require correlation of anesthetic drug concentrations, EEG parameters, and clinical measures of depth of anesthesia for, first, individual anesthetic drugs, and then, combinations of anesthetic drugs.

Evoked Responses

Sensory or nerve stimulation produces a low-amplitude signal, or evoked response, within the CNS. This evoked response can be separated by means of special computer techniques from the underlying, spontaneous electroencephalogram. The ability to evoke a response is a measure of the functional integrity of the sensory receptors and the pathways between the sensory receptor and neural generator of peaks in the evoked response waveform. The evoked responses are used primarily to monitor the functional integrity of the neural structures, to identify neural structures, and to diagnose neurophysiologic conditions. Because evoked responses are sensitive to anesthetic drugs, they have been investigated as possible measures of anesthetic drug effect and depth of anesthesia.[96]

The sensory stimulation most commonly used in recording of evoked responses consists of somatosensory (electrical) stimulation of peripheral nerves; auditory stimulation, in which noises (clicks) are applied to the auditory canal; visual stimulation using flashing lights; or electrical stimulation of the tooth pulp.

Recording of evoked responses involves recording EEG epochs and time-referencing them to sensory stimuli that have been applied in a repeated fashion. Computer techniques for processing EEG signals extract the evoked potential from the underlying electroencephalogram after repetitive stimuli; the evoked potential represents 100 to 1,000 stimuli. Therefore, the evoked response represents a time versus voltage relationship that can be quantitated by measuring the poststimulus latency and interpeak amplitudes in the waveform. Evoked response methodology has been reviewed by Grundy.[117,118]

Using evoked potentials to monitor anesthetic drug effect and depth of anesthesia entails both advantages and disadvantages. The electrophysiologic response to sensory nerve stimulation seems to be an attractive variable to monitor when assessing depth of anesthesia. As discussed earlier, the body's response to some form of stimulation is the key to assessing depth of anesthesia. Monitoring of evoked potentials uses a noninvasive continuous EEG measurement and the response to appropriate stimuli. However, the limitations of measuring evoked potentials are significant. Although all anesthetics affect the evoked response to some degree, as with the electroencephalogram itself, there exist no standard measures of drug effect that enable one to identify or characterize drug effect or depth of anesthesia. The issue of choosing the best evoked response parameters to measure is in approximately the same state of uncertainty as the choice of parameters to characterize the processed electroencephalogram.

The technical, clinical, and practical complexities of recording evoked responses are significantly greater than those of recording spontaneous EEGs. Many confounding artifacts can alter evoked potentials: stimulus characteristics (intensity, duration, interstimulus interval), electrode placement, recording equipment, technique, and age and gender of the subject. Anesthetic factors include choice of anesthetic drug, arterial blood gas tensions, and body temperature.[117,118]

As with the electroencephalogram and depth of anesthesia, initial investigations have sought to characterize the effects of anesthetics on different evoked responses[96] and to describe the relationship between drug concentration and response. For example, as the concentration of potent inhaled anesthetic (halothane, enflurane, isoflurane) increases, several changes in evoked responses occur. The latencies of somatosensory, visual, and auditory evoked potentials increase. A generalized increase occurs in conduction time between different neural generators. Also, in general, the amplitude of somatosensory and visual potentials decreases.[119] In contrast, nitrous oxide produces a dose-related decrease in the amplitude of visual and somatosensory evoked responses but no effect on latency.[120]

The most comprehensive assessment of anesthetic drug effect on evoked potentials used the auditory evoked response.[121-125] The auditory evoked response can be divided into the brain-stem response, which is obtained in the first 10 milliseconds after stimulation; the early cortical response (from 15 to 80 milliseconds); and the late cortical response (from 80 to 100 milliseconds). The potent inhaled anesthetics have been found to have similar effects on the early cortical waves of the auditory evoked response. Halothane, enflurane, etomidate, and Althesin (the combination of alphadolone and alphaxolone) all increase the latency and decrease the amplitude of the early cortical waves in the auditory evoked response in a reversible dose- and concentration-related manner. The change in evoked potential appears to be similar and uniform for potent inhaled anesthetics and intravenously administered anesthetics. This similarity and uniformity contrast with the previous description of EEG waveform analysis, in which different parameters must be examined, depending on the intravenous or inhaled anesthetic being used.

Thornton et al.[126] examined the effects of surgical stimulation on the early cortical auditory evoked response in 11 patients anesthetized with nitrous oxide (70 percent) and halothane (at an end-tidal concentration of 0.3 percent). Baseline auditory evoked responses were recorded before and after surgical stimulation. In 6 of 11 patients, the amplitude of early cortical waves increased progressively and significantly, resembling what would be expected from a lower end-tidal concentration of volatile anesthetic, despite the fact that the end-tidal concentration of halothane was being held constant throughout. Surgical stimulation seems to have antagonized the effect of halothane on the auditory evoked response. Only 3 of the 11 patients showed a clear autonomic response, as judged by blood pressure and pulse response. The authors concluded that surgical stimulation partially reverses the change in early cortical waves brought about by halothane anesthesia. These changes affected only the amplitude of the early cortical waves. This study demonstrates the complex effect of noxious surgical stimulation on the auditory evoked response. More detailed examination is necessary before the usefulness of the auditory evoked response in monitoring anesthetic can be determined in relation to the potent inhaled anesthetics.

Hill and colleagues[127] studied the relationships of the plasma concentration of alfentanil, subjective pain report, and brain evoked responses after repeated painful stimulation of tooth pulp stimulation in volunteers. The study demonstrates the significant complexities of monitoring evoked potentials. In a careful crossover study using saline (control) and intravenous bolus injections of alfentanil, the investigators examined recordings of evoked potentials, visual analogue scores of the individual's degree of pain, and measurements of venous plasma concentrations of alfentanil. After administration of alfentanil, the peak-to-peak amplitude of the waveforms from 150 milliseconds (negative peak) to 250 milliseconds (positive peak) increased markedly. This change in evoked potential dissipated, however, within 6 to 10 minutes. The time course of subjective scores of pain relief differed from that of the evoked responses, lasting significantly longer.

This study involved several difficulties. The authors attempted to relate plasma concentration of alfentanil to both evoked response and verbal pain response. Unfortunately, their sampling of venous plasma during the rapid redistribution phase and lack of any pharmacodynamic modeling prevent reasonable interpretation of their results. Also, the authors document the significant adaption or "learning effect" that occurs with the repeated stimulation of tooth pulp in volunteers given a placebo. This effect must be distinguished from the drug effect. Finally, the study shows that the significant amount of signal processing and averaging necessary to obtain evoked responses can prevent identification of meaningful measures of drug effect.

Which electrophysiologic modality (electroencephalogram versus evoked responses) might be useful for measuring depth of anesthesia? The physical and technical complexity of monitoring evoked responses makes this method less practical in clinical anesthesia. Although both modalities still require a great deal more research, the processed electroencephalogram appears to have greater promise and potential as a noninvasive, continuous measure of depth of anesthesia.

Contractility of the Lower Esophagus

Measuring lower esophageal contractility is a novel method of assessing depth of anesthesia. The human esophagus is composed of striated muscle in the upper quarter, smooth muscle in the lower quarter, and both types of muscle in the middle portion. The striated portion of the esophagus is innervated by the reticular formation of the brain stem. Three different types of esophageal contraction have been identified: (1) primary contractions initiated by swallowing, (2) secondary propulsive contractions that occur in response to esophageal dilatation, and (3) tertiary or spontaneous nonpropulsive contractions that occur only in the lower quarter of the esophagus.

Evans and colleagues[128,129] were the first to propose that depth of anesthesia might be measured by the degree of spontaneous contraction of the lower esophagus. Their two relatively uncontrolled studies demonstrated that increasing concentrations of potent inhaled anesthetics decreased lower esophageal contractility. A recent controlled study by Sessler et al.[130] investigated the hypothesis that the frequency of such contractions can predict movement in response to skin incision during anesthesia with either nitrous oxide or alfentanil. Tourniquets placed around both lower extremities and inflated before muscle paralysis isolated the lower extremities and allowed measurement of movement in response to skin incision. Increasing concentrations of halothane and/or increasing doses of alfentanil were found to decrease the probability of movement to skin incision. With one exception, the absence of spontaneous contractions of the lower esophageal sphincter contractility in the 6 minutes before skin incision correlated with no movement in nine subjects given halothane. With one exception, all patients having more than two contractions also moved on skin incision. In contrast, no correlation existed between spontaneous contraction of the lower esophageal sphincter and movement in patients given alfentanil and nitrous oxide. The authors concluded that the correlation of lower esophageal contractility and movement in response to skin incision depends on the type of anesthetic given. Monitoring of lower esophageal contractility appears to be applicable to potent inhaled anesthetics but not to nitrous oxide/opioid anesthesia.

SUMMARY

It is important to separate the definition of anesthesia from that of depth of anesthesia. As discussed by Prys-Roberts,[15] these are two different entities that are frequently confused because of the sharing of the common word. *Anesthesia* can be defined as the lack of response and recall to noxious stimuli. Anesthesia does not include paralysis, nor does it include analgesia where consciousness is present. The anesthetic state can be created by a broad range of drugs that have "anesthetic" effects, some relatively specific (i.e., opioids), others diffuse or multiple (i.e., inhaled anesthetics, barbiturates). All of the drugs used to create the anesthetic state demonstrate relationships of dose, plasma concentration, and degree of drug effect. For some drugs the effect can be quantal (all or none) as seen with movement. Other effects can be continuous and allow some resolution of measurement. Continuous effects can appear quantal if the concentration–response relationship is very steep. Increasing concentrations of a drug that causes an anesthetic state will generally increase the degree of effects to some maximum.

Adequate *depth of anesthesia* occurs when the concentrations of agent(s) is (are) sufficient to produce a collage of effects needed for the comfort of the patient and the conduct of surgery. There is no simple, unifying definition of depth of anesthesia because the anesthesia state is produced by a number of pharmacologic effects that are not necessarily produced by all drugs or may be produced by different concentrations of the same drug. *Depth of anesthesia* is a clinical term that accounts for both diverse drug effects and diverse clinical needs. It involves a complex interaction of multiple drug concentration–response relationships for both direct anesthetic effects and side effects. From a scientific perspective, depth of anesthesia can be defined for very specific drugs alone or in combination using specific defined stimuli and response measurements. The specific scientific definition, however, may not resemble the clinical reality seen in the practice of anesthesia.

REFERENCES

1. Cullen DJ: Anesthetic Depth and MAC. p. 553. In Miller RD (ed): Anesthesia. 2nd Ed. Vol. 1. Churchill Livingstone, New York, 1986
2. Cullen SC, Larson CP: Evaluation of anesthetic depth. p. 77. In Essentials of Anesthetic Practice. Year Book, Chicago, 1974
3. White DC: Anaesthesia: A privation of the senses. An historical introduction and some definitions. p. 1. In Rosen M, Lunn JN (eds): Consciousness, Awareness, and Pain in General Anaesthesia. Butterworths, London, Boston, 1987
4. Plomley F: Operations upon the eye (letter). Lancet 1:134, 1847
5. Snow J: On the Inhalation of the Vapors of Ether in Surgical Operations. Containing a Description of the Various Stages of Etherization, and a Statement of the Result of Nearly Eighty Operations in Which Ether has been Employed in St. George's and University College Hospitals. John Churchill, London, 1847. Reproduced by Lea & Febiger, Philadelphia, 1959
6. Snow J: On Chloroform and Other Anesthetics. John Churchill, London, 1858
7. Gillespie NA: The signs of anaesthesia. Anesth Analg 22:275, 1943
8. Guedel AE: Inhalational Anesthesia, A Fundamental Guide. Macmillan, New York, 1937
9. Artusio JF, Jr: Di-ethyl ether analgesia: A detailed description of the first stage of ether analgesia in man. J Pharmacol Exp Ther 111:343, 1954
10. Robson JG: Measurement of depth of anaesthesia. Br J Anaesth 41:785, 1969
11. Curare in anaesthesia (editorial). Lancet 2:81, 1945
12. Winterbottom EH: Insufficient anaesthesia (letter). Br Med J 1:247, 1950
13. Woodbridge PD: Changing concepts concerning depth of anesthesia. Anesthesiology 18:536, 1957
14. Pinsker MC: Anesthesia: A pragmatic construct (letter). Anesth Analg 65:819, 1986
15. Prys-Roberts C: Anaesthesia: A practical or impossible construct? (editorial) Br J Anaesth 59:1341, 1987
16. Eger EI II, Saidman LJ, Brandstater B: Minimum alveolar anesthetic concentration: A standard of anesthetic potency. Anesthesiology 26:756, 1965
17. Robertson HR: Without benefit of anesthesia: George Wilson's amputation and Fanny Burney's mastectomy. Ann R Coll Physicians Surg Can 22:27, 1989
18. Vickers MD: Detecting consciousness by clinical means. p. 12. In Consciousness, Awareness, and Pain in General Anesthesia. Butterworth's, London, Boston, 1987
19. Bogetz MS, Katz JA: Recall of surgery for major trauma. Anesthesiology 61:6, 1984
20. On being aware (editorial). Br J Anaesth 51:711, 1979
21. Wilson J, Turner DJ: Awareness during caesarean section under general anaesthesia. Br Med J 1:280, 1969
22. Mainzer J, Jr: Awareness, muscle relaxants and balanced anaesthesia. Can Anaesth Soc J 26:386, 1979
23. Breckenridge JL, Aitkenhead AR: Awareness during anaesthesia: A review. Ann R Coll Surg Engl 65:93, 1983
24. Wilson SL, Vaughan RW, Stephen CR: Awareness, dreams, and hallucinations associated with general anesthesia. Anesth Analg 54:609, 1975
25. Hutchinson R: Awareness during surgery. A study of its incidence. Br J Anaesth 33:463, 1961
26. Saucier N, Walts LF, Moreland JR: Patient awareness during nitrous oxide, oxygen, and halothane anesthesia. Anesth Analg 62:239, 1983
27. Bahl CP, Wadwa S: Consciousness during apparent surgical anaesthesia: A case report. Br J Anaesth 40:289, 1968
28. Mark JB, Greenberg LM: Intraoperative awareness and hypertensive crisis during high-dose fentanyl-diazepam-oxygen anesthesia. Anesth Analg 62:698, 1983
29. Mummaneni N, Rao TLK, Montoya A: Awareness and recall with high-dose fentanyl-oxygen anesthesia. Anesth Analg 59:948, 1980
30. Hilgenberg JC: Intraoperative awareness during high dose fentanyl-oxygen anaesthesia. Anesthesiology 54:341, 1981
31. Tunstall ME: Detecting wakefulness during general anaesthesia for caesarean section. Br Med J 1:1321, 1977
32. Tunstall ME: The reduction of amnesic wakefulness during Caesarean section. Anaesthesia 34:316, 1979
33. Schultetus RR, Hill CR, Dharmaraj CM, et al: Wakefulness during cesarean section after anesthetic induction with ketamine, thiopental, or ketamine and thiopental combined. Anesth Analg 65:723, 1986
34. Russell IF: Balanced anesthesia: Does it anesthetize? (letter) Anesth Analg 64:941, 1985
35. Russell IF: Comparison of wakefulness with two anaesthetic regimens. Total I.V. v. balanced anaesthesia. Br J Anaesth 58:965, 1986
36. Breckenridge J, Aitkenhead AR: Isolated forearm technique for detection of wakefulness during general anaesthesia (abstract). Br J Anaesth 53:665P, 1981
37. Abouleish E, Taylor FH: Effect of morphine-diazepam on signs of anesthesia, awareness, and dreams of patients under N_2O for cesarean section. Anesth Analg 55:702, 1976
38. Levinson BW: States of awareness during general anaesthesia. Preliminary communication. Br J Anaesth 37:544, 1965
39. Blacher RS: Awareness during surgery (editorial). Anesthesiology 61:1, 1984
40. Bennett HL, Davis HS, Giannini JA: Non-verbal response to intraoperative conversation. Br J Anaesth 57:174, 1985
41. Woo R, Seltzer JL, Marr A: The lack of response to suggestion

under controlled surgical anesthesia. Acta Anaesthesiol Scand 31:567, 1987

42. Eich E, Reeves JL, Katz RL: Anesthesia, amnesia, and memory/awareness distinction. Anesth Analg 64:1143, 1985

43. Blacher RS: On awakening paralyzed during surgery. A syndrome of traumatic neurosis. JAMA 234:67, 1975

44. Larson CP: On awakening paralyzed during surgery (letter). JAMA 235:1209, 1976

45. Pandit SK, Heisterkamp DV, Cohen PJ: Further studies on the anti-recall effect of lorazepam: A dose-time-effect relationship. Anesthesiology 45:495, 1976

46. Holford NHG, Sheiner LB: Understanding the dose-effect relationship: Clinical application of pharmacokinetic-pharmacodynamic models. Clin Pharmacokinet 6:429, 1981

47. Sheiner LB, Stanski DR, Vozeh S, et al: Simultaneous modeling of pharmacokinetics and pharmacodynamics: Application to d-tubocurarine. Clin Pharmacol Ther 25:358, 1979

48. Stanski DR, Sheiner LB: Pharmacokinetics and dynamics of muscle relaxants (editorial). Anesthesiology 51:103, 1979

49. Eger EI II, Bahlman SH: Is the end-tidal anesthetic partial pressure an accurate measure of the arterial anesthetic partial pressure? Anesthesiology 35:301, 1971

50. Waud BE, Waud DR: On dose-response curves and anesthetics (editorial). Anesthesiology 33:1, 1970

51. Waud DR: On biological assays involving quantal responses. J Pharmacol Exp Ther 183:577, 1972

52. Merkel G, Eger EI II: A comparative study of halothane and halopropane anesthesia: Including the method for determining equipotency. Anesthesiology 24:346, 1963

53. Quasha AL, Eger EI II, Tinker JH: Determination and applications of MAC. Anesthesiology 53:315, 1980

54. Cullen DJ: Drugs and anesthetic depth. p. 287. In Smith NT, Miller RD, Corbascio AN (eds): Drug Interactions in Anesthesia. Lea & Febiger, Philadelphia, 1981

55. Stoelting RK, Longnecker DE, Eger EI II: Minimum alveolar concentrations in man on awakening from methoxyflurane, halothane, ether and fluroxene anesthesia: MAC awake. Anesthesiology 33:5, 1970

56. Yakaitis RW, Blitt CD, Angiulo JP: End-tidal halothane concentration for endotracheal intubation. Anesthesiology 47:386, 1977

57. Roizen MF, Horrigan RW, Frazer BM: Anesthetic doses blocking adrenergic (stress) and cardiovascular responses to incision—MAC BAR. Anesthesiology 54:390, 1981

58. Saidman LJ, Eger EI II: Effect of nitrous oxide and of narcotic premedication on the alveolar concentration of halothane required for anesthesia. Anesthesiology 25:302, 1964

59. de Jong RH, Eger EI II: MAC expanded: AD_{50} and AD_{95} values of common inhalation anesthetics in man. Anesthesiology 42:384, 1975

60. Torri G, Damia G, Fabiani ML: Effect of nitrous oxide on the anaesthetic requirement of enflurane. Br J Anaesth 46:468, 1974

61. Cullen DJ, Eger EI II, Stevens WC, et al: Clinical signs of anesthesia. Anesthesiology 36:21, 1972

62. Eger EI II: Monitoring the depth of anesthesia. p. 1. In Saidman LJ, Smith NT (eds): Monitoring in Anesthesia. 2nd Ed. John Wiley & Sons, New York, 1983

63. Neff W, Mayer EC, de la Luz Percales M: Nitrous oxide and oxygen anesthesia with curare relaxation. Calif Med 66:67, 1947

64. Lowenstein E, Hallowell P, Levine FH, et al: Cardiovascular response to large doses of intravenous morphine in man. N Engl J Med 281:1389, 1969

65. Lowenstein E: Morphine "anesthesia"—a perspective (editorial). Anesthesiology 35:563, 1971

66. Stanley TH, Webster LR: Anesthetic requirements and cardiovascular effects of fentanyl-oxygen and fentanyl-diazepam-oxygen anesthesia in man. Anesth Analg 57:411, 1978

67. Waller JL, Hug CC, Jr, Nagle DM, Craver JM: Hemodynamic changes during fentanyl-oxygen anesthesia for aortocoronary bypass operation. Anesthesiology 55:212, 1981

68. Wynands JE, Wong P, Townsend GE, et al: Narcotic requirements for intravenous anesthesia. Anesth Analg 63:101, 1984

69. Hynynen M, Takkunen O, Salmenperä M, et al: Continuous infusion of fentanyl or alfentanil for coronary artery surgery. Plasma opiate concentrations, haemodynamics and postoperative course. Br J Anaesth 58:1252, 1986

70. Murphy MR, Hug CC, Jr: The anesthetic potency of fentanyl in terms of its reduction of enflurane MAC. Anesthesiology 57:485, 1982

71. Hall RI, Murphy MR, Hug CC, Jr: The enflurane sparing effect of sufentanil in dogs. Anesthesiology 67:518, 1987

72. Hall RI, Szlam F, Hug CC, Jr: The enflurane-sparing effect of alfentanil in dogs. Anesth Analg 66:1287, 1987

73. Murphy MR, Hug CC, Jr: The enflurane sparing effect of morphine, butorphanol, and nalbuphine. Anesthesiology 57:489, 1982

74. Bailey PL, Port JD, McJames S, et al: Is fentanyl an anesthetic in the dog? Anesth Analg 66:542, 1987

75. Ardnt JO, Bednarski B, Parasher C: Alfentanil's analgesic, respiratory, and cardiovascular actions in relation to dose and plasma concentration in unanesthetized dogs. Anesthesiology 64:345, 1986

76. Ardnt JO, Mikat M, Parasher C: Fentanyl's analgesic, respiratory, and cardiovascular actions in relation to dose and plasma concentration in unanesthetized dogs. Anesthesiology 61:355, 1984

77. de Lange S, de Bruijn NP: Alfentanil-oxygen anaesthesia: Plasma concentrations and clinical effects during variable-rate continuous infusion for coronary artery surgery. Br J Anaesth 55:183S, 1983

78. Ausems ME, Hug CC, Jr, Stanski DR, Burm AGL: Plasma concentrations of alfentanil required to supplement nitrous oxide anesthesia for general surgery. Anesthesiology 65:362, 1986

79. Ausems ME, Vuyk J, Hug CC, Jr, Stanski DR: Comparison of computer-assisted infusion versus intermittent bolus administration of alfentanil as a supplement to nitrous oxide for lower abdominal surgery. Anesthesiology 68:851, 1988

80. Scott JC, Ponganis KV, Stanski DR: EEG quantitation of narcotic effect: The comparative pharmacodynamics of fentanyl and alfentanil. Anesthesiology 62:234, 1985

81. King BD, Harris LC, Jr, Greifenstein FE, et al: Reflex circulatory responses to direct laryngoscopy and tracheal intubation performed during general anesthesia. Anesthesiology 12:556, 1951

82. Stoelting RK: Circulatory changes during direct laryngoscopy and tracheal intubation: Influence of duration of laryngoscopy with or without prior lidocaine. Anesthesiology 47:381, 1977

83. Brett CM, Fisher DM: Thiopental dose-response relations in unpremedicated infants, children, and adults. Anesth Analg 66:1024, 1987

84. Sear JW, Prys-Roberts C, Phillips KC: Age influences the minimum infusion rate (ED_{50}) for continuous infusions of Althesin and methohexitone. Eur J Anaesthesiol 1:319, 1984

85. Sear JW, Phillips KC, Andrews CJH, Prys-Roberts C: Dose-re-

sponse relationships for infusions of Althesin or methohexitone. Anaesthesia 38:931, 1983

86. Becker KE, Jr: Plasma levels of thiopental necessary for anesthesia. Anesthesiology 49:192, 1978

87. Tammisto T, Aromaa U, Korttila K: The role of thiopental and fentanyl in the production of balanced anaesthesia. Acta Anaesthesiol Scand 24:31, 1980

88. Brazier MAB: The effect of drugs on the electroencephalogram of man. Clin Pharmacol Ther 5:102, 1964

89. Caton R: The electrical currents of the brain (abstract). Br Med J 2:278, 1875

90. Berger H: Über das Elektrenkephalogramm des Menschen. Arch Psychiatr 101:452, 1933

91. Gibbs FA, Gibbs EL, Lennox WG: Effect on the electro-encephalogram of certain drugs which influence nervous activity. Arch Intern Med 60:154, 1937

92. Faulconer A, Jr: Correlation of concentrations of ether in arterial blood with electro-encephalographic patterns occurring during ether-oxygen and during nitrous oxide, oxygen and ether anesthesia of human surgical patients. Anesthesiology 13:361, 1952

93. Kuramoto T, Oshita S, Takeshita H, Ishikawa T: Modification of the relationship between cerebral metabolism, blood flow, and electroencephalogram by stimulation during anesthesia in the dog. Anesthesiology 51:211, 1979

94. Levy WJ, Shapiro HM, Maruchak G, Meathe E: Automated EEG processing for intraoperative monitoring: A comparison of techniques. Anesthesiology 53:223, 1980

95. Gregory TK, Pettus DC: An electroencephalographic processing algorithm specifically intended for analysis of cerebral electrical activity. J Clin Monit 2:190, 1986

96. Clark DL, Rosner BS: Neurophysiologic effects of general anesthetics. I: The electroencephalogram and sensory evoked responses in man. Anesthesiology 38:564, 1973

97. Galla SJ, Rocco AG, Vandam LD: Evaluation of the traditional signs and stages of anesthesia: An electroencephalographic and clinical study. Anesthesiology 19:328, 1958

98. Levy WJ: Intraoperative EEG patterns: Implications for EEG monitoring. Anesthesiology 60:430, 1984

99. Berezowskyj JL, McEwen JA, Anderson GB, Jenkins LC: A study of anaesthesia depth by power spectral analysis of the electroencephalogram (EEG). Can Anaesth Soc J 23:1, 1976

100. Winter WD: Effects of drugs on the electrical activity of the brain: Anesthetics. Annu Rev Pharmacol Toxicol 16:413, 1976

101. Homer TD, Stanski DR: The effect of increasing age on thiopental disposition and anesthetic requirement. Anesthesiology 62:714, 1985

102. Arden JR, Holley FO, Stanski DR: Increased sensitivity to etomidate in the elderly: Initial distribution versus altered brain response. Anesthesiology 65:19, 1986

103. Scott JC, Stanski DR: Decreased fentanyl and alfentanil dose requirements with age. A simultaneous pharmacokinetic and pharmacodynamic evaluation. J Pharmacol Exp Ther 240:159, 1987

104. Prior PF: The EEG and detection of responsiveness during anaesthesia and coma. p. 34. In Rosen M, Lunn JN (eds): Consciousness, Awareness, and Pain in General Anesthesia. Butterworths, London, Boston, 1987

105. Bimar J, Bellville JW: Arousal reactions during anesthesia in man. Anesthesiology 47:449, 1977

106. Miyauchi Y, Sakabe T, Maekawa T, et al: Responses of EEG, cerebral oxygen consumption and blood flow to peripheral nerve stimulation during thiopentone anaesthesia in the dog. Can Anaesth Soc J 32:491, 1985

107. Rampil IJ, Matteo RS: Changes in EEG spectral edge frequency correlate with the hemodynamic response to laryngoscopy and intubation. Anesthesiology 67:139, 1987

108. Schwilden HJ, Schüttler J, Stoeckel H: Quantitation of the EEG and pharmacodynamic modeling of hypnotic drugs: Etomidate as an example. Eur J Anaesthesiol 2:121, 1985

109. Schüttler J, Stanski DR, White PF, et al: Pharmacodynamic modeling of the EEG effects of ketamine and its enantiomers in man. J Pharmacokinet Biopharm 15:241, 1987

110. Schwilden H, Stoeckel H: Quantitative EEG analysis during anaesthesia with isoflurane in nitrous oxide at 1.3 and 1.5 MAC. Br J Anaesth 59:738, 1987

111. Schwilden H, Schüttler J, Stoeckel H: Closed-loop feedback control of methohexital anesthesia by quantitative EEG analysis in humans. Anesthesiology 67:341, 1987

112. Smith NT, Rampil IJ: The use of computer generated numbers in interpreting the EEG. p. 214. In Prakash O (ed): Computing in Anesthesia and Intensive Care. Martinus Nijhoff, Boston, 1983

113. Hudson RJ, Stanski DR, Saidman LJ, Meathe E: A model for studying depth of anesthesia and acute tolerance to thiopental. Anesthesiology 59:301, 1983

114. Smith NT, Dec-Silver H, Sanford TJ, Jr, et al: EEGs during high-dose fentanyl-, sufentanil-, or morphine-oxygen anesthesia. Anesth Analg 63:386, 1984

115. Smith NT, Westover CJ, JR, Quinn M, et al: An electroencephalographic comparison of alfentanil with other narcotics and with thiopental. J Clin Monit 1:236, 1985

116. Bührer M, Maitre PO, Ebling WF, Stanski DR: Defining thiopental's steady state plasma concentration – EEG effect relationship (abstract). Anesthesiology 67:A399, 1987

117. Grundy BL: Evoked potential monitoring. p. 345. In Monitoring in Anesthesia and Critical Care Medicine. Churchill Livingstone, New York, 1985

118. Grundy BL: Intraoperative monitoring of sensory-evoked potentials. Anesthesiology 58:72, 1983

119. Sebel PS, Ingram DA, Flynn PJ, et al: Evoked potentials during isoflurane anaesthesia. Br. J Anaesth 58:580, 1986

120. Sebel PS, Flynn PJ, Ingram DA: Effect of nitrous oxide on visual, auditory and somatosensory evoked potentials. Br J Anaesth 56:1403, 1984

121. Thornton C, Catley DM, Jordan C, et al: Enflurane anaesthesia causes graded changes in the brainstem and early cortical auditory evoked response in man. Br J Anaesth 55:479, 1983

122. Thornton C, Heneghan CPH, James MFM, Jones JG: Effects of halothane or enflurane with controlled ventilation on auditory evoked potentials. Br J Anaesth 56:315, 1984

123. Thornton C, Heneghan CPH, Navaratnarajah M, et al: Effect of etomidate on the auditory evoked response in man. Br J Anaesth 57:554, 1985

124. Thornton C, Heneghan CPH, Navaratnarajah M, Jones JG: Selective effect of Althesin on the auditory evoked response in man. Br J Anaesth 58:422, 1986

125. Heneghan CPH, Thornton C, Navaratnarajah M, Jones JG: Effect of isoflurane on the auditory evoked response in man. Br J Anaesth 59:277, 1987

126. Thornton C, Konieczko K, Jones JG, et al: Effect of surgical stimulation on the auditory evoked response. Br J Anaesth 60:372, 1988

127. Hill H, Walter MH, Saeger L, et al: Dose effects of alfentanil in human analgesia. Clin Pharmacol Ther 40:178, 1986

128. Evans JM, Davies WL, Wise CC: Lower oesophageal contractility: A new monitor of anaesthesia. Lancet 1:1151, 1984
129. Evans JM, Bithell JF, Vlachonikolis IG: Relationship between lower oesophageal contractility, clinical signs and halothane concentration during general anaesthesia and surgery in man. Br J Anaesth 59:1346, 1987
130. Sessler DI, Støen R, Olofsson CI, Chow F: Lower esophageal contractility predicts movement during skin incision in patients anesthetized with halothane, but not with nitrous oxide and alfentanil. Anesthesiology 70:42, 1989
131. Ebling WF, Lee EN, Stanski DR: Understanding pharmacokinetics and pharmacodynamics through computer simulation: The comparative chemical profiles of fentanyl and alfentanil. Anesthesiology (in press)

31
CARDIOVASCULAR MONITORING

Thomas E. Stanley III
J. G. Reves

HISTORIC PERSPECTIVES

On January 28, 1848, less than 2 years after the first public demonstration of anesthesia, 15-year-old Hannah Greener, while undergoing excision of an ingrown toenail, died as a result of chloroform administration. An account of this incident, the first known anesthesia-related mortality, is found in Robinson's *Victory over Pain* and quickly captures the attention of any practitioner of this speciality[1]:

> She was placed in a chair in an upright posture. It was the infancy of modern anesthesia: the operation was minor, but the error was major. A teaspoonful of chloroform was poured on a handkerchief and the inhalation began. . . . In half a minute, the anesthetist lifted the girl's arm, and found it rigid; he looked at her pupil and pinched her cheek, and found them insensible. . . . [The surgeon] made a semilunar incision, whereupon the girl gave a kick. Thinking that not enough chloroform had been given, the anesthetist was about to pour more on the handkerchief. Instead, he threw down the fatal handkerchief, for the girl's lips suddenly blanched, and there was froth at her mouth. The operation was abandoned for resuscitation. . . . They laid her on the floor, opened a vein in her arm, and then the jugular vein; no blood flowed. Two minutes sufficed for the tragedy of inhalation, operation, venesection, and extinction.

Nearly a century and a half later, one may speculate that even a rudimentary awareness of the patient's cardiovascular status may have averted this mishap.

1031

Clearly, anesthesiologists today realize the advantages of drugs far less toxic than chloroform. However, we now provide anesthesia for much longer, more complex and invasive surgical procedures in patients with far less capacity to tolerate such interventions. Adequate monitoring of the cardiovascular system is no less necessary or important today than it was at the time of the invention of anesthesia.

The remainder of the 19th century saw little advance in the development of objective monitoring during anesthesia. Assessment of a patient's cardiac status was entirely qualitative and subjective. This is not to say that such observational practices have no value in modern times. On the contrary, the development of these skills is an important part of an anesthesiologist's training and expertise. The continued employment of and reliance on the precordial stethoscope, first put into wide use by Guedel in the 1930s,[2] bear witness to this fact.

In 1903, largely on the recommendation of Harvey Cushing, an important new form of quantitative cardiac monitoring was first placed into routine use in anesthetic practice in this country. This was the measurement of systemic blood pressure using Riva-Rocci's sphygmomanometer, a cuff that occludes then slowly releases a major peripheral artery, a technique reported 7 years previously.[3] Cushing's first report of blood pressure measurement in surgical patients described readings as high as 355 mmHg systolic,[4] which likely represents the error now known to be associated with undersized cuffs then in use. The principle of this technique has persisted to the present, as most modern noninvasive blood pressure monitors depend on the Riva-Rocci method, varying only in the means by which the points of systolic and diastolic pressure are chosen during cuff deflation. The best recognized of these is the simple auscultation of the sounds associated with changes in blood flow, first described by Korotkoff in 1905,[5] which remains a standard technique for arterial blood pressure measurement in all facets of medical care. The oscillotonometer, developed by von Recklinghausen in 1931,[6] utilized a second cuff to sense changes in arterial pulsations. Most of today's automated blood pressure devices rely on this methodology. More recently, Doppler techniques and infrared photoplethysmography have been used in noninvasive blood pressure measurement.

Although the first direct intra-arterial measurement of blood pressure was made in 1733 by Stephen Hales, the routine application of this practice in humans awaited the development of safe percutaneous arterial cannulation, which was achieved by Peterson and Dripps in 1949.[7] Enthusiastic use of this modality grew in the next decade not only as a result of improvements in transducer technology but also because arterial catheters provided the means of fully exploiting the simultaneously evolving science of arterial blood gas measurement.[2] Invasive blood pressure monitoring is now widely used in all areas of critical care and is an accepted standard for measurement of this parameter.

However, it is important to realize that this technique also has shortcomings and inaccuracies that must be understood completely to prevent misuse of the data that it provides.

Deep venous cannulation for the purpose of cardiovascular monitoring was pioneered by the efforts of Werner Forssman,[8] who performed the first human cardiac catheterization on himself in 1929 (Fig. 31-1). This landmark achievement allowed the subsequent completion of many important investigations in cardiac physiology and pathophysiologic states, which have formed a basis of understanding for our current use of venous pressure monitoring tools. Lagerlof and Werko first reported the value of the pulmonary capillary "wedge" pressure as a reflection of left ventricular filling,[9] a finding that was later magnified in importance by several investigators who described poor correlation between the wedge pressure and central venous pressure in victims of myocardial infarction and in surgical patients.[10,11] The measurement of cardiac output using Fick's principle[12] was promoted by the work of Cournand.[13] Dexter and colleagues published oxygen saturation data for the right heart and pulmonary artery.[14] Finally, the routine implementation of pulmonary artery catheterization for continuous pressure monitoring was made possible with the development of a flexible, balloon-tipped, flow-directed catheter by Swan and Ganz et al. in 1970.[15] Moreover, the guide-wire-directed technique for deep vascular cannulation described by Seldinger[16] has added significantly to the ease and safety of establishing this form of cardiac monitoring. Modern pulmonary artery catheters provide a variety of additional diagnostic and therapeutic tools, such as thermodilution determinations of cardiac output, mixed venous oxygen saturation, and atrial and ventricular pacing, and have thus become the hallmark of "full" invasive cardiac monitoring in anesthesia and critical care.

The most recent addition to the armamentarium of intraoperative cardiac monitors is transesophageal echocardiography (TEE), which represents a modification of a well-established cardiac diagnostic tool. The use of ultrasound in cardiology began in 1954 with publication of the work of Edler and Hertz,[17] who used their "reflectoscope" to detect movement of cardiac structures. This unidimensional motion (M) mode analysis has largely given way to two-dimensional (2-D) echocardiography, which displays cardiac anatomy in various planes and images its motion in real time. Development of a transesophageal transducer was first established for 2-D examination by Hisanaga et al.[18] in 1980 and improved to phased array technology by Schluter 2 years later.[19] Although the original purpose of transesophageal imaging was simply to enhance cardiac *diagnostic* efforts by overcoming the limitations in image quality of the standard precordial position, TEE has gained significant popularity in anesthesia as a platform for stable, continuous, noninvasive, high-quality intraoperative monitoring of global and regional car-

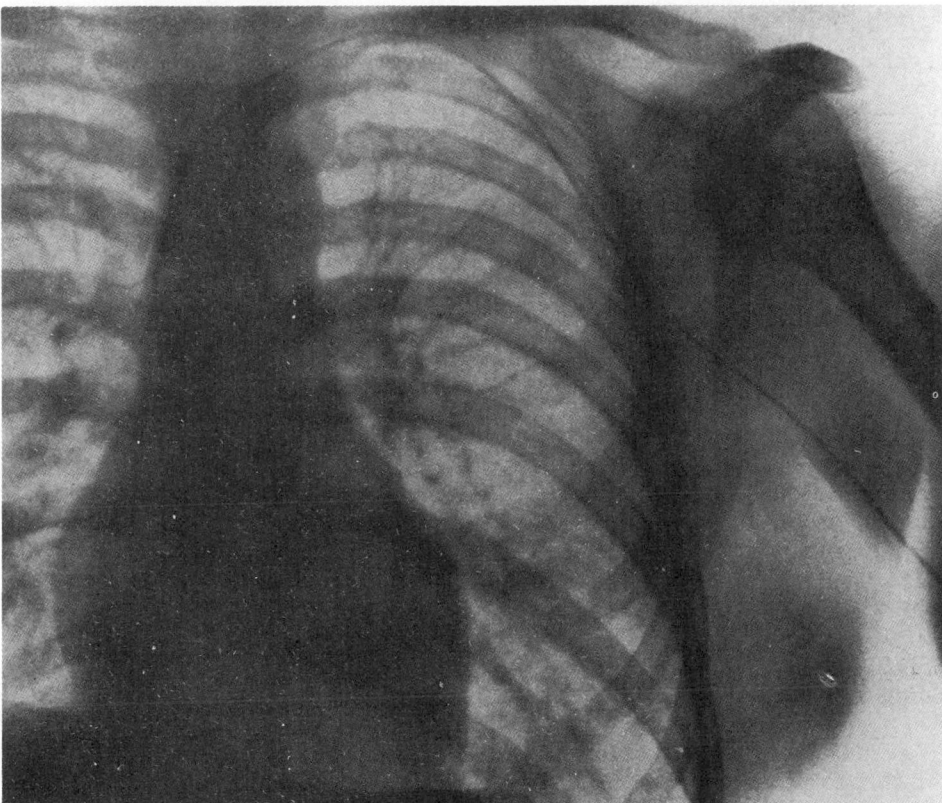

Fig. 31-1. Forsmann's original chest radiograph of himself demonstrating the passage of a catheter from the left cephalic vein into the right atrium. (From Forssman,[8] with permission.)

diac function. Moreover, the addition of Doppler technology and color flow imaging, which allows simultaneous imaging of blood flow along with 2-D cardiac anatomy, has further established TEE as an important tool in modern anesthesia practice.

These historic perspectives on cardiovascular monitoring provide an outline and introduction to the topics that will now be discussed in detail. An obvious omission from this section has been the development and use of the electrocardiogram (ECG), which is discussed in Chapter 32.

SELECTION OF CARDIAC MONITORS

The cardiovascular system is responsible for the transport of chemicals to and from all organ systems (including itself) in order to support their continued normal function. It stands to reason, therefore, that monitoring of end-organ function might provide a reflection of the adequacy of the cardiovascular system performance. This is in fact a well-known principle, an example of which is the measurement of urine output as an index of intravascular volume status and cardiac output. Skin color and turgor can also reflect levels of perfusion. Finally, the differential diagnosis of syncope and altered cerebral perfusion includes several possibilities of cardiac pathophysiology. An obvious caveat to the *exclusive* use of these kinds of measures is that they require the absence of intrinsic end-organ dysfunction, such as primary renal insufficiency. Also, the anesthetic state removes from consideration the use of cerebral indices, such as mentation and sensory or motor function.

Direct assessment of various facets of the cardiovascular system is therefore the more practical method of providing this aspect of patient care in the anesthesia environment. The complexity and level of invasiveness to which this monitoring is indicated for a given patient are dependent on many variables. The nature of the surgical procedure, the "fragility" of the patient's cardiovascular system, and the risks and costs of the various monitoring techniques all play roles in making this decision. Thus, no uniform approach or formula for choosing cardiac monitors can be recommended. Monitoring decisions are a function of the judgment of the anesthesiologist to choose the techniques that will provide sufficient information to optimize the management of a particular patient.

HEART RATE MONITORING

Probably the simplest and least invasive form of cardiac monitoring is the measurement of heart rate. The gauging of this parameter predates any form of objective cardiac assessment and remains an important guide in determining the influences of anesthetics and reaction to surgical stimulus, as well as signifying baseline cardiovascular status. One's ability to determine heart rate quickly by a "finger on the pulse" is a skill as important as this expression is ubiquitous. However, under most circumstances in anesthesia practice, other monitoring devices can provide a continuous numerical display of heart rate. Any monitor that senses the period of the cardiac cycle can be used to present heart rate. Electrocardiography, a standard monitor in nearly every anesthetic setting, is the most common technique used for this purpose, measuring QRS intervals on a beat-to-beat basis. Automatic noninvasive blood pressure devices usually display heart rate as the result of counting the cuff oscillations, and many direct blood pressure monitoring systems provide a heart rate value derived from arterial or pulmonary artery waveforms. Finally, most commercially available pulse oximeters compute and display heart rate.

A theme that will recur in this chapter is the pitfalls of a monitoring method, and heart rate measurement is no exception. All of the automatic monitors of heart rate are subject to errors from artifact, pathologic states, or other therapies. ECG monitors often count pacemaker artifacts (especially atrial) or exceptionally tall T waves as an additional QRS, causing a doubling of the actual heart rate. Intra-aortic balloon pump (IABP) counterpulsation can effect the same doubling error in blood-pressure-derived heart rate; presence of pulsus alternans may falsely divide these heart rate values by a factor of 2. Electrocautery invariably interferes with most ECG monitors and pulse oximeters, rendering their data transiently invalid. Prevention of these errors is limited by current technology, and the anesthesiologist must recognize their cause(s) and ensure that the patient's actual heart rate is within an acceptable range.

ARTERIAL BLOOD PRESSURE MONITORING

The frequent measurement and recording of arterial blood pressure are also fundamental parts of patient monitoring during anesthesia care. Like heart rate, arterial blood pressure is a fundamental cardiovascular parameter. It not only represents the force that drives perfusion of the body but also reflects in part the workload of the heart.

Techniques for measuring arterial blood pressure fall into two major categories: indirect (Riva-Rocci cuff devices) and direct (arterial cannulation and pressure transduction) methods. These differ in nearly every respect, notably in terms of the physical process being monitored and the level of "invasiveness" of their application. Significant variance in arterial blood pressure data exists both within and between these different techniques.[20] So common are these inconsistencies that Bruner et al. stated, "Blood pressure is a function of the way it is measured."[21] In the following discussion, studies comparing different blood pressure monitoring techniques are cited, and some allude to the data of intra-arterial cannulae as the standards against which those of another method should be judged. In fact, there are very many ways in which direct arterial pressure transduction can itself yield spurious blood pressure information, and comparisons of techniques should be read with this in mind. In a review of this subject, Gorback writes, "It is preferable to understand the strengths and weaknesses of the various techniques and expected relative values, since they do not measure the same event."[22] Again, the anesthesiologist must acquire sufficient understanding of the characteristics of these monitors in order to become the arbiter of discrepancies and to use the *total* information presented to the patient's advantage.

Indirect Methods of Blood Pressure Measurement

Intermittent Techniques

As mentioned in the historical introduction, all indirect methods of blood pressure determination rely on the Riva-Rocci sphygmomanometer. This device involves inflating a pneumatic cuff that encloses a peripheral artery to the point of occluding blood flow, then sensing a sequence of physical changes occurring in or around the artery as the pressure is released.

Manual Methods

The simplest technique is a manual intermittent estimate using auscultation of Korotkoff sounds. These sounds are a complex series of audible frequencies that are produced by turbulent flow, instability of the arterial wall, and shock wave formation created as external occluding pressure on a major artery is reduced.[22] The pressure at which the first sound (phase I) is heard is usually taken as the systolic value. The sound character changes (phases II and III), then becomes muffled (phase IV) and finally absent (phase V). Diastolic pressure is recorded at phase IV or V, but phase V may never occur in certain pathophysiologic states, such as aortic regurgitation.[23]

The errors in the auscultatory method occur as a result of deficiencies in the transmission of sound, such as long or loose stethoscope tubing, or of poor hearing sensitivity of the observer. Aneroid manometers are subject to calibration errors and should be checked periodically.

A more basic shortcoming of auscultation is the reliance of blood *flow* to generate the Korotkoff sounds.

Pathologic or iatrogenic causes for decreased peripheral blood flow, such as cardiogenic shock or use of vasopressors, can result in delayed sound generation and a significant underestimation of blood pressure.[24] In contrast, low compliance of the tissues underlying the cuff, encountered, for example, in a shivering patient, will require an excessively high occluding pressure and produce a "pseudohypertension." [22]

Other factors that apply to all methods of sphygmomanometer use involve proper cuff size and deflation rate. The width of the cuff should be 20 to 30 percent of the circumference of the limb. The pneumatic bladder should span at least one-half of this circumference and should be centered over the artery. Excessively narrow cuffs yield erroneously high blood pressure values, as demonstrated by Cushing's early data[4]; overly wide cuffs underestimate the pressure.

Cuff deflation rate is another important feature of precise blood pressure recording, especially when deflation is performed manually. Decreasing occlusion pressure should proceed slowly enough for the sensing process to detect the appropriate changes and to assign them to the current pressure of the cuff. Failure to do so will result in falsely low pressures. A deflation rate of 3 mmHg/s limits this source of error. Coupling the deflation rate to heart rate (2 mmHg/beat) has been found to further improve accuracy.[25]

Automatic Methods

Many of the problems discussed are minimized by the use of automated noninvasive blood pressure (ANIBP) devices. The advantages of ANIBP technology have resulted in its expanding use in many areas of medical care. By complying with a single algorithm or method of data interpretation, ANIBP devices provide consistent, reliable blood pressure information. Also, many of these machines compute an accurate value for mean arterial pressure (MAP), a valuable hemodynamic parameter. They free the operator to perform other duties, provide alarm systems to draw attention to extreme blood pressure values, and have the capacity to transfer data to an automated trending device or record keeper. Allowing machines to act independently can be hazardous, however, as anyone with an erroneous bank account statement will confirm. Care must be taken that the automated inflation-deflation cycling of the cuff not occur so frequently as to limit perfusion of the distal extremity. Cases of ulnar nerve paraesthesia, superficial thrombophlebitis, and compartment syndrome have been reported to result from ANIBP devices' repeatedly attempting to determine blood pressure in the presence of an artifact-producing condition, such as involuntary muscle tremors.[26] Fortunately, these are rare occurrences.

The technique most commonly incorporated in ANIBP devices is the oscillometric principle. In this method, variations in cuff pressure resulting from arterial pulsations during deflation are sensed by the device and are used to determine arterial blood pressure values. The peak amplitude of pulsations approximates mean arterial pressure. Values for systolic and diastolic pressure are derived by using various formulas that examine the rate of change of the pressure pulsations (Fig. 31-2). The systolic point is generally chosen as the pressure at which pulsations are increasing and are 25 to 50 percent of maximum. Diastolic pressure is more difficult to determine but is commonly placed at the point of 80 percent decline of pulse amplitude.[22]

Keeping in mind the aforementioned caveat regarding comparisons of vastly different methods of blood pressure measurement, multiple studies have suggested that the oscillometric technique correlates well with the direct arterial approach and provides an acceptable measurement of arterial blood pressure.[20,27,28] Specific attention has been paid to the use of these noninvasive devices in pediatric patients, with favorable comparisons to direct arterial pressure found in most investigations.[29-31]

Other ANIBP devices use ultrasonic technology in the detection of arterial activity during cuff deflation. One type uses the Doppler principle to determine blood flow distal to the cuff, and another senses the motion of the arterial wall (Arteriosonde). Both provide acceptable blood pressure data,[32,33] but besides having the general problems of auscultatory techniques, they also require explicit attention to placement and securing of the ultrasound transducer. Dislodgment of the transducer leads to sudden loss of information and a disturbing experience for the clinician, who must quickly decide whether the failure is within the machine or within the patient. For these reasons, widespread use of these devices has not occurred.

Continuous Techniques

Until recently, the need for continuous blood pressure monitoring required direct arterial cannulation. Modern advances in microprocessor and servomechanical control technology have enabled noninvasive techniques to provide at least a respectable representation of the arterial pressure waveform and a nearly continuous assessment of blood pressure variables. The better known of these devices is the servoplethysmomanometer, designed and first reported by Penaz[34] in 1973, which is now available commercially (Finapres, Ohmeda). The device consists of a small cuff secured around the middle phalanx of the (usually middle) finger. Within the cuff is built an infrared photoplethysmograph. The cuff and photoplethysmograph interact through a sophisticated servo-controlled mechanism strapped to the hand (Fig. 31-3). The plethysmograph continually measures the size (diameter) of the digital arteries using transillumination. To begin monitoring, a "locking" calibration procedure is performed by varying the cuff pressure in order to establish the vessel size at which oscillometric pressure variation is maximal. An electromechanical feedback loop is then estab-

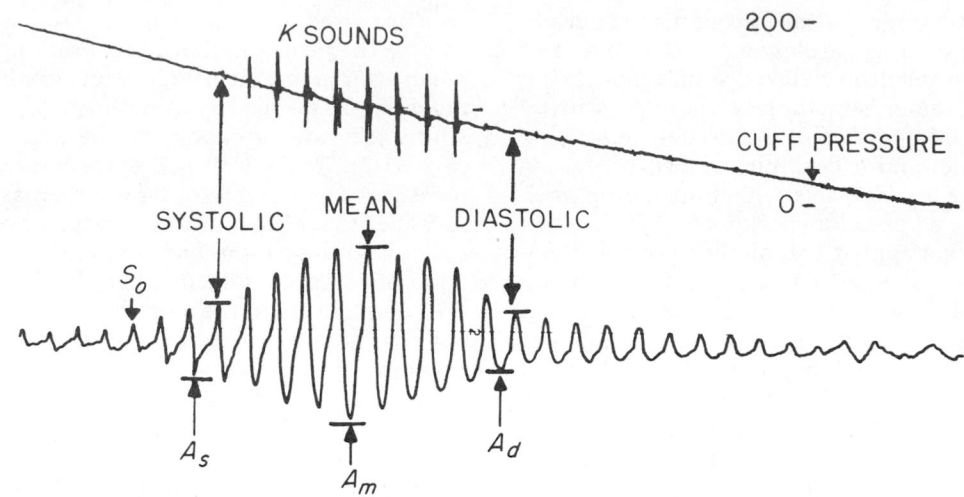

Fig. 31-2. Cuff pressure with superimposed Korotkoff sounds (above) and amplified cuff pressure oscillations (below). S_0, point where cuff pressure oscillations start to increase; A_s, amplitude corresponding to auscultatory systolic pressure; A_d, amplitude corresponding to auscultatory diastolic pressure; A_m, maximum oscillation amplitude, which signals mean pressure. (From Geddes,[45] with permission.)

lished, and external pressure applied to the cuff is continuously varied to keep the measured vessel size constant at this setpoint. Thus, the cuff pressure tracks arterial pressure throughout the cardiac cycle and is displayed on the monitor screen as a continuous waveform. Systolic, mean, and diastolic pressures are computed and trends are recorded. Periodic "locking" recalibrations are necessary and are automatically performed by the device.[35,36]

Comparison studies have demonstrated reasonable correlation of data from the Penaz device with that of direct arterial catheters, with the former method resulting in slightly lower absolute pressures, especially the systolic.[35-38] Placement of the cuff on the thumb has provided superior results.[37] There is a tendency for downward pressure drift that is thought to be the result of progressive changes in interstitial fluid under the cuff, causing alteration of the plethysmograph signal. Repeated calibration usually corrects this problem.[36] The blood pressure measured is necessarily that of the finger, which does not easily allow movement of this "transducer" to different positions, such as to the cerebral level in the sitting position. One study reported that for 5 to 12 percent of the time, the pressure information was found to be unacceptable, probably because of peripheral arterial blood flow limitation secondary to arterial spasm.[38] Finally, the potential for circulatory impairment of the distal finger caused by the constantly inflated cuff has been investigated. Gravenstein and colleagues demonstrated mild hypoxemia in the capillary blood of the fingertip after 10 minutes of Penaz device use.[39] This decrease in PO_2 stabilized before becoming alarming, and no adverse outcome was noted in any patient. Other investigators have applied the instrument for 7 to 12 hours with no untoward sequelae.[38]

An even more recently developed technology that provides continuous noninvasive blood pressure is a monitor of changes in arterial elasticity (APM 770, Cortronic). This device uses a standard size upper arm cuff inflated to a constant, low pressure (typically 30 mmHg) and incorporates complex proprietary algorithms to interpret instantaneous changes in cuff pressure. These data are used to derive information regarding arterial distension, a reflection of phasic intraluminal blood pressure. Further information about clinical evaluation of this device is presently unavailable.

The role that these new continuous noninvasive blood pressure monitors will ultimately assume in anesthesia practice is unclear at this time. Although it is doubtful that they will entirely supplant direct arterial pressure monitoring, there certainly will be a population of patients in whom this technique will find a niche and become an important part of the monitoring armamentarium.

Direct Arterial Blood Pressure Monitoring

Intra-arterial cannulation with continuous blood pressure transduction and display remains the accepted standard for comprehensive arterial blood pressure monitoring. Moreover, the use of indwelling arterial catheters solves another problem frequently encountered in anesthesia and critical care: the need for repeated sampling of arterial blood for blood gas or other analyses. Extensive experience with this technique over the years has demonstrated its value and safety, so that the current indications for its use have become numerous and the threshold for applying it lowered to encompass nearly any seriously ill patient or compli-

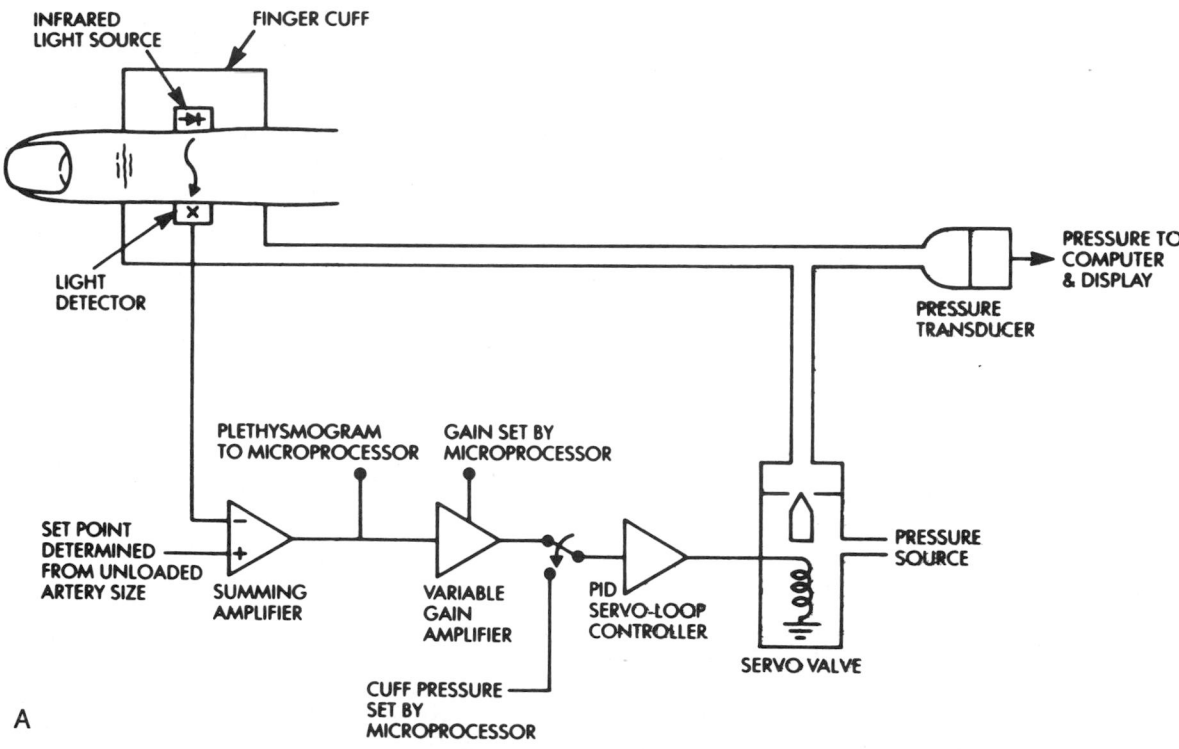

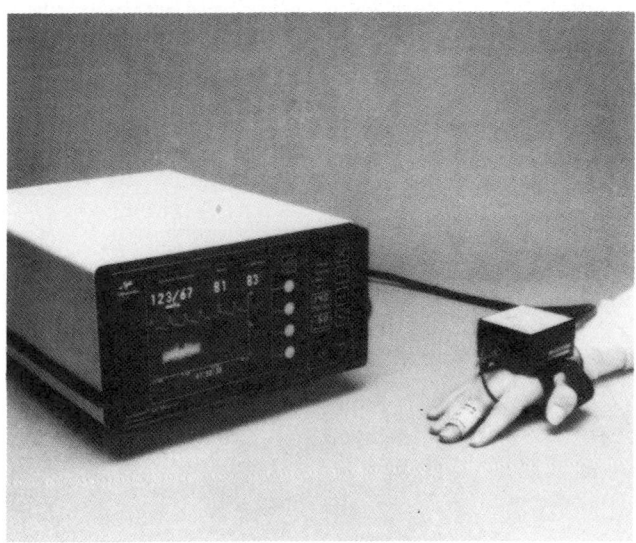

Fig. 31-3. (A) Schematic of the feedback loop of the servocontrol system of the Penaz finger blood pressure monitor. When the monitor is in a closed-loop mode (as shown), it tracks arterial blood pressure. When the loop is open during calibration, the monitor determines the artery size at a transmural blood pressure of zero (unloaded artery size). **(B)** Penaz blood pressure device in place. (Adapted from Boehmer,[35] with permission.)

cated surgical procedure. A list of indications for arterial catheterization is provided in Table 31-1.

Several peripheral arteries are available for percutaneous cannulation. The radial artery is most commonly used because of its accessibility, the presence of collateral circulation to the hand, and because extensive experience in its use and safety has been gained.[40,41]

Technique for Percutaneous Radial Artery Cannulation

Like any procedural skill, percutaneous arterial cannulation is best learned by observing and emulating the methods of other, more experienced personnel. Although many successful variations in technique exist, the following technique and tips for cannulation of the radial artery are given.

Exposure of the radial artery is usually optimized by gentle, but not excessive dorsiflexion and securing of the wrist across a pad, folded towel, or stack of sponges. The artery is palpated along its course over several centimeters to the point that it enters the flexor retinaculum. Tracing this path on the skin with a pen may assist one in developing a good bearing on the vessel's position. The area should be prepared widely with multiple layers of povidone iodine or other antiseptic solution. Local anesthetic (typically 1 percent lidocaine) solution should be injected intradermally using a 25-gauge needle. A wheal that blanches the skin, as well as a generous subcutaneous infiltration on each side of the artery, has several advantages. First, satisfactory local anesthesia is imperative in this and all invasive monitoring techniques. Also, the anesthetic solution may prevent arterial spasm at the time of puncture. Finally, the dermis becomes somewhat softened, and the volume of the subcutaneous space is expanded, increasing both the control over the catheter and one's "working room" in the tissues. A nick in the skin wheal with a #11 surgical blade or large hypodermic needle will further smooth the entry of the catheter. A 20-gauge (smaller in pediatric patients) Teflon catheter first should be checked for frictionless movement of the catheter over the stylet. Many commercial catheters are

TABLE 31-1. Indications for Arterial Catheterization

Continuous BP measurement
Anticipated cardiovascular instability
   Massive fluid shifts
   Intracranial surgery
   Trauma
   Known or suspected significant cardiovascular
     disease
     Previous myocardial infarction, history of
      angina
     Left ventricular hypertrophy
     Valvular disease
     Diabetes
   Cardiac arrest and resuscitation
Direct manipulation of cardiovascular system
   Cardiac surgery
   Major vascular surgery
   Deliberate hypotension
   Deliberate hypothermia
Inability to accurately measure pressure indirectly
   Obesity

Frequent arterial blood samplings
Arterial blood gas measurement
   History of pulmonary disease
   Thoracic surgery, especially involving single lung
     ventilation
   Surgery on the airway
   Other major surgery
Acid-base derangements
   Sepsis
Severe electrolyte or glucose abnormalities
Coagulopathies

encased in a plastic sleeve that can be inserted into the stylet hub and act as a reservoir for the blood that pulses out when the artery is entered. This may help prevent spilling blood on the patient's or one's own hands. The catheter is introduced at a fairly steep angle (typically 30 degrees) to the skin (Fig. 31-4A). Smooth insertion through the tissues and a tactile sense of nearing the artery are important aspects of this step. When the stylet pierces the vessel and blood begins to flow vigorously into the stylet hub and reservoir, the angle of the catheter should be decreased somewhat (typically to 10 degrees). At this point, carefully advancing the stylet another 1/2 millimeter may insure that the *catheter* tip is in the lumen of the vessel. The catheter is then gently slipped off of the stylet and up into the artery (Fig. 31-4B).

If the stylet punctures the back wall of the artery, it is not a grievous error. Studies have shown no influence of arterial puncture technique (single wall versus transfixion) on the incidence of postcannulation arterial thrombosis.[42-44] The stylet should be retracted into the catheter and the catheter slowly pulled back until pulsatile blood flow is restored. Then, the cannula usually can be advanced into the artery. Difficulty may arise if the tip of the plastic catheter is bent or frayed. Under no circumstances should the catheter be advanced against a resistance in the artery. This may lead to intimal damage of the artery and subsequent thrombosis. If one is unsuccessful in passing the catheter, repeated attempts can be made, but excessive punctures of the artery increase the risk of damage to the vessel. If the catheter appears to be in the lumen of the artery, but there is difficulty in advancing further into the vessel, a sterile guide wire may be passed up the artery in order to direct insertion. Some arterial cannulation kits have integrated stylet-guide wire-catheter assemblies for this purpose. Once the catheter is fully advanced into the vessel lumen, occlusive pressure is held transiently on the proximal artery to limit blood loss and the stylet removed. Narrow bore, low-compliance pressure tubing is then fastened to the catheter, an appropriate sterile dressing is applied, and the apparatus is securely taped to the wrist.

Pressure Transducer Systems (Also See Ch. 29)

The pressure tubing is attached to a transduction system, which consists of a fluid-filled electromechanical strain gauge, with stopcocks attached for flushing the catheter to prevent thrombus formation. Many systems incorporate an automatic mechanism for continuous, slow (1 to 3 ml/h) infusion of heparinized saline (1 unit/ml) and a spring-loaded valve that allows periodic high-pressure flushing for clearing the line after a blood sample.

The accuracy with which a transducer system measures arterial pressure is dependent on many interrelated physical factors. A complete description of the

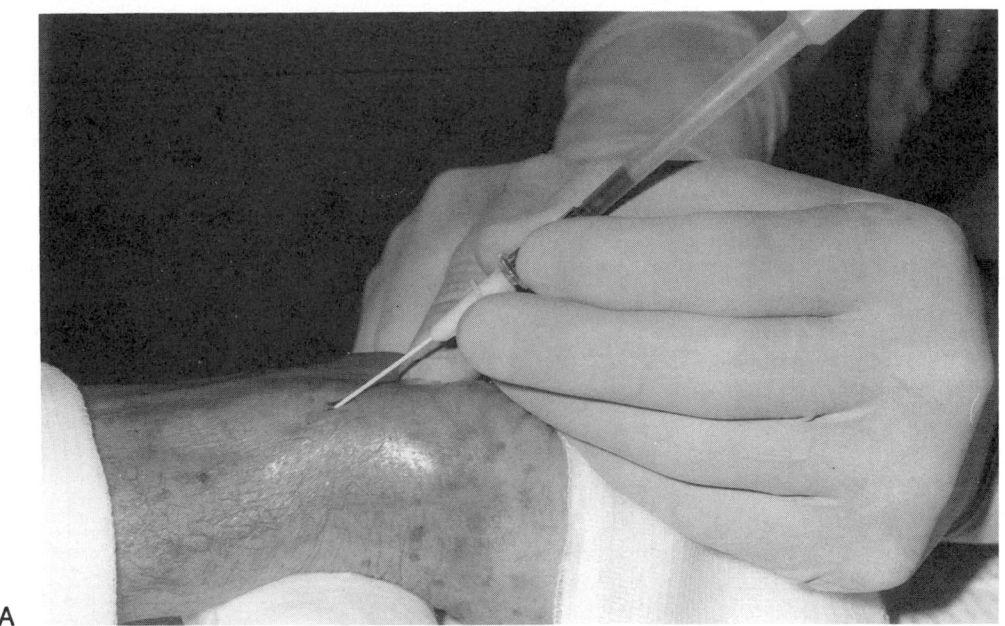

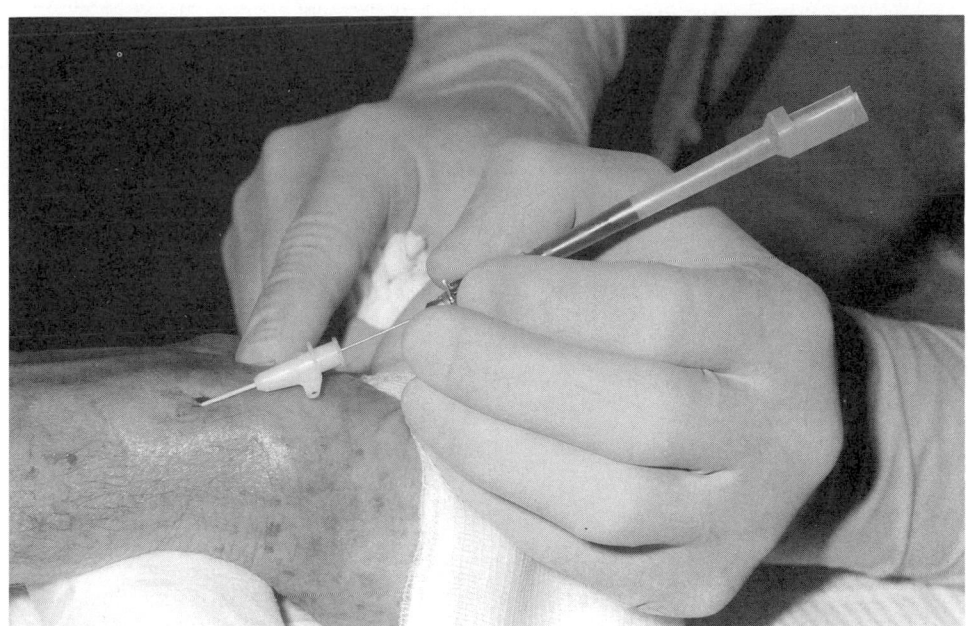

Fig. 31-4. Percutaneous radial artery cannulation. **(A)** The catheter assembly is inserted at a 30-degree angle to puncture the artery. Note the blood in the attached reservoir. **(B)** The angle is then decreased to 10 degrees and the catheter advanced off of the needle.

theoretical basis of this process is beyond the scope of this chapter but is readily available from other sources.[22,45–47] Sufficient understanding of the mechanical characteristics of transducer systems can be gained by comprehension of two descriptive parameters. The first is the *natural frequency* (f_n) of the integrated apparatus. This is the frequency at which the system will resonate or "ring." Physiologic frequencies occurring near f_n are spuriously amplified by the system. Thus, it is preferable for f_n to exceed the maximum significant frequency that exists in a blood pressure signal, which is generally considered to be about 20 Hz.[22] The other parameter is the *damping coefficient* (ζ), which describes the tendency of the apparatus to extinguish oscillations through viscous and frictional forces. The mechanical characteristics of the system that combine to produce these variables are given in the following equations[45]

$$f_n = \frac{d}{8} \sqrt{\frac{3}{\pi L \rho V_d}} \qquad (1)$$

$$\zeta = \frac{16n}{d^3} \sqrt{\frac{3LV_d}{\pi \rho}} \qquad (2)$$

where d = tubing diameter
L = tubing length
ρ = density of the fluid
V_d = transducer fluid volume displacement
n = viscosity of the fluid

Factors that decrease f_n, such as increased tubing length (L), predispose to oscillation in the range of physiologic frequencies, with resulting overshoot of the pressure waveforms. A system with an adequate f_n of 45 Hz using 6-inch tubing is compromised to a f_n of 7 Hz if 6-foot tubing is substituted.[48] Thus, it is preferable to limit the length of the pressure tubing. However, this is often not possible in clinical practice, and it therefore becomes important to be able to assess the amount of the distortion existing in a system. This can be accomplished by "snapping" the flush valve to perturb the system transiently with a high-frequency pulse and observing the response (Fig. 31-5). Ideally, the pressure trace should resolve to the original waveform with a slight overshoot (Fig. 31-5C). Excessive ringing (Fig. 31-5A) may be compensated by increasing the damping coefficient ζ. A *small* air bubble in the line serves this purpose by increasing the elastic components of the system. However, care must be taken not to overdamp the system by excessive increases in ζ, which cause loss of detail in the waveform and underestimation of pressures (Fig. 31-5D). Also, placing an air bubble in the line runs the risk of subsequently flushing it retrograde in the arterial tree, possibly causing cerebral embolization.[49] Commercial devices that allow fine tuning of system damping, avoiding the risks of air bubbles, are available (Accudynamic, CorrecTORR).[50]

Another consideration in transducer system use that applies to all invasive pressure monitoring includes maintenance of sterility. This has largely been answered by increasing use of prepackaged disposable units. Baseline drift of the transducer's electrical circuits can occur, necessitating periodic checks and re-zeroing. Proper placement of the transducer relative to the patient's position (usually at the level of the right atrium) is important for the correct interpretation of blood pressure data. One should keep in mind that the zero reference point for the transducer is the tip of the *stopcock* that is turned out to atmospheric pressure during zero calibration, not necessarily the transducer dome or strain gauge head. These factors are clearly of increased importance during the measurement of low-pressure parameters such as central venous pressure.

Improper damping and calibration account for a large percentage of the errors in direct arterial pressure monitoring. Another cause of these errors is the auto-

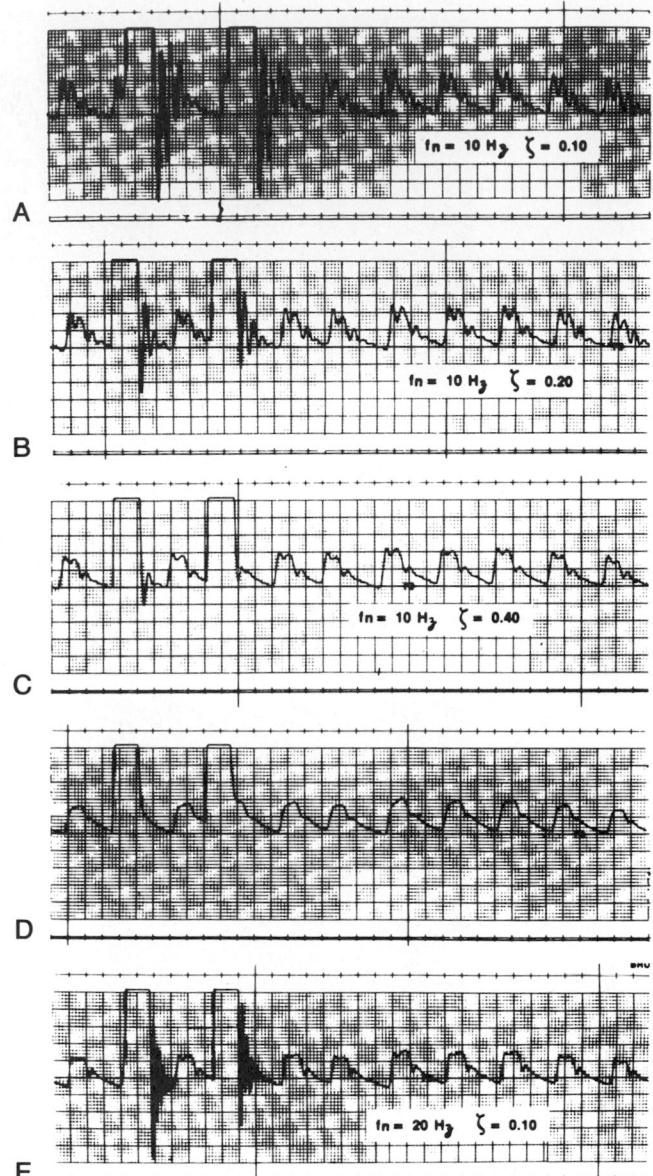

Fig. 31-5. Five pressure tracings showing the method of optimizing transducer fidelity using the flush technique and a damping adjustment device. **(A)** Pressure waveform with two flushes that shows a low f_n of 10 Hz and a low z of 0.1. Note overshoot and ringing in the pressure waveform. **(B)** Damping increased to z = 0.2, f_n unchanged. Ringing after flushing decays more quickly. **(C)** Near-optimum damping (z = 0.4). Note that here is little ringing on the flush signals. **(D)** Over-damping of the transducer system. From the flush, f_n and z are not easily determined; however the flush clearly indicates over-damping because there is no ringing. **(E)** F_n is increased to 20 Hz by shortening the interconnecting tubing length; however, z = 0.1. Note that the pressure waveform is much less distorted than in tracing A. (From Gardner,[47] with permission.)

matic numerical display of pressure values on the monitor screens. The algorithm usually implemented in these monitors dutifully determines whatever maxima and minima are present in the waveform and displays these as the systolic and diastolic values, respectively. Resonance and artifactual amplification in an underdamped system are usually not recognized automatically and result in an erroneous pressure display. Moreover, low-frequency variation in blood pressure caused by ventilation is not accounted for in the numerical presentation. Thus, the use of strip chart recordings of pressure waveforms is often an important part of accurate blood pressure interpretation.

Other blood pressure discrepancies have more physiologic etiologies. Pulse pressure undergoes a natural amplification during transit through the arterial tree. Accurately measured radial arterial systolic pressure is normally greater and diastolic pressure lower than that found in the central aorta. However, under certain circumstances, this relationship is reversed. It has been demonstrated in both adult[51,52] and pediatric patients[53] that after cardiopulmonary bypass (CPB), systolic and mean radial artery pressures were significantly lower than corresponding central aortic values. This phenomenon is thought to result from transient vascular resistance changes induced by CPB.

Complications of Invasive Arterial Blood Pressure Monitoring

The Allen Test

Invasive arterial pressure monitoring carries with it the risk of limiting blood flow in that vessel and causing ischemia distally. Since the risk of this complication is diminished by the presence of collateral blood supply, it is appropriate to take steps to ensure the adequacy of this source of reserve perfusion. In 1929, E.V. Allen reported a technique to determine the site and severity of arterial stenoses distal to the wrist in cases of thromboangiitis obliterans.[54] His original description of this method, largely unchanged in present use, follows:

> The patient closes his hand as tightly as possible for a period of one minute in order to squeeze blood out of the hand; the examiner compresses [the] wrist between his thumb and fingers; thus occluding the radial artery; the patient quickly extends his fingers partially while compression of the radial artery is maintained by the examiner. The return of color to the hand and fingers is noted. In individuals with an intact arterial tree the pallor is quickly replaced by rubor of a higher degree than normal, which gradually fades to the normal color. If the ulnar artery is occluded, pallor is maintained for a variable period, due to obstruction to arterial inflow in the two main channels. . . . Repetition of the test with the examiner's thumb compressing the ulnar artery demonstrates the presence or absence of such a lesion in the radial artery.

Allen's test has become a popular technique for bed-side assessment of ulnar artery patency prior to radial artery cannulation. A common deviation from the technique is to compress both radial and ulnar arteries after exsanguination of the palm, then release the ulnar occlusion. Scoring of this test is made in terms of time to complete return of original color. Normally, full blushing is complete at 7 seconds; 8 to 14 seconds is borderline; 15 seconds is considered abnormal. If ulnar flow is sluggish, then poor ulnar collateral flow is suggested, and radial cannulation is avoided.

The Allen test is meant to identify patients at high risk for ischemic complications during or after radial artery catheterization. In recent years, the predictive value of this test has been questioned. Many reports reviewing permanent ischemic sequelae noted normal Allen tests prior to these catheterizations.[55–58] Moreover, cannulations performed in spite of abnormal Allen tests developed no ischemic complications.[41,43,59] Allen tests of *radial* artery patency bore no relationship to distal blood flow assessment by fluorescein dye injection[60] or photoplethysmography.[61] Other authors have found the Allen test useful and have encouraged its full implementation to assess arterial blood flow of the forearm.[42,62] Although it is obviously of great importance that the clinician minimize the chances of significant distal ischemia from this monitoring technique, it appears that the Allen test per se cannot be relied upon to predict this adverse outcome.

Factors Affecting Thrombosis with Arterial Cannulation

In several studies of percutaneous placement of radial arterial cannulae, other factors have been identified as contributors to the formation of potentially damaging arterial thrombi after cannulation. The incidence of thrombosis increases with duration of catheterization[40,59] and catheter size (18-gauge versus 20-gauge).[63] Tapered Teflon catheters cause significantly *less* radial artery thrombosis than those made of polypropylene.[64,65] Proximal emboli, prolonged shock, and pre-existing vascular disease may also contribute to thrombotic complications at catheter sites.[55] In a study of 1,699 patients, Slogoff and Keats found a 25 percent incidence of diminished arterial flow after removal of percutaneous radial artery catheters.[41] Two-thirds of these became normal after 4 to 7 days. Abnormal flow was correlated only with the presence of hematoma, female gender, and use of extracorporeal circulation. Despite acute flow reductions or occlusions in the radial artery as a result of cannulation, the great majority of vessels recanalized over a period of days or weeks. Thus, the incidence of serious ischemic complications is low (0 to 4 percent).[41,42,55,66] Studies of radial artery catheters in neonates and infants have shown the same low complication rates.[67,68]

Hematoma formation and catheter site infection with possible systemic sepsis are other complications of arterial catheter placement. The incidence of these complications is decreased by meticulous attention to insertion techniques and subsequent sterile dressing and care.

Alternative Arterial Cannulation Sites

Ulnar Artery

If the radial arteries are unavailable for catheterization, alternative sites may be chosen. The ulnar artery is often an appropriate choice, especially if it appears to provide the nondominant arterial supply to the hand. The technique for its cannulation is very similar to that for the radial artery.

Brachial Artery

Cannulation of the brachial artery does not carry with it the potential benefit of collateral circulation that exists at the radial or ulnar site. However, studies have proved the safety of this technique in both intraoperative[69] and long-term outpatient settings.[70] Larger, longer brachial artery catheters (placed for chronic hepatic artery infusions) were associated with increased incidence of ischemic symptoms but no permanent sequelae.[71]

Axillary Artery

The axillary artery is advocated as a cannulation site when more peripheral locations are inaccessible, such as that seen with Buerger's disease,[72] or for pressure monitoring over extended periods of time.[73,74] Catheterization approach is very similar to that of a brachial plexus nerve block, and a 15-cm-long, 20- or 18-gauge Teflon catheter is placed using a Seldinger guide wire technique. It is preferable to use the left axillary artery, since it has a decreased risk of carotid artery obstruction or embolization. Vertebral artery impingement may occur on either side, however. Advantages of this approach include increased patient comfort and mobility during long-term monitoring, availability of a more "central" arterial pressure waveform, and ability to insert large, secure cannulae that can be used for hemodialysis outflow.[73] Complications (infections, bleeding, nerve plexus injury) are very infrequent.[73-76]

Femoral Artery

The femoral artery is another large vessel easily accessible for pressure monitoring. This is usually accomplished by using a percutaneous technique just below the inguinal ligament. A short (7.5-cm) catheter is placed directly or a longer (15-cm) catheter inserted over a guide wire. This site offers particular advantages in certain surgical circumstances. Arterial pressure distal to the aortic cross-clamp during aortic aneurysm or dissection repair is occasionally monitored. This may be especially important during surgery on the thoracic aorta, since during aortic cross-clamp the femoral artery pressure also reflects the perfusion pressure to the kidneys and to a large portion of the spinal cord via the

spinal artery of Adamkiewicz. Femoral artery catheters are sometimes placed in anticipation of later need for an intra-aortic balloon pump (IABP) and act as quick access sites for this device. However, monitoring femoral arterial blood pressure is of little value in the presence of an IABP, since the physiologic parameters of interest exist proximal to the balloon.

Femoral artery catheters have a record of safety similar to that for other sites,[77] although there may be a slightly higher risk for infectious complications with this approach than for the radial arterial site.[74,78,79] Glenski et al. found a low rate of complications in pediatric patients, with the exception of a 25 percent incidence of ischemic symptoms with 20-gauge femoral arterial cannulae in a group of neonates.[80]

Dorsalis Pedis and Posterior Tibial Arteries

Except for being absent in up to one-eighth of the population,[81] the dorsalis pedis artery is an acceptable choice for cannulation under most circumstances but should be limited to a 20-gauge or smaller cannula. Together with the posterior tibial artery and its branches, the dorsalis pedis artery forms the same loop collateral circulation for the foot as the radial and ulnar arteries do for the hand. Collateral circulation is therefore usually adequate for its safe cannulation.[82] Despite this, a history of peripheral vascular disease, especially in diabetics, is a contraindication to the use of either the dorsalis pedis or the posterior tibial artery. A test analogous to the Allen test can be performed for these vessels, using a pinch of the great toe to provide an exsanguinated tissue bed. The test is considered abnormal if the time to return of color exceeds 10 seconds.

The posterior tibial artery is a similarly useful vessel for arterial pressure monitoring. Catheters placed in this artery may be less susceptible to kinking or dorsiflexion of the foot than in the dorsalis pedis artery and may be especially valuable in neonates and infants.[67]

Superficial Temporal Artery

The superficial temporal artery provides an arterial monitoring site that originates at the aortic arch but is not a branch of a subclavian artery. Certain cases demand special attention to arterial pressure monitoring site choice because of specific derangements of vascular anatomy. The right radial site is the first choice in repair of aortic coarctation, since the left subclavian artery may be incorporated into the surgical repair. If the right upper extremity sites are unusable or are distal to an aberrant right subclavian artery,[83] the superficial temporal artery may be used. This vessel is palpable between the lateral margin of the maxilla and the superior anterior edge of the pinna. Randel and colleagues have reported the safety of cannulating this artery in a series of 21 neonates, in whom there were no complications of this technique.[67] However, the risks of ischemia of the scalp and face, as well as the possibility of cerebral embolization by flushing air or particulate matter retrograde to the carotid artery, have been described[84] and should be born in mind when considering this site for pressure monitoring.

CARDIAC FILLING PRESSURE MONITORING

The fact that overall cardiac performance depends in part on the filling of the heart during diastole is the foundation for the practice of monitoring cardiac filling pressure (see Ch. 16). This monitoring is applied by using a number of techniques that provide this information from specific locations of the heart. These methods include monitoring of central venous pressure, pulmonary artery pressure, and left atrial pressure. Table 31-2 summarizes the values for these and other pressures normally encountered in the cardiovascular system. The following section describes the indications, methodology, measurement, and complications of each of these techniques.

Central Venous Cannulation

Establishment of cardiac filling pressure monitoring requires the invasive procedure of central venous cannulation. There are several other indications for central venous cannulation (Table 31-3), such as the need for a secure line for administration of vasoactive drugs or agents that might irritate and injure smaller peripheral veins. Also, central placement of large cannulae provides excellent intravenous access for rapid infusion of fluids to correct severe hypovolemia. Often the central venous location is the only site available for adequate IV access of any kind. Patients at risk for venous air

TABLE 31-3. Indications for Central Venous Cannulation

Cardiac filling pressure monitoring
Central venous pressure
Pulmonary artery pressure

Drug administration
Secure access for administration of vasoactive or peripherally caustic drugs
Chronic drug administration
   Hyperalimentation
   Chemotherapy
   Long-term antibiotics

Rapid infusion of fluids (via large cannulae)
Massive trauma
Major vascular surgery
Liver transplantation

Aspiration of air emboli

Inadequate peripheral IV access

emboli (those having sitting position craniotomies or surgery involving major abdominal veins) often have central venous catheters placed for aspiration of entrained air. Finally, pulmonary artery catheterization for more comprehensive cardiac monitoring obviously requires central venous access.

The invasive nature of central venous cannulation raises the question of the proper timing for catheter placement. In certain patient populations, such as those with known or suspected ischemic heart disease, the cardiovascular consequences of stimulation, from either pain or anxiety, may be detrimental. For this reason, some authors advocate postponing pulmonary artery catheterization in cardiac surgical patients until after induction of anesthesia.[85] Although investigators have shown that central venous cannulation (including placement of pulmonary artery [PA] catheters) in the awake patient can result in unwanted increases in heart rate and blood pressure,[86] other studies have failed to confirm these findings and in fact support the opposite view.[87-90] In addition, the use of adequate local anesthesia and judicious preoperative sedation or β-adrenergic blockade largely prevents the problem. Therefore, the many benefits of cardiac filling pressure monitoring for anesthesia induction and the dubious contraindications to its establishment in the awake state clearly support its preinduction implementation.

The locations and techniques for placing central venous cannulae are numerous. Among anesthesiologists especially, a popular site for this procedure is the internal jugular vein (IJV).[91] The reasons for this preference relate to its consistent, predictable anatomic location within palpable landmarks; its short, straight (right IJV), valveless course to the superior vena cava (SVC) and right atrium; and its position at the patient's head providing easy access by the anesthesiologist in most intraoperative settings. Finally, the success rate for its use exceeds 90 percent in most series of

TABLE 31-2. Normal Cardiovascular Pressures

Cardiac Chamber	Pressures (mmHg)	
	Average	Range
Right atrium, $\overline{M}$	4	0–8
Right ventricle, $\frac{S}{D}$	$\frac{24}{4}$	$\frac{15-28}{0-8}$
Pulmonary artery, $\frac{S}{D} \overline{M}$	$\frac{24}{10}$ 16	$\frac{15-28}{5-16}$ 10–22
PCWP, $\overline{M}$	9	6–15
Left atrium, $\overline{M}$	7	4–12
Left ventricle, $\frac{S}{D}$	$\frac{130}{7}$	$\frac{90-140}{4-12}$
Brachial artery, $\frac{S}{D} \overline{M}$	$\frac{130}{70}$ 85	$\frac{90-140}{60-90}$ 70–105

Abbreviations and symbols: $\frac{S}{D} \overline{M}$, $\frac{systolic}{diastolic}$ mean; PCWP, pulmonary capillary wedge pressure.
(From Schlant et al.,[290] with permission.)

adults[92-94] and children.[92,94] Other locations for central venous cannulation, such as the subclavian veins, also have advantages and proponents.[95] The right IJV will be used here as the example of a technique for placement of central venous catheters.

Technique for Internal Jugular Vein Cannulation

Careful positioning of the patient for IJV cannulation is important, not only to afford the greatest chance of success of the procedure but also to ensure optimal patient comfort. For the right IJV, the patient's head should be turned to the left and the neck slightly extended. A small pillow rest at the left of the patient's head may allow for greater relaxation of neck musculature and lessened anxiety. Placement of the patient in the Trendelenburg position is not an absolute requirement and is necessary only when there is evidence that the patient is hypovolemic. Clinical history and observation of the external jugular vein (EJV) can be of value in determining the need for a slight degree of Trendelenburg angle. Patients with a history of congestive heart failure (who are frequent candidates for central venous cannulation) may be best managed by using some degree of *reverse* Trendelenburg during the procedure.

Most instruction given for determining the position of the IJV in adult patients focuses on the relationship of the IJV to the sternocleidomastoid muscle (SCM). A typical "central" approach starts at the apex of the triangle formed by the two heads of the SCM as the insertion site, with the needle directed toward the ipsilateral nipple. This is generally a useful guide, which leads to a successful IJV cannulation in most cases. However, a patient's body habitus (obesity, short neck) can obscure or distort the usual association of the IJV and SCM. An anatomic relationship that is not distorted is that between the IJV and the *carotid artery*.[96,97] In the neck, both of these vessels, along with the vagus nerve, are enclosed in a fibrous sheath that allows no separation of its contents. At the point of emergence of this sheath from the thoracic inlet, the IJV is positioned laterally and slightly anteriorly to the carotid artery. Moving cephalad, the IJV maintains a lateral position but swings posteriorly, crossing behind the carotid artery at the level of the thyroid cartilage. The most commonly used IJV cannulation techniques (more than 15 have been described[98]) use an insertion site caudad to the thyroid cartilage. Palpation of the carotid artery at the level of the cricoid cartilage will define the position of the IJV (just lateral and anterior to the carotid) in every instance. All approaches based on SCM anatomy (central, posterior, anterior) converge on this location of the IJV (Fig. 31-6). The important feature of this approach is that the carotid artery must be well defined. The commonly used tactic of instructing the patient to lift his or her head transiently in order to tense and better distinguish the SCM, is therefore counterproductive, as well as inconvenient for the patient. Instead, full relaxation of the muscles of the neck should be encouraged at the outset to provide easy and complete palpation and definition of the carotid artery. This assists both in locating the IJV and in preventing puncture of the artery.

In performing any type of central venous cannulation, attention to sterility is exceedingly important. Infection at the puncture site or of the catheter itself is a serious complication. The chosen insertion site should be prepared widely and gently scrubbed with multiple layers of povidone iodine or other antiseptic solution. For the IJV, the preparation area should include the entire side of the neck from the earlobe to the clavicle and suprasternal notch. Most central venous catheter kits include a sterile fenestrated paper drape. This should be applied lightly and centered over the puncture site. At this juncture, it is especially important to communicate one's actions to the patient, since the drape may contribute to unwanted anxiety. Supplemental oxygen administration via nasal cannulae may not only be therapeutic but also offer a psychological advantage in allaying possible fears of "smothering."

The significance of an excellent local anesthetic preparation of the cannulation site for any central venous catheterization cannot be overstated. The arguments favoring preinduction placement of these monitoring devices depend largely on this aspect of the procedure. It is not unreasonable to use the entire allotment of local anesthetic solution (typically 5 ml of 1 percent lidocaine) found in most kits for IJV cannulation. If a 25-gauge needle is used and the anesthetic is injected slowly in a mildly sedated patient, the intradermal skin wheal can often be established without being noticed (Fig. 31-7A). A large skin wheal is advised, so that an area of anesthetized skin will be available for later suturing of the catheter. The 3/4-inch 25-gauge needle is then inserted toward the predetermined IJV location and aspirated gently. In nonobese patients, the length of this needle may be sufficient to "find" the IJV. Several milliliters of anesthetic solution is slowly injected into the subcutaneous tissue; the needle is extracted slightly if blood is aspirated. Changing to a 1 1/2-inch 22-gauge needle may be necessary to locate the IJV and to anesthetize the entire tract to the skin.

Keeping in mind the orientation of the "finder" needle, a 1 3/4-inch 18-gauge catheter-over-needle assembly is used to cannulate the IJV. A small skin nick in the anesthetic wheal may make this step easier and less noticeable to the patient. Also, gentle countertraction on the skin with one's nondominant hand may make this puncture smoother (Fig. 31-7B). This larger, slightly less sharp needle may not puncture the encasing sheath as easily as did the smaller finder needle, and when it does, its force may cause it to pierce quickly both walls of the IJV. Thus, a perceived "miss" with no blood return may actually be a "hit," and extracting the needle slowly with gentle aspiration may demonstrate this to be the case.

With the needle in the IJV, the catheter is advanced carefully into the vessel and the needle is removed. Cov-

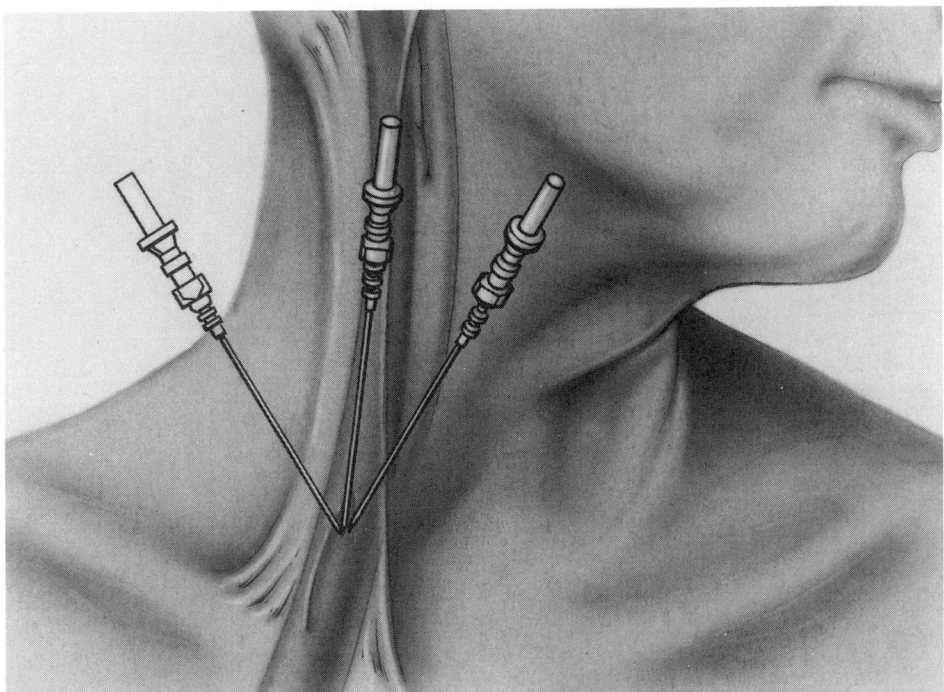

Fig. 31-6. Common approaches to the right internal jugular vein (IJV) for central venous cannulation. Note the relationship of the IJV (darker structure) to the common carotid artery (lighter, more medial vessel). The heads of the sternocleidomastoid muscle can be seen overlying these vessels. The needles demonstrate three commonly used techniques for IJV cannulation (from left to right): posterior approach, central approach, and anterior approach. See text for further description. Note that all approaches converge on the IJV at the same point, just lateral and anterior to the carotid artery.

ering the tip of the catheter with one's thumb will limit the risk of air entrainment. One should attach the syringe to the catheter and aspirate to ensure free blood return. If this maneuver fails, careful adjustment of the catheter while aspirating and having the patient perform a gentle Valsalva maneuver may be necessary to place the cannula properly.

A small amount of blood should flow from the catheter when the syringe is removed. If it does not, a slight increase in the Trendelenburg angle should be used so that air embolus may be prevented. A Seldinger guide wire, typically having a J-shaped end or a *soft*, flexible straight end, is inserted into the cannula. The wire should advance easily into the IJV with little resistance. The electrocardiogram (ECG) should be continuously monitored in order to observe arrhythmias that can occur during these steps,[99] and if direct arterial pressure monitoring is planned, it should be established prior to central venous cannulation. These additional monitors are especially important if a pulmonary artery catheter is to be advanced. The 18-gauge catheter is then removed, leaving the wire in place.

The guide wire is then used to place the final IJV cannula, which is determined by the type of monitoring anticipated. For CVP monitoring, an 8 to 10-inch single- or multilumen catheter is chosen. Sheath introducers used for placement of PA catheters are typically of size

8.5 French. The skin nick at the puncture site should be enlarged to accommodate the size of the catheter used. One should be careful to ensure that control of the guide wire is never lost. This is done by leaving a sufficient amount of wire extending beyond the length of the catheter (Fig. 31-7C). The catheter should be inserted smoothly, maintaining firm countertraction on the skin. Failure to stabilize the skin against the pressure of the advancing catheter can result in "bunching up" of the skin, distortion of the established tract to the IJV, damage to the catheter tip, and *significant* discomfort to the patient. Gently twisting the catheter during insertion also may help to prevent these problems.

With the catheter inserted to the appropriate distance (typically 18 to 20 cm to reach the junction of the SVC and RA), the wire is gently extracted, and the catheter is connected to the monitoring tubing (Fig. 31-7D). The system is aspirated to remove any air before use. The catheter is usually secured with a suture passed behind the puncture site in the original skin wheal. Placing a drop of antibiotic ointment on the puncture site and adding an occlusive dressing complete the procedure.

Other approaches to the IJV differ in the position of the neck for the skin puncture (Fig. 31-6). A "posterior" approach begins at the lateral edge of the clavicular head of the SCM, coursing medially underneath the muscle to arrive at the IJV. The carotid artery is just

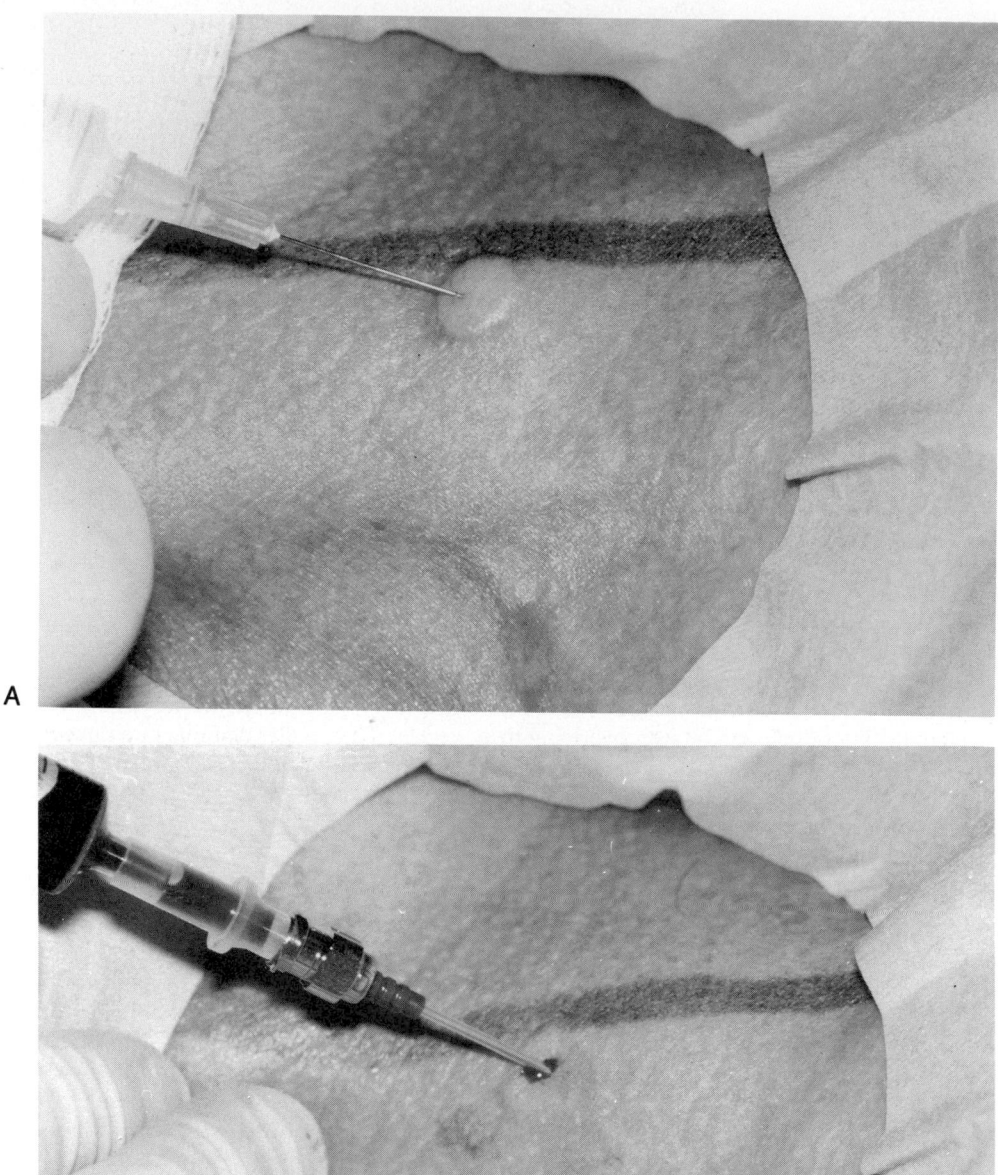

Fig. 31-7. Technique for cannulation of the right internal jugular vein (IJV). **(A)** The right side of the neck has been sterilely prepared and draped. The patient's head is to the left of the photo, and the line on the neck indicates the position of the palpated carotid artery. Local anesthetic is injected subdermally, raising a large wheal that blanches the skin. **(B)** An 18-gauge needle-catheter assembly punctures the IJV located lateral and slightly anterior to the carotid artery. *(Figure continues).*

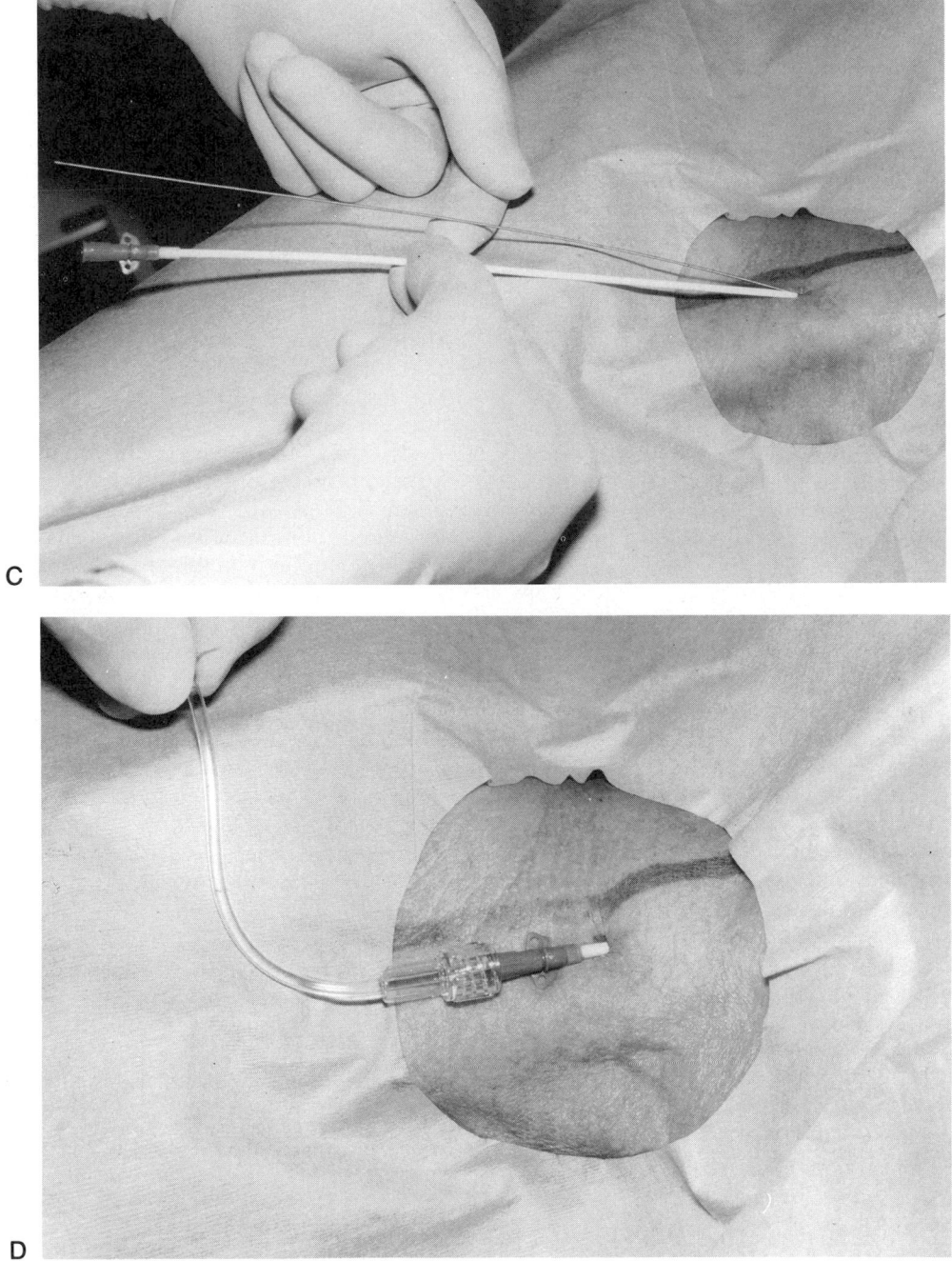

C

D

Fig. 31-7 *(Continued).* **(C)** After passing the guide wire and removing the short catheter, the CVP pressure monitoring catheter is prepared for insertion. Note that sufficient length of guide wire is left exposed to retain control over its position when this longer catheter is placed. **(D)** CVP catheter in place with pressure monitoring tubing attached.

beyond this path, albeit slightly posterior, and may be at increased risk for puncture. The "anterior" approach starts medially and somewhat cephalad, coursing laterally in line with the ipsilateral nipple, and engages the IJV at its anteromedial surface.

Alternative Central Venous Cannulation Sites

External Jugular Vein

Besides the internal jugular veins, either external jugular vein (EJV) may be cannulated for central venous access. The smaller and more tortuous EJV is cannulated with an 18-gauge catheter in a fashion similar to that for a peripheral vein. A guide wire is then passed into the central circulation. This wire should be of the J type with a small radius of curvature of the J, as these have been found to be advanced more successfully.[100,101] Because the external jugular vein is a superficial vessel, EJV cannulation carries less risk of damage to neck anatomy. However, there are venous valves within its course that may impede catheter placement. Moreover, the large-sheath introducers for PA catheters should not be inserted fully, as there is risk of the stiff introducer's tearing the vessel where it joins the subclavian vein.

Subclavian Vein

The subclavian vein still enjoys popularity as a site for central venous access.[95] The fact that the point of insertion is in a broad, flat area of the chest makes it ideal for use in chronic central venous cannulation by affording increased patient comfort and longevity of the occlusive dressing. The infraclavicular approach to this vein is the most commonly taught technique.[102] Beginning in the skin and subcutaneous tissue inferior to the clavicle, a 16-gauge needle is advanced medially so that it passes behind the clavicle just lateral to the curvature at its midpoint. The angle of the needle should be low (tangential to the ribs, if possible) in order to prevent perforation of the pleura. Passage of a guide wire is performed in the usual fashion, followed by the catheter. The subclavian artery is posterior to the vein and in line with this approach. Its puncture may result in significant hemothorax or hemomediastinum because it is more difficult to apply direct pressure to this artery if it is punctured.

Antecubital Vein

The basilic and cephalic veins provide the least risk of complications in central venous catheterization. However, the difficulty in reliably passing these catheters into the SVC makes them a less popular technique in routine practice. Studies report meager success rates, ranging from 25 to 67 percent.[103,104] Moreover, there may be an increased risk of thrombosis and thrombophlebitis with long-term cannulation of these vessels.

Complications of Central Venous Cannulation

Complications of central venous cannulation are infrequent but can result in serious morbidity when they occur (Table 31-4). They may be divided into complications of the puncture and insertion technique and those relating to the catheter itself. Trauma to structures adjacent to the targeted vein is the most commonly recognized error during the cannulation process. Puncture of the carotid artery (1.9 to 3.6 percent incidence[105-107]), the pleural cavity, and the branchial plexus or stellate ganglion is seen during IJV cannulation. Subclavian vein catheterization can result in subclavian artery puncture, pleural injury, and damage to the thoracic duct (left-side approaches). Entrainment of air during catheter placement can be prevented with careful cannulation technique but may also occur if the catheter becomes disconnected at a later time. Catheter shearing and embolization of fragments are serious complications sometimes seen with catheter-through-the-needle sets.

Arrhythmias are occasionally noted when the guide wire or central venous catheter is excessively advanced into the right atrium (RA) or right ventricle (RV) and are typically self-limited when these objects are withdrawn. Infectious complications may involve a superficial inflammation at the insertion site or more serious contamination of the catheter with the possibility of

---

TABLE 31-4. Complications of Cardiac Filling Pressure Monitoring

Complications of cannulation
Arterial puncture
   Carotid artery
   Subclavian artery
Hematoma, hemothorax, chylothorax
Mediastinal, pleural effusion
Pneumothorax
Nerve injury
   Brachial plexus
   Stellate ganglion (Horner syndrome)
Emboli
   Air
   Catheter shearing

Complications of catheter insertion
General
   Cardiac perforation
   Arrhythmias, heart block
PA catheters
   Knotting
   Tricuspid, pulmonic valve injury

Complications of catheter presence
General
   Thrombosis, thromboembolism
   Infection
      Sepsis
      Endocarditis
   Arrhythmias
PA catheters
   Pulmonary artery rupture
   Pulmonary infarction
   Valve trauma

generalized sepsis. The presence of infection necessitates removal of the catheter.

Central Venous Pressure Monitoring

Strictly speaking, central venous pressure (CVP) is the blood pressure at the junction of the vena cavae and the RA. It reflects the driving force for filling the RA and RV. The large veins of the thorax, abdomen, and proximal extremities form a compliant reservoir for a sizable percentage of the total blood volume. CVP is therefore highly dependent on intravascular volume status, as well as the intrinsic tone of these vessels. The functional capacity of the right heart is another determinant of CVP. Thus, CVP monitoring is used for assessment of blood volume as well as right heart function.

CVP monitoring can be accomplished by using an aqueous-fluid-filled manometer connected via stopcock to a running fluid line. This is the simplest, least expensive monitoring system and is sufficient in many cases for a general assessment of intravascular volume status. However, a wealth of information exists in the waveform of the CVP, which can be observed most easily by electronic transduction and display. Most of these monitor devices display the pressure data in millimeters of mercury, not centimeters of water (used on manometers). One should bear in mind the conversion factor for these units (1.36 cmH$_2$O = 1 mmHg) when interpreting pressure data. Also, it is very important when monitoring this low-pressure system that the transducer be placed and zeroed at the correct (right atrial) level.

The normal sequence of mechanical events of the cardiac cycle is responsible for the waves in a typical CVP trace (Fig. 31-8). The a wave is a positive deflection caused by atrial contraction and is quickly followed by a smaller c wave, which represents the initial bulging of the tricuspid valve (TV) into the atrium with the onset of ventricular systole. The x descent follows this wave as the atrium relaxes and the TV is pulled downward. A late, positive v wave occurs as blood accumulates in the vena cavae and RA with the TV closed. Finally, the y descent results from opening of the TV and right ventricular filling.

Several pathophysiologic conditions may be diagnosed or confirmed by examination of the CVP waveform. Atrial fibrillation results in ineffective atrial contraction, therefore an absence of the a wave. Giant (cannon) a waves occur when the atrium contracts against a closed TV and can assist in diagnosing arrhythmias such as heart blocks or nodal rhythms (Fig. 31-9). Tricuspid regurgitation from ventricular overfilling or failure causes distortion and increased size of the v wave.[108]

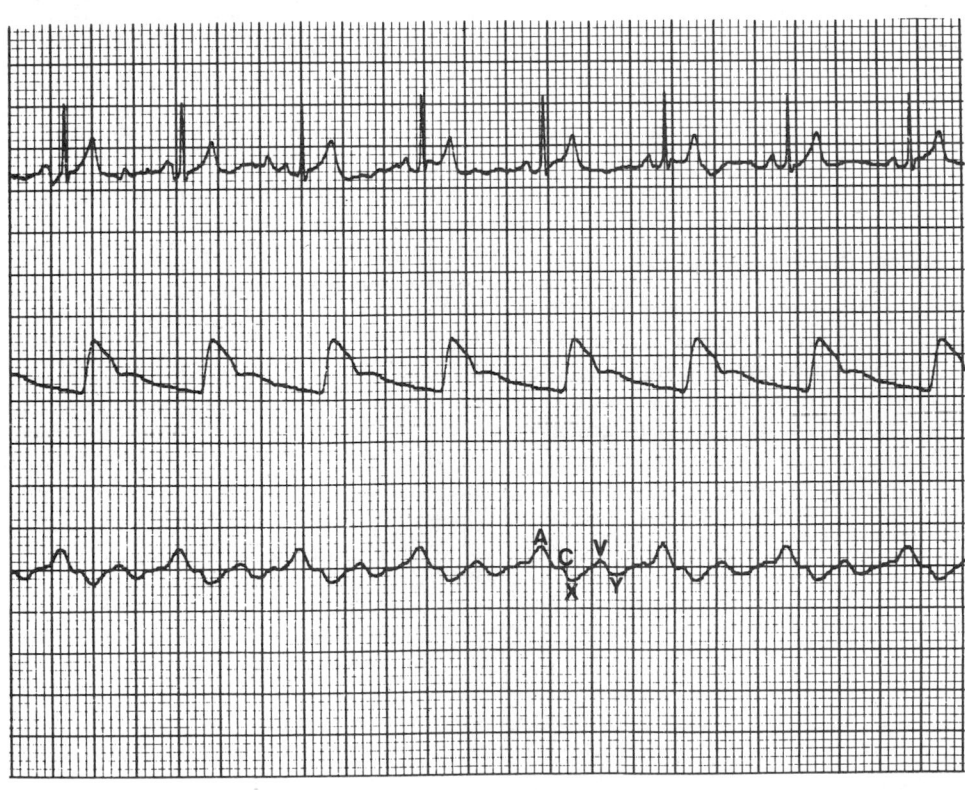

Fig. 31-8. Central venous pressure waves (lower trace) with their temporal relationship to the ECG (upper trace) and arterial pressure waveform (middle trace). See text for description of the a, c, and v waves, and x and y descents.

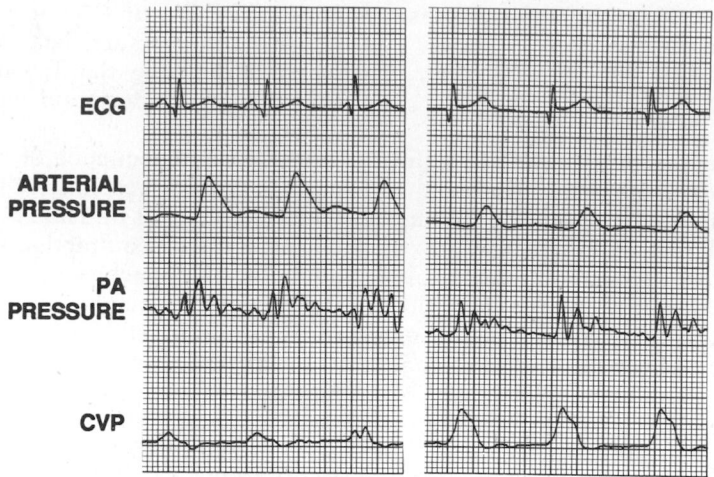

Fig. 31-9. Development of a nodal rhythm. The last cardiac cycle of the left panel shows the beginning of this arrhythmia. The CVP trace at this beat starts to demonstrate an abnormality. In the right panel, the nodal rhythm is established, and the CVP has a giant "cannon" A wave. Note the arterial and pulmonary artery hypotension caused by the lack of atrial contribution to ventricular filling.

The value recorded for CVP is typically a single reading of the mean of the wave at end-exhalation. Ventilation, either spontaneous or controlled, has a significant effect on CVP and should be accounted for in one's interpretation of these data. Trends in CVP during anesthesia and surgery are very useful in determining the effect of fluid or blood loss and in guiding replacement therapy. The response of the CVP to fluid boluses can provide information about overall fluid volume status, venous compliance, and function and efficiency of the right heart. CVP monitoring is commonly used in situations involving large fluid shifts, such as cardiovascular surgery, major abdominal cases, and massive trauma.

Pulmonary Artery Pressure Monitoring

The introduction of the flow-directed pulmonary artery catheter (PAC) two decades ago[15] represented a quantum advance in our ability to define and monitor the hemodynamic status of a patient. With this catheter, pulmonary artery pressures, as well as CVP, can be measured easily. Cardiac output determination using the thermodilution technique is an equally important use of this monitor. The pulmonary capillary wedge pressure (PCWP) or pulmonary artery occlusion pressure (PAOP) under most circumstances provides an accurate estimate of the diastolic filling (preload) of the left heart. This inference is based on the proportionality of pulmonary artery pressures with left atrial pressure (LAP) and left ventricular end-diastolic pressure (LVEDP) (Fig. 31-10). A complete understanding of this concept requires a knowledge of the mechanical factors that influence these relationships.

If left ventricular compliance is normal, LVEDP can be used as an indicator of left ventricular end-diastolic volume (LVEDV), the best overall measure of preload.

Unless an abnormal pressure gradient exists across the mitral valve, LAP and pulmonary venous pressure (PVP) reflect LVEDP. PCWP is used as an estimate of PVP and LAP. "Wedging" the catheter tip into a small pulmonary artery causes the phasic blood flow and pressure in that artery and all distal branches to cease, leaving a static column of blood between the catheter tip and the pulmonary veins and left atrium. Thus, this fraction of the pulmonary vascular bed becomes a simple conduit, "extending" the catheter and tubing to the left heart, and can therefore approximate LAP. However, an important caveat to this concept is the influence of alveolar pressure (P_A) on the capillary bed. West described the pulmonary vasculature as a group of zones (I, II, III) based on the gravitationally determined relationships among pulmonary artery pressure (PAP), PVP, and P_A.[109] As depicted in Figure 31-10, the PA must be in a pulmonary segment within zone III, in which PVP exceeds P_A, for the capillary conduit to be completely open and capable of transmitting blood pressure information. In the supine position, a large portion of the lung is in zone III. However, significant increases in P_A caused by positive end-expiratory pressure (PEEP) may "convert" an area of zone III to zone II or I, possibly causing discrepancies between PCWP and LAP. This source of error has been demonstrated by Lorzman and co-workers, who found that PCWP-LAP correlation was lost when PEEP exceeded 10 cmH_2O.[110] However, decreased pulmonary compliance often seen in critically ill patients may limit this influence of PEEP on pulmonary vascular pressures.[111] Several studies of simultaneous PCWP and direct LAP in cardiac surgical patients have shown good correlation between these measurements,[112,113] except when LAP exceeds 15 mmHg, during which time PCWP may be a poor predictor of LAP.[114]

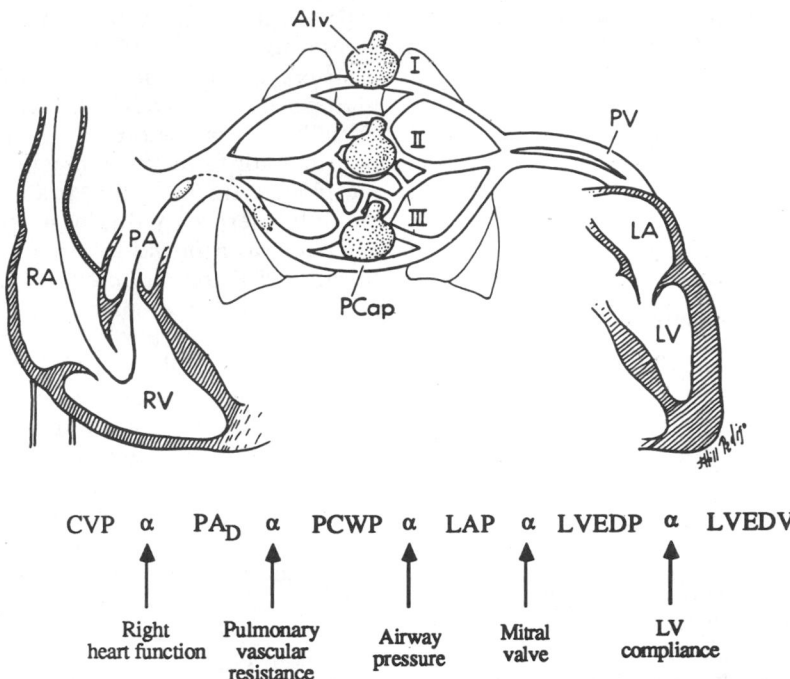

CVP α PA$_D$ α PCWP α LAP α LVEDP α LVEDV

Right heart function

Pulmonary vascular resistance

Airway pressure

Mitral valve

LV compliance

Fig. 31-10. The course of a PAC through the right heart and its normal position in a proximal pulmonary artery. With the balloon inflated, the PAC floats (dotted line) to the "wedge" position, in this case to a segment of zone III lung. The lower panel indicates the relationships of cardiac filling pressures to left ventricular end-diastolic volume (LVEDV) and the mechanical factors that influence them. RA, right atrium; RV, right ventricle; PA, pulmonary artery; P$_{Cap}$, pulmonary capillary; Alv, alveolus, PV, pulmonary vein; LA, left atrium; LV, left ventricle; I, II, III, zones of pulmonary vasculature as described by West (see text). CVP, central venous pressure; PA$_D$, pulmonary artery diastolic pressure; PCWP, pulmonary capillary wedge pressure; LAP, left atrial pressure, LVEDP, left ventricular end-diastolic pressure. (Adapted from Vender,[115] with permission.)

Pulmonary artery diastolic pressure (PADP) is often used as an indicator of PCWP. However, PADP is measured during *phasic* pulmonary artery blood flow and is therefore subject to the influences of pulmonary vascular impedance on the pressure wave. Pulmonary vascular resistance (PVR), normally low, is increased by hypoxia, hypercarbia, and hypothermia, as well as many forms of chronic lung disease. Under these conditions, PADP may not correlate well with PCWP. Also, tachycardia will limit the time for diastolic "runoff" of blood flow, so that at a high heart rate (>120 beats/min), PADP may exceed PCWP.[115]

In contrast to the generally good agreement of PADP and PCWP with LAP, there is ample evidence to suggest that CVP is an unreliable index of left ventricular filling pressure.[10,11,116-119] CVP not only is influenced by the pulmonary impedance parameters just described but also is largely determined by the functional capacity or contractility of the right heart. Thus, only in situations in which left heart function is thought to match that of the right heart *and* there is no condition suggesting grossly abnormal PVR should the CVP be trusted as the sole indicator of overall cardiac filling pressures. For cases in which this degree of normality exists, PA catheters are probably not needed.[120]

Indications and Uses of Pulmonary Artery Catheterization

The indications for placement of a PAC thus center on the presence of significant left ventricular dysfunction or the suspicion that dysfunction may develop or be uncovered as a result of the planned surgical procedure or an ongoing medical condition (Table 31-5). Similarly, known or suspected lung disease that could affect the pulmonary vasculature is considered an indication for PA pressure monitoring in patients undergoing major procedures. Kaplan and Wells found PAC highly useful in detecting myocardial ischemia in patients with known coronary artery disease.[121] They found that over half of the patients who developed ischemia had this diagnosis made by changes in PCWP alone and that ECG changes were less sensitive markers of ischemia. In a study of myocardial reinfarction rates in the postoperative period in 733 patients, Rao et al. found that the incidence of this complication was higher in patients who had hemodynamic instability intraoperatively.[122] They suggested that aggressive hemodynamic monitoring in the perioperative period was indicated in these patients. On the other hand, it has been suggested by Robin that PACs are highly overused and that their

**TABLE 31-5. Indications for
Pulmonary Artery Catheterization**

Left ventricular dysfunction (present or anticipated)
Dilated cardiomyopathy
Valvular heart disease
Ventricular aneurysm
Severe ischemic heart disease
   Global or regional dysfunction
   Recent myocardial infarction
   Ischemia-related valve dysfunction
Idiopathic hypertrophic subaortic stenosis

Aortic surgery (requiring aortic cross-clamp)
Aortic aneurysmectomy
   Thoracic
   Abdominal
Aortic dissection repair

Severe pulmonary disease
Pulmonary hypertension
Pulmonary emboli

justification is based on "semiscientific" information at best.[123] He advocated that routine use of PACs be suspended until an appropriate clinical trial is performed to delineate fully their benefit/risk ratio. Tuman and colleagues recently attempted to perform such a trial by examining outcome variables in a series of 1,094 patients undergoing coronary artery revascularization matched for preoperative risk factors who did or did not receive PAC monitoring perioperatively.[124] They found no influence of the use of PAC on such variables as in-hospital mortality, postoperative myocardial infarction rate, and length of intensive care unit stay. However, assignment to PAC or non-PAC groups was not randomized. Moreover, 7 percent of the non-PAC patients had a PA catheter placed during the study period because, in the opinion of the anesthesiologist, a clinical need for more comprehensive monitoring existed. As the authors acknowledge, it is unclear what influence the continuation of CVP monitoring only in these patients might have had on outcome results. Clearly, the decision to implement monitoring by using a PAC rests on the clinical judgment of the physician, who must consider and weigh all facets of this process in the context of the condition of the particular patient.

Technique for Placement of a Pulmonary Artery Catheter

Pulmonary artery catheters can be successfully placed from all of the central venous cannulation sites previously described, but for the reasons already mentioned, the right internal jugular vein is preferred by most anesthesiologists. External jugular veins may also be used, but the success rate in passing a large catheter centrally via this route is lower than that for the IJV. If the neck veins are unavailable, the left subclavian vein is the best alternative choice for PAC placement, since its course to the SVC is a more gradual turn than the right subclavian vein.

Cannulation of the right IJV for PAC placement is similar to that for CVP monitoring up through the step of inserting the guide wire into the IJV (Fig. 31-7A–C). Modern PAC introducer kits contain a 8.0 or 8.5 French, 15-cm Teflon sheath introducer with a side-port adaptor for central infusion of fluids. A dilator stylet placed through the adaptor and sheath allows smooth insertion of this larger cannula. This approach is passed over the guide wire into the IJV, and the dilator and wire are extracted. Excellent local anesthesia, adequate enlargement of the skin nick, and careful, gentle insertion technique are very important to this step of the procedure (Fig. 31-11A & B). Because the PAC is a longer, more cumbersome catheter, one's attention to maintaining a wide sterile field is very important. In most situations, an assistant handles the nonsterile aspects of PAC placement.

Modern PA catheters are available in a variety of sizes (typically 7.0 to 7.5 French for adults) and often incorporate additional diagnostic or therapeutic features. All have a distal port for PA pressure monitoring, a proximal port (typically at the 30 cm mark) for CVP monitoring or intravenous fluid infusion, and a balloon at the catheter tip for flow-directed placement. This balloon should be inflated with no more than 1.5 ml of air. The syringe included with the PAC is usually restricted to this maximum inflation volume. Special PACs include extra venous infusion ports, fiberoptic bundles for blood oxygen saturation measurement, a lumen for passage of a ventricular pacing wire, and externally mounted electrodes for ventricular and atrial pacing or ECG recording. Smaller, 5.0 French PACs are available for pediatric patients.

Whichever PAC is chosen, all lumens are flushed, and the distal port is connected to a transducer system with a continuous waveform display, and preferably a strip chart recorder. The catheter is passed through a sterile plastic sheath then inserted into the introducer. The balloon is tested by inflation to the full 1.5 ml volume. It should inflate evenly without becoming eccentric, because eccentricity can result in erroneous PCWP readings. Although the PAC is a flexible catheter, most are manufactured with a slight stiffness over the distal 10 cm in the shape of a gentle curve. This curve is very helpful in directing the catheter, especially from more awkward insertion sites such as the left IJV.

The PAC is inserted through the valved port of the introducer to approximately 20 cm. As it is inserted into a right IJV cannula, the curvature of the PAC should be oriented so that it will point just leftward of true anterior (the 11 o'clock position as viewed from the head) (Fig. 31-11C). The balloon is then inflated, and the catheter is advanced toward the right atrium and tricuspid valve. At this point, ECG monitoring for arrhythmias (and arterial pressure monitoring to note their significance) is very important, since premature ventricular complexes (PVCs) are often seen during PA catheter insertion and may require intervention. The location of the tip of the PAC is determined by identify-

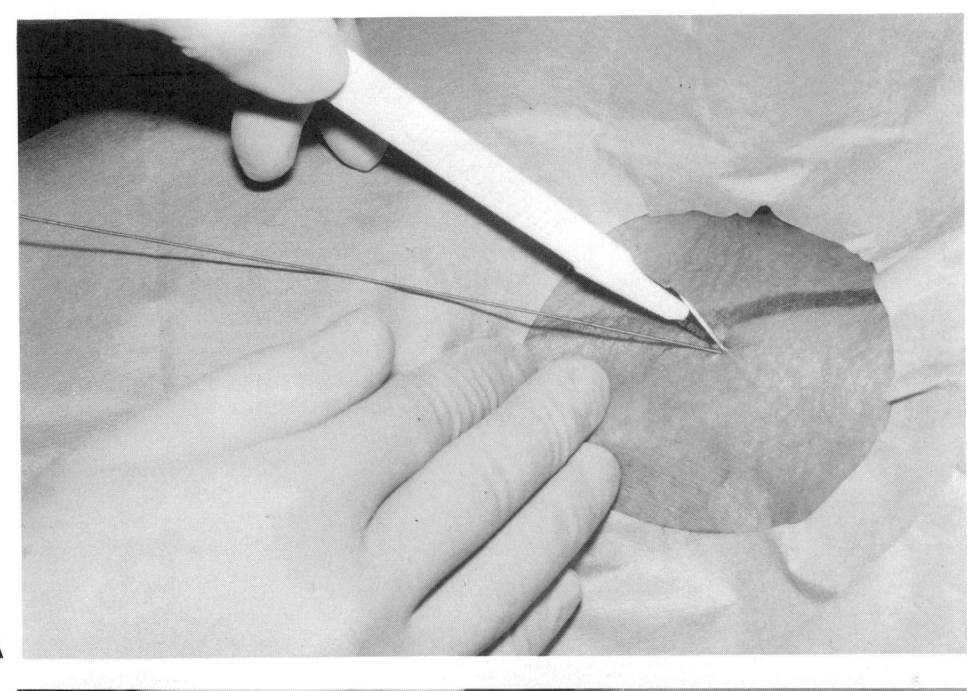

A

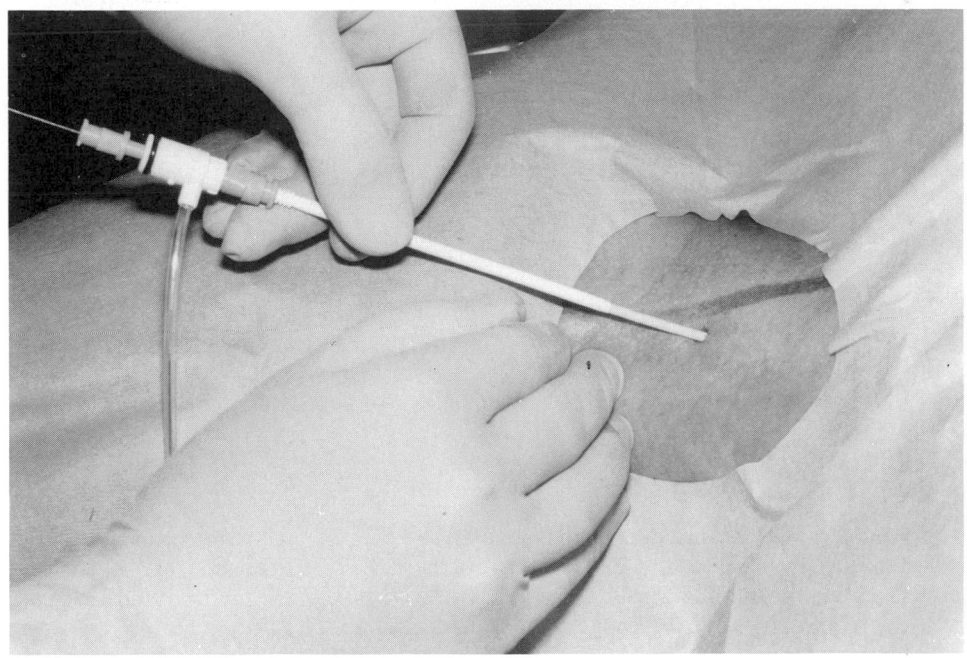

B

Fig. 31-11. Preparation for placement of a pulmonary artery catheter (PAC) via the right internal jugular vein. The initial steps for establishing central venous access and placement of the guide wire are similar to those for CVP monitoring (Fig. 31-7). **(A)** Enlarging the puncture site slightly with a #11 scalpel blade in order to accommodate the larger inducer used for a PAC. **(B)** The introducer sheath and dilator assembly are inserted using the wire guide. Note the counter traction applied with the nondominant hand to prevent the skin's "bunching up" and distorting the insertion tract. *(Figure continues).*

ing the characteristic pressures of the cardiac chambers and vessels encountered (Fig. 31-12). Typically, the tricuspid valve is encountered at 35 to 45 cm from a right IVJ approach, and the wide pulse of the right ventricular (RV) trace is observed. The pulmonic valve is crossed at the 45- to 55-cm mark, and the higher diastolic pressure of the PA is noted, typically with some additional high-frequency artifact from catheter "fling." Although the RV and PA traces are usually easily distinguished, they may be confused when large res-

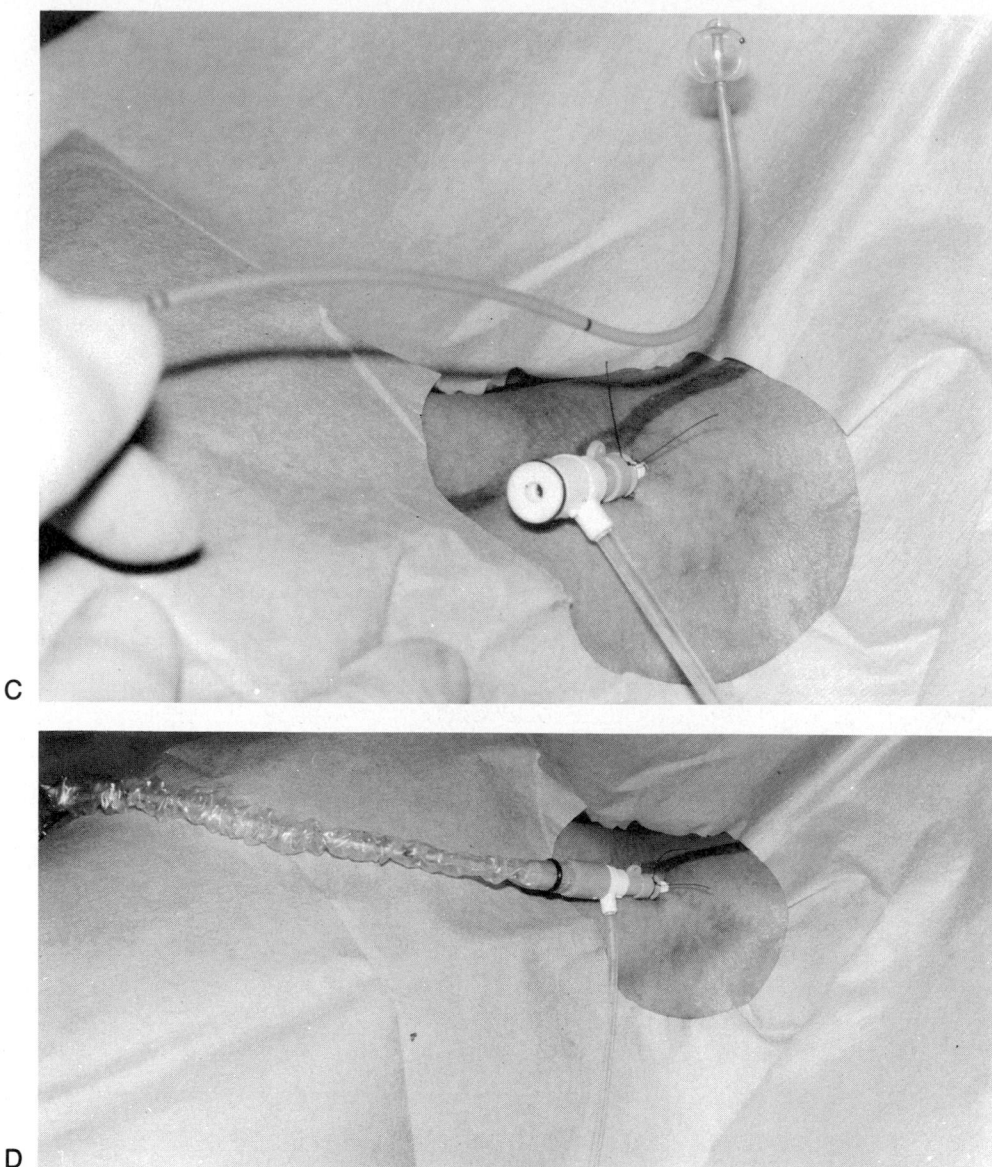

Fig. 31-11 *(Continued).* **(C)** The introducer is in place and the PAC balloon is tested before insertion. The PAC has been passed through the sterile sheath. Note the curve of the PAC pointing the tip at an "11 o'clock" position. Maintaining this orientation during insertion facilitates the passage through the anteriorly located tricuspid valve. **(D)** The PAC in place with the sterile sheath extended and locked onto the introducer.

piratory variation is present, adding significant artifact to the pressure traces. An observation that can often solve this dilemma is to note that just before the rapid pressure upswing of the next systole, the diastolic pressure in the PA is decreasing (as a result of continued forward blood flow and a closed pulmonic valve); in the RV, pressure at end-diastole is increasing (with progressive RV filling and atrial contraction). If the PA waveform is not observed after inserting the catheter 60 cm, chances are good that coiling in the RV has occurred, predisposing to catheter knotting. Careful extraction after balloon deflation, redirecting (twisting), and readvancing of the catheter are used to prevent this

complication. The catheter is advanced farther through the pulmonary artery until the "wedge" position is reached (usually at 50 to 60 cm), with a lower mean pressure and loss of much of the pulsatile character seen in the PA. The balloon is then deflated, and the PA waveform should be restored. Repeated inflation of the balloon should demonstrate the PCWP only at the full extent of the inflation (or shortly afterward as the balloon is gently guided by forward flow into the wedge position). Wedging at lower balloon inflation volumes not only predisposes to "overwedged" traces and erroneous data but also increases the risk of pulmonary artery rupture. PACs often migrate distally during the

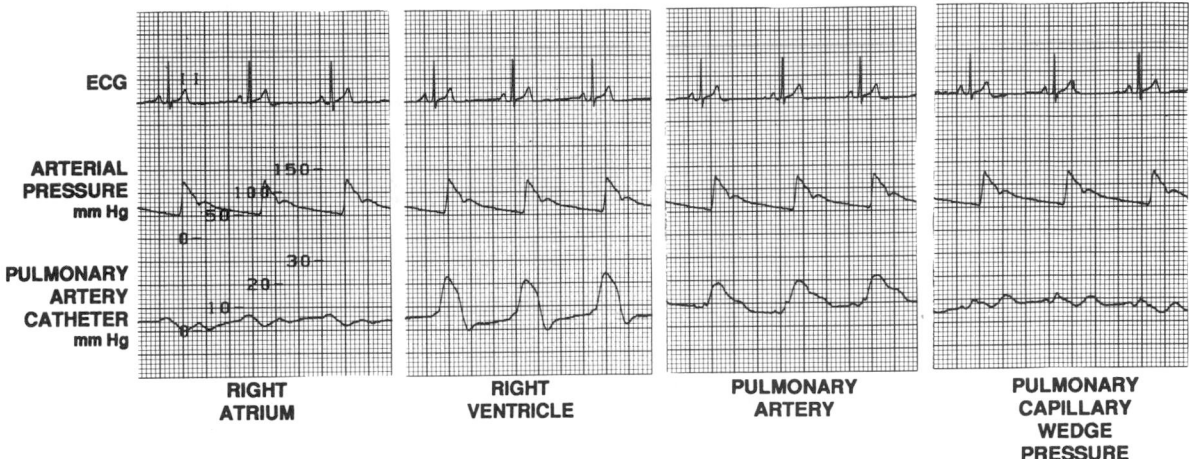

Fig. 31-12. Characteristic waveforms encountered during normal passage of the pulmonary artery catheter. Note the progressive increase in diastolic pressure in the right ventricle, as opposed to a decrease during diastole in the pulmonary artery pressure (see text). Note also the mild respiratory variation in all of these pressures.

course of their use[125] and may have to be checked periodically (by radiograph or *careful* balloon inflation) and pulled back as appropriate. Adjustment of the catheter position is made possible by the sterile protective sleeve covering the PA catheter outside the introducer, although it is debatable whether this device offers significant protection from contamination.[126]

The natural curve of the catheter and the course defined by its passage through the right heart most frequently place the catheter tip in the arteries to the right middle or lower lobe of the lung.[127] This is fortunate, since this location will likely represent zone III pulmonary vasculature and will therefore provide a useful PCWP measurement as explained earlier. If possible, a chest radiograph should be obtained immediately to confirm the satisfactory position of the catheter.

Measurement of Pulmonary Artery Pressure

Although the PAC can provide information that may be invaluable to the care of the critically ill patient, there are several pitfalls in the measurement and interpretation of these data that can make the PAC a counterproductive and even hazardous tool. The catheter balloon for PCWP measurement is inflated "blindly," observing only the PA pressure trace to determine the catheter's position. The waveform can be distorted by artifacts, altering the expected normal progression of the PA pulse wave to the "wedge" trace. This confusion can result in erroneous information or dangerous balloon overinflation.[128]

The effects of PA catheter movement ("whip" or "fling") during the cardiac cycle can result in significant high-frequency artifact in the displayed waveform. The low natural frequency f_n and resonance amplification of these necessarily long catheters are responsible for these erroneous data (see previous discussion of transducer systems). Automatic numeric display moni-

tors are generally not to be trusted to interpret these waveforms accurately, and monitoring of PAP and PCWP is performed optimally by examining a strip chart recording of these pressures. The mode of ventilation (spontaneous or controlled) also must be accounted for in interpreting the effects of respiratory variation on PA pressures and the appropriate information chosen at *end-exhalation*.

If the PAC balloon is inflated excessively, then "overwedging" can occur. This is generally the result of the overfilled balloon's either herniating over the tip of the catheter or driving the tip into the wall of the pulmonary artery. An overwedged trace appears as a ramplike increase in pressure to the top of the display scale. Often a failure to recognize the PCWP trace results in overinflation. The presence of a significant v wave, as a result of mitral regurgitation, for example, can cause the PCWP tracing to resemble the normal PA waveform, and the unsuspecting clinician may continue to inflate the balloon after the wedge position has been obtained (Fig. 31-13). Careful attention to subtle changes in the waveforms during PCWP measurement is thus required to prevent this error.

Complications of Pulmonary Artery Catheterization

Clearly, PAC use is associated with a variety of potential complications that must be considered in one's decision to implement this type of cardiac monitor. Problems can be roughly categorized as those associated with catheter insertion and those seen later as a result of catheter presence (Table 31-4). One study of 211 PAC patients in an intensive care ward found a 51 percent incidence of complications when all problems, major and minor, were considered.[129] In 4 percent of cases, the complications were considered life-threatening, and 2 PACs (0.9 percent) were thought to result in patient demise. In a review of 6,245 undergoing pulmo-

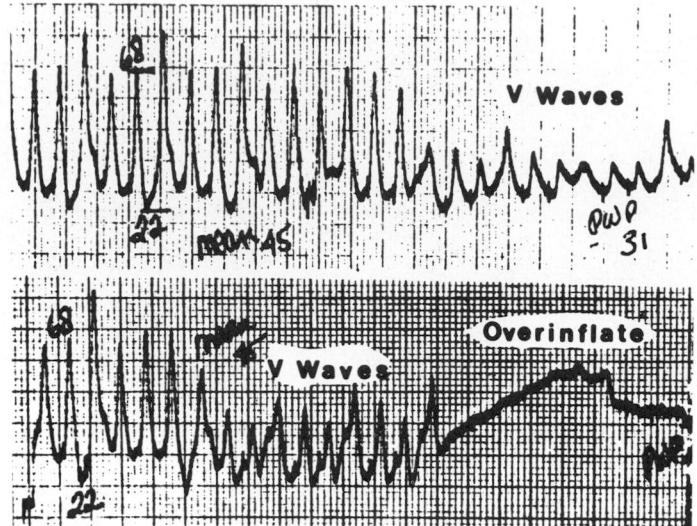

Fig. 31-13. Tracings show V waves and results of a dangerous attempt to compensate for them by overinflation of the catheter balloon. The balloon is deflated in the left half of the upper tracing and inflated in the right half. In the lower tracing the balloon is deflated in the left third of the tracing, inflated during the middle third, and overinflated in the right third. (From Schmitt and Brantigan,[128] with permission.)

nary artery catheterization, Shah et al. reported extremely low rates of morbidity resulting from the PAC itself.[105]

Tachyarrhythmias

Studies have reported a 45 to 69 percent incidence of premature ventricular complexes (PVCs) during PAC insertion or removal.[130,131] However, only 3 percent of these arrhythmias required intervention.[105] Although PVCs rarely may progress to ventricular tachycardia, the vast majority are transient and have been shown not to cause significant morbidity.

Complete Heart Block

Case reports of PAC passage causing complete heart block (CHB) in patients with pre-existing left bundle branch block (LBBB) have led to suggestions that a temporary pacing catheter be used in this population of patients.[132,133] More recently, Morris et al.[134] reported a total of 82 PAC placements in 47 patients with either chronic (> 1-month history) or newly diagnosed LBBB. There were five episodes of CHB in the chronic LBBB group, but each of these occurred either before the PAC was placed or after it was removed. Two episodes of CHB occurred in patients with new LBBB, but neither could be attributed to the presence of the PAC. They concluded that PAC placement was associated with a very low risk of CHB in LBBB patients and suggested that temporary pacing capability is unnecessary in these patients.

Infectious Complications

Catheter-related infections are a well-recognized complication of all types of invasive hemodynamic monitoring. Initial studies of the incidence of positive cultures of PA catheters indicated an association of this complication with duration of catheterization (10 percent at > 72 hours) and with pre-existing sepsis (25 to 50 percent).[135] Subsequent studies have corroborated these findings, placing the overall incidence of PA catheter tip infection at 2.1 to 5.8 percent in cardiac surgical and other intensive care patients.[136,137] However, systemic infection caused by PACs was extremely infrequent.

Catheter Knotting

Catheter knotting is a rare complication, but when it occurs, is a difficult problem to solve and can add significantly to patient morbidity.[138,139] Predisposing factors for development of PAC kinks and knots include excessive catheter insertion and coiling in the right ventricle. Incomplete inflation of the balloon during insertion may increase the chance of the catheter's passing around a papillary muscle or chordae tendinae.[139] The best therapy for this PAC knotting includes awareness of these risk factors and early recognition of the problem (damped PA pressure trace or difficulty in flushing the distal lumen), with subsequent confirmation by chest radiograph. If the knot has not already been drawn tight, it may be untied under fluoroscopy by using a combination of intravascular snares.[140] Otherwise, removal under direct surgical exposure of the venous cannulation site may be required.[141]

Pulmonary Infarction

Another infrequent, but serious complication of PAC management is pulmonary infarction.[142] This results from advancing the catheter in the pulmonary artery to an excessive extent, causing persistent wedging of the catheter tip and ischemia of the lung segment distal to this vessel. This problem highlights the need for careful, frequent assessment of catheter location, since it is known that the PAC will migrate distally in the artery.

Hemodynamic and Respiratory Effects of Balloon Inflation

PAC balloon inflation transiently occludes blood flow through a major pulmonary artery. Hypotension[143] and decreased PaO_2[144] during inflation of the balloon have been reported.

Pulmonary Artery Rupture

The most devastating complication of PAC use is rupture of a pulmonary artery. It is fortunate that this is an uncommon event (0.2 to 0.5 percent)[129,145] because its occurrence carries an extremely high mortality (45 percent).[146] PA rupture can be caused by chronic erosion of a catheter tip or by an eccentrically inflated balloon's driving an exposed catheter tip through the artery.[147,148] More often, however, mismanagement of the balloon inflation itself causes this complication. Hardy et al., studying cadaveric specimens, determined that the pressure required to rupture the pulmonary artery was well within the range of pressures normally exerted by balloon inflation when patient age exceeded 60 years.[146] Pulmonary arteries of younger patients were able to withstand significantly higher inflation pressures. They also found that the presence of pulmonary artery atheromas (taken as an indicator of pulmonary hypertension) had no influence on the susceptibility of these pulmonary arteries to rupture. This is in contrast with reports citing pulmonary hypertension as a risk factor for this complication.[145,148] Atheromatous changes were minimal in the middle or distal pulmonary artery where PAC balloons are typically inflated.[146] It may be that pulmonary hypertension is simply one of the characteristics frequently seen in patients in whom PA catheterization is performed. Thus, considering pulmonary hypertension a contraindication for PAC use is probably questionable.[147]

The hallmark of PA rupture is hemoptysis, which may occur acutely in small amounts or as massive exsanguination. Signs in less obvious cases include hypoxia, hypertension, bronchospasm, and pulmonary artery air emboli. A chest radiograph may show infiltration around the catheter tip. Injection of radiopaque dye

through the PA port will help differentiate pulmonary infarction from PA rupture by demonstrating extravasation into the pulmonary parenchyma in cases of the latter diagnosis. Klibaner et al. reported fatal pulmonary hemorrhage from PA rupture that was not manifested until 14 days after PAC removal.[149]

Treatment of PA rupture will depend on the rate of blood loss and cardiorespiratory stability of the patient. Anticoagulation, if present and not absolutely required, should be reversed. Steps should be taken to lower pulmonary artery pressure. Ventilatory support requirements range from oxygen supplementation to endobronchial intubation to protect the unaffected lung. Only after such intubation should the patient be turned laterally to place the bleeding lung up in order to decrease effective pulmonary artery pressure at that site and slow the hemorrhage.[147] PEEP may be of use in tamponading the bleeding site.[150] In severe cases, emergent surgical intervention is required, with procedures ranging from simple vascular repair to lobectomy or pneumonectomy. The best treatment for this potentially catastrophic complication, however, is prevention, which is best achieved by adhering to several guidelines for safe balloon inflation (Table 31-6).

Left Atrial Pressure Monitoring

Because of its method of placement, direct left atrial pressure (LAP) monitoring is usually restricted to patients undergoing a cardiac surgical procedure. This technique affords a more definitive assessment of left heart filling pressure for patients for whom this information is critically important to their care (notably cardiac valve surgery)[151] and for whom PCWP pressures may be inaccurate (see discussion of PCWP). Diagnosis of a malfunctioning mitral valve prosthesis was reported to be aided by LAP monitoring.[152] Access to the left atrium is typically accomplished by passing a thin catheter through a secure purse-string suture in the right superior pulmonary vein, although a trans-septal approach from the right atrium has been described.[153]

TABLE 31-6. Guidelines for PA Catheter Balloon Inflation

Never use fluid to inflate balloon.

Never use more than the recommended inflation volumes.

Always inflate balloon slowly, watching trace for signs of an "early" wedge pressure trace that may signify peripheral migration of the catheter tip.

Withdraw PA catheter several centimeters just before instituting cardiopulmonary bypass.

Be especially aware of risk of PA rupture in elderly patients.

The catheter is then brought out through the infraxiphoid chest wall and securely connected to a closed pressure monitoring system.

This direct access to the left heart chambers carries the obvious risk of air and particulate embolization to the systemic circulation. LAP monitoring systems therefore require close attention to proper management of periodic or continuous heparin flushes.[154] Also, removal of these lines can result in mediastinal bleeding or catheter shearing.[155] The risk of bleeding generally dictates that the LAP catheter be discontinued before removal of the mediastinal drainage tubes.

CARDIAC PERFORMANCE MONITORING

The primary purpose of the cardiovascular system is to supply adequate blood flow to the tissues, to deliver oxygen and other nutrients and remove waste products. Comprehensive cardiovascular monitoring should provide information about the performance and efficiency of the heart as a pump that supplies this tissue perfusion.

Invasive Cardiac Output Measurement

The most straightforward technique for assessing cardiac performance is the direct measurement of cardiac output (CO). Cardiac output is the total blood flow generated by the heart; in a normal adult at rest, it ranges from 5 to 6 L/min. Under normal conditions, the body regulates cardiac output to meet tissue metabolic requirements, making CO a revealing indicator of the entire cardiovascular system, including the neural and humoral control influences. It is possible for cardiac output to increase by a factor of 5 or more during strenuous exercise. In combination with the measurement of arterial and venous pressures, determination of cardiac output allows computation of other useful hemodynamic parameters, such as systemic vascular resistance, which can assist greatly in the management of patients in the intraoperative and critical care environment.

Fick Cardiac Output Measurement

Measurement of flow in any fluid system can be performed by injecting a measurable indicator into the flow stream and determining the changes in its concentration at various points over time. This principle states that flow is directly proportional to the amount of substance entering a stream of flow during the measurement period divided by the difference between the concentrations of the substances at upstream and downstream measurement sites:

$$\text{Flow} = \frac{\text{indicator amount/time}}{\text{downstream-upstream indicator concentration difference}} \quad (3)$$

This method was first proposed in 1870 by the German physiologist Adolph Fick, who described a means to determine blood flow by measuring overall oxygen uptake and content in blood[12,156]:

> One determines how much oxygen an animal takes out of the air in a given time. . . . During the experiment one obtains a sample of arterial and a sample of venous blood. In both the content of oxygen are to be determined. The difference in oxygen contents tells how much oxygen each cubic centimeter of blood takes up in its course through the lungs, and since one knows the total quantity of oxygen absorbed in a given time, one can calculate how many cubic centimeters of blood passed through the lungs in this time.

In this case, oxygen is the indicator whose uptake in the lungs and extraction by the tissues cause a difference in its content in arterial and venous blood. For this direct Fick method, equation (3) thus becomes:

$$\dot{Q} = \frac{\dot{V}O_2}{(CaO_2 - C\bar{v}O_2 \cdot 10} \quad (4)$$

where
$\dot{Q}$ = cardiac output (L/min)
$\dot{V}O_2$ = oxygen consumption (ml O_2/min)
CaO_2 = oxygen content of arterial blood (ml O_2/100 ml blood)
$C\bar{v}O_2$ = oxygen content of mixed venous blood (ml O_2/100 ml blood)

The direct Fick method is limited by (1) errors in sampling and analysis of the oxygen, (2) changing cardiac output over the usual 2- to 3-minute sampling time, and (3) changes in the respiratory conditions.[157] Moreover, cumbersome equipment (exhaled gas collection bag) is required to measure the oxygen consumption accurately, and blood gases must be analyzed from invasively sampled arterial and mixed venous (preferably pulmonary artery) sites. However, provided that steady-state hemodynamics is present, the Fick method provides highly reproducible measurements of cardiac output.[158,159] In addition, the development of continuous respiratory gas analysis using infrared and mass spectroscopy, as well as continuous arterial and mixed venous oximetry, has rekindled an interest in Fick methodology for cardiac output measurement during anesthesia and in the intensive care unit.

Indicator Dilution Cardiac Output Measurement

The indicator dilution method is a variant of the Fick technique in which a known amount of a substance is injected into the blood stream and its concentration change measured at a downstream location. The Stewart-Hamilton equation, named for two investigators who were instrumental in the development of this technique,[160,161] relates these quantities to blood flow:

$$\dot{Q} = \frac{I}{\int_0^\infty C_I dt} \qquad (5)$$

where

$\dot{Q}$ = cardiac output
I = amount of indicator
$\int_0^\infty C_I dt$ = integral of indicator concentration over time

This method offers the advantage of relatively rapid cardiac output determinations. However, continuous withdrawal of arterial blood is required to plot the concentration curve, and the indicator dye (e.g., indocyanine green) can gradually build up with repeated injections. Computer-assisted equipment can be used to calculate the area under the concentration curve and to generate a cardiac output value quickly. Recirculation of dye is usually not a problem during routine cardiac output determination but will greatly influence the results of this method if an intracardiac shunt is present. In fact, indicator dilution has been used expressly for the diagnosis of such shunts. The normal curve (Fig. 31-14A) is easily distinguished from abnormal curves (Fig. 31-14B–D). Shunt detection by dye dilution curves has largely given way to use of Doppler echocardiographic techniques, especially Doppler color flow imaging.

Thermodilution Cardiac Output

Two developments have had significant impact on the routine measurement of cardiac output in clinical practice. The first was the introduction of thermal indicators (iced or room temperature saline or dextrose in water) by Fegler[162] in 1954. The second was the incorporation of the necessary temperature measurement capability (thermistor) in the tip of standard flow-directed pulmonary artery catheters. Thus, cardiac output measurement is immediately available when pulmonary artery catheterization is implemented and can be performed repeatedly with a nontoxic, nonaccumulating, nonrecirculating indicator. In pediatric patients undergoing cardiac surgical procedures in whom PA catheter placement is not possible because of size constraints, thermodilution cardiac output can still be measured by placing a small thermistor directly into the pulmonary artery during surgery and making injections through a central venous catheter. Because of its ease of implementation and long clinical experience, the thermodilution technique has become the de facto standard for clinical cardiac output determination.

For thermal indicators, the Stewart-Hamilton equation requires some alterations, becoming:

$$\dot{Q} = \frac{V(T_B - T_I)K}{\int_0^\infty \Delta T_B(t)dt} \qquad (6)$$

where

$\dot{Q}$ = cardiac output (L/min)
V = volume of the injectate (ml)
$T_B - T_I$ = initial blood-injectate temperature difference
K = computation constant
$\int_0^\infty \Delta T_B(t)dt$ = integral of temperature change over time.

The computation constant K, which is a function of catheter size, injectate specific heat, rate of injection, and injectate volume, is entered manually by the operator into the cardiac output computer. Moreover, the constant also accounts for injectate temperature T_I, unless this term is directly measured. It is very important, therefore, that the constant K be the correct value for the particular catheter and injectate characteristics and that the chosen injection technique be adhered to during measurements, or significant errors in derived cardiac output may occur. Many thermodilution systems automatically measure injectate temperature. This is a useful feature that corrects for occasional variability in T_I but requires close attention so that the additional thermistor at the injection port does not become disconnected. If this occurs, T_I will be read as room temperature and, when using an iced injectate, the $T_B - T_I$ term will be erroneously low, resulting in artificially decreased cardiac output values. Finally, it is very useful to have a display of the temperature curve during the injection. This allows the user to detect artifact in this curve that may result from baseline temperature drift or recirculation peaks from intracardiac shunts, both of which cause errors in the measurement.

Studies comparing thermodilution cardiac output determination to controlled in vitro measurements[163] and to other in vivo techniques,[164] such as direct electromagnetic flow measurements or other indicator dilution, have demonstrated a 3 to 13 percent variability in its overall accuracy. This variance is primarily the result of discrepancies between the injection technique or injectate characteristics and the computation constant. The precision or reproducibility of this method is also dependent on these factors. In clinical practice, multiple cardiac output determinations are performed in order to arrive at an average value, since measurements made in triplicate have been shown to improve the confidence limits of the value nearly twofold.[165] It would be expected that the use of a large volume of colder injectate, which results in the largest temperature curve area, would add to the precision of the integral term of the cardiac output equation. It is true that 10-ml injectate volumes result in better reproducibility of cardiac output values, but studies have shown little if any added precision with the use of iced versus room temperature injectate.[163,166] Moreover, cardiac arrhythmias and bradycardia have been shown to result from the rapid injection of iced indicator.[167,168] Finally, the effects of respiration on instantaneous cardiac out-

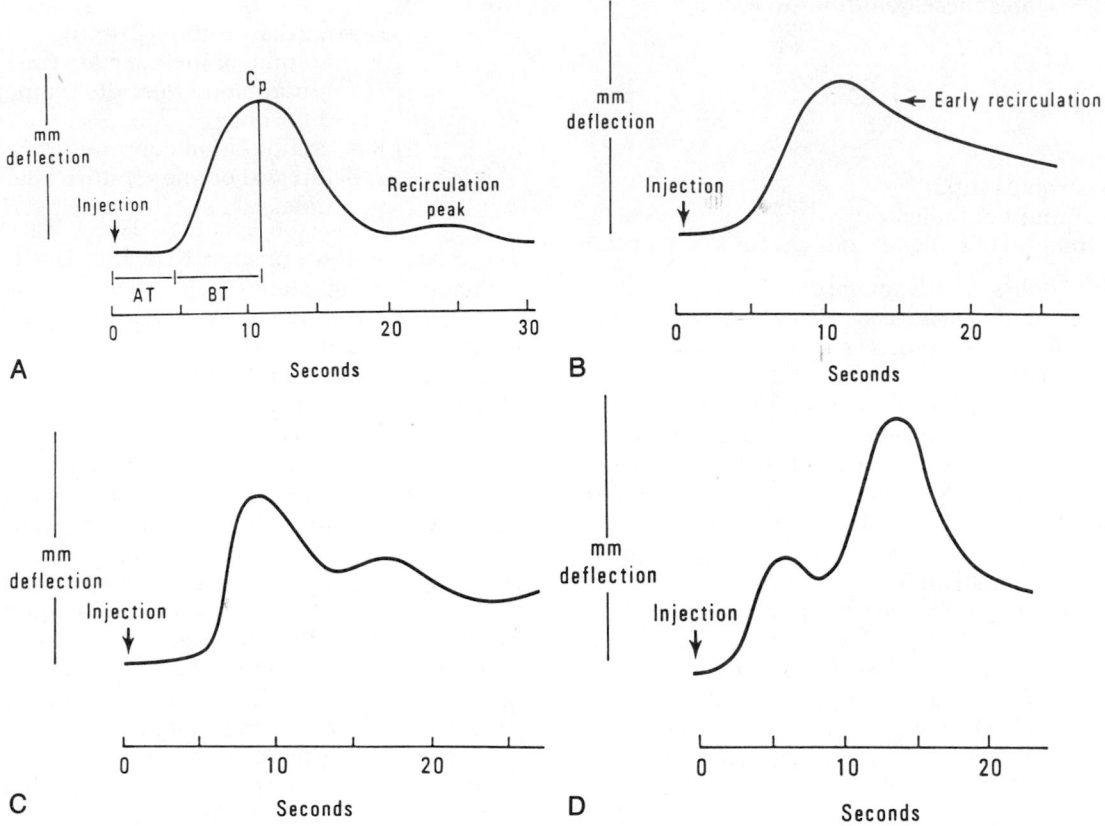

Fig. 31-14. Indicator dye dilution curves typically seen in the computation of cardiac output and the diagnosis of intracardiac shunt. **(A)** Normal curve of indicator concentration (photometric absorbance) versus time. The concentration peak (C_p) is followed by a normal, lesser recirculation peak. **(B)** Early recirculation with a large left-to-right shunt produces a curve with a gradual downstroke, since the normal primary peak and recirculation peak are essentially merged. **(C)** A smaller left-to-right shunt demonstrates an early but more recognizable recirculation peak. **(D)** A large right-to-left shunt causes a reversal of the size and timing of the dual peaks, with an early small initial peak followed by a larger second peak because the right sided injection crosses into the left heart prematurely. (Adapted from Rorie,[291] with permission.)

put can be standardized by making repeated injections during the same phase of the respiratory cycle (typically end-exhalation) in order to improve the precision of the measurement.

Noninvasive Cardiac Output

The applicability of Fick principle-based techniques for cardiac output measurement is limited somewhat by the degree of invasiveness and expense necessary to implement them. This is especially true for the popular thermodilution method, since pulmonary artery catheterization, along with its attendant risks, is required. This consideration has been a significant factor in the recent exploration and development of noninvasive methods for determining cardiac output.

Doppler Cardiac Output

The capacity of Doppler ultrasound to quantitate blood velocity has stimulated the development of devices that use this principle to measure blood flow in the thoracic aorta and to provide a relatively noninvasive monitor of cardiac output. (For a full description of the Doppler principle and the technology surrounding its use in monitoring, see the section, *Doppler Ultrasound.*) The various methods of Doppler-derived cardiac output differ in the anatomic location from which the blood flow measurements are obtained. However, all techniques require that several steps be completed: (1) A value for the cross-sectional area of the ascending aorta ($Area_{Ao}$) must be obtained. (2) An ultrasonic transducer is placed in such a position that its beam falls in a line closely parallel to the direction of aortic blood flow. (3)

The ultrasound device must integrate measured blood flow velocity over the period of ejection (T_{ej}) to determine an average velocity value (V_{avg}) for each heart beat. (4) V_{avg}, $Area_{Ao}$, T_{ej}, and heart rate (HR) are multiplied to derive cardiac output:

$$CO = V_{avg} \cdot Area_{Ao} \cdot T_{ej} \cdot HR \qquad (7)$$

Suprasternal Doppler Cardiac Output

The suprasternal Doppler cardiac output method has been implemented by using either a continuous wave (CW) or pulse wave (PW) Doppler ultrasound probe from a suprasternal location to measure blood flow velocity at the aortic valve.[169-171] An advantage of the suprasternal technique is that it allows positioning of the ultrasound beam parallel to the direction of measured blood flow (Fig. 31-15C). This limits error due to misalignment of the beam and blood flow jet, since the cosine of this angle θ is a part of the Doppler formula for velocity measurement. The total cardiac output (minus coronary artery blood flow) is also assessed from this vantage point. The diameter of the aortic root is measured by using standard precordial echocardiographic imaging (Fig. 31-15A), but is alternatively estimated from a nomogram using patient's height and weight.

This technique allows intermittent, noninvasive measurements of cardiac output under most circumstances. Errors in these determinations are dependent in part on the type of Doppler technique used. Continuous wave Doppler has the capability of measuring a limitless range of flow velocities but cannot be focused or "gated" to a specific area. The returning Doppler signal therefore contains flow information from all sites along the beam path, making this technique highly dependent on proper beam direction. Pulse wave Doppler can sample velocity information from discrete locations (volumes) along its path, thus adding another dimension to one's ability to "steer" the measurement to the proper anatomic position. Unfortunately, PW Doppler is restricted in the maximum velocity that it can measure by a phenomenon called *aliasing* (see the section, *Doppler Ultrasound*). This limitation is especially severe if, as in this situation, the location of the sample volume is at some distance from the transducer. If aliasing occurs, huge errors in measured maximal flow velocity result. Thus, probe positioning is critically important to this technique in either case. Since the

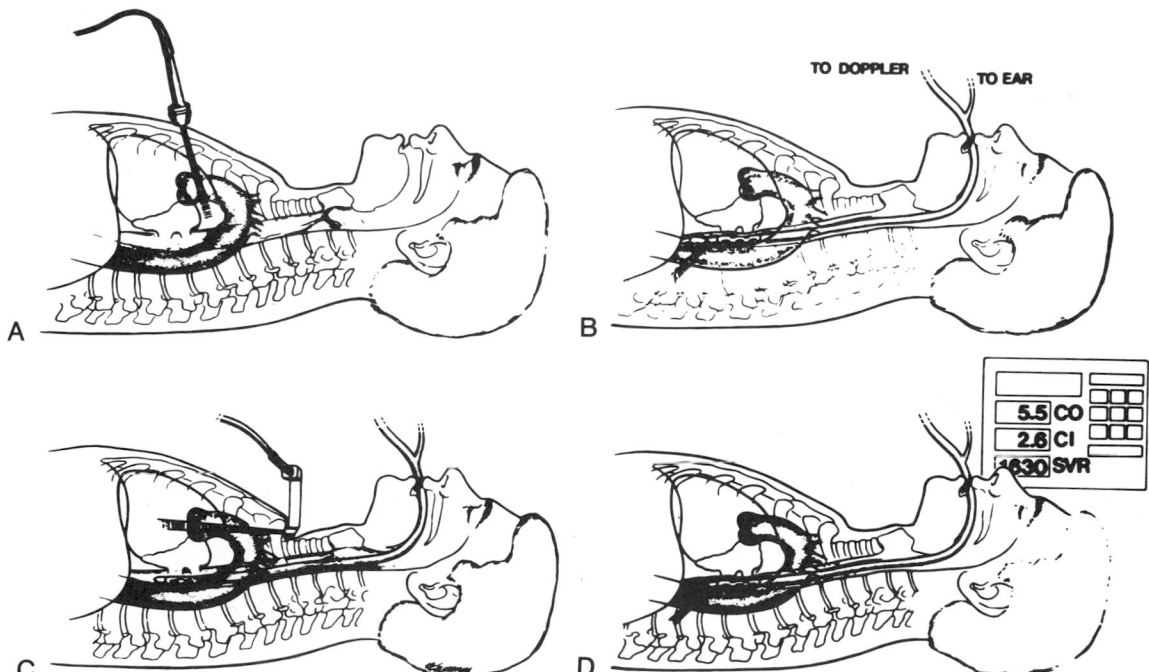

Fig. 31-15. Steps in cardiac output determination by suprasternal and esophageal Doppler systems. **(A)** Preliminary determination of aortic diameter is made above the sinus of Valsalva by pulsed A-mode ultrasonography. **(B)** The esophageal Doppler probe is inserted and adjusted for optimal ultrasonic signal. Descending aortic blood velocity is continuously determined. **(C)** Cardiac output is determined by measuring with a suprasternal Doppler probe the ascending aortic blood velocity. This method is used either as an outright intermittent monitor of cardiac output or as a means of establishing a proportionality constant for continuous determination of cardiac output using the esophageal probe (see text). **(D)** Calibrated esophageal probe in place displaying rapidly updated estimation of cardiac output. (From Freund,[174] with permission.)

suprasternal approach is used intermittently, a certain amount of training and expertise in handling the device are required to obtain repeated measurements consistently and objectively. Significant rates of failure to obtain acceptable data have been reported with this method.[169,172] Abnormalities of the aortic valve (stenosis, regurgitation, or other anatomic derangement) cause inaccuracies with this technique. Also, certain surgical procedures (e.g., median sternotomy for cardiac surgery) can make this approach difficult if not impossible in the intraoperative environment.

Comparisons of suprasternal Doppler-derived cardiac output (CO_{ssd}) data to those measured by thermodilution (CO_{td}) have yielded generally favorable results. Using CW mode Doppler, Nishimura et al. demonstrated reasonable correlation of CO_{ssd} and CO_{td} in medical intensive care and postcardiac surgical patients ($r = 0.94$, 0.85, respectively).[171] Chandraratna and colleagues found CO_{ssd} closely tracked CO_{td} over a wide range of values (1.86 to 10.1 L/min).[173] Huntsman et al. also reported good agreement of these measurement techniques ($r = 0.94$) in 85 percent of patients studied.[169] For technical reasons, the remaining 15 percent of these patients produced unacceptable CO_{ssd} data.

In contrast to these favorable results, a similar study of critically ill patients using a pulse wave Doppler instrument revealed significant underestimation of CO_{td} by CO_{ssd} ($r = 0.53$; regression slope, 0.66).[170] This may have resulted from an error in velocity measurements due to aliasing or imprecise positioning of the transducer.

Transesophageal Doppler Cardiac Output

In an effort to provide continuous, unattended measurements of cardiac output using Doppler techniques, an ultrasound transducer that has been fitted to the tip of a standard esophageal stethoscope has been developed to determine blood flow velocity in the descending thoracic aorta (Fig. 31-15B). Obviously, this requires some form of calibration in order to provide a conversion factor that relates this fraction of the aortic blood flow to true cardiac output. This is accomplished by using a suprasternal probe built into the same unit that provides a value for total cardiac output at the same moment that the esophageal probe reports descending aortic flow (Fig. 31-15C). The suprasternal probe is then removed, and the stored proportionality factor is used to extrapolate the cardiac output measurement from the constantly monitored esophageal transducer (Fig. 31-15D). This, of course, assumes that this blood flow relationship remains constant over the range of cardiac output reported. This may be an unwarranted premise, given the autoregulation of cerebral blood flow. Moreover, the esophageal ultrasound beam is directed at a 45-degree angle to aortic blood flow. Deviations from this prescribed angle of incidence result in relatively greater errors in velocity measurement than when beam and flow are more parallel. The somewhat large size of this device in the esophagus precludes its being considered *completely* noninvasive, and it is therefore used primarily in anesthetized patients.

Comparison of the esophageal approach for cardiac output measurement (CO_{ed}) to CO_{td} by Freund demonstrated only fair correlation of these techniques ($r = 0.67$).[174] However, cases studied later in the investigation showed improved agreement ($r = 0.85$), possibly indicating a learning curve for proper instrument utilization. Another study by Mark et al.,[175] using esophageal Doppler-derived cardiac output during cardiac surgery, reported that tracking of cardiac output trends by the esophageal instrument was generally good (multiple regression analysis $R^2 = 0.95$), but the absolute difference between CO_{ed} and CO_{td} was significant in many cases. This was most likely the result of inaccurate initial calibration using the suprasternal ultrasound probe. Moreover, comparison of the aortic diameter measurement by ultrasound showed poor correlation to direct surgical measurements ($r = 0.31$), which may have contributed to the calibration error.

Transtracheal Doppler Cardiac Output

Intratracheal placement of the ultrasound probe is the most recent development in Doppler-derived cardiac output determination. This device (ABCOM 1, Applied Biometrics) uses a special endotracheal tube incorporating a pulse wave Doppler ultrasound transducer in its tip. The tube cuff has an ellipsoid shape that, when inflated, holds the probe against the anterior wall of the trachea at a point that places the ultrasound beam in the path of ascending aortic blood flow (Fig. 31-16). Aortic diameter is measured automatically by using Doppler range gating and requires no other instrumentation. Cardiac output is then determined as described previously. This technique has the advantage of providing a continuous measurement of ascending (total) aortic blood flow. There is no need for a calibration step as in the esophageal approach. Disadvantages include its obvious restriction to intubated patients. The angle of incidence of the ultrasound beam and the blood flow vector is roughly 52 degrees,[176] making the range gate measurement of aortic diameter as well as tube movement during monitoring an extremely sensitive source of error in this technique. Even though pulse wave Doppler is used, aliasing is probably not a serious problem because of the close proximity of the transducer to the sample volume. Data correlating transtracheal Doppler cardiac output with thermodilution values are preliminary but appear to indicate a reasonable agreement of these techniques ($R^2 = 0.83$).[176,177]

Impedance Plethysmography

An interest in studying cardiovascular function during space flight initially prompted investigations of impedance plethysmography as a noninvasive method of determining cardiac output. This technique was first re-

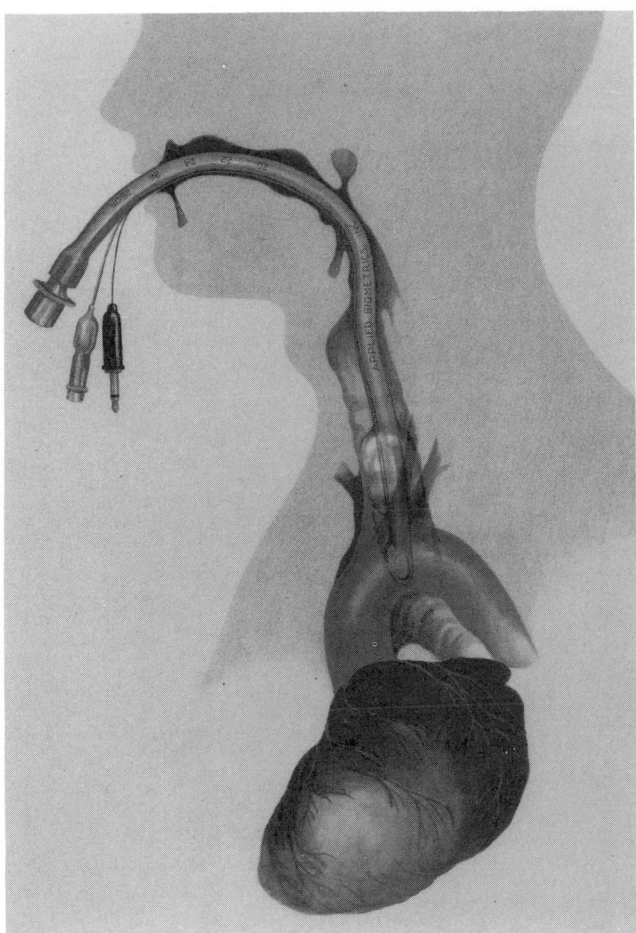

Fig. 31-16. Sketch of an endotracheal tube-transtracheal Doppler cardiac output transducer in position to detect ascending aortic blood flow velocity. The trapezoidal shape of the cuff holds the transducer (just above and to the left of the Murphy eye of the endotracheal tube) fast against the anterior trachea to allow adequate sound conduction. The electrical plug connects to the cardiac output computer. (Courtesy of Applied Biometrics Inc.)

ported by Kubicek and co-workers[178] and is based on characterizing the changes in the electrical impedance of thoracic cavity that occur with the ejection of blood during cardiac systole. Their original formula relates these bioimpedance measurements to stroke volume as follows:

$$SV = \frac{\rho L^2}{Z_0^2} \cdot VET \cdot \max \frac{dZ}{dt} \tag{8}$$

where ρ = specific resistivity of blood
L = thoracic length
Z_0 = basal thoracic impedance
VET = ventricular ejection time
$\max \frac{dZ}{dt}$ = maximum rate of impedance change during systolic upstroke

From this information, computation of cardiac output is straightforward. Initial studies in healthy volunteers comparing bioimpedance cardiac output (CO_{bi}) with thermodilution measurements (CO_{td}) revealed good correlation between the techniques.[178] With subsequent improvements to this algorithm[179] and computerization of the analysis process, a commercial noninvasive monitor of cardiac output based on this methodology has been produced (NCCOM 3, BoMed Medical Manufacturing). Four pairs of standard skin electrodes are applied to the neck and lower thorax (Fig. 31-17), and impedance measurements are made by applying a continuous small electrical current across the chest. Patient height, weight, and gender are entered by the operator to allow an accurate computation of the volume of the thoracic cavity. CO_{bi} is computed for each cardiac cycle and continuously displayed as an average value over several heart beats.

Using this device, studies have compared CO_{bi} and CO_{td} in both cardiac surgical and intensive care unit (ICU) patients. Appel et al.[180] found reasonable agreement of these methods in 16 of 21 ICU patients. In 4 of the other 5 patients, CO_{bi} could not be determined because of inadequate impedance measurements. The same good correlation (r = 0.97) was found in a study of 10 critically ill children (age 4 months to 15 years).[181] However, 3 of these patients were excluded because of technical difficulties in obtaining CO_{bi}. Also, Spinale and co-workers measured bioimpedance cardiac output in patients after cardiac surgery.[182] The linear relation to CO_{td} was less robust (r = 0.71) in this population of patients, with CO_{bi} generally underestimating CO_{td}. Additionally, CO_{bi} data were unobtainable in the presence of atrial pacemaker artifacts. Overall, CO_{bi} was found to diverge from CO_{td} at increased heart rates (> 140 beats/min).[180,182] Also, since the bioimpedance system estimates the *pulsatile* component of the stroke volume during the systolic time interval, conditions in which blood flow assumes a more continuous quality (sepsis, hemodilution) may result in falsely low CO_{bi}.[180] However, with progressive improvements in instrumentation that overcome these confounding factors, bioimpedance cardiac output determination, by virtue of its highly noninvasive implementation, may find significant applicability in the intraoperative and critical care environments.

Venous Oxygen Saturation

Knowledge of the importance of venous oxygen saturation has its origin very early in the history of medicine, when Hippocrates observed that dark veins indicated a poor prognosis.[183] Venous oxygen saturation (SvO_2) is possibly a more comprehensive measure of cardiac performance than cardiac output itself, since it reflects whether or not cardiac output is adequate to meet tissue metabolic needs (Fig. 31-18). However, several other important factors influence SvO_2 and must be accounted for when interpreting this measurement.

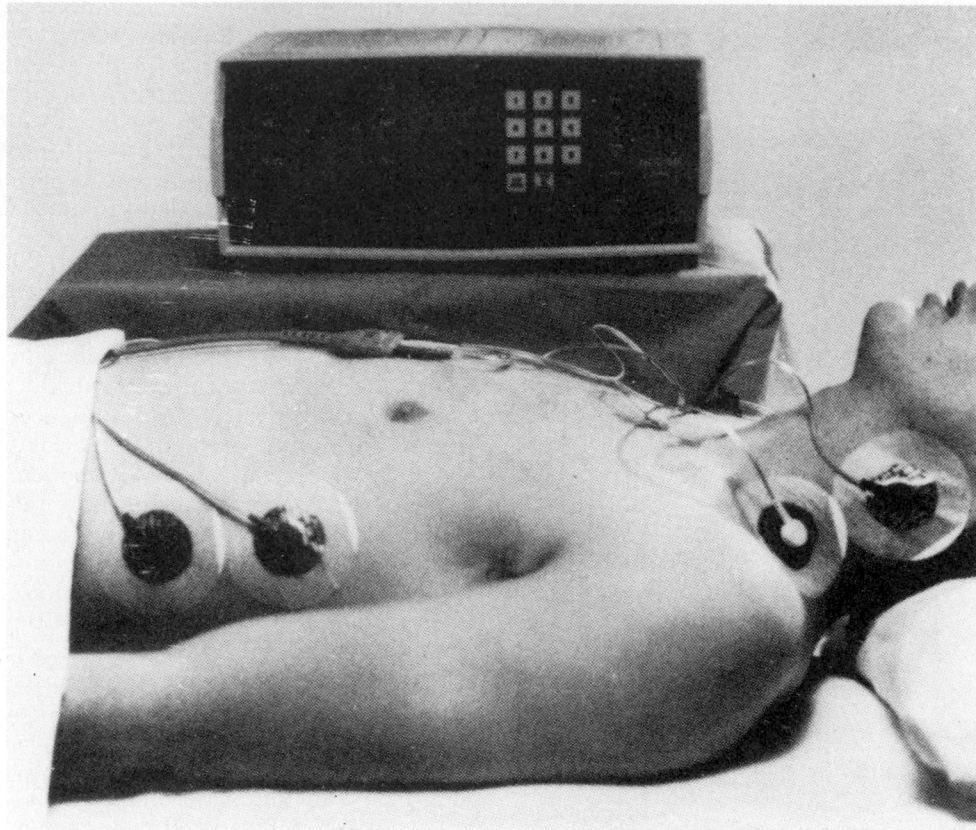

Fig. 31-17. The bioimpedance cardiac output computer with electrodes attached to a patient. Four additional electrodes are placed in similar positions on the patient's right side. (From Spinale et al.,[182] with permission.)

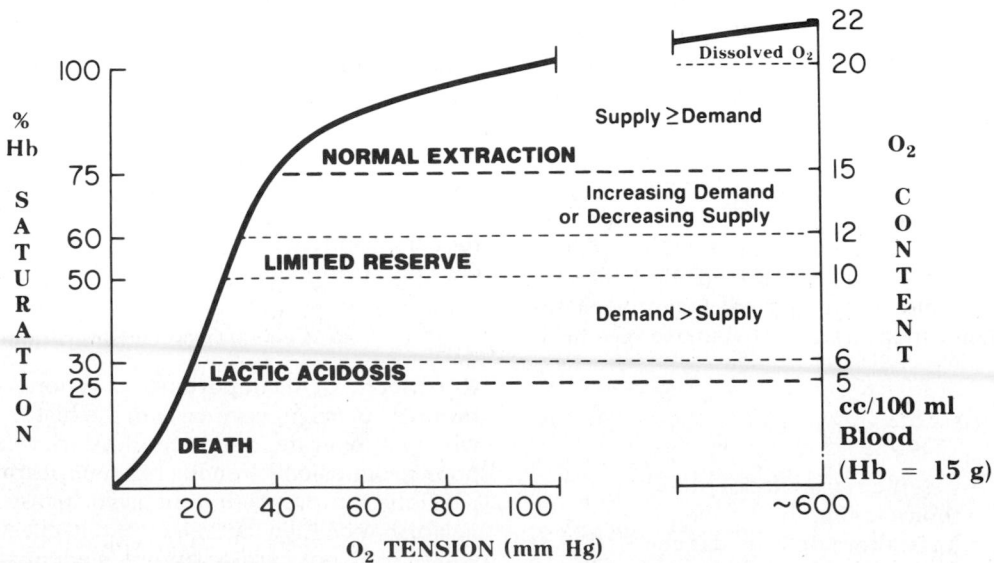

Fig. 31-18. The relationships between oxygen saturation, tension, and content are shown by the familiar oxyhemoglobin dissociation curve. The oxygen balance profile illustrates the clinical importance of changes in mixed venous oxygen saturation (SvO₂). (From Norfleet and Watson,[186] with permission.)

These factors can be easily understood by deriving the formula for SvO_2, substituting oxygen saturation terms for oxygen content in the Fick equation and rearranging to yield:

$$SvO_2 = SaO_2 - \frac{\dot{V}O_2}{CO \cdot 1.34\, Hb} \qquad (9)$$

Thus, SvO_2 is a function of (1) the level of arterial oxygen saturation, SaO_2; (2) the rate of oxygen consumption, $\dot{V}O_2$; (3) the cardiac output, CO; and (4) the concentration of hemoglobin, Hb. The amount of oxygen physically dissolved in blood is considered to be a negligible factor in this equation at normal atmospheric pressures.

Correlation of SvO_2 with cardiac performance was demonstrated by Boyd et al.[184] in 1959, and early studies of SvO_2 in critically ill patients demonstrated this parameter "to be the earliest sign of hemodynamic competence or failure."[185] Improvements in reflective photometric oximetry techniques and advances in fiberoptic design have resulted in incorporation of this technology within a pulmonary artery catheter (PAC), providing the capability of continuously determining mixed venous oxygen saturation. A specialized computer connected to this PAC collects and displays trends in SvO_2 and also performs thermodilution CO measurements. These modern devices take advantage of multiwavelength technology and reflection intensity algorithms that avoid measuring reflectance from a wall of the pulmonary artery. They also incorporate both in vitro and in vivo methods of calibration to provide accurate SvO_2 data.[186]

An advantage of this method is its ability to provide *continuous* assessment of cardiac performance. SvO_2 monitoring allows an immediate quantitative appraisal of the influence of a physiologic event or intervention on the cardiovascular system. The disadvantage of this form of monitoring is apparent in equation (9). Multiple independent parameters have equal influence in determining SvO_2. Rapid changes in hemoglobin level, arterial oxygenation, or oxygen consumption quickly dissociate SvO_2 from the parameter it is most often compared with, cardiac output. Even as a more general index of oxygen delivery/consumption ratio, SvO_2 has pitfalls. In septic shock or in the presence of anatomic arteriovenous shunts, SvO_2 monitoring clearly loses diagnostic value.[186] Moreover, the addition of SvO_2 measurement capability adds greatly to the cost of the PAC itself.

This mix of advantages and disadvantages of SvO_2 monitoring has led to many studies of its clinical usefulness and cost-effectiveness. An early study by Waller et al. in cardiac surgical patients demonstrated the sensitivity of decreased SvO_2 in predicting parallel changes in cardiac output.[187] A 5 percent decrease in SvO_2 had an 86 percent chance of being associated with a significant lowering of cardiac output. A subsequent study in a similar patient population made exclusively during the postoperative period reported a poorer correlation

of SvO_2 and CO.[188] This probably resulted from instability of other factors involved in the SvO_2 equation during this period, such as hemoglobin level (resolution of intraoperative hemodilution) and oxygen consumption (shivering after hypothermic cardiopulmonary bypass). In studies of other critically ill patients, investigators have reported both favorable[189-191] and unfavorable[192,193] conclusions as to the overall effectiveness of SvO_2 monitoring.

Derived Cardiac Performance Variables

Vascular Resistance Measurement

The obvious similarity of the cardiovascular system to an electrical circuit has allowed development of a relationship between blood pressure and blood flow that is analogous to Ohm's law, E (voltage) = I (current) × R (resistance). The decrease in arterial blood pressure across a vascular bed is equal to the product of the blood flow through it and the resistance to flow that it imparts. Rearranging this equation allows the derivation of a resistance term for the cardiovascular system. Although this formula can be used for any regional vascular bed, its most common application is determining overall systemic vascular resistance (SVR) and pulmonary vascular resistance (PVR) (Table 31-7).

The validity of this analogy between Ohm's law for electrical circuits and the cardiovascular system depends on several requirements of the latter (hydraulic) system. Blood flow is assumed to be at a steady state, continuous and laminar, and carried through rigid conduits.[194,195] These criteria are met to some degree in the systemic vascular circulation, and estimation of SVR is thus useful in determining the influence of vascular tone on cardiac performance. Knowledge of SVR is important in directing the use of the many potent drugs, such as phenylephrine and sodium nitroprusside, that alter vascular tone and resistance.

Carrying the same analysis to the pulmonary vascular bed is less straightforward, since many of the required

TABLE 31-7. Derived Hemodynamic Parameters

	Units	Normal Range
$CI = \dfrac{CO}{BSA}$	L/min/m²	2.8–4.2
$SV = \dfrac{CO}{HR}$	ml/beat	60–90
$SVR = \dfrac{MAP - CVP}{CO}\ (\times 80)$	Wood units dyne/s/cm⁵	11–17.5 900–1400
$PVR = \dfrac{\overline{PAP} - PCWP}{CO}\ (\times 80)$	Wood units dyne/s/cm⁵	2–4 150–250

Abbreviations and symbols: CO, cardiac output L/min); BSA, body surface area (m²); HR, heart rate (beats/min); MAP, mean arterial pressure (mmHg); CVP, central venous pressure (mmHg); PAP, mean pulmonary artery pressure (mmHg); PCWP, pulmonary capillary wedge pressure (mmHg); [× 80], factor to convert Wood units (mmHg/L/min) to dyne/s/cm⁵).
(From Schlant et al.,[290] with permission.)

blood flow characteristics are not present.[196] At end-diastole, pulmonary blood flow may cease transiently, since pulmonary artery diastolic pressure (PADP) and pulmonary venous pressure (as reflected by the "wedge" pressure, PCWP) are often similar. Also, pulmonary vascular compliance is very high, making these vessels easily distensible and compressible. The influence of alveolar pressure in generating a "critical closing pressure" in the pulmonary vasculature cannot be ignored.[194,197] (See preceding discussion of West's[109] zones of pulmonary vasculature.) Finally, the relative importance of direct pulmonary vascular abnormalities versus left ventricular functional indices in establishing overall right ventricular afterload remains unclear. Moreover, intrinsic changes in left ventricular function usually simultaneously affect two variables in the formula for PVR (both CO and PCWP) often to disparate, asymmetric degrees. Thus, it is probably not valid to make assumptions about the pulmonary vasculature based on changes in calculated PVR when radical changes in LV performance have occurred. Some researchers have recommended excluding cardiac output and examining only the mean PAP — PCWP difference in estimating actual pulmonary vascular impedance.[196]

Cardiac Index

Another common derivation of a directly measured hemodynamic parameter is the cardiac index (CI), which is the cardiac output divided by the body surface area of the patient (BSA) (Table 31-7). Cardiac index has been used to "normalize" the wide range of cardiac outputs measured in the average population. Body surface area is derived from a complex formula using patient height and weight. This value is used to represent the body size or mass and, theoretically, also the amount of blood flow that is needed for adequate overall perfusion. Interestingly, Reeves and co-workers, in a study of cardiac output in normal volunteers published in 1961, reported cardiac index to be an insensitive standard of normal blood flow.[198] Instead, they found a relatively constant arteriovenous oxygen difference over a range of cardiac output and oxygen uptake levels. This was taken as evidence that cardiac output is autoregulated. They felt that cardiac index "does not take into account the large variations in predicted basal oxygen uptake resulting from differences in age and sex, or the variation between individuals in metabolic rate," and that it is "based on body surface area, a biometric measurement whose fundamental relationship to blood flow is obscure." Clearly, it is important to be aware of a patient's body habitus and medical history in interpreting and treating changes in cardiac performance. However, use of an arbitrary "normal" value for cardiac index as a universal indicator of cardiovascular well-being for all patients is probably unwarranted.

Other Cardiac Performance Measurement Techniques

Systolic Time Intervals

The temporal relationship of the mechanical and electrical events of the cardiac cycle forms the basis for the use of systolic time intervals (STIs) as an index of cardiac contractility and performance. The interval from the time of the QRS complex to the end of left ventricular ejection (occurrence of S_2, the second heart sound) is considered total electromechanical systole (QS_2) (Fig. 31-19). This period can be divided between the left ventricular ejection time (LVET) and the pre-ejection period (PEP). The ratio PEP/LVET (normal: 0.35) has been correlated favorably with other indices of cardiac contractility.[199] This is an inverse relationship, since PEP decreases and LVET increases with increases in the contractile state.

The advantage of STI measurement is that it is a noninvasive means of assessing cardiac performance. All that it requires are an ECG and a simultaneously recorded phonocardiogram. During surgery involving the chest, an esophageal phonocardiogram can be used. The first heart sound (S_1) of the phonocardiogram represents the separation of PEP and LVET. Obviously, the QS_2 is determined by the Q wave of the ECG and the second heart sound.

Other hemodynamic parameters have influences on STI values. Clearly, tachycardia diminishes QS_2, PEP, and LVET. PEP is lengthened by increased afterload and shortened by increased preload. These factors must be considered when using STI in clinical monitoring. Nonetheless, STIs have been used in clinical studies of anesthetic and other drug effects on the cardiovascular system.[200,201]

Radionuclide Angiography

Nuclear imaging of the heart has provided a useful means of assessing cardiovascular performance status by a noninvasive technique. This form of measurement relies on the detection of gamma emission from an intravenously injection radiopharmaceutical, such as technecium 99m, as it passes through the heart and great vessels. A scintillation counter or "gamma camera" is used to detect radiation from specific locations over a wide area, providing two-dimensional images of emission patterns. Two basic techniques of nuclear imaging are used for cardiac performance measurements. The first is multigated blood pool imaging (MUGA), which is performed by radiolabeling albumin or a sample of the patient's red blood cells and injecting this bound tracer into the circulation. The radionuclide, equilibrated in the blood stream, is detected over hundreds of cardiac cycles, with particular images (end-diastole and end-systole) "gated" by the R wave of the ECG. By averaging counts over many gated images

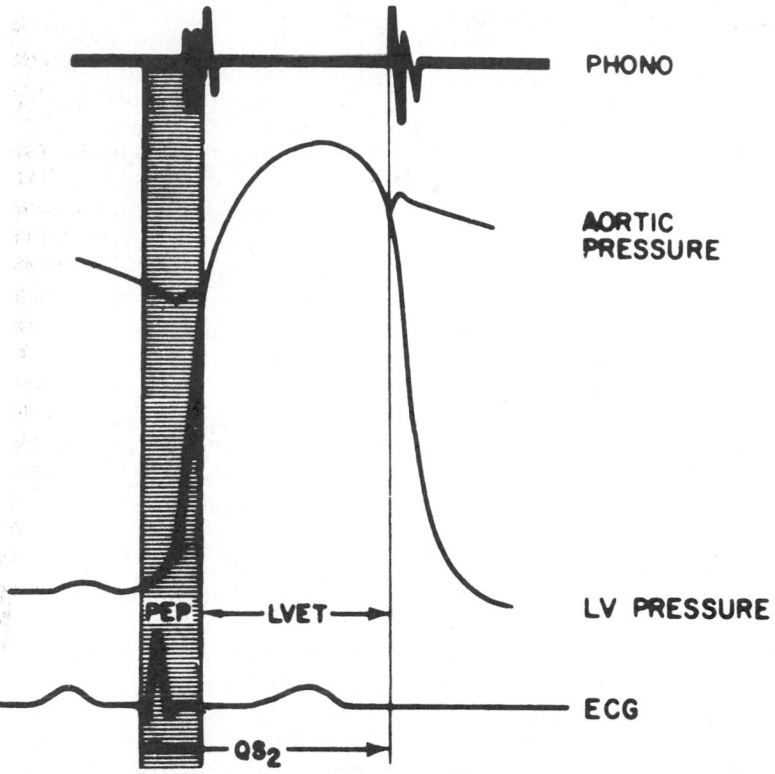

PHONO

AORTIC
PRESSURE

LV PRESSURE

←PEP→ ←LVET→

ECG

←QS₂→

Fig. 31-19. A schematic representation of the left ventricular events that constitute the systolic time interval (STI). PEP, pre-ejection period; QS₂, total electromechanical systole; LVET, left ventricular ejection time. (From Lewis et al.,[200] with permission.)

and subtracting background (lung) counts, images representing relative ventricular volumes are obtained.[202] This allows accurate computation of global indices of cardiac function, such as ejection fraction, as well as estimation of regional cardiac wall motion. Moreover, the gated equilibration method allows examination to be extended over a long period (up to several hours), providing the opportunity to perform exercise testing and other maneuvers during a single examination period.[203]

The other commonly used radionuclide imaging technique is first-pass radionuclear angiography (RNA). In this method, a single bolus of a radiopharmaceutical is injected either peripherally or centrally, and detection of its first passage through the heart and lungs is performed over 15 to 20 seconds. A rapid-response gamma camera capable of measuring high radioactive count rates is necessary for this technique. Identification of the radionuclide bolus as it passes through the right and left sides of the heart allows independent computations of performance indices of each ventricle. First-pass RNA is particularly useful in measuring cardiac function at discrete moments, such as in response to an intervention or exercise. Purut et al. described a use for RNA in the perioperative period using simultaneous left ventricular pressure measurements to con-

struct pressure-volume "loops" to describe the cardiac contractile state of patients at various stages of coronary artery bypass grafting.[204] These investigators used a sophisticated, relatively compact digital gamma camera (Scinticor) to obtain RNA data. However, the instrumentation needed for nuclear imaging is still bulky and costly to the degree that its use in the intraoperative setting is restricted to clinical research applications.

Magnetic Resonance Imaging

A relatively new medical diagnostic tool is magnetic resonance imaging (MRI). This complex technology uses a combination of high-strength magnetic fields and radio frequency electrical signals both to stimulate and to detect changes in magnetic alignment of certain asymmetric atomic nuclei in tissues, notably hydrogen (^{1}H).[205] By spatial analysis of multiple signals, a high-resolution tomographic image is constructed that rivals or exceeds the clarity of radiographic computed tomography (CT) scans, without the use of ionizing radiation. Moreover, the tomographic "slice" can be oriented in a variety of planes (sagittal, transverse), providing an improved means of assessing structures in all three dimensions. Recently, increases in MRI imaging speed to near real time (cine MRI) have allowed this technique to provide a noninvasive means of demonstrating cardiac function as well as an anatomic description.[206] This may not only provide an improved method of characterization of acquired cardiac disease but also allow congenital cardiac malformations to be visualized more completely. Furthermore, the ability of MRI to selectively detect other paramagnetic elements, such as carbon (^{13}C), allows the tracing of metabolic activity in selected tissues by labeling substrates with these materials. Unfortunately, the requirement of MRI for large, high-powered magnetic fields precludes its use in the intraoperative environment. However, its preoperative cardiac diagnostic capabilities will be of increasing value to the anesthesiologist.

ECHOCARDIOGRAPHY

Of the many technologies to be introduced recently to the field of intraoperative cardiac monitoring, none has provided as much new and previously unattainable information as echocardiography. Of course, echocardiography is not a new diagnostic tool. The new development has been the introduction of a transesophageal approach for ultrasound imaging of the heart. With this technique, continuous echocardiographic assessment of the patient during anesthesia and surgery is possible. Popularity of transesophageal echocardiography in this environment is growing rapidly. Thus, in order to take full advantage of this sophisticated monitoring technique, it is important that the anesthesiologist acquire a clear understanding of the background and methods of echocardiography.

Cardiac Imaging

Physics of Ultrasound

Sound energy behaves according to the principles of longitudinally propagating waves, with alternating compression and rarefaction of the transmitting medium. Sound is characterized by the frequency (f) of the waves in cycles per second or hertz (Hz) and by wavelength (λ). These terms are related to the velocity of sound (V) as follows:

$$\lambda = \frac{V}{f} \qquad (10)$$

Ultrasound is defined as sound whose frequency exceeds the maximum audible frequency of 20,000 Hz. In clinical applications, ultrasound frequencies in the range of several million hertz (megahertz [MHz]) are used.

In order to produce ultrasound with these frequencies, special piezoelectric (pressure electric) crystals are utilized. These materials have the property of mechanically expanding when stimulated by an electrical potential. With removal of the applied voltage, the crystal returns to its previous shape. The energy of this me-

chanical process is then propagated as ultrasound through the surrounding medium. The frequency of this ultrasound is a function of the physical characteristics (composition and resonance properties) of the crystal itself.[207] Most crystals used in echocardiography are designed to produce frequencies of 2.5, 3.5, or 5.0 MHz.

The characteristics of sound waves are greatly affected by the physical properties of the media through which they travel. The velocity of the propagated sound is determined by the density and elasticity of the conducting medium. In soft tissues, this velocity is 1540 m/s (1.54 mm/μs)[208]; in air it is significantly slower (0.381 mm/μs).[209] With the velocity fixed by the medium and frequency determined by the transducer material, equation (10) correctly denotes wavelength as the dependent variable. Thus, higher-frequency ultrasound transducers are needed to provide shorter wavelengths and increased resolution of imaging.

Other physical properties of ultrasound are important in understanding its transmission characteristics. Because the sound is propagated by oscillations of the conducting medium, part of its energy is lost in this process. The degree of this attenuation is determined by the type of medium and is most significant in air. Also, the amount of attenuation of ultrasound is directly proportional to its frequency.[207] This tends to limit the maximum distance that higher-frequency ultrasound can penetrate before it is completely absorbed.

The principal characteristic of ultrasound that forms the basis for its use in imaging is its reflection from surfaces encountered in its path. A *surface* can be defined as the interface between two media of differing acoustic impedance (Z), which is determined by the density and velocity of sound conductance of the individual materials. If the surface is large with respect to the wavelength of the sound, then the reflection is *specular*, or mirrorlike (Fig. 31-20A) and the angle of reflection is equal to the angle of incidence of the wave. The intensity of a specularly reflected wave (I_r) is proportional to that of the incident wave (I_i) and to the difference in impedances (Z_1, Z_2) of the adjacent media:[207]

$$I_r = I_i \left(\frac{Z_2 - Z_1}{Z_2 + Z_1} \right)^2 \qquad (11)$$

The proportion of the wave that is transmitted through the second medium is refracted according to Snell's law (Fig. 31-20).[209]

If, on the other hand, the reflecting surface is small in comparison to the sound wavelength, specular reflection is not observed, but the waveform is *scattered*, with only a small portion of its energy being reflected to the source (Fig. 31-20b). Also, irregularities in a large surface can act as individual small surfaces and cause significant scattering of the ultrasound beam. Thus, desirable specular reflection is enhanced by using higher-frequency, shorter-wavelength ultrasound.

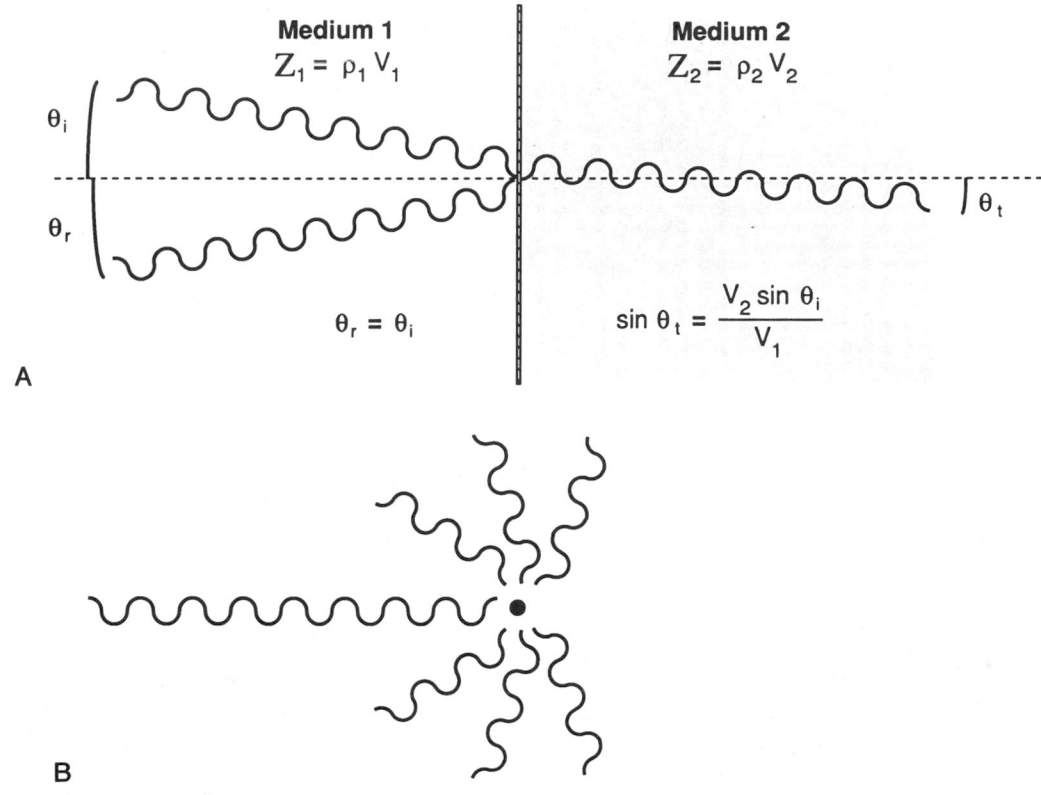

Fig. 31-20. Behavior of a sound wave contacting surfaces of various sizes. **(A)** Specular reflection caused by a surface that is large in comparison to the wavelength. The angle of incidence θ_i equals the angle of reflection θ_r. The intensity of the reflected wave is a function of the difference in acoustic impedance (Z) between the media forming the surface. Acoustic impedance of a material is the product of its density (r) and the velocity of sound conduction (V). **(B)** Scattering of a wave occurs when the reflecting surface is small in comparison to its wavelength. The angles of reflection are many and unpredictable.

When the reflected ultrasonic waves reach the transducer, an energy transfer process that is the inverse of sound transmission results. An electrical signal proportional to the received sound intensity is generated by the piezoelectric crystal and can be detected by the imaging system circuits. As noted, a reflected wave indicates that a surface exists between different media. Knowing the velocity of the ultrasound (V) and the time (t) required for transmission and reflection determines the distance (d) of the surface from the transducer:

$$d = \frac{Vt}{2} \qquad (12)$$

The reflected ultrasound waves thus determine the location of the surfaces of objects in the field being examined.

Ultrasound Instrumentation

Transducers

The construction of the transducer crystal element plays an important role in the control of ultrasound propagation. A small single piezoelectric element creates waves that emanate in a spherical fashion in three dimensions (Fig. 31-21). A larger single element produces multiple waves that combine and reinforce each other to create a planar wavefront parallel to the transducer face and moves along a line perpendicular to these planes. This effect can be imitated by using an array of small elements all electrically pulsed at the same instant. At a certain distance, however, the wave front begins to diverge from this straight course. The length (L) of this *near* field that follows this linear propagation is determined by the radius (r) of the transducer element(s) and the wavelengths of the ultrasound[209]:

$$L = \frac{r^2}{\lambda} \qquad (13)$$

Thus, high-frequency, short-wavelength ultrasound devices have an extended near-field distance.

Most ultrasound transducers are constructed as an array of small crystal elements. With this design, a number of advantages are realized. By controlling the timing of electrical impulses to the individual elements, the ultrasound waves can be created in such a way that the resulting wave front can be manipulated to correct

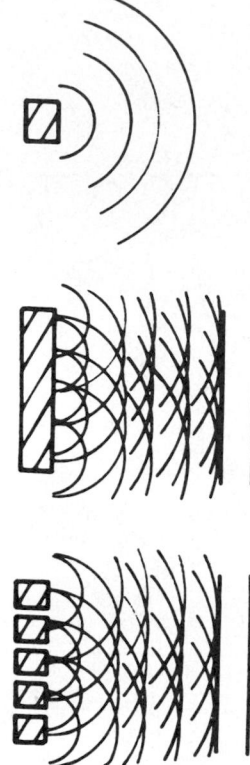

Fig. 31-21. Wave fronts produced by single- and multiple-element transducers. (See text for description.) (From Hill,[209] with permission.)

for the natural divergence of the beam or purposefully steered in a direction other than perpendicular to the plane of the transducer face. This process forms the basis for electronic phased array two-dimensional ultrasound scanning. Transducers generally have an acoustic insulation behind the piezoelectric elements to absorb spuriously directed sound and to sharpen the ultrasound pulse that is emitted. On the front of the transducer is a specially designed face plate that is of the precise thickness (one quarter-wavelength) and acoustic impedance to facilitate transmission of the fullest possible intensity of ultrasound across the transducer/tissue interface. Typically, a transmitted pulse of ultrasound has a duration of 1 μs, after which the transducer is placed in receive or "listen" mode for up to 250 μs. This process can be repeated several thousand times per second. When the reflected ultrasound is received, the multiple-element array can be used again to fine-tune this incoming signal, allowing adjustable or dynamic focusing of reception on many points along the beam.

Because of the attenuation of ultrasound during its transit through tissues, objects at greater distances will return diminished signals relative to those of nearer objects even though their surfaces may be equally dis-

tinct. To correct for this problem, circuits within the imaging system allow selective amplification of late-arriving, more-distant signals. This time-gain compensation (TGC) is usually provided by a series of slide potentiometers that allow the user to make these adjustments easily and to improve image clarity.

Imaging Systems

Figure 31-22 demonstrates a summary of the methods by which ultrasound information has been displayed. In **A-** (amplitude) mode display, the actual returned ul-

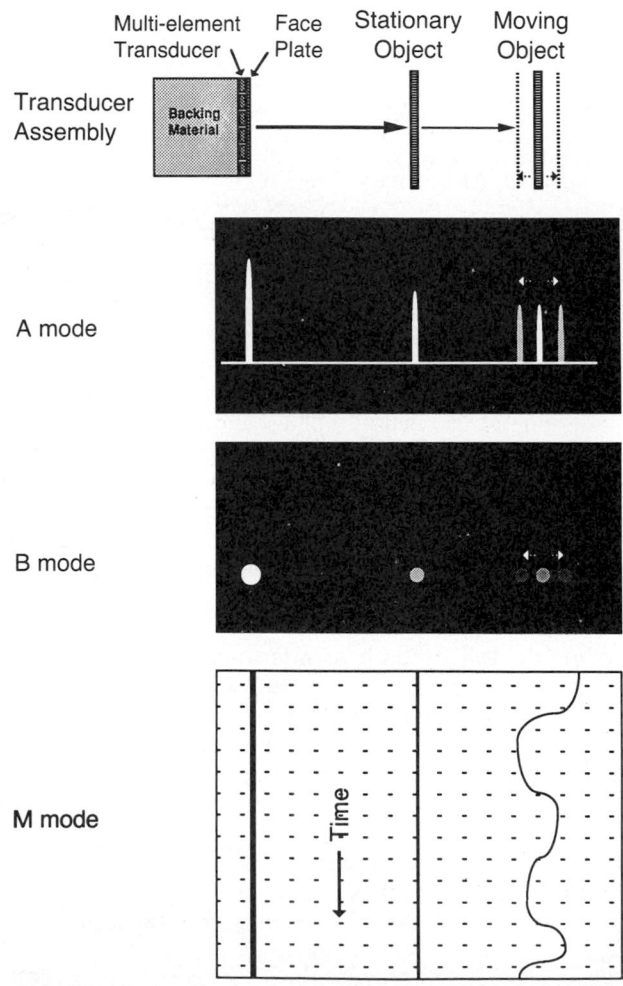

Fig. 31-22. Diagram of an echocardiography transducer imaging two objects of similar densities, one stationary and one moving. The transducer is constructed of a multielement piezoelectric crystal assembly with face plate and backing material. The A-mode display represents the surfaces as "peaks" of ultrasound intensity. Note that the more distant object has a lower peak than the nearer one due to ultrasound attenuation. Time gain compensation is applied to correct for this effect. B-mode displays the objects using points (dots) of varying brightness. The M-mode display charts the motion of the B-mode dots over time.

trasound intensity peaks representing objects are displayed on an oscilloscope. The height of a peak is influenced not only by the difference in the media that define the particular surface but also by the distance of the object from the transducer. This points to the importance of time-gain compensation to correct for ultrasound attenuation. **B-** (brightness) mode displays convert these peaks to dots of an intensity that is proportional to the amplitude of the signal. **M-** (motion) mode display uses B-mode information displayed continuously over time to provide a representation of the extent and velocity of movement of objects in the line of sight of the ultrasound beam. None of these techniques can be truly termed an *imaging* method, since the displays do not resemble the anatomy that they describe. Of these, only M mode is still used clinically. Since M mode focuses repeated interrogations of a single unidimensional "view," it offers very good assessment of rapidly moving objects, such as mitral valve leaflets. However, the preponderance of clinical echocardiographic monitoring uses two-dimensional scanning.

Two-Dimensional Scanning Systems

Two-dimensional (2-D) ultrasound scanning represents a significant advance in complexity and sophistication of this technology, because it provides a recognizable image of the objects being examined. In essence, 2-D imaging is composed of multiple B-mode interrogations performed over a sweeping arc of scan lines. The resulting information is displayed on a video screen as a series of lines emanating radially from a single location, with the intensities of the surfaces along the lines indicated by a particular brightness or "gray level." The time needed for performing an entire sweep of the sector arc is sufficiently short that the resulting image is considered a still frame of a moving object. Moreover, the 2-D scan can be repeated 30 to 60 times/s, so that the resulting video image is seen by the human eye as a continuous real-time monitor, with essentially all movement of the examined objects displayed.

Two types of 2-D scanning transducers are used. The mechanical scanner is a unidirectional transducer that is physically rotated to sweep the sector being interrogated. These somewhat bulky transducers have been replaced for the most part by smaller, phased array scanners that take advantage of the ability of multielement transducers to "steer" the beam across the scan area electronically.

The resolution of a 2-D scanning system, that is, its ability to discriminate objects in close proximity, is measured for each of the two dimensions. The axial or depth resolution is a function of the wavelength of the ultrasound beam and the number of wave periods generated in a single transmitted pulse. For modern, high-frequency scanning systems, this resolution is 0.5 to 1.0 mm. The lateral resolution, or discrimination between adjacent scan lines, is a function of the precision of beam steering and focusing by the phased array transducer. Generally, a larger number of individual array elements improves this resolution. Phased array transducers today are made with 32 to 64 elements.

Other methods of improving 2-D imaging are built into the circuits of modern ultrasound systems. A number of analog filters are used to improve the ultrasound signal (Fig. 31-23). Digital microprocessors have advanced in speed and sophistication to the point that they are now incorporated extensively in this type of image processing application. Ultrasound information from individual scan lines is typically converted to a numeric representation, which is used to perform image enhancement processes that would otherwise be difficult to implement. For instance, at increasing distances, individual scan lines begin to separate to the degree that gaps would be left in the 2-D representation. The digitized scan information at these distances can be used to interpolate the intermediate points, creating a smooth image.[207] Other image optimizing steps include modifications of echo information based on data from adjacent scan lines (spatial processing) or from previous images (temporal processing).

Transesophageal Echocardiography

Implementation

Diagnostic echocardiographic examinations have typically used several standard views of the heart from a transthoracic vantage point. These views are often limited by the presence of only a few acoustic windows into the mediastinum, since adjacent anatomic structures, such as bone and lung, present overwhelming obstacles to the conduction of ultrasound. Common pathologic states, such as obesity and emphysema, compound this already difficult problem. Because of these limitations, the *transesophageal* approach became an attractive means of improving the quality of imaging in selected circumstances. Esophageal placement of the ultrasound transducer results in its close proximity to the heart, separated only by the soft tissues of the mediastinum, offering the benefits of near-field scanning and avoiding the problems of image degradation. An additional advantage of transesophageal echocardiography (TEE) is its ability to provide continuous, stable views of the heart for protracted periods. In an intraoperative setting, TEE thus becomes a *monitor* of the cardiovascular system, rather than an intermittently applied diagnostic tool.

The development of TEE followed the same evolutionary course as standard echocardiography. The first esophageal transducers were M mode only. Two-dimensional TEE first used a mechanical scanning system.[18] Modern 2-D TEE devices, however, use the smaller phased array transducer developed by Schluter.[19] The first of these instruments to be made commercially available was manufactured by Diasonics. Its 3.5-MHz transducer contains 32 array elements. Other companies have developed improved

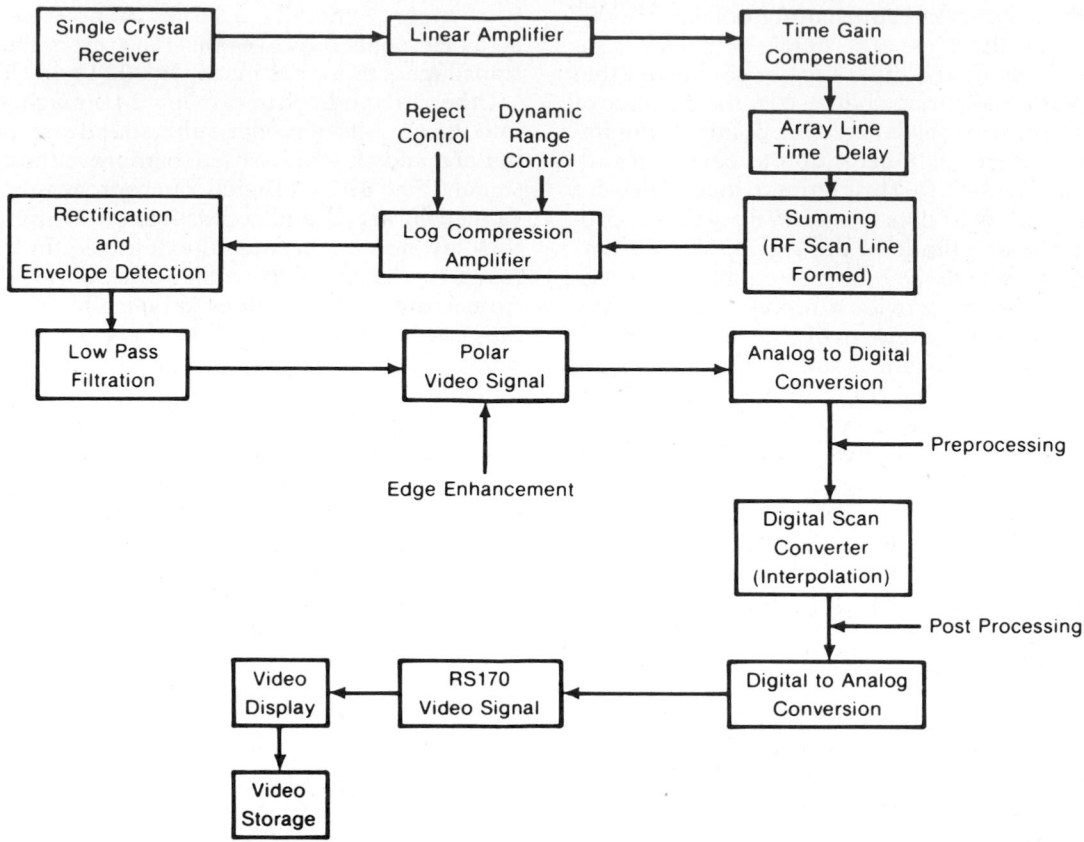

Fig. 31-23. Block flow diagram of the steps involved in reception of the reflected ultrasound and formation of the image. (From Geiser and Oliver,[207] with permission.)

TEE devices. These transducers are higher-frequency devices (5.0 MHz) that contain 64 array elements and offer generally improved axial and lateral image resolution. Moreover, most units incorporate Doppler blood flow velocity measurement capability (see following section). The basic designs for these instruments are similar. The transducer, typically 1.2 by 1.0 by 3.0 cm in size, is placed at the tip of a standard 110-cm-long flexible gastroscope. The distal 10 cm of the shaft is especially flexible and can be deflected 180 degrees in two planes, providing a variety of echocardiographic views (Fig. 31-24).

Although TEE is often used in awake patients with mild sedation and topical oropharyngeal anesthesia, it is more eminently suitable for use during general anesthesia. Only after securing the anesthetized patient's airway by tracheal intubation should the TEE device be placed. Gastric air that may have been introduced previously should be evacuated. A water-soluble acoustic jelly is usually placed on the end of the transducer, which is introduced orally. The presence of the endotracheal tube tends to push the larynx down over the esophagus. This may require gently lifting the mandible in order to open the posterior pharynx. Alternatively, careful visualization using a laryngoscope can expose the opening of the esophagus. A bite block should be

used to protect both the patient's teeth and the TEE instrument. Once the device has passed the upper pharynx, its positioning is guided by observing the ultrasound image. There are very few risks associated with this procedure. Pharyngeal trauma is prevented by careful attention to gentle placement of the instrument. The transducer itself generates some heat, but the problem of thermal injury to the esophagus has been prevented in the newer transducers by incorporation of a thermistor that guards against overheating. TEE use is contraindicated in cases of abnormal esophageal anatomy (Table 31-8).

A variety of different views may be obtained from the transesophageal position. The long or major axis view shown in Figure 31-25 allows examination of all four cardiac chambers and atrioventricular valves. From this basic position, small adjustments in longitudinal, angular, and rotational position of the transducer can demonstrate the left ventricular outflow tract (LVOT), a cross-section of the aortic valve annulus, or a close examination of the interatrial septum. Advancing the transducer and applying a more cephalad angulation yield the shorter or minor axis view (Fig. 31-26). This view affords an examination of a cross-section of the ventricles at any of several "slices" from base to apex. However, the most commonly monitored site is the

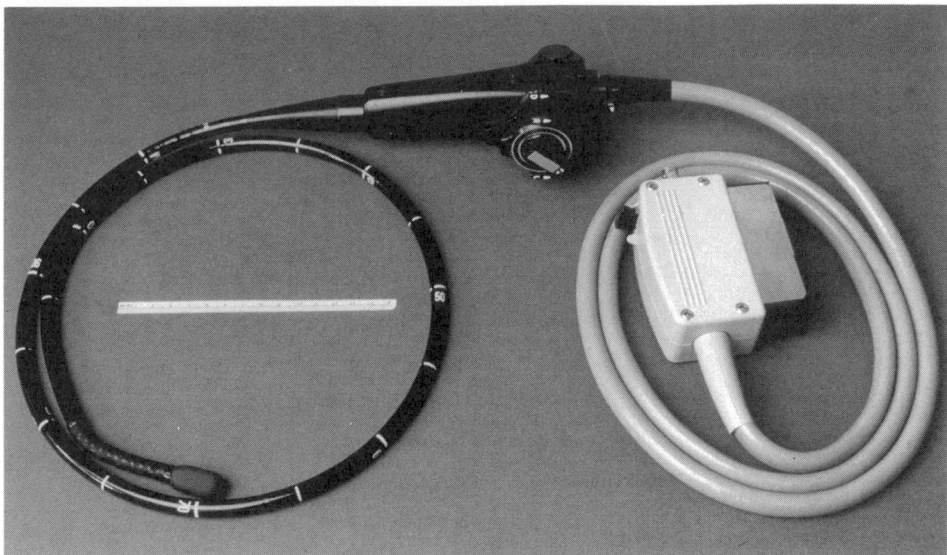

Fig. 31-24. Transesophageal echocardiography (TEE) probe. The transducer element is fitted into the tip of a modified gastroscope and can be steered by manipulating the wheels in the handle.

minor axis at the midpapillary muscle level. Here, all coronary vascular beds are represented,[210] making it an ideal position for assessment of regional myocardial ischemia.

TABLE 31-8. Transesophageal Echocardiography

Advantages
Noninvasive, low-risk procedure in anesthetized patients
Excellent image quality
No impingement on surgical field
Stable, continuous cardiac monitoring

Uses
Global cardiac function measurement
Assessment of *regional* cardiac function
    Early monitoring for myocardial ischemia
Diagnosis of abnormal cardiac anatomy
    Calcific, infectious valve abnormalities
    Cardiac myxomas
    Mural thrombi
Visualization of intracardiac air emboli
Contrast perfusion studies

Indications
History of poor myocardial or cardiac valve function
Risk of intraoperative myocardial ischemia
History of intracardiac shunts
Monitoring for intracardiac air
    Open chamber cardiac surgery
    Venous air emboli
        Sitting position
        Inferior vena cava surgery

Contraindications
Esophageal pathology
    Stricture
    Masses
    Large varices
    Previous surgery (esophageal or upper gastric)

Clinical Uses of TEE

Global Cardiac Function. Like other important cardiac monitors, TEE provides a means of assessing overall cardiac performance, by allowing the clinician to evaluate the global function of the heart, with focus usually directed on the left ventricle (LV). TEE is, however, constrained to a two-dimensional view of heart at any given instant. It is important, therefore, that information from the "slice" of the heart being examined provide an accurate reflection of cardiac function in all three dimensions. Typically, the minor axis view is chosen for this type of monitoring, since its approximately circular view of the LV cavity is more suited to computations of area changes. It is obviously important that a reliable description of the endocardial border of the LV be available. Providing this description is fortunately an easy task with the high-quality imaging afforded by TEE. By freezing the 2-D image at end-diastole (ED) and end-systole (ES), it is possible to outline LV cavity areas using the tracing features built into most ultrasound imaging systems. A cross-sectional area (A) measurement is computed, and area ejection fraction (EF_{area}) can be derived by using the following equation:

$$EF_{area} = \frac{A_{ED} - A_{ES}}{A_{ED}} \cdot 100\% \qquad (14)$$

Konstadt et al. demonstrated excellent correlation of LV dimensions and area changes of the LV cavity as measured by both TEE and direct on-heart echocardiography.[211] Echocardiographic measurements have been shown to predict overall left ventricular ejection fraction as estimated from angiograms performed at cardiac catheterization.[212] These investigations were performed using ultrasound images from two perpen-

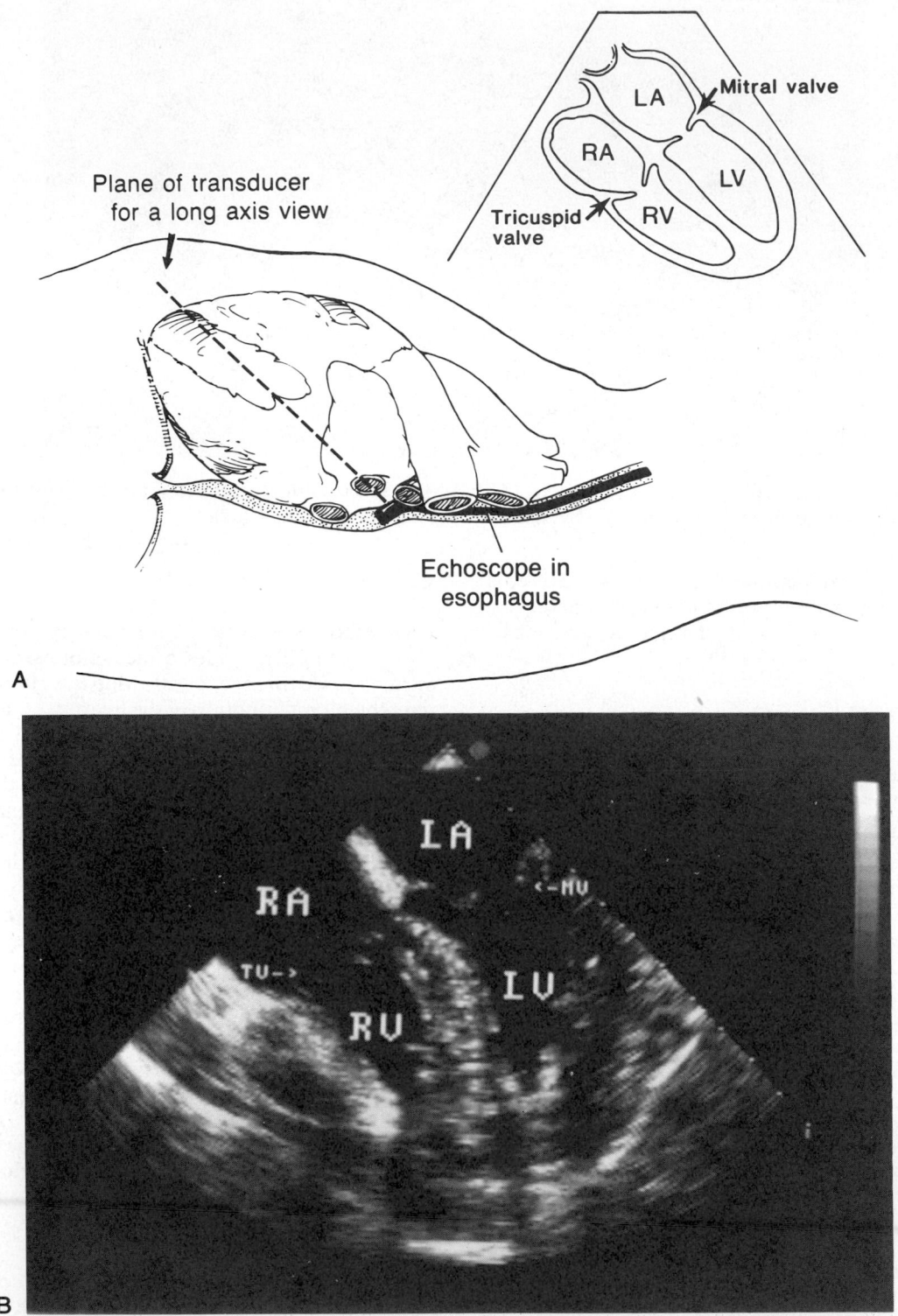

Fig. 31-25. (A) Sagittal section of the thorax demonstrating the TEE probe positioned in the esophagus for examination of the cardiac long axis. The inset shows the configuration of the four-chamber view typically seen. **(B)** Actual TEE image of the long axis view. RA, right atrium; RV, right ventricle; LA, left atrium; LV, left ventricle; TV, tricuspid valve; MV, mitral valve.

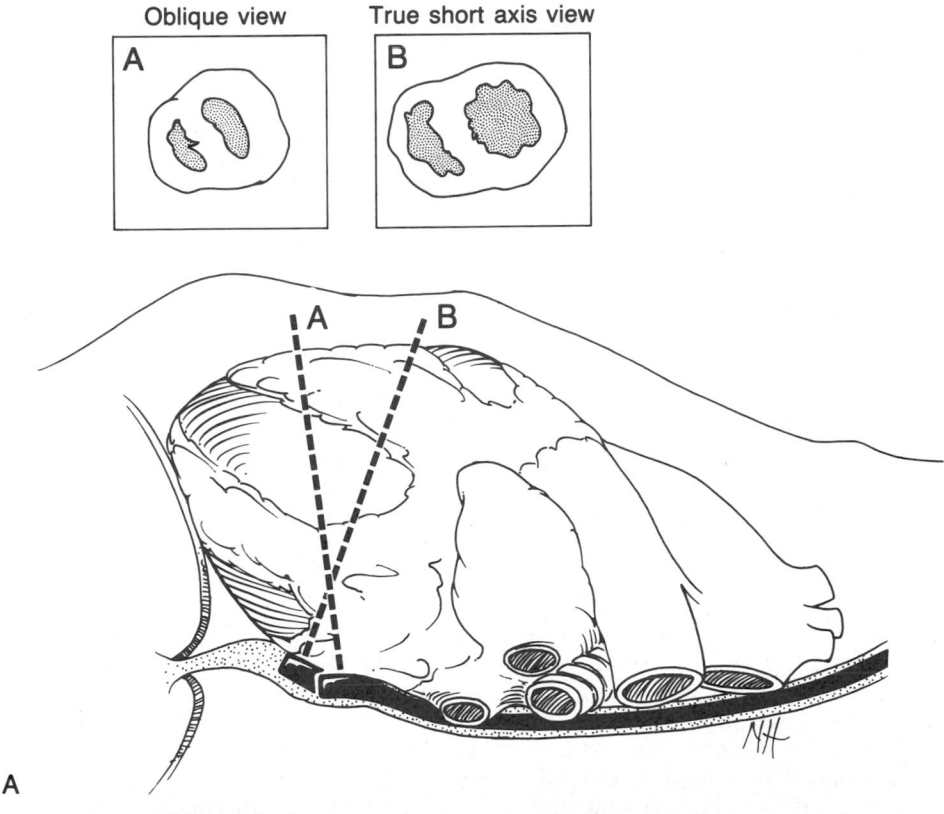

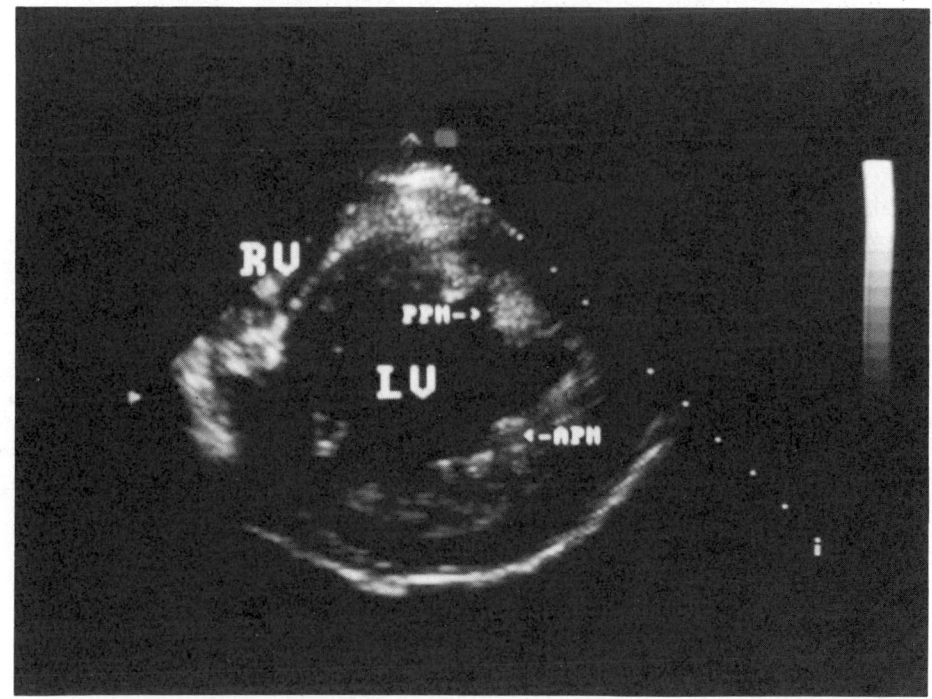

Fig. 31-26. **(A)** Diagrammatic view of thorax similar to Figure 31-25 with the TEE probe positioned for a short (minor) axis view of the ventricles. The image in plane A shows an oblique view, in which the ventricular walls appear falsely thick. The true short axis (plane B) is the preferable view and may require some anterior flexion of the transducer element. **(B)** Actual TEE minor axis image. RV, right ventricle; LV, left ventricle; PPM, posterior papillary muscle; APM, anterior papillary muscle.

dicular planes. Thys and co-workers used single-plane (minor axis) echocardiographic information to derive LV volumes using a truncated ellipsoidal model and computed an estimate of cardiac output.[213] They demonstrated a strong correlation between this approximation of LV volume changes and thermodilution cardiac output. Moreover, pulmonary capillary wedge pressure was poorly associated with calculated LV end-diastolic volumes, pointing to the importance of considering LV compliance when relating pressure measurements to volume changes. Clements et al. performed simultaneous 2D TEE and first-pass RNAs on patients undergoing major vascular surgery.[214] They reported that the TEE-derived minor axis area ejection fraction provided a reasonable prediction of actual ejection fraction determined by RNA (r = 0.96).

Regional Cardiac Function. It has been known since 1935 that the contractile function of the heart is exquisitely sensitive to the adequacy of its perfusion. Tennant and Wiggers published what has become a classic work demonstrating an immediate decrease in the force of contraction in hearts after occlusion of a coronary artery.[215] Detection of regional cardiac dysfunction in response to acute ischemia constitutes an important role for echocardiography. Moreover, the concept that intraoperative myocardial ischemia may lead to postoperative myocardial infarction[216] provides significant

impetus for using TEE to diagnose ischemic changes during anesthesia and surgery.

Many studies in both experimental and clinical settings have demonstrated the sensitivity of regional functional disturbances in indicating inadequate myocardial perfusion. Moreover, the occurrence of regional wall motion abnormalities (RWMAs) with the onset of acute ischemia has been found to precede the development of characteristic electrocardiographic changes (Fig. 31-27). Waters et al. noted RWMA after 50 percent reduction in coronary blood flow; ECG changes were not apparent until flow reduction reached 75 percent.[217] Similarly, Battler and co-workers reported a dissociation in onset of RWMA versus ECG changes in graded reductions in coronary blood flow in conscious animals.[218] The differences in time of onset were most apparent when partial coronary artery stenoses were applied.

In clinical investigations, Horowitz and colleagues demonstrated that echocardiographic determination of cardiac dysfunction at the time of initial evaluation of angina correctly identified 31 of the 33 patients in the study who developed acute myocardial infarction (MI).[219] Smith et al. studied a group of patients undergoing major vascular surgery who were considered to be at high risk for perioperative ischemia.[220] Intraoperative episodes of RWMA were present in 100 percent of those patients who later developed MI in the postopera-

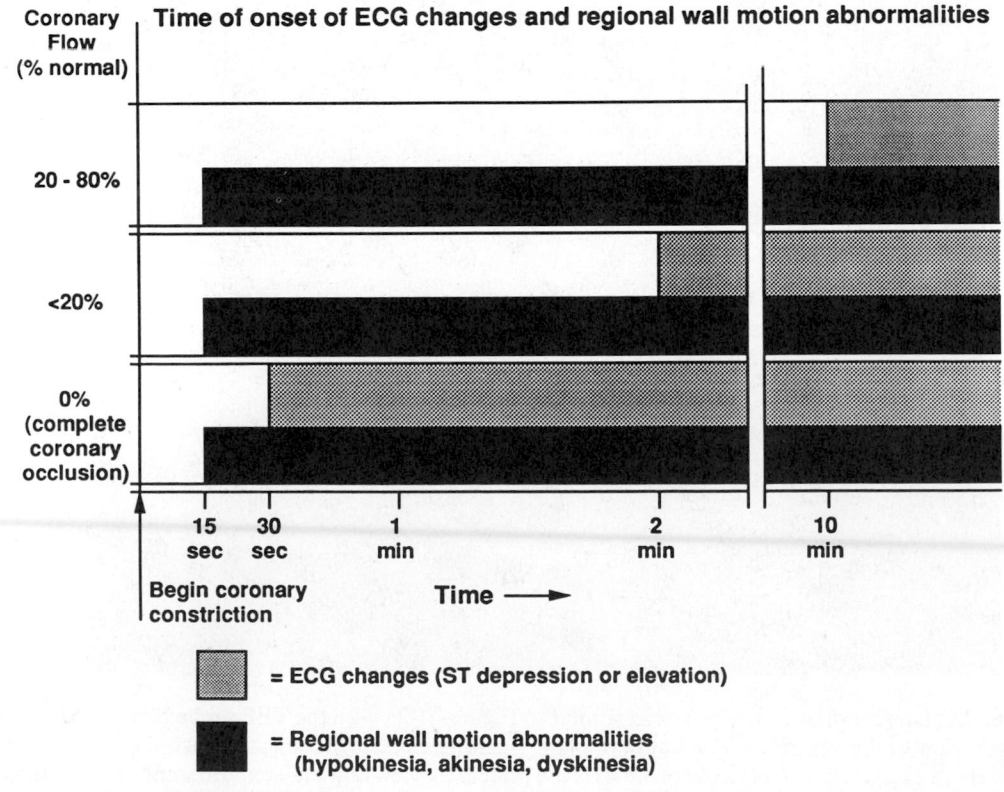

Fig. 31-27. Temporal relationship between acute coronary constriction and the onset of ECG and regional wall motion abnormalities. (From Clements and de Bruijn,[292] with permission.)

tive period. ECG changes were seen during surgery in only one-third of this subset of patients.

Not all myocardium found to be dysfunctional by echocardiographic monitoring is necessarily ischemic. Lima described a "tethering" phenomenon, by which areas of normal myocardium adjacent to ischemic regions may show diminished contractile activity as a result of simply being attached to the truly hypoperfused areas.[221] Moreover, the presence of cardiac dysfunction, either global or regional, does not *absolutely* indicate an ischemic etiology. Other hemodynamic factors, such as afterload, heart rate, and effects of anesthetic or vasoactive drugs, can play a significant role in altering the functional profile from one moment to the next. These factors must be born in mind when considering a diagnosis of ischemia during these evaluations.

Interpretation of Regional Cardiac Function by Echocardiography. An important caveat in the use of echocardiographic techniques is the reliance on qualitative evaluation of images. Unlike other intraoperative cardiac monitors that provide numeric results and have well-established ranges of normal values, TEE monitoring currently requires a subjective interpretation, which is possible only after a period of supervised training of the observer. Clements et al. demonstrated that training for recognition of regional wall motion abnormalities is fairly easily achieved[222]; Hillel et al. reported slightly less favorable results in the subjective estimation of LV ejection fraction.[223] Terminology used to score cardiac ultrasound images reflects the qualitative nature of these assessments. A decrease in regional function is evaluated as mild, moderate, or severe *hypokinesis*, and is further identified by its location within the ventricle (Fig. 31-28). Absence of movement is termed *akinesis*, while outward systolic bulging or thinning of the ventricular wall is designated *dyskinesis*. Other terms, *asyneresis* and *asynchrony*, describe deviations from the normally symmetric contraction of all areas of the

ventricle during systole. Moreover, these descriptions must be applied with respect to a baseline examination of the particular patient in order to diagnose an intraoperative change in function. This step is often best accomplished by recording TEE images on videotape at selected periods to facilitate a quick review of the patient's previous status. Newer imaging systems incorporate a built-in memory or "cine loop" feature that offers simultaneous observation of moving images recorded at separate time periods.

A quantitative approach to echocardiographic analysis of regional cardiac function has been a goal of investigators for a number of years. Today, the need for a more objective treatment of this information is even more apparent during TEE examinations in the intraoperative setting, where rapid changes in a patient's cardiovascular status and effects of therapeutic intervention are best followed with numeric, trendable information. Were it not for significant obstacles to this form of processing, this obviously needed development would have been in common use long ago.

Quantitation of cardiac wall motion in the past has suffered from poor overall image quality, inability to obtain stable standard cardiac views between examinations, and inadequate means by which to base or "reference" sequential comparisons of the altered ventricular wall motion. TEE largely corrects the problems of image quality and stability, but the referencing problem has remained. In addition to contracting, the heart rotates and shifts (translates) in the thorax between diastole and systole. Failure to correct for these motion artifacts may result in a misleading analysis of cardiac contraction. However, in examining only the motion of the endocardial outline, such correction is difficult to perform.[224] An example of this problem is seen in the use of the "floating" axis system, which aligns end-diastolic and end-systolic images by superimposing their computed "centers of mass" (Fig. 31-29). A dyskinetic bulge at end-systole results in a shift of the computed

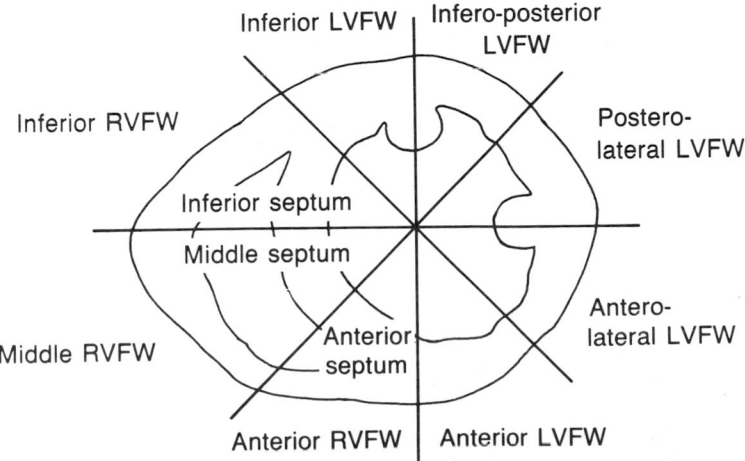

Fig. 31-28. Diagram of the midventricular minor (short) axis view with segmentation and nomenclature for specification in regional functional examination. (From de Bruijn and Clements,[293] with permission.)

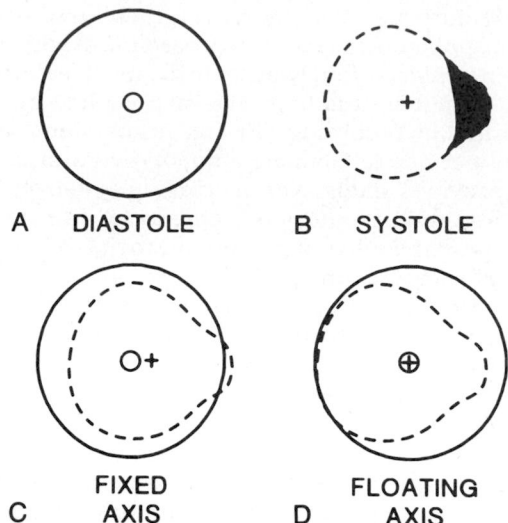

A   DIASTOLE   B   SYSTOLE

C   FIXED
AXIS   D   FLOATING
AXIS

Fig. 31-29. Demonstration of the shortcomings of endocardial wall motion referencing systems in evaluating regional cardiac contraction. **(A & B)** End-diastolic (solid contour) and end-systolic (dotted contour) are shown for a cardiac cycle in which dyskinesis (shaded bulge) has occurred. The fixed axis method **(C)** allows recognition of this dyskinetic segment but cannot identify true translational or rotational artifact. The floating axis system **(D)** superimposes the centers of each image; this may cause the dyskinetic area to appear more normal and the normal wall to appear hypokinetic or akinetic. (From Skorton et al.,[224] with permission.)

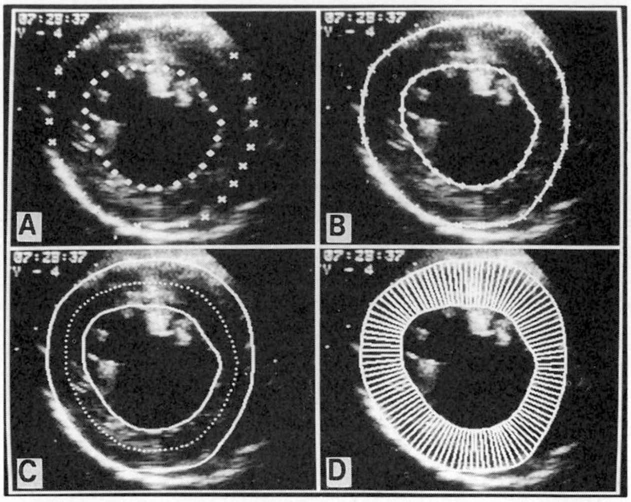

Fig. 31-30. Steps in centerline wall thickness determination. **(A)** Endocardial and epicardial points are chosen around the circumference of a minor axis image. **(B)** Remaining points of outlines are interpolated by using a cubic polynomial algorithm. **(C)** A set of 100 points equidistant from the two outlines is computed as a centerline. **(D)** Wall thickness chords are constructed as perpendiculars to tangents around the centerline and intersect the original outlines. (From Stanley et al.,[225] with permission.)

center toward the abnormal segment. Alignment of the centers of the two images, supposedly to correct for a translational artifact, in fact falsely minimizes the amount of dyskinesis actually present. Using a "fixed" axis system prevents this kind of error but does not account for translational or rotational movement when it truly occurs.

Measurement of systolic wall thickening (SWT) is a means by which analysis errors such as these may be prevented. By encompassing the epicardial outline in the quantitation process and examining the entire mass of the myocardium in the short axis view, much of the overall cardiac motion artifact can be corrected without losing sight of pathophysiologic motion changes[225] (Fig. 31-30). Moreover, SWT may be a more accurate descriptor of ischemic changes than simple endocardial wall motion. Ren et al. described SWT abnormalities in 92 to 100 percent of patients who had ventricular dysfunction documented by angiography.[226] Endocardial wall motion abnormalities were present in only 46 to 60 percent of these patients. Gallagher and colleagues demonstrated significant decreases in SWT with progressive reductions in coronary blood flow.[227] Laboratory[228] and clinical[229] studies have shown excellent correlation of echocardiographically measured SWT changes with the onset of myocardial ischemia.

A serious impediment to the routine use of any pres-

ently available quantitative analysis scheme in echocardiography is the requirement for a significant amount of user interaction. The operator must trace cardiac outlines on a frozen video image in order for measurements to be made. This consumes too much time to be a practical part of intraoperative monitoring with TEE. Computer analysis and image processing in echocardiography are also well established fields of research, and on-line automatic computerized image recognition and processing is the ultimate goal that will solve this problem.[224] However, progress in this area has been restrained by poor image resolution and lack of a mathematically clear, comprehensive understanding of the interaction of ultrasound with biologic tissue. Improvements in overall image quality by enhanced TEE technology and development of powerful, portable computer resources may finally allow implementation of the complex algorithms that will be needed to replicate objectively what the observer's eye and brain subjectively perform.

Assessment of Cardiac Anatomy. Another important application for TEE is the ability to visualize anatomic abnormalities of the heart and their potential influence on cardiac performance. The long axis 2-D view using TEE offers excellent perspectives of the mitral and aortic valves, which can be used to diagnose the presence and severity of calcific changes. These appear as dense, highly reflective ultrasound targets. Masses or vegetations on the valve structures, such as those occurring with endocarditis, can often be visualized.

Inspection of the left atrial cavity is very easy using TEE, since this is the closest cardiac chamber to the esophageal transducer. Cardiac myxomas, which most frequently occur in the left atrium, can be easily diagnosed with this monitoring technique.[230] Thrombus formation in the atria, which is seen in patients with chronic atrial fibrillation or after large myocardial infarction, is another type of cardiac mass that can be assessed using echocardiography. Care must be taken to prevent excessive manipulation of the heart by the TEE device in these patients, as this could dislodge the suspected cardiac masses. Since the esophageal probe does not extend significantly behind the heart in a long axis view (Fig. 31-25), the chance of its impacting on an intracardiac mass is small.

Intracardiac Air. The introduction of air bubbles into the systemic circulation can result in significant morbidity. Monitoring for massive venous air embolization is an important part of anesthesia care in patients undergoing procedures in the sitting position. Moreover, open chamber cardiac surgical procedures necessarily result in intracardiac air introduction. The extreme difference in acoustic impedance between air and blood causes air bubbles to be strongly reflective of ultrasound (see discussion of ultrasound physics). Exceptionally small bubbles (2 to 100 μm) can be visualized by echocardiography, making this technique a most sensitive means of diagnosing air bubbles in the circulation.

Cucchiara et al. found TEE superior to precordial Doppler techniques in the diagnosis of venous air embolization in 9 of 15 neurosurgical patients in the sitting position.[231] Moreover, TEE was able to demonstrate the more ominous occurrence of paradoxical air emboli via a patent foramen ovale in one of these patients. Topol and colleagues studied the incidence of air emboli diagnosed by TEE in patients undergoing various types of cardiac surgical procedures.[232] Not surprisingly, air was present in a much greater percentage of patients undergoing open chamber procedures (74 percent) than extracardiac operations (12 percent). Interestingly, there was no association of the severity of air emboli and postoperative focal neurologic abnormalities, although detailed prospective neuropsychiatric testing was not performed. Neurologic sequelae after cardiac surgery can be quite subtle. One may speculate, therefore, that using TEE to judge the adequacy of air evacuation after cardiac surgery may have a positive effect on efforts to minimize neurologic complications.

Contrast Echocardiography. The intense reflectivity of air bubbles can be put to use safely to provide a "contrast agent" in echocardiography, provided that the bubbles are of sufficiently small size. By vigorously agitating saline or other injectable vehicle, cavitation and mixing with surrounding air cause the formation of *microbubbles*. Injection of this solution during echocardiographic imaging results in an easily visualized bolus of fluid passing through the cardiac chambers. The microbubbles created by hand agitation are slightly larger than red blood cells ($\sim 15 \mu$m diameter) but have a short half-life in the circulation (2 to 3 minutes).[233]

Echocardiographic imaging of microbubble injections has been used to diagnose abnormal blood flow across cardiac valves or lesions such as septal defects.[234,235] However, the incorporation of Doppler technology in the ultrasound imaging systems, especially the recent development of Doppler color flow imaging, has largely supplanted the microbubble technique for assessing intracardiac blood flow.

Direct coronary artery injection of microbubble solutions during cardiac catheterization[236] and coronary artery bypass surgery[237] has provided ultrasonic visualization of regional myocardial perfusion. This technique requires more carefully prepared microbubbles, usually using sonicated renografin solution to provide smaller bubble diameter (5 μm), which has been used safely in cardiac surgical patients. Echocardiographic contrast measurement of myocardial perfusion is at a preliminary stage of development, but the rapid growth of intraoperative echocardiography using TEE provides a fertile environment for continued research in this area.

Doppler Ultrasound

An extension of the diagnostic and monitoring capabilities of clinical ultrasound is the measurement of blood flow velocities using the Doppler principle. This physical law relating velocities of objects to changes in the frequency of reflected wave energy has been incorporated in a variety of applications, from monitoring the weather to establishing the speed of automobiles on the highways. The use of Doppler ultrasound in echocardiography is not a recent development: Light[238] and Wells[239] described clinical application over 20 years ago. However, the difficulties in implementing and interpreting the data of early Doppler techniques restrained growth of its popularity relative to standard echocardiographic imaging, which provides more recognizable information. Recent improvements in electronic processing technology, especially the advent of Doppler color flow imaging, have provided greater facility for understanding Doppler-derived blood flow information. Finally, the incorporation of Doppler capability in the newer TEE devices has brought this means of blood flow analysis to the intraoperative environment.

Basic Principles

The Doppler principle takes its name from the Austrian mathematician and physicist Johann Christian Doppler, who presented the principle in 1842 at a scientific meeting.[240] Unfortunately, he used an erroneous suggestion to describe his idea, that the movement of stars relation to earth caused their altered coloration. He was roundly criticized by his peers, one of whom, Buys Ballot, in seeking to disprove this theory, performed an experiment in 1845 that actually verified the principle. He placed a trumpeter on a train moving past an observer who was trained to recognize perfect musical pitch. Other stationary trumpets were placed nearby and played the same note to provide a reference. As the train approached, the pitch of the trumpet moving toward the observer was perceived to be higher than that of the stationary trumpets. As the train went by, the pitch heard immediately dropped below the reference note.[241]

The differences in this easily understandable example and the application of the principle to echocardiography are several, but are not difficult to comprehend. In Doppler ultrasound, the transducer instrument is both the source of sound energy and the "observer" or receiver of the frequency-shifted *reflected* sound signal. The moving objects that reflect the ultrasound are red blood cells in the vessels or cardiac chambers being interrogated. Figure 31-31 demonstrates this effect for blood cells moving toward the transducer. Movement away from the transducer results in a lower reflected frequency than that originally emitted. Another difference in this application from the classic example is that there are millions of these objects (red blood cells) whose potentially different velocities are assessed simultaneously. Thus, a more complex set of reflected frequencies is actually returned to the transducer, especially when blood flow loses its laminar characteristics and becomes turbulent.

To use this frequency shift phenomenon, there must be a means of quantitating the velocities that the frequency changes represent. Fortunately, a relatively simple equation fulfills this requirement. The original Doppler equation to predict the reflected frequency can be rearranged for the velocity (V) of the object(s):

$$V = \frac{c \cdot f_r}{2f_t \cdot \cos\theta} \qquad (15)$$

where c = speed of sound in blood
f_r = frequency of the reflected sound wave
f_t = frequency of the transmitted sound wave
θ = angle between the sound wave direction and the direction of blood flow

All of these factors are known or measured during a Doppler examination, with the exception of the angle of incidence θ, which must be estimated. This angle should be as close to zero as possible, so that the cosine of θ approaches unity and errors resulting from beam misalignment will be minimal. Generally, angles greater than 25 degrees yield clinically unacceptable quantitative estimates of velocity.[242] Much of the error in the techniques for Doppler-derived cardiac output is the result of an inability to optimize or standardize this alignment angle (see the section, *Doppler Cardiac Output*).

The next required step is to display the velocity information in a meaningful format. The difficult aspects of this process, which have been resolved by the use of modern, high-speed digital technology, are the separation and quantitation of all the velocities (frequencies) acquired. A spectral analysis in real time using fast Fourier transformation (FFT) separates the complex ultrasound waveform into its component frequencies and displays the computed velocities on the y axis of a screen or strip chart as a function of time on the x axis. The relative power of a particular velocity (analogous to the "amount" of blood traveling at that speed) is the third variable, which is represented by the intensity or darkness of the spectral trace (Fig. 31-32). An analog or amplitude display traces maximal and mean velocity values over time. The spectral display is useful in showing the distribution of various velocities, since a wide range of flows may suggest turbulence resulting from a pathologic condition.

Doppler Instrumentation

Continuous Wave Doppler

To this point, the discussion of Doppler techniques has assumed that the velocity measurement is uninterrupted. In fact, continuous wave (CW) Doppler does provide constant blood flow information by using separate transmit and receive transducer elements (Fig. 31-33). Normal blood flow velocity in humans does not exceed 1.5 m/s. However, in pathologic conditions such as aortic stenosis, a jet of blood flow can exceed 5 m/s. Continuous wave Doppler can measure a limitless range of blood flow velocities, making it very useful in quantitating these jets. The main disadvantage of CW Doppler is its inability to determine the anatomic posi-

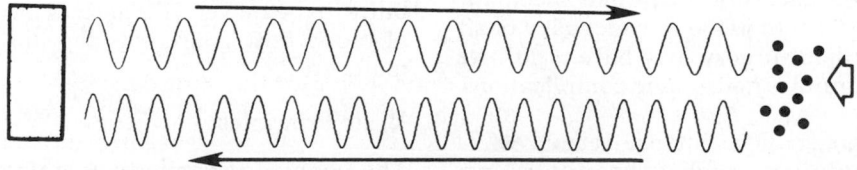

Fig. 31-31. Example of the Doppler effect resulting from red blood cells traveling toward the transducer at the left. A burst of ultrasound is sent into the tissue at a given frequency and is reflected off the red cells moving toward the transducer at a higher frequency. This is a positive Doppler shift. (From Kisslo et al.,[242] with permission.)

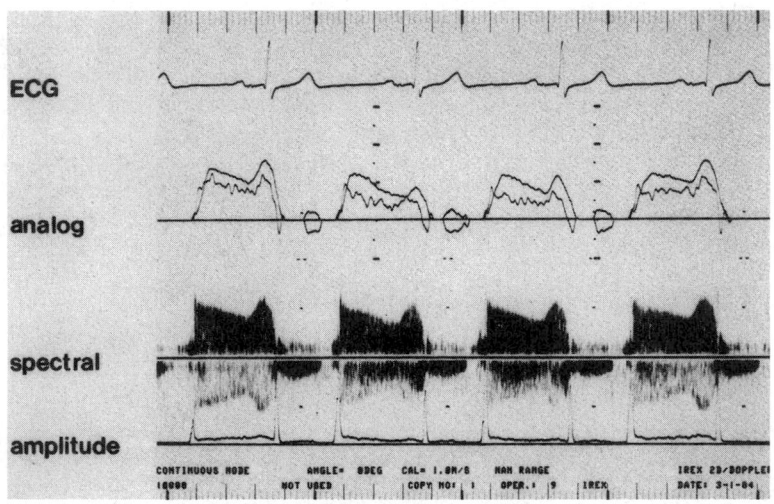

Fig. 31-32. An example of the various Doppler displays from a patient with mitral stenosis with the transducer held at the apex. Flow in diastole is toward the transducer. The ECG is at the top. The analog outputs are of maximum and mean velocities. The spectral recording shows spectral broadening toward the transducer in diastole, indicating turbulent flow. Because the diastolic signal is so strong, there is some "mirroring" into the opposite channel. (From Kisslo et al.,[242] with permission.)

tion from which the abnormal jet arises. In other words, CW Doppler has no capacity for *range* discrimination but displays a mix of velocity data from all points along its beam. Moreover, CW Doppler is a "blind" technique, since there can be no other echocardiographic imaging taking place while the transducer is continually in the Doppler mode. One method designed to correct this problem is to shift ultrasound modes of a phased array scanner periodically between 2-D imaging

and CW Doppler. In this way, the benefits of both anatomic display and high-velocity measurement are provided in a nearly simultaneous fashion.[242]

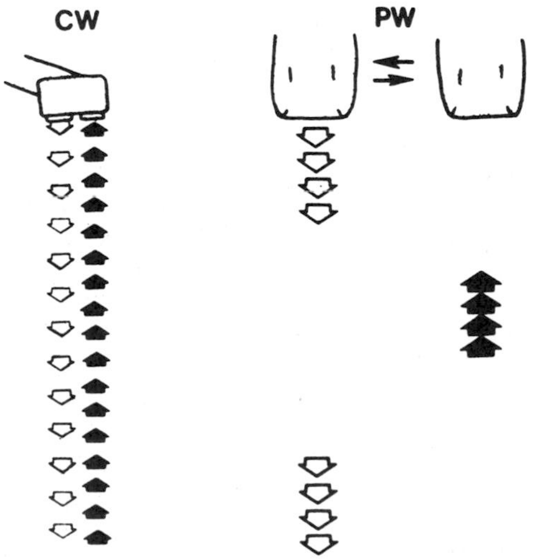

Pulse Wave Doppler

A more common technique for providing range (location) information for the velocity being measured is pulse wave (PW) Doppler. In this method, short bursts or pulses of ultrasound are emitted by a single transducer, which then switches to a "listen" mode and waits for a returning signal (Fig. 31-33). By selecting or "gating" this listening process to a particular elapsed time (T_e) after transmission and knowing the velocity of sound in tissues (c), the distance (D) of the sample volume from the transducer is derived:

$$D = \frac{c \cdot T_e}{2} \qquad (16)$$

Thus velocity information from a specific site is available. The remainder of the returning Doppler signal outside this gate is ignored. This allows the ultrasound system to perform standard imaging during the intervening time. Concurrent imaging is of great advantage, since one can "see" where the PW Doppler sampling is taking place within the field of view. With most phased array systems, the operator may "steer" the PW beam to a particular point in the 2-D image and view the spectral Doppler display simultaneously (Fig. 31-34).

The major disadvantage of pulse wave Doppler techniques is that the maximum measurable velocity is limited, often to a significant degree. The reason for this problem is a phenomenon called *aliasing*, which is the result of a mismatching of the Doppler frequency shift being measured and the rate at which PW samples are

Fig. 31-33. Modes of transmission and reception. In CW there is constant transmission and reception, whereas in PW the system must alternate between transmit and receive functions using the same transducer. (From Kisslo et al.,[242] with permission.)

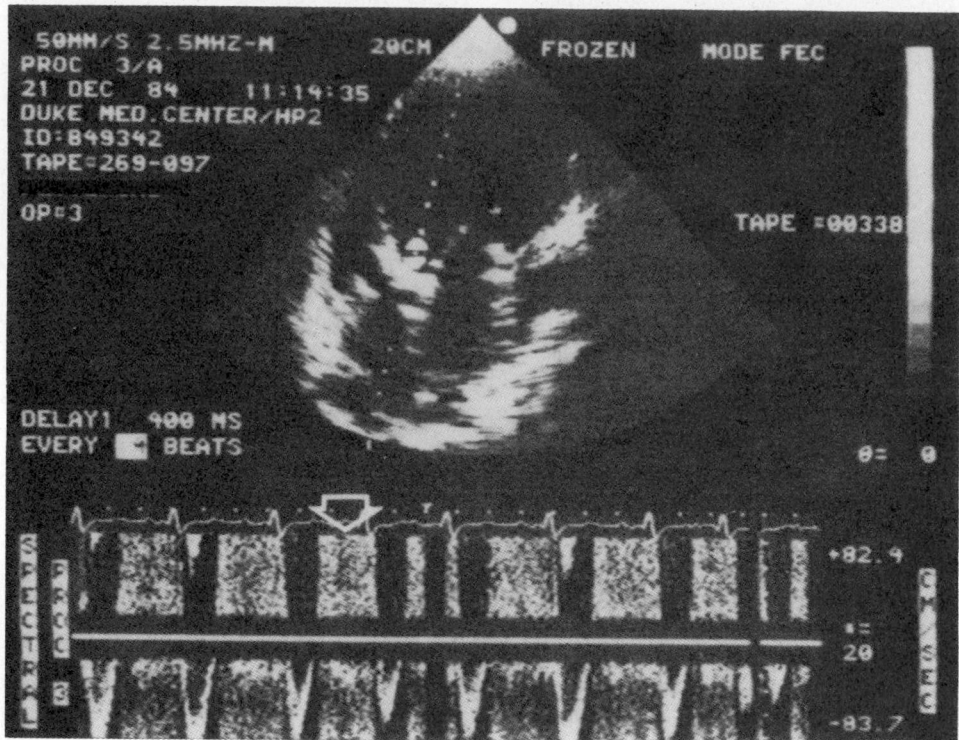

Fig. 31-34. Concurrent display of 2-D echocardiographic image and PW Doppler spectral analysis. The PW cursor is located on the dotted line just below the aortic valve in a transthoracic examination of a patient with aortic insufficiency, which is seen on the spectral display as a high-velocity, severely aliased jet directed toward the transducer during diastole (arrow). (Adapted from Kisslo et al.,[242] with permission.)

repeated. The analogy commonly used to explain aliasing is that of a mark on a wheel rotating at fixed rate. If the position of the mark is not viewed (sampled) frequently enough, its movement will be misrepresented and the mark may appear to be turning in the opposite direction (Fig. 31-35). The maximum Doppler shift ($f_{Doppler}$) value that can be accurately measured by PW Doppler is one-half the sampling frequency (f_{sample}). This maximum velocity cutoff is called the Nyquist limit:

$$f_{Doppler} = \frac{f_{sample}}{2} = \text{Nyquist limit} \qquad (17)$$

Aliasing appears on the spectral plot as a velocity contour that "wraps around" the display and appears to be directed oppositely (Fig. 31-36). One method to prevent aliasing is to shift the reference baseline of velocity measurement, so that only unidirectional flow will be demonstrated but the Nyquist limit will be extended twofold (Fig. 31-36C). Physical factors that affect the Nyquist limit include the distance (D) of the sample volume from the transducer and the reference ultrasound frequency (f_t) being used:

$$\text{Nyquist limit} = \frac{c^2}{8 f_t D} \qquad (18)$$

where c is the speed of sound in blood. Thus, using low-frequency transducers (2.5-MHz) and interrogating sample volumes close to the transducer allow PW Doppler to measure blood flow velocity most accurately.

Color Flow Imaging

Doppler color flow imaging (CFI) is the most recent enhancement in Doppler echocardiography, providing real-time images of blood flow velocity in *two dimensions* superimposed on a standard 2-D echocardiogram.[241,243] This allows an immediate and relatively straightforward identification and qualitative assessment of many intracardiac lesions that affect blood flow patterns. Color flow imaging is the product of very sophisticated high-speed electronic processing, which separates Doppler frequency shift information from reflected ultrasound signals from multiple points along most or all of the scan lines of a 2-D ultrasound image. In essence, color flow systems perform *multigated* pulse wave Doppler analyses on literally hundreds of sample volumes over a two-dimensional space. In order to present a recognizable display of the direction and velocity of these many individual flow measurements, a color scheme is utilized. Typically, blood flow

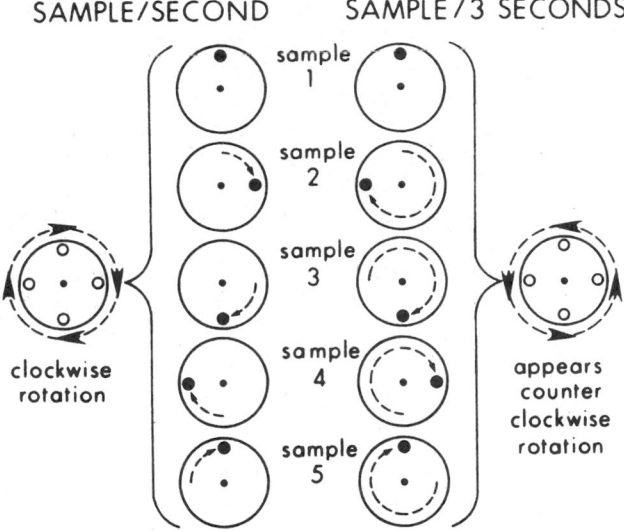

SAMPLE/SECOND   SAMPLE/3 SECONDS

sample 1

sample 2

sample 3

sample 4

sample 5

clockwise rotation

appears counter clockwise rotation

Fig. 31-35. Schematic explanation of aliasing. The marked wheel is turning clockwise at the rate of one full rotation every 4 seconds. This represents the velocity (Doppler shift) being measured. If the sampling rate is 1/s, then the true movement of the mark is accurately determined. However, if the samples are taken only once per 3 seconds, the mark appears to turn counterclockwise. (Adapted from Kisslo et al.,[242] with permission.)

directed toward the transducer is colored red, and flow away is blue.* The velocity is indicated by the shade of the color, with higher velocities causing the red hue to become lighter or even turn yellow and blue colors to reach a light cyan appearance. Because of the use of PW Doppler methods with a necessarily low pulse repetition frequency, aliasing occurs to a significant degree in CFI. However, aliasing is actually somewhat advantageous in this method, because it has the effect of "wrapping" the color around to the opposite hue (bright red aliases immediately to bright blue), creating a "mosaic" color pattern on the display of aliased and unaliased velocity measurements when high-velocity turbulent flows are imaged. This makes abnormal blood flow jets more recognizable, since these are most likely to attain velocities high enough to cause aliasing. Some of the newer generation of transesophageal echocardiography transducers incorporate color flow capability,[244] making this technology available for monitoring in the intraoperative setting.

---

* A clear understanding of Doppler CFI is best accomplished by examining actual color images. A full complement of color figures demonstrating both normal and pathologic cardiac flow is found in Kisslo J, Adams DB, Belkin RN: Doppler Color Flow Imaging. New York, Churchill Livingstone, 1988.

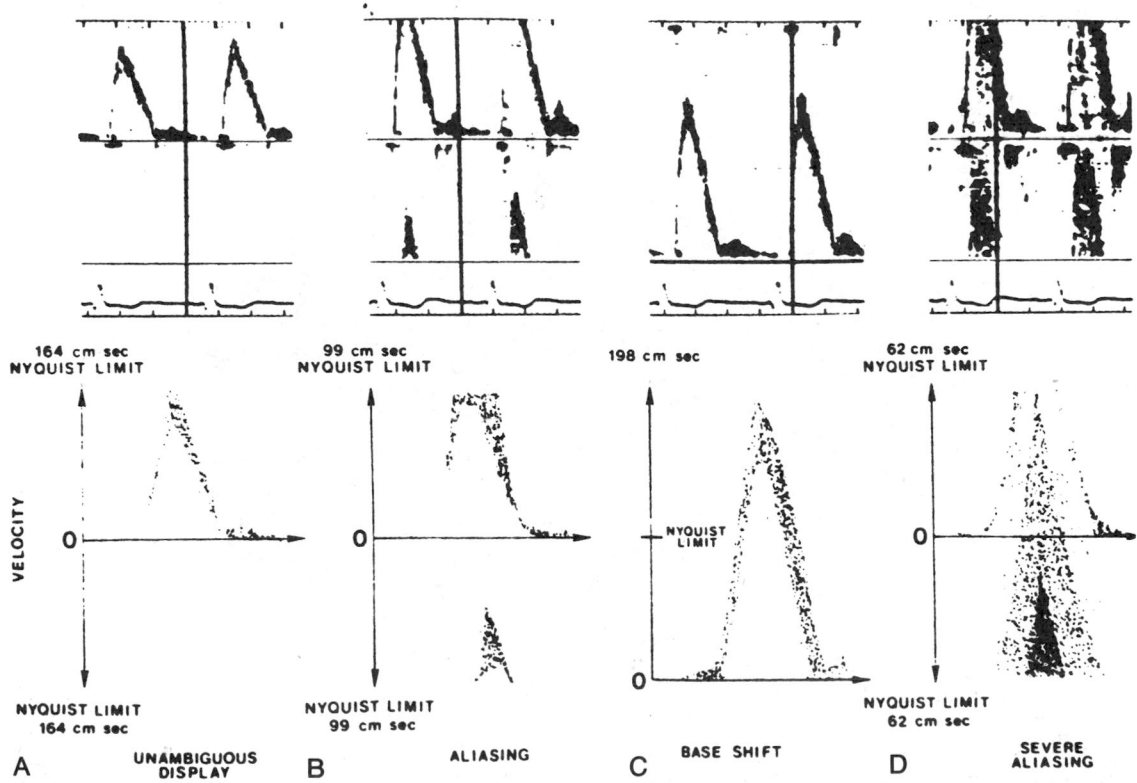

164 cm sec NYQUIST LIMIT

99 cm sec NYQUIST LIMIT

198 cm sec

62 cm sec NYQUIST LIMIT

VELOCITY

0

0

NYQUIST LIMIT

0

0

NYQUIST LIMIT 164 cm sec

NYQUIST LIMIT 99 cm sec

NYQUIST LIMIT 62 cm sec

A   UNAMBIGUOUS DISPLAY

B   ALIASING

C   BASE SHIFT

D   SEVERE ALIASING

Fig. 31-36. Diagrammatic and spectral illustration of normal **(A)** and aliased PW Doppler **(B)** displays. **(C)** A baseline shift allows flow to be shown above the Nyquist limit. **(D)** Severe aliasing with more than one wraparound is seen. (From American Society of Echocardiography,[296] with permission.)

Clinical Applications of Doppler Ultrasound

Despite the limitations imposed by the physical principles of Doppler ultrasound, many applications for this technology exist in anesthesia. The previous discussion of cardiac output monitoring outlines the variety of methods that use Doppler ultrasound to estimate aortic blood flow velocity and to compute cardiac output. These techniques have formed the basis for much of the recent interest and development of continuous cardiac output monitoring.

Identification and quantitation of abnormal blood flow is another major use of Doppler echocardiography. Once an abnormal flow jet is characterized, other important anatomic information can often be derived. The Bernoulli equation is a complex formula relating the velocity (V) of a jet of blood flow to the pressure difference ($P_1 - P_2$) on each side of the orifice creating the jet. For practical purposes, the formula can be simplified to:

$$P_1 - P_2 = 4V^2 \qquad (19)$$

If an accurate measurement of peak flow velocity can be made in a Doppler examination (best done with CW Doppler), then the pressure gradient can be estimated. This is very useful in assessing stenotic valve lesions and for judging whether a septal defect is restrictive or unrestrictive.

The diastolic function of the left ventricle (LV) can be assessed by using Doppler measurements of flow across the mitral valve during diastole. From the apical long axis view during a transthoracic examination or from an equivalent plane during TEE monitoring, interrogation of transmitral valve flow can be accomplished accurately because the angle of incidence, θ, is nearly zero. Under normal conditions, Doppler flow recording reveals a large early diastolic velocity peak (E), corresponding to rapid ventricular filling. A lesser peak (A) occurs just after the P wave of the ECG, which represents atrial contraction (Fig. 31-37). Under conditions of diminished LV compliance (LV hypertrophy, myocardial ischemia), the E peak is decreased, since diastolic filling is impaired. Investigators have used the ratio of E to A peaks to determine the severity of these pathophysiologic states. Ryan et al. demonstrated reductions in E/A ratio after coronary artery occlusions in an experimental animal model.[245] In the clinical setting, Visser and co-workers measured E/A ratio in patients admitted for acute myocardial infarction and found this Doppler examination a useful method for identifying patients at risk for congestive heart failure.[246]

Doppler color flow imaging during intraoperative cardiac monitoring with TEE can offer valuable information regarding a number of cardiac abnormalities that can impact greatly on anesthesia care. De Bruijn and colleagues reported that intraoperative identification of valvular abnormalities, especially mitral and aortic regurgitation, was easily accomplished by using TEE-based CFI.[244] Interestingly, a high incidence of

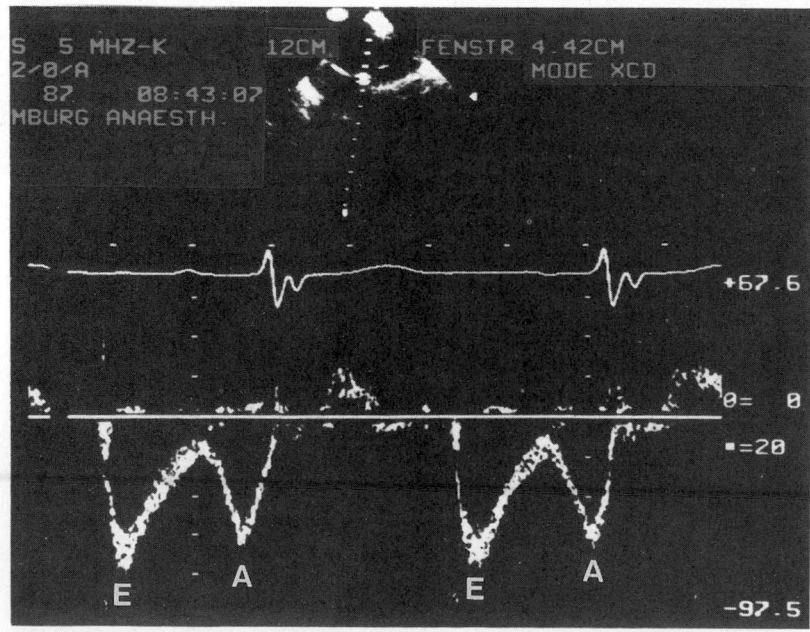

Fig. 31-37. Simultaneous recording (from top to bottom) of 2-D TEE long axis image with PW Doppler sample volume position at the mitral valve, the electrocardiogram, and the Doppler velocity spectrum (recording speed 100 mm/s). In sinus rhythm, the transmitral Doppler spectrum showed a biphasic velocity curve with a flow away from the transducer. The first peak (E) is the velocity of early diastolic filling, the second represents an increase in velocity after atrial contraction (A). (Adapted from Roewer et al.,[294] with permission.)

asymptomatic mitral regurgitation was seen in patients presenting for coronary artery bypass grafting in this study. A particular advantage of the transesophageal approach to cardiac imaging is its use in diagnosing prosthetic valve dysfunction. From the transthoracic perspective, paravalvular leaks around mitral or aortic prostheses often cannot be imaged, since the metal or plastic parts of the prosthesis block transmission of ultrasound, casting a "shadow" in the areas where regurgitant flow would be apparent. This problem is prevented by the use of TEE, since the heart is imaged from the opposite direction.

The growing popularity of cardiac valve repair is greatly assisted by the ability of CFI to provide intraoperative assessment of the effectiveness of the surgery and to allow immediate revision of the procedure if necessary. For the same reasons, Doppler CFI is extremely valuable during repair of congenital cardiac defects, since abnormal blood flow patterns are commonly the primary indication for these procedures, and visualization of corrected blood flow after the repair is highly advantageous. Several recent investigations have documented the usefulness of CFI in this setting.[247-249] Typically, imaging is accomplished by using a direct on-heart approach with a sterile ensheathed transducer, since more viewing angles than TEE can provide are necessary in examining these patients. Further developments in Doppler CFI may include means of quantitating flows, although this will be difficult, largely because aliasing may misrepresent actual flow velocities. At present, evaluation of these images depends on the qualitative interpretation of well-trained clinicians.

SPECIAL TOPICS

Right Ventricular Function Monitoring

As suggested in the previous discussion, cardiac function monitoring has focused primarily on status of the left ventricle. The potential consequences of right ventricular ((RV) dysfunction have been recognized for many years.[250] Several patient populations are at increased risk of right ventricular dysfunction, including those with chronic obstructive pulmonary disease (COPD) and adult respiratory distress syndrome (ARDS). Furthermore, patients with long-standing left heart failure, such as those awaiting cardiac transplantation, have a high incidence of increased right heart afterload. In fact, failure of the donor right ventricle after cardiac transplantation accounts for up to 30 percent of the early mortality from this procedure.[251]

Unfortunately, the geometric configuration of the RV (highly variable crescent shape) has not lent itself well to mathematical modeling and derivation of the functional parameters commonly applied to the left ventricle. Monitoring of right ventricular filling pressure (central venous pressure [CVP]) and afterload (pulmonary vascular resistance [PVR]) is easy to perform and offers a perspective of RV functional performance. However, the previously discussed concerns about the usefulness of PVR as an accurate hemodynamic measurement casts some doubt on the validity of its application to this problem. Electrocardiographic measurements that are more specific to the right ventricle have been used to diagnose right ventricular ischemic changes. Special electrode configurations (V_4R, CR_4R) have been recommended for this purpose.[252]

Some of the new imaging techniques described here have the capacity to define more fully RV geometry and changes in its function. If the appropriate viewing plane is used, nuclear imaging can detect the passage of tracer specifically through the RV and can determine its ejection fraction and rates of contraction.[253] Similarly, advances in rapid imaging using magnetic resonance techniques provide a means for measuring right heart function.[254]

In the intraoperative environment, neither nuclear imaging nor MRI can be applied on a routine basis. Transesophageal echocardiography can determine the movement of a portion of the RV, although the anterior position of the right ventricle makes it a less easily visualized chamber from the transesophageal perspective. Moreover, the limitation of echocardiography to a two-dimensional sampling of RV wall motion results in significant errors when this information is extrapolated to the poorly understood three-dimensional characteristics of the RV.[252]

Another means of assessing RV function during anesthesia and surgery is the measurement of right ventricular ejection fraction (RVEF) using a thermodilution technique.[254a] This method uses a standard pulmonary artery catheter that has a rapid response thermistor. The ability to detect more subtle changes in temperature with this more sensitive thermistor allows the computation of right ventricular stroke volume and ejection fraction (Fig. 31-38). The thermodilution RVEF method loses accuracy when cardiac arrhythmias occur or when there is a significant amount of tricuspid valve incompetence.[252] Comparison studies of this technique with angiographic or nuclear imaging counterparts have yielded mixed results in terms of accuracy,[255,256] probably reflecting the fact that a true "gold standard" for this technique does not exist. Nonetheless, thermodilution RVEF has been reported to be a useful intraoperative monitoring method.[257]

Anticoagulation Monitoring

Many cardiovascular surgical procedures involve practices that predispose to blood coagulation, such as stasis of blood flow with arterial cross-clamping or contact of blood with nonendothelial surfaces during cardiopulmonary bypass (CPB). To prevent blood coagulation during these periods, the patient must be anticoagulated. Heparin was introduced in 1938 as an effective anticoagulant[258] and is the drug of choice to

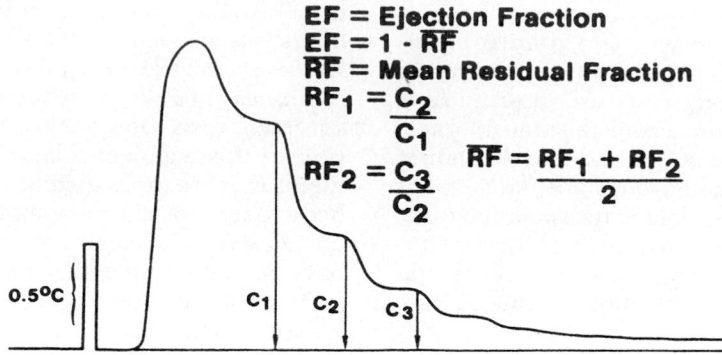

$$EF = \text{Ejection Fraction}$$
$$EF = 1 - \overline{RF}$$
$$\overline{RF} = \text{Mean Residual Fraction}$$
$$RF_1 = \frac{C_2}{C_1}$$
$$RF_2 = \frac{C_3}{C_2} \qquad \overline{RF} = \frac{RF_1 + RF_2}{2}$$

Fig. 31-38. Thermal dilution cardiac output curve obtained with a rapid response pulmonary artery catheter. After 0.5°C calibration spikes, a thermal bolus is injected. Plateaus represent diastolic C_1, C_2, and C_3 temperature differences between respective diastolic plateaus. (From Kay et al.,[254a] with permission.)

prevent coagulation. Heparin acts by binding to and activating antithrombin III. Since antithrombin III inactivates coagulation proteins throughout the entire coagulation cascade, heparin is a very effective and nonspecific anticoagulant. Heparin is prepared commercially from bovine lung or porcine intestine or lung and is composed of sulfated mucopolysaccharides that are highly variable in structure and activity. Despite great variability in heparin source and content and imprecise standardization, the drug is associated with few complications and its use is routine for all patients who require anticoagulation during surgery. It is important to monitor anticoagulation during and after cardiac surgery, since it is crucial that there be adequate heparinization during CPB and appropriate reversal of heparin with protamine after CPB. There are a number of methods used to monitor coagulation during cardiac surgery and the ones commonly used will be discussed. Table 31-9 contains the normal value of intraoperative coagulation variables.

Activated Coagulation Time (Also See Ch. 51)

The activated coagulation time (ACT) was introduced in 1966 by Hattersley.[259] The test is simple, reproducible, accurate, cost-effective, and rapid. The ACT involves placing 2 ml of blood in a glass test tube that contains 12 mg of diatomaceous earth, mixing the contents of the test tube, and observing the beginning of clot formation signified by thickening of the blood upon gentle inversion. Diatomaceous earth is a fine powder that provides a large surface area, thus accelerating the conversion of factor XII to factor XIIa.[260] Alternatively, the test can be conducted with an automated system such as the Hemochron. This device uses a special test tube that contains a small cylindrical magnet. After addition of the blood and thorough mixing with the diatomaceous earth, the tube is inserted into the device, which rotates the tube in such a way that the magnet rolls through the blood, maintaining the contacts of a proximity switch located in the base of the machine. A heating unit provides a constant blood temperature of 37°C. As the blood clots, the magnet is pulled along with the clot and is eventually rotated away from the proximity switch, breaking its contacts. This halts the timer that was started on initial mixing of the blood, an audible alarm is sounded, and the elapsed time (the ACT) is displayed in seconds. Normal ACT is 106 ± 13 seconds with a coefficient of variation of 4.5 to 7.0 percent.[259] The ACT is extremely sensitive to temperature and care must be taken to warm hypothermic blood samples. Even with automatic warming, the manufacturers of the Hemochron advise correcting for hypothermia. Hemodilution is another factor that will prolong the ACT.[261]

The ACT is linearly prolonged by the administration of heparin according to dose administered. Although the precise range of the linearity is not known, it is generally considered to extend from the normal value (100 seconds) to approximately 60 seconds. Marked variation in heparin effect in patients monitored with the ACT was reported by Bull et al.[262] in 1975. In a study of 100 patients they found a fourfold variability in heparin sensitivity and threefold range in the rate at which heparin is degraded.[262,263] Because this enormous variability in the patient response to heparin could result in possible under- or overdosing with heparin, Bull et al.

TABLE 31-9. Normal Values of Intraoperative Coagulation Studies[a]

aPTT	25–49 s
ACT	70–110 s
TEG R	7–15 min
TEG MA	50–60 mm
TEG A60	(MA-5) mm

Abbreviations: aPTT, activated partial thromboplastin time; ACT, activated clotting time performed with a Hemochron; TEG, thromboelastogram. (See text and Fig. 31-41 for definition of TEG R, TEG MA, and TEG A60.)
(From Spiess and Ivankovich,[285] with permission)

devised an individual heparin dose-effect management strategy.[264]

The quantitative method to heparin and protamine dosing involves (1) defining the individual heparin dose and ACT response, (2) achieving and maintaining an adequate prolongation of the ACT, and (3) reversing residual heparin with protamine. The patient dose-response determination requires administering 200 units heparin/kg and plotting the ACT response on a graph along with the baseline ACT for the patient (Fig. 31-39). If the initial dose of heparin does not prolong the ACT to an acceptable level, a second dose is calculated and given. A safe ACT value for undergoing CPB is generally considered to be greater than 400 seconds, although there are few data to support this value. There is one report of a small number (N = 9) of monkeys and pediatric patients (N = 5), which demonstrated that only with an ACT ≥ 400 seconds was there no evidence of coagulation in the oxygenator reservoir filter.[265] However, in another report, fibrin deposition on the arterial perfusate line in 6 patients was not encountered with ACT values in the range of 286 to 1,000 seconds.[266] The dose of heparin usually required to attain an ACT ≥ 480 seconds for adults is 300 units/kg and for children is 430 units/kg according to one investigation.[267] Children and infants do require more heparin to

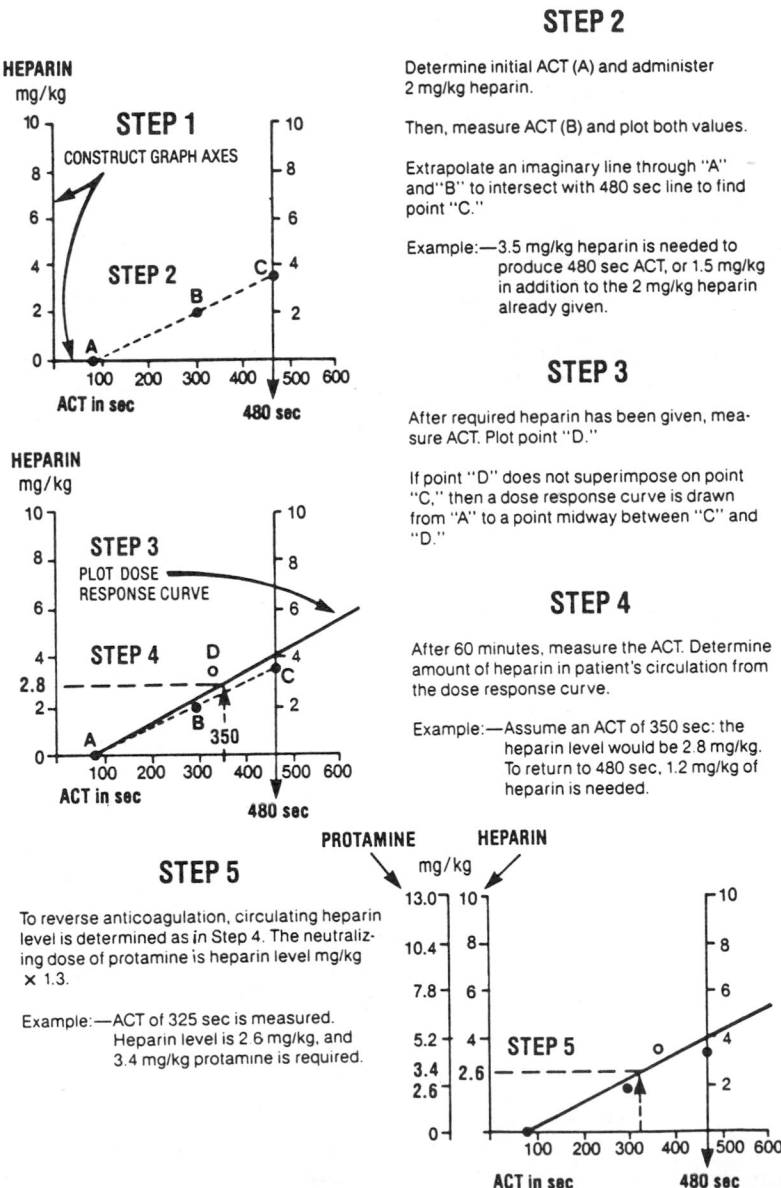

Fig. 31-39. Procedure for construction and use of the dose-response curve in heparin therapy. ACT, activated clotting time. (From Bull et al.,[264] with permission.)

achieve a prolonged ACT.[268] In general, there is a Gaussian distribution of heparin response in patients.[267,269] Since heparin requires the presence of antithrombin III, it will not be effective in patients with a deficiency of this factor. There also are data that show that the effect of heparin is less when given to patients receiving nitroglycerin infusion,[270] and since this drug is commonly used in cardiovascular surgery patients, the ACT should be carefully monitored in patients receiving both drugs. Causes of heparin resistance are listed in Table 31-10.[271]

The intervals at which the ACT should be measured during CPB are not known but probably should vary, depending on the speed of the patient's biotransformation of heparin. A repeated measurement protocol of between 30 and 90 minutes should be adequate. Sampling is required less often during hypothermia than during rewarming or at normothermia, presumably because there is less metabolism of the heparin. The ACT is not considered linearly related to heparin at values greater than 500 or 600 seconds, and there appears to be no reason to attempt to obtain these prolonged values. However, there is no evidence to show that prolonged values are harmful. The greatest danger during surgery is inadequate heparinization, which can precipitate catastrophic clotting or initiate disseminated intravascular coagulation.[263,271]

Heparin anticoagulation is reversed by protamine, another nonhomogeneous protein extracted from the cell nuclei of salmon sperm. The amount of protamine that will neutralize the heparin is generally given in the ratio of 1.3 mg protamine/100 units heparin. Heparin is highly acidic and combines stoichiometrically with the base protamine, resulting in a neutral inactive salt. Thus, it is appropriate to give protamine on a fixed-weight (milligrams) dose of residual heparin.[267] The heparin dose and ACT response diagram (Fig. 31-39)

TABLE 31-10. Etiology of Marked Heparin Resistance

Specific disease states
Antithrombin III deficiency
  Congenital
  Secondary
Hypereosinophilia
Coronary artery disease

Drug interaction
Previous heparin therapy
Oral contraceptives

Errors of administration[a]
Improper product
Incorrect dose
Errors of route (infiltrated intravenous line)

Miscellaneous
Ongoing active coagulation
Advanced age

[a] Not truly a resistance but in the differential diagnosis.
(Adapted from Ellison et al.,[271] with permission.)

can be used to predict the amount of residual heparin and to determine the appropriate amount of protamine. With this protocol the ACT will return to within about 7 percent of the control value.[266] If the protamine does not return the ACT to the baseline value, a second protamine dose should be calculated. Heparin rebound, defined as a significant increase in the ACT after a documented correction using protamine, has been reported in 0 to 50 percent of patients.[261,271] More protamine should be administered if heparin rebound occurs. If bleeding persists in the presence of a normal ACT, it probably is a manifestation of inadequate surgical hemostasis, platelet dysfunction, or factor deficiency (none of which is detected by the ACT).

Heparin Protamine Titration

Heparin protamine titration (HPT) can be performed to calculate the theoretical circulating level of heparin and to determine precisely the amount of protamine required to neutralize residual heparin. These titrations are based on the theory that each individual patient has a linear heparin protamine neutralization during the conduct of surgery. Titration curves can then be used in subsequent analysis (after heparin) to maintain the desired "amount of heparin" based on the HPT reaction.[272] A theoretical heparin level can be maintained with this method of monitoring. This technique has not been validated by actual measurement of heparin levels in blood or plasma.

Since there is a direct proportionality of the amount of heparin neutralized to the amount of protamine present, titration methods can be used to quantify the needed protamine dose. In such procedures, increasing concentrations of protamine are added to a heparinized blood specimen and the degree of heparin neutralization is measured. The most common method of monitoring this interaction is the shortening of the ACT of the heparinized blood. This curve of heparin neutralization is characterized by three phases.[273-275] In the linear first phase, as increasing amounts of protamine are added there is a proportional shortening of the clotting time until complete neutralization is achieved. With further increases of protamine amount the clotting time remains unchanged (second phase) until a third phase of response, in which protamine exerts an anticoagulant effect and the ACT prolongs, is reached.

Since introduction of the first clinically useful method of HPT[274] in the mid 1950s, various methods of performing titrations have been described.[275-277] Currently the most commonly used protocols are employed in automated systems. These are the Hemochron Protamine Dose Assay (PDA) and the Hepcon System. Both methods employ test tubes or test wells containing different concentrations of protamine. Heparinized blood is added to these vessels, and the amount of protamine required to neutralize the heparin is determined. These systems differ in the phase of the heparin/protamine interaction used in the titration and in the way that a neutralizing protamine dose is calculated. Reports have shown that neutralization is achieved with a ratio of protamine to heparin to be 1.25 mg/100 units using the Hepcon system[277] and 0.57 mg/100 units using the PDA system.[278] Controlled comparative studies of the two titration systems have not been performed to evaluate the significantly diminished predicted protamine dose using the PDA method.

Interestingly, there is, in general, a poor correlation between the ACT and plasma heparin assays.[279,280] Moreover, it is the effect of heparin on blood coagulation, not the absolute plasma heparin level, that is of concern when monitoring anticoagulation for cardiopulmonary bypass. The ACT has proved to be a reliable guide to adequate heparin anticoagulation and neutralization with protamine, but the role of HPT methods in clinical management is not yet fully defined.

Activated Partial Thromboplastin Time

The activated partial thromboplastin time (aPTT) is another measure of the intrinsic clotting system and, like the ACT, is a useful measure of the effect of heparin given in low doses. It is not a useful monitor of heparin during cardiopulmonary bypass because it loses its linearity with heparin doses greater than 200 units/kg.[281] The aPTT measures the time necessary to initiate fibrin clot formation along the intrinsic pathway; it requires 4.5 ml of whole blood, which must be centrifuged for 15 minutes to obtain plasma for the test. Because multiple reagents and instrumentation are required, the test is best performed in a laboratory and not at the bedside.[282] The aPTT is almost always prolonged more than 600 seconds during heparinization for bypass and therefore is a poor guide of heparin effect during cardiac surgery.[268]

Viscoelastic Measurement of Clot Formation

The thromboelastograph (TEG) is the descendent technology of the use of viscosimeters to measure the continuous formation of whole blood clots.[283] The role of TEG in monitoring coagulation in cardiovascular surgery is the prediction and perhaps diagnosis of the cause of excessive postoperative hemorrhage.[282,284,285] The method involves placing 0.35 ml of whole blood in a rotating metal cuvette heated to 37°C. A piston is suspended in the sample, and the rotational motion is transferred to the piston as fibrin strands form between the wall of the cuvette and the piston (Fig. 31-40).[284] Electronic devices record the clot on a continuously moving paper so that various measurements of the tracing can be made (Fig. 31-41). Abnormalities in the measurement depict deficiencies in the coagulation system. Prolonged R values reflect heparinization or absence of some coagulation factors. The MA represents maximum clot strength, and reductions signify hypofibrinogenemia, thrombocytopenia, or platelet dysfunction. The A60 demonstrates clot destruction, and small

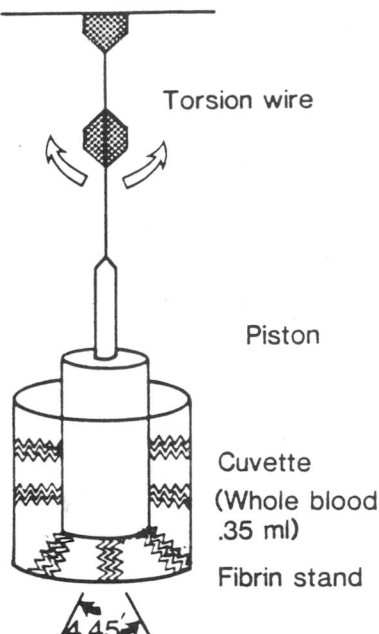

Fig. 31-40. The functional components of the TEG consist of a rotating metal cuvette and a suspended piston. As blood in the cuvette coagulates, a connection is completed between the cuvette and the piston, revealing a characteristic tracing over time. (From Tuman et al.,[295] with permission.)

values at this time can represent fibrinolysis as with fibrinolytic therapy (Fig. 31-42)[285] or with spontaneous fibrinolysis. Use of the TEG has been reported to reduce overall blood product utilization in pediatric cardiac patients by as much as 72 percent.[286] As a bedside guide to component blood product therapy the TEG is promising, since it can distinguish between the treatable common bleeding causes (heparinization, platelet dysfunction, and fibrinolysis) and results are available within an hour.[285]

Another device that uses viscoelastic clot properties to predict coagulation status is the Sonoclot. This instrument uses a rapidly vibrating plastic probe immersed to a fixed depth in 0.4 ml of either whole blood or plasma.[283] As the blood clots, movement of the probe is impeded, altering an electrical signal in direct proportion to the fluid's viscoelasticity. This signal is recorded on a strip chart that over time demonstrates the formation, retraction, and lysis of the clot. A "signature" of each clot, which can be compared to normal curves,[287] is thus formed. The sonoclot signature gives qualitative information similar to the thromboelastograph. Both record clot formation, clot strength, and clot lysis. Data regarding platelet activity may be obtained with both; such information is not available with the ACT.

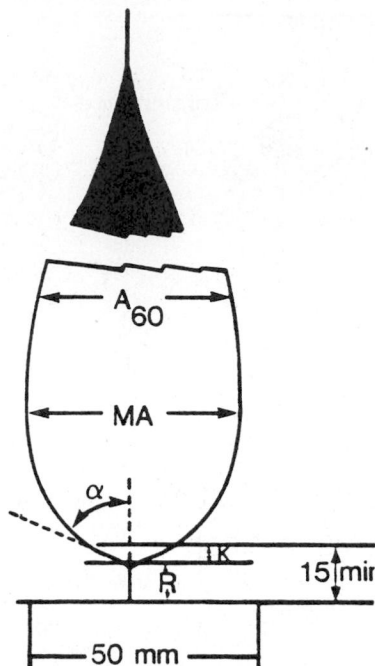

Fig. 31-41. A characteristic TEG tracing and standard measurements. Normal values: R = 10 to 15 minutes, K = 6 to 12 minutes, a° = 45 degrees, MA = 50 to 60 mm, A_{60} = MA − 5 mm; all measurements at 2 mm/min paper speed. (From Tuman et al.,[295] with permission.)

In summary, despite multiple alternatives, the best method of determining heparin anticoagulation is use of the ACT. It is simple, reliable, and inexpensive and linearly reflects the heparin effect on coagulation. It is significantly prolonged by hypothermia, however. For the diagnosis of excessive hemorrhage after the reversal of heparin with protamine, the TEG seems most promising, although there are limited data on its use. More specific coagulation tests are generally available in most hospitals to determine causes of a bleeding diathesis. They should be used when nonsurgical bleeding is excessive and bedside tests are uninformative.

Automated Anesthesia Record Keeping

The use of numerous cardiac monitors in conjunction with other standard anesthesia monitors can result in the generation of huge amounts of monitoring data during the course of an anesthetic. One of the responsibilities of the anesthesiologist is to create a record that chronicles the anesthetic management and clinical course of the patient in the perioperative period. However, recording all of the information produced in complex, and highly monitored cases can become a burdensome clerical task and can actually detract from patient care by diverting the anesthesiologist's attention. The use of automated anesthesia record keeping devices to address this problem has received increasing attention in the last decade. Obviously, the organization of vital sign data from monitors is only a part of the input into an anesthetic record. Patient demographics, a history of operative events, fluid and anesthetic agent administration, and various text notes are all important additional features of this document. The automated device must perform all of these functions efficiently and completely in order to replace the manual anesthesia record.

A secondary benefit of automated record keeping is the ability to collect anesthesia-related data in a unified format across many cases. Analysis of this "data base" of comprehensive information would allow efficient management of quality assurance issues, operating room efficiency, as well as procurement of data for clinical research.

Automated record keeping devices fall into two basic categories: custom-designed units assembled by and for the specific needs of the particular institution and commercial products designed for general use in a large number of settings. The development of commercial devices has been based largely on the successes and failures observed in the earlier custom installations. A good example of early research in this area is the Duke Automatic Monitoring Equipment (DAME) System. DAME was an outgrowth of previous work in patient monitoring at Duke University Medical Center, expanding the existing set of custom-designed ECG, blood pressure, EEG, and temperature monitors to allow automatic collection, display, and printing of these data within a unified system.[288] First put into service in 1980, DAME suffered from several major problems. First, the size and weight of the monitoring units severely restricted their positioning in the operating room. Second, DAME was designed as a network system, with all operating room units dependent on the function of a central controlling computer. Malfunctions of this host computer affected monitoring in all operating rooms served by the system. Finally, the human interface factor proved to be unsatisfactory for most users of the system. The primary reason for this latter problem was the relative inflexibility of the computer in its interaction with the user, resulting in the clinician's being required to pay more attention to the monitor and less to the patient, exactly the opposite of the purpose of an automated monitoring system.

The benefit that the DAME system provided was an unprecedented amount of information regarding the requirements for viable automated anesthesia monitoring and data recording systems. Commercial manufacturers have been able to use the DAME experience to optimize the features of their own monitors and anesthesia record keeping devices. Today, nearly all direct patient monitors use some form of built-in digital microprocessor technology, often relying heavily on the capabilities of this type of data processing. As a result,

TEG Tracings – Examples

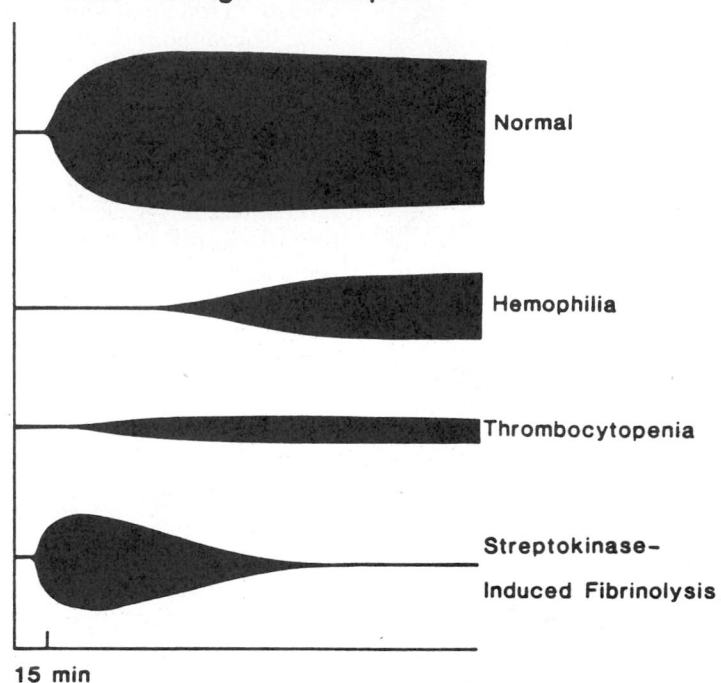

Fig. 31-42. Representative abnormal TEG tracings. (From Speiss and Ivankovitch,[285] with permission.)

most of these new "computerized" monitoring devices have the capacity to relay their information to another data collection computer in a digital format. Recently introduced anesthesia record keepers thus act as "background" computers, assimilating information from a number of other monitors, rather than being responsible for the entire monitoring process, as the DAME system had attempted. The great advances made over the last decade in the power and miniaturization of microcomputers allow the record system not only to perform this function but also to provide a more suitable user interface that allows other requirements of the anesthesia record to be more easily completed. Finally, these computers are small enough to be designed as individual stand-alone units for each location, preventing the problems of a network-based system. The DAME system was therefore a valid concept but was developed years ahead of the ability of technology to fully meet its intended goal.

Because a variety of patient monitors are now built directly into anesthesia machines, it has been a natural extension of this development for the manufacturer to include an integrated record keeping device as well. Several manufacturers have produced anesthesia machines with this capability. These provide a printed record of automatically acquired intraoperative patient monitor data and can be annotated with other anesthesia information either manually or via a touch screen interface.

Other record keeping systems exist as separate units. The ARKIVE system (Diatek, Inc.) is an example of such a device. This multiple microprocessor system has the advantage of directly interfacing with a wide variety of patient monitors from various manufacturers (Fig. 31-43). The Arkive touch screen display resembles an anesthesia record, with patient vital sign data updated at frequent intervals automatically. The display screen doubles as the input device, with the user's touching the position on the "record" where a change or entry of new information is to be made. Alternatively, a voice recognition module can be used to "tell" the system of events when they occur. A standard computer printer built into the system prints a complete document that can be used as the official anesthesia record for the case. In addition, all patient data are written to a computer file for long-term storage. Files for all cases can be analyzed together on a desktop personal computer, facilitating the data base aspects of the record keeping process.[289]

Another anesthesia record keeper is the CARIN system (Computerized Anesthesia Systems, Inc.). This device uses a standard commercial microcomputer (Apple Macintosh) with special hardware to interface to patient monitors. Interaction with the operator is effected by taking advantage of the easy user interface design of the Macintosh computer. The Carin system also prints a formal anesthesia record and stores this information for later examination and analysis.

Devices such as these have made great strides toward the goals set out by early systems such as the DAME. Problems with these new systems are both unique to their modern designs and similar to those of the older

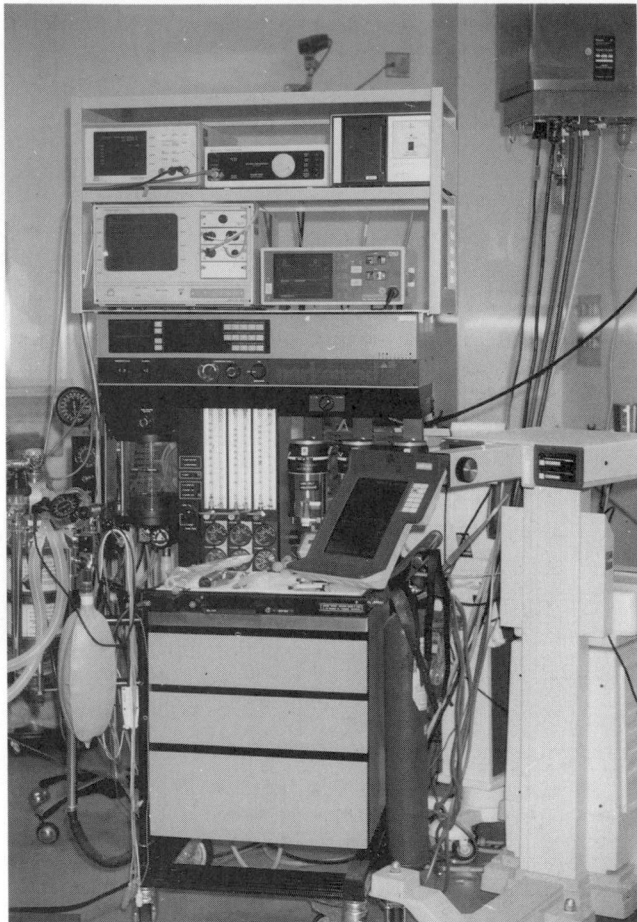

Fig. 31-43. Arkive automated anesthesia record keeping device (to the right of the anesthesia machine) in a cardiac surgical operating room. All of the patient monitors utilized for cardiac surgery are directly connected to the Arkive unit, which collects and organizes this large array of information into a formal anesthesia record.

systems. The human interface to the computer continues to be a problem that prevents a more universal application of these devices. Development of larger, faster-acting, and more comprehensive displays will be necessary to allow the computer record to replace manual records totally. In gathering patient data that are entered by the user, the computer must be "friendly" enough to allow an easy interaction, yet "demanding" enough to require this information unconditionally for all cases. Failure of this process negates the system's usefulness as a data base system for administration, quality assurance, or research. Finally, the commitment of vital sign data entry to an automatic process places this facet of the anesthesia record at the mercy of data artifacts that invariably occur in the generation of these parameters. This is especially applicable to electrocardiographs and pulse oximeters, which are subject to electrocautery interference, and direct

blood pressure monitors, which frequently display obviously erroneous data during transducer manipulation. Throughout this chapter, there have been examples of the need for the human observer to interpret the information being presented by cardiac monitors, applying a knowledge of the large set of factors that can influence the data, in order to reveal the true state of the patient's cardiovascular system. The use of direct, unalterable transcription of monitor data to the anesthesia record severely inhibits this important step. Automated record systems, in conjunction with improvements in direct patient monitors, must somehow overcome this obstacle in order to represent the patient's condition accurately.

REFERENCES

1. Robinson V: Victory over Pain. Henry Schuman, New York, 1946
2. Harmel MH: Monitoring, past, present, future. Int J Clin Monit Comput 3:147, 1986
3. Riva-Rocci S: Un nuovo sfigmomanometro. Gaz med Torino, 47:981, 1896
4. Cushing HW: On routine determinations of arterial tension in operating room and clinic. Boston Med Surg J 148:250, 1903
5. Korotkof NS: On the subject of methods of determining blood pressure. Bull Imp Med Acad St. Petersburg 11:365, 1905
6. von Recklinghausen H: Neue Wege zur Blutdruckmessung. Springer-Verlag, Berlin, 1931
7. Peterson LH, Dripps RD, Risman GC: A method for recording the arterial pressure pulse and blood pressure in man. Am Heart J 37:771, 1949
8. Forssman W: Die Sondierung des rechten Herzens. Klin Wochenschr 8:2085, 1929
9. Lagerlof H, Werko L: Studies on the circulation of blood in man. VI: The pulmonary capillary venous pressure pulse in man. Scand J Clin Lab Invest 1:147, 1949
10. Forrester JS, Diamond G, McHugh TJ, et al: Filling pressures in right and left sides of the heart in acute myocardial infarction: A reappraisal of central venous pressure monitoring. N Engl J Med 285:190, 1971
11. Civetta JM, Gabel JC: Flow-directed pulmonary artery catheterization in surgical patients: Indications and modification of technique. Ann Surg 176:753, 1972
12. Fick A: Uber die Messung des Blutquantuns in den Herzventrikeln. Verh Dtsch Phys-med Ges Wurzburg 2:16, 1870
13. Cournand A: Measurement of cardiac output in man using the right heart catheterization: Description of technique, discussion of validity and of place in the study of circulation. Fed Proc 4:207, 1945
14. Dexter L, Haynes FW, Burwell CS, et al: Studies of congenital heart disease. II: The pressure and oxygen content of blood in the right auricle, right ventricle, and pulmonary artery in control patients, with observations on the oxygen saturation and source of pulmonary "capillary" blood. J Clin Invest 26:554, 1947
15. Swan HJC, Ganz W, Forrester J, et al: Catheterization of the heart in man with use of a flow directed balloon-tipped catheter. N Engl J Med 283:447, 1970
16. Seldinger SI: Catheter replacement of the needle in percutaneous arteriography. Acta Radiologica 39:368, 1953

17. Edler I, Hertz CH: Use of the ultrasonic reflectoscope for continuous recording of movement of heart walls. Kung Fysiogr Sallsk Lund Fordhandl 24:1, 1954

18. Hisanaga K, Hisanaga A, Nagata K, et al: Transesophageal cross-sectional echocardiography. Am Heart J 100:605, 1980

19. Schluter M, Langenstein BA, Polster J, et al: Transesophageal cross-sectional echocardiography with a phased-array transducer system. Br Heart J 48:67, 1982

20. Davis RF: Clinical comparison of automated auscultatory and oscillometric and catheter-transducer measurements of arterial pressure. J Clin Monit 1:114, 1985

21. Bruner JMR, Krenis LJ, Kunsman JM, et al: Comparison of direct and indirect methods of measuring arterial pressure. Med Instrum 15:183, 1981

22. Gorback MS: Considerations in the interpretation of systemic pressure monitoring. In Lumb PD, Bryan-Brown CW (eds.): Complications in Critical Care Medicine. Yearbook Medical Publishers, Chicago, 1988

23. Goldstein S, Killip T: Comparison of direct and indirect arterial pressures in aortic regurgitation. N Engl J Med 267:1121, 1962

24. Cohn JN: Blood pressure measurement in shock. JAMA 199:118, 1967

25. Yong PG, Geddes LA: The effect of cuff pressure deflation rate on accuracy in indirect measurement of blood pressure with the auscultatory method. J Clin Monit 3:155, 1987

26. Celoria G, Dawson JA, Teres D: Compartment syndrome in a patient monitored with an automated blood pressure cuff. J Clin Monit 3:139, 1987

27. Yelderman M, Ream AK: Indirect measurement of mean blood pressure in the anesthetized patients. Anesthesiology 59:349, 1979

28. Borow KM, Newburger JW: Noninvasive estimate of central aortic pressure using the oscillometric method for analyzing systemic artery pulsatile bliood flow: Comparative study of indirect systolic, diastolic, and mean brachial artery pressure with simultaneous direct ascending aortic pressure measurements. Am Heart J 103:879, 1982

29. Cullen PM, Dye J, Hughes DG: Clinical assessment of the neonatal Dinamap 847 during anesthesia in neonates and infants. J Clin Monit 3:229, 1987

30. Friesen RH, Lichtor JL: Indirect measurement of blood pressure in neonates and infants utilizing an automatic non-invasive oscillometric monitor. Anesth Analg 60:742, 1981

31. Kimble KJ, Darnall RA, Yelderman M, et al: An automated oscillometric technique for estimating mean arterial pressure in critically ill newborns. Anesthesiology 54:423, 1981

32. Kazamias TM, Gander MP, Franklin DL, et al: Blood pressure measurement with Doppler ultrasonic flowmeter. J Appl Physiol 30:585, 1971

33. Zahed B, Sadove MS, Hatano S, et al: Comparison of automated Doppler ultrasound and Korotkoff measurements of blood pressure. Anesth Analg 50:699, 1971

34. Penaz J; Photoelectric measurement of blood pressure, volume, and flow in the finger. p. 104. In Digest of the 10th International Conference on Medical and Biological Engineering. Dresden, 1973

35. Boehmer RD: Continuous, real-time, non-invasive monitor of blood pressure: Penaz methodology applied to the finger. J Clin Monit 3:282, 1987

36. Molhoek GP, Wesseling KH, Settels JJM, et al: Evaluation of the Penaz servople-thysmomanometer for continuous, non-invasive measurement of finger blood pressure. Basic Res Cardiol 79:598, 1984

37. Kurki T, Smith NT, Head H, et al: Noninvasive continuous blood pressure measurement from the finger. Optimal measurement condition and factors affecting reliability. J Clin Monit 3:6, 1987

38. Smith NT, Wesseling KH, de Wit B: Evaluation of two prototype devices producing noninvasive, pulsatile, calibrated blood pressure measurement from a finger. J Clin Monit 1:17, 1985

39. Gravenstein JS, Paulus DA, Feldman J, et al: Tissue hypoxia distal to a Penaz blood pressure cuff. J Clin Monit 1:120, 1985

40. Mandel MA, Dauchot PJ: Radial artery cannulation in 1000 patients: Precautions and complications. J Hand Surg 2:482, 1977

41. Slogoff S, Keats AS, Arlund C: On the safety of radial artery cannulation. Anesthesiology 59:42, 1980

42. Cederholm I, Sorensen J, Carlsson C: Thrombosis following percutaneous radial artery cannulation. Acta Anaesthesiol Scand 30:227, 1986

43. Davis FM, Stewart JM: Radial artery cannulation: A perspective study in patients undergoing cardiothoracic surgery. Br J Anaesth 52:42, 1980

44. Jones RM, Hill AB, Nahrwold ML, et al: The effect of method of radial artery cannulation on post-cannulation blood flow and thrombus formation. Anesthesiology 55:76, 1981

45. Geddes LA: Cardiovascular Devices and Their Applications. John Wiley & Sons, New York, 1984

46. Prys-Roberts C: Invasive monitoring of the circulation. pp. 79. In Saidman LJ, Smith NT (eds): Monitoring in Anesthesia. 2nd Ed. Butterworth (Publishers), Boston 1984

47. Gardner RM: Direct blood pressure measurement — dynamic response requirements. Anesthesiology 54:227, 1981

48. Boutros A, Albert S: Effect of dynamic response of transducer tubing system on accuracy of direct blood pressure measurement. Crit Care Med 11:124, 1983

49. Lowenstein E, Little JW, Lo HH: Prevention of cerebral embolization from flushing radial artery cannulae. N Engl J Med 285:1414, 1971

50. Abrams JH: Damping devices in clinical practice. p. 133. In Cerra FB (ed: Perspectives in Critical Care. Vol. 1, No. 1. Quality Medical Publishing, St. Louis, 1988.

51. Stern DH, Gerson JI, Allen FB, et al: Can we trust the direct radial artery pressure immediately after cardiopulmonary bypass? Anesthesiology 62:557, 1985

52. Beker B, LaFontaine E, Lin CY: Accuracy of radial artery pressure monitoring. In Proceedings of the Society of Cardiovascular Anesthesiologists, 5th Annual Meeting (abstract). San Diego, April 1983

53. Gallager JD, Moore RA, McNicholas KW, et al: Comparison of radial and femoral arterial pressures in children after cardiopulmonary bypass. J Clin Monit 1:168, 1985

54. Allen EV: Thromboangiitis obliterans: Methods of diagnosis of chronic obstructive lesions distal to the wrist with illustrative cases. Am J Med Sci 178:237, 1929

55. Wilkins RG: Radial artery cannulation and ischaemic damage: A review. Anaesthesia 40:896, 1985

56. Baker RJ, Chunprapaph B, Nyhus LM: Severe ischaemia of the hand following radial artery catheterization. Surgery 80:449, 1976

57. Mangano DT, Hickey RF: Ischemic injury following uncomplicated radial artery catheterization. Anesth Analg 58:55, 1979

58. Thompson SR, Hirshberg A: Allen's test re-examined (letter). Crit Care Med 16:915, 1988

59. Bedford RF, Wollman H: Complications of percutaneous radial artery cannulation: An Objective prospective study in man. Anesthesiology 38:228, 1973

60. McGregor AD: The Allen test—an investigation of its accuracy by fluorescein dye. J Hand Surg 12:82, 1987

61. Stead SW, Stirt JA: Assessment of digital blood flow and palmar collateral circulation. Int J Clin Monit Comput 2:29, 1985

62. Meyer RM, Katele GV: The case for a complete Allen's test. Anesth Analg 62:947, 1983

63. Bedford RF: Radial artery function following percutaneous cannulation with 18-gauge and 20-gauge catheters. Anesthesiology 47:37, 1977

64. Bedford RF: Percutaneous radial artery cannulation—increased safety using Teflon catheters. Anesthesiology 42:219, 1975

65. Kin JM, Arakawa K, Bliss J: Arterial cannulation: Factors in the development of occlusion. Anesth Analg 54:836, 1975

66. Russell JA, Joel M, Hudson RJ, et al: Prospective evaluation of radial and femoral artery catheterization sites in critically ill adults. Crit Care Med 11:936, 1983

67. Randel SN, Tsang BH, Wung JT, et al: Experience with percutaneous indwelling peripheral arterial catheterization in neonates. Am J Dis Child 141:848, 1987

68. Sellden H, Nilsson K, Larsson LE, et al: Radial artery catheterization in children and neonates: A prospective study. Crit Care Med 15:1106, 1987

69. Barnes RW, Foster EJ, Jansen GA, et al: Safety of brachial artery catheterization as monitors in the intensive care unit—prospective evaluation with the Doppler ultrasonic velocity detector. Anesthesiology 44:260, 1976

70. Moran KT, Halpin DP, Zide RS, et al: Long-term brachial artery catheterization: Ischemic complications. J Vasc Surg 8:76, 1988

71. Mann S, Jones RI, Millar-Craig MW, et al: The safety of ambulatory intra-arterial pressure monitoring: A clinical audit of 1000 studies. Int J Cardiol 5:585, 1984

72. Yacoub OF, Bacaling JH, Kelly M: Monitoring of the axillary arterial pressure in a patient with Buergers disease requiring clipping of an intracerebral aneurysm. Br J Anaesth 59:1056, 1987

73. Adler DC, Bryan-Brown CW: Use of the axillary artery for intravascular monitoring. Crit Care Med 1:148, 1973

74. Gurman GM, Kriemerman S: Cannulation of big arteries in critically ill patients. Crit Care Med 13:217, 1985

75. Brown M, Gordon LH, Brown OW, et al: Intravascular monitoring via the axillary artery. Anaesth Intensive Care 13:38, 1985

76. Bryan-Brown CW, Kwun KB, Lumb PD, et al: The axillary artery catheter. Heart Lung J 12:492, 1983

77. Ersoz CJ, Hedden M, Lain L: Prolonged femoral artery catheterization for intensive care. Anesth Analg 49:160, 1973

78. Singh S, Nelson N, Acosta I, et al: Catheter colonization and bacteremia with pulmonary and arterial catheters. Crit Care Med 10:736, 1982

79. Soderstrom CA, Wasserman DH, Ransom KJ, et al: Infected false femoral artery aneurysms secondary to monitoring catheters. J Cardiovasc Surg 24:63, 1983

80. Glenski JA, Beynen FM, Bracy J: A prospective analysis of femoral artery monitoring in pediatric patients. Anesthesiology 66:227, 1987

81. Huber JF: The arterial network supplying the dorsum of the foot. Anat Rec 80:373, 391, 1941

82. Youngberg JA, Miller ED: Evaluation of percutaneous cannulation of the dorsalis pedis artery. Anesthesiology 44:80, 1976

83. Sweeney MF, Estrin JA, Stanley TE III: Coarctation and systemic hypertension. p. 130. In Reves JG, Hall KD (eds): Common Problems in Cardiac Anesthesia. Year Book Medical Publishers, Chicago, 1987

84. Bull MJ, Schriner RL, Garg BP, et al: Neurologic complications following temporal artery catheterization. J Pediatr 93:115, 1980

85. Dzelzkalns R, Stanley TH: Placement of the pulmonary artery catheter before anesthesia for cardiac surgery: A stressful, painful, unnecessary crutch. J Clin Monit 1:197, 1985

86. Lunn JK, Stanley TH, Webster LR, et al: Arterial blood pressure and pulse-rate responses to pulmonary and radial artery catheterization prior to cardiac and major vascular operations. Anesthesiology 51:265, 1979

87. Waller JL, Zaidan JR, Kaplan JA, et al: Hemodynamic responses to preoperative vascular cannulation in patients with coronary artery disease. Anesthesiology 56:219, 1982

88. Pyles ST, Scher KS, Vega ET, et al: Cannulation of the dorsal radial artery: A new technique. Anesth Analg 61:876, 1982

89. Quintin L, Whalley DG, Wynands JE, et al: The effects of vascular catheterization upon heart rate and blood pressure before aortocoronary bypass. Can Anaesth Soc J 28:244, 1981

90. Streisand JB, Clark NJ, Pace NL: Placement of the pulmonary artery catheter before anesthesia for cardiac surgery: Safe, intelligent, and appropriate use of invasive hemodynamic monitoring. J Clin Monit 1:193, 1985

91. Sanford TJ: Internal jugular vein cannulation versus subclavian vein cannulation: An anesthesiologist's view: The right internal jugular vein. J Clin Monit 1:58, 1985

92. English JC, Frew RM, Pigott JF, et al: Percutaneous catheterization of the internal jugular vein. Anaesthesia 24:521, 1969

93. Tyden HE: Cannulation of the internal jugular vein—500 cases. Acta Anaesthesiol Scand 26:485, 1982

94. Vaughan RW, Weyjandt GR: Reliable percutaneous central venous pressure measurement. Anesth Analg 52:709, 1973

95. Hoyt DB: Internal jugular vein cannulation versus subclavian vein cannulation: A surgeon's view: The subclavian vein. J Clin Monit 1:58, 1985

96. Oda M, Fukushima Y, Hirota T, et al: The para-carotid approach for internal jugular vein catheterization. Anaesthesia 36:896, 1981

97. Horrow JC, Metz S, Thickman D, et al: Prior carotid surgery does not affect the reliability of landmarks for location of the internal jugular vein. Anesth Analg 66:452, 1987

98. Rosen M, Latto IP, Shang W: The internal jugular vein. In Handbook of Percutaneous Vein Catheterizations. WB Saunders, London, 1981

99. Royster RL, Johnson WE, Gravlee GP, et al: Arrhythmias during venous cannulation prior to pulmonary artery catheter insertion. Anesth Analg 64:1214, 1985

100. Blitt CD, Carlson GL, Wright WA, et al: J-wire versus straight wire for central venous system cannulation via the external jugular vein. Anesth Analg 61:536, 1982

101. Nordstrom L, Fletcher R: Comparison of two different J-wires for central venous cannulation via the external jugular vein. Anesth Analg 62:365, 1983

102. Borja AR, Hinhaw JR: A safe way to perform infraclavicular subclavian vein catheterization. Surg Gynecol Obstet 130:673, 1970

103. Kellner GA, Smart JF: Percutaneous placement of catheters to measure "central venous pressure." Anesthesiology 36:515, 1972

104. Webre DR, Arens JF: Use of cephalic and basilic veins for introduction of cardiovascular catheters. Anesthesiology 38:389, 1973

105. Shah KB, Rao TLK, Laughlin S, et al: A review of pulmonary

artery catheterization in 6,245 patients. Anesthesiology 61:271, 1984

106. Davies MJ, Cronin KD, Domaingue CM: Pulmonary artery catheterization: An assessment of risks and benefits in 220 surgical patients. Anaesth Intensive Care 10:9, 1982

107. Sise MJ, Hollingsworth P, Brimm JE, et al: Complications of the flow-directed pulmonary-artery catheter: A prospective analysis in 219 patients. Crit Care Med 9:315, 1981

108. O'Rourke RA: Physical examination of the arteries and veins. p. 188. In Hurst JW, et al (eds): The Heart. 5th Ed. McGraw-Hill, New York 1982

109. West JB, Dollery CT, Naimark A: Distribution of blood flow in isolated lung: Relation to vascular and alveolar pressures. J Appl Physiol 19:713, 1964

110. Lorzman J, Powers SR, Older T, et al: Correlation of pulmonary wedge and left atrial pressure in man. Arch Surg 109:270, 1974

111. Berryhill RE, Benumof JL: PEEP-induced discrepancy between pulmonary artery wedge pressure and left atrial pressure: The influence of controlled vs. spontaneous ventilation and compliant vs. non-compliant lungs. Anesthesiology 46:383, 1979

112. Humphrey CB, Oury JH, Virgilo RW, et al: An analysis of direct and indirect measurement of left atrial filling pressures. J Thorac Cardiovasc Surg 41:643, 1976

113. Lappas D, Lell WA, Gabel JC, et al: Indirect measurement of left atrial pressure in surgical patients — pulmonary capillary wedge pressure and pulmonary artery diastolic pressure compared with left atrial pressure. Anesthesiology 38:394, 1973

114. Walston A, Kendall ME: Comparison of pulmonary wedge and left atrial pressure in man. Am Heart J 86:159, 1973

115. Vender JS: Pulmonary artery catheter monitoring. p. 743. In Barash PG (ed): Cardiac Monitoring. WB Saunders, Philadelphia, 1988

116. Swan HJC: Central venous pressure monitoring is an outmoded procedure of limited practical value. p. 185. In Ingelfinger FJ, Ebert RV, Finland M, et al (eds): Controversies in Internal Medicine. WB Saunders, Philadelphia, 1974

117. Samii K, Conseiller C, Viars P: Central venous pressure and pulmonary wedge pressure. Arch Surg 111:1122, 1976

118. Bell H, Stubbs D, Pugh D: Reliability of central venous pressure as an indicator of left atrial pressure. Chest 59:169, 1971

119. Toussaint GPM, Burges JS, Hampson LG: Central venous pressure and pulmonary capillary wedge pressure in critical surgical illness. Arch Surg 109:265, 1974

120. Bashein G, Johnson PW, Davis KB, et al: Elective coronary bypass surgery without pulmonary artery catheter monitoring. Anesthesiology 64:451, 1985

121. Kaplan JA, Wells PH: Early diagnosis of myocardial ischemia using the pulmonary artery catheter. Anesth Analg 60:789, 1981

122. Rao TLK, Jacobs KH, El-Etr AA: Reinfarction following anesthesia in patients with myocardial infarction. Anesthesiology 59:499, 1983

123. Robin ED: Overuse and abuse of Swan-Ganz catheters. Int J Clin Monit Comput 4:5, 1987

124. Tuman KJ, McCarthy RJ, Spies BD, et al: Effect of pulmonary artery catheterization on outcome in patients undergoing coronary artery surgery. Anesthesiology 70:199, 1989

125. Johnston WE, Royster RL, Choplin RH, et al: Pulmonary artery catheter migration during cardiac surgery. Anesthesiology 64:258, 1986

126. Heard SO, Davis RF, Sherertz RJ, et al: Influence of sterile

protective sleeves on the sterility of pulmonary artery catheters. Crit Care Med 15:499, 1987

127. Benumof JL, Saidman LJ, Arkin DB, et al: Where pulmonary artery catheters go: Intrathoracic distribution. Anesthesiology 46:336, 1977

128. Schmitt EA, Brantigan CO: Common artifacts of pulmonary artery wedge pressure: Recognition and interpretation. J Clin Monit 2:44, 1986

129. Horst HM, Obeid FN, Vij D, et al: The risks of pulmonary artery catheterization. Surg Gynecol Obstet 159:229, 1984

130. Damen J: Ventricular arrhythmias during insertion and removal of pulmonary artery catheters. Chest 88:190, 1985

131. Patel C, Laboy V, Venus B, et al: Acute complications of pulmonary artery catheter insertion in critically ill patients. Crit Care Med 14:195, 1986

132. Abernathy WS: Complete heart block caused by the Swan-Ganz catheter. Chest 65:349, 1974

133. Thomson IR, Dalton BC, Lappas DG, et al: Right bundle branch block and complete heart block caused by the Swan-Ganz catheter. Anesthesiology 51:359, 1979

134. Morris D, Mulvihill D, Lew WY: Risk of developing complete heart block during bedside pulmonary artery catheterization in patients with left bundle branch block. Arch Intern Med 147:2005, 1987

135. Applefield JJ, Caruthers TE, Reno DJ, et al: Assessment of the sterility of long-term cardiac catheterization using the thermodilution Swan-Ganz catheter. Chest 74:377, 380, 1978

136. Damen J, Verhoef J, Bolton DT, et al: Microbiologic risk of invasive hemodynamic monitoring in patients undergoing open-heart operations. Crit Care Med 13:548, 1985

137. Myers ML, Austin TW, Sibbald WJ: Pulmonary artery catheter infections: A prospective study. Ann Surg 201:237, 1985

138. Lipp H, O'Donoghue K, Resnekov L: Intra-cardiac knotting of a flow-directed balloon catheter. N Engl J Med 284:220, 1971

139. Fibuch EE, Tuohy GF: Intracardiac knotting of a flow-directed balloon-tipped catheter. Anesth Analg 59:217, 1980

140. Dumesil JG, Proulx G: A new nonsurgical technique for untying tight knots in flow-directed balloon catheters. Am J Cardiol 53:395, 1984

141. Michel L, Installe E, Joucken K: Knotting of intracardiac flow-directed balloon catheter: Simple surgical method for removal. Chest 83:147, 1983

142. Foote GA, Schabel SI, Hodges M: Pulmonary complications of the flow-directed balloon-tipped catheter. N Engl J Med 290:927, 1973

143. Willis C, Wight D, Zidulka A: Hypertension secondary to balloon inflation of a pulmonary artery catheter. Crit Care Med 12:915, 1984

144. Kainuma M, Shimada Y: Decreased partial pressure of oxygen in arterial blood secondary to inflation of a pulmonary artery flow-directed balloon. Anesthesiology 66:214, 1987

145. McDaniel DD, Stone JF, Faltas AN, et al: Catheter-induced pulmonary artery hemorrhage: Diagnosis and management in cardiac operations. J Cardiovasc Surg 82:1, 1981

146. Hardy J-F, Morissette M, Taillefer J, et al: Pathophysiology of rupture of the pulmonary artery by pulmonary artery balloon-tipped catheters. Anesth Analg 62:925, 1983

147. Muller BJ, Gallucci A: Pulmonary artery catheter induced pulmonary artery rupture in patients undergoing cardiac surgery. Can Anaesth Soc J 32:258, 1985

148. Barash PG, Nardi D, Hammond G, et al: Catheter-induced pulmonary artery perforation: Mechanisms, management, and modifications. J Thorac Cardiovasc Surg 82:5, 1981

149. Klibaner MI, Hayes JA, Dobnick D: Delayed fatal pulmonary

hemorrhage complicating use of a balloon flotation catheter. Angiology 36:358, 1985

150. Scuderi PE, Prough DS, Price JD, et al: Cessation of pulmonary artery catheter-induced endobronchial hemorrhage associated with the use of PEEP. Anesth Analg 62:236, 1983

151. Sarin CL, Yalav E, Clement AJ, et al: The necessity for measurement of left atrial pressure after cardiac valve surgery. Thorax 25:185, 1970

152. Reves JG, Schonlau E: Use of a left atrial pressure monitor to diagnose a malfunctioning mitral valve prosthesis. Anesthesiology 50:247, 1979

153. Wolpowitz A: Trans-septal monitoring of left atrial pressure after cardiac surgery: An alternative method. S Afr Med J 53:185, 1978

154. Taylor T: Monitoring left atrial pressures in the open-heart surgical patient. Crit Care Nurse 6:62, 1986

155. Akl BF, Pett SB, Wernly JA, et al: Unusual complication of direct left atrial pressure monitoring line. J Thorac Cardiovasc Surg 88:1033, 1984

156. Hoff HE, Scott HJ: Physiology. N Engl J Med 239:120, 1948

157. Guyton AC, The Fick principle. p. 21. In: Guyton A, Jones CE, Coleman TG (eds): Circulatory Physiology: Cardiac Output and Its Regulation. 2nd Ed. WB Saunders, Philadelphia, 1973

158. Selzer A, Sudrann RB: Reliability of the determination of cardiac output in man by means of the Fick principle. Circ Res 6:485, 1958

159. Thomasson B: Cardiac output in normal subjects under standard basal conditions: The repeatability of measurements by the Fick method. Scand J Clin Lab Invest 9:365, 1957

160. Stewart GN: Researches on the circulation time and on the influences which affect it. IV: The output of the heart. J Physiol 22:159, 1897

161. Hamilton WF, Moore JW, Kinsman JM, et al: Studies on the circulation. IV: Further analysis of the injection method, and changes in hemodynamics under physiologic and pathological conditions. Am J physiol 99:534, 1932

162. Fegler G: Measurement of cardiac output in anesthetized animals by a thermodilution method. Q J Exp Physiol 39:153, 1954

163. Bilfinger TV, Lin CY, Anagnostopoulos CE: In vitro determination of accuracy of cardiac output measurements by thermal dilution. J Surg Res 33:409, 1982

164. Levitt JM, Replogle RL: Thermodilution cardiac output: A critical analysis and review of the literature. J Surg Res 27:392, 1979

165. Stetz CW, Miller RG, Kelly GE, et al: Reliability of the thermodilution method in the determination of cardiac output in clinical parctice. Am Rev Respir Dis 126:1001, 1982

166. Nelson LD, Anderson HB: Patient selection for iced versus room temperature injectate for thermodilution cardiac output determination. Crit Care Med 13:182, 1986

167. Weisel RD, Berger RL, Hechtman RB: Measurement of cardiac output by thermodilution. N Engl J Med 292:682, 1975

168. Nishikawa T, Dohi S: Slowing of the heart during cardiac output measurement by thermodilution. Anesthesiology 57:538, 1982

169. Huntsman LL, Steward DK, Barnes SR, et al: Noninvasive Doppler determination of cardiac output in man. Circulation 67:593, 1983

170. Donovan KD, Dobb GJ, Newman MA, et al: Comparison of pulsed Doppler and thermodilution methods for measuring cardiac output in critically ill patients. Crit Care Med 15:853, 1987

171. Nishimura RA, Callahan MJ, Schaff HA, et al: Noninvasive measurement of cardiac output by continuous-wave doppler echocardiography: Initial experience and review of the literature. Mayo Clin Proc 59:484, 1984

172. Levy BI, Payen DM, Tedgui A: Noninvasive ultrasonic cardiac output in intensive care unit. Ultrasound Med Biol 11:841, 1985

173. Chandraratna PA, Nanna M, McKay C: Determination of cardiac output by transcutaneous continuous-wave Doppler computer. Am J Cardiol 53:234, 1984

174. Freund PR: Transesophageal Doppler scanning versus thermodilution during general anesthesia: An initial comparison of cardiac output techniques. Am J Surg 153:490, 1987

175. Mark JB, Steinbrook RA, Gugino LD, et al: Continuous noninvasive monitoring of cardiac output with esophageal doppler ultrasound during cardiac surgery. Anesth Analg 65:1013, 1986

176. Abrams JH, Weber RE, Holmen KD: Continuous cardiac output determination using transtracheal Doppler: Initial results in humans. Anesthesiology 71:11, 1989

177. Pierpont GL, Weber RE, Kan FK, et al: Continuous cardiac output monitoring by transtracheal Doppler ultrasound (abstract). Circulation 78:II-351, 1988

178. Kubicek WG, Karnegis JN, Patterson RP, et al: Development and evaluation of an impedance cardiac output system. Aerospace Med 37:1208, 1966

179. Bernstein DP: A new stroke volume equation for thoracic electrical bioimpedance: Theory and rationale. Crit Care Med 14:904, 1986

180. Appel PL, Kram HB, MacKabee J: Comparison of measurements of cardiac output by bioimpedance and thermodilution in severly ill surgical patients. Crit Care Med 14:933, 1986

181. McKinley DF, Pollack MM: A comparison of thoracic bioimpedance to thermodilution cardiac output in critically ill children (abstract). Crit Care Med 15:358, 1987

182. Spinale FG, Reines HD, Crawford FA: Comparison of bioimpedance and thermodilution methods for determining cardiac output: Experimental and clinical studies. Ann Thorac Surg 45:421, 1988

183. Hippocrates: The book of prognostics. In Major RH (ed): Classic Descriptions of disease. 6th Ed. Charles C. Thomas, Springfield, IL, 1965

184. Boyd AD, Tremblay RE, Spencer FC, et al: Estimation of cardiac output soon after intra-cardiac surgery with cardiopulmonary bypass. Ann Surg 150:613, 1959

185. McArthur KT, Clark LC, Lyons C, et al: Continuous recording of blood oxygen saturation in open heart operations. Surgery 51:121, 1962

186. Norfleet EA, Watson CB: Continuous mixed venous oxygen saturation measurement: A significant advance in hemodynamic monitoring? J Clin Monit 1:245, 1985

187. Waller JL, Kaplan JA, Bauman DI, et al: Clinical evaluation of a new fiberoptic catheter oximeter during cardiac surgery. Anesth Analg 61:676, 1982

188. Magilligan DJ, Teasdall R, Eisinminger R, et al: Mixed venous oxygen saturation as a predictor of cardiac output in the postopertive cardiac surgical patient. Ann Thorac Surg 44:260, 1987

189. Orlando R: Continuous mixed venous oximetry in critically ill surgical patients. Arch Surg 121:470, 1986

190. Birman H, Haq A, Hew E, et al: Continuous monitoring of mixed venous oxygen saturation in hemodynamically unstable patients. Chest 86:753, 1984

191. Divertie MB, McMichan JC: Continuous monitoring of mixed venous oxygen saturation. Chest 85:423, 1984

192. Vaughn S, Puri VK: Cardiac output changes and continuous mixed venous oxygen saturation measurements in the critically ill. Crit Care Med 16:495, 1988

193. Pearson KS, Gomez MN, Carter JG, et al: A cost/benefit analysis of randomized invasive monitoring in cardiac surgery (abstract). Anesth Analg 66:S138, 1987

194. McGregor M, Sniderman A: On pulmonary vascular resistance: The need for more precise definition. Am J Cardiol 55:217, 1985

195. Harvey RM, Enson Y: Pulmonary vascular resistance. Adv Intern Med 15:73, 1969

196. Hilgenberg JC: Pulmonary vascular impedance: Resistance versus pulmonary artery diastolic-pulmonary artery occluded pressure gradient. Anesthesiology 58:484, 1983

197. Mitzner W: Resistance of the pulmonary circulation. Clin Chest Med 4:127, 1983

198. Reeves JT, Grover RF, Filley GF, et al: Cardiac output in normal resting man. J Appl Physiol 16:276, 1961

199. Martin CE, Shaver JS, Thompson ME: Direct correlation of external systolic time intervals with internal indices of left ventricular function in man. Circulation 44:419, 1971

200. Lewis RP, Rittgers SE, Forester WF, et al: A critical review of systolic time intervals. Circulation 56:146, 1977

201. Dauchot PJ, Rasmussen JP, Nicholson DH, et al: On-line systolic time intervals during anesthesia in patients with and without heart disease. Anesthesiology 44:472, 1976

202. Mangano DT: Preoperative assessment. p. 341. In Kaplan JA (ed): Cardiac Anesthesia. 2nd Ed. Grune & Stratton, Orlando, 1987

203. Slutsky R, Karliner J, Ricci D, et al: Response of left ventricular volume to exercise in man assessed by radionuclide equilibrium angiography. Circulation 60:565, 1979

204. Purut CM, Sell TL, Jones RJ: A new method to determine left ventricular pressure-volume loops in the clinical setting. J Nucl Med 29:1492, 1988

205. Cassarella WJ, Berger HJ: Magnetic resonance imaging of the heart and great vessels. p. 188. In Hurst JW, et al (eds): The Heart 6th Ed. McGraw-Hill, New York, 1985

206. Higgins CB, Holt W, Pflugfelder P, et al: Functional evaluation of the heart with magnetic resonance imaging. Magn Reson Med 6:121, 1988

207. Geiser EA, Oliver LH: Echocardiography: Physics and instrumentation. p. 3. In Collins SM, Skorton DJ (eds): Cardiac Imaging and Image Processing. McGraw-Hill, New York, 1986

208. Wells PNT: Absorption and dispersion of ultrasound in biological tissue. Ultrasound Med Biol 1:369, 1975

209. Hill RF: Principles of ultrasound. p. 9. In de Bruijn NP, Clements FM (eds): Transesophageal Echocardiography. Martinus Nijhoff, Boston, 1987

210. Heger JJ, Weyman AE, Wann LS, et al: Cross-sectional echocardiography in acute myocardial infarction: detection and localization of regional left ventricular asynergy. Circulation 60:531, 1979

211. Konstadt SN, Thys D, Mindich BP, et al: Validation of quantitative intraoperative transesophageal echocardiography. Anesthesiology 65:418, 1986

212. Ren JF, Panidis IP, Kotler MN, et al: Effect of coronary bypass surgery and valve replacement on left ventricular function: Assessment by intraoperative two-dimensional echocardiography. Am Heart J 109:281, 1985

213. Thys DM, Hillel Z, Goldman ME, et al: A comparison of hemodynamic indices derived by invasive monitoring and two-dimensional echocardiography. Anesthesiology 67:630, 1987

214. Clements FM, Harpole D, Quill TJ, et al: Simultaneous measurement of cardiac volumes, area and ejection fractions by transesophageal echocardiography and first pass radionuclide angiography (abstract). Anesthesiology 69:A4, 1988

215. Tennant R, Wiggers CJ: Effects of coronary occlusion of myocardial contraction. Am J Physiol 112:351, 1935

216. Slogoff S, Keats AS: Does perioperative myocardial ischemia lead to postoperative myocardial infarction? Anesthesiology 62:107, 1985

217. Waters DD, da Luz P, Wyatt HL, et al: Early changes in regional and global left ventricular function induced by graded reductions in regional coronary perfusion. Am J Cardiol 39:537, 1977

218. Battler A, Froelicher VF, Gallagher KP, et al: Dissociation between regional myocardial dysfunction and ECG changes during ischemia in the conscious dog. Circulation 62:735, 1980

219. Horowitz RS, Morganroth J, Parrotto C, et al: Immediate diagnosis of acute myocardial infarction by two-dimensional echocardiography. Circulation 65:323, 1982

220. Smith J, Cahalan M, Benefiel D, et al: Intraoperative detection of myocardial ischemia at high-risk patients: Electrocardiography versus two-dimensional transesophageal echocardiography. Circulation 72:1015, 1985

221. Lima JAC, Becker LA, Melin JA, et al: Impaired thickening of non-ischemic myocardium during acute regional ischemia in the dog. Circulation 71:1048, 1985

222. Clements FM, Hill R, Kisslo J, et al: How easily can we learn to recognize regional wall motion abnormalities with 2D-transesophageal echocardiography (abstract). Anesthesiology 65:A478, 1986

223. Hillel Z, Thys D, Ali J: Can left ventricular ejection fraction be estimated by visual inspection of 2D-echocardiographic images? Proceedings of the Society of Cardiovascular Anesthesiologists, 11th Annual Meeting, Seattle, 1989

224. Skorton DJ, Collins SM, Kerber RE: Digital image processing and analysis in echocardiography. p. 171. In Collins SM, Skorton DJ (eds): Cardiac Imaging and Image Processing. McGraw-Hill, New York, 1986

225. Stanley TE III, Skelton TN, de Bruijn NP: Centerline systolic wall thickening: A method for quantitating regional cardiac function using transesophageal echocardiography (abstract). Anesth Analg 68:S275, 1989

226. Ren JF, Kotler M, Hakki A, et al: Quantitation of regional left ventricular function by two-dimensional echocardiography in normals and patients with coronary artery disease. Am Heart J 110:552, 1985

227. Gallagher KP, Kumada T, Koziol JA, et al: Significance of regional wall thickening abnormalities relative to transmural myocardial perfusion in anesthetized dogs. Circulation 62:1266, 1980

228. Pandian NG, Kerber RE: Two-dimensional echocardiography in experimental coronary stenosis. I: Sensitivity and specificity in detecting transient myocardial dyskinesis: Comparison with sonomicrometers. Circulation 66:597, 1982

229. Kerber RE, Taylor AL, Hiratzka LF, et al: Transient myocardial ischemia: Experimental echocardiographic demonstration and evaluation of myocardial contraction abnormalities. Can J Cardiol Supplement A:136A, 1986

230. Moses HW, Nanda NC: Real-time two dimensional echocardiography in the diagnosis of left atrial myxoma. Chest 78:788, 1980

231. Cucchiara RF, Nugent M, Seward JB, et al: Air embolism in upright neurosurgical patients: Detection and localization

by two-dimensional transesophageal echocardiography. Anesthesiology 60:353, 1984

232. Topol EJ, Humphrey LS, Borkon AM, et al: Value of intraoperative left ventricular microbubbles detected by transesophageal 2-dimensional echocardiography in predicting neurologic outcome after cardiac operations. Am J Cardiol 56:773, 1985

233. Kort A, Kronzon I: Microbubble formation: In vitro and in vivo observations. J Clin Ultrasound 10:117, 1982

234. Kerber RE, Kioschos DT, Lauer RM: Use of ultrasonic contrast method in the diagnosis of valvular regurgitation and intracardiac shunts. Am J Cardiol 34:722, 1974

235. Valdez-Cruz LM, Sahn DJ: Ultrasonic contrast studies for the detection of cardiac shunts. J Am Coll Cardiol 3:978, 1984

236. Cheirif J, Zoghbi WA, Raizner AE, et al: Assessment of myocardial perfusion in humans by contrast echocardiography. I: Evaluation of regional coronary reserve by peak contrast intensity. J Am Coll Cardiol 11:735, 1988

237. Goldman ME, Mindich BP: Intraoperative cardioplegic contrast echocardiography for assessing myocardial perfusion during open heart surgery. J Am Coll Cardiol 4:1029,1984

238. Light H: Non-injurious ultrasonic technique for observing flow in the human aorta. Nature 224:1119, 1969

239. Wells PNT: A range-gated ultrasonic Doppler system. Med Biol Eng 7:641, 1969

240. Doppler JC: Uber das farbige Licht der Doppelsterne. Abhandlungen der Koniglishen Bohmischen Gesellschaft der Wissenschaften 2:465, 1842

241. Kisslo J, Adams DB, Belkin RN: Doppler Color Flow Imaging. Churchill Livingstone, New York, 1988

242. Kislo J, Adams DB, Marks DB (eds): Basic Doppler Echocardiography. Churchill Livingstone, New York, 1986

243. Sahn DJ: Real-time two dimensional Doppler echocardiographic flow mapping. Circulation 71:849, 1985

244. de Bruijn NP, Clements FM, Kisslo J: Intraoperative transesophageal color flow mapping: Initial experience. Anesth Analg 66:386, 1987

245. Ryan T, Armstrong WF, Feigenbaum H: Doppler assessment of left ventricular filling during experimental myocardial ischemia. Circulation 72:III, 1985

246. Visser CA, deKonig H, Delemarre B, et al: Pulsed Doppler-derived mitral inflow velocity in acute myocardial infarction: An early prognostic indicator. J Am Coll Cardiol 7:136A, 1986

247. Hagler DJ, Tajik AJ, Seward JB, et al: Intraoperative two-dimensional Doppler echocardiography: A preliminary study for congenital heart disease. J Thorac Cardiovasc Surg 95:516, 1988

248. Greeley WJ, Ungerleider RM, Stanley TE, III: Intraoperative echocardiography and color flow imaging during pediatric cardiovascular anesthesia and surgery (abstract). Anesthesiology 69:A778, 1988

249. Greeley WJ, Stanley TE, III, Ungerleider RM, et al: Intraoperative hypoxemic spells in Tetralogy of Fallot: An echocardiographic analysis of diagnosis and treatment. Anesth Analg 68:815, 1989

250. Isner JM, Roberts WC: Right ventricular infarction complicating left ventricular infarction secondary to coronary heart disease. Am J Cardiol 42:885, 1978

251. Bhatia SJS, Kirshenbaum JM, Shemin RJ, et al: Time course of resolution of pulmonary hypertension and right ventricular remodeling after orthotopic cardiac transplantation. Circulation 76:819, 1987

252. Hines R: Monitoring right ventricular function. p. 851. In

253. Barash PG (ed): Cardiac Monitoring. WB Saunders, Philadelphia, 1988

253. Dehmer GJ, Firth BG, Hills LO, et al: Nongeometric determination of RV volume from equilibration blood pool scans. Am J Cardiol 49:78, 1982

254. Machiewicz W, Sechtem V, Higgins C: Evaluation of the right ventricle by magnetic resonance imaging. Am Heart J 113:8, 1987

254a. Kay H, Afshan M, Barash PG, et al: Measurement of ejection fraction by thermal dilution techniques. J Surg Res 34:337, 1983

255. Urban P, Scheidegger D, Gabathuler J, et al: Thermodilution determination of right ventricular volume and ejection fraction. Crit Care Med 15:652, 1987

256. Morrison DA, Stovall R, Sensecqua J, et al: Thermodilution measurement of the right ventricular ejection fraction. Cathet Cardiovasc Diagn 13:167, 1987

257. Hines R, Barash PG: Intraoperative right ventricular dysfunction detected with a right ventricular ejection fraction catheter. J Clin Monit 2:206, 1986

258. Chargoff F, Olson KB: Studies on the chemistry of blood coagulation. VI: Studies on the action of heparin and other anticoagulants: The influence of protamine on the anticoagulant effect in vivo. J Biol Chem 122:153, 1937

259. Hattersley PG: Activated coagulation time of whole blood. JAMA 196:440, 1966

260. Kopriva CJ: The activated coagulation time (ACT). p. 155. In Ellison N, Jobes DR (eds): Effective Hemostasis in Cardiac Surgery. WB Saunders, Philadelphia, 1988

261. Fiser WP, Read RC, Wright FE, et al: A randomized study of beef lung and pork mucosal heparin in cardiac surgery. Ann Thorac Surg 35:615, 1983

262. Bull BS, Korpman RA, Huse WM, et al: Heparin therapy during extracorporeal circulation. I: Problems inherent in existing heparin protocols. J Thorac Cardiovasc Surg 69:674, 1975

263. Bull BS: Heparin anticoagulation. Ann Thorac Surg 30:204, 1980

264. Bull BS, Huse WM, Brauer FS, et al: Heparin therapy during extracorporeal circulation. II: The use of a dose-response curve to individualize heparin and protamine dosage. J Thorac Cardiovasc Surg 69:685, 1975

265. Young JA, Kisker CT, Doty DB: Adequate anticoagulation during cardiopulmonary bypass determined by activated clotting time and the appearance of fibrin monomer. Ann Thorac Surg 26:231, 1978

266. Cohen JA: Activated coagulation time method for control of heparin is reliable during cardiopulmonary bypass. Anesthesiology 60:121, 1984

267. Doty DB, Knott HW, Hoyt JL, et al: Heparin dose for accurate anticoagulation in cardiac surgery. J Cardiovasc Surg 20:597, 1979

268. Dauchot PJ, Berzina-Moettus L, Rabinovitch A, et al: Activated coagulation and activated partial thromboplastin times in assessment and reversal of heparin-induced anticoagulation for cardiopulmonary bypass. Anesth Analg 62:710, 1983

269. Esposito RA, Culliford AT, Colvin SB, et al: The role of the activated clotting time in heparin administration and neutralization for cardiopulmonary bypass. J Thorac Cardiovasc Surg 85:174, 1983

270. Habbab MA, Haft JI: Heparin resistance induced by intravenous nitroglycerin. Arch Intern Med 147:857, 1987

271. Ellison N, Jobes DR, Schwartz AJ: Heparin therapy during

cardiac surgery. p. 1. In: Ellison N, Jobes DR (eds): Effective Hemostasis in Cardiac Surgery. WB Saunders, Philadelphia, 1988

272. Donahoo KM, Taylor CA, Soloway HB: A promising new multi-function instrument for monitoring heparin therapy. Adv Ther 2:150, 1985

273. Goto H, Katayama H, Benson K, et al: PTT-protamine dose-response curve with and without heparin in vitro (abstract). Anesthesiology 61:A48, 1984

274. Perkins H, Osborn J, Hurt R, et al: Neutralization of heparin in vivo with protamine: A simple method of estimating the required dose. J Lab Clin Med 48:223, 1956

275. LaDuca F, Mills D, Thompson S, et al: Neutralization of heparin using a protamine titration assay and the activated clotting time test. J Extra-Corp Tech Proc 19:358, 1987

276. Dutton D, Hothersall A, McLaren A, et al: Protamine titration after cardiopulmonary bypass. Anesthesia 38:264, 1983

277. Pifarre R, Babka R, Sullivan H, et al: Management of postoperative heparin rebound following cardiopulmonary bypass. J Thorac Cardiovasc Surg 81:378, 1981

278. LaDuca F, Thompson S, Reitz B: Optimization of the protamine dose to neutralize heparin: Use of a titration assay to individualize dosage requirements. (In press)

279. Thomas SJ, Gitel SN, Starr NJ, et al: Activated clotting time and heparin levels during hypothermic cardiopulmonary bypass (abstract). Anesthesiology 53:S115, 1980

280. Culliford AT, Gitel SN, Starr N, et al: Lack of correlation between activated clotting time and plasma heparin during cardiopulmonary bypass. Ann Surg 193:105, 1981

281. Congdon JE, Kardinal CG, Wallin JD: Monitoring heparin: Therapy in hemodialysis. JAMA 226:1529, 1973

282. Howland WS, Schweizer O, Gould P: A comparison of intraoperative measurements of coagulation. Anesth Analg 53:657, 1974

283. Shenaq SA, Saleem A: Viscoelastic measurement of clot formation: The Sonoclot. p. 183. In: Ellison N, Jobes DR (eds): Effective Hemostasis in Cardiac Surgery. WB Saunders, Philadelphia, 1988

284. Spiess BD, Tuman KJ, McCarthy RJ, et al: Thromboelastography as an indicator of post-cardiopulmonary bypass coagulopathies. J Clin Monit 3:25, 1987

285. Spiess BD, Ivankovich AD: Thromboelastography: A coagu-

lation-monitoring technique applied to cardiopulmonary bypass. p. 163. In: Ellison N, Jobes DR (eds): Effective Hemostasis in Cardiac Surgery. WB Saunders, Philadelphia, 1988

286. Greeley WJ, Quill TJ, Greenberg CS: Blood coagulation and thromboelastogram changes during and after pediatric cardiovascular surgery. In Proceedings of the Society of Cardiovascular Anesthesiologists, 9th Annual Meeting, (abstract).146, 1987

287. Saleem A, Blifeld C, Saleh SA, et al: Viscoelastic measurement of clot formation: A new test of platelet function. Ann Clin Lab Sci 13:115, 1983

288. Block FE, Jr, Burton LW, Rafal MD, et al: Two computer-based anesthetic monitors: The Duke Automatic Monitoring Equipment (DAME) System and the MicroDame. J Clin Monit 1:30, 1985

289. Smith LR, Stanley TE, III, White WD, et al: Automated continuous recording of anesthesia data during cardiac surgery: Opportunities and problems. Proceedings of the Society of Cardiovascular Anesthesiologists, 11th Annual Meeting. Seattle, 1989

290. Schlant RC, Sonnenblick EH, Gorlin R: Normal physiology of the cardiovascular system. p. 93. In Hurst JW (ed): The Heart. 5th edition. McGraw-Hill, New York, 1982

291. Rorie DK: Monitoring during cardiovascular surgery. p. 55. In Tarhan S (ed): Cardiovascular Anesthesia and Postoperative Care. Year Book Medical Publishers, Chicago, 1982

292. Clements FM, de Bruijn NP: Perioperative evaluation of regional wall motion by transesophageal two-dimensional echocardiography. Anesth Analg 66:249, 1987

293. de Bruijn NP, Clements FM. Transesophageal Echocardiography. Martinus Nijhoff, Boston, 1987

294. Roewer N, Bednarz F, Sculte am Esch J: Continuous measurement of intracardiac and pulmonary blood flow velocities with transesophageal pulsed Doppler echocardiography: Technique and initial clinical experience. J Cardiothorac Anesth 1:418, 1987

295. Tuman K, Speiss B, McCarthy, et al: Effects of progressive blood loss on coagulation as measured by thromboelastography. Anesth Analg 66:856, 1987

296. American Society of Echocardiography: Recommendations for Terminology and Display for Doppler Echocardiography. American Society of Echocardiography, Raleigh, NC, 1984

32
ELECTROCARDIOGRAPHY

Joel A. Kaplan
Daniel M. Thys

INTRODUCTION

The electrocardiogram (ECG) is used as a routine monitor during anesthesia and surgery. Cannard and associates[1] showed the value of the ECG in diagnosing rhythm disturbances during anesthesia in 1960. Standard limb lead II was used at that time and is still often used to diagnose arrhythmias, since its electrical axis parallels the electrical axis of the heart and the P wave is usually easily observed. In recent years, coronary artery disease has become the number one health problem in the United States. Patients coming for all types of surgical procedures have significant coronary artery disease, and in these patients, the ECG should be used to identify myocardial ischemia as well as to recognize arrhythmias. Since many patients are now coming to surgery with pacemakers in place, the ECG also enables the physician to evaluate the function of the pacemaker during the surgical procedure. The major uses of the ECG during the perioperative period may be divided into its role during the preoperative, intraoperative, and postoperative periods.

APPLICATIONS OF ECG

Diagnostic Uses of ECG

Rate and Rhythm Disturbances

Bradycardias and tachycardias can be diagnosed as to their site of origin, possible etiologies, and clinical importance.[2] Supraventricular rhythms can be separated from ventricular rhythms and decisions about therapeutic interventions made preoperatively.

Ischemic Heart Disease

Previous myocardial infarction or myocardial ischemia can be diagnosed from the QRS complex and the ST segments of the ECG.[3] Acute changes indicating ischemia must always be sought during the preoperative period.

Chamber Enlargement

Atrial and ventricular hypertrophy can easily be diagnosed from the preoperative ECG. Specific chamber enlargements tend to be associated with certain diseases, such as left ventricular hypertrophy with hypertension and left atrial hypertrophy with mitral stenosis.[4]

Heart Block

Both sinoatrial (SA) and atrioventricular (AV) conduction blocks can be diagnosed.[5] Especially important are combinations of bundle branch blocks of the conduction system. First-degree, second-degree, and third-degree heart block, as well as different types of hemiblocks, can be diagnosed and may even lead to insertion of a pacemaker during the preoperative period.

Electrolyte and/or Drug Effects

Electrolyte and/or drug effects can frequently be diagnosed from the preoperative ECG.[6] For example, a tentative diagnosis of hypokalemia and digitalis effect may be important in the anesthetic management of the patient.

Pericardial Disease

Occasionally, pericardial disease may be diagnosed from the preoperative ECG, since pericarditis and pericardial effusions are associated with characteristic ECG abnormalities.[7]

Exercise Tolerance Tests

Many variations of the original stress test protocols are used to diagnose ischemic heart disease or rhythm disturbances.[8]

Ambulatory Preoperative ECG Monitoring

Prolonged monitoring for 24 to 72 hours is often used to help diagnose cardiac problems.[9] The new Q-Med system has been used to look for ST-segment changes of ischemia.

Intraoperative Uses of ECG

Arrhythmia Detection

Arrhythmia detection is still the most important use of the intraoperative ECG.[10] The abilities to separate supraventricular from ventricular arrhythmias and to assess therapeutic interventions are extremely important uses of the ECG. Common arrhythmias, such as wandering atrial pacemaker or AV dissociation under halogenated anesthetics, may explain hemodynamic changes that occur during the anesthetic procedure.

Ischemia Detection

Ischemia detection has become much more important since patients with severe coronary artery disease are routinely undergoing major surgical procedures.[11] Differentiation of inferior wall ischemia from anterior or lateral wall ischemia is easily accomplished during the intraoperative period.

Electrolyte Changes

Electrolyte changes, frequently occur during anesthesia and mechanical ventilation.[12] Significant changes in potassium as well as calcium levels occur and can be diagnosed with the ECG.

Pacemaker Function

Pacemaker function requires continuous evaluation during surgical procedures in patients with permanent pacemakers.[13] This is especially important when the surgical procedure will be done near the pacemaker wires or unit or when the electrocautery will be used during surgery.

Postoperative Uses of ECG

There are two major postoperative uses of the ECG:

1. Detection of significant arrhythmias, with associated changes in blood gases or electrolytes that may be a result of the anesthetic procedure.[14]
2. Diagnosis of myocardial ischemia or infarction that may occur during the postoperative period.[15]

PROBLEMS SPECIFIC TO THE SURGICAL ENVIRONMENT

Basic Requirements of ECG Monitoring

Although monitoring of the ECG has become routine intraoperatively, particular problems pertain to its use in the surgical environment. During surgery, the ECG is read off the oscilloscope and may be recorded if indicated. All operating rooms in which cardiac surgery is performed should have permanent ECG-recording capabilities, and recorders should be available to all other operating rooms for interesting diagnostic problems. It would be ideal to have a single-channel ECG recorder on all operating room oscilloscope monitors. The recorder is needed to make accurate diagnoses of complex arrhythmias as well as to permit precise evaluation of changes in the P wave, QRS complex, ST segment, and T wave. In addition, a recorder is frequently needed to ensure that artifacts are not being seen on the oscilloscope. The presence of a written record of the arrhythmia is preferable to the storage, nonfade oscilloscopes that have been employed on some operating room monitors. The ability to store the tracing on the oscilloscope adds little to the capability of diagnosis in the operating room. It certainly does not provide written documentation and a legal record, both of which are provided by a written ECG trace when added to the patient's hospital record. The ECG recorder in the operating room should meet all the standards of accepted cardiology ECG recorders, including types of paper, paper speeds, and markers.

Changes in the ST segment indicative of myocardial ischemia can be evaluated visually or analyzed by a computer. Computerized ST-segment analysis has been increasingly incorporated into operating room ECG systems. Both individual lead analysis systems and multilead trend lines can be obtained.[16] The value of computerized ST-segment analysis is still being evaluated in the operating rooms, but it may be a significant advance for making early diagnosis of myocardial ischemia.

Artifacts on the Oscilloscope

Artifacts on the oscilloscope can be a major problem because they can lead to incorrect diagnosis during the intraoperative period. The ECG may simulate arrhythmias under the following conditions:

1. Tremors of various types, as when the patient is awake and shivering in the operating room
2. Hiccuping or movements of the diaphragm
3. Artifacts in the ECG machine
4. Poor ECG connections
5. Interference from other electrical apparatus, especially the electrocautery or heart-lung machine
6. Interference from contact with other people

The ECG may produce several types of artifacts as a result of either malfunction or improper adjustment.[17] Loose electrodes may simulate many types of arrhythmias. Broken electrode wires, as well as hypothermia with shivering, have been reported to produce an ECG pattern easily mistaken for atrial flutter.[18] Artifacts produced by the roller pumps on the heart–lung machine can also create an ECG pattern that resembles atrial flutter (Fig. 32-1).

The biggest electrical problem with ECG monitoring in the operating room is the electrocautery. When the cautery is used, the standard ECG is totally lost as a result of electrical interference. This interference is a combination of radiofrequency current (800 to 2,000 kHz), alternating current (ac)-line frequency (60 Hz), and low-frequency current (0.1 to 10 Hz). Doss et al.[19] have shown that it is possible to modify the ECG preamplifiers so that they will function well in the presence of the electrocautery. This is now being done to more monitoring units designed for use in the operating room.

In addition to the above causes of ECG changes that may occur during surgery, purely mechanical factors can also affect the ECG.[20] Respiratory variation can affect the height of the QRS complex, which is most marked in leads III and aVF. This is due to either a shift

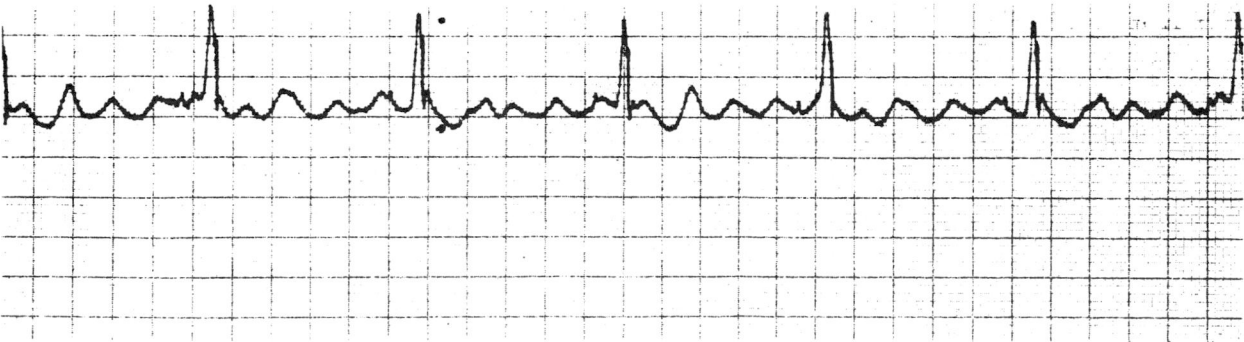

Fig. 32-1. The electrocardiogram of the patient shortly after he was placed on cardiopulmonary bypass. He is in a regular sinus rhythm; however, the ECG appears to show atrial flutter because of an artifact created by the roller pump on the heart–lung machine.

of the mediastinum with respirations or a change in volume of the heart with the respiratory effects on venous return. Studies have shown that increases in the ventricular end-diastolic volume lead to increased height of the QRS complex and that hemorrhage leads to a decreased height of the QRS complex.[21]

ECG telemetry has been tried in a few institutions, but most authorities believe that it is not necessary in the modern operating room setting. The advantages of having no hard wires are balanced against disadvantages with technical problems and limitations in capabilities and modifications. However, there are some situations in which it could be extremely useful, such as during neurodiagnostic radiologic procedures (e.g., pneumoencephalography or computed tomography [CT] scan). In these cases, access to the patient is lim-

ited; wires are in the way, easily twisted, and dislodged; and telemetry may be a useful method of monitoring.

ECG LEAD SYSTEMS

The standard leads are bipolar leads, since they record the potential difference between two electrodes. Additional information can be obtained by placing electrodes closer to the heart or around the thorax. If the three standard leads are connected through resistances of 5,000 Ω, a common central terminal with zero potential is obtained. When this common electrode is used with another active electrode, the potential difference between them represents the actual potential. This is the basis of unipolar lead systems, with a neutral electrode formed by the standard leads and an additional

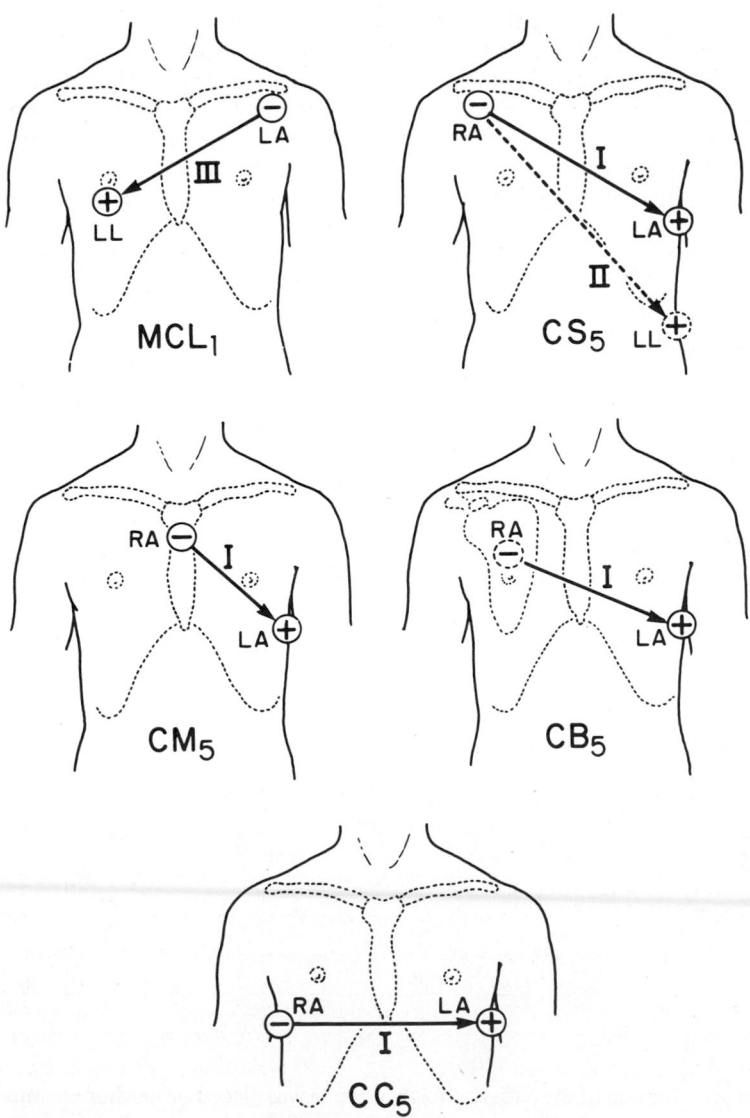

Fig. 32-2. Modified bipolar standard limb lead systems including MCL₁ CS₅, CM₅, CB₅, and CC₅. See text for details. (From Thys and Kaplan,[3] with permission.)

electrode called the exploring electrode. The exploring electrode will theoretically give an accurate representation of electrical activity, since it is referred to a zero potential. Unipolar leads that have proved most useful are the precordial leads designated by a letter V and a numeral that corresponds to the location of the electrode on the chest wall:

V_1 just to the right of the sternum in the fourth intercostal space

V_2 just to the left of the sternum in the fourth intercostal space

V_3 midway between V_2 and V_4

V_4 in the midclavicular line in the fifth intercostal space

V_5 in the anterior axillary line lateral to V_4

V_6 in the midaxillary line lateral to V_5

Precordial leads are more sensitive than the standard leads in detecting myocardial ischemia. The multiple-lead ECG system recommended by Kaplan and King[11] consists of four electrodes on the extremities and a fifth electrode in the V_5 position, which allows for selection of any of seven different ECG leads (I, II, III, aVR, aVL, aVF, or V_5). Leads II and V_5 are usually displayed simultaneously, allowing for observation of both inferior wall and anterolateral myocardial ischemia. This system has become the standard way of monitoring patients with significant coronary artery disease. The use of the unipolar precordial exploring lead (true V_5) requires a five-electrode system to produce the common central terminal. However, many operating room ECG monitors still have only a three-electrode system. These three-electrode systems can be adapted so that similar ECG information can be obtained with modified bipolar standard limb leads.

The Modified Bipolar Standard Limb Leads

To look at one particular area of the heart more closely, several modifications of the basic three-electrode bipolar chest leads have been devised (Fig. 32-2). The nomenclature and classification of these lead systems have evolved over time and can be confusing. Table 32-1 gives the principal bipolar leads useful in the operating room and intensive care setting. The nomenclature of these lead systems is based on that used for the precordial leads.

CS₅ Lead (Central Subclavicular Lead)

The central subclavicular lead, CS_5, may be more correctly described as the MCR_5 lead. The right arm (negative) electrode is placed under the right clavicle, the left arm (positive) electrode is placed in the V_5 position, and the left leg electrode remains in the usual position to serve as the ground (Figs. 32-2 and 32-3). Lead I is then selected. During stress test studies, this lead has been shown to be excellent for detection of anterior ischemia.[22] In the operating room, this CS_5 lead is the best and easiest alternative to the true V_5 lead for monitoring myocardial ischemia. One particular advantage of the CS_5 lead is that lead II can also be monitored by using the same configuration of electrodes, since the left leg electrode is in its usual position. This enables periodic monitoring of the inferior wall of the heart for the development of ischemia as well as using lead II for arrhythmia detection.

CB₅ Lead (Central Back Lead)

The central back lead, CB_5, is obtained by placing the right arm (negative) electrode over the center of the right scapula and the left arm (positive) electrode in the V_5 position. The vector monitored by this lead is in the same direction as that monitored by the true V_5 lead (i.e., downward, leftward, and anterior). The P wave may not be seen on the true V_5 lead, since a certain proportion of the atria may lie to the right or posterior of the origin of the V_5 vector. However, the CB_5 lead, since it originates to the right of the atrium, produces a good P-wave deflection in addition to providing a QRS complex similar to that of the V_5 lead for detection of ischemia. A study comparing CB_5 and V_5 leads in patients with closed and open chests demonstrated a good correlation between ventricular deflections in both leads.[23] The ventricular deflection was 20 percent larger in the CB_5 lead, and more significantly, the P wave was 90 percent larger. Therefore, with this one lead, monitoring for supraventricular arrhythmias and ischemia can be obtained. This may be useful in certain patients with ischemic heart disease who may be especially susceptible to the development of arrhythmias during the perioperative period.

INVASIVE ELECTROCARDIOGRAPHIC MONITORING

In addition to recording the electrical potentials of the heart from the surface of the body, they may also be obtained from body cavities adjacent to the heart (i.e., the esophagus and trachea) or from within the heart itself. This type of ECG monitoring is useful in the anesthetized patient.

The Esophageal ECG

The concept of placing an electrode in the esophagus adjacent to the heart to monitor the ECG is not new. Numerous studies have confirmed the value of the esophageal lead in nonsurgical patients to facilitate the diagnosis of complex arrhythmias. The principal advantage of the esophageal ECG compared with the surface leads is the ability to record a prominent P wave and thus identify the presence of atrial depolarization and its temporal relationship to ventricular activity. In addition, the esophageal ECG has been shown to be a

TABLE 32-1. Bipolar Leads for Use with Three Electrodes

Lead System	MCL_1	CS_5	CM_5	CB_5	CC_5
Right arm electrode	Ground	Under right clavicle (−) (subclavicular)	Manubrium sternum (−)	Center of right scapula (−)	Right anterior axillary line $(V_5R)(−)$
Left arm electrode	Under left clavicle (−)	V_5 (+)	V_5 (+)	V_5 (+)	V_5 (+)
Left leg electrode	V_1 (+)	Ground	Ground	Ground	Ground
Lead selected	III	I	I	I	I
Advantages and indications	Good P-wave and QRS complex; useful for diagnosis of arrhythmias	Monitoring for anterior ischemia	Monitoring for anterior ischemia	Monitoring for anterior ischemia; good P wave for diagnosis of arrhythmias	Monitoring for ischemia

Symbols: +, positive electrode; −, negative electrode.
(From Thys and Kaplan,[3] with permission.)

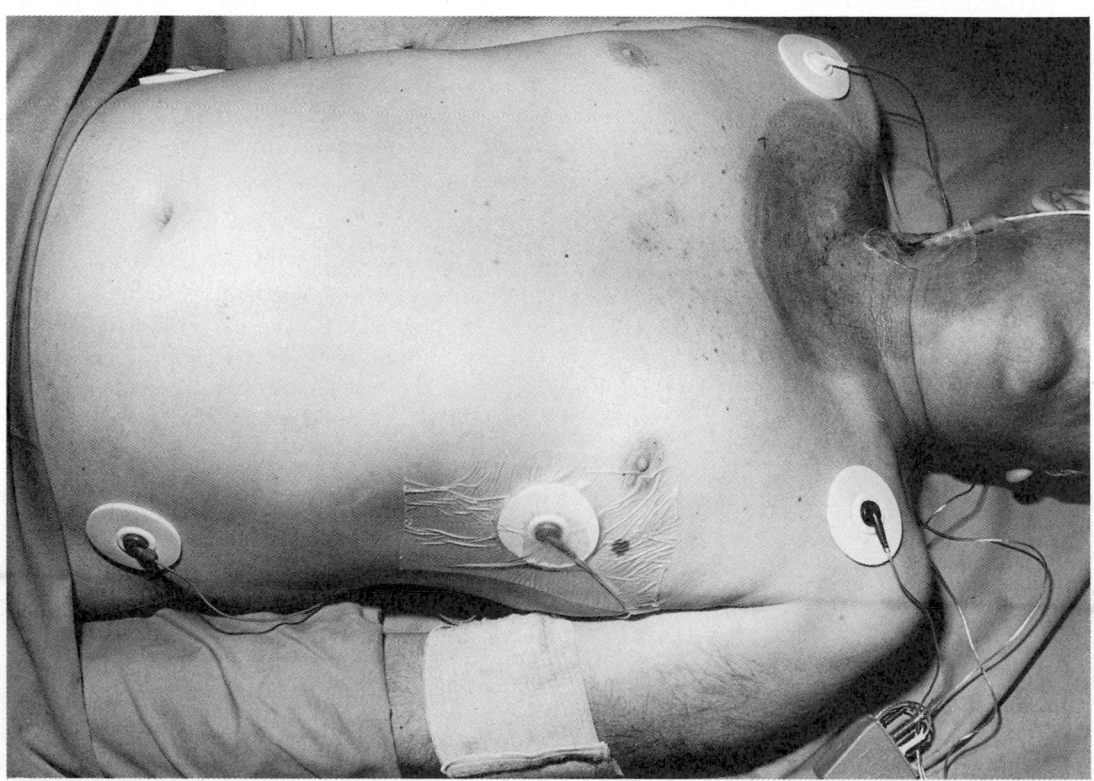

Fig. 32-3. A modified CS_5 lead is demonstrated in which the left arm lead has been moved down to the V_5 position. Lead I can then be turned on to measure from the right arm to the V_5 position (CS_5), and lead II can be used to look at the inferior wall.

useful monitor of posterior ischemia owing to its close anatomic location to the posterior aspect of the left ventricle.

An esophageal ECG electrode system is commercially available that is suitable for use during anesthesia, in the recovery room, or in the intensive care unit. This esophageal ECG monitor consists of an 18-French esophageal stethoscope with two external electrodes 7 and 20 cm from the distal end. The wires from the electrodes are extruded through the wall of the stethoscope and welded to conventional ECG lead wires at the proximal ends. To observe a bipolar esophageal ECG, the leads are connected to the right and left arm terminals and lead I is selected on the monitor. A typical esophageal ECG tracing is shown in Figure 32-4, with lead V_5 for comparison.[24] To minimize the risk of electrocution or esophageal burn injury, strict electrical safety precautions must be followed. All ECG-monitoring equipment should be incapable of delivering more than 10 μA of leakage current to a patient. In addition, when electrocautery is used, a properly applied ground plate of sufficient surface area should be used, and as an extra precaution, an electrocautery protection filter capable of filtering radiofrequencies greater than 20 kHz can be inserted between the ECG cable and the esophageal lead.

Pulmonary Artery Pacing Catheters

The multipurpose pulmonary artery catheter that is available has five electrodes: two intraventricular electrodes situated 18.5 and 19.5 cm from the distal end, and three intra-atrial electrodes situation 28.5, 31.0, and 33.5 cm from the distal end. Incorporation of a third intra-atrial electrode has enabled the electrodes to be properly positioned in heart chambers and great vessels of various sizes. The multipurpose pulmonary artery catheter provides for comprehensive hemodynamic monitoring (pulmonary artery pressure, wedge pressure, central venous pressure, and cardiac output), stable intra-atrial and intraventricular ECG monitoring, and the capability of atrial, AV sequential, or ventricular pacing, if necessary. The high-fidelity tracings obtained from intracardiac electrodes are particularly suitable for computer analysis and reliable, consistent operation of any device requiring QRS triggering mechanisms (e.g., the intraventricular ECG provides a large voltage spike that can be used for triggering an intraaortic balloon pump).[25] The application of the multipurpose pacing catheter, however, should not be limited to cardiac surgical patients and should be considered whenever critically ill patients with serious cardiac disease present for noncardiac surgery.

The Edwards Paceport catheters allow an atrial or ventricular wire to be passed through a small lumen into the appropriate chamber. The wire can be used for pacing or ECG diagnostic purposes.[26]

ARRHYTHMIA DETECTION

Arrhythmia detection has been and still is the most important use of the ECG during and after surgery. Intraoperative arrhythmias were reported during the early 1900s, but the first large series of ECG studies during anesthesia was reported in 1936 by Kurtz et al.[27] In more than 100 patients, they found that sinus arrhythmias, premature ventricular contractions (PVCs), and downward displacement of the pacemaker site predominated. Bertrand et al.[28] studied 100 patients, using continuous electromagnetic tape recording during surgery, and reported an 84 percent incidence of supraventricular and ventricular arrhythmias. Arrhythmias were most common at times of endotracheal intubation and extubation. Patients with pre-existing cardiac disease had a higher incidence of ventricular arrhythmias than did patients without known heart disease (60 percent versus 37 percent). Twenty-four of 25 patients with heart disease had a rhythm disturbance during surgery. In a further study of patients undergoing cardiac surgery, Angelini et al.[14] reported that in 29 of 50 patients (58 percent) having valve surgery and in 35 of 78 patients (45 percent) undergoing coronary revascularization, significant postoperative arrhythmias developed.

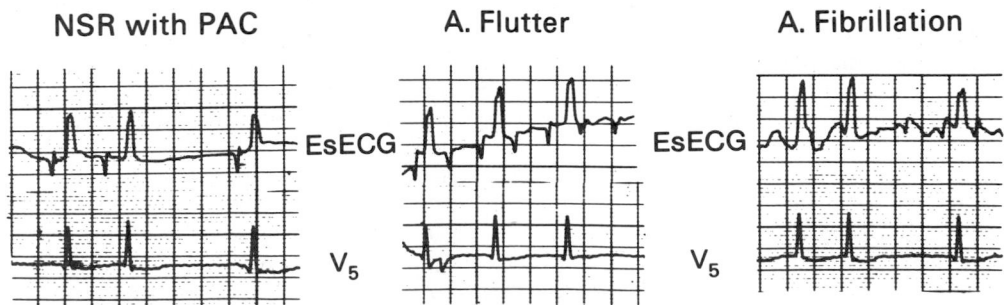

Fig. 32-4. Arrhythmia progression in one patient is shown. Esophageal ECG (EsECG) distinctly reflects changes in atrial rhythm from normal sinus rhythm (NSR) with one premature atrial contraction (PAC) to atrial flutter (A. Flutter) and atrial fibrillation (A. Fibrillation). Lack of information about atrial activity from lead V_5 made definitive diagnosis impossible.

These arrhythmias tended to correlate with the severity of the heart disease, led to a prolonged hospital stay, and were responsible for up to 80 percent of the surgical mortality in the series.

The following factors have been shown to be possible contributors to the etiology of arrhythmias during the perioperative period.

1. *Anesthetics.* Volatile anesthetics such as halothane or enflurane have been shown to produce arrhythmias, probably by a reentrant mechanism.[29] In addition, these agents, especially halothane, have been shown to sensitize the myocardium to both endogenous and exogenous catecholamines. Drugs such as cocaine and ketamine, which block the reuptake of norepinephrine, can facilitate the development of epinephrine-induced arrhythmias.[30]

2. *Abnormal arterial blood gases or electrolytes.* Edwards et al.[12] showed that hyperventilation to a $PaCO_2$ or 30 or 20 mmHg lowered a normal serum potassium to 3.64 or 3.12 meq/L, respectively. If serum potassium and total body potassium start at low levels, it is possible to decrease the serum potassium to the 2 meq/L range by hyperventilation and thus precipitate severe cardiac arrhythmias. Alterations of blood gases or electrolytes may lead to arrhythmias either by producing reentrant mechanisms or by altering phase 4 depolarization of conduction fibers.

3. *Endotracheal intubation.* Endotracheal intubation may be the most common cause of arrhythmias during surgery. These arrhythmias are occasionally associated with severe hypertension.[31] Several investigators have emphasized the hemodynamic alterations that may occur during endotracheal intubation.

4. *Reflexes.* Vagal stimulation may produce sinus bradycardias and permit ventricular escape mechanisms to occur. In addition, specific reflexes such as the oculocardiac reflex can produce severe rhythm disturbances during surgery.

5. *Central nervous system stimulation.*[32] Many ECG abnormalities have been reported with intracranial pathology, especially subarachnoid hemorrhage, including changes in QT intervals, development of Q waves, ST-segment changes, and the occurrence of U waves. The mechanism of these arrhythmias appears to be due to changes in the autonomic nervous system.[32]

6. *Location of surgery.* Dental surgery is often associated with arrhythmias, since profound stimulation of both the sympathetic and parasympathetic nervous systems often occurs.[33] Junctional rhythms commonly occur and may be due to stimulation of the autonomic nervous system via the 5th cranial nerve.

7. *Pre-existing cardiac disease.* Studies by Angelini et al.[14] have shown that patients with known cardiac disease have a much higher incidence of arrhythmias during anesthesia than do patients without known cardiac disease.

8. *Insertion of catheters or wires in the heart.* Arrhythmias may be induced by the placement of a pulmonary artery catheter, often leading to premature ventricular contractions (Fig. 32-5).

Arrhythmias may also be attenuated or eliminated by general anesthesia. This could be due to relief of anxiety and loss of sympathetic stimulation, to an antiarrhythmic property of the anesthetic agent itself, or to the correction of abnormalities of respiration, blood gases, and electrolytes.

The diagnosis and treatment of important intraoperative arrhythmias can be simplified by using the following six questions as a checklist when looking at a rhythm strip or oscilloscope and attempting to decide whether treatment is necessary[34]:

1. What is the heart rate?
2. Is the rhythm regular?
3. Is there one P wave for each QRS complex?
4. Is the QRS complex normal?
5. Is the rhythm dangerous?
6. Does the rhythm require treatment?

The following are common intraoperative arrhythmias that require diagnosis and treatment to which the six key questions should be applied.

Sinus Bradycardia

The pacemaker site is in the sinus node, but the rate is slower than normal. Etiologic factors include drug effects, acute inferior myocardial infarction, hypoxia, vagal stimulation, and high sympathetic blockade (Fig. 32-6). Sinus bradycardia accounts for 11 percent of intraoperative dysrhythmias.[35]

1. *Heart rate*—40 to 60 beats/min. In patients on chronic β-adrenergic blocking therapy, the arrhythmia is defined as a heart rate of less than 50 beats/min.[36]

2. *Rhythm*—The rhythm is regular except for occasional escape beats from other pacemaker sites.

3. *P:QRS*—There is a 1:1 relationship between the P waves and the QRS complexes.

4. *QRS complex*—Normal.

5. *Significance*—Heart rates below 40 beats/min are poorly tolerated even in healthy patients and should be evaluated on the basis of their effect on cardiac output. Treatment is recommended if hypotension, ventricular arrhythmias, or signs of poor peripheral perfusion are observed. A sinus bradycardia may be part of the sick sinus syndrome in which sinus node dysfunction can precipitate bradycardias, heart block, tachyarrhythmias, or alternating bradytachyarrhythmias.[37]

6. *Treatment*—There is usually none necessary, but a progression from atropine (0.4 to 2 mg IV) to ephedrine (5 to 25 mg IV) to isoproterenol (1 to 4 μg IV) to

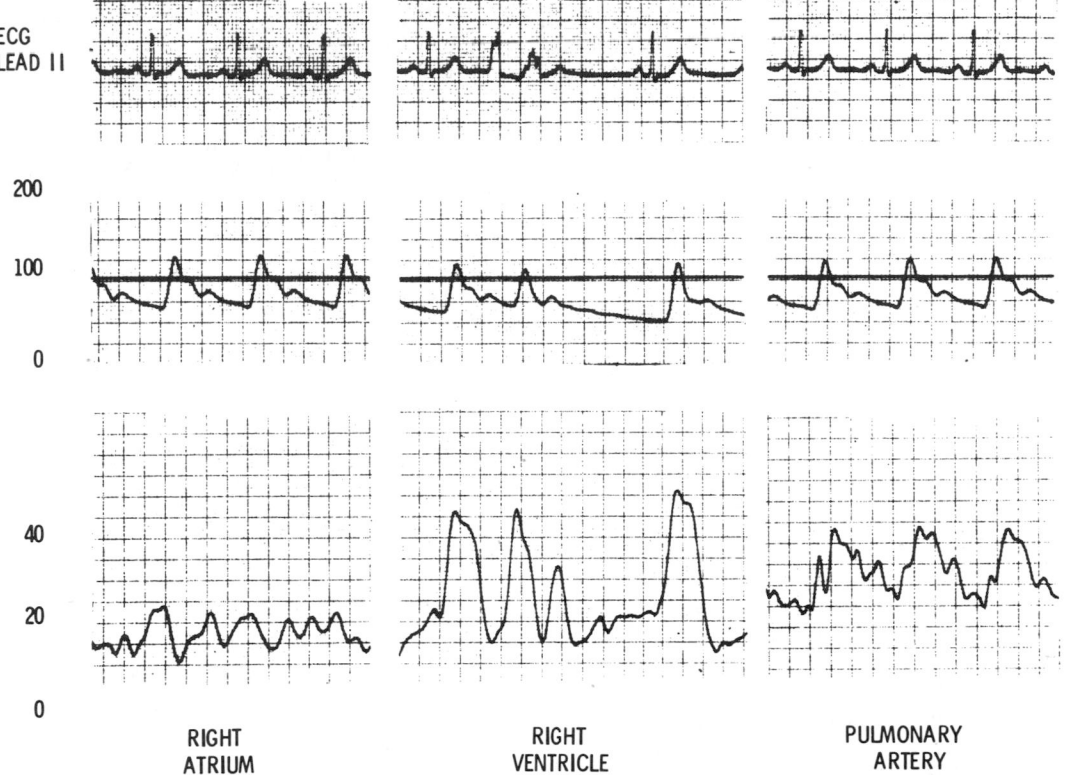

Fig. 32-5. Multifocal premature ventricular contractions are demonstrated on lead II of the ECG. These occurred with passage of the Swan-Ganz catheter from the right atrium into the right ventricle and then disappeared upon entrance of the catheter into the pulmonary artery. The arterial tracing demonstrates the systemic hemodynamic effects of these premature contractions.

temporary transvenous pacemaker insertion may be necessary for severe or refractory sinus bradycardias.

Sinus Tachycardia

The pacemaker site is in the SA node, but the rate is faster than normal. Sinus tachycardia is the most commonly occurring arrhythmia in the perioperative period. It occurs with such frequency that it is not included in most incidence studies. Common causes include pain, inadequate anesthesia, hypovolemia, fever, hypoxia, hypercarbia, heart failure, and drug effects.

1. *Heart rate* — The rate is greater than 100 beats/min and can go up to 170 beats/min, which may be seen with a severe episode of hyperpyrexia (Fig. 32-7).
2. *Rhythm* — Regular.
3. *P:QRS* — 1:1.

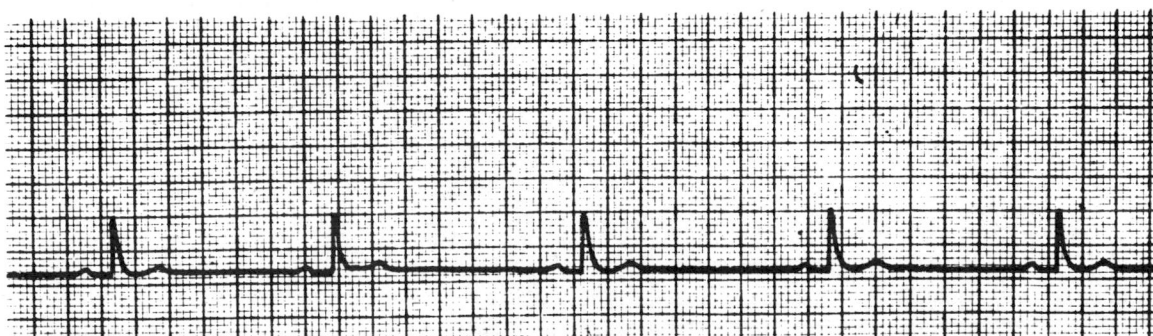

Fig. 32-6. A sinus bradycardia with an intrinsic rate of about 45 beats/min is demonstrated. Also notice that the patient has a mild sinus arrhythmia with variations in heart rate associated with respirations.

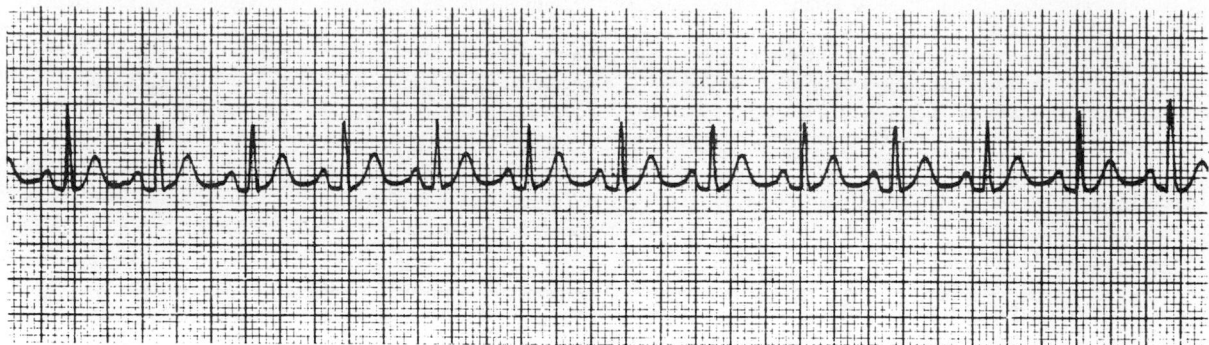

Fig. 32-7. A sinus tachycardia is demonstrated with an intrinsic heart rate over 100 beats/min.

4. *QRS complex*—Normal. There may be associated ST-segment depression with severe increases in heart rate and resulting myocardial ischemia.
5. *Significance*—Prolonged tachycardias in patients with underlying heart disease can precipitate congestive heart failure owing to the increased myocardial work required. The tachycardia decreases coronary perfusion time, which can cause secondary ST-T wave changes and can precipitate angina pectoris in patients with coronary artery disease. A major diagnostic problem is encountered when the heart rate is 150 beats/min since this is a common rate for a sinus tachycardia, a paroxysmal atrial tachycardia (PAT), or an atrial flutter with a 2:1 block.[38] These three arrhythmias can sometimes be separated by the use of carotid sinus massage, intravenous administration of edrophonium, or atrial or esophageal ECG leads to identify the P waves on the ECG more accurately.
6. *Treatment*—The underlying disorder should be treated. If necessary, while determining the cause, esmolol or propranolol should be used in patients with ischemic heart disease who develop ST-segment changes to prevent further myocardial ischemia.

Sinus Arrhythmia

The pacemaker impulse arises from the SA node, but the arrhythmia is manifested by alternating periods of slower and more rapid heart rates. The PR interval is normal, as is the QRS complex (Fig. 32-8). Most commonly but not invariably the rate increases with inspiration and decreases with expiration. It occurs more often in children than in adults.

1. *Heart rate*—60 to 100 beats/min.
2. *Rhythm*—Irregular.
3. *P:QRS*—1:1.
4. *QRS complex*—Normal.
5. *Significance*—Normal finding.
6. *Treatment*—None.

Premature Atrial Contractions

An ectopic pacemaker site in either the left or right atrium initiates the premature atrial contraction (PAC). The shape of the P wave is abnormal and possibly inverted. The PR interval may be shorter or longer than normal, depending on the site of the ectopic focus and the refractoriness of the AV nodal pathway. The PAC spreads not only through the AV node and ventricular conduction system but also in a retrograde fashion reaches the SA node, thus resetting the sinus pacemaker. The interval from the PAC to the next sinus beat is therefore a normal sinus cycle (i.e., no compensatory pause). The absence of a compensatory pause is an important distinguishing feature between PACs and PVCs. Occasionally, PACs may find part of the ventricular conduction system refractory. In that case, they will travel down an aberrant pathway and create an abnormal QRS complex. They are then called PACs with ventricular aberration and can very easily be confused with PVCs. Since the recovery period of the right ventricular

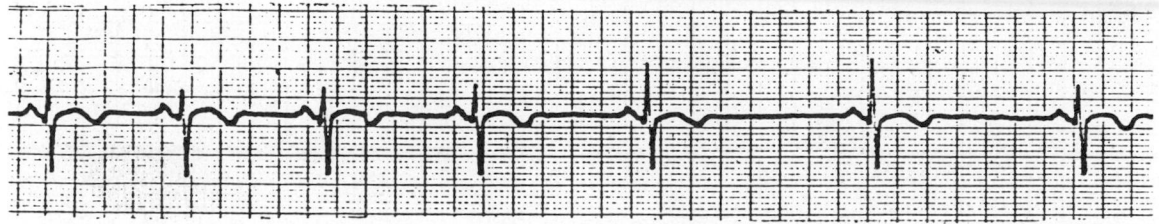

Fig. 32-8. Sinus arrhythmia. Note the normal PR interval and QRS complex. (From Thys and Kaplan,[3] with permission.)

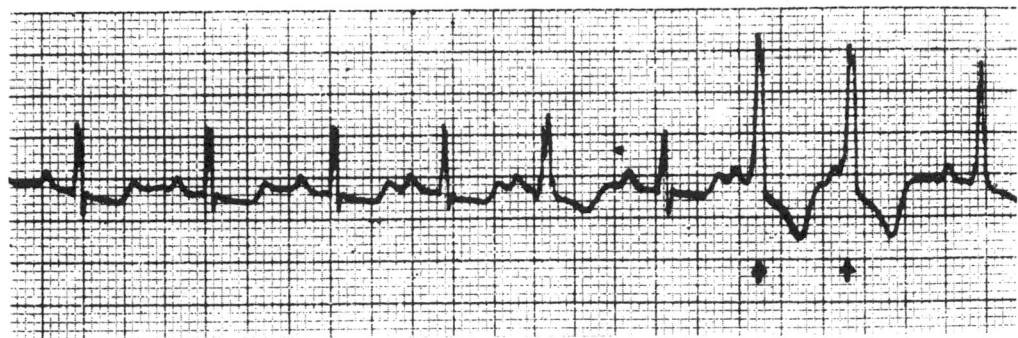

Fig. 32-9. ECG tracing with multiple premature atrial contractions. The fourth beat shows no aberration, while the fifth beat shows partial aberration and the seventh and eighth beats, with arrows, show marked aberration.

(RV) conduction system outlasts that of the left, the most common form of aberration appears as a right bundle branch block (RBBB). Helpful points in separating a PAC with aberration from a PVC are the following: (1) there is a preceding P wave, usually abnormally shaped; (2) the QRS complex has an RBBB configuration; (3) there is an rSR' in V_1; and (4) the initial vector forces are identical with the preceding beat but are usually the opposite with a PVC (Fig. 32-9). Other characteristics of PACs are as follows:

1. *Heart rate* — Variable, depending on frequency of PACs.
2. *Rhythm* — Irregular.
3. *P:QRS* — Usually 1:1. The P waves have various shapes and may even be lost in the QRS or T waves. Occasionally, the P wave will be so early as to find the ventricle refractory and a nonconducted beat will occur.
4. *QRS complex* — Usually normal unless there is ventricular aberration, as mentioned above (Fig. 32-9).
5. *Significance* — PACs represented 10 percent of the total intraoperative arrhythmias seen in one study.[35] They have little clinical significance, but frequent PACs may lead to other more serious supraventricular arrhythmias or be a sign of digitalis intoxication.
6. *Treatment* — Rarely necessary, but digitalis, β-adrenergic blocking agents, or verapamil may be considered if hemodynamic function is impaired.

Paroxysmal Atrial Tachycardia

A run of rapidly repeated supraventricular premature beats from a site other than the SA node characterizes PAT. The inclusion of tachycardias originating in the AV node allows for the useful classification of paroxysmal supraventricular tachycardia (SVT). The rhythm is usually abrupt in both its onset and termination.

1. *Heart rate* — 150 to 250 beats/min.
2. *Rhythm* — Usually regular unless the impulse originates from multiple atrial foci.
3. *P:QRS* — There is a 1:1 relationship, although the P wave is often hidden in the QRS complex or T wave.
4. *QRS complex* — Generally normal, but ST-T changes indicative of ischemia may be noted (Fig. 32-10). Aberration of ventricular conduction may occur, thus complicating the differential diagnosis with ventricular tachycardia. SVT may also be confused with sinus tachycardia, atrial flutter, and atrial fibrillation. In differentiating these rhythms, carotid sinus massage and edrophonium (5 to 10 mg IV) may be used to slow the rate. Esophageal ECG leads to better define atrial activity may also be helpful.
5. *Significance* — Paroxysmal SVT can be seen in 5 percent of normal young adults and in patients with Wolff-Parkinson-White syndrome or other aberrant conduction pathway syndromes. During anesthesia, it makes up 2.5 percent of all arrhythmias,[35] and it

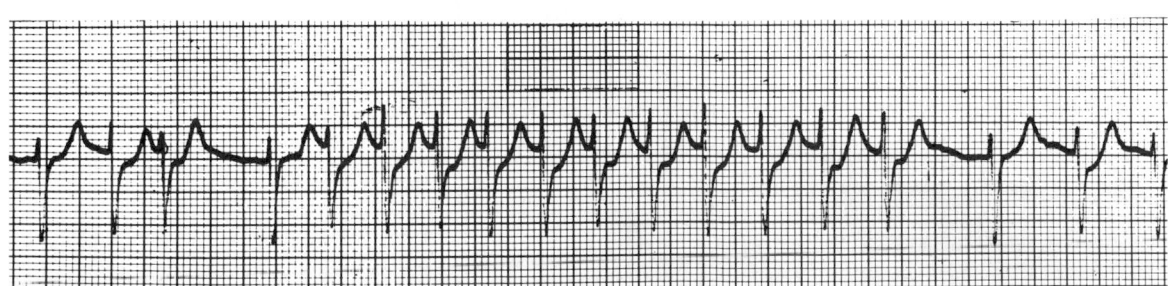

Fig. 32-10. Paroxysmal atrial tachycardia. (From Thys and Kaplan,[3] with permission.)

has been associated with intrinsic heart disease, systemic illness, thyrotoxicosis, digitalis toxicity, pulmonary embolism, and pregnancy.[39] Under anesthesia, it can be precipitated by changes in the autonomic nervous system, drug effects, or volume shifts and can produce severe hemodynamic deterioration.[40] At times, the PAT may be associated with AV block owing to the fast atrial rate and slow AV conduction. PAT with 2:1 block represents digitalis intoxication in many patients.

6. *Treatment* — This arrhythmia often must be treated because of its rapid rate and associated poor hemodynamic function. Several steps can be taken to treat this dysrhythmia[41]:

   a. Vagal maneuvers such as carotid sinus massage, which should only be applied to one side.
   b. Verapamil (5 to 10 mg IV) terminates AV nodal reentry successfully in about 90 percent of cases and has become the drug of choice.[42] (It should be avoided in patients with known Wolff-Parkinson-White syndrome since it may lead to increased conduction through the abnormal pathway.)
   c. Esmolol (1 mg/kg bolus and 50 to 200 μg/kg/min infusion) has been shown to be very effective in treating postoperative SVTs.[43]
   d. Propranolol in 0.5 mg IV bolus doses.
   e. Edrophonium (Tensilon) in 5 to 10 mg IV bolus doses.
   f. Phenylephrine, if the patient is hypotensive; use 100 μg IV bolus doses in an effort to increase the blood pressure and achieve a reflex vagal slowing of the heart rate.
   g. Intravenous digitalization with one of the short-acting digitalis preparations: ouabain (0.25 to 0.5 mg IV) or digoxin (0.5 to 1.0 mg IV).[44]
   h. Rapid overdrive pacing, in an effort to capture the ectopic focus.[45]
   i. Cardioversion with appropriate synchronization.[46]

Atrial Flutters

Atrial flutters represent a faster discharge from an irritable focus in the atria than does a rapid atrial tachycardia. Since it is so fast, it is usually associated with AV block. Classic sawtooth flutter waves (F waves) are usu-

ally present (Fig. 32-11). The characteristics of atrial flutter are as follows:

1. *Heart rate* — The atrial heart rate is 250 to 350 beats/min, with a ventricular rate of about 150 beats/min.
2. *Rhythm* — The atrial rhythm is regular. The ventricular rhythm may be regular if a fixed AV block is present or irregular if a variable block exists.
3. *P:QRS* — Usually there is a 2:1 block with an atrial rate of 300 beats/min and a ventricular rate of 150 beats/min, but it may vary between 2:1 and 8:1. F waves are best seen in leads V_1, II, or the esophageal lead.
4. *QRS complex* — Normal. T waves are lost in the F waves.
5. *Significance* — It usually indicates the presence of severe heart disease. It is seen with increased incidence in patients with coronary artery disease, mitral valve disease, pulmonary embolism, hyperthyroidism, cardiac trauma, malignant cancers of the heart, and myocarditis.
6. *Treatment:*
   a. The initial treatment of choice is synchronous direct current (dc) cardioversion with very low voltage (10 to 40 W-s), which is effective in more than 90 percent of cases.[47]
   b. Rapid atrial pacing effectively terminates atrial flutter in many patients and results in a return to sinus rhythm or atrial fibrillation with a slow ventricular rate.[48]
   c. Esmolol (50 to 200 $\mu$is very effective in slowing the rate.[43]
   d. Verapamil (5 to 10 mg IV).[42]
   e. Digitalis, with or without propranolol.

Atrial Fibrillation

Atrial fibrillation is an excessively rapid and irregular atrial focus with no P waves appearing on the ECG but, instead, a fine fibrillatory activity called f waves. This is the most irregular rhythm; it is called irregularly irregular and may be associated with a pulse deficit (Fig. 32-12). The characteristics are as follows:

1. *Heart rate* — The atrial rate is 350 to 500 beats/min and the ventricular rate is between 60 and 170 beats/min.

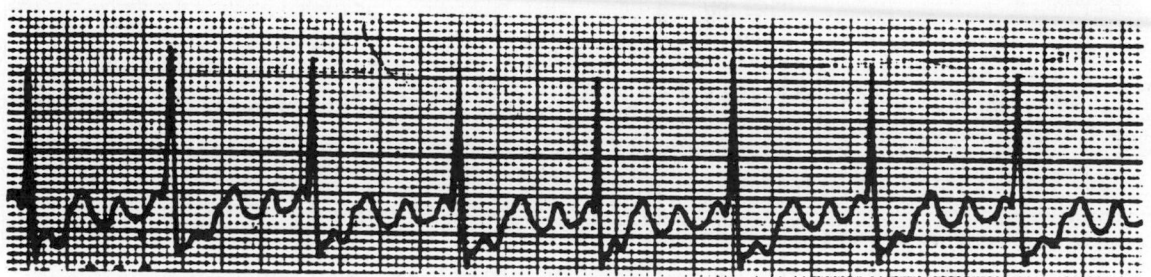

Fig. 32-11. Classic sawtoothed flutter waves (F waves) are seen in this patient with atrial flutter.

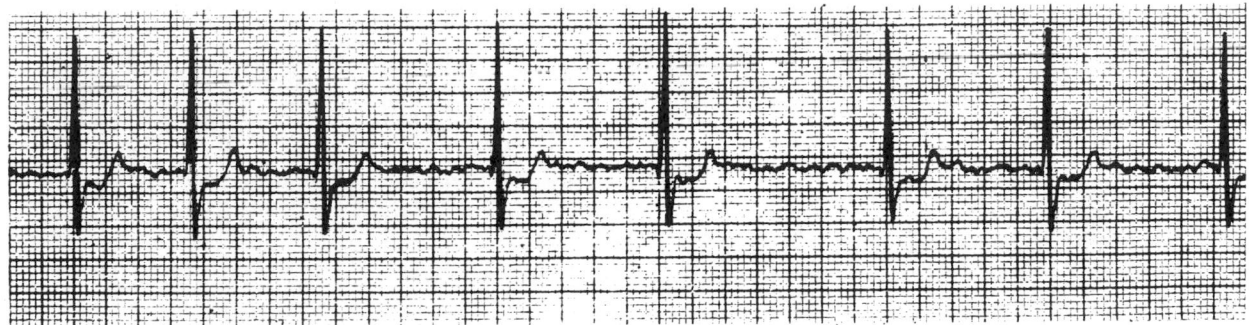

Fig. 32-12. Atrial fibrillation with fine fibrillatory activity is demonstrated. Note the irregularly irregular pattern of the QRS complexes.

2. *Rhythm*—Irregularly irregular.
3. *P:QRS*—P wave is absent and replaced by f waves or no obvious atrial activity at all.
4. *QRS complex*—Normal.
5. *Significance*—The etiologic factors of atrial fibrillation are similar to those of atrial flutter. This rhythm is almost invariably associated with significant cardiac disease. The clinical significance and treatment of atrial fibrillation are also similar to those of atrial flutter except for two important considerations. The loss of an atrial kick secondary to inefficient contraction of the atria will reduce ventricular filling and may significantly compromise cardiac output. In addition, atrial fibrillation may lead to the formation of atrial thrombi with resultant pulmonary and systemic embolization.
6. *Treatment*—Digitalis is most commonly used to slow the ventricular rate on a chronic basis. Esmolol is very effective in the perioperative period and may lead to a higher conversion rate to sinus rhythm then is seen with verapamil.[49]

Junctional Rhythms

The AV node itself shows no intrinsic phase 4 depolarization. Therefore, cells in the node cannot act as pacemakers. Ectopic activity, however, may be initiated from sites just above and below the node. It would make sense to consider these arrhythmias as AV junctional in nature. The resultant P wave will be abnormal and, depending on the position of the ectopic pacemaker, may be very close to, buried in, or following the QRS complex. Depending on the rate of fire of the ectopic pacemaker, the resultant rhythm will be nodal premature; nodal quadrigeminy, trigeminy, or bigeminy; nodal rhythm; or nodal tachycardia.

1. *Heart rate*—Variable, 40 to 180 beats/min (nodal bradycardia to tachycardia) (Fig. 32-13).
2. *Rhythm*—Regular.
3. *P:QRS*—1:1, but there are three varieties[50]:
   a. High-nodal rhythm—The impulse reaches the atrium before the ventricle; therefore, the P wave precedes the QRS but has a shortened PR interval (less than 0.1 second).
   b. Mid-nodal rhythm—The impulse arrives in the atrium and the ventricle at the same time, and the P wave is lost is the QRS.
   c. Low-nodal rhythm—The impulse reaches the ventricle first and then the atrium so that P wave follows the QRS complex.
4. *QRS complex*—Normal, unless altered by the P wave.
5. *Significance*—Junctional rhythms are common under anesthesia (about 20 percent of the cases), especially with halogenated anesthetic agents. The junctional rhythms frequently decrease blood pressure and cardiac output by about 15 percent but can

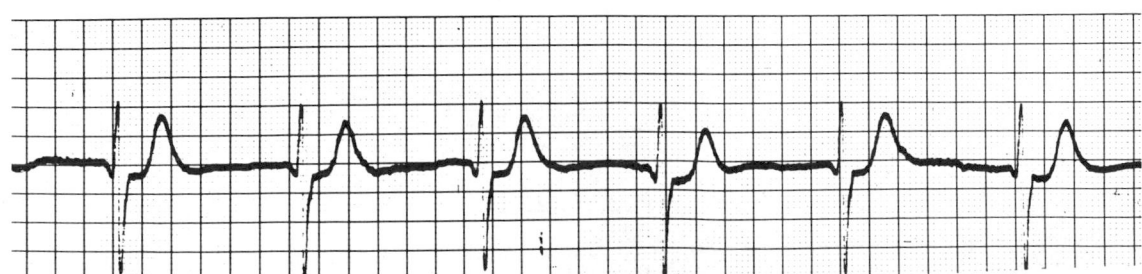

Fig. 32-13. Junctional rhythm. Note that the P waves are buried in the QRS complex. (From Thys and Kaplan,[3] with permission.)

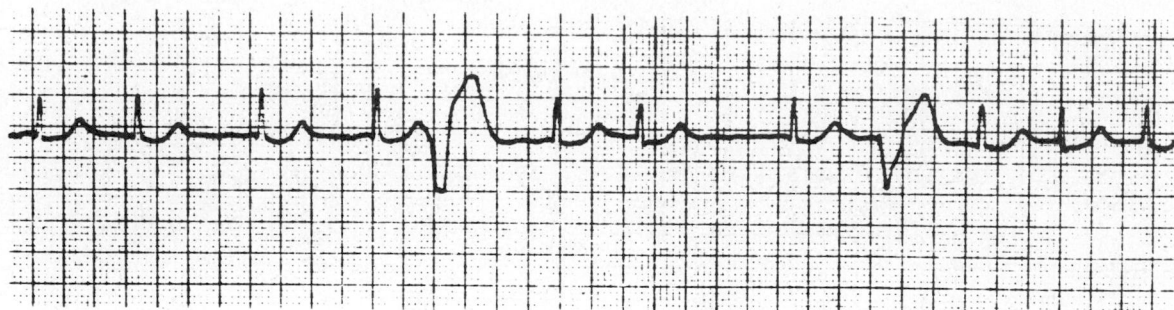

Fig. 32-14. Premature ventricular contractions are identified by the fact that they are premature, have a wide QRS complex, and an ST segment that slopes in the opposite direction. They may also have a compensatory pause.

decrease cardiac output by up to 30 percent in patients with heart disease.[51]

6. *Treatment*—Usually no treatment is required, and the rhythm reverts spontaneously. If hypotension and poor perfusion are associated with the rhythm, treatment is indicated. Atropine, ephedrine, or isoproterenol can be used in an effort to increase the activity of the SA node so it will take over as the pacemaker. A small dose of succinycholine (10 mg IV) may revert a nodal rhythm to a sinus rhythm during anesthesia with halothane or enflurane.[52] This probably works as a result of the effect of succinylcholine as a sympathetic ganglionic stimulator. In some cases, propranolol may correct the rhythm disturbance if it is due to sympathetic stimulation.[53]

Premature Ventricular Contractions

PVCs result from ectopic pacemaker activity arising from below the AV junction. The PVC originates in and spreads through the myocardium or ventricular conducting system, resulting in a wide (0.12 second), bizarre QRS complex. The ST segment usually slopes in the opposite direction to the main deflection of the QRS complex. There is no P wave associated with a PVC, but retrograde depolarization of the atria or blocked sinus beats may obscure the diagnosis (Fig. 32-14).

The most important entity in the differential diagnosis is PACs with aberrant ventricular conduction.

The distinction should be made whenever possible. While a PAC will normally reach the SA node and reset the sinus rhythm, such an occurrence is rare when the ectopic pacemaker is in the ventricle. Therefore, a PVC will block the next depolarization from the SA node, but the following sinus beat occurs on time. The result is a compensatory pause, consisting of the interval from the PVC to the expected normal QRS, which is blocked at the AV node, plus a normal sinus interval. PVCs are common during anesthesia, accounting for 15 percent of observed arrhythmias.[35] They are much more common in anesthetized patients with pre-existing cardiac disease. Other than heart disease, known etiologic factors include electrolyte and blood gas abnormalities, drug interactions, brain stem stimulation, and trauma to the heart.

1. *Heart rate*—Depends on the underlying sinus rate and frequency of the PVCs.
2. *Rhythm*—Irregular.
3. *P:QRS*—No P wave with the PVCs.
4. *QRS complex*—Wide and bizarre with a width of more than 0.12 second.
5. *Significance*—The new onset of PVCs must be considered life threatening because in certain clinical situations it may progress to ventricular tachycardia or fibrillation. These situations include coronary artery insufficiency, myocardial infarction, digitalis

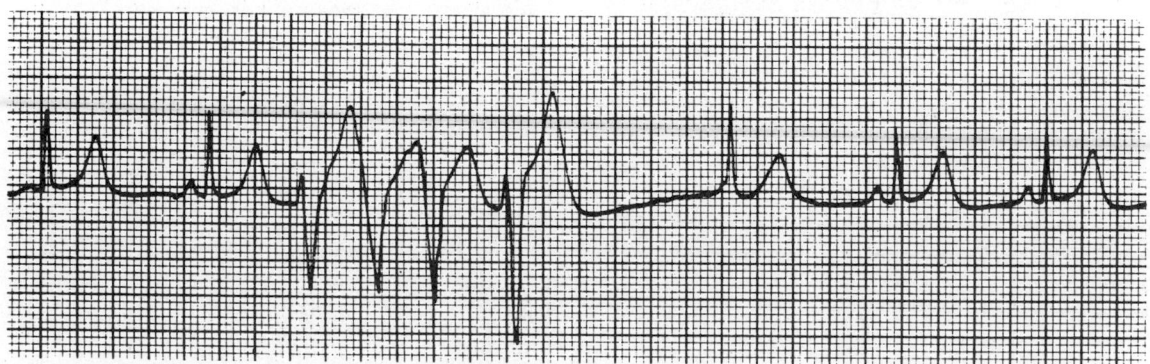

Fig. 32-15. Three or more PVCs in a row is defined as a run of ventricular tachycardia. A fusion beat, capture beat, or AV dissociation seen on the trace helps make the specific diagnosis of ventricular tachycardia.

toxicity with hypokalemia, and hypoxemia. PVCs are more likely to lead to fibrillation if they are multiple, multifocal, bigeminal, or occur near the vulnerable period of the preceding ventricular depolarization (the so-called R-on-T phenomenon).[54]

6. *Treatment*—The first step is to correct any underlying abnormalities such as decreased serum potassium or low arterial oxygen tension. Lidocaine is then usually the treatment of choice with an initial bolus dose of 1.5 mg/kg IV. Recurrent PVCs can be treated with a lidocaine infusion of 1 to 4 mg/min; additional therapy can be supplied with esmolol, propranolol, bretylium, procainamide, quinidine, verapamil, disopyramide, atropine, or overdrive pacing.

Ventricular Tachycardia

Ventricular tachycardia is a run of rapidly repeated ectopic beats arising from the ventricle that are potentially life threatening. Diagnostic criteria include the presence of fusion beats, capture beats, and AV dissociation (Fig. 32-15).[55] The characteristics of ventricular tachycardia are as follows:

1. *Heart rate*—100 to 200 beats/min.
2. *Rhythm*—Usually regular but may be irregular if the ventricular tachycardia is paroxysmal.
3. *P:QRS*—No fixed relationship, since ventricular tachycardia is a form of AV dissociation in which the P waves can be seen marching through the QRS complex.
4. *QRS complex*—Wide, more than 0.12 second in width.
5. *Significance*—Acute onset is life threatening and requires immediate treatment.
6. *Treatment*—Lidocaine and/or immediate cardioversion is usually required. Recurrent episodes may require therapy with any or all of the drugs listed under the treatment of PVCs.

Ventricular Fibrillation

Ventricular fibrillation is an irregular rhythm resulting from a rapid discharge of impulses from one or more foci in the ventricles. The ventricular contractions are erratic and are represented on the ECG by bizarre patterns of various sizes and configurations. P waves are not seen (Fig. 32-16). Important causes of the arrhyth-

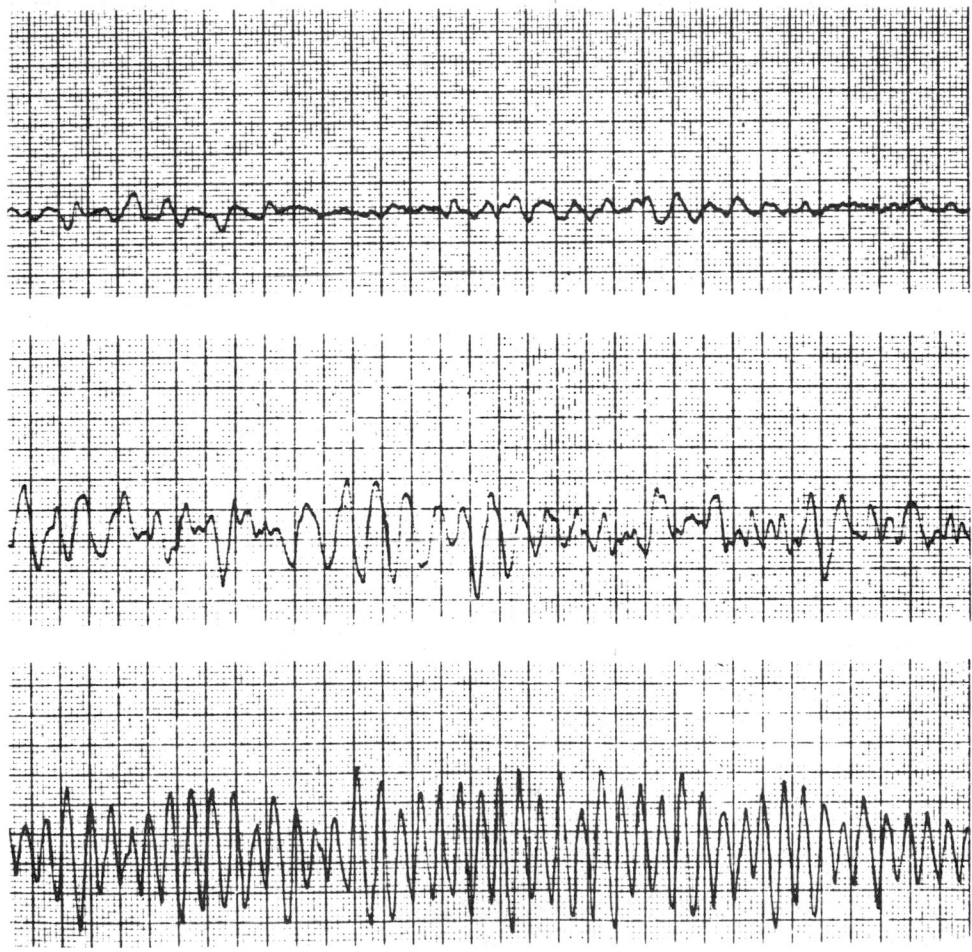

Fig. 32-16. Ventricular fibrillation can occur in a very fine, moderate, or coarse pattern, as demonstrated on the ECGs.

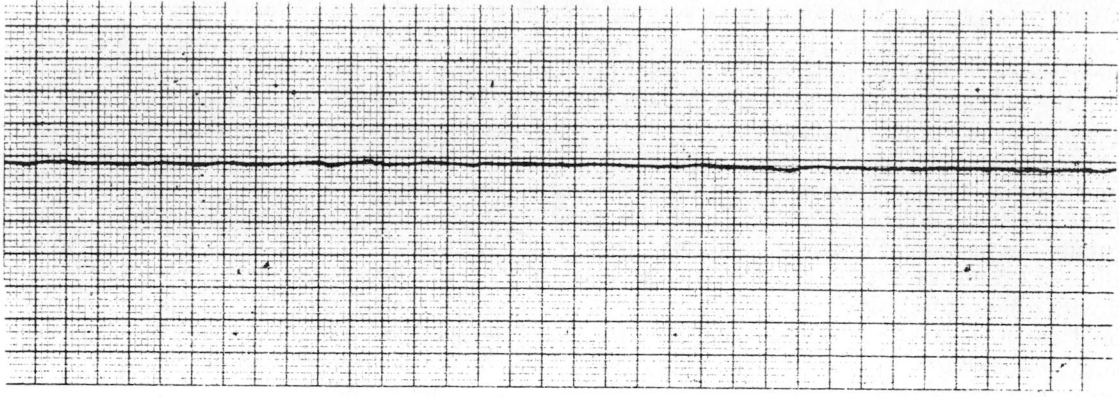

Fig. 32-17. Asystole is diagnosed by the straight line on the ECG. It must be ascertained that this is not an ECG strip taken with a lead or cable disconnected from the patient.

mia include myocardial ischemia, hypoxia, hypothermia, electric shock, electrolyte imbalance, and drug effects. The characteristics are as follows:

1. *Heart rate* — Rapid and grossly disorganized.
2. *Rhythm* — Totally irregular.
3. *P:QRS* — None seen.
4. *QRS complex* — Not present.
5. *Significance* — There is no effective cardiac output, and life must be sustained by artificial means, such as external cardiac massage.
6. *Treatment* — Cardiopulmonary resuscitation must be initiated immediately and then defibrillation performed as rapidly as possible. External defibrillation should be performed with a dc defibrillator, using 200 to 400 W-s.[56] Supportive pharmacologic therapy may include propranolol, bretylium, or lidocaine. In some instances, epinephrine is used to coarsen the fibrillation in an attempt to defibrillate the patient.[54]

Asystole

During asystole, no ventricular activity is present. Asystole is the second most common rhythm disorder (after ventricular fibrillation) during cardiac arrests. The characteristics are as follows:

1. *Heart rate* — None present.
2. *Rhythm* — Straight line on the ECG (Fig. 32-17).
3. *P:QRS* — None present.
4. *QRS complex* — Absent.
5. *Significance* — Difficult to treat; an attempt should be made to convert it to ventricular fibrillation.
6. *Treatment* — Maintain cardiopulmonary resuscitation while administering isoproterenol, epinephrine, sodium bicarbonate, and, if necessary, inserting a transvenous pacemaker.

CONDUCTION ABNORMALITIES

Three types of conduction system block are possible: SA block, AV heart block, and intraventricular conduction block (Table 32-2). Bundle of His electrograms

have greatly improved the understanding of conduction through the heart.[57] In SA block, the block occurs at the sinus node. Since atrial excitation is not initiated, P waves are not found on the ECG. The next beat can be a normal sinus beat, a nodal escape beat, or a ventricular escape beat.

The second type of heart block is an AV heart block, or AV block, which may be either incomplete or complete.[58] First- and second-degree AV blocks are usually considered incomplete, while a third-degree AV block is considered to be complete heart block. First-degree AV block is often found in normal hearts but is also associated with coronary artery disease or digitalis administration. It is characterized by a PR interval longer than 0.21 second. All atrial impulses progress through the AV node to the Purkinje system. This form of heart block ordinarily requires no treatment (Fig. 32-18).

Second-degree AV block is associated with the con-

TABLE 32-2. Conduction Defects

A. Sinus node block
B. Atrioventricular conduction defects
  1. First degree
  2. Second degree
    a. Mobitz I
    b. Mobitz II
  3. Third degree (complete)
C. Intraventricular conduction defects
  1. Right bundle branch block (RBBB)
    a. Complete
    b. Incomplete
  2. Left bundle branch block (LBBB)
    a. Complete
    b. Incomplete
  3. Left fascicular block
    a. Left anterior hemiblock (LAHB)
    b. Left posterior hemiblock (LPHB)
  4. Bifascicular block
    a. RBBB + LAHB
    b. RBBB + LPHB
    c. Alternative LBBB/RBBB
    d. AV conduction defect + LBBB or RBBB
  5. Trifascicular block
  6. Indeterminate (bizarre conduction defect, not possible to allocate to above categories)

(From Thys and Kaplan,[3] with permission.)

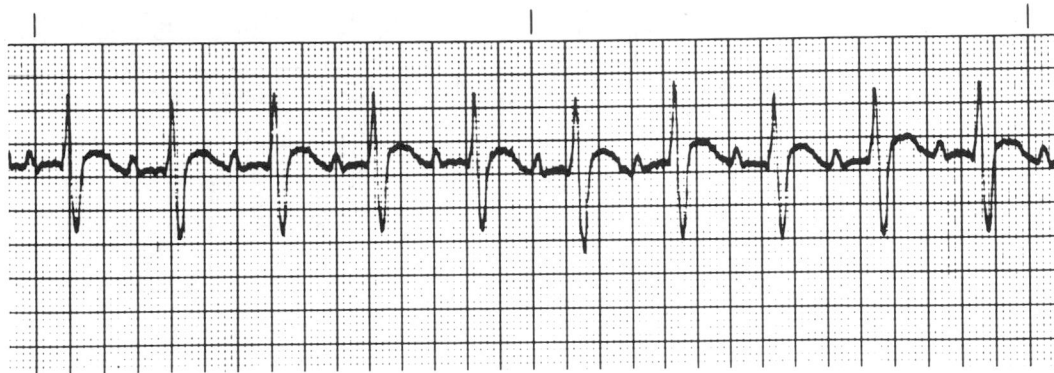

Fig. 32-18. First-degree heart block is diagnosed by the presence of a PR interval of longer than 0.21 second.

duction of some, but not all, of the atrial impulses to the AV node and into the Purkinje system. It is further subdivided into two specific types.[59] Mobitz type 1, or Wenckebach block, is characterized by progressive lengthening of the PR interval until an impulse is not conducted and the beat is dropped (Fig. 32-19). This form of block is relatively benign and often reversible and does not require a pacemaker. It may be caused by digitalis toxicity or myocardial infarction and is usually transient in nature. The Mobitz type 1 block reflects disease of the AV node. The other form of second-degree heart block is a Mobitz type 2 block, which reflects disease of the bundle of His Purkinje tissues. In this, the less common and more serious form of second-degree heart block, dropped beats occur without any progressive lengthening of the PR interval. This type of block has a serious prognosis, since it frequently progresses to complete heart block and may require pacemaker insertion prior to major surgical procedures (Fig. 32-20).

Third-degree AV block, also called complete heart block, occurs when all electrical activity from the atria fails to progress into the Purkinje system. The atrial and ventricular contractions have no relationship to each other, although each can regularly contract. The ventricular rate will be approximately 40 beats/min. The QRS complex may be normal if the pacemaker site is in the AV node, but it is usually widened to longer than 0.12 second when the pacemaker site is located in the ventricle. The heart rate is usually too slow to maintain adequate cardiac output, and syncope or Adams-Stokes syndrome may occur, as well as heart failure. These patients usually require insertion of either a transvenous endocardial or epicardial pacemaker to increase their heart rate and cardiac output (Fig. 32-21).

The third type of block is an intraventricular conduction disturbance, which is usually classified as either a left bundle branch block (LBBB), RBBB, or hemiblock.

The LBBB is the most serious of these conduction disturbances. Impulses reach the ventricles exclusively through the right bundle branch, hence the wide QRS complex of more than 0.12 second and a wide-notched R wave in leads I, aVL, and V_6. The most important leads to study in bundle branch blocks are I, V_1, and V_6. The pattern of LBBB in V_6 is similar to left ventricular (LV) hypertrophy, but exaggerated. An LBBB pattern is always associated with significant cardiac disease (Fig. 32-22).

In an RBBB, the QRS complex exceeds 0.11 second and leads V_1 to V_3 have broad rSR' complexes, while leads I and V_6 have wide S waves. An RBBB may be of no clinical significance, as opposed to the LBBB. However, it is frequently associated with chronic lung disease or atrial septal defects (Fig. 32-23).

Hemiblock is a term used when one of two divisions of the left bundle is blocked, since if both divisions are blocked a complete LBBB exists. Even though hemiblocks are a form of intraventricular block, the QRS complex is not prolonged. Marriott's[60] criteria for left anterior hemiblock are as follows (Fig. 32-24): (1) left axis deviation (usually −60 degrees); (2) small Q in lead I and aVL and small R in II, III, and aVF; (3) a normal QRS duration; (4) a late intrinsicoid deflection in aVL (>0.045 second); and (5) an increased QRS voltage in

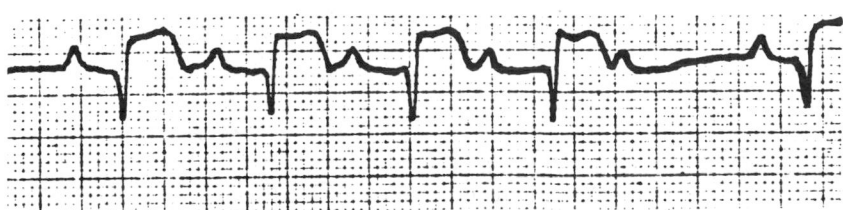

Fig. 32-19. Mobitz type 1 (or Wenckebach) block is diagnosed by the progressive lengthening of the PR interval until an impulse is not conducted and a dropped beat occurs.

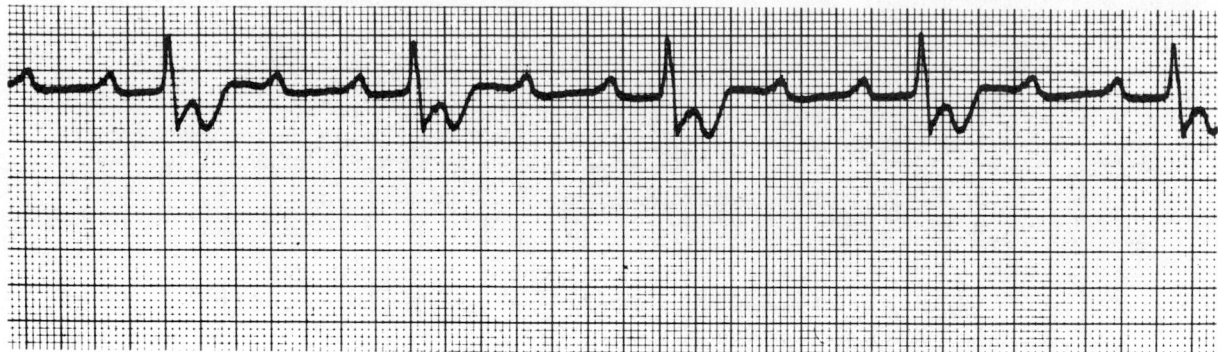

Fig. 32-20. Mobitz type 2 second-degree heart block is demonstrated in which dropped beats occur without a progressive lengthening of the PR interval.

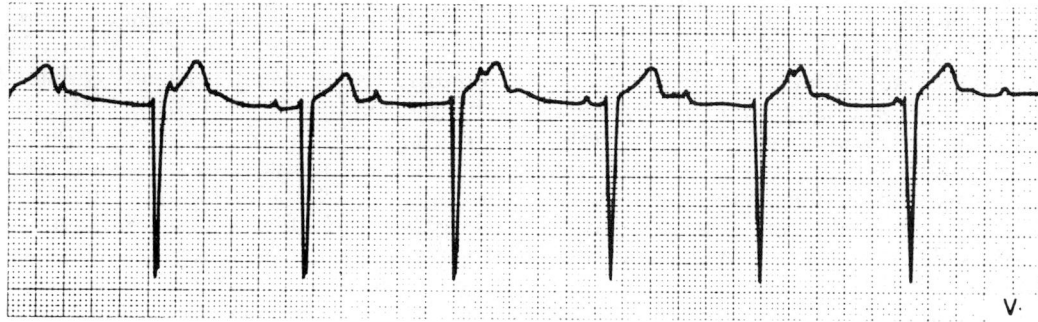

Fig. 32-21. Complete, or third-degree, heart block is diagnosed by the total dissociation between the atrial and the ventricular complexes with a ventricular rate of about 40 beats/min.

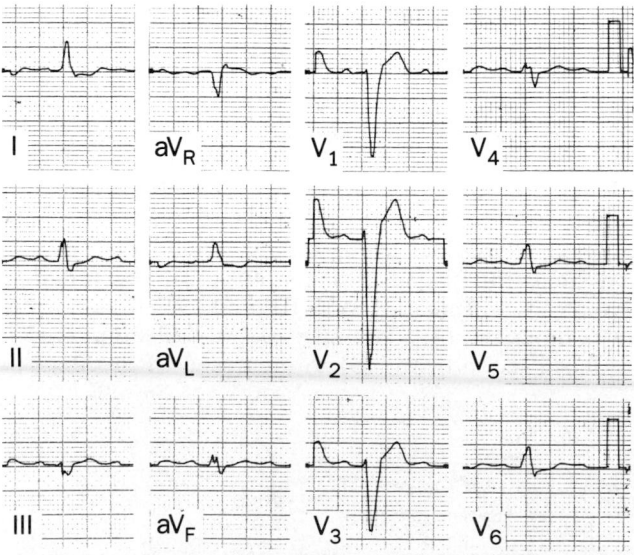

Fig. 32-22. Left bundle branch block. Note the rS pattern in V_1 and the notched rR′ pattern in V_6. In V_5 and V_6 a moderate depression of the ST segment is noted. (From Thys and Kaplan,[3] with permission.)

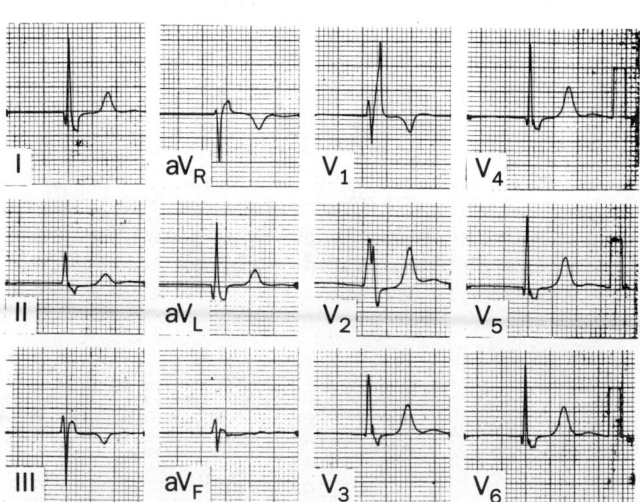

Fig. 32-23. Right bundle branch block. Note the rSR′ pattern in V_1 with slurring of R′ reflecting late right ventricular depolarization. (From Thys and Kaplan,[3] with permission.)

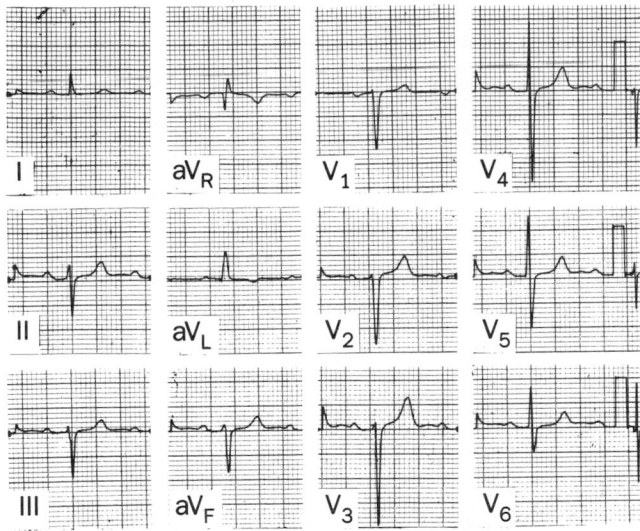

Fig. 32-24. Left anterior hemiblock. Note the left axis deviation and the terminal S in the inferior leads. (From Thys and Kaplan,[3] with permission.)

limb leads. By contrast, the criteria for a left posterior hemiblock are as follows (Fig. 32-25): (1) right axis deviation (usually +120 degrees); (2) small R in leads I and aVL, and small Q in II, III, and aVF; (3) a normal QRS duration; (4) a late intrinsicoid deflection in aVF (>0.045 second); (5) an increased QRS voltage in limb leads; and (6) no evidence of RV hypertrophy. The hemiblocks can occur by themselves but are often associated with an RBBB to form a bilateral bundle branch block. Patients with RBBB and a left anterior hemiblock progress to complete heart block only 10 percent of the time, while patients with RBBB and a left posterior hemiblock usually proceed to complete heart block (Figs. 32-26 and 32-27).

Trifascicular blocks are usually said to consist of one of the above bilateral bundle branch blocks (i.e., RBBB plus a left fascicular block) in addition to a prolonged PR interval (Fig. 32-28). As above, bundle of His electrograms would be necessary to determine whether the AV conduction disturbance was in fact localized in the AV node or whether it was distal, possibly representing an incomplete fascicular block in the last remaining fascicle.

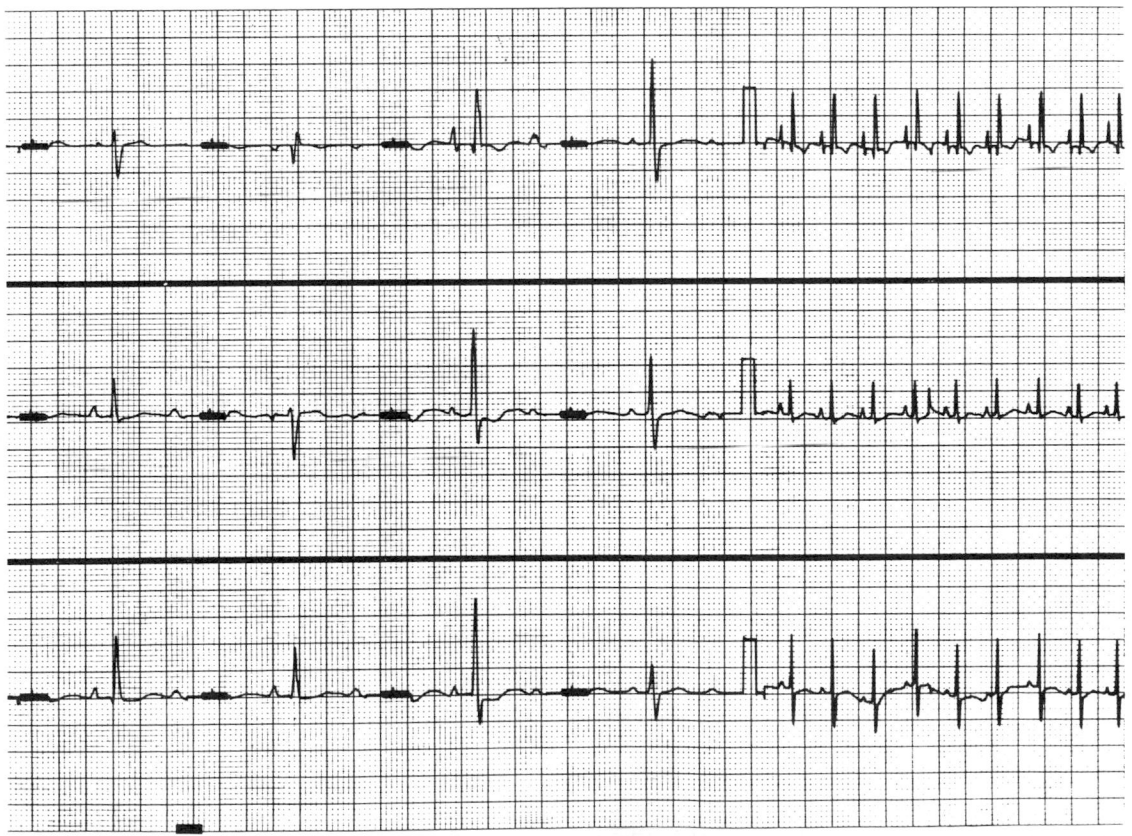

Fig. 32-25. Left posterior hemiblock in association with biatrial enlargement and nonspecific ST- and T-wave abnormalities.

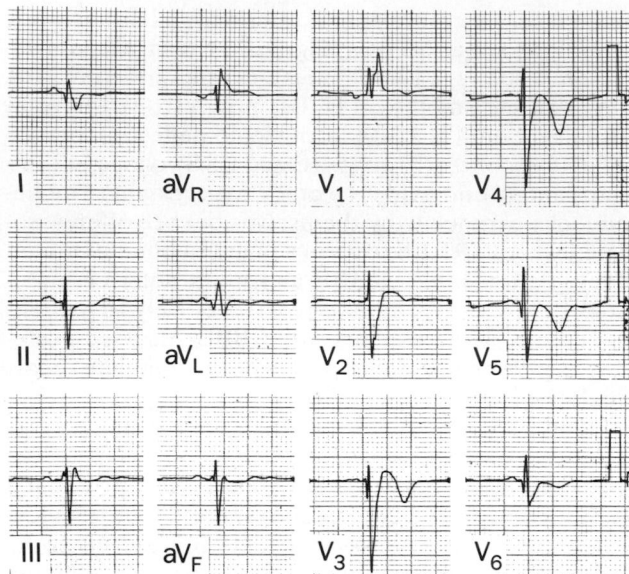

Fig. 32-26. Right bundle branch block with left anterior hemiblock. Note the RsR′ pattern in V_1 and the wide S in the lateral leads. The axis of the initial QRS vector is −88 degrees. (From Thys and Kaplan,[3] with permission.)

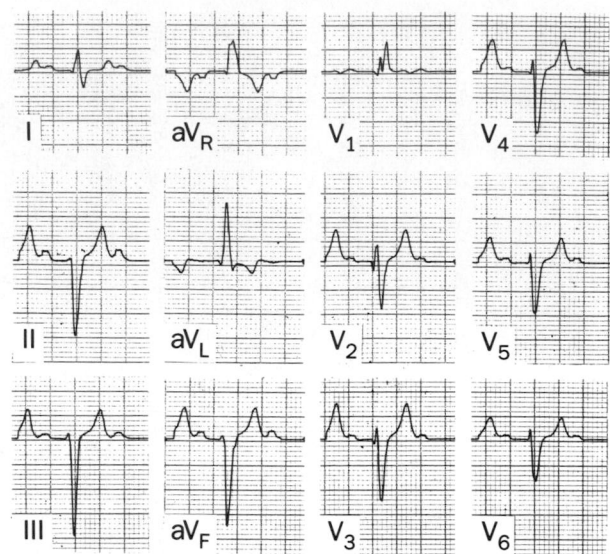

Fig. 32-28. Trifascular block. The PR interval is 232 ms and a right bundle branch block is noted. The axis of the QRS vector is −85 degrees, indicating a left anterior hemiblock. (From Thys and Kaplan,[3] with permission.)

MYOCARDIAL ISCHEMIA

Factors Predisposing to the Development of Ischemia

It is important to identify those factors that may cause perioperative ischemia and myocardial infarction to define appropriate measures for their prevention and treatment. The presence of pre-existing coronary artery disease (CAD) is a major risk factor for the subsequent

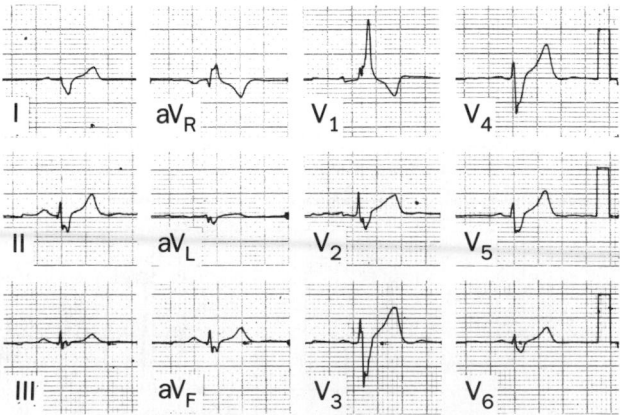

Fig. 32-27. Right bundle branch block with left posterior hemiblock. Note the wide S in the lateral leads and the rR′ pattern in V_1. The axis of the initial QRS vector is +166 degrees. (From Thys and Kaplan,[3] with permission.)

development of perioperative ischemia.[61] Coriat et al.[62] found that patients with disabling angina (class III and IV) had the highest incidence of myocardial ischemia. Many groups have studied the incidence of perioperative myocardial infarction in patients with CAD with or without previous coronary artery bypass grafting (CABG).[63] Patients without prior CABG who developed perioperative infarction usually had three-vessel CAD. The infarction rate in the CABG group has been very low, supporting the protective effect of prior CABG before noncardiac surgery.

Anesthesia, especially during induction, periods of surgical stress, and emergence, may produce adverse hemodynamic changes that affect the myocardial oxygen balance. Hypertension and tachycardia during intubation may produce myocardial ischemia in healthy patients[64] and in those with CAD.[65] Intraoperative hypotension in patients with ischemic heart disease has been associated with the development of postoperative ECG changes and postoperative infarction in patients with preoperative myocardial infarction.[66] Rao et al.[66] found a higher incidence of reinfarction in patients who developed episodes of intraoperative hypotension or hypertension (with or without tachycardia). Slogoff and Keats[61] found that tachycardia (heart rate over 100 beats/min), but not hypotension or hypertension, correlated best with myocardial ischemia and infarction.

Although the concept is attractive that a particular anesthetic technique may affect the incidence of perioperative myocardial ischemia and infarction, numerous studies have failed to demonstrate any benefits of different anesthetic regimens.[66,67] In the prospective study conducted by Rao et al.,[66] patients receiving nitrous oxide, oxygen, a muscle relaxant, and a narcotic had a higher incidence of infarction compared with those receiving other anesthetic drugs, but for no apparent reason. However, the pitfalls of subjecting such data to multiple retrospective analysis has thrown some doubt on these findings.[68] The retrospective study by Steen et al.[67] included two groups of patients who had transurethral resections of the prostate under either general (50 patients) or spinal (44 patients) anesthesia. The incidence of perioperative myocardial infarction was similar in both groups, and it appears that regional or general anesthesia is equally safe if properly conducted with maintenance of normal hemodynamic parameters.

The effect of the type and duration of surgery on the development of perioperative infarction and ischemia has also been extensively studied. Several studies have demonstrated an increased risk of reinfarction after intrathoracic or abdominal surgery.[66,67] Rao et al.[66] showed that surgery longer than 4 hours increased the incidence of reinfarction in the retrospective group but had no influence on the prospective group of patients. This finding may reflect the advantages of intensive hemodynamic monitoring with prompt treatment of hemodynamic aberrations during prolonged surgery, which may be associated with major physiologic and hemodynamic changes.

ECG Lead Systems for the Detection of Ischemia

The ECG was originally used in the operating room to diagnose rhythm disturbances. For this purpose, standard limb lead II was used, since its axis paralleled the electrical axis of the heart, thereby producing a large P-wave deflection. However, it has long been known that the precordial leads are superior to the standard leads for the detection of myocardial ischemia.[69] With the development of the exercise ECG test for the detection of latent coronary insufficiency, many lead systems were introduced for simplicity and good performance during muscular effort. In a comparative study of different chest lead configurations, Blackburn[69] found that for the detection of ischemia the most sensitive exploring electrode position was at the V_5 position. Furthermore, of all the lead configurations tested, the CM_5 lead was superior for the detection of significant ischemia and least affected by variations in body build, electrical frontal plane position, and noise. However, these results were not confirmed in another study of postexercise ECG testing utilizing visual and computerized techniques.[70] ST-segment depression and slope were compared by using standard lead V_5 and the bipolar leads CM_5 and CC_5 in two groups of subjects, one with known CAD and one without. Lead CM_5 was found to be less sensitive than V_5 for the detection of ischemia, and lead CC_5 was more comparable to V_5. Both bipolar leads were less affected by noise than standard lead V_5.

Dalton[71] reported use of lead V_5 monitoring during cardiac surgery by attaching the exploring precordial lead to a sterile spinal needle inserted subcutaneously after skin preparation. Kaplan and King[11] first demonstrated the value of monitoring lead V_5 with a modern multilead system during both cardiac and noncardiac surgery. These investigators were able to monitor leads I, II, II, aVR, aVL, aVF, and V_5 using a five-wire system and demonstrated that significant ST-segment depression in V_5 could occur in the absence of any changes in the standard leads.

In 1976, Kaplan[11] recommended that a five-electrode ECG system be used during all cardiac surgery. Four disposable ECG pads are placed on the extremities, with a fifth pad placed in the V_5 position and covered with Steri-drape. The electrodes are positioned before the induction of the anesthesia, and the V_5 electrode is included in the skin preparation without detrimental effect on the ECG tracing. Standard and augmented limb leads can be displayed in addition to lead V_5 by using an ECG monitor with a lead selector switch. Before surgery, all seven leads are displayed and recorded to serve as a baseline reference. During induction of anesthesia and surgery, leads II and V_5 can be displayed simultaneously to monitor anterior and inferior ischemic changes, respectively.

Many operating room ECG monitors are equipped with a three-electrode system and therefore are unable to monitor a true lead V_5. Modified bipolar lead CM_5 or CS_5 can be employed in this case, as described above. Although the comparability of ST-segment changes obtained with various bipolar leads and those recorded with a true V_5 lead during stress testing is disputed,[70] any of these leads is satisfactory during anesthesia[72] (Fig. 32-29). Blackburn[69] showed that 89 percent of significant ST-segment depression after exercise was found in precordial lead V_5 of a 12-lead ECG. Further-

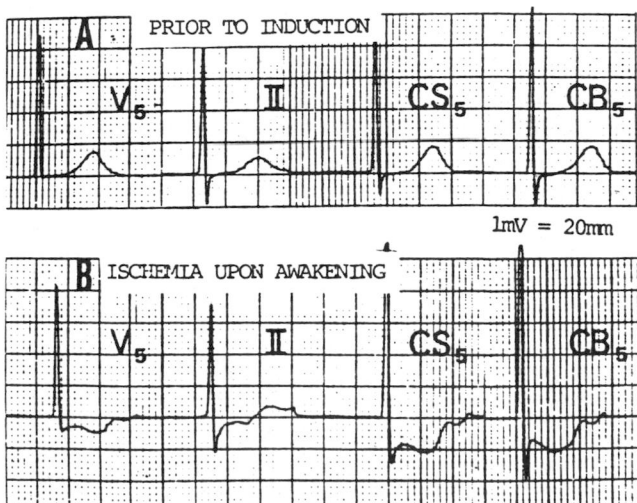

Fig. 32-29. Leads V_5, II, CS_5, and CB_5 during surgery. **(A)** Prior to ischemia. **(B)** During ischemia. (From Thys and Kaplan,[3] with permission.)

more, Blackburn[69] showed that 100 percent of the ST-segment changes could be detected by recording leads II, aVF, and anterior precordial leads V_3 to V_6. Mason et al.[73] demonstrated the value of multiple-lead ECG recording during and after exercise. Nineteen of 67 patients with angina showed a positive test in only one lead. Overall, 30 patients showed anterior ischemia (leads I and V_3 to V_6), and 8 showed inferior ischemia (leads II, III, and aVF). Multiple-lead ECGs are usually not used during anesthesia for routine monitoring since the anesthesiologist may not be able to assimilate the amount of information provided by the continuous simultaneous display of 12 ECG leads. Nonetheless, especially in high-risk cases, the anterior, inferior, and posterior surfaces of the heart should be monitored for the development of ischemia. The inferior surface of the heart overlies the diaphragm, and ischemia is seen in leads II, III, and aVF. Lead II is most often used to detect inferior ischemia, which may remain undetected if only anterior leads are employed,[74] since it is also helpful in detecting rhythm problems. Recently, London et al.[75] showed that leads V_5, V_4, and II showed the highest incidence of ischemia during surgery. Unfortunately, current operating room monitors cannot measure leads V_4 and V_5 simultaneously. Thus, the best routine lead combinations are still V_5 and II, CS_5 and II, or CB_5.

True posterior or right-sided ischemia may not be detected by leads looking at the inferior or the anterolateral surface of the heart. Anatomically, the posterior wall of the left ventricle lies adjacent to the esophagus. An esophageal ECG lead inserted 40 to 50 cm into the esophagus will reflect the electrical potential of the posterior surface of the heart and, therefore, may be used for the detection of posterior myocardial ischemia and infarction.[24,76]

Analysis of the ST Segment

The patterns of ST-segment change that fulfill the criteria of myocardial ischemia have been extensively studied in subjects with and without CAD undergoing exercise stress testing in the laboratory. Since anesthesia and surgery may be regarded as a potentially stressful situation, these criteria may be applied to anesthetized patients.

For the accurate diagnosis of ischemia, a knowledge of the normal morphology of the ST segment and the response to exercise is essential. The J point is the junction between the S wave and the ST segment. Exercise causes a downward displacement of the J point, such that the baseline is depressed below the isoelectric line in the resting tracing. The ST segment normally becomes upsloping and slightly concave and returns to the baseline (PR junction) within 0.04 to 0.06 second after the J point. J-point depression with an upsloping ST segment may be the earliest indication of myocardial ischemia. Stuart and Ellestad[77] concluded that an upsloping ST segment was indicative of ischemia if the

ST segment was depressed at least 2.0 mm below the baseline of the PR segment at 0.08 second from the J point (Fig. 32-30). With ongoing ischemia, the J-point depression evolves into progressive horizontal depression of the ST segment. Significant myocardial ischemia is present when there is greater than 1 mm of ST-segment depression measured 0.06 second from the J point.[78] The ST-segment depression may be convex in form or downsloping. The magnitude of ST-segment depression correlates with the amount of myocardium involved and the extent that is made ischemic. There is also a relationship between the severity of CAD and the ST-segment configuration induced. Robb and Marks[79] were able to demonstrate an increased mortality and worse prognosis for patients with downsloping ST-segment depression compared with horizontal depression. Goldshlager et al.[80] compared ST-segment depression with extent of disease as demonstrated by coronary angiography and found a correlation between downsloping ST-segment depression and increasing number of diseased vessels. Downsloping ST-segment depression represents profound myocardial ischemia and possibly even transmural ischemia. ST-segment elevation greater than 1 mm is also indicative of severe transmural ischemia. When ST-segment elevation occurs in the absence of any obvious hemodynamic or rhythm disturbances, coronary artery spasm (Prinzmetal's angina) should be suspected as the cause of the myocardial ischemia.

Intraoperative Analysis of the ST Segment

For the accurate evaluation of ST-segment changes, the ECG monitor should be properly calibrated before use so that a signal of 1 mV will produce a vertical deflection of 10 mm. It is also important that the ECG signal displayed on the oscilloscope be an accurate representation of the true signal. This becomes a major consideration when the ST segment is subject to computer analysis. Many of the oscilloscopes currently used in the operating room can distort the ST segment and T wave of the ECG. This is largely the result of electronic filtering circuits used to remove artifacts from the ECG, such as baseline wandering and 60-cycle interference. The lower end of the normal frequency response of the ECG is 0.14 cycles/s, below which electrical signals are attenuated by low-frequency filters. On some monitors, this filter may be selected as the diagnostic mode and should be used to evaluate ST-segment changes. However, in this mode the ECG is very susceptible to baseline wandering caused by respiration, movement, or electrode artifact. The baseline may be stabilized by further filtering of low-frequency signals up to 4 cycles/s in the monitor mode. Unfortunately, the addition of more filtration may cause spurious shifts in the ST segment owing to the absence of the usual low-frequency components.[51,52] An isoelectric ST segment may become elevated or depressed, resembling ischemia (Fig. 32-31). Moreover, elevated or depressed ST

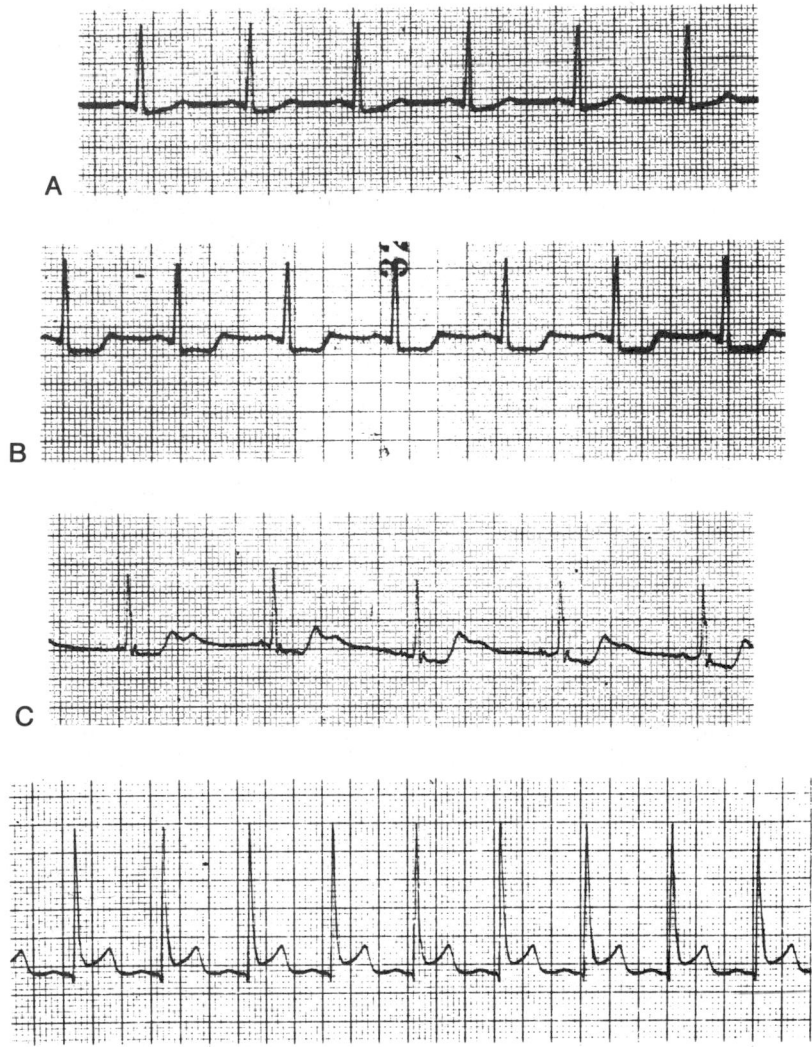

Fig. 32-30. Significant myocardial ischemia is defined as > 1 mm of horizontal or downsloping ST-segment depression, or as an ST-segment elevation > 1 mm. ST-segment changes of myocardial ischemia are demonstrated. **(A)** J-point depression and upsloping ST-segment depression of possible ischemia. **(B)** Horizontal ST-segment depression of ischemia. **(C)** Downsloping ST-segment depression of ischemia. **(D)** ST-segment elevation of ischemia.

segments may be shifted toward the isoelectric line, effectively masking ongoing ischemia.

Computer analysis was first applied to stress testing as an alternative to close scrutiny of tracings that may inevitably introduce an element of human error. Accurate computer analysis of changes in ST-segment configuration depends on selection of ECG complexes that are unaffected by artifact. Development of computer averaging techniques over several beats with the rejection of ectopic beats has reduced the amount of random noise and enabled studies of the ECG during and after graded exercise.[81] Computer analysis of the ECG has also established precise numerical measurements for the objective ECG diagnosis of ischemia.[82]

The technology of computerized segment monitoring is equally applicable to conscious and anesthetized patients. Roy et al.[83] first described the use of a computerized exercise testing system to detect ischemia during anesthesia. During induction, leads V_4, V_5, and V_6 were continuously recorded on paper; for the remainder of the procedure, leads V_5 and II were continuously displayed and leads II, aVF, V_3, V_4, V_5, and V_6 were recorded on paper every 3 minutes. The diagnosis of ischemia was aided by a continuous digital readout of the magnitude of ST-segment depression and an averaged picture of the last 16 QRST complexes in lead V_5. Every 20 minutes, a written histogram retrospectively demonstrated the amount of ST-segment displacement over 1-minute intervals.

Kotrly et al.[84] reported the use of a modified microcomputer-based ECG that displayed, as a trend line, the summed ST-segment deviations from the isoelectric

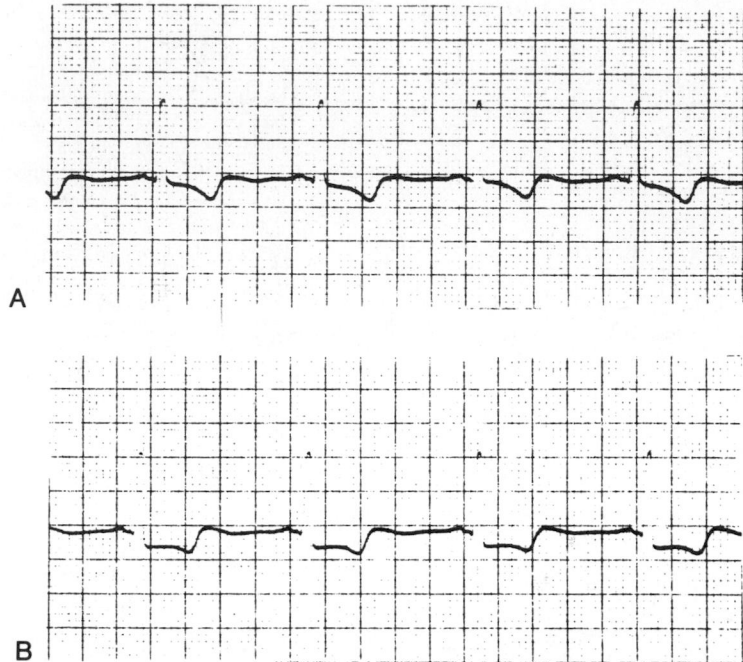

Fig. 32-31. An artifact on the ECG can be demonstrated by switching from the diagnostic filter mode (**A**) to the monitoring filter mode (**B**). Significant changes in the ST segments can be produced by altering these filters, as demonstrated.

line in leads V_5, aVF, and $-V_1$. The trend line is continuously displayed for 20 minutes and thereafter may be retained in hard-copy form. In addition, the three ECG complexes can be electronically stored every 10 minutes. The ST-segment analyzer has been recently updated and currently analyzes leads I, II, and V_5.

Holter monitoring has been utilized by a number of investigators to document the perioperative incidence of dysrhythmias and ischemia. In Holter monitoring, ECG information from one or two bipolar leads is recorded by a miniature magnetic tape recorder. Up to 48 hours of ECG signals can be collected. Subsequently, the tape is processed by a playback system and the ECG signals are analyzed. On most modern systems, the playback unit includes a dedicated computer for rapid analysis of the data and automatic recognition of arrhythmias.

Although one of Holter's initial publications[85] described the recording of ST-T changes during an anginal attack, the use of this method for the recording of ischemic changes has not been widely applied. Particularly, in the early days of Holter monitoring, a number of authors voiced their concern about the reliability of this technique for the recognition of ST-segment changes. One of the reasons was that on early instruments narrow bandwidth recordings were utilized to eliminate artifacts and to provide a stable baseline. Since ST-segment changes often have a low frequency, the narrow bandwidth that stabilized the baseline produced considerable ST-segment distortion. The intro-

duction of frequency modulated (FM) recording systems partially solved this problem. Balasubramanian et al.,[86] comparing various recording systems, demonstrated the FM recorders were able to accurately detect ST-segment changes at rest and during exercise.

Bragg-Remschel et al.[87] studied the frequency response characteristics of ambulatory ECG-recording equipment from eight manufacturers. They established that none of the systems fully met the American Heart Association low-frequency and high-frequency response values and that only three systems were able to reproduce accurately the actual degree of ST depression, as well as provide flat ST-segment depression. Even FM systems did not always faithfully reproduce the ST segment. However, Tzivoni et al.[88] have recently compared ECG findings recorded simultaneously by two-lead Holter and 12-lead ECGs in 144 patients undergoing a Bruce protocol treadmill exercise test. The two exploring electrodes of the Holter system were attached to the V_3 and V_5 positions, while the two negative electrodes were placed at the right side of the upper sternum. They found that in 96 percent of the patients, the results of the two recording techniques were concordant and concluded that V_3, V_4, and V_5 Holter recordings were as accurate as 12-lead ECG systems for the detection of ischemic changes during exercise.

Intraoperatively, Coleman and Jordan[89] obtained continuous ECG recordings from 36 healthy patients undergoing elective general surgical procedures. They observed ST-segment changes around the time of induction and intubation in six of these patients, while two others exhibited ST-segment changes at the end of surgery. Coriat et al.,[90] studying 51 patients with ischemic heart disease undergoing vascular surgery, recorded ST-segment changes in 20 of these patients. The Holter recording was started 30 minutes before induction of anesthesia and lasted 24 hours. In 11 of the patients, the ischemic changes occurred during induction, while in two patients, they first appeared 2 hours after extubation.

In a different study, but with a similar group of patients, Coriat et al.[91] further observed that continuous administration of nitroglycerin did not prevent a high incidence of myocardial ischemia. They continuously monitored lead CM$_5$ for 24 hours and defined as an ischemic episode ST-segment depression greater than 1 mm lasting for more than 10 beats. Ischemic changes occurred in 18 of the 45 patients, but in only eight of these episodes were the changes detected by the anesthesiologist. Thomson et al.[92] used Holter monitoring of leads II and CS$_5$ to study ischemic changes in 20 patients undergoing CABG. They also observed a high incidence of myocardial ischemia and were unable to demonstrate a reduction in ischemic episodes with the prophylactic administration of nitroglycerin.

Most recently, the Q-Med continuous ECG monitoring system has been used in numerous studies to demonstrate a high incidence of myocardial ischemia preoperatively and postoperatively in patients undergoing both cardiac and noncardiac surgery.[75] The incidence of ischemia is much higher in the postoperative period than during the operation. Most episodes of ischemia before and after surgery have been shown to be silent and are only detectable by continuous ECG monitoring.

REFERENCES

1. Cannard TH, Dripps RD, Helwig J, et al: The ECG during anesthesia and surgery. Anesthesiology 21:194, 1960
2. Atlee JL: Perioperative Cardiac Dysrhythmias. Year Book Medical Publishers, Chicago, 1985
3. Thys D, Kaplan JA: The ECG in Anesthesia and Critical Care. Churchill Livingstone, New York, 1987
4. Hurst JW: The Heart. 6th Ed. McGraw-Hill, New York, 1986
5. Rooney S, Goldiner P, Muss E: Relationship of right bundle branch block and marked left axis deviation to complete heart block during general anesthesia. Anesthesiology 44:64, 1976
6. Vitez TS, Soper E, Wong KC, Soper PG: Chronic hypokalemia and intraoperative dysrhythmias. Anesthesiology 63:130, 1985
7. Spodick DH: Acute pericardial tamponade, pathologic physiology, diagnosis and management. Prog Cardiovasc Dis 10:64, 1967
8. Detrano R, Froelicher VF: Exercise testing: Uses and limitations. Prog Cardiovasc Dis 31:173, 1988
9. Kennedy HL, Wiens RD: Ambulatory electrocardiography and myocardial ischemia. Am Heart J 117:164, 1989
10. Katz RL, Bigger JT: Cardiac arrhythmias during anesthesia and operation. Anesthesiology 33:193, 1970
11. Kaplan JA, King SB: The precordial electrocardiographic lead (V$_5$) in patients who have coronary artery disease. Anesthesiology 45:570, 1976
12. Edwards R, Winnie AL, Ramamurthy S: Acute hypocapnic hypokalemia: An iatrogenic anesthetic complication. Anesth Analg 56:786, 1977
13. Atlee J: Pacemakers and cardioversion. p. 855. In Kaplan JA (ed): Cardiac Anesthesia. 2nd Ed. Grune & Stratton, Orlando, FL, 1987
14. Angelini L, Feldman MI, Lufschonowski R, et al: Cardiac arrhythmias during and after heart surgery: Diagnosis and management. Prog Cardiovasc Dis 16:469, 1974
15. Kennedy FB, Ticzon AR, Duffy FC, et al: Disappearance of ECG pattern of inferior wall myocardial infarction after aortocoronary bypass surgery. J Thorac Cardiovasc Surg 74:585, 1977
16. Kotter GS, Kotrly KJ, Kalbfleisch JH, et al: Myocardial ischemia during cardiovascular surgery as detected by an ST segment trend monitorial system. J Cardiothorac Anesth 1:190, 1987
17. Arbeit SR, Rubin IL, Gross H: Dangers in interpreting the ECG from the oscilloscope monitor. JAMA 211:453, 1970
18. Borrello G: ECG artifacts simulating atrial flutter. JAMA 223:439, 1973
19. Doss JD, McCabe CW, Weiss GK: Noise free ECG data during electrosurgical procedures. Anesth Analg 52:156, 1973
20. Goldberg E: Mechanical factors and the ECG. Am Heart J 93:629, 1977
21. Voukydis PC: Effect of intracardiac blood on the ECG. N Engl J Med 291:612, 1974
22. Froelicher VF, Wolthius R, Kelser N, et al: A comparison of two bipolar exercise ECG leads to lead V$_5$. Chest 70:611, 1976
23. Bazaral MG, Norfleet EA: Comparison of CB$_5$ and V$_5$ leads for intraoperative electrocardiographic monitoring. Anesth Analg 60:849, 1981
24. Kates RA, Zaidan JR, Kaplan JA: Esophageal lead for intraoperative electrocardiographic monitoring. Anesth Analg 61:781, 1982
25. Lichtenthal PR, Wade L, Collins JT: Multipurpose pulmonary artery catheter. Ann Thorac Surg 36:493, 1983
26. Trankina MF, White RD: Perioperative cardiac pacing using an atrioventricular pacing pulmonary artery catheter. J Cardiothorac Anesth 3:154, 1989
27. Kurtz CM, Bennett JH, Shapiro HH: ECG studies during surgical anesthesia. JAMA 106:434, 1936
28. Bertrand CA, Steiner NV, Jameson AG, et al: Disturbances of cardiac rhythm during anesthesia and surgery. JAMA 216, 1615, 1971
29. Atlee JL, Rusy BF: Ventricular conduction times and AV nodal conductivity during enflurane anesthesia in dogs. Anesthesiology 47:498, 1977
30. Koehntop DE, Liao JC, Van Bergen FH: Effects of pharmacologic alterations of adrenergic mechanisms by cocaine, tropolone, aminophylline, and ketamine on epinephrine-induced arrhythmias during halothane-nitrous oxide anesthesia. Anesthesiology 46:83, 1977
31. Fox EJ, Sklar GS, Hill CH, et al: Complications related to the pressor response to endotracheal intubation. Anesthesiology 47:524, 1977
32. Smith M, Ray CT: Cardiac arrhythmias, increased intracranial pressure, and the autonomic nervous system. Chest 61:125, 1972
33. Alexander JP: Dysrhythmia and oral surgery. Br J Anesth 43:773, 1971
34. Manos J, Thys DM: A practical approach to the detection of

dysrhythmias. p. 155. In Thys DM, Kaplan JA (ed): The ECG in Anesthesia and Critical Care. Churchill Livingstone, New York, 1987

35. Kuner J, Enescu V, Utsu F, et al: Cardiac arrhythmias during anesthesia. Dis Chest 52:580, 1967

36. Kaplan JA, Dunbar RW, Bland JW, et al: Propranolol and cardiac surgery: A problem for the anesthesiologist? Anesth Analg 54:571, 1975

37. Slapa WJ: The sick sinus syndrome. Am Heart J 92:648, 1976

38. Moe GK, Mendez C: Physiologic basis of premature beats and sustained tachycardia. N Engl J Med 288:250, 1973

39. Jones RM, Broadbeht MP, Adams AB: Anaesthetic considerations in patients with paroxysmal supraventricular tachycardia. Anaesthesia 39:307, 1984

40. Sprague DH, Mandel SD: Paroxysmal supraventricular tachycardia during anesthesia. Anesthesiology 46:75, 1977

41. Chung EK: Tachyarrhythmias in Wolff-Parkinson-White syndrome: Antiarrhythmia therapy. JAMA 237:376, 1977

42. Rinkenberger RL, Prystowsky EN, Heger JJ: Effects of intravenous and chronic oral verapamil administration in patients with supraventricular tachyarrhythmias. Circulation 62:996, 1980

43. Morganroth J, Horowitz L, Anderson J, et al: Comparative efficacy and tolerance of esmolol to propanolol for control of supraventricular tachyarrhythmias. Am J Cardiol 56:33F, 1985

44. Zipes DP: Specific arrhythmias, diagnosis and treatment. p. 709. In Braunwald E (ed): Heart Disease. WB Saunders, Philadelphia, 1984

45. Escher DJW, Furman S: Emergency treatment of cardiac arrhythmias: Emphasis on use of electrical pacing. JAMA 214:2028, 1970

46. Kleiger RE: Cardioversion of paroxysmal arrhythmias. JAMA 213:107, 1970

47. Glassman E: Direct current cardioversion. Am Heart J 82:128, 1971

48. Camm J, Ward D, Spunell R: Response of atrial flutter to overdrive atrial pacing and intravenous disopyramide phosphate, singly and in combination. Br Heart J 44:240, 1980

49. Michaelson EL, Porterfield JK, Das G, et al: A comparison of esmolol and verapamil in the treatment of atrial fibrillation/flutter. J Am Coll Cardiol 7:157A, 1986

50. Scherlag BJ, Lazzara R, Helfant RH: Differentiation of "AV junctional rhythms." Circulation 48:304, 1973

51. Haldemann G, Schoer H: Haemodynamic effects of transient atrioventricular dissociation in general anesthesia. Br J Anaesth 44:159, 1972

52. Galindo A, Wyte SR, Wetherhold JW: Junctional rhythm induced by halothane anesthesia—treatment with succinylcholine. Anesthesiology 37:261, 1972

53. Hill R: Treatment of isorhythmic A-V dissociation during general anesthesia with propranolol. Anesthesiology 70:141, 1989

54. Cranefield PF: Ventricular fibrillation. N Engl J Med 289:732, 1973

55. Pietras RJ, Mautner R, Denes P, et al: Chronic recurrent right and left ventricular tachycardia: Comparison of clinical, hemodynamic and angiographic findings. Am J Cardiol 40:32, 1977

56. Geddes LA, Tacker WA, Rosborough J, et al: The electrical doses for ventricular defibrillation with electrodes applied directly to the heart. J Thorac Cardiovasc Surg 68:593, 1974

57. Hecht HH, Kossman EC, Childers RW, et al: Atrioventricular and intraventricular conduction: Revised nomenclature and concepts. Am J Cardiol 31:232, 1973

58. Kastor JA: Atrioventricular block. N Engl J Med 292:462, 572, 1976

59. Wynands JE: Anesthesia for patients with heart block and artificial cardiac pacemakers. Anesth Analg 55:626, 1976

60. Marriott HJL: Practical Electrocardiography. 7th Ed. Williams & Wilkins, Baltimore, 1983

61. Slogoff S, Keats AS: Does perioperative myocardial ischemia lead to postoperative myocardial infarction? Anesthesiology 62:107, 1985

62. Coriat P, Harari A, Daloz M, Viars P: Clinical predictors of intraoperative myocardial ischemia in patients with coronary artery disease undergoing non-cardiac surgery. Acta Anaesthesiol Scand 26:287, 1982

63. Crutchley P, Kaplan JA, Hug CC, et al: Non-cardiac surgery in patients with prior myocardial revascularization. Can Anaesth Soc J 30:629, 1983

64. Kaplan JA: Cardiac Anesthesia. 2nd Ed. Grune & Stratton, Orlando, FL, 1987

65. Roy WL, Edelist G, Gilbert B: Myocardial ischemia during non-cardiac surgical procedures in patients with coronary artery disease. Anesthesiology 51:393, 1979

66. Rao TLK, Jacobs KH, El-Etr AA: Reinfarction following anesthesia in patients with myocardial infarction. Anesthesiology 59:499, 1983

67. Steen PA, Tinker JH, Tarhan S: Myocardial reinfarction after anesthesia and surgery. JAMA 239:2566, 1978

68. Lowenstein E, Yusef S, Teplick R: Perioperative myocardial reinfarction: A glimmer of hope - a note of caution. Anesthesiology 59:493, 1983

69. Blackburn H: The exercise electrocardiogram: Technological, procedural, and conceptual development. In Blackburn H (ed): Measurements in Exercise Electrocardiography. Charles C Thomas, Springfield, IL, 1967

70. Fortuin NJ, Weiss JL: Exercise stress testing. Circulation 56:699, 1976

71. Dalton B: A precordial ECG lead for chest operations. Anesth Analg 55:740, 1976

72. Griffin RM, Kaplan JA: Comparison of ECG leads V$_5$, CS$_5$, CB$_5$, and II by computerized ST segment analysis. Anaesthesia 42:155, 1987

73. Mason RE, Likar I, Biern RO, Ross RS: Multiple lead electrocardiography. Circulation 36:517, 1967

74. Kistner JR, Miller ED, Epstein RM: More than V$_5$ is needed. Anesthesiology 47:75, 1977

75. London MJ, Hollenberg M, Wong MG, et al: Intraoperative myocardial ischemia: Localization by continuous 12-lead electrocardiography. Anesthesiology 69:232, 1988

76. Trager M, Feinberg BI, Kaplan JA: Right ventricular ischemia diagnosed by an esophageal ECG and right atrial tracing. J Cardiothorac Anesth 1:123, 1987

77. Stuart RJ, Ellestad MH: Upsloping ST segments in exercise stress testing. Am J Cardiol 37:19, 1976

78. Ellestad MH, Cooke BM, Greenberg PS: Stress testing: Clinical application and predictive capacity. Prog Cardiovasc Dis 21:431, 1979

79. Robb GP, Marks H: Post-exercise ECG in arteriosclerotic heart disease. JAMA 200:918, 1967

80. Goldshlager N, Selzer A, Cohn K: Treadmill stress tests as indicators of presence and severity of coronary artery disease. Ann Intern Med 85:277, 1976

81. Davies CT, Kitchin AH, Knibbs AV: Computer quantitation of ST segment response to graded exercise in untrained and trained normal subjects. Cardiovasc Res 5:201, 1971

82. Sheffield LT, Holt JH, Lester FM, et al: On-line analysis of the exercise ECG. Circulation 40:935, 1969

83. Roy WL, Edelist G, Gilbert B: Myocardial ischemia during non-cardiac surgical procedures in patients with coronary artery disease. Anesthesiology 51:393, 1979

84. Kotrly KJ, Kotter GS, Montana D, et al: Intraoperative detection of myocardial ischemia with an ST segment trend monitoring system. Anesth Analg 63:343, 1984

85. Holter NJ: New method for heart studies. Continuous electrocardiography of active subjects over long periods is now practical. Science 134:1214, 1961

86. Balasubramanian V, Lahini A, Green HL, et al: Ambulatory ST segment monitoring problems, pitfalls, solutions and clinical applications. Br Heart J 44:419, 1980

87. Bragg-Remschel DA, Anderson CM, Winkle RA: Frequency response characteristics of ambulatory ECG monitoring systems and their implications for ST segment analysis. Am Heart J 103:20, 1982

88. Tzivoni D, Benhorin J, Gavish A, et al: Holter recording during treadmill testing in assessing myocardial ischemic changes. Am J Cardiol 55:1200, 1985

89. Coleman AJ, Jordan C: Cardiovascular responses to anaesthesia. Influence of beta-adrenoreceptor blockade with metoprolol. Anaesthesia 35:972, 1980

90. Coriat P, Harari A, Daloz M, et al: Clinical predictors of intraoperative myocardial ischemia in patients with coronary artery disease undergoing non-cardiac surgery. Acta Anaesthesiol Scand 26:287, 1982

91. Coriat P, Daloz M, Bousseau D, et al: Prevention of intraoperative myocardial ischemia during noncardiac surgery with intravenous nitroglycerin. Anesthesiology 61:193, 1984

92. Thomson IR, Mutch WAC, Culligan JD: Failure of intravenous nitroglycerin to prevent intraoperative myocardial ischemia during fentanyl-pancuronium anesthesia. Anesthesiology 61:385, 1984

33

RESPIRATORY MONITORING

Richard E. Moon
Enrico M. Camporesi

INTRODUCTION

The *Oxford English Dictionary* defines a monitor as "something that reminds or gives warning." Another definition is "an instrument used to measure continuously or at intervals a condition that must be kept within prescribed limits."[2] If the discussion of monitors were to be confined to the latter definition, then perhaps only self-contained instruments (e.g., pulse oximeters) should be discussed in this chapter. However, a wider view is more appropriate. For example, intermittent, though not necessarily at fixed intervals, analysis of arterial blood gases is often an important monitor of a patient's condition. We will therefore discuss respiratory physiology as it applies to assessment of patient well-being as well as appropriate measures that may be either continuously or intermittently obtained.

Eichhorn et al.[3] outlined minimal recommended standards for patient monitoring during anesthesia at hospitals within Harvard Medical School. In addition to monitors of cardiovascular function and patient temperature, these authors suggested that mandatory respiratory monitors include methods of continuous monitoring of patient ventilation (including a breathing system disconnection monitor) and a monitor of oxygen concentration within the patient breathing system. A strong recommendation was made for monitoring end-tidal carbon dioxide concentrations. These recommendations should be considered as only minimal acceptable standards. More sophisticated monitoring is required in many instances, and new technology has allowed the development of useful monitors for the operating room, the intensive care unit, the hospital ward, and the home that are well outside the range of the Harvard standards.

The limited ability of human organ systems to metabolize anaerobically dictates a functioning transport system that can maintain oxygen delivery to peripheral tissues. The monitoring of one component of this system, the cardiovascular system, will be discussed in Chapter 31. This chapter will discuss the other component, the respiratory system, and the appropriate monitoring necessary to detect malfunction in its gas exchange properties and other conditions that may lead to impaired gas exchange.

GAS EXCHANGE
(Also See Ch. 15)

The major function of the lung is gas exchange: the addition of O_2 into blood and the elimination of CO_2 from blood. Because of the close relationship between the partial pressure of CO_2 in blood (PCO_2) and arterial (and hence tissue) pH it is important to ensure that arterial PCO_2 remain within an appropriate physiologic range. Adequate oxygen delivery must also be maintained. Figure 33-1 shows the O_2 cascade from atmospheric gas to the intracellular site of utilization. Assessment of the adequacy of this delivery system may be made at any step of the cascade. For example, common clinical practice dictates that arterial O_2 content (PaO_2) should be sufficient. One should generally aim to keep Hb-O_2 saturation ($SaO_2 > 90$ percent). This level is rea-

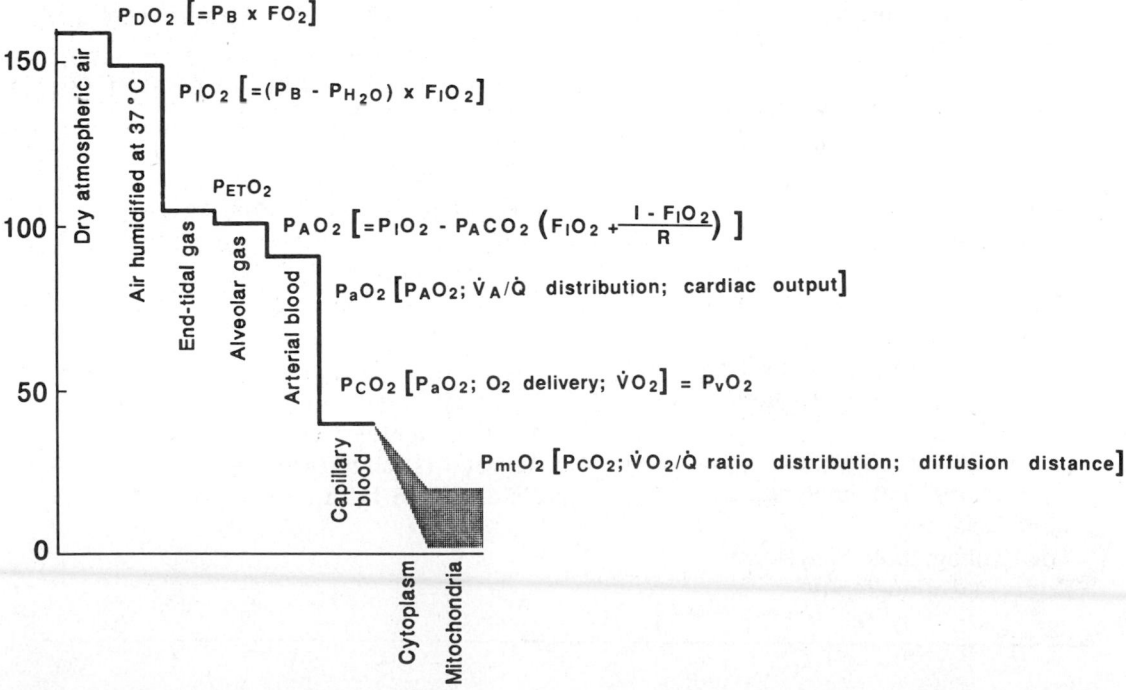

Fig. 33-1. Oxygen transport cascade. A schematic view of the steps in oxygen transport from the atmosphere to the site of utilization in the mitochondrium is shown here. Approximate PO_2 values are shown for each step in the cascade, and factors determining those partial pressures are shown within the square brackets. There is a distribution of tissue PO_2 values depending on local capillary blood flow, tissue oxygen consumption, and diffusion distances. Mitochondrial PO_2 values are depicted as a range because reported levels vary widely. (Adapted from Nunn,[4] with permission.)

sonable for two reasons: First, clinical experience supports the notion that maintenance of hemoglobin at 90 percent saturation with O_2 in the presence of adequate cardiac output will provide sufficient O_2 delivery to the tissues. Second, since the Hb-O_2 dissociation curve becomes abruptly steeper at O_2 saturation levels below 90 percent, further decreases in PaO_2 may result in sharp diminution of O_2 content and hence O_2 delivery.

Alveolar Gases

Before attempting to understand respiratory gas exchange monitoring it is imperative to understand the basis of gas exchange physiology. The lung consists of a heterogeneous collection of gas exchange units (alveoli), with a range of O_2 and CO_2 gas tensions. It is therefore totally erroneous to speak of *the* alveolar PO_2 or PCO_2. However, the concept of a homogeneous lung, in which all alveoli have the same gas tensions, is a useful one. The alveolar partial pressures calculated by using such a model may be thought of as averages for the O_2 and CO_2 partial pressures in the real (nonhomogeneous) lung. Equations for alveolar PO_2 and PCO_2 (PAO_2 and $PACO_2$) or alveolar gas equations are as follows:

$$PACO_2 = k \frac{\dot{V}CO_2}{\dot{V}A} \qquad (1)$$

$$PAO_2 = PIO_2 - PACO_2 \cdot \left[FIO_2 + \frac{1 - FIO_2}{R} \right] \qquad (2)$$

where

$\dot{V}O_2 = O_2$ consumption
$\dot{V}A = $ alveolar ventilation
$k = $ constant
$FIO_2 = $ fractional inspired O_2 concentration
$PIO_2 = $ inspired $PO_2 = (P\text{barometric} - PH_2O) \cdot FIO_2$
$R = $ respiratory quotient $= \dfrac{\dot{V}CO_2}{\dot{V}O_2}$ (usually ≈ 0.8)

The equation for $PACO_2$ is a function of only two variables. Since, in clinical medicine, $\dot{V}CO_2$ is relatively constant, $PACO_2$ is therefore mainly a function of alveolar ventilation to which it is inversely proportional. Since

$$\dot{V}A = \dot{V}E - \dot{V}D \qquad (3)$$

where:

$\dot{V}E = $ respiratory minute ventilation
$\dot{V}D = $ dead space ventilation

And since in fact, alveolar ventilation is usually a constant fraction of minute ventilation:

$$\dot{V}A = k' \cdot \dot{V}E \qquad (4)$$

The alveolar gas equation for CO_2 may be rewritten

$$PACO_2 \approx c \cdot \left[\frac{1}{\dot{V}E} \right] \qquad (5)$$

where $c = $ constant derived from k and k'.

This approximation may not hold if $\dot{V}CO_2$ is substantially elevated, for example, during a major motor seizure, shivering, or fever. $\dot{V}CO_2$ may decrease as a result of general anesthesia or hypothermia. $\dot{V}CO_2$ is altered by approximately 7 percent for each degree Celsius (°C) change in body temperature and may increase approximately threefold during violent shivering.

The alveolar gas equation for O_2 (equation [2]) can be examined to delineate the factors that will result in low alveolar PO_2. The major factors are

1. Low PIO_2.
   a. Decreased barometric pressure (high altitude).
   b. Breathing a gas mixture with FIO_2 less than 0.21.
2. Elevation in $PACO_2$, usually due to hypoventilation.
3. Changes in respiratory quotient (R) will also affect PAO_2 but only to a minor extent since the physiologic range of R is on the order of 0.7 to 1.2, the latter seen during metabolic acidosis.

Arterial Gases

The parameters that determine alveolar gas tension have been described. Additional factors that determine the gas tensions in arterial blood include the following:

1. Diffusion nonequilibrium
2. Ventilation/perfusion ($\dot{V}A/\dot{Q}$) mismatching
3. Right-to-left shunting

Diffusion nonequilibrium is the situation that would exist if the gas tensions in the pulmonary capillary erythrocyte ($Pc'O_2$, $Pc'CO_2$) are not equal to the alveolar gas tensions. This can occur under two physiologic conditions: either (1) increased pulmonary blood flow such that the erythrocyte does not have sufficient time in the alveoli to enable gas tensions to reach equilibrium, or (2) a thickening of the alveolar-capillary membrane such that the rate of diffusion of gas from alveolus to capillary or vice versa is slowed. For CO_2 diffusion nonequilibrium would result in arterial PCO_2 ($PaCO_2$) higher than $PACO_2$. For O_2 it would mean that PaO_2 would be less than PAO_2. In practice, there has never been any evidence for diffusion nonequilibrium of CO_2. Despite much discussion of O_2 diffusion nonequilibrium, it probably rarely exists in clinical medicine. There is evidence for its existence during moderate exercise in patients with interstitial fibrosis and in severe exercise in normal individuals, particularly at altitude.[5] In anesthesia it would probably occur only under very unusual circumstances, for example, a septic patient's breathing room air at the top of Pike's Peak (altitude 14,000 ft), a situation in which the high cardiac output due to sepsis might simulate exercise.

In order to understand the role of $\dot{V}A/\dot{Q}$ in determining arterial gas tensions it is necessary to discard the homogeneous lung model and consider a model with multiple parallel units of gas exchange and blood flow. The resulting arterial gas tension is determined by the mixing of different proportions of blood from each gas exchange unit. The gas tensions in each unit will de-

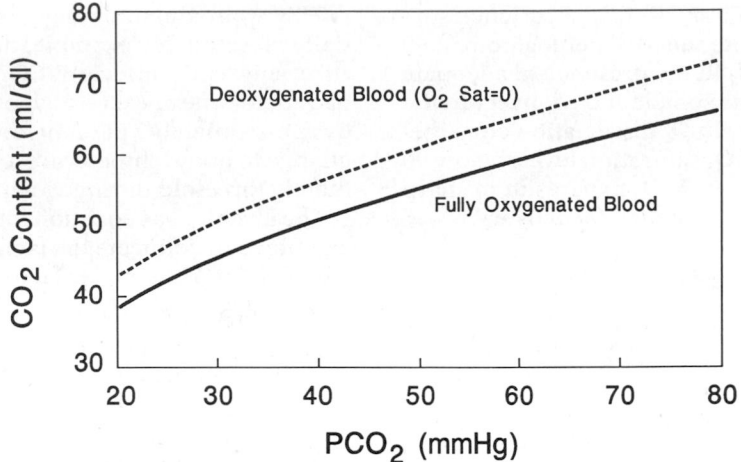

Fig. 33-2. CO_2 content of arterial blood as a function of PCO_2. For a given PCO_2 deoxygenated blood has a higher CO_2 content than oxygenated blood (Haldane effect). Unlike the $Hb\text{-}O_2$ saturation curve (Fig. 33-10) the CO_2 content curve has no plateau and in the clinically useful range can be approximated by a straight line. (Data from Christiensen et al.[6])

pend upon the regional ventilation, perfusion, and diffusion.

The effect of $\dot{V}_A/\dot{Q}$ mismatching on $PaCO_2$ is often erroneously assumed to be negligible. The CO_2-blood dissociation curve (Fig. 33-2) is a monotonically increasing one. Moreover, the variability of $Pc'CO_2$ is relatively small. Venoarterial PCO_2 difference is usually only 5 mmHg under resting conditions and rarely exceeds 10 mmHg. Therefore, it is possible for lung units with low $PaCO_2$ (and hence $Pc'CO_2$) to "compensate" for units with high PCO_2, producing a normal $PaCO_2$ even in the face of substantial $\dot{V}_A/\dot{Q}$ abnormality. Unlike the CO_2-blood dissociation curve, the O_2-blood dissociation curve has a plateau at the point at which Hb is fully saturated (see Fig. 33-9). Therefore, $\dot{V}_A/\dot{Q}$ mismatching always results in arterial hypoxemia. Although $\dot{V}_A/\dot{Q}$ mismatching affects CO_2 exchange to the same degree as it does O_2 exchange, this is often not reflected in the blood gases since, as pointed out above, compensatory hyperventilation can maintain arterial PCO_2 within the normal range.

Right-to-left shunting is a special case of $\dot{V}_A/\dot{Q}$ mismatch, with a $\dot{V}_A/\dot{Q}$ ratio of zero. Blood flowing through a right-to-left shunt, whether intrapulmonary or intracardiac, will have gas tensions equal to mixed venous values. The net effect on arterial PO_2 and PCO_2 will depend upon the magnitude of the shunt (Fig. 33-3) and the mixed venous and pulmonary capillary gas tensions. Since a major determinant of mixed venous PO_2 (and to a lesser extent PCO_2) is cardiac output ($\dot{Q}$), changes in $\dot{Q}$ may alter arterial PO_2 independently of lung gas exchange. (Fig. 33-4).

It follows that the most likely causes of low PaO_2 are

Low inspired PO_2
Hypoventilation

$\dot{V}_A/\dot{Q}$ mismatching, including right-to-left shunt (effect modified by mixed venous PO_2)

A common measurement used to assess the adequacy of pulmonary gas exchange is the A-a gradient:

$$\text{A-a gradient} = PAO_2 - PaO_2 \qquad (6)$$

Calculation of the A-a gradient takes into account any degree of hypoventilation or low inspired PO_2 such that an abnormally high A-a gradient reflects either $\dot{V}_A/\dot{Q}$ mismatch (more specifically, low $\dot{V}_A/\dot{Q}$ units) or shunt. The normal value for a child or young adult is less than 10 mmHg. A-a gradient has been related to age in years[8] according to the following formula:

$$\text{A-a gradient} = 0.21 \cdot (\text{Age} + 2.5) \qquad (7)$$

There is considerable scatter of the data around the mean values predicted by this relationship, with individual values for A-a gradient exceeding 30 mmHg. A-a gradient also increases with abnormalities of pulmonary gas exchange. The utility of A-a gradient may be demonstrated by an example. The interpretation of the following arterial blood gases in an unconscious individual in an emergency room (breathing room air) may be aided by calculating the A-a gradient:

$$PaO_2 = 50 \text{ mmHg}$$
$$PaCO_2 = 76 \text{ mmHg}$$
$$pH = 7.17$$

Assuming barometric pressure = 760 mmHg, body temperature = 37°C (therefore $PH_2O = 47$ mmHg), and respiratory quotient = 0.8, in this case using equation (2), $PAO_2 = 59$ mmHg. The A-a gradient therefore equals $59 - 50 = 9$ mmHg, a normal value. Since the impairment of arterial oxygenation is associated with a normal A-a gradient, there is no intrinsic abnormality

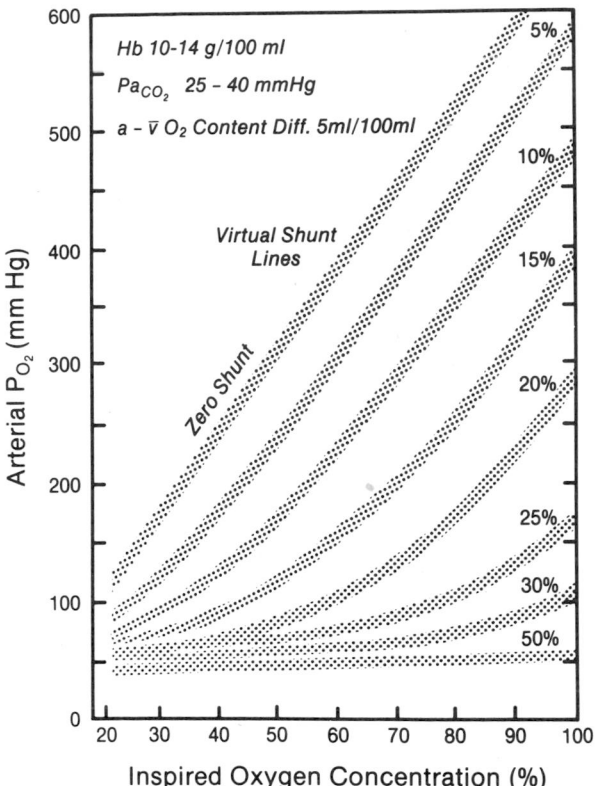

Fig. 33-3. Arterial PO_2 as a function of FIO_2 and shunt fraction ($\dot{Q}s/\dot{Q}T$). Assumptions are shown on the upper left hand section of the figure. The presence of shunt decreases arterial PO_2 for a given FIO_2. As $\dot{Q}s/\dot{Q}T$ increases, supplemental O_2 has progressively less effect on arterial PO_2. (From Benumof,[7] with permission.)

of pulmonary gas exchange. The diagnosis is most likely central respiratory depression.

One problem with the clinical use of A-a gradient is that the normal value is highly dependent on inspired O_2 concentration. As FIO_2 increases, A-a gradient becomes larger. In a normal individual breathing 100 percent O_2 the A-a gradient can exceed 70 mmHg. The interpretation of A-a gradient in a patient breathing supplemental O_2 can therefore be difficult. A more useful parameter is a/A ratio = PaO_2/PAO_2. Empirically a/A ratio was shown by Gilbert and Keighley[9] to be relatively invariant with FIO_2. This observation of constant a/A ratio is also valid in a hyperbaric chamber up to an ambient pressure of 3 ATA (see Ch. 67). Normal a/A ratio is ≥ 0.85. Lower values indicate impairment of pulmonary gas exchange.

If mixed venous blood is available for analysis, a solution can be found for a simplified but clinically useful compartmental model of the lung. This three-compartment model assumes the following division of gas exchange units within the lung:

A compartment with $\dot{V}A/\dot{Q} = 1$ (optimal matching of ventilation and perfusion)
A compartment with $\dot{V}A/\dot{Q} = 0$ (shunt compartment)
A compartment with $\dot{V}A/\dot{Q} = \infty$ (dead space compartment)

Shunt fraction (venous admixture) is the proportion of total blood flow perfusing the shunt compartment and can be calculated from the following equation:

$$\dot{Q}s/\dot{Q}T = \frac{Cc'O_2 - CaO_2}{Cc'O_2 - C\bar{v}O_2} \qquad (8)$$

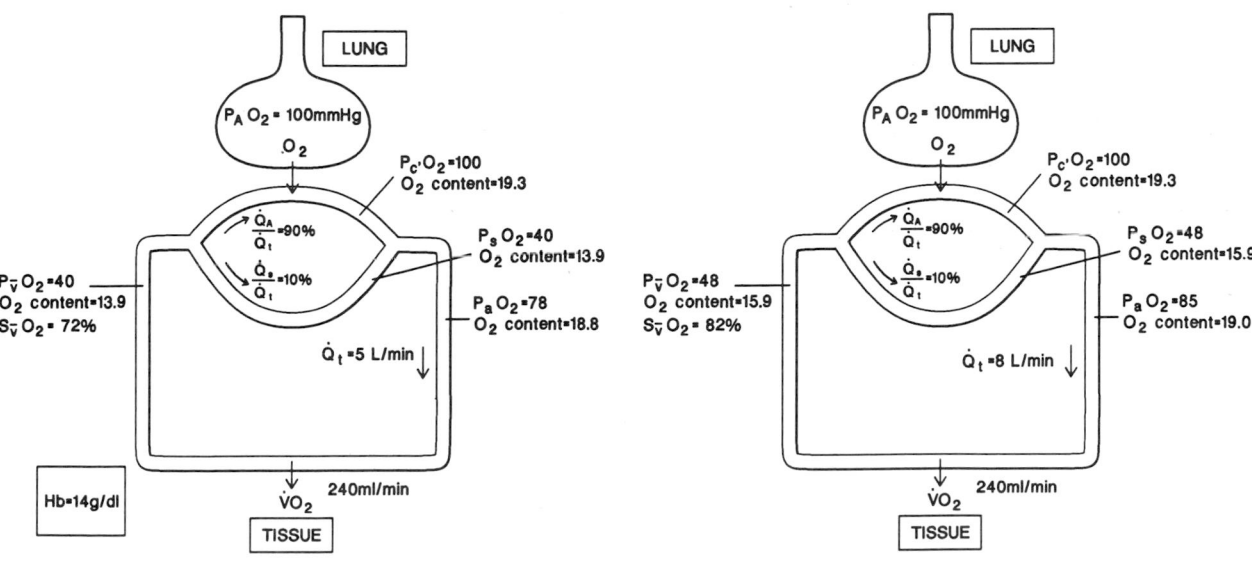

Fig. 33-4. Effect of cardiac output on PO_2. **(A)** Arterial and mixed venous O_2 tension and content are shown at a cardiac output of 5 L/min. Assuming the same $\dot{V}O_2$ it can be seen that an increase in cardiac output to 8 L/min **(B)** will increase the PaO_2 from 78 to 85 mmHg. The reason for this is that at higher cardiac output $S\bar{v}O_2$ increases. The resulting increase in O_2 content of the shunted blood (here assumed to be 10 percent of cardiac output) then raises arterial O_2 content and hence PaO_2. PO_2 is in mmHg; O_2 content is in ml/dl.

where

$$\dot{Q}s = \text{shunt blood flow}$$
$$\dot{Q}_T = \text{cardiac output}$$
$$Cc'O_2, CaO_2, C\bar{v}O_2 = O_2 \text{ content in the alveolar capillary,}$$
arterial, and mixed venous blood,
respectively

CaO_2 and $C\bar{v}O_2$ can be measured directly. $Cc'O_2$ must be calculated from PaO_2 and the Hb-O_2 dissociation curve. $\dot{Q}s/\dot{Q}_T$ calculated in this way normally includes units of low $\dot{V}A/\dot{Q}$ in addition to pure shunt. Breathing 100 percent O_2, however, eliminates the contribution of low $\dot{V}A/\dot{Q}$ units to $\dot{Q}s/\dot{Q}_T$ since any lung unit with nonzero $\dot{V}A/\dot{Q}$ will fully saturate with O_2 the capillary blood perfusing it. Some clinicians routinely measure blood gases in patients breathing 100 percent O_2 in order to estimate the shunt. Unfortunately, the measurement is compounded by the fact that 100 percent O_2 breathing results in the progressive development of resorption atelectasis, and a parallel increase in shunt is observed.[10]

Whereas normal a/A ratio and hence PaO_2 must imply the absence of low $\dot{V}A/\dot{Q}$ ratios or shunt, a normal $PaCO_2$ does not. Regional hypercapnea may occur in pulmonary capillaries perfusing lung units that are relatively underventilated. A unit may be underventilated because of local airway obstruction or because of a high proportion of underperfused or nonperfused units (dead space) that consume a disproportionate amount of total ventilation. In either case, $PaCO_2$ can be restored to normal by increasing total ventilation. $\dot{V}A/\dot{Q}$ abnormalities that affect pulmonary CO_2 exchange therefore may not be detectable simply by inspection of the arterial blood gases. The way in which to find the most common type of abnormality affecting CO_2 exchange (high $\dot{V}A/\dot{Q}$ units) is to measure the dead space by using the Bohr equation:

$$V_D = V_T \left[1 - \frac{P_ECO_2}{P_ACO_2} \right] \quad (9)$$

where

$$P_ECO_2 = \text{mixed expired } PCO_2$$
$$V_T = \text{tidal volume}$$

Frequently it is assumed that $P_ACO_2 = PaCO_2$ (Enghoff modification). In order to measure P_ECO_2 expired gas must be analyzed in a mixing box or a bag used to collect several expired breaths. Although there is a slight increase of dead space with increasing age, as a rule of thumb the normal dead space (in milliliters) is equal to the patient weight (in pounds).

Mixed expired gas analysis is often not clinically available. An assessment of dead space ventilation may therefore be made by examining the relationship between minute ventilation ($\dot{V}E$) and $PaCO_2$. $\dot{V}E$ is continuously displayed by modern ventilators and can also be measured in spontaneously breathing individuals by using a spirometer. Assuming normal $\dot{V}CO_2$, the following equation describes an empirical relationship.[11]

$$\dot{V}E \cdot PaCO_2 \leq 8 \cdot W \quad (10)$$

where W = body weight (kg)

In other words, if $\dot{V}E$ (L/min) times $PaCO_2$ (mmHg) exceeds eight times body weight (kg), an increase in dead space exists, indicating that in order to maintain a normal $PaCO_2$ higher than usual ventilation is required. This product may also be elevated by increased $\dot{V}CO_2$ (shivering, fever, metabolic acidosis).

Using the respiratory gases to assess pulmonary gas exchange has some drawbacks. First, the relationship between partial pressure and gas content is nonlinear for both O_2 and CO_2. Alterations in cardiac output, hemoglobin concentration (resulting in altered venous blood gas tensions), or inspired gas composition may lead to different calculated values of $\dot{Q}s/\dot{Q}_T$ or V_D/V_T even if actual $\dot{V}A/\dot{Q}$ ratios in the lung are unchanged.[12] Second, changes in O_2 or CO_2 exchange can only provide information on a limited portion of the spectrum of $\dot{V}A/\dot{Q}$ ratios. For instance, an increase in calculated $\dot{Q}s/\dot{Q}_T$ (equation [8]) cannot distinguish between a shift to lower $\dot{V}A/\dot{Q}$ ratios and an increase in true shunt.

A more sophisticated technique has been described by Wagner et al.[13] in which a dilute mixture of several "inert" (not metabolically active) tracer gases is infused intravenously. The ratio of partial pressures $Pa/P\bar{v}$ or $P_E/P\bar{v}$ at a gas exchange unit is described by the following equation:

$$Pa/P\bar{v} = P_A/P\bar{v} = \frac{\lambda}{\lambda + \dot{V}A/\dot{Q}} \quad (11)$$

where

$$Pa, P\bar{v}, P_A = \text{partial pressures of the gas in arterial blood,}$$
venous blood, and alveolar gas, respectively
$$\lambda = \text{blood/gas partition coefficient of the gas}$$
$$\dot{V}A/\dot{Q} = \text{ventilation/perfusion ratio of the gas exchange}$$
unit

In this technique (multiple inert gas elimination [MIG]), six gases are usually chosen (SF_6, ethane, cyclopropane, enflurane, diethyl ether, and acetone) spanning a range of λ of around 70,000. Each gas provides information about a particular region in the spectrum of $\dot{V}A/\dot{Q}$, permitting a 50-compartment model to be calculated. Dueck et al.[14] have used the MIG method to demonstrate the development of both $\dot{V}A/\dot{Q}$ mismatching and shunt under halothane anesthesia. Shunt fraction assessed by using MIG has been correlated with atelectatic areas in dependent lung regions visible on chest computed tomography (CT) scan[15] (Fig. 33-5). Although this technique cannot yet be used as an online monitor, future development of rapid, inexpensive gas analyzers could conceivably allow continuous monitoring of $\dot{V}A/\dot{Q}$.

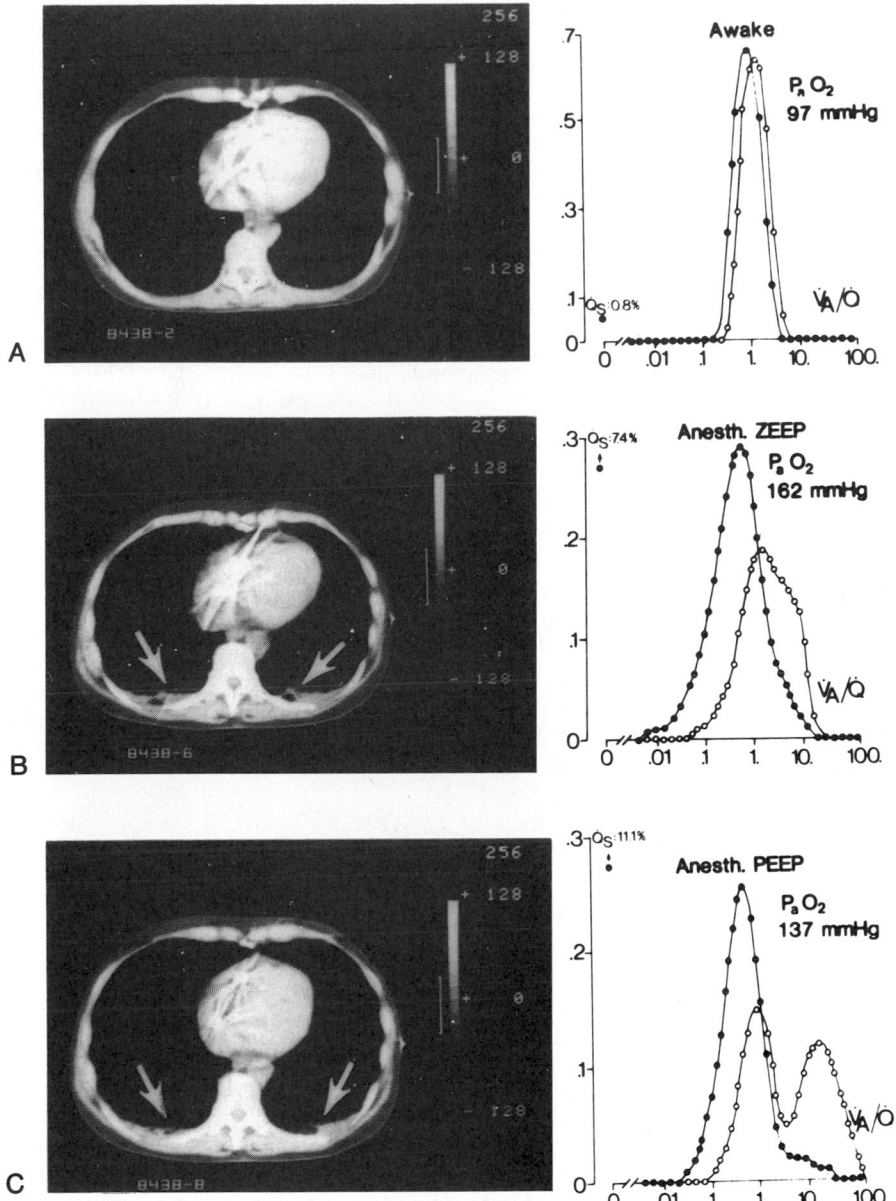

Fig. 33-5. Effect of anesthesia on pulmonary atelectasis and gas exchange. **(A)** CT scan through the chest of an awake patient. Adjacent to it is the distribution of ventilation (open circles) and perfusion (solid circles) in a 50-compartment lung model, determined by using the multiple inert gas method. A unimodal distribution is shown for the awake individual with a $\dot{Q}s/\dot{Q}T$ of 0.8 percent. **(B)** After a period of general anesthesia with positive-pressure ventilation crescent shaped areas of increased tissue density (arrows) appear in posterior lung regions. Corresponding to these changes is a widening of both $\dot{V}A$ and $\dot{Q}$ distributions and an increase in $\dot{Q}s/\dot{Q}T$ to 7.4 percent. **(C)** The same individual after the application of 10 cmH$_2$O PEEP. Very little change is observed in the areas of atelectasis, and $\dot{V}A/\dot{Q}$ matching is further worsened, with the development of a bimodal ventilation distribution and a further increase in $\dot{Q}s/\dot{Q}T$ to 11.1 percent. These changes are accompanied by a drop in PaO$_2$ from 162 to 137 mmHg. (From Tokics et al.,[15] with permission.)

MEASUREMENT OF BLOOD GAS TENSIONS
(Also See Ch. 29)

The most straightforward method of ascertaining arterial PO_2 is to measure it directly from a blood sample. Arterial O_2 tension is usually measured by using a Clark electrode. The principle of its operation is that O_2 molecules in solution are reduced by electrons from the electrode.

The electrons from the cathode react as follows:

$$O_2 + 2H_2O + 2e^- \rightarrow H_2O_2 + 2OH^-$$
$$H_2O_2 + 2e^- \rightarrow 2OH^- \qquad (12)$$

Each molecule of O_2 is reduced to two hydroxyl ions by four electrons. The electrode current is proportional to local PO_2. In the Clark electrode the cathode and anode (or reference electrode) are enclosed within an electrolyte solution and separated from the fluid being measured (e.g., blood) by a thin oxygen-permeable membrane. The current generated is proportional to PO_2 within the adjacent liquid (usually blood sample).

PCO_2 electrodes work by measuring the change in pH induced when blood equilibrates with a $KCl/NaHCO_3$ solution.[16] The history of the development of blood gas analysis has been described by Severinghaus and Astrup[17] and that of oxygen monitoring in general by Severinghaus.[18] An excellent treatment of the electrochemistry and mathematics of blood gas electrodes can be found in Ref. 19 and Chapter 29.

To obviate the need to withdraw blood samples for PO_2 analysis, intra-arterial PO_2 monitors are being developed. Initial attempts to use a Clark-type electrode were confounded by problems of drift and blood coagulation. More recently a fiberoptic technique has been developed, based on the property of oxygen to absorb energy from excited electrons in a fluorescent dye. Incident light is used to elevate electrons in the dye to a higher energy state. These excited electrons may then return to a lower energy level, emitting a photon in the process. Alternatively, molecular oxygen can absorb the energy, therefore inhibiting the photon emission. The process, fluorescence quenching, is related to the PO_2. Barker et al.[20] correlated PaO_2 measured in this way ($OpPO_2$) with conventionally measured PaO_2 with a blood gas analyzer in four dogs. The investigators found an excellent correlation coefficient in 290 pairs of observations ($r = 0.956$) over a range of PaO_2 from 40 to 650 mmHg.

In situations in which arterial puncture cannot be achieved or may be technically difficult (for example, in neonates) capillary PCO_2 may approximate the arterial value. This is particularly true if the sampling site (e.g., heel) is prewarmed, causing an abundance of local blood flow relative to local tissue O_2 consumption. Although capillary PO_2 tends to be significantly lower than the arterial value, capillary O_2 saturation approximates arterial O_2 saturation (capillary value is usually slightly lower) because of the shallow slope of the upper part of the Hb-O_2 dissociation curve.

Temperature Correction of Blood Gases
(Also See Ch. 38)

Conventionally, blood gas electrode temperature is maintained at 37 °C in most hospital laboratories. Rarely is a patient's body temperature exactly 37 °C. Obtaining a blood gas sample at any other temperature and then either warming or cooling the sample to 37 °C will therefore result in a change in the blood gas tensions inside the syringe. Heating of a sample of blood will result in decreased gas solubility in plasma as well as decrease in O_2 affinity for hemoglobin. Therefore, if a syringe of blood is gas-tight and no bubbles are present, heating of the syringe will elevate blood gas tension. The reverse is true for cooling a blood sample. Therefore, PO_2 (and PCO_2) values obtained from a hypothermic patient will be artifactually elevated. Algorithms exist for temperature correction, such that the true partial pressure, predictive of physical and chemical activity at the tissue, can be calculated. The algorithm commonly used in clinical instruments[21] is shown in equation (13):

$$\Delta \log_{10} PO_2 = \left[\frac{5.49 \times 10^{-11} \cdot PO_2^{3.88} + 0.071}{9.72 \times 10^{-9} \cdot PO_2^{3.88} + 2.3} \right] \cdot \Delta T \quad (13)$$

The application of this equation is shown in Figure 33-6. The PO_2 derived from a 37 °C electrode is overestimated when the patient is hypothermic and underestimated if the patient is febrile. At high PO_2 values (> 400 mmHg) the effect is small, since hemoglobin is fully saturated in this region. At PO_2 values below 100 mmHg, however, the degree of overestimation may be severe. For example, at a patient temperature of 30 °C, and a PO_2 below 80 mmHg, the true PO_2 is overestimated by about 60 percent unless temperature correction is applied. We therefore recommend temperature correction of PO_2 values.[22]

A simpler equation[21] exists for temperature correction of PCO_2:

$$\Delta \log_{10} PCO_2 = 0.019 \cdot \Delta T \quad (14)$$

This correction is of less importance because intrinsic changes in PCO_2 are generally of lesser physiologic importance than the resulting alteration in pH. Temperature correction of pH[21] can be accomplished by using equation (15):

$$\Delta pH = [-0.0147 + 0.0065(7.4 - pH)] \cdot \Delta T \quad (15)$$

Temperature correction of pH is discussed in Chapter 38.

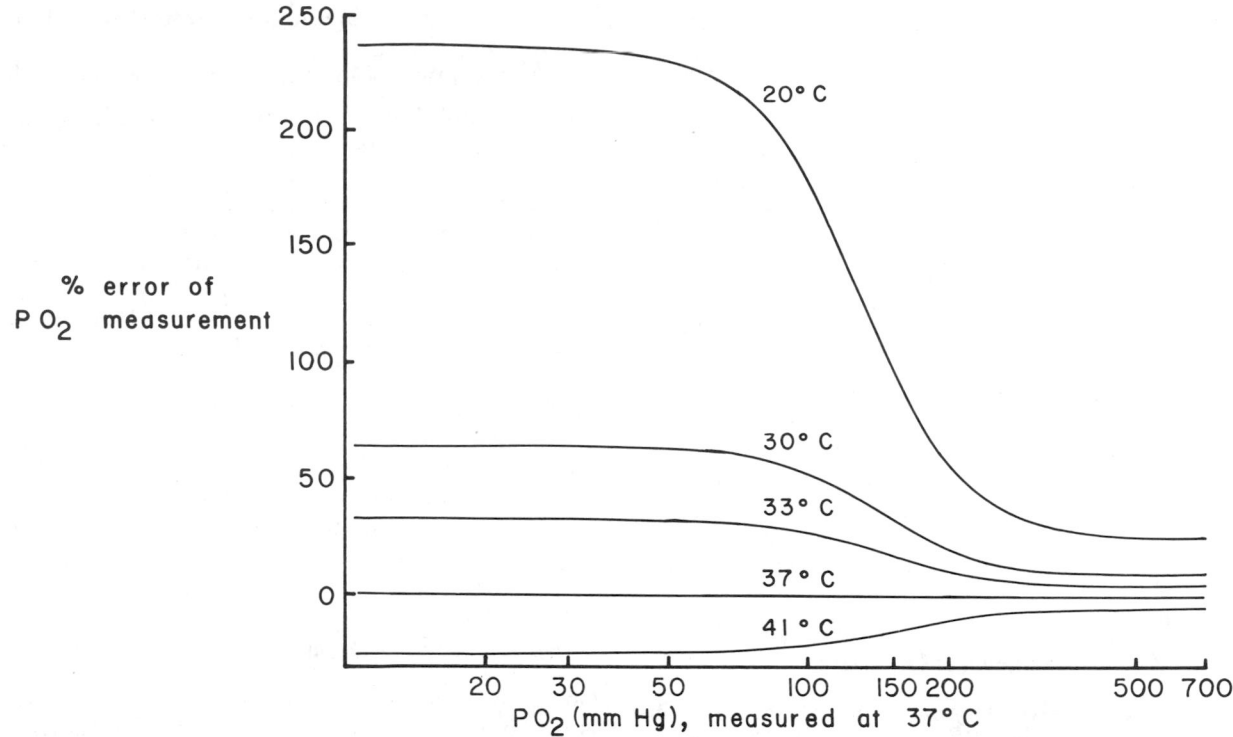

Fig. 33-6. Temperature correction of blood PO_2: percentage error of PO_2 measurement at various body temperatures, with blood gas electrode at 37 °C. If patient temperature is 20 °C a PO_2 measurement performed at 37 °C would overestimate the true value by more than 200 percent. The curves demonstrate that the percentage of error is greater for venous values ($PO_2 < 100$ mmHg) than for arterial measurements ($PO_2 > 300$ mmHg). (From Camporesi and Moon,[22] with permission.)

Artifactual Effects on Gas Tension Measurement

Handling of arterial blood samples for measurement in a laboratory removed from the patient is important in order to maintain stability of gas tensions. Gas bubbles in the syringe will allow diffusion of O_2 and CO_2 between the blood sample and the bubbles, usually lowering the values in the blood. This is particularly true for O_2 at high PO_2 values, since in this region O_2 is less soluble in blood than is CO_2. Removal of all air bubbles before capping the syringe and placement of the syringe in ice water can maintain stability of blood gas samples for several hours. Erythrocytes do not contain mitochondria and therefore do not consume oxygen. However, leukocytes and platelets contain the necessary apparatus for oxygen use, and in the presence of extreme leukocytosis or thrombocytosis significant O_2 consumption by the blood sample may occur.[23] This may be suspected when PO_2 values are inexplicably low in the presence of high leukocyte or platelet counts. Inhibition of cellular O_2 consumption may be accomplished by adding to the sample sodium fluoride[24] available in evacuated tubes used for collection of blood for glucose measurement. Cyanide may also be used in this manner.

MEASUREMENT OF OXYGEN SATURATION

An alternative method of assessing blood oxygenation is to measure Hb-O_2 saturation. The traditional method for monitoring arterial O_2 saturation is to observe the skin and mucous membranes for cyanosis. In 1947 a systematic comparison of the clinical detection of cyanosis by medical staff and blood O_2 saturation measurement with an ear oximeter in normal volunteers demonstrated the poor accuracy of cyanosis as an indicator of hypoxemia.[25] In this study a total of 7,204 observations of skin and mucous membrane color were made in normal volunteers breathing air or hypoxic gas over a measured range of arterial O_2 saturation from 71 to 100 percent. False-positive diagnosis of cyanosis was common: cyanosis was diagnosed in 37 percent of 4,587 observations despite a measured SaO_2 from 91 to 100 percent. On the other hand, in 1,723 observations of hypoxic volunteers with a measured SaO_2 between 71 and 80 normal color was said to be present 12 percent of the time. Lundsgaard and Van Slyke[26] had suggested that in order for cyanosis to be detectable, 5 g/dl of deoxygenated Hb must be present in the arterial blood, although lower amounts of arterial deoxygenated Hb were associated with cyanosis in the study of Stadie[27] (Fig. 33-7). Using this fact, if $SaO_2 \leq 70$ percent is arbitrarily considered clinically dangerous, then simple calculation can demonstrate that this degree of hypoxemia could be difficult to detect if the Hb concentration is less than 16 g/dl. Conceivably some of the false-negative observations in Comroe's study[25] were due to a lack of sufficient circulating Hb. In the operating room or intensive care unit, conditions may not be optimally favorable for observation of skin color. Application of oximeter technology in the critical care setting therefore may be expected to yield increased accuracy in assessing arterial oxygenation, compared to clinical assessment.

Transcutaneous Oximetry

The principles of oximetry have been discussed in Chapter 29. The fact that different species of hemoglobin, particularly Hb and Hb-O_2, have different absorption spectra suggests the possibility of using absorption of light in vivo to calculate arterial Hb-O_2 saturation (SaO_2). A dual wavelength system can be used to estimate SaO_2 if the following conditions are met:

The light is transilluminating arterial blood.
There are no significant quantities of other hemoglobin species (e.g., methemoglobin [MetHb], carboxyhemoglobin [COHb]).

The absorption of light due to tissue is negligible.

The first condition may be met, for example, by transilluminating the earlobe, provided the tissue is kept warm. Under these circumstances the ratio of blood flow to tissue O_2 consumption is relatively high and the capillary blood is therefore predominantly arterial. The second condition is met under most clinical circumstances, in which the total of other Hb species is usually less than 5 percent of the total. The third condition can occur by appropriate choice of wavelength.

Dual wavelength oximeters became available in the 1940s. Because of their rather cumbersome size and the necessity to calibrate them for each individual patient, they never attained widespread use. An eight-wavelength instrument was designed by Hewlett-Packard.[28] Active heating of the earlobe by the sensor maintained a high proportion of arterial blood in the capillary bed.

Principles of Pulse Oximetry

One of the major objections to the use of ear oximeters is that one can never be totally sure that the earlobe contains predominantly arterial blood, since this instrument has no means of differentiating between arterial and venous hemoglobin. The pulse oximeter is able to make this differentiation by assuming that the pulsatile portion of the signal is entirely arterial blood. This is almost always true except under unusual clinical circumstances (high venous pulsation, tricuspid regurgitation).

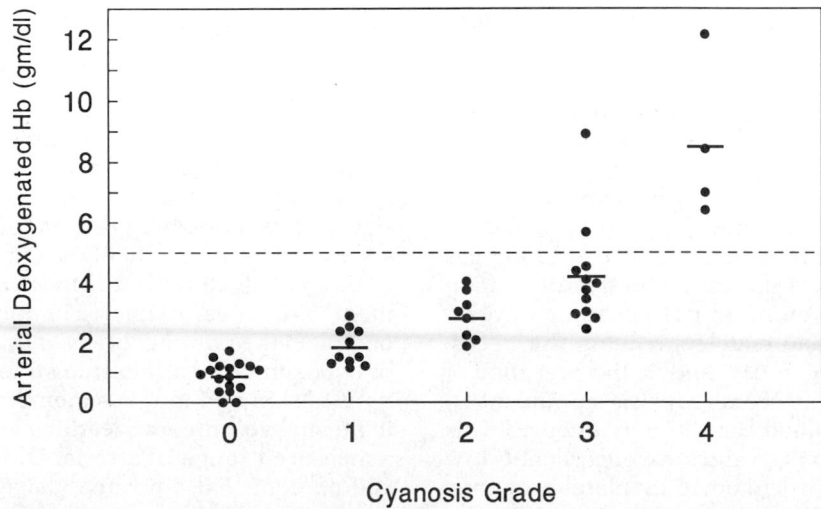

Fig. 33-7. Quantity of deoxygenated Hb in arterial blood as a function of degree of cyanosis. Although traditionally it has been assumed that 5 g/dl of deoxygenated hemoglobin is required for the detection of cyanosis, mild cyanosis can clearly be observed at lower values. (Data plotted from Stadie.[27])

The principle of pulse oximetry is shown schematically in Figure 33-8. The light passing through tissue is absorbed by tissue, as well as venous and arterial blood. The following ratio (S) is calculated at two wavelengths of light, usually around 660 nm and 940 nm:

$$S = \frac{AC_{660}/DC_{660}}{AC_{940}/DC_{940}} \qquad (16)$$

where

AC_{660}, AC_{940} = pulsatile components of absorbances at 660 and 940-nm wavelengths
DC_{660}, DC_{940} = corresponding steady-state components

S is then empirically related to O_2 saturation and incorporated into the design of the instrument.

In practice, pulse oximeters use two light-emitting diodes (LEDs) and one photo diode as transmitting and sensing transducers, usually placed on opposite sides of a digit. The two LEDs are activated alternatively. The ratio S is calculated electronically; from it SaO_2 is then derived from an internally stored algorithm. Although in principle the light absorbance technology for monitoring oxyhemoglobin (O_2Hb) saturation has been in existence for almost 50 years, the use of the pulse principle has increased substantially the reliability of such monitors and resulted in their extremely widespread use. The main drawback of oximetry is that it is rather insensitive to large changes in arterial PO_2 at the high end of the Hb-O_2 dissociation curve.

Errors in Pulse Oximetry

Since pulse oximeters are dual-wavelength devices the presence of Hb species other than Hb and O_2Hb must therefore result in erroneous readings.

Carboxyhemoglobin

The effect of carboxyhemoglobin (COHb) may be discerned by examining its absorption spectrum. At 920 nm COHb has an extremely low absorbance and therefore does not contribute to the total absorbance at this wavelength. At 660 nm, however, COHb has an absorbance very similar to that of O_2Hb. The O_2 saturation will therefore be falsely high. This effect has been measured in a canine study in which the actual pulse oximeter reading of Nellcor and Ohmeda pulse oximeters was approximated by the following formula[30]:

$$SaO_2^* \approx \frac{[O_2Hb] + 0.9 \cdot [COHb]}{[Hb]} \cdot 100 \qquad (17)$$

where

$$SaO_2^* = \text{pulse oximeter reading}$$

A falsely high pulse oximeter reading therefore occurs in the presence of COHb. When COHb was 50 percent, the measured SaO_2 by the pulse oximeters was about 95 percent.

Methemoglobin

Methemoglobin (MetHb) has a larger absorbance than either of the two major species of Hb at 940 nm but simulates Hb at 660 nm. Therefore, at high SaO_2 levels (>85 percent) the reading underestimates the true value; at low SaO_2 (<85 percent) the value is falsely high.[31] In the presence of high MetHb concentrations the measured SaO_2 approaches 85 percent, independent of the actual arterial oxygenation.

Hemoglobin F

In neonates there is a large proportion of hemoglobin F. Since hemoglobin F has almost the same absorption spectrum as hemoglobin A there is no major effect on pulse oximetry.[29]

Dyes

Clinically used dyes may also have an effect on pulse oximetry. Methylene blue results in a severe decrease in measured SaO_2.[32] Indocyanine green has a smaller

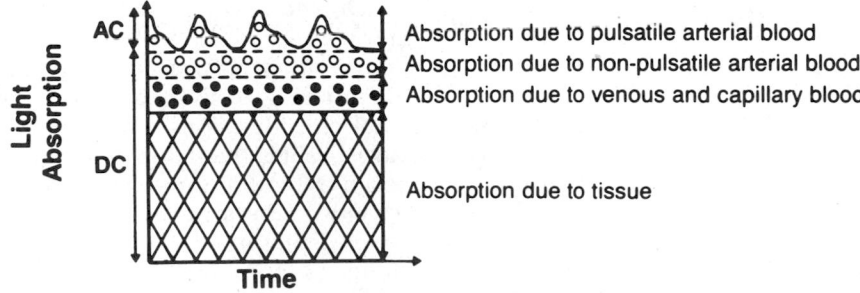

Fig. 33-8. Principle of pulse oximetry. Light passing through tissue containing blood is absorbed by tissue as well as arterial, capillary, and venous blood. Usually only the arterial blood is pulsatile, however. Light absorption may therefore be split into a pulsatile component (AC) and a constant or nonpulsatile component (DC). Hb-O_2 saturation may be obtained by application of equation (16) in text. (From Tremper and Barker,[29] with permission.)

effect,[33] with the smallest decrease noted with indigo carmine.[33,34] Fluorescein injection has no measurable effect.[33,34] Administration of methylene blue may result in methemoglobinemia, which can alter SaO_2 reading. Additionally, alterations in cardiac output (increase, then decrease) can occur after injection. In the presence of $\dot{V}A/\dot{Q}$ mismatch this may result in a transient increase and then a decrease in actual SaO_2. The presence of high concentrations of methylene blue in blood can also alter co-oximeter readings such that an artifactual decrease in measured O_2 saturation may result, although quantitative information is lacking.

Nail Polish

Effects of nail polish have also been measured. Blue nail polish, with absorbance near 660 nm, has the greatest effect on SaO_2 reading, an artifactual decrease. Other colors have smaller effects.[35]

Bilirubin

High levels of bilirubin have no significant effect on pulse oximeter readings although nonpulsatile oximetry may measure a falsely low value.[28]

Skin Pigment

Deeply pigmented skin can result in inability to pick up arterial pulsations by a pulse oximeter. Small errors in SaO_2 reading from black individuals have been reported by some investigators, with others' finding no significant effect.[34]

Tape

Four varieties of transparent tape have been shown not to alter SaO_2 measurements from 85 to 100 percent.[36] However, smeared adhesive caused by reusing a disposable oximeter probe has been reported to cause falsely low SaO_2 readings.[37]

Low Oxygen Saturation

Routine in vivo calibration of pulse oximeters at low O_2 saturation can be difficult and potentially dangerous. Animal data may not be applicable to humans. Therefore, clinical pulse oximetry may provide erroneous measurements when O_2 saturation is less than 70 percent. Severinghaus et al.[38] tested pulse oximeters from 14 manufacturers while inducing hypoxemia for periods up to 30 seconds in normal volunteers. Arterial O_2 saturation as low as 40 percent was achieved. There was considerable variation among manufacturers. At 75 percent O_2 saturation the bias (systematic error) was scattered uniformly around zero, with individual units' either overestimating or underestimating the true SaO_2 by as much as 7 percent. Below 60 percent O_2 saturation most units underestimated the actual O_2 saturation

(false low measurement). The largest underestimate at this low saturation was approximately 13 percent.

Pulse oximetry has been well reviewed by Alexander et al.,[39] Kelleher,[34] and Tremper and Barker.[29]

MIXED VENOUS OXYGEN MONITORING

Mixed venous O_2 saturation ($S\bar{v}O_2$) is related to a number of factors, as shown in equation (22):

$$S\bar{v}O_2 = SaO_2 - \frac{\dot{V}O_2}{13.9 \cdot \dot{Q} \cdot [Hb]} \qquad (18)$$

where

[Hb] = hemoglobin concentration
13.9 = constant (O_2 combining power of Hb [ml/10 g])
$\dot{Q}$ = cardiac output

It can be seen that low SaO_2, low cardiac output, low [Hb], or elevated $\dot{V}O_2$ may result in a decrease in $S\bar{v}O_2$. All of these conditions could produce impairment of O_2 delivery to the tissues. Therefore, this single measurement ($S\bar{v}O_2$) may be uniquely helpful in detecting any condition that might result in impaired tissue oxygenation. $S\bar{v}O_2$ can be monitored by intermittent measurement of blood withdrawn through a pulmonary artery catheter or may be continuously monitored by using a pulmonary artery catheter equipped with fiberoptic bundles. These catheters (American Edwards Laboratories, Santa Ana, California, and Oximetrix Inc., Mountain View, California) have two fiberoptic bundles carrying an incident light beam and a reflected light beam. Using the fact that the reflected spectrum of Hb is dependent upon the degree of oxygenation, the appropriate calculations can be performed by the instrument and a continuous display of $S\bar{v}O_2$ provided. Low $S\bar{v}O_2$ (usually less than 60 percent) may sensitively reflect an abnormality of one or more of the factors on the right-hand side of equation (22). Several factors may artifactually elevate $S\bar{v}O_2$, however. These include wedging of the catheter and mitral regurgitation (which tend to bring the catheter tip into contact with arterialized blood), as well as sepsis and left-to-right shunts (either intracardiac or peripheral).

Monitoring of $P\bar{v}O_2$ instead of $S\bar{v}O_2$ requires additional considerations. Although $S\bar{v}O_2$ is a function of four variables (equation [22]), other factors acting on the Hb-O_2 binding curve may alter $P\bar{v}O_2$ independently. In Figure 33-9 a normal curve is shown adjacent to curves depicting both increased and decreased Hb-O_2 affinity. For the same SaO_2 and $S\bar{v}O_2$ (and hence arteriovenous O_2 content difference) substantially different values for $P\bar{v}O_2$ will occur under the three conditions. Correct interpretation of mixed venous oxygen tension values must therefore depend on the position of the Hb-O_2 dissociation curve, as dictated by pH, PCO_2, body temperature, and erythrocyte diphosphoglycerate concentration.

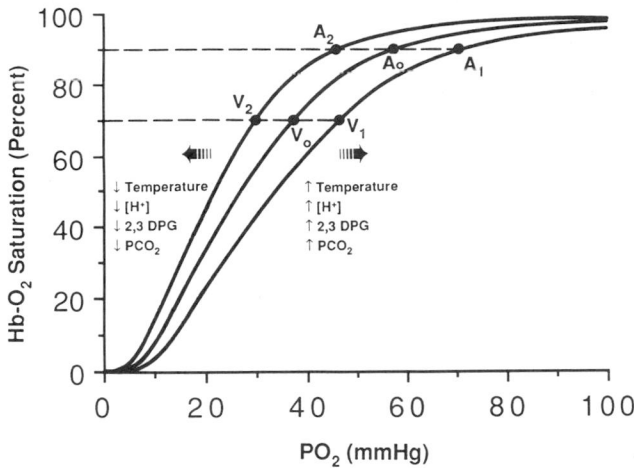

Fig. 33-9. Hb-O$_2$ saturation curves. Dotted lines indicate common arterial and venous values: SaO$_2$ = 90 percent and S$\bar{v}$O$_2$ = 70 percent. The middle curve (A$_0$, V$_0$) represents the relationship with pH = 7.40, body temperature = 37 °C. The right-hand curve (A$_1$, V$_1$) would occur if pH were 7.20 or T = 41 °C. The left-hand curve (A$_2$, V$_2$) represents the relationship when T = 33 °C. Raised levels of any of the four factors shown (temperature, [H$^+$], erythrocyte 2,3-diphosphoglycerate, PCO$_2$) will decrease Hb-O$_2$ affinity (rightward shift); decreased levels will raise Hb-O$_2$ affinity (leftward shift). The same arterial and venous Hb-O$_2$ saturation under different conditions can therefore result in a wide range of arterial and venous gas tension values.

S$\bar{v}$O$_2$ measurement has been carried one step further by Räsänen et al.,[40] who have used this instrument (to measure S$\bar{v}$O$_2$) and a pulse oximeter (to measure SaO$_2$) to calculate shunt fraction continuously according to the following modification of the standard equation:

$$\frac{\dot{Q}s}{\dot{Q}T} \approx \frac{1 - SaO_2}{1 - S\bar{v}O_2} \qquad (19)$$

This approximation is correct if end-capillary blood is fully saturated with oxygen. The authors demonstrated that their instrument, producing a continuous reading of $\dot{Q}s/\dot{Q}T$ using this principle, could be used as a guide to providing an optimum level of CPAP in a group of patients whose tracheas were intubated in whom lowest $\dot{Q}s/\dot{Q}T$ was desired. The authors found that the on-line method was cost-effective and concluded that CPAP therapy could be accurately titrated in the majority of patients with acute respiratory failure by using this noninvasive method to calculate shunt fraction.

TISSUE OXYGENATION

Arterial oxygenation as an indicator of respiratory function may in fact be controversial, since an acceptable arterial O$_2$ content may not necessarily be associated with adequate tissue oxygenation, because of abnor-

malities of blood flow. A more appropriate monitor of oxygen delivery would in fact measure tissue oxygenation. Tissue PO$_2$ electrodes have been designed and implemented but have associated problems of sampling bias and tissue destruction. In addition, because of heterogeneity of local tissue blood flow and $\dot{V}$O$_2$ there exists a distribution of tissue PO$_2$ values, rather than a single value as in blood PO$_2$. Nevertheless, changes in tissue oxygenation have been demonstrated under varying clinical conditions[41] (Fig. 33-10).

Another approach is the noninvasive monitoring of cytochrome redox state using infrared laser technology. Reduction of O$_2$ to water occurs at the terminal end of the cytochrome chain. Measurement of cytochrome redox state would therefore provide a better estimate of O$_2$ availability at the cellular level than presently available monitors. Instruments have been designed and used for monitoring of brain and skeletal muscle in experimental situations.[42,43] It is highly likely that this technology will ultimately be used for clinical monitoring in the operating room and intensive care settings.

EXPIRED GAS ANALYSIS

Mass Spectrometry
(Also See Ch. 29)

Mass spectrometers are devices that measure concentrations of gases depending largely on their molecular weight. Gas samples are passed through an ionizer, typically an electron beam, which strips the individual molecules of one or more electrons, giving them a positive charge. The ionizing beam also splits some molecules, creating molecular fragments. After ionization the gas mixture to be measured is accelerated through a magnetic field. In the *sector* type the ionized gas molecules are passed through magnetic and electric fields at right angles to each other. The paths of the ions become curved by the action of these two fields, in a manner dependent upon the charge/mass ratio. Detectors placed at specific locations allow individual gas concentrations to be measured proportionally to the counts per minute. The *quadrupole* type of mass spectrometer uses both radio frequency and constant electric fields to force ions of a fixed charge to mass ratio to pass through selectors into a detector, usually a photomultiplier tube. After ionization the gas molecules can then be accelerated by an electric field toward a target after first being focused into a narrow beam. On the way to the target the ion beam passes through an arrangement of rods, the quadrupole. The quadrupole's electrostatic field is changed in a stepwise fashion such that only ions of a single charge/mass ratio may reach the target area (Fig. 33-11). The rate at which ions hit the target is proportional to the concentration of that particular gas in the original mixture. The electrostatic field settings appropriate for a given charge/mass ratio

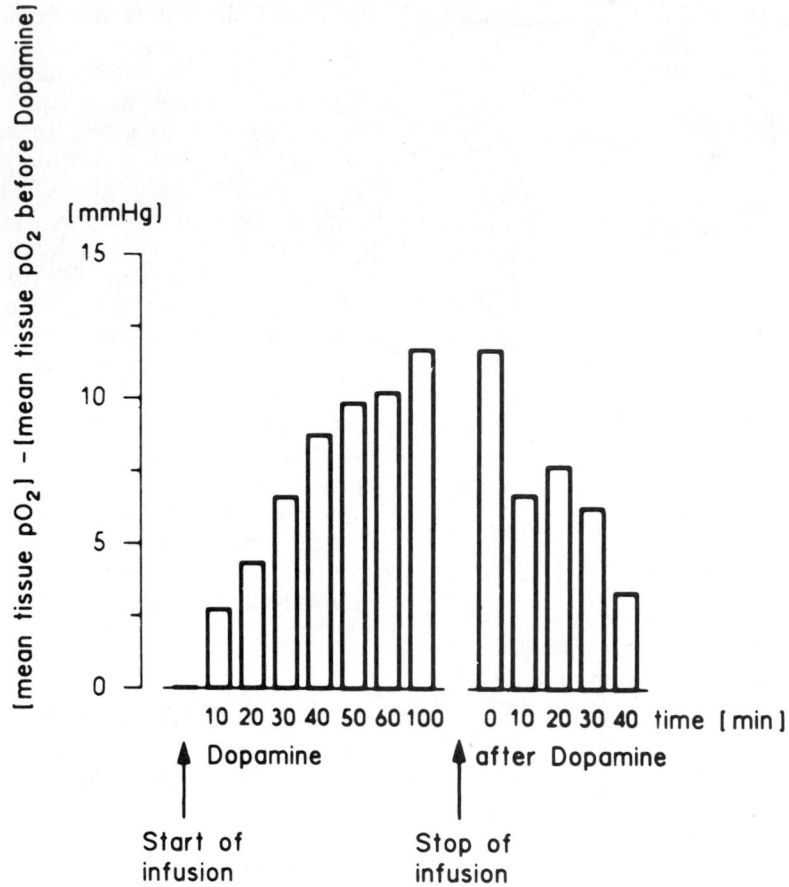

Fig. 33-10. Changes in muscle PO$_2$ during dopamine infusion. Displayed values represent the mean of seven septic patients treated in an intensive care unit. Dopamine infusion results in an increase in tissue PO$_2$ of around 12 mmHg after 100 minutes. (From Kersting et al.,[41] with permission.)

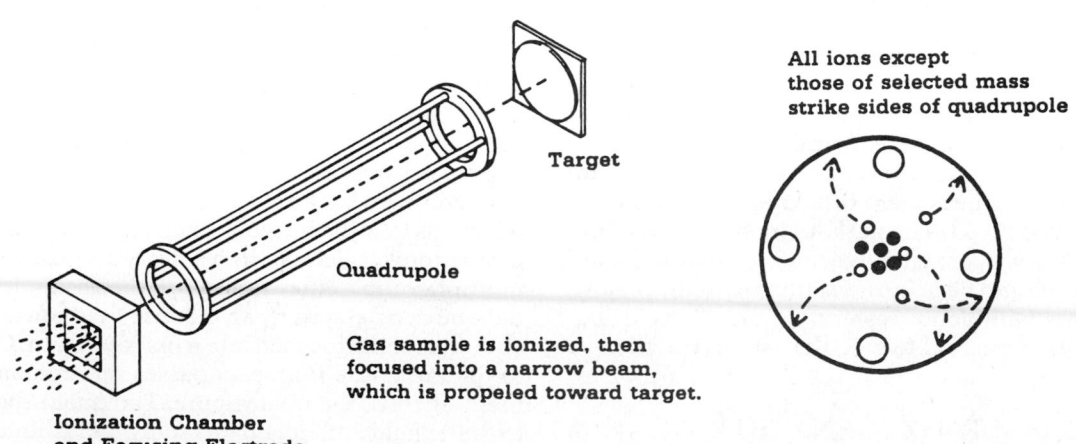

Fig. 33-11. Quadrupole mass spectrometer. The gas sample passes through the ionization chamber and focusing electrode. Ions then pass through the quadrupole. Rapid changes in the applied electric fields cause all ions except those with the chosen charge to mass ratio to hit the sides of the instrument. Only the ions of interest will strike the target and be detected. (From Ohmeda,[44] with permission.)

are alternated in order to measure in turn each of the gases of interest in the mixture (multiplexing). These instruments are reliable and relatively rugged, with delay time typically on the order of 100 to 200 msec.[44]

The ability of the mass spectrometer to measure individually different concentrations of gases depends upon charge/mass ratio. Since most of the ions created by the ionizer are singly charged (missing a single electron), the most important variable is therefore the molecular weight. Two different molecules of the same molecular weight (for example, CO_2 and N_2O) are therefore not ordinarily distinguishable by a mass spectrometer using the principles outlined. In order to surmount this difficulty, empirical algorithms that distinguish particular pairs of molecules by analyzing molecular fragments created by the ionizing beam have been designed.

Since mass spectrometers have traditionally been large and expensive instruments, the original implementation of their use in anesthesia placed them in a remote location. Samples would be conducted to the instrument from a large number of operating rooms, and analysis was performed on a time-sharing basis.[45] This time-sharing approach increased the delay time because of the necessary length of tubing necessary between the patient and the instrument. Another disadvantage was that each patient could only be analyzed for a fraction of the total time available. Presently a number of instruments are available for individual operating room use (e.g., the Ohmeda 6000 Multigas Monitor: Ohmeda, Madison, Wisconsin). These instruments typically can measure CO_2, O_2, N_2, Ar, N_2O, enflurane, halothane, and isoflurane simultaneously.

Raman Gas Analysis

When a photon from a light source collides with a molecule of gas it may be re-emitted (scattered light) with no loss of energy *(Rayleigh scattering)*. Alternatively, there may be absorption of some of the kinetic energy from the photon, resulting in the scattered photon's having a lower energy level and hence longer wavelength *(Raman scattering)*. In Raman scattering the degree of energy absorption by a molecule from incident photons depends upon molecular weight and structure. Spectral analysis of the scattered light may therefore be used to measure simultaneously the individual concentrations of a mixture of gases. The light source is usually an argon laser with a wavelength of 488 nm. Samples of gas are conducted through a cell and the scattered light passed through a spectrometer. The peaks are then detected with a photomultiplier tube. Anesthetic gases and respiratory gases can be simultaneously measured.[46] A clinical instrument based upon the Raman principle (RASCAL, Albion Instruments, Salt Lake City, Utah) has been tested on patients undergoing general anesthesia.[47] Comparison with a mass spectrometer revealed similar accuracy for CO_2, N_2, O_2, and anesthetic gases.

Infrared Absorption

In the infrared absorption method an infrared (IR) light beam is projected through the gas sample and the intensity of the transmitted light is measured. CO_2 absorbs light with a characteristic peak at a wavelength close to 4,300 nm. Several other molecules, such as nitrous oxide, water vapor, carbon monoxide, and O_2 also absorb light in this area of the spectrum, interfering with CO_2 measurement, especially if the incident light composition includes wavelengths other than those in a very narrow region around the CO_2 absorption peak. In practical use the fixed geometry of the gas-sampling cell, a narrow-band IR light source, and compensating electronic circuits can often automatically correct for interference by other gases.

TRANSCUTANEOUS GAS TENSION MEASUREMENT

In areas of the skin where local blood flow exceeds the amount required for local O_2 consumption, as mentioned previously, capillary PO_2 may approximate PaO_2. This may be particularly true if the local area is warmed. This principle has been exploited by manufacturers of transcutaneous PO_2 ($PtcO_2$) measuring devices. These devices usually consist of a small electrode that is attached with adhesive to the skin. The skin is locally warmed to 40 or 41 °C. O_2 from capillaries diffuses through the intact skin into a Clark-type electrode that measures PO_2 directly. This value usually correlates well with PaO_2. However, in the presence of peripheral vasoconstriction or thick (adult) skin the measurement may be erroneous. A reduction in cardiac output tends to result in an artifactual decrease in $PtcO_2$ because of the ensuing cutaneous hypoxia. However, the technique is particularly useful in infants, in whom local skin blood flow tends to be high and in whom repeated withdrawals of arterial blood may cause anemia. Unfortunately, these instruments tend to be somewhat unstable, requiring direct arterial measurements to calibrate the transcutaneous instrument. Furthermore, the time constant of measurement is on the order of minutes, and a sudden decrease in arterial PO_2 may not be detectable quickly enough so that a therapeutic response can be made.[48] Also, skin burns have sometimes resulted from prolonged application of these devices.

An approach to minimize the problems associated with slow diffusion time of respiratory gases across skin has been made by designing an instrument to measure conjunctival PO_2 (Orange 1 Oxygen Monitoring System: Orange Medical Instruments, Costa Mesa, California). The Clark-type PO_2 electrode in this instrument is embedded in a polymethylmethacrylate ring-shaped scleral conformer that is contoured to fit the eye. The conformer is placed under the upper and lower eyelids such that the electrode rests against the palpebral conjunctiva. These devices may be kept in place for 24 hours or longer in unanesthetized individuals. Testing in normal volunteers was reported by Chapman et al.[49] Over a range of PaO_2 from 28 to 205 mmHg conjunctival PO_2 ($PcjO_2$) correlated well with PaO_2 ($r = 0.94$). Moreover, the time to 90 percent response to an abrupt change in inspired PO_2 was relatively fast (38 to 96 seconds). However, $PcjO_2$ was uniformly lower than PaO_2, with $PcjO_2/PaO_2$ ratios' varying among individuals (range 0.47 to 0.79). Patient-specific calibration is therefore required to estimate absolute PaO_2.

WAVEFORM ANALYSIS OF EXPIRED RESPIRATORY GASES

Capnography, the measurement of CO_2 in expired gases, has evolved in the last few years into a commonly used procedure. Whereas a variety of techniques can be used for CO_2 measurement (mass spectrometry, Raman analysis), the majority of capnographs rely on IR absorption.[50] Use of this technique can reliably and quantitatively provide vital respiratory monitoring information in the operating room and in all critical care areas.

End-tidal PO_2 ($ETPO_2$) may be used as an estimate of alveolar and hence arterial PO_2. Whereas end-tidal CO_2 ($ETCO_2$) analysis has achieved a high degree of popularity, this has not occurred for PO_2 monitoring because of the variable alveolar-arterial gradient. In normal individuals this gradient may be less than 10 mmHg; however, in patients with severe $\dot{V}A/\dot{Q}$ mismatching the gradient may be substantially increased. Furthermore, the A-a gradient is increased at high inspired O_2 concentration even with normal lungs. $ETPO_2$ therefore almost always overestimates PaO_2. For example, the $ETPO_2$ of a dead person being ventilated with 100 percent O_2 would be approximately 700 mmHg. (Pbarometric − PH_2O)! An example of a continuous tracing of expired PO_2 in an anesthetized patient is shown in Figure 33-12.

According to the gas sampling technique, infrared CO_2 monitors can be separated into two categories: *sidestream monitors*, which draw a continuous sample of the gas from the respiratory circuit into the measuring cell, and *mainstream monitors*, which directly straddle the airway with a reading cell placed at the attachment between respiratory circuit and endotracheal tube or breathing mask. The key difference in use between the two types of capnographs depends on details of practical importance and on the type of monitoring environment and duration.

Sidestream Capnographs

Of importance is the concept that sidestream capnographs depend crucially on a sampling flow that continuously aspirates from the "side" of the main respiratory gas flow a fixed amount of gas. The rate of gas sampling can be usually adjusted from 50 to 500 ml/min and at times up to 2 L/min. This continuous bias flow can be

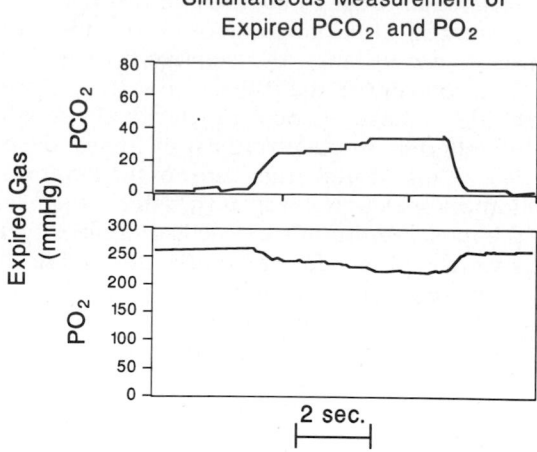

Simultaneous Measurement of Expired PCO_2 and PO_2

Fig. 33-12. Simultaneous measurement of expired PCO_2 and PO_2. These tracings were obtained with $PaO_2 = 153$ mmHg and $PaCO_2 = 32$ mmHg. Whereas $ETPCO_2$ is close to $PaCO_2$, $ETPO_2$ substantially overestimates the arterial value.

the source of significant methodologic error. If the sampling flow ever exceeds the expired gas flow then contamination from the fresh gas flow source will occur. The sampling gas pump, flow regulator, sampling system (including the connector to the sampling port), and the water trap or water separator constitute multiple sites for gas leak or breakage. Additionally, depending upon size and length of the sampling tube and rate of gas flow, a certain delay in gas detection is introduced (CO_2 flight time), which can amount to several seconds when the sampling rate is low and the sampling dead space is high (e.g., long tubes). After measurement in the gas cell, the sampled gas may be exhausted into the atmosphere or retrieved and reinjected through a second tube into the breathing circuit in order to restore breathing circuit volume. This variable may be of great importance in closed-circuit and precise metabolic gas volume measurements. The analytic core of the instrument, the IR measuring cell, must be carefully protected so that liquids and particulate matter do not enter it and cause erroneous readings of CO_2 due to their high IR absorbance. The major problem is caused by water vapor, which is invariably present in expired air (at 37 °C) with a saturated vapor pressure of 47 mmHg. This condenses at lower (room) temperature on sampling tube walls. In critical care settings and often in the operating room the inspired gas is kept warm and humid during long cases. This increases the load on water separation systems applied to capnographs. Water traps and filters have been designed to protect the measuring chamber. Several clever designs have been tested, but all work best when periodic cleaning and maintenance are provided.

Monitoring of $ETCO_2$ in the spontaneously breathing patient whose trachea is not intubated requires some improvisation. Nasotracheal cannulae connected to a sidestream monitor usually provide a usable waveform but frequently become obstructed with saliva or mucus and are uncomfortable. Turner et al.[51] described a method to prevent this problem in which an intravenous catheter is threaded into the common lumen of a pair of nasal O_2 cannulae such that the tip lies midway between the two nasal prongs. The extension tube normally connected to the O_2 source is tied off and the IV catheter connected to a sidestream capnometer.

Mainstream Capnometers

In a mainstream capnometer, with the measuring head placed in close proximity to the endotracheal tube, the measuring chamber is usually heated up to about 40 °C to prevent water condensation on the chamber window. The heated sensing head must be kept away from direct contact with the patient's skin; it is relatively heavy and must be supported to prevent endotracheal tube kinking. In addition, the sensor's window must be kept clean of mucus and particles to prevent false reading; calibration may be problematic. Despite all these problems the response time is faster: no gas is subtracted from the breathing circuit, no sampling pumps or other suction devices add complexities to the mechanical system, and there is no uncertainty caused by the rate of gas sampling.

Calibration of capnographs must be accomplished periodically, at different intervals in various models but often at least daily. Equipment drift is most often due to accumulation of saliva or other extraneous materials accumulating in the light path of the analyzer. Calibration can usually be performed by periodic use of calibrated gases. Mainstream capnometers are often equipped with calibration sample cells sealed with mixtures of CO_2 and N_2. In some instruments, room air is sampled in the mainstream curvette to "zero" the CO_2 level automatically.

A useful analysis range varies from 0 to 10 percent (76 mmHg) for $ETCO_2$ to an extended range up to 100 mmHg, which may be useful in rare cases of hypoventilation or malignant hyperthermia. The inspired CO_2 range must include 0 and extend up to 15 mmHg for cases when rebreathing must be detected and determination of peak values is needed.

Time Delays

A capnogram is produced by the sequential analysis of inspired and expired gas, either flowing by the mainstream window, usually positioned just proximal to the endotracheal tube or breathing mask, or sampled from a sidestream sampling site connected to the breathing circuit. In the case of sidestream sampling, a definite time delay is introduced by the length and volume of the tubing carrying the sampled gas to the detector. This holds equally true for a capnogram produced by an IR sensing device or a respiratory mass spectrometer or other gas-sensing device based on a different principle.

This delay time caused by the transfer of the sampled gas into the reading cell can be minimized by using high flow rates for the sampling flow and narrow, short tubing assemblies compatible with the position of the equipment with respect to the patient breathing circuit. Once the sampled gas reaches the sensing cell, an additional delay is introduced by the rise time of each instrument. The rise time is a characteristic delay induced by the exponential response to a square front of changing gas concentration, in which CO_2 changes instantaneously from zero to a steady-state level (I). Most often this is described by the following exponential equation:

$$S = I(1 - e^{t/\tau}) \qquad (20)$$

where

S = signal at time t
e = base of natural logarithms (≈ 2.718)
τ = time constant

When $t = \tau$ (one time constant), it is possible to calculate that $S = 0.63 \cdot I$. This is frequently used to measure the response of the circuitry. It is often presented in clinical instruments as a different fraction of the response, such as the 10 to 90 percent response time ($\approx 2\tau$).

If we assume a square-wave capnogram, for argument's sake only, as the most difficult for an instrument to follow, and a time constant of 100 milliseconds (a frequent value for a clinical instrument), it is usually theoretically possible to follow respiratory profiles of CO_2 within 5 percent of the real value (accuracy better than 5 percent) up to respiratory rates of 100 breaths/min. In practice, most clinical capnographs display this accuracy up to 60 breaths/min.[50] A shared mass-spectrometer, with the usually longer sampling line used in the shared configuration, may display significant inaccuracy at respiratory rates around 40 breaths/min.[52] The relative duration of inspiration and expiration (I/E ratio) can also affect the accuracy of the recording instrument. Standardized respiratory cycle profiles have been used to compare the most commonly employed clinical instruments.[53]

When quantitative results are expected to be collected through CO_2 sampling lines, the solubility of CO_2 in the tubing materials used must be taken into account, as polyethylene and Teflon tubing are much more permeable to CO_2 than nylon. The composition of sampling lines has been shown to affect significantly mass-spectrometry readings for CO_2.[54] Whereas *radial diffusion* of CO_2 out of the sampling line is mainly affected by the tubing material and the length of exposure of the sample inside the tubing (related to the flow rate of sampling), *axial diffusion* across the fronts of CO_2-rich boluses traveling along sampling lines can also smear both the upstrokes and the downstrokes of waveforms. This type of diffusion has a significant effect on the interpretation of $ETPCO_2$ at higher respiratory frequencies.

The Capnographic Waveform

Traditionally, several phases are distinguished in the capnograph trace during expiration (see Fig. 33-13). The first expired gas during a normal exhalation presents to the sample site gas exhaled from the anatomic dead-space, usually warm and humidified, but devoid of CO_2. As the expiration continued, a short second phase of the capnograph is recognized, with a rapid upstroke toward the alveolar plateau: this represents the rising front of CO_2. The boundary of this front can be smeared by a variety of causes, but most notably by uneven mixing in the airways of the alveolar CO_2 bolus. The third portion of the capnograph is also called alveolar plateau, and it represents the constant or slowly upsloping part of the capnogram, reaching a peak, usually attained only during the final phase of exhalation, and therefore called end-tidal CO_2 value ($ETPCO_2$). $ETPCO_2$ in the normal individual is usually 2 to 3 mmHg lower than arterial PCO_2. Chronic pulmonary disease and acute disturbances in $\dot{V}A/\dot{Q}$ usually widen this difference to several mmHg. When expiration is prolonged and progresses to a lung volume below closing capacity, expired CO_2 concentration may rise sharply at the end of the alveolar plateau, in a fashion analogous to that of N_2 concentration after washout with 100 percent O_2 (phase IV, see Fig. 33-13).[55] The reason for this is that lung units subtended by airways predisposed to closure, at least in the spontaneously breathing patient, tend to have lower $PaCO_2$. Closure of these airways

allows a greater proportion of CO_2-rich gas to reach the upper airway, producing the sharp upswing in CO_2 concentration.

In the usual capnograph representation, where CO_2 concentration during tidal breathing is plotted versus time, the alveolar plateau lasts for the greater part of the trace (see Fig. 33-14*A1*), although the expiratory flow is highest at the beginning of the expiration and tapers off in exponential fashion during the last third of expiratory time. Most of the exhaled volume of a passive expiration, therefore, exits the trachea (and the tracheal tube or the anesthetic mask) during the first half of exhalation time.

Several causes are responsible for the frequent appearance of the gentle upslope observed in the alveolar plateau. Most can be traced to uneven emptying of different alveolar regions with different time constants and varying $\dot{V}A/\dot{Q}$ ratios. An additional important cause is that the alveolar gas that is sampled later in expiration is, in fact, richer in CO_2 than the early fraction, since CO_2 excretion from pulmonary capillaries into the alveoli continues at nearly constant rate during expiration, but CO_2 molecules are diluted into a lung volume made progressively smaller by the exhalation process. Slow exhalation, as during an acute asthmatic attack, or

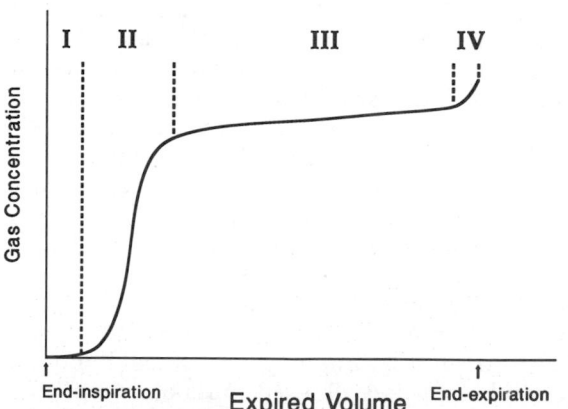

Fig. 33-13. Phases of a single breath gas washout. Gas concentration is shown on the ordinate as a function of exhaled gas volume. This curve may represent CO_2 concentration, or any other resident gas (e.g., N_2) after taking a breath of 100 percent O_2. Phase I consists of gas exhaled from the large airways. Phase II consists of a rapid increase in resident gas concentration to the alveolar plateau (phase III), which consists of "alveolar" gas. An upslope in phase III may occur because of uneven mixing within the lung. Closure of lung units, usually in the lung bases (in the upright patient), or posteriorly (in the supine position) is accompanied by a sharp increase in resident gas exhaled concentration (phase IV).

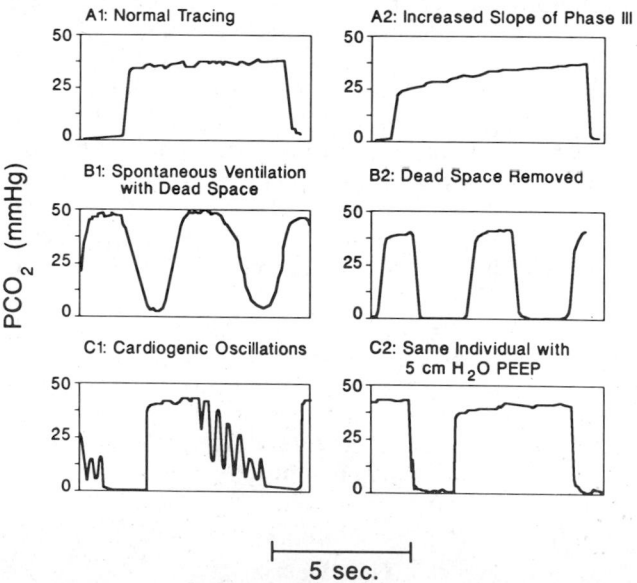

Fig. 33-14. Examples of capnograph waveforms. **(A1)** A normal tracing. **(A2)** An increased slope of phase III, usually representing uneven gas mixing within the lung. **(B1)** Spontaneous ventilation with added dead space. After removal of the dead space inspired CO_2 concentration decreases to 0 and the upstroke and downstroke of the waveforms become sharper because of less mixing **(B2)**. **(C1)** Rapid oscillations of expired CO concentration due to cardiac action. **(C2)** The same patient after application of 5 cmH$_2$O PEEP. The abolition of cardiogenic oscillations by PEEP is probably due to an effect of increased lung volume. (See text for details.)

in patients with chronic obstructive pulmonary disease (COPD), with reduced lung recoil, usually induces a steeper alveolar plateau (Fig. 33-14*A2*).

When patients are anesthetized in the lateral position, uneven ventilation of the dependent lung and lesser perfusion of the nondependent lung increase the range of alveolar gas disparity and hence the upslope of the alveolar plateau. This can be verified by alternating sampling sites between the two lungs when ventilating a patient in the lateral position with separate endobronchial tubes.

The last segment of a capnograph is represented by the rapidly decreasing value of CO_2 toward the inspired value, which is caused by the inspired gas being suctioned into the sampling area. The capnogram value during inspiration represents the concentration of CO_2 in the inspirate and is dependent mostly on the breathing circuit used and inspiratory flow and fresh gas flow values. Rebreathing of dead space volume is often the cause of an inspired level above baseline (see Fig. 33-14*B1*): this can be promptly corrected by removing the dead space (Fig. 33-14*B2*). Exhaustion of the CO_2 absorber may also result in elevated P_ICO_2. The sampling flow rate of sidestream monitors must be taken into account when interpreting many features of the capnogram profile. Usually, sampling flow rates vary, and they can be set between 50 ml/min and 400 ml/min, with an average optimal value for an adult patient of about 200 ml/min. As soon as the respiratory gas flows decrease below the sidestream gas sampling rate, the characteristics of the sampling vary: in lieu of "sampling" a portion of the main-stream flow, the equipment contributes significantly to bulk flow in and out of the respiratory circuit. This is of great importance in the pediatric setting, during low-flow anesthesia, and when interpreting capnograms obtained during very low respiratory rates. For example, during a prolonged expiration, or a end-expiratory pause, while the gas flow exiting the trachea approaches zero, the sampling of the monitor may aspirate gas alternatively from the trachea and the inspiratory limb. A profile that illustrates this effect is shown in Fig. 33-14*C1*; it is called cardiogenic oscillation, referring to the cause of the alteration. Synchronous changes in pulmonary blood flow during slow expiration and mechanical agitation of different lung regions induced by cardiac activity and pulmonary blood flow contribute to the creation of ripples often observed in a repetitive pattern during the alveolar plateau in synchrony with the heartbeat. The usual interpretation of cardiogenic oscillatory ripples is a mechanical agitation of deep lung regions that expel CO_2-rich gas in synchrony with the heartbeat. Waveforms due to cardiogenic oscillation are more pronounced when sampling of gas is obtained from deeper tracheal and bronchial areas. Such fluctuations are often smoothed over when the sampling port is more distal to the airways or when lung volume is increased by the application of PEEP (see Fig. 33-14*C2*).

Inspection of the whole curve rather than measurement of just peak expired and peak inhalation values, which may be reported digitally, improves the scope and interpretation of the trace. When a capnographic trace is displayed such that all characteristics of the various stages of the waveform are visible, on a rapidly scrolling oscilloscope or on fast-moving paper, it is possible to recognize several features that may be of diagnostic value. When capnograms are plotted on slow-moving paper or trends of only inspired and $ETCO_2$ values are produced, it is still possible to recognize important clinical information regarding rising or falling concentrations of CO_2 both inspired and expired.

Normal end-expiratory CO_2 partial pressure ranges between 35 and 45 mmHg. An increase above this level (hypercapnia) must be interpreted in the light of additional information, as it depends on a variety of factors:

1. Increased CO_2 production, such as during an acute attack of malignant hyperpexia or developing fever
2. Depression of the respiratory center, with concomitant reduction of total ventilation and elevation of $ETPCO_2$
3. Reduction of ventilation induced by partial paralysis, neurologic disease, high spinal anesthesia, weakened respiratory muscle, or acute respiratory distress

If ventilation is controlled, inadequate mechanical ventilation must be the first interpretation of increased $ETCO_2$. If an increasing trend in $ETCO_2$ is observed while total ventilation remains constant, it is essential to verify the patient's temperature in order to exclude the diagnosis of hyperpexia. Additional causes frequently observed for transient increases in $ETCO_2$ are induced by release of tourniquets with reperfusion of ischemic areas, release of aortic clamps, intravenous administration of bicarbonate (Fig. 33-15), insufflation

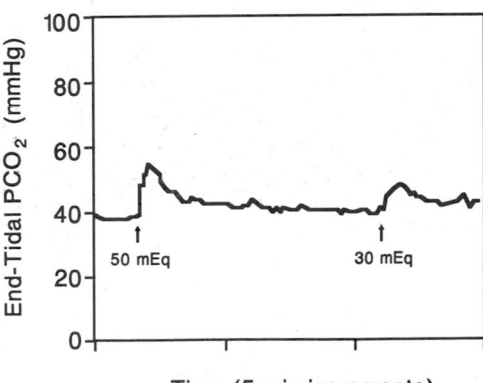

Time (5 min increments)

Fig. 33-15. The effect of sodium bicarbonate administration on $ETPCO_2$. A continuous tracing of $ETPCO_2$ is shown as a function of time. Intravenous administration of 50 mEq then 30 mEq of $NaHCO_3$ results in an abrupt increase in expired CO_2 due to neutralization of bicarbonate by hydrogen ion.

of carbon dioxide in the peritoneal cavity as during laparoscopy, and acute defects in mechanical ventilation systems.

Abnormally low end-tidal values (below 35 mmHg) most often reflect hyperventilation but may also be caused by increased dead space with normal $PaCO_2$. For example, alveolar gas emanating from a lung region with no blood flow (and hence no local CO_2 transfer) dilutes exhaled gas and decrease $ETPCO_2$ relative to $PaCO_2$. Hypocapnea may also be artifactually induced by high sampling rate of the sidestream monitor, in the face of an elevated fresh gas flow rate. In addition, low $ETPCO_2$ may reflect decreased $\dot{V}CO_2$ ($ETPCO_2$ during cardiac arrest may equal 0).

Similarly, areas of lung that are perfused but unventilated (e.g., in atelectasis), due to shunting of mixed venous blood, will have high regional $PaCO_2$ and hence high $PaCO_2 - ETPCO_2$. Arterial minus $ETPCO_2$ has been used as a criterion for optimizing PEEP in ventilated patients.[56] Increasing levels of PEEP would be expected to resolve atelectasis and hence decrease $PaCO_2 - ETPCO_2$ in these areas. In normal areas, overdistension will impair perfusion and therefore increase regional $PaCO_2 - ETPCO_2$. Optimum PEEP will be attained when a balance is reached.

Irregularities in the alveolar plateau are often observed when mechanical factors acutely alter the pattern of alveolar emptying, such as when the arm of a surgeon compresses the chest at midexpiration. A cleft or a dip may indicate a spontaneous breath of small tidal volume, able to move just a small bolus of inspired gas past the sampling site. This has been often interpreted as an indication of activation of respiratory centers by a patient recovering from anesthesia or an activation of respiration induced by sudden increasing stimulation in the surgical field. It may also indicate inadequate inspiratory power during switching from mechanical to spontaneous ventilation and can be the first sign of the need of reversal of neuromuscular blockade; or it may just indicate the opposite, the need for increased total ventilation in order to induce apnea in the patient. The dip in the plateau of the capnogram must be interpreted with care, therefore, depending on the surgical stage, the drug exposure history of the patient, and the anesthetic plan.

The main use of the capnographic signal in anesthesia is the immediate verification of tracheal intubation beyond doubt by the immediate and continuous presence of metabolic CO_2 in the expired gas. Esophageal intubation may produce one or a few breaths containing CO_2 during expiration, but the concentration of this gas in exhalations from the stomach cavity rapidly decreases to zero. In this fashion the continuous appearance of expired CO_2 is rapidly being adopted as a criterion for correct tracheal intubation. Another major use of this signal has been to determine the correct ventilatory needs ($\dot{V}E$) during controlled ventilation. This use is easily extended to continuous monitoring of spontaneous ventilation and to monitoring of appropriate ventilation during titration of anesthetic agents that de-

press ventilation. In partial rebreathing circuits and in low-flow anesthesia, capnometry facilitates the adjustment of fresh gas flow, which is a major determinant of carbon dioxide levels insofar as it may increase minute ventilation. The shape of a partial rebreathing capnogram may vary greatly, depending on the ventilatory frequency and tidal volume. In all these utilization modes, the sensing head of the capnograph or the site of gas sampling is best kept close to the tracheal tube, connected with the minimal dead space assembly. In this mode, for instance, it is easy to reveal disconnection of the breathing system or inappropriate functioning of mechanical ventilators. Partial rebreathing circuit systems include a carbon dioxide absorber, whose exhaustion is manifested by hypercarbia. Clinical signs of hypercarbia may be only slowly recognized, whereas increase in inspired CO_2 is immediately observable with a capnograph. Rapid alterations in $ETPCO_2$ can be recognized within a single exhalation. In a different setting, capnography has been used on the exhaust side of a cardiopulmonary bypass oxygenator to track CO_2 excretion at different body temperatures.

Errors in Capnography

Because water vapor is often the major source of error, several "water trap" devices or heated suction tubes are used to deliver moisture-free gas to the reading cell.

The effect of gas temperature is as follows. Assume body temperature is 37 °C and $PaCO_2 = ETPCO_2 = 40$ mmHg. If the sampling tube and detector are maintained at a temperature greater than 37° C there will be no condensation or "rain out" of water, and the measured PCO_2 will be 40 mmHg. On the other hand, if the expired gas is allowed to cool to room temperature (say 20 °C) then water will condense in the tubing, such that the new water vapor pressure (PH_2O) decreases to the saturated water vapor pressure at room temperature. If a drying agent is used in the sample line PH_2O will drop to zero. In either case the measured PCO_2 will change, as shown in Table 33-1.

TABLE 33-1. Effect of Water Condensation or Gas Sample Drying on End-Tidal CO_2 Measurement at Sea Level and 15,000 Ft Altitude[a]

	Mouth	Cell (20°C)	Cell (Active Drying)
Sea level ($P_B = 760$ mmHg)			
PH_2O	47.0	17.5	0
$ETFCO_2$	0.053	0.055	0.056
$ETPCO_2$	40.0	41.7	42.6
15,000 ft altitude ($P_B = 429$ mmHg)			
PH_2O	47.0	17.5	0
$ETFCO_2$	0.093	0.100	0.105
$ETPCO_2$	40.0	43.1	44.9

[a] Since barometric pressure remains constant throughout the system, the removal of water vapor either partially (tubing and cell at room temperature) or completely (active drying) will elevate the fractional concentraion, and hence partial pressure, of remaining gases. The magnitude of the effect is greater at high altitude, where PH_2O is a larger fraction of barometric pressure. Note that the fractional concentraton of CO_2 in end-tidal gas is considerably higher at 15,000 ft than at sea level despite a constant $ETPCO_2$.

OXYGEN AND CARBON DIOXIDE EXCHANGE MONITORING
(Also See Ch. 15)

The most direct method of measuring oxygen consumption ($\dot{V}O_2$) and CO_2 production ($\dot{V}CO_2$) is by analysis of inspired and expired gas concentrations. If one can measure the minute volume along with inspired and expired O_2 and CO_2 concentrations, then $\dot{V}CO_2$ can be calculated by using the following equation:

$$\dot{V}CO_2 = \dot{V}E \cdot FECO_2 - \dot{V}I \cdot FICO_2 \qquad (21)$$

where

$\dot{V}E, \dot{V}I$ = expired and inspired minute volumes, respectively

$FECO_2, FICO_2$ = expired and inspired CO_2 concentrations, respectively

$\dot{V}I$ and $\dot{V}E$ differ slightly because $\dot{V}O_2$ rarely equals $\dot{V}CO_2$. Since $FICO_2$ usually is zero, equation (25) can be simplified to

$$\dot{V}CO_2 = \dot{V}E \cdot FECO_2 \qquad (22)$$

Similarly, an equation can be written for the calculation of oxygen consumption:

$$\dot{V}O_2 = \dot{V}I \cdot FIO_2 - \dot{V}E \cdot FEO_2 \qquad (23)$$

In practice, it is difficult to measure minute ventilation with the necessary degree of accuracy to be able to distinguish small differences between $\dot{V}I$ and $\dot{V}E$. Since inert (i.e., gas in the breathing mixture that is not either CO_2 or O_2) gas exchange generally equals 0, $\dot{V}I$ can be calculated as follows:

$$\dot{V}I = \dot{V}E \cdot \frac{FE\text{inert}}{FI\text{inert}} \qquad (24)$$

where:

$FI\text{inert} = 1 - FIO_2$
$FE\text{inert} = 1 - (FEO_2 + FECO_2)$

Therefore, equation (27) can be rewritten as

$$\dot{V}O_2 = \dot{V}E \left[FIO_2 \frac{FE\text{inert}}{FI\text{inert}} - FEO_2 \right] \qquad (25)$$

$\dot{V}O_2$ measurement using this equation is usually accurate. However, an error develops at high FIO_2 values because $FI\text{inert}$ becomes small. Errors in the measurement of $FI\text{inert}$ result in correspondingly large errors in $\dot{V}O_2$. In fact, if $FIO_2 = 1$ then this equation cannot be used.

Open circuit measurement of $\dot{V}O_2$ and $\dot{V}CO_2$ under anesthesia using this method have been described by Viale et al.[57] Self-contained analyzers have been designed (e.g., the MGM/TWO system [Utah Medical Products, Midvale, Utah],[58] and the Sensormedics Horizon System [Sensormedics, Anaheim, California]).[59] These instruments have proved to be extremely satisfactory for gas exchange monitoring in patients in the critical care environment. One practical problem, at least with the MGM system, is that the zirconium oxide O_2 sensor is extremely sensitive to small concentrations of fluorinated anesthetic gases, which may cause severe malfunction of the system.

Another method of measuring O_2 consumption is to monitor the arteriovenous O_2 content difference and multiply by cardiac output:

$$\dot{V}O_2 = (CaO_2 - C\overline{v}O_2) \cdot \dot{Q}T \qquad (26)$$

where

$CaO_2, C\overline{v}O_2$ = arterial and mixed venous O_2 contents, respectively (ml/L)
$\dot{Q}T$ = cardiac output

Blood O_2 content may be calculated as

$$CaO_2, C\overline{v}O_2 = SaO_2, S\overline{v}O_2 \cdot [Hb] \cdot 13.9 + 0.03 \cdot PaO_2, P\overline{v}O_2 \qquad (27)$$

This method of calculation of $\dot{V}O_2$ is reasonably satisfactory for clinical purposes, although it becomes less accurate in the setting of high cardiac output and low arteriovenous O_2 content differences.

RESPIRATORY CENTER DRIVE

Measurement of the respiratory drive is particularly important in assessment of the effects of anesthetic agents on the respiratory system and in particular in the process of weaning patients from mechanical ventilation. Of the various causes of respiratory failure, including pulmonary mechanical abnormalities and impairment of respiratory gas exchange, depressed ventilatory drive is a common cause of failure to wean after general anesthesia. Experimentally, the drive to breathe has been mesured as the ventilatory output ($\dot{V}E$) as a function of varying levels of elevated $PaCO_2$ or decreased levels of $PaCO_2$ (see Ch. 15). These measurements are difficult to obtain in the clinical situation, and various measures of neural respiratory center output have been sought.

Partitioning the respiratory wavform into inspiratory and expiratory components can provide further information. Mean inspiratory flow (tidal volume/inspiratory time, VT/TI) is an index of respiratory drive.[60] However, it is possible for a patient to have a high respiratory drive but not be able to translate that drive into respiratory output because of impaired ventilatory mechanics.

A low ventilation rate (VF) is considered to be a reasonably accurate assessment of respiratory depression caused by anesthetic agents, particularly narcotics. Although parenteral narcotics usually produce a slowing of VF, there are pitfalls in the reliance on bradypnea as a sign of respiratory depression. Camporesi et al.[61] demonstrated that the predominant mode of ventilatory depression in normal volunteers given epidural morphine was a reduction in tidal volume, with little change in respiratory rate. Rawal and Wattwil[62] showed in both normal volunteers and postoperative cholecystectomy patients no change or increase in VF after epidural morphine despite a significant reduction in V̇E. Sandler and Chovaz[63] monitored six patients receiving epidural morphine after elective thoracotomy. Two of the six patients experienced periods of apnea that were not preceded by slow respirations. Ready et al.[64] described four cases of marked respiratory depression after epidural morphine. All had $PaCO_2$ values of 63 mmHg or higher; one patient developed a $PaCO_2$ of 95 mmHg. Respiration rates in all four patients were 8/min or greater. The patients with a $PaCO_2$ of 95 had a respiration rate of 12/min. Clearly bradypnea does not predict apnea, and severe respiratory depression can exist in patients with acceptable respiration rates.

A more sophisticated measure is the maximum negative inspiratory airway pressure (P_{100} or $P_{0.1}$) obtained 100 milliseconds after a temporary occlusion of the airway in a spontaneously breathing patient. Periodic transient airway occlusion that occurs in this way is not appreciably noticed by the patient. Furthermore, chemosensitivity, determined in volunteers by CO_2 responsiveness, is not significantly affected by intermittent (every 30 seconds) P_{100} maneuvers.[65] The normal value for P_{100} during resting ventilation is 1 to 2 cmH_2O. P_{100} is a useful index of respiratory drive, requiring no voluntary effort on the part of the subject and being minimally affected by changes in respiratory mechanics. The technique is well described by Milic-Emili et al.[66] Under anesthesia P_{100} is depressed.[67] However, the effect of anesthesia is highly dependent upon $PaCO_2$, with methoxyflurane actually causing an elevation in P_{100} at high $PaCO_2$. Possibly one could use P_{100} as a guide to the discontinuation of mechanical ventilation after general anesthesia. We are unaware of any systematic studies in this setting, however. In acute respiratory failure due to other causes P_{100} is generally elevated; Herrera et al.[68] and Sassoon et al.[69] found values of P_{100} above 6 cmH_2O and 4.2 cmH_2O, respectively, during T-tube trials to be correlated to lack of success in weaning. Montgomery et al.[70] found a similar relationship but reported a better prediction of weaning successes using the P_{100} response after breathing of 3 percent CO_2 (P_{100H}). Mean P_{100H}/P_{100} ratio was 2.04 in seven successful weans and 1.17 in seven failures.

PULMONARY AND CHEST WALL MECHANICAL FUNCTION (Also See Ch. 15)

Principles of Gas Flow Measurement

Monitoring of inspiratory and expiratory flow can be useful for a variety of reasons. First, measures of resistance (discussed later) require both pressure and flow measurement. Second, flow may be integrated to provide a monitor of inspired or expired volume. Several types of flow meters exist. Possibly the most commonly used flow meter in anesthesia is the rotameter. In this type of instrument gas flow imparts movement to a series of vanes connected to a wheel. The Wright spirometer integrates this movement, providing the user with a measure of volume. The Fleisch pneumotachograph consists of a bundle of small-diameter tubes in parallel. Flow within these capillary tubes is laminar, and pressure drop is therefore linearly related to gas flow.[71] Screen-type pneumotachographs work by measurement of the pressure drop across a mesh screen. These devices are usually smaller and lighter than Fleisch-type pneumotachographs; however, they are inherently nonlinear. Moreover, their practical implementation is often limited by their tendency to collect moisture and debris, which changes the operating characteristics. Vortex-type pneumotachographs are frequently used in modern mechanical ventilators. These devices work by measurement of interruptions in an ultrasonic beam placed across a tube in which struts disrupt the laminar flow, resulting in vortices.[71] Ultrasonic flow meters measure the speed of ultrasonic waves propagated parallel to the direction of flow.[72] Hot wire anemometers consist of electrically heated wires placed in the gas flow, which tend to cool the wire and change the electrical conductivity. Flow is measured by the amount of additional electrical current necessary to maintain the wire at constant temperature. These devices characteristically have an extremely high frequency response, but their behavior is highly dependent on gas temperature and contamination of the gas stream with mucus and water droplets.[71]

Respiratory Output

The mechanical output of the respiratory system may be assessed by measuring respiratory muscle activity and resulting gas flow.

Electrical activity of the diaphragm, the most important inspiratory muscle, has been measured with needle electrodes inserted into the eighth or ninth intercostal spaces in the midaxillary line in adults[73] or in neonates by surface electrodes, applied subcostally at the nipple line.[74] Diaphragmatic EMG can be obtained in this manner in neonates but in adults is frequently contaminated by the simultaneous electrical activity of the overlying intercostals. A cleaner diaphragmatic EMG signal may be obtained by using an esophageal electrode.[75] Electrical gating of the much larger ECG signal may allow relatively pure diaphragmetic EMG signals to be recorded.[76] Fatiguing muscle tends to produce EMG potentials at lower frequencies, allowing diaphragmatic fatigue in a variety of situations to be diagnosed by frequency analysis of the signal obtained in this way.[75] Mechanical activity of the diaphragm cannot be assessed directly. However, because of its shape (approximately hemiellipsoidal) contraction of the diaphragm must result in a transdiaphragmatic pressure (Pab − Ppl). Esophageal and gastric pressure simultaneously measured may be used to calculate transdiaphragmatic pressure. A nasogastric tube with esophageal and gastric balloons specifically manufactured for this purpose can be purchased (Nasogastric Esophageal Balloon: Sheridan Catheter Corp., Argyle, New York). Transdiaphragmatic pressure measurement has been used to assess diaphragmatic function[77] and loss of diaphragmatic contraction demonstrated in the early postoperative period after upper abdominal surgery.[78] Loss of transdiaphragmatic pressure generation implies lack of diaphragmatic contraction (Fig. 33-16).[79]

Diaphragm motion can be assessed somewhat more indirectly by observing or monitoring thoracic and abdominal movements during inspiration. The normal outward movement of both chest and abdomen during inspiration is replaced by paradoxical inward movement of the abdomen in the presence of diaphragmatic inaction,[80] which may be due to phrenic nerve paresis or diaphragmatic fatigue.[81] External movement of the thorax and abdomen can be monitored in this way by using magnetometers, which can monitor anteroposterior and lateral thoracic and abdominal dimensions,[80,82] or strain gauge displacement transducers.[83] Another method uses two coils of wire that encircle the torso at the thorax and abdomen. The self-inductances of the coils change in proportion to the encircled areas and can be calibrated to provide continuous monitoring of ventilation.[84] Unfortunately these methods are rather sensitive to changes in posture or body position[85] and furthermore cannot be used intraoperatively during surgery on the thorax or abdomen.

The final mechanical output of the respiratory system (gas flow) can be assessed by monitoring minute ventilation ($\dot{V}E$) directly or monitoring its components: VF and VT.

Monitoring of breath sounds provides a low-cost, high-reliability semiquantitative measure of the gas flow into and out of the lung. Continuous monitoring of breath sounds using an earpiece connected to a precor-

dial or esophageal stethoscope allows immediate detection of breathing circuit disconnection in mechanically ventilated patients. It facilitates early detection of decreased tidal volume, changes in respiration rate, and endotracheal tube cuff leaks. It also provides qualitative data that may indicate changes in pulmonary mechanics. Wheezes (rhonchi) are produced when gas flow and airways interact such that airway walls become apposed. Oscillation of the airways between open and nearly closed produces the sound heard as wheezing. Airway vibration then results in sound production detected as wheezing. Wheezes may occur when airway diameter is narrowed as a result of smooth muscle contraction (bronchospasm), mucosal thickening or edema, buildup of secretions, extrinsic compression, or endobronchial mass such as tumor or foreign body. Although severe generalized airways obstruction may occur without wheezing, for example, in emphysema, the presence of wheezes correlates with *reversibility* of airways obstruction.[86] Crackles (rales) are discontinuous sounds produced by the sudden opening of small airways during inspiration. These are indicative of airway closure and subsequent reopening, which may occur in interstitial fibrosis or in any situation resulting in premature closure of small airways (pneumonia, pulmonary edema, low lung volumes). In patients with large amounts of airway secretions, particularly in the large airways, crackles may also be caused by gas bubbling through airway secretions. The origin of lung sounds has been reviewed.[87,88]

$\dot{V}E$ and VT are easy to measure directly in patients whose tracheas are intubated and are indeed routinely measured by modern mechanical ventilators. However, in the patient whose trachea is not intubated, these parameters can only be obtained somewhat inaccurately by monitoring external dimensions of the thorax and abdomen either "clinically" by direct obser-

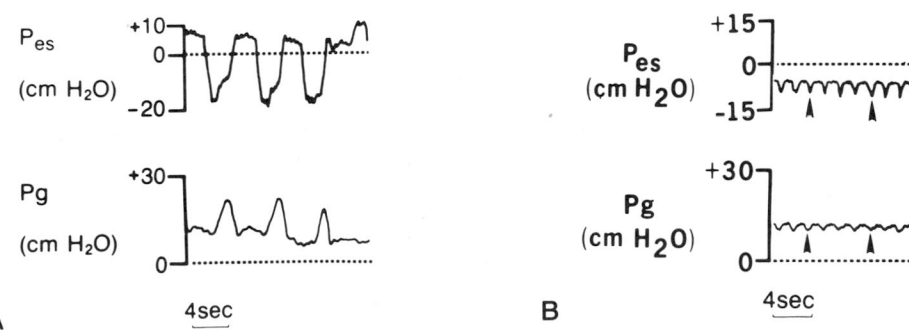

Fig. 33-16. Examples of transdiaphragmatic pressure monitoring. **(A)** Simultaneous esophageal and gastric pressure waveforms during tidal breathing in the normal individual. Negative esophageal (and hence pleural) pressure swings are accompanied by positive gastric pressure waves, indicating the development of transdiaphragmatic pressure during inspiration. **(B)** The same waveforms in a patient with phrenic nerve palsy (and hence absent diaphragmatic contraction). Negative intrathoracic pressure swings (arrows) are accompanied by gastric pressure swings in the same direction. Intrathoracic pressure changes are therefore being directly transmitted through a passive diaphragm. These changes can also be observed in the early postoperative period in patients who have had upper abdominal surgery. (From Brown et al.,[79] with permission.)

vation or by using one of the techniques noted. Subjective assessment in particular is extremely inaccurate,[89] commonly with overestimation of V_T by up to 60 percent. Alternatively, $\dot{V}_E$ can be monitored directly by using a head tent.[90] These methods are difficult to apply for routine clinical use. Therefore, mesurement of V_F remains the mainstay of respiratory output monitoring. Mechanical measures of gas flow such as these provide combined assessments of both respiratory drive and mechanical function of the respiratory system. However, in the presence of relatively normal thoracic mechanics, respiratory gas movement is considered to be a reasonable monitor of respiratory output.

Measurement of Respiratory Mechanics (See Ch. 15)

Principles

Mechanical properties of the respiratory system include the passive mechanical properties of *resistance*, *elastance*, and *inertance*, in addition to the motor properties of the muscles of respiration. Resistance (R), in pulmonary mechanical terms, is the increment in pressure (ΔP) applied to the system divided by the increment in flow or rate of change of volume ($\dot{V}$):

$$R = \frac{\Delta P}{\Delta \dot{V}} \qquad (28)$$

Normal resistance is 1.5 centimeters of H_2O per liter per second ($cmH_2O \cdot L^{-1} \cdot sec$). Under anesthesia R may be as high as 9 $cmH_2O \cdot L^{-1} \cdot sec$. Most of the resistance of the respiratory system is due to the flow resistance of the major conducting airways. A small portion of the resistance is due to the tissue viscosity. *Conductance* (G) is the reciprocal of resistance:

$$G = \frac{1}{R} \qquad (29)$$

Elastance (E) is the applied pressure divided by the resulting static change in volume:

$$E = \frac{\Delta P}{\Delta V} \qquad (30)$$

A more commonly used variable is *compliance* (C), the reciprocal of elastance:

$$C = \frac{1}{E} \qquad (31)$$

A commonly used unit for compliance is ml/cmH_2O. Since the lung and chest wall are mechanically in series,

$$\frac{1}{C_{TH}} = \frac{1}{C_L} + \frac{1}{C_{CW}} \qquad (32)$$

Where C_{TH}, C_L, and C_{CW} are the thoracic, lung, and chest wall compliances, respectively. *Inertance* (I) is the applied pressure divided by the gas acceleration, or

the second derivative of volume with respect to time:

$$I = \frac{\Delta P}{\Delta \ddot{V}} = \frac{P}{(d\dot{V}/dt)} \qquad (33)$$

Inertance is analogous to the mass of tissue and gas within the lung. Normal thoracic inertance is .02 to .04 $cmH_2O \cdot L^{-1} \cdot sec^2$. Ordinarily, because acceleration of gas flow and mass of gas and tissue are low, inertance plays a minor part in the mechanical behavior of the respiratory system. However, under conditions of high-frequency ventilation or high inspired gas density, inertance may play a major role in determining gas flow.

Practical Measurement of Passive Respiratory Mechanical Properties

Estimates of compliance and resistance in the respiratory system may be obtained by inspection of the airway pressure-volume (or time) relationships. Thoracic compliance may be obtained by inflating the lungs with known increments of volume and measuring the static pressure at each point. Under normal circumstances the lung and chest wall have approximately equal compliance of approximately 200 ml/cmH$_2$O, resulting in a total thoracic compliance of 100 ml/cmH$_2$O. Individual measurements of chest wall and lung components to the total respiratory compliance cannot be made without some estimate of pleural pressure. Conventionally, pleural pressure is measured by inserting a pressure monitoring balloon within the esophagus. Unfortunately, in the supine patient the weight of the mediastinum results in a falsely high estimate of pleural pressure when using this technique. Direct pleural pressure measurement must therefore be obtained in order to measure lung and chest wall compliance accurately in this position. A noninvasive method of pleural pressure measurement using a flat loop of Teflon insulated wire attached to the skin of the suprasternal fossa has been described.[91] The skin movement that accompanies changes in intrapleural pressure is transduced by the coil of wire by continuous measuring of its self-inductance. Measurements of pulmonary compliance using this technique correlated well with similar measurements using an esophageal balloon to estimate intrapleural pressure. However, the technique is time-consuming and measurements cannot be obtained in some individuals.

Estimation of thoracic compliance can be made on a breath-by-breath basis by monitoring the inspiratory pressure-time curve. If a constant tidal volume is being used to ventilate a patient, then the thoracic compliance will be inversely related to the inspiratory pressure. It is important that the pressure used to calculate thoracic compliance be at end inspiration ("plateau pressure"), since during the period of inspiratory gas flow there is an additional component of pressure due to airways resistance. The changes in peak airway pressure (related to both airways resistance and thoracic compliance) and the plateau pressure (related only to compliance) may quickly identify pulmonary mechanical abnormalities in ventilated patients (see Fig. 33-17). An empirically defined measurement, peak inspiratory pressure change divided by tidal volume, is defined as *dynamic compliance:*

$$Cdyn = \frac{Ppk - PEEP}{V_T} \qquad (34)$$

The normal value is 40 to 80 ml/cmH$_2$O.

Plateau pressure change (Pplat − PEEP) divided by tidal volume is called *static compliance:*

$$Cstat = \frac{Pplat - PEEP}{V_T} \qquad (35)$$

The normal value is 50 to 100 ml/cmH$_2$O.

It is important to note that in order to make these compliance calculations the end-expiratory pressure (if any) must be subtracted from Ppk or Pplat. The PEEP value can usually be read directly from the airway pressure monitor at end expiration. However, when insufficient expiratory time prevents complete emptying of the lungs, significant end-expiratory elevation of alveolar pressure that is not detected at the airway pressure monitor *(auto-PEEP)* may occur. Auto PEEP is most likely to exist when elevation of airway resistance or compliance cause prolongation of expiratory time or when high ventilation rates are required.[92] Auto-PEEP can result in decreased cardiac output, hypotension, and electromechanical dissociation in mechanically ventilated patients. It also affects compliance measurements. Detection of auto-PEEP can be accomplished by occluding the exhalation port of the ventilator while delaying the onset of the next ventilator breath. Alveolar pressure will then equilibrate with the ventilator circuit and auto-PEEP can be read on the airway pressure monitor (Fig. 33-18). During this temporary occlusion maneuver it is important to prevent supplementary gas flow (e.g., fresh gas flow) from entering the circuit and falsely elevating the auto-PEEP value.

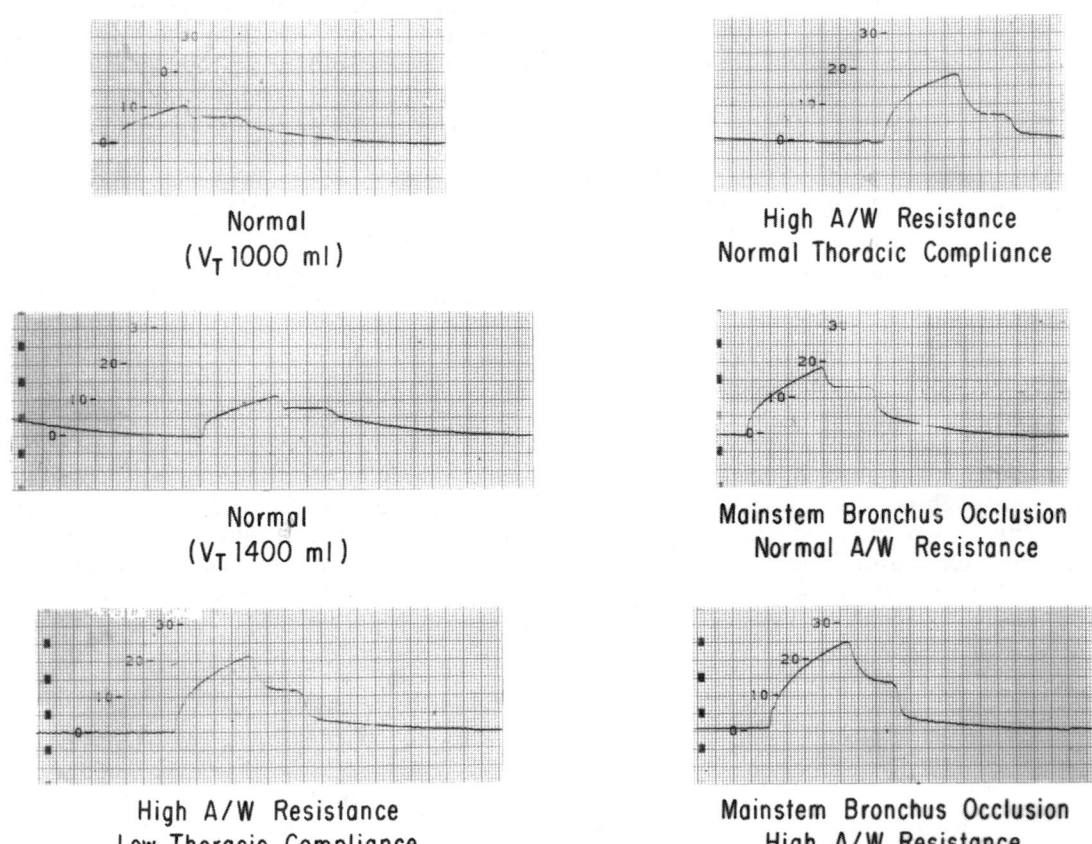

Fig. 33-17. Examples of airway pressure waveforms. Airway pressure is plotted versus time. Decreased static thoracic compliance results in an increase in *plateau* pressure; increases in airway resistance cause increased *peak* airway pressure and hence decreased dynamic compliance. (See text for details.)

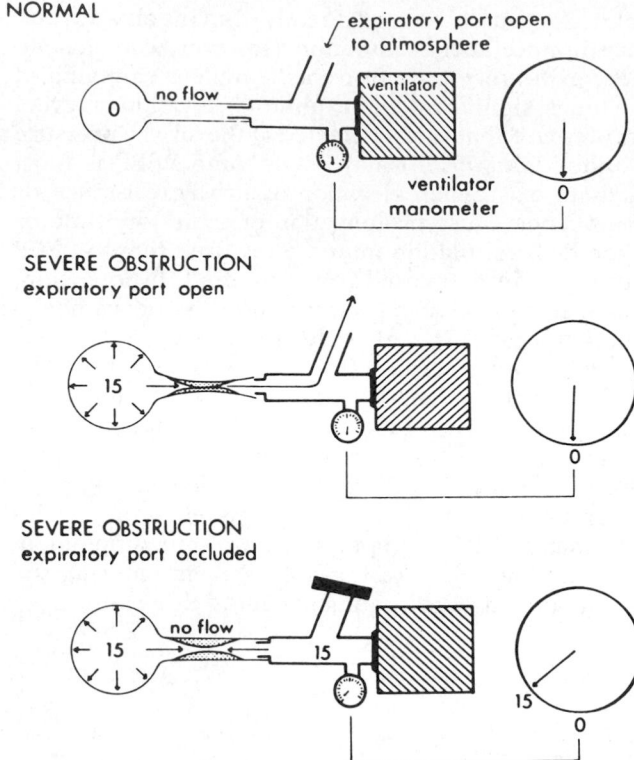

NORMAL

expiratory port open
to atmosphere

SEVERE OBSTRUCTION
expiratory port open

SEVERE OBSTRUCTION
expiratory port occluded

Fig. 33-18. Auto-PEEP. Severe airway obstruction may result in high alveolar gas pressure at end expiration that can exert the same effect on hemodynamics as externally applied PEEP. This is not usually detectable unless the expiratory port of the ventilator circuit is occluded. Auto-PEEP may then be read directly from the airway pressure monitor. (From Pepe and Marini,[92] with permission.)

An increase in static compliance may be caused by atelectasis, pulmonary edema, pneumothorax, external compression of the chest (e.g., intra-abdominal hemorrhage; in the operating room abdominal packing or because of the surgeon's leaning on the torso), or accumulation of pleural fluid. Increases in dynamic compliance may be caused by elevated airways resistance (e.g., due to bronchospasm, mucus accumulation) or obstruction or kinking of the endotracheal tube.

It is important to realize that in parallel with the patient's thoracic compliance are the internal compliance of the breathing circuit and any associated humidification or gas warming systems. Circuit compliance may be as high as 10 ml/cmH$_2$O and must be accounted for if an accurate measurement of thoracic compliance is required.

Decreased thoracic compliance places an additional load on the patient's respiratory muscles. Thoracic compliance less than 25 ml/cmH$_2$O is unlikely to result in successful weaning from mechanical ventilation.[93]

Thoracic resistance (R$_{TH}$) can be measured in the intubated patient by oscillating the airway with a sinusoidal or randomly varying flow with simultaneous measurement of flow and pressure. Significant increases in R$_{TH}$ have been observed in anesthetized patients after reversal of neuromuscular blockade with edrophonium 0.43 mg/kg.[94] An indirect estimate of airways resistance may also be obtained by monitoring the flow/time or volume/time relationship of a passive exhalation after manual inflation of a lung.[95] If a constant thoracic compliance is assumed, then the time constant of exhalation is related to airways resistance.

APNEA MONITORING

Most of the principles of apnea monitoring have already been discussed. In practice, the appropriateness of a particular apnea monitor will depend upon the situation in which it is to be used. For example, a head canopy monitor of ventilation[90] may be appropriate in an intensive care unit but entirely inappropriate for use at home in a young child. Apnea monitors are usually based on one of three general principles: detection of gas flow, chest wall movement, and gas exchange (monitors of either arterial PCO$_2$ or O$_2$ saturation). Guyatt et al.[96] described a method in which a pressure transducer was connected to a nasal O$_2$ cannula. Periodic fluctuations of around 1 cmH$_2$O due to cyclical respiratory flow were observed during nose breathing. Respiratory rates could easily be obtained with this technique even when oxygen was flowing through the cannula. Direct monitoring of ventilation can be obtained easily in a patient whose trachea is intubated. Use of a rigid air-tight canopy that encases the subject's head with a neck seal has been described by Sorkin et al.[90] The canopy is continuously flushed with fresh gas. A subject's respiration produces a net flow in and out of the canopy, which is unaffected by the fresh gas flow. The system could comfortably be worn while either awake or asleep. Another method of airflow detection was described by Werthammer et al.[97]; in it an acoustic monitor encapsulated in silicone rubber was taped 0.25 cm inside an external naris. Eight premature infants were continuously monitored for 1 to 2 hours. Twenty-six episodes of apnea lasting 15 seconds or more were detected and confirmed by direct observation. An impedance monitor (see below) detected only seven of these episodes.

Chest wall movement may be detected in a variety of ways. Inductive plethysmography (e.g., Respitrace and Respigraph: Non-Invasive Monitoring Systems, Miami, Florida) has been described.[84] It consists of two coils, encircling the abdomen and thorax, respectively. Respiratory movements are detected as changes in the self-inductance of the coils. A more commonly used method is transthoracic impedance. This method of monitoring is frequently used concurrently with ECG monitoring. In this technique, a small alternating current (typically 100 μA) at around 100 kHz is passed through a pair of ECG leads. Transthoracic electrical impedance can therefore be continuously measured and is proportional to the measured 100-kHz voltage. Low-frequency changes in respiratory impedance can easily be demodulated from the signal.[97] Electromyogram of the respiratory muscles has also been used.[74] EMG monitoring is somewhat more difficult because of contamination of the EMG signal with a much higher voltage ECG potential. Another monitor of chest wall movement makes use of a detector placed under the bed mattress (RE-134 Apnea/Respiration Monitor: Electronic Monitors, Inc., Euless, Texas). This monitor detects changes in the patient's center of gravity that occur because of respiration. Algorithms are used to exclude ballistocardiographic artifacts that may otherwise be interpreted as respiratory movements. The main disadvantage of patient movement monitors is that they may fail to detect obstructive apnea, when ventilatory effort or movement can occur without gas flow.

Since apnea per se may not result in any physiologic abnormality, a measure of its possible adverse effects (hypoxia or hypercapnia) may be preferable. Continuous measurement of ETCO$_2$, although easy in a patient whose trachea is intubated, is more difficult in a patient whose trachea is not intubated, because of discomfort from the catheter placement and clogging with mucus and saliva. This problem frequently accompanies a direct placement of a cannula into the nasopharynx. Some improvements may be obtained if a catheter is placed inside a nasal airway. A more satisfactory solution has been described by Turner.[51] Another approach is to use O$_2$ saturation. George[98] compared arterial desaturation with manually detected events using a variety of monitors, including chin EMG, airflow measurement, and respiratory movement measured by inductance plethysmography. Apnea was defined as cessation of respiration for more than 10 seconds. Nine overnight records from six patients with sleep apnea were analyzed and compared with SaO$_2$ measurement using an ear oximeter. Decreases in SaO$_2$ > 3 percent from baseline were considered significant. Using this criterion only 1.32 percent of 4,008 apneic episodes were undetected. Ear oximetry and respiratory inductive plethysmography have been used to monitor patients postoperatively.[99] Using these techniques the authors demonstrated that morphine analgesia, compared to regional analgesia with local anesthetic, was associated with a high incidence of hypoxemia and associated obstructive apnea, central apnea, paradoxic breathing, and slow respiratory rate.

Given the proven reliability of pulse oximetry it would seem that this method, perhaps in association with capnography, may provide an excellent method of apnea monitoring. Principles of apnea monitoring have been reviewed in detail by Sackner and Krieger.[100]

LUNG WATER

The frequent occurrence of pulmonary edema in clinical medicine has led to a variety of techniques for the early detection of increased lung water. Bedside estimation of lung water would be clinically useful. A variety of techniques exist at present.

Chest Radiography

The most commonly used technique clinically is the standard chest radiograph. Radiographic signs of pulmonary edema are well described. An animal study demonstrated that an approximately 35 percent increase in extravascular lung water was required for the diagnosis of "definite pulmonary edema." However, the absence of radiographic evidence of pulmonary edema virtually rules out significant increases in lung water.[101]

Computed tomography (CT) of the lung may provide more detailed information about regional lung density changes that correlate with localized edema.[102] As in plain radiography, the changes seen on CT are not specific. Moreover, the radiation dose is higher and the cost is significantly greater than those of plain radiography.

Compton scattering has also been used for lung water measurement. Rather than using the attenuation of transmitted x-ray photons as the monitor, the Compton technique measures photons scattered at 90 degrees to the incident beam. As lung water increases, the number of scattered photons increases. Webber and Cortes[103] have described a portable instrument based on this technology.

Magnetic Resonance Imaging

Magnetic resonance imaging (MRI) has significant theoretical advantages over radiographic techniques.[104] Clinical devices operate by measurement of protons in water, with no interference from other molecules. It requires no radiation and it has resolution at least as good as that of CT scanning. Disadvantages are the cost and the long image acquisition time. Extravascular water cannot be distinguished from intravascular water, though the blood contained in large vessels can be subtracted.

Positron Emission Tomography

Positron emission tomography (PET) can be used to provide tomographic images of the lung by use of radioactive tracers.[105] Intravenous administration of radioactive tracer (^{15}O-labeled water) provides a marker for lung water. Extravascular water can be separated from total water by subtracting the intravascular signal for ^{15}O-labeled carbon monoxide administered by inhalation. Disadvantages include high cost and necessity of an on-site cyclotron to produce the necessary short-lived isotopes.

Double Indicator Dilution

Injection of ice cold indocyanine green dye solution into the pulmonary artery and simultaneous thermal and green dye densitometry detection by constant withdrawal of blood from the femoral artery constitute another technique that has been developed for measurement of lung water.[106] Green dye passes undisturbed through the lung, whereas heat, primarily from lung water, diffuses into the bolus, tending to warm it up to a degree that is dependent upon the thermal mass within the lung (primarily lung water). Animal studies have revealed excellent correlation between double dye dilution and postmortem wet/dry ratio measurement of lung water. Using the same technique in human organ donors, the thermal dye estimate consistently overestimated gravimetric measurement of extravascular lung water post mortem.[107] The error is probably due to warming of the bolus by the heart and blood vessels. More recent use of single thermal indicator has been shown to have approximately the same sensitivity as double dilution.[108] All thermodilution techniques depend upon physical contiguity of the lung water to the pulmonary vessels. Unperfused areas of edema are not measured.

Multiple Gas Technique

Inhalation of a mixture of an insoluble gas (e.g., helium) with a gas that is soluble in water (e.g., acetylene) allows another method of lung water estimation.[109,110] In one application of this method a mixture of gases is rebreathed. The rate of disappearance of the soluble gas is related to lung water and pulmonary blood flow. Corrections can be made for blood flow by adding to the gas mixture carbon monoxide (which is highly soluble in blood but has low solubility in extravascular lung water not containing hemoglobin). This method is noninvasive and relatively inexpensive. However, in a fashion analogous to that of thermal measurement of lung water, the method of gas dilution measures only lung water that is accessible to the airways.

Impedance Plethysmography

Electrical impedance of the chest is inversely related to the amount of lung water. Four band-shaped electrodes are applied. One pair of excitation electrodes (placed at the neck and lower thorax) is used to pass an alternating current of approximately 0.5 mA longitudinally through the thorax. Two inner electrodes (at the base of the neck and at the diaphragm, cephalad to the lower excitation electrode) detect the induced voltage, which is proportional to the thoracic electrical impedance (Z). Increases in air volume or intrathoracic fluid accumulation cause a decrease in impedance. Absolute water measurement cannot be obtained; however, each patient can serve as his or her own control. Moreover, the technique is sensitive to changes in any intrathoracic water. Van De Water et al.[111] have reported an experience using this technique in over 200 patients. In cases in which a decrease in intrathoracic water could be observed (radiographic clearance of pulmonary edema; thoracentesis; pericardiocentesis) the expected increase in Z occurred.

None of these methods has attained routine clinical use although the value of lung water measurements has been demonstrated by a number of studies. For example, in one study Shires et al.[112] showed that perioperative use of crystalloid, rather than colloid, does not increase lung water in patients undergoing aortic surgery. Future developments will undoubtedly result in clinical applicability for lung water measurement.

MONITORING OF HIGH-FREQUENCY VENTILATION

High-frequency ventilation has been variously defined but in general represents mechanical ventilation at high rates (usually > 60 breaths/min). Several means of ventilating in this manner have been used experimentally and clinically. The use of conventional positive-pressure ventilators at high rates and small tidal volumes is called high-frequency positive pressure ventilation (HFPV). Tidal volumes are usually on the order of 3 to 4 ml/kg body weight, with a frequency from 60 to 100/min. The use of an oscillator, providing both positive and negative pressure fluctuations (e.g., a loudspeaker), is called high-frequency oscillatory ventilation (HFOV). Higher frequencies, upward of 3,000/min, have been used with this modality. A "bias flow" of fresh gas at the level of the oscillator provides the source of the respiratory gas and washes out CO_2. Injection of a high-velocity pulse of gas into the airway through a narrow cannula, entraining with it fresh gas, is termed high-frequency jet ventilation (HFJV).

In all of these forms of high-frequency ventilation instantaneous gas flows and pressure fluctuations cannot usually be monitored using conventional transducers. Moreover, since the system is basically open, a portion of the gas flow directed into the airway may leak out and not participate in intrapulmonary gas exchange. High-frequency ventilatory fluctuations generated by these ventilators may also in part do nothing more than compress and decompress the compliance of the ventilatory circuit and large conducting airways. Conventional mechanical monitoring is therefore difficult. Furthermore, capnography is difficult or impossible to apply, since dilution of expired gas may render end-tidal measurements, even assuming a high-fidelity, high-frequency capnograph, artificially low.

Monitoring of patients receiving high-frequency ventilation requires ability to monitor O_2 and CO_2 exchange as well as mechanical safety, including airway disconnection and obstruction.

Whereas patient oxygenation can readily be monitored with pulse oximetry, there is no reliable noninvasive monitor of CO_2 exchange. One way of monitoring CO_2 is to measure the mean waste gas CO_2 concentration by placing a capnograph in the expired circuit. If any condition that interferes with CO_2 exchange develops, the mean expired CO_2 decreases. Although this method provides a fairly gross measure of adequacy of CO_2 exchange, the expired CO_2 concentration is highly dependent upon fresh gas flow rate. A more satisfactory monitor might multiply fresh gas flow by $FECO_2$ to obtain $\dot{V}CO_2$. Changes in $\dot{V}CO_2$ could then reflect a mechanical problem with the ventilator. Unfortunately there are other factors that may alter $\dot{V}CO_2$, such as anesthesia or hypothermia. One cannot obtain a measure of alveolar or arterial PCO_2 using this method. The best currently available method is to interject a conventional breath periodically, in order to measure $ETPCO_2$.

Monitoring of airway pressure is extremely important in high-frequency ventilation. HFJV in particular uses high pressures and gas flows. Expiratory port occlusion can therefore result in extremely high airway pressures. Commonly, gas pressures are measured on both sides of the jet valve (drive pressure and jet pressure), along with an independent pressure measurement in the airway (Fig. 33-19). An automated feedback

loop is required to interrupt the jet ventilation by closing the solenoid valve in the event of excessively high pressures either in the airway or on the jet side of the valve. Low pressures can be used as indications of airway disconnection or ventilator malfunction.

In addition to safety concerns, airway pressure in a number of studies has been shown to correlate with gas exchange efficiency during HFJV.[113] Increasing peak airway pressures result in lower $PaCO_2$. A superior indicator of $PaCO_2$ is actually the difference between peak airway pressure and end-expiratory airway pressure.[114] However, there is no unique relationship, and the actual $PaCO_2$ obtained for a given patient depends on properties of the lung. Position of the monitoring transducer may be critical since proximal airway pressures may be artifactually low.[114]

Jet ventilation for prolonged periods of time should ideally be performed on patients with the ability to monitor arterial blood gases directly. Periodic measurement of $PaCO_2$ may provide greater assurance of adequate pulmonary gas exchange than simple reliance on noninvasive measures.

WEANING FROM MECHANICAL VENTILATION

Mechanical ventilation may be instituted for a variety of reasons, including

  Impaired respiratory drive
  Increased mechanical load
  Impaired respiratory motor function
  Impaired gas exchange

The most common reason for mechanical ventilation during and after anesthesia is impaired respiratory drive. However, components of increased mechanical load and impaired neuromuscular function may contribute to an abnormally low ventilatory function. Patients with severe chronic obstructive lung disease usually are mechanically intubated because of transient increases in mechanical load superimposed upon a chronic increase in airways resistance. Impaired respiratory drive and abnormal respiratory muscle mechanics may also play a role, however. Abnormal arterial oxygenation may exist despite what would appear to be adequate ventilatory effort. Therefore, ventilatory support may be required mainly to support arterial oxygenation or CO_2 elimination. Assessment of the patient with regard to possible discontinuation of mechanical ventilation may therefore vary somewhat, depending upon the reason for mechanical ventilatory support. Weaning ventilatory support from a patient whose only reason for mechanical ventilation is residual anesthesia is generally straightforward. A different approach is often required for a patient who has had prolonged ventilatory support for chronic respiratory disease.[115] Postoperative patients may have components of both im-

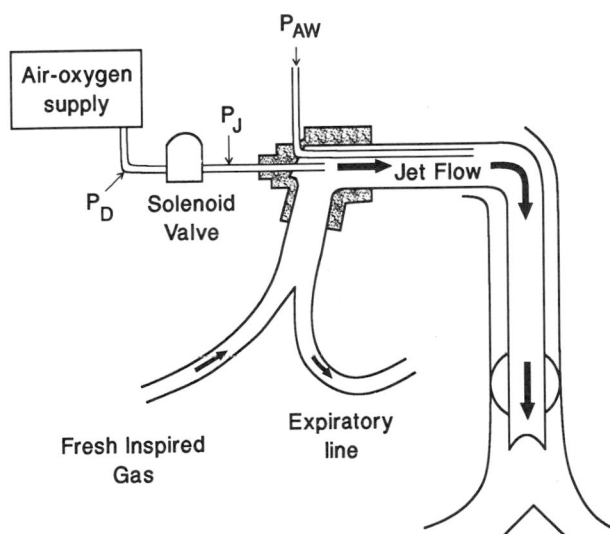

Fig. 33-19. High-frequency jet ventilation. The jet is created when high-pressure air-O_2 supply is rapidly modulated by the solenoid valve. Fresh inspired gas is from a low-pressure source, typically an anesthesia circuit. Drive pressure (PD) and jet pressure (PJ) are customarily monitored in order to detect solenoid or jet malfunction. An independent monitor of airway pressure (PAW), which will reliably detect overpressurization of the airway, circuit disconnection, or ventilator malfunction, should also be available.

paired respiratory drive (residual anesthesia) and abnormal pulmonary mechanics (stiff lungs due to edema; surgical trauma to respiratory muscles). Criteria that have been used are shown in Table 33-2. The most commonly used weaning criteria have included a vital capacity ≥ 10 ml/kg, maximum inspiratory pressure (MIP) ≤ -25 cmH$_2$O, respiratory rate ≤ 20/min, and $\dot{V}_E \leq 10$ to 20 L/min in the face of normal PaCO$_2$. Arterial oxygenation should also be maintained with an inspired O$_2$ concentration ≤ 50 percent, with 5 cmH$_2$O or less of PEEP.

Frequently a trial of spontaneous ventilation is recommended (T-tube trial). There is a potential fall in functional residual capacity during T-tube trials, which may further add to an increased respiratory load after extubation. Therefore, some clinicians advocate extubation while the patient is being supported with intermittent mandatory ventilation. For example, Gorback[122] considered general surgical patients postoperatively for extubation when the synchronized intermittent mandatory ventilation (SIMV) rate was 4/min, PaO$_2$ was ≥ 60 mmHg with FiO$_2$ ≤ 0.4, and PEEP ≤ 5 cmH$_2$O. Lack of inotropic support was also required. The investigators then proceeded to extubate patients if they matched three of the following five criteria:

Maximum inspiratory pressure ≤ -30 cmH$_2$O
Arterial pH ≥ 7.30
Respiratory rate ≤ 30/min (including IMV breaths)
Vital capacity ≥ 10 ml/kg
Tidal volume ≥ 5 ml/kg

One hundred and twenty consecutive extubations were performed using these criteria. Only 1 of the 120 patients required reintubation.

The individual approach used depends on the clinical situation. Since there is no single monitor available to facilitate rapid weaning, a combination of measures that will assess respiratory mechanical function as well as gas exchange is generally implemented.

EXTUBATION AFTER COMPROMISE OF AIRWAY

Protection of the airway with potential encroachment by hemorrhage, edema, infection, or tumor using an endotracheal tube often engenders uncertainty at the time of extubation. Airway patency after extubation may not be assured, and sudden loss of airway may occur. Reintubation may then be difficult or impossible.

Steps that should be taken at the time of extubation include the following: First, direct inspection of the upper airway, either directly or with a fiberoptic instrument, should be performed. Residual swelling of the oropharynx or nasopharynx may be detectable. Second, the endotracheal tube cuff should be deflated and the patient asked to breathe with the endotracheal tube occluded. If the patient is able to breathe around the tube in this way it is less likely that critical airway compromise will occur after extubation. It is possible that if the endotracheal tube is too large the patient may not be able to breathe around it even in the presence of a

TABLE 33-2. Possible Criteria for Ventilator Weaning

Test	Criterion for Weaning
Mechanical function	
Vital capacity (FVC)	$> 10-15$ ml/kg
FEV$_1$	> 10 ml/kg
Tidal volume (V$_T$)	> 5 ml/kg
Peak inspiratory pressure (PIP)	< -20 cmH$_2$O
Maximum voluntary ventilation (MVV)	> 2 times resting $\dot{V}_E$
Respiratory rate (V$_F$)	< 25/min
Inspiratory effort quotient $= \dfrac{(0.75 \cdot V_T/C_{dyn}) \cdot (T_I/T_{TOT})}{PIP}$	< 0.15
Functional residual capacity (FRC)	$> 50\%$ predicted
Transdiaphragmatic pressure (Pdi)/Pdi$_{max}$	< 0.4
Gas exchange function	
A-a gradient (FiO$_2$ = 1.0)	< 350 mmHg
Shunt fraction (Q̇s/Q̇T)	< 0.2
Deadspace/tidal volume ratio (V$_D$/V$_T$)	< 0.6
Minute ventilation with normal PaCO$_2$ ($\dot{V}_E$)	< 10 L/min
	< 180 ml/kg/min
Respiratory quotient (RQ)	< 0.9
Respiratory drive	
P$_{100}$	< 6 cmH$_2$O
Other	
Urine output	> 500 ml/6 h
Arterial pH	> 7.30

Abbreviations: C$_{dyn}$, dynamic thoracic compliance; T$_I$, inspiratory time; T$_{TOT}$, respiratory cycle length.
(Data from Refs. 11, 69, 70, and 115–122.)

normal airway. Replacement of the tube with a smaller-sized one may be accomplished over a rigid introducer. Third, when a trial of extubation has been definitely decided upon, a rigid introducer should be inserted and the tube removed slowly. Abrupt loss of the airway may then be treated immediately with reinsertion. A nasogastric tube with the bulbous end cut off may be used, but a more rigid plastic introducer is preferable. Alternatively, a fiberoptic bronchoscope may be introduced into the endotracheal tube. If the patient is able to breathe after removal of the tube from the larynx and lower pharynx, then direct inspection of the airway may be accomplished during removal of the fibroptic instrument.

These measures should be undertaken while someone with the necessary skills to perform an emergency tracheostomy is available. Before removal of the endotracheal tube the patient should be preoxygenated with 100 percent O_2 providing a margin of safety in the event of loss of airway.

TRANSPORTATION OF THE PATIENT

Movement of the patient between various critical care units (operating room, intensive care unit, postanesthesia care unit) or between the intensive care unit and diagnostic radiology presents special problems. Planning for such a move should include preparing for a "worse-case scenario." Movement of the patient from the operating room to the postanesthesia care unit may engender problems of hypoxemia, loss of airway, hemodynamic instability or vomiting, and aspiration. After an uncomplicated anesthetic the most likely untoward event is arterial hypoxemia and loss of airway. Since the patient is at risk for hypoxemia due to a variety of causes, including hypoventilation, atelectasis, impaired $\dot{V}_A/\dot{Q}$ matching, residual second gas effect (N_2O), shivering, and resulting decrease in mixed venous PO_2 and airway obstruction, it would appear safest to transport the patient with supplemental oxygen unless the distance between OR and PACU is short. Respirations should be continuously monitored. If supplemental O_2 is not used, a hand held under the chin may be used to detect respirations by directly feeling the airflow. Alternatively, a precordial stethoscope, or if the patient is still intubated, an esophageal stethoscope, can be used. Patients at higher risk of hypoxemia during transport include children, patients with baseline gas exchange abnormality, or obese individuals. Particularly in these types of patients relatively rapid desaturation may occur, even if the patient has been ventilated with 100 percent O_2 immediately before transport.[123]

A worst-case scenario for a patient undergoing transportation a long distance, particularly in an elevator, would include accidental extubation or inability to ventilate. Therefore, in addition to the monitoring techniques described, "long-distance" transportation within the hospital should always occur with the ability to provide

1. Emergency positive-pressure ventilation
2. Emergency endotracheal intubation

A laryngoscope, endotracheal tube, and muscle relaxant should be available. Patients at increased risk for hypoxemia or hypoventilation should ideally not be tracheally extubated immediately before transportation for more than a short distance within the hospital.

EPIDURAL AND INTRATHECAL OPIATES (Also See Ch. 69)

Discovery that narcotics may act selectively upon receptors in the spinal cord has led to their clinical use epidurally and intrathecally within the last decade. A large number of clinical reports suggest that spinal opiate administration may result in prolonged superior analgesia postoperatively compared to parenteral administration in the traditional fashion. Moreover, clinical investigation suggested that respiratory function, particularly after upper abdominal surgery,[124] may be improved with epidural administration of morphine compared to intravenous administration. However, early reports of delayed respiratory depression after epidural and intrathecal morphine administration have led to tremendous scrutiny of the respiratory depressant effect of narcotics given by this route. An excellent review has been written by Etches et al.[125] Several detailed clinical investigations of blood gases, ventilation, and chemosensitivity have shown acceptable degrees of depression after spinal narcotic administration. However, assessment of the mean response in small numbers of individuals may not predict the likelihood of an extreme response, which may occur infrequently. Few large-scale surveys are available. Rawal et al.[126] reported on a survey of 93 departments of anesthesia in Sweden. As reported by that study, during 1984 approximately 12,000 patients received epidural narcotics perioperatively and 1,000 patients received intrathecal narcotics. The vast majority of these patients received morphine; 0.04 percent of patients showed clinical signs of ventilatory depression within 1 hour of epidural morphine injection, and 0.09 percent demonstrated delayed ventilatory depression. Delayed ventilatory depression occurred in 0.36 percent of patients who received intrathecal morphine. This occurred within 7 to 9 hours after injection. All patients with ventilatory depression were successfully treated, and there were no deaths from this complication. Unfortunately, it is not known to what extent ventilatory depression occurs in patients given parenteral narcotics either intravenously or intramuscularly. Thus it is uncertain whether spinal narcotics are intrinsically more dangerous. However, one study has indeed confirmed episodes of episodic hypoxemia in patients given continuous intravenous infusions of morphine.[99] Earlier reports suggested that apnea monitoring should be used routinely on patients given spinal narcotics. More recent clinical experience has suggested that this may not be necessary, particularly in low-risk patients.[64,127]

Respiratory depression appears to be dose-related. Several other factors may predispose to respiratory depression. Table 33-3 lists some reported predisposing factors.

Ready et al.[64] suggested that respiratory monitor usage is not required when constant nursing surveillance is available (e.g., intensive care unit) or when all of the following criteria are met:

Age <50 years
ASA physical status I or II
Surgical site excluding thorax or upper abdomen
Duration of surgery <4 hours
Anesthetic technique using little or no narcotics or other long-acting CNS depressant before or during surgery
Epidural morphine dose 6 mg or less: subarachnoid morphine dose 0.5 mg or less

Apnea monitors are often associated with false alarms and are therefore frequently ignored. Most instances of respiratory depression are associated with sedation. Therefore, a frequent check of mental status may be as sensitive as more mechanical monitors in detecting clinical respiratory depression and is an important part of monitoring patients who have received epidural narcotics.

In conclusion, the widespread clinical use of epidural narcotics, particularly morphine, would suggest that it may be safe for most patients. An order sheet for use in patients receiving narcotics via this route has been suggested by Ready et al.[64] and includes the following:

1. Maintain IV access (drip, heparin lock) for 24 hours after last dose of epidural narcotic.

TABLE 33-3. Factors Predisposing to the Development of Respiratory Depression Following Epidural Opioids

Drug factors
   Hydrophilic drug (i.e., morphine)
   Large doses
   Repeated doses
   Concomitant administration of parenteral
     opioids or other CNS depressants

Patient factors
   Elderly or debilitated
   Coexisting respiratory disease
   Thoracic epidural
   High sensitivity to opioids (i.e., no previous
     exposure to opioids)
   Intrathecal administration
   Raised intrathoracic pressure (e.g., controlled
     ventilation, coughing, vomiting)

(From Etches et al.,[125] with permission.)

2. Naloxone 0.4 mg at bedside.
3. No systemic narcotics to be given except as ordered by acute pain service.
4. Monitoring
  a. Respiratory rate and sedation scale q1h for first 24 hours; Sedation scale q1h for second 24 hours; after 48 hours, sedation scale q4h.
  b. Respiratory monitor for first 24 hours (at the discretion of acute pain service).
5. Nausea/vomiting prophylaxis: metoclopramide 10 mg IV slowly q8h × 3; then q8h prn for nausea/vomiting.
6. Treatment of side effects
  a. Respiratory rate <10/min; call Acute Pain Service. Respiratory rate <8/min: naloxone 0.4 mg IV stat; may repeat prn. Call acute pain service.
  b. Naloxone 0.1 mg IV for severe itching; may repeat q10min × 5
  c. Droperidol 0.25 mg IV if metoclopramide ineffective for nausea/vomiting; may repeat ×1.
  d. Naloxone 0.1 mg IV for urinary retention; may repeat q10min × 5; if ineffective, "in and out" bladder catheter.

Until contrary information is available, patients who may be at higher risk of respiratory depression based on risk factor assessment should be monitored in a setting where constant nursing surveillance is available or on a general hospital floor with reliable mechanical or electrical apnea monitoring.

REFERENCES

1. The Oxford English Dictionary. Oxford University Press, Oxford, 1933
2. McGraw-Hill Dictionary of Scientific and Technical Terms. McGraw-Hill, New York, 1989
3. Eichhorn JH, Cooper JN, Cullen DJ, et al: Standards for patient monitoring during anesthesia at Harvard Medical School. JAMA 256:1017, 1986
4. Nunn JF: Applied Respiratory Physiology. Butterworths, London, 1987
5. Wagner PD, Gale GE, Moon RE, et al: Pulmonary gas exchange in humans exercising at sea level and simulated altitude. J Appl Physiol 61:260, 1986
6. Christiensen J, Douglas CG, Haldane JS: The absorption and dissociation of carbon dioxide by human blood. J Physiol 48:244, 1914
7. Benumof JL: Anesthesia for Thoracic Surgery. WB Saunders, Philadelphia, 1987
8. Mellemgaard K: The alveolar-arterial oxygen difference: Its size and components in normal man. Acta Physiol Scand 67:10, 1966
9. Gilbert R, Keighley JF: The arterial/alveolar oxygen tension ratio. An index of gas exchange applicable to varying inspired oxygen concentrations. Am Rev Respir Dis 109:142, 1974
10. Wagner PD, Laravuso RB, Uhs RR, West JB: Continuous distribution of ventilation-perfusion ratios in normal subjects breathing air and 100% O_2. J Clin Invest 54:54, 1974

11. Sahn SA, Lakshminarayan S, Petty TL: Weaning from mechanical ventilation. JAMA 235:2208, 1976
12. West JB: Ventilation-perfusion inequality and overall gas exchange in computer models of the lung. Respir Physiol 7:88, 1969
13. Wagner PD, Saltzman HA, West JB: Measurement of continuous distributions of ventilation-perfusion ratios: Theory. J Appl Physiol 36:588, 1974
14. Dueck R, Young I, Clausen J, Wagner PD: Altered distribution of pulmonary ventilation and blood flow following induction of inhalational anesthesia. Anesthesiology 52:113, 1980
15. Tokics L, Hedenstierna G, Strandberg A, et al: Lung collapse and gas exchange during general anesthesia: Effects of spontaneous breathing, muscle paralysis, and positive end-expiratory pressure. Anesthesiology 66:157, 1987
16. Severinghaus JW: Blood gas concentrations. p. 1475. In Fenn WO, Rahn H (eds.): Handbook of Physiology. Section 3. Vol. 2. American Physiological Society, Washington, 1965
17. Severinghaus JW, Astrup PB: History of blood gas analysis. Int Anesthesiol Clin 25:1, 1987
18. Severinghaus JW: Historical development of oxygenation monitoring. p. 1. In Payne JP, Severinghaus JW (eds): Pulse Oximetry. Springer-Verlag, New York, 1986
19. Cobbold RSC: Transducers for Biomedical Measurements. John Wiley, New York, 1974
20. Barker SJ, Tremper KK, Hyatt J, et al: Continuous fiberoptic arterial oxygen tension measurements in dogs. J Clin Monit 3:48, 1987
21. National Committee for Clinical Laboratory Standards: Tentative standard for definitions of quantities and conventions related to blood pH and gas analysis. NCCLS. Publ. 2:329, 1982
22. Camporesi EM, Moon RE: Arterial blood gas values should be corrected for temperature during hypothermic cardiopulmonary bypass. p. 35. In Gotta A (ed): Controversies in Anesthesiology. Martinus Nijhoff, New York, 1988
23. Hess CF, Nichols AB, Hunt WB, Suratt PM: Pseudohypoxemia secondary to leukemia and thrombocytosis. N Engl J Med 301:361, 1979
24. Schmaier AH: Pseudohypoxemia due to leukemia and thrombocytosis (letter). N Engl J Med 302:584, 1980
25. Comroe JH, Jr, Botelho S: The unreliability of cyanosis in the recognition of arterial hypoxemia. Am J Med Sci 214:1, 1947
26. Lundsgaard C, Van Slyke DD: Cyanosis. Medicine 2:1, 1923
27. Stadie WC: The oxygen of the arterial and venous blood in pneumonia and its relation to cyanosis. J Exp Med 30:215, 1919
28. Chaudhary BA, Burki NK: Ear oximetry in clinical practice. Am Rev Respir Dis 117:173, 1978
29. Tremper KK, Barker SJ: Pulse oximetry. Anesthesiology 70:98, 1989
30. Barker SJ, Tremper KK: The effect of carbon monoxide inhalation on pulse oximetry and transcutaneous PO_2. Anesthesiology 66:677, 1987
31. Eisenkraft JB: Pulse oximeter desaturation due to methemoglobinemia. Anesthesiology 68:279, 1988
32. Kessler MR, Eide T, Humayun B, Poppers PJ: Spurious pulse oximeter desaturation with methylene blue injection. Anesthesiology 65:435, 1986
33. Sidi A, Paulus DA, Rush W, et al: Methylene blue and indocyanine green artifactually lower pulse oximetry readings of oxygen saturation. Studies in dogs. J Clin Monit 3:249, 1987
34. Kelleher JF: Pulse oximetry. J Clin Monit 5:37, 1989
35. Coté CJ, Goldstein EA, Fuchsman WH, Hoaglin DC: The effect of nail polish on pulse oximetry. Anesth Analg 67:683, 1988
36. Read MS: Effect of transparent adhesive tape on pulse oximetry. Anesth Analg 68:701, 1989
37. Racys V, Nahrwold ML: Reusing the Nellcor pulse oximeter probe: Is it worth the savings? Anesthesiology 66:713, 1987
38. Severinghaus JW, Naifeh KH, Koh SO: Errors in 14 pulse oximeters during profound hypoxia. J Clin Monit 5:72, 1989
39. Alexander CM, Teller LE, Gross JB: Principles of pulse oximetry: Theoretical and practical considerations. Anesth Analg 68:368, 1989
40. Räsänen J, Downs JB, DeHaven B: Titration of continuous positive airway pressure by real-time dual oximetry. Chest 92:853, 1987
41. Kersting T, Reinhart K, Fleckenstein W, et al: Tissue PO_2 measurements in critical care: The effects of dopamine on muscular oxygen pressure fields. p. 109. In Ehrly AM, Hauss J, Hach R (eds): Clinical Oxygen Pressure Measurement. Springer-Verlag, New York, 1985
42. Jöbsis FF: Noninvasive, infrared monitoring of cerebral and myocardial oxygen sufficiency and circulatory parameters. Science 198:1264, 1977
43. Hampson NB, Camporesi EM, Stolp BW, et al: Cerebral oxygen availability by NIR spectroscopy during transient hypoxia in man. J Appl Physiol (in press)
44. Ohmeda 6000 Multi-Gas Monitor Service Manual. Madison: Ohmeda. Ref. #0178-0174-000, 1988
45. Gillbe CE, Heneghan CPH, Branthwaite MA: Respiratory mass spectrometry during general anesthesia. Br J Anaesth 53:103, 1981
46. Van Wagenen RA, Westenskow DR, Benner RE, et al: Dedicated monitoring of anesthetic and respiratory gases by Raman scattering. J Clin Monit 2:215, 1986
47. Westenskow DR, Smith KW, Coleman DL, et al: Clinical evaluation of a Raman scattering multiple gas analyzer for the operating room. Anesthesiology 70:350, 1989
48. Schachter EN, Rafferty TD, Knight C, et al: Transcutaneous oxygen and carbon dioxide monitoring: Use in adult surgical patients in an intensive care unit. Arch Surg 116:1193, 1981
49. Chapman KR, Liu FLW, Watson RM, Rebuck AS: Conjunctival oxygen tension and its relationship to arterial oxygen tension. J Clin Monit 2:100, 1986
50. Gravenstein JS, Paulus DA, Hayes TJ: Capnography in clinical practice. Butterworths, Boston, 1989
51. Turner KE, Sandler AN, Vosu HA: End-tidal CO_2 monitoring in spontaneously breathing adults. Can J Anaesth 36:248, 1989
52. Meny RG, Bhat AM, Aranas E: Mass spectrometer monitoring of expired carbon dioxide in critically ill neonates. Crit Care Med 13:1064, 1985
53. Brunner JX, Westenskow DR: How the rise time of carbon dioxide analyzers influences the accuracy of carbon dioxide measurements. Br J Anaesth 61:628, 1988
54. Scamman FL, Fishbaugh JK: Frequency response of long mass-spectrometer sampling catheters. Anesthesiology 65:422, 1986
55. Bindslev LB, Hedenstierna G, Santesson J, et al: Airway closure during anaesthesia, and its prevention by positive end expiratory pressure. Acta Anaesth Scand 24:199, 1980
56. Murray IP, Modell JH, Gallagher TJ, Banner MJ: Titration of PEEP by the arterial minus end-tidal carbon dioxide gradient. Chest 85:100, 1984
57. Viale JP, Annat G, Bertrand O, et al: Continuous measure-

ment of pulmonary gas exchange during general anaesthesia in man. Acta Anaesthesiol Scand 32:691, 1988

58. Westenskow DR, Cutler CA, Wallace WD: Instrumentation for monitoring gas exchange and metabolic rate in critically ill patients. Crit Care Med 12:183, 1984

59. Lewis WD, Chwals W, Benotti PN, et al: Bedside assessment of the work of breathing. Crit Care Med 16:117, 1988

60. Schoene RB: The control of ventilation in clinical medicine: To breathe or not to breathe. Respir Care 34:500, 1989

61. Camporesi EM, Nielsen CH, Bromage PR, Durant PAC: Ventilatory CO_2 sensitivity after intravenous and epidural morphine in volunteers. Anesth Analg 62:633, 1983

62. Rawal N, Wattwil M: Respiratory depression after epidural morphine—an experimental and clinical study. Anesth Analg 63:8, 1984

63. Sandler AN, Chovaz P: Respiratory depression following epidural morphine: A clinical study. Can Anaesth Soc J 33:542, 1986

64. Ready LB, Oden R, Chadwick HS, et al: Development of an anesthesiology-based postoperative pain management service. Anesthesiology 68:100, 1988

65. Camporesi EM, Feezor M, Fortune J, Salzano J: An electromagnetic valve for inspiratory occlusion pressures. J Appl Physiol 45:481, 1978

66. Milic-Emili J, Grassino AE, Whitelaw WA: Measurement and testing of respiratory drive. p. 675. In Hornbein TF (Ed): Regulation of Breathing. Part II. Marcel Dekker, New York, 1981

67. Derenne J-Ph, Couture J, Iscoe S, et al: Occlusion pressures in men rebreathing CO_2 under methoxyflurane anesthesia. J Appl Physiol 40:805, 1976

68. Herrera M, Blasco J, Venegas J, et al: Mouth occlusion pressure ($P_{0.1}$) in acute respiratory failure. Intensive Care Med 11:134, 1985

69. Sassoon CSH, Te TT, Mahutte CK, Light RW: Airway occlusion pressure: An important indicator for successful weaning in patients with chronic obstructive lung disease. Am Rev Respir Dis 135:107, 1987

70. Montgomery AB, Holle RHO, Neagley SR, et al: Prediction of successful ventilatory weaning using airway occlusion pressure and hypercapnic challenge. Chest 91:496, 1987

71. Sullivan WJ, Peters GM, Enright PL: Pneumotachographs: Theory and clinical application. Respir Care 29:736, 1984

72. Blumenfeld W, Turney SZ, Denman RJ: A coaxial ultrasonic pneumotachometer. Med Biol Eng 13:855, 1975

73. De Troyer A, Bastenier J, Delhez L: Function of respiratory muscles during partial curarization in humans. J Appl Physiol 49:1049, 1980

74. O'Brien MJ, Van Eykern LA, Oetomo SB, Van Vught HAJ: Transcutaneous respiratory electromyographic monitoring. Crit Care Med 15:294, 1987

75. Schweitzer TW, Fitzgerald JW, Bowden DA, Lynne-Davies P: Spectral analysis of human inspiratory diaphragmatic electromyograms. J Appl Physiol 46:152, 1979

76. Block R: Subtraction of electrocardiographic signal from respiratory electromyogram. J Appl Physiol 55:619, 1983

77. Rochester DF: Tests of respiratory muscle function. Clin Chest Med 9:249, 1988

78. Ford GT, Whitelaw WA, Rosinal WT, et al: Diaphragm function after upper abdominal surgery in humans. Am Rev Respir Dis 127:431, 1983

79. Brown KA, Hoffstein V, Byrick RJ: Bedside diagnosis of bilateral diaphragmatic paralysis in a ventilator-dependent patient after open-heart surgery. Anesth Analg 64:1208, 1985

80. Stagg D, Goldman M, Newsom Davis J: Computer-aided measurement of breath volume and time components using magnetometers. J Appl Physiol 44:623, 1978

81. Roussos C, Fixley M, Gross D, Macklem PT: Fatigue of inspiratory muscles and their synergic behavior. J Appl Physiol 46:897, 1979

82. Mead J, Peterson N, Grimby G, Mead J: Pulmonary ventilation measured from body surface movements. Science 156:1383, 1967

83. Faithfull D, Jones JG, Jordan C: Measurement of the relative contributions of rib cage and abdomen/diaphragm to tidal breathing in man. Br J Anaesth 51:391, 1979

84. Cohn MA, Rao ASV, Broudy M, et al: The respiratory inductive plethysmograph: A new non-invasive monitor of respiration. Bull Eur Physiopathol Respir 18:643, 1982

85. Stradling JR, Chadwick GA, Quirk C, Phillips T: Respiratory inductance plethysmography: Calibration techniques, their validation and the effects of posture. Bull Eur Physiopathol Respir 21:317, 1985

86. Marini JJ, Pierson DJ, Hudson LD, Lakshminarayan S: The significance of wheezing in chronic airflow obstruction. Am Rev Respir Dis 120:1069, 1979

87. Forgacs P: Lung sounds. Baillière Tindall, London, 1978

88. Loudon R, Murphy RLH, Jr: Lung sounds. Am Rev Respir Dis 130:663, 1984

89. Semmes BJ, Tobin MJ, Snyder JV, Grenvick A: Subjective and objective measurement of tidal volume in critically ill patients. Chest 87:577, 1985

90. Sorkin B, Rapoport DM, Falk DB, Goldring RM: Canopy ventilation monitor for quantitative measurement of ventilation during sleep. J Appl Physiol 48:724, 1980

91. Tobin MJ, Jenouri GA, Watson H, Sackner MA: Noninvasive measurement of pleural pressure by surface inductive plethysmography. J Appl Physiol 55:267, 1983

92. Pepe PE, Marini JJ: Occult positive end-expiratory pressure in mechanically ventilated patients with airflow obstruction. Am Rev Respir Dis 126:166, 1982

93. Tobin MJ: Respiratory monitoring in the intensive care unit. Am Rev Respir Dis 138:1625, 1988

94. Carle KA, Camporesi EM, Moon RE: Edrophonium-induced bronchoconstriction during reversal of muscle relaxants. Anesthesiology suppl., 65:A495, 1986

95. Wakakuri H, Camporesi EM: Peak expiratory flow during a passive exhalation: An index of expiratory resistance during anesthesia. Acta Anaesth Scand 23:207, 1979

96. Guyatt AR, Parker SP, McBride MJ: Measurement of human nasal ventilation using an oxygen cannula as a Pitot tube. Am Rev Respir Dis 126:434, 1982

97. Werthammer J, Krasner J, DiBenedetto J, Stark AR: Apnea monitoring by acoustic detection of airflow. Pediatrics 71:53, 1983

98. George CF, Millar TW, Kryger MH: Identification and quantification of apneas by computer-based analysis of oxygen saturation. Am Rev Respir Dis 137:1238, 1988

99. Catley DM, Thornton C, Jordan C, et al: Pronounced episodic oxygen desaturation in the postoperative period: Its association with ventilatory pattern and analgesic regimen. Anesthesiology 63:20, 1985

100. Sackner MA, Krieger BP: Noninvasive respiratory monitoring. p. 663. In Scharf SM, Cassidy SS (eds): Heart-Lung Interactions in Health and Disease. Marcel Dekker, New York, 1989

101. Laggner A, Kleinberger G, Haller J, et al: Bedside estimation of extravascular lung water in critically ill patients: Compari-

son of the chest radiograph and the thermal dye technique. Intensive Care Med 10:309, 1984

102. Hedlund LW, Vock P, Effman EL, et al: Hydrostatic pulmonary edema: An analysis of lung density changes by computed-tomography. Invest Radiol 19:254, 1984

103. Webber CE, Cortes G: A clinical system for the *in vivo* measurement of lung density. Med Phys 9:473, 1982

104. Cutillo AG, Morris AH, Ailion DC, et al: Determination of lung water content and distribution by nuclear magnetic resonance imaging. J Thorac Imag 1:39, 1986

105. Schuster DP, Mintun MA, Green MA, Ter-Pogossian MM: Regional lung water and hematocrit determined by positron emission tomography. J Appl Physiol 59:860, 1985

106. Sivak ED, Wiedemann HP: Clinical measurement of extravascular lung water. Crit Care Clin 2:511, 1986

107. Mihm FG, Feeley TW, Jamieson SW: Thermal dye double indicator dilution measurement of lung water in man: Comparison with gravimetric measurements. Thorax 42:72, 1987

108. Baudendistel LJ, Kaminski DL, Dahms TE: Evaluation of extravascular lung water by single thermal indicator. Crit Care Med 14:52, 1986

109. Overland ES, Gupta RN, Huchon GJ, Murray JF: Measurement of pulmonary tissue volume and blood flow in persons with normal and edematous lungs. J Appl Physiol 51:1375, 1981

110. Petrini MF, Norman JR: Soluble gas uptake from alveolar gas. Respir Care 34:470, 1989

111. Van De Water JM, Mount BE, Barela JR, et al: Monitoring the chest with impedance. Chest 64:597, 1973

112. Shires GT, III, Peitzman AB, Alberts SA, et al: Response of extravascular lung water to intraoperative fluids. Ann Surg 197:515, 1983

113. Waterson CK, Quan SF: Delivery equipment and monitoring techniques for high frequency ventilation. p. 90. In Hamilton LH, Neu J, Calkins JM (eds): High-Frequency Ventilation. CRC Press, Boca-Raton, 1986

114. Waterson CK, Militzer HW, Quan SF, Calkins JM: Airway

115. Hall JB, Wood LDH: Liberation of the patient from mechanical ventilation. JAMA 257:1621, 1987

116. Hodgin JE, Bowser MA, Burton GG: Respirator weaning. Crit Care Med 2:96, 1974

117. Tahvanainen J, Salmenperä M, Nikki P: Extubation criteria after weaning from intermittent mandatory ventilation and continuous positive airway pressure. Crit Care Med 11:702, 1983

118. Karpel JP, Aldrich TK: Respiratory failure and mechanical ventilation: Pathophysiology and methods of promoting weaning. Lung 164:309, 1986

119. Milic-Emili, J: Is weaning an art or a science? Am Rev Respir Dis 134:1107, 1986

120. Tobin MJ, Peres W, Guenthen SM, et al: The pattern of breathing during successful and unseccessful trials of weaning from mechanical ventilation. Am Rev Respir Dis 134:1111, 1986

121. Sporn PHS, Morganroth ML: Discontinuation of mechanical ventilation. Clin Chest Med 9:113, 1988

122. Gorback MS, Kantor K: Extubation without a trial of spontaneous ventilation in the general surgical population. Respir Care 32:178, 1987

123. Chripko D, Bevan JC, Archer DP, Bherer N: Decreases in arterial oxygenation in paediatric outpatients during transfer to the postanaesthetic recovery room. Can J Anaesth 36:128, 1989

124. Bromage PR, Camporesi EM, Chestnut D: Epidural narcotics for postoperative analgesics. Anesth Analg 59:473, 1980

125. Etches RC, Sandler AN, Daley MD: Respiratory depression and spinal opioids. Can J Anaesth 36:165, 1989

126. Rawal N, Arner S, Gustafsson LL, Allvin R: Present state of extradural and intrathecal opioid analgesia in Sweden. Br J Anaesth 59:791, 1987

127. Brodsky JB, Brose WG, Vivenzo K: A postoperative pain management scrvice. Anesthesiology 70:719, 1989

pressure as a measure of gas exchange during high frequency jet ventilation. Crit Care Med 12:742, 1984

34

MONITORING OF RENAL FUNCTION

David J. Cullen

INTRODUCTION

Although renal function can be assessed in various ways, the most practical test is measurement of the rate of urinary output. This procedure entails only minimal expense. The patient undergoes Foley catheterization, after which urine is collected and its volume recorded intraoperatively, usually on a 15- to 30-minute basis. However, the catheter must be irrigated at regular intervals with aseptic techniques, as the most common cause of low urinary output (<0.5 ml/kg/min) is occlusion of the catheter. The rate of urinary output is a reasonable measure of perfusion of the kidney, provided the patient has adequate blood volume and no pre-existing renal disease. During resuscitation from acute injury, decreased urinary flow may reflect low blood volume, poor perfusion of the kidney, or onset of acute renal failure (ARF). This chapter discusses the conditions leading to ARF and ways to prevent them.

As described in the following, urinary output provides a good estimate of the adequacy of renal perfusion. The specific gravity of urine indicates the concentrating ability of the kidneys. Traditionally, determination of serum levels of creatinine and blood urea nitrogen (BUN) has been used to monitor renal function. However, because these values are not abnormal until 70 percent of renal function is lost, other less frequently used tests may also be helpful. For example, a decreasing concentration of sodium in urine (<10 to 20 mEq/L) and/or rising urinary osmolarity (>450

1165

mOsm/L) may be an early sign of hypovolemia. Urinary levels of sodium exceeding 40 mEq/L indicate acute tubular necrosis, and urinary osmolarity less than 300 mOsm/L suggests antetubular necrosis. Later sections discuss these conditions in detail.

Acute renal failure is a clinical condition characterized by rapid and progressive increases in BUN and creatinine that are not immediately reversible by manipulation of extrarenal factors.[1] In surgical patients, ARF is a highly lethal complication, the mortality rate being 60 to 90 percent for oliguric or anuric ARF, and 40 to 50 percent for nonoliguric ARF. Furthermore, because of the many complications that prove so devastating in surgical patients, recovery of patients with ARF has not improved significantly over the past 50 years.[2,3] Consequently, prevention of ARF is extremely important.

Nonoliguric, oliguric, and anuric renal failure constitute a progression of increasingly severe injury to the kidney. That is, injury is minor in nonoliguric renal failure, moderate in oliguric renal failure, and severe in anuric renal failure. The anesthesiologist should take whatever steps possible to prevent the occurrence of ARF. Conditions likely to cause ARF should be minimized and severity of renal injury reduced as much as possible. Preoperative preparation of high-risk patients, intraoperative management of critical variables (particularly intravenous fluid administration and cardiovascular function), and postoperative monitoring and therapy are all extremely important in preventing or ameliorating ARF. Such attempts to reduce the incidence or severity of ARF depend on a thorough understanding of the pathophysiology of ARF.

PATHOGENESIS OF ACUTE RENAL FAILURE

Acute renal failure develops in two phases, an initiating phase and a perpetuating phase. In most instances, ARF is caused by renal vasoconstriction and ischemia. Several processes mediate renal ischemia, including the renin-angiotensin system, activation of sympathetic innervation of renal vasculature, and possibly swelling of endothelial cells leading to obstruction of the microvasculature. Once renal vasoconstriction has caused ischemic damage, however, restoration of renal blood flow does not promptly return renal function to normal. Renal failure persists because swelling of cells and accumulation of debris obstruct the tubules. Thus, less glomerular filtration takes place and ischemia damages the tubular epithelium. The small amount of glomerular filtrate that does form has increasing difficulty passing through the tubular lumen.

Pathogenesis of Decreased Glomerular Filtration in Acute Renal Failure

Several conditions decrease glomerular filtration rate (GFR): (1) A reduction in renal blood flow decreases afferent arteriolar blood flow to individual glomeruli. (2) During renal vasoconstriction, renal blood flow decreases to a greater extent in the cortex than in the medulla. Because most glomeruli are located in the renal cortex, renal blood flow is preferentially redistributed toward the medulla and away from the glomeruli. (3) The glomerular capillary ultrafiltration coefficient decreases as the glomerular capillary endothelium tightens its junctions. (4) Intratubular obstruction increases pressure in the glomerulus, thereby reducing the gradient favoring filtration. (5) As glomerular filtrate moves through the nephron, it leaks back through the cell membranes of damaged tubular cells and returns to the circulation. The degree to which each of these conditions contributes to diminished glomerular filtration depends on the type of injury and the time at which each condition is studied. Obviously, many of these conditions not only coexist but also change independently of each other. For example, despite the fact that renal blood flow decreases in almost all models of ARF, restoration of renal blood flow may not improve GFR, as intratubular obstruction has developed in all models of ARF studied to date, and back leakage has usually been related to the severity of tubular cell injury.

Renal Blood Flow during Hypovolemia

Although the kidneys constitute less than 0.5 percent of body mass, they receive 20 percent of cardiac output. Essentially all blood to the kidney passes through glomeruli (80 to 90 percent passes through the cortical glomeruli). Beyond the glomeruli, the vascular pattern is very complex.

Because oliguria most commonly results from reduced cardiac output secondary to hypovolemia, it is essential to understand how hypovolemia affects distribution of renal blood flow. Activation of the sympathetic nervous system and possibly the renin-angiotensin system reduces renal blood flow and GFR. Despite well-maintained arterial blood pressure, blood flow may decrease to one-third its normal level. Constriction of afferent arterioles becomes sufficient to reduce the hydrostatic pressure in glomerular capillaries to levels inadequate for maintenance of normal filtration levels. Thus, oliguria is initially caused by a decrease in GFR from reduced renal blood flow. This condition occurs before the metabolic function of the kidney itself becomes inadequate. As decreased renal blood flow progresses, arteriolar vasoconstriction leads to actual ischemia and morphologic damage.

Renal arteriographic and xenon washout studies in patients with ARF have shown selected profound reduction in renal blood flow[4-6] (Fig. 34-1). Arteriography revealed severe attenuation of the intrarenal arterial tree, inability to visualize cortical vessels, absence of a normal cortical nephrogram, and striking reduction in the velocity of contrast dye as it passed through the kidney. These same patients had no bleeding from the cortex during open renal biopsy. Also, xenon washout studies show that the usual rapid transit of xenon

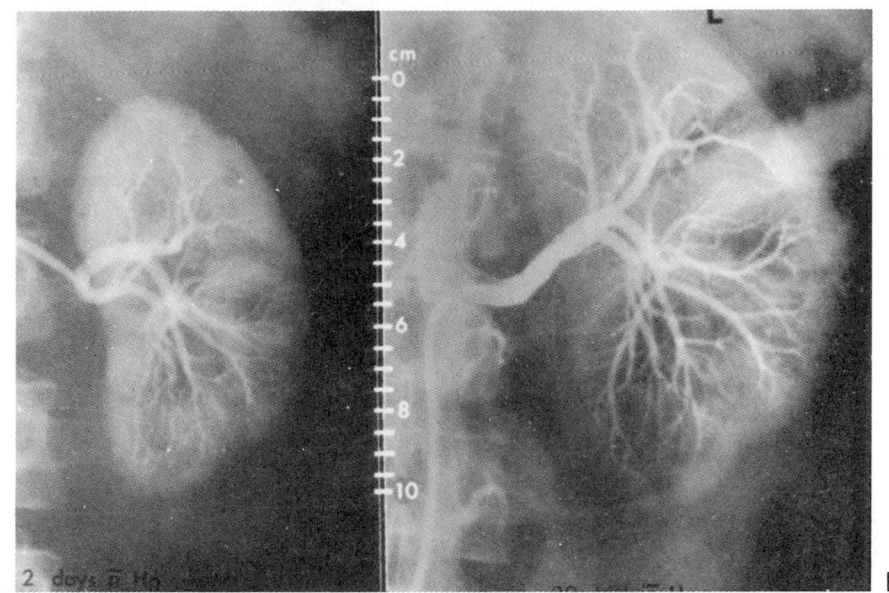

Fig. 34-1. Selective renal arteriogram in a patient during oliguric renal failure: **(A)** after the ingestion of bichloride of mercury; **(B)** during early recovery when creatinine clearance was 22 ml/min. Note the greatly diminished renal blood flow, particularly cortical blood flow, early in renal failure (Fig. A), and the improvement in both the size of renal vessels and the extent of cortical blood flow during recovery (Fig. B). (From Hollenberg et al.,[4] with permission.)

through the cortex (indicating cortical perfusion) in the normal kidney is absent in acute oliguria. Renal cortical perfusion that is reduced to one-third its normal level and involves constriction of the afferent arterioles is a condition more than sufficient to stop renal functioning.

Renal Vasoconstriction

Renal ischemia interferes with normal aerobic metabolism. Because the renal cortex contains most of the glomeruli and depends on oxidative metabolism for energy, ischemic hypoxia will injure the renal cortical structures, particularly the pars recta of the proximal tubules. As ischemia persists, the supply of glucose and substrates continues to decrease; glycogen is consumed; and the medulla, which depends to a greater extent on glycolysis for its energy sources, becomes more adversely affected. *Interruption of blood flow to the kidneys for more than 30 to 60 minutes results in acute renal failure and irreversible cell damage.* Very early changes,which are reversible, include swelling of cell organelles, especially the mitochrondria. As ischemia progresses, lack of adenosine triphosphate (ATP) interferes with the sodium pump mechanism, water and sodium accumulate in the endoplasmic reticulum of tubular cells, and the cells begin to swell.

In experimental ARF, the following pathologic changes occur: (1) swelling of tubular epithelial cells, leading to formation of bullae, which protrude into the tubular lumen distal to the cell; (2) necrosis of tubular cells, with subsequent abnormal membrane permeabil-

ity; (3) structural changes in the glomerular epithelium, which may decrease glomerular filtration; and (4) constriction of intrarenal arteries and arterioles, with subsequent further reduction in glomerular blood flow.

The time course of tubular damage in experimental models is as follows. Within 25 minutes of ischemia, the microvilli of the proximal tubular cell brush borders change. Within an hour, they slough into the tubular lumen and membrane bullae protrude into the straight portion of the proximal tubule. After a few hours, intratubular pressure rises and passive backflow of tubular fluid occurs. Within 24 hours, obstructing casts are seen in the distal tubular lumen. Despite complete restoration of renal blood flow after 60 to 120 minutes of ischemia, GRF does not improve[7] (Fig. 34-2).

In ischemia-induced ARF, lesions are spotty in distribution, probably reflecting variability in blood flow. In contrast, in nephrotoxin-induced ARF, the proximal tubular cells become necrotic and obstruct the tubular lumen with castlike material; also, lesions are more evenly distributed among all nephrons.[8] After restoration of blood flow, intrarenal vascular resistance is high because of cell swelling and ischemic damage, and blood flow will be as much as 50 percent below control values.[9]

The way in which the nephron processes labeled inulin illustrates the functional deficits of renal ischemia. After 60 minutes of occlusion of the left renal artery in rats, labeled inulin was microinjected into a tubule and remained sequestered in the ischemic kidney. In control animals (no renal ischemia), recovery of radioac-

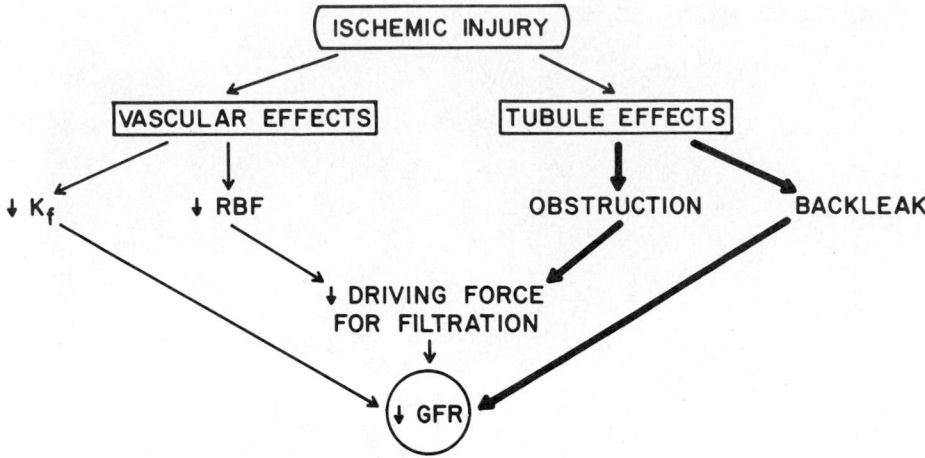

Fig. 34-2. Schematic representation of the mechanisms that initiate and maintain the defect in glomerular filtration rate (GFR) seen in experimental ischemia-induced acute renal failure. K_f, glomerular capillary ultrafiltration coefficient; RBF, renal blood blow. (From Hostetter et al.,[105] with permission.)

tive inulin was virtually complete from the ipsilateral kidney. Also, after 15, 25, and 60 minutes of renal artery occlusion, increasing amounts of radioactive inulin were recovered from urine of the contralateral kidney, meaning that back leakage and reabsorption from the ischemic kidney led to recirculation and excretion through the normal contralateral kidney. When horseradish peroxidase was microinjected into a proximal tubule, it penetrated the cytoplasm of isolated cells into the interstitium and vasculature of ischemic kidneys; no penetration occurred in the control kidney. The ability of large molecules to pass through damaged epithelial cells supports the concept that passive backflow of glomerular filtrate across such epithelium is a significant feature of postischemic renal failure.[7,9,10]

Histopathologic examination of biopsy and autopsy material from patients with postischemic oliguric ARF suggests a focal rather than a diffuse loss of brush border or intraluminal cast formation. However, recurrent episodes of hypotension in human ARF are accompanied by a proportionate decrease in renal blood flow. Such recurrent renal ischemia may induce fresh episodes of tubular necrosis or prevent healing of established pre-existing lesions. Thus, therapeutic efforts to prevent protracted or even permanent loss of renal function should be directed at stabilizing renal perfusion early in the course of ARF.[11] Renal angiography during xenon washout studies has demonstrated a decrease in renal cortical blood flow after ischemic damage in humans. The angiograms show marked cortical hypoperfusion and slowing of the normally rapid transit of inert gas through the cortex.[4,6]

In humans, the medullary thick ascending limb (mTAL) of the loop of Henle is selectively vulnerable to injury from ischemia or anoxia. A specific lesion (consistently observed within minutes and confined to the mTAL) progresses from mitochondrial swelling to nu-

clear pyknosis and complete cellular disruption.[12] The mTAL is extremely sensitive to ischemic or hypoxic damage because its low oxygen supply, imposed by the medullary countercurrent exchange system, is accompanied by a high rate of metabolism mandated by active reabsorption of sodium and chloride. Injury to the mTAL accompanied by complete arterial occlusion is less severe than hypoxic injury imposed during perfusion. This fact suggests that the process of tubular reabsorption aggravates the ischemic injury because the increase in oxygen demand is not met by adequate supply. Precipitation of Tamm-Horsfall mucoprotein, localized uniquely to the mTAL and released by damaged and leaking mTAL cells, may obstruct distal tubules. A reduction in renal medullary blood flow after ischemic injury of more than 50 percent elicits quantitative damage to the mTAL cells. As prerenal azotemia (i.e., azotemia caused by inadequate renal perfusion) progresses, the cortical-to-medullary redistribution of blood flow probably fails to provide enough oxygen to the outer medulla. Inhibiting cell transport activity with furosemide or abolishing glomerular filtration can protect the mTAL and consistently prevents injury to the mTAL in the isolated perfused kidney. Diversion of cortical blood flow to the medulla during hypotension probably protects the kidney from medullary ischemia directly, by increasing medullary oxygen delivery, and indirectly, by decreasing oxygen demand for solute reabsorption.

In summary, vascular and tubular factors interact in the pathogenesis of ARF. Ischemia, which initially triggers intrinsic renal vasoconstriction, leads to more ischemia, tubular cell damage, protrusion of cytoplasmic bullae, and perpetuation of ARF. Changes in glomerular membrane permeability and excessive back leakage across damaged tubular cells may contribute to continuation of ARF. The degree to which any of these pathogenic factors occurs depends on the nature, severity, and duration of the initial injury. These differences account for the various manifestations of ARF (nonoliguric, oliguric, and anuric).

Physiology of Glomerular Ultrafiltration

The mechanics of glomerular ultrafiltration involve several factors.[13,14] A positive hydraulic pressure gradient from the afferent arteriole to the glomerular capillary favors ultrafiltration. Opposing this force is the hydraulic pressure within the Bowman space. The difference between these two pressures at any point along the glomerular network is a measure of the net hydraulic pressure favoring ultrafiltration at that single point. The plasma oncotic pressure at the efferent end of the glomerulus is opposed by the oncotic pressure in the Bowman space. Because virtually all colloid remains within the vessel as plasma is filtered, the plasma oncotic pressure increases as plasma passes through the capillary bed. Thus, the hydraulic force favoring ultrafiltration is increasingly offset by the oncotic force opposing ultrafiltration. At some point in the glomerulus, an equal pressure point is reached and ultrafiltration ceases.[14] The mean hydraulic pressure at the afferent end of the glomerulus is approximately 40 percent of mean aortic pressure (Fig. 34-3).

Events and conditions that reduce renal plasma flow rate will reduce the hydraulic pressure and shift the filtration pressure equilibrium point toward the afferent end of the glomerular capillary. Increases in plasma flow rate will displace the point of filtration pressure equilibrium toward the efferent end of the capillary, thereby increasing the ultrafiltration pressure and the filtration rate (Fig. 34-3). Thus, hypovolemia and its accompanying renal vasoconstriction or hypotension lower the hydraulic pressure and reduce GFR.

Of theoretical interest is the effect of varying concentrations of proteins in plasma as the plasma enters a single nephron. As the concentration of proteins in the plasma decreases, the afferent oncotic pressure and the oncotic force opposing ultrafiltration also decrease. Thus, in the absence of other change, the net driving pressure for filtration increases. Conversely, a rise in afferent arterial oncotic pressure reduces the rate of glomerular filtration. What effect this relationship would have during normal renal functioning is not clear. However, it is interesting to speculate why patients resuscitated with albumin after massive transfusion had more renal dysfunction than those resuscitated with saline.[15] Perhaps maintaining oncotic pressure at a high level and possibly reducing the rate of glomerular filtration aggravated injury in an already stressed kidney.[14]

Role of the Renin-Angiotensin System

Autoregulation of renal blood flow is the mechanism by which renal blood flow and GFR are kept relatively constant, despite changes in mean arterial blood pres-

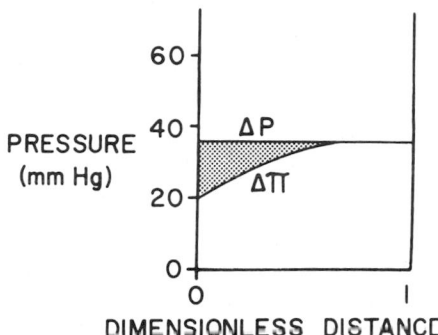

(mm Hg)

	Afferent End	Efferent End
P_{GC}	45	45
P_T	10	10
π_{GC}	20	35
$P_{UF} = P_{GC} - P_T - \pi_{GC}$	15	0

Fig. 34-3. Hydraulic and colloid osmotic pressure profiles along an idealized glomerular capillary in the rat. $\Delta P = P_{GC} - P_T$, and $\Delta_\pi = \pi_{GC} - \pi_T$, where P_{GC} and P_T are the hydraulic pressures in the glomerular capillary and Bowman space, respectively, and π_{GC} and π_T are the corresponding colloid osmotic pressures. P_{UF}, net ultrafiltration pressure. (From Brenner et al.,[14] with permission.)

sure of approximately 30 mmHg. Such autoregulation is accomplished by changes in afferent arteriolar resistance.[16] Sympathetic activation causes intense vasoconstriction and, more important, release of renin, which converts angiotensinogen to angiotensin I. Converting enzyme (located in the endothelium of the lung) converts angiotensin I to angiotensin II, which stimulates vasoconstrictor receptors (and thus raises blood pressure) and increases proximal reabsorption of sodium and secretion of aldosterone. Maximal sodium reabsorption and water retention result.

Release of renin is affected by several factors. The presence of epinephrine or a low-sodium diet results in renin release by lower-than-usual stimuli; that is, smaller changes in renal blood pressure result in release of renin. Conversely, a high-sodium diet delays renin release until renal blood pressure decreases to very low levels. Because a high-salt diet or sodium load attenuates impairment of renal function in experimental ARF and a high-salt diet also depresses plasma renin activity, suppression of renin release may be a major determinant in protecting renal function.[17] Although the precise cellular mechanisms governing renin release are as yet speculative, release of renin is known to be regulated by changes in both renal perfusion pressure and concentration/amount of sodium in the distal tubule.

The possibility that angiotensin II is implicated in the pathogenesis of ARF has been questioned, as experimental studies have not been able to demonstrate that suppression of renin release protects against ARF. It is agreed that volume depletion predisposes the kidneys to ARF and that the presence of some conditions (e.g., severe hemorrhage, crush injury, septic shock) makes ARF more likely to occur. In addition, the severity of experimental ARF can be attenuated by ingestion of sodium chloride, indirectly suggesting that suppression of the renin-angiotensin system is helpful. Although activation of renin is probably one mechanism by which profound renal vasoconstriction occurs, the evidence is not clear.

Perhaps one reason for this uncertainty is that prostaglandin E_2 (PGE_2) opposes the vasoconstriction caused by angiotensin. Angiotensin, a powerful stimulus to prostaglandin secretion, allows the opposing effects of angiotensin II, bradykinin, and PGE_2 to modulate the degree of renal vasoconstriction.[18] When renal vasoconstriction is induced by renal artery constriction, angiotensin I, angiotensin II, or infusions of norepinephrine or epinephrine, efflux of renal venous PGE_2 increases. This effect is unmasked when prostaglandin synthesis is inhibited by nonsteroidal anti-inflammatory drugs such as indomethacin.

For example, when indomethacin was administered in various studies, renal blood flow declined,[19-22] but only in animals subjected to the additional stress of laparotomy. The authors concluded that in the acutely stressed dog, support of renal circulation is an important effect of prostaglandins. Increased renin release and generation of angiotensin also increased PGE_2 production, which in turn helped restore renal blood flow toward normal levels during stimulation activating the renin-angiotension system. Unmasking this effect with indomethacin indicates the degree to which vasodilation by PGE_2 is responsible for antagonizing the effects of angiotensin. Similar results have been demonstrated in patients with congestive heart failure and prerenal azotemia.[23] Other drugs having a similar effect on renal function include aspirin, ibuprofen, naproxen, and fenoprofen, all of which reduce renal function in patients with systemic lupus erythematosus associated with reduced excretion of urinary prostaglandin-E-like compounds.[24-26]

Other patients having reduced renal function after administration of indomethacin include those with cirrhosis of the liver and ascites, those with nephrotic syndrome undergoing restricted sodium intake, those with Bartter's syndrome, and premature infants given prostaglandin synthetase inhibitors for closure of a patent ductus arteriosus.[18] Also, five cases of acute but reversible deterioration in renal function have been reported for patients given indomethacin for acute gout. Hyperkalemia also occurred and was attributed to decreases in renin and aldosterone secretion, distal tubular delivery of sodium, and urinary flow.[27]

Left Atrial Distention

Another powerful stimulus to renal vasoconstriction is left atrial hypotension.[28] Even after the return of normal left atrial pressure, renal pressure-flow relationships remain depressed for up to 1 hour. Renal blood flow appears to decrease much less during experimental cardiogenic shock in which left atrial pressures increase than during hemorrhagic shock in which left atrial pressures decrease, despite similar reductions in cardiac output and arterial blood pressure.[28] The mechanism may involve receptors located at the bifurcation of the main pulmonary artery, at the junction of the left atrium and pulmonary veins, and in the wall of the left atrium. It is postulated that when a decrease in cardiac output is accompanied by left atrial hypotension, reduction in systemic arterial blood pressure is followed by the normal response of renal vasoconstriction. In contrast, with left atrial distention, renal vasoconstriction is prevented. Because acute tubular necrosis often occurs during clinical hemorrhagic shock but rarely during cardiogenic shock, the difference in renal effects between these two sources of hypotension may be attributable to the severity of renal ischemia, which in turn is determined by the degree of left atrial distention. The mechanism by which the left atrial receptors connect to the renal circulation is not known.[29]

Recently, two biologically active peptides that exert profound effects on sodium excretion, urinary volume, and smooth muscle tone have been isolated from mammalian cardiac atria.[30,31] Although both peptides (atriopeptin I and atriopeptin II) have natriuretic and diuretic effects, the first compound selectively relaxes intestinal smooth muscle but not vascular smooth muscle, whereas the second relaxes both. Intravenous administration of 3 μg of atriopeptin I or 1 μg of atriopeptin II increases excretion of urinary sodium 10- to 15-fold. If changes in extracellular fluid volume and sodium trigger peptide release, this ability to produce renal vasodilation, natriuresis, and diuresis would then reduce atrial distention and stop release of the biologically active peptide.

Deliberate Hypotension

Deliberate hypotension (see also Ch. 43) induced by nitroglycerin or nitroprusside affects renal blood flow in different ways. Infusion of nitroprusside decreases renal blood flow significantly, and renal vascular resistance stays the same. In contrast, infusion of nitroglycerin keeps renal blood flow at control levels, and renal vascular resistance decreases.[32,33]

Positive End-Expiratory Pressure and Positive-Pressure Ventilation

Because positive-pressure ventilation and positive end-expiratory pressure reduce cardiac output and renal blood flow, the kidney responds to a "perceived" hypovolemic condition by increasing renal vasoconstriction (also see Ch. 71). As a result, retention of sodium and water increase, as does the secretion of hormones responsible for fluid retention. The decrease in renal function associated with respiratory support is usually attributed to a decrease in total renal blood flow,[34] to a redistribution of intrarenal blood flow from the outer cortex to the inner cortex and medulla,[35] and to an increase in sympathetic tone as a result of diminished "effective" intravascular volume.[36] Neither antidiuretic hormone levels nor prostaglandin levels change in response to positive-pressure ventilation.[37-40] Whether one of the biologically active peptides from the atria of the heart is responsible for the changes that occur remains speculative.

CAUSES AND DIAGNOSIS OF ACUTE RENAL FAILURE

The most frequent precipitating causes of ARF are profound shock, trauma, intravascular hemolysis, generalized sepsis, and exposure to toxic substances. The wide variety of substances that are nephrotoxic includes aminoglycoside antibiotics, iodinated dyes, and pigments. Drug interactions may involve cephalosporins that interact with other drugs such as furosemide or gentamicin to increase the likelihood of acute renal damage. By themselves, cephalosporins are rarely nephrotoxic.

Factors Predisposing the Kidney to Injury

Several factors predispose the kidney to injury. First, high blood flow delivers more potentially toxic substances per gram of tissue to the kidney than to any other organ in the body. The kidney has a moderately high basal oxygen consumption and, when actively involved in sodium and water reabsorption, has an even higher energy requirement. Second, the methods by which the kidney handles toxic materials cause these substances to accumulate within the cell and to produce direct damage. For example, for those substances not reabsorbed, reabsorption of water concentrates toxins in the tubular lumen. Gradients that may increase the concentration of certain drugs such as analgesics are established between cortex and medulla. Finally, glomerular ultrafiltration may separate toxins bound to plasma proteins and further concentrate their effects.

Mechanisms of Renal Damage

The most important mechanism by which the kidney is damaged is ischemia of sufficient duration to produce cellular disruption. Currently, the second most common cause of ARF in hospitalized patients is the use of aminoglycoside antibiotics. These drugs are transported to the kidney, filtered in the glomerulus, and reabsorbed to some extent in the proximal tubule. A third cause of ARF is the pigment in hemoglobin and myoglobin. These pigments are transported to the kidney and filtered but not reabsorbed; they cause cellular toxicity and tubular obstruction. Contrast dyes are also filtered but not reabsorbed; they accumulate in the renal tubule and may cause obstruction and local toxicity.

Importance of Urinary Volume

An important etiologic, diagnostic, and therapeutic consideration is the amount of urine produced by the damaged kidney. One study investigated nonoliguric ARF in 54 patients whose daily urinary volume averaged 1,280 ml.[41] Although there were many different causes of ARF for both medical and surgical patients, toxin-induced ARF occurred much more frequently in nonoliguric patients than in their oliguric counterparts. Nonoliguric patients had a significantly lower fractional excretion of sodium than oliguric patients, despite similar levels of BUN and creatinine. Nonoliguric patients also had significantly higher urine/plasma ratios of urea nitrogen. However, other test results were similar for the two groups. Nonoliguric patients with renal failure were azotemic for shorter periods of time, were hospitalized for a shorter duration, and had a lower incidence of complications. Mortality rate was half that for oliguric patients with ARF. Most of the deaths among oliguric patients with ARF (73 percent) were caused by prolonged intravascular volume depletion, low cardiac output, or sepsis. Only 8 percent of nonoliguric patients who had these conditions died. In the immediate postoperative period, mortality was 58 percent for patients with oliguric ARF and 27 percent for patients with nonoliguric ARF.

In addition, patients who became nonoliguric after administration of furosemide were compared with those who were unresponsive to furosemide. Although no differences existed in the dose of furosemide administered, the age of the patients, or the cause of ARF, patients responsive to furosemide appeared to have less impairment of renal function from the onset of renal failure. That is, BUN, serum creatinine, urinary concentration of sodium, and fractional excretion of sodium were lower; also, the urine/plasma ratio of urea was higher.

Several factors may account for the fact that more instances of nonoliguric renal failure are now being recognized. For one thing, seriously ill patients are monitored more carefully. Use of antibiotics has increased, and antibiotic-induced ARF is usually nonoliguric. In addition, potent diuretics and mannitol may convert some cases of oliguric ARF to nonoliguric ARF. On the other hand, in the study of nonoliguric ARF just discussed,[41] it is possible that even more seriously ill patients were prevented from becoming oliguric by superior medical management. Although the causes of nonoliguric ARF are similar to those for oliguric ARF, urinary diagnostic indices of the severity of renal failure in this study and in other studies suggest that impairment of renal function is less in nonoliguric ARF. Because patients responsive to furosemide appeared to have less impairment of renal function than those who were not responsive, and because other studies have shown no value in treating oliguric ARF with furosemide, it is likely that the severity of renal injury in furosemide-responsive patients was less than that in unresponsive patients. Thus, furosemide itself was not therapeutic; responsiveness to the drug was merely indicative of a lesser injury.

Another large series of consecutive medical and surgical patients indicated that some degree of renal insufficiency occurred in 5 percent of patients.[42] The most common causes were decreased renal perfusion, postoperative renal dysfunction, exposure to radiographic contrast dyes, and use of aminoglycoside antibiotics. The mortality rate for patients who had an increase in serum creatinine of 3 mg/dl or more was 64 percent. Iatrongenic factors accounted for 55 percent of all episodes of ARF. Among patients who had postoperative renal insufficiency, hypotension was documented in approximately half of the episodes. Twelve percent of these occurrences followed cardiac operations. An important prognostic indicator was severity of renal insufficiency: that is, the rate of rise of serum creatinine and the initial creatinine level. Also, oliguria was an important discriminant of mortality, death occurring in 52 percent of oliguric patients and in 17 percent of nonoliguric patients.

Differential Diagnosis of Acute Renal Failure

Attention to urinary flow facilitates the differential diagnosis of ARF. For example, if urinary flow suddenly ceases, the cause is probably mechanical obstruction of the urinary catheter. Kinking, clotting, mucous plugs, and tissue obstruction should be sought. Observation of urinary output is also helpful. Anuria is most often associated with complete urinary tract obstruction, a bilateral renal-vascular catastrophe, cortical necrosis, or severe proliferative glomerular nephritis. If urinary output varies widely from anuria to polyuria, intermittent obstructive uropathy may be the cause. Intravascular fluid status must be evaluated, as almost invariably, hypovolemia is in some way responsible for oliguria. If no diuretic has been administered within 12 to 18 hours, urinalysis to establish urinary osmolarity, sodium concentration, and perhaps fractional excretion of sodium may be helpful. Even though appropriate intravenous fluid challenges should increase urinary output, persistent oliguria indicates incipient renal failure. The common practice of administering "loop diuretics" (those acting primarily in the loop of Henle) is probably counterproductive, as such drugs may increase renal damage, interfere with urinary diagnostic indices, worsen hypovolemia, and cause hypokalemia.

For diagnostic purposes, the causes of acute renal failure are said to be "prerenal" (inadequate renal perfusion), "intrinsic" (most commonly, ischemia or the presence of nephrotoxins), or "postrenal" (obstruction). Of all instances of hospital-acquired ARF, approximately half are classified as prerenal ARF, followed closely by intrinsic ARF; only a small fraction (approximately 2 percent) are classified as postrenal ARF.

Prerenal Acute Renal Failure

During hypovolemia, renal blood flow decreases and compensatory mechanisms begin to increase solute and water retention. As a result, sodium and water reabsorption are maximal, and the normal kidney produces urine that is low in volume and highly concentrated. Thus, prerenal ARF is the result of a prolonged deficit in renal blood flow caused by (1) primary decreases in cardiac output resulting from acute or chronic cardiac dysfunction; (2) intravascular volume depletion from multiple causes such as hemorrhage, vomiting, diarrhea, drainage of a fistula, diuresis, or excessive dehydration; or (3) redistribution of the functional extracellular fluid volume. The last condition occurs in hypoalbuminema, in inflammatory states such as peritonitis and burns, or as a result of profound vasodilation.

Postrenal Acute Renal Failure

Postrenal ARF is caused by obstruction of urinary flow, a condition that increases intratubular pressure. The three main categories of postrenal ARF are (1) ureteral and pelvic obstruction from clots, stones, necrotic papillae, or extrinsic obstruction of the ureters; (2) bladder obstruction; and (3) prolonged urethral obstruction.

Intrinsic Acute Renal Failure

Intrinsic ARF is caused by many acute parenchymatous diseases that damage the kidney. Such diseases may attack the glomeruli or the vasculature of the tubules in various ways to produce medically rather than surgically induced types of ARF. In surgical patients, intrinsic ARF may accompany hepatic failure, prolonged hypovolemic shock, renal infection such as pyelonephritis, or acute papillary necrosis associated with intravascular hemolysis. This last condition may result from an incompatible blood transfusion or an allergic reaction to a variety of drugs.

Specific Causes of Acute Renal Failure

Radiographic Contrast Agents

Acute renal failure caused by exposure to radiographic contrast dyes has become an increasingly common cause of oliguria, morbidity, and mortality in surgical patients. Although this complication occurs in fewer than 2 percent of normal patients,[43] vascular surgery patients often undergo more than one radiographic study before surgery; the addition of the various causative conditions and events already mentioned may induce ARF. Patients undergoing less invasive radiographic studies (computed tomography [CT] with contrast medium or digital subtraction studies using intravenous injection for visualization of arteries) may receive very large amounts of contrast medium. In digital subtraction studies, inadequate visualization often necessitates a second study, thereby increasing the risk of dye-induced ARF.

The clinical course consists of oliguria that occurs within 24 hours, is usually self-limiting, and improves in 3 to 7 days. However, the severity of ARF often depends on the severity of the underlying renal disease, and 25 to 50 percent of patients require some form of dialysis. Renal injury is related to the dose of dye administered.

The pathologic changes in dye-induced ARF are similar to those for acute tubular necrosis on renal biopsy. Urinary excretion of lysozyme increases, and the urine may look like gel because of its viscosity and proteinuria. By the time renal blood flow is studied, renal vasoconstriction is usually intense. The crenation and clumping of red blood cells as sludge in the microcirculation lead to tissue ischemia.

Factors that predispose patients to dye-induced ARF include pre-existing renal disease (creatinine levels greater than 3 mg/dl), diabetes, hypovolemia, proteinuria, and multiple myeloma. Although diabetic patients with normal renal function are at minimal risk, those with moderate to severe renal dysfunction are at high risk.[43] Patients with pre-existing renal dysfunction (creatinine levels of 1.5 to 4.5 mg/dl) who then undergo dye studies may have an incidence of ARF as high as 50 percent; those having creatinine levels greater than 4 mg/dl may have an incidence exceeding 80 percent.[44,45]

There are very few reports of patients with dye-induced renal failure who have been given a second dose of dye. In three such patients, however, renal function ceased.[46,47] Advanced age is not a separate risk factor, because renal function deteriorates with time. Neither proteinuria nor uricosuria is a separate risk factor; again, the severity of ARF is related to the degree of renal disease.

Methods of preventing ARF induced by exposure to contrast agents include identifying high-risk patients, providing hydration, administering mannitol to promote diuresis, and minimizing the amount of dye given. Patients with mild renal insufficiency (creatinine levels ≤2.8 mg/dl) had a much lower incidence of ARF after dye studies when mannitol or furosemide was given with hydration.[48]

Nephrotoxic Antibiotics

Intrinsic ARF is often caused by aminoglycoside antibiotics[41,42] and can be partially or completely abolished by withdrawing the antibiotic. Such ARF is more likely to be nonoliguric than oliguric, thus facilitating management of fluids and electrolytes. Careful monitoring of renal function and antibiotic blood levels is required to limit the development of ARF in these patients. However, given the severity of illness among critical care patients requiring these potent antibiotics, drug-induced renal insufficiency is likely to continue.

Mild histologic changes almost invariably occur in patients given gentamicin,[49] and serum creatinine levels increase in approximately 10 to 20 percent of representative studies. Critically ill patients, elderly individuals, and those taking aminoglycosides in combination with other drugs such as cephalosporins or diuretics are also at greater risk of ARF. Although renal function often recovers on discontinuation of the drug, renal dysfunction occasionally persists. In the early stages, a vasopressin-resistant concentrating defect with increased fractional excretion of sodium may occur.[50] As a result of nephrotoxicity, excretion of gentamicin may diminish, further increasing the likelihood of ARF. Pathologic changes are typical of acute tubular necrosis, with focal degeneration involving the proximal tubular cells.[49] When kidney function is normal, gentamicin is excreted unchanged by the kidney, its half-life being approximately 2 hours.[51] However, concentrations of the drug are 20 to 30 times higher in the renal cortex than in plasma, as gentamicin is not reabsorbed effectively.[52] Therefore, the kidney is specifically at greater risk of toxicity than other tissues in the body. After filtration into the renal tubule, gentamicin is taken up by the renal tubular cell, and concentrated within the cell, and damage begins. Addition of cephalosporins enhances the toxicity of aminoglycosides.

Of the drugs in the aminoglycoside category, neomycin is not used systemically because of its excessive nephrotoxicity. Although tobramycin and amikacin are supposedly less nephrotoxic, the evidence is not yet certain. Preventing those conditions and events leading to prerenal ARF is paramount in minimizing nephrotoxic damage. Intravascular volume depletion is an important risk factor, and drug combinations such as cephalosporins and aminoglycosides should be avoided when possible. Nonsteroidal anti-inflammatory drugs, which inhibit prostaglandin synthesis, further enhance toxicity, as do diuretics, presumably by depleting intravascular volume. In high-risk patients, monitoring of antibiotic blood levels may be essential, as the trough level appears to be the best indicator of the risk of toxicity. Aminoglycosides are able to be dialyzed, and if renal failure and a high systemic level of the drug occur, the drug can be removed by dialysis.

Amphotericin B, a potent systemic antifungal drug, predictably causes renal dysfunction. Although oliguria is not common, the kidney is unable to concentrate urine. The presence of urinary casts indicates tubular damage, and BUN and creatinine rise.

Cyclosporine

Cyclosporine is an immunosuppressive drug approved for prevention of graft rejection by organ graft recipients. It inhibits activation of T-helper cells, decreases release of lymphokines by these cells, and induces long-term graft tolerance without prolonged, generalized immunosuppression. Because cyclosporine is not toxic to bone marrow, patients are less likely to have opportunistic infections. However, cyclosporine is nephrotoxic because it reduces renal blood flow and GFR. It may act through the renin-angiotensin-aldosterone system, causing direct renal vasoconstriction of preglomerular afferent arterioles.[53,54]

Atheromatous Embolization of Renal Vasculature

Autopsy examinations of 22 patients who died after surgery for an abdominal aortic aneurysm revealed atheroemboli in 17 patients. Of these patients 4 had acute anuric renal failure after an apparently uncomplicated elective surgical procedure. Once obstruction and renal failure had occurred, treatment was ineffective and the prognosis was very poor. This problem has continued since it was first described in 1957,[55] and even today an occasional patient undergoing elective abdominal aortic surgery experiences irreversible ARF during or very soon after surgery.

Hepatorenal Syndrome

Progressive renal failure often complicates the course of patients with advanced liver disease, leading to what is commonly known as the hepatorenal syndrome. Surprisingly few renal abnormalities appear at autopsy. Successful allografting of kidneys from cirrhotic patients dying with oliguric renal failure further suggests the intrinsic normality of the kidneys.[56] Xenon washout and angiographic studies that have assessed the renal vasculature of patients with renal insufficiency, oliguria, and severe cirrhosis have shown that profound vasoconstriction was present.[57] Angiograms revealed cortical ischemia and renal vasospasm in patients with the most severe degree of renal failure, supporting the concept of reduced renal cortical perfusion and decreased mean renal blood flow. Infusion of phentolamine into the renal artery in four patients did not change intrarenal hemodynamics significantly. Postmortem angiographic analysis of the kidneys of five patients who had been studied before death revealed filling of the peripheral vasculature and smooth and regular interlobar and arcuate arteries. Postmortem histologic examination of the kidneys of six patients showed normal intrarenal vessels and changes similar to those reported elsewhere. The failure of phentolamine to increase renal blood flow significantly suggests that factors other than sympathomimetic activity were involved. Regardless of the mechanism, active renal vasoconstriction leads to renal failure in patients with severe liver disease.

Although the hepatorenal syndrome resembles severe prerenal ARF, it does not respond to volume repletion and has a very poor prognosis. The precipitating causes are not specific, as many patients with the same problems do not later have the syndrome. Associated causes include surgery, gastrointestinal hemorrhage, sepsis, paracentesis, and diuresis. Although these patients usually have low systemic vascular resistance, high cardiac output, and elevated plasma volume, their kidneys are actively vasoconstricted. Prognosis is poor and therapy usually ineffective. However, potentially reversible causes of ARF should be ruled out and nephrotoxic agents discontinued if possible.

Prerenal ARF is not unusual in patients with severe liver disease, as such patients often have problems with fluid loss, redistribution of intravascular fluid to other spaces, or cardiac failure. Excessive diuresis may produce dehydration, and reabsorption of sodium in the distal tubule may be impaired. Also, ARF may occur more frequently in patients with jaundice, perhaps because increased bilirubin levels reduce systemic blood pressure and renal perfusion.

Hemoglobin- and Myoglobin-Induced Acute Renal Failure

Hemoglobin- and myoglobin-induced ARF usually occur after trauma and release of myoglobin from damaged muscles; in hypovolemic or hemoconcentrated patients after strenuous exercise; after arterial embolization causing ischemic myopathy; during states of excessive muscle contraction such as status epilepticus, status asthmaticus, or prolonged labor and delivery; and during malignant hyperthermia and other forms of severe fever.[58]

Seven patients who had traumatic crush injuries and severe rhabdomyolysis were treated by rapid expansion of extracellular fluid volume with half-normal saline and 5 percent dextrose, mannitol as needed, and sodium bicarbonate, with serum sodium and potassium held at normal levels.[59] Although one therapeutic goal was to maintain diuresis of 300 ml/h, urinary output averaged over 500 ml/h for 60 hours. The patients had marked fluid retention and were edematous, yet pulses remained palpable, no leg pain occurred, and decompression fasciotomies were not required.

Hemoglobin-induced ARF may occur during acidosis, dehydration, shock, or decreased renal blood flow. The most feared cause is a hemolytic blood reaction after incompatible transfusion (also see Ch. 48). In any case, prevention is essential, and dehydration or renal ischemia must be avoided to minimize or prevent renal damage. Otherwise, tubular obstruction by pigmented casts, a prominent finding in pigment-induced ARF, will occur. Osmotic diuresis with mannitol may help prevent intratubular precipitation of pigments.[60,61] Furosemide does not have a consistently beneficial effect on experimental ARF of this type.[62] Unfortunately, no controlled trials have demonstrated the usefulness of mannitol *after* injury has occurred, only before. As the risks of mannitol administration are minimal compared with its possible benefits, mannitol is currently recommended.

Because the overall mortality rate from ARF has not improved significantly in the last several decades, prevention of these many inciting factors is crucial. Clinicians should attempt to keep levels of nephrotoxic drugs below toxic thresholds. Adequate hydration and attention to the circulation are important, particularly for patients undergoing radiographic studies with contrast media. Also, one must recognize high-risk categories of patients (e.g., those with proteinuria, pre-existing renal insufficiency, hepatic dysfunction, hypolabuminemia, diabetes mellitus, and jaundice). Shock from any cause (especially rupture of an abdominal aortic aneurysm), massive trauma, open heart surgery, and peripheral vascular surgery are all events entailing a high possibility of renal failure. Therefore, appropriate measures should be taken.

CLINICAL DIAGNOSIS OF OLIGURIA

Figure 34-4 provides a clinical and laboratory approach to the diagnosis of ARF. *Oliguria*, the most important clinical symptom, is defined as urinary output of less than 400 ml/24 h or 0.5 to 1 ml/kg/h. As mentioned earlier, treatment of ARF in the surgical patient is still so unsatisfactory that prevention is most important. Careful review of the patient's history and physical examination should be followed by determination of perioperative circumstances and, in particular, drug administration, blood and fluid loss and replacement, and intravascular volume status.

Importance of Urinalysis

Urinalysis is of great value, as oliguria with low sodium concentration (less than 20 mEq/L), urine of high specific gravity (greater than 1.020), and a urine/serum osmolarity ratio greater than 1.5:1 indicate that the kidney is attempting to conserve fluid volume maximally in response to reduced renal blood flow. Moreover, the fractional excretion of sodium is an accurate prognosticator of tubular dysfunction.[63] A fractional excretion of sodium of more than 1 percent indicates acute tubular necrosis, nonoliguric acute tubular necrosis, and urinary tract obstruction. If it is less than 1 percent, the problem is usually prerenal azotemia or acute glomerulonephritis. The fractional excretion of sodium (FE_{Na}) is calculated as follows:

$$FE_{Na} (\%) = [(U_{Na}/S_{Na}) \times 100]/[U_{Cr}/S_{Cr}]$$

where U_{Na} = urine sodium, S_{Na} = serum sodium, U_{Cr} = urine creatinine, and S_{Cr} = serum creatinine.

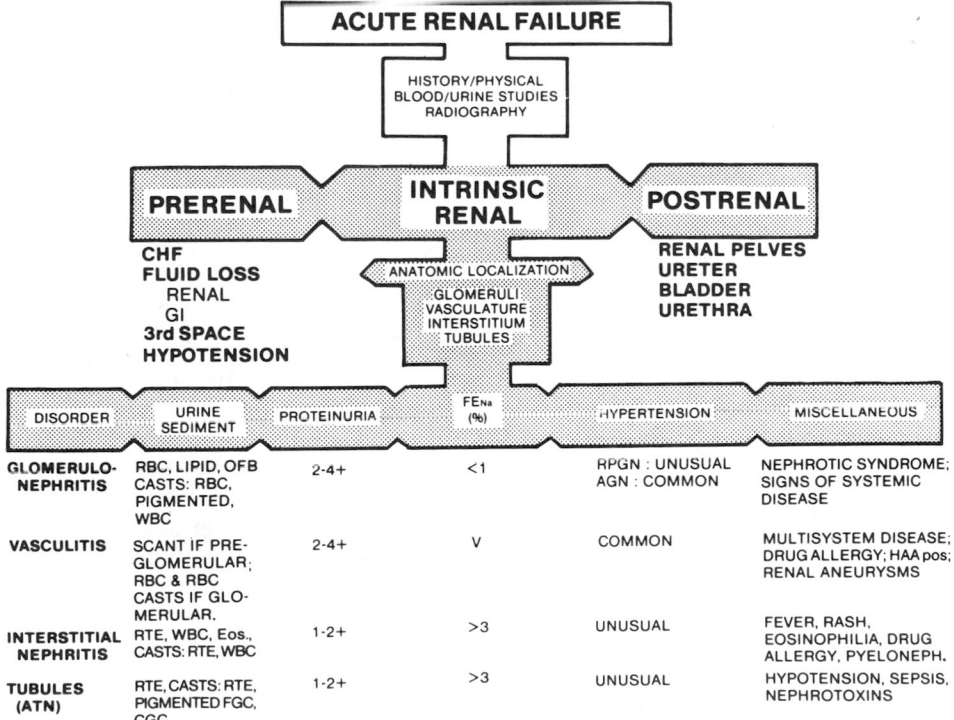

Fig. 34-4. A clinical and laboratory approach to the diagnosis of acute renal failure. AGN, acute glomerulonephritis; ATN, acute tubular necrosis; CGC, coarsely granular cast; CHF, congestive heart failure; Eos, eosinophil; FE_{Na} fractional excretion of sodium; FGC, finely granular cast; GI, gastrointestinal; HAA pos, positive test for hepatitis-associated antigen; OFB, oval fat body; RBC, red blood cell; RPGN, rapidly progressive glomerulonephritis; RTE, renal tubule epithelial cell; V, variable; WBC, white blood cell. (From Rudnick et al.,[106] with permission.)

Under defined clinical conditions, the fractional excretion of filtered sodium can precisely measure disease-induced changes in tubular reabsorption of sodium, a sensitive measure of renal tubular function. Because both creatinine and sodium clearances are considered, both filtration and reabsorption of sodium are related to the measurement. In one study of acute tubular necrosis (which is characterized by restriction of sodium reabsorption), the fractional excretion of sodium was high and, except for one patient, was always more than 1 percent.[64] A value of more than 3 percent is definitely diagnostic of acute tubular necrosis. In contrast, in prerenal azotemia and acute glomerulonephritis (conditions characterized by avid reabsorption of filtered sodium by the renal tubule), a fractional excretion of sodium of less than 1 percent indicates normal tubular function. Obviously, use of diuretics that affect sodium transport will affect these results. As with other tests of renal function, urine should be tested before administration of diuretics.

Urinalysis yields other useful diagnostic information. The pH of urine tends to be more acidic (<6) in prerenal ARF than in intrinsic or postrenal ARF. The existence of glucosuria without hyperglycemia indicates proximal tubular damage. A positive urine test for blood in the absence of red cells suggests the presence of free hemoglobin or myoglobin in the urine. A large amount of proteins in the urine indicates renal parenchymal disease.

Microscopic examination of urinary sediment may show increased numbers of hyaline and finely granular casts in patients with prerenal azotemia. Absence of sediment frequently occurs in patients with obstructive uropathy but is rare in acute tubular necrosis or renal parenchymal disease. In acute tubular necrosis, urinary sediment contains cellular casts, large numbers of tubular epithelial cells, and numerous brown cellular casts. In contrast, red cell casts occur in acute glomerular nephritis but rarely in acute tubular necrosis. In postrenal ARF, oxalate or uric acid crystals may be seen, as well as fungi, renal papillae, clots, and other elements. Also, in intrinsic ARF, one may see pigmented, coarsely granular casts and many tubular epithelial cells. Interstitial nephritis produces urine rich in eosinophils. In methicillin-induced nephropathy, eosinophila may account for one-third of the white cells in the urinary sediment.

Additional Tests

Once the urine has been analyzed, more invasive tests may be indicated to determine the cause of ARF. Such tests include hemodynamic evaluation, intravenous fluid challenge, and radiologic studies. Anuria (urinary output of < 100 ml/d) is unusual in prerenal azotemia but common in postrenal ARF or severe forms of intrinsic ARF. Vascular occlusion, severe acute glomerulonephritis, and renal cortical necrosis may be associated with anuria.

When urinary osmolarity is below 350 mOsm/L, ARF (whether intrinsic or postrenal) is likely. When osmolarity exceeds 450 to 500 mOsm/L, the kidney is capable of concentrating enough solutes to suggest that prerenal ARF is present. Values between these two extremes are indeterminant.

Similarly, when urinary sodium is less than 20 mEq/L, prerenal insufficiency is likely. If urinary sodium exceeds 40 mEq/L, intrinsic or postrenal failure is more common. Between 20 and 40 mEq/L, much overlap exists.

With greater use of the measurement of fractional excretion of sodium, more false-negative results have been observed, because classic acute tubular necrosis is seen with a low fractional excretion of sodium (less than 1 percent).

If GRF ceased completely in the average patient, the serum concentration of creatinine would rise 1 to 3 mg/dl/d. Greater increases would indicate muscle breakdown, whereas smaller increases would indicate some glomerular filtration. A rise in BUN is less diagnostic of ARF as is a rise in creatinine, as BUN is modified by many factors: a high-protein diet, gastrointestinal bleeding, fever, sepsis, crush injuries, and other conditions associated with hypercatabolism. Normally, BUN rises 10 to 20 mg/dl/d, but during hypercatabolism, it can increase much faster. In prerenal azotemia, BUN may increase more than serum creatinine because urea clearance decreases more than does creatinine clearance, and the BUN/creatinine ratio may rise beyond 20:1. Creatinine clearance measured in the first 24 hours after admission to the intensive care unit (ICU) significantly correlated with the in-hospital death rate for 379 consecutive postoperative ICU patients.[65] Specifically, the death rate was 70 percent for patients with creatinine clearance of less than 20 mg/min on admission.

Another study described creatinine clearance in 40 patients with multiple trauma.[66] Acute renal dysfunction developed in 7 patients, all of whom had creatinine clearance of less than 25 ml/min. The 33 patients who had normal renal function had creatinine clearance greater than 25 ml/min for more than 4 hours after surgery. Free-water clearance and fractional excretion of sodium did not differ between the two groups.

One study analyzed the value of several urinary diagnostic indices in ascertaining the cause of early ARF, defined as being an acute rise in serum creatinine levels (from less than 1.4 to more than 2 mg/dl).[67] Urinary osmolarity was significantly higher in prerenal azotemia than in all other diagnostic categories. Considerable overlap of diagnoses occurred when urinary osmolarity was 350 to 500 mOsm/L; when osmolarity was below 350 mOsm/L, prerenal azotemia was uncommon. The concentration of sodium in urine was significantly lower in prerenal azotemia and glomerulonephritis than in other categories. A sodium level less than 20 mEq/L strongly suggested intrinsic ARF. Considerable overlap in diagnoses existed when values were 20 to 40 mEq/L. Urine/plasma ratios of BUN and creatinine were higher in patients with prerenal azotemia and glomerulonephritis. The fractional excretion of sodium showed very little overlap, particularly when oliguric patients were compared. That is, 27 of 30 patients with prerenal azotemia, but only 1 of 24 patients with oliguric ARF, had values for fractional excretion of sodium of less than 1 percent. Therefore, when urinary test results are clear-cut, prerenal ARF can be differentiated from acute tubular necrosis with some degree of accuracy. However, when tests produce intermediate values, such distinctions are not always possible.

PREVENTION OF ACUTE RENAL FAILURE

Given all of the mechanisms involved in ARF, therapeutic interventions that improve cardiovascular function are most important.

Intravascular Fluid Administration

The first major step toward improving cardiovascular function is to ensure adequate intravascular volume. Therefore, the possibility of hypovolemia is determined by history and clinical examination. The latter includes taking note of central venous pressure and, if possible, pulmonary artery pressure and pulmonary capillary wedge pressure (PCWP) or observing a paradoxical arterial pulse with each positive-pressure inspiration.[68,69] A useful test is to infuse 250 ml of fluid rapidly and to observe the changes in central venous pressure or PCWP. If hypovolemia exists, fluids must be given intravenously in the form of blood, colloid, and/or crystalloid replacement.

The issue of administration of colloids versus crystalloids for intravascular volume expansion has been studied as it pertains to renal function[70] (also see Ch. 47). Baboons subjected to hemorrhagic shock and resuscitated with intravenous saline had normal levels of urinary output and compared favorably with those resuscitated with colloid solutions. Also, during return of shed blood, urinary output was higher than in animals resuscitated with colloid. Tubular dysfunction was apparent only in animals resuscitated with colloid.

Another report described patients given an average of 15 units of blood for resuscitation following hemorrhagic shock.[15] Those given albumin to maintain a normal serum albumin concentration had lower GRF, sodium and osmolar clearances, and slightly lower urinary output than patients resuscitated with crystalloid. Renal failure (serum creatinine greater than 3 mg/dl) occurred in 4 of 27 patients resuscitated with albumin and blood and in 1 of 25 patients resuscitated with crystalloid and blood. Thus, intravascular fluid administration attempts to raise left atrial filling pressures to levels that will maximize cardiac output. For patients with previously normal cardiac function who have acute myocardial infarction, it may be necessary to raise left atrial filling pressure or PCWP to 18 mmHg to achieve this goal.[71] For patients with septic shock, a lower left atrial filling pressure (approximately 12 mmHg) will provide optimal cardiac output.[72]

Because of the importance of protecting renal function by aggressive intravascular fluid administration, endotracheal intubation and controlled ventilation with positive end-expiratory pressure may be necessary to maintain sufficient oxygenation and elimination of carbon dioxide.

Inotropic Support

In some instances, intravascular volume therapy alone is not sufficient to improve low cardiac output, because the maximal filling pressure, beyond which cardiac output cannot increase, has been reached. Inotropic support may become necessary when either left atrial pressure is excessively high from left ventricular failure or volume therapy has pushed left atrial pressures to maximal levels without improving renal function (see also Ch. 14).

Dopamine is the current inotropic drug of choice because it augments renal blood flow and usually increases arterial pressure and cardiac output, depending on the dose administered.[73] The increase in renal blood flow is attributed to the effect of dopamine (DA) on a specific dopamine receptor subtype, DA_1, which vasodilates renal and mesenteric vascular beds. However, the natriuretic effect of dopamine has only recently been clarified by the use of selective DA_1 or DA_2 antagonists. Antagonism of the DA_1 receptor reduces renal blood flow and sodium and potassium excretion, whereas blockade of the DA_2 receptor has no effect.[74,75] Undesirable side effects (which may occur at any dose level of dopamine) include tachycardia and, on rare occasion, ventricular irritability.

Very low doses (1 to 3 μg/kg/min) of dopamine primarily stimulate dopaminergic receptors in the renal vasculature, thereby increasing renal blood flow and shifting renal perfusion toward the renal cortex.[76] In this low-dose range, dopamine often improves urinary output even without increasing cardiac output. Doses of 4 to 6 μg/kg/min began to exert a β-adrenergic effect, increasing heart rate and contractility, occasionally with a fall in peripheral vascular resistance. At high doses (approximately 7 to 10 μg/kg/min or more), dopamine resembles norepinephrine, in that both produce primarily α-adrenergic vasoconstriction. In a group of postcardiac surgical patients at risk of progressive renal failure who were initially oliguric for 2 hours, administration of low doses of dopamine increased urinary output and improved renal tubular function.[77] Other studies have demonstrated the beneficial effects of dopamine on renal blood flow in animals and humans.[78,79]

Improving inotropy with administration of digitalis

at this point in the patient's clinical course is unwise for several reasons. First, acute administration of digitalis in unstable patients may cause serious, prolonged, and irreversible arrhythmias. Second, potassium balance is often unstable in these critically ill patients. If hypokalemia ensues, the level of digitalis that was once therapeutic may become toxic. Third, almost any arrhythmia occurring in the presence of digitalis must be considered a product of digitalis toxicity until proved otherwise. Fourth, treating digitalis-induced arrhythmias is very difficult. Fifth, if creatinine clearance decreases and renal failure develops, less digitalis is excreted and digitalis toxicity occurs sooner. Because we do not know the toxic dose threshold or the protein binding of digitalis in a given patient, and because the patient may lose renal function despite one's best efforts, digitalis toxicity may develop and be exceedingly difficult to manage. Furthermore, catecholamine stimulation offers more inotropic support than digitalis.[80]

Use of the inotropic drug digoxin entails another consideration. One study suggests that in many patients with renal insufficiency the presence of an endogenous substance having digoxinlike immunoactivity may seriously compromise the accuracy of measurements of digoxin concentration. Specifically, patients in renal failure who were known to be free of digoxin had false-positive results ("apparent" digoxin concentrations as high as 1 ng/ml) on most assays (Fig. 34-5).[81] Measured digoxin concentration in a single serum specimen can vary greatly between immunoassays for patients with renal impairment, whereas patients with normal renal function show good interassay agreement.

Identification of High-Risk Patients

Prevention of ARF relies on identification of high-risk patients and procedures; reversal, if possible, of preoperative renal dysfunction; prompt replacement of fluid losses; and use of invasive hemodynamic monitoring when appropriate. Many conditions incur a high risk of postoperative ARF: patient age in excess of 50 years (renal reserve falls progressively with age), pre-existing renal dysfunction, cardiac or hepatic failure associated with abnormal renal hemodynamics, cardiac surgery, and abdominal aortic surgery in which aortic cross-clamping may alter distribution of renal blood flow. Other high-risk, conditions include obstructive jaundice; presence of an abscess and/or septic shock; obstetric problems such as severe postpartum hemorrhage, amniotic fluid embolism, and toxemia; rhabdomyolysis and myoglobinuria after crush injury; prolonged immobilization; coma; and malignant hyperthermia. When hypovolemia is treated successfully before surgery, use of salt-containing solutions rather than low-sodium solutions helps prevent aldosterone-induced hyponatremia, oliguria, and hypokalemic alkalosis. During surgery, urinary output of 0.5 to 1 ml/kg/h is usually adequate. Hemodynamic management emphasizes the need to maintain adequate arterial blood pressure and cardiac output to minimize the stress response on renal blood flow and to prevent secondary release of renin-angiotensin, which can further alter renal blood flow. Preload should be maintained, as left atrial hypotension is a potent renal vasoconstrictor.[28]

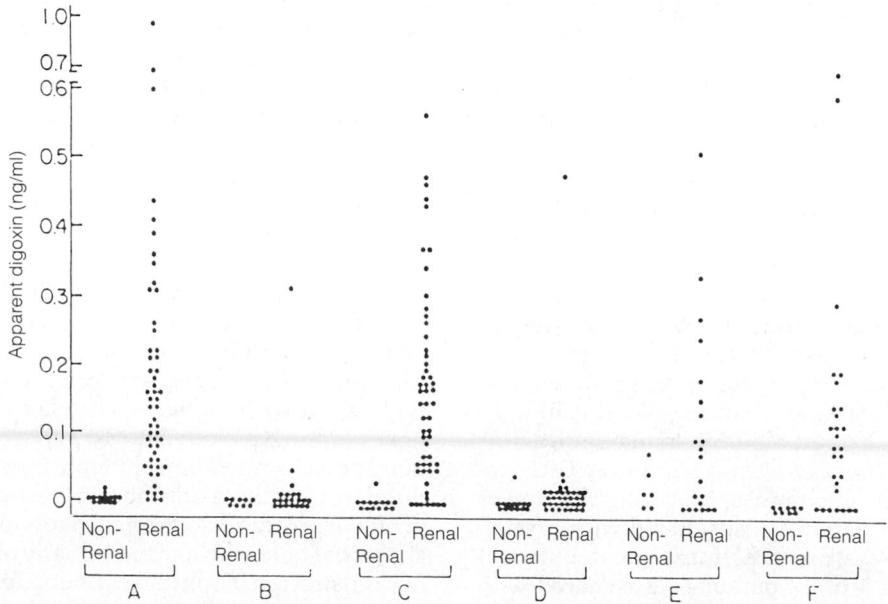

Fig. 34-5. False-positive results for concentrations of digoxin (as measured by six different assays) for 54 patients with renal impairment who were known to be free of digoxin. This "apparent" digoxin concentration (as high as 1 ng/ml, depending on the assay used) is attributed to the presence of an endogenous digoxinlike substance in many patients who have renal insufficiency. (From Graves et al.,[81] with permission.)

Normothermic Ischemia

Normothermic ischemic renal damage is an occasional complication of vascular surgery. Preservation of kidneys during extracorporeal storage of these organs for transplantation consists of flushing of the kidneys with special solutions, followed by cold storage. If these flushing solutions could also protect the kidney against normothermic ischemic damage in situ, the risk of ischemic injury during vascular reconstructive surgery would decrease.

One study investigated this possibility by comparing currently available solutions with a sucrose solution buffered with phosphate, with and without the additive ATP-magnesium chloride.[82] These solutions were also compared with pretreatment with mannitol, the most effective standard method of reducing the severity of normothermic postischemic ARF.[83,84] Rat kidneys were subjected to 1 hour of ischemia in vivo, followed by morphologic and renal function studies at 48 hours. Rats whose ischemic kidneys were flushed with standard solutions became anuric and had high creatinine levels and severe morphologic damage. The degree of damage was at least as great as that occurring in control rats whose ischemic kidneys were not flushed. Rats whose ischemic kidneys were flushed with phosphate-buffered sucrose solution had almost normal morphologic characteristics, with few focal spots of damage. There resulted a small rise in creatinine, some brush border degeneration, and presence of cytoplasmic debris in the tubular lumen. Animals whose ischemic kidneys were flushed with phosphate-buffered sucrose containing ATP-magnesium chloride had the best results. Their kidneys appeared normal (i.e., essentially the same as the kidneys of nonischemic control rats). Very few proximal tubules were missing brush borders; serum creatinine and urinary volume were normal. Interestingly, rats pretreated with only mannitol before ischemia had functional and morphologic damage that was approximately midway in severity between that manifested by normal and severely damaged kidneys.

Thus, 1 hour of normothermic ischemia in rat kidneys caused severe renal damage that could be prevented entirely by flushing of the kidneys with special preservative solutions. These solutions counteract the swelling and subsequent rupturing of tubular cells. The additive ATP-magnesium chloride is believed to augment reparative processes.

Use of Diuretics

Because oliguria is an important clinical feature of ARF and management of ARF is more difficult in surgical patients who are oliguric, diuretics are often used to reverse oliguria. Both mannitol, an osmotic diuretic, and ethacrynic acid and furosemide, potent loop diuretics, have been used to increase urinary output. The rationales for using these drugs include the belief that diuretics not only increase urinary flow but also improve renal function (i.e., reverse renal failure itself). In addition, clinicians believe that management of oliguric patients is facilitated when these patients are made nonoliguric. In the absence of supporting evidence for these two rationales, clinicians also use diuretics because "increased urine flow helps in relieving the psychological tension of both the patient and the physician involved."[85]

Mannitol

Although the mechanisms are unknown, prophylactically administered mannitol protects renal function.[83,84,86] Given parenterally after renal artery occlusion, mannitol does not overcome the "no-reflow phenomenon," in which vascular endothelial cells swell after ischemia. Despite this swelling, renal blood flow returns to normal quite promptly after vascular occlusion. In addition, a study on rats given mannitol and controls given saline showed that the favorable effect of mannitol on GFR after arterial occlusion is also not the result of an increase in renal blood flow in the rats given mannitol.[87] During partial occlusion of the renal artery, renal blood flow and filtration were greater in rats given mannitol than in control animals given isotonic saline.[88] There were a large decrease in afferent arteriolar resistance and a small decrease in efferent arteriolar resistance; glomerular capillary pressure also increased. This improvement with mannitol was blunted by prior treatment with indomethacin or infusion of prostaglandin, which may interfere with prostaglandin-induced vasodilation.[89] Mannitol given either before or after the intrarenal infusion of norepinephrine has also improved renal function in this vasoconstriction model of ARF.[90] The mechanism seems related to both increase in renal blood flow and osmolar clearance.

When norepinephrine-induced vasoconstriction was used to produce ischemic injury in one kidney, pretreatment with mannitol attenuated the decrease in GFR 1 hour and 24 hours after ischemia (Fig. 34-6).[91] Mitochondrial oxygen consumption, calcium uptake, and calcium release rates were also preserved. On the other hand, pretreatment with mannitol did not prevent cessation of blood flow to a norepinephrine-infused kidney.[92] However, recovery from 40 minutes of norepinephrine-induced ischemia was greater in kidneys pretreated with mannitol than in those perfused with saline, in that the adenine nucleotide profile was better preserved. In addition, pathologic changes associated with ischemia were minimized as a result of pretreatment with mannitol.

Thus, prophylactic administration of mannitol improves but does not restore normal renal function in many experimental models of renal failure. The mechanism of action is not yet well understood.

One study investigated the effects of mannitol during abdominal aortic aneurysm resection. Aggressive intravascular fluid administration followed by mannitol be-

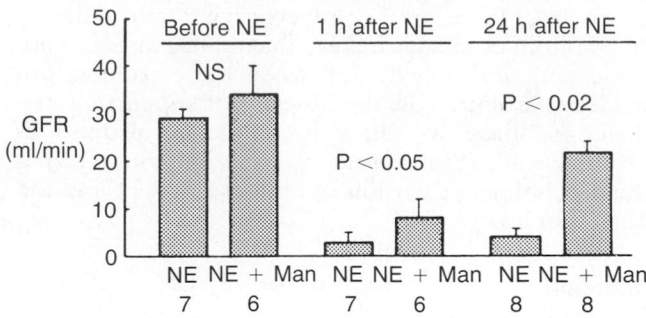

Fig. 34-6. Glomerular filtration rate (GFR) before norepinephrine (NE) and at 1 hour and 24 hours after norepinephrine in untreated dogs (striped bars) and in dogs infused intrarenally with isotonic mannitol prior to norepinephrine (crosshatched bars). Mannitol improved GFR at 1 hour and 24 hours after norepinephrine (P<0.05 and P<0.02, respectively). Numbers below each bar represent the number of animals studied. (From Schrier et al.,[91] with permission.)

fore aortic cross-clamping resulted in dramatic and sustained diuresis.[93] However, intraoperative urinary output probably does not predict postoperative renal function in patients undergoing abdominal aortic revascularization surgery.[94] That is, when mannitol and/or furosemide was given to patients undergoing this procedure, no relationship existed between intraoperative urinary output (or the lowest hourly urinary output) and changes from preoperative to postoperative levels of BUN or creatinine.[94] The crucial issue in this study was maintenance of intraoperative arterial blood pressure and PCWP (by means of appropriate intravenous fluid administration) prior to cross-clamping of the aorta. In all likelihood, intraoperative urinary output and postoperative renal function did not correlate because urinary output was maintained by adequate hydration, the most important method of preventing renal vasoconstriction.

In another study, use of mannitol plus dopamine infusion either after induction of anesthesia or for a 40-minute period after release of the aortic cross-clamp produced no significant difference in mean GFR between the control group and the two groups of patients given mannitol and dopamine.[95] However, once again, urinary flow rates in all three groups were kept above 1 ml/min at all times during the study.

Loop Diuretics

Loop diuretics may help prevent ARF. Several tubular mechanisms are possible: inhibition of salt reabsorption within the distal tubule, prevention of tubular obstruction by maintenance of high flow and pressure within the tubule, vasodilation or reversal of intrinsic renal vasoconstriction, or increase in flow to the macula densa because of damage to the reabsorptive capacity of more proximal segments (a high flow to the macula densa would reduce GFR). If furosemide were

to inhibit this feedback mechanism, more urine would be produced. There is no evidence that diuretics improve the problem of back leakage and glomerular damage itself. The most favorable results with furosemide have been obtained in the vasoconstriction model of ARF induced by infusion of norepinephrine into the canine renal artery. Furosemide, given before or within 30 minutes of norepinephrine infusion, improved GFR, an effect related to elevation of osmolar clearance, not renal blood flow.[90,96] However, as determined by extrapolation of data, the dose of furosemide required to protect renal function in humans would be enormous, being several grams for intravenous bolus administration. The results for both mannitol and furosemide regarding nephrotoxin-induced ARF vary but are generally discouraging.

Clinical studies describing the value of mannitol and loop diuretics in preventing ARF are less well controlled because of the many more variables involving patient population, dose levels, timing of drug administration, and so forth. Over the past 25 years, numerous studies have provided little evidence that high-risk surgical patients receive greater clinical benefit from prophylactic administration of diuretics than from routine intravenous fluid replacement. No important prophylactic benefit of loop diuretics for open heart surgery, vascular surgery, or surgical shock has been apparent.[97] Pretreatment of dogs subjected to ARF induced by norepinephrine did not prevent abolishment of renal blood flow but did enable recovery of the adenine nucleotide profile; this did not occur in control animals.[92] Similar results were obtained with bradykinin and mannitol. Phenoxybenzamine also prevented damage caused by norepinephrine but (unlike bradykinin, mannitol, and furosemide) did so by preventing a decrease in renal blood flow.[92] Despite the logical conclusion that diuretics can be useful in preventing at least intratubular precipitation of hemoglobin or uric acid, no data support this idea. Levinsky and Bernard[97] suggests that prevention of ARF with diuretics may be beneficial if any of the following risk factors is present: (1) jaundice in surgical patients, (2) excessive exposure to contrast media, (3) hyperuricemia, (4) deposition of pigment in urine, or (5) administration of methotrexate, cisplatin, or amphotericin B. There is no evidence that prophylactic diuretics are of any benefit in other surgical situations, and fluid administration is still crucial.

Identifying "early" acute renal failure, such as might occur between the prerenal phase and the established oliguric phase of ARF, is difficult. However, this is a time in which some response to diuretics might be expected, and such a response may account for some of the variable results that have been reported. Patients with oliguria of short duration seem to respond to diuretics. Moreover, the Levinsky-Bernard[97] summary suggests that patients with early ARF whose urinary flow can be increased with diuretics may be more likely to survive. However, the ability to respond to diuretics may merely identify ARF that is intrinsically less severe. The other possibility is that diuretics alter the natural history of ARF and thereby improve survival.

The use of loop diuretics to treat established ARF has been unsuccessful. Furosemide administered directly into the renal artery of 6 patients with ARF showed no favorable effects on total renal blood flow or intrarenal distribution of blood flow.[98] In a larger study of 66 patients with established oliguric ARF, 33 received intravenous furosemide, 1.5 to 6 mg/kg every 4 hours; the other 33 patients (controls) received no furosemide.[99] Five treated and 2 control patients had persistent diuresis, although hemodialysis was required in most patients. Furosemide did not significantly alter the course of ARF. In another study, patients given large doses of furosemide (up to 3,200 mg/d) had higher urinary output and a shorter duration of oliguria, required less dialysis, and had a more rapid decrease in serum creatinine and BUN levels than did patients not given diuretics.[100] However, overall mortality was similar for both groups.

Administration of furosemide (a bolus, 1 mg/kg, followed by an infusion at the rate of 1 mg/kg/h) with or without dopamine (3 μg/kg/min) was tested in dogs subjected to ARF induced by uranyl nitrate.[101] Neither furosemide nor dopamine alone was protective, but the combination of the two improved creatinine clearance and renal blood flow and enabled a brisk and persistent diuresis.

In conclusion, diuretics can increase urinary flow in some types of experimental ARF, particularly when given prophylactically. However, this effect is not necessarily synonymous with improvement or protection of renal function. The risk of mannitol therapy is very low, especially in surgical patients in whom intravascular volume and fluid shifts are unlikely to be excessive. The risks of furosemide relate primarily to ototoxicity. Also, loop diuretics in particular interfere with the ability to use the urine for diagnostic purposes. Diuretic-induced urine has high sodium content, is isosmolar, and is indistinguishable from urine produced during ARF. Therefore, urine must be tested before administration of diuretics, or 12 to 24 hours after the last administered dose. Use of diuretics may also divert the physician's attention from the real problems involved in the pathophysiologic changes of incipient ARF. After all other means of reversing ARF have failed, mannitol, furosemide, or thiazides (alone or in combination) may be tried to establish sustained diuresis or to reverse oliguria. Occasional patients may even respond, rendering their management easier.

DRUG CONSIDERATIONS

Recent studies concerning interaction between acute renal failure and drug administration should be mentioned. The pharmacokinetics and pharmacodynamics of atracurium do not differ between anephric patients and those with normal renal function.[102] However, renal failure may prolong the effect of morphine, as the kidney plays an important role in elimination of morphine. After a bolus administration of morphine, the mean plasma concentration of unchanged morphine is similar in normal patients and in those with renal failure. However, morphine metabolites remain in the circulation of patients with renal failure long after they have been eliminated from normal patients. Some of the morphine glucuronides act directly on central nervous system function and may prolong respiratory depression and other clinical signs of morphine retention.[103,104]

CONCLUSIONS

Acute renal failure, a highly lethal complication in critically ill surgical patients, is better prevented than treated. A variety of mechanisms are responsible for its development. Early and active intervention in the perioperative period, which is facilitated by proper monitoring, is administered in the hope of reducing the incidence and severity of ARF.

REFERENCES

1. Schrier RW: Acute renal failure. JAMA 247:2518, 1982
2. Stott RB, Cameron JS, Ogg CS, Bewick M: Why the persistently high mortality in acute renal failure? Lancet 2:75, 1972
3. Kleinknecht D, Ganeval D: Preventive hemodialysis in acute renal failure: Its effect on mortality and morbidity. p. 165. In Friedman EA, Eliahou HE (eds): Proceedings, Acute Renal Failure Conference. Publication No. (NIH) 74-608, Washington, D.C., 1973
4. Hollenberg NK, Epstein M, Rosen SM, et al: Acute oliguric renal failure in man: Evidence for preferential renal cortical ischemia. Medicine 47:455, 1968
5. Hollenberg NK, Adams DF, Oken DE, et al: Acute renal failure due to nephrotoxins: Renal hemodynamics and angiographic studies in man. N Engl J Med 282:1329, 1970
6. Hollenberg NK, Sandor T, Conroy M, et al: Xenon transit through the oliguric human kidney: Analysis by maximum likelihood. Kidney Int 3:177, 1973
7. Donohoe JF, Venkatachalam MA, Bernard DB, Levinsky NG: Tubular leakage and obstruction after renal ischemia: Structural-functional correlations. Kidney Int 13:208, 1978
8. Kreisberg JI, Venkatachalam MA: Morphologic factors in acute renal failure. p. 45. In Brenner BM, Lazarus JM (eds): Acute Renal Failure. 2nd Ed. New York, Churchill Livingstone, 1988
9. Arendshorst WJ, Finn WF, Gottschalk CW: Pathogenesis of acute renal failure following temporary renal ischemia in the rat. Circ Res 37:558, 1975
10. Tanner GA, Steinhausen M: Tubular obstruction ischemia-induced acute renal failure in the rat. Kidney Int 10:S-65, 1976
11. Myers BD, Moran SM: Hemodynamically mediated acute renal failure. N Engl J Med 314:97, 1986
12. Brezis M, Rosen S, Silva P, Epstein FH: Renal ischemia: A new perspective (editorial). Kidney Int 26:375, 1984

13. Brenner BM, Humes HD: Mechanics of glomerular ultrafiltration. N Engl J Med 297:148, 1977
14. Brenner BM, Deen WM, Robertson CR: Glomerular filtration. p. 251. In Brenner BM, Rector FR, Jr (eds): The Kidney. Vol. 1. Philadelphia, WB Saunders, 1976
15. Lucas CE, Weaver D, Higgins RF, et al: Effects of albumin versus non-albumin resuscitation on plasma volume and renal excretory function. J Trauma 18:564, 1978
16. Wright FS: Intrarenal regulation of glomerular filtration rate. N Engl J Med 291:135, 1974
17. Stein JH, Lifschitz MD, Barnes LD: Current concepts on the pathophysiology of acute renal failure (editorial). Am J Physiol 234:F171, 1978
18. Epstein M, Lifschitz MD: Volume status as a determinant of the influence of renal PGE on renal function (editorial). Nephron 25:157, 1980
19. Fox DA, Jick H: Nonsteroidal anti-inflammatory drugs and renal disease. JAMA 251:1299, 1984
20. Oken DE: Role of prostaglandins in the pathogenesis of acute renal failure. Lancet 1:1319, 1975
21. Schrier RW, Henrich WL: Nonsteroidal anti-inflammatory drugs: Caution still indicated (editorial). JAMA 251:1301, 1984
22. Terragno NA, Terragno DA, McGiff JC: Contribution of prostaglandins to the renal circulation in conscious, anesthetized, and laparotomized dogs. Circ Res 40:590, 1977
23. Walshe JJ, Venuto RC: Acute oliguric renal failure induced by indomethacin: Possible mechanism. Ann Intern Med 91:47, 1979
24. Kimberly RP, Bowden RE, Keiser HR, Plotz PH: Reduction of renal function by newer nonsteroidal anti-inflammatory drugs. Am J Med 64:804, 1978
25. Schrier RW: Acute renal failure. Kidney Int 15:205, 1979
26. Lonigro AJ, Terragno NA, Malik KU, McGiff JC: Differential inhibition by prostaglandins of the renal actions of pressor stimuli. Prostaglandins 3:595, 1973
27. Galler M, Folkert VW, Schlondorff D: Reversible acute renal insufficiency and hyperkalemia following indomethacin therapy. JAMA 246:154, 1981
28. Gorfinkel HJ, Szidon JP, Hirsch LJ, Fishman AP: Renal performance in experimental cardiogenic shock. Am J Physiol 222:1260, 1972
29. Kahl FR, Flint JF, Szidon JP: Influence of left atrial distention on renal vasomotor tone. Am J Physiol 226:240, 1974
30. Ballermann BJ, Brenner BM: Biologically active atrial peptides. J Clin Invest 76:2041, 1985
31. Currie MG, Geller DM, Cole BR, et al: Purification and sequence analysis of bioactive atrial peptides (atriopeptins). Science 223:67, 1984
32. Colley PS, Sivarajan M: Regional blood flow in dogs during halothane anesthesia and controlled hypotension produced by nitroprusside or nitroglycerin. Anesth Analg 63:503, 1984
33. Leighton KM, Bruce C, MacLeod BA: Sodium nitroprusside-induced hypotension and renal blood flow. Can Anaesth Soc J 24:637, 1977
34. Priebe H-J, Hedley-Whyte J: Respiratory support and renal function. Int Anesthesiol Clin 22(1):203, 1984
35. Hall SV, Johnson EE, Hedley-Whyte J: Renal hemodynamics and function with continuous positive-pressure ventilation in dogs. Anesthesiology 41:452, 1974
36. Fewell JE, Bond GC: Role of sinoaortic baroreceptors in initiating the renal response to continuous positive-pressure ventilation in the dog. Anesthesiology 52:408, 1980
37. Annat G, Viale JP, Xuan BB, et al: Effect of PEEP ventilation on renal function, plasma renin, aldosterone, neurophysins and urinary ADH, and prostaglandins. Anesthesiology 58:136, 1983
38. Kaukinen S, Eerola R: Positive end expiratory pressure ventilation, renal function and renin. Ann Clin Res 11:58, 1979
39. Priebe H-J, Heinmann JC, Hedley-Whyte J: Mechanisms of renal dysfunction during positive end-expiratory pressure ventilation. J Appl Physiol 50:643, 1981
40. Mullin RJ, Dawe EJ, Lucas CE, et al: Mechanisms of impaired renal function with PEEP. J Surg Res 37:189, 1984
41. Anderson RJ, Linas SL, Berns AS, et al: Nonoliguric acute renal failure. N Engl J Med 296:1134, 1977
42. Hou SH, Bushinsky DA, Wish JB, et al: Hospital-acquired renal insufficiency. A prospective study. Am J Med 74:243, 1983
43. Coggins CH, Fang LS-T: Acute renal failure associated with antibiotics, anesthetic agents, and radiographic contrast agents. p. 295. In Brenner BM, Lazarus JM (eds): Acute Renal Failure. 2nd Ed. New York, Churchill Livingstone, 1988
44. Harkonen S, Kjellstrand CM: Exacerbation of diabetic renal failure following intravenous pyelography. Am J Med 63:939, 1977
45. Van Zee BE, Hoy WE, Talley TE, Jaenike JR: Renal injury associated with intravenous pyelography in nondiabetic and diabetic patients. Ann Intern Med 89:51, 1978
46. Feldman HA, Goldfarb S, McCurdy DK: Recurrent radiographic dye-induced acute renal failure. JAMA 229:72, 1974
47. Alexander RD, Berkes SL, Abuelo G: Contrast media-induced oliguric renal failure. Arch Intern Med 138:381, 1978
48. Anto HR, Cho S-Y, Porush JG, Shapiro WB: Intravenous infusion pyelography and renal function: Effects of hypertonic mannitol in patients with chronic renal insufficiency. Arch Intern Med 141:1652, 1981
49. Houghton DC, Campbell-Boswell MV, Bennett WM, et al: Myeloid bodies in the renal tubules of humans: Relationship to gentamicin therapy. Clin Nephrol 10:140, 1978
50. Gary NE, Buzzeo L, Salaki J, Einsinger RP: Gentamicin-associated acute renal failure. Arch Intern Med 136:1101, 1976
51. Chiu PJS, Brown A, Miller G, Long JF: Renal extraction of gentamicin in anesthetized dogs. Antimicrob Agents Chemother 10:277, 1976
52. Edwards CQ, Smith CR, Baughman KL, et al: Concentrations of gentamicin and amikacin in human kidneys. Antimicrob Agents Chemother 9:925, 1976
53. Keown PA, Stiller CR, Wallace AC, et al: Cyclosporine nephrotoxicity: Exploration of the risk factors and prognosis of the renal injury. Transplant Proc 17:suppl. 1, 247, 1985
54. Humes HD, Jackson NM, O'Connor RP, et al: Pathogenetic mechanisms of nephrotoxicity. Transplant Proc 17:suppl. 1, 51, 1985
55. Thurlbeck WM, Castleman B: Atheromatous emboli to the kidneys after aortic surgery. N Engl J Med 257:442, 1957
56. Koppel MH, Coburn JW, Mims MM, et al: Transplantation of cadaveric kidneys from patients with hepatorenal syndrome: Evidence for the functional nature of renal failure in advanced liver disease. N Engl J Med 280:1367, 1969
57. Levenson DJ, Skorecki KL, Newell GC, Narins RG: Acute renal failure associated with hepatobiliary disease. p. 535. In Brenner BM, Lazarus JM (eds): Acute Renal Failure. 2nd Ed. New York, Churchill Livingstone, 1988
58. Dubrow A, Flamenbaum W: Acute renal failure associated with myoglobinuria and hemoglobinuria. p. 279. In Brenner BM, Lazarus JM (eds): Acute Renal Failure. 2nd Ed. New York, Churchill Livingstone, 1988
59. Ron D, Taitelman U, Michaelson M, et al: Prevention of acute

renal failure in traumatic rhabdomyolysis. Arch Intern Med 144:277, 1984

60. Teschan PE, Lawson NL: Studies in acute renal failure: Prevention by osmotic diuresis, and observations on the effect of plasma and extracellular volume expansion. Nephron 3:1, 1966

61. Wilson DR, Thiel G, Arce ML, Oken DE: Glycerol induced hemoglobinuric acute renal failure in the rat. III: Micropuncture study of the effects of mannitol and isotonic saline on individual nephron function. Nephron 4:337, 1967

62. Bailey RR, Natale R, Turnbull DI, Linton AL: Protective effect of frusemide in acute tubular necrosis and acute renal failure. Clin Sci Mol Med 45:1, 1973

63. Espinel CH, Gregory AW: Differential diagnosis of acute renal failure. Clin Nephrol 13:73, 1980

64. Espinel CH: The FE$_{Na}$ test: Use in the differential diagnosis of acute renal failure. JAMA 236:579, 1976

65. Shin B, Richards W, Howridge M, et al: Outcome prediction of intensive care in postoperative patients (abstract). Anesthesiology 59:A131, 1983

66. Shin B, Mackenzie CF, Helrich M: Creatinine clearance for early detection of posttraumatic renal dysfunction. Anesthesiology 64:605, 1986

67. Miller TR, Anderson RJ, Linas SL, et al: Urinary diagnostic indices in acute renal failure: A prospective study. Ann Intern Med 89:47, 1978

68. Coyle JP, Teplick RS, Long MC, Davison JK: Respiratory variations in systemic arterial pressure as an indicator of volume status (abstract). Anesthesiology 59:A53, 1983

69. Perel A, Pizov R, Cotev S: Systolic blood pressure variation is a sensitive indicator of hypovolemia in ventilated dogs subjected to graded hemorrhage. Anesthesiology 67:498, 1987

70. Siegel DC, Cochin A, Geocaris T, Moss GS: Effects of saline and colloid resuscitation on renal function. Ann Surg 177:51, 1973

71. Crexells C, Chatterjee K, Forrester JS, et al: Optimal level of filling pressure in the left side of the heart in acute myocardial infarction. N Engl J Med 289:1263, 1973

72. Packman MI, Rackow EC: Optimum left heart filling pressure during fluid challenge of patients with septic shock (abstract). Crit Care Med 9:234, 1981

73. Goldberg LI: Cardiovascular and renal actions of dopamine: Potential clinical applications. Pharmacol Rev 24:1, 1972

74. Frederickson ED, Bradley T, Goldberg LI: Blockade of renal effects of dopamine in the dog by the DA$_1$ antagonist SCH 23390. Am J Physiol 249:F236, 1985

75. Goldberg LI: Dopamine and new dopamine analogs. Receptors and clinical application. J Clin Anesth 1:66, 1988

76. Hollenberg NK, Adams, DF, Mendell P, et al: Renal vascular responses to dopamine: Haemodynamic and angiographic observations in normal man. Clin Sci Mol Med 45:733, 1973

77. Davis RF, Lappas DG, Kirklin JK, et al: Acute oliguria after cardiopulmonary bypass: Renal functional improvement with low-dose dopamine infusion. Crit Care Med 10:852, 1982

78. Bennett D, Hynd J, Tighe D: The effects of dopamine on renal function in hypovolaemic shock (abstract). Crit Care Med 9:253, 1981

79. Hemmer M, Suter PM: Treatment of cardiac and renal effects of PEEP with dopamine in patients with acute respiratory failure. Anesthesiology 50:399, 1979

80. Spann JF, Jr, Buccino RA, Sonnenblick EH, Braunwald E: Contractile state of cardiac muscle obtained from cats with experimentally produced ventricular hypertrophy and heart failure. Circ Res 21:341, 1967

81. Graves SW, Brown B, Valdes R, Jr: An endogenous digoxin-like substance in patients with renal impairment. Ann Intern Med 99:604, 1983

82. Andrews PM, Coffey AK: Protection of kidneys from acute renal failure resulting from normothermic ischemia. Lab Invest 49:87, 1983

83. Green RD, Boyer D, Halasz NA, Collins GM: Pharmacological protection of rabbit kidneys from normothermic ischemia. Transplantation 28:131, 1979

84. Collins GM, Green RD, Boyer D, Halasz NA: Protection of kidneys from warm ischemic injury: Dosage and timing of mannitol administration. Transplantation 29:83, 1980

85. Borirakchanyavat V, Vongsthongsri M, Sitprija V: Furosemide in acute renal failure. Postgrad Med J 54:30, 1978

86. Selkurt EE: The changes in renal clearance following complete ischemia of the kidney. Am J Physiol 144:395, 1945

87. Kashgarian M, Siegel NJ, Ries AL, et al: Hemodynamic aspects in development and recovery phases of experimental postischemic acute renal failure. Kidney Int 10:S-160, 1976

88. Johnston PA, Bernard DB, Donohoe JF, et al: Effect of volume expansion on hemodynamics of the hypoperfused rat kidney. J Clin Invest 64:550, 1979

89. Johnston PA, Bernard DB, Levinsky NG: Mechanism of vasodilatory effect of mannitol (M) in the hypoperfused rat kidney: Role of renal hormones (abstract). Kidney Int 16:774, 1979

90. Patak RV, Fadem SZ, Lifschitz MD, Stein JH: Study of factors which modify the development of norepinephrine-induced acute renal failure in the dog. Kidney Int 15:227, 1979

91. Schrier RW, Arnold PE, Gordon JA, Burke TJ: Protection of mitochondrial function by mannitol in ischemic acute renal failure. Am J Physiol 247:F365, 1984

92. Sinsteden TD, O'Neill TJ, Hill S, Lifschitz MD: The role of high-energy phosphate in norepinephrine-induced acute renal failure in the dog. Circ Res 59:93, 1986

93. Mazze RI, Barry KG: Prevention of functional renal failure during anesthesia and surgery by sustained hydration and mannitol infusion. Anesth Analg 46:61, 1967

94. Alpert RA, Roizen MF, Hamilton WK, et al: Intraoperative urinary output does not predict postoperative renal function in patients undergoing abdominal aortic revascularization. Surgery 95:707, 1984

95. Paul MD, Mazer CD, Byrick RJ, et al: Influence of mannitol and dopamine on renal function during elective infrarenal aortic clamping in man. Am J Nephrol 6:427, 1986

96. de Torrente A, Miller PD, Cronin RE, et al: Effects of furosemide and acetylcholine in norepinephrine-induced acute renal failure. Am J Physiol 235:F131, 1978

97. Levinsky NG, Bernard DB: Mannitol and loop diuretics in acute renal failure. p. 841. In Benner BM, Lazarus JM (eds): Acute Renal Failure. 2nd Ed. New York, Churchill Livingstone, 1988

98. Epstein M, Schneider NS, Befeler B: Effect of intrarenal furosemide on renal function and intrarenal hemodynamics in acute renal failure. Am J Med 58:510, 1975

99. Kleinknecht D, Ganeval D, Gonzalez-Duque LA, Fermanian J: Furosemide in acute oliguric renal failure: A controlled trial. Nephron 17:51, 1976

100. Cantarovich F, Locatelli A, Fernandez JC, et al: Frusemide in high doses in the treatment of acute renal failure. Postgrad Med J 47:April suppl., 13, 1971

101. Lindner A, Cutler RE, Goodman WG: Synergism of dopamine plus furosemide in preventing acute renal failure in the dog. Kidney Int 16:158, 1979

102. Fahey MR, Rupp SM, Fisher DM, et al: The pharmacokinetics

and pharmacodynamics of atracurium in patients with and without renal failure. Anesthesiology 61:699, 1984

103. Chauvin M, Sandouk P, Scherrmann JM, et al: Morphine pharmacokinetics in renal failure. Anesthesiology 66:327, 1987

104. Osborne RJ, Joel SP, Slevin ML: Morphine intoxication in renal failure: The role of morphine-6-glucuronide. Br Med J 292:1548, 1986

105. Hostetter TH, Wilkes BM, Brenner BM: Renal circulatory and nephron function in experimental acute renal failure. p. 108. In Brenner BM, Lazarus JM (eds): Acute Renal Failure. 2nd Ed. New York, Churchill Livingstone, 1988

106. Rudnick MR, Bastl CP, Elfinbein IB, Narins RG: The differential diagnosis of acute renal failure. p. 177. In Brenner BM, Lazarus JM (eds): Acute Renal Failure. 2nd Ed. New York, Churchill Livingstone, 1988

35
NEUROLOGIC MONITORING

Susan Black
Roy F. Cucchiara

INTRODUCTION

The evaluation of neurologic signs was one of the earliest scientific approaches to judging the effects of anesthetics on the brain. Guedel in the 1940s proposed the use of pupillary signs as a guide to determining the depth of anesthesia. As the patient passes through the stages of anesthesia, the pupils change from normal when awake to dilated during the excitement phase of stage II. In early stage III the pupils constrict secondary to the loss of cortical inhibitory effects on the Edinger-Westphal nucleus. In deeper planes of stage III the pupils progressively dilate as paralysis of the fibers of the pupiloconstrictor muscles ensues (also see Ch. 30).

Modern anesthetics are usually combined with intravenously administered drugs (see Chs. 8 to 10) or supplemental drugs (e.g., narcotics) so that eye signs are no longer as helpful in determining anesthetic depth as they once were. The development of modern elec-

tronics and microprocessors has made possible the rapid evaluation of electrical data from the body to allow nearly real-time evaluation of nervous system function.

In this chapter we focus on monitoring of the intact nervous system utilizing electronic instruments, examine some of the electroneurophysiologic and pathologic changes that occur acutely in the operating room, and see how these signals are altered by commonly used anesthetics.

MONITORING MODALITIES

Those techniques most available in sophisticated operating rooms today include the electroencephalogram (EEG), evoked potentials, and electromyogram.

The EEG is used to help identify pathologic brain findings, define clinical problems, and predict outcome of brain insults. This is the result of correlation of pattern recognition with clinical states over nearly half a century of experience. The encephalographer can accurately identify consciousness, unconsciousness, epilepsy, sleep, and coma. The correlation between EEG pattern and anesthetic depth is less clear, perhaps because of the variety of types of drugs used in anesthesia and the subtle loss of awareness. The electrode records activity from the brain tissue nearest it, and all areas of the brain do not respond identically to the same anesthetic drug level. Precise assessment of anesthetic depth by EEG is possible with certain specific drugs at specific levels of anesthesia. The steps in the continuum from awake to deeply anesthetized are not all equally clear, but some general patterns are described. Computer advances have made possible high-speed mathematical manipulation of the EEG signal to present it in a more readable fashion. Interpretation of the raw EEG is still largely dependent on the experience of the reader (also see Ch. 30).

Evoked potentials are measurements of electrical potential changes that pass along stimulated nervous tissue. The voltages generated in this process are quite small and are obscured by the higher voltages produced by the EEG. Repeated sampling and sophisticated electronic summation and averaging techniques are needed to extract the evoked potential signal from the background EEG.

For practical purposes today it is convenient to consider all evoked potential monitoring as evaluation of sensory pathways. There are three basic types of sensory evoked potentials: somatosensory (SSEP), auditory (BAEP), and visual (VEP). The SSEP is used to assess a peripheral nerve to central nervous system pathway. The BAEP is a measure of conduction through cranial nerve VIII, through brain stem structures, and out to the cortex. The VEP utilizes stimulation of the light receptors of the retina to evaluate pathways from the optic nerve to the occipital cortex.

THE STANDARD EEG

The Signal

The technical goal of the EEG is to provide a clear signal free of electrical noise and permit anatomic localization of the various signals generated. The recording electrode impedance should be about 5 kΩ to permit clear EEG signals in the 10- to 50-μV range. As electrode impedance increases, the signal to noise ratio decreases. This permits the background electrical "noise" to obscure the EEG signal. Impedance is kept low by using silver electrodes with electrolyte gel between the scalp and electrode and holding the electrode tightly to the scalp with colloidin. When wick electrodes are applied directly to the brain surface, impedance is decreased by saturation of the wick with an electrolyte solution.

The recording montage permits anatomic localiza-

tion of the signal. The standard EEG montage is the 10-20 system. This system is a symmetric array of scalp electrodes 10 percent of the circumferential distance above the inion and external auditory meatus and 20 percent of the circumferential distance apart. A total of 20 recording electrodes is used with one or more reference electrodes placed outside the recording field. This permits the encephalographer to select a pair of electrodes with a discrete anatomic location from which to record. The standard is a 16-channel recording.

Recordings of electrical activity of the brain may be made directly from microelectrodes to measure activity from an individual unit or from larger electrodes to record from the brain surface or from the scalp. The conventional EEG is recorded from the scalp; the recording from the surface of the brain is the electrocorticogram (ECoG). The generators of these waveforms are not clearly defined, although the patterns have been well described and correlated with clinical and pathologic conditions.

The EEG signal contains three basic parameters: amplitude, frequency, and time. Amplitude is the electrical height of the wave in μV. Frequency can be thought of simply as the number of times per second the wave crosses the zero voltage line. Time is the duration of the sampling of the signal. This is continuous and is real time in the standard EEG but is a sample epoch in the processed EEG.

The Normal EEG

The patterns seen on the EEG vary somewhat among individuals but are consistent enough to allow for accurate recognition. The usual base frequency in the awake patient is the β-range (>13 Hz). This high-frequency and usually low-amplitude signal is common from the alert attentive brain. With the action of closing the eyes, the tracing immediately adds signals from the α-range (8 to 13 Hz) with a slightly higher amplitude (Fig. 35-1). This range is usually used as a reference signal during anesthesia. When events that lead the brain to produce higher frequencies occur, the EEG is described as "activated," and when slower frequencies are produced (θ at 4 to 7 Hz and δ at <4 Hz) the EEG is "depressed." The sleep EEG may contain all of these frequencies at various times. The slower frequencies occur during deep natural sleep with sleep spindles (Fig. 35-2), but during light sleep (rapid eye movement [REM] sleep) the EEG becomes activated and the eye muscle EMG appears on the EEG.

General characteristics of the normal EEG are that it is symmetric, the patterns are predictable, spike waveforms are absent, and it cannot be used to predict normal brain function.

The Abnormal EEG

General characteristics of the "abnormal" EEG are asymmetry and patterns of amplitude and frequency that are not predictable or expected in the usual recording. These reflect either anatomic or metabolic alter-

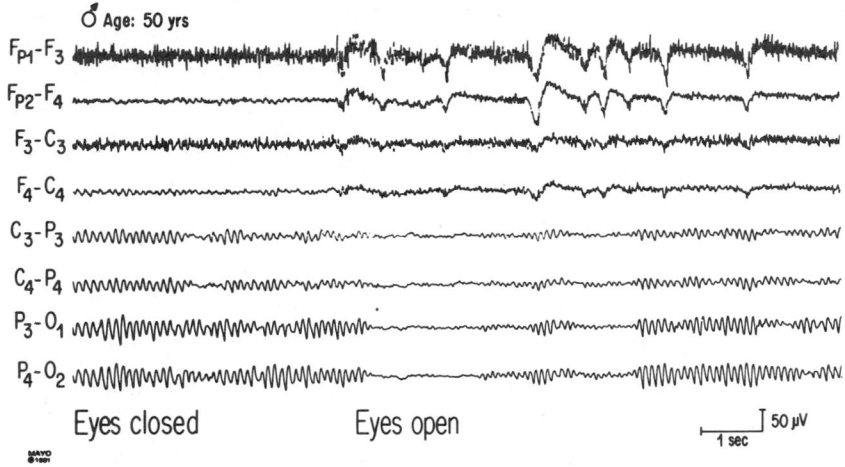

Fig. 35-1. The loss and return of α-activity as the eyes open and close can be seen. The large spikes are muscle artifact. (By permission of the Mayo Foundation.)

ation in the underlying brain. Regional asymmetry can be seen with tumor, epilepsy, and cerebral infarction. Epilepsy may be recognized by high-voltage spike waves, whereas cerebral infarction may appear as low voltage and low frequency pattern, as compared to the rest of the brain tracing. Global distortions of the EEG are not asymmetric because there is no normal side with which to compare the tracing. The clinical situation is very important in identification of "abnormality" in global EEG patterns that deviate from normal. Epilepsy, hypoxia, and anesthetic effects are examples.

Processed EEG

The interpretation of the standard written EEG record is both a science and an art. The waveforms are the data base for the interpretation; qualitative overall impression of the record is the experience. Both are important in arriving at a diagnosis. Until recent years the latter

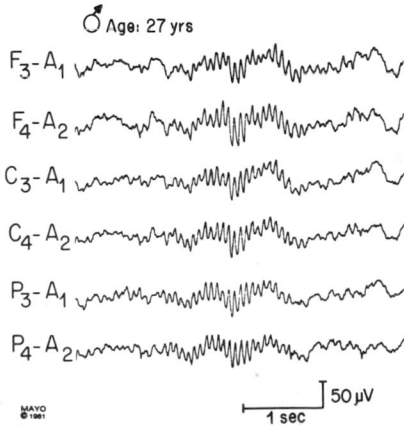

Fig. 35-2. Characteristic "sleep spindles" in normal sleep are shown in the center of the figure. (By permission of the Mayo Foundation.)

approach was dominant, simply because the waveforms could not be described mathematically in a time frame that would make such a data base of any use. Mainframe computers then began to be used to convert the analog signal of the EEG to a digital signal and mathematically manipulate the data. The process was complex and expensive and still had little relevance to the clinician. Early techniques took 1 hour to digitize and analyze 1 second of EEG data. The hardware capability of computers has exploded in the last decade and thus caught up with the mathematical potential available in analysis of complex waveforms. Real time, online processing previously requiring mainframe computer capability began to appear as the EEG processor "black box" developed.

In general, five assumptions can be made when moving to the processed EEG. First we assume that the changes we are looking for will be in either amplitude or frequency or both. Any system that emphasizes either frequency or amplitude preferentially can be expected to fail to display changes that occur primarily in the other parameter. Second, as the processed EEG signal becomes more electronically remote (more processed), there will be a point where it will be increasingly difficult or even impossible to relate what we know about the raw EEG to comprehension of the processed signal. Third, the standard 16-channel EEG montage provides more information than can consistently be utilized in processed EEG and more than is needed for intraoperative diagnostic use. Fourth, since the processed EEG is derived from the raw EEG, it will not contain information that is not in the original signal. Derivations of the original signal may include computational displays and algorithms, but the data base can only be the original signal. Fifth, some of the diagnostic changes will be unilateral and some bilateral. Display of the activity of both hemispheres is necessary to delineate unilateral from bilateral changes. An appropriate number of leads is needed. The gold standard for EEG analysis remains the continuous visual inspection of a 16- to 20-channel ink-on-paper EEG by an experienced electroencephalographer.[1,2]

Devices

There are specific frequency and amplitude ranges that seem to be important in the EEG under anesthesia. The simplest way to remove artifact and accentuate the waves of interest is to use a system of filters and amplifiers so that frequencies above 20 Hz are filtered out and waves between 4 and 10 Hz are selectively amplified. The power (amplitude squared) can be displayed for each hemisphere. This concept is the basis for the cerebral function monitor (CFM) and the power spectrum analyzer (PSA-1). A *power spectrum analysis* uses a computer to perform a Fourier transformation converting the irregular EEG waves to equivalent sine waves of known frequency and amplitude. The three-dimensional display may show time and amplitude (as power) as one axis and frequencies on the horizontal axis; this is the compressed spectral array (CSA), as is seen on the Neurotrac (Fig. 35-3). The same data can be displayed in two dimensions distinguishing the relative amplitude by increasing the density of dots at various frequencies, the density modulated spectral array

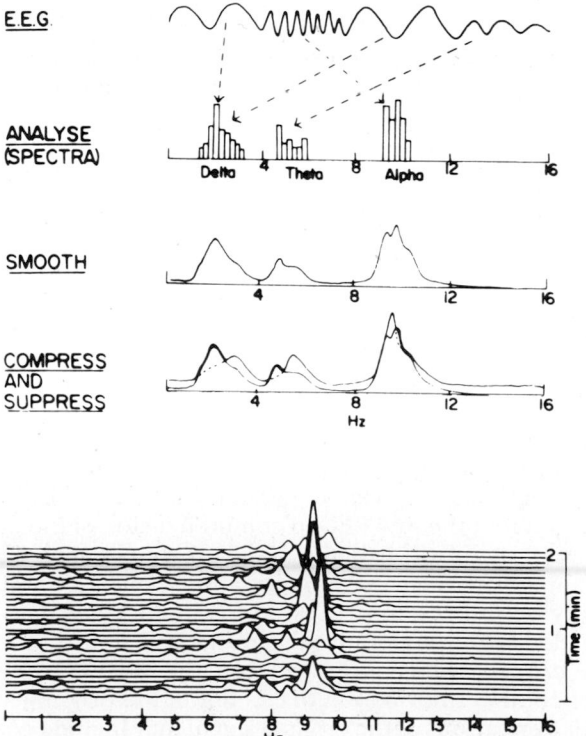

Fig. 35-3. Diagram of technique used to generate compressed spectral array. Example below shows compressed spectra of the α-rhythm from a normal subject. (From Stockard and Bickford,[13] with permission.)

(DSA). Another technique for processed EEG is *aperiodic analysis*, in which each waveform is analyzed without an averaging technique. The signal is broken into four component frequencies (α- through δ-waves), with the amplitudes at each frequency in each hemisphere. A commercial algorithm that emphasizes the amplitude is displayed in the Lifescan brain monitor; a unit that uses power emphasis to "map" brain areas in the Cerebral Tracer. A variety of creative display techniques are available to simplify or enhance the data from the processed EEG.[3-7]

Data Acquisition Period

An important consideration in the processed EEG is the element of time. The standard EEG is continuous in real time. The processed EEG usually obtains its data over a given time period (epoch), processes the data, and then displays them. There is a relationship between epoch length and spectral resolution.[8] If an infinite epoch length is chosen, the waveform can be described precisely. If a short length is chosen, three main factors mitigate against mathematical precision: the epoch sampled may not be representative of the overall activity, the nature of the data window becomes increasingly important, and there may be insufficient data points for Fourier transformation. This issue, as related to the intraoperative EEG for anesthetic depth, has been studied by Levy.[8] A longer epoch may produce less epoch-to-epoch variability and allow more precise description of frequency and power. However, the longer epoch increases the delay before new information is processed and displayed, thereby reducing the amount of information available for clinical decision making. In studying EEG epochs of 2 to 32 seconds, Levy concluded that 2-second epochs are appropriate during general anesthesia. However, burst suppression is an exception because of the possibility of sampling primarily during burst or suppression periods. This is not a major shortcoming since this pattern is easily identified on raw EEG and is expected with use of barbiturates in anesthesia.

Anesthesia and the EEG

With the advent of the then "high-tech" EEG in 1950, Courtin, Bickford, and Faulconer sought to monitor the brain and devise a servo-controlled system that could adjust the anesthetic concentration administered on the basis of the EEG pattern.[9] It was an ingenious idea, but, despite descriptions of the EEG during anesthesia, knowledge and technology were not adequate at that time. In general, as the patient goes to sleep with general anesthesia, the brain waves become larger in amplitude and slower in frequency. These higher-amplitude waves increase the calculated integrated total power of the EEG, and this increase in power was used as an indicator of depth of anesthesia. However, since all anesthetics do not produce exactly the same changes in EEG pattern as anesthesia ensues, generic correlation of the EEG with depth of anesthesia has been an elusive goal. During increasing anesthetic depth with volatile agents the fast activity of the EEG "shifts" anteriorly as consciousness is lost.[10] This anatomic localization can be more readily identified on the standard EEG because of the multitude of leads but cannot easily be seen on the processed EEG with a limited number of leads (Table 35-1).

Intravenous Anesthetic Drugs

Barbiturates
(Also See Ch. 8)

The barbiturates used clinically appear to yield very similar neuroelectric activity. However, differences do exist among the barbiturates with regard to potency and duration of action.

Barbiturates initially produce fast waves in the EEG in the range of 20 to 30 Hz (Fig. 35-4). This pattern is known as the *initial rapid sequence* to barbiturates (Fig. 35-4A).[11,12] This fast activity is initiated in the frontal area, where it is most prominent, and spreads toward the occiput. The frequency of these fast waves decreases as the total cumulative dose of barbiturate rises. Next, spindle-shaped bursts are superimposed on the fast activity with these waves in the 5- to 12-Hz range. This pattern is generally referred to as "barbiturate spindles," and it is at this point that the patient generally loses consciousness (Fig. 35-4B). Further increase in the total dose of barbiturate yields a decline in the spindle bursts of the 5- to 12-Hz waves and EEG then develops large polymorphic waves of 1 to 3 Hz (Fig. 35-4C). If the barbiturate is injected rapidly, the slow-wave activity is produced with only a few traces of the fast-wave activity and barbiturate spindles preceding.[13] It is when this slow-wave polymorphic activity becomes dominant that the patient tolerates skin incision. With increasing concentrations, periods of suppression begin to appear on the EEG (Fig. 35-4D). Each of these periods is followed by "bursts" of renewed activity that contains high-frequency components. The burst period

TABLE 35-1. Factors Affecting the EEG in Relation to Anesthesia

Anesthetic agents
Surgery
Cardiopulmonary bypass
Carotid endarterectomy
Epilepsy
Pathophysiologic
Hypoxia
Hypotension
Hypothermia
Hypercarbia and hypocarbia
Untoward events
Brain death

subsides as the next period of suppression arises. Therefore, barbiturates produce this burst suppression pattern with the burst activity starting in the 8-Hz range and decelerating to 2 to 6 Hz. The suppression period progressively lengthens with increasing dose until total electrical silence occurs.

Narcotics
(Also See Ch. 10)

The EEG changes produced by fentanyl are fairly consistent. The effects of high-dose fentanyl (30 to 70 μg/kg) have been studied in patients receiving lorazepam (4 to 5 μg) and morphine (10 μg) as premedicants. Approximately 1 minute after induction with fentanyl, the α-rhythm becomes slower and broader. In 1 to 2 minutes, diffuse θ-waves (4 to 8 Hz) are seen with some δ-activity (<3 Hz). This is followed by irregular diffuse slow δ-waves, which can become more synchronous with a monomorphic EEG picture. At lower doses of fentanyl (30 μg/kg) the EEG exhibits significantly faster activity.

At times, patients show isolated sharp wave activity after induction of anesthesia with fentanyl. This phenomenon is more evident with increasing doses, being present in 20 percent of patients at 30 μg/kg, 60 percent at 50 μg/kg, 58 percent at 60 μg/kg, and 80 percent at 70 μg/kg. This activity is mainly noted in the frontotemporal region.[14]

Ketamine
(Also See Ch. 9)

Ketamine produces a "dissociative state" of analgesia and altered awareness in humans with intravenous doses of 0.25 to 0.5 mg/kg, and unconsciousness at 1 to 2 mg/kg.[15] The EEG changes appear to represent activation of thalamic and limbic structures, producing hypersynchronous δ-waves. No information is available about the relationship between emergence reactions and the EEG.

Benzodiazepines
(Also See Ch. 9)

Midazolam produces dose-related EEG changes, with initial increased amplitude with predominantly θ-wave (4 to 8 Hz) activity. Increasing dose produces high-amplitude activity below 8 Hz. Burst suppression does not appear to occur, and the EEG does not appear to become isoelectric.[16–18]

Volatile Anesthetic Drugs
(Also See Ch. 30)

Isoflurane

Subanesthetic concentrations of isoflurane yield 15- to 30-Hz activity, predominantly in the frontal areas. At the minimum alveolar anesthetic concentration (MAC)

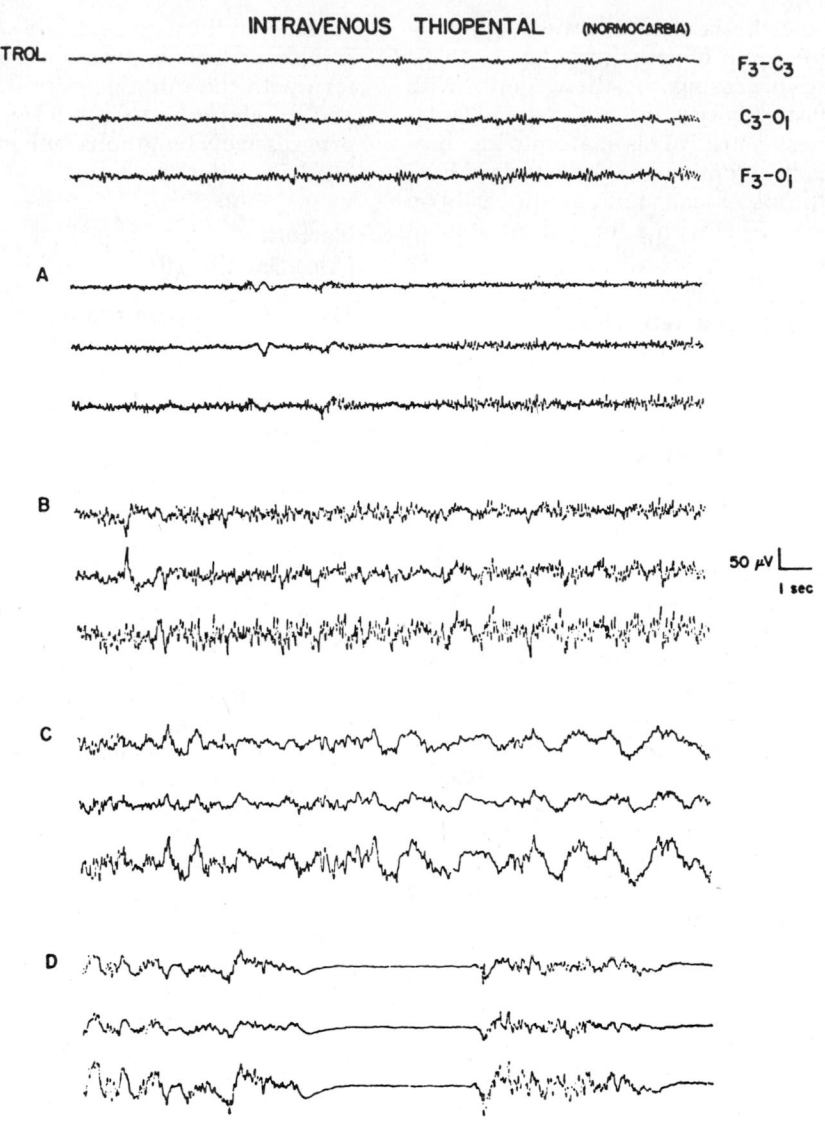

Fig. 35-4. EEG effects of intravenous administration of thiopental in humans. (**A**) Rapid activity; (**B**) barbiturate spindles; (**C**) slow waves; (**D**) burst suppression. (From Clark and Rosner,[105] with permission.)

of isoflurane (1 to 2 percent) 4- to 8-Hz waves dominate the EEG. At 1.5 MAC the waves on the EEG increase in amplitude and slow to the 1- to 4-Hz range. It is at 1.5 MAC that suppressions first appear and become longer until electrical silence commences at 2 to 2.5 MAC. At times an isolated spike wave can be seen with intersuppression activity at 1.5 to 2.0 MAC isoflurane.[19]

Enflurane

At subanesthetic concentrations, enflurane induces rapid activity in the EEG. The patient generally loses consciousness while this activity is prominent. At approximately 1 MAC (1.7 percent) large 7- to 12-Hz

waves appear. When the concentration of enflurane approaches 1.5 MAC, spikes and spike waves appear, to be followed by burst suppression. As the concentration of enflurane is increased to 2 to 3 MAC the EEG consists of groups of two or three 400- to 800-μV spike and wave discharges separated by 5 to 15 seconds of isoelectricity. Electrographic seizures can be seen with end-tidal concentrations of 3 percent enflurane with hypocapnia. Decreasing the $PaCO_2$ increases the length of suppression, decreases the duration of bursts, but increases their amplitude and main frequency components.[20] In dogs the cerebral metabolic effects of seizure activity during deep enflurane anesthesia was the same as that induced by pentylenetetrazol, a known convulsant.[21]

Halothane

At subanesthetic concentrations, halothane produces fast sinusoidal activity in the 10- to 20-Hz range. This pattern persists until loss of consciousness occurs. At 1 MAC halothane (0.84 percent) and normocarbia, the dominant frequencies in the EEG are between 10 and 15 Hz. As the concentration of halothane is increased, the EEG continues to slow. At 2 MAC and 2.5 MAC the predominant background rhythm is at 7.5 and 6 Hz, respectively. The slowing of the background rhythm continues with increasing halothane concentrations (4 to 5 Hz at 3.5 MAC) until at 4 MAC almost all activity is in the 0.5-Hz range. One must be careful to separate the direct effects of halothane on suppression of cortical electrical activity from the attenuation in cortical electrical activity that may be the result of decreased cerebral blood flow secondary to the cardiovascular depressant effects of halothane.[22]

Surgery

Cardiopulmonary Bypass
(Also See Ch. 51)

In humans there are always several circumstances that occur with the institution of cardiopulmonary bypass (CPB). For example, the level of anesthesia may be altered by CPB, alterations in arterial carbon dioxide tension and blood pressure may occur, and hemodilution with hypothermic perfusate may be used. These make it difficult to isolate the effects of CPB, brain perfusion, and anesthetic level on EEG. Profound EEG changes occur, sometimes asymmetrically, and interpretation is difficult at best. Levy has tried to distinguish the effects of hypothermia from other events occurring at the institution of bypass.[23] Assessment of anesthetic level during narcotic-based anesthesia suggests a shift to lower frequencies with production of an anesthetic state without recall.[24] Much work remains to be done in utilization of the processed EEG to provide information for clinical management of patients during CPB.

Carotid Endarterectomy
(Also See Ch. 53)

Of all of the uses of the processed EEG it seems clear that the easiest to read are those events that are linked to a known event at a specific time and are unilateral, involving a large part of the hemisphere. These are the fortunate circumstances that are present when monitoring the brain of a patient undergoing carotid endarterectomy. The primary reason to monitor the brain during carotid endarterectomy is to acquire data to use as a basis for therapeutic intervention (e.g., placement of a shunt). We may fortuitously see changes in the processed EEG when a shunt becomes kinked or displaced or when cerebral emboli occur during dissection of the plaque, during hypotension, or even after the repair should a patient suffer intracerebral hemorrhage. But

these are uncommon events. The main thrust of brain monitoring in carotid procedures is to aid in identifying the patient who needs a shunt. The concept of selective shunting is not agreed upon by all surgeons. There are those who never place a shunt and claim results that are nearly flawless. There are those who always place a shunt with similar results. If the processed EEG is not going to be utilized to provide information for selective shunting, its usefulness is drastically reduced. If the processed EEG is to be used as a guide for shunting, then it must accurately identify those patients who are made critically ischemic by temporary unilateral occlusion of their carotid system.

In an attempt to explore the effectiveness of both the equipment and the anesthesiologist in interpreting the tracings we studied the Cerebral Function Monitor (CFM) and the Lifescan during carotid occlusion for carotid endarterectomy. They are presented as representative instruments. The findings were compared to the full EEG and CBF measurements.

The CFM used in the study was a single-channel model. It has become apparent that a view of the activity of both hemispheres is important for comparison, so all manufacturers now provide at least 2 channels for bilateral use. In this study of 55 patients the full EEG changed at carotid occlusion in 11 patients.[25] The anesthesiologist saw changes in the CFM in 9 of these. The remaining 2 had subtle changes in the full EEG. In all of the 11 the regional cerebral flow was below the critical level for halothane (less than 18 ml/100 g/min). Figure 35-5 shows a typical case. It can be seen that the tracing decreases as the carotid is occluded to place the shunt and again to remove the shunt. Note that at the end of the case the anesthetic level lightens and the EEG again decreases much as it does during occlusion, except that the change is due to changing anesthetic depth rather than ischemia. This demonstrates the importance of the clinical picture in interpretation of the tracing. The tracing of the newer CFM has a somewhat different appearance.

The Lifescan is a more sophisticated device that uses aperiodic analysis of the EEG. It maps each waveform in relation to its frequency, amplitude, and time of occurrence rather than averaging a large number of waveforms over a given epoch. Fifty patients undergoing carotid endarterectomy were studied to compare the Lifescan to the full 16-channel EEG and regional cerebral blood flow measurements as indicators of cerebral ischemia.[26] Three anesthesiologists with different levels of experience with EEG interpreted the tracings without knowledge of the case. They were presented only the written trace with an indication of the point at which the carotid was clamped (Fig. 35-6). The accuracy of interpretation hinges on the false-negative result. If a false-negative finding is read the surgeon might fail to shunt an ischemic patient. A false-positive result is less of a problem because that patient is not ischemic but is given a shunt anyway.

The predictive value of the anesthesiologist's being

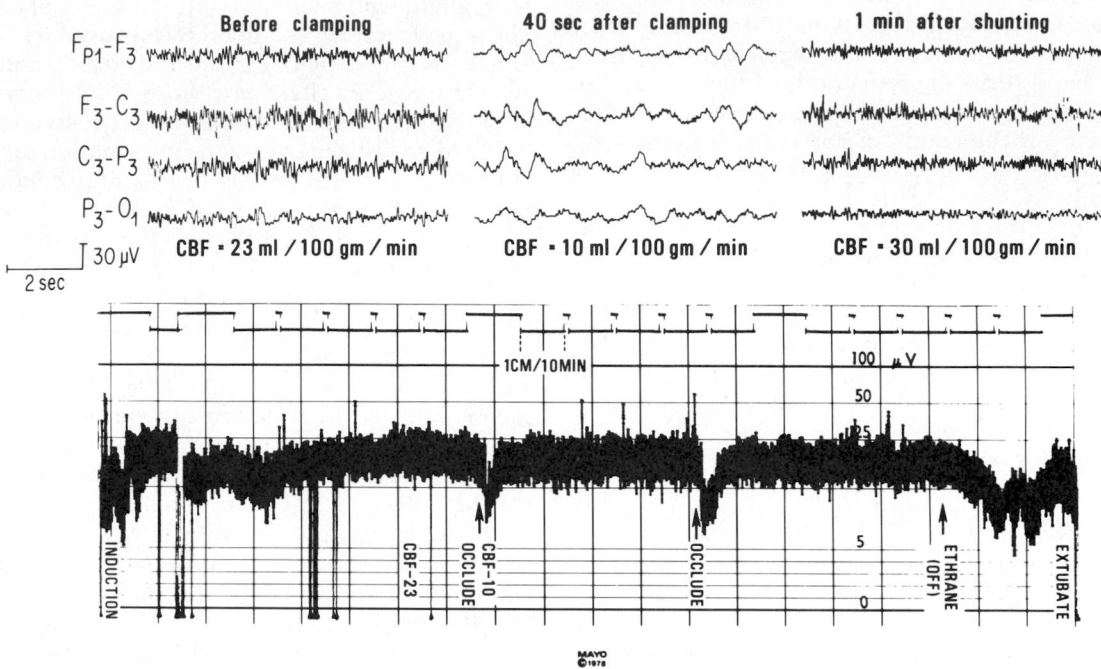

Fig. 35-5. Changes in the cerebral function monitor (an electronic filter processor device [EFP]), EEG, and CBF during carotid occlusion. (From Cucchiara et al.,[6] with permission.)

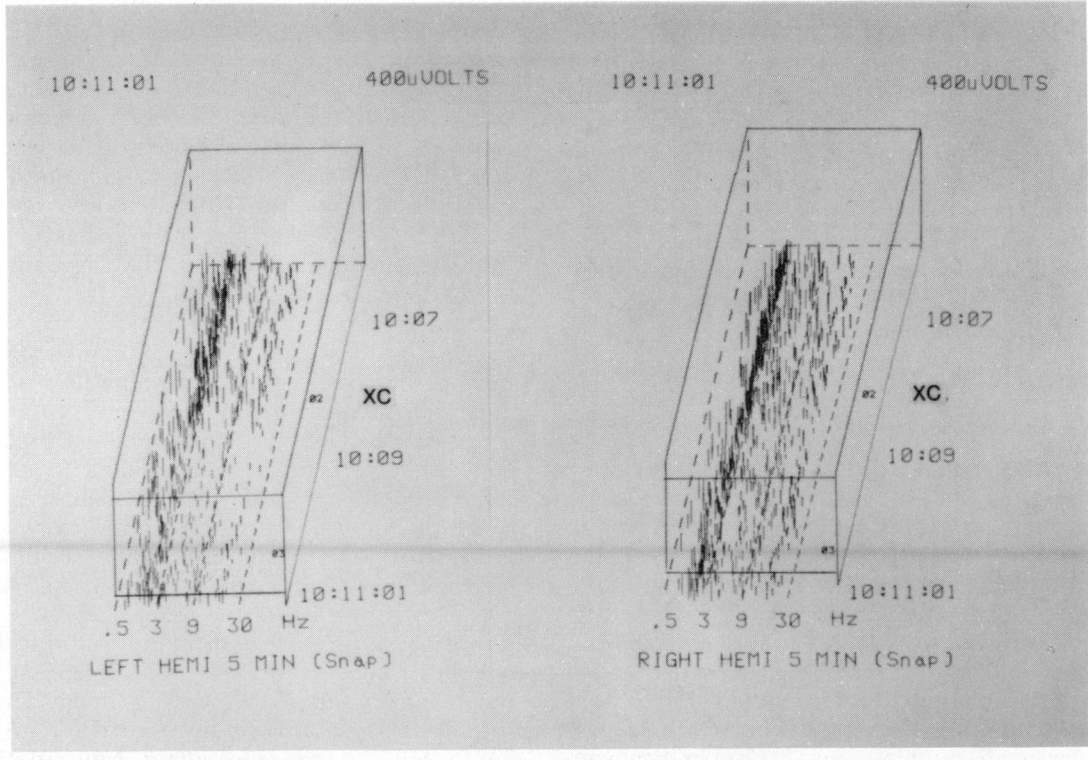

Fig. 35-6. This Lifescan printout was obtained approximately 3 minutes after occlusion *(XC)* of the left carotid artery. It shows attenuation of activity on the left with occlusion. The EEG showed a similar change. The rCBF with occlusion was 9 ml/100 g/min. (From Spackman et al.,[26] with permission.)

correct in interpreting the trace as unchanged after clamping was 91 to 98 percent. This indicates that the device can be used by relatively novice interpreters with fair accuracy to determine the presence of cerebral ischemia at the time of carotid occlusion.

Surgery for Epileptic Foci

It has long been recognized that seizures can begin with a focus of electrical synchrony that spreads to include the remainder of the cortex. Localization of such a focus at the operating table is an important part of present-day surgery for drug-resistant seizures. This localization is performed by provocation during general anesthesia with recording electrodes on or in the brain. The anesthetic level is minimized, and a provocative technique such as hyperventilation, small-dose barbiturate administration, or addition of enflurane, can be employed to trigger the focus so as to aid on its localization. If the cortex is excessively depressed pharmacologically seizure activity cannot be provoked.

Pathophysiologic Effects on the EEG

Hypoxia

"Slowing" of the EEG during hypoxia is a nonspecific global effect. Fast frequencies are lost and low frequencies dominate. Eventually the EEG is abolished as cerebral metabolic activity is severely reduced, depending upon the severity of the hypoxic event.

Hypotension

Significant levels of hypotension seem to be needed to cause the earliest of central nervous system (CNS) signs, as measured by discrimination tests such as the flicker-fusion test. This test examines the flicker rate at which the observer perceives the light to be continuous. In the early days of deliberate hypotension this test was part of the preoperative evaluation to judge how far the pressure could be reduced for operation. Clear signs of confusion and inability to concentrate or respond properly to simple commands must represent very low levels of cerebral perfusion when due to hypotension because the cerebral vasculature is maximally dilated at that time. The EEG changes associated with even this level of hypotension are not dramatic, although they are clear by comparison with a previously active recording. Herein lies the problem with using the processed EEG to determine whether the level of hypotension has resulted in brain ischemia. The changes on processed EEG are not very pronounced and are bilateral. Such changes can be detected, but when the hypotension is induced slowly the changes are gradual and harder to read. Changes associated with acute hypotension as caused by sudden arrhythmia are easier to read. A tracing of the effect of hypotension on the CSA is shown in Figure 35-7.[13] In our opinion EEG changes due to hypotension really do

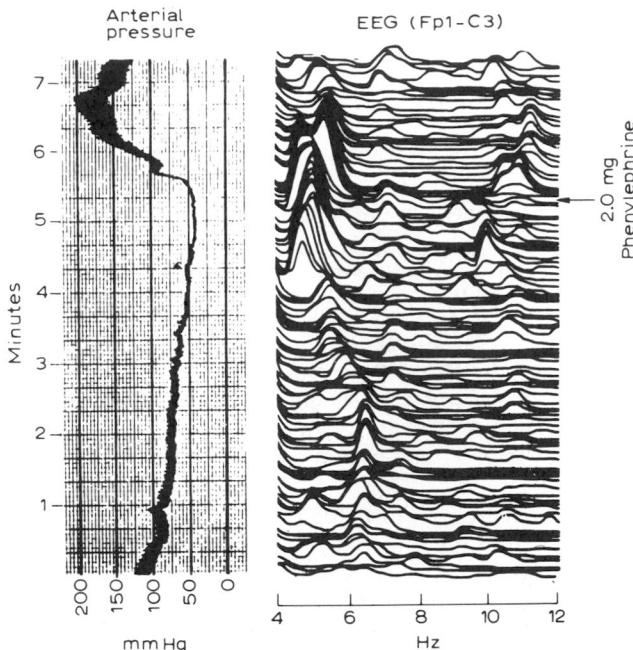

Fig. 35-7. Changes in the compressed spectral array during hypotension. (From Stockard and Bickford,[13] with permission.)

represent cerebral ischemia of a significant degree and should be considered an important finding.

Hypothermia

During cooling on CPB the total power and peak power frequency of the high-frequency band were highly correlated with temperature using Fourier analysis and spectral edge data. However, there was significant variability between subjects, especially during cooling.[23]

Hypercarbia and Hypocarbia

Hyperventilation is known to activate excitable seizure foci. Hypoventilation with accumulation of carbon dioxide has subtle effects similar to increasing the end-tidal tension of the volatile anesthetics.[27]

Untoward Events

One of the suggested reasons for monitoring the brain is to enable us to detect "untoward events" during anesthesia. This suggests that there are CNS insults that, if detected early, could be rapidly reversed or treated to prevent permanent injury. We have already considered hypoxia, hypotension, and cerebral ischemia due to carotid artery occlusion. What "untoward event" may have occurred when a patient awakens from general anesthesia with an unexpected neurologic deficit? Most such problems are due to peripheral nerve injuries and with a sufficiently detailed neurologic examination can be identified as such. It is unlikely that any routine

TABLE 35-2. Criteria for Determination of Brain Death

1. Absent cerebral and brain stem function

2. Well-defined irreversible etiology

3. Persistent absence of all brain function after observation and/or treatment

4. Hypothermia, drug intoxication, metabolic encephalopathy, and shock excluded

(From Darby et al.,[30] with permission.)

TABLE 35-3. Clinical Tests of Brain Death

Cerebral unresponsiveness

No spontaneous motor activity

Absent pupillary, corneal, and oculocephalic/oculovestibular reflexes

Absent cough reflex with deep tracheal suctioning

No increase in heart rate in response to intravenous administration of atropine (2 mg)

No respiratory efforts on apnea testing ($PaCO_2 > 60$ mmHg)

Electrocerebral silence documented by electroencephalography (desirable)

(From Darby et al.,[30] with permission.)

brain monitor is going to help us identify such injuries. Although somatosensory evoked potentials measured from the distribution of the nerve at risk might very well do so, this level of monitoring is not routine and would probably be used only when one expects a nerve injury to occur.

We had an opportunity to describe three patients who demonstrated an unexpected focal neurologic deficit on emergence from anesthesia.[28] On the basis of what we know about the processed EEG let us speculate on whether it would have been useful in these cases. An older man with chronic atrial fibrillation underwent percutaneous ultrasonic lithotripsy under enflurane anesthesia. He awakened slowly and was found to have right hemiplegia and aphasia. The diagnosis was thromboembolism of cardiac origin to the distribution of the middle cerebral artery. This intraoperative event probably would have been detected on the processed EEG because it would have been acute and unilateral. On the other hand, there was little in the way of definitive treatment for this problem so the value of making the diagnosis is reduced. Another patient was a middle-aged woman undergoing vaginal hysterectomy under enflurane anesthesia. She was lethargic in the recovery room for some time before it was realized that she was hemiplegic. She had suffered an intracerebral bleed intraoperatively. Again the processed EEG would be expected to show a fairly definitive picture in this kind of case because the changes would be hemispheric and rather acute. That information might have raised the level of suspicion and led to earlier diagnosis. Treatment consisted of evacuation of the hematoma. The sooner this therapy could be implemented the better the result expected. Perhaps this patient's residual deficit would have been reduced if such monitoring had been used. Finally, a young woman was undergoing laparoscopic tubal ligation under enflurane anesthesia. During the procedure she had multifocal ventricular ectopy and elevated airway pressures. She entered the recovery room unusually lethargic and hemiplegia was noted shortly thereafter. She probably sustained paradoxical carbon dioxide embolism to her coronary and cerebral circulation. This type of global cerebral event probably would not be evident on the processed EEG because even though it is acute, the changes would have to be very dramatic to be noticed since they would be bilateral. These cases occurred in a surgical case load of nearly 60,000 general anesthetics. The routine use of

the processed EEG thus could have been expected to contribute rarely to the overall care of this patient group. It is for the reader to decide whether this information applies to his or her practice.

Brain Death

The clinical diagnosis of brain death is made when there is demonstration of the absence of all cerebral and brain stem function (Table 35-2). Various clinical tests have been devised to diagnose brain death (Table 35-3). Apnea testing is accepted as an essential component of the evaluation. However, electrocerebral silence on the EEG, when not confounded by the presence of high-dose barbiturates, metabolic encephalopathy, or very young age, supports the diagnosis of brain death.[29,30]

INTRAOPERATIVE MONITORING OF SENSORY EVOKED POTENTIALS

Intraoperative monitoring of sensory evoked potentials (SEPs) has gained increasing popularity over the last several years because it provides the ability to monitor the functional integrity of sensory pathways in the anesthetized patient undergoing surgical procedures placing these pathways at risk. Evoked potentials are electrical manifestations of the central nervous system's response to external stimuli. Sensory evoked potentials are recorded by stimulating a peripheral sensory nerve and recording the resulting electrical potential at various sites along the sensory pathway to the cerebral cortex. Because of the very low amplitude of evoked potential (0.1 to 20 μV) it is not possible to distinguish them from background brain-wave activity and artifacts in the routine electroencephalogram. To extract the evoked potential from the background EEG activity, computer signal averaging or summation is utilized. With this technique the electrical activity both evoked and spontaneous after a repetitive sensory stimulus is averaged. The sensory evoked potential occurs at a constant time after the sensory stimulus; the spontaneous brain activity (the EEG) occurs at random intervals after the sensory stimulus. The sum of the nonrandom evoked response (SEP) increases directly with the number of responses added. The sum of the random EEG activity increases by the square root of the number of samples obtained. The averaged response of two electrical activities, SEP and spontaneous EEG, increases at different rates and the SEP is revealed above the spontaneous electrical activity of the brain.[31] The resolution of the evoked potentials increases as the square root of the responses recorded.

Sensory evoked potentials are of two general types determined by the distance of the recording electrode from the neural generator of the evoked response. Evoked potentials recorded from electrodes close to the neural generators (within approximately 3 to 4 cm in the average adult) are termed near field potentials.[32] Near field potentials are transmitted to the recording electrode by propagated conduction along a discrete length of nerve,[33] and the morphology is directly affected by electrode locations.[32] Far field potentials are recorded from electrodes located a greater distance from the neural generator and are conducted to the recording electrode through a volume conductor (brain, cerebrospinal fluid, and membranes). As a result it is more difficult to locate the source of the active tissue (the current spreads diffusely throughout the conducting medium) and the electrode position has little effect on the morphology of the recorded evoked potential.[32,33] As the distance between the recording electrode and the neural generator increases, the recorded SEP becomes smaller and slower. More signals have to be averaged to record far field potentials (up to several thousand) than near field potentials (as few as 50 to 100).[32,33] Evoked potentials are also defined as cortical or subcortical (which arise from the spinal cord and brain stem). With evoked potentials recorded from scalp electrodes (standard 10–20 system for EEG) cortical evoked responses are near field potentials and brain stem responses are far field potentials.

In evaluating evoked potentials the latency and amplitude of the generated waveforms are measured. Deflections below the baseline are labeled positive (P) and those above the baseline negative (N). Standard identification of waveforms is by letter designating the direction of the deflection followed by a number representing the latency of that waveform (e.g., N14). Because amplitude and latency change with recording circumstances normal values must be established for each lab and differ somewhat from values recorded in other labs. Sensory evoked potentials utilized for diagnostic evaluation of patients with suspected neurologic abnormalities as well as those monitored intraoperatively are somatosensory evoked potentials (SSEPs), brainstem auditory evoked potentials (BAEPs), and visual evoked potentials (VEPs). For all these modalities recording electrodes are placed on the scalp, using the International 10–20 system as for recording the standard EEG.

Intraoperative changes in evoked potentials, such as decreased amplitude, increased latency, or complete loss of the waveform, are considered to be indications of surgical trespass or ischemia. When these changes are detected and considered to be significant the anesthesiologist and/or surgeon can make changes to relieve or lessen the insult to the monitored pathway. Interventions by the anesthesiologist are directed at improving perfusion to the nervous tissue at risk and include increasing arterial blood pressure, especially if induced hypotension is being used or the patient's pressure has fallen to below the preoperative level; transfusion if significant anemia is present; volume expansion; and normalization of arterial blood gas tensions if indicated. Alterations in evoked potentials may, for example, warn the surgeon of excessive retractor pressure or surgical dissection in the vicinity of otherwise undetected cranial or peripheral nerves or correction of scoliosis to a degree that is compromising blood supply to the cord. Appropriate changes in the operative procedure may result in avoidance or lessening of postoperative neurologic dysfunction. Tolerance limits for degree of change in evoked potentials or duration of complete loss of waveform before permanent neurologic dysfunction occurs are unknown.

SSEPs are recorded after stimulation of a peripheral sensory nerve usually with electrical stimulation via a surface electrode on the skin or fine needle electrodes. A square wave stimulus of 0.2- to 2-millisecond duration is delivered to the peripheral nerve and the intensity is adjusted to produce a minimal muscle contraction. Increasing the stimulus intensity beyond the sum of the motor and sensory threshold does not influence the amplitude or latency of the recorded evoked potential.[34] Rate of stimulation varies from 1 to 2 Hz.[32] The common sites of stimulation include median nerve at the wrist, common peroneal nerve at the knee, and posterior tibial nerve at the ankle.[34] The tongue, trigeminal nerve, and pudendal nerve have also been studied.[34]

SSEPs consist of both short- and long-latency evoked potentials. The short-latency SSEPs are the ones most commonly studied intraoperatively because they are less influenced by factors that may vary during the perioperative period such as anesthetic depth. The pathways involved in the generation of short-latency SSEPs include large-fiber sensory nerves with their cell bodies in the dorsal root ganglia and central processes traveling rostrally in the ipsilateral posterior column of the spinal cord synapsing in the dorsal column nuclei at the cervicomedullary junction (first-order fibers), second-order fibers crossing and traveling to the contralateral thalamus via the medial lemniscus, and third-order fibers from the thalamus to the frontoparietal sensorimotor cortex.[34] Primary cortical evoked responses result from the earliest electrical activity generated by the cortical neurons and are thought to arise from the postcentral sulcus parietal neurons. The secondary cortical potentials (longer-latency) are thought to arise in the association cortex, are less stable, have greater variability of waveform than primary cortical responses,[33] and habituate rapidly on repetitive stimulation.[32] Nonspecific cortical responses occur widely across the frontal and temporal cortex regardless of the sensory stimulation, show marked habituation with repetitive stimulation, but are enhanced when the stimulation is meaningful or when the subject concentrates.[32] Cortical evoked potentials other than the primary cortical response are not recorded intraoperatively because they are severely altered by general anesthesia or extremely difficult to record in the operating room environment.[32]

For recording SSEPs after upper limb stimulation, recording electrodes are placed at Erb's point above the clavicle overlying the brachial plexus, at the posterior midline of the neck at the second cervical vertebra (over the gracile and cuneate nuclei), and on the scalp overlying the sensory (parietal) cortex contralateral to the stimulated limb. For recording evoked potentials after lower limb stimulation electrodes are placed over the lower lumbar spine.[34] Intraoperatively cortical SSEPs may also be recorded from electrodes placed directly on the cerebral cortex and subcortical potentials with electrodes placed invasively into bone, ligament, or the epidural space in the operative site.[32] Proported generators for short-latency SSEPs are listed in Table 35-4, and Figure 35-8.[32,34] After lower limb stimulation absolute latencies are increased because of the greater distance the stimulation must travel along the peripheral sensory nerve. The first cortical response occurs at approximately 27 milliseconds after stimulation. Interpeak latencies are also evaluated to assess specific conduction times such as N9 to N14 conduction time reflecting transmission in the proximal brachial plexus, the cervical roots, and the dorsal columns; the N14 to N19 conduction represents pure central conduction time between the dorsal column nuclei and the primary sensory cortex.[35]

Intraoperative recording of SSEPs has been used to assess the functional integrity of the sensory pathways during operative procedures that place these pathways at risk as a result of surgical trespass either along the course of the peripheral nerve, within the spinal canal, or in the brain or when there is potential for compromise of the vascular supply to the sensory pathways. SSEP monitoring has also been used to assess the integ-

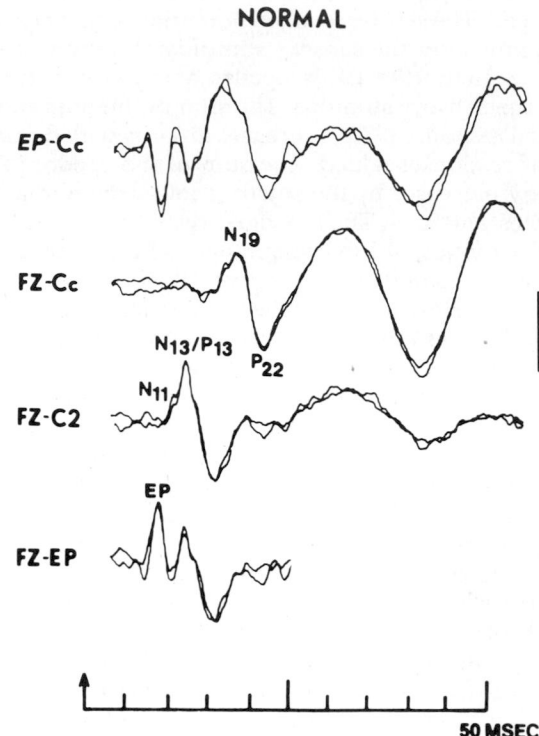

NORMAL

50 MSEC

Fig. 35-8. Short-latency somatosensory evoked potentials produced by stimulation of the median nerve at the wrist. (From Chiappa and Ropper,[34] with permission.)

rity of adjacent structures that are more difficult to monitor directly, such as the motor tracts. Intraoperative SSEP monitoring has been described for a wide variety of procedures, including correction of scoliosis with Harrington rod instrumentation[36,37]; spinal cord decompression and stabilization after acute spinal cord injury[38,39]; spinal fusion[40]; brachial plexus exploration after injury to the plexus[41]; resection of spinal cord tumor, cyst, or vascular lesion[42]; correction of cervical spondylosis[42]; resection of fourth ventricular cyst;[42] release of a tethered cord[42]; resection of acoustic neuroma[42]; resection of intracranial vascular lesions involving the sensory cortex[42]; resection of thalamic tumor[43]; surgical correction after thoracic spine fracture[44]; and abdominal and thoracic aortic aneurysm repair.[32] Intraoperative monitoring of SSEPs has been used most extensively in patients undergoing surgical procedures involving the spinal column and/or spinal cord. Extensive experience has been gained in patients having decompressive laminectomies or undergoing corrective procedures for scolosis such as Harrington rod placement. Intraoperative changes in SSEPs have been noted in 2.5 to 65 percent of patients undergoing surgical procedures on the spine or spinal cord.[37,40,44,45] When these changes reversed either spontaneously or with interventions by the surgeon or anesthesiologist such as lessening the degree of spine straightening in scolosis surgery or increasing arterial blood pressure,

TABLE 35-4. Generators of SSEPs after Median Nerve Stimulation

Peak	Generator
N9 (EP)	Brachial plexus
N11	Posterior columns or spinal roots
N13/P13	Dorsal column nuclei
N14,15	Brain stem and/or thalamus
N19/P22	Parietal sensory cortex

Abbreviation: SSEPs, somatosensory evoked potentials.

the patients most often have preserved neurologic function postoperatively. However, when these changes persisted, the patients most often awakened with worsened neurologic deficit. Both false-negative and false-positive results have been reported with SSEP monitoring during spine surgery. Patients with intact SSEPs throughout the procedure have awakened with a new significant neurologic deficit. On the other hand, patients with significant changes in intraoperative SSEPs have suffered no change in neurologic function postoperatively.[45] Overall the reliability of adequate SSEP monitoring to predict the postoperative somatic sensory function has been reported to be excellent.[32,42,44] However, because the motor tracts are not monitored and the blood supply to the dorsal columns of the somatosensory tracts monitored is primarily from the posterior spinal arteries and that to the motor tracts is primarily from the anterior spinal artery, it is possible for a significant motor deficit to develop postoperatively in patients with intact SSEPs throughout the operative course. Indeed such events have been reported.[38,46] In operations on the spine and after acute spinal cord injury the sensory and motor changes usually follow closely.[32] However, in patients suffering neurologic dysfunction after abdominal aortic aneurysm repair, frequently proprioception is intact when motor and other sensory functions are impaired. This occurred in 32 percent of patients with neurologic injury after aortic aneurysm repair in one series.[47] Clearly intraoperative SSEP monitoring in these patients carries a significant risk for false-negative results. In addition, significant difficulties in intraoperative recording of SSEPs have been reported. Technically inadequate intraoperative SSEP recordings are reported to occur in 0 to 41 percent of patients monitored.[42-44,48] These difficulties arise from the electrically hostile environment of the operating room, a high incidence of artifact, abnormal preoperative SSEPs in patients with abnormal neurologic function, inaccessible electrodes during the operative procedure, and sensitivity of the evoked potential, especially the cortical components, to factors that may fluctuate in the intraoperative period, such as temperature, blood gas tensions, anesthetic depth, and blood pressure. Indeed, one author found the SSEPs to be the most difficult of sensory evoked potentials to monitor intraoperatively.[44]

Evaluation of central conduction time during SSEP monitoring has also been used in acute settings other than the perioperative period. Prolongation of central conduction in comatose patients has been associated with a worse long-term prognosis.[49] Prolongation of central conduction time in patients after subarachnoid hemorrhage is associated with transient neurologic deficits and precedes the development of these deficits. The changes in central conduction time are likely related to cerebral ischemia.[50]

Brain stem auditory evoked potentials (BAEPs) are recorded by delivering clicks repeatedly to one ear. Stimulus intensity is usually set at 60 to 70 dB above the patient's click-hearing threshold. The duration of the click is approximately 100 microseconds and the frequency 10 Hz. Use of different click polarity (the direction of the initial movement of the tympanic membrane) to cause either rarefaction or condensation produces different waveforms, amplitudes, and latencies. BAEP may be recorded with one or the other click polarity, but not usually both. Intraoperatively clicks of alternating polarity may be used to decrease stimulus artifact, but the waveforms produced are an average of those produced by either one alone. Rate and intensity of stimulus delivery affect the BAEP.[32,51] Monaural stimulation is used because responses from a normal ear obscure any abnormal responses from the other ear. The stimuli are delivered by acoustically shielded headphones when not used in the operation room. Intraoperatively inserted earphones on molded earpieces are used. Although they admit more extraneous noise, they do not interfere with access to the surgical field and are preferable for intraoperative monitoring.[32,51] Recording electrodes are placed on the lobe of the stimulated ear and on the top of the head (vertex).[51] White noise is delivered to the contralateral ear. Five hundred to 2,000 repetitions are required on average because BAEPs recorded from the scalp are far field potentials.[32,51]

Peaks in recordings of BAEP are labeled I through VII and the purported neural generators for these peaks are listed in Table 35-5 (Fig. 35-9). As with SSEP, amplitude, absolute latencies, and interpeak latencies are evaluated to assess integrity of the auditory system, localize the functional defect, and assess peripheral and central conduction times. Because waves VI and VII are inconsistent they are not routinely studied,[51] and most papers reporting use of BAEP in the operating room use waves up to wave V.[52-54]

TABLE 35-5. Correlation between Various BAEPs with Area from Which These Potentials are Generated

Wave	Generator
I	Nerve VII contiguous with the spinal ganglia in the mastoid bone
II	Intracranial acoustic nerve and/or cochlear nucleus (low pons)
III	Superior olive (low pons)
IV	Lateral lemniscus (middle pons)
V	Inferior colliculus (midbrain)
VI	Medial geniculate (thalamus)
VII	Thalamocortical radiations

Abbreviation: BAEPs, brain stem auditory evoked potentials.

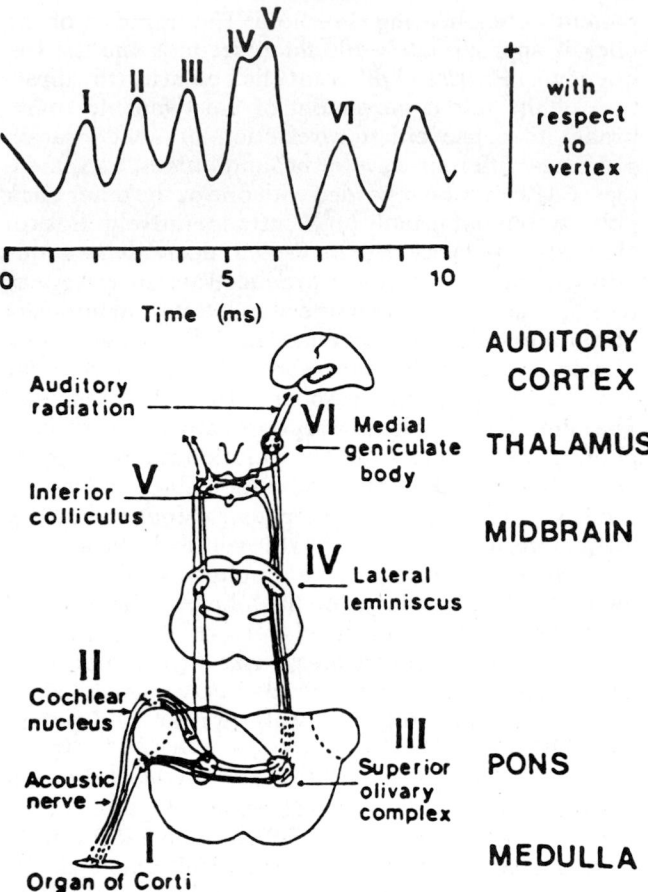

Fig. 35-9. *(Top)* Brain stem auditory evoked response. *(Bottom)* Different levels of the auditory pathway. Roman numerals indicate sites of origin of the brain stem waves. (From Maurer et al.,[106] with permission.)

BAEPs have been monitored intraoperatively during procedures involving or near the auditory pathway as well as in posterior fossa procedures when brain stem function might be compromised. Cases in which BAEPs are commonly monitored include microvascular decompression of cranial nerves (especially V and VII), resection of acoustic neuroma, posterior fossa exploration for vascular or neoplastic lesions, clipping of basilar artery aneurysm, and section of nerve VIII for intractable tinnitus.[42,52,53] During microvascular decompression of the facial nerve in patients with hemifacial spasm, hearing loss has been reported in 15 percent of cases, and this incidence can be greatly decreased with BAEP monitoring.[55,56] Intraoperative changes noted included transient or permanent latency increases on the operative side, obliteration of waveform distal to the operative site that was either transient or permanent, and, rarely, obliteration of BAEP contralateral to the operative side.[43,44,52,53] These changes were associated with a variety of perioperative events, including section of nerve VIII (deliberate or unintentional); retraction on nerve VIII, cerebellum, or brain stem; operative manipulation of nerve VIII; hypotension and hypocarbia; drilling around the internal auditory canal; irrigation of nerve VIII; severe cerebellar edema; and positioning of the head for retromastoid craniotomy[43,52,53] (see Table 35-6). Patients with transient or persistent increases in latency and/or decreases in amplitude can be expected to have unchanged or only slight worsening of hearing postoperatively. Patients with complete but reversible loss of BAEP will also have unchanged or mild worsening of hearing postoperatively. Patients with complete irreversible loss of BAEP will most likely have complete or near complete loss of hearing in the ipsilateral ear postoperatively.[42–44,53] One series had a single false-positive result. One patient had complete loss of BAEP with intact hearing postoperatively.[43] False-negative results are extremely rare. In one series BAEPs were monitored in a patient undergoing resection of a meningioma in the lateral ventricle and were unchanged intraoperatively and postoperatively. However, this patient did not regain consciousness postoperatively.[44] This case illustrates the lack of cortical function monitoring with intraoperative monitoring of BAEP through wave V. BAEPs are considered the easiest of the sensory evoked potentials to monitor intraoperatively and are least sensitive to changes in perioperative variables. Ability to record technically adequate BAEP has been reported in 90 to 100 percent of cases in which monitoring was attempted.[42,43,52,53] Preoperative deafness on the operative side eliminates the possibility of recording intraoperative BAEPs. Preservation of BAEP intraoperatively indicates preserved hearing postoperatively and persistent changes indicate significant risk for injury.

TABLE 35-6. Correlation between BAEP Changes and Associated Clinical Events

BAEP Change	Associated Events
Transient latency increase	Drilling, irrigation, retraction, surgical irritation, hypocarbia and hypotension, positioning
Persistent latency increases	Retraction or pressure on auditory tract
Transient loss of EP	Retraction, pressure, surgical distention
Permanent loss of ipsilateral EP	Surgical interruption of auditory pathway
Loss of contralateral EP	Cerebellar edema

Abbreviations: BAEP, brain stem auditory evoked potential; EP, evoked potential.

Visual evoked potentials (VEPs) are recorded after monocular stimulation with recording electrodes over the occipital, parietal, and central scalp.[51] Shift reversal of a checkerboard pattern with constant luminance is the preferred stimulus because the generated evoked potentials have a narrower range of normal variation and are more sensitive to conduction defects. However, it is currently not possible to deliver this type of stimulation intraoperatively. Instead flash stimulation with a change in luminance is utilized. The stimuli are produced by light-emitting diodes placed in a goggle over a closed lid. The flash rate is 1 to 3 Hz with a duration of 3 to 5 milliseconds. The sample time is 250 to 500 milliseconds, and 64 to 128 samples are averaged per recording.[32,43,44,51] For some operative procedures, such as operations on the anterior cranial fossa, the goggles interfere with approach to the operative field. Light-emitting diodes mounted on a contact lens have been used in these situations.[42] VEPs are cortical evoked potentials, which vary with the type of stimulus, part of the retina stimulated, degree of pupil dilation, and patient's attention level.[32] Two positive peaks at approximately 100 and 200 milliseconds are observed[32] (Fig. 35-10).

Intraoperative VEP monitoring has been advocated for procedures placing the visual system at risk, especially for those in the area of the optic chiasm. Procedures in which VEP monitoring has been used include resection of pituitary tumors, craniopharyngioma, optic glioma, orbital pseudotumor, occipital arteriovenous malformation, meningioma impinging on the optic chiasm, chondrosarcoma of the sphenoid wing, drainage of pituitary abscess, clipping of internal carotid artery and basilar artery aneurysms, surgical correction of CSF rhinorrhea, and treatment of orbital fracture.[42-44] Changes in evoked potential latency and amplitude were used to guide operative manipulations or to indicate adequate systemic blood pressure in patients in whom induced hypotension was being used.[32,44] Satisfactory intraoperative recordings can be recorded in 88 to 100 percent of patients.[42-44] However, intraoperative variability unrelated to changes in neu-

rologic function may be as high as 68 to 81 percent.[43,44] In addition, in one large series there was a relatively high incidence of both false-positive and false-negative results. Thirteen percent of patients with intraoperative loss of VEPs had unchanged vision postoperatively, and 7 percent had intact VEPs with significant visual defects.[44] VEPs are sensitive to a number of factors that cannot be controlled intraoperatively, such as luminance, since the flash must pass through the closed eyelid; pupil size and direction; and attention to the stimulus. In addition, improved systems to deliver the stimulus intraoperatively have to be developed.[44] In the opinion of the author of one of the largest series of patients studied with intraoperative VEP monitoring with current techniques, VEPs cannot be reliably interpreted intraoperatively.[44] VEPs have enjoyed the least popularity of all forms of intraoperative evoked potential monitoring.

Pharmacologic Factors Influencing Sensory Evoked Potentials

There are multiple drugs used in the perioperative period that can influence the intraoperative monitoring of SEPs (Table 35-7). Different classes of drugs have differing effects. In addition, the sensitivity of evoked responses to drug effects varies with the sensory modality monitored. In general, VEPs are the most sensitive and BAEPs the most resistant to drug effects. In addition, early waves (brain stem) are less affected by drugs than late potentials (cortical).

The volatile anesthetics isoflurane, enflurane, and halothane have similar effects in differing degrees on the SEPs. As with most drugs, VEPs are the most sensitive to the effects of volatile anesthetics and the BAEPs are the most resistant to anesthetic-induced changes. The spinal and subcortical waves are less affected than the cortical potentials.[57,59]

The effects of the currently used volatile agents on SSEPs are dose-dependent increases in latency and conduction times and decrease in amplitude.[57-61] The relative effects of different volatile agents on SSEPs are somewhat controversial: some evidence suggests that halothane has a greater impact on SSEPs than either isoflurane or enflurane[59]; other evidence supports a greater effect by enflurane and isoflurane than halothane.[57] Up to 0.5 to 1 MAC isoflurane in the presence of nitrous oxide is compatible with adequate monitoring of cortical SSEPs (Fig. 35-11).[57-61] Preservation of the ability to monitor cortical SSEPs has been reported with similar levels (0.5 to 1 MAC) of both halothane and enflurane in nitrous oxide (Figs. 35-12 and 35-13).[57,59]

The volatile anesthetics result in increases in latency of BAEPs without affecting the amplitude.[61-64] However, volatile anesthetics cause both increases in latency and decreases in amplitude in the early cortical responses after auditory stimulation.[63] Adequate monitoring of BAEPs is possible with the volatile agents in

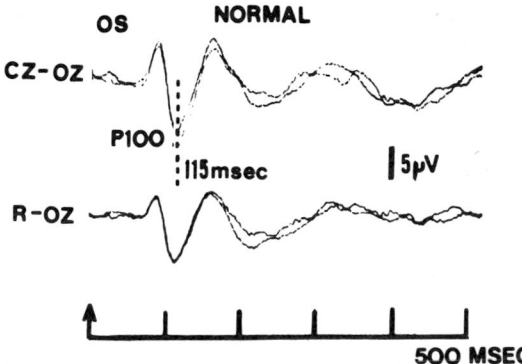

Fig. 35-10. Pattern-shift visual evoked potentials. (From Chiappa and Ropper,[51] with permission.)

TABLE 35-7. Drug Effects on Sensory Evoked Potentials

Drug	SSEPs		BAEPs		VEPs	
	LAT	AMP	LAT	AMP	LAT	AMP
Isoflurane	↑	↓	↑	0	↑	↓
Enflurane	↑	↓	↑	0	↑	↓
Halothane	↑	↓	↑	0	↑	0
Nitrous oxide	0	↓	0	0	↑	↓
Barbiturates	↑	↓	↑	0		
Etomidate	↑	↑	↑	↓		
Droperidol	↑	↓				
Diazepam	↑	↓	0	0		
Midazolam	0	↓				
Fentanyl	↑	↓	0	0		
Morphine	↑	↓				
Meperidine	↑	↑/↓				

Abbreviations: SSEPs, somatosensory evoked potentials; BAEPs, brain stem auditory evoked potentials; VEPs, visual evoked potentials; LAT, latency; AMP, amplitude.

concentrations up to and exceeding 1 MAC (with and without nitrous oxide) (Figs. 35-14 and 35-15).[61-65]

Use of the volatile agents during monitoring of VEPs results in dose-dependent increases in latency with or without changes in amplitude.[61,66-69] Isoflurane results in dose-dependent increases in latency and decreases in amplitude up to 1.8 percent in 100 percent oxygen, at which time the waveform is lost.[61,66] Enflurane in the absence of hypocarbia also leads to decrease in amplitude.[69] Halothane causes increases in latency without changes in amplitude (Fig. 35-16).[67,68]

Although the volatile anesthetics cause significant changes in the waveforms of sensory evoked potential, it is possible to provide adequate monitoring intraoperatively in the presence of a volatile agent. Doses of agents causing obliteration of the response to be monitored must be prevented. Equally important, anesthetic concentration should not be changed during the critical periods of intraoperative monitoring, those in which surgical interventions are most likely to result in damage to neurologic tissue and changes in the SEPs. Because the volatile anesthetic-induced changes in SEPs are dose-dependent, increasing anesthetic depth at a crucial point in the operative procedure can result in confusing changes in the SEPs that may be due to either the anesthetic or the surgical procedure. The appropriate intervention is then difficult to determine.

As with the volatile anesthetics, nitrous oxide causes differing effects on the SEPs depending on the sensory system monitored. It causes decreases in amplitude without changes in latency in SSEPs when used alone or when added to a narcotic based or volatile anesthetic.[57,58,70] Addition of 50 percent nitrous oxide to a fentanyl-based anesthetic results in greater decreases in amplitude than administration of up to 1 percent isoflurane or enflurane, especially in patients with abnormal preoperative SSEPs.[58] The addition of nitrous oxide to a maintenance volatile anesthetic during the

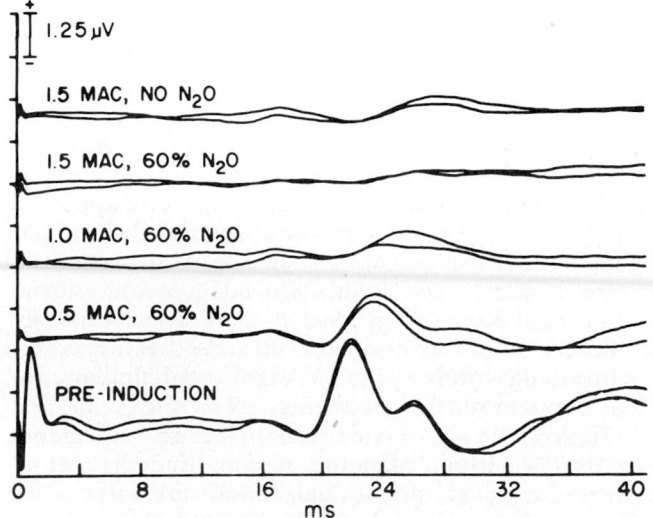

Fig. 35-11. Representative SSEP cortical responses (C-3, C-4-FPz) at various MAC levels of isoflurane. (From Peterson et al.,[57] with permission.)

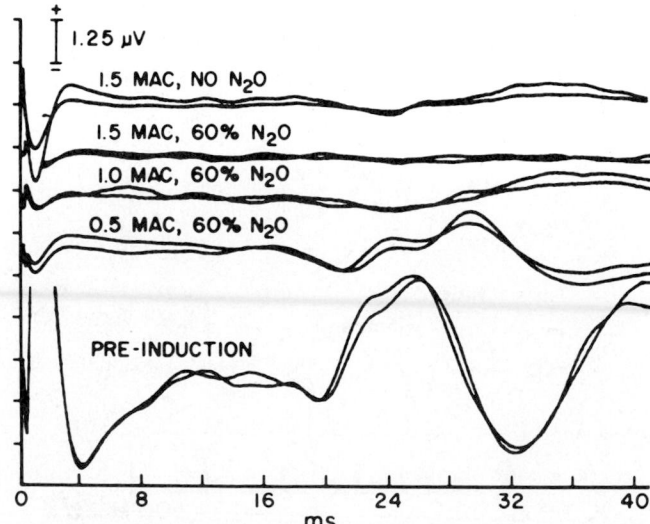

Fig. 35-12. Representative SSEP cortical responses (C-3, or C-4-FPz) at various MAC levels of enflurane. (From Peterson et al.,[57] with permission.)

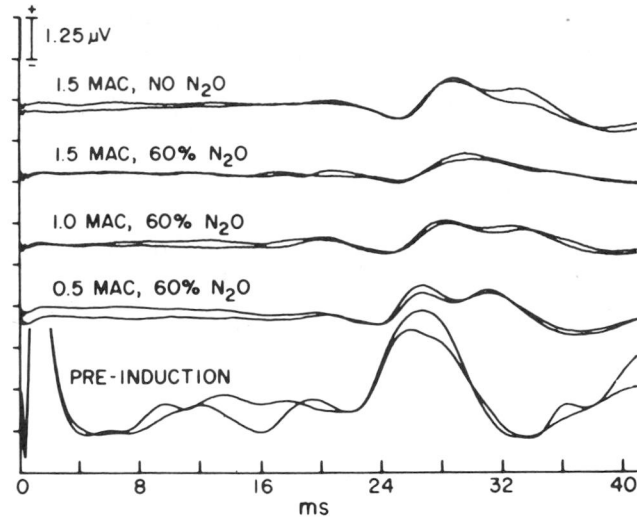

Fig. 35-13. Representative SSEP cortical responses (C-3, C-4-FPz) at various MAC levels of halothane. (From Peterson et al.,[57] with permission.)

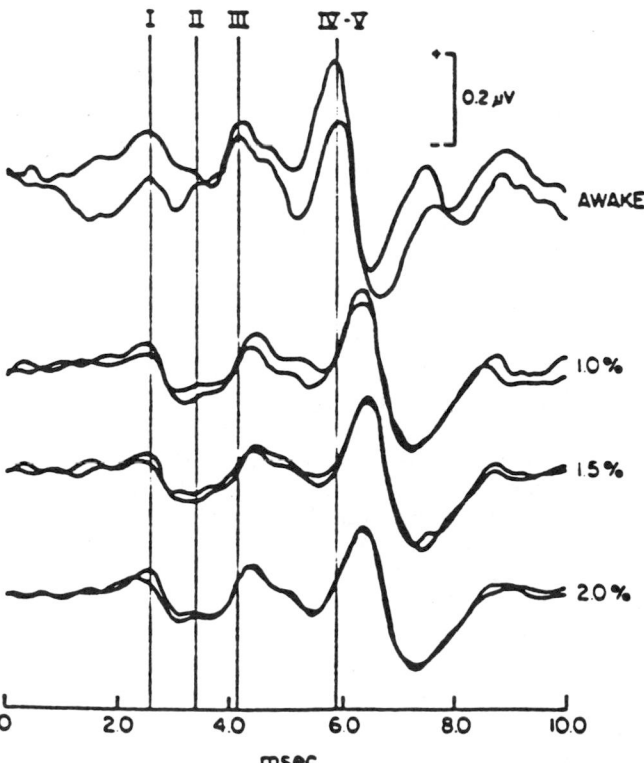

Fig. 35-14. Influence of isoflurane alone on BAEP in a typical subject. Latency of peaks III and IV to V increased at 1.0 percent but plateaued with increasing anesthetic depth. (From Manninen et al.,[62] with permission.)

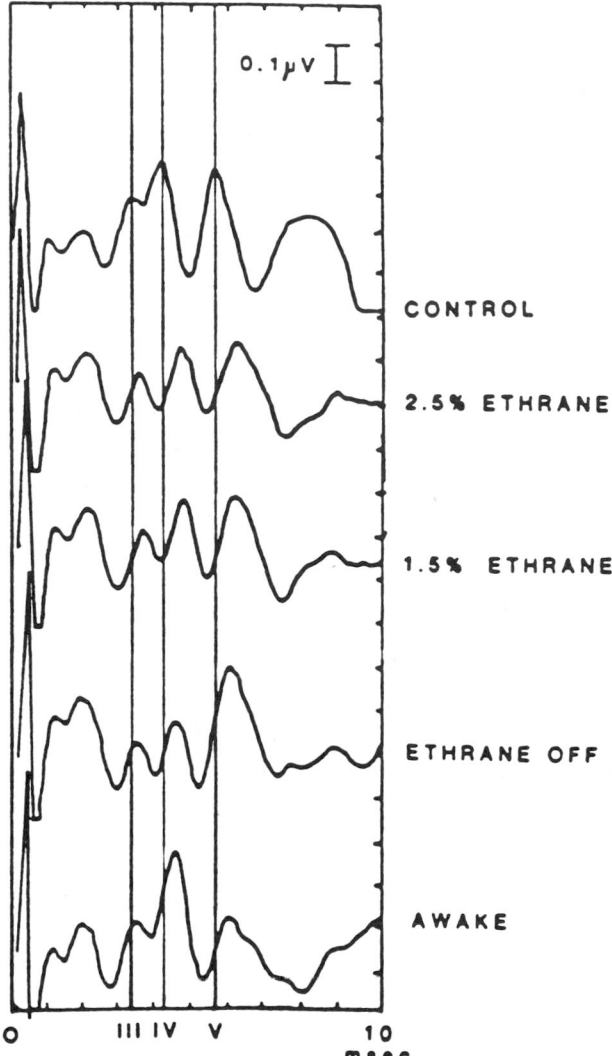

Fig. 35-15. BAER recording obtained in one patient at different enflurane inspired concentrations. (From Dubois et al.,[64] with permission.)

monitoring of BAEPs caused no further change.[62] Likewise use of nitrous oxide alone causes no change in BAEPs.[70] Use of nitrous oxide alone results in an increase in latency and a decrease in amplitude in VEPs, but when it is added to a volatile anesthetic technique it causes no further changes in VEPs.[66,70]

The effects of barbiturates on evoked potentials have been studied both in animal models and in humans. Increasing doses of thiopental in patients result in progressive dose-dependent increases in latency and decreases in amplitude in median nerve SSEPs and progressive increases in latency in BAEPs. The changes in SSEPs are more pronounced than the changes in BAEPs, and changes in later wave forms exceeded those in the earlier waveforms. This is consistent with the theories that barbiturates affect synaptic transmission more than axonal conduction, that the early waveforms in SEPs are due more to axonal transmission, and

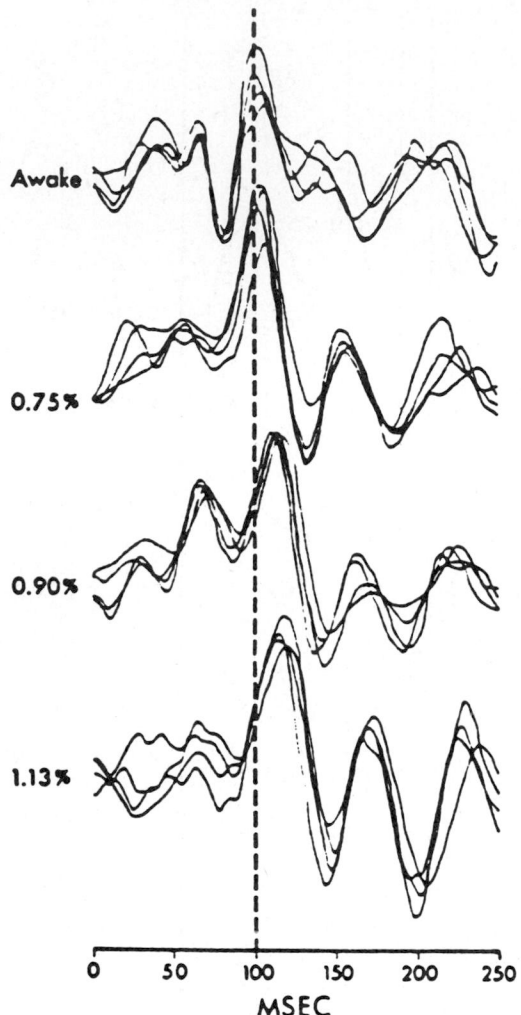

Awake

0.75%

0.90%

1.13%

| 0 | 50 | 100 | 150 | 200 | 250 |

MSEC

Fig. 35-16. Waveforms of visual evoked responses from one patient, elicited when awake and anesthetized at three end-expired levels of halothane. Four separate tracings obtained during each condition have been superimposed. (From Uhl et al.,[67] with permission.)

that later waves are dependent on multisynaptic pathways. At doses of thiopental far in excess of those producing an isoelectric EEG, adequate monitoring of SSEPs and BAEPs was preserved.[71] The effects of pentobarbital in cats have also been evaluated. The effects on SSEPs and BAEPs observed are similar to those of thiopental in humans. Increases in latency of both BAEPs and SSEPs were seen. The waveforms were never obliterated even at doses above those causing complete suppression of spontaneous EEG activity. VEPs were more sensitive, in that at low doses all except the earliest waveforms were obliterated. The early potentials persisted with increases in latency even to very high pentobarbital doses.[72] Similar increases in latency and decreases in amplitude of both spinal and cortical SSEPs were seen in humans with thiamylal sodium.[73] Preserved ability to monitor SSEPs in head injured patients receiving therapeutic thiopental infusions has been

demonstrated.[74] Adequate perioperative monitoring of sensory evoked potentials is possible even in the presence of high-dose barbiturate therapy as long as the effects of the drug (increased latency with or without decreased amplitude) are considered.

After both bolus administration and intravenous infusions etomidate causes increases in latency of all waves and prolongation of central conduction time in SSEPs as well as increases in amplitude of the cortical waves but slight decreases in amplitude of cervical potentials.[75] This effect may be due to an alteration in the balance of inhibitory and excitatory influences or an increase in the irritability of the neural system. The effects seem to be present in the cortex but not in the spinal cord.[76] Etomidate infusions have been used to enhance SSEP recording in patients in whom it was not possible to obtain reproducible responses at the beginning of intraoperative monitoring because of the patients' pathologies. The infusions provided adequate monitoring and detection of intraoperative events leading to compromise of the spinal cord.[76] The effects of etomidate on BAEPs are dose-dependent increases and decreases in amplitude.[77]

Droperidol in premedicant doses has been demonstrated to have varying effects on SSEPs. In most patients decreases in amplitude were noted as well as loss of late waves. However, in a few patients increases in amplitude were noted. In all patients conduction time was prolonged.[78] The benzodiazepenes also can cause changes in SEPs.[25,79,80] Diazepam causes increases in latency and decreases in amplitude of SSEPs, increases in latency in the cortical response after auditory stimulation, and no change in BAEPs.[79,80] Midazolam causes decreases in amplitude without changes in latency of SSEPs.[75] Phenothiazines, diphenylhydantoin, phenobarbital, and ethosuximide in therapeutic doses do not result in consistent changes in BAEPs.[81] Acute alcohol ingestion results in dose-dependent increases in latency and decreases in amplitude in VEPs in healthy patients.[82]

The narcotics in general cause dose-dependent increases in latency and decreases in amplitude of somatosensory evoked potentials. Fentanyl causes dose-dependent increases in latency of all waves, with the cortical or late waves affected more than earlier waves. It also causes a decrease in amplitude. The amplitude changes are more variable than the latency increases.[83,84] Even at high doses of fentanyl (up to 60 μg/kg) reproducible SSEPs can be recorded.[84] Morphine causes similar dose-dependent changes in SEPs to fentanyl.[83] Meperidine causes increases in latency but may also result in increases in amplitude of SSEPs.[85] Narcotics even in relatively high doses can be used in patients requiring intraoperative SSEP monitoring without impairment of ability to monitor neurologic function adequately. However, narcotic-induced changes must be taken into account when evaluating the recordings. Bolus dosing of narcotics should be avoided at times of potential surgical compromise to neurologic function to prevent confusing the interpretation of SEP changes if they develop. BAEPs were resistant to doses of fentanyl up to 50 μg/kg with no changes observed in absolute latency, interpeak latency, or amplitude.[86]

Physiologic Factors Influencing Sensory Evoked Potentials

A number of physiologic variables, including systemic blood pressure, temperature, and blood gas tensions, can influence SEP recordings. With decreases in mean arterial blood pressure to below levels of cerebral autoregulation due to either blood loss or vasoactive agents progressive changes in SEPs have been noted. SSEP changes observed are progressive decreases in amplitude until loss of the waveform with no changes in latency.[87,88] BAEPs are relatively resistant to even profound levels of hypotension (MAP of 20 mmHg in dogs).[87] Cortical (synaptic) function appears to be more sensitive to ischemia than spinal cord transmission.[88] Rapid decreases in blood pressure to levels above the lower limit of autoregulation have also been associated with transient SSEP changes of decreased amplitude that resolve after several minutes of continued hypotension at the same level.[89] Reversible SSEP changes at systemic pressures within the normal range have been observed in patients undergoing Harrington rod placement after spinal distraction. These changes resolved with increases of systemic blood pressure to slightly above the patient's normal pressure, suggesting that the combination of surgical manipulation with levels of hypotension generally considered "safe" could result in spinal cord ischemia.[90] Changes in temperature also effect SEPs. Hypothermia causes increases in latency and decreases in amplitude with loss of the waves at 25 to 27°C in VEPs[91] and increases in latency and alterations in morphology of BAEPs with late waves more affected than early ones.[92] Hyperthermia also alters SEPs, with increases in temperature leading to decreases in amplitude in SSEPs and loss of EPs at 42°C during induced hyperthermia.[93] Changes in arterial blood gas tensions have been reported to alter SEPs, probably in relation to changes in blood flow or oxygen delivery to neural structures.[94,95] SSEP changes (decreased amplitude) resulting from hypoxia have been reported.[95] Isovolemic hemodilution results in progressive increases in latency of SSEPs and VEPs that become significant at hematocrits below 15 percent. Changes in amplitude were variable until very low hematocrits (less than 7 percent) were reached when amplitude of all waveforms decreased.[96]

MONITORING OF MOTOR TRACTS AND NERVES

Intraoperative monitoring of cranial and peripheral motor nerves is used in a number of operative procedures to allow early detection of surgical trespass of the nerve and to assess level of nerve function intraopera-tively. Intraoperative electromyographic monitoring of motor nerve function can include evaluation of three types of motor nerve and muscle activity. Neurotonic discharges are recorded from fine wires placed in muscles innervated by the motor nerve and are spontaneous bursts of activity resulting from operative stimulation of the nerve by either irrigating fluids or operative instruments.[97] Occurrence of neurotonic discharges warns the surgeon of the presence of the nerve within the operative area and can help prevent unintentional damage to the nerve during the procedure. Density and frequency of neurotonic discharges are correlated with degree of postoperative nerve dysfunction.[98] Compound muscle action potentials (CMAPs) are the muscle activity recorded from either fine wires within muscles innervated by the motor nerve or surface electrodes over the muscle after direct stimulation of the nerve within the operative field by the surgeon using a hand-held stimulating electrode. Stimulation of the nerve proximal to the operative area or tumor can be used to assess functional integrity of the nerve.[97] Nerve action potentials (NAPs) are recorded after direct stimulation of the nerve either within or outside the operative field and recording of the summated activity of the axons within the operative field. NAP monitoring allows for localization of slowing or block of nerve impulse conduction within the operative field.[97]

Intraoperative monitoring of facial nerve function has been used in patients undergoing surgical procedures placing the facial nerve at risk, such as acoustic neuroma resection, microvascular decompression for hemifacial spasm, resection of cerebellopontine angle meningiomas, removal of temporal bone neoplasms and cerebellar hemangiomblastoma, and surgical treatment of glomus tympanicum and traumatic facial nerve paralysis.[97,99] Much of the experience with intraoperative facial nerve monitoring is during acoustic neuroma resection. Improved preservation of facial nerve function after acoustic neuroma resection by intraoperative facial nerve EMG monitoring has been demonstrated especially in patients with medium- to large-size tumors.[98] In patients with hemifacial spasm two abnormal responses are seen during EMG monitoring: autoexcitation and lateral spread response. Autoexcitation refers to late responses lasting 50 to 100 milliseconds that follow the normal motor response to facial nerve stimulation. Electrical stimulation of one branch of the facial nerve results in muscle response not only in the muscle innervated by that branch but also in those innervated by other branches of the facial nerve; this is termed the lateral spread response. Both of these responses are abnormal and have been demonstrated to disappear intraoperatively when the facial nerve is adequately decompressed. During microvascular decompression for hemifacial spasm intraoperative monitoring of the facial nerve provides both warning of surgical encroachment on the nerve and information on the adequacy of the operative procedure to relieve the patient's symptoms intraoperatively.[100]

Intraoperative monitoring of the motor component

of other cranial nerves has been performed. EMG monitoring of the trigeminal nerve can be accomplished with wires placed in the temporalis or masseter muscles or surface electrodes over these muscles. Fifth cranial nerve monitoring has been used during nerve section for tic douloureux to ensure preservation of the motor branch of the trigeminal nerve. It is also used in conjunction with facial nerve monitoring during resection of large posterior fossa lesions.[97] The spinal accessory nerve can be monitored with recording electrodes in the trapezius or sternocleidomastoid muscles, for example, during resection of large meningiomas, glomus jugular tumors, and neck carcinomas.[97] EMG monitoring of the hypoglossal nerve with electrodes in the tongue has been infrequently used for large posterior fossa lesions and clivus tumors.[97] Although EMG monitoring of the eye muscles can be performed, it is rarely used.

Monitoring of peripheral motor nerves has been performed in a number of operative procedures by placing wire electrodes in the muscles innervated by nerves that may traverse the operative area. EMG monitoring can warn the surgeon of unexpected surgical trespass of the nerve, help locate a nerve within the field, and localize the level of conduction block or delay. EMG of peripheral nerves has been used in patients undergoing spine surgery to decrease the risk of nerve root injury during the procedure as radiculopathies have been reported to occur after these procedures.[97] Monitoring of peripheral nerves has also been performed in patients undergoing nerve plexus or single-nerve explorations to locate areas of injury and assess axonal continuity in order to help guide the operative procedure.[97]

In patients undergoing EMG monitoring of cranial or peripheral motor nerves anesthetic management is not influenced, except that muscle relaxants should be avoided or limited during the period of monitoring. Although the most common approach is to avoid neuromuscular blocking agents completely during the period of monitoring, adequate monitoring of the facial nerve is possible during partial neuromuscular blockade (decrease of the CMAP by 50 percent). This level of blockade is associated with clinical weakness.[101] In patients undergoing selective dorsal rhizotomy for relief of spasticity the EMG is monitored to determine which rootlets to section. These patients have abnormal muscle responses, and in some volatile anesthetics and nitrous oxide may impair the ability to monitor adequately and narcotics tend to influence the ability to monitor less.[102,103]

Monitoring of the integrity of the motor tracts within the spinal cord is a technique with great potential benefit. Loss of motor function during spinal or vascular surgery without loss of sensory function or change in SSEPs can occur because of the different location and blood supply of the motor tracts from the dorsal columns monitored by SSEP. Transcranial stimulation of the motor tract with monitoring of nerve impulse in the spinal cord and peripheral nerve as well as muscle response has been performed and loss of motor transmission without loss of SSEP demonstrated.[104] This technique has applications in spinal surgery in which transmission across the operative field can be assessed as well as in aortic surgery with the potential for impairment of the blood supply to the anterior cord. To monitor muscle function, neuromuscular blocking agents should be avoided. However, these agents can be used if only nerve transmission in the cord or peripheral nerves is to be monitored. The effects of anesthetic agents on these tracts are largely unreported. Our early clinical experience with transcortical magnetic stimulation of the motor tracts suggests that narcotics have less effect than volatile anesthetics on the recording of motor evoked potentials.

REFERENCES

1. Martin JT, Faulconer A, Jr, Bickford RG: Electroencephalography in anesthesiology. Anesthesiology 20:359, 1959
2. Sharbrough FW, Messick JM, Jr, Sundt TM: Correlation of continuous electroencephalograms with cerebral blood flow measurements during carotid endarterectomy. Stroke 4:674, 1973
3. Bickford RG, Fleming NI, Billinger TW: Compression of EEG data by isometric power spectral plots. Electroencephalogr Clin Neurophysiol 31:632, 1971
4. Fleming RA, Smith NT: Density modulations: A technique for the display of three-variable data in patient monitoring. Anesthesiology 50:543, 1979
5. Fleming RA, Smith NT: An inexpensive device for analyzing and monitoring the electroencephalogram. Anesthesiology 50:456, 1979
6. Cucchiara RF, Sharbrough FW, Messick JM, Tinker JH: An electroencephalographic filter-processor as an indicator of cerebral ischemia during carotid endarterectomy. Anesthesiology 51:77, 1979
7. Klein FF: A waveform analyzer applied to the human EEG. IEEE Trans Biomed Eng 23:246, 1976
8. Levy WJ: Effect of epoch length on power spectrum analysis of the EEG. Anesthesiology 66:489, 1987
9. Courtin RF, Bickford RG, Faulconer A, Jr: The classification and significance of electroencephalographic patterns produced by N_2O/ether anesthesia during surgical operations. Proc Staff Meet Mayo Clin 25:197, 1950
10. Tinker JH, Sharbrough FW, Michenfelder JD: Anterior shift of the dominant EEG rhythm during anesthesia in the Java monkey: Correlation with anesthetic potency. Anesthesiology 46:252, 1977
11. Brazier MAB: The effect of drugs on the electroencephalogram of man. Clin Pharmacol Ther 5:102, 1964
12. Brechner VL: Current status of electroencephalography in the practice of clinical anesthesia. Clin Anesth 2:87, 1964
13. Stockard JJ, Bickford RG: The neurophysiology of anaesthesia. p. 3. In Gordon E (ed): A Basis and Practice of Neuroanesthesia. New York, Elsevier, 1981
14. Sebel PS, Bovill JG, Wauquier A, Pieternella R: Effects of high dose fentanyl anesthesia on the electroencephalogram. Anesthesiology 55:203, 1981
15. White PF, Way WL, Trevor AJ: Ketamine — its pharmacology and therapeutic uses. Anesthesiology 56:119, 1982

16. Reves JG, Fragen RJ, Vinik HR, Greenblatt DJ: Midazolam: Pharmacology and uses. Anesthesiology 62:310, 1985
17. Fleischer JE, Milde JH, Moyer TP, Michenfelder JD: Cerebral effects of high-dose midazolam and subsequent reversal with RO 15-1788 in dogs. Anesthesiology 68:234, 1988
18. Nugent M, Artru AA, Michenfelder JD: Cerebral metabolic, vascular and protective effects of midazolam maleate. Anesthesiology 56:172, 1982
19. Clark DL, Hosick EC, Neigh JL: Neurophysiologic effects of isoflurane in man. Anesthesiology 39:261, 1973
20. Clark DL, Hosick EC, Rosner BS: Neurophysiological effects of different anesthetics in unconscious man. J Appl Physiol 31:884, 1971
21. Michenfelder JD, Cucchiara RF: Canine cerebral oxygen consumption during enflurane anesthesia and its modification during induced seizures. Anesthesiology 40:575, 1974
22. Backman LE, Loefstroem B, Widen L: Electroencephalography in halothane anesthesia. Acta Anaesthesiol Scand 8:115, 1964
23. Levy WJ: Quantitative analysis of EEG changes during hypothermia. Anesthesiology 60:291, 1984
24. Smith NT, Dec-Silver H, Sanford TJ, Jr, et al: EEGs during high-dose fentanyl-, sufentanil-, or morphine-oxygen anesthesia. Anesth Analg 63:386, 1984
25. Cucchiara RF, Sharbrough FW, Messick JM, Tinker JH: An electroencephalographic filter-processor as an indicator of cerebral ischemia during carotid endarterectomy. Anesthesiology 51:77, 1979
26. Spackman TN, Faust RJ, Cucchiara RF, Sharbrough FW: A comparison of aperiodic analysis of the EEG with standard EEG and cerebral blood flow for detection of ischemia. Anesthesiology 66:229, 1987
27. Clowes GHA, Jr, Kretchmer HE, McBurney RW, et al: The electroencephalogram in the evaluation of the effects of anesthetic agents and carbon dioxide accumulation during surgery. Ann Surg 138:558, 1953
28. Oliver SB, Cucchiara RF, Warner MA, Muir JJ: Unexpected focal neurologic deficit on emergence from anesthesia. Anesthesiology 67:823, 1987
29. Report of the Medical Consultants on the Diagnosis of Death to the President's Commission for the Study of Ethical Problems in Medicine and Biomedical and Behavioral Research: Guidelines for the determination of death. JAMA 246:2184, 1981
30. Darby JM, Stein K, Grevnik A, Stuart SA: Approach to management of the heart beating "brain dead" organ donor. JAMA 261:2222, 1989
31. Kelly DL, Goldring S, O'Leary JL: Averaged evoked somatosensory responses from exposed cortex of man. Arch Neurol 13:1, 1965
32. Grundy BL: Monitoring of sensory evoked potentials during neurosurgical operation methods and applications. Neurosurgery 11:556, 1982
33. Greenberg RP, Ducker TB: Evoked potentials in the clinical neurosciences. J Neurosurg 56:1, 1982
34. Chiappa KH, Ropper AH: Evoked potentials in clinical medicine. N Engl J Med 306:1205, 1982
35. Ganes T: A study of peripheral, cervical, and cortical evoked potentials and afferent conduction times in the somatosensory pathway. Electroencephalogr Clin Neurophysiol 49:446, 1980
36. Engler GL, Spielholz NI, Bernhard WN, et al: Somatosensory evoked potentials during Harrington instrumentation for scoliosis. J Bone Joint Surg 60A:528, 1978
37. Maccabee PJ, Pinkhasov EI, Tsairis P, Levine DB: Spinal and short latency scalp derived somatosensory evoked potentials during corrective spinal column surgery. Electroencephalogr Clin Neurophysiol 53:P32, 1982
38. Spielholz NI, Benjamin MV, Engler GL, Ransohoff J: Somatosensory evoked potentials during decompression and stabilization of the spine: Methods and findings. Spine 4:500, 1979
39. Spielholz NI, Benjamin MV, Engler G, Ransohoff J: Somatosensory evoked potentials and clinical outcome in spinal cord injury. p. 217. In Popp AJ, Bourke RS, Nelson LR, Kimelberg HK (eds): Neural Trauma. New York, Raven Press, 1979
40. Luederes H, Gurd A, Hahn J, et al: A new technique for intraoperative monitoring of spinal cord function: Multichannel recording of spinal cord and subcortical evoked potentials. Spine 7:110, 1982
41. Landi A, Copeland SA, Wynn-Parry CB, Jones SJ: The role of somatosensory evoked potentials and nerve conduction studies in the surgical management of brachial plexus injuries. J Bone Joint Surg 62B:492, 1980
42. Grundy BL: Intraoperative monitoring of sensory evoked potentials. p. 624. In Nodar RH, Barber C (eds): Evoked Potentials II. Boston, Butterworth, 1984
43. Allen A, Starr A, Nudleman K: Assessment of sensory function in the operating room utilizing cerebral evoked potentials: A study of fifty-six surgically anesthetized patients. Clin Neurosurg 28:457, 1981
44. Raudzens PA: Intraoperative monitoring of evoked potentials. Ann NY Acad Sci 388:308, 1982
45. McCallum JE, Bennett MH: Electrophysiologic monitoring of spinal cord function during intraspinal surgery. Surg Forum 26:469, 1975
46. Halliday AM, Wakefield GS: Cerebral evoked potentials in patients with dissociated sensory loss. J Neurol Neurosurg Psychiatry 26:211, 1963
47. Szilagyi DE, Hageman JH, Smith RF, Elliott JP: Spinal cord damage in surgery of the abdominal aorta. Surgery 83:38, 1978
48. Grundy BL: Intraoperative monitoring of sensory-evoked potentials. Anesthesiology 58:72, 1983
49. Hume AI, Cant BR, Shaw NA: Central somatosensory conduction time in comatose patients. Ann Neurol 5:379, 1979
50. Symon L, Hargadine J, Zawirshi M, Branston N: Central conduction time as an index of ischaemia in subarachnoid haemorrhage. J Neurol Sci 44:95, 1979
51. Chiappa KH, Ropper AH: Evoked potentials in clinical medicine. N Engl J Med 306:1140, 1982
52. Grundy BL, Jannetta PJ, Procopio PT, et al: Intraoperative monitoring of brain-stem auditory evoked potentials. J Neurosurg 57:674, 1982
53. Raudzens PA, Shetter AG: Intraoperative monitoring of brain-stem auditory evoked potentials. J Neurosurg 57:341, 1982
54. Duncan PG, Sanders RA, McCollough DW: Preservation of auditory-evoked responses in anaesthetized children. Can Anaesth Soc J 26:492, 1979
55. Auger RG, Piepgras DG, Laws ER: Hemifacial spasm: Results of microvascular decompression of the facial nerve in 54 patients. Mayo Clin Proc 61:640, 1986
56. Møller AR, Janetta PJ: Monitoring auditory functions during cranial nerve microvascular decompression operations by direct recording from the eighth nerve. J Neurosurg 59:493, 1983
57. Peterson DO, Drummond JC, Todd MM: Effects of halothane, enflurane, isoflurane, and nitrous oxide on somato-

sensory evoked potentials in humans. Anesthesiology 65:35, 1986

58. McPherson RW, Mahla M, Johnson R, Traystman RJ: Effects of enflurane, isoflurane, and nitrous oxide on somatosensory evoked potentials during fentanyl anesthesia. Anesthesiology 62:626, 1985

59. Pathak KS, Amaddio BS, Scoles PV, et al: Effects of halothane, enflurane, and isoflurane in nitrous oxide on multilevel somatosensory evoked potentials. Anesthesiology 70:207, 1989

60. Samra SK, Vanderzant CW, Domer PA, Sackellares JC: Differential effects of isoflurane on human median nerve somatosensory evoked potentials. Anesthesiology 66:29, 1987

61. Sebel PS, Ingram DA, Flynn PJ: Evoked potentials during isoflurane anaesthesia. Br J Anaesth 58:580, 1986

62. Manninen PH, Lam AM, Nicholas JF: The effects of isoflurane-nitrous oxide anesthesia on brainstem auditory evoked potentials in humans. Anesth Analg 64:43, 1985

63. Thornton C, Catley DM, Jordan C, et al: Enflurane anaesthesia causes graded changes in the brainstem and early cortical auditory evoked response in man. Br J Anaesth 55:479, 1983

64. Dubois MY, Sato S, Chassy J, Macnamara TE: Effects of enflurane on brainstem auditory evoked responses in humans. Anesth Analg 61:898, 1982

65. Cohen MS, Britt RH: Effects of sodium pentobarbital, ketamine, halothane, chloralose on brainstem auditory evoked responses. Anesth Analg 61:338, 1982

66. Chi OZ, Field C: Effects of isoflurane on visual evoked potentials in humans. Anesthesiology 65:328, 1986

67. Uhl RR, Squires KC, Bruce DL, Starr A: Effect of halothane anesthesia on the human cortical visual evoked response. Anesthesiology 53:273, 1980

68. Domino EF, Corssen G, Sweet RB: Effects of various general anesthetics on the visually evoked response in man. Anesth Analg 42:735, 1963

69. Burchiel KG: Stockard JJ, Myers RR, Bickford RG: Visual and auditory evoked responses during enflurane anesthesia in man and cats. Electroencephalogr Clin Neurophysiol 39:434P, 1973

70. Sebel PS, Flynn PJ, Ingram DA: Effect of nitrous oxide on visual, auditory, and somatosensory evoked potentials. Br J Anaesth 56:1403, 1984

71. Drummond JC, Todd MM, Sang H: The effect of high dose sodium thiopental on brain stem auditory and median nerve somatosensory evoked responses in humans. Anesthesiology 63:249, 1985

72. Sutton LN, Frewen T, Marsh R, et al: The effects of deep barbiturate coma on multimodality evoked potentials. J Neurosurg 57:178, 1982

73. Shimoji K, Kano T, Nakashima H, Shimizu H: The effects of thiamyl sodium on electrical activities of the central and peripheral nervous systems in man. Anesthesiology 40:234, 1974

74. Ganes T, Lundar T: The effect of thiopentone on somatosensory evoked responses and EEGs in comatose patients. J Neurol Neurosurg Psychiatry 46:509, 1983

75. Koht A, Schütz W, Schmidt G, et al: Effects of etomidate, midazolam, and thiopental on median nerve somatosensory evoked potentials and the additive effects of fentanyl and nitrous oxide. Anesth Analg 67:435, 1988

76. Sloan TB, Ronai AK, Toleikis JR, Koht A: Improvement of intraoperative somatosensory evoked potentials by etomidate. Anesth Analg 67:582, 1988

77. Navaratnarajah M, Thornton C, Heneghan CPH, et al: Effect

of etomidate on the auditory evoked response in man. Proceedings of the Anaesthetic Research Society 55:1157P, 1983

78. Grundy BL, Brown RH, Clifton PC: Effect of droperidol on somatosensory cortical evoked potentials. Electroencephalogr Clin Neurophysiol 50:158, 1980

79. Doring WH, Daub D: Akustisch evozierte Hirstamm und Rindepotentiale bei sedierung mit diazepam. Arch Otorhinolaryngol 227:522, 1980

80. Grundy BL, Brown RH, Greenbergh BA: Diazepam alters cortical potentials. Anesthesiology 51:538, 1979

81. Stockard JJ, Rossiter VS, Jones TA, Sharbrough FW: Effects of centrally acting drugs on brainstem auditory responses. Electroencephalogr Clin Neurophysiol 43:550, 1977

82. Erwin CW, Linnoila M: Effect of ethyl alcohol on visual evoked potentials. Alcoholism 5:49, 1981

83. Pathak KS, Brown RH, Cascorbi HF, Nash CL: Effects of fentanyl and morphine on intraoperative somatosensory cortical-evoked potentials. Anesth Analg 63:833, 1984

84. Schubert A, Peterson DO, Drummond JC, Saidman LJ: The effect of high-dose fentanyl on human median nerve somatosensory evoked responses. Anesth Analg 65:S136, 1986

85. Grundy BL, Brown RH: Meperidine enhances somatosensory cortical evoked potentials. Electroencephalogr Clin Neurophysiol 50:177, 1980

86. Samra SK, Lilly DJ, Rush NL, Kirsh MM: Fentanyl anesthesia and human brain-stem auditory evoked potentials. Anesthesiology 61:261, 1984

87. Eng DY, Dong WK, Bledsoe SW, et al: Electrical and pathological correlates of brain hypoxia during hypotension. Anesthesiology 53:S92, 1980

88. Kobrine AI, Evans DE, Rizzoli HV: Relative vulnerability of the brain and spinal cord to ischemia. J Neurol Sci 45:65, 1980

89. Bunegin L, Albin MS, Helsel P, et al: Evoked responses during trimetaphan hypotension. Anesthesiology 55:A232, 1981

90. Grundy BL, Nash CL, Brown RH: Arterial pressure manipulation alters spinal cord function during correction of scoliosis. Anesthesiology 54:249, 1981

91. Russ W, Kling D, Loesevitz A, Hempelmann G: Effect of hypothermia on visual evoked potential (VEP) in humans. Anesthesiology 61:207, 1984

92. Stockard JJ, Sharbrough FW, Tinker JA: Effects of hypothermia on the human brainstem auditory response. Ann Neurol 3:368, 1978

93. Dubois M, Loppola R, Buchsbaum MS, Lees DE: Somatosensory evoked potentials during whole body hyperthermia in humans. Electroencephalogr Clin Neurophysiol 52:157, 1981

94. Nakagawa Y, Ohtsuka T, Tsura M, Nakamura N: Effects of mild hypercapnia on somatosensory evoked potentials in experimental cerebral ischemia. Stroke 25:275, 1984

95. Grundy BL, Heros RC, Tung AS, Doyle E: Intraoperative hypoxia detected by evoked potential monitoring. Anesth Analg 60:437, 1981

96. Nagao S, Roccaforte P, Moody RA: The effects of isovolemic hemodilution and reinfusion of packed erythrocytes on somatosensory and visual evoked potentials. J Surg Res 25:S30, 1978

97. Harper CM, Daube RJ: Surgical monitoring with evoked potentials: The Mayo Clinic experience. p. 275. In Desmedt JE (ed): Neuromonitoring in Surgery. Elsevier Science Publishers, New York, 1989

98. Harner SG, Daube JR, Beatty CW: Improved preservation of facial nerve function with use of electrical monitoring dur-

ing removal of acoustic neuromas. Mayo Clin Proc 62:92, 1987

99. Harner SG, Daube JR, Ebersold MJ: Electrophysiologic monitoring of facial nerve during temporal bone surgery. Laryngoscope 96:65, 1986

100. Møller AR, Jannetta PJ: Microvascular decompression in hemifacial spasm: Intraoperative electrophysiological observations. Neurosurgery 16:612, 1985

101. Welna JO, Oliver SB, Daube JR, Lennon RL: Effect of partial neuromuscular blockade on intraoperative electromyography in patients undergoing resection of acoustic neuroma. Anesthesiology 69:A636, 1988

102. Zentner J, Kiss I, Ebner A: Influence of anesthetics—nitrous oxide in particular—on electromyographic response evoked by transcranial electrical stimulation of the cortex. Neurosurgery 24:253, 1989

103. Zentner J, Abner A: Nitrous oxide suppresses the electromyographic response evoked by electrical stimulation of the motor cortex. Neurosurgery 24:60, 1989

104. Levy WJ, York DH, McCaffrey M, Tanzer F: Motor evoked potentials from transcranial stimulation of the motor cortex in humans. Neurosurgery 15:287, 1984

105. Clark DL, Rosner BS: Neurophysiologic effects of general anesthetics. Anesthesiology 38:564, 1973

106. Maurer K, Schafer E, Leitner H: The effect of varying stimulus polarity (rarefaction versus condensation) on early auditory potentials (EPs). Electroencephalogr Clin Neurophysiol 50:332, 1980

INDEX

Note: Page numbers followed by f denote figures; those followed by t denote tables.

1